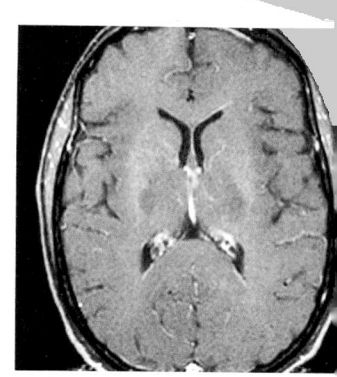

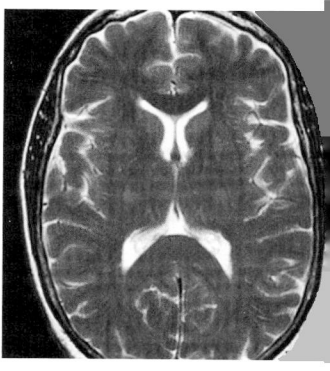

OSBORN'S BRAIN
IMAGING, PATHOLOGY, AND ANATOMY

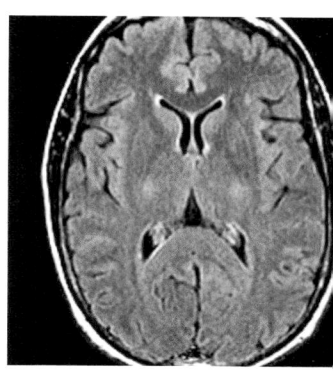

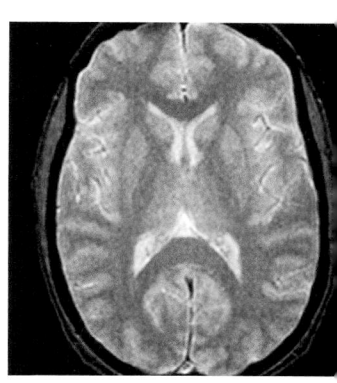

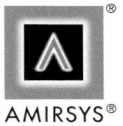

AMIRSYS®

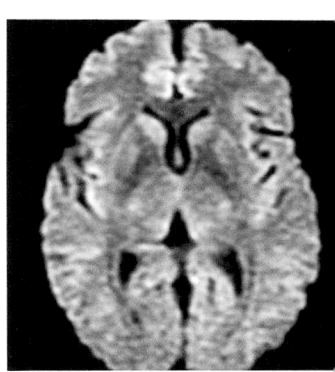

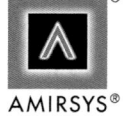

AMIRSYS®

iii

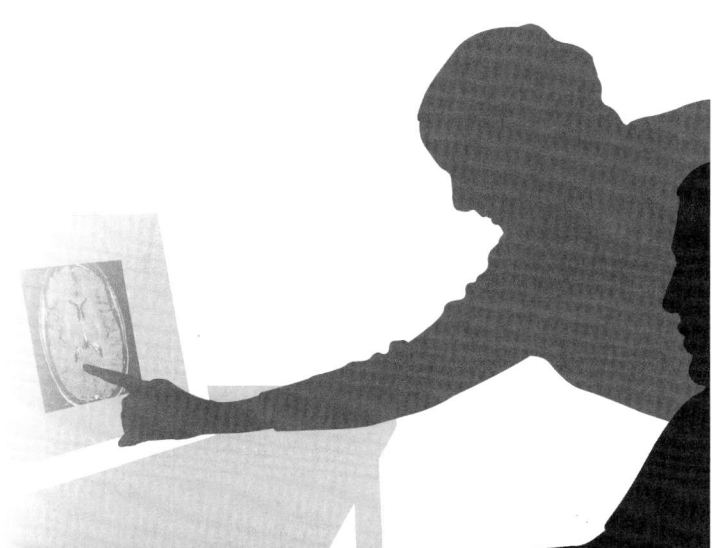

University Distinguished Professor
Professor of Radiology

William H. and Patricia W. Child
Presidential Endowed Chair in Radiology

University of Utah School of Medicine
Salt Lake City, Utah

Anne G. Osborn, MD, FACR

iv

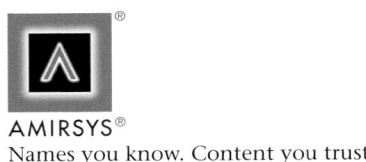

AMIRSYS®
Names you know. Content you trust.®

First Edition

Second Printing - January 2013

© 2013 Amirsys, Inc.

Compilation © 2013 Amirsys Publishing, Inc.

All rights reserved. No part of this publication may be reproduced, stored in a retrieval system, or transmitted, in any form or media or by any means, electronic, mechanical, photocopying, recording, or otherwise, without prior written permission from Amirsys, Inc.

Printed in Canada by Friesens, Altona, Manitoba, Canada

ISBN: 978-1-931884-21-1

Notice and Disclaimer

Library of Congress Cataloging-in-Publication Data

Osborn, Anne G., 1943-
  Osborn's brain : imaging, pathology, and anatomy / Anne G. Osborn. -- 1st ed.
    p. ; cm.
  Includes bibliographical references.
  ISBN 978-1-931884-21-1
  I. Title.
  [DNLM: 1. Brain--physiopathology. 2. Central Nervous System Diseases--pathology. 3. Neuroimaging--methods. WL 301]

616.8--dc23
                    2012031063

FOR RON

Beloved sweetheart and eternal companion, you didn't live to see the book completed. Nevertheless, your unconditional love and supportive spirit sustained me throughout the process—from beginning to the very end. I hope it makes you proud! Until we meet again, all my love and devotion right back at you!

PREFACE

With the publication of *Osborn's Brain*, I'm breaking a longstanding promise to myself: I swore I'd never, *EVER*, write another prose-based book. And yet here it is. But let me tell you, this isn't just "another prose book." Far from it! When my colleagues and I published the first edition of *Diagnostic Imaging: Brain*, Dr. Michael Huckman said in his Foreword to the book, "[Osborn] has decided to abandon the usual conventions of medical textbooks." Amirsys's now-classic bulleted format does indeed deliver more information in less space than traditional prose. And I do love those efficiencies! However, I want to give more than, "Just the facts, ma'am." I want to show the thinking *behind* the facts. The reasoning. The framework that facilitates understanding a tough, complex subject.

That's why I've structured the book as a learning curriculum. We start with the most immediate "must know" topics, beginning with trauma. We next discuss nontraumatic hemorrhage, stroke, and vascular lesions. In other words, we jump right into emergent imaging issues before delving into infections, demyelinating and inflammatory diseases, neoplasms, toxic-metabolic-degenerative disorders, and congenital brain malformations.

If you're just starting your residency in radiology, neurosurgery, or neurology, I suggest you begin at the beginning. Read the first three chapters and digest them. Then go part by part, chapter by chapter, straight through the book. If you are a senior resident or fellow, this is a great way to review what you think you already know pretty well. I guarantee you, there's stuff in here that will be new to you. If you're a practicing general radiologist, neuroradiologist, or neurosurgeon, consider this a neuroimaging refresher course. And if you are an honest-to-goodness neuroradiologist, I've tucked a number of cool tidbits into every chapter that I hope you will find intriguing and thought-provoking.

Many of you have asked, emailed, and even written (yes, old-fashioned written) me with your pleas for a new "Osborn." So here it is. I wrote every word of it myself, so the style is mine alone and the approach is therefore consistent from chapter to chapter. I've combined essential anatomy together with gross pathology and imaging to show you just why diseases appear the way they do. The book is illustration-rich, with loads of high definition state-of-the-art imaging and glorious color. My trademark summary boxes are scattered throughout the text, allowing for quick review of the essential facts.

I've drawn on an entire career of accumulated knowledge and intense interest in neuropathology, neurosurgery, and clinical neurosciences to select the very most relevant information for you. It's been fun to do this, the culmination of my decades of continued learning in our beloved subspecialty. I hope you enjoy the journey!

Best regards and good reading!

Anne G. Osborn, MD, FACR
University Distinguished Professor
Professor of Radiology
William H. and Patricia W. Child Presidential Endowed Chair in Radiology
University of Utah School of Medicine
Salt Lake City, Utah

Editor in Chief
Ashley R. Renlund, MA

Text Editing
Kellie J. Heap, BA
Dave L. Chance, MA
Arthur G. Gelsinger, MA
Lorna Kennington, MS
Rebecca L. Hutchinson, BA
Angela M. Green, BA
Kalina K. Lowery, MS

Image Editing
Jeffrey J. Marmorstone, BS
Lisa A. M. Steadman, BS

Medical Editing
Pieter Janse van Rensburg, MB, ChB, FRCR
Donald V. La Barge, MD
Karen L. Salzman, MD
Brian Chin, MD
Paula J. Woodward, MD
Kevin R. Moore, MD

Illustrations
Lane R. Bennion, MS
Richard Coombs, MS
Laura C. Sesto, MA
James A. Cooper, MD

Art Direction and Design
Laura C. Sesto, MA

Software Development
R. J. Sargent, BS

Publishing Lead
Katherine L. Riser, MA

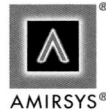

AMIRSYS®
Names you know. Content you trust.®

ACKNOWLEDGEMENTS

No one truly ever produces a text of this magnitude alone. While I am the sole author, there are many individuals who have contributed everything from images to suggestions, opinions, and ideas. Thank you from the bottom of my heart. You know who you are.

Several individuals and groups deserve special mention. First of all, thanks to our neuroradiology colleagues at the University of Utah for their support. A big one to Brian Chin, my 2011-12 clinical neuroradiology research fellow who tirelessly searched out cases and references for the book. Couldn't have done it without you!

Ever since my sabbatical as Distinguished Scientist at the world-renowned Armed Forces Institute of Pathology in Washington, D.C. (which alas is no more, a victim of government downsizing), pathology has formed the foundation of how I view and teach neuroradiology. It's a big part of this text. Special thanks to Richard H. Hewlett and his colleague, the late Stuart Rutherfoord, whose elegant gross photographs make the book sing. Thanks also to Peter Burger, the late Bernd Scheithauer, and their wonderful neuropathology colleagues. Some of the images reproduced here come from their wonderful synoptic text, *Diagnostic Pathology: Neuropathology* (Amirsys Publishing, 2012).

Thanks to the entire Amirsys team. Special mention and profound thanks goes to our inimitable, indomitable, and beloved colleague Paula Woodward, MD. Paula stepped into the editing and production wherever needed. At the end, she jumped in to do a bunch of heavy lifting with the medical edits to keep us on a very tight, unforgiving schedule. Ashley Renlund, our chief editor, made invaluable suggestions, polishing the text and layout. She worked tirelessly to fit almost all the images on the same or facing pages with the referenced text.

Thanks to the international Amirsys Brain, Spine, and Head and Neck case teams. You guys have contributed amazing stuff over the years to the Amirsys database, which now reaches tens of thousands of radiologists and trainees through STATdx™ and RadPrimer™. You have enhanced teaching and improved patient care around the world. Thanks for your superb work...and prompt response when any of us emailed an urgent "request for cases" for one of our many projects. It didn't matter how common or obscure the diagnosis, someone somewhere (and often several of you) sent a perfect case.

Thanks also to the many colleagues who have generously given me fascinating cases over the years. I've tried to keep track of which case came from whom and to acknowledge you appropriately in the captions. Special thanks to all of the image contributors.

-Anne G. Osborn

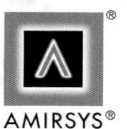

AMIRSYS®

IMAGE CONTRIBUTORS

AFIP Archives

N. Agarwal, MD

B. Alvord, MD

S. Andronikou, MD

J. Ardyn, MD

M. Ayadi, MD

S. Aydin, MD

C. Baccin, MD

R. Bert, MD

S. Blaser, MD

J. Boxerman, MD

P. Burger, MD

S. Candy, MD

M. Castillo, MD

P. Chapman, MD

S. Chung, MD

M. Colombo, MD

J. Comstock, MD

J. Curé, MD

A. Datir, MD

B. K. DeMasters, MD

M. Edwards-Brown, MD

H. Els, MD

A. Ersen, MD

N. Foster, MD

S. Galetta, MD

L. Ginsberg, MD

C. Glastonbury, MD

S. Harder, MD

H. R. Harnsberger, MD

B. Hart, MD

M. Hartel, MD

E. T. Hedley-Whyte, MD

G. Hedlund, DO

S. Hetal, MD

R. Hewlett, MD

P. Hildenbrand, MD

C. Y. Ho, MD

S. S. M. Ho, MBBs

B. Horten, MD

M. Huckman, MD

T. Hutchins, MD

A. Illner, MD

D. Jacobs, MD

B. Jones, MD

J. A. Junker, MD

B. Krafchik, MD

D. Kremens, MD

W. Kucharczyk, MD

P. Lasjaunias, MD

S. Lincoff, MD

L. Loevner, MD

S. Ludwin, MD

T. Markel, MD

M. Martin, MD

V. Mathews, MD

A. Maydell, MD

S. McNally, MD

T. Mentzel, MD

M. Michel, MD

K. Moore, MD

K. Morton, MD

S. Nagi, MD

N. Nakase, MD

K. Nelson, MD

R. Nguyen, MD

G. P. Nielsen, MD

M. Nielsen, MS

K. K. Oguz, MD

G. Oliveira, MD

J. P. O'Malley, MD

N. Omar, MD

J. Paltan, MD

G. Parker, MD

C. D. Phillips, MD

R. Ramakantan, MD

C. Robson, MBChB

F. J. Rodriguez, MD

P. Rodriguez, MD

A. Rosenberg, MD

E. Ross, MD

A. Rossi, MD

L. Rourke, MD

E. Rushing, MD

M. Sage, MD

B. Scheithauer, MD

P. Shannon, MD

D. Shatzkes, MD

A. Sillag, MD

P. Sundgren, MD

C. Sutton, MD

E. T. Tali, MD

M. Thurnher, MD

T. Tihan, MD

K. Tong, MD

J. Townsend, MD

S. van der Westhuizen, MD

P. J. van Rensburg, MD

M. Warmuth-Metz, MD

S. Yashar, MD

Table of Contents

Toxic, Metabolic, Degenerative, and CSF Disorders

Congenital Malformations of the Skull and Brain

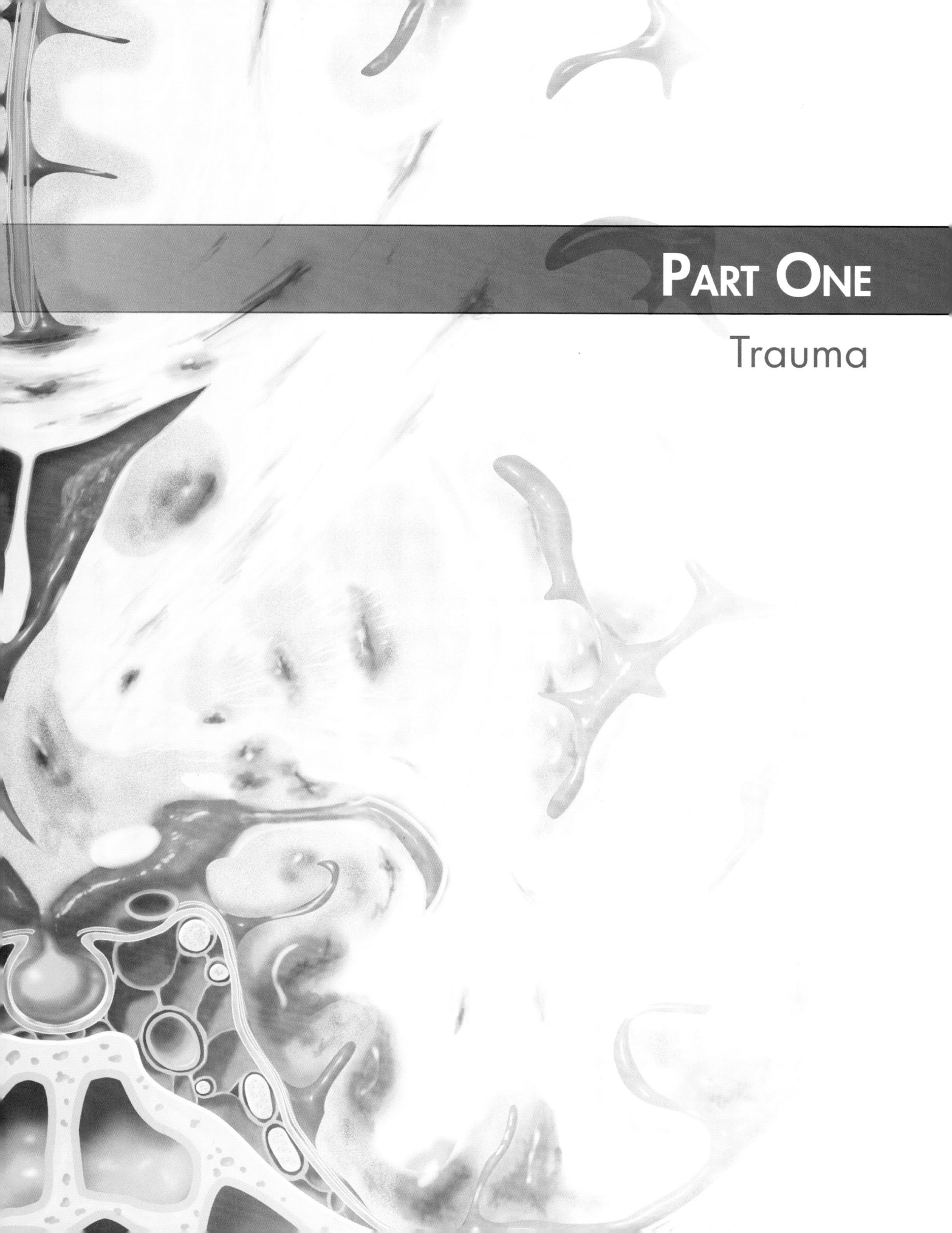

PART ONE

Trauma

1

Trauma Overview

Trauma is one of the most frequent indications for emergent neuroimaging. Because imaging plays such a key role in patient triage and management, we begin this book by discussing skull and brain trauma.

We start with a brief consideration of epidemiology. Traumatic brain injury (TBI) is a worldwide public health problem that has enormous personal and societal impact. The direct medical costs of caring for acutely traumatized patients are huge. The indirect costs of lost productivity and long-term care for TBI survivors are even larger than the short-term direct costs.

We then briefly discuss the etiology and mechanisms of head trauma. Understanding the different ways in which the skull and brain can be injured provides the context for understanding the spectrum of findings that can be identified on imaging studies.

Introduction

Epidemiology of Head Trauma

Trauma—sometimes called the "silent epidemic"—is the most common worldwide cause of death and disability in children and young adults. Neurotrauma is responsible for the vast majority of these cases. In the USA alone, more than two million people annually suffer a traumatic brain injury. Of these, 500,000 require hospital care. At least 10 million people worldwide sustain TBI each year.

Of all head-injured patients, approximately 10% sustain fatal brain injury, and an additional 5-10% have serious permanent neurologic deficits. Even more have subtle deficits ("minimal brain trauma"), while 20-40% of TBI survivors have moderate disability.

Etiology and Mechanisms of Injury

Trauma can be caused by missile or non-missile injury. Missile injury results from penetration of the skull, meninges, and/or brain by an external object such as a bullet.

Non-missile closed head injury (CHI) is a much more common cause of neurotrauma than missile injury. High-speed motor vehicle collisions exert significant acceleration/deceleration forces, causing the brain to move suddenly within the skull. Forcible impaction of the brain against the unyielding calvaria and hard, knife-like dura results in gyral contusion. Rotation and sudden changes in angular momentum may deform, stretch, and damage long vulnerable axons, resulting in axonal injury.

The etiology of TBI also varies according to patient age. Overall, almost 30% of TBIs are caused by falls. Falls are the leading cause of TBI in children younger than four years and in elderly patients older than 75. Gunshot wounds are most common in adolescent and young adult males but relatively rare in other groups. Motor vehicle and auto-pedestrian collisions occur at all ages without gender predilection.

Classification of Head Trauma

The most widely used *clinical* classification of brain trauma, the Glasgow Coma Scale (GCS), depends on the assessment of three features: Best eye, verbal, and motor responses. Using the GCS, TBI can be designated as mild, moderate, or severe injury.

TBI can also be divided chronologically and *pathoetiologically* into primary and secondary injury, the system used in this text. **Primary injuries** occur at the time of initial trauma. Skull fractures, epi- and subdural hematomas, contusions, axonal injury, and brain lacerations are examples of primary injuries.

Secondary injuries occur later and include cerebral edema, perfusion alterations, brain herniations, and CSF leaks. Although vascular injury can be immediate (blunt impact) or secondary (vessel laceration from fractures, occlusion secondary to brain herniation), for purposes of discussion, it is included in the chapter on secondary injuries.

CLASSIFICATION OF HEAD TRAUMA
Primary Effects
- Scalp and skull injuries
- Extraaxial hemorrhage/hematomas
- Parenchymal injuries
- Miscellaneous injuries

Secondary Effects
- Herniation syndromes
- Cerebral edema
- Cerebral ischemia
- Vascular injury (can be primary or secondary)

Imaging Acute Head Trauma

Imaging is absolutely critical to the diagnosis and management of the patient with acute traumatic brain injury. The goal of emergent neuroimaging is twofold: (1) identify treatable injuries, especially emergent ones, and (2) detect and delineate the presence of secondary injuries such as herniation syndromes and vascular injury.

How to Image?

A broad spectrum of imaging modalities can be used to evaluate patients with TBI. These range from outdated, generally ineffective techniques (i.e., skull radiographs) to very sensitive but expensive studies (e.g., MR). Techniques that are still relatively new include CT and MR perfusion, diffusion tensor imaging (DTI), and functional MRI (fMRI).

Skull Radiography

For decades, skull radiography (whether called "plain film" or, more recently, "digital radiography") was the only noninvasive imaging technique available for the assessment of head injury.

Skull radiography is reasonably effective in identifying calvarial fractures. Yet skull x-rays cannot depict the far more important presence of extraaxial hemorrhages and parenchymal injuries.

Between one-quarter and one-third of autopsied patients with fatal brain injuries have no identifiable skull fracture! Therefore, skull radiography obtained solely for the purpose of identifying the presence of a skull fracture has no appropriate role in the current management of the head-injured patient. With rare exceptions, it's the brain that matters—not the skull!

NECT

CT is now accepted as the worldwide screening tool for imaging acute head trauma. Since its introduction almost 40 years ago, CT has gradually but completely replaced skull radiographs as the "workhorse" of brain trauma imaging. The reasons are simple: CT depicts both bone and soft tissue injuries. It is also widely accessible, fast, effective, and comparatively inexpensive.

Nonenhanced CT (NECT) scans (four or five millimeters thick) from just below the foramen magnum through the vertex should be performed. Two sets of images should be obtained, one using brain and one with bone reconstruction algorithms. Viewing the brain images with a wider window width (150-200 HU, the so-called subdural window) should be performed on PACS (or film, if PACS is not available). The scout view should always be displayed as part of the study (see below).

Because delayed development or enlargement of both extra- and intracranial hemorrhages may occur within 24-36 hours following the initial traumatic event, repeat CT should be obtained if there is sudden unexplained clinical deterioration, regardless of initial imaging findings.

Multidetector Row CT and CT Angiography

Because almost one-third of patients with moderate to severe head trauma also have cervical spine injuries, multidetector row CT (MDCT) with both brain and cervical imaging is often performed. Soft tissue and bone algorithm reconstructions with multiplanar reformatted images of the cervical spine should be obtained.

CT angiography (CTA) is often obtained as part of a whole-body trauma CT protocol. Craniocervical CTA should also specifically be considered (1) in the setting of penetrating neck injury, (2) if a fractured foramen transversarium or facet subluxation is identified on cervical spine CT, or (3) if a skull base fracture traverses the carotid canal or a dural venous sinus. Arterial laceration or dissection, traumatic pseudoaneurysm, carotid-cavernous fistula, or dural venous sinus injury are nicely depicted on high-resolution CTA.

MR

There is general agreement that NECT is the procedure of choice in the initial evaluation of brain trauma. With one important exception—suspected child abuse—using MR as a routine screening procedure in the setting of *acute* brain trauma is uncommon. Standard MR together with new techniques such as diffusion tensor imaging is most useful in the subacute and chronic stages of TBI. Other modalities such as fMRI are playing an increasingly important role in detecting subtle abnormalities, especially in patients with mild cognitive deficits following minor TBI.

Who and When to Image?

Who to image and when to do it is paradoxically both well-established and controversial. Patients with a GCS score indicating moderate (GCS = 9-12) or severe (GCS ≤ 8) neurologic impairment are invariably imaged. The real debate is about how best to manage patients with GCS scores of 13-15.

GLASGOW COMA SCALE

Best eye response (maximum = 4)
- 1 = no eye opening
- 2 = eye opening to pain
- 3 = eyes open to verbal command
- 4 = eyes open spontaneously

Best verbal response (maximum = 5)
- 1 = none
- 2 = incomprehensible sounds
- 3 = inappropriate words
- 4 = confused
- 5 = oriented

Best motor response (maximum = 6)
- 1 = none
- 2 = extension to pain
- 3 = flexion to pain
- 4 = withdrawal to pain
- 5 = localizing to pain
- 6 = obedience to commands

Sum = "coma score" and clinical grading
- 13-15 = mild brain injury
- 9-12 = moderate brain injury
- ≤ 8 = severe brain injury

In an attempt to reduce CT overutilization in emergency departments, several organizations have developed clinical criteria that help separate "high-risk" from "low-risk" patients. (Several of these are delineated in the boxes below.) Yet the impact on the emergency department physician ordering behavior has been inconsistent. In places with high malpractice rates, many emergency physicians routinely order NECT scans on every patient with head trauma regardless of GCS score or clinical findings.

Whether—and when—to obtain follow-up imaging in trauma patients is also controversial. In a large study of children with GCS scores of 14 or 15 and a normal initial CT scan, only 2% had follow-up CT or MR performed. Of these, only 0.05% had abnormal results on the follow-up study, and *none* required surgical intervention. The negative predictive value for neurosurgical intervention for a child with an initial GCS of 14 or 15 and normal CT was 100%. From this, the authors concluded that children with a GCS of 14 or 15 and a normal initial head CT are at very low risk for subsequent traumatic findings on neuroimaging and extremely low risk of needing neurosurgical intervention. Hospitalization of children with minor head trauma after normal CT scan results for neurologic observation was deemed unnecessary.

Appropriateness Criteria

Three major and widely used Appropriateness Criteria for Imaging Acute Head Trauma have been published: The American College of Radiology (ACR) Appropriateness Criteria, the New Orleans Criteria (NOC), and the Canadian Head CT Rule (CHCR).

ACR CRITERIA. Emergent NECT in mild/minor CHI with the presence of a focal neurologic deficit and/or other risk factors is deemed "very appropriate," as is imaging all traumatized children under 2 years of age. While acknowledging that NECT in patients with mild/minor CHI (GCS ≥ 13) without risk factors or focal neurologic deficit is "known to be low yield," the ACR still rates it as 7 out of 9 in appropriateness.

NOC AND CHCR. Both the New Orleans Criteria and Canadian Head CT Rule attempt to triage patients with minimal/mild head injuries in a cost-effective manner. A GCS score of 15 (i.e., normal) without any of the NOC indicators is a highly sensitive negative predictor of clinically important brain injury or need for surgical intervention.

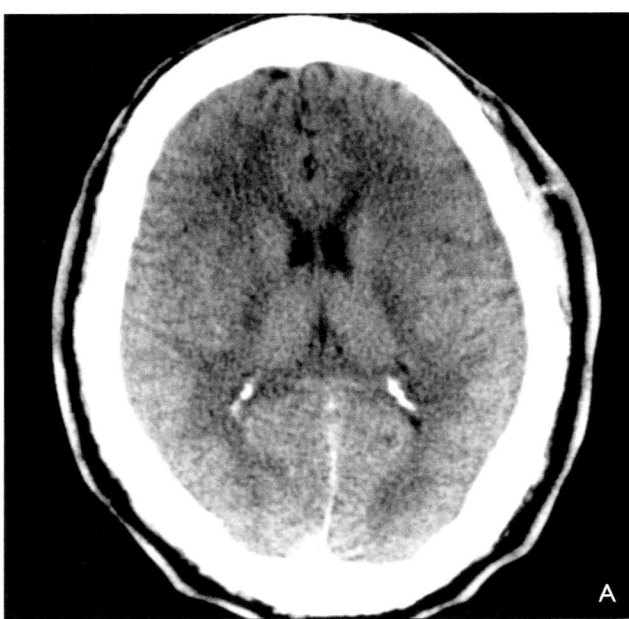

1-1A. *Axial NECT scan of a prisoner imaged for head trauma shows no gross abnormality.*

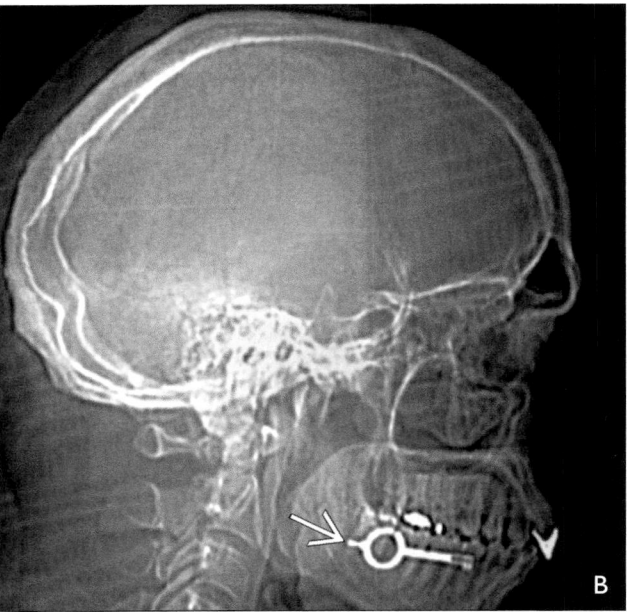

1-1B. *Scout view in the same case shows a foreign object ➔ (a handcuff key!) in the prisoner's mouth. He faked the injury and was planning to escape, but the radiologist alerted the guards and thwarted the plan. (Courtesy J. A. Junker, MD.)*

NEW ORLEANS CRITERIA IN MINOR HEAD INJURY

CT indicated if GCS = 15 plus any of the following
- Headache
- Vomiting
- Patient > 60 years old
- Intoxication (drugs, alcohol)
- Short-term memory deficits (anterograde amnesia)
- Visible trauma above clavicles
- Seizure

Adapted from Stiell IG et al: Comparison of the Canadian CT head rule and the New Orleans criteria in patients with minor head injury. JAMA 294(12):1511-1518, 2005

CANADIAN HEAD CT RULE IN MINOR HEAD INJURY

CT if GCS = 13-15 and witnessed LOC, amnesia, or confusion

High risk for neurosurgical intervention
- GCS < 15 at 2 hours
- Suspected open/depressed skull fracture
- Clinical signs of skull base fracture
- ≥ 2 vomiting episodes
- Age ≥ 65 years

Medium risk for brain injury detected by head CT
- Antegrade amnesia ≥ 30 minutes
- "Dangerous mechanism" (i.e., auto-pedestrian, ejection from vehicle, etc.)

Adapted from Stiell IG et al: Comparison of the Canadian CT head rule and the New Orleans criteria in patients with minor head injury. JAMA 294(12):1511-1518, 2005

According to the CHCR, patients with a GCS score of 13-15 and witnessed loss of consciousness (LOC), amnesia, or confusion are imaged, along with those deemed "high risk" for neurosurgical intervention or "medium risk" for brain injury.

Between 6-7% of patients with minor head injury have positive findings on head CT scans. Most also have headache, vomiting, drug or alcohol intoxication, seizure, short-term memory deficits, or physical evidence of trauma above the clavicles. CT should be used liberally in these cases as well as in patients over 60 years of age and in children under the age of two.

Trauma Imaging: Keys to Analysis

Four components are essential to the accurate interpretation of CT scans in patients with head injury: The scout image plus brain, bone, and subdural views of the NECT dataset. Critical information may be present on just one of these four components.

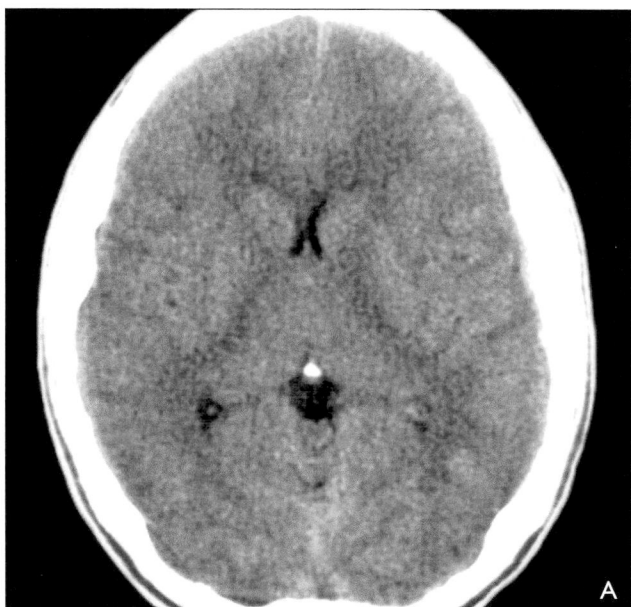

1-2A. *NECT scan at standard brain windows (80 HU) shows no definite abnormality.*

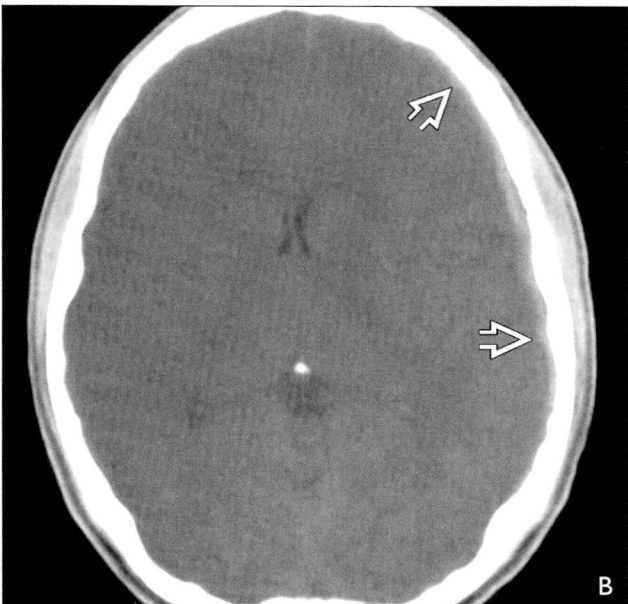

1-2B. *Intermediate window width (175 HU) shows a small left subdural hematoma* ▶. *Thin subdural hematomas may be visible only with wider window widths.*

Suggestions on how to analyze NECT images in patients with acute head injury are delineated below.

Scout Image

Before you look at the NECT scan, examine the digital scout image! Look for cervical spine abnormalities such as fractures or dislocations, jaw and/or facial trauma, and the presence of foreign objects **(1-1)**. If there is a suggestion of cervical spine fracture or malalignment, MDCT of the cervical spine should be performed before the patient is removed from the scanner.

Brain Windows

Methodically and meticulously work your way from the outside in. First evaluate the soft tissue images, beginning with the scalp. Look for scalp swelling, which usually indicates the impact point. Carefully examine the periorbital soft tissues.

Next look for extraaxial blood. The most common extraaxial hemorrhage is traumatic subarachnoid hemorrhage (tSAH), followed by sub- and epidural hematomas. The prevalence of traumatic SAH in moderate to severe TBI approaches 100%. tSAH is usually found in the sulci adjacent to cortical contusions, along the sylvian fissures, and around the anteroinferior frontal and temporal lobes. The best place to look for subtle tSAH is the interpeduncular cistern, where blood collects when the patient is supine.

Any hypodensity within an extraaxial collection should raise suspicion of rapid hemorrhage with accumula-

tion of unclotted blood or (especially in alcoholics or older patients) an underlying coagulopathy. This is an urgent finding that mandates immediate notification of the responsible clinician.

Look for intracranial air ("pneumocephalus"). Intracranial air is always abnormal and indicates the presence of a fracture that traverses either the paranasal sinuses or mastoid.

Now move on to the brain itself. Carefully examine the cortex, especially the "high-yield" areas for cortical contusions (anteroinferior frontal and temporal lobes). If there is a scalp hematoma due to impact (a "coup" injury), look 180° in the opposite direction for a classic "contre-coup" injury. Hypodense areas around the hyperdense hemorrhagic foci indicate early edema and severe contusion.

Move inward from the cortex to the subcortical white and deep gray matter. Petechial hemorrhages often accompany axonal injury. If you see subcortical hemorrhages on the initial NECT scan, this is merely the "tip of the iceberg." There is usually a *lot* more damage than what is apparent on the first scan. A general rule: The deeper the lesion, the more severe the injury.

Finally, look inside the ventricles for blood-CSF levels and hemorrhage due to choroid plexus shearing injury.

Subdural Windows

Look at the soft tissue image with both narrow ("brain") and intermediate ("subdural") windows **(1-2)**. Small subtle subdural hematomas can sometimes be overlooked on standard narrow window widths (75-100 HU) yet are readily apparent when wider windows (150-200 HU) are used.

Bone CT

Bone CT refers to bone algorithm reconstruction viewed with wide (bone) windows. If you can't do bone algorithm reconstruction from your dataset, widen the windows and use an edge enhancement feature to sharpen the image. Three-dimensional shaded surface displays (3D SSDs) are especially helpful in depicting complex fractures (1-3).

Even though standard head scans are four to five millimeters thick, it is often possible to detect fractures on bone CT. Look for basisphenoid fractures with involvement of the carotid canal, temporal bone fractures (with or without ossicular dislocation), mandibular dislocation ("empty" condylar fossa), and calvarial fractures. And remember: Nondisplaced linear skull fractures that don't cross vascular structures (such as a dural venous sinus or middle meningeal artery) are in and of themselves basi-

cally meaningless. It's the brain and blood vessels that matter!

The most difficult dilemma is deciding whether an observed lucency is a fracture or a normal structure (e.g., suture line or vascular channel). Keep in mind: It is virtually unheard of for a calvarial fracture to occur in the absence of overlying soft tissue injury. If there is no scalp "bump," it is unlikely that the lucency represents a nondisplaced linear fracture.

Bone CT images are also very helpful in distinguishing low density from air vs. fat. While most PACS stations have a region of interest (ROI) function that can measure attenuation, fat fades away on bone CT images and air remains very hypodense.

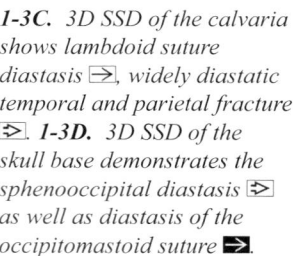
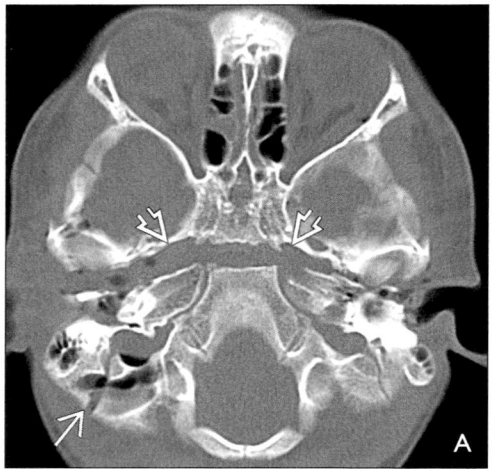
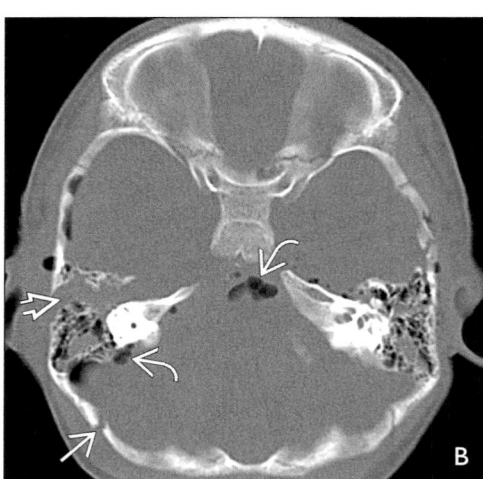

1-3A. Bone CT in a 3-year-old boy with severe head trauma shows multiple linear skull base fractures. Fracture through the right occipital bone ➡ crosses the jugular foramen. There is a severe diastatic fracture through the sphenooccipital synchondrosis ➡. 1-3B. More cephalad bone CT scan shows transverse temporal bone fracture ➡, diastasis of the right lambdoid suture ➡, and extensive pneumocephalus ➡.

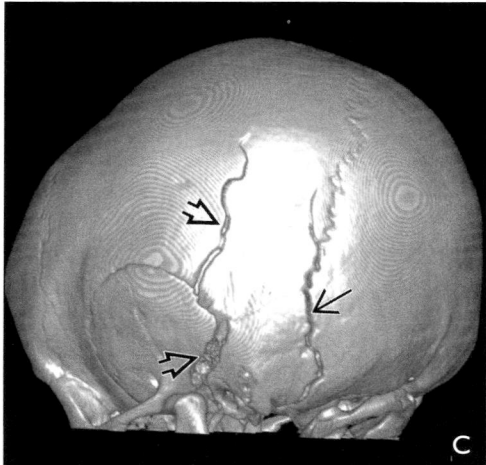
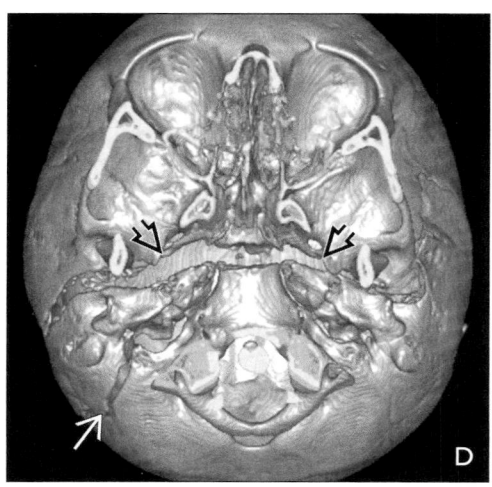

1-3C. 3D SSD of the calvaria shows lambdoid suture diastasis ➡, widely diastatic temporal and parietal fracture ➡. 1-3D. 3D SSD of the skull base demonstrates the sphenooccipital diastasis ➡ as well as diastasis of the occipitomastoid suture ➡.

HEAD TRAUMA: CT CHECKLIST

Scout Image
- Evaluate for
  - Cervical spine fracture-dislocation
  - Jaw dislocation, facial fractures
  - Foreign objects

Brain Windows
- Scalp swelling (impact point)
- Extraaxial blood (focal hypodensity in clot suggests rapid bleeding)
  - Epidural hematoma
  - Subdural hematoma (SDH)
  - Traumatic subarachnoid hemorrhage
- Pneumocephalus
- Cortical contusion
  - Anteroinferior frontal, temporal lobes
  - Opposite scalp laceration/skull fracture
- Hemorrhagic axonal injury
- Intraventricular hemorrhage

Subdural Windows
- 150-200 HU (for thin SDHs under skull)

Bone CT
- Bone algorithm reconstruction > bone windows
- Any fractures cross a vascular channel?

CT Angiography

CT angiography (CTA) is generally indicated if (1) basilar skull fractures cross the carotid canal or a dural venous sinus, (2) if a cervical spine fracture-dislocation is present, especially if the transverse foramina are involved, or (3) if the patient has stroke-like symptoms or unexplained clinical deterioration. Both the cervical and intracranial vasculature should be visualized.

While it is important to scrutinize both the arterial and venous sides of the circulation, a CTA is generally sufficient. Standard CTAs typically show both the arteries and the dural venous sinuses well whereas a CT venogram (CTV) often misses the arterial phase.

Examine the source images as well as the multiplanar reconstructions and maximum-intensity projection (MIP) reformatted scans. Traumatic dissection, vessel lacerations, intimal flaps, pseudoaneurysms, carotid-cavernous fistulas, and dural sinus occlusions can generally be identified on CTA.

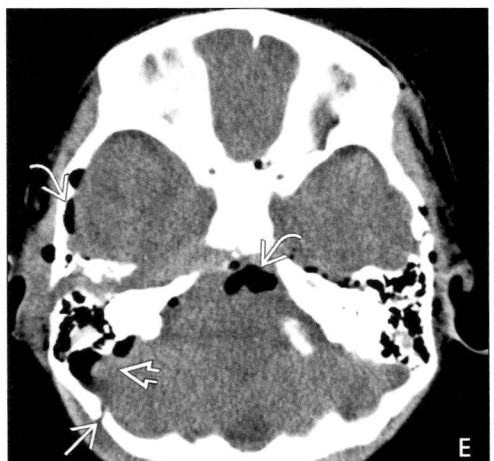

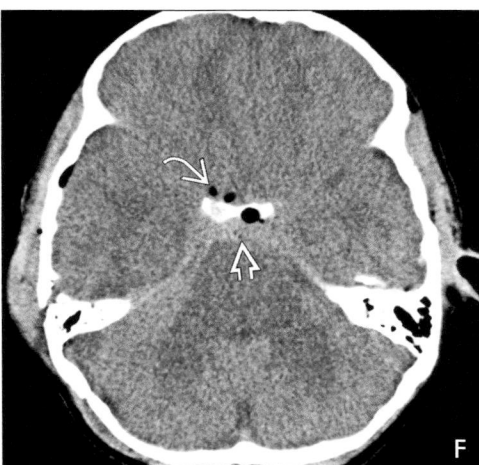

1-3E. Soft tissue windows in the same patient show the extensive pneumocephalus ➡. The occipitomastoid fracture ➡ is seen adjacent to air, which seems to outline a displaced sigmoid sinus ➡. 1-3F. More cephalad NECT scan shows diffuse brain swelling with obliteration of all basal cisterns. Note pneumocephalus ➡ and traumatic subarachnoid hemorrhage ➡.

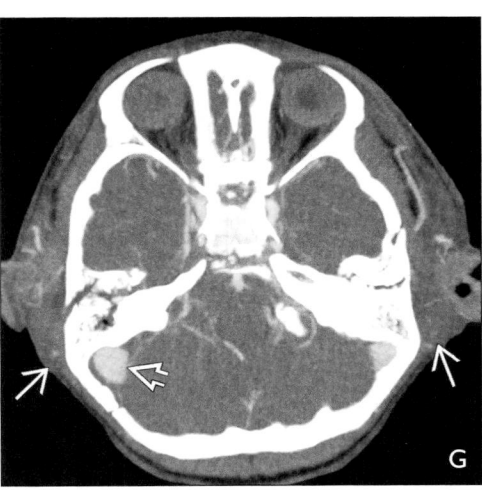

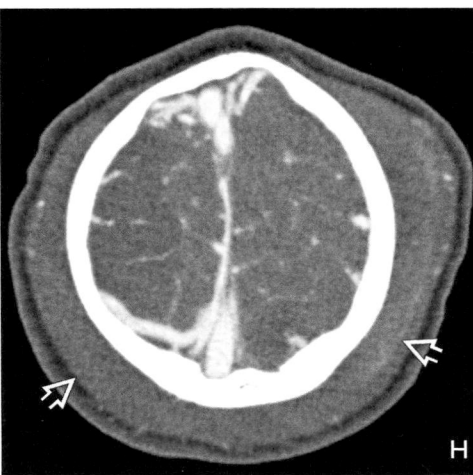

1-3G. CTA was obtained because of the multiple basilar skull fractures, one of which appeared to traverse the right jugular foramen. The sigmoid sinus ➡ is intact but displaced medially. Massive scalp bleeding is apparent as seen by the rapidly enlarging extracranial soft tissues ➡ compared to the CTA scan obtained a few minutes earlier. 1-3H. More cephalad scan shows a massive subgaleal hematoma ➡.

Selected References

- Holmes JF et al: Do children with blunt head trauma and normal cranial computed tomography scan results require hospitalization for neurologic observation? Ann Emerg Med. 58(4):315-22, 2011
- Gean AD et al: Head trauma. Neuroimaging Clin N Am. 20(4):527-56, 2010
- Stiell IG et al: Comparison of the Canadian CT Head Rule and the New Orleans Criteria in patients with minor head injury. JAMA. 294(12):1511-8, 2005

2

Primary Effects of CNS Trauma

Primary head injuries are defined as those that occur at the time of initial trauma even though they may not be immediately apparent on initial evaluation.

Head injury can be caused by direct or indirect trauma. **Direct trauma** involves a blow to the head and is usually caused by automobile collisions, falls, or injury inflicted by an object such as a hammer or baseball bat. Scalp lacerations, hematomas, and skull fractures are common. Associated intracranial damage ranges from none to severe.

Significant forces of acceleration/deceleration, linear translation, and rotational loading can be applied to the brain *without* direct head blows. Such **indirect trauma** is caused by angular kinematics and typically occurs in high-speed motor vehicle collisions (MVCs). Here the brain undergoes rapid deformation and distortion. Depending on the site and direction of the force applied, significant injury to the cortex, axons, penetrating blood vessels, and deep gray nuclei may occur. Severe brain injury can occur in the absence of skull fractures or visible scalp lesions.

We begin our discussion with a consideration of scalp and skull lesions as we work our way from the outside to the inside of the skull. We then delineate the spectrum of intracranial trauma, starting with extraaxial hemorrhages. We conclude this chapter with a detailed discussion of injuries to the brain parenchyma (e.g., cortical contusion, diffuse axonal injury, and the serious deep subcortical injuries).

Scalp and Skull Injuries

Scalp and skull injuries are common manifestations of cranial trauma. While brain injury is usually the most immediate concern in managing traumatized patients, superficial lesions such as scalp swelling and focal hematoma can be helpful in identifying the location of direct head trauma. On occasion, these initially innocent-appearing "lumps and bumps" can become life-threatening. Before turning our attention to intracranial traumatic lesions, therefore, we briefly review scalp and skull injuries, delineating their typical imaging findings and clinical significance.

Scalp Injuries

Scalp injuries include lacerations and hematomas. Scalp **lacerations** are seen as focal discontinuities in the skin. Soft tissue swelling, foreign bodies, and subcutaneous air are commonly identified in more extensive scalp injuries.

It is important to distinguish between the two distinctly different types of scalp **hematomas**: Cephalohematomas and subgaleal hematomas. The former are usually of no clinical significance, whereas the latter can cause hypovolemia and hypotension.

Cephalohematomas are *subperiosteal* blood collections that lie between the outer surface of the skull and elevate the periosteum **(2-1)**. Cephalohematomas occur in 1% of newborns and are more common following instrumented delivery.

Cephalohematomas are the extracranial equivalent of an intracranial epidural hematoma. Cephalohematomas do not cross suture lines and are typically unilateral. Because they are anatomically constrained by the tough fibrous periosteum, cephalohematomas rarely attain large size.

Cephalohematomas are often diagnosed clinically but infrequently imaged. NECT scans show a somewhat lens-shaped soft tissue mass that overlies a single bone (usually the parietal or occipital bone) **(2-2)**. If more than one bone is affected, the two collections are separated by the intervening suture lines.

Complications from cephalohematoma are rare, and most resolve spontaneously over a few days or weeks. The elevated periosteum at the periphery of a chronic cephalohematoma may undergo dystrophic calcification, creating a firm palpable mass.

Subgaleal hematomas are *subaponeurotic* collections and are common findings in traumatized patients of all ages. Here blood collects under the aponeurosis (the "galea") of the occipitofrontalis muscle **(2-3)**. Because a subgaleal hematoma lies external to the periosteum, it is not anatomically limited by suture lines.

Bleeding into the subgaleal space can be very extensive. Subgaleal hematomas are usually bilateral lesions that often spread diffusely around the entire calvaria. NECT scans show a heterogeneous scalp mass that crosses one or more suture lines **(2-4)**.

Most subgaleal hematomas resolve without treatment. In contrast to benign self-limited cephalohematomas, however, expanding subgaleal hematomas in infants and small children can cause significant blood loss.

Facial Injuries

Facial fractures are commonly overlooked on initial imaging (typically head CT scans). Important soft tissue markers can be identified that correlate with facial fractures and may merit a dedicated CT evaluation of the facial bones. These include periorbital contusions and

2-1. Graphic shows the skull of a newborn, including the anterior fontanelle, coronal, metopic, sagittal sutures. Cephalohematoma ⇒ is subperiosteal, limited by sutures. Subgaleal hematoma ⇒ is under the scalp aponeurosis, not bounded by sutures. 2-2. Bone CT in newborn with traumatic delivery shows skull fracture ⇉, cephalohematoma ⇒ overlying parietal bone. Note that the cephalohematoma does not cross the sagittal suture ⇉.

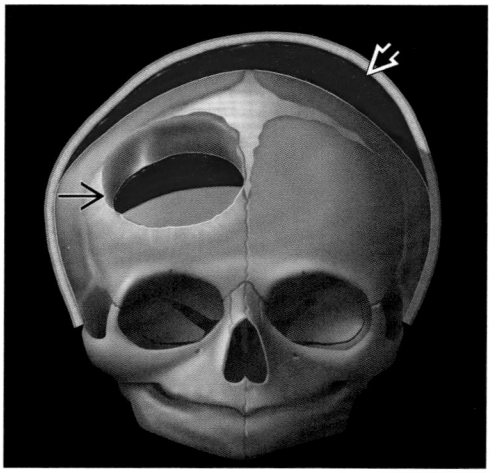
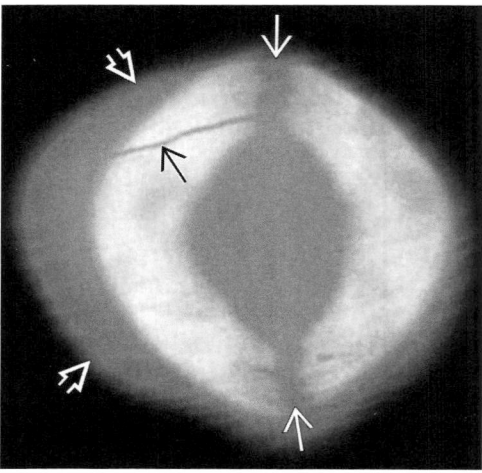

2-3. Autopsy case from a traumatized infant shows a massive biparietal subgaleal hematoma ⇒. The galea aponeurotica has been partially opened ⇒ to show the large biparietal hematoma that crosses the sagittal suture ⇗. 2-4. NECT scan through the vertex of an infant with severe head injury shows an enormous mixed-density acute subgaleal hematoma ⇒ that surrounds the entire skull, crossing the sagittal suture ⇒.

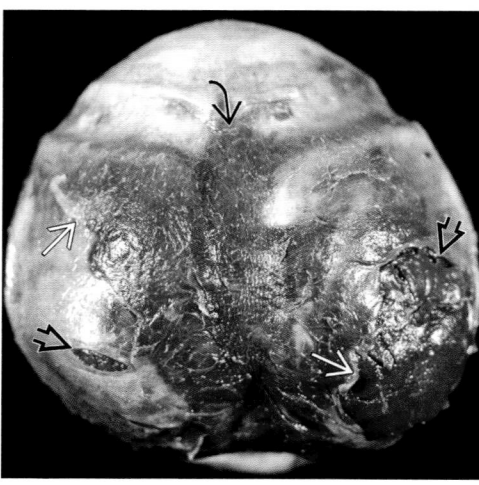
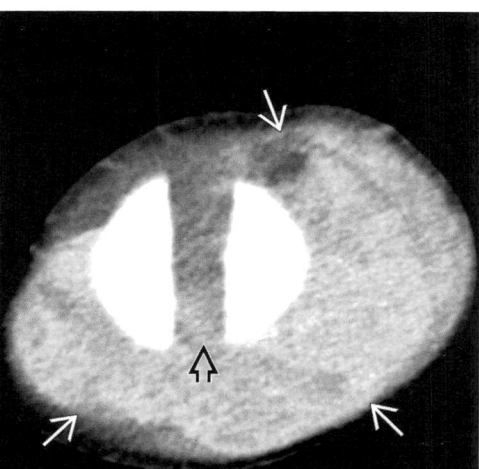

subconjunctival hemorrhage as well as lacerations of the lips, mouth, and nose.

Holmgren et al. have proposed the mnemonic LIPS-N (**l**ip laceration, **i**ntraoral laceration, **p**eriorbital contusion, **s**ubconjunctival hemorrhage, and **n**asal laceration) be used in conjunction with physical examination. If any of these is present, a traumatized patient should have a dedicated facial CT in addition to the standard head CT.

Skull Fractures

Calvarial fractures rarely—if ever—occur in the absence of overlying soft tissue swelling or scalp laceration. Skull fractures are present on initial CT scans in about two-thirds of patients with moderate head injury, although 25-35% of severely injured patients have no identifiable fracture even with thin-section bone reconstructions.

Skull fractures can be simple or comminuted, closed or open. In open fractures, skin laceration results in communication between the external environment and intracranial cavity. Infection risk is high in this type of fracture, as it is with fractures that cross the mastoids and paranasal sinuses.

Several types of acute skull fracture can be identified on imaging studies: Linear, depressed, elevated, and diastatic fractures. Fractures can involve the calvaria, skull base, or both. Another type of skull fracture, a "growing" skull fracture, is a rare but important complication of skull trauma.

Linear Skull Fractures

A **linear skull fracture** is a sharply marginated linear defect that typically involves both the inner and outer tables of the calvaria (2-5).

Most linear skull fractures are caused by relatively low-energy blunt trauma that is delivered over a relatively wide surface area. Linear skull fractures that extend into and widen a suture become diastatic fractures (2-6).

Depressed Skull Fractures

A **depressed skull fracture** is a fracture in which the fragments are displaced inward (2-7). Comminution of the fracture fragments starts at the point of maximum impact

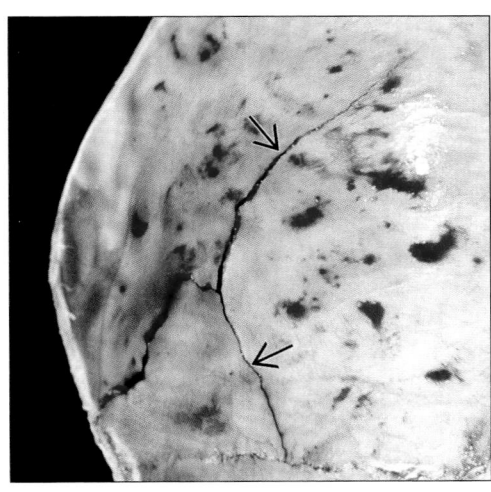

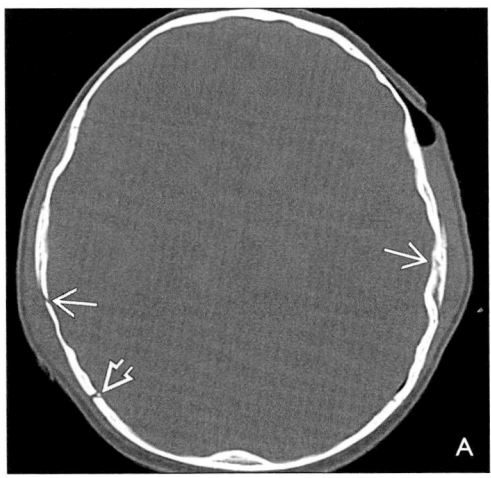

2-5. Autopsy case with calvaria viewed from the endocranial aspect. Note the nondepressed linear temporoparietal skull fracture ➡. (Courtesy E. T. Hedley-Whyte, MD.) 2-6A. Bone CT in a severely traumatized patient shows scalp swelling overlying bilateral linear skull fractures ➡. The right lambdoid suture ➡ is diastatic.

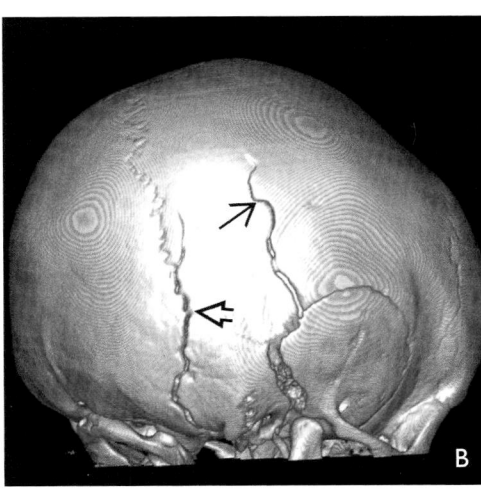

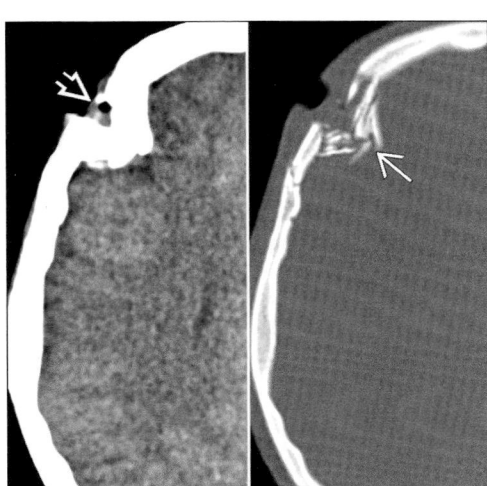

2-6B. 3D SSD shows the right calvarial linear skull fracture ➡ and diastatic fracture involving the lambdoid suture ➡. 2-7. (Left) NECT scan with soft tissue windows shows a depressed skull fracture ➡ with normal-appearing underlying brain. (Right) Bone algorithm shows the severely comminuted, deeply depressed fracture fragments ➡.

and spreads centrifugally. Depressed fractures are most often caused by high-energy direct blows to a small surface with a blunt object (e.g., hammer, baseball bat, or metal pipe).

Depressed skull fractures typically tear the underlying dura and arachnoid and are associated with cortical contusions and potential leakage of CSF into the subdural space. Fractures extending to a dural sinus or the jugular bulb are associated with venous sinus thrombosis in 40% of cases.

Elevated Skull Fractures

An **elevated skull fracture**—often combined with depressed fragments—is uncommon. Elevated fractures are usually caused by a long, sharp object (such as a machete or propeller) that fractures the calvaria, simultaneously lifting and rotating the fracture fragment (2-8).

Diastatic Skull Fractures

A **diastatic skull fracture** is a fracture that widens a suture or synchondrosis (2-9). Diastatic skull fractures

usually occur in association with a linear skull fracture that extends into an adjacent suture.

Traumatic diastasis of the sphenooccipital, petrooccipital, and/or occipitomastoid synchondroses is common in children with severely comminuted central skull base fractures. As it typically does not ossify completely until the mid-teens, the sphenooccipital synchondrosis is the most common site.

"Growing" Skull Fractures

A **"growing" skull fracture** (GSF), also known as "post-traumatic leptomeningeal cyst" or "craniocerebral erosion," is a rare lesion that occurs in just 0.3-0.5% of all skull fractures. Most patients with GSF are under three years of age.

GSFs develop in stages and slowly widen over time. In the first "prephase," a skull fracture (typically a linear or comminuted fracture) lacerates the dura, and brain tissue or arachnoid membrane herniates through the torn dura. Stage I extends from the time of initial injury to just before the fracture enlarges. Early recognition and dural repair of stage I GSFs produce the best results.

2-8A. Axial NECT scan shows severe scalp laceration ⬅ with a combination of elevated ⬈ and depressed ↘ skull fractures. 2-8B. Bone CT in the same case shows that the elevated fracture is literally "hinged" away from the calvaria.

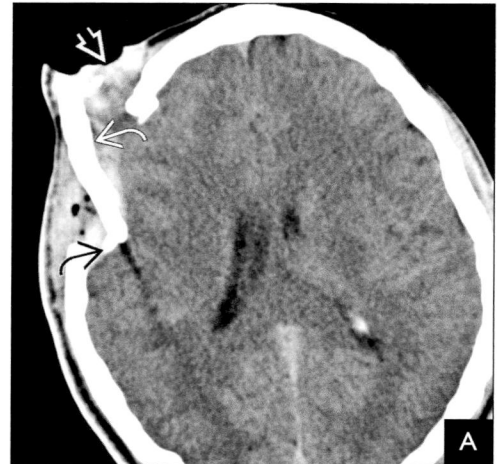
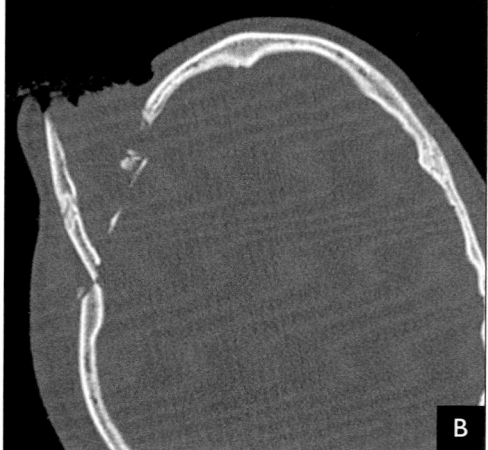

2-9A. NECT scan shows a large subgaleal hematoma ⬈ crossing the sagittal suture. Hyperdense vertex hematoma ↘ also crosses the midline, suggesting that the blood is in the epidural space. 2-9B. Bone CT in the same case shows a diastatic fracture of the sagittal suture ↘. The superior sagittal sinus has been torn; the intracranial blood seen on soft tissue windows is a vertex venous epidural hematoma.

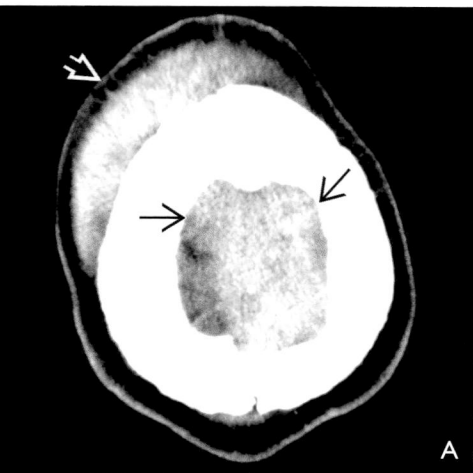
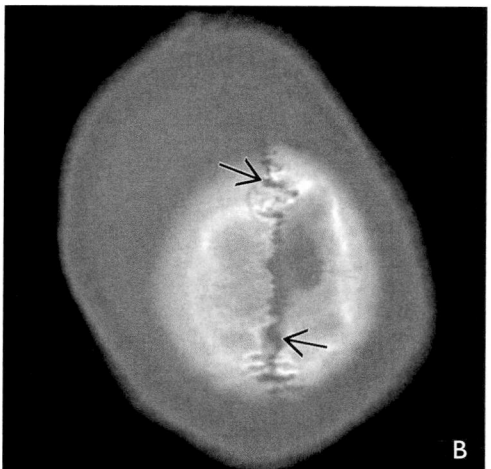

Stage II is the early phase of GSF. Stage II lasts for approximately two months following initial fracture enlargement. At this stage, the bone defect is small, the skull deformity is relatively limited, and neurologic deficits are mild. Nevertheless, the entrapped tissue prevents normal fracture healing.

Stage III represents late-stage GSF and begins two months after the initial enlargement begins. During this stage, the bone defect becomes significantly larger. Brain tissue and CSF extend between the bony edges of the fracture through torn dura and arachnoid.

Patients with late-stage GSFs often present months or even years after head trauma. Stage III GSFs can cause pronounced skull deformities and progressive neurologic deficits if left untreated.

Imaging

GENERAL FEATURES. Plain skull radiographs have no role in the modern evaluation of traumatic head injury. One-quarter of patients with fatal brain injuries have no skull fracture at autopsy. CT is fast, widely available, sensitive for both bone and brain injury, and the worldwide diagnostic standard of care for patients with head injuries. Both bone and soft tissue reconstruction algorithms should be used. Soft tissue reconstructions should be viewed with both narrow ("soft tissue") and intermediate ("subdural") windows.

New generations of multisection CT scanners offer excellent spatial resolution. Three-dimensional reconstruction and curved MIPs of the skull have been shown to improve fracture detection over the use of axial sections alone.

CT FINDINGS. While fractures can involve any part of the calvaria or skull base, the middle cranial fossa is most susceptible because of its thin "squamous" bones and multiple foramina and fissures.

NECT scans demonstrate *linear* skull fractures as sharply marginated lucent lines (2-6). *Depressed* fractures are typically comminuted and show inward implosion of fracture fragments (2-7). *Elevated* fractures show an elevated, rotated skull segment. Diastatic fractures appear as widened sutures or synchondroses (2-9) and are usually associated with linear skull fractures (2-2).

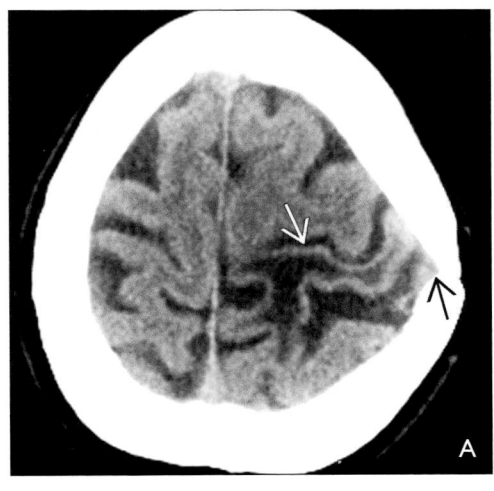
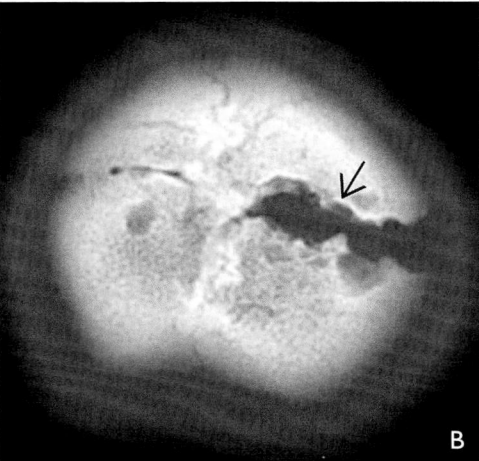

2-10A. Axial NECT scan in a patient with progressive right hemiparesis following prior head trauma shows left parietal encephalomalacia ➡. The overlying skull appears focally deformed and thinned ➡. *2-10B.* Bone CT in the same patient shows a wide lucent skull lesion with rounded, scalloped margins ➡.

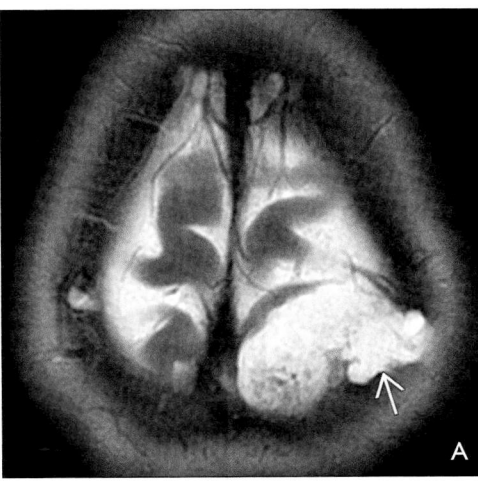
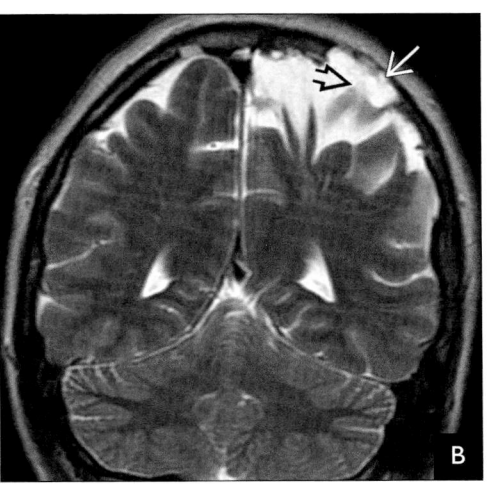

2-11A. Axial T2WI in the same patient shows a lobulated CSF collection ➡ that extends into and almost completely through the calvarial vault. *2-11B.* Coronal T2WI shows the intradiploic CSF collection ➡ with encephalomalacic brain stretched and tethered into the lesion ➡. Classic "growing" skull fracture (leptomeningeal cyst).

Stage I *"growing"* fractures are difficult to detect on initial NECT scans as scalp and contused brain are similar in density. Identifying torn dura with herniated brain tissue is similarly difficult although cranial ultrasound can be more helpful.

Later stage GSFs demonstrate a progressively widening and unhealing fracture. A lucent skull lesion with rounded, scalloped margins and beveled edges is typical (2-10). CSF and soft tissue are entrapped within the expanding fracture (2-11). Most GSFs are directly adjacent to post-traumatic encephalomalacia, so the underlying brain often appears hypodense.

MR FINDINGS. MR is rarely used in the setting of acute head trauma because of high cost, limited availability, and lengthy time required. Compared to CT, bone detail is poor although parenchymal injuries are better seen. Adding T2* sequences, particularly SWI, is especially helpful in identifying hemorrhagic lesions.

In some cases, MR may be indicated for early detection of potentially treatable complications. A young child with neurologic deficits or seizures, a fracture larger than four

millimeters, or a soft tissue mass extending through the fracture into the subgaleal space is at risk for developing a GSF. MR can demonstrate the dural tear and differentiate herniated brain from contused, edematous scalp.

ANGIOGRAPHY. If a fracture crosses the site of a major vascular structure such as the carotid canal or a dural venous sinus (2-12), (2-13), CT angiography is recommended. Sagittal, coronal, and MIP reconstructions help delineate the site and extent of vascular injuries.

Clival fractures are strongly associated with neurovascular trauma, and CTA should always be obtained in these cases (2-14). Cervical fracture-dislocations, distraction injuries, and penetrating neck trauma also merit further investigation. Uncomplicated asymptomatic soft tissue injuries of the neck rarely result in significant vascular injury.

Differential Diagnosis

The major differential diagnoses of skull fracture are normal structures such as vascular grooves and sutures. **Vascular grooves** have well-corticated margins and are not

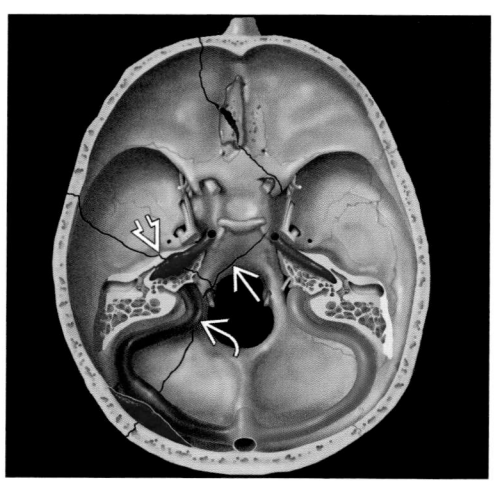
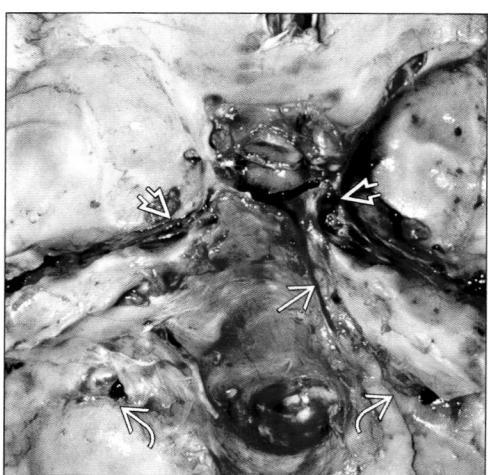

2-12. Axial graphic depicts different basilar skull fractures crossing the petrous apex and clivus ➡, as well as extending into the jugular foramen ➡ and carotid canal ➡. 2-13. Autopsy case shows multiple skull base fractures that involve the clivus ➡, both carotid canals ➡, and both jugular foramina ➡. (Courtesy E. T. Hedley-Whyte, MD.)

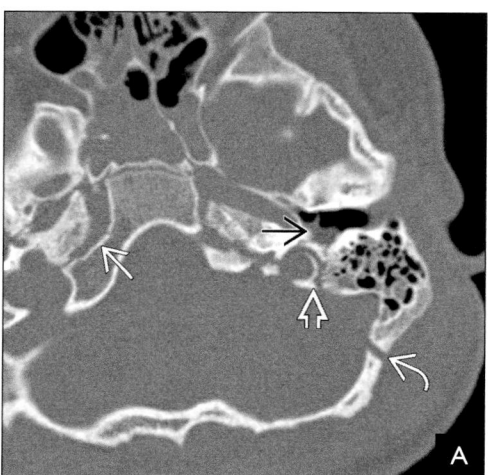
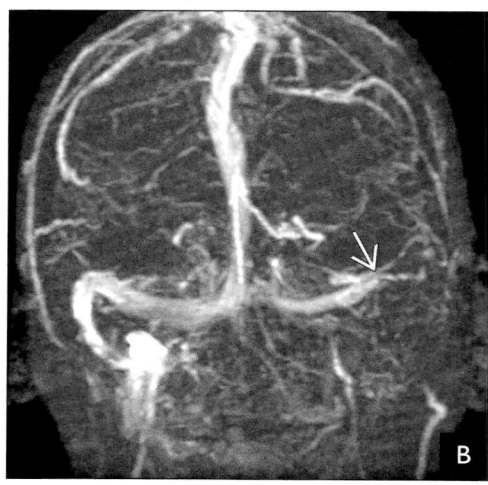

2-14A. Axial bone CT shows skull base fractures that involve the clivus ➡, left sigmoid sinus ➡, and jugular foramen ➡. Note hemotympanum ➡. 2-14B. AP view of MR venogram in the same patient shows occlusion ➡ of the distal left transverse and sigmoid sinuses, jugular bulb.

typically as sharp or lucent as linear skull fractures. Overlying soft tissue swelling is absent. **Sutures** occur in predictable locations (i.e., coronal, sagittal, and mastoid), are densely corticated, and are less distinct than fractures. Sutures wider than two millimeters in the presence of a linear skull fracture are probably diastatic.

Venous lakes and **arachnoid granulations** are smooth, corticated, and occur in predictable locations (i.e., parasagittal and adjacent to or within dural venous sinuses).

SCALP AND SKULL INJURIES

Scalp Injuries
- Cephalohematoma
  - Usually in infants
  - Subperiosteal, limited by sutures
  - Typically small, unilateral; resolves spontaneously
- Subgaleal hematoma
  - Between galea, periosteum of calvaria
  - Not limited by sutures
  - Bilateral, can be extensive

Skull Fractures
- Linear
  - Sharp lucent line
- Depressed
  - Internally displaced fragments
  - Often lacerates dura-arachnoid
- Elevated
  - Rare; fragment rotated outward
- Diastatic
  - Widens suture or synchondrosis
- "Growing"
  - Rare; usually in young children
  - Fracture lacerates dura-arachnoid
  - Brain tissue or arachnoid herniates through torn dura
  - Trapped tissue prevents bone healing
  - CT shows rounded edges, scalloped margins
  - MR shows CSF ± brain

Extraaxial Hemorrhages

Extraaxial hemorrhages and hematomas are common manifestations of head trauma. They can occur in any intracranial compartment, within any space (potential or actual), and between any layers of the cranial meninges. Only the subarachnoid spaces exist normally; all the other spaces are potential spaces and occur only under pathological conditions.

Epidural hematomas arise between the inner table of the skull and outer (periosteal) layer of the dura. **Subdural hematomas** are located between the inner (meningeal) layer of the dura and the arachnoid. **Traumatic sub-**

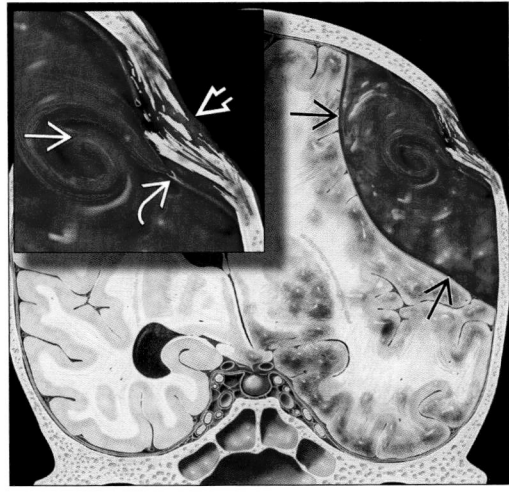

2-15. EDH ➡ with depressed skull fracture ➡ lacerating the middle meningeal artery ➡. Inset shows rapid bleeding, "swirl" sign ➡.

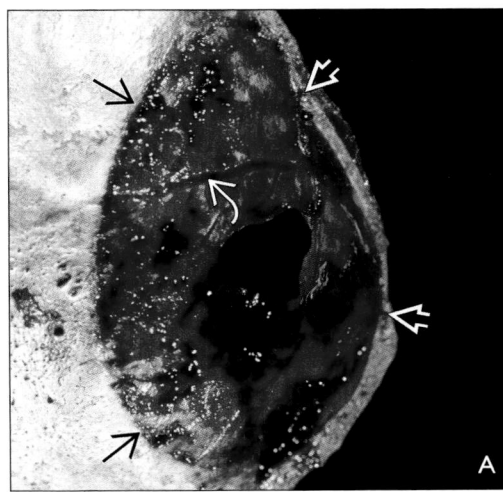

2-16A. Endocranial view shows temporal bone fracture ➡ crossing the middle meningeal artery groove ➡. Note biconvex margins of EDH ➡.

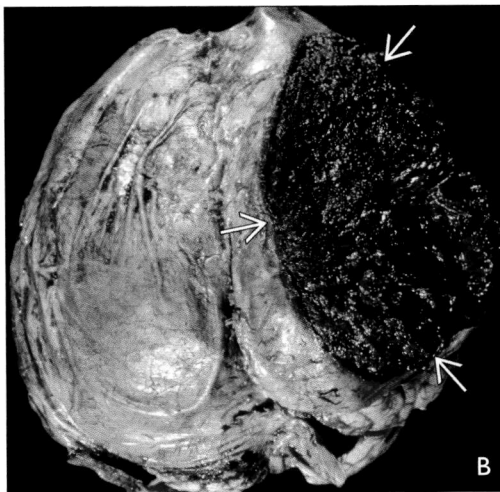

2-16B. Dorsal view of the dura-covered brain shows the biconvex EDH ➡ on top of the dura. (Courtesy E. T. Hedley-Whyte, MD.)

arachnoid hemorrhage is found within the sulci and subarachnoid cisterns, between the arachnoid and the pia.

To discuss extraaxial hemorrhages, we work our way from the outside to inside. We therefore begin this section with a discussion of epidural hematomas, then move deeper inside the cranium to the more common subdural hematomas. We conclude with a consideration of traumatic subarachnoid hemorrhage.

Acute Epidural Hematoma

Epidural hematomas (EDHs) are uncommon but potentially lethal complications of head trauma. If an EDH is promptly recognized and appropriately treated, mortality and morbidity can be minimized.

Terminology

An epidural hematoma is a collection of blood between the calvaria and outer (periosteal) layer of the dura.

Etiology

Most EDHs arise from direct trauma to the skull that lacerates an adjacent artery or dural venous sinus. The vast majority (90%) are caused by arterial injury, most commonly to the middle meningeal artery. Approximately 10% of EDHs are venous, usually secondary to a fracture that crosses a dural venous sinus.

Pathology

LOCATION. Over 90% of EDHs are unilateral and supratentorial. Between 90-95% are found directly adjacent to a skull fracture (2-15). The squamous portion of the temporal bone is the most common site.

GROSS PATHOLOGY. EDHs are biconvex in shape (2-16A). Adherence of the periosteal dura to the inner calvaria explains this typical configuration. As EDHs expand, they strip the dura away from the inner table of the skull, forming the classic lens-shaped hematoma (2-16B), (2-17), (2-18), (2-19). Because the dura is especially tightly attached to sutures, EDHs rarely cross suture lines.

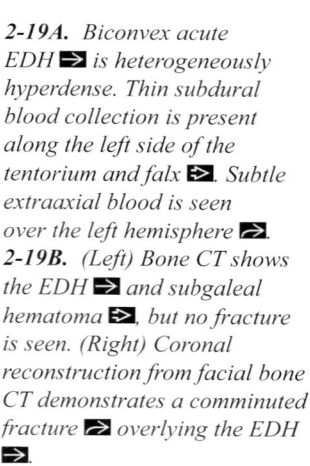

2-17. NECT scan shows classic hyperdense biconvex appearance of acute epidural hematoma ⮕ over the temporal, parietal lobes. 2-18. Axial NECT scan in a child with acute head trauma shows that the gray-white matter interface is displaced medially ⮕ by an actively bleeding EDH with "swirl" sign ⮕. Linear skull fracture is not seen, but hemorrhage under the periosteum has produced a focal cephalohematoma ⮕.

2-19A. Biconvex acute EDH ⮕ is heterogeneously hyperdense. Thin subdural blood collection is present along the left side of the tentorium and falx ⮕. Subtle extraaxial blood is seen over the left hemisphere ⮕. 2-19B. (Left) Bone CT shows the EDH ⮕ and subgaleal hematoma ⮕, but no fracture is seen. (Right) Coronal reconstruction from facial bone CT demonstrates a comminuted fracture ⮕ overlying the EDH ⮕.

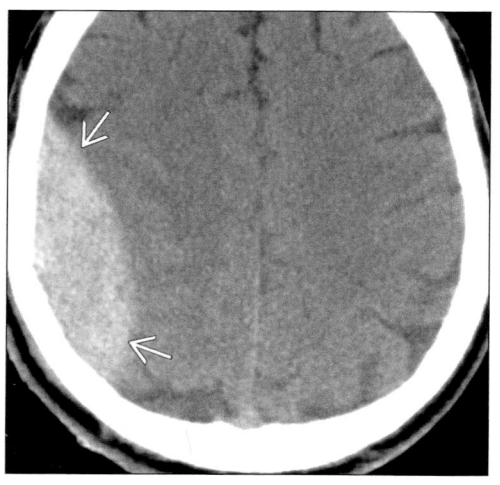

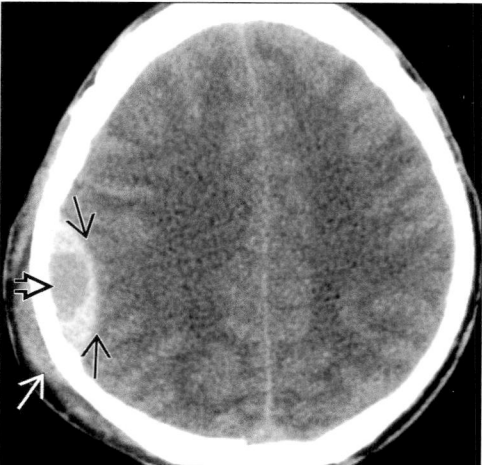

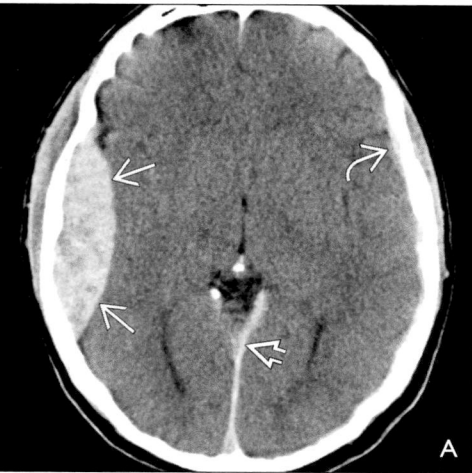

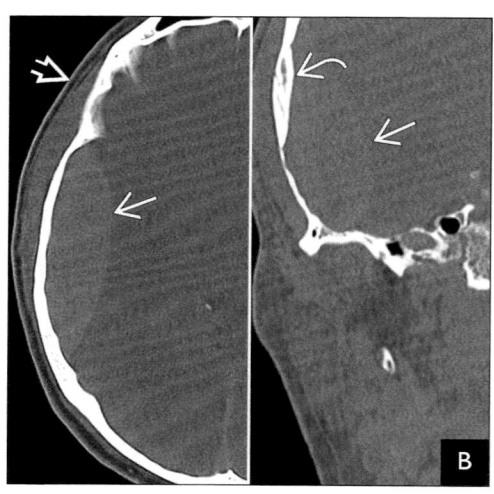

The typical gross or intraoperative appearance of an acute EDH is a dark purple ("currant jelly") lentiform clot.

Clinical Issues

EPIDEMIOLOGY. EDHs are much less common than either traumatic subarachnoid hemorrhage (tSAH) or subdural hematoma (SDH). Although EDHs represent up to 10% of fatal injuries in autopsy series, they are found in only 1-4% of patients imaged for craniocerebral trauma.

DEMOGRAPHICS. EDHs are uncommon in infants and the elderly. Most are found in older children and young adults. The M:F ratio is 4:1.

PRESENTATION. The prototypical "lucid interval," during which a traumatized patient has an initial brief loss of consciousness followed by an asymptomatic period of various length prior to onset of coma and/or neurologic deficit, occurs in only 50% of EDH cases. Headache, nausea, vomiting, symptoms of intracranial mass effect (e.g., pupil-involving third cranial nerve palsy) followed by somnolence and coma are common.

NATURAL HISTORY. Outcome depends on size and location of the hematoma, whether the EDH is arterial or venous, and if there is active bleeding (see below). Overall mortality rate with prompt recognition and treatment is under 5%.

Patients with mixed-density EDHs tend to present earlier than patients with hyperdense hematomas and have lower Glasgow Coma Scores, larger hematoma volumes, and poorer prognosis.

Delayed development or enlargement of an EDH occurs in 10-15% of cases, usually within 24-36 hours following trauma.

TREATMENT OPTIONS. Most EDHs are surgically evacuated. Mixed-density EDHs expand rapidly in size and require even earlier and more aggressive treatment.

Occasionally, a small hyperdense EDH that does not exhibit a "swirl" sign and has minimal or no mass effect is managed nonoperatively with close clinical observation and follow-up imaging **(2-20)**.

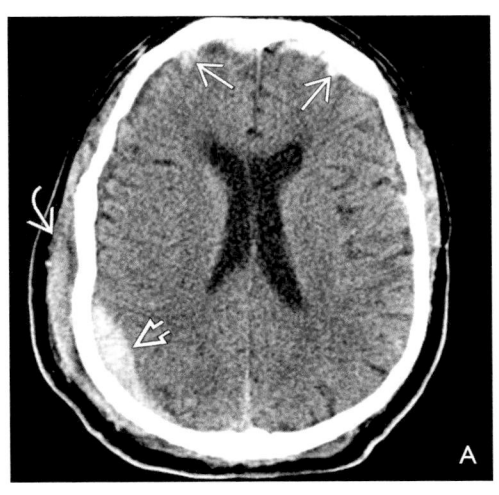

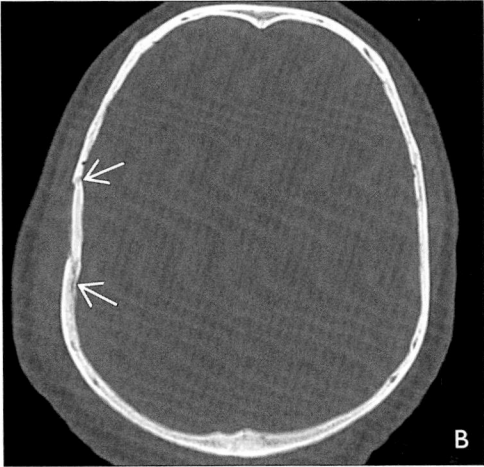

2-20A. Series of imaging studies demonstrates temporal evolution of a small EDH. Initial NECT scan shows a right parietal EDH ➤, subgaleal hematoma ➤, and bifrontal contusions with some traumatic subarachnoid hemorrhage ➤. 2-20B. Bone CT in the same patient shows a slightly depressed right temporoparietal skull fracture ➤. The patient was managed conservatively.

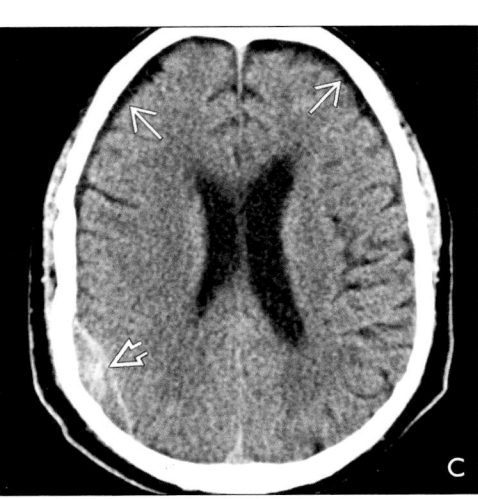

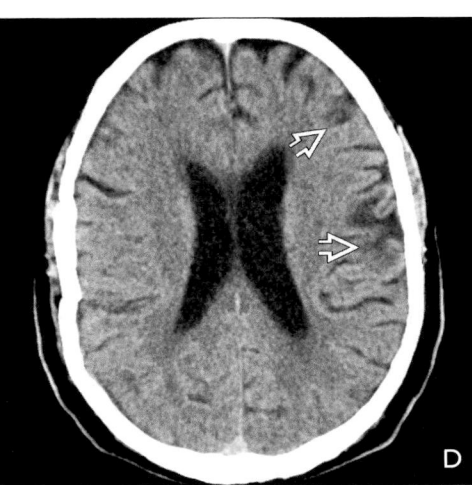

2-20C. Repeat NECT scan 10 days later shows that the density of the EDH ➤ has decreased significantly. Small bifrontal hypodense subdural hygromas ➤ are now seen. 2-20D. Repeat study 6 weeks after trauma shows that the EDH has resolved. Foci of left hemisphere encephalomalacia ➤ from "contre-coup" injury are now evident.

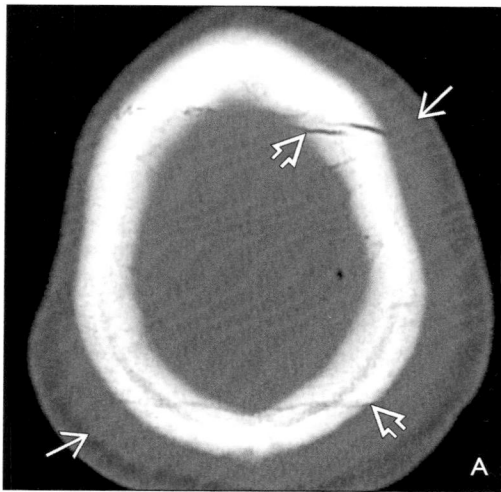

2-21A. Axial bone CT shows extensive subgaleal hematoma ➡ and linear skull fractures ⬛➡ crossing the sagittal suture.

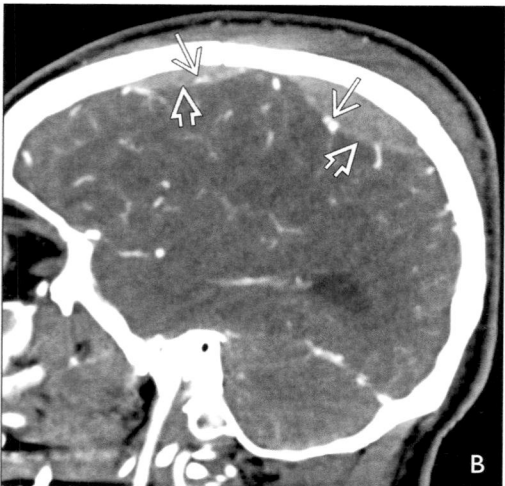

2-21B. Sagittal reformatted image from CTA shows biconvex extrasagittal reformat hematomas ⬛➡ displacing the cortical veins inward ⬛➡.

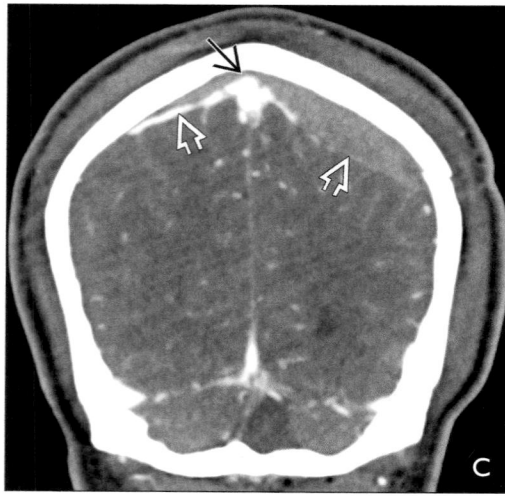

2-21C. Coronal scan shows that vertex epidural hematomas ⬛➡ cross the midline, displacing the superior sagittal sinus ⬛➡ away from the skull.

Imaging

GENERAL FEATURES. EDHs, especially in adults, typically do not cross sutures unless a fracture with sutural diastasis is present. In children, 10% of EDHs cross suture lines, usually the coronal or sphenosquamous suture.

Look for other comorbid lesions such as "contre-coup" injuries, tSAH, and secondary brain herniations, all of which are common findings in patients with EDHs.

CT FINDINGS. NECT scan is the procedure of choice for initial imaging in patients with head injury. Both soft tissue and bone reconstruction algorithms should be obtained. Multiplanar reconstructions are especially useful in identifying vertex epidural hematomas, which may be difficult to detect if only axial images are obtained.

The classic imaging appearance of **arterial EDHs** is a hyperdense (60-90 HU) lentiform extraaxial collection **(2-17)**. Presence of a hypodense component ("swirl" sign) is seen in about one-third of cases and indicates active, rapid bleeding with unretracted clot **(2-18)**.

EDHs compress the underlying subarachnoid space and displace the cortex medially, "buckling" the gray-white matter interface inward.

Air in an EDH occurs in approximately 20% of cases and is usually—but not invariably—associated with a sinus or mastoid fracture.

The much less common **venous EDHs** are often smaller and develop more slowly than arterial EDHs. Most are caused by a skull fracture that crosses a dural venous sinus and therefore occur near the vertex (superior sagittal sinus) or skull base (transverse/sigmoid sinus). In contrast to their arterial counterparts, venous EDHs can "straddle" intracranial compartments, crossing both sutures and lines of dural attachment **(2-21)**, **(2-22)**.

Venous EDHs—especially "vertex" hematomas—are easily overlooked. Coronal and sagittal reformatted imaging is helpful in their detection and delineation.

MR FINDINGS. Acute EDHs are typically isointense with underlying brain, especially on T1WI. The displaced dura can be identified as a displaced "black line" between the hematoma and the brain.

ANGIOGRAPHY. DSA may show a lacerated middle meningeal artery with "tram-track" fistulization of contrast from the middle meningeal artery into the paired middle meningeal veins. Mass effect with displaced cortical arteries and veins is seen.

Differential Diagnosis

In the appropriate setting, imaging findings of EDH are pathognomonic.

The major differential diagnosis is **subdural hematoma**, which is usually crescentic and frequently crosses suture lines but is confined by dural attachments of the falx or tentorium. Coexistence of an EDH and an SDH is common.

Other hyperdense extraaxial collections on NECT scan include both primary and metastatic **neoplasms** such as meningioma, lymphoma, and metastases. Occasionally, infections (such as dural **tuberculoma**), inflammatory masses (e.g., **pseudotumors**, histiocytoses), and **extramedullary hematopoiesis** present as hyperdense extraaxial masses.

ACUTE EPIDURAL HEMATOMA

Terminology
- EDH = blood between skull, dura

Etiology
- Associated skull fracture in 90-95%
  - Skull fracture lacerates vessel
- Arterial (90%), venous (10%)

Pathology
- Unilateral, supratentorial (> 90%)
- Biconvex shape (dura stripped away from skull)
- Usually does not cross suture lines
- Can cross sites of dural attachment

Clinical Issues
- Relatively rare (1-4% of head trauma)
- Older children, young adults; M:F = 4:1
- Classic "lucid interval" in only 50%
- Delayed deterioration common
- Prompt recognition and treatment = low mortality

Imaging
- Hyperdense lens-shaped clot
- Hypodensity ("swirl" sign) = rapid bleeding
- "Vertex" EDH usually venous, can cross midline

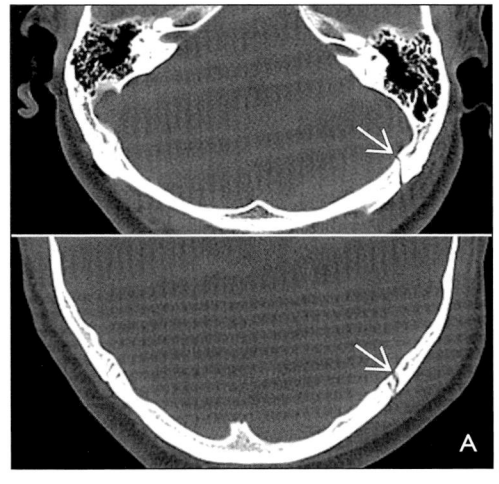

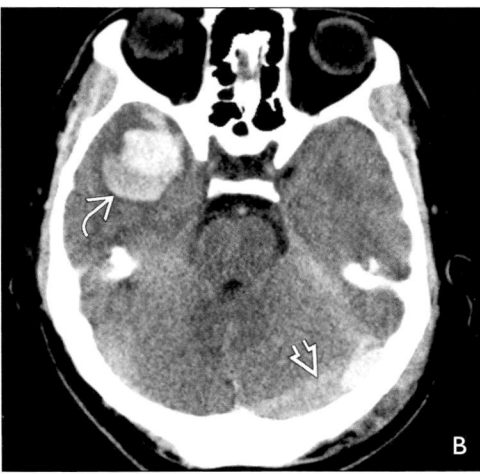

2-22A. (Top) Bone CT in a 26-year-old man who fell 25 feet onto his head shows a diastatic fracture ➡ of the left lambdoid suture. (Bottom) The fracture continues superiorly, following the lambdoid suture above the insertion of the tentorium. 2-22B. NECT scan shows a mixed-density posterior fossa EDH ➡. Note "contre-coup" contusion of the right temporal lobe with mixed attenuation hematoma ➡ suggesting rapid bleeding.

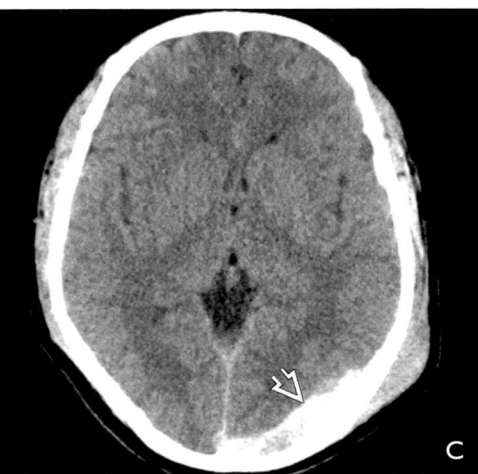

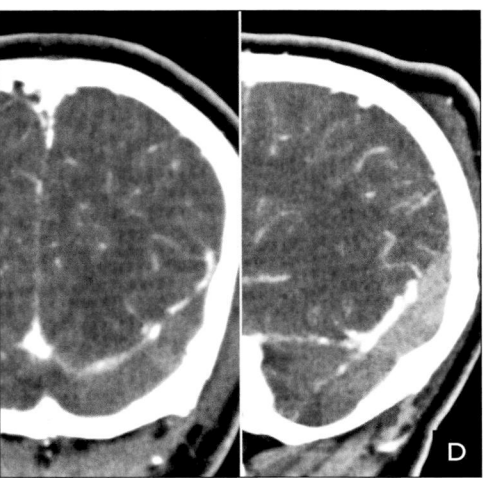

2-22C. More cephalad scan in the same patient shows that the EDH ➡ extends above the tentorium behind the left occipital lobe. 2-22D. CTA was obtained because CT findings suggested venous EDH with laceration of the left transverse sinus. (Left) Coronal, (right) sagittal reformatted images nicely show that the EDH extends below and above the tentorium, displacing cortical veins as well as elevating and compressing the left transverse sinus.

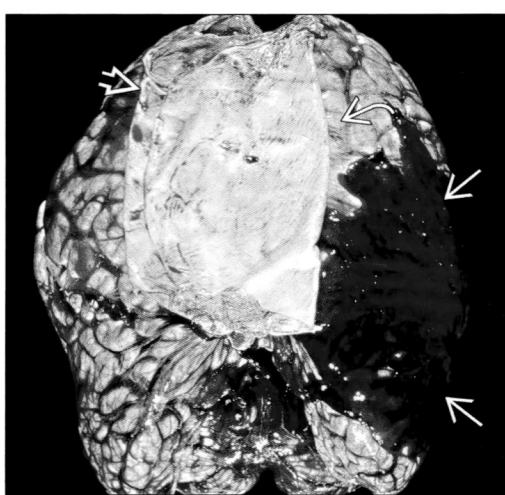

2-23. Graphic depicts crescent-shaped acute SDH ➡ with contusions and "contre-coup" injuries ➡, diffuse axonal injuries ➡.

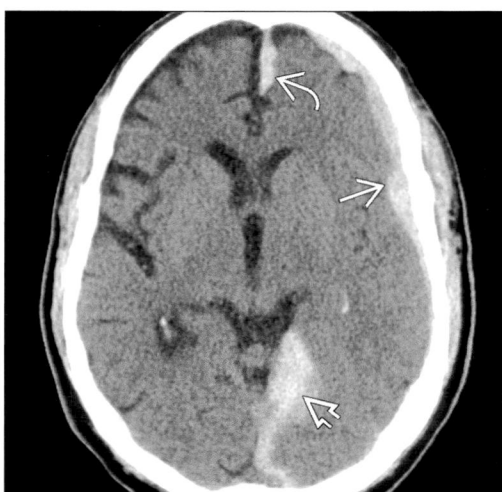

2-24. Autopsy shows acute SDH ➡ spreading over the brain between dura ➡, thin veil-like arachnoid ➡. (Courtesy E. T. Hedley-Whyte, MD.)

2-25. Acute SDH spreads over left hemisphere ➡, along tentorium ➡, into interhemispheric fissure ➡ but does not cross midline.

Acute Subdural Hematoma

Acute subdural hematomas are one of the leading causes of death and disability in patients with severe traumatic brain injury. Subdural hematomas (SDHs) are much more common than epidural hematomas (EDHs). Most do not occur as isolated injuries; the vast majority of SDHs are associated with traumatic subarachnoid hemorrhage as well as significant parenchymal injuries such as cortical contusions, brain lacerations, and diffuse axonal injuries.

Terminology

An acute subdural hematoma (aSDH) is a collection of acute blood products that lies in or between the inner border cell layer of the dura and the arachnoid (2-23).

Etiology

Trauma is the most common cause of aSDH. Both direct blows to the head and non-impact injuries may result in formation of an aSDH. Tearing of bridging cortical veins as they cross the subdural space to enter a dural venous sinus (usually the superior sagittal sinus) is the most common etiology. Cortical vein lacerations can occur with either a skull fracture or the sudden changes in velocity and brain rotation that occur during non-impact closed head injury.

Blood from ruptured vessels spreads quickly through the potential space between the dura and the arachnoid. Large SDHs may spread over an entire hemisphere, extending into the interhemispheric fissure and along the tentorium.

Tearing of cortical arteries from a skull fracture may also give rise to an aSDH. The arachnoid itself may also tear, creating a pathway for leakage of CSF into the subdural space, resulting in admixture of both blood and CSF.

Less common causes of aSDH include aneurysm rupture, skull/dura-arachnoid metastases from vascular extracranial primary neoplasms, and spontaneous hemorrhage in patients with severe coagulopathy.

Rarely, an acute spontaneous SDH of arterial origin occurs in someone without any traumatic history or vascular anomaly. These patients usually have sudden serious disturbance of consciousness and have a poor outcome unless the aSDH is recognized and treated promptly.

Pathology

GROSS PATHOLOGY. The gross appearance of an aSDH is that of a soft, purplish, "currant jelly" clot beneath a tense bulging dura (2-24). More than 95% are supratentorial. Most aSDHs spread diffusely over the affected hemisphere and are therefore typically crescent-shaped.

Clinical Issues

EPIDEMIOLOGY. An aSDH is the second most common extraaxial hematoma, exceeded only by traumatic subarachnoid hemorrhage (tSAH). An aSDH is found in 10-20% of all patients with head injury and is observed in 30% of autopsied fatal injuries.

DEMOGRAPHICS. An aSDH may occur at any age from infancy to the elderly. There is no gender predilection.

PRESENTATION. Even relatively minor head trauma, especially in elderly patients who are often anticoagulated, may result in an acute SDH. In such patients, a definite history of trauma may be lacking.

Clinical findings vary from none to loss of consciousness and coma. Most patients with aSDHs have low Glasgow Coma Scores on admission. Delayed deterioration, especially in elderly anticoagulated patients, is common.

NATURAL HISTORY. An aSDH may remain stable, grow slowly, or rapidly increase in size causing mass effect and secondary brain herniations. Prognosis varies with hematoma thickness, midline shift, and the presence of associated parenchymal injuries. An aSDH that is thicker than two centimeters correlates with poor outcome (35-90% mortality). An aSDH that occupies more than 10% of the total available intracranial volume is usually lethal.

TREATMENT OPTIONS. Presence of an aSDH in a traumatized patient is generally considered a neurosurgical emergency. Evacuation of an aSDH that has significant mass effect is typical. Small collections are sometimes managed with close clinical observation and follow-up imaging. Any sudden deterioration in the patient's condition should be evaluated with repeat CT scan.

Imaging

GENERAL FEATURES. The classic finding of an aSDH is a supratentorial crescent-shaped extraaxial collection that displaces the gray-white matter interface medially. SDHs are typically more extensive than EDHs, easily spreading along the falx, tentorium, and around the anterior and middle fossa floors (2-25). SDHs may cross suture lines but generally do not cross dural attachments. Bilateral

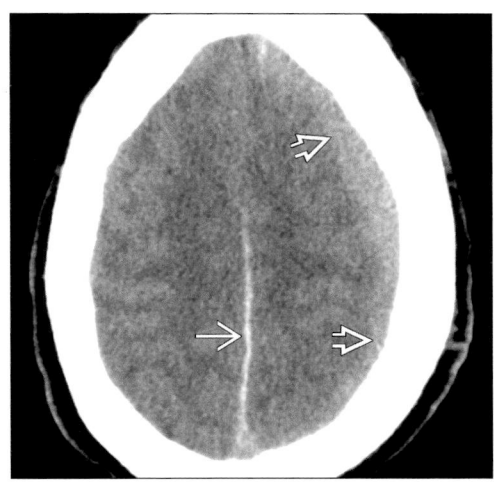

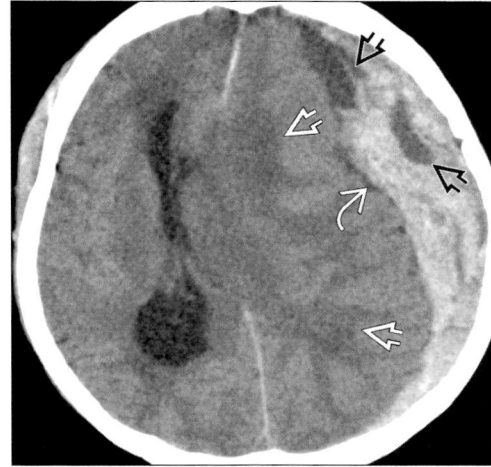

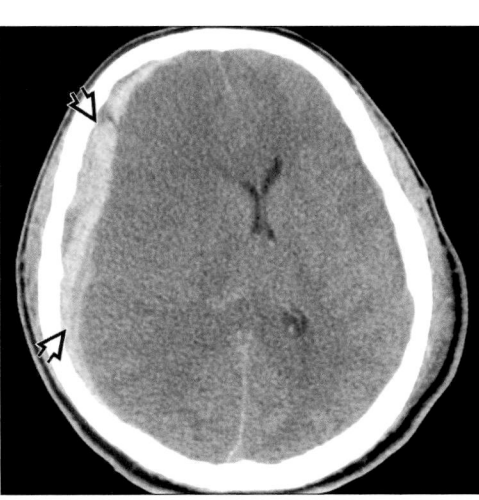

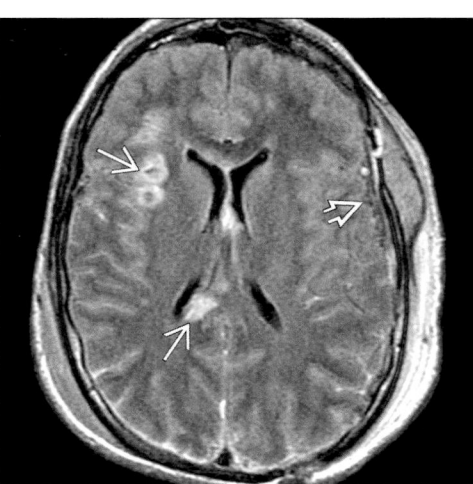

2-26. Axial NECT shows typical hyperdense interhemispheric aSDH ➡. SDH over the left hemisphere ⮞ is less dense, probably because an arachnoid tear is allowing CSF to intermix with blood. The patient's hematocrit was normal.
2-27. Mixed-density aSDH with rapid bleeding and hypodense unretracted clots ⮡ compresses the underlying CSF-filled subarachnoid space ➡. The gray-white matter interface ⮞ is displaced medially.

2-28. NECT shows mixed-density aSDH ⮡ with a disproportionately large subfalcine herniation of the lateral ventricles. The entire right hemisphere is hypodense, indicating diffuse holohemispheric brain swelling. This life-threatening complication of an aSDH may require emergent decompressive craniectomy. 2-29. FLAIR scan in a patient 2 days after closed head trauma shows a small hypodense SDH ⮞ and multiple axonal injuries ➡.

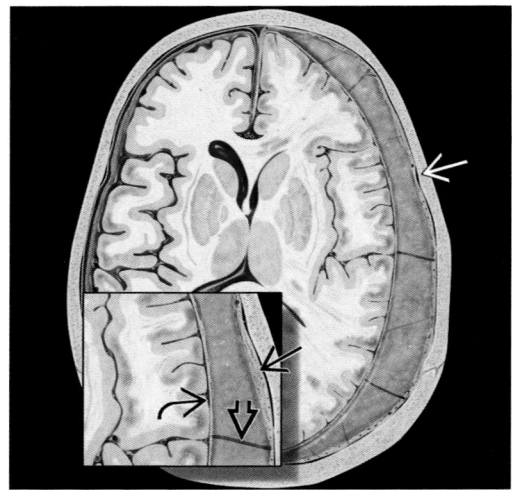

2-30. Graphic depicts sSDH ➡. *Inset shows bridging vein* ⏩ *and thin inner* ⤳, *thick outer* ➡ *membranes.*

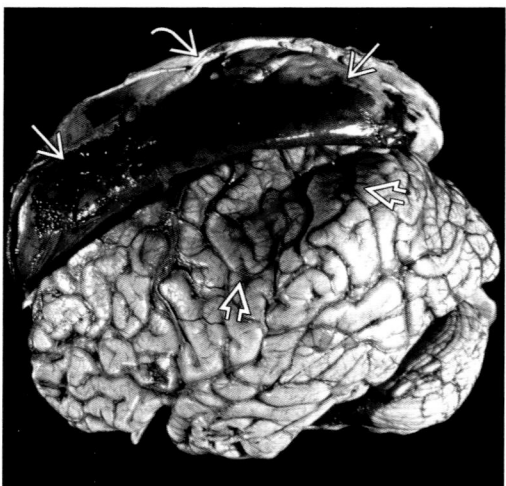

2-31. Autopsy case shows sSDH with organized hematoma ➡, *thick outer membrane* ⤴, *deformed brain* ➡. *(Courtesy R. Hewlett, MD.)*

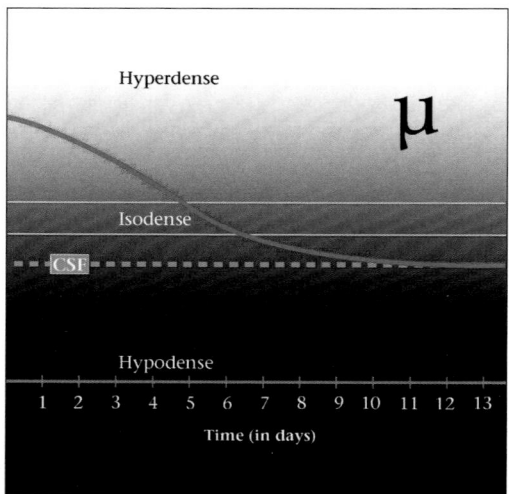

2-32. SDHs decrease approximately 1.5 HU/day. By 7-10 days, blood in hematoma is isodense with cortex. By about 10 days, it is hypodense.

SDHs occur in 15% of cases. "Contre-coup" injuries such as contusion of the contralateral hemisphere are common.

Both standard soft tissue and intermediate ("subdural") windows should be used in all trauma patients as small, subtle aSDHs can be obscured by the density of the overlying calvaria.

CT FINDINGS.

NECT. Approximately 60% of aSDHs are hyperdense on NECT scans **(2-25)**, **(2-26)**. Mixed attenuation lesions are found in 40% of cases **(2-27)**. Pockets of hypodensity within the larger hyperdense collection ("swirl" sign) usually indicate rapid bleeding **(2-28)**. "Dots" or "lines" of CSF trapped within compressed, displaced sulci are often seen underlying an aSDH **(2-27)**.

Mass effect with an aSDH is common. In some patients, especially athletes with repeated head injury, brain swelling with unilateral hemisphere vascular engorgement occurs. Here the mass effect is disproportionate to the size of the SDH, which may be relatively small. This entity, the "second impact syndrome," is probably caused by vascular dysautoregulation (see Chapter 3).

Occasionally, an aSDH is nearly isodense with the underlying cortex **(2-26)**. This unusual appearance is found in extremely anemic patients (Hgb under 8-10 g/dL) and sometimes occurs in patients with coagulopathy. In rare cases, CSF leakage through a torn arachnoid may mix with—and dilute—the acute blood that collects in the subdural space.

CECT. CECT scans are helpful in detecting small isodense aSDHs. The normally enhancing cortical veins are displaced inward by the extraaxial fluid collection.

Perfusion CT. CT or xenon perfusion scans may demonstrate decreased cerebral blood flow (CBF) and low perfusion pressure, which is one of the reasons for the high mortality rate of patients with aSDHs. The cortex underlying an evacuated aSDH may show hyperemic changes with elevated rCBF values. Persisting hyperemia has been associated with poor outcome.

MR FINDINGS.
MR scans are rarely obtained in acutely brain-injured patients. In such cases, aSDHs appear isointense on T1WI and hypointense on T2WI. Signal intensity on FLAIR scans is usually iso- to hyperintense compared to CSF but hypointense compared to the adjacent brain **(2-29)**. aSDHs are hypointense on T2* scans.

DWI shows heterogeneous signal within the hematoma but may show patchy foci of restricted diffusion in the cortex underlying the aSDH.

ANGIOGRAPHY.
CTA may be useful in visualizing a cortical vessel that is actively bleeding into the subdural space.

Differential Diagnosis

In the setting of acute trauma, the major differential diagnosis is **epidural hematoma** (EDH). Shape is a helpful feature as most aSDHs are crescentic while EDHs are biconvex. EDHs are almost always associated with skull fracture; SDHs frequently occur in the absence of skull fracture. EDHs may cross sites of dural attachment; SDHs do not cross the falx or tentorium.

Subacute Subdural Hematoma

With time, subdural hematomas (SDHs) undergo organization, lysis, and neomembrane formation. Within two to three days, the initial soft, loosely organized clot of an acute subdural hematoma becomes organized. Breakdown of blood products and the formation of organizing granulation tissue change the imaging appearance of subacute and chronic SDHs.

Terminology

A subacute subdural hematoma (sSDH) is between several days and several weeks old.

Pathology

A collection of partially liquified clot with resorbing blood products is surrounded on both sides by a "membrane" of organizing granulation tissue (2-30). The outermost membrane adheres to the dura and is typically thicker than the inner membrane, which abuts the thin, delicate arachnoid (2-31).

In some cases, repetitive hemorrhages of different ages arising from the friable granulation tissue may be present. In others, liquefaction of the hematoma over time produces serous blood-tinged fluid.

Clinical Issues

EPIDEMIOLOGY AND DEMOGRAPHICS. SDHs are common findings at imaging and autopsy. In contrast to acute SDHs, subacute SDHs show a distinct bimodal distribution with children and the elderly as the most commonly affected age groups.

PRESENTATION. Clinical symptoms vary from asymptomatic to loss of consciousness and hemiparesis caused by sudden rehemorrhage into an sSDH. Headache and seizure are other common presentations.

NATURAL HISTORY AND TREATMENT OPTIONS. Many sSDHs resolve spontaneously. In some cases, repeated hemorrhages may cause sudden enlargement and mass effect. Surgical drainage may be indicated if the sSDH is enlarging or becomes symptomatic.

Imaging

GENERAL FEATURES. Imaging findings are related to hematoma age and the presence of encasing membranes. Evolution of an untreated, uncomplicated SDH follows a very predictable pattern on CT. Density of an extraaxial hematoma decreases approximately 1-2 HU each day (2-32). Therefore, an SDH will become nearly isodense with the underlying cerebral cortex within a few days following trauma.

CT FINDINGS. sSDHs are typically crescent-shaped fluid collections that are iso- to slightly hypodense compared to the underlying cortex on NECT (2-33). Medial displacement of the gray-white interface ("buckling") is often present, along with "dot-like" foci of CSF in the trapped, partially effaced sulci underlying the sSDH (2-34), (2-35). Mixed-density hemorrhages are common.

Bilateral sSDHs may be difficult to detect because of their "balanced" mass effect (2-34). Sulcal effacement with displaced gray-white matter interfaces is the typical appearance.

CECT scans show the enhanced cortical veins are displaced medially. The encasing membranes, especially the thicker superficial layer, may enhance.

MR FINDINGS. MR can be very helpful in identifying sSDHs, especially small lesions that are virtually isodense with underlying brain on CT scans.

Signal intensity varies with hematoma age but is less predictable than on CT, making precise "aging" of subdural collections more problematic. In general, early subacute SDHs are isointense with cortex on T1WI and hypointense on T2WI but gradually become more hyperintense as extracellular methemoglobin increases (2-36A), (2-37A), (2-37B). Most late-stage sSDHs are T1/T2 "bright-bright." A linear T2 hypointensity representing the encasing membranes that surround the SDH is sometimes present.

FLAIR is the most sensitive standard sequence for detecting sSDH as the collection is typically hyperintense (2-37C). Because FLAIR signal intensity varies depending on the relative contribution of T1 and T2 effects, early subacute SDHs may initially appear hypointense due to their intrinsic T2 shortening.

T2* scans are also very sensitive as sSDHs show distinct "blooming" (2-36B).

Signal intensity on DWI also varies with hematoma age. DWI commonly shows a crescentic high intensity area with a low intensity rim closer to the brain surface ("double layer" appearance) (2-36C). The low intensity area corresponds to a mixture of resolved clot and CSF whereas the high intensity area correlates with solid clot.

2-33. Axial NECT scan shows right sSDH ➡ that is isodense with the underlying cortex. The right GM-WM interface is displaced and buckled medially ➡ compared to the normal left side ➡. *2-34.* NECT scan in another patient shows bilateral "balanced" isodense subacute SDHs ➡. Note that both GM-WM interfaces are inwardly displaced. A "dot" of CSF in the compressed subarachnoid space is seen under the left sSDH ➡.

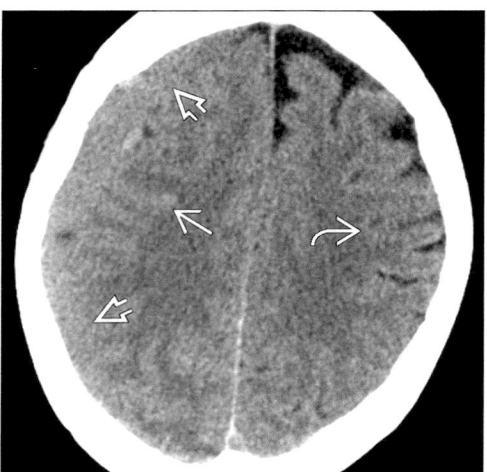

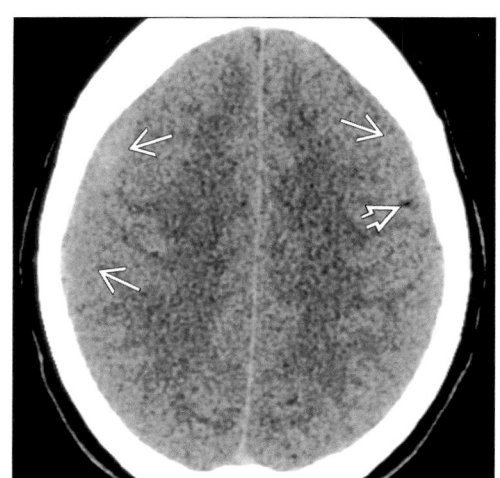

2-35. NECT in an elderly patient with sSDH, moderate cortical atrophy shows the difference between the nearly isodense SDH and CSF in the underlying compressed subarachnoid space, sulci ➡. *2-36A.* Axial T1WI in a patient with a late-stage aSDH shows a crescent-shaped hyperintense collection ➡ that extends over the entire surface of the left hemisphere. Note gyral compression with almost completely obliterated sulci compared to the normal-appearing right hemisphere.

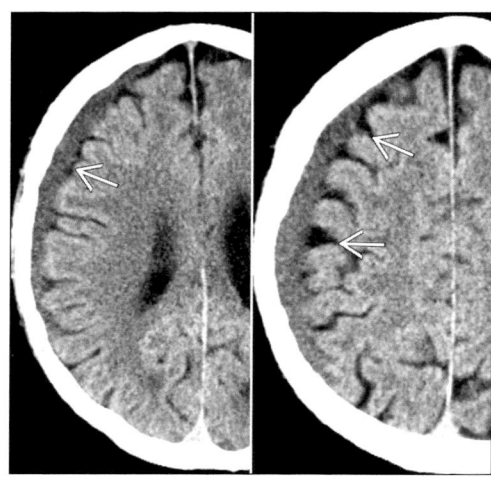

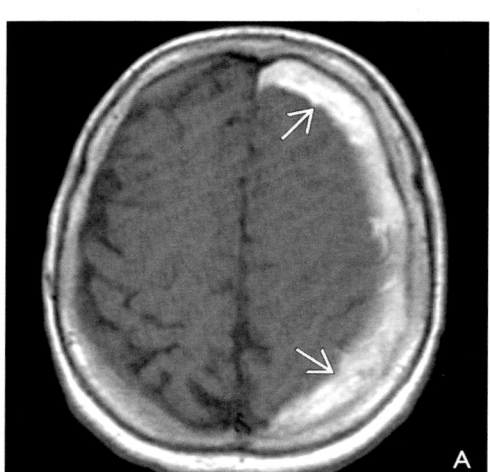

2-36B. T2* GRE scan shows some "blooming" ➡ in the sSDH. *2-36C.* DWI shows the classic "double layer" appearance of an sSDH with hypointense rim on the inside ➡ and mildly hyperintense rim on the outside ➡ of the clot.

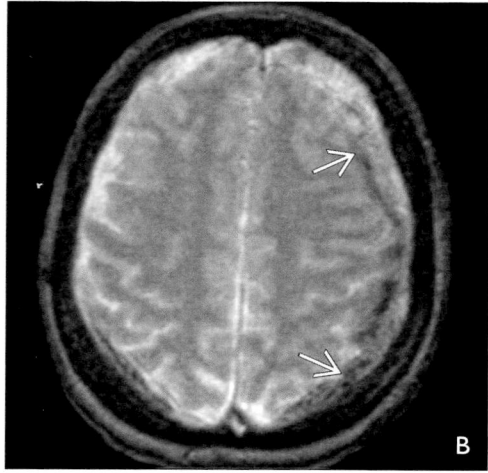

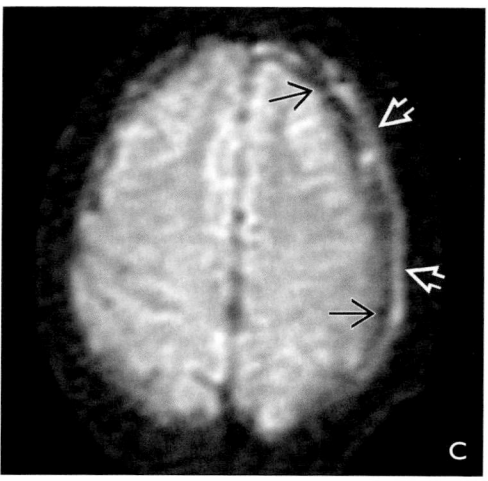

T1 C+ scans demonstrate enhancing, thickened, encasing membranes (2-37D). The membrane surrounding an sSDH is usually thicker on the dural side of the collection. Delayed scans may show gradual "filling in" and increasing hyperintensity of the sSDH.

Differential Diagnosis

The major differential diagnosis of an sSDH is an **isodense acute SDH**. These are typically seen only in an extremely anemic or anticoagulated patient. A **subdural effusion** that follows surgery or meningitis or that occurs as a component of intracranial hypotension can also mimic an sSDH. A **subdural hygroma** typically is isodense/isointense with CSF and does not demonstrate enhancing, encapsulating membranes.

Chronic/Mixed Subdural Hematoma

Terminology

A chronic subdural hematoma (cSDH) is an encapsulated collection of sanguineous or serosanguineous fluid confined within the subdural space. Recurrent hemorrhage(s)

into a preexisting cSDH are common and produce a mixed-age SDH (mSDH).

Etiology

With continued degradation of blood products, a subdural hematoma becomes progressively more liquified until it is largely serous fluid tinged with blood products (2-38). Rehemorrhage, either from vascularized encapsulating membranes or rupture of stretched cortical veins crossing the expanded subdural space, occurs in 5-10% of cSDHs and is considered "acute-on-chronic" SDH.

Pathology

GROSS PATHOLOGY. Blood within the subdural space incites tissue reaction around its margins. Organization and resorption of the hematoma contained within the "membranes" of surrounding granulation tissue continues. These neomembranes have fragile, easily disrupted capillaries and easily rebleed, creating an mSDH. Multiple hemorrhages of different ages are common in mSDHs (2-39), (2-40).

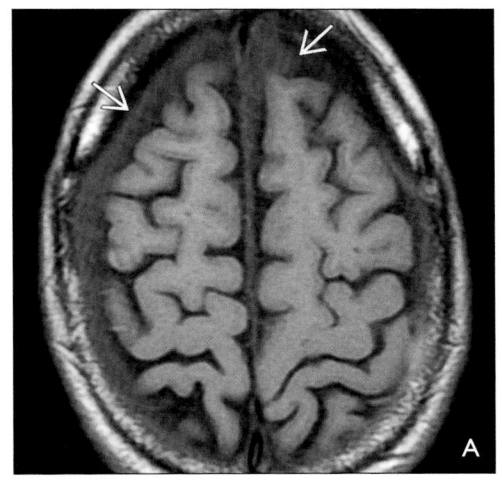
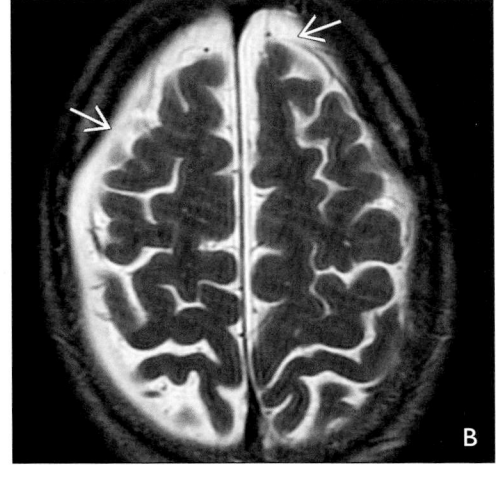

2-37A. *T1WI in a 59-year-old man with seizures shows bilateral subdural collections ➡ that are slightly hyperintense to CSF.* 2-37B. *T2WI shows that both collections ➡ are isointense with CSF in the underlying subarachnoid cisterns.*

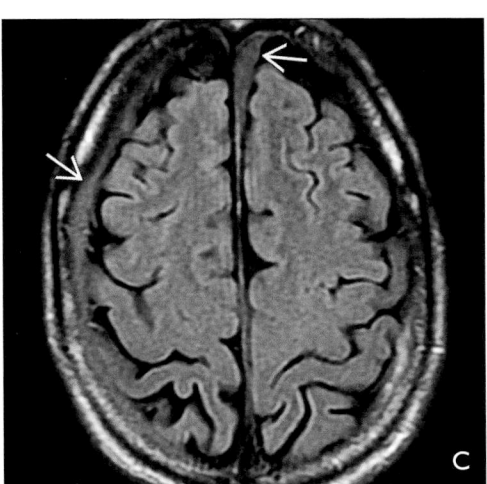
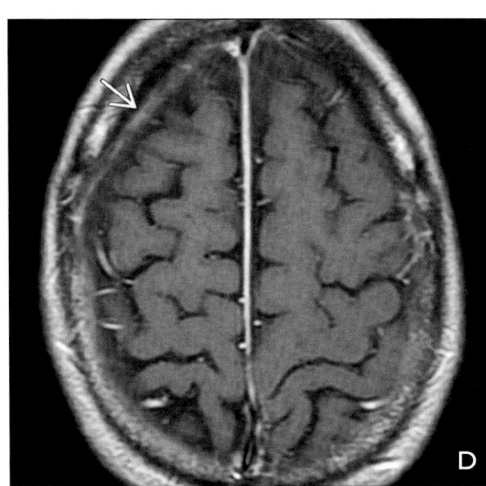

2-37C. *The fluid collections ➡ do not suppress on FLAIR and are hyperintense to CSF in the underlying cisterns.* 2-37D. *T1 C+ shows that the outer membrane of the SDH enhances ➡. Findings are consistent with late subacute/early chronic subdural hematomas.*

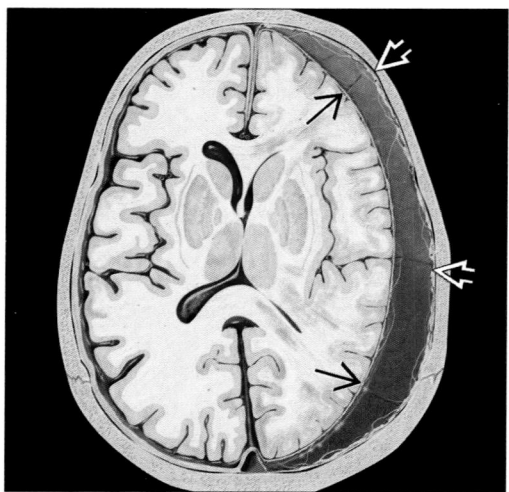

2-38. Uncomplicated cSDHs contain serosanguineous fluid with hematocrit effect & thin inner ⇨, thick outer ⇨ encapsulating membranes.

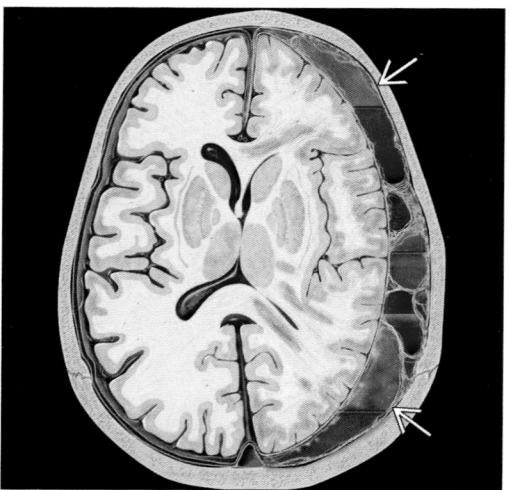

2-39. Complicated cSDHs contain loculated pockets of old and new blood, seen as fluid-fluid levels ⇨ within septated cavities.

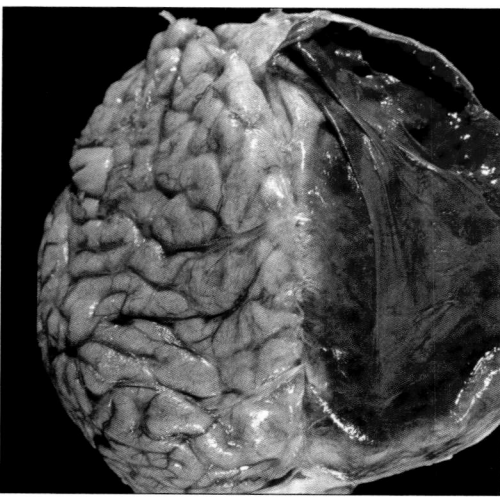

2-40. Autopsy case shows loculated collections with old and new blood, characteristic of mixed chronic SDH. (Courtesy R. Hewlett, MD.)

Eventually, most of the liquified clot in a cSDH is resorbed. Only a thickened dura-arachnoid layer remains with a few scattered pockets of old blood trapped between the inner and outer membranes.

Clinical Issues

EPIDEMIOLOGY. Unoperated, uncomplicated subacute SDHs eventually evolve into cSDHs. Approximately 5-10% will rehemorrhage, causing multiloculated mixed-age SDHs.

DEMOGRAPHICS. Chronic SDHs may occur at any age. Mixed-age SDHs are much more common in elderly patients.

PRESENTATION. Presentation varies from no/mild symptoms (e.g., headache) to sudden neurologic deterioration if a preexisting cSDH rehemorrhages.

NATURAL HISTORY. In the absence of repeated hemorrhages, cSDHs gradually resorb and largely resolve, leaving a residue of thickened dura-arachnoid that may persist for months or even years. Older patients, especially those with brain atrophy, are subject to repeated hemorrhages.

TREATMENT OPTIONS. If follow-up imaging of a subacute SDH shows expected resorption and regression of the cSDH, no surgery may be required. Surgical drainage with evacuation of the cSDH and resection of its encapsulating membranes is performed if significant mass effect or repeated hemorrhages cause neurologic complications.

Imaging

GENERAL FEATURES. Chronic SDHs have a spectrum of imaging appearances. **Uncomplicated cSDHs** show relatively homogeneous density/signal intensity with slight gravity-dependent gradation of their contents ("hematocrit effect").

Mixed SDHs with acute hemorrhage into a preexisting cSDH show a hematocrit level with distinct layering of the old (top) and new (bottom) hemorrhages. Sometimes, septated pockets that contain hemorrhages of different ages form. Dependent layering of blood within the loculated collections may appear quite bizarre.

Extremely old, **longstanding cSDHs** with virtually complete resorption of all liquid contents are seen as pachymeningopathies with diffuse dura-arachnoid thickening.

CT FINDINGS.

NECT. A hypodense crescentic fluid collection extending over the surface of one or both cerebral hemispheres is the classic finding in cSDH. Uncomplicated cSDHs approach CSF in density. The hematocrit effect creates a slight gradation in density that increases from top to bottom (2-41).

Trabecular or loculated cSDHs show internal septations, often with evidence of repeated hemorrhages **(2-42)**, **(2-43)**. With age, the encapsulating membranes surrounding the cSDH become thickened and may appear moderately hyperdense. Eventually, some cSDHs show peripheral calcifications that persist for many years. In rare cases, a cSDH may densely calcify or even ossify, a condition aptly termed "armored brain" **(2-44)**.

CECT. The encapsulating membranes around a cSDH contain fragile neocapillaries that lack endothelial tight junctions. Therefore, the membranes show strong enhancement following contrast administration **(2-45)**.

MR FINDINGS. As with all intracranial hematomas, signal intensity of a cSDH or mSDH is quite variable and depends on age of the blood products. On T1 scans, uncomplicated cSDHs are typically iso- to slightly hyperintense compared to CSF **(2-46A)**. Depending on the stage of evolution, cSDHs are iso- to hypointense compared to CSF on T2 scans.

Most cSDHs are hyperintense on FLAIR and may show "blooming" on T2* scans if subacute-chronic blood clots are still present. In about one-quarter of all cases, superficial siderosis can be identified over the gyri underlying a cSDH **(2-47)**.

The encapsulating membranes of a cSDH enhance following contrast administration. Typically, the outer layer is thicker than the inner layer **(2-46B)**.

Uncomplicated chronic SDHs do not restrict on DWI. With cSDHs, a "double layer" effect—a crescent of hyperintensity medial to a nonrestricting fluid collection—indicates acute rehemorrhage **(2-48)**.

Differential Diagnosis

A mixed-age SDH is difficult to mistake for anything else. In older patients, a small uncomplicated cSDH may be difficult to distinguish from simple **brain atrophy** with enlarged bifrontal CSF spaces. However, cSDHs exhibit mass effect; they flatten the underlying gyri, often extending around the entire hemisphere and into the interhemispheric fissure. The increased extraaxial spaces in patients with cerebral atrophy are predominantly frontal and temporal.

A traumatic **subdural hygroma** is an accumulation of CSF in the subdural space after head injury, probably secondary to an arachnoid tear. Subdural hygromas are sometimes detected within the first 24 hours after trauma; however, the mean time for appearance is nine days after injury.

A classic uncomplicated subdural hygroma is a hypodense, CSF-like, crescentic extraaxial collection that consists purely of CSF, has no blood products, lacks encap-

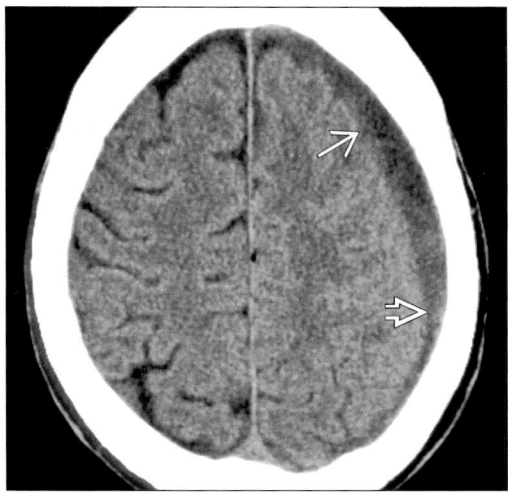

2-41. NECT shows cSDH with graduated hypodensity ("hematocrit effect") from more hypodense (top) ➡ to less hypodense (bottom) ➡.

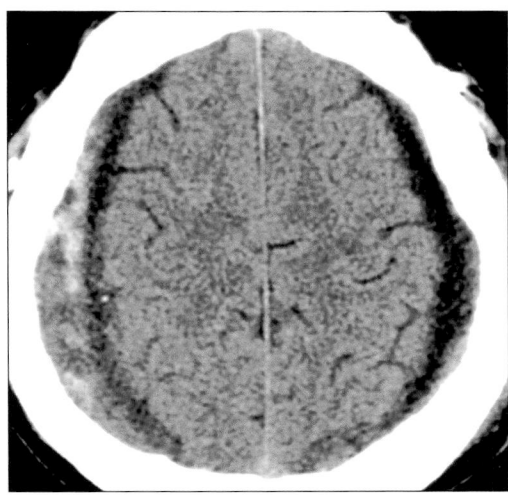

2-42. NECT shows bilateral mixed-density chronic SDHs.

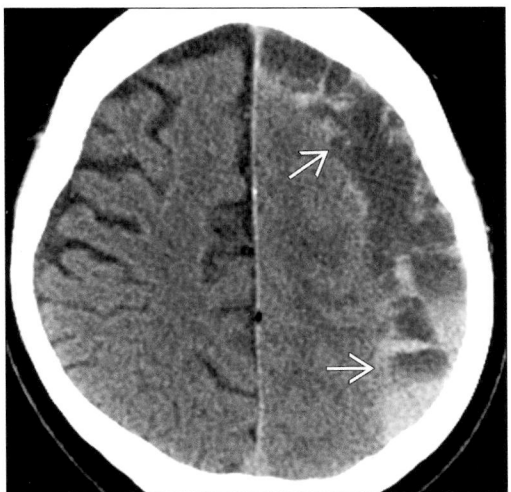

2-43. NECT shows mixed cSDH ➡ that features multiple loculated pockets of blood with old blood layered on top of recent hemorrhages.

2-44. *Gallery of different cases shows the broad spectrum of imaging findings in cSDH. Here, NECT scan in a patient with a history of multiple shunts and drains for very longstanding cSDHs shows densely calcified bifrontal subdural hematomas ➡, the "armored brain" appearance.*

2-45. *CECT scan shows cSDH with an intensely enhancing internal membrane ➡.*

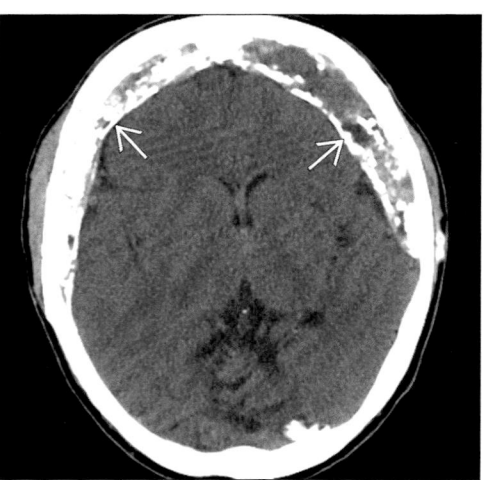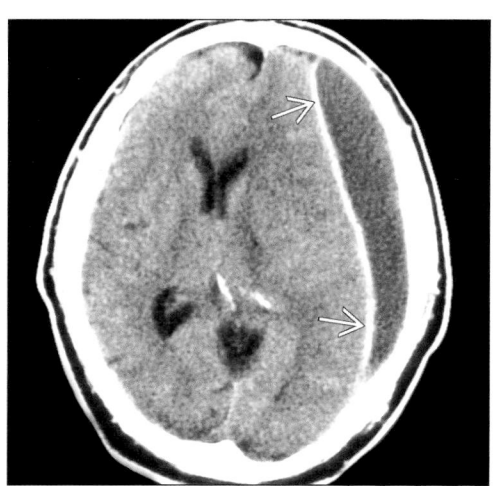

2-46A. *Mixed-age SDHs are common. Axial T1WI shows a subacute right, early chronic left SDH. The chronic collection ➡ is isointense to brain, while the more subacute SDH ➡ appears isointense with the underlying brain.*

2-46B. *Coronal T1 C+ scan in a different patient shows almost completely resorbed bilateral cSDHs with diffuse dura-arachnoid thickening ➡. A small residual loculated fluid collection ➡ is all that remains of the formerly very extensive cSDHs.*

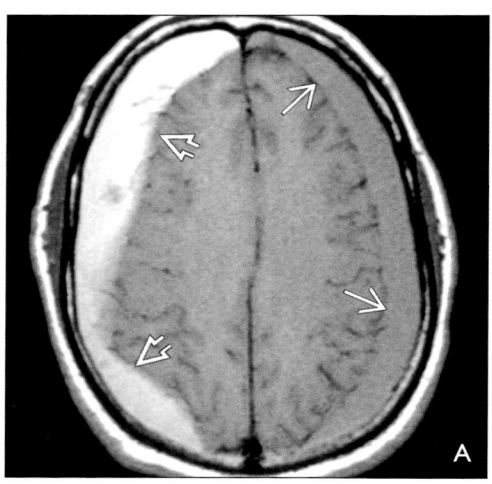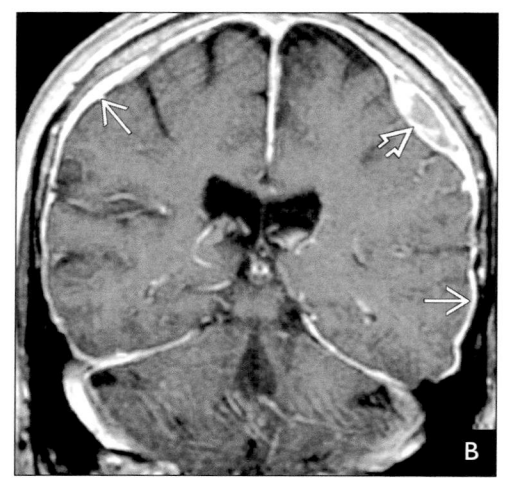

2-47. *T2* GRE scan in a patient with mixed cSDH and multiple loculated pockets of old and new hemorrhage shows dramatic "blooming" with distinct fluid-fluid levels ➡.*

2-48. *DWI in a patient with chronic right SDH shows the "double layer" effect of a large nonrestricting cSDH ➡ and a thinner area of rehemorrhage with diffusion restriction ➡.*

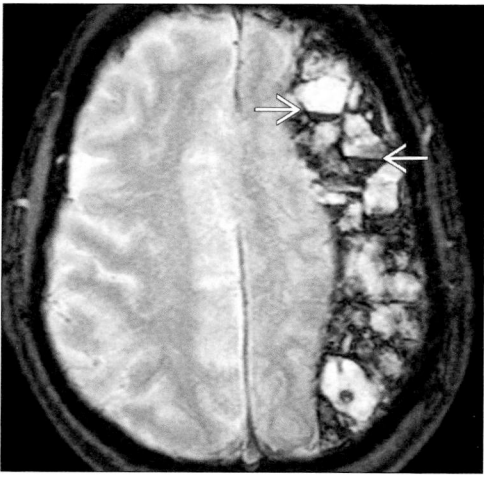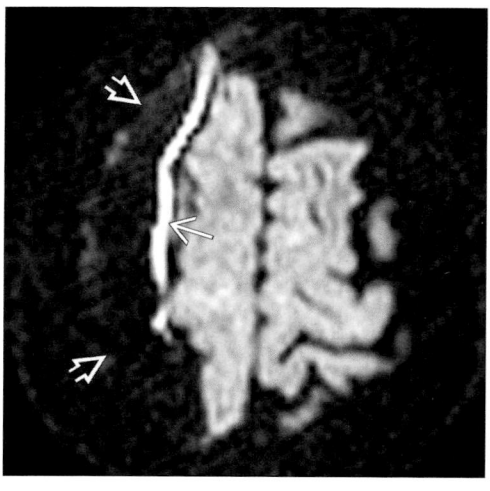

sulating membranes, and shows no enhancement following contrast administration. CSF leakage into the subdural space is also present in the vast majority of patients with cSDH. Therefore, many—if not most—cSDHs contain a mixture of *both* CSF and blood products.

A **subdural effusion** is an accumulation of clear fluid over the cerebral convexities or in the interhemispheric fissure. Subdural effusions are generally complications of meningitis; a history of prior infection, not trauma, is typical.

A **subdural empyema** (SDE) is a hypodense extraaxial fluid collection that contains pus. Most SDEs are secondary to sinusitis or mastoiditis, have strongly enhancing membranes, and often coexist with findings of meningitis. A typical SDE restricts strongly and uniformly on DWI.

Traumatic Subarachnoid Hemorrhage

Traumatic subarachnoid hemorrhage (tSAH) is found in virtually all cases of moderate to severe head trauma. Indeed, trauma—*not* ruptured saccular aneurysm—is the most common cause of intracranial subarachnoid hemorrhage.

Etiology

Traumatic SAH can occur with both direct trauma to the skull and non-impact closed head injury. Tearing of cortical arteries and veins, rupture of contusions and lacerations into the contiguous subarachnoid space, and choroid plexus bleeds with intraventricular hemorrhage may all result in blood collecting within the subarachnoid cisterns. Less commonly, tSAH arises from major vessel lacerations or dissections, with or without basilar skull fractures.

While tSAH occasionally occurs in isolation, it is usually accompanied by other manifestations of brain injury. Subtle tSAH may be the only clue on initial imaging studies that more serious injuries lurk beneath the surface....

Pathology

Location. tSAHs are predominantly found in the perisylvian regions, in the anteroinferior frontal and temporal sulci, and over the hemispheric convexities **(2-49)**. In very severe cases, tSAH spreads over most of the brain. In mild cases, blood collects in a single sulcus or the dependent portion of the interpeduncular fossa.

Gross Pathology. With the exception of location and associated parenchymal injuries, the gross appearance of tSAH is similar to that of aneurysmal SAH (aSAH). Curvilinear foci of bright red blood collect in cisterns and surface sulci **(2-50)**.

Traumatic SAH typically occurs adjacent to cortical contusions. tSAH is also commonly identified under acute epi- and subdural hematomas.

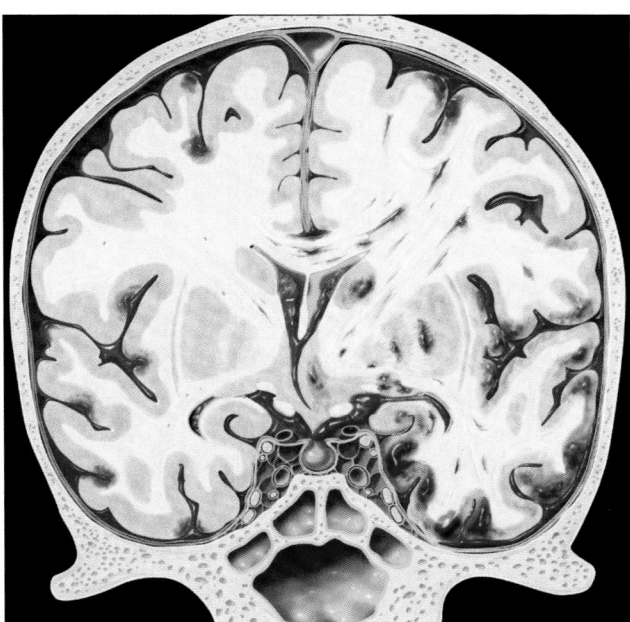

2-49. Graphic depicts traumatic subarachnoid hemorrhage. tSAH is most common around the sylvian fissures and in the sulci adjacent to contused gyri.

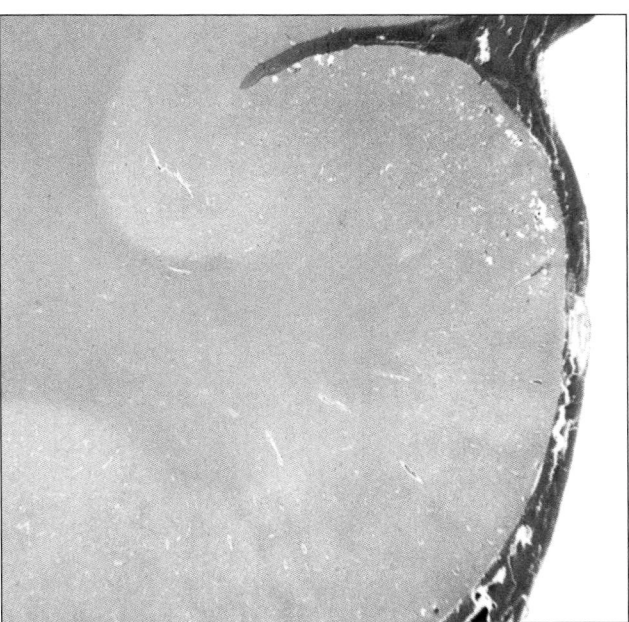

2-50. Low-power photomicrograph shows an autopsied brain of a boxer who collapsed and expired after being knocked unconscious. Typical tSAH covers the gyri and extends into the sulci. (Courtesy J. Paltan, MD.)

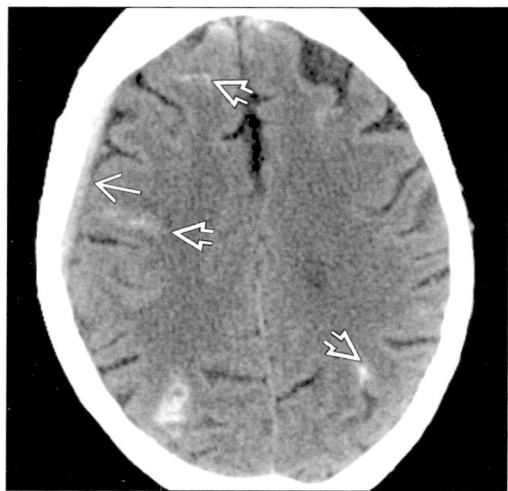

2-51. *NECT shows a small right SDH* ➡, *multiple scattered foci of tSAH* ➡ *in the sulci over the convexities.*

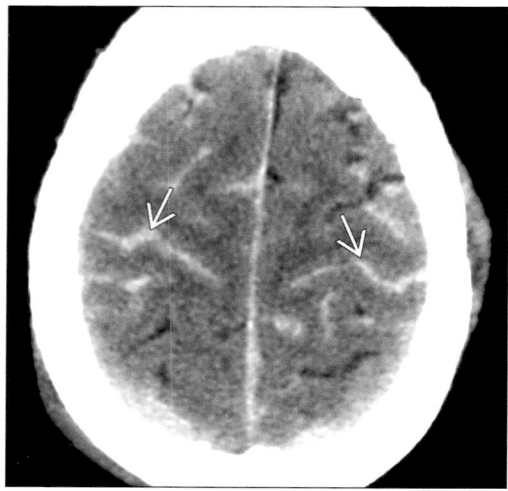

2-52. *NECT scan in another case shows more extensive tSAH, seen as diffuse hyperdensity filling most of the convexity sulci* ➡.

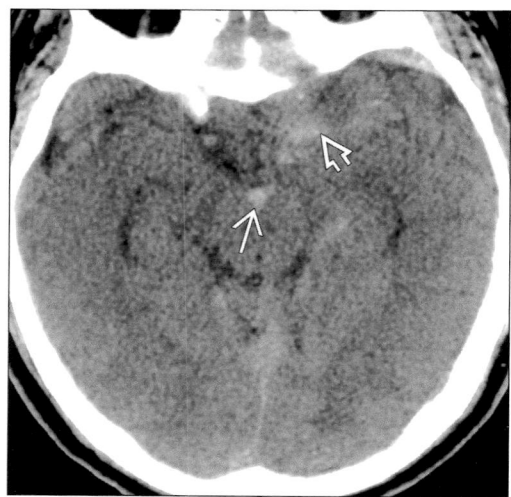

2-53. *Subtle tSAH in a patient with closed head injury is present in the interpeduncular fossa* ➡, *left sylvian fissure* ➡.

Clinical Issues

EPIDEMIOLOGY. Traumatic SAH is found in most cases of moderate trauma and is identified in virtually 100% of fatal brain injuries at autopsy.

DEMOGRAPHICS. The prevalence of tSAH generally follows that of other traumatic brain injuries, i.e., it is bimodal and most commonly occurs in young adults (especially males) and the elderly.

PRESENTATION. Clinical symptoms are primarily related to other traumatic injuries such as extraaxial hematoma, contusions, and axonal injury. In some cases, tSAH may cause delayed vasospasm and secondary ischemic symptoms.

NATURAL HISTORY. Breakdown and resorption of tSAH occurs gradually. Outcome is generally dictated by other injuries and is related to the initial Glasgow Coma Score as well as the amount of blood in the subarachnoid cisterns at initial imaging.

TREATMENT OPTIONS. Supportive therapy is the primary treatment. In some cases, infusion of nimodipine or other calcium channel blockers such as verapamil may prevent vasospasm and its attendant complications.

Imaging

GENERAL FEATURES. With the exception of location, the general imaging appearance of tSAH is similar to that of aSAH, i.e., sulcal-cisternal hyperdensity/hyperintensity. Traumatic SAH is typically more focal or patchy than the diffuse subarachnoid blood indicative of aneurysmal hemorrhage (2-51).

CT FINDINGS. Acute tSAH appears as linear hyperdensities in sulci adjacent to cortical contusions or under epi- or subdural hematomas (2-52). Occasionally, isolated tSAH is identified within the interpeduncular fossa (2-53). Posttraumatic interpeduncular or ambient cistern hemorrhage is a good marker for possible brainstem lesions in patients with otherwise unexplained coma and may warrant further investigation.

Some cases of mild tSAH may have hemorrhage in a single convexity sulcus. In severe cases, tSAH spreads diffusely in the subarachnoid cisterns and layers over the tentorium. Chronic tSAH may appear as hypodense fluid that expands the affected sulci.

MR FINDINGS. As acute blood is isointense with brain, it may be difficult to detect on T1WI. "Dirty" sulci with "smudging" of the perisylvian cisterns is typical. Subarachnoid blood is hyperintense to brain on T2WI and appears similar in signal intensity to cisternal CSF. FLAIR scans show hyperintensity in the affected sulci (2-54).

"Blooming" with hypointensity can be identified on T2* scans, typically adjacent to areas of cortical contusion. tSAH is recognized on GRE or SWI sequences as very hypointense signal intensity surrounded by hyperintense CSF.

tSAH also exhibits a unique morphology. Compared with smooth linear veins, SAH has a "triangle" shape with rough irregular boundaries and inhomogeneous signal intensity. Chronic tSAH causes focal superficial siderosis that appears as curvilinear hypointensity along gyral crests and sulci.

DWI in tSAH may show foci of restricted diffusion in areas of frank ischemia or trauma-induced cytotoxic edema.

ANGIOGRAPHY. CTA is typically normal for the first several days after tSAH. Vasospasm may ensue from two to three days to two weeks after trauma and is identified as multifocal areas of vessel narrowing or "beading."

DSA is rarely performed in acute brain trauma unless vascular injury such as dissection or pseudoaneurysm is suspected. Vasospasm with acute tSAH is unusual but may develop several days after the initial traumatic event.

Differential Diagnosis

The major differential diagnosis of tSAH is **nontraumatic SAH** (ntSAH). Aneurysmal rupture causes 80-90% of all ntSAHs. In contrast to tSAH, aSAH is concentrated in the basal cisterns. CTA can identify a saccular aneurysm in most cases with aSAH.

Arteriovenous malformations account for 10-15% of ntSAHs and are easily identified on both CT and MR. Dissections and dissecting aneurysms, especially of the vertebrobasilar system, are less common but important causes of ntSAH.

Sulcal-cisternal hyperintensity on FLAIR is nonspecific and can be caused by **meningitis, neoplasm, artifact** (incomplete CSF suppression), **contrast** leakage into the subarachnoid space (e.g., with renal failure), and **high inspired oxygen** during general anesthesia **(2-55)**.

The term **pseudosubarachnoid hemorrhage** has been used to describe the CT appearance of a brain with severe cerebral edema. Hypodense brain makes circulating blood in arteries and veins look relatively hyperdense. The hyperdensity seen here is smooth and conforms to the expected shape of the vessels, not the subarachnoid spaces, and should not be mistaken for either tSAH or ntSAH **(2-56)**.

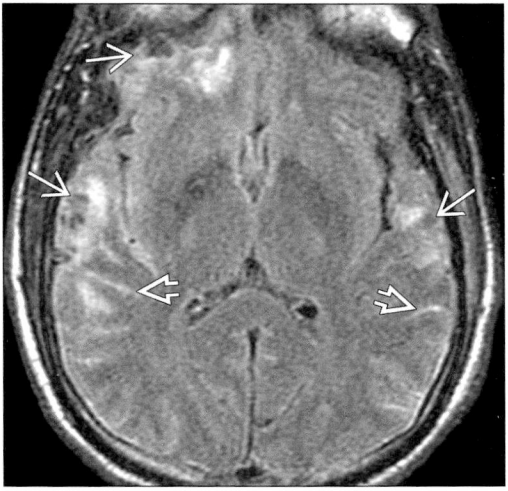

2-54. *Axial FLAIR shows multifocal cortical contusions* ➡️ *with traumatic SAH, seen as sulcal hyperintensities adjacent to the lesions* ⇨.

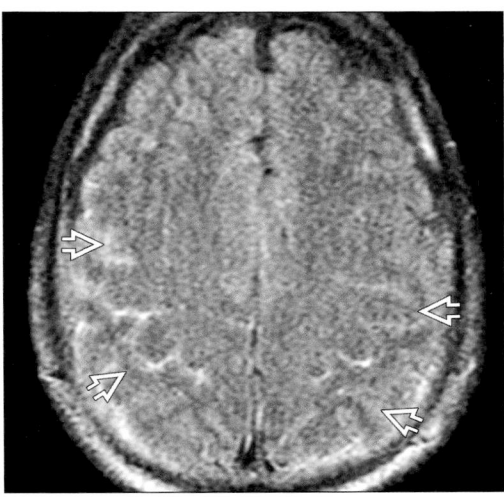

2-55. *FLAIR scan with artifactual sulcal hyperintensity* ⇨ *caused by incomplete water suppression. Repeat scan (not shown) was normal.*

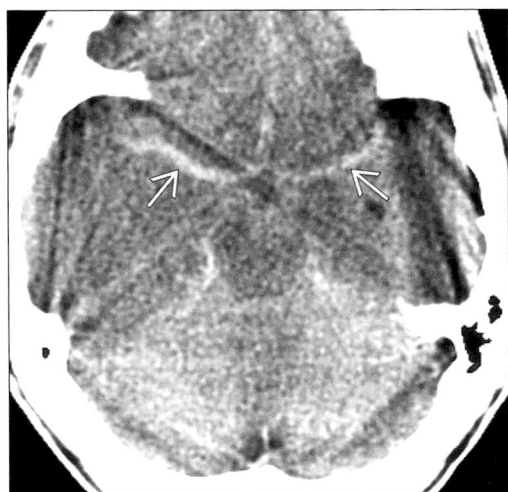

2-56. *NECT in severe cerebral edema shows pseudosubarachnoid hemorrhage caused by low-density brain adjacent to normal blood vessels* ⇨.

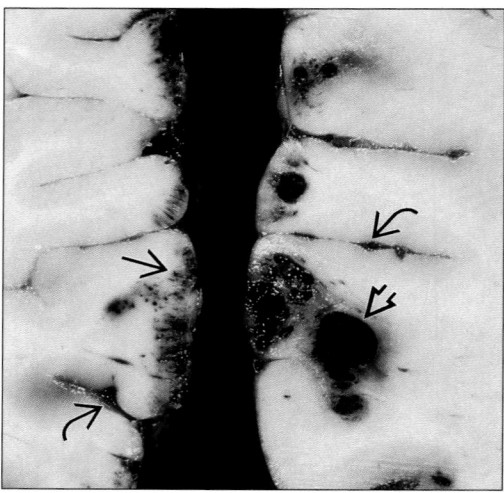

2-57. *Cortical contusions are located primarily along gyral crests ▷, around a sylvian fissure. tSAH is common in adjacent sulci ▷.*

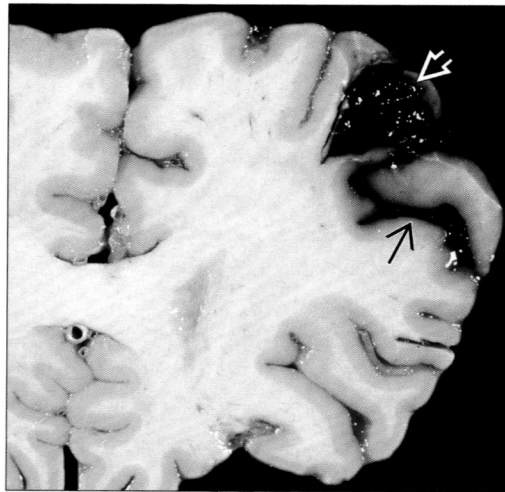

2-58. *Autopsy shows petechial ▷ and larger confluent cortical contusions ▷, tSAH in adjacent sulci ▷. (Courtesy R. Hewlett, MD.)*

2-59. *Autopsy shows large frontal contusion ▷ with focal traumatic SAH enlarging the adjacent sulcus ▷. (Courtesy J. Townsend, MD.)*

SUBDURAL AND SUBARACHNOID HEMORRHAGE

Acute SDH (aSDH)
- Second most common traumatic extraaxial hemorrhage
  - Acute SDH > > epidural hematoma
- Crescentic collection of blood between dura, arachnoid
  - Supratentorial (95%), bilateral (15%)
  - SDHs cross sutures but not dural attachments
- CT
  - Hyperdense (60%), mixed (40%)
  - Isodense aSDH rare (anemia, coagulopathy, CSF mixture)

Subacute SDH (sSDH)
- Clot organizes, lyses, forms "neomembranes"
- CT
  - Density decreases 1-2 HU/day
  - Isodense with cortex in 7-10 days
  - Look for displaced "dots" of CSF under SDH
  - Gray-white interface "buckled" inward
  - Displaced cortical veins seen on CECT
- MR
  - Signal varies with clot age
  - T2* (GRE, SWI) shows "blooming"
  - T1 C+ shows clot inside enhancing membranes

Chronic/Mixed SDH (cSDH)
- Serosanguineous fluid
  - Hypodense on NECT
  - Rehemorrhage (5-10%)
  - Loculated blood "pockets" with fluid-fluid levels common
- Differential diagnosis of uncomplicated cSDH
  - Subdural *hygroma* (arachnoid tear → subdural CSF)
  - Subdural *effusion* (clear fluid accumulates after meningitis)
  - Subdural *empyema* (pus)

Traumatic Subarachnoid Hemorrhage (tSAH)
- Most common traumatic extraaxial hemorrhage
- tSAH > > aneurysmal SAH
- Adjacent to cortical contusions
- Superficial sulci > basilar cisterns

Parenchymal Injuries

Intraaxial traumatic injuries include cortical contusions and lacerations, diffuse axonal injury (DAI), subcortical injuries, and intraventricular hemorrhages. In this section, we again begin with the most peripheral injuries—cortical contusions—and work our way inward, ending with the deepest (subcortical) injuries. *In general, the deeper the abnormalities, the more serious the injury.*

Cerebral Contusions and Lacerations

Cerebral contusions are the most common of the intraaxial injuries. True brain lacerations are rare and typically occur only with severe (often fatal) head injury.

Terminology

Cerebral contusions are basically "brain bruises." They evolve with time and often are more apparent on delayed scans than at the time of initial imaging. Cerebral contusions are also called gyral "crest" injuries **(2-57)**. The term "gliding" contusion is sometimes used to describe parasagittal contusions.

Etiology

Most cerebral contusions result from non-missile or blunt head injury. Closed head injury induces abrupt changes in angular momentum and deceleration. The brain is suddenly and forcibly impacted against an osseous ridge or the hard, knife-like edge of the falx cerebri and tentorium cerebelli. Less commonly, a depressed skull fracture directly damages the underlying brain.

Pathology

LOCATION. Contusions are injuries of the brain surface that involve the gray matter and contiguous subcortical white matter **(2-57)**, **(2-58)**, **(2-59)**. They occur in very characteristic, highly predictable locations. Nearly half involve the temporal lobes. The temporal tips, as well as the lateral and inferior surfaces and the perisylvian gyri, are most commonly affected **(2-60)**. The inferior (orbital) surfaces of the frontal lobes are also frequently affected **(2-61)**.

Convexity gyri, the dorsal corpus callosum body, dorsolateral midbrain, and cerebellum are less common sites of cerebral contusions. The occipital poles are rarely involved, even with relatively severe closed head injury.

SIZE AND NUMBER. Cerebral contusions vary in size from tiny lesions to large confluent hematomas **(2-59)**. They are almost always multiple and often bilateral **(2-62)**. Contusions that occur at 180° opposite the site of direct impact (the "coup") are common and are called "contre-coup" lesions.

GROSS PATHOLOGY. Contusions range in appearance from small petechial to large confluent hemorrhages. Cortical contusions are usually associated with traumatic subarachnoid hemorrhage in the adjacent sulci.

MICROSCOPIC FEATURES. Perivascular micro-hemorrhages rapidly form and coalesce over time into more confluent hematomas. Edema surrounding the hemorrhages develops. Activation and proliferation of astrocytes together with macrophage infiltration ensues.

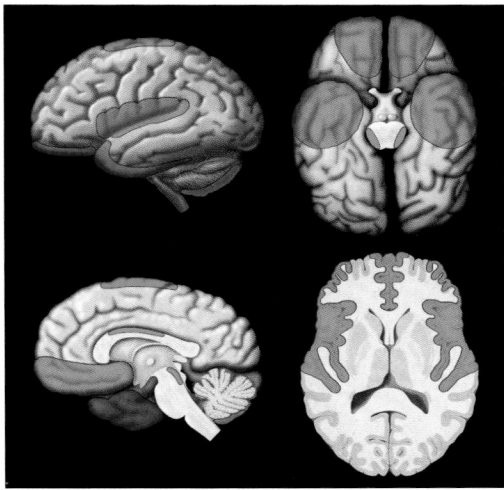

2-60. *Graphics depict the most common sites of cerebral contusions in red. Less common sites are shown in green.*

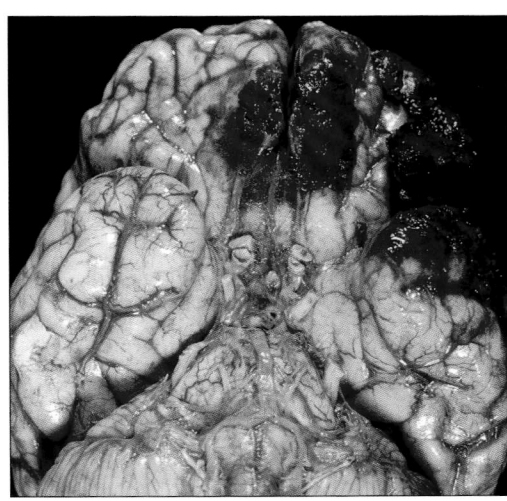

2-61. *Autopsied brain shows typical locations of contusions, i.e., the anteroinferior frontal and temporal lobes. (Courtesy R. Hewlett, MD.)*

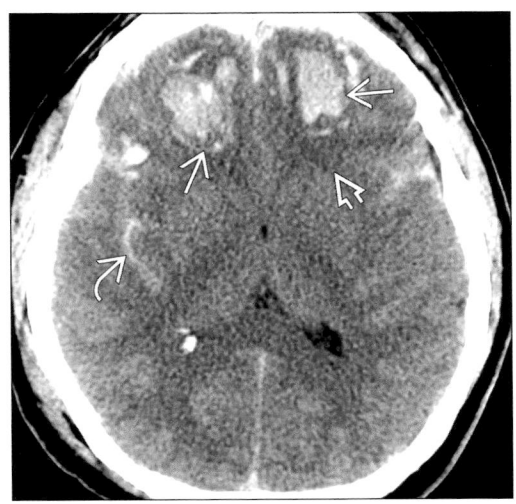

2-62. *NECT scan shows bilateral inferior frontal confluent contusions ➡, perilesional edema ➡, traumatic SAH ➡.*

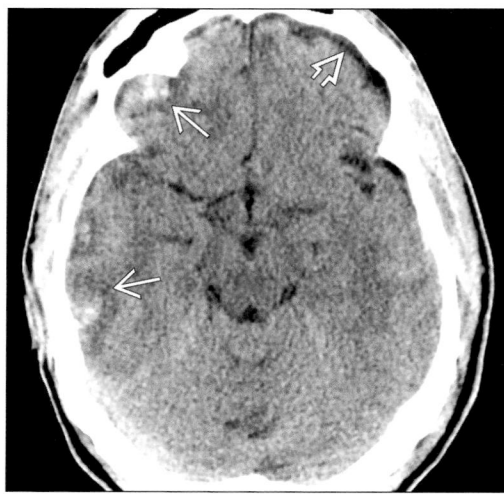

2-63. NECT scan 24 hours after trauma shows frontotemporal contusions ➡, *left inferior frontal subdural hygroma* ➡.

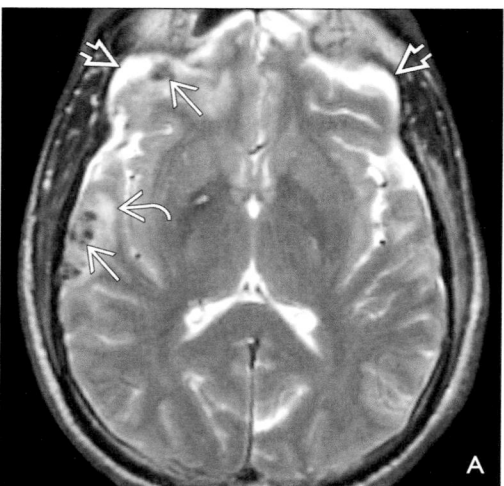

2-64A. T2WI obtained immediately after the CT scan above shows contusions ➡ *with perilesional edema* ➡, *bilateral subdural hygromas* ➡.

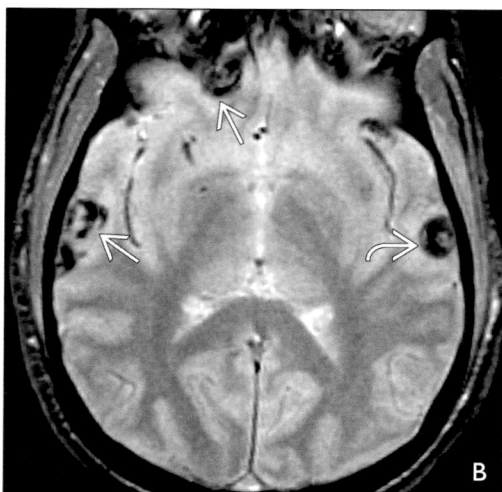

2-64B. T2* GRE shows "blooming" of right frontotemporal contusions ➡. *A left temporal contusion* ➡ *is seen that was not evident on T2WI.*

Necrosis with neuronal loss and astrogliosis as well as hemosiderin-laden macrophages are present in subacute and chronic lesions.

Clinical Issues

EPIDEMIOLOGY AND DEMOGRAPHICS. Cerebral contusions account for approximately half of all traumatic parenchymal lesions. They occur at all ages, from infants to the elderly. The peak age is from 15-24 years, and the M:F ratio is 3:1.

PRESENTATION. Initial symptoms vary from none to confusion, seizure, or obtundation. Compared to diffuse axonal injuries (see below), cerebral contusions are less frequently associated with immediate loss of consciousness unless they are extensive or occur with other traumatic brain lesions (e.g., brainstem trauma or axonal injury).

NATURAL HISTORY. Neurologic deterioration is more common in older patients. Patients with large contusions, initial low Glasgow Coma Scores (GCS), coagulopathy, and presence of a coexisting subdural hematoma are prone to clinical deterioration. Those with small contusions, good initial GCS, and absence of clinical deterioration in the first 48 hours are unlikely to require surgery.

Hematoma expansion requiring surgical intervention occurs in approximately 20% of conservatively managed patients. Patients with unexplained clinical deterioration should have repeat imaging.

TREATMENT OPTIONS. Treatment options vary from conservative (observation with repeat imaging if the patient deteriorates) to surgical evacuation of large focal hematomas. Craniectomy is performed in patients with severe brain swelling to prevent fatal brain herniation.

Imaging

GENERAL FEATURES. With time, cortical contusions become more apparent on imaging studies. Radiologic progression is the rule, not the exception. Nearly half of all patients show increase in lesion size and number over the first 24-48 hours. In the absence of clinical deterioration, though, the relevance of documenting this progression is debatable.

CT FINDINGS. Initial scans obtained soon after a closed head injury may be normal. The most frequent abnormality is the presence of petechial hemorrhages along gyral crests immediately adjacent to the calvaria (2-63). A mixture of petechial hemorrhages surrounded by patchy ill-defined hypodense areas of edema is common.

Lesion "blooming" over time is frequent and is seen with progressive increase in hemorrhage, edema, and mass effect. Small lesions may coalesce, forming larger focal

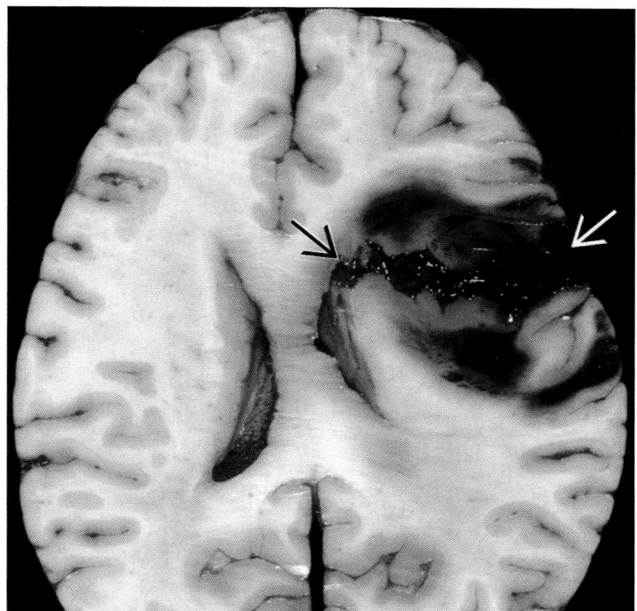

2-65. Autopsy shows a "burst" lobe with a "full thickness" laceration extending from the pial surface ➡ to the ventricle ⟶. (Courtesy R. Hewlett, MD.)

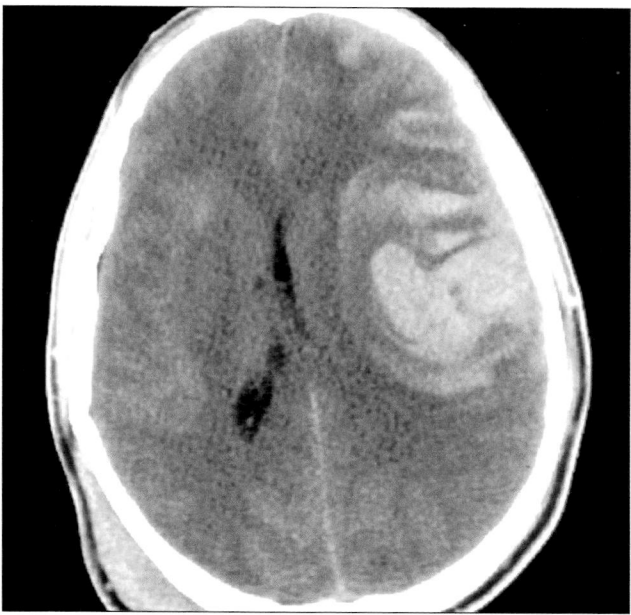

2-66. NECT scan shows a "burst" lobe with rapid parenchymal hemorrhage extending deep into the brain. The patient died shortly after this scan was obtained.

hematomas. Development of new lesions that were not present on initial imaging is also common.

MR FINDINGS. MR is much more sensitive than CT in detecting cerebral contusions but is rarely obtained in the acute stage of traumatic brain injury. T1 scans may show only mild inhomogeneous isointensities and mass effect. T2 scans show patchy hyperintense areas (edema) surrounding hypointense foci of hemorrhage **(2-64A).**

FLAIR scans are most sensitive for detecting cortical edema and associated traumatic subarachnoid hemorrhage, both of which appear as hyperintense foci on FLAIR. T2* (GRE, SWI) is the most sensitive sequence for imaging parenchymal hemorrhages. Significant "blooming" is typical in acute lesions **(2-64B).**

Hemorrhagic contusions follow the expected evolution of parenchymal hematomas, with T1 shortening developing over time. Atrophy, demyelination, and microglial scarring are seen on FLAIR and T2WI. Parenchymal volume loss with ventricular enlargement and sulcal prominence is common.

DWI in patients with cortical contusion shows diffusion restriction in areas of cell death. DTI may disclose coexisting white matter damage in minor head trauma even when standard MR sequences are normal.

Differential Diagnosis

The major differential diagnosis of cortical contusion is **diffuse axonal injury** (DAI). Both cerebral contusions and DAI are often present in patients who have sustained

moderate to severe head injury. Contusions tend to be superficial, located along gyral crests. DAI is most commonly found in the corona radiata and along compact white matter tracts such as the internal capsule and corpus callosum.

Severe cortical contusion with confluent hematomas may be difficult to distinguish from brain laceration on imaging studies. **Brain laceration** occurs when severe trauma disrupts the pia and literally tears the underlying brain apart.

A "burst lobe" is the most severe manifestation of frank brain laceration **(2-65), (2-66).** Here the affected lobe is grossly disrupted, with large hematoma formation and adjacent traumatic subarachnoid hemorrhage. In some cases, especially those with depressed skull fracture, the arachnoid is also lacerated and hemorrhage from the burst lobe extends to communicate directly with the subdural space, forming a coexisting subdural hematoma.

Diffuse Axonal Injury

Diffuse axonal injury (DAI) is the second most common parenchymal lesion seen in traumatic brain injury, exceeded only by cortical contusions. Patients with DAI often exhibit an apparent discrepancy between clinical status (often moderately to severely impaired) and initial imaging findings (often normal or minimally abnormal).

Terminology

Diffuse axonal injury is also known as traumatic axonal stretch injury. As most DAIs are stretch—not frank

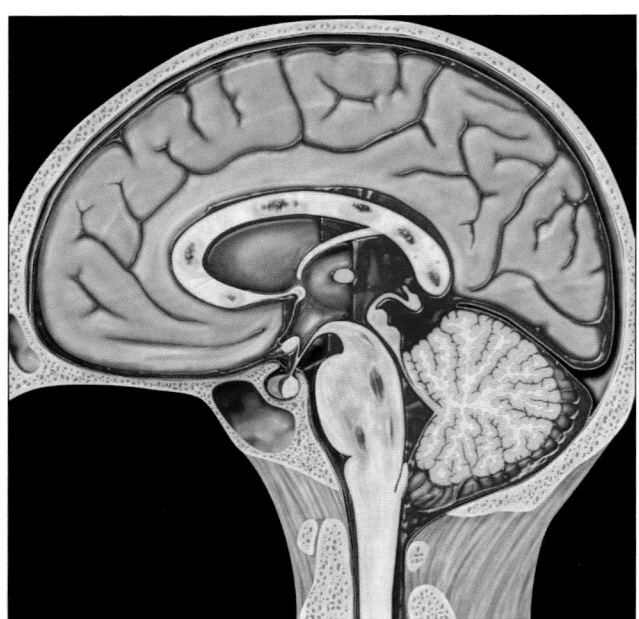

2-67. *Sagittal graphic depicts common sites of axonal injury in the corpus callosum and midbrain. Traumatic intraventricular and subarachnoid hemorrhage is present.*

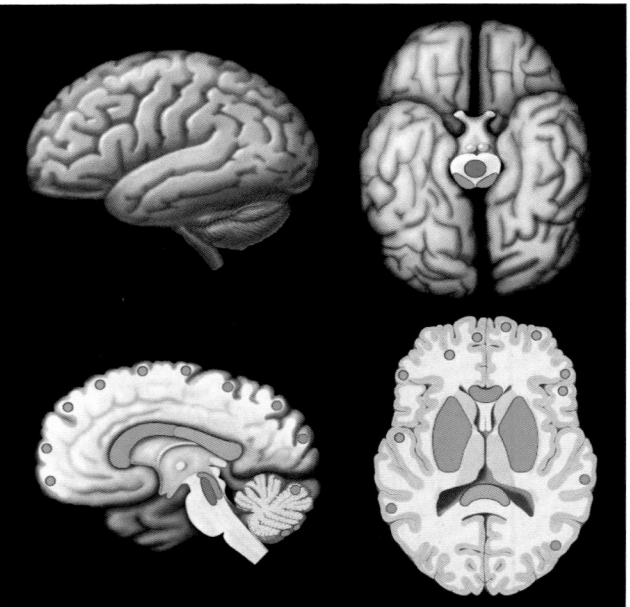

2-68. *Graphics depict the most common sites of axonal injury in red. Frequent but relatively less common locations are shown in green. Injury to the midbrain/upper pons (purple) is uncommon but often lethal.*

shearing—lesions, the term "shearing lesion" should be avoided. True "shearing" injury with frank axonal disconnection is uncommon and typically occurs only with very severe trauma.

Etiology

Direct head impact is not required to produce DAI. Most DAIs are not associated with skull fracture.

Most DAIs are caused by high-velocity auto accidents and are non-impact injuries resulting from the inertial forces of rotation generated by sudden changes in acceleration/deceleration. The cortex moves at different speed in relationship to underlying deep brain structures (white matter, deep gray nuclei). This results in axonal stretching, especially where brain tissues of different density intersect, i.e., the gray-white matter interface.

Traumatic axonal stretching causes impaired axoplasmic transport, depolarization, ion fluxes, spreading depression, and release of excitatory amino acids. Cellular swelling with cytotoxic edema ensues, altering anisotropy of the brain. Significant and widespread alterations of brain metabolites occur as a result of traumatic brain injury (TBI).

Pathology

LOCATION. DAI occurs in highly predictable locations. The cortex is typically spared; it is the subcortical and deep white matter that is most commonly affected. Lesions in compact white matter tracts such as the corpus callosum, especially the genu and splenium, fornix, and

internal capsule, are frequent. The midbrain and pons are less common sites of DAI **(2-67)**, **(2-68)**.

GROSS PATHOLOGY. The vast majority of DAIs are microscopic and nonhemorrhagic. Tears of penetrating vessels may cause small round to ovoid or linear hemorrhages that sometimes are the only gross indications of underlying axonal injury **(2-69)**. These visible lesions are truly just the "tip of the iceberg."

MICROSCOPIC FEATURES. Axonal swellings or "retraction balls" form, leaving microscopic gaps in the white matter **(2-70)**. Neuronal apoptosis and microglial reaction ensue. Chronic upregulation of activated microglia immunoreactive for galectin-3/Mac-2 and nerve growth factor has been demonstrated following DAI.

STAGING, GRADING, AND CLASSIFICATION. The Adams and Gennarelli classification defines mild, moderate, and severe grades of TBI.

In mild TBI, lesions are seen in the frontotemporal gray-white matter interfaces. Injury is designated as moderate when the lobar white matter and corpus callosum are affected. In severe TBI, lesions are present in the dorsolateral midbrain and upper pons. More than half of all TBI cases with DAI are designated as moderate to severe.

Clinical Issues

EPIDEMIOLOGY AND DEMOGRAPHICS. DAI is present in virtually all fatal TBIs and is found in almost three-quarters of patients with moderate or severe injury who survive the acute stage.

DAI may occur at any age, but peak incidence is in young adults (15-24 years old). Males are at least twice as often afflicted with TBI as females.

PRESENTATION. DAI typically causes much more significant impairment compared to extracerebral hematomas and cortical contusions. DAI often causes immediate loss of consciousness (LOC). LOC may be transient (in the case of mild TBI) or progress to coma (with moderate to severe injury).

NATURAL HISTORY. Mild TBI may result in persisting headaches, mild neurocognitive impairment, and memory difficulties. DAI is more common in moderate to severe injuries. While DAI itself rarely causes death, severe DAI may result in persistent vegetative state. Prognosis correlates with the number and severity of lesions as well as the presence of other abnormalities such as cortical contusions and herniation syndromes.

TREATMENT OPTIONS. Management of intracranial pressure is the most serious issue. In some cases with impending herniation, craniectomy may be a last resort.

Imaging

GENERAL FEATURES. One of the most striking features of DAI is the discrepancy between clinical symptoms and imaging findings. NECT scans are almost always the initial imaging study obtained in TBI **(2-71)**, although MR is much more sensitive in detecting changes of DAI. CT is very useful in detecting comorbid injuries such as extracerebral hemorrhage and parenchymal hematomas.

DAI typically evolves with time, so lesions are usually more apparent on follow-up scans. Between 10-20% evolve to gross hemorrhages with edema and mass effect.

CT FINDINGS. Initial NECT is often normal or minimally abnormal **(2-72A)**. Mild diffuse brain swelling with sulcal effacement may be present. Gross hemorrhages are uncommon immediately following injury. A few small round or ovoid subcortical hemorrhages may be visible **(2-71)**, but the underlying damage is typically much more diffuse and much more severe than these relatively modest abnormalities would indicate.

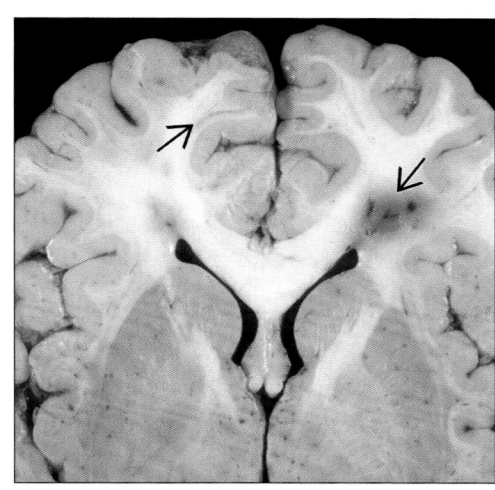

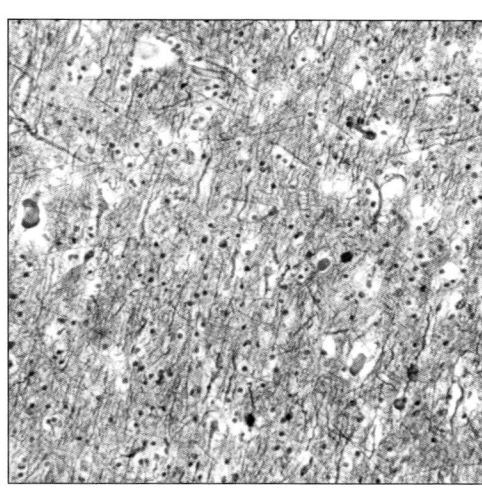

2-69. Autopsy case shows typical findings of diffuse axonal injury with linear hemorrhages ➡ in the subcortical and deep periventricular white matter. 2-70. H&E microscopy shows numerous white gaps or "bare" areas caused by axonal injury. (Courtesy R. Hewlett, MD.)

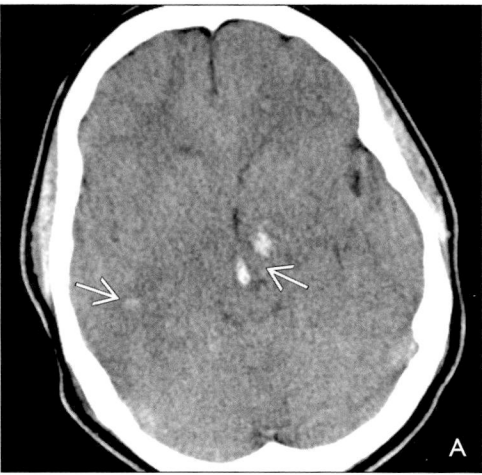

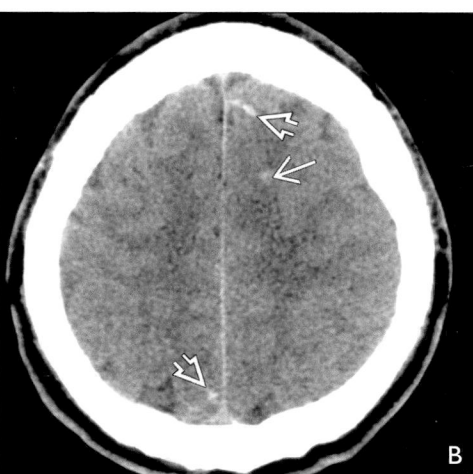

2-71A. NECT in a patient with severe nonimpact head injury shows diffuse brain swelling with small ventricles, effaced sulci and cisterns. DAI is present, seen as several punctate and linear hemorrhagic foci in the subcortical WM, midbrain, and left thalamus ➡. 2-71B. More cephalad scan in the same patient shows additional hemorrhagic foci in the corona radiata ➡, subcortical WM ➡.

MR FINDINGS. As most DAIs are nonhemorrhagic, T1 scans are often normal, especially in the early stages of TBI. T2WI and FLAIR may show hyperintense foci in the subcortical white matter and corpus callosum. Multiple lesions are the rule, and a combination of DAI and contusions or hematomas is very common.

T2* scans are very sensitive to the microbleeds of DAI and typically show multifocal ovoid and linear hypointensities **(2-72B)**. SWI sequences typically demonstrate more lesions than GRE. Residua from DAI may persist for years following the traumatic episode.

DWI may show restricted diffusion, particularly within the corpus callosum **(2-73)**. DTI tractography may be useful in depicting white matter disruption. MRS shows widespread decrease of NAA with increased Cho.

Differential Diagnosis

Cortical contusions often coexist with DAI in moderate to severe TBI. Cortical contusions are typically superficial lesions, usually located along gyral crests.

Multifocal hemorrhages with "blooming" on T2* (GRE, SWI) scans can be seen in numerous pathologies, including DAI. **Diffuse vascular injury** (see below) appears as multifocal parenchymal "black dots." Pneumocephalus may cause multifocal "blooming" lesions in the subarachnoid spaces. Parenchymal lesions are rare.

Several nontraumatic lesions also appear as multifocal T2* parenchymal hypointensities. **Cerebral amyloid angiopathy** and **chronic hypertensive encephalopathy** are common in older patients. Zabramski type 4 cavernous malformations are also seen as "black dots" on T2* MR scans.

Diffuse Vascular Injury

Terminology

Diffuse vascular injury (DVI) probably represents the extreme end of the diffuse axonal injury continuum.

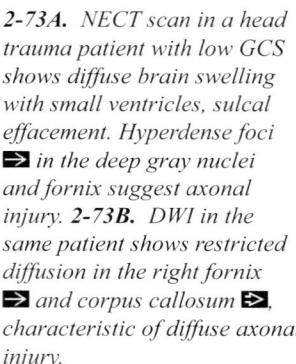

2-72A. NECT scan in a patient with closed head injury from high-speed motor vehicle collision shows no definite abnormalities. 2-72B. Because of the discrepancy between imaging findings and the patient's clinical status (GCS = 8), MR was obtained. T2 GRE scan shows multiple "blooming" foci in the subcortical/deep white matter and corpus callosum ⇨, characteristic of hemorrhagic axonal injury.*

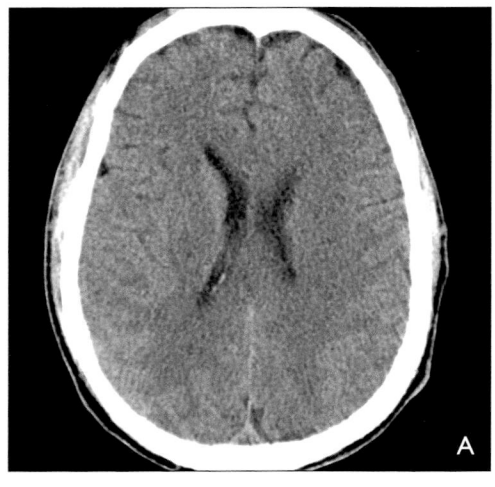

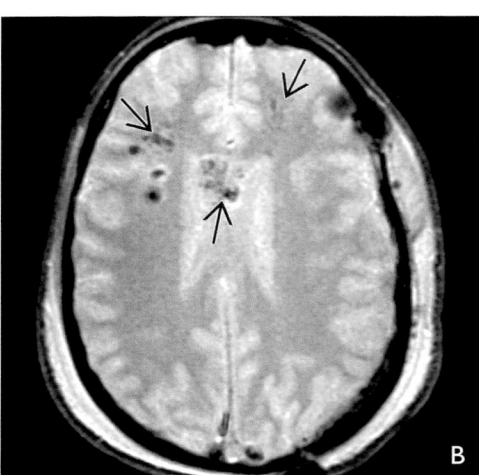

2-73A. NECT scan in a head trauma patient with low GCS shows diffuse brain swelling with small ventricles, sulcal effacement. Hyperdense foci ⇨ in the deep gray nuclei and fornix suggest axonal injury. 2-73B. DWI in the same patient shows restricted diffusion in the right fornix ⇨ and corpus callosum ⇨, characteristic of diffuse axonal injury.

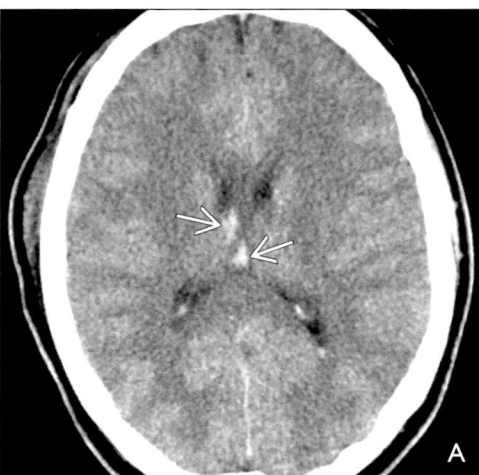

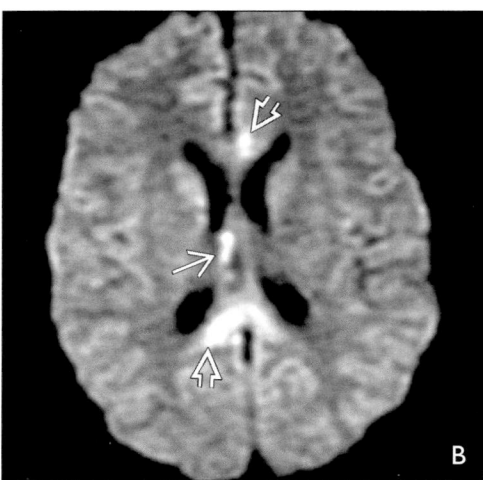

Etiology

DVI is caused by the extreme acceleration/rotational forces that are incurred in high-velocity motor vehicle collisions (MVCs). The brain microvasculature is disrupted by high tensile forces, resulting in numerous small parenchymal hemorrhages.

Pathology

GROSS PATHOLOGY. Autopsied brains of patients with DVI show numerous small hemorrhages in the subcortical and deep white matter as well as in the deep gray nuclei **(2-74)**.

MICROSCOPIC FEATURES. Many more hemorrhages are detected on microscopic examination than are seen in the gross appearance of the brain. Blood is identified along periarterial, perivenous, and pericapillary spaces with focal hemorrhages in the adjacent parenchyma.

Clinical Issues

EPIDEMIOLOGY. Autopsy series suggest DVI is present in 1-2% of fatal MVC victims and 15% of cases with diffuse brain injury.

DEMOGRAPHICS. While DVI can occur at any age, most occur in adults.

PRESENTATION. Immediate coma from the moment of impact is typical. A very low GCS, often less than 6-8, is typical in patients who survive the initial impact.

NATURAL HISTORY. Death within minutes or a few hours following injury is typical although some long-term survivors have been reported.

Imaging

GENERAL FEATURES. Many patients with DVI do not survive long enough for imaging. In those who do, the most striking feature is the dissociation between clinical severity and imaging findings.

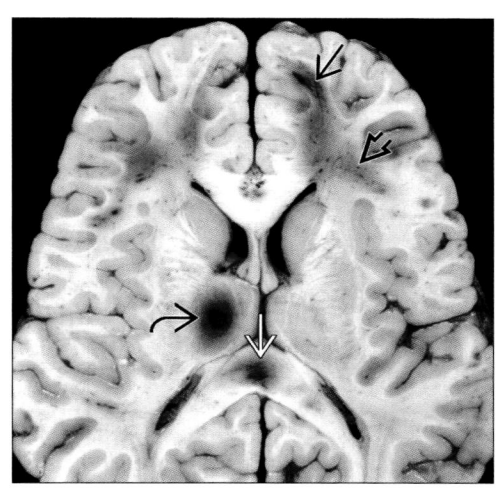

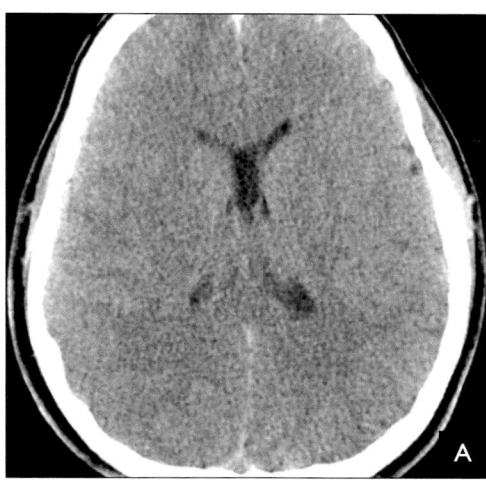

2-74. Autopsy case shows findings of diffuse vascular injury with multiple petechial ➢ and linear ⮕ subcortical WM hemorrhages. Note subcortical injury to thalamus ⮡, corpus callosum splenium ⮕. (Courtesy R. Hewlett, MD.) 2-75A. NECT in a male patient involved in a high-speed, high-impact MVC shows only diffuse brain swelling. GCS was 8 at the scene; by the time he reached the emergency department, the GCS had decreased to 3.

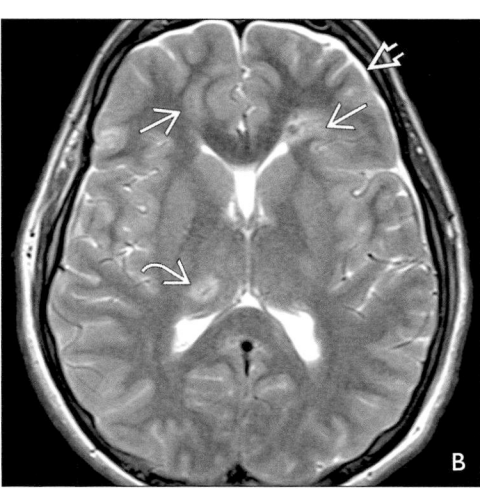

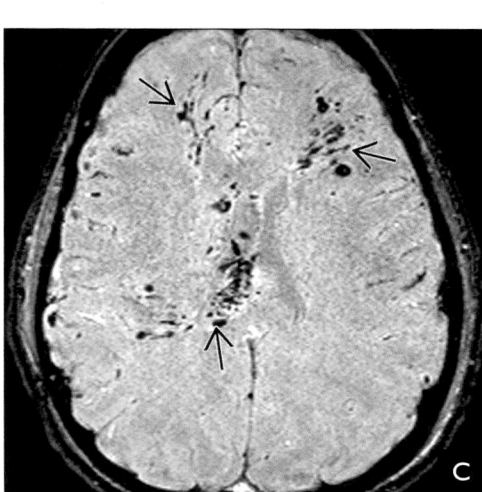

2-75B. MR was obtained because of the gross discrepancy between clinical and imaging findings. T2WI shows hyperintensities in the right thalamus ⮕ and WM of both frontal lobes ⮕. Torn arachnoid is probably responsible for the small bifrontal hygromas ⮕. 2-75C. SWI in the same patient shows innumerable linear and ovoid "blooming" hypointensities in the subcortical and deep WM ⮕ consistent with diffuse vascular injury.

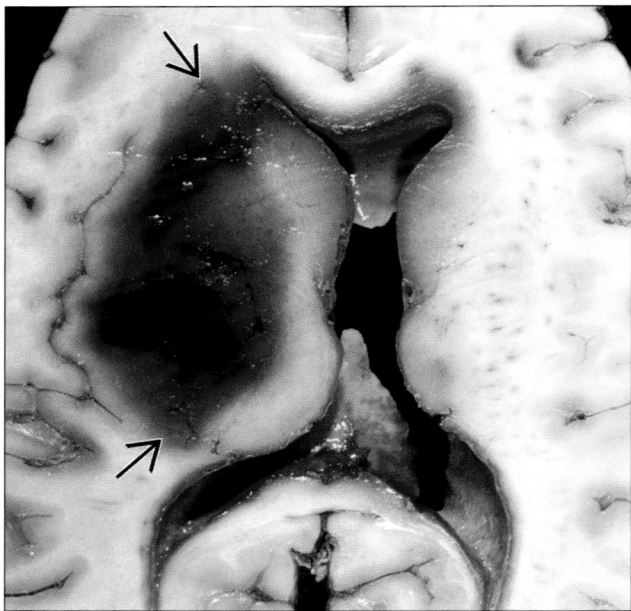

2-76. Autopsy specimen from a patient who died in a high-speed MVC shows a large hemorrhage ⮕ in the deep gray nuclei, characteristic of severe subcortical injury. (Courtesy R. Hewlett, MD.)

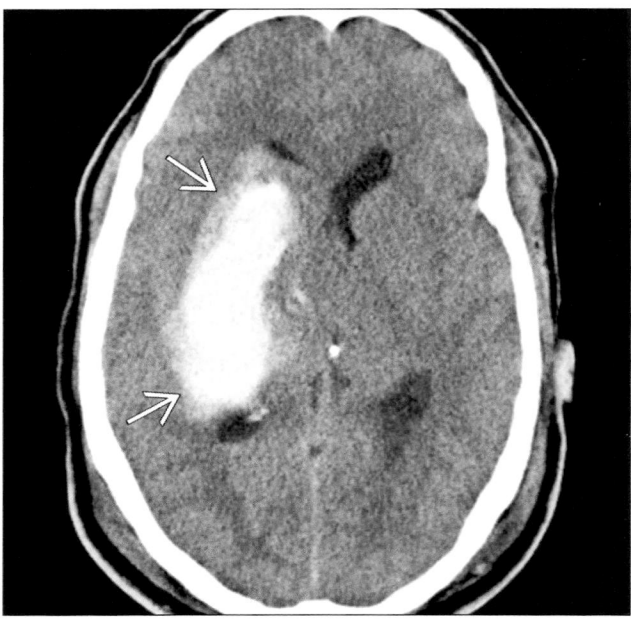

2-77. NECT scan in a patient with post-traumatic subcortical injury shows a large expanding basal ganglia hematoma ⮕.

CT FINDINGS. NECT scans may show only diffuse brain swelling with effaced superficial sulci and small ventricles **(2-75A)**. A few small foci of hemorrhage in the white matter and basal ganglia can sometimes be identified. Bone CT shows multiple skull fractures in unrestrained passengers, but fractures are absent in one-third of individuals wearing seat belts.

MR FINDINGS. T1WI shows only mild brain swelling. T2WI and FLAIR scans may demonstrate a few foci of hyperintensity in the white matter **(2-75B)**. Occasionally, scattered hypointensities can be identified within the hyperintensities, suggesting the presence of hemorrhage.

T2* scans, especially susceptibility-weighted sequences, are striking. Punctate and linear "blooming" hypointensities are seen oriented perpendicularly to the ventricles, predominantly in the subcortical and deep white matter, especially the corpus callosum **(2-75C)**. Additional lesions in the basal ganglia, thalami, brainstem, and cerebellum are often present.

DWI may demonstrate a few foci of restricted diffusion consistent with ischemia caused by the vascular injuries.

Differential Diagnosis

The major differential diagnosis is **diffuse axonal injury** (DAI). While some lesions in DAI are hemorrhagic, the majority are not. DVI is characterized by the presence of innumerable petechial hemorrhages on T2* imaging. It is the number, severity, and extent of the hemorrhages that distinguishes DVI from DAI.

Subcortical (Deep Brain) Injury

Terminology

Subcortical injuries (SCIs) are traumatic lesions of deep brain structures such as the brainstem, basal ganglia, thalami, and ventricles. Most represent severe shear-strain injuries that disrupt axons, tear penetrating blood vessels, and damage the choroid plexus of the lateral ventricles.

Etiology

SCIs are caused by the violent acceleration/deceleration and brain rotation that occurs with severe, often fatal, motor vehicle collisions. Sudden craniocaudal displacement or lateral impaction of the midbrain against the tentorial incisura is common with these injuries.

Pathology

GROSS PATHOLOGY. Manifestations of SCI include deep hemorrhagic contusions, nonhemorrhagic lacerations, intraventricular bleeds, and traumatic subarachnoid hemorrhage (tSAH) **(2-76)**. SCIs usually occur with other traumatic lesions such as cortical contusions and diffuse axonal injury (DAI).

Clinical Issues

EPIDEMIOLOGY. Between 5-10% of patients with moderate to severe brain trauma sustain subcortical injuries. SCIs are the third most common parenchymal brain injury, after cortical contusions and DAI.

DEMOGRAPHICS. As with most traumatic brain injuries, SCIs are most common in males between the ages of 15 and 24.

PRESENTATION. Immediate loss of consciousness with profound neurologic deficits is typical. Obtundation is the rule, not the exception. As with DAI, gross discrepancy between immediate imaging findings (often minimal) and GCS (low) is common.

NATURAL HISTORY. Prognosis is poor in these severely injured patients. Many do not survive; those who do typically have profound neurologic impairment with severe long-term disability.

TREATMENT OPTIONS. Controlling intracranial pressure is the most pressing issue. Craniectomy may be an option in exceptionally severe cases of brain swelling.

Imaging

GENERAL FEATURES. Minimal abnormalities may be present on initial imaging but show dramatic increase on follow-up scans.

SCI typically exists with numerous comorbid injuries. Lesions ranging from subtle traumatic SAH to gross parenchymal hemorrhage are common (2-77). Mass effect with cerebral herniation and gross disturbances in regional blood flow may develop.

CT FINDINGS. NECT scans often show diffuse brain swelling with punctate and/or gross hemorrhage in the deep gray nuclei and midbrain. Intraventricular and choroid plexus hemorrhages are common and may form a "cast" of the lateral ventricles. Blood-fluid levels are common.

MR FINDINGS. MR is much more sensitive than CT even though acute hemorrhage is isointense with brain on T1 scans. FLAIR and T2* are the most sensitive sequences. DWI may show foci of restricted diffusion. DTI mapping delineates the pattern of white matter tract disruption.

Differential Diagnosis

Secondary midbrain ("Duret") hemorrhage may occur with severe descending transtentorial herniation. These hemorrhages are typically centrally located within the midbrain whereas contusional SCIs are dorsolateral.

PARENCHYMAL BRAIN INJURIES

Cerebral Contusions
- Most common intraaxial injury
  - Brain impacts skull and/or dura
  - Causes "brain bruises" in gyral crests
  - Usually multiple, often bilateral
  - Anteroinferior frontal, temporal lobes most common sites
- Imaging
  - Superficial petechial, focal hemorrhage
  - Edema, hemorrhage more apparent with time
  - T2* (GRE, SWI) most sensitive imaging

Diffuse Axonal Injury
- Second most common intraaxial injury
  - Spares cortex, involves subcortical/deep WM
- Imaging
  - GCS low; initial imaging often minimally abnormal
  - Subcortical, deep petechial hemorrhages ("tip of iceberg")
  - T2* (GRE, SWI) most sensitive technique

Diffuse Vascular Injury
- Rare, usually fatal
- High-speed, high-impact MVCs
- May represent extreme end of DAI spectrum
- Imaging
  - CT shows diffuse brain swelling
  - T2 and FLAIR show a few scattered hyperintensities
  - SWI shows innumerable linear hypointensities

Subcortical Injury
- "The deeper the injury, the worse it is"
- Basal ganglia, thalami, midbrain, pons
  - Hemorrhages, axonal injury, brain tears
  - Gross intraventricular hemorrhage common

Miscellaneous Injuries

A broad spectrum of miscellaneous primary injuries occurs in head trauma. Some such as pneumocephalus are relatively common. Other lesions are rare. We conclude this chapter with a consideration of these miscellaneous lesions, as well as the topics of child abuse and gunshot wounds.

Pneumocephalus

Terminology

Pneumocephalus simply means the presence of gas or air within the skull; intracranial air does not exist under normal conditions. In pneumocephalus, air can be found anywhere within the cranium, including blood vessels, and within any compartment. While intracranial air is never normal, it can be an expected and therefore routine finding (e.g., after surgery). **Tension pneumocephalus** is a collection of intracranial air that is under pressure and causes mass effect on the brain **(2-78)**. Intracerebral pneumatocele or "aerocele" is a less commonly used term and refers specifically to a focal gas collection within the brain parenchyma **(2-79)**.

Etiology

Intracranial air is most often associated with trauma and surgery. Infection by gas-forming organisms is a rare cause of pneumocephalus.

Any breach in integrity of the calvaria, central skull base, mastoid, or paranasal sinuses that also disrupts the dura and arachnoid can allow air to enter the cranium. A ball-valve mechanism may entrap the air, which can be exacerbated by forcible sneezing, coughing, straining, or Valsalva maneuver.

Intravascular air is usually secondary to intravenous catheterization, most commonly found in the cavernous sinus, and of no clinical importance. Intraarterial air is seen only with air embolism (transient) or brain death.

Clinical Issues

EPIDEMIOLOGY. Trauma is the most common cause of pneumocephalus. It is present in 3% of all patients with skull fractures and 8% of those with paranasal sinus fractures.

Virtually all patients who have supratentorial surgery have some degree of pneumocephalus on imaging studies obtained within the first 24-28 hours. **Tension pneumocephalus (2-78)** is a relatively uncommon complication of surgery, usually seen after subdural hematoma evacuation. Occasionally, **spontaneous pneumocephalus** can occur with primary defects in the temporal bone (**"otogenic pneumocephalus"**). Rarely, defects in or rupture of an enlarged paranasal sinus air cell ("pneumosinus dilatans") results in intracranial air.

PRESENTATION. The most common presentation is nonspecific headache. Less commonly, neurologic deficit and disturbances of consciousness are observed.

NATURAL HISTORY AND TREATMENT OPTIONS. Unless it is under tension, most intracranial air resolves

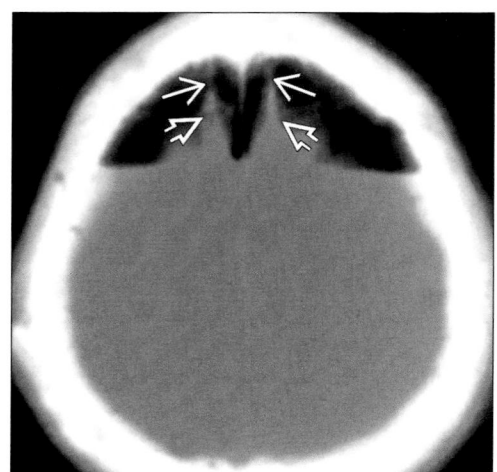

2-78. NECT scan shows subdural air with "pointing" of the frontal lobes. This "Mount Fuji" sign is caused by cortical veins ➡ tethering the frontal lobes ➡, and it indicates tension pneumocephalus.
2-79. NECT scan shows a focal pneumatocele in the right frontal lobe ➡. Some air is also present in the frontal horn of the left lateral ventricle ➡.

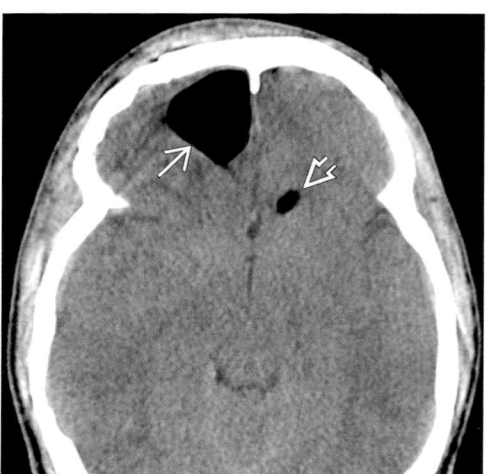

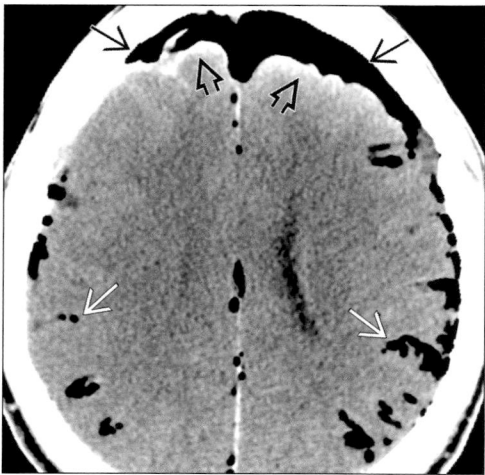

2-80. NECT shows bifrontal subdural air ➡. Note that "overshoot" artifact from the air creates the appearance of increased attenuation in the underlying brain ➡. "Spots" and "dots" of air are in the subarachnoid spaces ➡.
2-81. Bone CT in a child with multiple fractures ➡ shows air in the arteries that comprise the circle of Willis ➡.

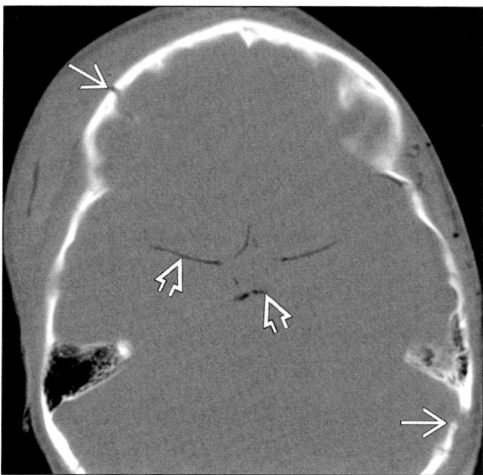

spontaneously within a few days after trauma or surgery. Occasionally, air collections increase and may require evacuation with duraplasty.

Imaging

GENERAL FEATURES. Intracranial air can exist in any compartment and conforms to the shape of that compartment or potential compartment. **Epidural air** is typically unilateral, solitary, biconvex in configuration, and does not move with changes in head position.

Subdural air is confluent, crescentic, often bilateral, frequently contains air-fluid levels, moves with changes in head position, and surrounds cortical veins that cross the subdural space.

Subarachnoid air is typically seen as multifocal small "dots" or "droplets" of air within and around cerebral sulci **(2-80)**. **Intraventricular air** forms air-fluid levels, most often in the frontal horns of the lateral ventricles. **Intravascular air** conforms to the vascular structure(s) within which it resides **(2-81)**.

CT FINDINGS. Air is extremely hypodense on CT, measuring approximately -1,000 HU. The "Mount Fuji" sign of tension pneumocephalus is seen as bilateral subdural air collections that separate and compress the frontal lobes **(2-78)**. The frontal lobes are displaced posteriorly by air under pressure and are typically pointed where they are tethered to the dura-arachnoid by cortical veins, mimicking the silhouette of Mount Fuji.

Distinguishing air from fat on CT is extremely important. With typical narrow soft tissue windows, both appear similarly hypodense. Increasing window width or simply looking at bone CT algorithms (on which air is clearly distinct from the less hypodense fat) helps differentiate fat from air.

MR FINDINGS. Air is seen as areas of completely absent signal intensity on all sequences. On T2* GRE, intracranial air "blooms" and appears as multifocal "black dots."

Differential Diagnosis

Air is air and shouldn't be mistaken for anything else. If wide windows are not used, a ruptured dermoid cyst with fat droplets in the CSF cisterns can mimic subarachnoid air.

Reminder!

With the exception of tension pneumocephalus, air itself generally isn't the problem; figure out what's causing it!

Nonaccidental Trauma (Child Abuse)

Radiologists play a key role in the early diagnosis and imaging of suspected inflicted injury. Imaging must be performed with care, interpreted with rigor, and precisely described.

Terminology

The term "nonaccidental trauma" (NAT), also known as nonaccidental injury (NAI) or shaken-baby syndrome (SBS), refers to intentionally inflicted injury. Abusive head trauma (AHT) and acute inflicted head injury are more specific terms applied to brain injuries.

Etiology

NAT brain injuries can be divided into two major groups: Direct impact injuries and indirect or "shaking" injuries.

Direct injuries are inflicted by blows to the head or direct impact of the cranium on an object such as a wall. These generally result in skull fractures, subdural hematomas, contusions in the subjacent brain, and "contre-coup" injuries.

The precise pathoetiology of indirect injuries is unclear, as is the minimum force required to produce them. Shaking can result in violent "to and fro" motions of the head. The head of an infant or young child is relatively large compared to its body, and the cervical musculature is comparatively weak. Shaking causes rapid rotation of the head relative to the neck, resulting in a form of whiplash injury. The most common result is diffusely distributed subdural hematomas.

Pathology

Subdural hematomas of differing ages are the hallmark of inflicted brain injury **(2-82)**.

Clinical Issues

EPIDEMIOLOGY. The annual incidence of child abuse is estimated at 15-25 per 100,000. Between three and four million cases of suspected abuse are reported annually in the United States alone.

DEMOGRAPHICS. NAT is the most common overall cause of traumatic death in infants, and head trauma is the most common cause of morbidity and mortality. Most abused children are under two years old. The peak age is between two and five months. While the majority of victims are males, in some cultures, female infants are more common victims of NAT.

No nationality or demographic group is exempt, and NAT can be found in all socioeconomic groups. Some predisposing factors have been identified, including young age of the parents, domestic conflict, financial or emotional stress, and drug and alcohol abuse.

PRESENTATION. Clinical presentation of an abused child is variable. Discordance between stated history and severity of injury is common. Falls from a height less than around four feet (e.g., "falling off the couch") usually do not induce enough force to cause the types of brain injuries observed in NAT.

Irritability, apneic episodes, vomiting, and unarousability are common. Unusual bruises, patches of torn hair, lip lacerations, and retinal hemorrhages should raise the suspicion of NAT and prompt appropriate imaging.

NATURAL HISTORY. Finding evidence of repetitive violence indicates that the infant or child is at a high risk for further injury and death. Mortality in NAT ranges from 15-60%, and morbidity is high. Post-traumatic brain damage with seizures and retardation are common.

TREATMENT OPTIONS. The medical imperative is to protect the child. Radiologists must clearly communicate any suspicion of abuse and the degree of certainty to appropriate clinicians. Notifying Child Protective Services of any suspected case of child abuse is legally required in many countries. All 50 states in the USA have statutes that mandate reporting cases of suspected child abuse or neglect.

Imaging

GENERAL FEATURES. The Section on Radiology of the American Academy of Pediatrics recently updated its recommendations on diagnostic imaging in cases of suspected child abuse.

Initial imaging in cases of suspected child abuse should include a complete skeletal survey and brain CT as the initial screening procedures. MR is recommended for children two years or younger.

While some experts favor MR for medical-legal documentation, caution should be exercised in attempting to "time" intracranial bleeds. Many experts emphasize that, while dating of both brain and skeletal injuries is imprecise, the more important goal is determining whether the pattern is that of "differing age" lesions regardless of location.

CT FINDINGS. NECT using both soft tissue and bone algorithm with multiplanar reformatting is the primary tool in the initial evaluation of abusive head trauma. Skull

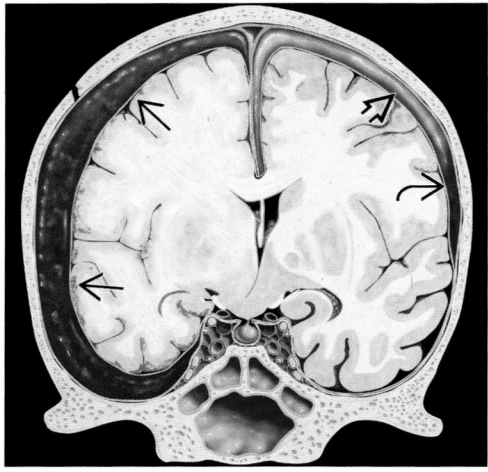
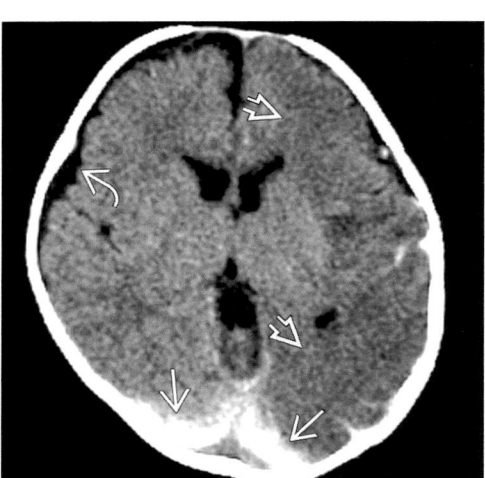

2-82. Graphic of NAT shows an acute SDH over the right hemisphere ⊟ and a smaller left sSDH ⊠ with "hematocrit effect" ⊠. Other injuries (e.g., traumatic SAH, cortical contusions) are illustrated and are common in NAT. 2-83. NECT scan in suspected NAT shows findings of "differing age" SDHs with chronic right ⊠, bilateral acute ⊟ SDHs. Note diffuse edema involving almost the entire left hemisphere ⊠.

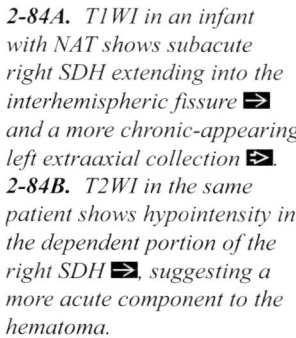
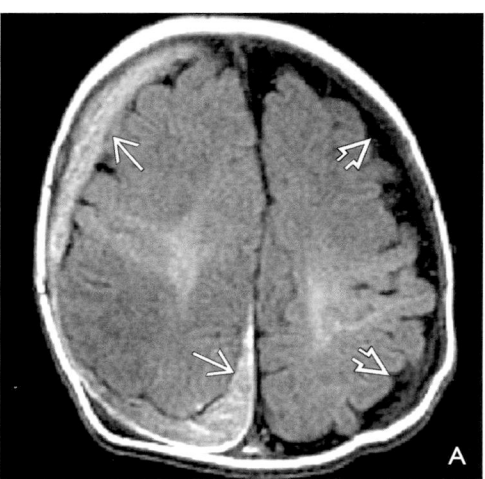
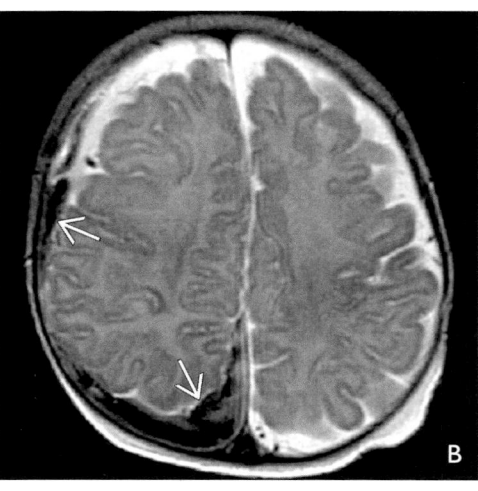

2-84A. T1WI in an infant with NAT shows subacute right SDH extending into the interhemispheric fissure ⊟ and a more chronic-appearing left extraaxial collection ⊠. 2-84B. T2WI in the same patient shows hypointensity in the dependent portion of the right SDH ⊟, suggesting a more acute component to the hematoma.

fractures are present in nearly half of all cases, and scalp hematomas can be readily detected.

The identification and characterization of intracranial hemorrhages, especially "differing age" subdural hematomas (SDHs), is critical **(2-83)**. Epidural hematomas are rare in NAT, but SDHs are seen in over half of all cases and are the dominant feature in shaking-type NAT.

Bifrontal, interhemispheric, and peritentorial subdural hematomas of differing ages strongly suggest inflicted injury. Traumatic subarachnoid hemorrhage, cortical contusions, and occasionally diffuse axonal injuries are common. Ischemic injury may also be present and varies from territorial infarcts to global hypoxic brain injury.

Hemispheric or diffuse brain swelling occurs in some infants with acute subdural hematomas. This has been dubbed the "big black brain" for its striking hypodensity on NECT scans. Mortality is high in these cases. When "differing age" SDHs occur in the presence of severe hemisphere swelling, a "second impact" type syndrome (see Chapter 3) from NAT should be considered **(2-83)**.

MR FINDINGS. "Differing age" SDHs on T1-weighted images with mixed hyper- and isointense components is highly suggestive of NAT **(2-84)**. FLAIR is helpful in detecting small extraaxial collections and white matter injury.

T2* (GRE, SWI) scans are very sensitive for chronic blood products, particularly subtle petechial cortical contusions and hemorrhagic axonal injuries. DWI is essential for evaluating foci of ischemic injury.

Spine and spinal cord injuries are common in infants and children with shaking injuries. MR is the procedure of choice as significant injuries can occur in the absence of fractures or subluxations.

PET FINDINGS. PET in conjunction with high-detail skeletal survey is helpful in the assessment of skeletal trauma but of limited utility in evaluating brain injury.

Differential Diagnosis

Rarely, an **inborn error of metabolism** (such as glutaric aciduria and Menkes kinky hair syndrome) can cause retinal hemorrhages and bilateral SDHs, mimicking NAT. **Bleeding dyscrasias** can cause recurrent subdural hematomas. **Metastatic neuroblastoma** with "raccoon eyes" can also mimic NAT.

Missile and Penetrating Injuries

The extent of tissue damage from a projectile depends on the type of bullet, its velocity and mass, and the physical characteristics of the affected tissues. Projectile craniocerebral injuries are qualitatively different from other traumatic brain injuries and from injuries in unconfined soft tissues with similar impact.

While a detailed discussion of projectiles and their ballistics is beyond the scope of this text, we will briefly

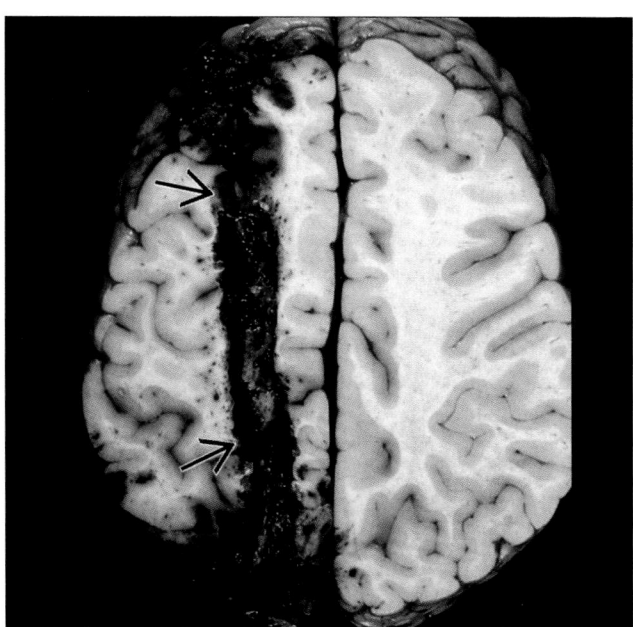

2-85. Autopsy specimen from a patient with a gunshot wound from a 9 mm bullet shows the typical findings of a relatively high-velocity projectile, namely hemorrhage and disrupted macerated brain along the bullet path ➥.

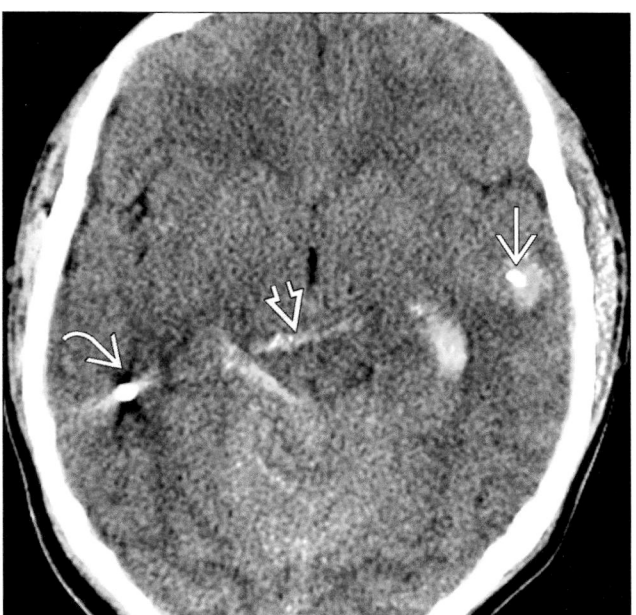

2-86. NECT scan shows a low-velocity injury with a bullet fragment ➘, *linear hemorrhage along a relatively narrow projectile path* ➘, *and a remaining fragment* ➘ *where the projectile slowed and then stopped.*

consider the ballistics of projectile injury and their craniocerebral consequences.

Readers interested in greater detail are referred to the definitive article by Jandial et al., Ballistics for the neurosurgeon. *Neurosurgery* 62(2): 472-80, 2008. Much of the information on ballistics and tissue injury summarized below is derived from this excellent source.

Terminology

The high-velocity projectile brain injuries seen in noncombatant populations are predominantly gunshot wounds. Stabbing injuries inflicted by sharp objects such as a knife, screwdriver, or ice-pick may also penetrate the calvaria and damage the underlying brain.

Etiology

The major factors that determine whether a projectile will penetrate the cranium are (1) its energy at impact on bone, (2) the contact area, and (3) the thickness of bone at the point of impact. Penetration by a ballistic projectile craters bone, punching it inward through the dura and into the brain.

The severity of tissue damage is proportional to the kinetic energy deposited in the tissue by the penetrating projectile *plus* a "rate effect" that is dependent on projectile size.

Pressure is very high at the tip of an advancing projectile. As a projectile penetrates brain, it leaves a temporary cavity in its wake. It also causes outward radial stretching of adjacent tissue, depositing energy at very high strain rates.

As a bullet penetrates the brain, it yaws (not tumbles). This explains why the entry wound is typically small and tissue damage expands as the bullet slows. The exit wound may be quite large.

Projectiles with high kinetic energy may transfer enough energy to the skull to transform the bone fragments themselves into tiny secondary missiles. In the aggregate, these fragments can be just as lethal as through-and-through penetration by the projectile itself.

2-87A. Series of NECT scans depicts findings from a patient with a large-caliber, high-velocity gunshot wound. The entrance wound is through the squamous portion of the right temporal bone. A mass of blood, imploded bone, and a few bullet fragments ⇨ is seen under the entrance wound. 2-87B. More cephalad scan shows the wide pathway ⇨ formed by fragments that penetrated the brain at high velocity and high energy.

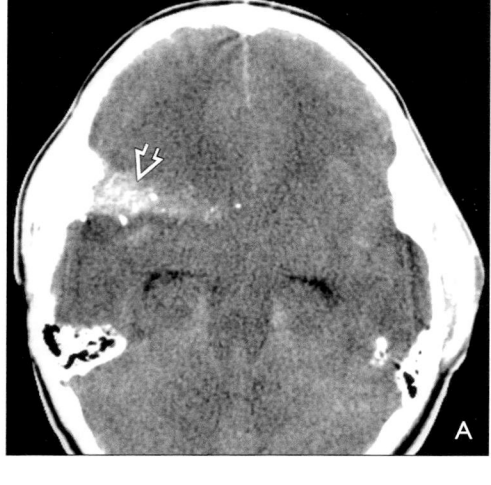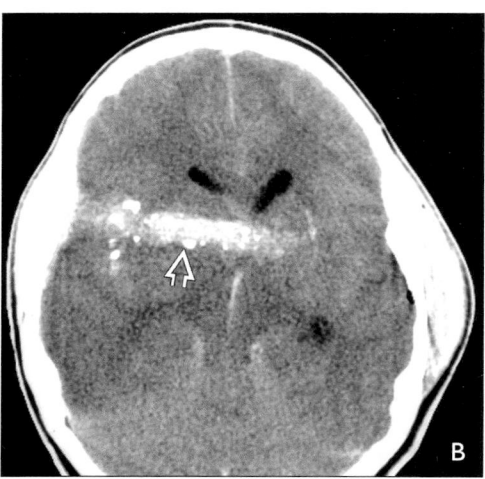

2-87C. Scan through the frontal horns shows continuation of the pathway ⇨ through the lateral ventricles. 2-87D. Image through the upper lateral ventricles shows intraventricular hemorrhage. Blood is seen along the rest of the projectile pathway ⇨. Enough kinetic energy was present to punch the remaining fragments through the left squamous temporal bone ➡, fracturing and exploding the skull outward ⇥.

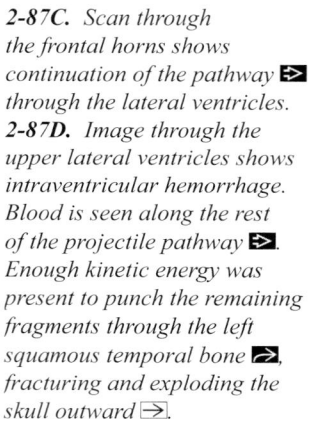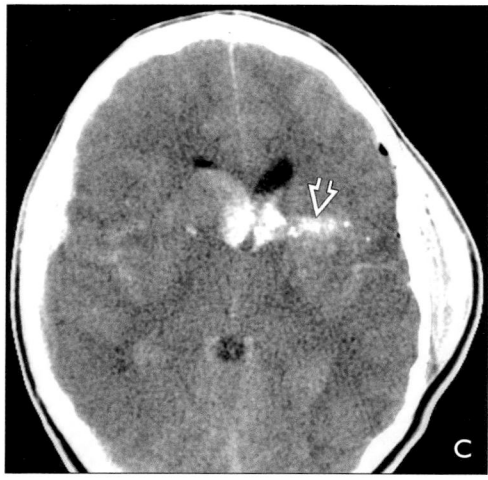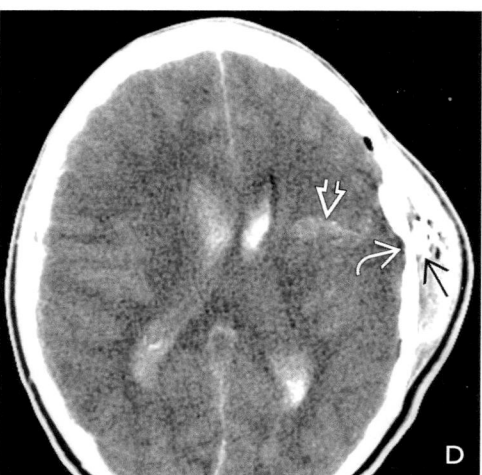

Pathology

The behavior of a projectile acting on tissue (the brain) that is anatomically constrained within a closed space (the skull) is different from injuries in unconfined soft tissue with similar impact.

Bullets passing through the firm brain tissue often take a slightly curved path between the entry point and final location. The trajectory is marked by macerated tissue, torn vessels, and disrupted axons **(2-85)**.

Clinical Issues

DEMOGRAPHICS. While patients at virtually any age can be affected, gunshot would patients tend to be overwhelmingly male and young.

PRESENTATION. Patients with gunshot wounds to the brain typically present with signs and symptoms of brain swelling and herniation, including apnea and bradycardia. The sudden increase in intracranial pressure caused by the cavitation and expansion of brain can cause coma or death, even if eloquent structures are not directly affected.

Patients with tangential gunshot wounds commonly present with a relatively good GCS and no loss of consciousness. In these cases, the bullet typically does not breach the skull, although the tangential gunshot wounds may transfer considerable force to the brain and result in extraaxial hematoma, cortical contusion, and/or traumatic subarachnoid hemorrhage.

NATURAL HISTORY. Prognosis is highly variable, ranging from death to full recovery. Gunshot wounds that have a central trajectory and are transventricular or bihemispheric have a high morbidity/mortality. Most fatalities occur within the first 24 hours after injury. Tangential gunshot wounds with smaller caliber, low-velocity bullets may have a better outcome.

Imaging

The morphology of gunshot wounds is extremely variable. Injuries are most severe with large-caliber missiles traveling at high velocity that fragment early on entry into the cranium.

GENERAL FEATURES. CT with both bone and soft tissue reconstruction is the diagnostic procedure of choice. The radiologist's report should identify the entry site, describe the missile path including bone fragmentation and ricochet paths, and evaluate for exit wound. Possible damage to critical blood vessels should be noted along with secondary effects such as ischemia and herniation syndromes.

In general, a small-caliber, low-velocity projectile will have a relatively small linear track through the brain **(2-86)**. The track is larger with large-caliber, high-velocity bullets.

CT FINDINGS. Entrance wounds are typically "punched-in" cones of bone. The bullet path is hyperdense and tends to curve slightly, broadening as the bullet yaws and slows. Bullet and bone fragments should be noted. The exit wound is typically either a ledge-shaped fracture or "punched-out" bone **(2-87)**. Pneumocephalus may be present.

ANGIOGRAPHY. CTA with multiplanar reconstruction and MIP images is helpful in evaluating vascular injuries such as pseudoaneurysm, dissection, traumatic dural arteriovenous fistula, and venous injury or thrombosis.

Selected References

- Hymel KP et al: Head injury depth as an indicator of causes and mechanisms. Pediatrics. 125(4):712-20, 2010

Scalp and Skull Injuries

Facial Injuries

- Holmgren EP et al: Facial soft tissue injuries as an aid to ordering a combination head and facial computed tomography in trauma patients. J Oral Maxillofac Surg. 63(5):651-4, 2005

Skull Fractures

- Liu XS et al: Growing skull fracture stages and treatment strategy. J Neurosurg Pediatr. 9(6):670-5, 2012
- Ochalski PG et al: Fractures of the clivus and traumatic diastasis of the central skull base in the pediatric population. J Neurosurg Pediatr. 7(3):261-7, 2011
- Ringl H et al: The skull unfolded: a cranial CT visualization algorithm for fast and easy detection of skull fractures. Radiology. 255(2):553-62, 2010

Extraaxial Hemorrhages

Acute Epidural Hematoma

- Huisman TA et al: Epidural hematoma in children: do cranial sutures act as a barrier? J Neuroradiol. 36(2):93-7, 2009
- Le TH et al: Neuroimaging of traumatic brain injury. Mt Sinai J Med. 76(2):145-62, 2009
- Pruthi N et al: Mixed-density extradural hematomas on computed tomography-prognostic significance. Surg Neurol. 71(2):202-6, 2009

Acute Subdural Hematoma

- Cantu RC et al: Second-impact syndrome and a small subdural hematoma: an uncommon catastrophic result of repetitive head injury with a characteristic imaging appearance. J Neurotrauma. 27(9):1557-64, 2010
- Dalfino JC et al: Visualization of an actively bleeding cortical vessel into the subdural space by CT angiography. Clin Neurol Neurosurg. 112(8):737-9, 2010
- Chieregato A et al: Hyperemia beneath evacuated acute subdural hematoma is frequent and prolonged in patients with an unfavorable outcome: a xe-computed tomographic study. Neurosurgery. 64(4):705-17; discussion 717-8, 2009
- Naama O et al: Acute spontaneous subdural hematoma: an unusual form of cerebrovacular accident. J Neurosurg Sci. 53(4):157-9, 2009
- Westermaier T et al: Clinical features, treatment, and prognosis of patients with acute subdural hematomas presenting in critical condition. Neurosurgery. 61(3):482-7; discussion 487-8, 2007

Subacute Subdural Hematoma

- Wind JJ et al: Images in clinical medicine. Bilateral subacute subdural hematomas. N Engl J Med. 360(17):e23, 2009
- Kuwahara S et al: Diffusion-weighted imaging of traumatic subdural hematoma in the subacute stage. Neurol Med Chir (Tokyo). 45(9):464-9, 2005

Chronic/Mixed Subdural Hematoma

- Lee KS et al: Acute-on-chronic subdural hematoma: not uncommon events. J Korean Neurosurg Soc. 50(6):512-6, 2011
- Kakeda S et al: Superficial siderosis associated with a chronic subdural hematoma: T2-weighted MR imaging at 3T. Acad Radiol. 17(7):871-6, 2010
- Kristof RA et al: Cerebrospinal fluid leakage into the subdural space: possible influence on the pathogenesis and recurrence frequency of chronic subdural hematoma and subdural hygroma. J Neurosurg. 108(2):275-80, 2008
- Zanini MA et al: Traumatic subdural hygromas: proposed pathogenesis based classification. J Trauma. 64(3):705-13, 2008

Traumatic Subarachnoid Hemorrhage

- Beretta L et al: Post-traumatic interpeduncular cistern hemorrhage as a marker for brainstem lesions. J Neurotrauma. 27(3):509-14, 2010
- Wu Z et al: Evaluation of traumatic subarachnoid hemorrhage using susceptibility-weighted imaging. AJNR Am J Neuroradiol. 31(7):1302-10, 2010
- Lee DJ et al: Intra-arterial calcium channel blocker infusion for treatment of severe vasospasm in traumatic brain injury: case report. Neurosurgery. 63(5):E1004-6; discussion E1006, 2008

Parenchymal Injuries

- Hymel KP et al: Head injury depth as an indicator of causes and mechanisms. Pediatrics. 125(4):712-20, 2010

Cerebral Contusions and Lacerations

- Alahmadi H et al: The natural history of brain contusion: an analysis of radiological and clinical progression. J Neurosurg. 112(5):1139-45, 2010
- Khan S et al: Evolution of traumatic intracerebral hemorrhage captured with CT imaging: report of a case and the role of serial CT scans. Emerg Radiol. 17(6):493-6, 2010

Diffuse Axonal Injury

- Al-Sarraj S et al: Focal traumatic brain stem injury is a rare type of head injury resulting from assault: a forensic neuropathological study. J Forensic Leg Med. 19(3):144-51, 2012
- Govind V et al: Whole-brain proton MR spectroscopic imaging of mild-to-moderate traumatic brain injury and correlation with neuropsychological deficits. J Neurotrauma. 27(3):483-96, 2010
- Skandsen T et al: Prevalence and impact of diffuse axonal injury in patients with moderate and severe head injury: a

cohort study of early magnetic resonance imaging findings and 1-year outcome. J Neurosurg. 113(3):556-63, 2010

- Venkatesan C et al: Chronic upregulation of activated microglia immunoreactive for galectin-3/Mac-2 and nerve growth factor following diffuse axonal injury. J Neuroinflammation. 7:32, 2010
- Li XY et al: Diffuse axonal injury: novel insights into detection and treatment. J Clin Neurosci. 16(5):614-9, 2009

Diffuse Vascular Injury

- Iwamura A et al: Diffuse vascular injury: convergent-type hemorrhage in the supratentorial white matter on susceptibility-weighted image in cases of severe traumatic brain damage. Neuroradiology. 54(4):335-43, 2012
- Hijaz TA et al: Imaging of head trauma. Radiol Clin North Am. 49(1):81-103, 2011
- Onaya M: Neuropathological investigation of cerebral white matter lesions caused by closed head injury. Neuropathology. 22(4):243-51, 2002

Subcortical (Deep Brain) Injury

- Mamere AE et al: Evaluation of delayed neuronal and axonal damage secondary to moderate and severe traumatic brain injury using quantitative MR imaging techniques. AJNR Am J Neuroradiol. 30(5):947-52, 2009

Miscellaneous Injuries

Pneumocephalus

- Abbati SG et al: Spontaneous intraparenchymal otogenic pneumocephalus: A case report and review of literature. Surg Neurol Int. 3:32, 2012
- Sinclair AG et al: Imaging of the post-operative cranium. Radiographics. 30(2):461-82, 2010
- Venkatesh SK et al: Clinics in diagnostic imaging (119). Post-traumatic intracerebral pneumatocele. Singapore Med J. 48(11):1055-9; quiz 1060, 2007

Nonaccidental Trauma (Child Abuse)

- Schwartz ES et al: Nonaccidental trauma (child abuse). In Barkovich AJ et al: Pediatric Neuroimaging. Philadelphia: Lippincott Williams & Wilkins. 344-51, 2012
- Adamsbaum C et al: How to explore and report children with suspected non-accidental trauma. Pediatr Radiol. 40(6):932-8, 2010
- Sato Y: Imaging of nonaccidental head injury. Pediatr Radiol. 39 Suppl 2:S230-5, 2009
- Section on Radiology; American Academy of Pediatrics: Diagnostic imaging of child abuse. Pediatrics. 123(5):1430-5, 2009
- Duhaime AC et al: Traumatic brain injury in infants: the phenomenon of subdural hemorrhage with hemispheric hypodensity ("big black brain"). Prog Brain Res. 161:293-302, 2007

Missile and Penetrating Injuries

- Farhat HI et al: A tangential gunshot wound to the head: case report and review of the literature. J Emerg Med. 43(2):e111-4, 2012
- Maiden N: Ballistics reviews: mechanisms of bullet wound trauma. Forensic Sci Med Pathol. 5(3):204-9, 2009
- Jandial R et al: Ballistics for the neurosurgeon. Neurosurgery. 62(2):472-80; discussion 480, 2008
- Oehmichen M et al: Gunshot injuries to the head and brain caused by low-velocity handguns and rifles. A review. Forensic Sci Int. 146(2-3):111-20, 2004

3

Secondary Effects and Sequelae of CNS Trauma

Traumatic brain injury (TBI) is not a single "one and done" event. TBI is a ongoing series of pathophysiological reactions that extends from the moment of injury for days, months, or even years into the future. Acute TBI is just the initial triggering insult.

A veritable "cascade" of adverse pathophysiologic events continues to develop after the initial injury. Some—such as progressive hemorrhagic injury—occur within the first 24 hours after trauma. Others (e.g., brain swelling and herniation syndromes) may take a day or two to develop. Delayed complications such as CSF leaks and intracranial hypotension may develop weeks or months later. Finally, there is a broad spectrum of post-traumatic encephalopathic syndromes that may manifest years or even decades later.

Secondary effects of CNS trauma are defined as those that occur after the initial injury. These secondary effects are often more devastating than the initial injury itself and can become life-threatening. While many of the primary effects of CNS trauma (e.g., cortical contusions and axonal injuries) are permanent injuries, some secondary effects are either preventable or treatable.

Many potentially serious secondary effects are at least partially reversible if recognized early and treated promptly. Aggressive management of elevated intracra-

nial pressure, perfusion alterations, and oxygenation deficits may help mitigate both the immediate and long-term effects of brain trauma.

Chapter 2 focused on the primary effects of TBI. In this chapter, we consider a broad spectrum of secondary effects that follow brain trauma, beginning with herniation syndromes.

Herniation Syndromes

Brain herniations occur when one or more structures is displaced from its normal or "native" compartment into an adjacent space. They are the most common secondary manifestation of *any* expanding intracranial mass regardless of etiology.

In this section, we briefly discuss the relevant anatomy and physiology that explain the pathology underlying brain herniations. We then delineate the spectrum of brain herniations and their imaging findings, beginning with the most common types (subfalcine and descending transtentorial herniation). Posterior fossa herniations (ascending transtentorial and tonsillar herniations) are then considered. We conclude the discussion with a brief consideration of rare but important types of herniations, such as transdural/transcranial herniations and brain displacements that occur across the sphenoid wing.

Relevant Anatomy

Bony ridges and dural folds divide the intracranial cavity into three compartments: Two supratentorial hemicrania (the right and left halves) and the posterior fossa (3-1).

The dura mater consists of 2 layers, an outer (periosteal) and an inner (meningeal) layer. The periosteal layer is tightly applied to the inner surface of the calvaria, especially at suture lines. The meningeal layer folds inward to

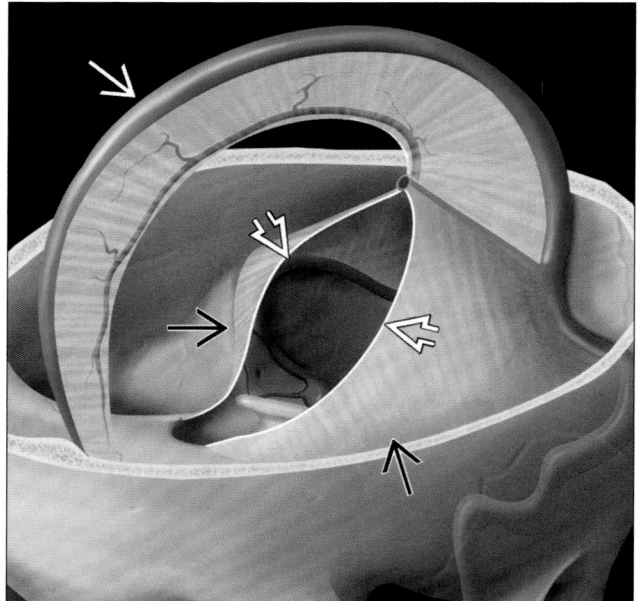

3-1. The falx cerebri ➡ divides the supratentorial compartment into 2 halves. The tentorium ⇨ separates the supra- from the infratentorial compartment. Medial borders of the tentorium form a U-shaped opening ➽, the tentorial incisura.

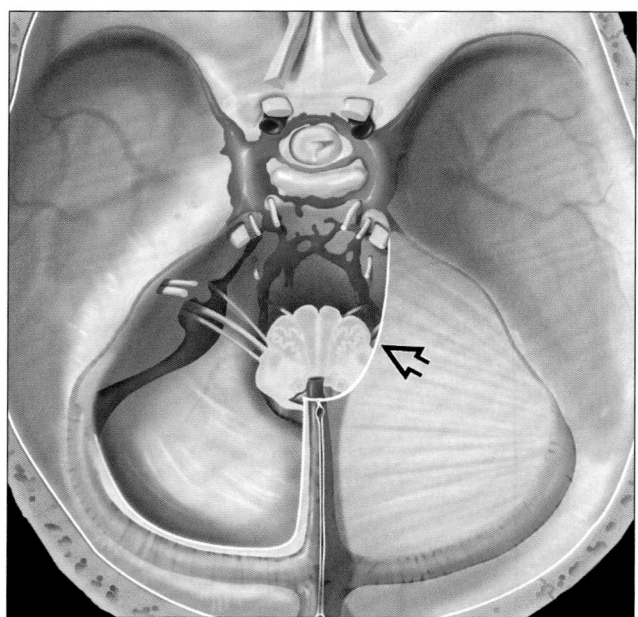

3-2. The right half of the tentorium has been removed to show the posterior fossa. The left half is shown forming the edge of the tentorial incisura ➽.

form 2 important fibrocollagenous sheets, the falx cerebri and tentorium cerebelli. The falx cerebri separates the right and left hemispheres from each other whereas the tentorium cerebelli separates the supratentorial from the infratentorial compartment.

The **falx cerebri** is a broad, sickle-shaped dural fold that attaches superiorly to the inside of the skull on either side of the midline, where it contains the superior sagittal sinus (SSS). The falx descends vertically within the interhemispheric fissure. It is shorter in front, where it is attached to the crista galli, and gradually deepens as it extends posteriorly.

The concave inferior "free" margin of the falx contains the inferior sagittal sinus. As it courses posteriorly, the inferior margin of the falx forms a large open space above the corpus callosum and cingulate gyrus. This open space allows potential displacement of brain and blood vessels from one side toward the other. The opening is largest in the front and becomes progressively smaller, ending where the falx joins the tentorium cerebelli at its apex.

The **tentorium cerebelli** is a tent-shaped dural sheet that extends inferolaterally from its confluence with the falx, where their two merging dural folds contain the straight sinus. The straight sinus courses posteroinferiorly toward the sinus confluence with the SSS and transverse sinuses.

The tentorium is attached laterally to the petrous ridges, anteroinferiorly to the dorsum sellae, and posteriorly to the occipital bone. It has two concave medial edges that contain a large U-shaped opening called the **tentorial incisura** (3-2). Displacement of brain structures

and accompanying blood vessels from the supratentorial compartment or posterior fossa can occur in either direction—up or down—through the tentorial incisura.

Relevant Physiology

Once the sutures fuse and the fontanelles close, brain, CSF, and blood all coexist in a rigid, unyielding "bone box." The cerebral blood volume (CBV), perfusion, and CSF volume exist in a delicate balance within this closed box. Under normal conditions, pressures within the brain parenchyma and intracranial CSF spaces are equal.

The **Monro-Kellie hypothesis** states: "The sum of volumes of brain, CSF, and intracranial blood is constant in an intact skull. An increase in one should cause a decrease in one or both of the remaining two." Accordingly, any increase in intracranial volume from whatever source (blood, edema, tumor, etc.) requires a compensatory and equal decrease in the other contents.

When extra volume (blood, edema, tumor, etc.) is added to a cranial compartment, CSF in the sulci and subarachnoid cisterns is initially squeezed out. The ipsilateral ventricle becomes compressed and decreases in size. As intracranial volume continues to increase, the mass effect eventually exceeds the brain's compensatory capacity, and intracranial pressure (ICP) begins to rise.

If a mass becomes sufficiently large, brain, CSF spaces, and blood vessels are displaced from one intracranial compartment into an adjacent one, resulting in one or more cerebral herniations.

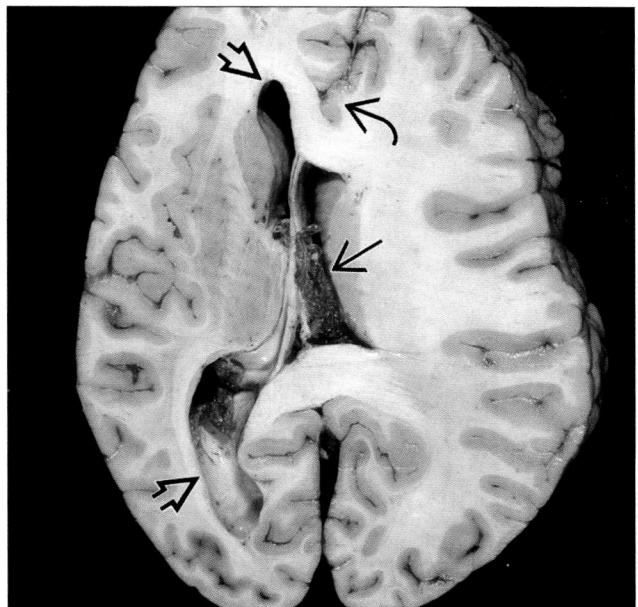

3-3. Autopsied brain shows subfalcine herniation. The left lateral ventricle is compressed ⊡ and shifted across the midline, as is the cingulate gyrus ⊡. The right lateral ventricle ⊡ is enlarged secondary to obstructed foramen of Monro.

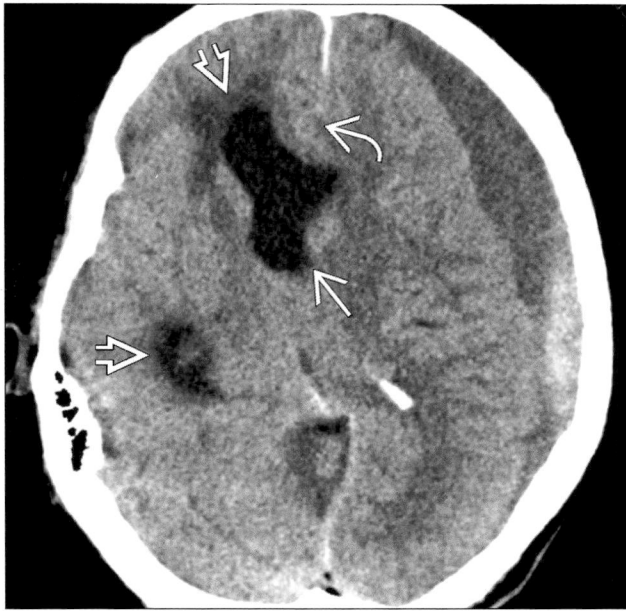

3-4. NECT shows subfalcine herniation of cingulate gyrus ⊡. The left lateral ventricle is compressed, shifted across the midline ⊡. The right ventricle is enlarged. Periventricular "halo" ⊡ is caused by accumulating extracellular fluid.

In turn, cerebral herniations may cause their own cascade of secondary effects. Parenchyma, cranial nerves, and/or blood vessels can become compressed against the adjacent unyielding bone and dura. Secondary ischemic changes, frank brain infarcts, cranial neuropathies, and focal neurologic deficits may develop.

If treatment is unavailable or unsuccessful, severe neurologic damage or even death is the result of what becomes, in essence, a brain "compartment syndrome."

Subfalcine Herniation

Terminology and Etiology

Subfalcine herniation (SFH) is the most common cerebral herniation and the easiest to understand. In a simple uncomplicated SFH, an enlarging supratentorial mass in one hemicranium causes the brain to begin shifting toward the opposite side. Herniation occurs as the affected hemisphere pushes across the midline under the inferior "free" margin of the falx, extending into the contralateral hemicranium **(3-3)**.

Imaging

Axial and coronal images show that the cingulate gyrus, anterior cerebral artery (ACA), and internal cerebral vein (ICV) are pushed from one side to the other under the falx cerebri. The ipsilateral ventricle appears compressed and displaced across the midline **(3-4)**.

Complications

Early complications of SFH include unilateral hydrocephalus, seen on axial NECT as enlargement of the contralateral ventricle. As the mass effect increases, the lateral ventricles become progressively more displaced across the midline. This displacement initially just deforms, then kinks, and eventually occludes the foramen of Monro.

The choroid plexus in the contralateral ventricle continues to secrete CSF. Because the foramen of Monro is obstructed, CSF has no egress, causing the lateral ventricle to enlarge. Severe unilateral obstructive hydrocephalus reduces drainage of extracellular fluid into the deep subependymal veins. Fluid accumulates in the periventricular white matter and is seen on NECT as periventricular hypodensity with "blurred" margins of the lateral ventricle.

If SFH becomes severe, the herniating ACA can become pinned against the inferior "free" margin of the falx cerebri and then occludes, causing secondary infarction of the cingulate gyrus.

3-5A. *Autopsied brain shows descending transtentorial herniation. The right uncus and hippocampus are displaced medially and demonstrate "grooving"* ⇨ *caused by impaction against the tentorial incisura. CN III is compressed* ⇨ *by the herniating temporal lobe.* **3-5B.** *Axial section in the same case shows uncal* ⇨*, hippocampal* ⇨ *herniation compressing midbrain against the opposite edge of the tentorium* ⇨ *("Kernohan notch"). (Courtesy R. Hewlett, MD.)*

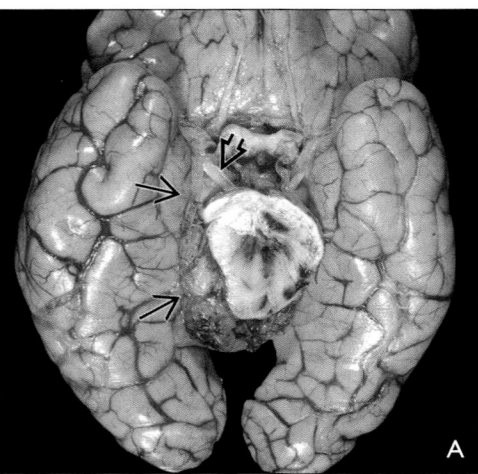

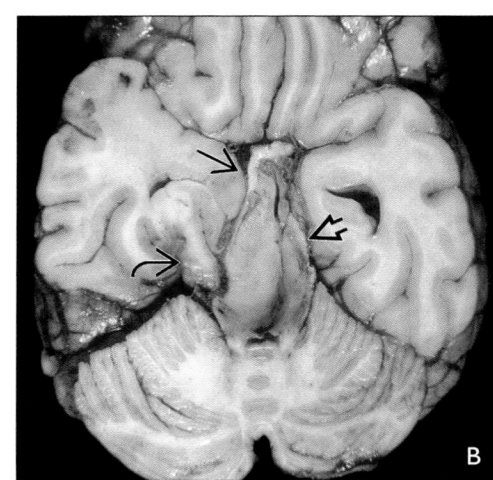

3-6. *NECT scan in acute trauma shows early herniation of the uncus* ⇨ *into the suprasellar cistern.* **3-7.** *NECT of mixed SDHs shows findings of more severe descending transtentorial herniation. The right temporal lobe is shifted medially* ⇨*, almost completely obliterating suprasellar cistern. The temporal horn* ⇨ *is displaced almost to midline. The MCA is elevated* ⇨ *over the sphenoid wing by the middle fossa fluid collection (ascending transalar herniation).*

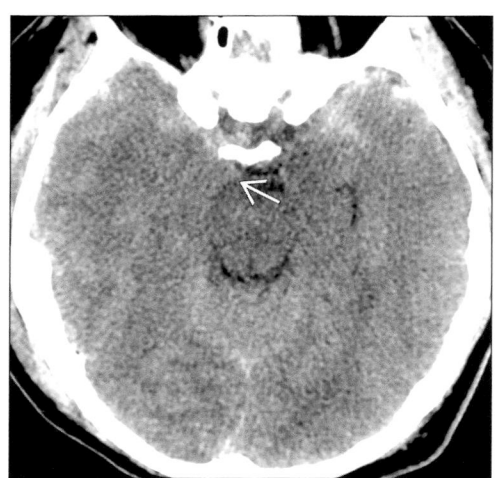

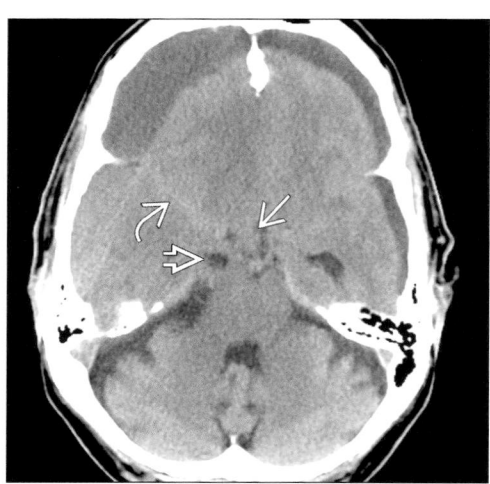

3-8. *Autopsy shows gross findings of complete bilateral ("central") descending transtentorial herniation. The suprasellar cistern is obliterated by the inferiorly displaced hypothalamus* ⇨*. The uncus* ⇨ *and hippocampus* ⇨ *of both temporal lobes are herniated medially and inferiorly into the tentorial incisura. (Courtesy R. Hewlett, MD.)* **3-9.** *NECT in a patient with severe trauma, diffuse brain swelling shows complete effacement of all basal cisterns.*

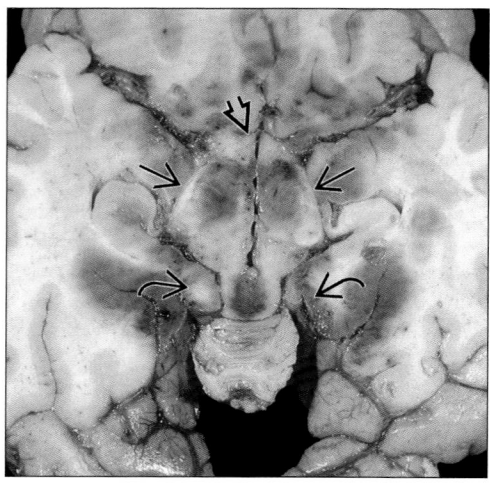

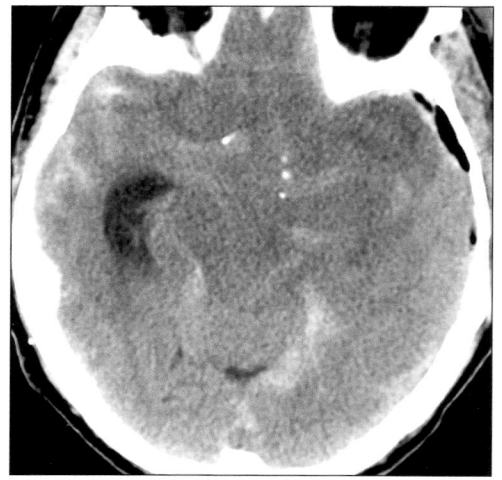

SUBFALCINE HERNIATION

Etiology and Pathology
- Unilateral hemispheric mass effect
- Brain shifts across midline under falx cerebri

Epidemiology
- Most common cerebral herniation

Imaging
- Cingulate gyrus, ACA, ICVs displaced across midline
- Foramen of Monro kinked, obstructed
- Ipsilateral ventricle small, contralateral enlarged

Complications
- Obstructive hydrocephalus
- Secondary ACA infarction (severe cases)

Descending Transtentorial Herniation

Transtentorial herniations are brain displacements that occur through the tentorial incisura. While these displacements can occur in both directions (from top down or bottom up), descending herniations from supratentorial masses are far more common than ascending herniations.

Terminology and Etiology

Descending transtentorial herniation (DTH) is the second most common type of intracranial herniation syndrome. DTH is caused by a hemispheric mass that initially produces side-to-side brain displacement (i.e., subfalcine herniation). As the mass effect increases, the uncus of the temporal lobe is pushed medially and begins to encroach on the suprasellar cistern. The hippocampus soon follows and starts to efface the ipsilateral quadrigeminal cistern.

With progressively increasing mass effect, both the uncus and hippocampus herniate inferiorly through the tentorial incisura (3-5).

Descending transtentorial herniation can be unilateral or bilateral. **Unilateral DTH** occurs when a hemispheric mass effect pushes the uncus and hippocampus of the ipsilateral temporal lobe over the edge of the tentorial incisura.

Bilateral DTH, sometimes called "complete" or "central" descending herniation, occurs when the supratentorial mass effect becomes so severe that *both* temporal lobes herniate into the tentorial incisura.

Imaging

Axial CT scans in early **unilateral DTH** show that the uncus is displaced medially and the ipsilateral aspect of the suprasellar cistern is effaced (3-6). As DTH increases, the hippocampus also herniates medially over the edge of the tentorium, compressing the quadrigeminal cistern and pushing the midbrain toward the opposite side of the incisura. In severe cases, entire suprasellar and

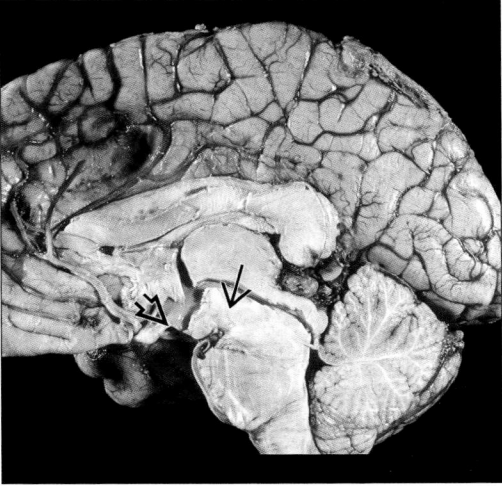

3-10. Complete DTH. Midbrain is kinked inferiorly ⇒, hypothalamus smashed down over dorsum sellae ⊵. (Courtesy R. Hewlett, MD.)

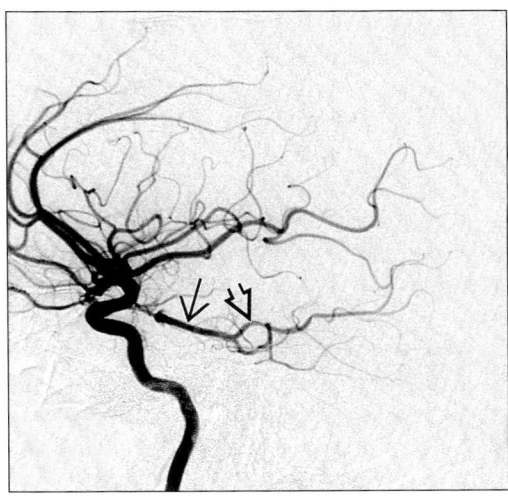

3-11. Vascular findings in DTH. Proximal PCA ⇒ is displaced inferiorly through incisura, "kinked" ⊵ as it passes over the edge of the tentorium.

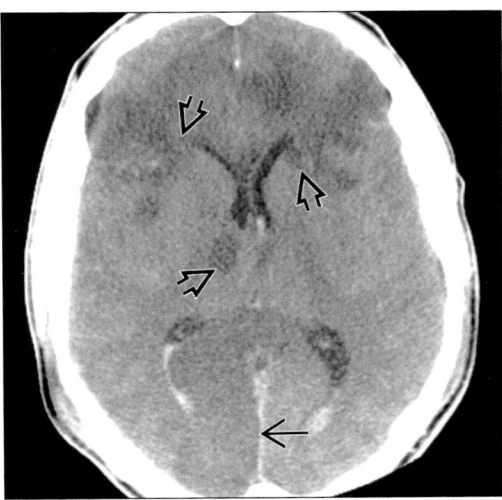

3-12. NECT in a surviving patient shows sequelae of severe bilateral DTH with right PCA ⇒, multiple penetrating artery infarcts ⊵.

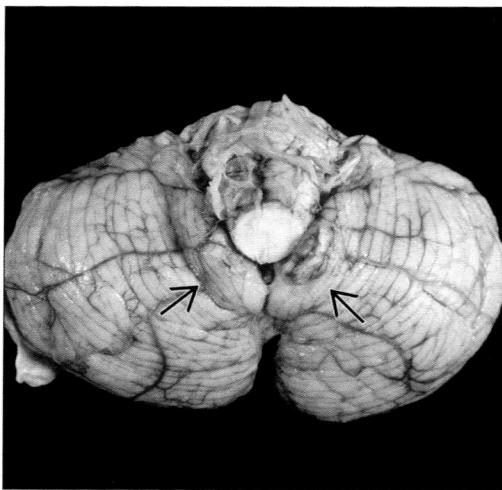

3-13. Tonsillar herniation. Tonsils are displaced inferiorly, "grooved" ⇨ *by bony margins of foramen magnum. (Courtesy R. Hewlett, MD.)*

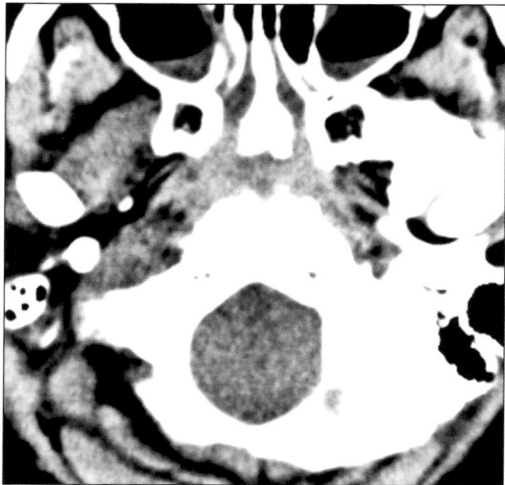

3-14. NECT in a patient with tonsillar herniation shows only effacement of CSF within the foramen magnum.

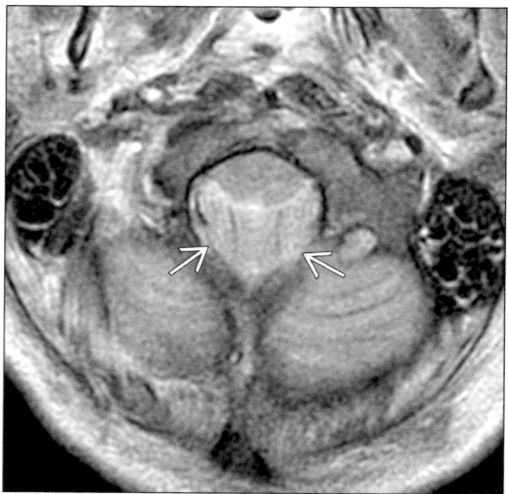

3-15. T2WI in the same patient shows tonsils ▶ *filling the foramen magnum, displacing the medulla anteriorly.*

quadrigeminal cisterns are effaced. The temporal horn can even be displaced almost into the midline **(3-7)**.

With **bilateral DTH**, both hemispheres become so swollen that the whole central brain is flattened against the skull base. All the basal cisterns are obliterated as the hypothalamus and optic chiasm are crushed against the sella turcica **(3-8)**, **(3-9)**.

In complete bilateral DTH, both temporal lobes herniate medially into the tentorial hiatus. The midbrain is compressed and squeezed medially from both sides. The midbrain is also displaced inferiorly through the tentorial incisura, pushing the pons downward. The angle between the midbrain and pons is progressively reduced from nearly 90° to almost 0° **(3-10)**.

Complications

Even mild DTH can compress the third cranial (oculomotor) nerve as it exits from the interpeduncular fossa and courses anterolaterally toward the cavernous sinus **(3-5A)**. This may produce a **pupil-involving third nerve palsy**.

Other, more severe complications may occur with DTH. As the temporal lobe is displaced inferomedially, it pushes the posterior cerebral artery (PCA) below the tentorial incisura. The PCA can become kinked and eventually even occluded as it passes back up over the medial edge of the tentorium **(3-11)**, causing a **secondary PCA (occipital) infarct**.

As the herniating temporal lobe pushes the midbrain toward the opposite side of the incisura, the contralateral cerebral peduncle is forced against the hard, knife-like edge of the tentorium, forming a **Kernohan notch (3-5B)**. Pressure ischemia leads to an ipsilateral (not contralateral) hemiplegia, the "false localizing" sign.

Severe uni- or bilateral DTH may cause pressure necrosis of the uncus and hippocampus. "Top-down" mass effect displaces the midbrain inferiorly and closes the midbrain-pontine angle. Perforating arteries that arise from the top of the basilar artery are compressed and buckled inferiorly, eventually occluding and causing a secondary hemorrhagic midbrain infarct known as a **Duret hemorrhage**.

With complete bilateral DTH, perforating arteries that arise from the circle of Willis are compressed against the central skull base and also occlude, causing **hypothalamic and basal ganglia infarcts (3-12)**.

In a vicious cycle, the hemispheres become more edematous, and intracranial pressure soars. If the rising intracranial pressure exceeds intraarterial pressure, perfusion is drastically reduced and eventually ceases, causing **brain death**.

DESCENDING TRANSTENTORIAL HERNIATION (DTH)

Terminology and Pathology
- Unilateral DTH
  - Temporal lobe (uncus, hippocampus) pushed over tentorial incisura
- Severe bilateral DTH = "complete" or "central" herniation
  - Hypothalamus, chiasm flattened against sella

Epidemiology
- Second most common cerebral herniation

Imaging
- Unilateral DTH
  - Suprasellar cistern encroached, then obliterated
  - Herniating temporal lobe pushes midbrain to opposite side
- Bilateral DTH
  - Basal cisterns completely effaced
  - Midbrain pushed down, compressed on both sides

Complications
- CN III compression → pupil-involving third nerve palsy
- Secondary occipital (PCA) ± hypothalamus, basal infarcts
- Compression of contralateral cerebral peduncle ("Kernohan notch")
- Midbrain ("Duret") hemorrhage

Tonsillar Herniation

Two types of herniations occur with posterior fossa masses: Tonsillar herniation and ascending transtentorial herniation (ATH). Tonsillar herniation is the more common of these two herniations (3-13).

Terminology and Etiology

In tonsillar herniation, the cerebellar tonsils are displaced inferiorly and become impacted into the foramen magnum. Tonsillar herniation can be congenital (e.g., Chiari 1 malformation) or acquired.

Acquired tonsillar herniation occurs in two different circumstances. The most common cause is an expanding posterior fossa mass *pushing* the tonsils downward into the foramen magnum.

Inferior tonsillar displacement also occurs with intracranial hypotension. Here the tonsils are *pulled* downward by abnormally low intraspinal CSF pressure (Chapter 34).

Imaging

Diagnosing tonsillar herniation on NECT scans may be problematic. The foramen magnum usually contains CSF that surrounds the medulla and cerebellar tonsils. Herniation of one or both tonsils into the foramen magnum obliterates most or all of the CSF in the cisterna magna (3-14).

Tonsillar herniation is much more easily diagnosed on MR. In the sagittal plane, the normally horizontal tonsillar folia become vertically oriented and the inferior aspect of

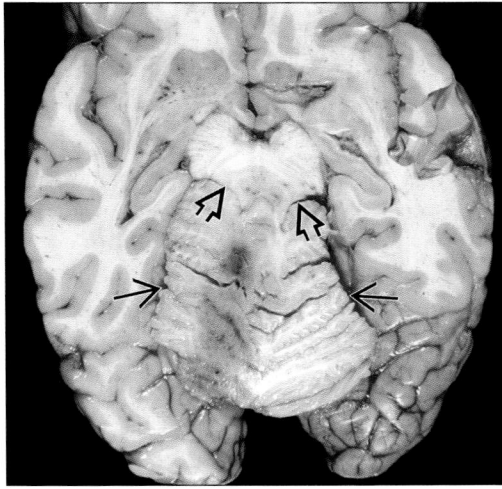
3-16. ATH with vermis, cerebellum ⟹ pushed upward through tentorial incisura, compressing midbrain/tectum ⟹. (Courtesy R. Hewlett, MD.)

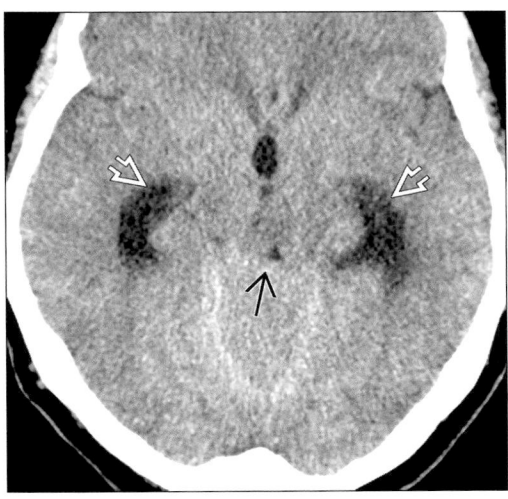
3-17. NECT shows moderate ATH with obliterated quadrigeminal cistern, compressed tectum ⟹. Note severe obstructive hydrocephalus ⟹.

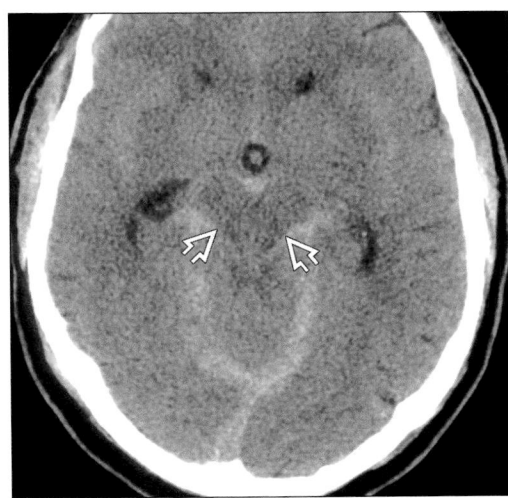
3-18. Severe ATH with midbrain deformity ⟹ caused by upward herniation of the cerebellum through the tentorial incisura.

the tonsils becomes pointed. Tonsils more than five millimeters below the foramen magnum are generally abnormal, especially if they are peg-like or pointed (rather than rounded).

In the axial plane, T2 scans show that the tonsils are impacted into the foramen magnum, obliterating CSF in the cisterna magna and displacing the medulla anteriorly **(3-15)**.

Complications

Complications of tonsillar herniation include obstructive hydrocephalus and tonsillar necrosis.

Ascending Transtentorial Herniation

Terminology and Etiology

In ascending transtentorial herniation (ATH), the cerebellar vermis and hemispheres are pushed upward ("ascend") through the tentorial incisura into the supratentorial compartment. The superiorly herniating cerebellum first flattens and displaces, then effaces the

quadrigeminal cistern and compresses the midbrain **(3-16)**.

Ascending transtentorial herniation is much less common than descending herniation. ATH can be caused by any expanding posterior fossa mass although neoplasms are a more common cause than trauma.

Imaging

Axial NECT scans show that CSF in the superior vermian cistern and cerebellar sulci is effaced **(3-17)**. The quadrigeminal cistern is first compressed and then obliterated by the upwardly herniating cerebellum. As the herniation progresses, the tectal plate becomes compressed and flattened. In severe cases, the dorsal midbrain may actually appear concave instead of convex **(3-18)**.

Eventually, the entire tentorial incisura becomes completely filled with soft tissue, and all normal anatomic landmarks disappear.

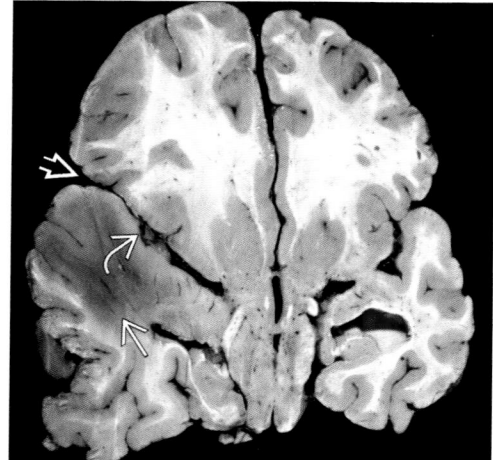
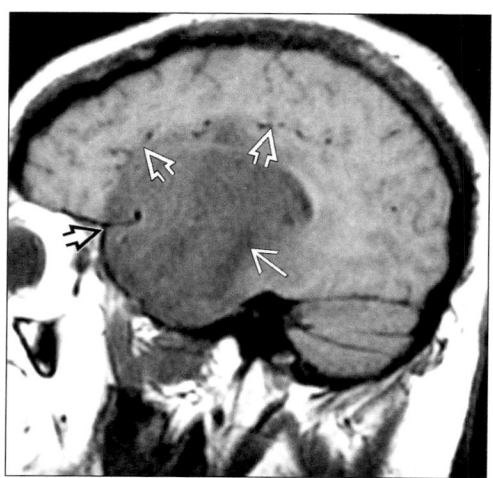

3-19. Autopsy demonstrates findings in ascending transalar herniation. A temporal lobe mass ➡ pushes the sylvian fissure and middle cerebral artery (MCA) ➡ up and over the site of greater sphenoid wing ➡. Compare to the normal left side. 3-20. Sagittal T1WI shows a large hypointense holotemporal lobe mass ➡ elevating the sylvian fissure and MCA ➡, pushing the temporal lobe up and over the greater sphenoid wing ➡.

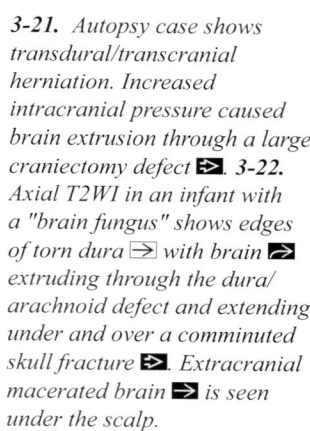
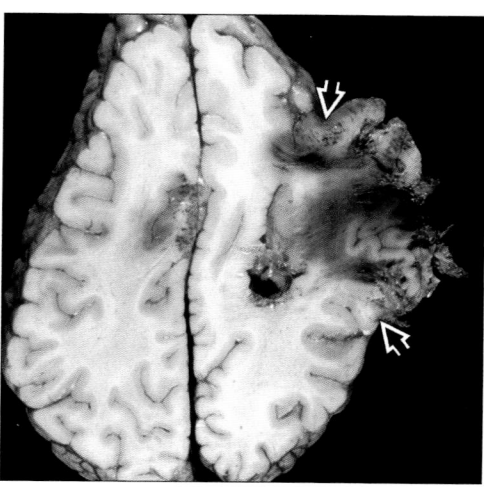
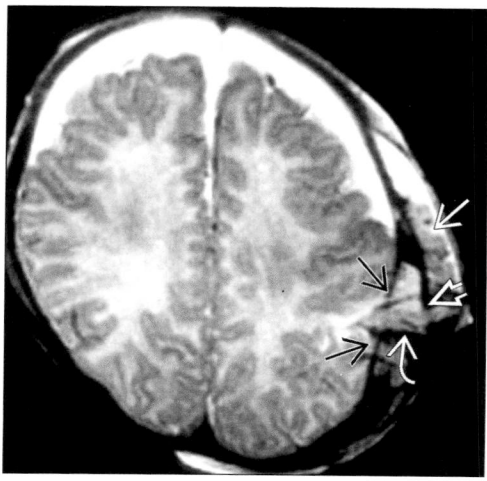

3-21. Autopsy case shows transdural/transcranial herniation. Increased intracranial pressure caused brain extrusion through a large craniectomy defect ➡. 3-22. Axial T2WI in an infant with a "brain fungus" shows edges of torn dura ➡ with brain ➡ extruding through the dura/ arachnoid defect and extending under and over a comminuted skull fracture ➡. Extracranial macerated brain ➡ is seen under the scalp.

Complications

The most common complication of ATH is acute intraventricular obstructive hydrocephalus caused by compression of the cerebral aqueduct.

POSTERIOR FOSSA HERNIATIONS

Ascending Transtentorial Herniation
- Relatively rare
  - Caused by expanding posterior fossa mass
  - Neoplasm > trauma
  - Cerebellum pushed upward through incisura
  - Compresses, deforms midbrain
- Imaging findings
  - Incisura filled with tissue, CSF spaces obliterated
  - Quadrigeminal cistern, tectal plate compressed/flattened
- Complications
  - Hydrocephalus (aqueduct obstruction)

Tonsillar Herniation
- Most common posterior fossa herniation
  - Can be congenital (Chiari 1) or acquired
  - 1 or both tonsils > 5 mm below foramen magnum
- Imaging findings
  - Foramen magnum appears tissue-filled on axial NECT, T2WI
  - Inferior "pointing" or peg-like configuration of tonsils on sagittal MR
- Complications
  - Obstructive hydrocephalus
  - Tonsillar necrosis

Other Herniations

The vast majority of cerebral herniations are subfalcine, descending/ascending transtentorial, and tonsillar herniations. Other less common herniation syndromes are transalar and transdural/transcranial herniations.

Transalar Herniation

Transalar herniation occurs when brain herniates across the greater sphenoid wing (GSW) or "ala." Transalar herniations can be either ascending (the most common) or descending.

Ascending transalar herniation is caused by a large *middle cranial fossa mass*. An intratemporal or large extraaxial mass displaces part of the temporal lobe together with the sylvian fissure and middle cerebral artery (MCA) up and over the greater sphenoid wing **(3-19)**.

Ascending transalar herniation is best depicted on off-midline sagittal MRs. The GSW is seen as the bony junction between the anterior and middle cranial fossae. The MCA branches and sylvian fissure are elevated, and the superior temporal gyrus is pushed above the GSW **(3-20)**.

Descending transalar herniation is caused by a large *anterior cranial fossa mass*. Here the gyrus rectus is forced posteroinferiorly over the GSW, displacing the sylvian fissure and shifting the MCA backward.

Transdural/Transcranial Herniation

This rare type of cerebral herniation, sometimes called a "brain fungus" by neurosurgeons, can be life-threatening. For transdural/transcranial herniation to occur, the dura must be lacerated, a skull defect (fracture or craniotomy) must be present, and intracranial pressure (ICP) must be elevated.

Traumatic transdural/transcranial herniations typically occur in infants or young children with a comminuted skull fracture that deforms inward with impact, lacerating the dura-arachnoid. When ICP increases, brain can herniate through the torn dura and across the skull fracture into the subgaleal space.

Iatrogenic transdural/transcranial herniations occur when a burr hole, craniotomy, or craniectomy is performed in a patient with severely elevated intracranial pressure. When the dura is opened, brain under pressure extrudes through the defect **(3-21)**.

MR best depicts these unusual herniations. The disrupted dura is seen as a discontinuous black line on T2WI. Brain tissue, together with accompanying blood vessels and variable amounts of CSF, is literally extruded through the dural and calvarial defects into the subgaleal space **(3-22)**.

OTHER HERNIATIONS

Ascending Transalar Herniation
- Most common transalar herniation
- Caused by middle fossa mass
- Sylvian fissure, MCA displaced up/over greater sphenoid ala
- Best appreciated on off-midline sagittal T1WI

Descending Transalar Herniation
- Anterior fossa mass
- Frontal lobe (gyrus rectus) pushed back, down over greater sphenoid ala
- MCA, sylvian fissure displaced backward

Transcranial/Transdural Herniation
- ↑ ICP + skull defect + dura-arachnoid tear
- Caused by
  - Comminuted, often depressed skull fracture
  - Craniectomy
- Brain extruded through skull, under scalp aponeurosis
- Best appreciated on axial T2WI

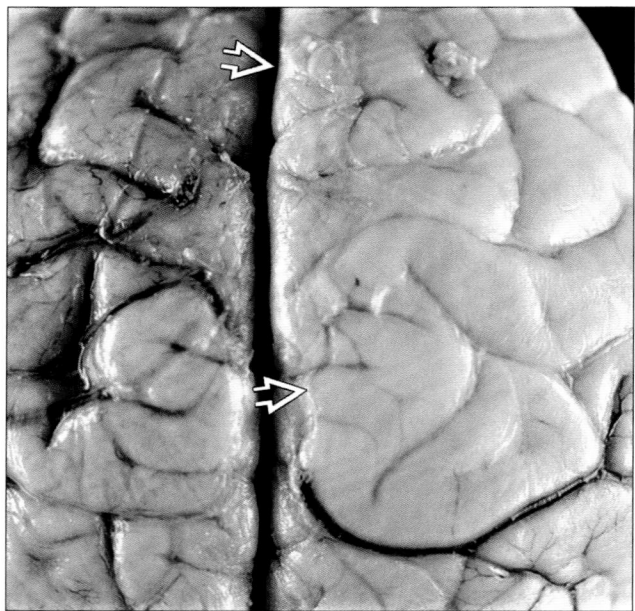

3-23. Autopsy specimen shows unilateral hemispheric swelling ⬿ that expands the gyri, compresses and obliterates the sulci.

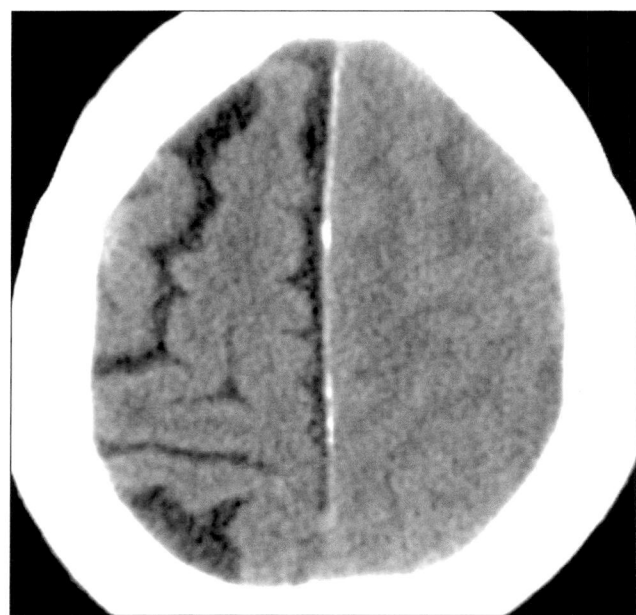

3-24. Axial NECT scan shows normal right sulci and obliterated ("disappearing") convexity sulci over the swollen left hemisphere.

Edema, Ischemia, and Vascular Injury

Traumatic brain injury (TBI) can unleash a cascade of physiologic responses that may adversely affect the brain more than the initial trauma. These responses include diffuse brain swelling, excitotoxic responses elicited by glutamatergic pathway activation, perfusion alterations, and a variety of ischemic events including territorial infarcts.

Post-Traumatic Brain Swelling

Massive brain swelling with severe intracranial hypertension is among the most serious of all secondary traumatic lesions. Mortality approaches 50%, so early recognition and aggressive treatment of this complication is imperative.

Etiology and Epidemiology

Focal, regional, or diffuse brain swelling develops in 10-20% of patients with traumatic brain injury (TBI) (3-23). Whether this is caused by increased tissue fluid (cerebral edema) or elevated blood volume (cerebral hyperemia) secondary to vascular dysautoregulation is unclear. While both are likely involved in post-traumatic brain swelling, the accumulation of intracellular fluid (cytotoxic edema) appears to be the major contributor.

Clinical Issues

Children and young adults are especially prone to developing post-traumatic brain swelling and are almost twice as likely as older adults to develop this complication. While gross enlargement of one or both hemispheres may occur relatively quickly after the initial event, delayed onset is typical. Severe cerebral edema generally takes between 24 and 48 hours to develop.

Imaging

The appearance of post-traumatic brain swelling evolves over time. Initially, mild hemispheric mass effect with sulcal/cisternal compression is seen on NECT scans (3-24).

During the early stages of brain swelling, gray-white matter differentiation appears relatively preserved (3-25), (3-26). While the ipsilateral ventricle may be slightly compressed, subfalcine displacement is generally minimal. However, if the mass effect is disproportionately large compared to the size of an extraaxial collection such as a subdural hematoma, early swelling of the underlying brain parenchyma should be suspected.

MR shows swollen gyri that are hypointense on T1WI and hyperintense on T2WI. Diffusion-weighted scans show restricted diffusion with low ADC values.

As brain swelling progresses, the demarcation between the cortex and underlying white matter becomes indistinct and eventually disappears. The lateral ventricles

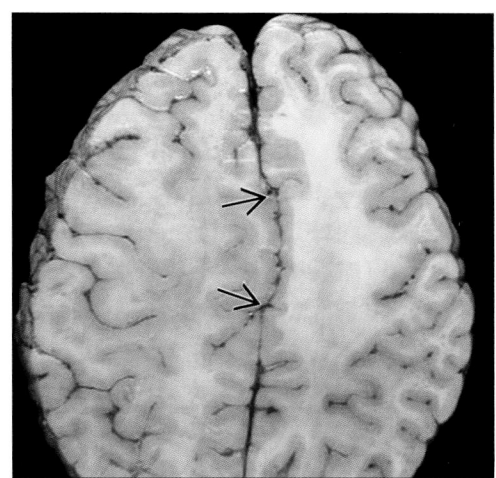

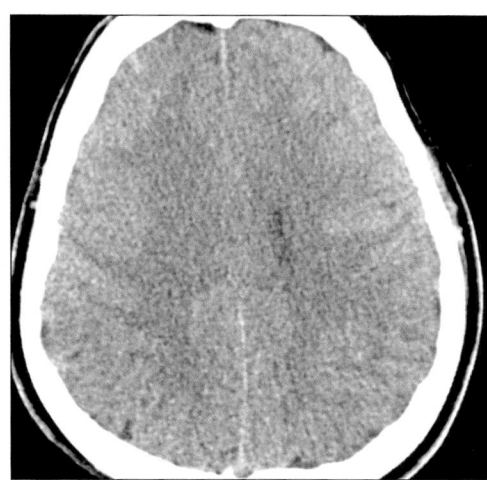

3-25. *Autopsy specimen shows mild to moderate right hemisphere edema, subfalcine herniation of the cingulate gyrus* ➡️. **3-26.** *NECT scan following closed head injury shows mild diffuse cerebral edema. The sulci are mostly effaced, but the gray-white matter interface is preserved.*

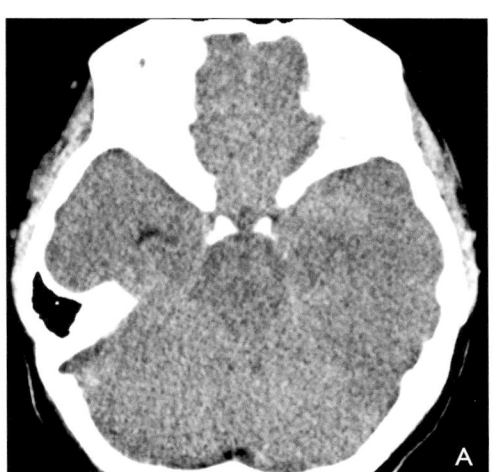

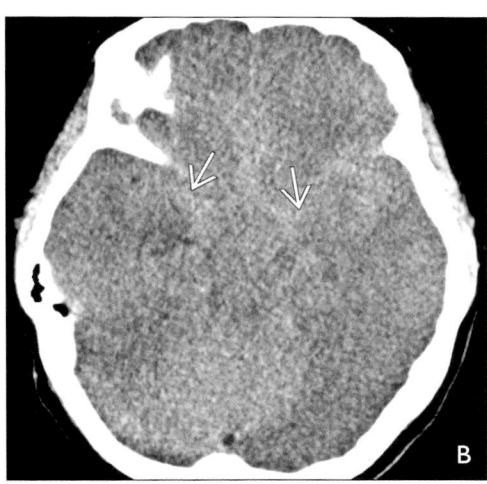

3-27A. *Series of NECT scans demonstrates severe post-traumatic cerebral edema. The middle and anterior cranial fossa sulci are obliterated, and the brain appears moderately hypodense.* **3-27B.** *More cephalad scan in the same patient shows complete obliteration of the suprasellar and basilar cisterns. In comparison to the hypodense swollen brain, circulating blood in the MCAs looks relatively hyperdense* ➡️.

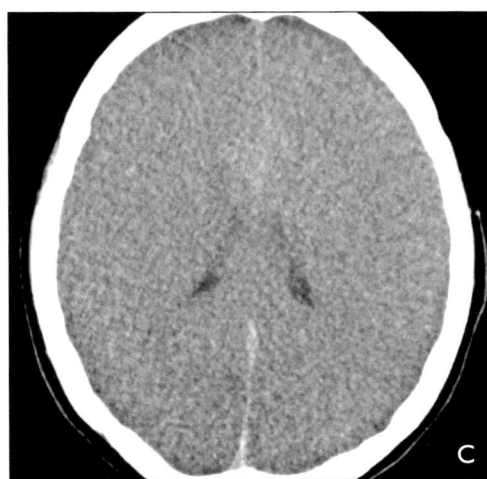

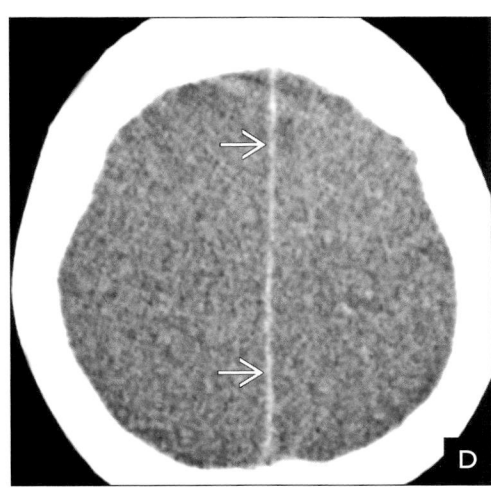

3-27C. *Scan through the mid-ventricular level in the same patient shows that the ventricles are small and that all gray-white interfaces have disappeared.* **3-27D.** *Scan through the vertex demonstrates no surface sulci. Both hemispheres are diffusely edematous, making the falx cerebri* ➡️ *appear abnormally dense.*

appear smaller than normal, and the superficial sulci are no longer visible (3-27).

Post-Traumatic Cerebral Ischemia and Infarction

Traumatic ischemia and infarction are uncommon but important complications of TBI. They have a variety of causes, including direct vascular compression, systemic hypoperfusion, vascular injury, vasospasm, and venous congestion. The most common cause of post-traumatic cerebral ischemia is mechanical vascular compression secondary to a brain herniation syndrome.

Post-Traumatic Infarcts

The most common brain herniation that causes secondary cerebral infarction is descending transtentorial herniation (DTH). Severe unilateral DTH displaces the temporal lobe and accompanying posterior cerebral artery (PCA) inferiorly into the tentorial incisura. As the herniating PCA passes posterior to the midbrain, it courses superiorly and is forced against the hard, knife-like edge of the

tentorial incisura. The P3 PCA segment occludes, resulting in occipital lobe infarction (3-28), (3-29).

Less commonly, subfalcine herniation presses the callosomarginal branch of the anterior cerebral artery against the undersurface of the falx cerebri and causes cingulate gyrus infarction. (3-30), (3-31).

With complete bilateral ("central") DTH, penetrating arteries that arise from the circle of Willis are crushed against the skull base, resulting in multiple scattered basal ganglia and hypothalamus infarcts. Pressure necrosis of the uncus and hippocampus can also occur as the herniated temporal lobes impact the free edge of the tentorial incisura.

Traumatic Cerebral Ischemia

Focal, regional, and generalized perfusion alterations also occur with TBI. Extraaxial hematomas that exert significant focal mass effect on the underlying brain may cause reduced arterial perfusion and cortical ischemia. They may also compress the underlying cortical veins, causing venous ischemia (3-32).

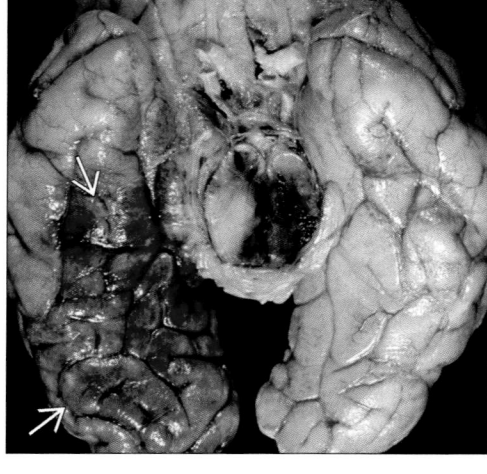 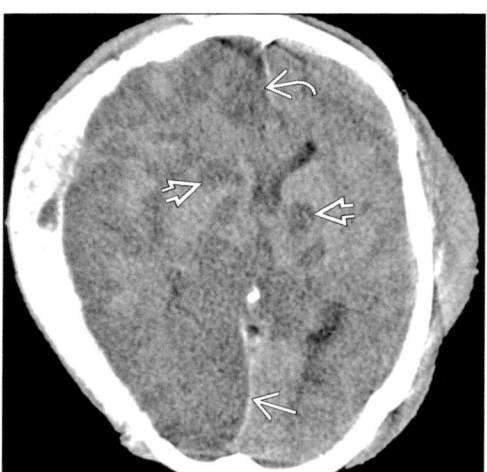

3-28. Descending transtentorial herniation can occlude the posterior cerebral artery against the tentorial incisura, causing a secondary PCA territorial infarction ➡. 3-29. A severely traumatized patient with diffuse brain swelling and right subfalcine plus descending transtentorial herniation. NECT obtained 5 days after the initial insult shows PCA ➡, ACA ➘, and multiple perforating artery ➯ infarcts.

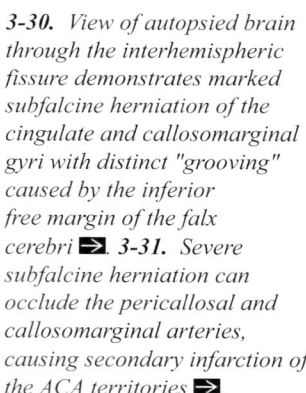 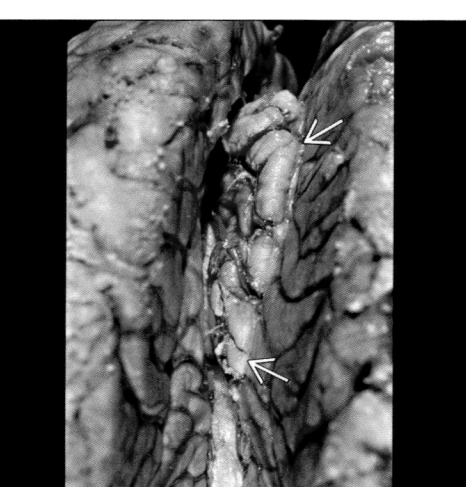 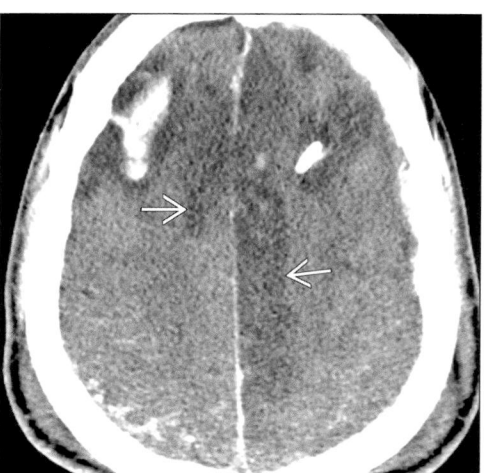

3-30. View of autopsied brain through the interhemispheric fissure demonstrates marked subfalcine herniation of the cingulate and callosomarginal gyri with distinct "grooving" caused by the inferior free margin of the falx cerebri ➡. 3-31. Severe subfalcine herniation can occlude the pericallosal and callosomarginal arteries, causing secondary infarction of the ACA territories ➡.

Global or generalized **cerebral ischemia** may result from hypoperfusion, hypoxia, membrane depolarization, or loss of cellular membrane integrity and ion homeostasis. Cellular energy failure may induce glutamate-mediated **acute excitotoxic brain injury.**

NECT scans show hypodensity with loss of gray-white differentiation in the affected parenchyma. CT perfusion may show decreased CBF with prolonged time to drain. In cases of excitotoxic brain injury, MR shows swollen, hyperintense gyri on T2/FLAIR that do not correspond to defined vascular territories (3-33).

Post-Traumatic Vasospasm

Post-traumatic vasospasm (PTV) is a potentially significant yet underrecognized cause of ischemic damage following traumatic brain injury. Transcranial Doppler studies detect vasospasm in more than one-third of patients with TBI.

Moderate to severe PTV develops in 10% of patients and is an independent predictor of poor outcome. PTV is especially common in younger, more severely injured patients. Patients with parenchymal contusions and fever are also at increased risk of developing PTV.

CEREBRAL EDEMA AND VASCULAR COMPLICATIONS

Post-Traumatic Brain Swelling
- Found in 10-20% of TBI
- Focal, regional, or diffuse
- Most common in children, young adults
- Early: Sulcal effacement
- Later: Indistinct gray-white interfaces
- End-stage: Brain uniformly low density

Cerebral Infarction
- Secondary PCA infarct most common
- ACA next most common
- Perforating artery infarcts with complete DTH

Cerebral Ischemia
- Common under subdural hematomas

Vasospasm
- Moderate/severe develops in 10%
- Independent predictor of poor outcome

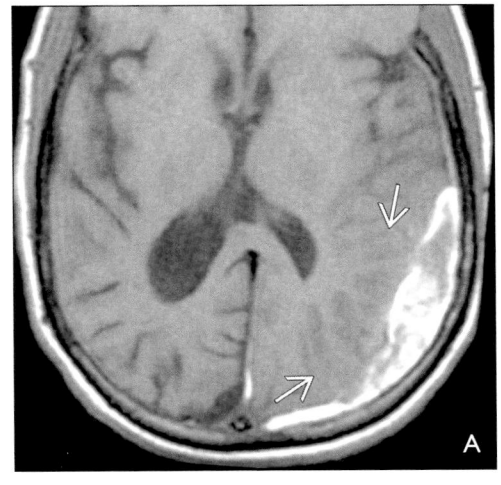 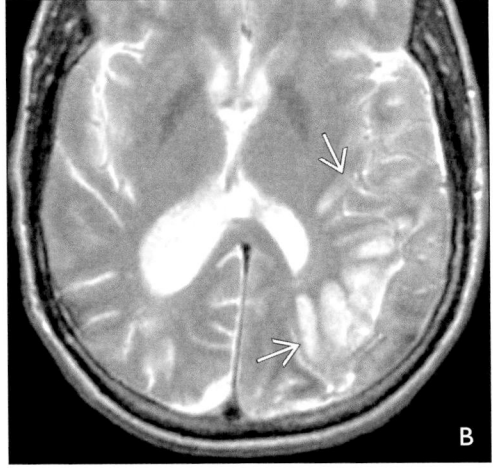

3-32A. T1WI in a patient with an early subacute subdural hematoma shows sulcal effacement, gyral swelling in the underlying parietooccipital cortex ➔. 3-32B. T2WI in the same patient shows cortical edema ➔ under the SDH. Regional perfusion alterations are common under subdural hematomas.

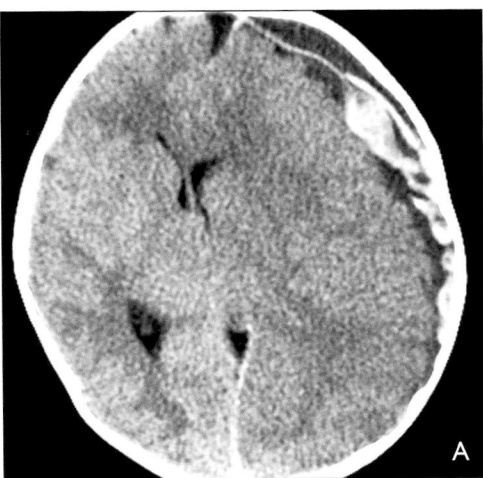 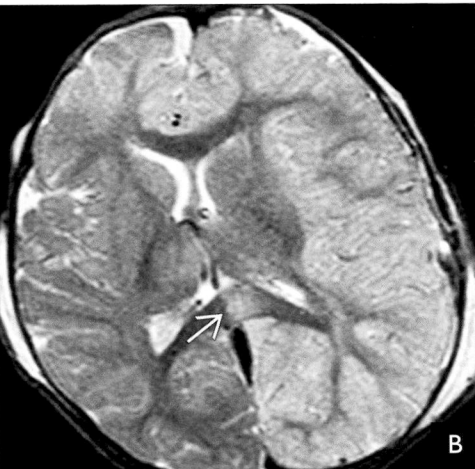

3-33A. NECT scan shows mixed-density SDHs in an infant with inflicted (nonaccidental) trauma. Note the left hemisphere hypodensity ("big black brain"). The mass effect and subfalcine herniation are much larger than would be expected from the SDHs themselves. 3-33B. T2WI shows marked hemispheric edema, sparing only the basal ganglia. Hyperintensity in the corpus callosum ➔, right frontal lobe may represent excitotoxic injury.

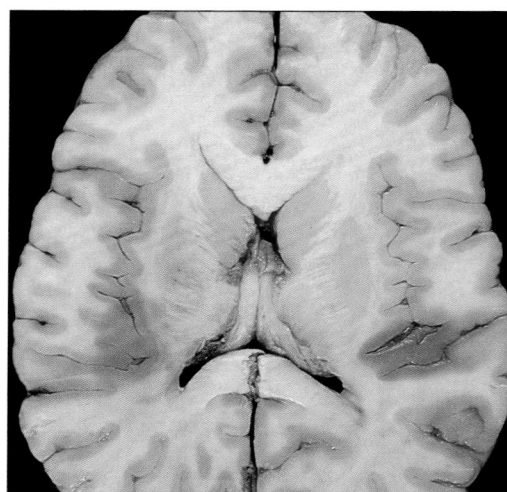

3-34. Brain death shows diffuse swelling, poor GM-WM discrimination, small ventricles, effaced surface sulci. (Courtesy R. Hewlett, MD.)

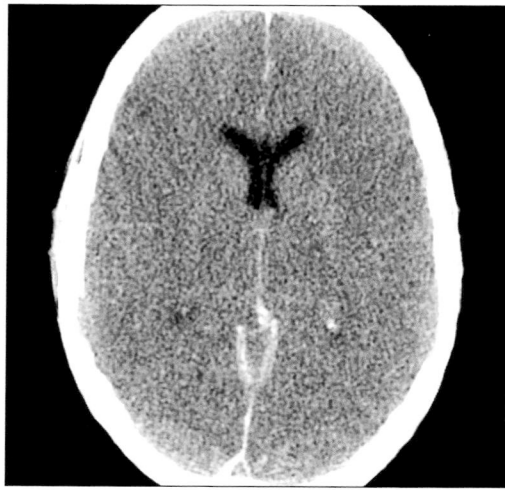

3-35. Axial NECT scan in a child with clinical evidence of brain death shows diffuse cerebral edema, no GM-WM differentiation.

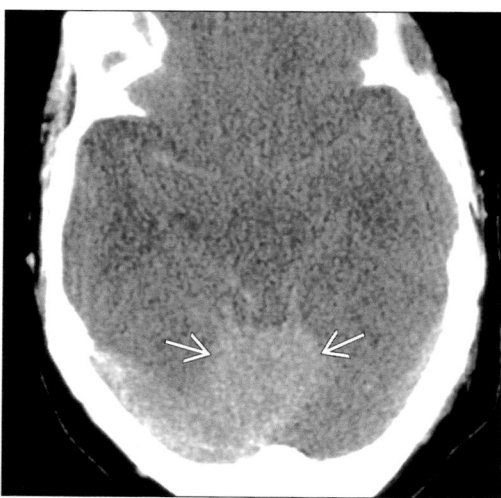

3-36. NECT shows "white cerebellum" ➡, hypodense featureless cerebral hemispheres ("big black brain"), total obliteration of CSF spaces.

Brain Death

Terminology

Brain death (BD) is defined pathophysiologically as complete, irreversible cessation of brain function (3-34). Some investigators distinguish between "whole brain death" (all intracranial structures above the foramen magnum), "cerebral death" (all supratentorial structures), and "higher brain death" (cortical structures).

The legal definition of brain death varies from country to country (e.g., the USA and the United Kingdom) and from state to state. Since adoption of the Uniform Determination of Death Act, all court rulings in the United States have upheld the medical practice of death determination using neurologic criteria according to state law.

Clinical Issues

Brain death is primarily a clinical diagnosis. Three clinical findings are necessary to confirm irreversible cessation of all functions of the entire brain, *including the brainstem*: (1) coma (with a known cause), (2) absence of brainstem reflexes, and (3) apnea.

Complex spontaneous motor movements and false-positive ventilator triggering may occur in patients who are brain dead, so expert assessment is crucial. Once reversible causes of coma (e.g., drug overdose, status epilepticus) are excluded, the clinical diagnosis of BD is highly reliable *if* the determination is made by experienced examiners using established, accepted criteria.

There are no published reports of recovery of neurologic function in adults after a diagnosis of BD using the updated 1995 American Academy of Neurology practice parameters.

Imaging

Imaging studies may be helpful in confirming BD but neither replace nor substitute for clinical diagnosis.

CT FINDINGS. NECT scans in BD show diffuse, severe cerebral edema (3-35). The superficial sulci, sylvian fissures, and basilar cisterns of both hemispheres are completely effaced. The normal attenuation relationship between gray and white matter is inverted, with gray matter becoming iso- or even hypodense relative to the adjacent white matter (the **"reversal" sign**).

In striking contrast to the hypodense hemispheres, density of the cerebellum appears relatively normal (the **"white cerebellum" sign**) (3-36). Density of the deep gray nuclei and brainstem may be initially maintained; however, all supratentorial structures eventually assume a featureless, uniform hypodensity.

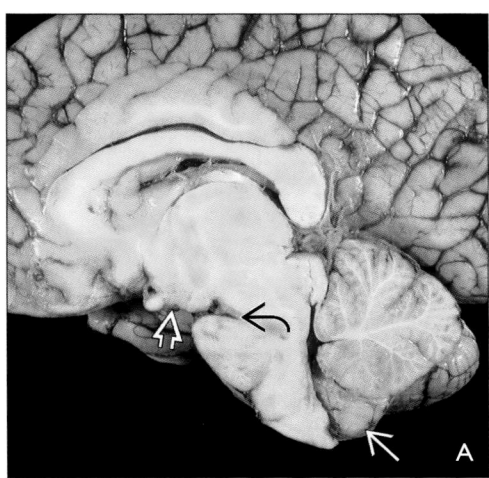

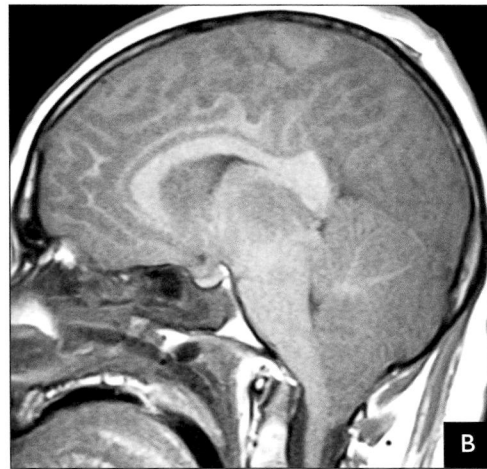

3-37A. Sagittal autopsy from a patient with brain death shows diffuse brain swelling, bilateral ⬌ severe descending transtentorial herniation with inferiorly displaced midbrain ⬌, and tonsillar herniation ⬌. *3-37B.* Sagittal T1WI was performed a few minutes before life support for this patient was discontinued. Note the findings of diffuse brain swelling and herniation similar to the autopsy case shown on the left.

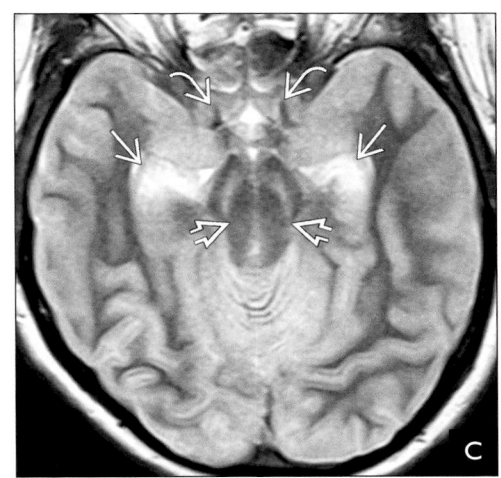

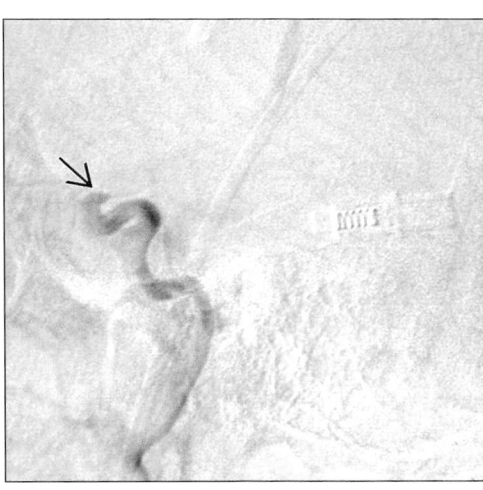

3-37C. T2WI in the same patient shows diffuse gyral swelling, hippocampal hyperintensity ⬌, bilateral DTH "squeezing" the midbrain medially and inferiorly ⬌. "Flow voids" in both intracranial internal carotid arteries are miniscule ⬌. *3-38.* Late phase DSA with selective injection of the internal carotid artery shows no evidence of circulation in the intracranial internal carotid artery ⬌. This constitutes angiographic evidence of brain death.

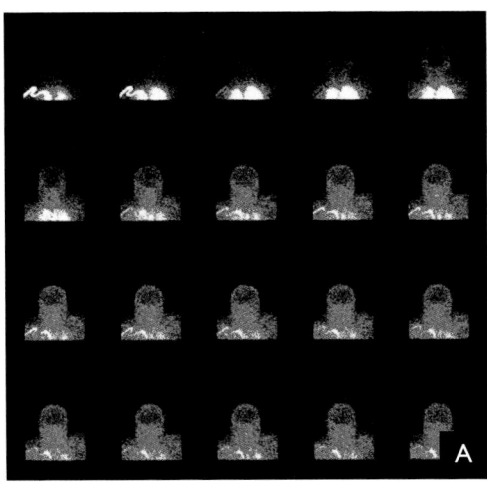

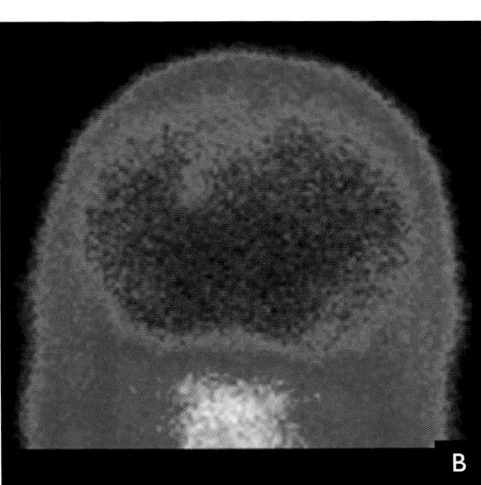

3-39A. Dynamic flow images from Tc-99m HMPAO-SPECT scan in a patient with clinical brain death show no brain activity. *3-39B.* Static image in the same patient shows no brain activity ("light bulb" sign) with increased uptake in the nose ("hot nose" sign).

MR FINDINGS. Sagittal T1WI shows complete descending central brain herniation with the optic chiasm and hypothalamus compressed against the skull base and the midbrain "buckled" inferiorly through the tentorial incisura **(3-37A), (3-37B)**. The hemispheres appear swollen and hypointense, with indistinct gray-white matter differentiation.

T2 scans show swollen gyri with hyperintense cortex **(3-37C)**. DWI in patients with brain death typically shows restricted diffusion with decreased ADC in both the cerebral cortex and white matter.

ANGIOGRAPHY. Ancillary tests are sometimes necessary to make a diagnosis of BD if the clinical examination cannot be completed or confounding factors are present. Lack of cerebral circulation is an important confirmatory test in such cases. When intracranial pressure exceeds intraarterial perfusion pressure, brain blood flow ceases.

Conventional digital subtraction angiography (DSA) shows severe, prolonged contrast stasis with filling of the external carotid artery. Although most BD patients show no intracranial flow **(3-38)**, almost 30% have some proximal opacification of intracranial arteries. The deep venous drainage remains unopacified throughout the examination.

CTA is emerging as an acceptable noninvasive alternative to DSA in many jurisdictions. Demonstrating lack of opacification in the MCA cortical segments and internal veins in CTA is an efficient and reliable method for confirming BD.

ULTRASOUND. Transcranial Doppler may show oscillating "to-and-fro" signal. Orbital Doppler shows absence or reversal of end-diastolic flow in the central retinal arteries together with markedly increased arterial resistive indices.

NUCLEAR MEDICINE. Tc-99m scintigraphy shows scalp uptake but absent brain activity (the "light bulb" sign). Together with increased extracranial activity (the "hot nose" sign), these findings are both highly sensitive and specific for BD **(3-39)**.

Differential Diagnosis

Potentially reversible causes of BD such as deep coma due to **drug overdose** or **status epilepticus** must be excluded clinically.

Technical difficulties with imaging studies that may mimic BD include a "missed bolus" on either CTA or nuclear medicine flow studies. Vascular lesions such as arterial dissection and vasospasm may also delay or even prevent opacification of intracranial vessels.

Massive cerebral infarction (especially "malignant MCA infarction") with severe edema can mimic BD but is typically territorial and does not involve the entire brain.

Brain death can also mimic other disorders. **End-stage brain swelling** from severe trauma or profound hypoxic encephalopathy (e.g., following cardiopulmonary arrest) makes the cranial arteries, dura, and dural venous sinuses all seem relatively hyperdense compared to the diffusely edematous low-density brain.

With very low-density brain, comparatively high-density areas are seen along the basal cisterns, sylvian fissures, tentorium cerebelli, and sometimes even within the cortical sulci. This appearance is sometimes termed **pseudo-subarachnoid hemorrhage** (pseudo-SAH). Pseudo-SAH should not be mistaken for "real" subarachnoid hemorrhage. The density of pseudo-SAH is significantly lower (between 30-40 HU) than the attenuation of "real" SAH (between 50-60 HU).

Chronic Effects of CNS Trauma

Patients surviving traumatic brain injury (TBI) may have long-term sequelae, from mild cognitive disorders and neuropsychiatric effects to devastating neurologic deficits. While a comprehensive discussion of all possible post-TBI effects is beyond the scope of this text, we will consider some of the more important sequelae of brain trauma in this section.

Post-Traumatic Encephalomalacia

Pathology

The pathologic residue of TBI varies from microscopic changes (e.g., axonal retraction balls and microglial clusters) to more extensive confluent areas of gross parenchymal loss and encephalomalacia. Focal areas of encephalomalacia are most commonly found in areas with a high incidence of cortical contusions, i.e., the anteroinferior frontal lobes and anterior temporal lobes **(3-40)**.

Imaging

Encephalomalacic changes generally appear as low-density foci on NECT. Hypointense areas on T1-weighted MR that appear hyperintense on T2WI and FLAIR are typical. T2* GRE scans may show hemorrhagic residua around the encephalomalacic foci. In patients with significant traumatic subarachnoid hemor-

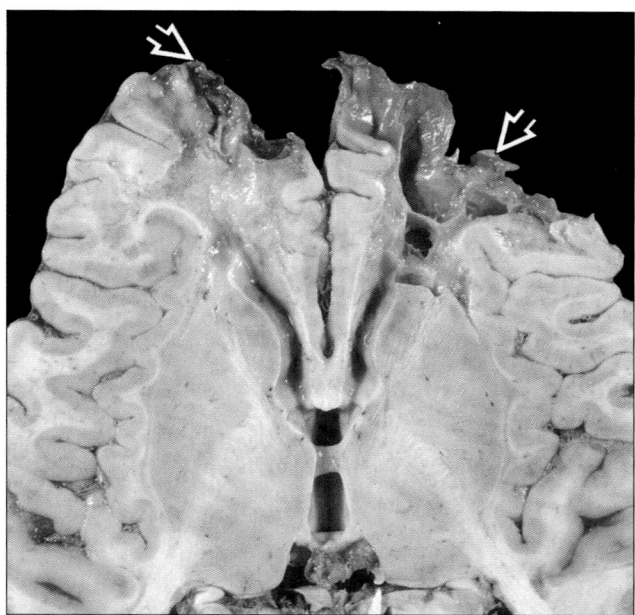

3-40. Autopsy specimen shows effects of remote trauma with bifrontal encephalomalacia ⮊.

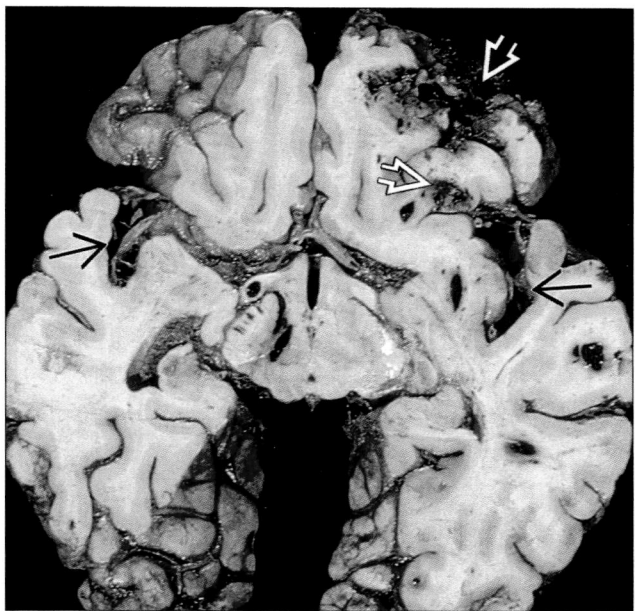

3-41. Autopsy specimen from a patient with remote trauma shows contusions ⮊ *and extensive superficial siderosis* ⮕.

rhage, superficial siderosis can sometimes be seen as curvilinear hypointense foci along the pial surfaces of the brain **(3-41), (3-42)**.

TBI often results in a variable amount of **generalized atrophy**. While overall parenchymal volume loss with increased ventricular size and prominent sulci can be seen on standard imaging studies, subtle cases of regional or global atrophy may require quantitative MR (qMRI) studies for detection.

Reduced cerebellar volume can be seen in some patients following TBI, possibly reflecting the high vulnerability of the cerebellum and its related projection areas to fiber degeneration.

Advanced imaging studies can be helpful adjuncts in assessing residua of TBI. MR spectroscopy may demonstrate reduced neurometabolites following TBI. NAA levels may be low, even in a normal-appearing brain. FDG PET may show focal or more widespread areas of regional glucose hypometabolism.

Diffusion tensor imaging (DTI) demonstrates low FA and high ADC in the corpus callosum of some patients with persistent cognitive deficits following mild TBI.

Chronic Traumatic Encephalopathy

Terminology

Initially reported in boxers and called "dementia pugilistica," the term **chronic traumatic encephalopathy** (CTE) has been recently introduced to describe a wide spectrum of chronic neurobehavioral abnormalities that result from multiple blows to the head.

Etiology

CTE represents a cumulative process of repetitive head blows. There is some clinical and epidemiological overlap of CTE with Alzheimer disease (AD). In addition, there is a close association of CTE and neurofibrillary tangle formation, suggesting a mixed pathology promoted by pathogenetic cascades that may result in both diseases. Both CTE and AD also have an overrepresentation of the *APOE*E3* allele.

Pathology

The gross findings in autopsied brains of deceased athletes suffering from CTE have been likened to that of an "octogenarian Alzheimer patient." Tearing of the septi pellucidi with frontotemporal volume loss, thalamic gliosis, substantia nigra degeneration, and cerebellar scarring are other common features.

Microscopic studies of CTE show variable histologic phenotypes predicated on the presence or absence of neurofibrillary tangles, neutrophil threads, amyloid plaques, and diffuse neuronal loss. In contrast to AD, the hippocampus is frequently spared in CTE.

Clinical Issues

DEMOGRAPHICS. Between 15-40% of former professional boxers have symptoms of chronic brain injury. While most cases of CTE have been reported in males,

3-42A. *NECT scan in an elderly patient with moderately severe head trauma shows left frontotemporal contusions* ➡. *3-42B.* *More cephalad scan shows diffuse left hemisphere swelling with interhemispheric* ➡, *convexity subdural hematomas* ➡. *Several foci of traumatic subarachnoid hemorrhage* ➡ *are present within the compressed sulci.*

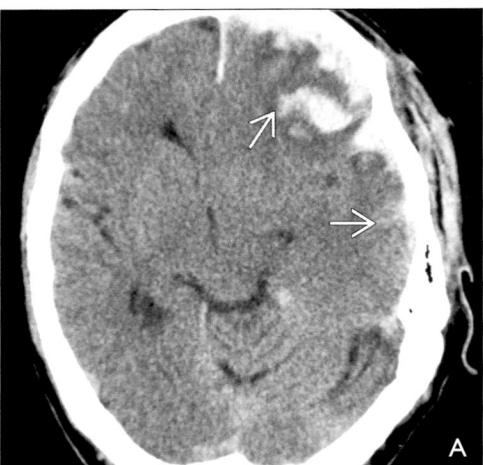

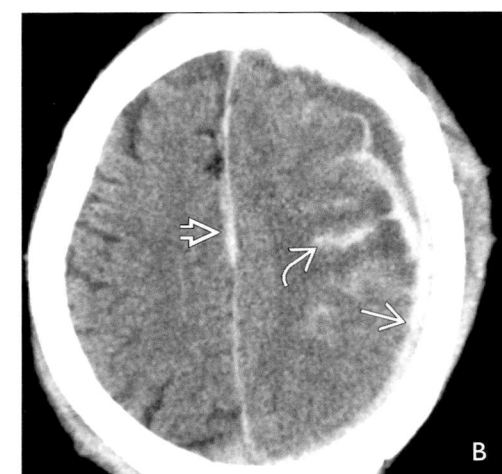

3-42C. *T2WI obtained 6 months later shows left frontal encephalomalacia* ➡. *3-42D.* *More cephalad T2WI shows several faint curvilinear hypointensities* ➡ *over some of the gyri and extending into the sulci.*

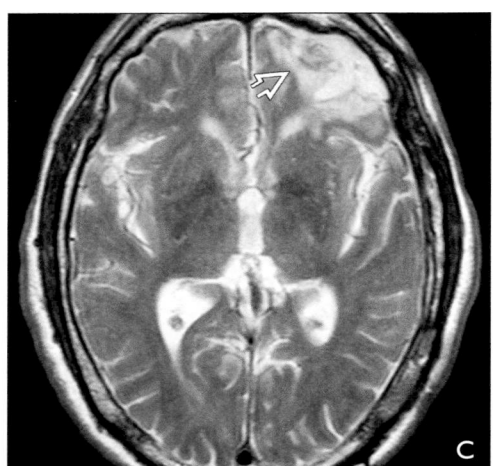

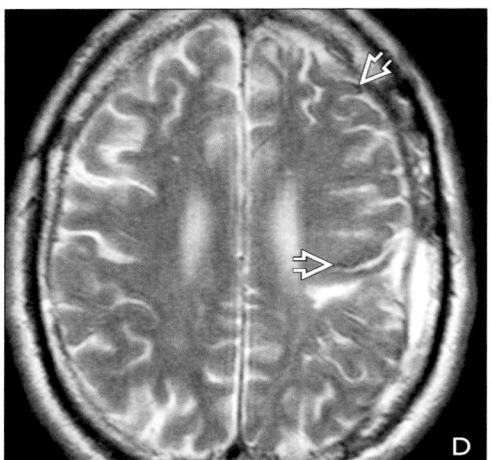

3-42E. *T2* GRE scan in the same patient shows "blooming" hemorrhagic residua around the left frontal encephalomalacia* ➡. *3-42F.* *More cephalad T2* GRE scan shows extensive post-traumatic superficial siderosis* ➡.

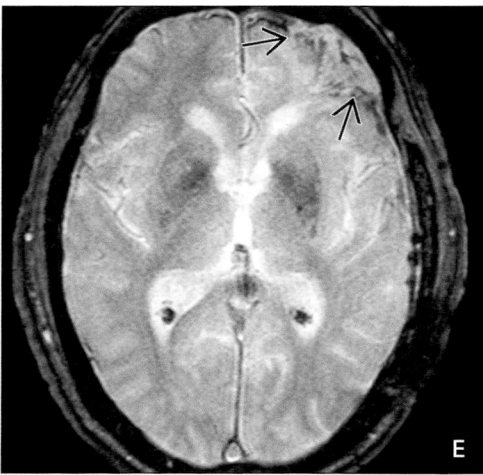

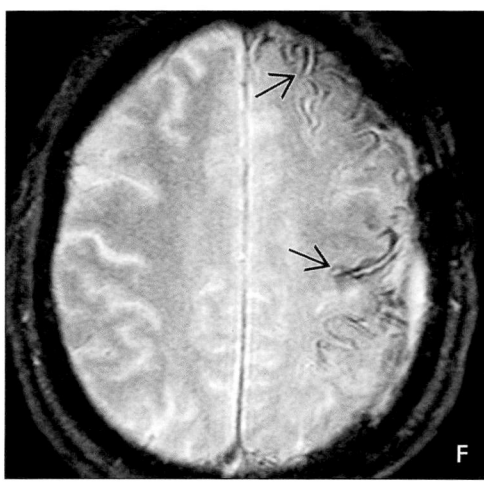

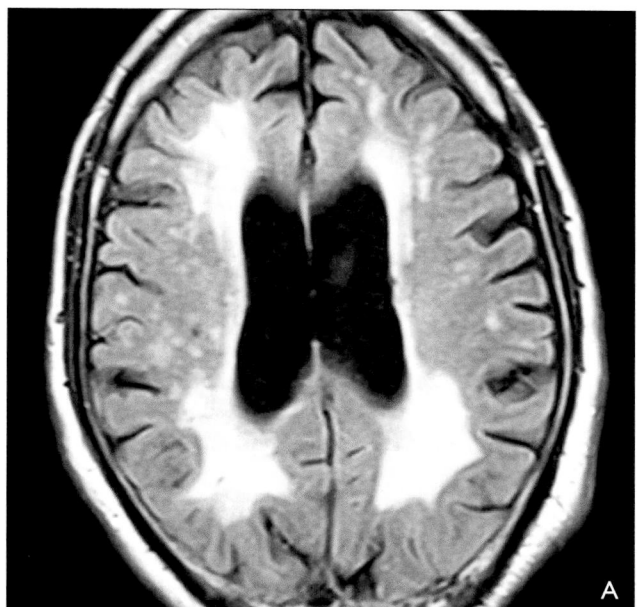

3-43A. Axial FLAIR scan in a middle-aged former professional athlete with early-onset dementia shows diffuse bihemispheric volume loss, extensive confluent and punctate WM hyperintensities.

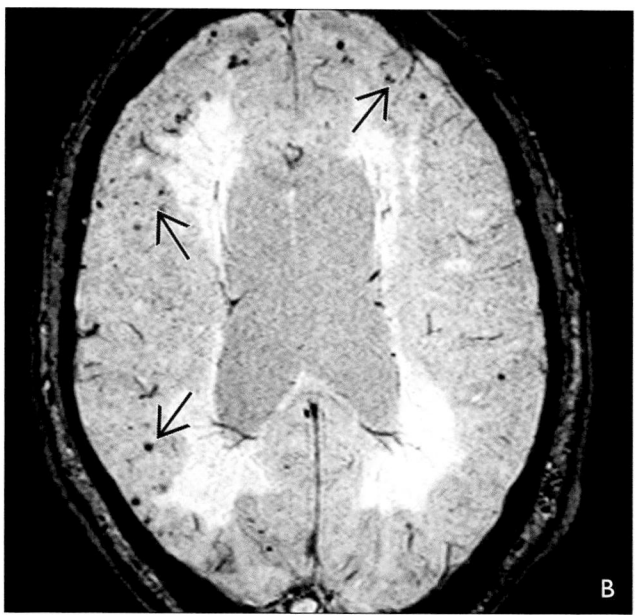

3-43B. T2* SWI scan in the same patient shows numerous blooming microbleeds ⊡. Imaging and clinical features are suggestive of chronic traumatic encephalopathy.

they have also been reported in battered women and abused children subjected to repetitive head injury. Elderly patients with repeated falls may also be at risk for CTE.

PRESENTATION. Impairments in memory, language, information processing, and executive function as well as cerebellar, pyramidal, and extrapyramidal symptoms are characteristic of CTE. Progressive cognitive deterioration, recent memory loss, and mood and behavioral disorders such as paranoia, panic attacks, and major depression are common.

Imaging

CT FINDINGS. In the largest series evaluating professional boxers with CTE, CT scans were normal in 93% and showed "borderline" atrophy in 6%. Increased prevalence of a cavum septi pellucidi (CSP) was present in those boxers with atrophy.

MR FINDINGS. Standard sequences in patients with CTE are often normal. Age-inappropriate volume loss and nonspecific white matter lesions are seen in 15% of cases **(3-43A)**. 3.0 T MR with susceptibility-weighted sequences (SWI) shows microhemorrhages in approximately 10% of patients with CTE **(3-43B)**.

Second-Impact Syndrome

Terminology

A more acute, potentially catastrophic complication of repetitive head injury has been recently recognized and dubbed **"second-impact syndrome"** (SIS) or **"dysautoregulation/second-impact syndrome."**

Etiology

Clinical studies show that a single concussive brain injury opens a "temporal window" of metabolic abnormality that can be exacerbated by repeated trauma.

In SIS, individuals (often, but not exclusively, athletes) who are still symptomatic from a prior head injury suffer a second injury. In most cases, a small acute subdural hematoma (aSDH) is associated with disproportionately large brain swelling.

Brain swelling in SIS is probably due to dysautoregulation rather than simply the mass effect of the subdural hematoma (SDH) on the underlying hemisphere. In SIS, loss of autoregulation of cerebral blood flow results in rapid cerebrovascular engorgement, increased ICP, and brain swelling.

Excitotoxic brain injury from either increased release and leakage or decreased reuptake of glutamate may also contribute to the unusually widespread cytotoxic edema seen in SIS patients.

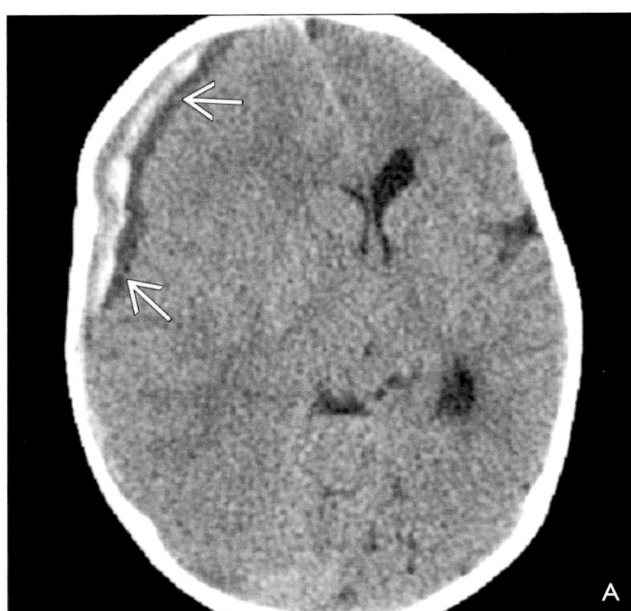

3-44A. *NECT scan in an infant with suspected nonaccidental trauma shows SDHs of 3 different ages* ➡. *Mass effect and subfalcine herniation are disproportionate to the size of the SDHs.*

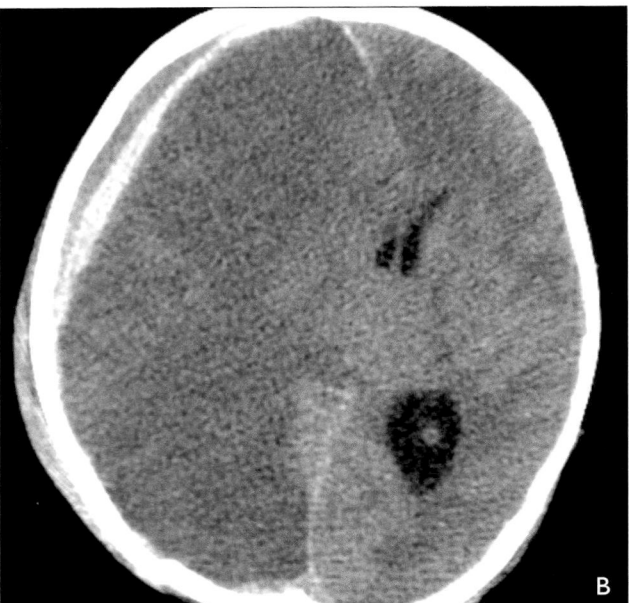

3-44B. *Repeat scan a few weeks later shows another mixed SDH with massive swelling, diffuse edema in the right hemisphere. Probable second-impact syndrome following multiple concussive injuries.*

Clinical Issues

DEMOGRAPHICS. Most reported SIS cases are in young male athletes. Another group that may be susceptible to SIS is elderly patients with recurrent SDHs and repeat episodes of mild to moderate head trauma. Some investigators have also postulated that children with nonaccidental trauma and repetitive brain injury share common pathophysiologic features with athletes suffering from SIS.

PRESENTATION. In SIS, the athlete is often suffering headaches and other symptoms from the initial concussion but returns to competition and sustains a second—often relatively minor—blow to the head. The athlete initially remains conscious but appears stunned and dazed ("got his bell rung") before collapsing and becoming semicomatose.

Recovery from a concussive event is nonlinear and does not coincide with the resolution of clinical symptoms.

NATURAL HISTORY. The clinical scenario of SIS is often catastrophic with rapid onset of coma and fixed, dilated pupils. Neurologic deterioration may occur within minutes. Mortality and morbidity are extremely high. Patients who survive, even with emergent decompressive craniectomy, often have multifocal ischemic infarcts with severe residual cognitive and neurologic deficits.

Imaging

NECT scans in patients with SIS show a small (usually < 0.5 cm) crescent-shaped, hyper- or mixed-density sub-

dural hematoma overlying a swollen, hypodense cerebral hemisphere. The extent of the mass effect and midline shift is disproportionate to the relatively small size of the aSDH **(3-44)**.

Initially, the gray-white matter interface is preserved but, as brain swelling progresses, the entire hemisphere becomes hypodense. The basal cisterns and cerebral sulci are totally effaced. Complete "central" descending herniation with brainstem compression ensues.

MR shows swollen T2/FLAIR hyperintense brain underlying a relatively small SDH. T2* (GRE, SWI) scans are usually negative for intraparenchymal hemorrhage. The swollen brain restricts strongly on DWI. MRS shows decreased NAA.

Post-Traumatic Pituitary Dysfunction

Between 25-40% of TBI survivors develop hormonal deficiencies within 6-12 months after injury. Approximately 20% are severe enough to warrant hormone replacement.

Endocrine dysfunction in patients with other complex medical and psychosocial issues is often overlooked. Hypothalamic-pituitary dysfunction may contribute to poor quality of life, exacerbate neurologic deficits, and even become life-threatening. It may cause growth hormone deficiency and short stature in children.

The diagnosis of post-traumatic hypopituitarism is based on clinical evaluation, laboratory testing, and neuroimaging. A spectrum of MR findings has been reported and

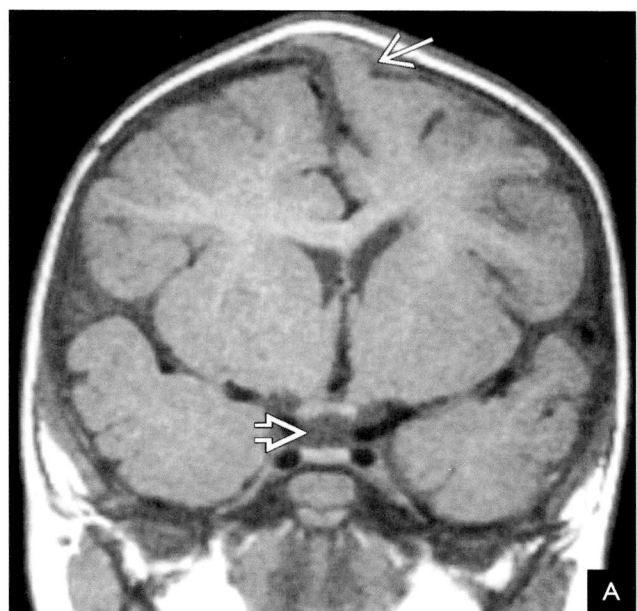

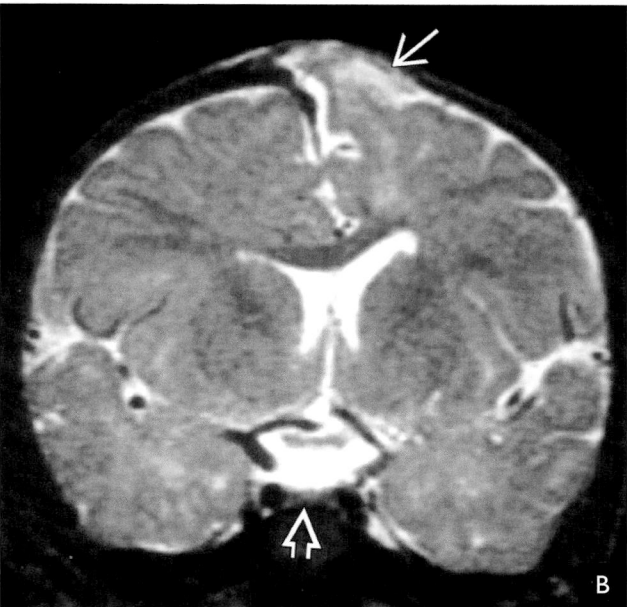

3-45A. Coronal T1WI in a child with post-traumatic hypopituitarism shows an absent infundibular stalk (probably secondary to traumatic transection) ➡, "growing" skull fracture over the vertex ➡.

3-45B. T2WI in the same patient shows partially empty sella ➡ and absent pituitary stalk. Encephalomalacic brain ➡ in the "growing" skull fracture is nicely demonstrated.

includes hypothalamic and/or posterior pituitary hemorrhage, anterior pituitary lobe infarction, and stalk transection. Traumatic pituitary stalk interruption shows a partially empty sella with a very thin or transected stalk (3-45). Decreased vascularization on dynamic contrast-enhanced sequences may be present.

Selected References

- Pitfield AF et al: Emergency management of increased intracranial pressure. Pediatr Emerg Care. 28(2):200-4; quiz 205-7, 2012
- Tong WS et al: Early CT signs of progressive hemorrhagic injury following acute traumatic brain injury. Neuroradiology. 53(5):305-9, 2011

Herniation Syndromes

- Figaji AA et al: Surgical treatment for "brain compartment syndrome" in children with severe head injury. S Afr Med J. 96(9 Pt 2):969-75, 2006
- Mokri B: The Monro-Kellie hypothesis: applications in CSF volume depletion. Neurology. 56(12):1746-8, 2001

Subfalcine Herniation

- Kubal WS: Updated imaging of traumatic brain injury. Radiol Clin North Am. 50(1):15-41, 2012

Edema, Ischemia, and Vascular Injury

Post-Traumatic Cerebral Ischemia and Infarction

- Shahlaie K et al: Risk factors for posttraumatic vasospasm. J Neurosurg. 115(3):602-11, 2011
- Moritani T et al: Diffusion-weighted imaging of acute excitotoxic brain injury. AJNR Am J Neuroradiol. 26(2):216-28, 2005

Brain Death

- Wijdicks EF: The transatlantic divide over brain death determination and the debate. Brain. 135(Pt 4):1321-31, 2012
- Burkle CM et al: Brain death and the courts. Neurology. 76(9):837-41, 2011
- Kim E et al: Patterns of accentuated grey-white differentiation on diffusion-weighted imaging or the apparent diffusion coefficient maps in comatose survivors after global brain injury. Clin Radiol. 66(5):440-8, 2011
- Savard M et al: Selective 4 vessels angiography in brain death: a retrospective study. Can J Neurol Sci. 37(4):492-7, 2010
- Wijdicks EF et al: Evidence-based guideline update: determining brain death in adults: report of the Quality Standards Subcommittee of the American Academy of Neurology. Neurology. 74(23):1911-8, 2010
- Frampas E et al: CT angiography for brain death diagnosis. AJNR Am J Neuroradiol. 30(8):1566-70, 2009
- Yuzawa H et al: Pseudo-subarachnoid hemorrhage found in patients with postresuscitation encephalopathy: characteristics of CT findings and clinical importance. AJNR Am J Neuroradiol. 29(8):1544-9, 2008
- Kavanagh EC: The reversal sign. Radiology. 245(3):914-5, 2007
- Practice parameters for determining brain death in adults (summary statement): The Quality Standards Subcommittee of the American Academy of Neurology. Neurology. 45(5):1012-4, 1995

Chronic Effects of CNS Trauma

Chronic Traumatic Encephalopathy

- Costanza A et al: Review: Contact sport-related chronic traumatic encephalopathy in the elderly: clinical expression and structural substrates. Neuropathol Appl Neurobiol. 37(6):570-84, 2011
- Hasiloglu ZI et al: Cerebral microhemorrhages detected by susceptibility-weighted imaging in amateur boxers. AJNR Am J Neuroradiol. 32(1):99-102, 2011
- Omalu B et al: Emerging histomorphologic phenotypes of chronic traumatic encephalopathy in American athletes. Neurosurgery. 69(1):173-83; discussion 183, 2011

Second-Impact Syndrome

- Cantu RC et al: Second-impact syndrome and a small subdural hematoma: an uncommon catastrophic result of repetitive head injury with a characteristic imaging appearance. J Neurotrauma. 27(9):1557-64, 2010

Post-Traumatic Pituitary Dysfunction

- Gasco V et al: Hypopituitarism following brain injury: when does it occur and how best to test? Pituitary. 15(1):20-4, 2012
- Maiya B et al: Magnetic resonance imaging changes in the pituitary gland following acute traumatic brain injury. Intensive Care Med. 34(3):468-75, 2008
- Makulski DD et al: Neuroimaging in posttraumatic hypopituitarism. J Comput Assist Tomogr. 32(2):324-8, 2008

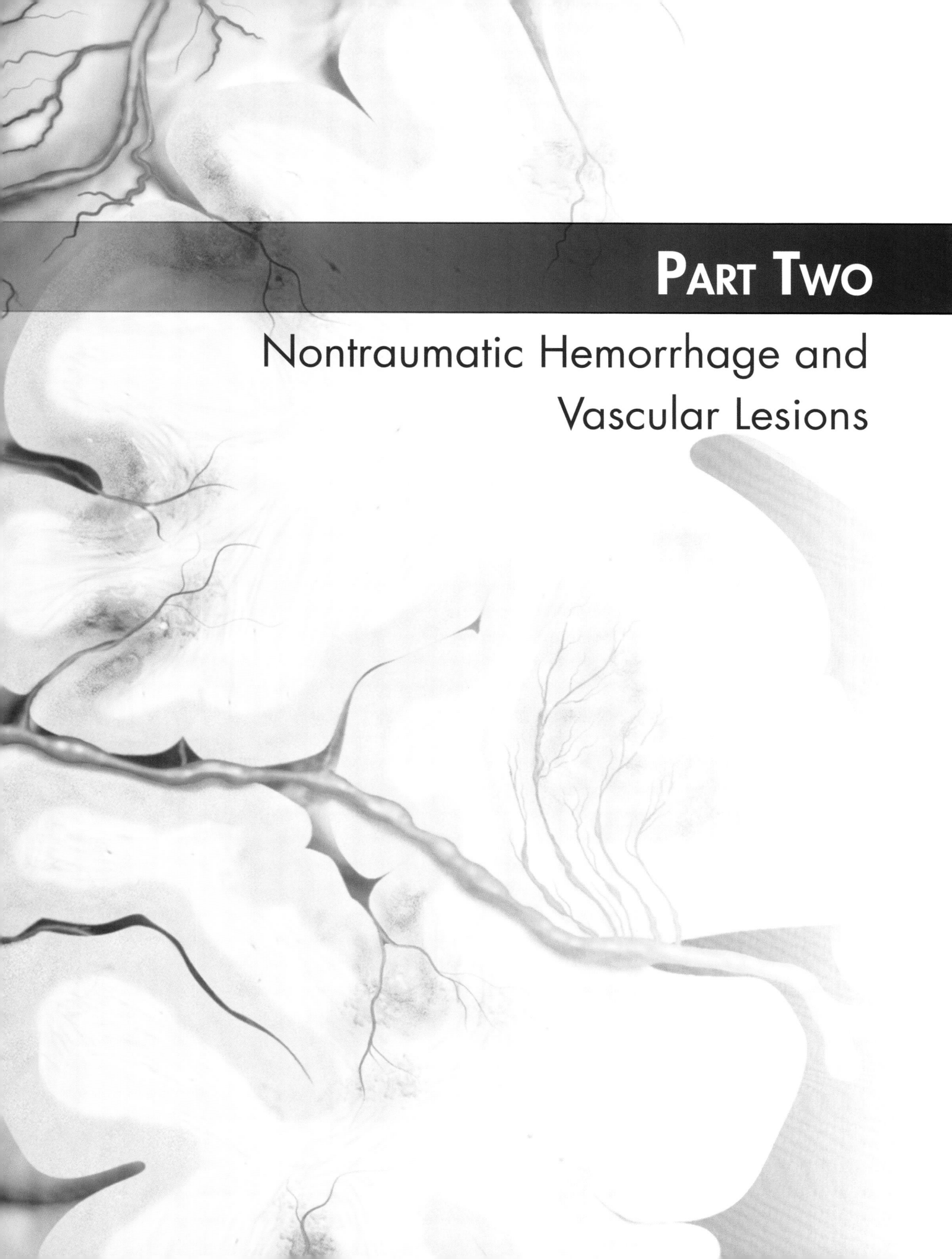

PART TWO

Nontraumatic Hemorrhage and Vascular Lesions

4

Approach to Nontraumatic Hemorrhage and Vascular Lesions

This part devoted to "spontaneous" (i.e., nontraumatic) hemorrhage and vascular lesions begins with a general discussion of brain bleeds. Subsequent chapters delineate a broad spectrum of vascular pathologies ranging from aneurysms/subarachnoid hemorrhage and vascular malformations to cerebral vasculopathy and strokes. Where appropriate, anatomic considerations and the pathophysiology of specific disorders are included.

Spontaneous (i.e., nontraumatic) intracranial hemorrhage (ICH) and vascular brain disorders are second only to trauma as neurologic causes of death and disability. Stroke or "brain attack"—defined as sudden onset of a neurologic event—is the third leading *overall* cause of death in industrialized countries and is the most common cause of neurologic disability in adults.

Significant public health initiatives aimed at decreasing the prevalence of comorbid diseases such as obesity, hypertension, and diabetes have only marginally decreased the incidence of strokes and brain bleeds. Therefore, it will continue to be important to understand the pathoetiology of intracranial hemorrhages and the various stroke subtypes together with their imaging manifestations.

We start this chapter with a brief overview of nontraumatic ICH and vascular diseases of the CNS, beginning with a short discussion of who, why, when, and how to image these patients. We then develop an anatomy-based approach to evaluating nontraumatic ICH. We close the discussion with a pathology-based introduction to the broad spectrum of congenital and acquired vascular lesions that affect the brain.

Imaging Hemorrhage and Vascular Lesions

Who and Why to Image?

Because of its widespread availability and speed, an emergent NECT scan is generally the first-line imaging procedure of choice in patients with sudden onset of an unexplained neurologic deficit. NECT imaging is also commonly obtained to evaluate for suspected subarachnoid hemorrhage, hydrocephalus, or intracranial mass in patients with severe headache but nonfocal neurologic examination.

If the initial NECT scan is negative and no neurologic deficit is apparent, further imaging is usually unnecessary. However, if the history and clinical findings suggest a thromboembolic stroke, additional imaging is indicated.

When and How to Image?

Some of the most challenging questions arise when screening NECT discloses parenchymal hemorrhage. What are the potential causes? Is the patient at risk for hematoma expansion? Should further emergent imaging be performed?

CT angiogram (CTA) is indicated in patients with sudden clinical deterioration and a mixed-density hematoma (indicating rapid bleeding or coagulopathy). A "bleeding globe" caused by rupture of a lenticulostriate microaneurysm (Charcot-Bouchard aneurysm) can sometimes be identified.

CTA is also an appropriate next step in children and young/middle-aged adults with spontaneous (nontraumatic) ICH detected on screening NECT. In contrast to elderly patients, vascular malformation is a common underlying etiology in younger age groups.

Emergency MR is rarely necessary if CTA is negative. However, follow-up MR without and with contrast enhancement can be very useful in patients with unexplained ICH. In addition to the standard sequences (i.e., T1WI, T2WI, FLAIR, DWI, and T1 C+), a T2* sequence—either GRE or susceptibility-weighted imaging (SWI)—should be obtained.

MR evidence for prior hemorrhage(s) can be very helpful in narrowing the differential diagnosis. Benign ICH typically follows an orderly, predictable evolution on MR scans. MR evidence of disordered or bizarre-looking hemorrhage should raise the possibility of neoplasm, underlying arteriovenous malformation, or coagulopathy.

If MR demonstrates multiple parenchymal hemorrhages of different ages, the underlying etiology varies with patient age. Multiple microbleeds in elderly patients are typically associated with chronic hypertension or amyloid angiopathy. Cavernous malformations or hematologic disorder are the most common causes in children and young adults.

Approach to Nontraumatic Hemorrhage

Hematoma location, age, and number (solitary or multiple) should be noted.

The differential diagnosis of spontaneous nontraumatic ICH varies widely with anatomic location. Because the brain parenchyma is the most common site, we begin

4-1. *Autopsy specimen from an elderly adult shows a parenchymal hematoma ➔ centered in the striatocapsular region. The external capsule/ putamen location is classic for hypertensive hemorrhage.* *4-2.* *Autopsy case from a middle-aged patient with metastatic renal cell carcinoma shows 2 hemorrhagic metastases ➔ at the gray-white matter interface, a typical location.*

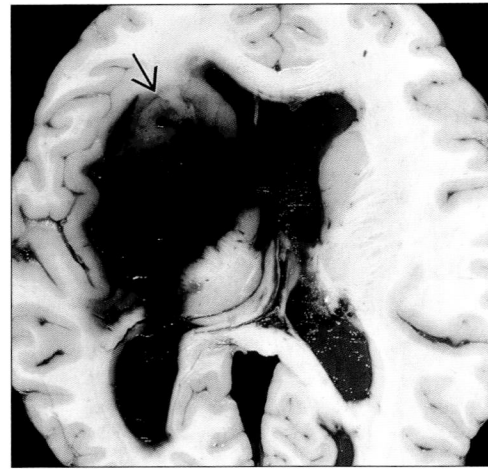

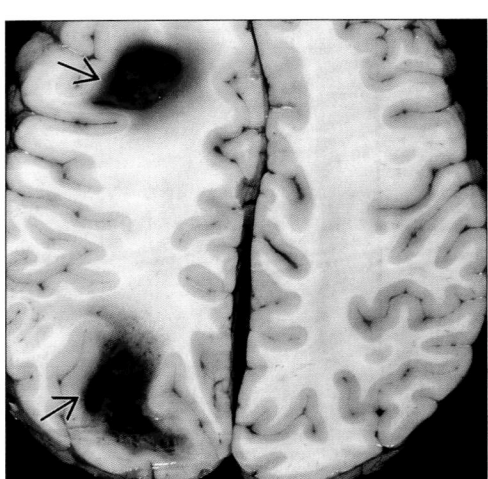

4-3. *Autopsy case from a young patient with a large hematoma ➔ centered in the hemispheric white matter with focal extension ➔ through the cortex. Underlying arteriovenous malformation was the cause of this fatal intracranial hemorrhage.* *4-4.* *Autopsy case of a child with multifocal parenchymal hemorrhages ➔ caused by leukemia. (Cases courtesy R. Hewlett, MD.)*

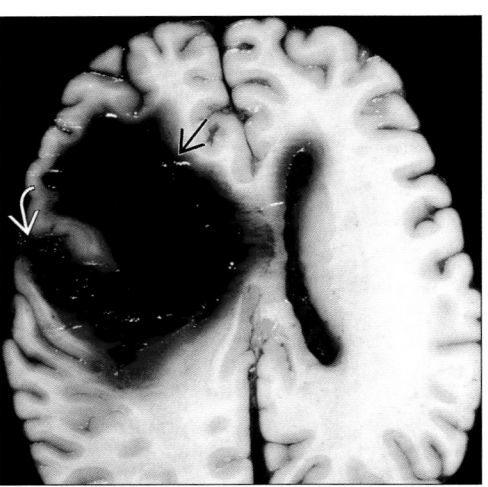

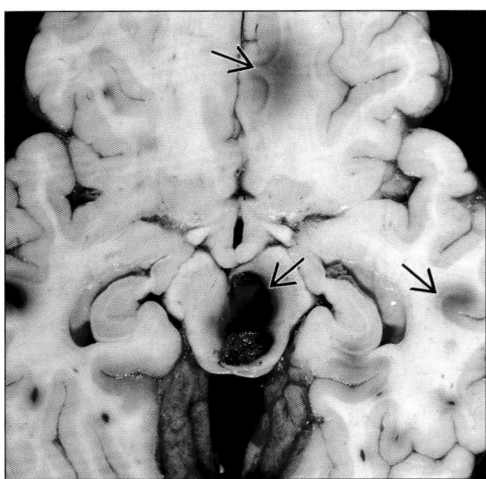

with a discussion of intraaxial hemorrhages, then turn our attention to extraaxial bleeds.

Intraaxial Hemorrhage

Clinical Issues

Parenchymal hemorrhage is the most devastating type of stroke. Although recent advances have improved the treatment of ischemic strokes, few evidence-based treatments exist for ICH. Strategies are largely supportive, aimed at limiting further injury as well as preventing associated complications such as hematoma expansion, elevated intracranial pressure, and intraventricular rupture with hydrocephalus.

Imaging

Parenchymal hematomas are easily recognized on NECT scans by their hyperdensity or, in the case of rapid bleeding or coagulopathy, mixed iso-/hyperdense appearance. Hematomas are focal lesions that expand the brain, displacing the cortex outward and producing mass effect on underlying structures such as the cerebral ventricles.

The sulci are often compressed, and the overlying gyri appear expanded and flattened. The surrounding brain may appear grossly edematous.

Hematoma signal intensity on standard MR varies with clot age and imaging sequence. T2* (GRE, SWI) scans are especially important in evaluating patients with brain hemorrhage. They should be like your favorite credit cards: "Don't leave home without them!"

Differential Diagnosis

Sublocation of an intraparenchymal clot is very important in establishing putative etiology.

If a classic **striatocapsular** or **thalamic** hematoma is found in a middle-aged or elderly patient, hypertensive hemorrhage is by far the most common etiology (4-1). Drug abuse should be suspected in a young adult with a similar-appearing lesion. Ruptured aneurysms rarely cause lateral basal ganglionic hemorrhage and neoplasms with hemorrhagic necrosis are far less common than hypertensive bleeds in this location.

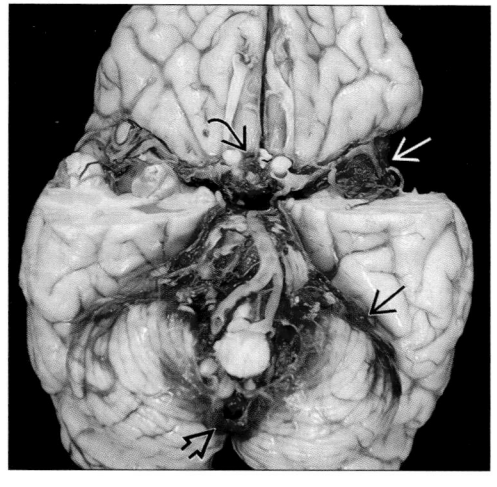

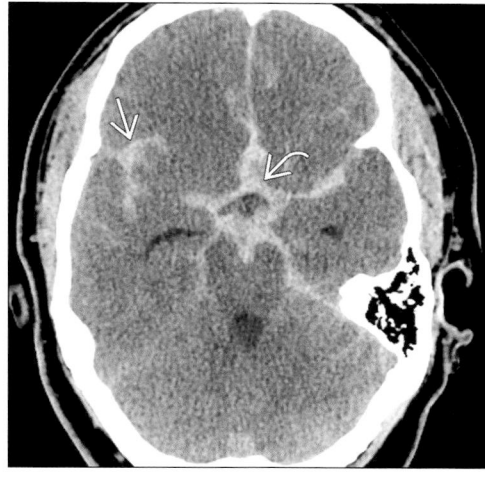

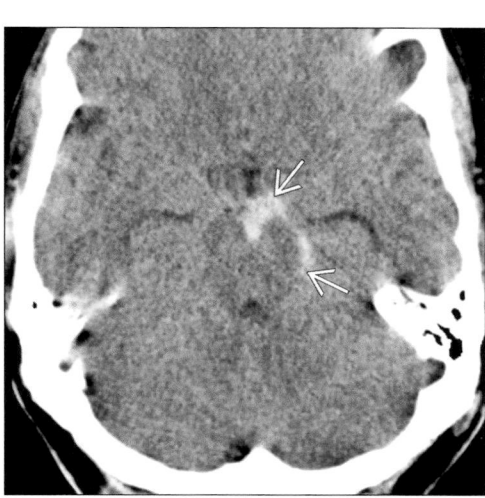

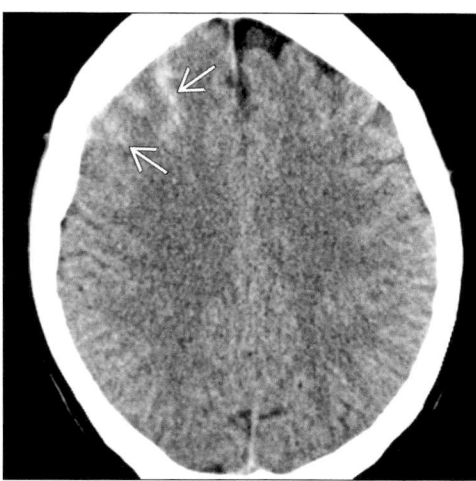

4-5. Autopsy case demonstrates diffuse acute subarachnoid hemorrhage in the basal cisterns. Blood fills the sylvian fissures ➡, *suprasellar cistern* ➡, *and cisterna magna* ➡. *Hemorrhage coats the surface of the pons and extends laterally into the cerebellopontine angle cisterns* ➡. *4-6. NECT scan in a patient with aneurysmal SAH. Diffuse hemorrhage fills the suprasellar cistern* ➡ *and sylvian fissures* ➡.

4-7. NECT scan shows classic perimesencephalic nonaneurysmal SAH ➡ *with subarachnoid blood localized around the midbrain, in the interpeduncular fossa, and in the ambient cistern. CTA was negative. 4-8. NECT scan in a young female with severe headache shows focal subarachnoid blood in the right frontal convexity sulci* ➡. *The basal cisterns (not shown) were normal. Proven reversible cerebral vasoconstriction syndrome.*

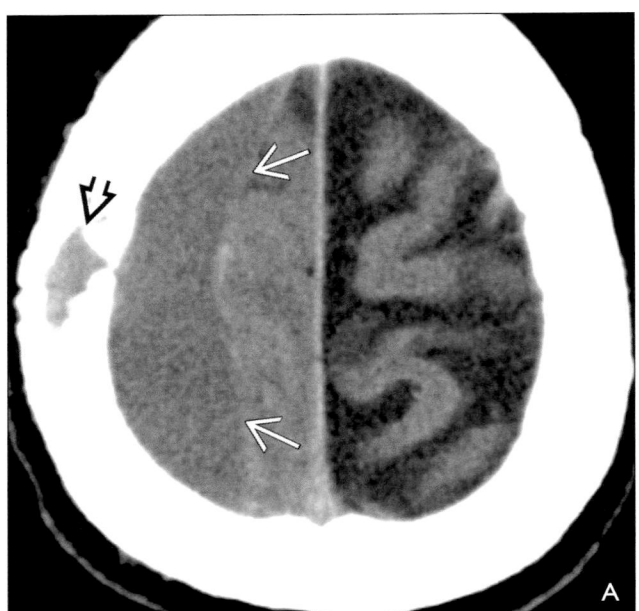

4-9A. NECT scan shows spontaneous nontraumatic subacute combined epi- and subdural hematoma ⮕ associated with a focal calvarial lesion ⮞.

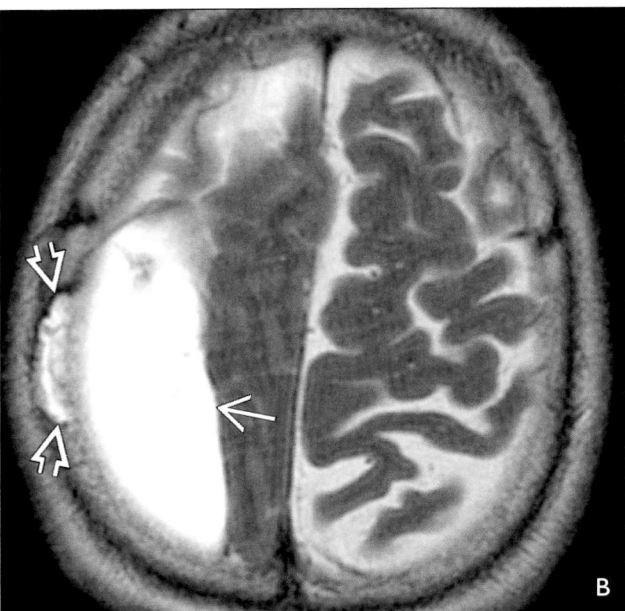

4-9B. T2WI in the same patient shows that the hematoma ⮕ is associated with a well-demarcated hyperintense lesion in the calvaria ⮞. Hemangioma was found at surgery.

Lobar hemorrhages present a different challenge as the differential diagnosis is much broader. In older patients, amyloid angiopathy, hypertension, and underlying neoplasm (primary or metastatic) are the most common causes (4-2). Vascular malformations (4-3) and hematologic malignancies (4-4) are more common in younger patients. Dural sinus and/or cortical vein thrombosis are uncommon but occur in patients of all ages.

Hemorrhages at the **gray-white matter interface** are typical of metastases, septic emboli, and fungal infection.

Multifocal hemorrhages confined to the **white matter** are rare. When they are identified in a patient with a history of a febrile illness followed by sudden neurologic deterioration, they are most likely secondary to a hemorrhagic form of acute disseminated encephalomyelitis called acute hemorrhagic leukoencephalopathy (also known as Weston-Hurst disease).

Clot age can likewise be helpful in suggesting the etiology of an intracranial hemorrhage. A hemosiderin-laden encephalomalacic cavity in the basal ganglia or thalamus of an older patient is typically due to an old hypertensive hemorrhage. The most common cause of a hyperacute parenchymal clot in a child is an underlying arteriovenous malformation.

Extraaxial Hemorrhage

Spontaneous extraaxial hemorrhages can occur into any of the three major anatomic compartments, i.e., the epidural space, subdural space, and the subarachnoid space. By far the most common are subarachnoid hem-

orrhages. In contrast to traumatic hemorrhages, spontaneous bleeding into the epi- and subdural spaces is uncommon.

Subarachnoid Hemorrhage

CLINICAL ISSUES. Patients with nontraumatic subarachnoid hemorrhage (ntSAH) usually present with sudden onset of severe headache ("worst headache of my life"). A "thunderclap" headache is very common.

IMAGING. Nontraumatic SAH is easily distinguished from a parenchymal hematoma by its location and configuration (4-5). Blood in the subarachnoid spaces has a feathery, curvilinear, or serpentine appearance as it fills the cisterns and surface sulci. It follows brain surfaces and rarely causes a focal mass effect.

SAH is hyperdense on NECT scans. Bloody sulcal-cisternal CSF appears "dirty" on T1WI, hyperintense on FLAIR, and "blooms" on T2*.

DIFFERENTIAL DIAGNOSIS. As with parenchymal bleeds, ntSAH sublocation is helpful in establishing an appropriate differential diagnosis. By far the most common cause of ntSAH is **aneurysmal subarachnoid hemorrhage** (aSAH). As most intracranial aneurysms arise from the circle of Willis and the middle cerebral bifurcation, aSAH tends to spread throughout the basal cisterns and extend into the sylvian fissures (4-6).

Two special, easily recognizable subtypes of subarachnoid hemorrhage are *not* associated with ruptured intracranial aneurysm. Blood localized to the subarachnoid spaces around the midbrain and anterior to the pons is called **perimesencephalic nonaneurysmal subarachnoid hemorrhage** (pnSAH) **(4-7)**. This type of SAH is self-limited, rarely results in vasospasm, and is probably secondary to venous hemorrhage. CTA is a reliable technique to rule out a basilar tip aneurysm. DSA and noninvasive follow-up imaging have had no demonstrable increased diagnostic yield in such cases.

Blood in one or more sulci over the upper cerebral hemispheres is called **convexal subarachnoid hemorrhage (4-8)**. This recently recognized type of SAH is associated with a number of diverse etiologies, including cortical vein thrombosis and amyloid angiopathy in older patients as well as reversible cerebral vasoconstriction syndrome in younger individuals.

Epidural Hemorrhage

The pathogenesis of extradural hematomas is almost always traumatic and arises from lacerated meningeal arteries, fractures, or torn dural venous sinuses.

Most are found in the spinal—not the cranial—epidural space and are an emergent condition that may result in paraplegia, quadriplegia, and even death. Elderly anticoagulated patients are most at risk.

Intracranial spontaneous epidural hemorrhages are very rare. Most reported cases are associated with bleeding disorders, craniofacial infection (usually mastoiditis or sphenoid sinusitis), dural sinus thrombosis, bone infarction (e.g., in patients with sickle cell disease), or a vascular lesion of the calvaria (e.g., hemangioma, metastasis, or intradiploic epidermoid cyst) **(4-9)**.

Subdural Hemorrhage

Trauma also causes the vast majority of subdural hematomas (SDHs). Nontraumatic SDHs represent less than 5% of all cases. Many occur with CSF volume depletion and intracranial hypotension, which can become life-threatening if sufficiently severe. Most cases of spontaneous intracranial hypotension are secondary to a dural tear following lumbar puncture, myelography, spinal anesthesia, or cranial surgery.

Nontraumatic SDHs have been reported in association with a number of other conditions including hyponatremic dehydration, inherited or acquired coagulation disorders, dural venous sinus thrombosis, and meningitis. A few cases of spontaneous SDH occur directly adjacent to a lobar peripheral hemorrhage and are associated with an underlying vasculopathy (such as cerebral amyloid disease with pseudoaneurysm formation) or vascular malformation. Others occur without an identifiable antecedent or predisposing condition.

Occasionally, a ruptured cortical artery or saccular aneurysm may result in a nontraumatic intracranial SDH. Dural hemangiomas have also been reported as causes of acute nontraumatic SDH. Elderly patients with intrinsic or iatrogenic coagulopathy can present with an SDH and either minor or no definite evidence for head trauma.

Approach to Vascular Disorders of the CNS

Here we discuss a general approach to vascular disorders in the brain, briefly introducing the major chapters in this part. Details regarding pathoetiology, clinical features, imaging findings, and differential diagnosis are delineated in each individual chapter.

Subarachnoid Hemorrhage and Aneurysms

Trauma is—by far—the most common cause of subarachnoid hemorrhage. Traumatic SAH is found in 100% of patients with fatal severe head injuries and is common in those with moderate to severe nonfatal closed head trauma.

Chapter 6 focuses on *nontraumatic* "spontaneous" SAH, which causes between 3-5% of all acute strokes. Of these, nearly 80% are caused by rupture of a saccular aneurysm. Aneurysmal SAH can generally be distinguished from nonaneurysmal SAH by its distribution on NECT scans (see above).

Classic saccular ("berry") aneurysms, as well as the less common dissecting aneurysms, pseudoaneurysms, fusiform aneurysms, and blood blister-like aneurysms, are discussed in this chapter.

Vascular Malformations

Cerebrovascular malformations (CVMs) are a fascinating, remarkably heterogeneous group of disorders with unique pathophysiology and imaging features. Chapter 7 discusses the four major types of vascular malformations, grouping them according to whether they shunt blood directly from the arterial to the venous side of the circulation without passing through a capillary bed.

CVMs that display AV shunting include arteriovenous malformations (AVMs) **(4-10)** and fistulas (AVFs). Included in this discussion is the newly described entity called cerebral proliferative angiopathy. Cerebral proliferative angiopathy can mimic AVM on imaging stud-

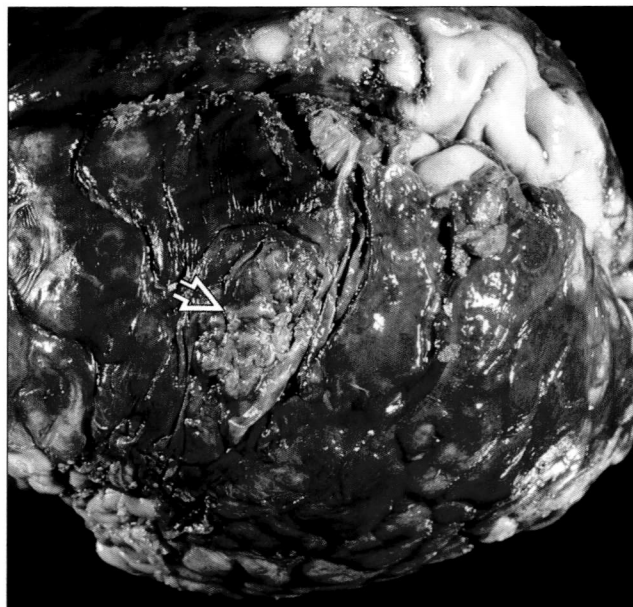

4-10. Autopsy case of an arteriovenous malformation causing massive intracranial hemorrhage. Note prominent draining veins ➡ over the surface of the hemisphere. (Courtesy R. Hewlett, MD.)

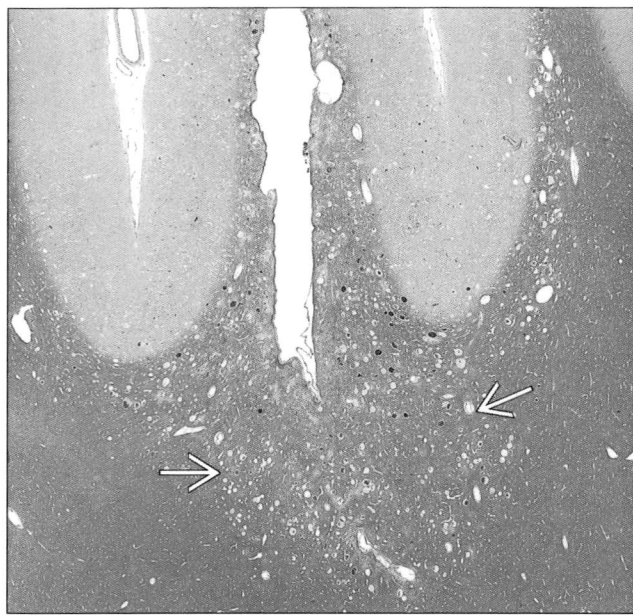

4-11. Low-power photomicrograph of a capillary telangiectasia found incidentally at autopsy. Note numerous "holes" ➡ caused by innumerable dilated capillaries and absence of mass effect or hemorrhage. (Courtesy P. Burger, MD.)

ies but has unique features that may influence treatment decisions.

With few exceptions, most CVMs that lack AV shunting—i.e., developmental venous anomalies (venous "angiomas") along with cavernous malformations and capillary telangiectasias **(4-11)**—are "leave me alone" lesions that are identified on imaging studies but generally do not require treatment.

Lastly, note that the topic of "occult" vascular malformation is not discussed. This is an outdated concept that originated in an era when angiography was the only available technique to diagnose brain vascular malformations prior to surgical exploration. Some vascular malformations such as cavernous angiomas and capillary telangiectasias are invisible (and therefore "occult") at angiography but are easily identified on MR imaging.

Arterial Anatomy and Strokes

Chapter 8 begins with a discussion of normal intracranial arterial anatomy and vascular distributions, an essential foundation for understanding the imaging appearance of cerebral ischemia/infarction.

The major focus of the chapter is thromboembolic infarcts in major arterial territories, as they are by far the most common cause of acute strokes **(4-12)**. Subacute and chronic infarcts are briefly discussed. While typically not amenable to intravascular treatment, they are nevertheless seen on imaging studies and should be recognized as residua from a prior infarct **(4-13)**.

The discussion of embolic infarcts includes cardiac and atheromatous emboli as well as lacunar infarcts and the distinct syndrome of fat emboli. The pathophysiology and imaging of watershed ("border zone") infarcts and global hypoxic-ischemic brain injury is also included. Miscellaneous strokes such as cerebral hyperperfusion syndrome are discussed.

The chapter concludes by illustrating strokes in unusual vascular distributions, including artery of Percheron and "top of the basilar" infarcts.

Venous Anatomy and Occlusions

The venous side of the cerebral circulation is—quite literally—"terra incognita" (an unknown land) to many physicians who deal with brain disorders. While many could sketch the major arterial territories with relative ease, few could diagram the intracranial venous drainage territories.

The brain veins and sinuses are unlike those of the body. Systemic veins typically travel parallel to arteries and mirror their vascular territories. Not so in the brain. Systemic veins have valves, and flow is generally in one direction.

The cerebral veins and dural sinuses lack valves and may thus exhibit bidirectional flow. Systemic veins have numerous collateral pathways that can develop in case of occlusion. Few such collaterals exist inside the calvaria.

Chapter 9 begins with a brief discussion of normal venous anatomy and drainage patterns before we con-

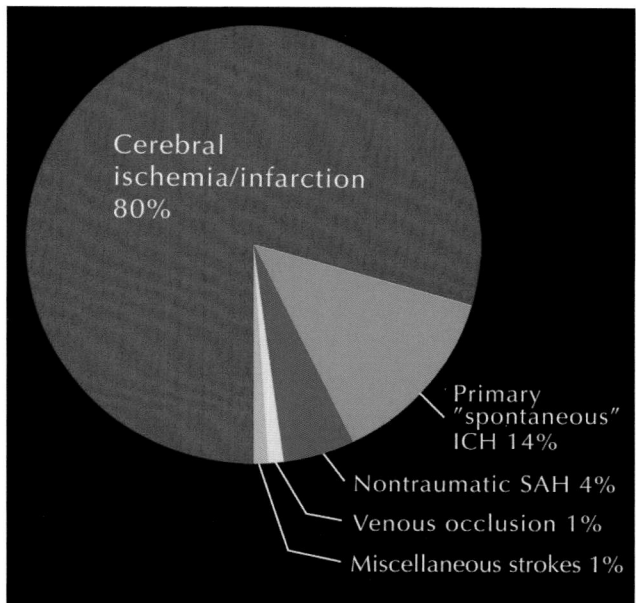

4-12. Diagram shows that cerebral ischemia-infarction represents the vast majority of strokes. The second most common is primary intracranial hemorrhage, followed by nontraumatic subarachnoid hemorrhage.

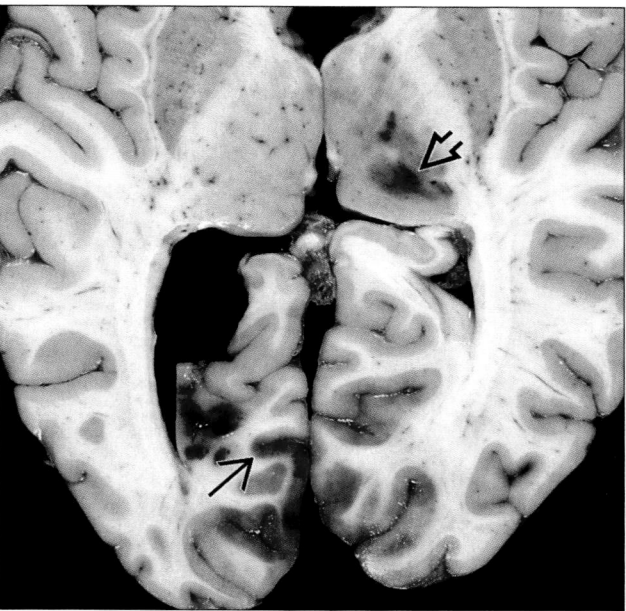

4-13. Autopsy of subacute cerebral infarct with hemorrhagic transformation in the occipital cortex ⮕ and contralateral thalamus ⮗. Anatomic distribution is that of a posterior (vertebrobasilar) territorial infarct. (Courtesy R. Hewlett, MD.)

sider the various manifestations of venous occlusion. Venous thrombosis causes just 1% of all strokes, and its clinical presentation is much less distinctive than that of major arterial occlusion. It is perhaps the type of stroke most frequently missed on imaging studies. Venous stroke can also mimic other disease (e.g., neoplasm), and in turn a number of disorders can mimic venous thrombosis.

Vasculopathy

Chapter 10, the final chapter in this part, is devoted to cerebral vasculopathy. This chapter begins with a review of normal extracranial arterial anatomy with special focus on the carotid arteries and their variants.

The bulk of the chapter is devoted to cerebral vasculopathy and is organized into two parts: Atherosclerosis **(4-14)** and nonatherosclerotic disease. The concept of the "vulnerable" or "at risk" atherosclerotic plaque is underscored. Indeed, while measuring the percent of internal carotid artery stenosis has been emphasized since the 1990s as a major predictor of stroke risk and the basis for treatment-related decisions, identifying a rupture-prone plaque is at least as important as determining stenosis.

The much-neglected but important topic of *intra*cranial atherosclerosis is also discussed. While major vessel and cardiac thromboemboli cause most arterial strokes, between 5-10% can be attributed to intracranial stenoocclusive disease **(4-15)**. The topic of arteriolosclerosis (i.e., small vessel vascular disease) is also considered here and again in the subsequent section on metabolic disease.

Nonatheromatous diseases of the cerebral vasculature are much less common than atherosclerosis and its sequelae. However, a number of vasculopathies can have serious consequences and should be recognized on imaging studies. This heterogeneous group of disorders includes fibromuscular dysplasia, dissection, vasospasm and the unusual but important cerebral vasoconstriction syndromes, and the often-confusing topic of vasculitis.

The vasculopathy chapter concludes with the intriguing topic of nonatheromatous microvascular diseases such as systemic lupus erythematosus, antiphospholipid syndrome, and amyloid angiopathy.

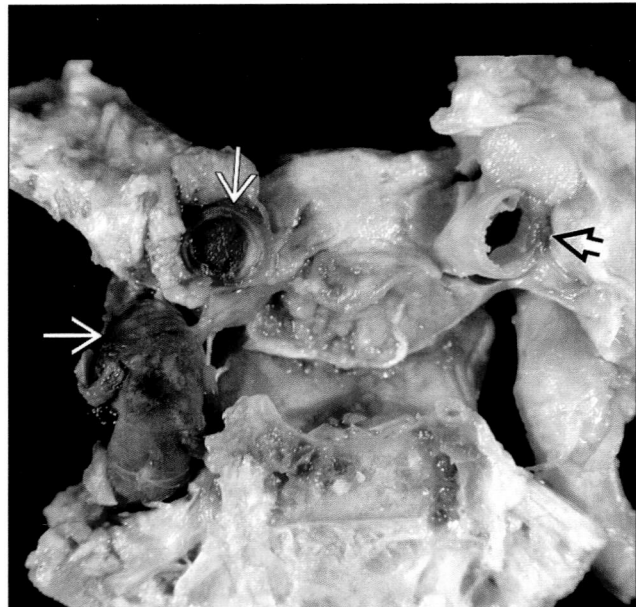

4-14. Autopsy case shows thrombosis of one cavernous/ supraclinoid internal carotid artery ➡ and atherosclerosis ⊵ in the other ICA. (Courtesy R. Hewlett, MD.)

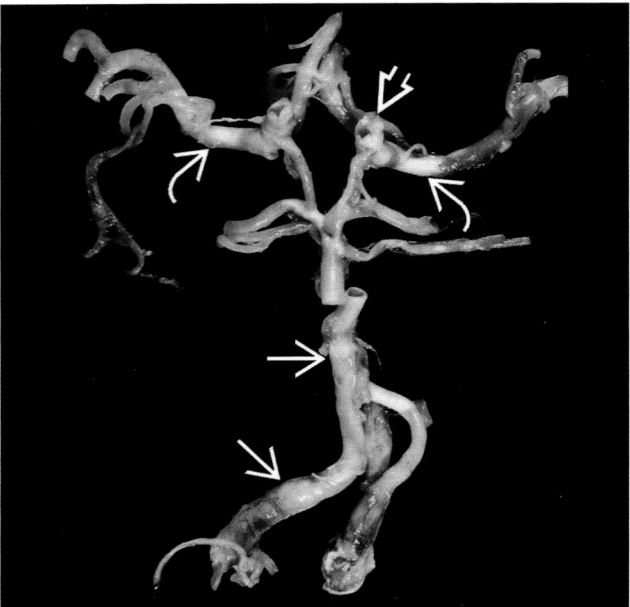

4-15. Yellowish discoloration and ectasia from ASVD is most prominent in the posterior circulation ➡, but the ICAs ⊵ and proximal MCAs ➢ are also affected. (Courtesy R. Hewlett, MD.)

Selected References

Approach to Nontraumatic Hemorrhage

- Fischbein NJ et al: Nontraumatic intracranial hemorrhage. Neuroimaging Clin N Am. 20(4):469-92, 2010

Intraaxial Hemorrhage

- Balami JS et al: Complications of intracerebral haemorrhage. Lancet Neurol. 11(1):101-18, 2012

Extraaxial Hemorrhage

- Cho KS et al: Epidural hematoma accompanied by oculomotor nerve palsy due to sphenoid sinusitis. Am J Otolaryngol. 32(4):355-7, 2011
- Cruz JP et al: Perimesencephalic subarachnoid hemorrhage: when to stop imaging? Emerg Radiol. 18(3):197-202, 2011
- Kaif M: Mastoiditis causing sinus thrombosis and posterior fossa epidural haematoma: case report. Sultan Qaboos Univ Med J. 11(1):108-11, 2011
- Kumar S et al: Atraumatic convexal subarachnoid hemorrhage: clinical presentation, imaging patterns, and etiologies. Neurology. 74(11):893-9, 2010
- Cohen MC et al: Histology of the dural membrane supports the theoretical considerations of its role in the pathophysiology of subdural collections in nontraumatic circumstances. Pediatr Radiol. 39(8):880-1, 2009

- Kocak A et al: Acute subdural hematomas caused by ruptured aneurysms: experience from a single Turkish center. Turk Neurosurg. 19(4):333-7, 2009

Approach to Vascular Disorders of the CNS

Vascular Malformations

- Marks MP et al: Cerebral proliferative angiopathy. J Neurointerv Surg. 4(5):e25, 2012
- de Champfleur NM et al: Magnetic resonance imaging evaluation of cerebral cavernous malformations with susceptibility-weighted imaging. Neurosurgery. 68(3):641-7; discussion 647-8, 2011
- Sayama CM et al: Capillary telangiectasias: clinical, radiographic, and histopathological features. Clinical article. J Neurosurg. 113(4):709-14, 2010
- Pham M et al: Radiosurgery for angiographically occult vascular malformations. Neurosurg Focus. 26(5):E16, 2009

5
Spontaneous Parenchymal Hemorrhage

In the absence of trauma, abrupt onset of focal neurological symptoms is presumed to be vascular in origin until proved otherwise. Rapid neuroimaging to distinguish ischemic stroke from intracranial hemorrhage (ICH) is crucial to patient management.

Epidemiology of Spontaneous ICH

Cerebral ischemia/infarction is responsible for almost 80% of all "strokes." Spontaneous (nontraumatic) primary intracranial hemorrhage (pICH) causes about 15% of strokes and is a devastating subtype with unusually high mortality and morbidity. In the United States alone, there are 70,000-80,000 new cases of ICH each year with an estimated lifetime cost for each case approaching US $120,000-150,000.

Natural History of Primary ICH

Early deterioration with pICH is common. More than 20% of patients experience a decrease in Glasgow Coma Scale (GCS) score of two or more points between initial assessment by paramedics and presentation in the emergency department.

Active bleeding with hematoma expansion occurs in 25-40% of patients and may continue for several hours after symptom onset. Hematoma expansion is predictive of clinical deterioration and carries significantly increased morbidity and mortality. Therefore, swift diagnosis is needed to direct treatment.

The prognosis is grave, even with prompt intervention. Between 20-30% of all patients die within 48 hours after the initial hemorrhage. The one-year mortality rate approaches 60%. Only 20% of patients who survive regain functional independence and recover without significant residual neurologic deficits.

Imaging Recommendations

The most recent American Heart Association/American Stroke Association (AHA/ASA) guidelines recommend emergent CT or MR as the initial screening procedure to distinguish ischemic stroke from intracranial hemorrhage.

If a parenchymal hematoma is identified, determining its etiology becomes critically important in patient triage. Detecting contrast extravasation within the clot can help identify patients at risk for hematoma expansion and who may be suitable candidates for surgical intervention. The AHA/ASA guidelines recommend considering CECT or CT angiography to look for a "bleeding globe" in these patients.

The management of unexplained brain bleeds also varies with patient age. If the patient is older than 45 years and has preexisting systemic hypertension, a putaminal, thalamic, or posterior fossa ICH is almost always hypertensive in origin and generally does not require additional imaging.

In contrast, lobar or deep brain bleeds in younger patients or normotensive adults—regardless of age—usually require further investigation. Contrast-enhanced CT/MR with angiography and/or venography may be helpful in detecting underlying abnormalities such as arteriovenous malformation, neoplasm, and cerebral sinovenous thrombosis.

In older patients with pICH, MR with T2* (GRE, SWI) is helpful in detecting the presence of "surrogate markers" of small vessel disease such as brain microbleeds, white matter hyperintensities, and lacunar infarcts.

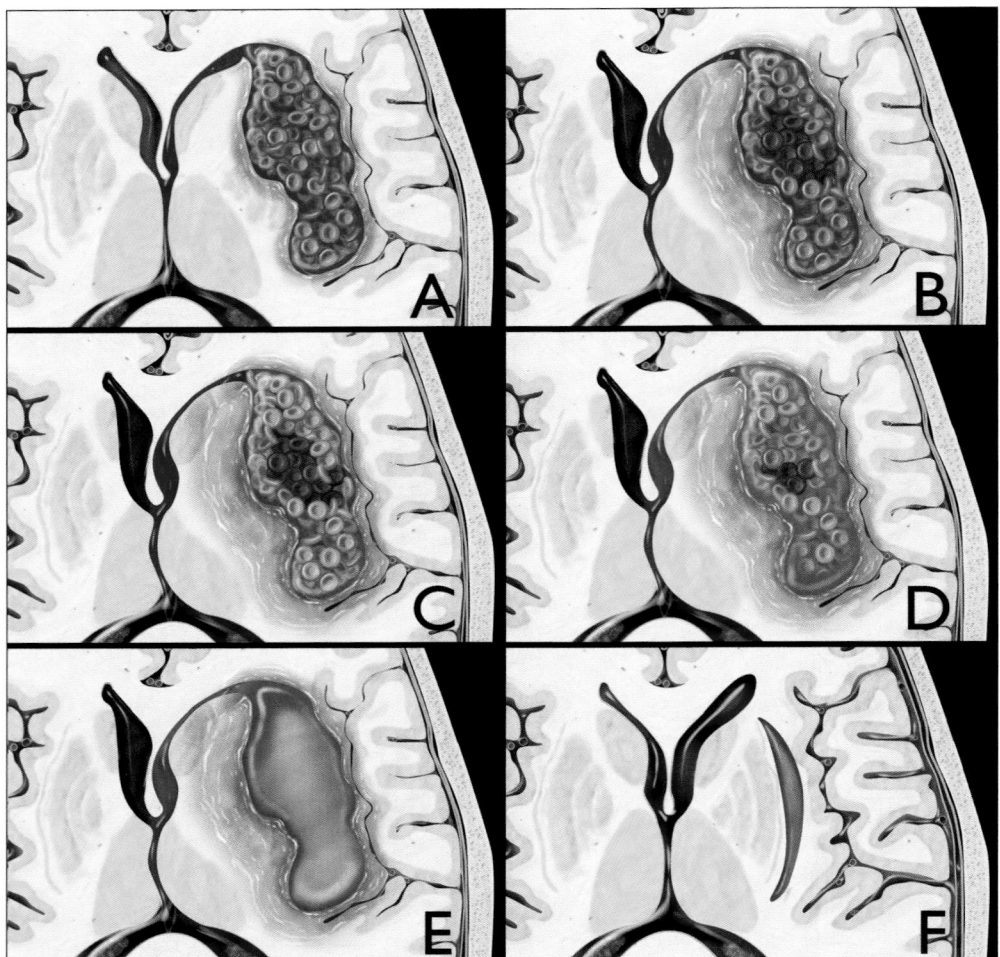

5-1. *(A) Hyperacute hemorrhage is a water-rich clot that is 95-98% oxy-Hgb. (B) Acute hemorrhage contains mostly oxy-Hgb. Some RBCs in the intensely hypoxic clot center may contain deoxy-Hgb. (C) Early subacute clots contain deoxy-Hgb in the center, intracellular met-Hgb in the periphery. (D) Late subacute clots contain mostly extracellular met-Hgb. (E) Chronic clots contain a yellowish pool of extracellular met-Hgb surrounded by a hemosiderin rim. (F) Only a slit-like scar remains.*

Overview of Primary ICH

We begin this chapter with a discussion of the pathophysiology of intracranial hemorrhage. This provides the basis for considering how pICH looks on imaging studies and why its appearance changes over time. We then consider some major causes of spontaneous ICH such as hypertension and amyloid angiopathy.

Solitary lesions comprise the vast majority of pICHs. The presence of more than one simultaneous *macro*scopic brain bleed is actually quite uncommon, accounting for just 2-3% of all pICHs. Multifocal brain *micro*bleeds are much more common. We therefore conclude this chapter with a discussion of multifocal brain microbleeds, their etiology, pathology, imaging appearance, and differential diagnosis.

Evolution of Intracranial Hemorrhage

Pathophysiology of Intracranial Hemorrhage

Clot Formation

Clot formation is a complex physiological event that involves both cellular (mainly platelet) and soluble protein components. Platelets are activated by vascular injury and aggregate at the injured site. Soluble proteins are activated by both intrinsic and extrinsic arms that merge into a common coagulation pathway, resulting in a fibrin clot.

Hemoglobin Degradation

Hemoglobin (Hgb) is composed of four protein (globin) subunits. Each subunit contains a heme molecule with an iron atom surrounded by a porphyrin ring.

Hgb within red blood cells (RBCs) that are extravasating into a pICH rapidly desaturates. Fully oxygenated Hgb (oxy-Hgb) contains nonparamagnetic ferrous iron. In a hematoma, oxy-Hgb is initially converted to deoxyhemoglobin (deoxy-Hgb).

With time, deoxy-Hgb is metabolized to methemoglobin (met-Hgb), which contains ferric iron. As red blood cells lyse, met-Hgb is released and eventually degraded and resorbed. Macrophages convert the ferric iron into hemosiderin and ferritin.

Ferritin is the major source of non-heme iron deposition in the human brain. Although iron is essential for normal brain function, iron overload may have devastating effects. Lipid peroxidation and free radical formation promote oxidative brain injury after ICH that may continue for weeks or months.

Stages of Intraparenchymal Hemorrhage

Five general stages in temporal evolution of hematomas are recognized: Hyperacute, acute, early subacute, late subacute, and chronic. Each has its own features that depend on three key factors: (1) clot structure, (2) red blood cell integrity, and (3) hemoglobin oxygenation status. In turn, imaging findings depend on hematoma stage (5-1), (Table 5-1).

Hematomas consist of two distinct regions: A central core and a peripheral rim or boundary. In general, hemoglobin degradation begins in the clot periphery and progresses centrally toward the core.

HYPERACUTE HEMORRHAGE. Hyperacute hemorrhage is minutes to under 24 hours old. Most imaged hyperacute hemorrhages are generally between four and six but less than 24 hours old. Initially, a loose fibrin clot that contains plasma, platelets, and intact red blood cells is formed. At this stage, diamagnetic intracellular oxyhemoglobin predominates in the hematoma.

In early clots, intact erythrocytes interdigitate with surrounding brain at the hematoma-tissue interface. Edema forms around the hematoma within hours after onset and is associated with mass effect, elevated intracranial pressure, and secondary brain injury.

ACUTE HEMORRHAGE. Acute ICH is defined as between one to three days old. Profound hypoxia within the center of the clot induces the transformation of oxy-Hgb to deoxy-Hgb. Iron in deoxy-Hgb is paramagnetic because it has four unpaired electrons.

Deoxyhemoglobin is paramagnetic, but as long as it remains within intact red cells, it is shielded from direct dipole-dipole interactions with water protons in the extracellular plasma. At this stage, magnetic susceptibility is induced primarily because of differences between the microenvironments inside and outside of the RBCs.

EARLY SUBACUTE HEMORRHAGE. Early subacute hemorrhage is defined as a clot that is from three days to one week old. Hemoglobin remains contained within intact RBCs. Hemoglobin at the hypoxic center of the clot persists as deoxy-Hgb. The periphery of the clot ages more rapidly and therefore contains intracellular met-Hgb. Intracellular met-Hgb is highly paramagnetic, but the intact RBC membrane prevents direct dipole-dipole interactions.

A cellular perihematomal inflammatory response develops. Microglial activation occurs as immune cells infiltrate the parenchyma surrounding the clot.

LATE SUBACUTE HEMORRHAGE. Late subacute hemorrhage lasts from one to several weeks. As RBCs lyse, met-Hgb becomes extracellular. Met-Hgb is now exposed directly to plasma water, reducing T1 relaxation time and prolonging the T2 relaxation time.

Imaging the Stages of Intraparenchymal Hemorrhage

Stage	Time (Range)	Blood Products	CT	T1	T2	T2*	DWI
Hyperacute	< 24 hours	Oxy-Hgb	Hyperdense	Isointense	Bright	Rim "blooms"	+
Acute	1-3 days	Deoxy-Hgb	Hyperdense	Isointense	Dark	↑ "blooming"	+
Early subacute	> 3 days to 1 week	Intracellular met-Hgb	Isodense	Bright	Dark	Very dark	+
Late subacute	1 week to months	Extracellular met-Hgb	Hypodense	Bright	Bright	Dark rim, variable center	-
Chronic	> 14 d (≥ months)	Hemosiderin	Hypodense	Dark	Dark	Dark	-

Table 5-1. *Deoxy-Hgb = deoxyhemoglobin; met-Hgb = methemoglobin; oxy-Hgb = oxygenated hemoglobin.*

5-2A. *NECT in a hypertensive patient shows a large heterogeneous hematoma in the left cerebellar hemisphere* ➡ *and a smaller, much less hyperdense clot in the right cerebellum* ➡. *Findings are consistent with a hyperacute (loose, largely unretracted) clot.* *5-2B.* *The patient suddenly deteriorated while still in the scanner. Repeat NECT scan now shows additional hemorrhage* ➡. *The patient died shortly after this scan was performed.*

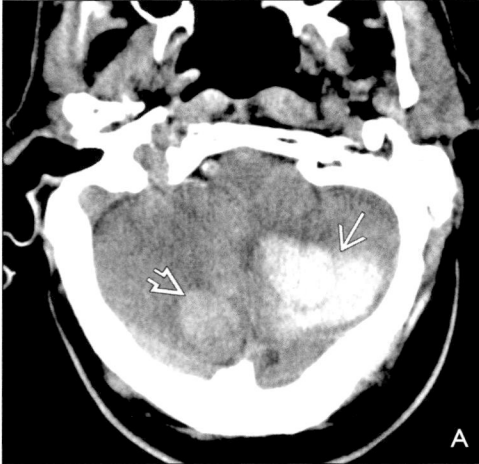

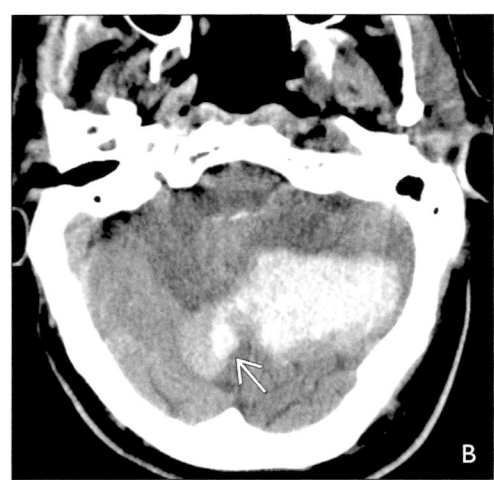

5-3A. *An adolescent male with acute myelogenous leukemia presented with acute onset of visual symptoms. Emergent NECT scan shows no abnormalities. Shortly after the scan was performed, sudden rapid clinical deterioration prompted MR.* *5-3B.* *T1WI obtained within minutes shows an ill-defined bifrontal mass* ➔ *that appears isointense with gray matter.*

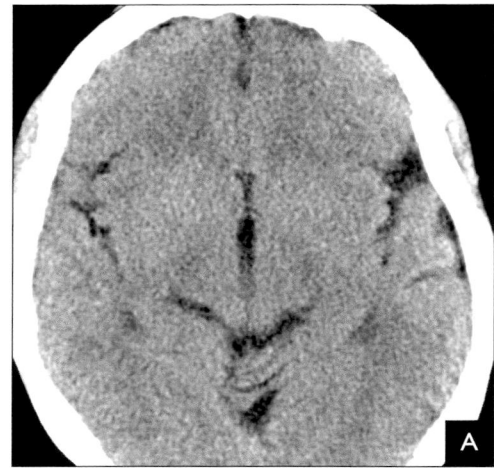

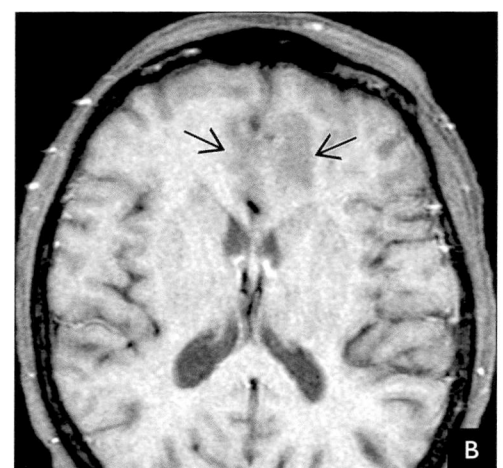

5-3C. *Obtained 5 minutes later, T2WI scan shows a mixed hypo-/iso-/hyperintense mass* ➡ *with fluid-fluid levels* ➡, *suggesting rapid bleeding.* *5-3D.* *The patient became decerebrate minutes after the MR was completed. Repeat NECT scan shows massive bifrontal mixed-density hemorrhage with diffuse brain swelling. Findings are those of hyperacute hemorrhage with rapid bleeding and underlying coagulopathy.*

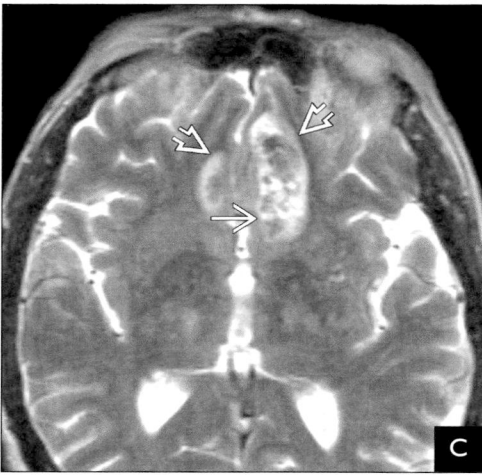

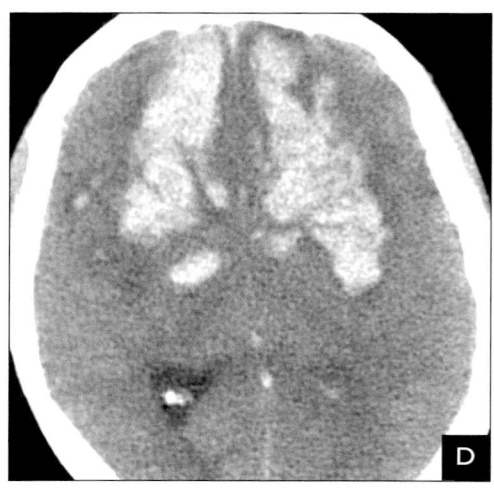

CHRONIC HEMORRHAGE. Parenchymal hemorrhagic residua persist for months to years. Heme proteins are phagocytized and stored as ferritin in macrophages. If the capacity to store ferritin is exceeded, excess iron is stored as hemosiderin. Intracellular ferritin and hemosiderin induce strong magnetic susceptibility.

Imaging of Intracranial Parenchymal Hemorrhage

The role of imaging in spontaneous ICH (sICH) is first to identify the presence and location of a clot (the easy part), to "age" the clot (harder), and then to detect other findings that may be clues to its etiology (the more difficult, demanding part).

The appearance of pICH on CT depends on just one factor, electron density. In turn, the electron density of a clot depends almost entirely on its protein concentration, primarily the globin moiety of hemoglobin. Iron and other metals contribute less than 0.5% to total clot attenuation and so have no visible effect on hematoma density.

In contrast, the imaging appearance of intracranial hemorrhage on MR is more complex and depends on a number of factors. Both intrinsic and extrinsic factors contribute to imaging appearance.

Intrinsic biologic factors that influence hematoma signal intensity are primarily related to macroscopic clot structure, red blood cell integrity, and hemoglobin oxygenation status. RBC concentration, tissue pH, arterial versus venous source of the bleed, intracellular protein concentration, and the presence and integrity of the blood-brain barrier also contribute to the imaging appearance of an intracranial hemorrhage.

Extrinsic factors include pulse sequence, sequence parameters, receiver bandwidth, and field strength of the magnet. Of these, pulse sequence and field strength are the most important determinants. T1- and T2-weighted images are the most helpful in estimating lesion age. T2* (GRE, SWI) is the most sensitive sequence in detecting hemorrhages (especially microhemorrhages).

Field strength also affects imaging appearance of ICH. The MR findings delineated below and in Table 5-1 are

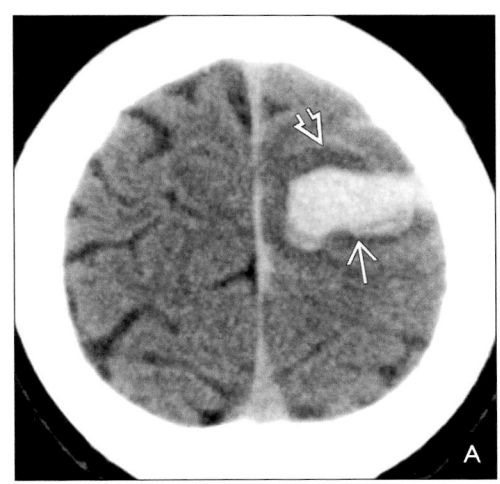
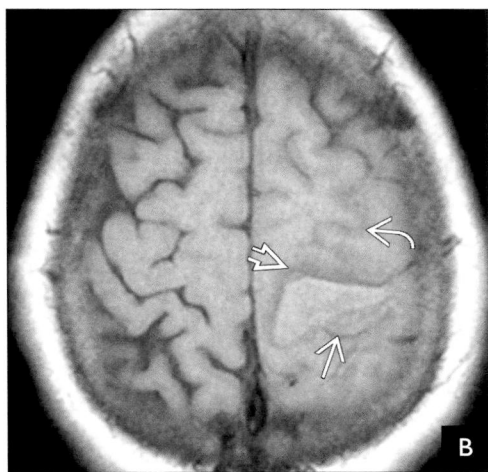

5-4A. NECT scan in a 45-year-old man shows acute pICH. A uniformly hyperdense clot ⇨ is surrounded by a small rim of hypodense edema ⇒.
5-4B. Because of the patient's age and normotensive status, MR was obtained to look for underlying pathology. T1WI shows that the hematoma itself is intermediate in signal intensity ⇨ and is surrounded by a rim of hypointense vasogenic edema ⇒. Note mass effect with adjacent sulcal effacement ⇨.

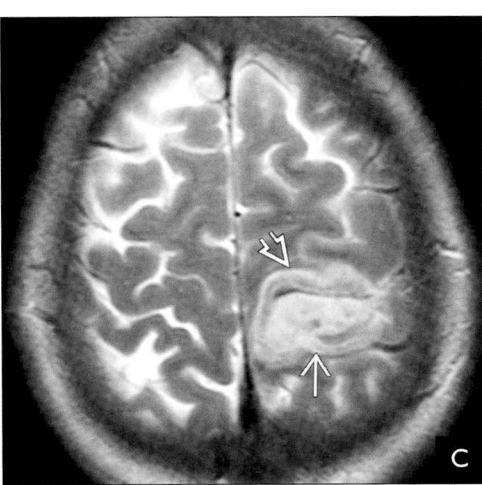
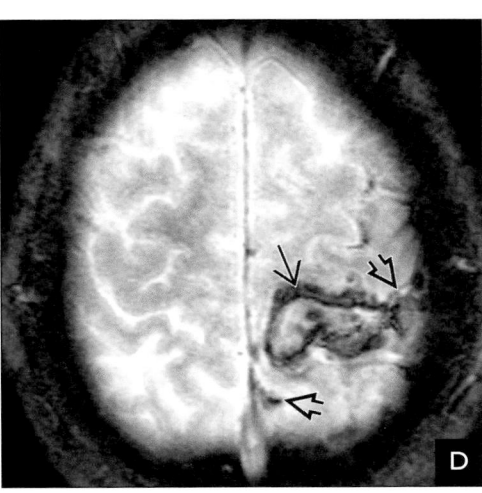

5-4C. T2WI shows that the clot is heterogeneously hyperintense ⇨ and is surrounded by hyperintense vasogenic edema ⇒. 5-4D. T2 GRE scan shows "blooming" around the periphery of the clot ⇨. Tubular hypointensity in adjacent cortical veins ⊳ suggests venous thrombosis.*

5-5A. T1WI obtained 4 days following ictus in a young patient with a spontaneous parenchymal ICH. The clot is mostly hyperintense ➡. 5-5B. The clot ➡ is profoundly hypointense on T2WI. The T1-T2 "bright-dark" appearance is consistent with late acute/early subacute hemorrhage. DSA (not shown) disclosed a mostly thrombosed arteriovenous malformation.

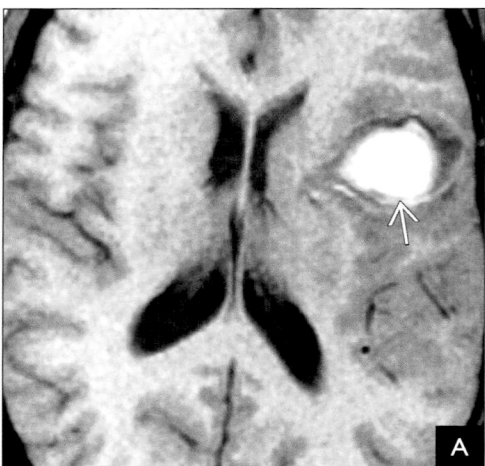
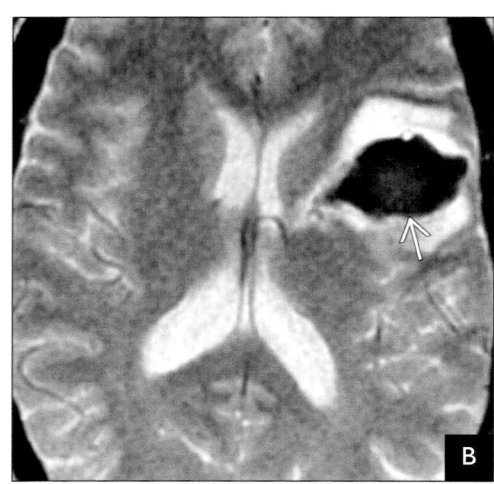

5-6A. Axial NECT scan in a patient with an acute lobar hypertensive hemorrhage shows relatively uniform hyperdense clot in the left parietal lobe ➡. 5-6B. Follow-up NECT scan was obtained 1 week later. Clot density has decreased significantly, especially around the periphery.

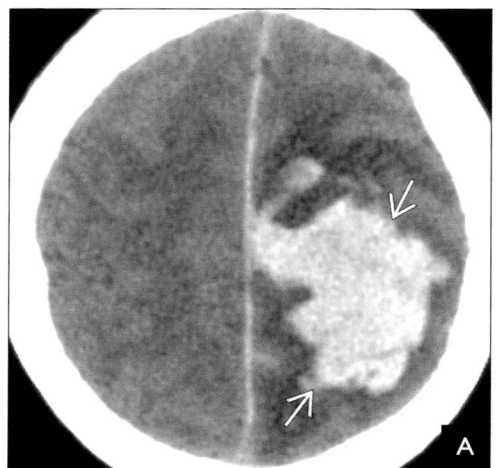
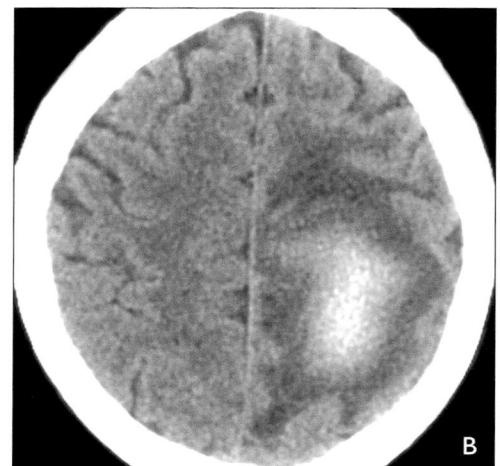

5-6C. MR scan was obtained immediately after the follow-up CT scan. T1WI shows the hematoma is hyperintense around the rim ➡, nearly isointense in the center ▷. 5-6D. T2WI shows that the clot is now mostly hyperintense ➡. A small area of lesser hyperintensity persists in the center, and a rim of hypointensity ➡ is beginning to appear around the periphery of the clot. Findings are consistent with late subacute hematoma.

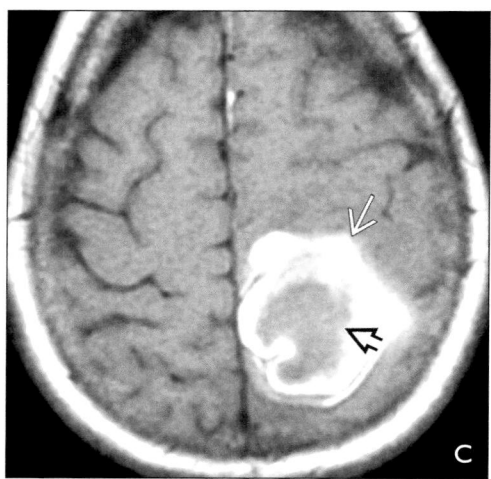
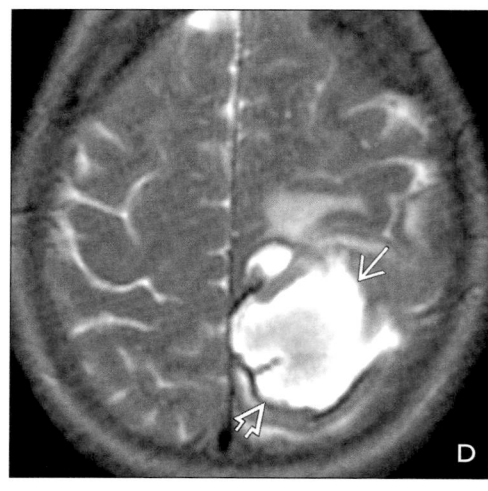

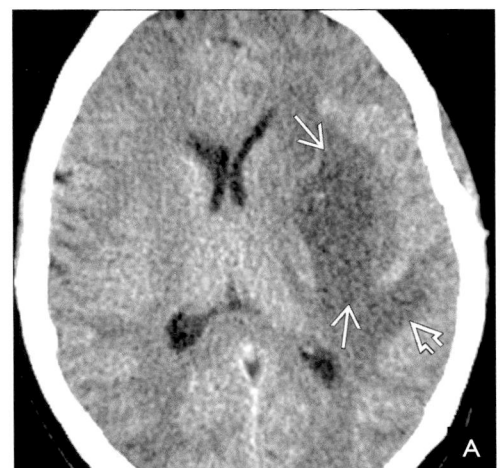

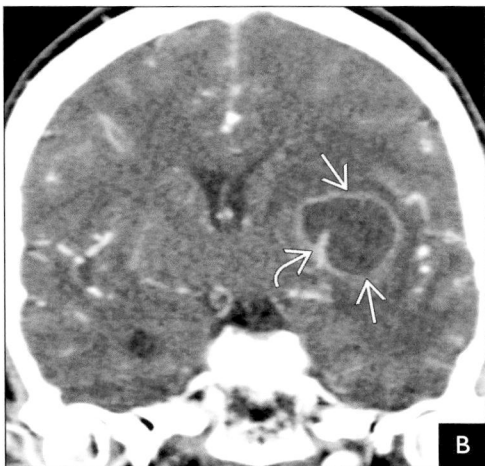

5-7A. *NECT scan in a hypertensive patient with striatocapsular hemorrhage 6 weeks prior to readmission to the hospital with headache shows a well-demarcated hypodense left putaminal/external capsule lesion* ➡ *with mass effect, edema* ⇉. **5-7B.** *CTA with coronal reformatted image shows enhancement around the periphery of the lesion* ⇉. *A linear enhancing focus* ➡ *within the resolving hematoma suggests a vascular structure.*

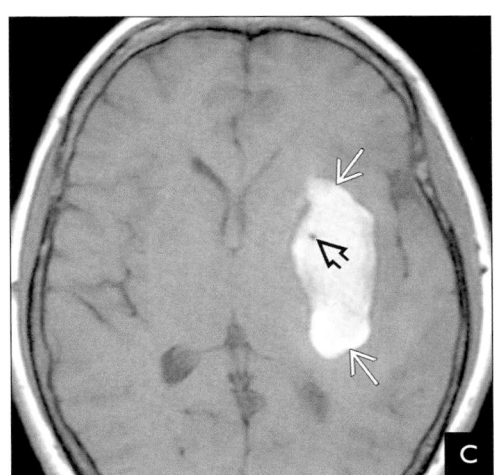

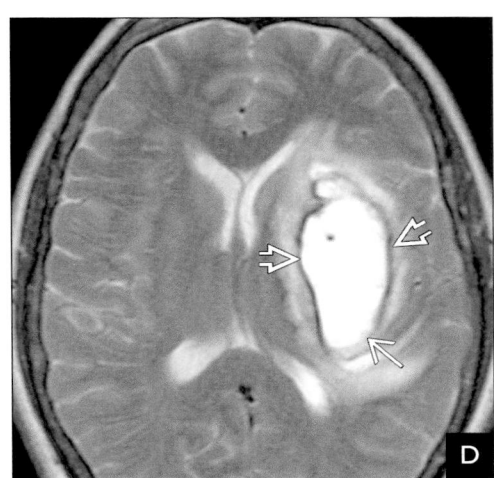

5-7C. *T1WI in the same patient shows an almost uniformly hyperintense late subacute hematoma* ➡ *with a central hypointensity* ⇉ *in the same region as the enhancing vessel seen on the CTA.* **5-7D.** *T2WI shows characteristics of late subacute hematoma with uniformly hyperintense fluid* ➡ *surrounded by a hypointense hemosiderin rim* ⇉.

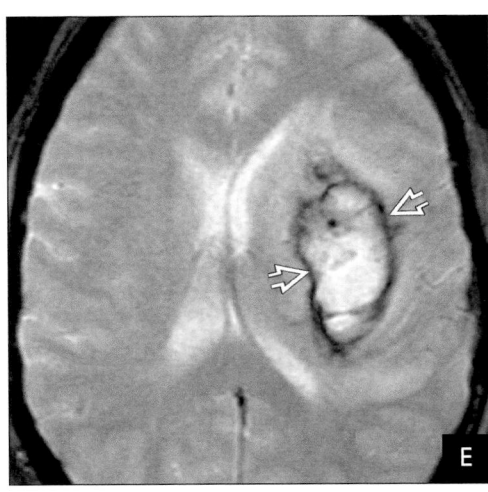

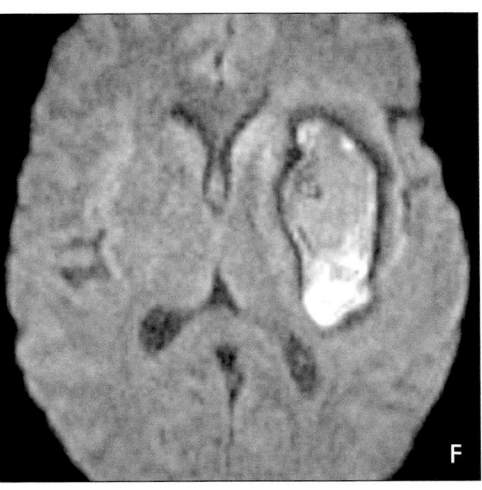

5-7E. *T2* GRE scan shows "blooming" around the rim of the clot* ⇉ *while the center is heterogeneously hyperintense.* **5-7F.** *DWI in the same patient shows no diffusion restriction; hyperintensity in the inferior portion of the clot is T2 "shine-through." Imaging findings are characteristic of a late subacute hypertensive hemorrhage with presumed remnant of "bleeding globe" lenticulostriate pseudoaneurysm.*

Hyperacute Hemorrhage

CT. If ICH is imaged within a few minutes of the ictus, the clot is loose, poorly organized, and largely unretracted **(5-2)**. Water content is still high, so a hyperacute hematoma may appear iso- or sometimes even hypodense relative to adjacent brain **(5-3A)**. If active hemorrhage is present, the presence of both clotted and unclotted blood results in a mixed-density hematoma with hypodense and mildly hyperdense components **(5-3D)**. Rapid bleeding and coagulopathy may result in fluid-fluid levels.

MR. Oxy-Hgb has no unpaired electrons and is diamagnetic. Therefore, signal intensity of a hyperacute clot depends mostly on its water content. Hyperacute clots are iso- to slightly hypointense on T1WI **(5-3B)**. Within minutes after hemorrhage begins, deoxy-Hgb begins to form around the clot periphery. A hyperacute clot generally has a hypointense rim and an iso- to slightly hyper-

calculated for 1.5 T scanners. At 3.0 T, all parts of acute and early subacute clots have significantly increased hypointensity on FLAIR and T2WI.

intense center (where oxy-Hgb still predominates) on T2 scans. **(5-3C)**.

Because the macroscopic structure of a hyperacute clot is so inhomogeneous, spin dephasing results in heterogeneous hypointensity ("blooming") on T2* sequences.

Acute Hemorrhage

CT. The hematocrit of a retracted clot approaches 90%. Therefore, an acute hematoma is usually hyperdense on NECT, typically measuring 60-80 HU **(5-4A)**. Exceptions to this general rule are found if hemorrhage occurs in extremely anemic patients with very low hematocrits or in patients with coagulopathies.

MR. Acute parenchymal hematomas are low to intermediate signal intensity on T1WI **(5-4B)**. Significant vasogenic edema develops around the clot and is hypointense on T1WI and hyperintense on T2/FLAIR **(5-4C)**. As the clot retracts, water content diminishes, and the hematoma becomes progressively less hyperintense on T2WI. The clot "ages" from outside to inside, so T2 hypointensity begins with its rim and gradually enlarges toward the cen-

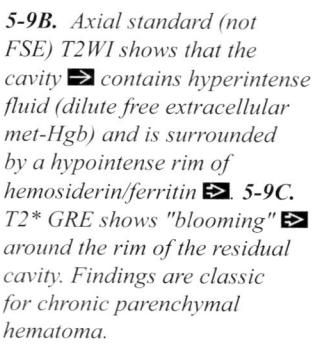
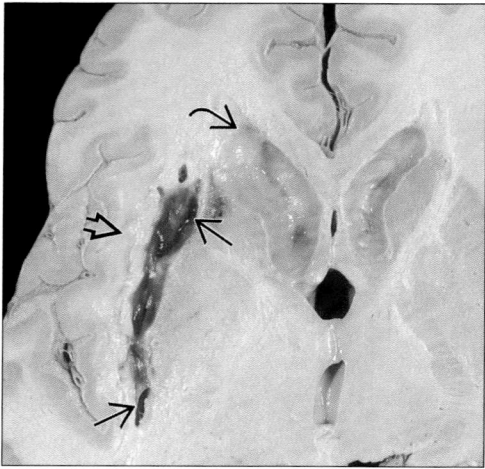
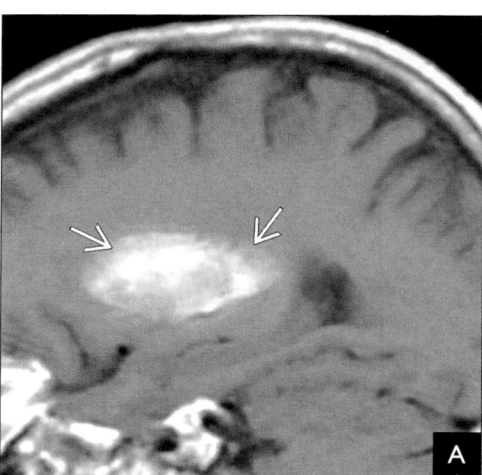
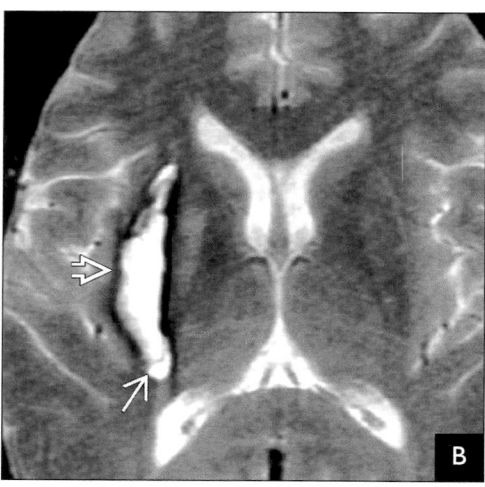
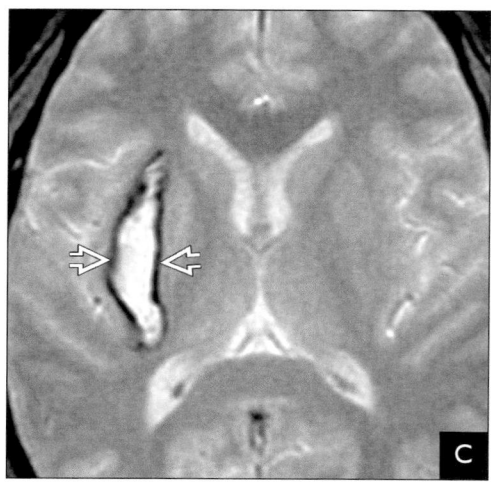

5-8. Gross autopsy case shows residua of remote striatocapsular hemorrhage. A slit-like cavity with a small amount of yellowish fluid is surrounded by dark hemosiderin staining ➡. Note volume loss with enlarged right frontal horn ➚, gliotic brain ➩ surrounding old hematoma. (Courtesy R. Hewlett, MD.) 5-9A. Sagittal T1WI in a patient 2 years following hypertensive hemorrhage shows ovoid hyperintense cavity ➡.

5-9B. Axial standard (not FSE) T2WI shows that the cavity ➡ contains hyperintense fluid (dilute free extracellular met-Hgb) and is surrounded by a hypointense rim of hemosiderin/ferritin ➩. 5-9C. T2 GRE shows "blooming" ➩ around the rim of the residual cavity. Findings are classic for chronic parenchymal hematoma.*

ter. Acute clots become progressively more hypointense on T2WI and "bloom" on T2* (GRE, SWI) **(5-4D)**.

Early Subacute Hemorrhage

CT. Hematoma density gradually decreases with time, beginning with the periphery of the clot. Clot attenuation diminishes by an average of 1.5 HU per day. At around seven to ten days, the outside of a pICH becomes isodense with the adjacent brain. The hyperdense center gradually shrinks, becoming less and less dense until the entire clot becomes hypodense. A subacute hematoma shows ring enhancement on CECT.

MR. Intracellular methemoglobin predominates around the clot periphery while deoxyhemoglobin persists within the center of the clot. A rim of T1 shortening (hyperintensity) surrounding an iso- to slightly hypointense core is the typical appearance on T1WI **(5-5A)**. Early subacute clots are generally hypointense on T2WI but are beginning to develop some hyperintensity around their rim **(5-5B)**. Profound hypointensity on T2* persists.

Late Subacute Hemorrhage

CT. With progressive aging, a pICH gradually becomes hypointense relative to adjacent brain on NECT scans **(5-6)**. Ring enhancement may persist for weeks up to two or three months **(5-7A)**, **(5-7B)**.

MR. Dilute free extracellular methemoglobin predominates at this stage of clot evolution. A late subacute hemorrhage is therefore typically hyperintense on both T1- and T2WI **(5-7C)**, **(5-7D)**, **(5-7E)**, **(5-7F)**. With the exception of minor susceptibility artifacts, late subacute clots appear similar on both 1.5 T and 3.0 T.

Chronic Hemorrhage

CT. A few very small healed hemorrhages **(5-8)** may become invisible on NECT scan. From 35-40% of chronic hematomas appear as a round or ovoid hypodense focus. Another 25% of patients develop slit-like hypodensities. Between 10-15% of healed hematomas calcify.

MR. Intracellular ferritin and hemosiderin are hypointense on both T1- and T2WI. A hyperintense cav-

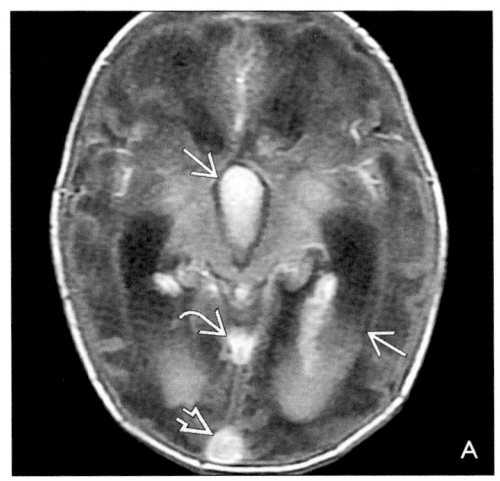
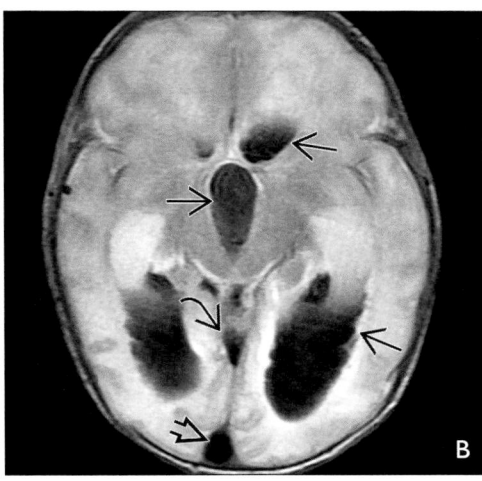

5-10A. Axial T1WI in a 34-week premature infant with sepsis shows hyperintense clot in the third and lateral ventricles → as well as thrombus in the straight sinus → and torcular herophili →. 5-10B. T2WI in the same patient shows the very hypointense acute blood within the ventricles → as well as an enlarged, thrombosed straight sinus → and venous sinus confluence →.

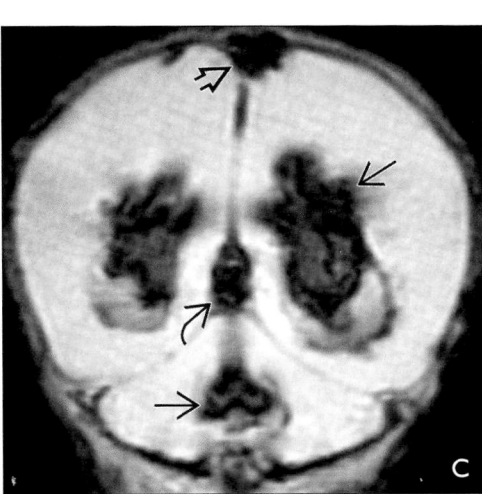
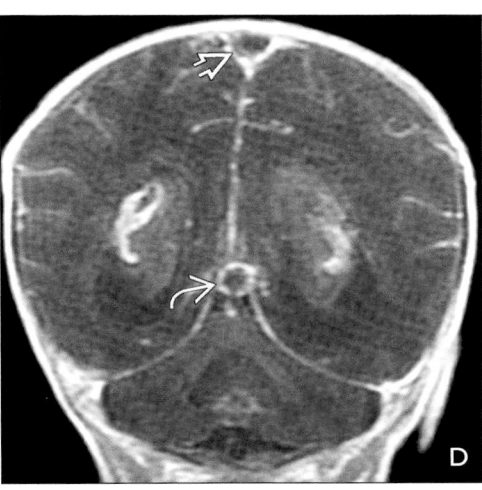

5-10C. Coronal T2 GRE scan shows "blooming" clot in both lateral ventricles and the fourth ventricle →. The superior sagittal sinus → and straight sinus → are thrombosed. 5-10D. Coronal T1 C+ scan shows the classic "empty delta" sign of dural sinus thrombosis in the superior sagittal → and straight sinuses →. In a term or near-term infant, dural venous sinus occlusion is the most common cause of intraventricular hemorrhage.*

ity surrounded by a "blooming" rim on T2* may persist for months or even years (5-9). Eventually, only a slit-like hypointense scar remains as evidence of a prior parenchymal hemorrhage.

Etiology of Nontraumatic Parenchymal Hemorrhages

There are many causes of nontraumatic ("spontaneous") or unexplained intracranial hemorrhage. The role of imaging in such cases is to localize the hematoma, estimate its age from its imaging features, and attempt to identify possible underlying causes.

The effect of age on the pathoetiology of sICH is profound. Knowing the patient's age is extremely important in establishing an appropriately narrowed differential diagnosis.

Patients with unexplained or atypical sICH on NECT may benefit from dual-energy CT, which can help distinguish between tumor bleeding and nonneoplastic ("pure") hemorrhage. Dual-energy CT can also help dif-

ferentiate ICH from extravasated contrast material staining.

MR imaging with standard sequences as well as fat-saturated contrast-enhanced scans can be very helpful. A T2* sequence (GRE and/or SWI) should always be included as the identification of other prior "silent" microhemorrhages affects both diagnosis and treatment decisions.

Newborns and Infants with sICH

ICH in the term newborn is most frequently associated with prolonged or precipitous delivery, traumatic instrumented delivery (e.g., forceps assistance or vacuum extraction), and primiparity. The most common cause of spontaneous ICH in *infants less than 34 gestational weeks* is **germinal matrix hemorrhage**.

The germinal matrix is a highly vascular, developmentally dynamic structure in the brain subventricular zone. The germinal matrix contains multiple cell types, including premigratory/migratory neurons, glia, and neural stem cells. Rupture of the relatively fragile germinal matrix capillaries may occur in response to altered cerebral blood flow, increased venous pres-

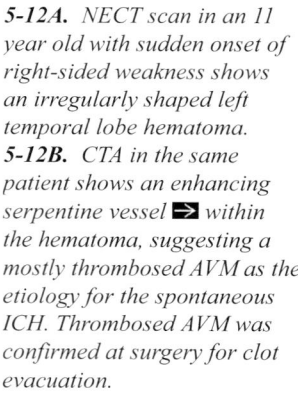

5-11A. NECT scan in a child with a family history of multiple cavernous malformations shows a small, solitary, calcified lesion in the right cerebral hemisphere ➡.
5-11B. Several weeks later, the child experienced sudden onset of severe headache and left-sided weakness. Acute rebleeding into the underlying cavernous malformation has produced a large parenchymal hematoma ➡.

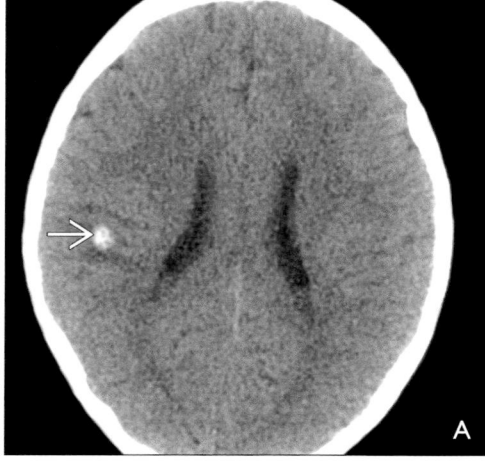

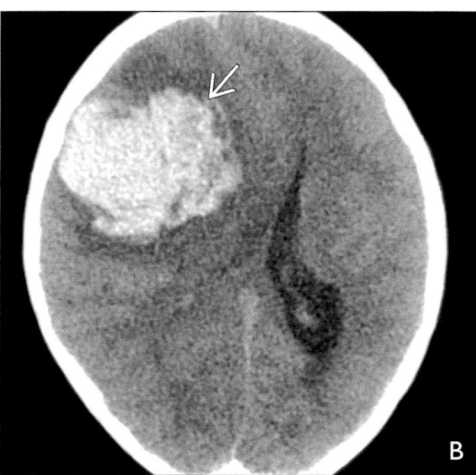

5-12A. NECT scan in an 11 year old with sudden onset of right-sided weakness shows an irregularly shaped left temporal lobe hematoma.
5-12B. CTA in the same patient shows an enhancing serpentine vessel ➡ within the hematoma, suggesting a mostly thrombosed AVM as the etiology for the spontaneous ICH. Thrombosed AVM was confirmed at surgery for clot evacuation.

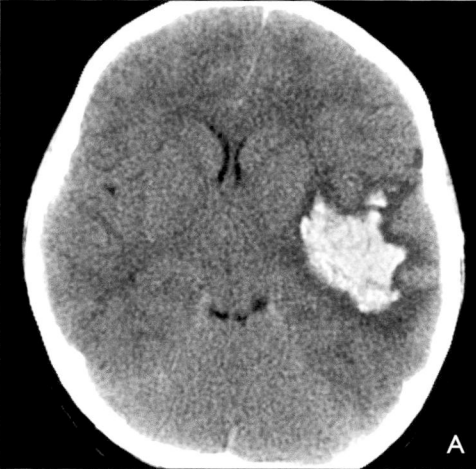

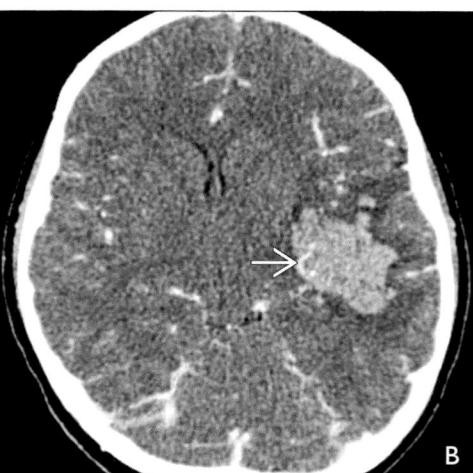

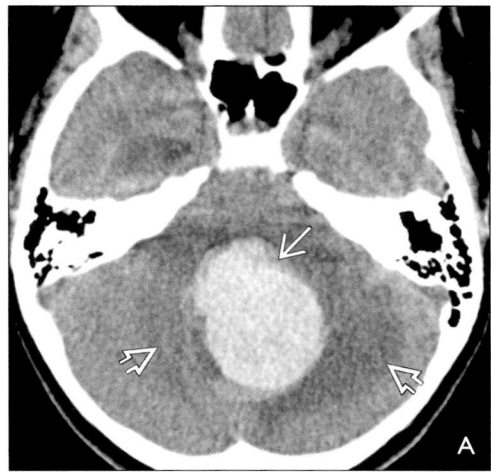

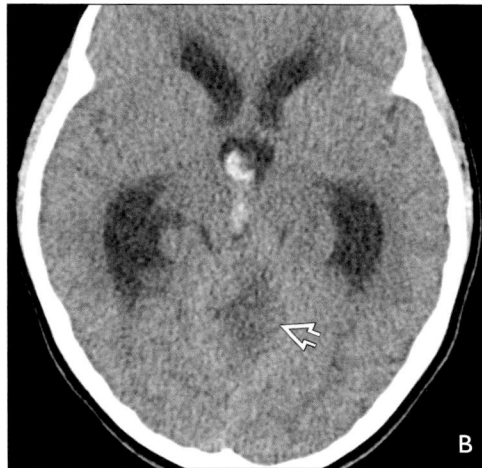

5-13A. *Axial NECT scan in a 10-year-old child with morning nausea and vomiting, sudden onset of severe headache, shows a large posterior fossa midline hemorrhage* ➡ *that involves the fourth ventricle and vermis. Moderate edema is seen in both cerebellar hemispheres* ⇨. **5-13B.** *Axial NECT scan in the same patient shows upward herniation of the edematous cerebellum* ⇨ *with acute obstructive hydrocephalus. Hemorrhagic pilocytic astrocytoma was found at surgery.*

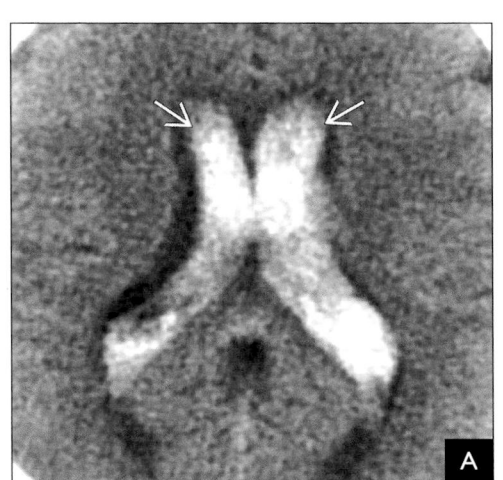

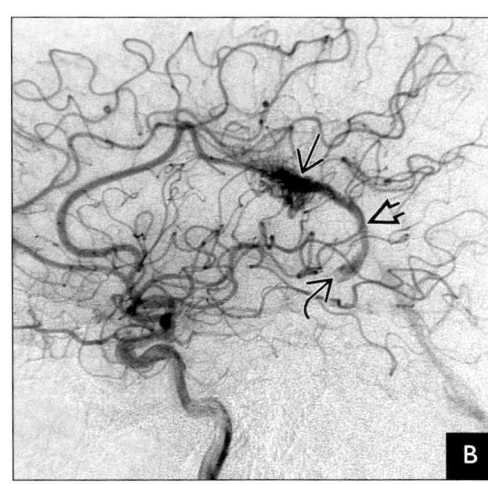

5-14A. *NECT scan in a young adult female with sudden severe headache followed by coma with no history of hypertension, drug abuse, or other predisposing factors. Both lateral ventricles are filled with acute clot* ➡. **5-14B.** *Lateral selective internal carotid DSA in the same patient shows a tangle of vessels* ➡ *in the cingulate gyrus with an "early draining vein"* ⇨ *and a contrast meniscus around a filling defect* ➔. *AVM with hemorrhage caused by draining vein occlusion.*

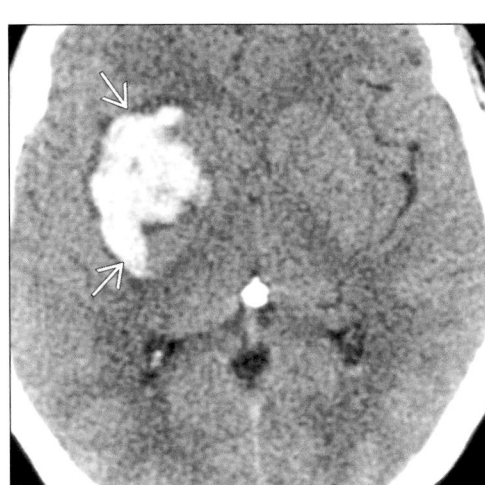

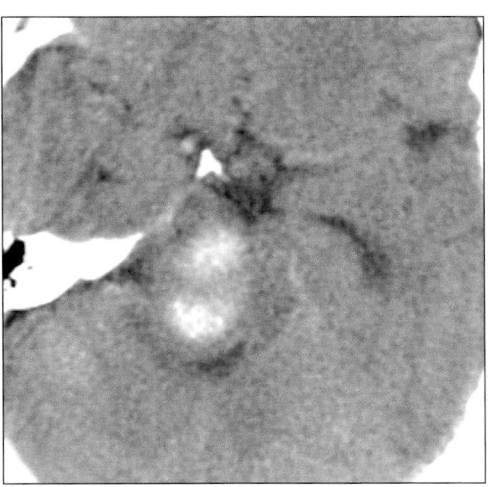

5-15. *NECT scan in a young adult with cocaine abuse, left-sided weakness, and altered mental status shows a classic hypertensive hemorrhage in the right putamen/external capsule* ➡. **5-16.** *NECT scan in another young patient with cocaine abuse and sudden onset of multiple cranial neuropathies shows a hypertensive hemorrhage in the upper pons and midbrain.*

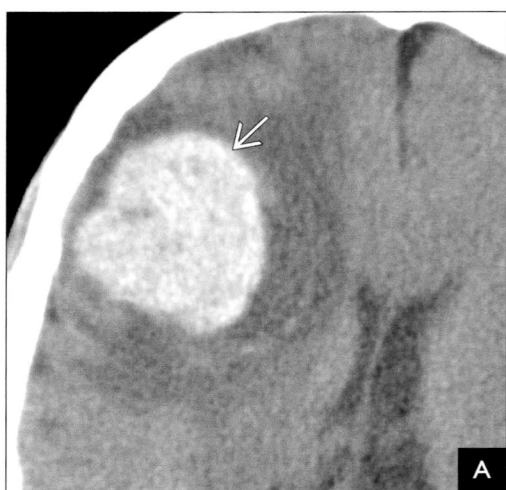

5-17A. NECT scan in an elderly normotensive patient with sudden headache, left hemiparesis. Note spontaneous right frontal ICH ➡.

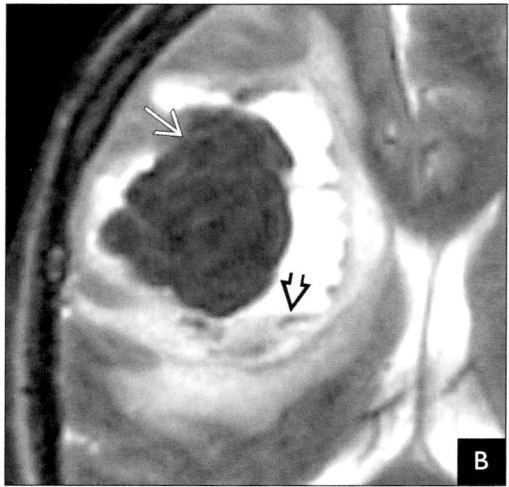

5-17B. Axial T2WI shows that the mass is mostly hypointense ➡ but has a definite fluid-fluid level ➡.

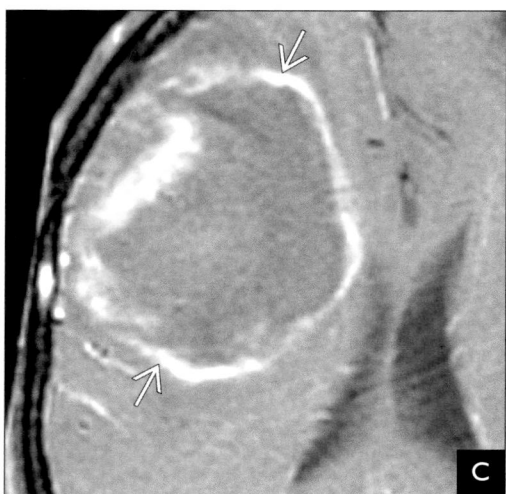

5-17C. T1 C+ scan shows irregular rim enhancement ➡. Surgery disclosed glioblastoma multiforme.

sure (e.g., with delivery), coagulopathy, or hypoxic-ischemic injury. Germinal matrix hemorrhage is discussed in greater detail later in this section (Chapter 8).

Isolated choroid plexus and **isolated intraventricular hemorrhage** do not involve the germinal matrix. **White matter injury of prematurity** generally does not show evidence of hemorrhage ("blooming") on T2* imaging.

The most common nontraumatic cause of spontaneous intraventricular hemorrhage (IVH) in *neonates beyond 34 gestational weeks* is **dural venous sinus thrombosis** (DVST) **(5-10)**. In contrast to older children and adults in whom the transverse sinus is most commonly affected, the straight sinus (85%) and superior sagittal sinus (65%) are the most frequent locations in infants. Multisinus involvement is seen in 80% of cases. Thalamic and punctate white matter lesions are common in infants with DVST.

Children with sICH

The most common cause of sICH in children ages one to 18 years is an underlying **vascular malformation**. Vascular malformations are responsible for nearly half of spontaneous parenchymal hemorrhages in this age group **(5-11)**.

At least 25% of all arteriovenous malformations (AVMs) hemorrhage by the age of 15 years **(5-12)**. Cavernous malformations, especially familial cavernous malformations ("cavernomas"), are a less common but important cause of sICH in children.

Other less common but important causes of pediatric sICH include **hematological disorders** and **malignancies**, **vasculopathy**, and **venous occlusion/infarction**.

Primary neoplasms are a relatively rare cause of sICH in children **(5-13)**. Infratentorial tumors are more common than supratentorial neoplasms.

Posterior fossa neoplasms that frequently hemorrhage include ependymoma and rosette-forming glioneuronal tumor (RGNT). Patchy or petechial hemorrhage is more common than large intratumoral bleeds.

Supratentorial tumors with a propensity to bleed include ependymoma and the spectrum of primitive neuroectodermal tumors. Malignant astrocytomas with hemorrhage occur but are rare. In contrast to middle-aged and older adults, hemorrhagic metastases from extracranial primary cancers are *very* rare in children.

Young Adults with sICH

An underlying **vascular malformation** is the most common cause of sICH in young adults as well **(5-14)**. **Drug abuse** is the second most common cause of unexplained hemorrhage. Cocaine may induce extreme sys-

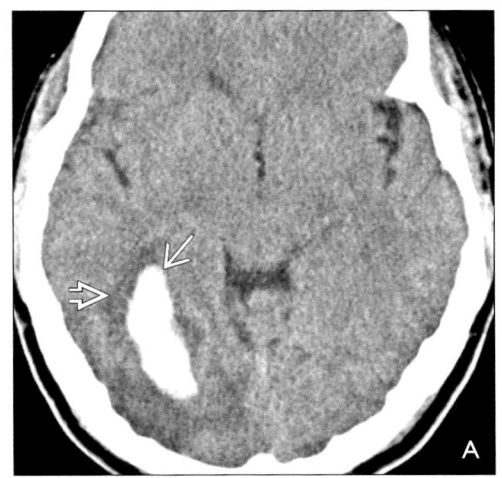 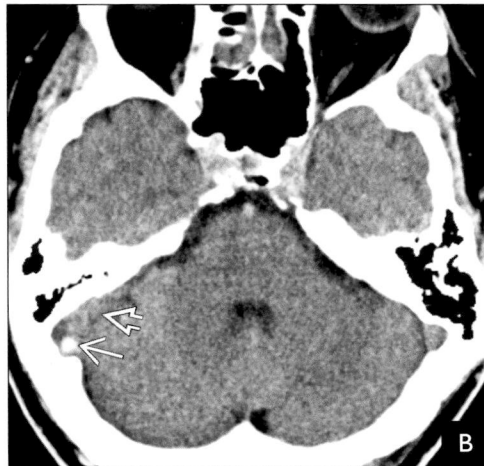

5-18A. *A 58 yo man had a severe headache 2 months prior to this scan. Outside NECT scan (not shown) was read as normal but had a hyperdense right transverse sinus. The patient came to the ED with worsening headache and acute onset of a left visual field defect. NECT scan shows right occipital parenchymal hematoma* ➡ *with mild edema* ➡. ***5-18B.** Posterior fossa NECT in the same case shows a round hyperdensity* ➡ *adjacent to an enlarged isodense right transverse sinus* ➡.

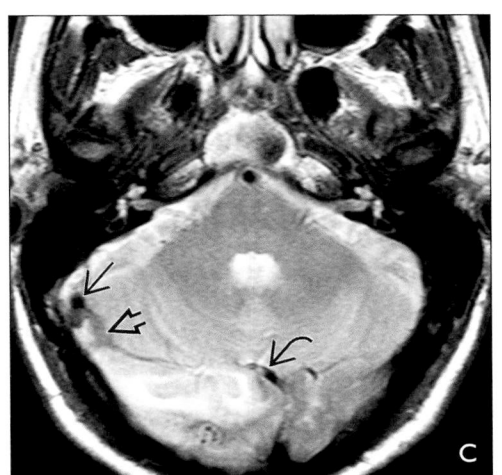 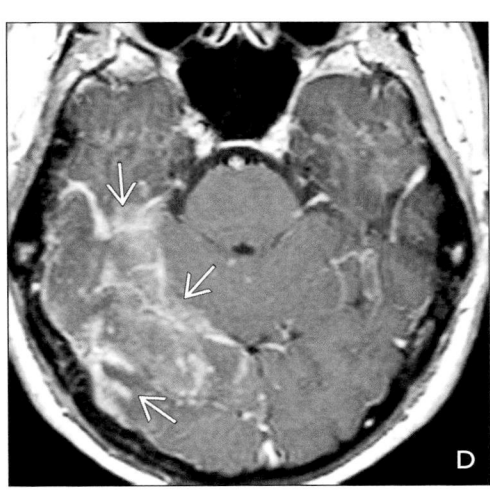

5-18C. *MR was obtained. Axial T2WI shows a round/ovoid hypointensity* ➡ *with what appears to be a thrombosed vessel* ➡. *Compare with the normal venous "flow void"* ➡. ***5-18D.** T1 C+ scan shows bizarre patchy, linear, and punctate enhancement in much of the posterior temporal and parietal lobes* ➡.

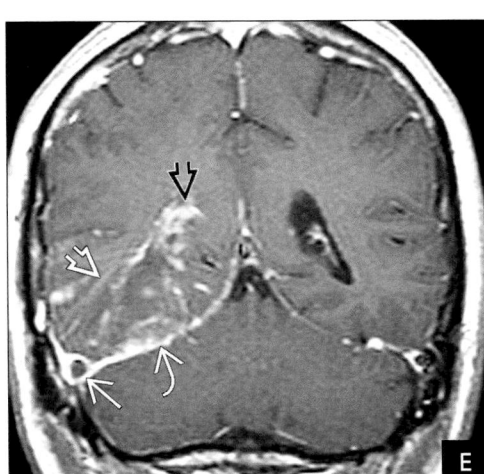 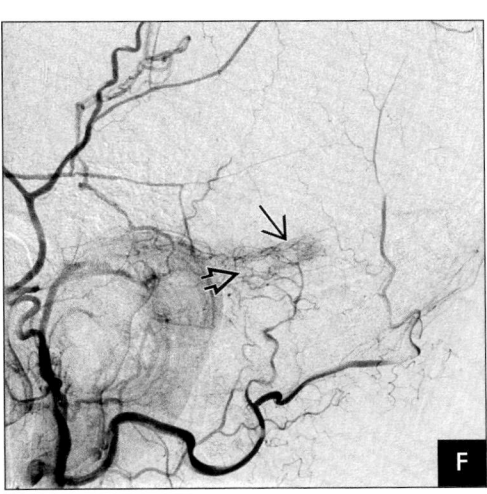

5-18E. *Coronal T1 C+ scan shows a thrombosed right TS* ➡ *("empty delta" sign). Bizarre enhancing vessels along the tentorium* ➡ *and in the occipital lobe* ➡ *represent venous stasis and retrograde venous drainage. Enlarged, intensely enhancing choroid plexus* ➡ *provides collateral venous drainage.* ***5-18F.** Lateral DSA shows a dAVF in the wall* ➡ *of the thrombosed left TS* ➡. *sICH was secondary to acute thrombosis of the outlet draining vein shown in Figure 5-18C.*

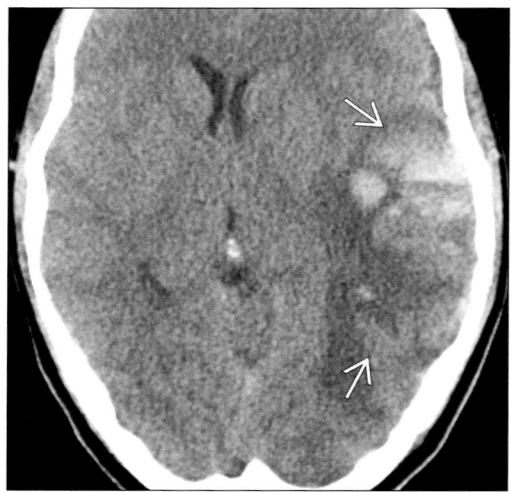

5-19. NECT scan in a 23 yo woman with headaches shows left temporoparietal hemorrhage ➡. CTV demonstrated occluded TS, vein of Labbé.

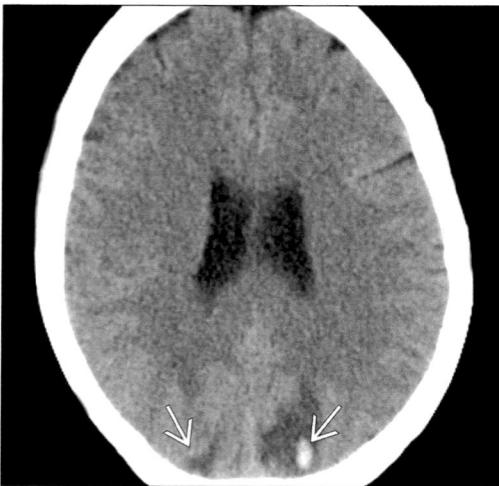

5-20. A 22 yo eclamptic woman has occipital lesions ➡ with edema and hemorrhage. Posterior reversible encephalopathy syndrome (PRES).

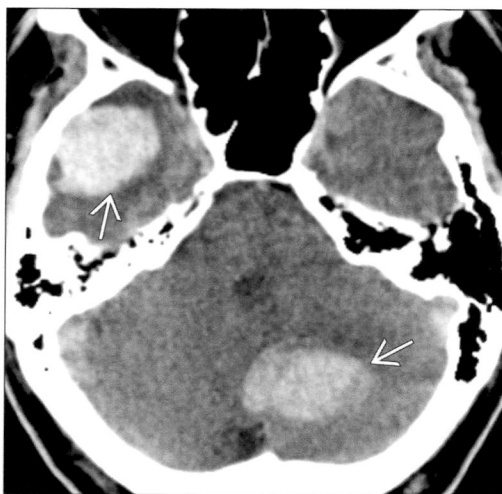

5-21. Axial NECT scan in an elderly patient with known renal cell carcinoma shows multiple hemorrhagic metastases ➡.

temic hypertension, resulting in a putaminal-external capsule bleed that looks identical to those seen in older hypertensive adults **(5-15)**, **(5-16)**.

Venous occlusion/infarction with or without **dural sinus occlusion** is also relatively common in this age group, especially in young women taking oral contraceptives. Severe **eclampsia/preeclampsia** with posterior reversible encephalopathy syndrome (PRES) may cause multifocal posterior cortical and subcortical hemorrhages.

Vasculitis occasionally causes pICH in young adults. Hemorrhagic neoplasms (both primary and metastatic) are rare.

SOLITARY SPONTANEOUS pICH

Newborns and Infants
- Common
  - Germinal matrix hemorrhage (< 34 gestational weeks)
  - Dural venous sinus thrombosis (≥ 34 gestational weeks)
- Rare
  - Congenital prothrombotic disorder
  - Thrombocytopenia
  - Hemophilia
  - Vitamin K deficiency bleeding

Children
- Common
  - Vascular malformations (~ 50%)
- Less common
  - Hematologic disorder
  - Vasculopathy
  - Venous infarct
- Rare
  - Primary neoplasm

Young Adults
- Common
  - Vascular malformation
  - Drug abuse
- Less common
  - Venous occlusion
  - PRES (eclampsia, preeclampsia)
- Rare
  - Neoplasm (primary, metastatic)
  - Vasculitis

Middle-aged and Elderly Adults
- Common
  - Hypertension
  - Amyloid angiopathy
  - Neoplasm (primary, metastatic)
- Less common
  - Venous infarct
  - Coagulopathy
- Rare
  - Aneurysm (usually anterior communicating artery)
  - Vascular malformation (usually dAVF)
  - Vasculitis

Middle-aged and Elderly Adults with sICH

The two most common causes of sICH in middle-aged and elderly patients are **hypertension** and **amyloid angiopathy**, both of which are discussed in detail below. Approximately 10% of spontaneous parenchymal hemorrhages are caused by bleeding into a brain **neoplasm**, generally either a high-grade primary tumor such as glioblastoma multiforme (5-17) or hemorrhagic metastasis from an extracranial primary such as renal cell carcinoma.

A less common but important cause of sICH in this age group is **venous infarct**. Venous infarcts are caused by cortical vein thrombosis, with or without dural sinus occlusion (5-18). Iatrogenic **coagulopathy** is also common in elderly patients as many take maintenance doses of warfarin for atrial fibrillation.

Occasionally a ruptured **saccular aneurysm** presents with a focal lobar hemorrhage rather than a subarachnoid hemorrhage. The most common source is an anterior communicating artery aneurysm that projects superolaterally and ruptures into the frontal lobe.

Underlying **vascular malformation** is a relatively rare cause of sICH in older patients. With a 2-4% per year cumulative rupture risk, a first-time AVM bleed at this age can occur but is unusual. So is hemorrhage from a cavernous malformation. However, **dural arteriovenous fistulas (dAVFs)** *do* occur in middle-aged and elderly patients. While dAVFs rarely hemorrhage unless they have cortical venous (not just dural sinus) drainage, spontaneous thrombosis of the outlet veins may result in sudden ICH.

Rare but important causes of sICH in this age group include **vasculitis** (more common in younger patients) and **acute hemorrhagic leukoencephalopathy**.

Multiple sICHs

Solitary spontaneous parenchymal hemorrhages are much more common than multifocal bleeds. Etiology varies with patient age.

Multifocal brain bleeds that occur at all ages include venous thrombosis (5-19), PRES (5-20), vasculitis (especially fungal), septic emboli, thrombotic microangiopathy, and acute hemorrhagic leukoencephalopathy.

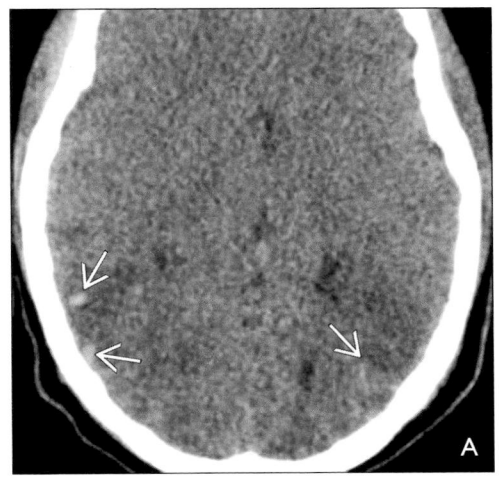

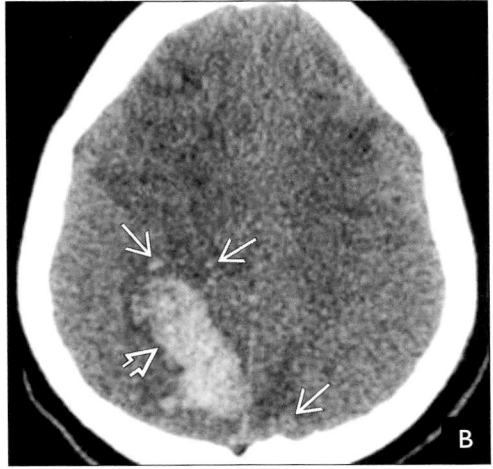

5-22A. NECT scan in a pregnant female with HELLP syndrome (hemolysis, elevated liver enzymes, low platelets) and thrombocytopenia shows bioccipital edema and multiple peripherally located small hemorrhages ➡. *5-22B.* More cephalad scan shows a single macro- ➡ and multiple microhemorrhages ➡.

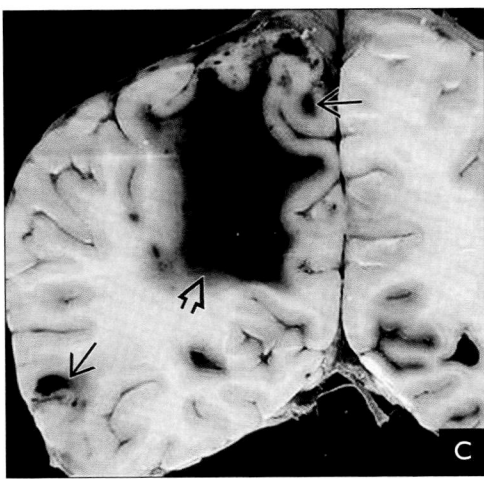

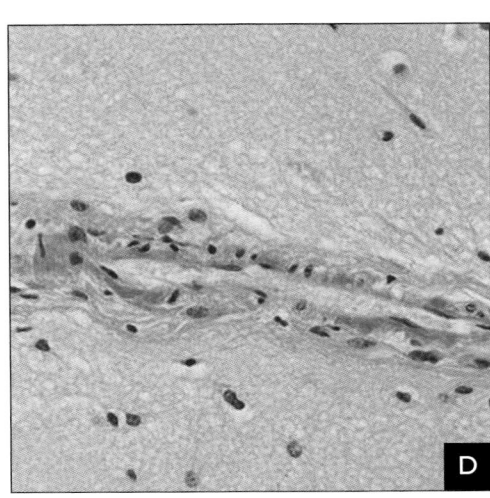

5-22C. The patient died. Coronal gross autopsy shows the gross hematoma ➡ as well as numerous small microbleeds ➡. *5-22D.* H&E microscopy shows intravascular fibrin deposition and fibrinoid necrosis of a brain arteriole. (Courtesy R. Hewlett, MD.)

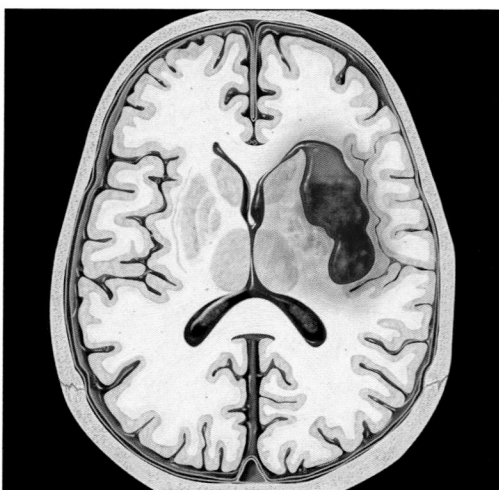

5-23. Graphic depicts acute hypertensive striatocapsular hemorrhage with edema, dissection into the lateral and third ventricles.

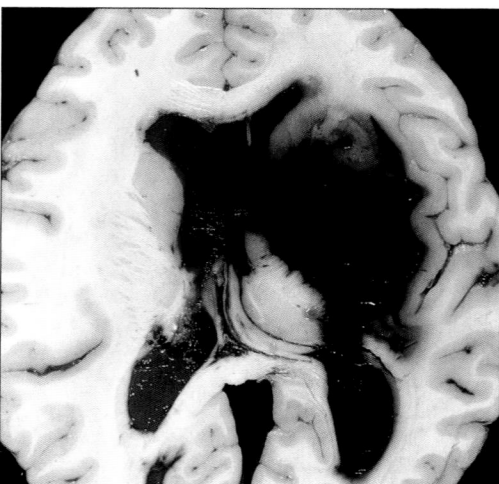

5-24. Autopsy demonstrates acute hypertensive ganglionic hemorrhage with intraventricular hemorrhage. (Courtesy R. Hewlett, MD.)

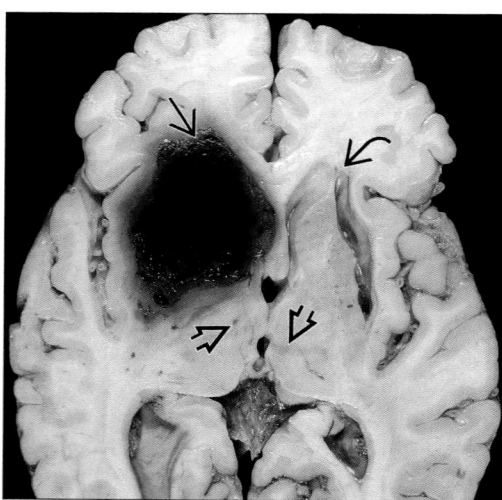

5-25. Autopsy shows acute ➡ and chronic ➔ hICH, together with several small old ganglionic microhemorrhages ➢. (Courtesy R. Hewlett, MD.)

Multiple *nontraumatic* brain bleeds in children and young adults are most often caused by multiple cavernous malformations and hematologic disorders (e.g., leukemia, thrombocytopenia) **(5-22)**.

The most common causes of multiple ICHs in middle-aged and older adults are hypertension, amyloid angiopathy, hemorrhagic metastases **(5-21)**, and impaired coagulation (either coagulopathy or anticoagulation).

MULTIPLE SPONTANEOUS ICHs

Children and Young Adults
- Multiple cavernous malformations
- Hematologic disorder/malignancy

Middle-aged and Older Adults
- Common
  - Chronic hypertension
  - Amyloid angiopathy
- Less common
  - Hemorrhagic metastases
  - Coagulopathy, anticoagulation

All Ages
- Common
  - Dural sinus thrombosis
  - Cortical vein occlusion
- Less common
  - PRES
  - Vasculitis
  - Septic emboli
- Rare but important
  - Thrombotic microangiopathy
  - Acute hemorrhagic leukoencephalopathy

Macrohemorrhages

The top two causes of spontaneous (nontraumatic) intraparenchymal hemorrhage in middle-aged and elderly adults are hypertension and amyloid angiopathy; they account for 78-88% of all nontraumatic ICHs. While both can cause extensive nonhemorrhagic "microvascular" disease, their most common manifestations are gross lobar and multifocal microbleeds. We therefore discuss them here.

Hypertensive ICH

Terminology

Hypertensive intracranial hemorrhage (hICH) is the *acute* manifestation of nontraumatic ICH secondary to systemic hypertension (HTN). *Chronic* hypertensive encephalopathy refers to the effects of longstanding HTN on the brain parenchyma and is mostly seen as subcortical white matter disease and/or multifocal microbleeds.

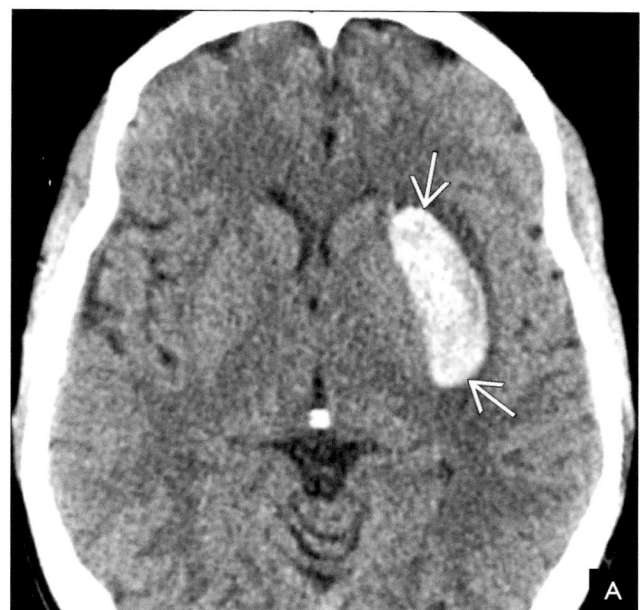

5-26A. Axial NECT scan in a 57-year-old hypertensive woman shows classic left striatocapsular hemorrhage ➡.

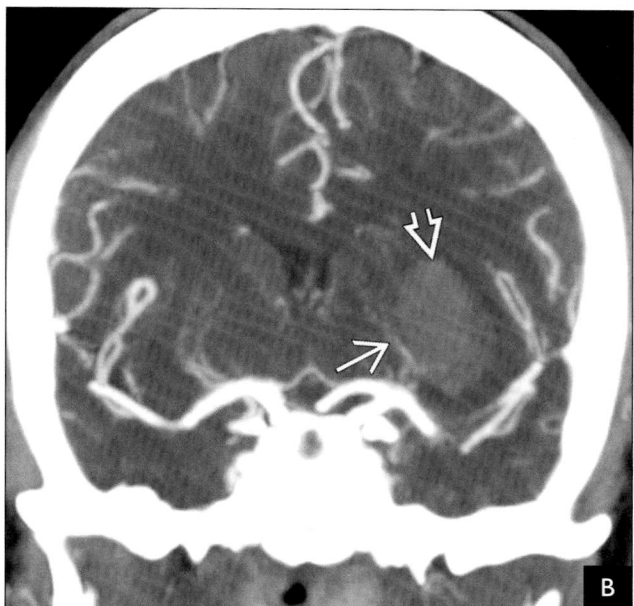

5-26B. Coronal MIP CTA shows that the left lenticulostriate arteries ➡ are displaced by the hematoma ⇥, but there is no evidence of contrast extravasation or "bleeding globe" to suggest increased risk of hematoma expansion.

Etiology

Hypertension accelerates atherosclerosis with lipohyalinosis and fibrinoid necrosis. Penetrating branches of the proximal middle and anterior cerebral arteries, primarily the lenticulostriate arteries (LSAs), are most severely affected, possibly because of their branching angle from the parent vessels.

Progressive weakening and accelerated degeneration of the LSA wall permits formation of small pseudoaneurysms ("Charcot-Bouchard aneurysms" or "bleeding globes"). Ruptured LSA pseudoaneurysm is thought to be the genesis of most striatocapsular hypertensive hemorrhages.

Pathology

LOCATION. The putamen/external capsule is the most common location (5-23), (5-24). These so-called striatocapsular hemorrhages account for nearly two-thirds of all hICHs. The thalamus is the next most common site, responsible for 15-25%. The pons and cerebellum are the third most common location and cause 10% of all hICHs. Lobar hemorrhages account for another 5-10%.

Multiple microbleeds are common in patients with chronic hypertension. Hypertension-related microbleeds tend to cluster in the basal ganglia and cerebellum with fewer lesions in the cortex and subcortical white matter.

SIZE AND NUMBER. Size varies from tiny submillimeter microbleeds to large macroscopic lesions that measure several centimeters in diameter (5-25). When T2*

sequences are used, the majority of patients with hICH have multiple lesions.

GROSS PATHOLOGY. The most common gross finding in hICH is a large ganglionic hematoma that often extends medially into the ventricles (5-24). Hydrocephalus and mass effect with subfalcine herniation are common complications.

MICROSCOPIC FEATURES. Generalized arteriosclerosis with lipohyalinosis and fibrinoid necrosis is common in patients with hICH. In some cases, small fibrosed pseudoaneurysms in the basal ganglia can be identified.

Clinical Issues

EPIDEMIOLOGY. Although the prevalence of hICH has declined significantly, hypertension still accounts for 40-50% of spontaneous "primary" intraparenchymal hemorrhages in middle-aged and older adults. hICH is from five to ten times less common than cerebral ischemia-infarction, accounting for approximately 10-15% of all strokes.

DEMOGRAPHICS. The overall risk of cardiovascular disease—including hypertensive ICH—is significantly increased with systolic-diastolic hypertension, isolated diastolic hypertension, and isolated systolic hypertension. Hypertension increases the risk of ICH four times compared to normotensive patients.

Elderly male patients are the demographic group most at risk for hICH, with peak prevalence between 45-70 years.

5-27A. *NECT scan in a 76-year-old hypertensive man shows acute pontine hematoma* ➡️. **5-27B.** *MR was obtained a few hours later. The clot* ➡️ *is somewhat heterogeneous but appears mostly iso- to mildly hyperintense on T1WI.*

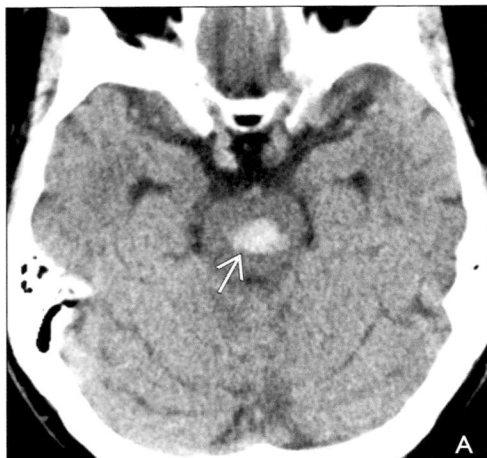

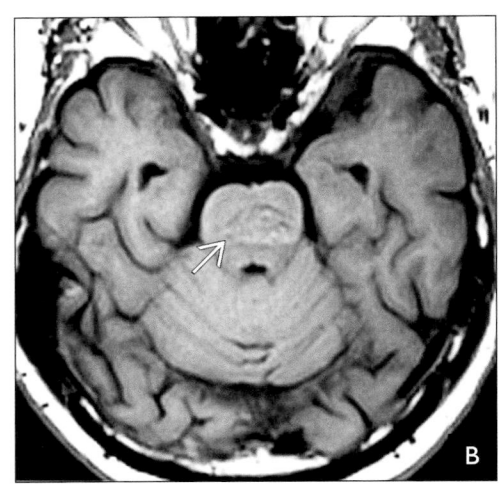

5-27C. *T2WI shows that the clot is hypointense* ➡️. *A thin rim of hyperintense edema* ⏩ *surrounds the hematoma.* **5-27D.** *T2* GRE scan shows "blooming" with profound hypointensity of the clot.*

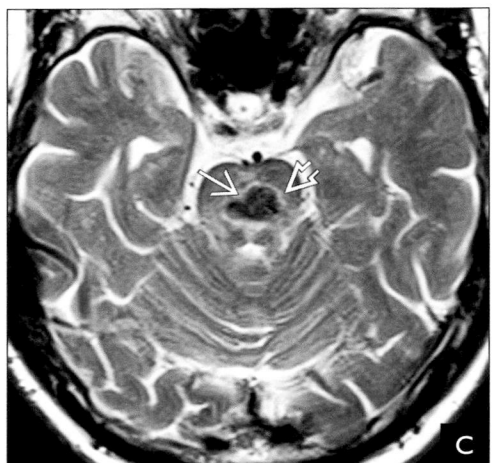

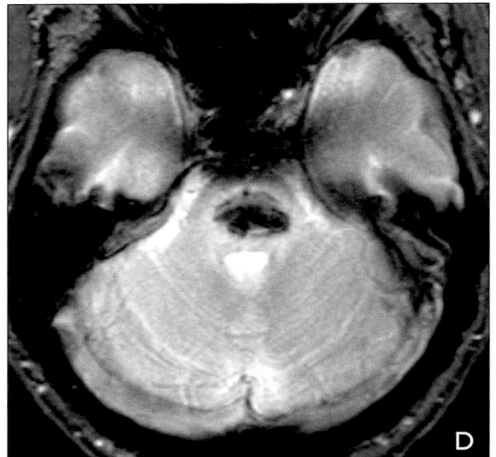

5-27E. *DWI shows that most of the clot* ⏩ *does not restrict; however, an area of hyperintensity* ➡️ *between the hematoma and the fourth ventricle suggests associated cytotoxic edema.* **5-27F.** *ADC in the same case shows that the hyperintense area seen on DWI is now hypointense* ➡️, *indicating the presence of true diffusion restriction.*

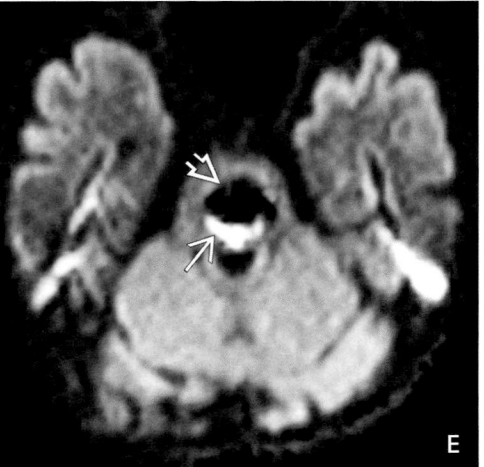

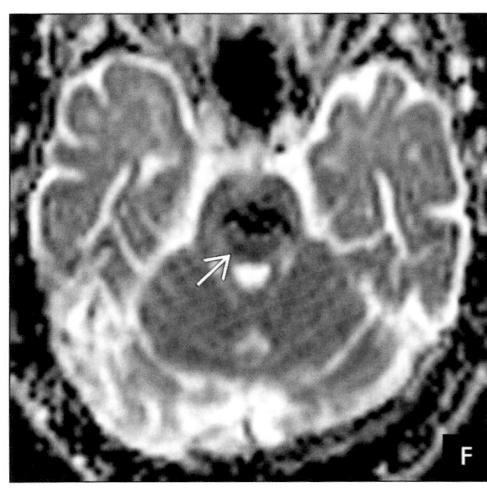

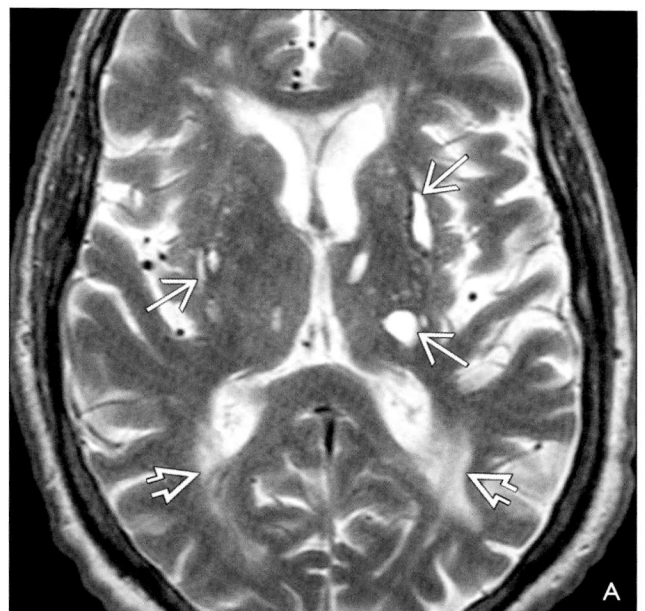

5-28A. T2WI in an elderly patient with longstanding hypertension shows confluent white matter hyperintensity ➡️ and multiple discrete hyperintense foci in both basal ganglia ➡️.

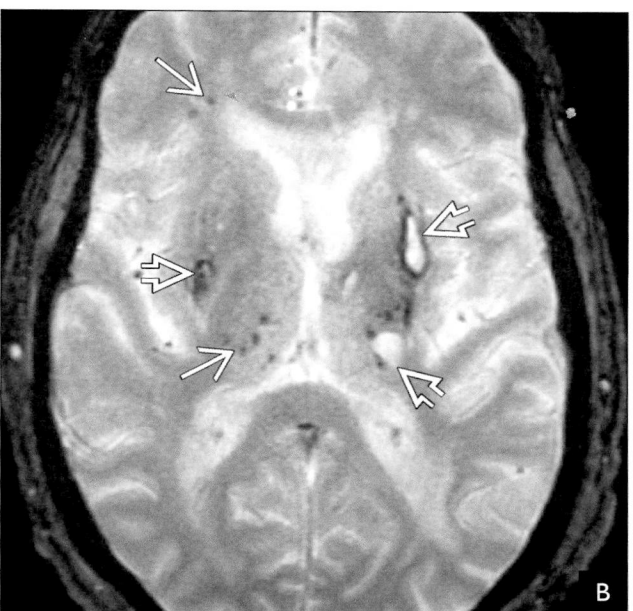

5-28B. T2* GRE shows multiple "blooming" microhemorrhages ➡️ as well as several old striatocapsular and thalamic bleeds ➡️.

African-Americans are the most commonly affected ethnic group in North America.

PRESENTATION. Large hICHs present with sensorimotor deficits and impaired consciousness. Patients may—or may not—have a history of longstanding untreated systemic hypertension.

NATURAL HISTORY. Neurologic deterioration after hICH is common. Hematoma expansion is frequent in the first few hours and is highly predictive of neurological deterioration, poor functional outcome, and mortality. For each 10% increase in ICH size, there is a 5% increase in mortality and an additional 15% chance of poorer functional outcome.

Mortality rate approaches 80% in patients with large hemorrhages. Of hICH survivors, between one-third and one-half are moderately or severely disabled.

TREATMENT OPTIONS. Control of intracranial pressure and hydrocephalus are standard. Hematoma evacuation and craniectomy for brain swelling are controversial.

Imaging

CT FINDINGS. NECT scans typically show a round or ovoid hyperdense mass centered in the lateral putamen/external capsule or thalamus (5-26A). In the presence of active bleeding or coagulopathy, the hemorrhage may appear inhomogeneously hyperdense with lower density areas and even fluid-fluid levels. Intraventricular extension is common. Acute hICH does not enhance on CECT.

MR FINDINGS. Signal intensity on MR changes with clot age (see above) and varies from a large acute hematoma (5-27) to a slit-like hemosiderin "scar." White matter hyperintensities (WMHs) on T2/FLAIR are common findings in patients with hICH. T2* sequences (GRE, SWI) frequently demonstrate multifocal "blooming black dots," especially in the basal ganglia and cerebellum (5-28).

ANGIOGRAPHY. Most hICHs are avascular on CTA (5-26B). However, an enhancing "spot" sign with contrast extravasation can sometimes be identified in actively bleeding lesions.

DSA in stroke patients with a classic striatocapsular hemorrhage and a history of hypertension is rarely required and usually does not contribute to patient management.

Differential Diagnosis

The major differential diagnosis for hICH is **cerebral amyloid angiopathy** (CAA). Patients with CAA are usually normotensive and have moderately impaired cognition. Although there is some overlap with hICH, the distribution of hemorrhages in CAA is typically lobar and peripheral more often than striatocapsular and central. Cerebellar hemorrhages are common in hICH but rare in CAA.

Hemorrhagic neoplasms (e.g., glioblastoma multiforme or metastasis) are more common in the white matter or gray matter-white matter junction and less common in the basal ganglia and cerebellum.

With the exception of dAVF, first-time hemorrhage from an underlying **vascular malformation** is unusual in middle-aged and elderly patients, the cohort most susceptible to hICH. **Coagulopathy** can cause or exacerbate spontaneous ICH. The majority of coagulation-related hemorrhages are usually lobar, not striatocapsular.

In younger patients, **drug abuse** (e.g., cocaine use) with extreme hypertension can cause putamen/external capsule hemorrhage. Drug-induced ganglionic hemorrhages can appear identical to the hICH seen in older patients.

Internal cerebral venous thrombosis can occur at all ages. These hemorrhages tend to be bilateral, thalamic, and more medially located than the striatocapsular bleeds of hICH.

HYPERTENSIVE INTRACRANIAL HEMORRHAGE (hICH)

Etiology
- Accelerated ASVD
  - Especially in lenticulostriate arteries
- Fibrinoid necrosis → tiny pseudoaneurysms
- Rupture → "bleeding globe" → striatocapsular hemorrhage

Location
- Putamen/basal ganglia (60-65%)
- Thalamus (15-25%)
- Pons/cerebellum (10%)
- Lobar hemispheric (5-10%)
- Multiple microbleeds common

Clinical Issues
- 10-15% of all "strokes"
- 40-50% of spontaneous hemorrhages in older adults

Imaging
- Classic = hyperdense clot in putamen/external capsule
- Look for old hemosiderin "scar," microbleeds on T2*

Differential Diagnosis
- Cerebral amyloid angiopathy
- Hemorrhagic neoplasm
- Internal cerebral vein thrombosis
- Drug abuse (e.g., cocaine use)

Cerebral Amyloid Angiopathy

Cerebral amyloid angiopathy (CAA) is one of three morphologic varieties of cerebral amyloid deposition disease (5-29A). Because CAA—also known as "congophilic angiopathy"—is a common cause of spontaneous lobar hemorrhage in elderly patients, we discuss it briefly here. The full spectrum of cerebral amyloid disease is discussed in greater detail in the chapter on vasculopathy (Chapter 10).

CAA causes approximately 1% of all strokes and 15-20% of primary intracranial bleeds in patients over the age of 60 years. Mean age at onset is 73 years. Patients with CAA are usually normotensive and moderately demented.

NECT scans show one or more lobar hematomas, often in different ages of evolution (5-29B). The parietal lobe is the most commonly affected site. A few patients with CAA —especially those with "thunderclap" headache—may demonstrate vertex ("convexal") subarachnoid hemorrhage.

MR is the most sensitive study to detect CAA. The vast majority of patients have multifocal and confluent areas of white matter hyperintensity on T2/FLAIR scans. At least one-third have evidence of old lobar or petechial microhemorrhages, seen as multifocal "blooming black dots" on T2* (GRE, SWI) sequences (5-29C), (5-29D).

Remote Cerebellar Hemorrhage

Terminology and Etiology

Remote cerebellar hemorrhage (RCH) is a less well-recognized and often misdiagnosed cause of spontaneous posterior fossa parenchymal hemorrhage in postoperative patients. Most reported cases occur a few hours following supratentorial craniotomy. RCH also occurs as a rare complication of foramen magnum decompression or spinal surgery.

The etiology of RCH is most likely CSF hypovolemia, with inferior displacement or "sagging" of the cerebellar hemispheres. Tearing or occlusion of bridging tentorial veins is thought to result in superficial cerebellar hemorrhage, with or without hemorrhagic necrosis.

Clinical Issues

RCH is relatively rare, occurring in 0.1-0.6% of patients with supratentorial craniotomies, most often for aneurysm clipping, temporal lobe epilepsy, or tumor resection. There is a slight male predominance. Median age is 51 years.

Many—if not most—cases of RCH are asymptomatic and discovered incidentally at postoperative imaging. The most common symptoms are delayed awakening from anesthesia, decreasing consciousness, and seizures.

Prognosis is generally excellent. Treatment is generally conservative as hematoma removal is rarely indicated.

Imaging

NECT demonstrates stripes of hyperdense blood layered over the cerebellar folia, the "zebra" sign. Hemorrhage can be uni- or bilateral, ipsi- or contralateral to the surgical site (5-30).

MR findings are variable, depending on the age/stage of hematoma evolution. "Blooming" black stripes are seen on T2* (GRE, SWI) **(5-31)**.

Microhemorrhages

For many years, pathologists have noted the presence of microhemorrhages in autopsied brains. While *macro*hemorrhages are easily detected on both CT and MR, until recently brain *micro*bleeds were invisible. With the advent of T2* (GRE, SWI) imaging, microsusceptibility changes in the brain can now be detected with relative ease.

Cerebral microbleeds (CMBs) represent perivascular collections of hemosiderin-containing macrophages. They indicate prior bleeds from an underlying hemorrhage-prone microangiopathy. CMBs are almost always multiple and have many etiologies, ranging from trauma

and infection to vasculopathy and metastases. Each is discussed in detail in the respective chapters that deal with the specific pathologic groupings.

In this section, we briefly summarize two distinct but related differential diagnoses: (1) entities that cause diffuse brain microbleeds and (2) the differential diagnosis of "black spots" or "blooming black dots" on T2* MR that often appear similar to but are *not* caused by microhemorrhages.

Multifocal Brain Microbleeds

A number of entities can cause diffuse brain microhemorrhages **(5-32)**, **(5-33)**, and the etiology of CMBs varies with age. Trauma with hemorrhagic axonal injury is the most common cause of CMBs in children and young adults. Chronic hypertension with arteriolar lipohyalinosis and amyloid angiopathy are the two most common pathologies responsible for CMBs in older adults.

In addition to age, a patient's history (i.e., trauma, hypertension, infection, treatment such as surgery or radiation therapy) is very helpful in narrowing the differential diag-

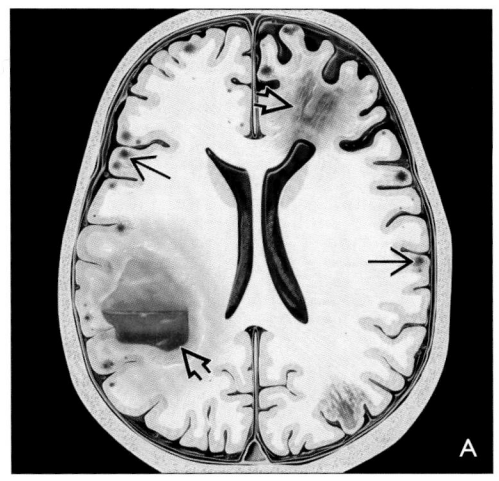
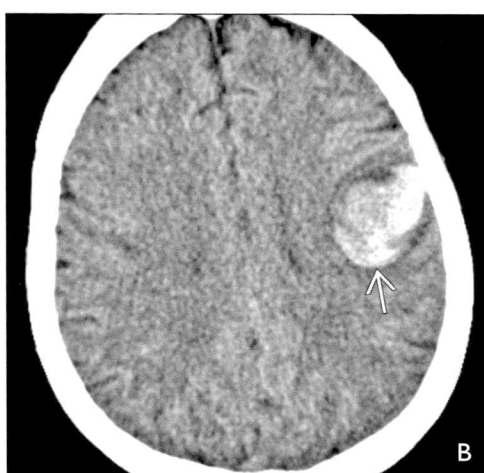

5-29A. *Graphic shows manifestations of cerebral amyloid angiopathy (CAA). Note lobar hemorrhages of different ages ⇨, multiple cortical/subcortical microbleeds ⇨.* **5-29B.** *Axial NECT in an elderly demented but normotensive patient with sudden onset of right-sided weakness shows a focal lobar hematoma ⇨.*

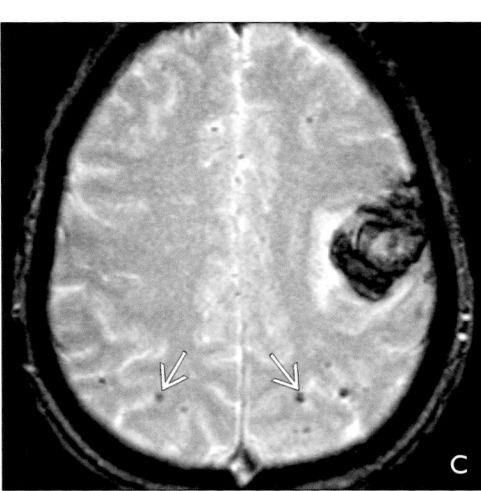
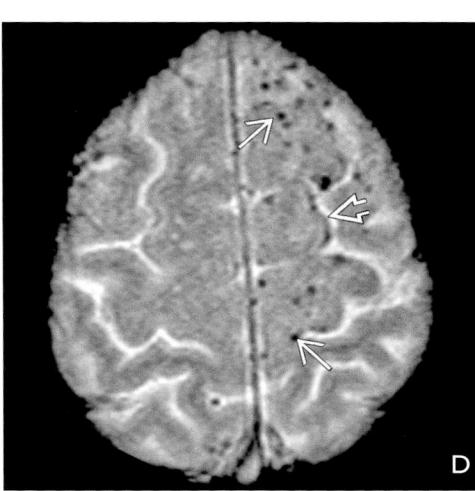

5-29C. *T2* GRE scan shows that the acute hematoma "blooms." Also note multiple small punctate hypointense foci in the cortex ⇨.* **5-29D.** *More cephalad SWI scan in the same patient shows innumerable punctate "blooming" foci ⇨ together with serpentine hypointensity over the pia ⇨ indicating superficial siderosis. These findings of acute lobar hemorrhage plus multiple cortical microbleeds and superficial siderosis are classic for CAA.*

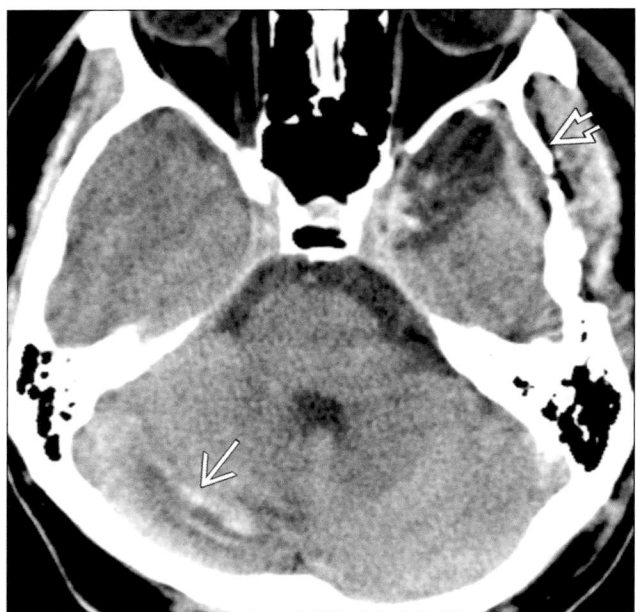

5-30. NECT scan after supratentorial craniotomy ➡ shows linear "zebra stripes" ➡ of alternating hyperdensity (blood) and low density (edema) in the right cerebellum, consistent with remote cerebellar hemorrhage.

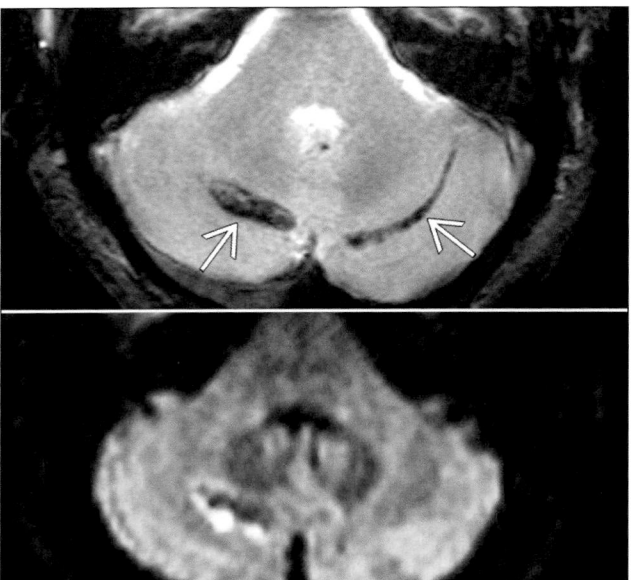

5-31. Bilateral remote cerebellar hemorrhage following resection of a supratentorial neoplasm. (Top) T2* GRE shows bilateral "blooming" lesions ➡. (Bottom) DWI shows some restriction in the right acute hemorrhage.

nosis of CMBs. The box below groups these different entities into common, less common, and rare but important disorders.

BRAIN MICROBLEEDS: ETIOLOGY

Common
- Diffuse axonal/vascular injury
- Cerebral amyloid angiopathy
  - Apolipoprotein E4 polymorphism
- Chronic hypertensive encephalopathy
- Hemorrhagic metastases

Less Common
- Multiple cavernous malformations
- Septicemia
- Fat emboli
- Vasculitis
  - Fungal
  - Sickle cell
- Coagulopathy

Rare but Important
- Acute hemorrhagic leukoencephalopathy
- Intravascular lymphoma
- Leukemia
- Radiation/chemotherapy
  - Radiation-induced telangiectasias
  - Mineralizing microangiopathy
- Thrombotic microangiopathy
  - Malignant hypertension
  - Disseminated intravascular coagulopathy
  - HUS/TTP
- High altitude cerebral edema

Nonhemorrhagic "Blooming Black Dots"

In addition to CMBs, a number of nonhemorrhagic entities cause the appearance of multifocal "black dots" on T2* imaging. These are summarized in the box below, again grouped by common, less common, and rare but important etiologies.

NONHEMORRHAGIC CAUSES OF "BLOOMING BLACK DOTS" ON T2*

Common
- Pneumocephalus

Less Common
- Multiple parenchymal calcifications
  - Neurocysticercosis
  - Tuberculomas

Rare but Important
- Extracorporeal membrane circulation
- Devices, complications
  - Metallic heart valves

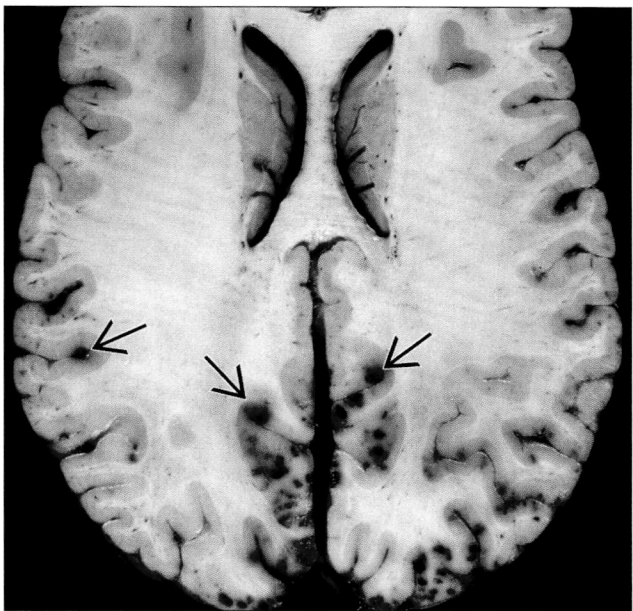

5-32. Autopsy in an immunocompromised patient shows multiple cortical microhemorrhages ⇥. (Courtesy R. Hewlett, MD.)

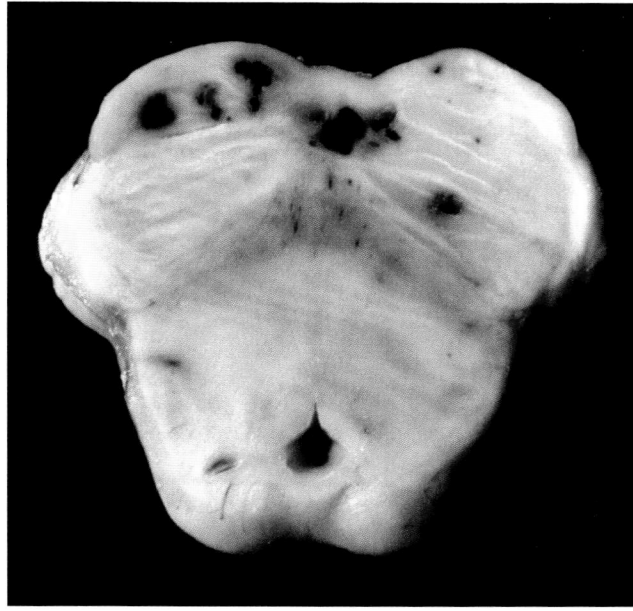

5-33. Autopsy shows multiple midbrain microhemorrhages from cavernous malformations. (Courtesy AFIP Archives.)

Selected References

- Jakubovic R et al: Intracerebral hemorrhage: toward physiological imaging of hemorrhage risk in acute and chronic bleeding. Front Neurol. 3:86, 2012
- Cordonnier C et al: Radiological investigation of spontaneous intracerebral hemorrhage: systematic review and trinational survey. Stroke. 41(4):685-90, 2010
- Morgenstern LB et al: Guidelines for the management of spontaneous intracerebral hemorrhage: a guideline for healthcare professionals from the American Heart Association/American Stroke Association. Stroke. 41(9):2108-29, 2010

Evolution of Intracranial Hemorrhage

Pathophysiology of Intracranial Hemorrhage

- Thomas B et al: Clinical applications of susceptibility weighted MR imaging of the brain - a pictorial review. Neuroradiology. 50(2):105-16, 2008
- Knight RA et al: Temporal MRI assessment of intracerebral hemorrhage in rats. Stroke. 39(9):2596-602, 2008

Imaging of Intracranial Parenchymal Hemorrhage

- Alemany Ripoll M et al: Detection and appearance of intraparenchymal haematomas of the brain at 1.5 T with spin-echo, FLAIR and GE sequences: poor relationship to the age of the haematoma. Neuroradiology. 46(6):435-43, 2004
- Allkemper T et al: Acute and subacute intracerebral hemorrhages: comparison of MR imaging at 1.5 and 3.0 T--initial experience. Radiology. 232(3):874-81, 2004

Etiology of Nontraumatic Parenchymal Hemorrhages

- Kim SJ et al: Dual-energy CT in the evaluation of intracerebral hemorrhage of unknown origin: differentiation between tumor bleeding and pure hemorrhage. AJNR Am J Neuroradiol. 33(5):865-72, 2012
- Phan CM et al: Differentiation of hemorrhage from iodinated contrast in different intracranial compartments using dual-energy head CT. AJNR Am J Neuroradiol. 33(6):1088-94, 2012
- Kersbergen KJ et al: The spectrum of associated brain lesions in cerebral sinovenous thrombosis: relation to gestational age and outcome. Arch Dis Child Fetal Neonatal Ed. 96(6):F404-9, 2011
- Beslow LA et al: Predictors of outcome in childhood intracerebral hemorrhage: a prospective consecutive cohort study. Stroke. 41(2):313-8, 2010
- Brouwer AJ et al: Intracranial hemorrhage in full-term newborns: a hospital-based cohort study. Neuroradiology. 52(6):567-76, 2010

Macrohemorrhages

- Kim SJ et al: Dual-energy CT in the evaluation of intracerebral hemorrhage of unknown origin: differentiation between tumor bleeding and pure hemorrhage. AJNR Am J Neuroradiol. 33(5):865-72, 2012

Hypertensive ICH

- Yakushiji Y et al: Clinical characteristics by topographical distribution of brain microbleeds, with a particular emphasis on diffuse microbleeds. J Stroke Cerebrovasc Dis. 20(3):214-21, 2011

Cerebral Amyloid Angiopathy

- Mehndiratta P et al: Cerebral amyloid angiopathy-associated intracerebral hemorrhage: pathology and management. Neurosurg Focus. 32(4):E7, 2012
- Hirohata M et al: Clinical features of non-hypertensive lobar intracerebral hemorrhage related to cerebral amyloid angiopathy. Eur J Neurol. 17(6):823-9, 2010

Remote Cerebellar Hemorrhage

- Park JS et al: Remote cerebellar hemorrhage complicated after supratentorial surgery: retrospective study with review of articles. J Korean Neurosurg Soc. 46(2):136-43, 2009

Microhemorrhages

- Poels MM et al: Improved MR imaging detection of cerebral microbleeds more accurately identifies persons with vasculopathy. AJNR Am J Neuroradiol. 33(8):1553-6, 2012

Multifocal Brain Microbleeds

- Liu T et al: Cerebral microbleeds: burden assessment by using quantitative susceptibility mapping. Radiology. 262(1):269-78, 2012
- Shoamanesh A et al: Cerebral microbleeds: histopathological correlation of neuroimaging. Cerebrovasc Dis. 32(6):528-34, 2011

6

Subarachnoid Hemorrhage and Aneurysms

Trauma is—by far—the most common cause of intracranial subarachnoid hemorrhage (SAH). Traumatic SAH (tSAH) occurs when blood from contused brain or lacerated vessels extends into adjacent sulci; it was discussed in connection with craniocerebral trauma (Chapter 2). This chapter focuses on nontraumatic SAH and aneurysms.

We begin with an overview of the brain subarachnoid spaces, which provides the context for our discussion of nontraumatic subarachnoid hemorrhage and aneurysms. We follow with detailed discussions of each topic.

Subarachnoid Space Overview

The subarachnoid spaces (SASs) are CSF-filled cavities that lie between the arachnoid and the pia. The SASs are crossed by numerous pia-covered trabeculae that extend between the brain and the inner surface of the arachnoid. It is the pia (*not* the arachnoid) that follows penetrating blood vessels into the brain parenchyma.

Prominent focal enlargements of the SASs, the cisterns, are found around the base of the brain, midbrain/pineal region, brainstem, and cerebellum. Most subarachnoid cisterns are named for their adjacent structures (e.g., suprasellar cistern, quadrigeminal cistern, cerebellopontine angle cistern). A few are named for their size (the great cistern or "cisterna magna"), shape, or sublocation.

The SASs are anatomically unique. They surround the entire brain, dipping into and out of the surface sulci and surrounding the cranial nerves. At some point, all major intracranial arteries and veins also pass through the SASs.

Nontraumatic Subarachnoid Hemorrhage

Nontraumatic "spontaneous" SAH causes 3-5% of all acute "strokes." Approximately 80% of these are caused by a ruptured intracranial saccular aneurysm. The remainder are caused by a variety of entities including dissections, venous hemorrhage or thrombosis, vasculitis, amyloid angiopathy, and reversible cerebral vasoconstriction syndrome.

Hemorrhage into the SAS can be limited and quite focal. More often, blood is extravasated into the SAS, mixes easily with CSF, and spreads diffusely throughout the cisterns and sulci. Sometimes, blood in the SAS is refluxed into the cerebral ventricles, producing secondary intraventricular hemorrhage (IVH).

Aneurysms

The word "aneurysm" comes from the combination of two Greek words meaning "across" and "broad." Indeed, brain aneurysms literally are widenings or dilatations of intracranial arteries.

Intracranial aneurysms are classified by their gross appearance. **Saccular** or **"berry" aneurysms** are the most common type and typically arise eccentrically at vessel branch points (6-1). **Pseudoaneurysms** often resemble "true" saccular aneurysms (SAs) in shape but are contained by cavitated clot, not components of arterial walls.

Blood blister-like aneurysms are thin-walled hemispheric bulges that—as the name suggests—resemble cutaneous blood blisters in appearance.

Fusiform aneurysms are focal dilatations that involve the entire circumference of a vessel, extend for relatively limited distances, and do not arise at branch points. Fusiform aneurysms are most often secondary to athero-

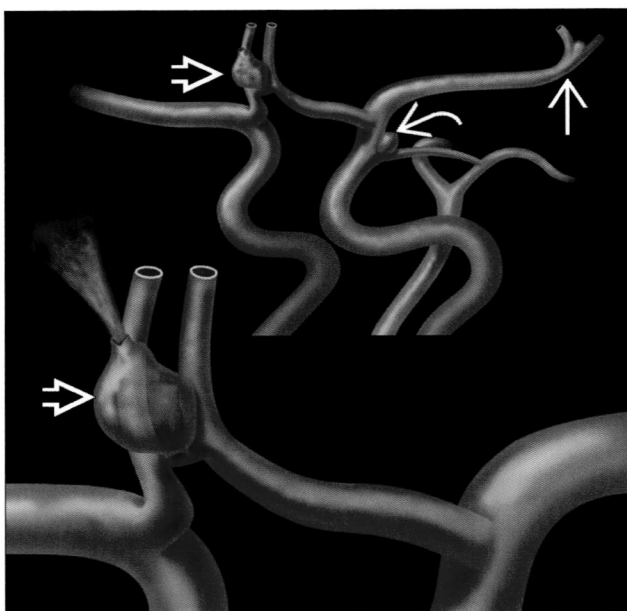

6-1. Graphic shows an SA of the anterior communicating artery ⮕ with active extravasation from a superiorly directed bleb ("teat"). Note additional PCoA SA ⮕, tiny bleb at the left MCA bifurcation ⮕.

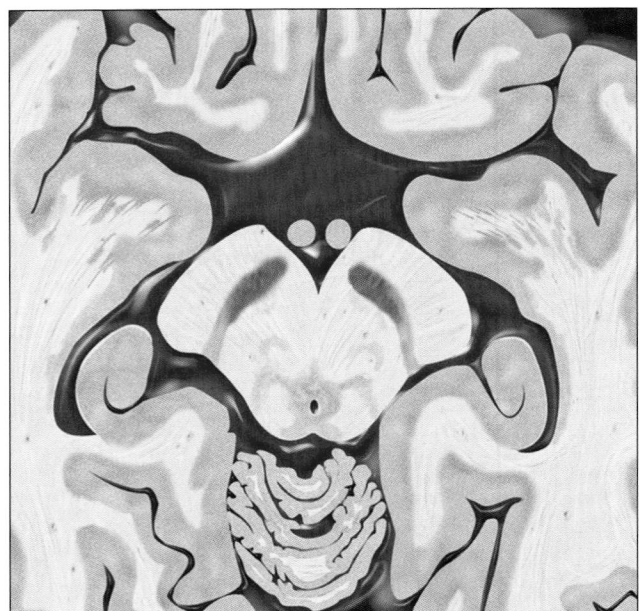

6-2. Axial graphic through the midbrain depicts SAH in red throughout the basal cisterns. Given the diffuse distribution of SAH without focal hematoma, statistically the most likely location of the ruptured aneurysm is the ACoA.

sclerosis but can also occur with nonatherosclerotic vasculopathies.

Ectasias refer to generalized arterial enlargement without focal ("aneurysmal") dilatation. While ectasias can affect any intracranial vessel, the most common site is the posterior circulation. Ectasias are not true aneurysms, so they are discussed in Chapter 10 on vasculopathy.

Subarachnoid Hemorrhage

Nontraumatic SAH (ntSAH) can be aneurysmal or nonaneurysmal in origin and acute or chronic in presentation. We begin this discussion with aneurysmal SAH and its most devastating complications, vasospasm and secondary cerebral ischemia.

We then review two special types of nontraumatic, nonaneurysmal SAH: Perimesencephalic SAH and a newly recognized pattern of SAH called convexal or convexity subarachnoid hemorrhage. Lastly, we discuss chronic repeated SAH and its rare but important manifestation, superficial siderosis.

Aneurysmal Subarachnoid Hemorrhage

Terminology

Aneurysmal SAH (aSAH) is an extravasation of blood into the space between the arachnoid and pia.

Etiology

Aneurysmal SAH is most often caused by rupture of a saccular ("berry") or (rarely) a blood blister-like aneurysm. Other less common causes of aSAH include intracranial dissections and dissecting aneurysms.

Pathology

LOCATION. Because most saccular aneurysms arise from the circle of Willis (COW) or the middle cerebral artery (MCA) bifurcation, the most common locations for aneurysmal SAH are the suprasellar cistern and sylvian fissures **(6-2)**, **(6-3)**.

Occasionally an aneurysm ruptures directly into the brain parenchyma rather than the subarachnoid space. This occurs most frequently when the apex of an anterior communicating artery (ACoA) aneurysm points upward and bursts into the frontal lobe.

GROSS PATHOLOGY. The gross appearance of aSAH is typically characterized by blood-filled basal cisterns. SAH may extend into the superficial sulci and ventri-

Subarachnoid Hemorrhage Grading

Grade	Hunt and Hess	WFNS	GCS	Modified Fisher CT
0	Unruptured/asymptomatic aneurysm	Unruptured aneurysm	Unruptured aneurysm	No visible SAH or IVH
1	Asymptomatic/minimal headache	GCS = 15	GCS = 15	≤ 1 mm SAH, no IVH
2	Moderate/severe headache + nuchal rigidity &/or cranial nerve palsy	GCS = 13-15, no neurologic deficit	GCS = 12-14	≤ 1 mm SAH + IVH
3	Drowsy, confused; mild neurologic deficit(s)	GCS = 13-15, focal neurologic deficit	GCS = 9-11	> 1 mm thick SAH, no IVH
4	Stupor, moderate/severe hemiparesis, early decerebration	GCS = 7-12	GCS = 6-8	> 1 mm thick SAH + IVH or parenchymal hemorrhage
5	Decerebrate, deeply comatose, moribund	GCS = 3-6	GCS = 3-5	N/A

Table 6-1. GCS = Glasgow Coma Score; IVH = intraventricular hemorrhage; N/A = not applicable; SAH = subarachnoid hemorrhage; WFNS = World Federation of Neurological Societies.

cles. Varying degrees of arterial narrowing caused by vasospasm may be present (see below).

Clinical Issues

EPIDEMIOLOGY. The overall prevalence of aSAH is approximately 10-12 per 100,000 per year.

DEMOGRAPHICS. The overall incidence of aSAH increases with age and peaks between the ages of 40 and 60 years. The M:F ratio is 1:2.

Aneurysmal SAH is rare in children. Regardless of their relative rarity, however, cerebral aneurysms cause the majority of spontaneous (nontraumatic) SAHs in children and account for approximately 10% of all childhood hemorrhagic "strokes."

PRESENTATION. Nonspecific headache is a common presenting complaint in emergency departments, accounting for approximately 2% of all visits. Subarachnoid hemorrhage accounts for just 1-3% of these headaches.

At least 75% of patients with aSAH present with sudden onset of the "worst headache of my life." The most severe form is a "thunderclap" headache, an extremely intense headache that comes on "like a boom of thunder" and typically peaks within minutes or even seconds. While there are many causes of "thunderclap" headache, the most serious and life-threatening is aSAH.

One-third of patients with aSAH complain of neck pain. Another third report vomiting.

Between 10-25% of patients experience symptoms days or even weeks before the onset of overt SAH. These "sentinel" or "warning" leaks may presage aneurysm rupture and should not be ignored.

CLINICALLY BASED GRADING OF SAH. While a number of different scales have been proposed to grade aSAH, none has gained universal acceptance. The two most commonly used systems are the Hunt and Hess and the World Federation of Neurological Societies (WFNS) scales. Both are based on clinical findings.

The **Hunt and Hess scale** grades aSAH from 0 to 5. An unruptured, asymptomatic aneurysm is designated grade 0. Patients who are either asymptomatic or have minimal headache are grade 1. Grade 2 represents moderate to severe headache with nuchal rigidity and/or cranial nerve palsy. Grades 3-5 designate more serious aSAH. Drowsy or confused patients with mild focal neurologic deficits are grade 3. Grade 4 equates to stupor, moderate to severe hemiparesis, and early decerebrate state. Grade 5 patients are decerebrate, deeply comatose, and moribund.

The **WFNS scale** also recognizes six scales of aSAH but is primarily based on the Glasgow Coma Score (GCS). Zero is an unruptured aneurysm. Grade 1 patients have a GCS of 15. Grade 2 patients have no neurologic deficits and a GCS of 13 or 14. Patients with GCS of 13-14 *with* a focal deficit are grade 3. GCS of 7-12 is grade 4. GCS scores of 3-6 are designated grade 5.

Recent studies have indicated that the best predictor of clinical outcome is based simply on the **Glasgow Coma Score**. As with the other scales mentioned, an unruptured aneurysm is designated Grade 0. Grades 1-5 differ slightly from the WFNS system. Grade 1 is GCS of 15. Grade 2 is 12-14, 3 is 9-11, 4 is 6-8, and 5 is a GCS of 3-5. Its simplicity, reliability, predictive power, and wide familiarity among health care personnel make the GCS the most logical system for grading aSAH and guiding patient treatment.

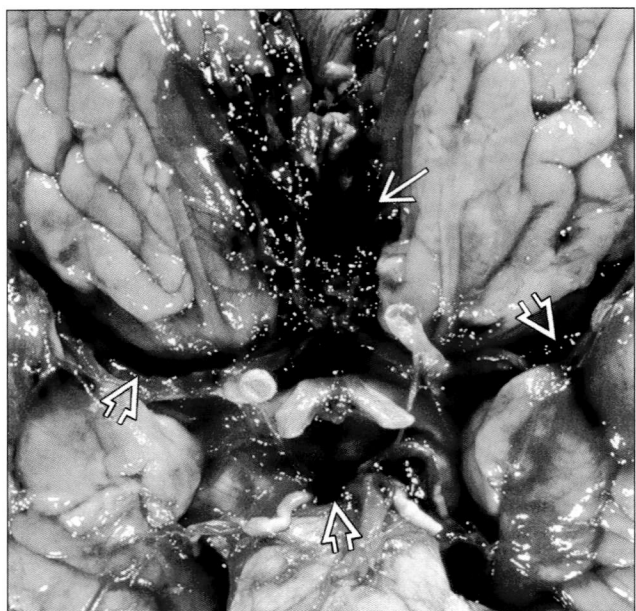

6-3. Autopsy shows diffuse basilar SAH ⮞ from a ruptured ACoA aneurysm. More focal clot is present in the interhemispheric fissure ➡. (Courtesy R. Hewlett, MD.)

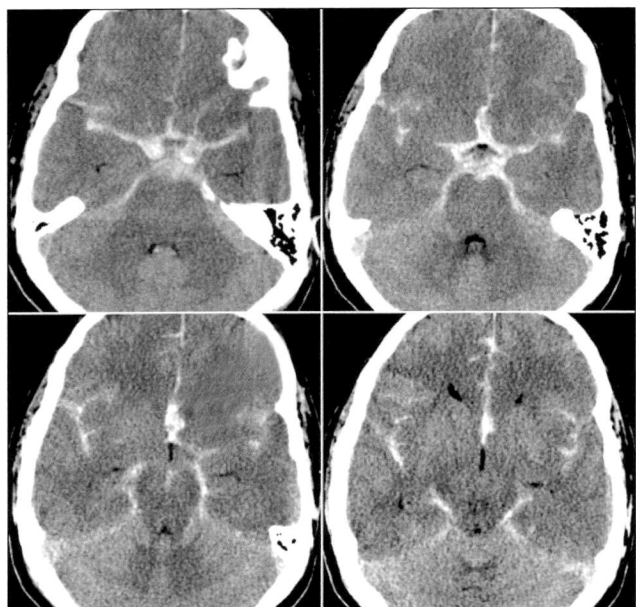

6-4. Series of axial NECT scans shows the typical appearance of aneurysmal SAH. Hyperdensity in the basilar cisterns and sylvian fissures is typical.

A fourth schema, the modified **Fisher scale**, is based on CT appearance (not clinical findings) but is included on the summary table for comparison **(Table 6-1)**.

NATURAL HISTORY. Although aSAH causes just 3-5% of all "strokes," nearly one-third of all stroke-related years of potential life lost before age 65 are attributable to aSAH. The mean age at death in patients with aSAH is significantly lower than in patients with other types of strokes.

Aneurysmal SAH is fatal or disabling in more than two-thirds of patients. Massive SAH can cause coma and death within minutes. Approximately one-third of patients with aSAH die within 72 hours; another third survive but with disabling neurologic deficits.

Despite advances in diagnosis and treatment, in-hospital mortality continues to exceed 25%. Without treatment, ruptured saccular aneurysms have a rebleed rate of 20% within the first two weeks following the initial hemorrhage.

Unfavorable outcome is associated with several factors including increasing age, worsening neurological grade, aneurysm size, large amounts of SAH on initial NECT scan, parenchymal hematoma, intraventricular hemorrhage, and vascular risk factors such as hypertension and myocardial infarction.

Patients who survive aSAH also have an increased lifetime risk of developing new ("de novo") intracranial aneurysms and new episodes of SAH, estimated at 2%

per year. They also carry an increased risk for other vascular diseases.

TREATMENT OPTIONS. The goals of aSAH treatment in patients who survive their initial bleed are to (1) obliterate the aneurysm (preventing potentially catastrophic rebleeding) and (2) prevent or treat vasospasm (see below).

Imaging

GENERAL FEATURES. NECT is an excellent screening examination for the diagnosis of suspected aSAH. Recent studies have shown that in the first three days after ictus, a negative CT scan is usually sufficient to exclude SAH. Lumbar puncture is generally unnecessary if the NECT is negative.

The best imaging clue to aSAH is hyperdense cisterns and sulci on NECT. In some cases, subarachnoid blood surrounds and outlines the comparatively hypodense-appearing aneurysm sac.

CT FINDINGS. The basal cisterns—especially the suprasellar cistern—are generally filled with blood **(6-4)**. While SAH distribution generally depends on location of the "culprit" aneurysm, it is also somewhat variable and not absolutely predictive of aneurysm location.

ACoA aneurysms tend to rupture superiorly into the interhemispheric fissure. MCA bifurcation aneurysms usually rupture into the sylvian fissure. Internal carotid-posterior communicating artery (IC-PCoA) aneurysms generally rupture into the suprasellar cistern. Verte-

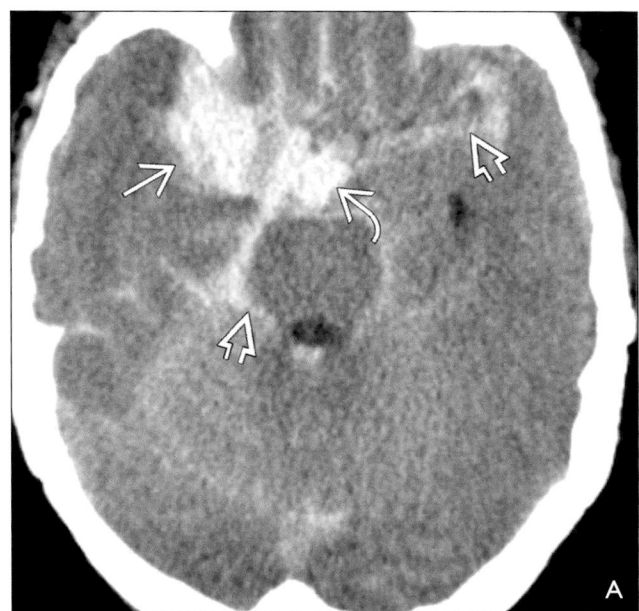

6-5A. NECT scan shows diffuse basilar SAH ➡ with more focal clot in the anteromedial temporal lobe ➡ and along the right side of the suprasellar cistern ➡.

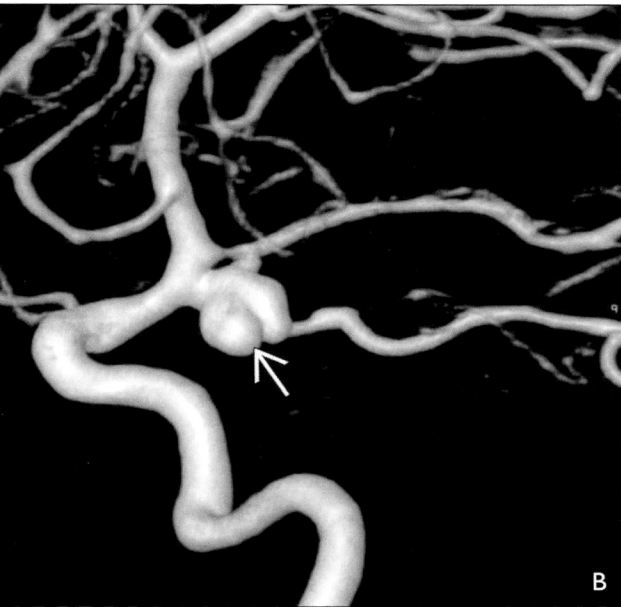

6-5B. 3D SSD of the right ICA angiogram in the same patient shows a large trilobed IC-PCoA aneurysm ➡.

brobasilar aneurysms often fill the fourth ventricle, prepontine cistern, and foramen magnum with blood.

Intraventricular hemorrhage (IVH) is present in nearly half of all patients with aSAH and is associated with a higher likelihood of in-hospital complications and poorer three-month post-SAH outcome.

Focal parenchymal hemorrhage is uncommon but, if present, is generally predictive of aneurysm rupture site **(6-5)**.

MR FINDINGS. Acute aSAH is isointense with brain on T1WI **(6-6A)**, **(6-6B)**. The CSF cisterns may appear smudged or "dirty." Because aSAH is hyperintense to brain on T2WI, it may be difficult to identify **(6-6C)**.

FLAIR is the best sequence to depict aSAH **(6-6D)**. Hyperintense CSF in the sulci and cisterns is present but nonspecific. Other causes of "bright" CSF on FLAIR include hyperoxygenation, meningitis, neoplasm, and artifact.

MR may also be a helpful additional examination when no structural cause for nontraumatic SAH is identified on screening NECT or CTA.

ANGIOGRAPHY. CTA is positive in 95% of aSAH cases if the "culprit" aneurysm is two millimeters or larger **(6-5B)**. While DSA is still considered the gold standard for detecting and delineating aneurysm angioarchitecture, many patients with aSAH and positive CTA undergo surgical clipping without DSA.

Standard DSA occasionally fails to demonstrate a "culprit" aneurysm. So-called angiogram-negative SAH is found in approximately 15% of cases. With the addition of three-dimensional rotational angiography and 3D shaded surface displays (SSDs), the rate of "angiogram-negative" SAH decreases to 4-5% of cases.

"Angiogram-negative" spontaneous SAH is not a benign entity, as there is a small but real risk of rehemorrhage and poor outcome. CTA is recommended in patients with diffuse-type SAH if the initial DSA is negative. A causative cerebral aneurysm is found in 9% of these cases.

IMAGING-BASED GRADING OF SAH. A simple scale based on NECT findings, the **modified Fisher scale**, has been proposed to grade aSAH. Grade 0 equates to no visible subarachnoid or intraventricular hemorrhage. A focal or diffuse thin (less than one millimeter) layer of subarachnoid blood without IVH is designated grade 1. If IVH is present, it is a Fisher grade 2. Focal or diffuse thick (more than one millimeter) SAH without IVH is designated grade 3. The presence of intraventricular blood together with thick SAH is designated a grade 4 bleed. Stepwise increases in modified Fisher grade have a moderately linear relationship with the risk of vasospasm, delayed infarction, and poor clinical outcome.

Computerized quantitative determination of subarachnoid hemorrhage volume is also a good predictor of delayed cerebral ischemia and functional outcome in aSAH but is not routinely available.

Differential Diagnosis

The major differential diagnosis of aSAH is **traumatic SAH**. Aneurysmal SAH is generally much more widespread, often filling the basal cisterns. tSAH typically occurs adjacent to cortical contusions or lacerations and is therefore most common in the superficial sulci.

Perimesencephalic nonaneurysmal SAH (pnSAH) is much more limited than aSAH and is localized to the interpeduncular, ambient, and prepontine cisterns. Occasionally, pnSAH spreads into the posterior aspect of the suprasellar cistern. It rarely extends into the sylvian fissures.

Convexal SAH is, as the name implies, localized to superficial sulci over the cerebral convexities. Often only a single sulcus is affected. Causes of convexal SAH are numerous and include cortical vein occlusion, amyloid angiopathy, vasculitis, and reversible cerebral vasoconstriction syndrome.

Pseudo-SAH is caused by severe cerebral edema. The hypodensity of the brain makes blood in the cerebral arteries and veins appear dense, mimicking the appearance of SAH.

Sulcal-cisternal FLAIR hyperintensity on MR is a nonspecific imaging finding and does not always denote subarachnoid hemorrhage. In addition to aSAH, FLAIR hyperintense CSF often occurs with flow disturbances and technical artifacts such as incomplete CSF nulling.

Pyogenic meningitis, meningeal carcinomatosis, and high inspired oxygen concentration may also cause CSF hyperintensity on FLAIR. Prior administration of gadolinium chelates (with or without decreased renal clearance) can result in diffuse delayed CSF enhancement.

Other etiologies of sulcal-cisternal FLAIR hyperintensity include hyperintense vessels with slow flow (e.g., acute arterial strokes, pial collaterals developing after cerebral ischemia-infarction, Sturge-Weber syndrome, moyamoya, and reversible cerebral vasoconstriction syndrome).

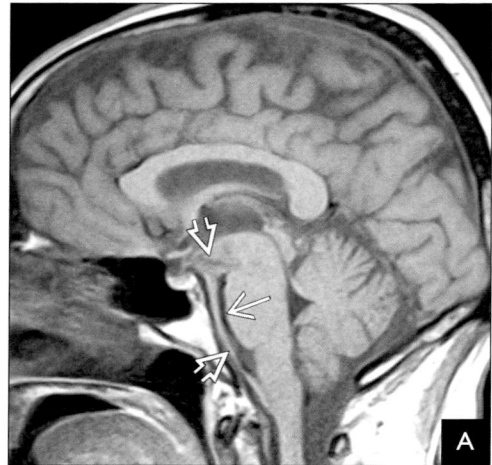 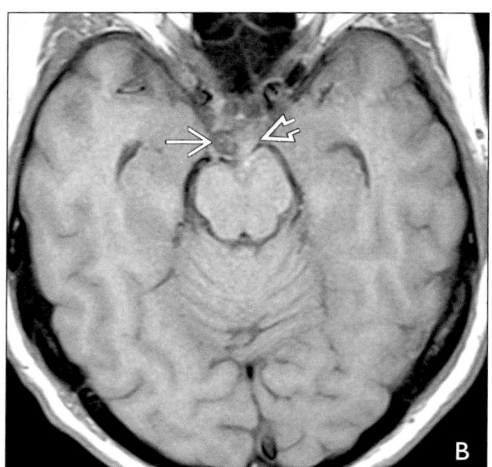

6-6A. Series of MR scans shows typical findings of acute aneurysmal SAH. Sagittal T1WI shows "dirty" CSF ➡ that appears isointense with adjacent brain. The basilar artery "flow void" ➡ is surrounded by the SAH.
6-6B. Axial T1WI in the same patient shows a nice contrast between the isointense "dirty" CSF ➡ and the more normal-appearing hypointense CSF ➡.

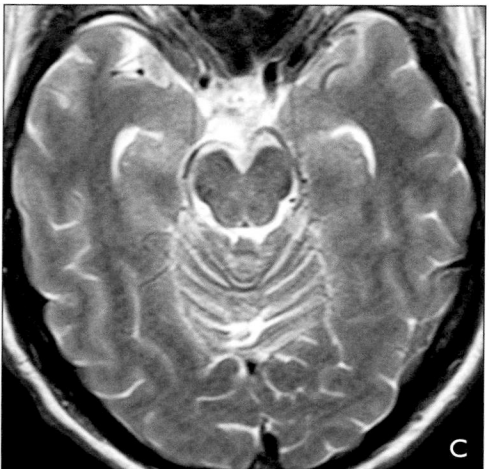 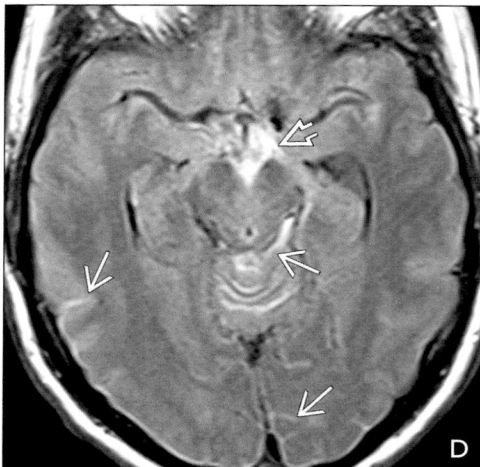

6-6C. T2WI in the same patient shows that the hyperintense SAH is difficult to distinguish from normal CSF. 6-6D. FLAIR scan shows the hyperintense CSF in the basilar cisterns ➡. Sulcal-cisternal hyperintensity is also evident in the left perimesencephalic and superior cerebellar cisterns, as well as the parietooccipital subarachnoid spaces ➡.

ANEURYSMAL SUBARACHNOID HEMORRHAGE

Etiology
- Ruptured saccular or blood-blister aneurysm
- Less common = intracranial dissection

Pathology
- Blood between arachnoid, pia
- Fills basal cisterns ± intraventricular heme

Clinical Issues
- Causes 3-5% of "strokes"
- "Thunderclap" headache
- Peak age = 40-60 years, M:F = 1:2
- Fatal or disabling in 2/3

Imaging
- NECT: Hyperdense basal cisterns, sulci
  - LP unnecessary if CT negative in first 3 days
  - Hydrocephalus common, onset often early
- MR
  - "Dirty" CSF on T1WI
  - Hyperintense cisterns, sulci on FLAIR
- Angiography
  - CTA positive in 95% if aneurysm ≥ 2 mm
  - DSA reserved for complex aneurysm, CTA negative
  - "Angiogram-negative" SAH (15%)
  - Negative 3D rotational DSA (only 5%)
  - Repeat "second look" DSA positive (5%)

Differential Diagnosis
- Traumatic SAH
  - Overall most common cause of SAH
- Perimesencephalic nonaneurysmal SAH
- Convexal SAH
- Pseudo-SAH

Aneurysmal SAH and Vasospasm

Cerebral vasospasm (CVS) is a common but poorly understood complication of aSAH **(6-7)**. CVS with delayed cerebral ischemia (DCI) is the major cause of morbidity and death in patients who survive the initial hemorrhage. Microcirculatory dysfunction related to endothelial damage, microvascular thrombosis, and loss of autoregulation have all been implicated in the pathogenesis of post-SAH DCI.

Aneurysmal SAH is complicated by vasospasm in two-thirds of all patients. Approximately 30% become symptomatic. More than half of these patients subsequently develop delayed infarcts. Patients with large volume SAH are at especially high risk for developing symptomatic vasospasm and its complications.

Noninvasive methods to detect early-stage CVS include color duplex ultrasound, transcranial Doppler ultrasound, CT angiography, CT perfusion (pCT), and MR. CTA with pCT is especially useful in evaluating critically ill patients. MR perfusion and diffusion weighted imaging (PWI, DWI) may be helpful in preangiographic determination of specific vessel segments "at risk" for subsequent development of cerebral infarction.

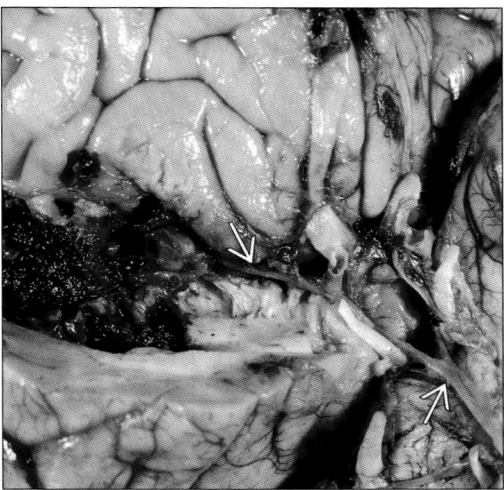

6-7. *Autopsy of ruptured MCA bifurcation aneurysm shows severe vasospasm with marked narrowing of the MCA and distal basilar artery* ➡.

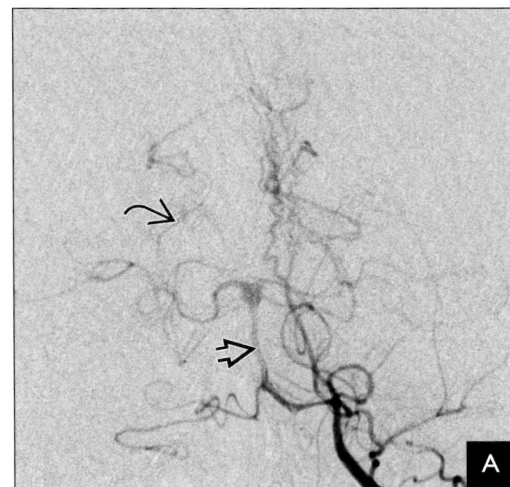

6-8A. *AP vertebral DSA shows severe vasospasm* ⊵ *from ruptured anterior circulation aneurysm. Distal vessels are barely opacified* ⊿.

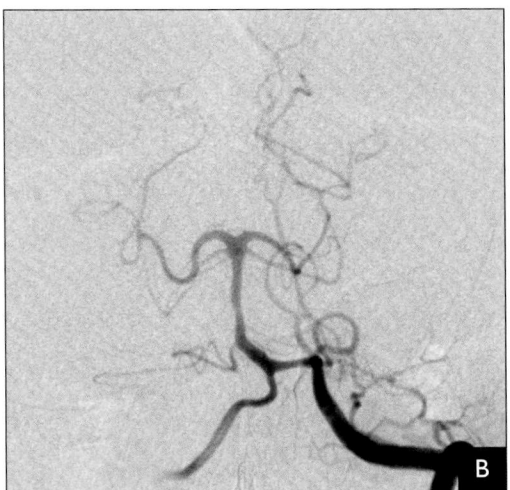

6-8B. *Fifteen mg of verapamil was infused. Repeat DSA 5 minutes later shows dramatic improvement in the vertebrobasilar circulation.*

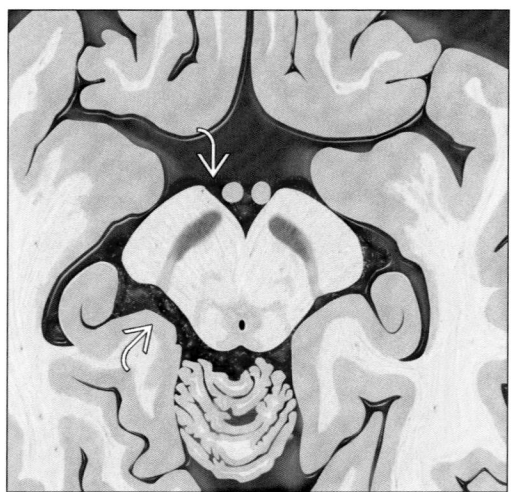

6-9. In pnSAH, hemorrhage is confined to the interpeduncular fossa and ambient (perimesencephalic) cisterns ➔.

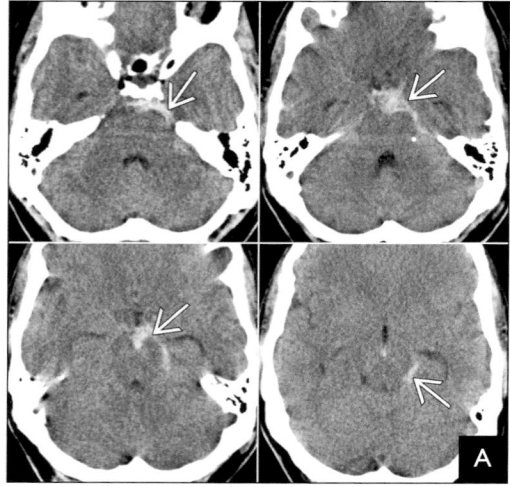

6-10A. NECT of pnSAH shows blood in prepontine, perimesencephalic cisterns ➔ but not anterior suprasellar cistern, sylvian fissures.

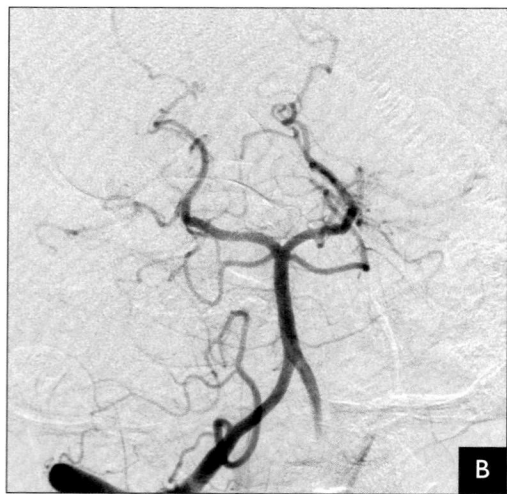

6-10B. AP DSA in the same patient is normal without evidence of basilar bifurcation aneurysm or dissection.

DSA is still considered the gold standard for the diagnosis of CVS **(6-8A)**. Angiographic vasospasm is strongly correlated with cerebral infarction. Multiple segments of vascular constriction and irregularly narrowed vessels are typical findings. DSA is often combined with endovascular treatment, usually transluminal balloon angioplasty and intraarterial nimodipine **(6-8B)**.

"Triple H" therapy (hypervolemia, hypertension, and hemodilution) has been used in combination with calcium antagonists in an attempt to increase cerebral perfusion and improve outcome following aSAH. However, recent controlled studies show no evidence of a positive effect of either "triple H" or its separate components on cerebral blood flow in SAH.

Differential Diagnosis

The differential diagnosis of vasospasm within the context of existing SAH is limited. If the patient has a known aneurysm with recent SAH, the findings of multisegmental vascular narrowing indicate CVS. However, if the SAH is convexal (see below), the differential diagnosis includes **reversible cerebral vasoconstriction syndrome** and **vasculitis**.

Other Complications of aSAH

Delayed cerebral ischemia (DCI) typically occurs 4-14 days after aSAH and is most commonly caused by vasospasm (see above). Other factors such as **oxidative stress** (including lipid peroxidation), activation of **inflammatory responses**, and production of inflammatory cytokines probably contribute to high mortality after SAH.

Obstructive hydrocephalus commonly develops in patients with aSAH, sometimes within hours of the ictus, and may be exacerbated by the presence of IVH. Imaging studies show increased periventricular extracellular fluid with "blurred" lateral ventricle margins.

Neurodegeneration biomarkers (e.g., calpain-derived proteolytic fragments, hypophosphorylated neurofilament H, ubiquitin ligase, and neuron-specific enolase) increase after severe aSAH and may be early predictors of pathophysiological complications and lasting brain dysfunction.

Terson syndrome (TS) is an intraocular hemorrhage that is found in 12-13% of patients with aSAH. TS is associated with more severe SAH grades and is probably caused by a rapid increase in intracranial pressure (ICP). The hemorrhage can be subhyaloid (most common), retinal, or vitreous.

Perimesencephalic Nonaneurysmal SAH

Terminology

Perimesencephalic nonaneurysmal SAH (pnSAH) is also known as benign perimesencephalic SAH. pnSAH is a clinically benign subarachnoid hemorrhage subtype that is anatomically confined to the perimesencephalic and prepontine cisterns **(6-9)**.

Etiology

The precise etiology of pnSAH is unknown, and the bleeding source in pnSAH is usually undetermined. Yet most investigators implicate venous—not aneurysmal—rupture as the most likely cause.

Clinical Issues

pnSAH is the most common cause of nontraumatic, nonaneurysmal SAH. The typical presentation is mild to moderate headache with Hunt and Hess grade 1-2. Occasionally patients experience severe "thunderclap" headache with meningismus.

The peak age of presentation in patients with pnSAH is between 40 and 60 years—identical to that of aneurysmal SAH. There is no gender predilection.

Most cases of pnSAH follow a clinically benign and uneventful course. Rebleeding is uncommon (< 1%). In contrast to aSAH, vasospasm and delayed cerebral ischemia are rare.

Imaging

pnSAH has well-defined imaging features. NECT scans show focal accumulation of subarachnoid blood around the midbrain (in the interpeduncular and perimesencephalic cisterns) and in front of the pons **(6-10)**.

Although more than 95% of patients with pnSAH have negative DSAs, a ruptured basilar bifurcation aneurysm or vertebrobasilar dissection occasionally causes a pattern of SAH that can mimic pnSAH. Therefore, imaging the cranial circulation is generally recommended **(6-11)**. High-resolution CTA is a reliable noninvasive alternative to catheter angiography in ruling out underlying aneurysm or dissection in such cases. If the initial CTA is negative, there is no significant additional diagnostic yield from DSA or MR.

Differential Diagnosis

The major differential diagnosis of pnSAH is **aneurysmal SAH**. Aneurysmal SAH is significantly more exten-

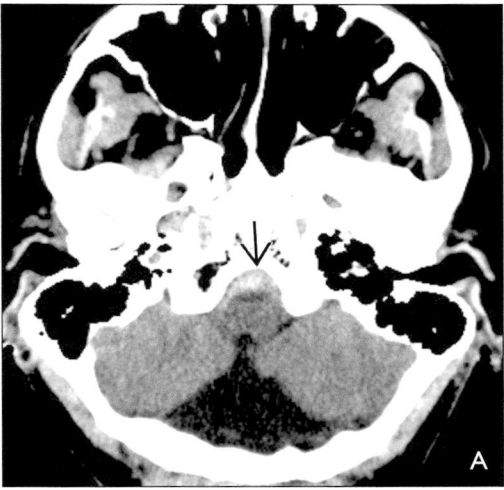

6-11A. Axial NECT scan in a 62-year-old man with sudden severe headache shows subarachnoid blood ⇨ anterior to the medulla.

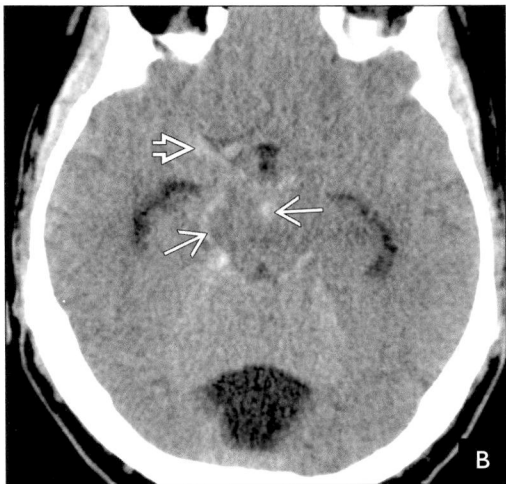

6-11B. More cephalad scan shows perimesencephalic, interpeduncular SAH ⇨ with minimal blood in the right sylvian fissure ⇨.

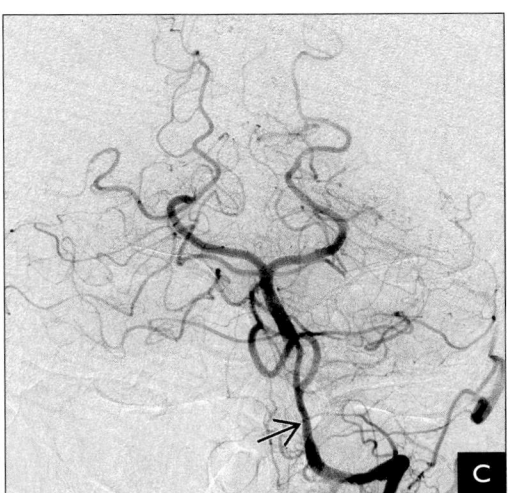

6-11C. DSA shows a dissected left vertebral artery ⇨. Intracranial dissections are an uncommon but important cause of pnSAH.

sive, spreading throughout the basal cisterns and often extending into the interhemispheric and sylvian fissures.

Traumatic SAH (tSAH) would be suggested both by history and imaging appearance. tSAH occurs adjacent to contused brain. It is usually more peripheral, lying primarily within the sylvian fissure and over the cerebral convexities. During closed head injury, the midbrain may be suddenly and forcibly impacted against the tentorial incisura. In such cases, the presence of perimesencephalic blood can mimic pnSAH. In contrast to pnSAH, interpeduncular and prepontine hemorrhage is usually absent.

Convexal SAH is found over the cerebral convexities, not in the perimesencephalic cisterns. Blood within a single sulcus or immediately adjacent sulci is common.

Convexal SAH

Terminology

Isolated spontaneous nontraumatic SAH that involves the sulci over the brain vertex is called convexal or convex-

ity subarachnoid hemorrhage (cSAH). cSAH is a unique type of subarachnoid hemorrhage with a very different imaging appearance from either aSAH or pnSAH: cSAH is restricted to the hemispheric convexities, sparing the basal and perimesencephalic cisterns **(6-12)**.

Etiology

A broad spectrum of vascular and even nonvascular pathologies can cause cSAH. These include dural sinus and cortical vein thrombosis (CoVT), arteriovenous malformations, dural AV fistulas, arterial dissection/stenosis/occlusion, mycotic aneurysm, vasculitides, amyloid angiopathy, coagulopathies, reversible cerebral vasoconstriction syndrome (RCVS), and PRES.

Clinical Issues

While cSAH can occur at virtually any age, most patients are between the fourth and eighth decades. Peak age is 70 years.

The clinical presentation of cSAH varies with etiology but is quite different from that of aSAH. Most patients with cSAH have nonspecific headache without nuchal

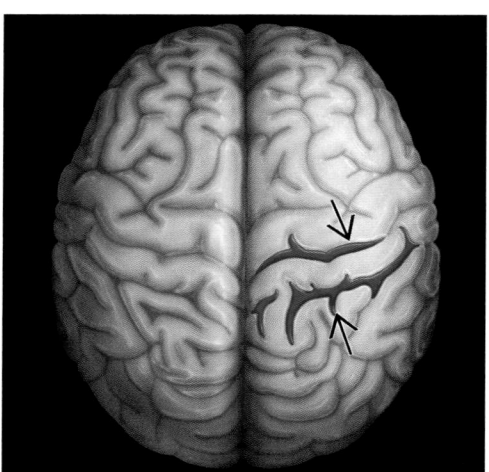
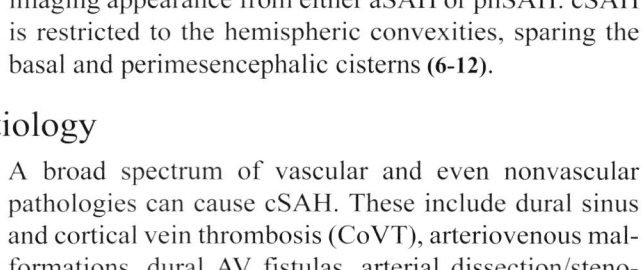
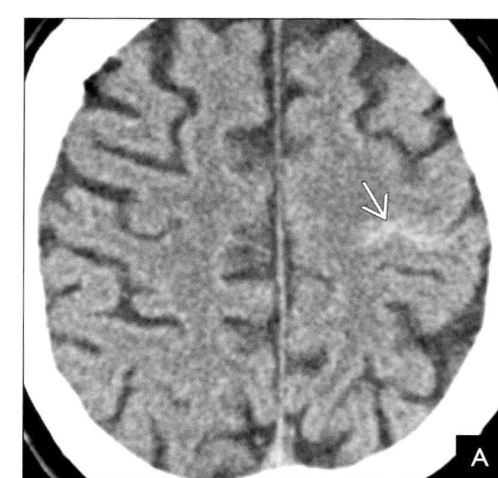

6-12. Graphic depicts convexal SAH with focal intrasulcal blood ⊟ over the vertex of the left hemisphere. **6-13A.** *NECT scan in patient with "thunderclap" headache shows isolated convexal SAH ➡.*

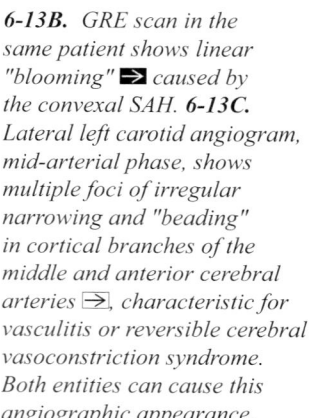
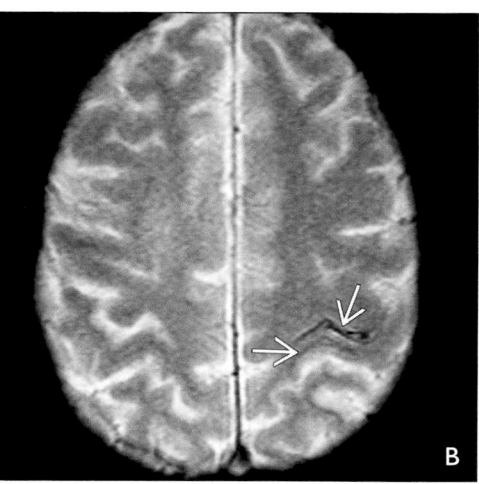
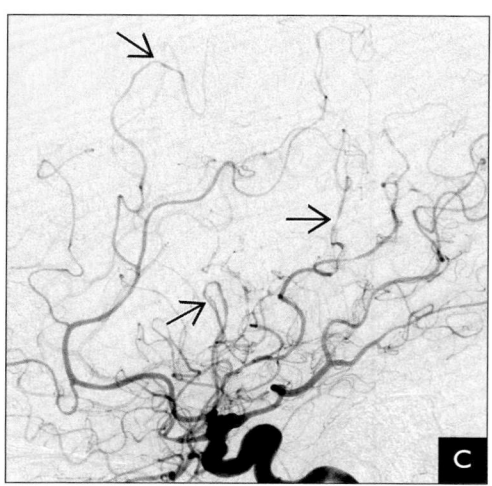

6-13B. GRE scan in the same patient shows linear "blooming" ➡ caused by the convexal SAH. **6-13C.** *Lateral left carotid angiogram, mid-arterial phase, shows multiple foci of irregular narrowing and "beading" in cortical branches of the middle and anterior cerebral arteries ➡, characteristic for vasculitis or reversible cerebral vasoconstriction syndrome. Both entities can cause this angiographic appearance.*

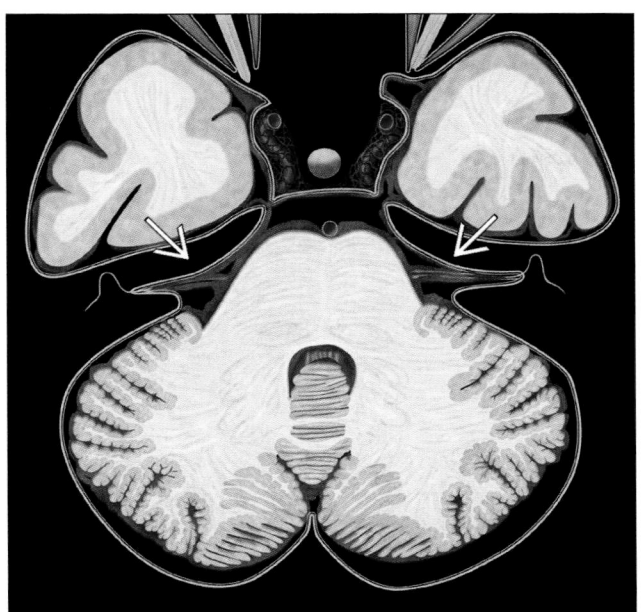

6-14. *Axial graphic shows darker brown hemosiderin staining on all surfaces of the brain, meninges, and cranial nerves. Notice that cranial nerves VII and VIII in the cerebellopontine angle-internal auditory canal* ➔ *are particularly affected.*

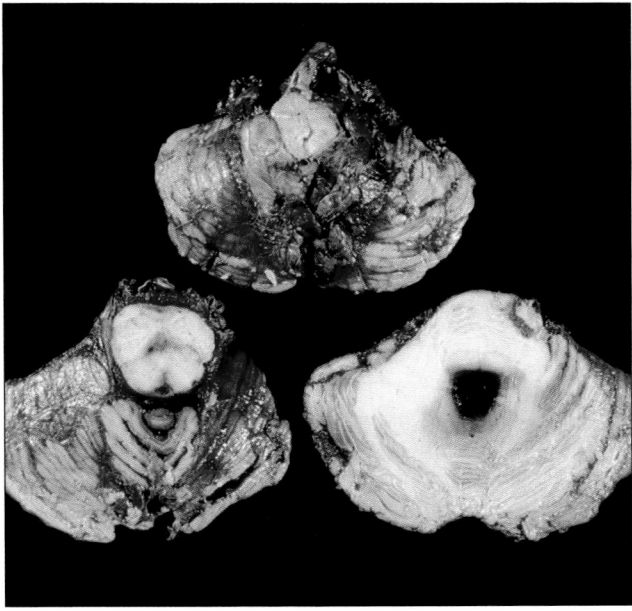

6-15. *Autopsy case shows superficial siderosis. The brainstem and cerebellum are covered with brown-staining hemosiderin deposits. (Courtesy E. T. Hedley-Whyte, MD.)*

rigidity. Some present with focal or generalized seizures or neurologic deficits.

Patients with cSAH secondary to RCVS may present with a "thunderclap" headache. The vast majority are middle-aged women. cSAH caused by venous thrombosis or vasculitis may have milder symptoms with more insidious onset. Mean age of CoVT accompanied by cSAH is 33 years.

Cerebral amyloid angiopathy (CAA) is the major cause of cSAH in elderly patients. Worsening dementia and headache are the common presentations.

The outcome of cSAH itself is generally benign and depends primarily on the underlying etiology. Vasospasm and delayed cerebral ischemia are rare.

Imaging

CT Findings. Most cases of cSAH are unilateral, involving one or several dorsolateral convexity sulci (6-13A). The basal cisterns are typically spared.

MR Findings. Focal sulcal hyperintensity on FLAIR is typical in cSAH. T2* (GRE, SWI) shows "blooming" in the affected sulci (6-13B). If the etiology of the cSAH is dural sinus or cortical vein occlusion, a hypointense "cord" sign may be present. Patients with CAA have multifocal cortical and pial microbleeds ("blooming black dots") on T2*. They may also show evidence of siderosis and prior lobar hemorrhages of differing ages.

Angiography. CTA, MRA, or DSA can be helpful in evaluating patients with convexal SAH secondary to vas-

culitis, dural sinus and/or cortical vein occlusion, and RCVS (6-13C).

Superficial Siderosis

Terminology

Hemosiderin deposition along brain surfaces, cranial nerves, and/or the spinal cord defines the condition known as superficial siderosis (SS) (6-14).

Etiology

SS is a consequence of chronic or intermittent hemorrhage into the subarachnoid space. Overall, trauma and surgery are the most common causes. Other reported etiologies include hemorrhagic neoplasm, vascular malformations, venous obstruction, and hemorrhagic vasculopathies such as amyloid angiopathy. SS due to repeated aneurysmal SAH is relatively uncommon.

Accelerated cerebellar ferritin synthesis and chronic intrathecal bleeding overload the ability of the microglia to biosynthesize ferritin, resulting in subpial iron excess. This facilitates free radical damage, lipid peroxidation, and neuronal degeneration.

Pathology

Location. Although it can occur anywhere in the CNS, SS has a predilection for the posterior fossa (cerebellar folia and vermis, CN VIII) and brainstem.

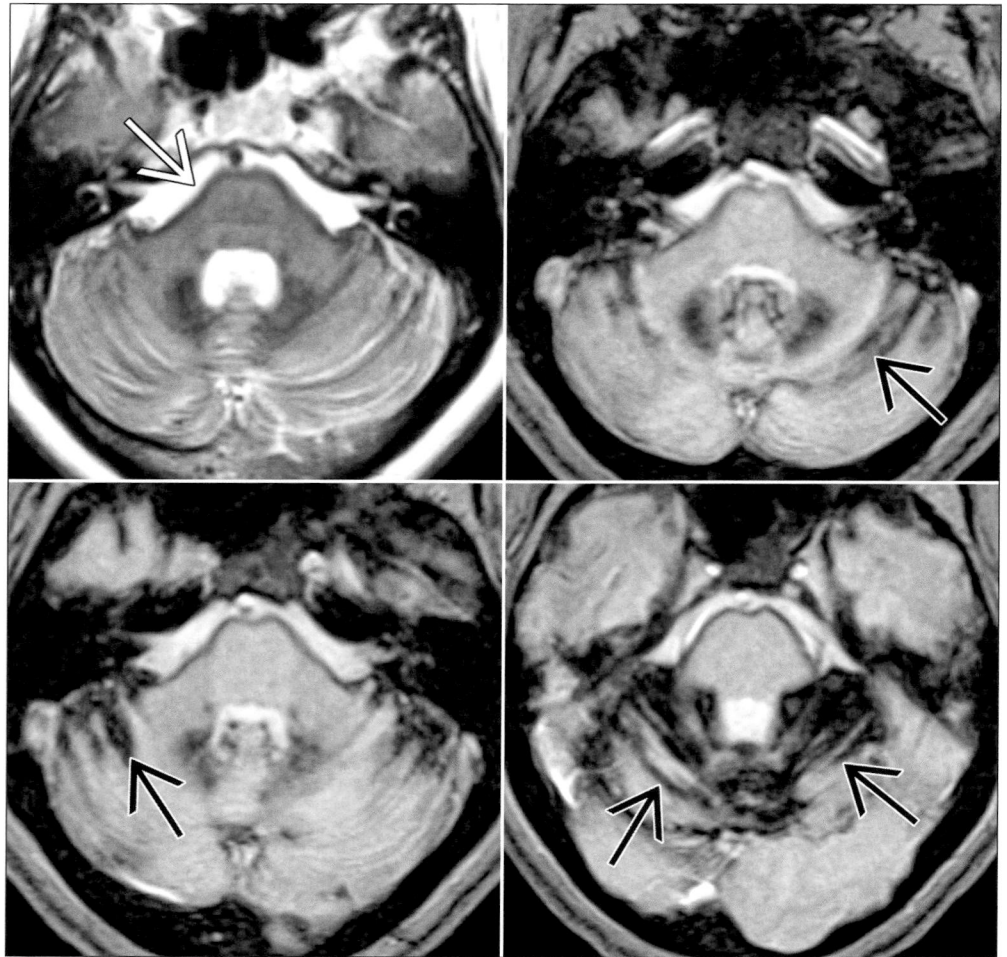

6-16. Series of MR images shows typical findings of superficial siderosis in a patient with bilateral sensorineural hearing loss and progressive ataxia. FSE T2WI shows linear hypointensity around the surfaces of the pons, cerebellum ➡. T2* GRE scans show marked "blooming" covering the pons and cerebellar hemispheres, extending into and along the folia ➡.

SS involving the cerebral convexities is seen in 60% of patients with cerebral amyloid angiopathy but is rare in non-CAA forms of intracerebral hemorrhages.

GROSS PATHOLOGY. Brownish yellow and blackish gray encrustations cover the affected structures, layering along the sulci and encasing cranial nerves **(6-15)**.

MICROSCOPIC FEATURES. Subpial hemosiderin depositions are the histologic hallmark of SS.

Clinical Issues

Patients often present with slowly progressive gait ataxia, dysarthria, and bilateral sensorineural hearing loss. Some patients present with progressive myelopathy. Often decades pass between the putative event that causes SS and the development of overt symptoms.

Imaging

CT is usually normal in patients with SS. Occasionally, iron deposition is severe enough to cause hyperattenuation along brain surfaces.

MR is the procedure of choice for evaluating patients with possible SS, both to establish the diagnosis and to identify the cause of repeated hemorrhage. In about one-third of cases, a bleeding source is not identified despite extensive investigation of the entire neuraxis.

SS is best identified on T2* (GRE, SWI) imaging and is seen as a hypointense rim (black "blooming") that follows along brain surfaces and coats the cranial nerves **(6-16)**. Despite extensive neuroimaging, the source of the SS often remains occult.

Differential Diagnosis

The major imaging differential diagnosis for superficial siderosis is **"bounce point" artifact**, reflecting a mismatch between repetition (TR) and inversion (TI) times on FLAIR and T1 IR sequences.

Occasionally, surface vessels such as **venous plexuses** with slow-flowing blood may cause focal linear hypointense areas along brain surfaces, especially on T2* imaging.

Rare causes of hypointensity and extensive "blooming" around the brain surfaces include two rare neurocutaneous syndromes: **Neurocutaneous melanosis** (typically hyperintense on T1WI) and **meningioangiomatosis** (thickened, enhancing, sometimes calcified and infiltrating proliferations of meningeal cells and blood vessels).

ANEURYSMAL vs. NONANEURYSMAL SAH

Aneurysmal SAH
- Widespread; basal cisterns
- Arterial origin
- Complications (vasospasm, ischemia) common

Perimesencephalic Nonaneurysmal SAH
- Focal; perimesencephalic, prepontine cisterns
- Probably venous origin
- Clinically benign; complications, recurrence rare

Convexal SAH
- Superficial (convexity) sulci
- Various causes (venous occlusion, vasculitis, amyloid)

Superficial Siderosis
- Posterior fossa > > supratentorial
- Chronic repeated SAH (cause often undetermined)
- Sensorineural hearing loss
- Brain, cranial nerves coated with hemosiderin

Aneurysms

Overview

Intracranial aneurysms are classified by their gross phenotypic appearance. The most common intracranial aneurysms are called **saccular** or **"berry" aneurysms** because of their striking sac- or berry-like configuration. Saccular aneurysms are acquired lesions that arise from branch points of major cerebral arteries where hemodynamic stresses are maximal. Saccular aneurysms lack some of the arterial layers (usually the internal elastic lamina and media) found in normal vessels. More than 90% of saccular aneurysms occur on the "anterior" (carotid) circulation.

Pseudoaneurysms are focal arterial dilatations that are not contained by any layers of the normal arterial wall. They are often irregularly shaped and typically consist of a paravascular, noncontained blood clot that cavitates and communicates with the parent vessel lumen. Intracranial pseudoaneurysms commonly arise from mid-sized arteries distal to the circle of Willis. Trauma, drug abuse, infection, and tumor are the usual etiologies.

Blood blister-like aneurysms (BBAs) are a special type of aneurysm recently recognized in the neurosurgical literature. BBAs are eccentric hemispherical arterial outpouchings that are covered by only a thin layer of adventitia. These dangerous lesions are both difficult to detect and difficult to treat. They have a tendency to rupture at a much smaller size and relatively younger age compared to saccular aneurysms. While BBAs can be found anywhere, they have a distinct propensity to occur along the supraclinoid internal carotid artery.

Fusiform aneurysms (FAs) are *focal* dilatations that involve the entire circumference of a vessel and extend for relatively short distances. FAs are more common on the vertebrobasilar ("posterior") circulation. FAs can be atherosclerotic (more common) or nonatherosclerotic in origin.

Saccular Aneurysm

Terminology

Saccular aneurysms (SAs) are sometimes called "true" aneurysms (to contrast them with pseudoaneurysms). A saccular ("berry") aneurysm is a focal arterial outpouching that affects only part of the parent artery circumference. Most SAs lack two important structural components of normal intracranial arteries, i.e., the internal elastic lamina and the muscular layer ("media").

Etiology

GENERAL CONCEPTS. The development and subsequent rupture of intracranial SAs reflects several complex interactions. SAs are *acquired* lesions that develop from abnormal vascular hemodynamics and wall shear stresses. Hemodynamic stresses are highest at arterial bifurcations or along the outer curves of major intracranial arteries. Abnormal wall shear stresses damage the internal elastic lamina, resulting in "bioengineering fatigue" and the arterial wall remodeling that precedes frank aneurysm formation.

GENETICS. Very few SAs are congenital (i.e., present at birth). However, many studies have demonstrated a genetic component to aneurysm development and rupture.

A number of genetic alterations have been associated with SAs although no single disease-causing gene variant has been identified. To date, most of the identified genes are moderators of cell cycle progression. They affect the

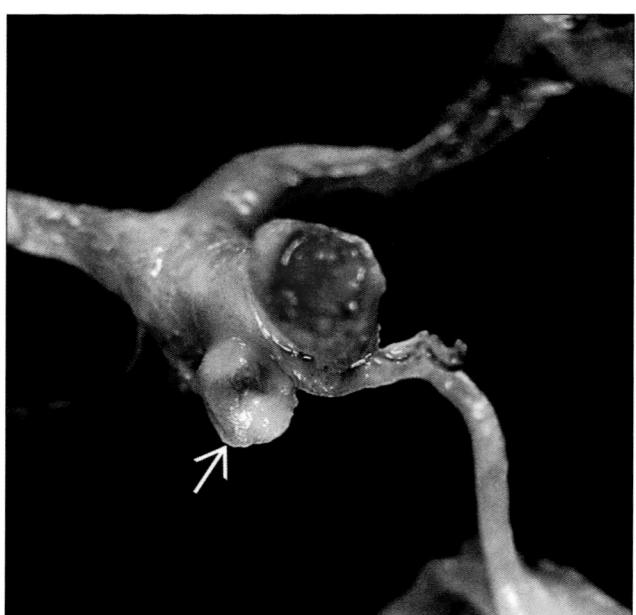

6-17. Autopsy specimen shows an incidental unruptured saccular aneurysm ➡ *at the IC-PCoA junction. (Courtesy B. Horten, MD.)*

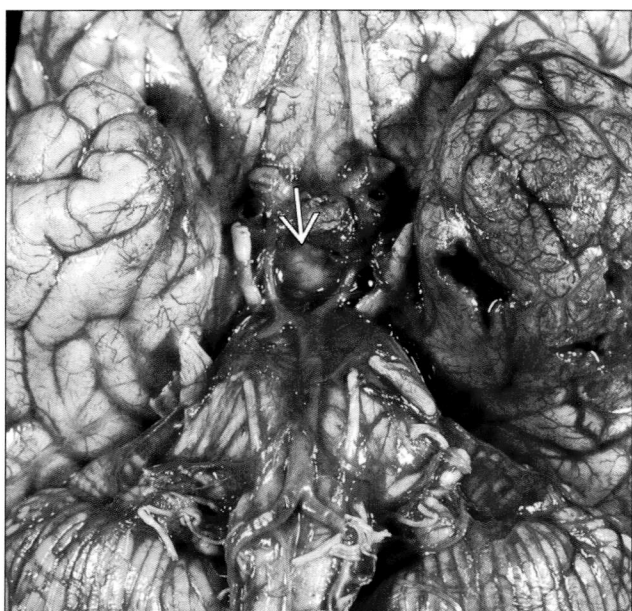

6-18. Autopsy demonstrates a ruptured basilar bifurcation aneurysm ➡ *with massive subarachnoid hemorrhage extending throughout all the basilar cisterns. (Courtesy R. Hewlett, MD.)*

proliferation and senescence of cell populations that are primarily responsible for vascular formation and repair.

Inherited vasculopathy, anomalous blood vessels, familial predisposition, and "high-flow" states (i.e., vessels supplying an arteriovenous malformation) all increase the risk of SA development.

Demographic studies have demonstrated that environmental factors such as systemic hypertension, smoking, and heavy alcohol consumption contribute significantly to the risk of developing SAs and may augment any underlying genetic propensities.

ANOMALOUS BLOOD VESSELS. A number of blood vessel asymmetries and some congenital vascular anomalies predispose to the development of an intracranial SA.

Bicuspid aortic valves, aortic coarctation, persistent trigeminal artery (TGA), and congenital anomalies of the anterior cerebral artery (i.e., A1 asymmetries or infraoptic course of the A1 segment) all carry an increased risk of SA. Whether arterial fenestrations (i.e., splitting and reuniting of a vessel such as the anterior communicating or basilar artery) are associated with an increased prevalence of SA is controversial.

INHERITED VASCULOPATHIES AND SYNDROMIC ANEURYSMS. Some multiorgan heritable connective tissue disorders (such as **Marfan** and **Ehlers-Danlos** syndromes or **fibromuscular dysplasia**) are associated with increased risk of intracranial aneurysms. Arteriopathy is common in patients with **neurofibromatosis type 1** (NF1). Although the vascular changes in NF1 primarily

affect the aorta and renal, coronary, and gastrointestinal arteries, some increased risk of developing intracranial aneurysms has been reported.

Autosomal dominant polycystic kidney disease carries an 8-10% lifetime risk of developing a saccular aneurysm.

FAMILIAL INTRACRANIAL ANEURYSMS. Up to 20% of patients with SAs have a family history of intracranial aneurysms. These intracranial SAs occur in "clusters" of related individuals without any known heritable connective tissue disorder and are termed **familial intracranial aneurysms** (FIAs). FIAs tend to occur in younger patients and rupture at a smaller size than sporadic SAs.

Patients with a first-order relative with aSAH have a 4-10 times higher risk of developing an SA. MR or CT angiography screening for asymptomatic, unruptured SAs in family members with two or more affected first-degree relatives is cost-effective and has been recommended by some investigators.

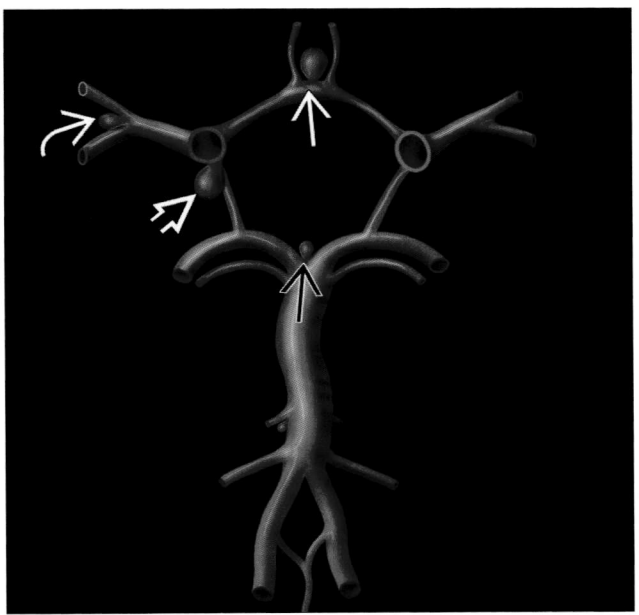

6-19. *The most common sites for saccular aneurysms are the ACoA* ➡ *and the IC-PCoA junction* ⮞. *Other locations include the MCA bifurcation* ⮚ *and the basilar tip* ➲.

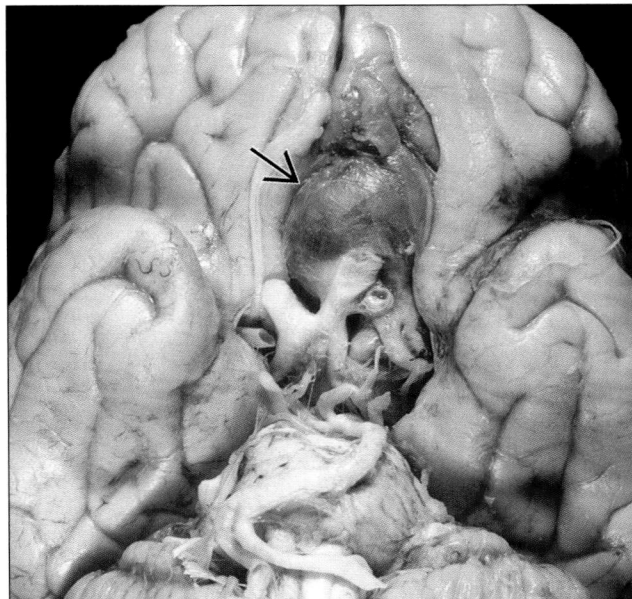

6-20. *Autopsy shows a giant aneurysm* ➲ *of the anterior communicating artery. (Courtesy R. Hewlett, MD.)*

SACCULAR ANEURYSM: ETIOLOGY

General Concepts
- Acquired, not congenital!
- Abnormal hemodynamics, shear stresses → weakened artery wall
- Underlying genetic alterations common

Increased Risk of SA
- Anomalous vessels
  ○ Persistent trigeminal artery
  ○ Fenestrated ACoA
- Vasculopathies, syndromes
  ○ Abnormal collagen (Marfan, Ehlers-Danlos)
  ○ Fibromuscular dysplasia
  ○ Autosomal dominant polycystic kidney disease
- Familial intracranial aneurysm
  ○ 4-10x ↑ risk if first-order family member with aSAH

Pathology

LOCATION. Most intracranial SAs occur at points of maximal hemodynamic stress. The vast majority arise from major blood vessel bifurcations or branches **(6-17)**. The circle of Willis (COW) and middle cerebral artery (MCA) bifurcations are the most common sites **(6-18)**. Aneurysms beyond the COW are uncommon as distal hemodynamic stresses are much lower. Many peripheral aneurysms are actually pseudoaneurysms secondary to trauma, infection, or tumor (see below).

Anterior circulation aneurysms. Ninety percent of SAs occur on the "anterior" circulation **(6-19)**. The anterior circulation consists of the internal carotid artery (ICA) and its terminal branches, the anterior (ACA) and

middle cerebral arteries. The ophthalmic artery, anterior (ACoA) and posterior communicating (PCoA) arteries, anterior choroidal artery (AChA), and hypophyseal arteries are all considered part of the anterior circulation.

Approximately one-third of SAs occur on the ACoA with another third arising at the junction of the ICA and the PCoA. Approximately 20% of SAs occur at the MCA bi- or trifurcation.

Posterior circulation aneurysms. Ten percent of SAs are located on the vertebrobasilar ("posterior") circulation. The basilar artery (BA) bifurcation is the most common site, accounting for about 5% of all SAs **(6-18)**. The posterior inferior cerebellar artery (PICA) is the second most common location.

SIZE AND NUMBER. SAs vary in size from tiny (two to three millimeters) to huge. SAs that are 2.5 cm or larger are called "giant" aneurysms **(6-20)**.

Between 15-20% of aneurysms are multiple. About 75% of patients with multiple aneurysms have two SAs, 15% have three, and 10% have more than three SAs. Multiple SAs are significantly more common in females.

GROSS PATHOLOGY. Intracranial SAs are dynamic—not static—lesions. Hemodynamic insults can elicit a pathological vascular response that leads to self-sustained aneurysmal remodeling. Persistence of the original inciting hemodynamic factors is not necessary for continued pathological progression.

The gross configuration of an SA changes with time as the arterial wall is remodeled in response to hemodynamic stresses. As it becomes progressively weakened, the wall begins to bulge outward, forming an SA **(6-21)**.

The opening (ostium) of an SA can be narrow or broad-based. Complex intraaneurysmal hemodynamics result in flow impinging on different parts of the aneurysm. Some impact the ostium, and others are most prominent at the dome. One or more lobules or an apical "tit" may develop as a result. Such outpouchings are usually the part of the aneurysm wall most vulnerable to rupture, resulting in aneurysmal SAH (aSAH).

MICROSCOPIC FEATURES. SAs demonstrate a disrupted or absent internal elastic lamina (IEL). The smooth muscle cell layer (media) is generally absent **(6-22)**. The delicate balance between the synthesis and degradation of the extracellular matrix (ECM)—a dynamic network of proteins and proteoglycans—is disrupted. Therefore, the wall of an SA is usually quite fragile, consisting of intima and adventitia in a degraded ECM. Variable

amounts of thrombus **(6-23)**, inflammation, and atherosclerotic changes may also be present.

Giant SAs often show mural calcification, laminated clot of different ages, and variable thrombosis.

Clinical Issues

EPIDEMIOLOGY. The overall incidence of intracranial SAs in the general population is 2-6%. Asymptomatic unruptured SAs are at least 10 times more prevalent than ruptured SAs.

DEMOGRAPHICS. Peak presentation is between 40 and 60 years of age. There is a definite female predominance, especially with multiple SAs.

SAs are rare in children, accounting for less than 2% of all cases, although they are the most common cause of spontaneous (nontraumatic) SAH in this age group.

In comparison to adult aneurysms, pediatric aneurysms have a predilection for the posterior circulation. They also attain larger size and frequently develop a more complex shape. Childhood aneurysms exhibit a relative lack

6-21A. Autopsy shows an ACoA aneurysm ➡ projecting superiorly between the A2 segments of both anterior cerebral arteries. *6-21B.* The aneurysm is dissected out and cut in coronal section. Reactive changes thicken the base of the aneurysm, but the dome ➡ is relatively thin. (Courtesy J. Townsend, MD.)

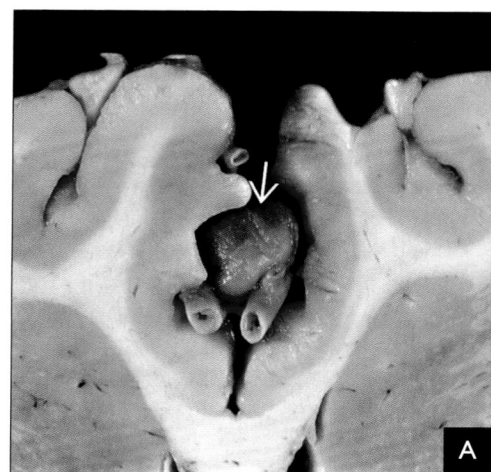

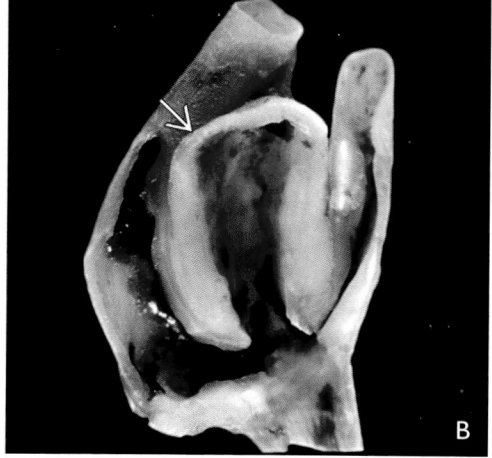

6-22. Cross section of an aneurysm shows normal internal elastic lamina, muscular layer in the parent artery wall ➡. The aneurysm sac ➡ lacks both these layers and is composed of only intima and adventitia. *6-23.* Close-up view of a mostly thrombosed aneurysm ➡ demonstrates organizing clots of different ages. (Courtesy R. Hewlett, MD.)

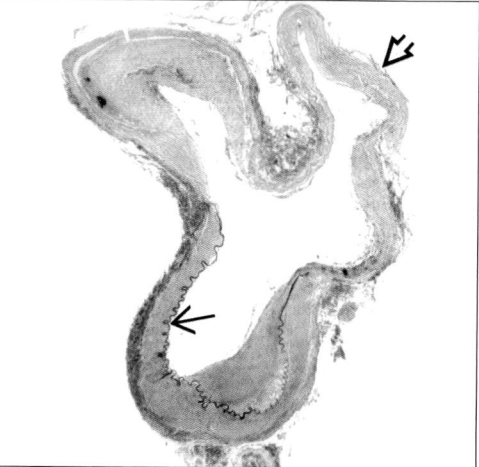

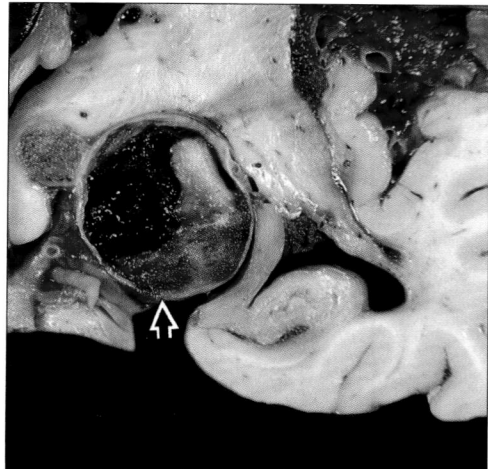

of female predominance and are more often associated with trauma or infection. Higher recurrence rates and de novo formation or growth are also common.

PRESENTATION. Between 80-90% of all nontraumatic SAHs are caused by ruptured SAs. The most common presentation is sudden onset of severe, excruciating headache ("thunderclap" or "worst headache of my life").

Cranial neuropathy is a relatively uncommon presentation of SA. Of these, a pupil-involving CN III palsy from a PCoA aneurysm is the most common. Occasionally, patients with partially or completely thrombosed aneurysms present with a transient ischemic attack or stroke.

NATURAL HISTORY. There are three stages in the natural history of SAs: (1) formation/initiation, (2) growth/enlargement, and (3) rupture.

No clear consensus exists as to whether aneurysm growth affects aneurysm behavior (i.e., rupture risk). SAs do not enlarge at a constant time-independent rate; their growth is highly variable and unpredictable. Enlarging aneurysms are more likely to rupture, but 10% of ruptures occur in the absence of detectable growth.

The overall annual rupture rate of SAs is 1-2%. However, the natural course of unruptured cerebral aneurysms varies according to size, location, and shape of the aneurysm. Larger size, location on either the anterior or posterior communicating arteries (vs. the MCA), and the presence of a "daughter" sac (irregular wall protrusion) all increase rupture risk. The "perianeurysmal environment" may also influence aneurysm geometry and rupture risk, especially at locations with contact restraint by bone or dura.

TREATMENT OPTIONS. There are three basic options for the treatment of SAs: (1) observation, (2) surgical clipping, and (3) endovascular occlusion. The management of unruptured SAs is controversial because of their unpredictable natural history. In contrast, virtually all ruptured SAs are treated. Ideally, management should be tailored to the individual patient with all options considered for optimum outcome.

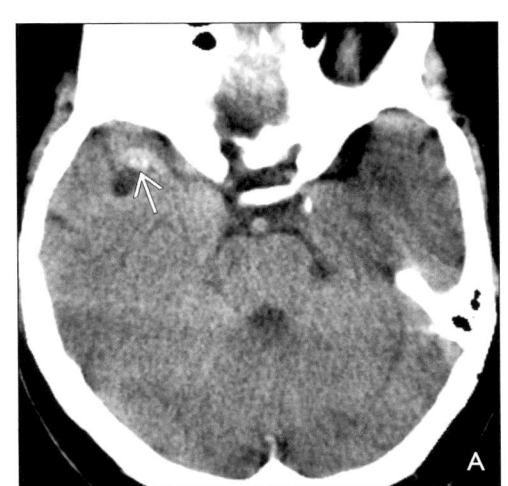

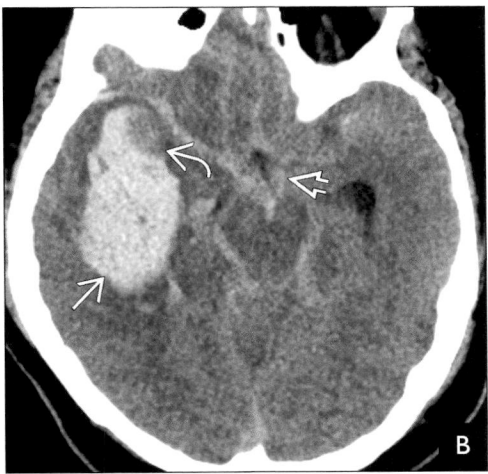

6-24A. NECT scan obtained in a patient following head trauma was called normal. In retrospect, a small rounded hyperdensity at the right middle cerebral artery bifurcation ➡ can be identified. 6-24B. Seven years later, the patient presented with sudden severe headache followed by collapse. NECT now shows diffuse basilar SAH ➡ and a right temporal hematoma ➡ with a focal round hypodense area in its superomedial border ➡.

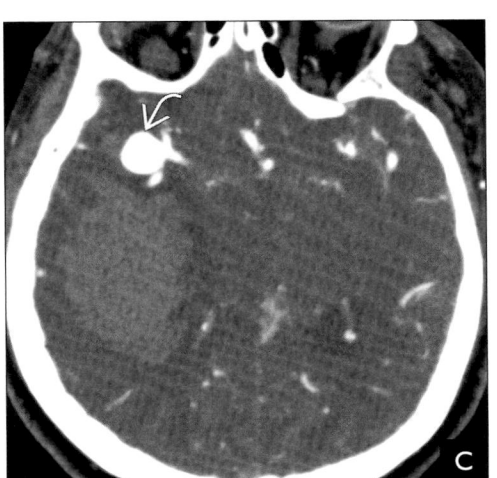

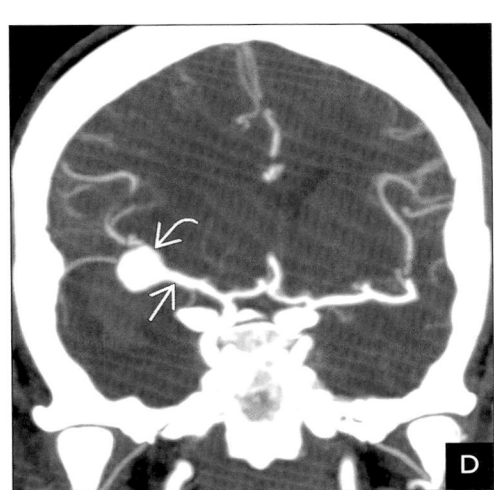

6-24C. CTA shows an intensely enhancing saccular aneurysm ➡ at the MCA bi-/trifurcation just anterior to the temporal lobe hematoma. 6-24D. Coronal MIP of the CTA nicely demonstrates the aneurysm ➡. The M1 MCA segment ➡ is elevated by the mass effect from the hematoma.

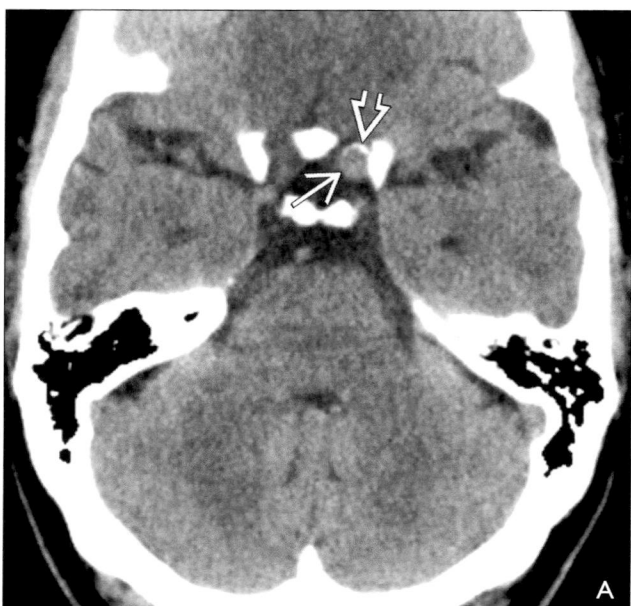

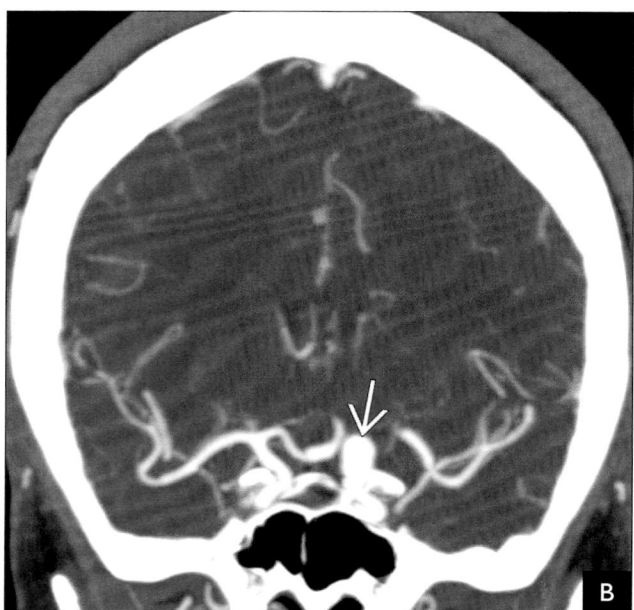

6-25A. NECT scan shows an incidentally discovered saccular aneurysm, seen here as a well-demarcated rounded hyperdensity ➡ with some peripheral calcification ➤.

6-25B. Coronal MIP of the CTA in the same patient shows a patent saccular aneurysm ➡ at the terminal bifurcation of the left ICA.

Aneurysmal SAH is a catastrophic event with high mortality and significant morbidity. Approximately one-third of patients die, and one-third survive with significant residual neurological deficits. Only one-quarter to one-third of patients with aSAH recover with good functional outcome.

Patients who survive the initial SAH are typically treated as soon as possible. Rebleeding risk is highest in the first 24-48 hours after the initial hemorrhage. Approximately 20% of ruptured but untreated SAs rebleed within two weeks. Half rehemorrhage within six months.

Observation. In 2000, the International Study of Unruptured Intracranial Aneurysms suggested that asymptomatic anterior circulation aneurysms seven millimeters or less in diameter rarely rupture. As a consequence, observation ("watchful waiting") with serial imaging of small, incidentally discovered unruptured aneurysms became a more common treatment approach.

However, more recent meta-analyses have demonstrated that 13% of ruptured intracranial SAs are less than five millimeters in diameter. Nearly half of all aneurysms under five millimeters in diameter rupture within five to ten years, suggesting that *there is no generally accepted "safe" minimum diameter threshold for rupture!*

Surgical clipping. SAs can be clipped, trapped, and/ or bypassed. Surgical clipping results in lower recurrence rates compared with endovascular treatment but is associated with higher complication rates, greater in-hospital mortality, and increased long-term morbidity.

Endovascular treatment. Endovascular treatment results in a 22.6% relative and 6.9% absolute decreased risk of complications compared to surgical clipping. Recovery is quicker, and in-hospital mortality/morbidity are generally lower.

Reopening occurs in approximately 20% of coiled aneurysms. While large aneurysm size and low coil packing are established risk factors, adequately occluded aneurysms smaller than 10 mm rarely recur within the first 5-10 years after coiling.

Imaging

GENERAL FEATURES. SAs are round or lobulated arterial outpouchings that are most commonly found along the COW and at the MCA bifurcation. Imaging features depend on whether the aneurysm is unruptured or ruptured (with aSAH) and whether the aneurysm sac is patent or partially or completely thrombosed.

CT FINDINGS. Very small unruptured SAs may be invisible on standard NECT scans. Larger lesions appear as well-delineated masses that are slightly hyperdense to brain (6-24). Rim or mural calcification may be present (6-25).

Acutely ruptured SAs present with aneurysmal SAH, which is often the dominant imaging feature and frequently obscures the "culprit" aneurysm. Occasionally, an SA appears as a well-delineated, relatively hypodense filling defect within a pool of hyperdense subarachnoid blood (6-24B).

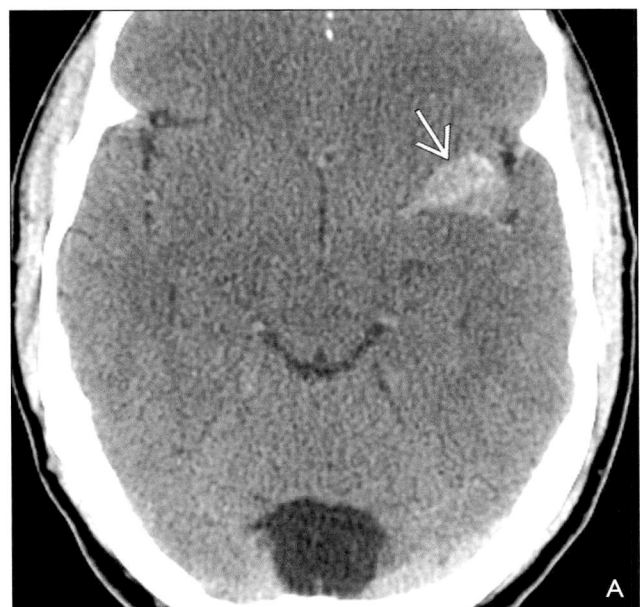

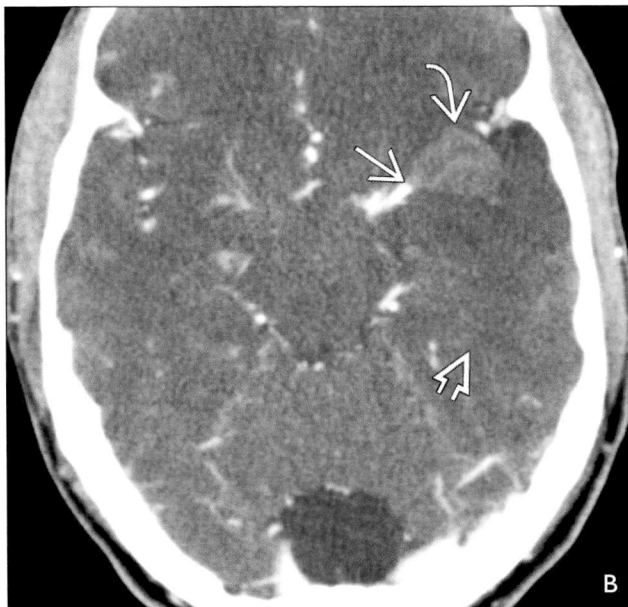

6-26A. NECT scan in a patient with sudden onset of right hemiparesis shows a large well-delineated ovoid hyperdensity along the left MCA ➡ suggesting acute thrombosis of a saccular aneurysm.

6-26B. CTA shows abrupt termination of the left MCA ➡ with nonfilling of the thrombosed aneurysm ➡. The paucity of normal vessels in the left temporal lobe ➡ is secondary to embolic occlusion of the distal MCA branches.

A partially or completely thrombosed SA is typically hyperdense compared to the adjacent brain on NECT scans **(6-26)**.

Patent SAs show strong, uniform enhancement of the aneurysm lumen **(6-24)**. A partially thrombosed SA shows enhancement of the residual lumen. Completely thrombosed SAs do not enhance although longstanding lesions may demonstrate rim enhancement secondary to reactive inflammatory changes.

MR FINDINGS. MR findings vary with pulse sequence, flow dynamics, and the presence as well as the age of associated hemorrhage (either in the subarachnoid cisterns or within the aneurysm itself).

About half of all patent SAs demonstrate "flow voids" on T1- and T2WI **(6-27)**. The other half exhibit heterogeneous signal intensity secondary to slow or turbulent flow, saturation effects, and phase dispersion. Propagation of pulsation artifacts in the phase-encoding direction is common. FLAIR scans may show hyperintensity in the subarachnoid cisterns secondary to aSAH.

If the aneurysm is partially or completely thrombosed, laminated clot with differing signal intensities is often present **(6-28)**. "Blooming" on susceptibility-weighted images (GRE, SWI) is common. Contrast-enhanced scans may show T1 shortening in intraaneurysmal slow-flow areas.

DWI sequences may show ischemic areas secondary to vasospasm or embolized thrombus.

ANGIOGRAPHY. High-resolution multidetector CTA is a common screening procedure in patients with suspected aSAH. The sensitivity of CTA is more than 95% for aneurysms larger than two millimeters in diameter. The overall sensitivity of MRA is 90% for aneurysms larger than two millimeters in diameter.

Although many patients with aSAH and an SA that has been demonstrated on either CTA or MRA go directly to surgery, conventional DSA is still considered the gold standard for detecting intracranial SAs—especially if endovascular treatment is considered.

All four intracranial vessels as well as the complete circle of Willis must be demonstrated in multiple projections. Rotational 3D DSA with shaded surface displays is helpful in delineating the precise relationship between the aneurysm and its parent vessels and branches.

Multiple intracranial aneurysms are demonstrated in 15-20% of cases. When more than one aneurysm is identified in patients with aSAH, determining which aneurysm ruptured is essential for presurgical planning. Contrast extravasation is pathognomonic of rupture but is rarely observed. Other angiographic features suggesting rupture include lobulation or the presence of an apical "tit," size (the largest aneurysm is generally—although not always—the one that ruptured), and the presence of focal perianeurysmal clot on CT or MR.

Computational analyses of intracranial aneurysms show that ruptured aneurysms are more likely to have complex and/or unstable flow patterns, concentrated inflows, and

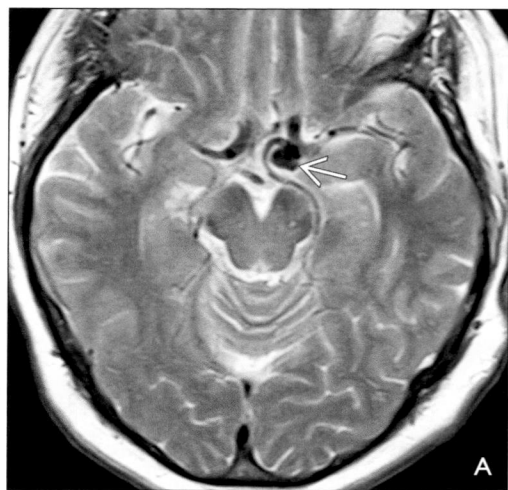

6-27A. *Axial T2WI shows a well-demarcated lobulated "flow void"* ➔ *consistent with a patent saccular aneurysm.*

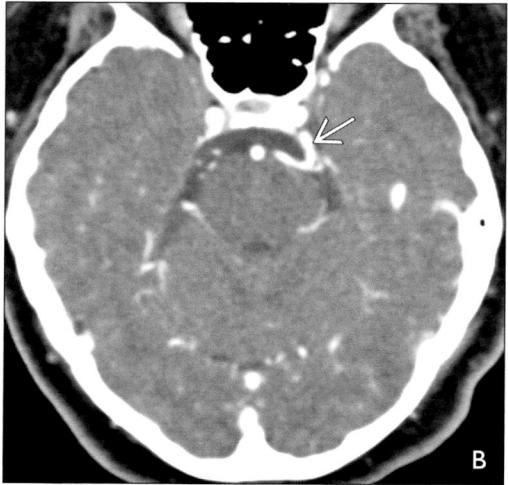

6-27B. *CTA source image in the same patient shows a classic persistent left trigeminal artery* ➔.

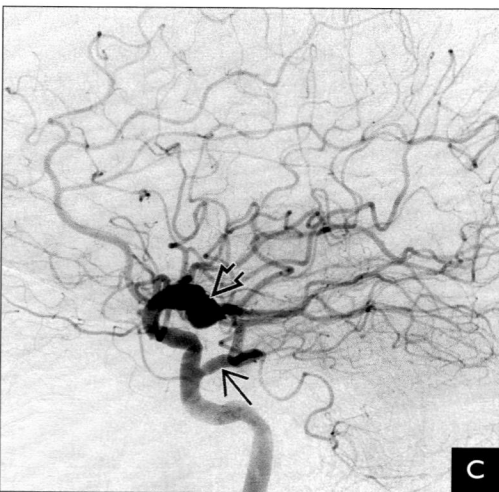

6-27C. *Lateral DSA shows the aneurysm* ⊳ *together with a classic "Neptune's trident" appearance of a persistent trigeminal artery* ➔.

small impingement regions from the "jet" of blood entering the lesion. Volume variations with the cardiac cycle may also influence rupture risk.

Differential Diagnosis

The major differential diagnosis of intracranial SA is a **vessel loop**. Intracranial arteries curve and branch extensively. On two-dimensional images (e.g., AP and lateral views of digital subtraction angiograms), overlapping or looping vessels may mimic the rounded sac of a small peripheral SA. Multiple projections and 3D shaded surface displays are helpful in sorting out overlapping or looping vessels from SA.

The second most common differential diagnosis is an **arterial infundibulum**. An infundibulum is a focal, symmetric, conical dilatation at the origin of a blood vessel that can easily be mistaken for a small saccular aneurysm. An infundibulum is small, typically less than three millimeters in diameter. The distal vessel typically arises from the apex—not the side—of the infundibulum. The PCoA is the most common location for an infundibulum.

While most infundibula are incidental anatomical variants without pathogenetic significance, occasionally an arterial infundibulum ruptures or, over time, even develops into a frank aneurysm. When these rare "aneurysm-like infundibula" rupture and cause subarachnoid hemorrhage, they are indistinguishable from classic saccular aneurysms.

A **pseudoaneurysm** may be difficult to distinguish from an SA. Pseudoaneurysms are more common on vessels distal to the circle of Willis and are often fusiform or irregular in shape. Focal parenchymal hematomas often surround intracranial pseudoaneurysms.

Fusiform aneurysms (FAs) are generally easily distinguished from SAs by their shape. FAs are long-segment, sausage-shaped lesions that involve the entire circumference of a vessel whereas SAs are round or lobulated lesions. Location is also a helpful feature in distinguishing an FA from an SA. FAs are more common in the vertebrobasilar ("posterior") circulation. SAs usually arise from terminal vessel bifurcations and are more common in the carotid ("anterior") circulation.

A **blood blister-like aneurysm** (BBA) may also be difficult to distinguish from a small, wide-necked SA. Although they can be found in virtually any part of the intracranial circulation, BBAs typically arise along the greater curvature of the supraclinoid internal carotid artery, not at its terminal bifurcation or PCoA origin.

An area of **signal loss** that mimics the "flow void" of an aneurysm on MR can be caused by an aerated ante-

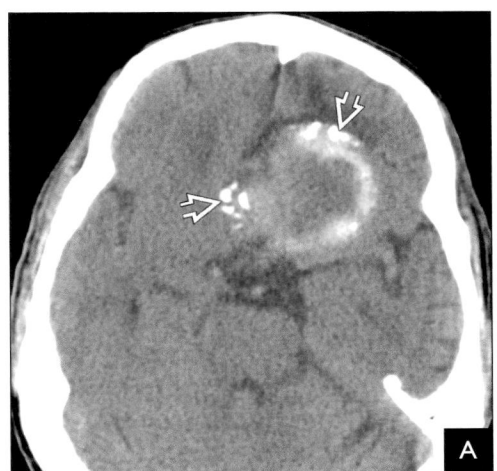

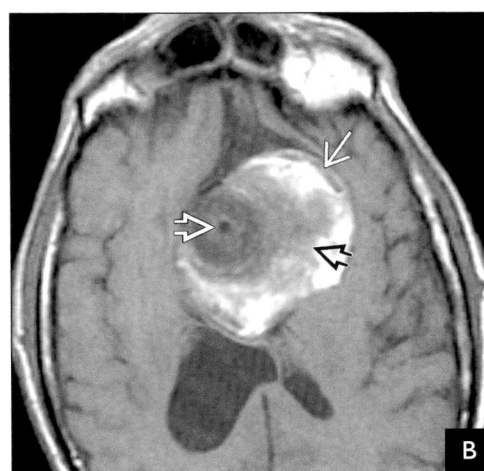

6-28A. NECT scan shows typical features of a giant saccular aneurysm with extensive calcified mural thrombus ⇨ surrounding an isodense central clot. 6-28B. T1WI in the same patient shows concentric rings of organized clot at different stages of evolution. The peripheral layer is hyperintense and older ➡ whereas the more central irregular isointense clot ⇱ is more recent. A small "flow void" ⇨ represents the residual patent lumen of the aneurysm.

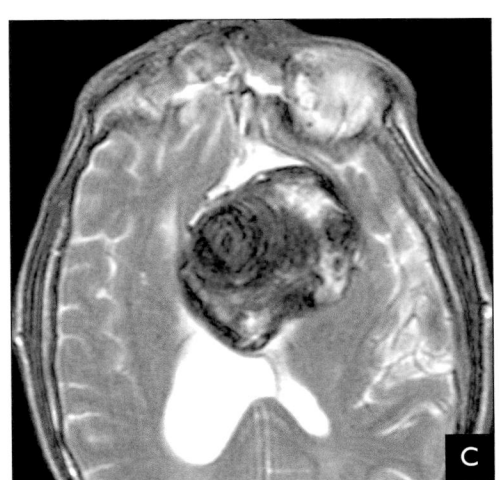

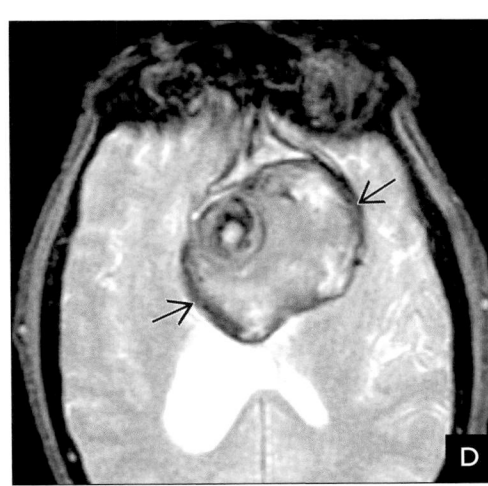

6-28C. T2WI in the same patient demonstrates multiple concentric rings of organized clot that resemble the layers of an onion. 6-28D. T2* GRE scan demonstrates hemosiderin deposition ➡ around the outer wall of the mostly thrombosed giant aneurysm.

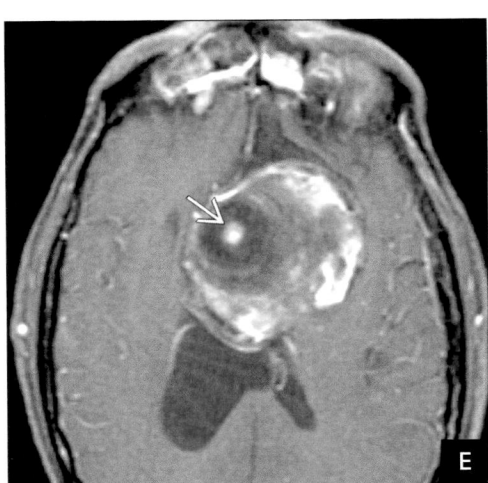

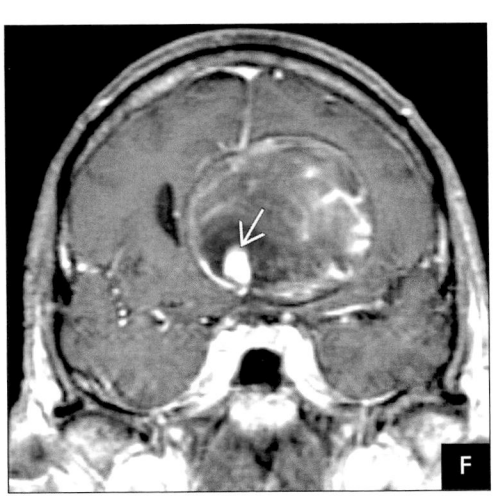

6-28E. T1 C+ FS scan shows that the small residual patent lumen of the aneurysm enhances ➡. 6-28F. Coronal T1 C+ shows that the small residual lumen ➡ is almost completely encased by thick layers of organized and organizing thrombus.

rior clinoid process or an aberrant supraorbital ethmoid or frontal sinus.

SACCULAR ANEURYSM

Location
- Anterior circulation (90%), posterior (10%)
- Circle of Willis, MCA bi-/trifurcation
- Multiple (15-30%)

Clinical Issues
- Overall prevalence = 2-6%
- Asymptomatic until rupture
- Risk generally correlates with size, but small lesions may bleed!
- Subarachnoid hemorrhage →"thunderclap" headache
- Peak age = 40-60 years (rare in children)

Imaging
- Round/lobulated arterial outpouching
- CTA 95% sensitive if aneurysm > 2 mm
- DSA with 3D SSD best delineates architecture

Differential Diagnosis
- Vessel loop
- Arterial infundibulum (conical, ≤ 2 mm)
- Blood blister-like aneurysm

Pseudoaneurysm

Pseudoaneurysm is a rare but important underdiagnosed cause of intracranial hemorrhage.

Terminology

Pseudoaneurysm—also sometimes called a "false" aneurysm to distinguish it from a "true" saccular aneurysm—is an arterial dilatation with complete disruption of the arterial wall.

Etiology

Pseudoaneurysms are usually caused by a specific inciting event—e.g., trauma, infection, drug abuse, neoplasm, or surgery—that initially weakens and then disrupts the normal arterial wall.

The weakened arterial wall expands and finally ruptures, forming a paravascular hematoma **(6-29)**. If the hematoma cavitates and communicates directly with the residual vessel lumen, a pseudoaneurysm is created.

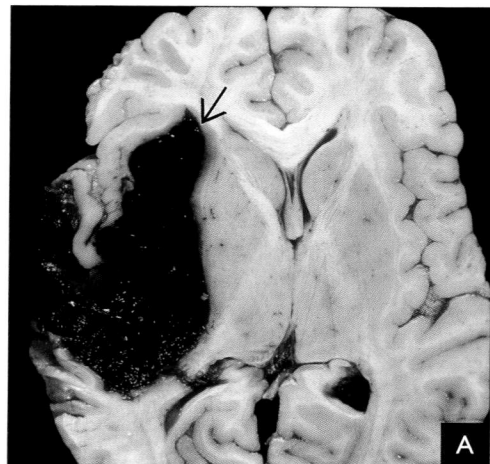
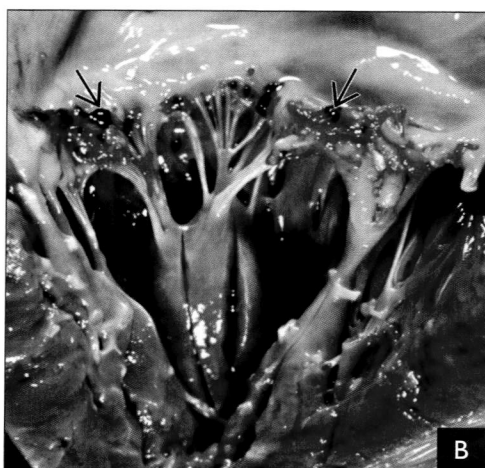

6-29A. Axial autopsy section from a patient with bacterial endocarditis shows a large focal right temporal lobe hematoma ⟶ *caused by a ruptured mycotic pseudoaneurysm of the middle cerebral artery. 6-29B. Sectioned heart from the same patient shows extensive hemorrhagic vegetations* ⟶ *covering much of the mitral valve.*

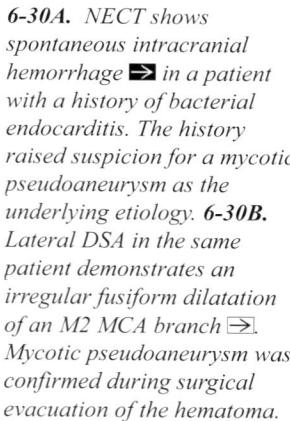
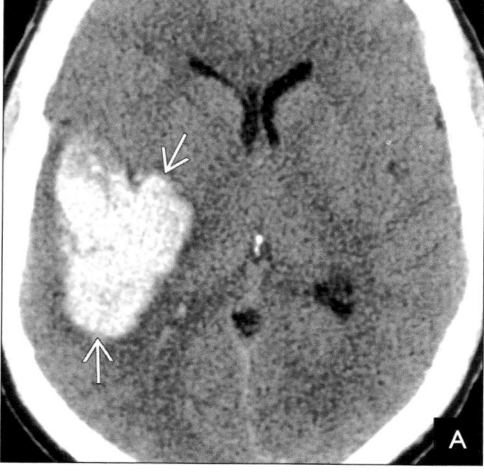
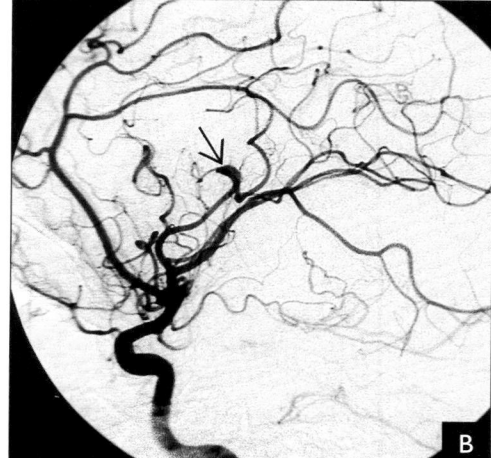

6-30A. NECT shows spontaneous intracranial hemorrhage ⟶ *in a patient with a history of bacterial endocarditis. The history raised suspicion for a mycotic pseudoaneurysm as the underlying etiology. 6-30B. Lateral DSA in the same patient demonstrates an irregular fusiform dilatation of an M2 MCA branch* ⟶*. Mycotic pseudoaneurysm was confirmed during surgical evacuation of the hematoma.*

Pseudoaneurysms are contained only by relatively fragile, cavitated clot and variable amounts of fibrous tissue. As they lack normal vessel wall components, pseudoaneurysms are especially prone to repeated hemorrhage.

Pathology

LOCATION. Traumatic pseudoaneurysms typically involve the proximal (cavernous or paraclinoid) intracranial ICA. Surgery and radiation therapy (typically for head and neck cancers) usually affect the extracranial carotid artery (carotid "blow-out" syndrome).

Infectious (mycotic), drug-related, and neoplastic (oncotic) pseudoaneurysms are typically located distal to the circle of Willis.

GROSS PATHOLOGY. Pseudoaneurysms are purplish masses typically contained only by thinned, discontinuous adventitia and organized hematoma. Hematomas associated with pseudoaneurysms are often large and may contain clots of varying ages.

MICROSCOPIC FEATURES. Wall disruption or necrosis is characteristic. Mycotic and oncotic pseudoaneurysms show extensive infiltration of the vessel wall by inflammatory or neoplastic cells, respectively. The parent vessel lumen is often occluded by thrombus, tumor, debris, or purulent exudate.

Clinical Issues

Patients with traumatic intracranial pseudoaneurysms often have skull base fractures. The interval between the initial injury and neurological deterioration varies from a few days up to several months. The major clinical presentations include sudden headache, loss of consciousness, recurrent epistaxis, and cranial nerve palsies.

Imaging

GENERAL FEATURES. Findings suggestive of cerebral pseudoaneurysm include unexplained enlargement of an existing parenchymal hematoma. In the appropriate clinical setting, unusual or delayed evolution of hematoma also suggests the possibility of an underlying pseudoaneurysm.

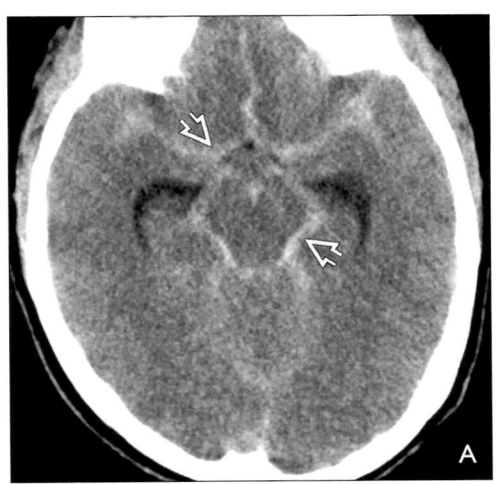
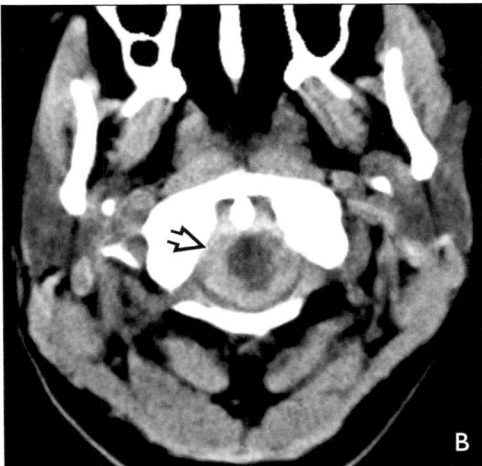

6-31A. Axial NECT scan in a 29-year-old woman with severe head and neck trauma shows typical aneurysmal SAH ➡ filling the basal cisterns. 6-31B. NECT scan of the craniovertebral junction shows unusually dense subarachnoid blood ➡ surrounding the upper cervical spinal cord.

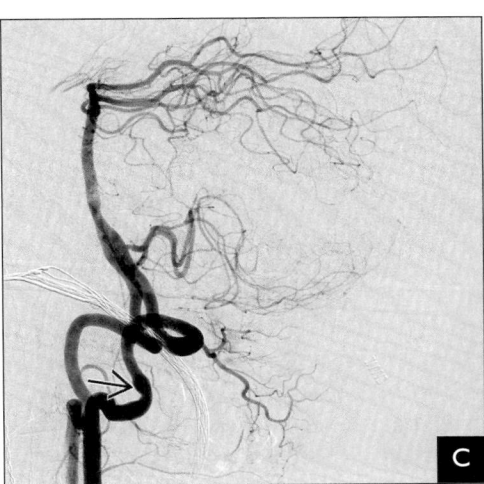
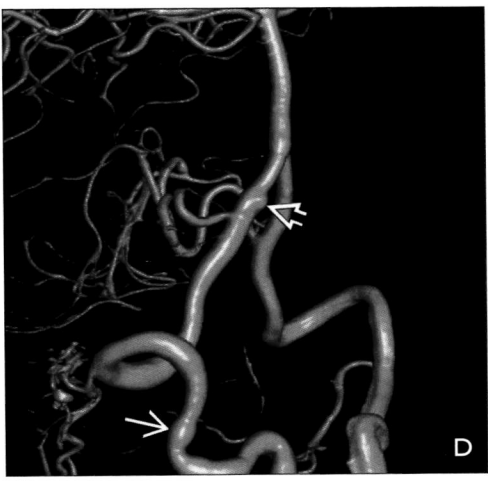

6-31C. Emergency DSA was obtained. Oblique lateral view of the selective right vertebral angiogram shows an irregularity of the vertebral artery between C1 and C2 ➡. 6-31D. 3D SSD shows a pseudoaneurysm of the distal extracranial right vertebral artery ➡. A second smaller pseudoaneurysm of the intracranial vertebral artery is seen ➡ just distal to the origin of the posterior inferior cerebellar artery.

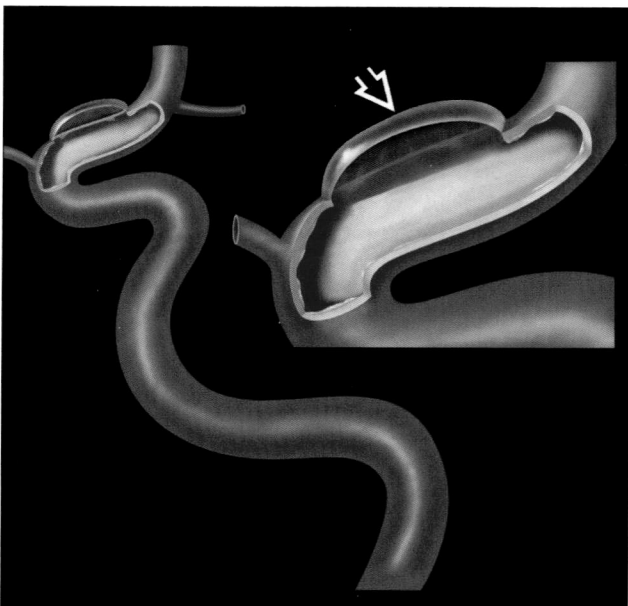

6-32. Graphic depicts blood blister-like aneurysm, seen here as a broad-based hemispheric bulge covered with a tissue-paper-thin layer of adventitia ➡.

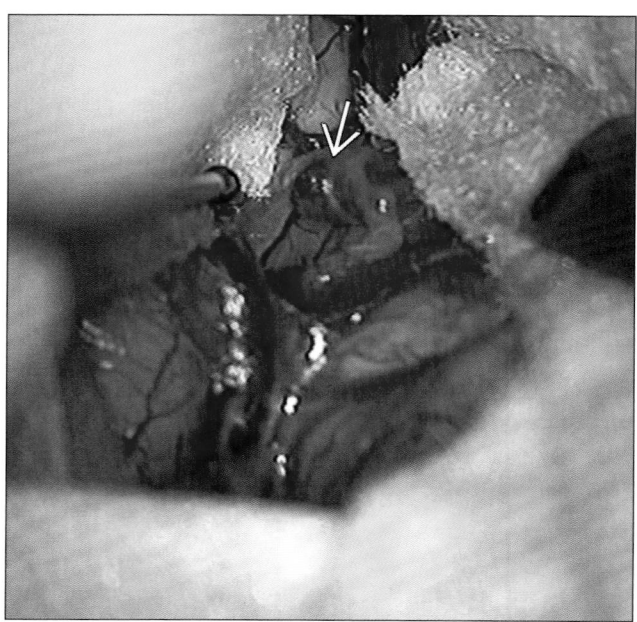

6-33. Intraoperative photograph shows a blood blister-like aneurysm ➡ with blood swirling under the thin, nearly transparent aneurysm wall.

CT FINDINGS. NECT scans are generally normal or nonspecific. A parenchymal hematoma is common (6-30). CTA sometimes shows a "spot" sign (focus of contrast enhancement) within a rapidly expanding hematoma.

MR FINDINGS. Hematoma signal varies with clot age and sequence. A "flow void" representing the residual lumen may be present within the hematoma. Intravascular enhancement represents the slow, delayed filling and emptying often seen with pseudoaneurysms.

ANGIOGRAPHY. Digital subtraction angiography shows a globular, fusiform, or irregularly shaped "neckless" aneurysm with delayed filling and emptying of contrast agent (6-31). Positional contrast stagnation is common.

Endovascular occlusion with coils, liquid embolics, or covered stent is the method of choice to treat intracranial pseudoaneurysms. Surgical options include trapping or sacrificing the parent artery with or without bypass graft.

Differential Diagnosis

The major differential diagnosis of pseudoaneurysm is a "true" or **saccular aneurysm**. Location is a helpful feature, as saccular aneurysms typically occur along the circle of Willis and at the MCA bifurcation.

Dissecting aneurysm most frequently occurs in the posterior circulation where the vertebral artery is the most common site. **Fusiform aneurysm** is also more common on the posterior circulation and typically involves the basilar artery.

PSEUDOANEURYSM

Terminology
- Also called "false" aneurysm
- Arterial wall completely disrupted

Pathology
- Often contained only by cavitated clot
- Caused by trauma, infection, drugs, tumor
- Delayed hematoma, sudden expansion common

Location
- Cavernous/paraclinoid ICA (trauma)
- Distal cortical branches (infection, drugs)

Imaging
- Fusiform, irregularly shaped vessel outpouching
- "Neck" usually absent
- ± surrounding avascular mass effect (hematoma)
- May show "spot" sign on CTA

Differential Diagnosis
- Saccular aneurysm
- Dissecting aneurysm
- Fusiform aneurysm

Blood Blister-like Aneurysm

Blood blister-like aneurysms (BBAs), also known as blister aneurysms, are an uncommon but potentially lethal subtype of intracranial pseudoaneurysm.

BBAs are small, broad-based hemispheric bulges that typically arise at nonbranching sites of intracranial arteries (6-32). BBAs have different clinical features and pose special diagnostic and treatment challenges in comparison with those of typical saccular aneurysms. Preoperative recognition of a BBA is essential for proper management.

Etiology and Pathology

Hemodynamic stress and atherosclerosis seem to be the most important factors in formation of a BBA. BBAs are often covered with only a thin friable cap of fibrous tissue, with or without a fragile layer of adventitia (6-33). Although BBAs can arise anywhere in the intracranial circulation, the anterosuperior (dorsal) wall of the supraclinoid ICA is the most common site.

Clinical Issues

BBAs tend to rupture at an earlier patient age and at significantly smaller size compared to typical saccular aneurysms.

Because they are extremely fragile lesions that lack a definable neck, treatment is difficult. BBAs easily tear during surgical clipping, which may result in fatal hemorrhage. Intraprocedural rupture is common, occurring in nearly 50% of cases.

Coiling BBAs is rarely successful because of their wide necks and fragile walls. Flow-diverting stents have been tried with some limited success. If sufficient collateral circulation is present, trapping and occluding the parent vessel may be an option. If endovascular treatment is unsuccessful, wrapping and revascularization have been recommended as potential surgical options.

Imaging

BBAs are small, often subtle lesions that are easily overlooked. A slight irregularity or small focal hemispherical bulge of the arterial wall may be the only finding. 3D DSA with shaded surface display has been helpful in identifying these difficult, dangerous lesions (6-34).

Fusiform Aneurysm

Fusiform aneurysms (FAs) can be atherosclerotic (common) or nonatherosclerotic (rare). In contrast to saccular aneurysms, FAs usually involve long, nonbranching vessel segments and are seen as focal circumferential outpouchings from a generally ectatic, elongated vessel.

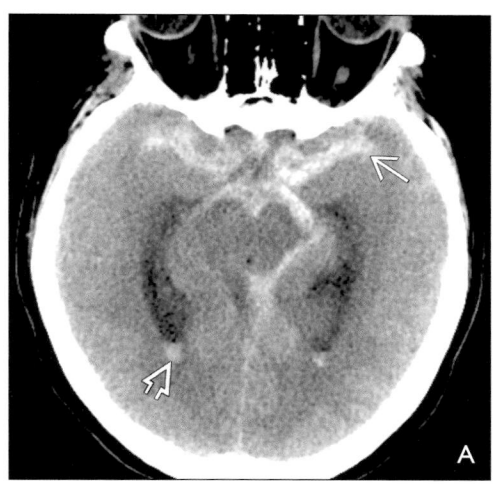

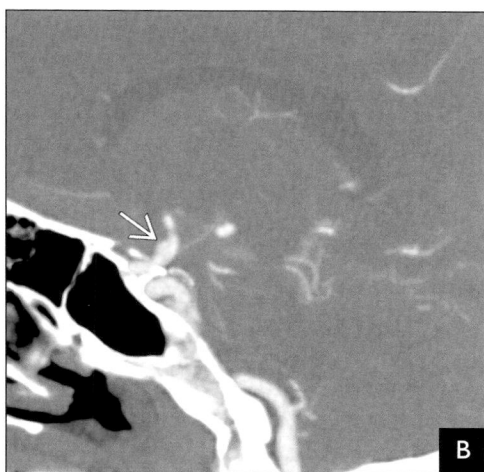

6-34A. *NECT scan in a young adult with sudden onset of severe "thunderclap" headache shows diffuse subarachnoid hemorrhage ➡, obstructive hydrocephalus with intraventricular hemorrhage ➡.* **6-34B.** *Reformatted lateral view of the CTA in the same patient shows a small broad-based contrast-filled hemispheric bulge ➡ along the greater curve of the ICA.*

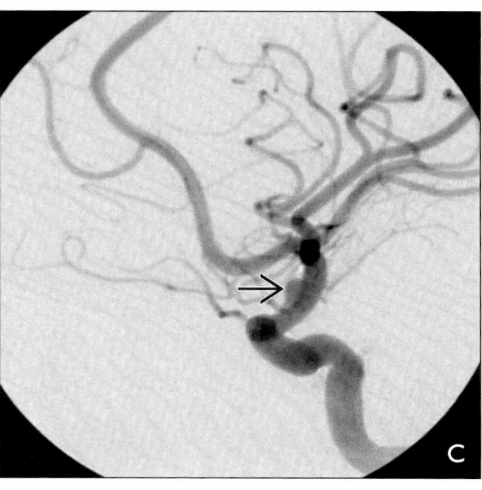

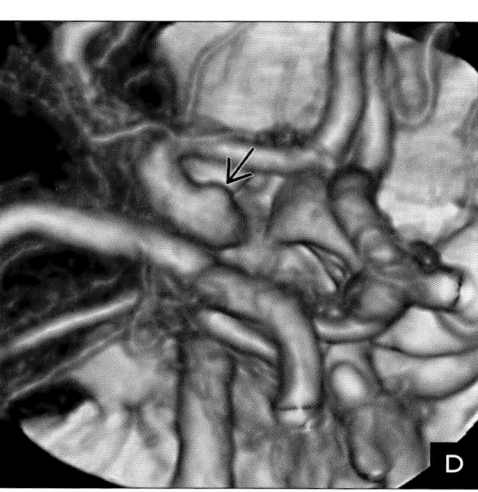

6-34C. *Lateral DSA in the same patient shows the classic appearance of a blood blister-like aneurysm and confirms the CTA finding of a focal broad-based hemispheric bulge ➡ along the greater curvature of the supraclinoid ICA.* **6-34D.** *CTA with 3D SSD nicely demonstrates the blood blister-like aneurysm ➡. (Courtesy C. D. Phillips, MD.)*

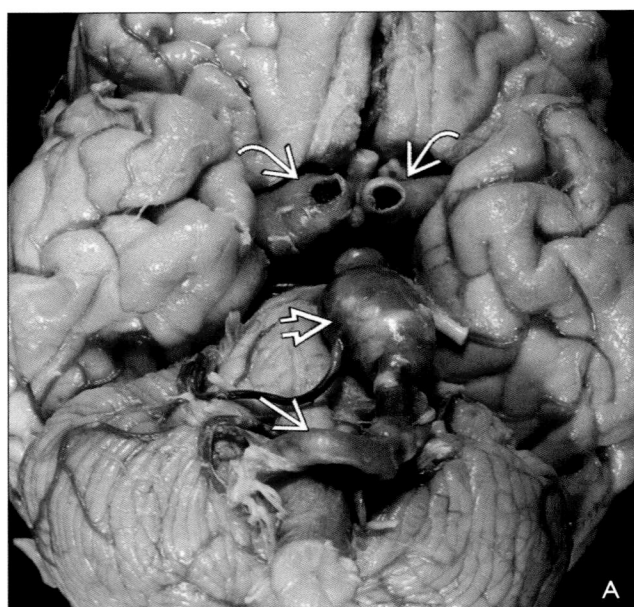

6-35A. Autopsy case shows generalized atherosclerotic dolichoectasia of the vertebrobasilar system ➡ and both internal carotid arteries ➡. A fusiform aneurysm involving the distal basilar artery ➡ is present.

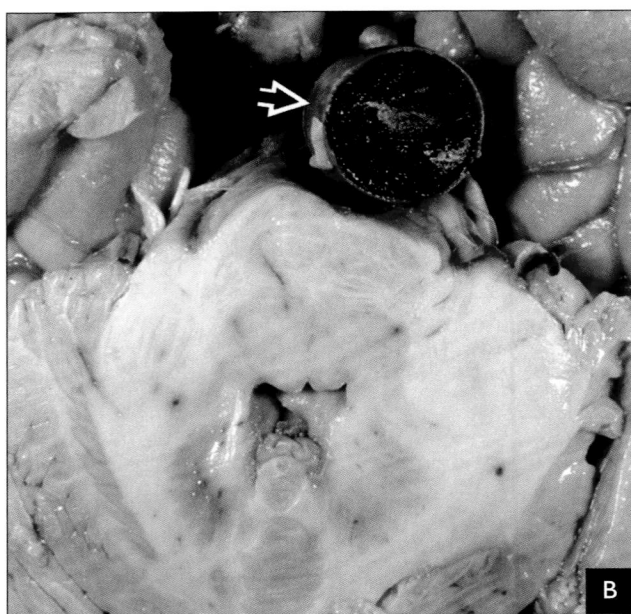

6-35B. Close-up view of axial section through the posterior fossa shows the fusiform aneurysm ➡. (Courtesy R. Hewlett, MD.)

Atherosclerotic Fusiform Aneurysm

Terminology

Atherosclerotic fusiform aneurysms (ASVD FAs) are also called aneurysmal dolichoectasias, distinguishing them from the more generalized nonfocal vessel elongations seen as a common manifestation of intracranial atherosclerosis.

Pathology

Arteriectasis is common with advanced atherosclerosis of the cerebral arteries. Fusiform dilatation is a frequent complication. Generalized ASVD with a focally dilated fusiform enlargement is the typical gross manifestation of an atherosclerotic FA (6-35).

ASVD FAs are more common in the vertebrobasilar (posterior) circulation and usually affect the basilar artery. Plaques of foam cells with thickened but irregular intima and extensive loss of elastica and media are present. Layers of organized thrombus surrounding a patent residual lumen are common.

Clinical Issues

Peak age of presentation is the seventh to eighth decade. Posterior circulation TIAs and stroke are the most common presentation. Cranial neuropathy is relatively uncommon.

Imaging

GENERAL FEATURES. ASVD FAs are often large (more than 2.5 cm in diameter) fusiform or ovoid dilatations that are superimposed on generalized vascular dolichoectasias.

CT FINDINGS. ASVD FAs are often partially thrombosed and frequently demonstrate mural calcification (6-36). Heterogeneously hyperdense clot is often present. The residual lumen enhances intensely following contrast enhancement.

MR FINDINGS. Similar to saccular aneurysms, the signal intensity of FAs also varies with pulse sequence, degree and direction of flow, and the presence and age of clot within the FA. Slow, turbulent flow in the residual lumen causes complex, sometimes bizarre signal (6-37).

FAs often are very heterogeneous on T1WI and strikingly hypointense on T2WI. The residual lumen can be seen as a rounded "flow void" surrounded by thrombus that varies from hypointense to hyperintense. Intense enhancement of the residual lumen with prominent phase artifact is common following contrast administration.

ANGIOGRAPHY. DSA shows generalized enlargement and ectasia of the parent vessel with a focal, round or fusiform, somewhat irregular contour that represents the residual lumen within a larger mass caused by mural thrombus.

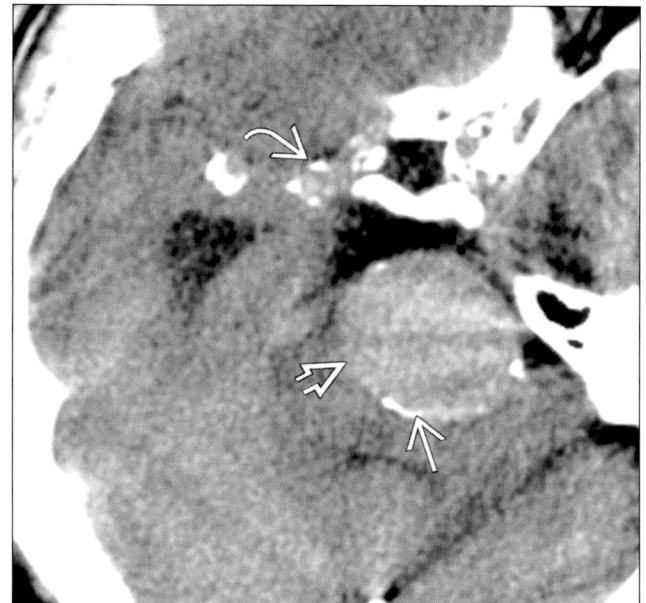

6-36. NECT scan shows typical hyperdense atherosclerotic fusiform aneurysm ⮞ with mural calcifications ➡. Note extensive calcification of the internal carotid, right middle cerebral arteries ⮞.

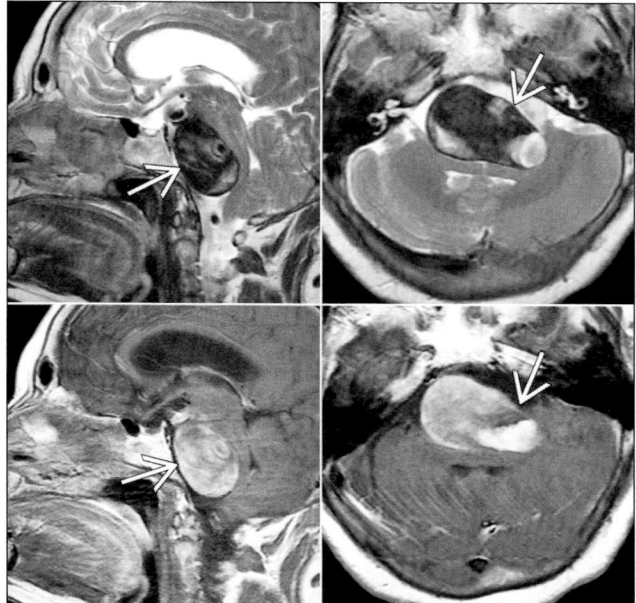

6-37. Series of MR images shows the bizarre appearance of classic atherosclerotic fusiform aneurysm ➡. (Courtesy M. Hartel, MD.)

Differential Diagnosis

The major differential diagnosis of an atherosclerotic FA is **dolichoectasia**. Dolichoectasias are fusiform elongations of vessels—usually in the posterior circulation—without focal fusiform or saccular dilatations. **Nonatherosclerotic fusiform aneurysms** are seen in younger patients who often have an inherited vasculopathy or immune deficiency. Like ASVD FAs, intracranial **dissecting aneurysms** are most common on the vertebrobasilar (posterior) circulation. Findings of generalized ASVD are usually absent.

Nonatherosclerotic Fusiform Aneurysm

Terminology

Nonatherosclerotic fusiform aneurysms (nASVD FAs) are fusiform elongations that occur in the absence of generalized intracranial ASVD.

Etiology

nASVD FAs occur with collagen vascular disorders (e.g., lupus), viral infections (varicella, HIV), and inherited vasculopathies (e.g., Marfan, Ehlers-Danlos, NF1).

Pathology

nASVD FAs are focally dilated fusiform arterial ectasias that often involve nonbranching segments of intracranial arteries **(6-38)**. Multiple lesions are common. The carotid

(anterior) and vertebrobasilar circulations are equally affected. Internal elastic lamina degeneration with myxoid changes and attenuation of the media are described findings at autopsy.

Clinical Issues

Patients are usually younger than those with ASVD FAs. Nonatherosclerotic FAs are common in children and young adults. Many are asymptomatic. TIAs and stroke are common in patients with HIV-associated vasculopathy. nASVD FAs may also cause subarachnoid hemorrhage.

Imaging

Long segments of tubular, fusiform, or ovoid arterial dilatations are seen in the absence of generalized ASVD **(6-39)**, **(6-40)**. Variable amounts of laminated thrombus may be present.

Differential Diagnosis

Fusiform intracranial dilatations in relatively young patients should suggest the possibility of nASVD vasculopathy and FA. **Vertebrobasilar dolichoectasia** (VBD) is seen in older patients with generalized changes of ASVD.

Pseudoaneurysms are common in patients with a history of trauma, infection, drug abuse, or neoplasm. The cavernous ICA, vessels distal to the circle of Willis, and vertebral arteries are the vessels most commonly affected by pseudoaneurysms.

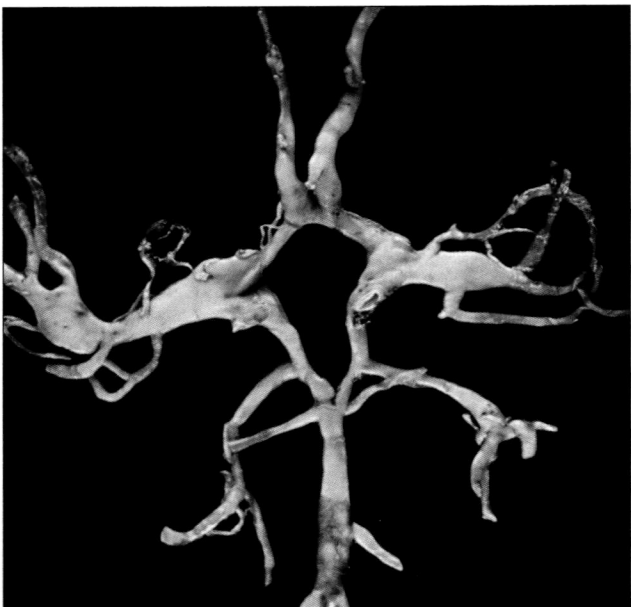

6-38. Dissected circle of Willis in a hemophiliac child with HIV shows nonatherosclerotic fusiform vasculopathy. (Courtesy L. Rourke, MD.)

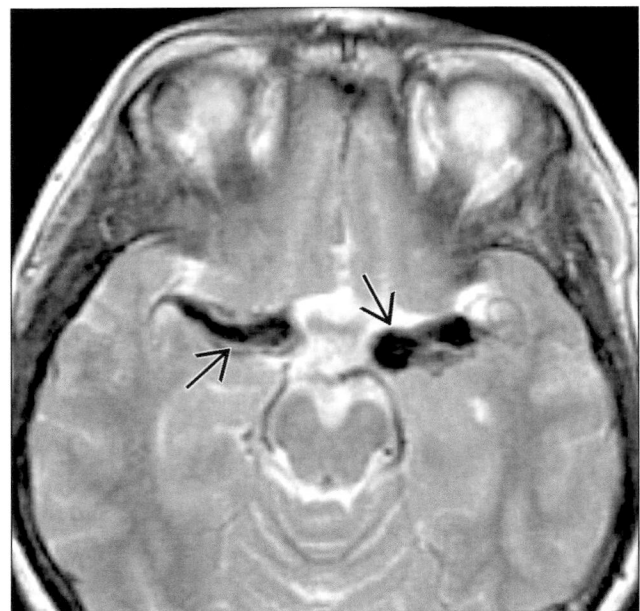

6-39. Axial T2WI in an HIV-positive child shows the fusiform "flow voids" ⇥ of HIV-related vasculopathy.

Selected References

Subarachnoid Hemorrhage

Aneurysmal Subarachnoid Hemorrhage

- Delgado Almandoz JE et al: Diagnostic yield of computed tomography angiography and magnetic resonance angiography in patients with catheter angiography-negative subarachnoid hemorrhage. J Neurosurg. 117(2):309-15, 2012
- Fountas KN et al: Terson hemorrhage in patients suffering aneurysmal subarachnoid hemorrhage: predisposing factors and prognostic significance. J Neurosurg. 109(3):439-44, 2008
- Ishihara H et al: Angiogram-negative subarachnoid hemorrhage in the era of three dimensional rotational angiography. J Clin Neurosci. 14(3):252-5, 2007
- Rosengart AJ et al: Prognostic factors for outcome in patients with aneurysmal subarachnoid hemorrhage. Stroke. 38(8):2315-21, 2007

Aneurysmal SAH and Vasospasm

- Zhang X et al: Factors responsible for poor outcome after intraprocedural rerupture of ruptured intracranial aneurysms: identification of risk factors, prevention and management on 18 cases. Eur J Radiol. 81(1):e77-85, 2012
- Sato T et al: Quantification of subarachnoid hemorrhage by three-dimensional computed tomography: correlation between hematoma volume and symptomatic vasospasm. Neurol Med Chir (Tokyo). 51(3):187-94, 2011
- Chen F et al: Neuroimaging research on cerebrovascular spasm and its current progress. Acta Neurochir Suppl. 110(Pt 2):233-7, 2011
- Ko SB et al: Quantitative analysis of hemorrhage volume for predicting delayed cerebral ischemia after subarachnoid hemorrhage. Stroke. 42(3):669-74, 2011
- Vatter H et al: Perfusion-diffusion mismatch in MRI to indicate endovascular treatment of cerebral vasospasm after subarachnoid haemorrhage. J Neurol Neurosurg Psychiatry. 82(8):876-83, 2011
- Dankbaar JW et al: Effect of different components of triple-H therapy on cerebral perfusion in patients with aneurysmal subarachnoid haemorrhage: a systematic review. Crit Care. 14(1):R23, 2010

Other Complications of aSAH

- Schneider UC et al: Functional analysis of pro-inflammatory properties within the cerebrospinal fluid after subarachnoid hemorrhage in vivo and in vitro. J Neuroinflammation. 9:28, 2012
- Siman R et al: Evidence that a panel of neurodegeneration biomarkers predicts vasospasm, infarction, and outcome in aneurysmal subarachnoid hemorrhage. PLoS One. 6(12):e28938, 2011

Perimesencephalic Nonaneurysmal SAH

- Kim YW et al: Nonaneurysmal subarachnoid hemorrhage: an update. Curr Atheroscler Rep. 14(4):328-34, 2012
- Cruz JP et al: Perimesencephalic subarachnoid hemorrhage: when to stop imaging? Emerg Radiol. 18(3):197-202, 2011
- Maslehaty H et al: Diagnostic value of magnetic resonance imaging in perimesencephalic and nonperimesencephalic

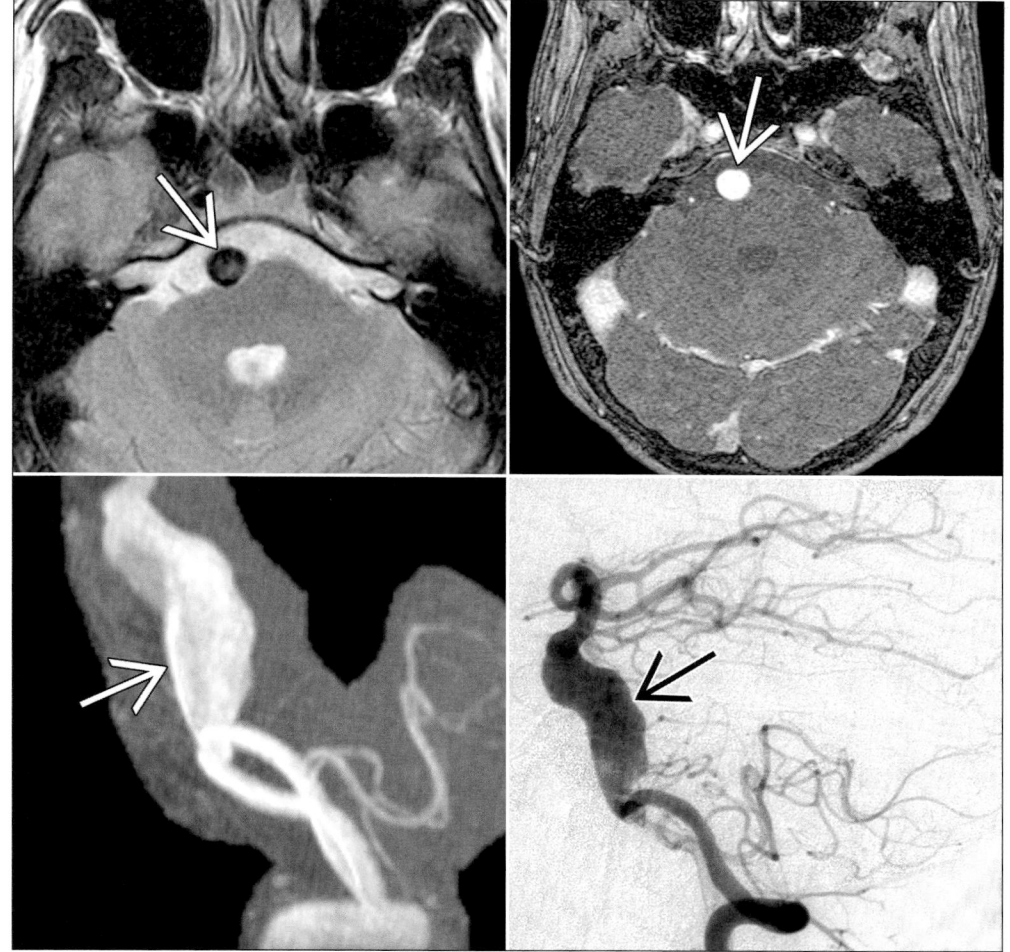

6-40. *(Upper left) T2WI in a 19-year-old man with collagen vascular disease shows an enlarged basilar "flow void"* ➜. *(Upper right) Source image from contrast-enhanced MRA shows the enlarged basilar artery* ➜. *(Lower left) MIP view of MRA shows a fusiform aneurysm* ➜ *that involves almost the entire basilar artery. (Lower right) DSA shows the nonatherosclerotic fusiform aneurysm* ➜.

subarachnoid hemorrhage of unknown origin. J Neurosurg. 114(4):1003-7, 2011

Convexal SAH

- Mas J et al: [Focal convexal subarachnoid hemorrhage: Clinical presentation, imaging patterns and etiologic findings in 23 patients.] Rev Neurol (Paris). Epub ahead of print, 2012

- Beitzke M et al: Clinical presentation, etiology, and long-term prognosis in patients with nontraumatic convexal subarachnoid hemorrhage. Stroke. 42(11):3055-60, 2011

- Oda S et al: Cortical subarachnoid hemorrhage caused by cerebral venous thrombosis. Neurol Med Chir (Tokyo). 51(1):30-6, 2011

- Singhal AB et al: Reversible cerebral vasoconstriction syndromes: analysis of 139 cases. Arch Neurol. 68(8):1005-12, 2011

- Finelli PF: Cerebral amyloid angiopathy as cause of convexity SAH in elderly. Neurologist. 16(1):37-40, 2010

- Kumar S et al: Atraumatic convexal subarachnoid hemorrhage: clinical presentation, imaging patterns, and etiologies. Neurology. 74(11):893-9, 2010

- Panda S et al: Localized convexity subarachnoid haemorrhage--a sign of early cerebral venous sinus thrombosis. Eur J Neurol. 17(10):1249-58, 2010

Superficial Siderosis

- Rodriguez FR et al: Superficial siderosis of the CNS. AJR Am J Roentgenol. 197(1):W149-52, 2011

- Kumar N: Neuroimaging in superficial siderosis: an in-depth look. AJNR Am J Neuroradiol. 31(1):5-14, 2010

- Linn J et al: Prevalence of superficial siderosis in patients with cerebral amyloid angiopathy. Neurology. 74(17):1346-50, 2010

Aneurysms

Saccular Aneurysm

- Firouzian A et al: Quantification of intracranial aneurysm morphodynamics from ECG-gated CT angiography. Acad Radiol. Epub ahead of print, 2012

- Sanchez M et al: Biomechanical assessment of the individual risk of rupture of cerebral aneurysms: a proof of concept. Ann Biomed Eng. Epub ahead of print, 2012

- Sforza DM et al: Effects of perianeurysmal environment during the growth of cerebral aneurysms: a case study. AJNR Am J Neuroradiol. 33(6):1115-20, 2012

- UCAS Japan Investigators et al: The natural course of unruptured cerebral aneurysms in a Japanese cohort. N Engl J Med. 366(26):2474-82, 2012

- Brinjikji W et al: Better outcomes with treatment by coiling relative to clipping of unruptured intracranial aneurysms in the United States, 2001-2008. AJNR Am J Neuroradiol. 32(6):1071-5, 2011

- Dolan JM et al: High fluid shear stress and spatial shear stress gradients affect endothelial proliferation, survival, and alignment. Ann Biomed Eng. 39(6):1620-31, 2011

- Kulcsár Z et al: Hemodynamics of cerebral aneurysm initiation: the role of wall shear stress and spatial wall shear stress gradient. AJNR Am J Neuroradiol. 32(3):587-94, 2011

- Meng H et al: Progressive aneurysm development following hemodynamic insult. J Neurosurg. 114(4):1095-103, 2011

- Menke J et al: Diagnosing cerebral aneurysms by computed tomographic angiography: Meta-analysis. Ann Neurol. 69(4):646-54, 2011

- Pritz MB: Cerebral aneurysm classification based on angioarchitecture. J Stroke Cerebrovasc Dis. 20(2):162-7, 2011

- Yurt A et al: Biomarkers of connective tissue disease in patients with intracranial aneurysms. J Clin Neurosci. 17(9):1119-21, 2010

- Broderick JP et al: Greater rupture risk for familial as compared to sporadic unruptured intracranial aneurysms. Stroke. 40(6):1952-7, 2009

Pseudoaneurysm

- Brzozowski K et al: The use of routine imaging data in diagnosis of cerebral pseudoaneurysm prior to angiography. Eur J Radiol. 80(3):e401-9, 2011

Blood Blister-like Aneurysm

- Yu-Tse L et al: Rupture of symptomatic blood blister-like aneurysm of the internal carotid artery: clinical experience and management outcome. Br J Neurosurg. 26(3):378-82, 2012

- Regelsberger J et al: Blister-like aneurysms--a diagnostic and therapeutic challenge. Neurosurg Rev. 34(4):409-16, 2011

- McLaughlin N et al: Surgical management of blood blister-like aneurysms of the internal carotid artery. World Neurosurg. 74(4-5):483-93, 2010

- Rasskazoff S et al: Endovascular treatment of a ruptured blood blister-like aneurysm with a flow-diverting stent. Interv Neuroradiol. 16(3):255-8, 2010

Nonatherosclerotic Fusiform Aneurysm

- Goldstein DA et al: HIV-associated intracranial aneurysmal vasculopathy in adults. J Rheumatol. 37(2):226-33, 2010

7

Vascular Malformations

Brain vascular malformations, also known as cerebrovascular malformations (CVMs), are a heterogeneous groups of disorders that exhibit a broad spectrum of biological behaviors. Some CVMs (e.g., capillary malformations) are almost always clinically silent and are found incidentally on imaging studies. Others, such as arteriovenous (AV) malformations and cavernous angiomas, may hemorrhage unexpectedly and without warning.

In this chapter, we begin with an overview of CVMs, starting with a discussion of terminology, etiology, and classification. CVMs are grouped according to whether or not they exhibit arteriovenous shunting, and then each type is discussed individually.

Terminology

Two major groups of vascular anomalies are recognized: Vascular *malformations* and vascular *hemangiomas*. All cerebrovascular malformations—the entities considered in this chapter—are malformative lesions and are thus designated as "malformations" or "angiomas." In contrast, vascular "hemangiomas" are true proliferating vasoformative neoplasms. Hemangiomas are classified as nonmeningothelial mesenchymal tumors and are discussed in Chapter 22 with meningiomas and other mesenchymal neoplasms.

Etiology

Most CVMs are congenital lesions and represent morphogenetic errors affecting arteries, capillaries, veins, or a combination of these elements.

Development of the human fetal vascular system occurs via two related processes: Vasculogenesis and angiogenesis. In **vasculogenesis**, capillary-like tubes develop first and constitute the primary vascular plexus. This primary capillary network is subsequently remodeled into large-caliber vessels (arteries, veins) and small capillaries.

Angiogenesis is regulated by a number of intercell signaling and growth factors. Mutations in various components of the angiogenetic system have been implicated in the development of various CVMs.

Classification

CVMs have been traditionally classified by histopathology into four major types: (1) arteriovenous malformations (AVMs), (2) venous angiomas (developmental venous anomalies), (3) capillary telangiectasias (sometimes simply termed "telangiectasia" or "telangiectasis"), and (4) cavernous malformations.

Many interventional neuroradiologists and neurosurgeons group CVMs by function, not histopathology. In this functional classification, CVMs are divided into two basic categories: (1) CVMs that display arteriovenous shunting and (2) CVMs without AV shunting (**Table 7-1**). The former are potentially amenable to endovascular intervention; the latter are either treated surgically or left alone.

In this book we use a combination of functional and histologic classifications. We begin with a discussion of CVMs that display arteriovenous shunting, i.e., AVMs and arteriovenous fistulas (AVFs). We then focus on CVMs that do not generally shunt blood from the arterial to the venous circulation. Nonshunting CVMs include developmental venous anomalies, capillary telangiectasias, and cavernous malformations.

Cerebrovascular Malformations

Type	Etiology	Pathology	Number	Location
CVMs with Arteriovenous Shunts				
AV malformations	Congenital (dysregulated angiogenesis)	Nidus + arterial feeders, draining veins; no capillary bed	Solitary (< 2% multiple)	Parenchyma (85%); supratentorial (15%); posterior fossa
Dural AV fistula	Acquired (trauma; dural sinus thrombosis)	Network of multiple AV microfistulas	Solitary	Skull base; dural sinus wall
Vein of Galen malformation	Congenital (fetal arterial fistula to primitive precursor of vein of Galen)	Large venous pouch	Solitary	Behind third ventricle
CVMs without Arteriovenous Shunts				
Developmental venous anomaly	Congenital (arrested fetal medullary vein development)	Dilated WM veins; normal brain in between	Solitary (unless BRBNS)	Deep WM, usually near ventricle
Sinus pericranii	Congenital	Bluish blood-filled subcutaneous scalp mass	Solitary	Scalp
Cavernous malformation	Congenital (*CCM*, *KRIT1* gene mutations in familial autosomal dominant syndrome; "de novo" lesions continue to form)	Collection of blood-filled "caverns" with no normal brain; complete hemosiderin rim	2/3 solitary (sporadic); 1/3 multiple (familial)	Throughout brain
Capillary telangiectasia	Congenital	Dilated capillaries; normal brain in between	Solitary > > > multiple	Anywhere but pons; medulla most common

Table 7-1. *AV = arteriovenous; BRBNS = blue rubber bleb nevus syndrome; CVM = cerebrovascular malformation; WM = white matter.*

CVMs with Arteriovenous Shunting

Arteriovenous Malformation

Terminology

An arteriovenous malformation (AVM) is a tightly packed "snarl" of thin-walled vessels with direct arterial to venous shunting. There is no intervening capillary bed. Most brain AVMs (BAVMs) are parenchymal lesions and are also called "pial AVMs," although mixed pial-dural malformations do occur.

Etiology

GENERAL CONCEPTS. AVMs are congenital defects of vascular development characterized by dysregulated angiogenesis. Endothelial cells in cerebral AVMs express GLUT1 (a protein in the embryonic microvasculature), matrix metalloproteinases (MMPs), proangiogenic growth factors such as vascular endothelial growth factor (VEGF). This results in "downstream" derangements in vascular function and integrity.

GENETICS. Recent studies suggest that genetic factors affect both susceptibility and disease progression. Transforming growth factor β (TGF-β) and functionally active polymorphisms of the *IL-1* complex have been associated with both increased risk of developing a BAVM and frequency of hemorrhage.

Most AVMs are solitary. Multiple AVMs are almost always syndromic. Common associations include **hereditary hemorrhagic telangiectasia** (HHT, also known as Rendu-Osler-Weber disease) and segmental neurovascular syndromes called **cerebrofacial arteriovenous metameric syndrome** (CAMS). Here somatic mutations of the neural crest occur along predefined migration paths, resulting in specific combinations of facial and intracranial vascular malformations. **Wyburn-Mason syndrome**, in which AVMs are found in both the retina and brain, is one example of a CAMS.

Prevalence	Age	Hemorrhage Risk	Best Imaging Clues
0.04-0.5% of population; 85-90% of CVMs with AV shunting	Peak = 20-40 years (25% by age 15 years)	Very high (2-4% per year, cumulative)	"Bag of worms," "flow voids" on MR
10-15% of CVMs with AV shunting	Peak = 40-60 years	Varies with venous draining (increased if cortical veins involved)	Enlarged meningeal arteries with network of tiny vessels in wall of thrombosed dural venous sinus
< 1% of CVMs with AV shunting	Newborn > > infant, older child	Low (but hydrocephalus brain damage common)	Large midline venous varix in neonate with high-output congestive heart failure
Most common CVM (60% of all), between 2-9% of the population	Any age	Extremely low unless mixed with cavernous malformation	"Medusa head" of dilated WM veins converging on enlarged collector vein
Rare	Any age (usually childhood)	Extremely low unless direct trauma	Vascular scalp mass connecting through skull defect to intracranial venous circulation
	Any age (peak = 40-60 years; younger in familial CCM syndrome)	High (0.25-0.75% per year; 1% per lesion per year in familial)	Varies; most common is solitary "popcorn ball" (locules with blood-fluid levels, hemosiderin rim); multifocal "black dots" in familial
15-20% of all CVMs	Any age (peak = 30-40 years)	Extremely low unless mixed with cavernous malformation	Faint brush-like enhancement, becomes hypointense on T2*

HHT is a genetically mediated hereditary disorder characterized by epistaxis, mucocutaneous telangiectases, and visceral AVMs. Two forms of HHT are recognized: HHT1 and HHT2. BAVMs are significantly more frequent in HHT1. A mutated endoglin (*ENG*) gene has been identified in HHT1. Some investigators have also linked *ACVRL1* (the *HHT2* gene) to formation of clinically sporadic AVM variants and dural AVFs in patients with HHT. HHT is discussed in greater detail in connection with neurocutaneous syndromes (Chapter 39).

Pathology

LOCATION. Over 85% of AVMs are supratentorial, located in the cerebral hemispheres. Only 15% are found in the posterior fossa.

SIZE AND NUMBER. Less than 2% of all brain AVMs are multiple. Almost all multiple AVMs are associated with vascular neurocutaneous syndromes (see above).

AVMs range in size from tiny ("micro" AVMs) to giant lesions that can occupy most of a cerebral hemisphere.

Most are intermediate in size, ranging from two to six centimeters in diameter.

GROSS PATHOLOGY. Most AVMs are compact ovoid or pyramidal lesions (7-2). Their broadest surface is at or near the cortex, and the apex points toward the ventricles.

The brain surrounding an AVM often appears abnormal. A "perinidal" capillary bed has been reported in some cases. Hemorrhagic residua in adjacent brain are common, as are gliosis and secondary ischemic changes.

MICROSCOPIC FEATURES. Vessels comprising the AVM nidus are of variable caliber and wall thickness. Some appear dysplastic and thin-walled without normal subendothelial support. Others exhibit intimal hyperplasia and fibrosis/hyalinization.

There are no capillaries and no normal brain parenchyma within an AVM nidus. Instead, varying amounts of laminated thrombus, dystrophic calcification, and hemorrhagic residua are often present. Small amounts of brain parenchyma within the nidus are occasionally identified but are typically gliotic and nonfunctional.

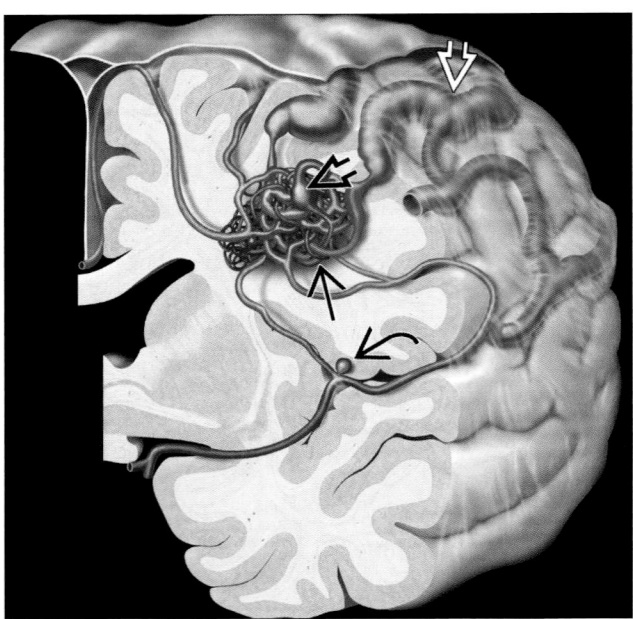

7-1. Graphic depicts AVM nidus ⇨ with intranidal aneurysm ⇨, feeding artery ("pedicle") aneurysm ⤳, and enlarged draining veins ⇨.

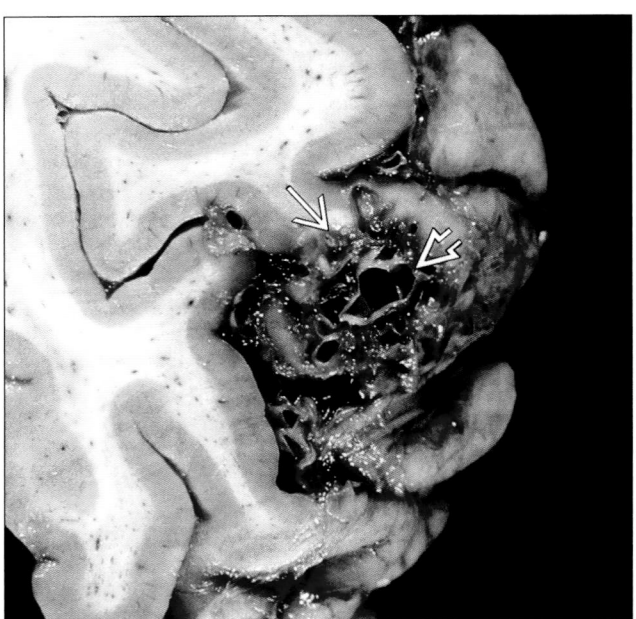

7-2. Autopsy case demonstrates a classic AVM. The nidus ⇨ contains no normal brain. An intranidal aneurysm ⇨ is present. (Courtesy R. Hewlett, MD.)

Clinical Issues

EPIDEMIOLOGY. Almost all AVMs are sporadic and solitary. With very rare exceptions ("de novo" AVMs), most are considered congenital lesions. Sporadic (nonsyndromic) AVMs are found in 0.02-0.14% of the general population.

DEMOGRAPHICS. Peak presentation occurs between 20-40 years of age, although 25% of patients harboring an AVM become symptomatic by age 15. There is no gender predilection.

PRESENTATION. Headache with parenchymal hemorrhage is the most common presentation, occurring in about half of all patients. Seizure and focal neurologic deficits are the initial symptoms in 25% each.

NATURAL HISTORY. The lifelong risk of hemorrhage is estimated at 2-4% per year, cumulative. Annual hemorrhage risk increases with increasing age, deep brain location, and deep venous drainage. Risk ranges from 1% per year (in patients whose initial presentation was nonhemorrhagic) to nearly 35% per year for patients harboring all three risk factors.

Several grading systems have been devised to characterize AVMs and estimate the risks of surgery. The most widely used is the **Spetzler-Martin scale**. Here AVMs are graded on a scale from 1-5 based on the sum of "scores" calculated from lesion size, location (eloquent vs. noneloquent brain), and venous drainage pattern (superficial vs. deep).

A simplified three-tier modification of the Spetzler-Martin scale combines grades 1 and 2 into class A, designates grade 3 AVMs as class B, and combines grades 4 and 5 into class C.

Other imaging findings besides size, location, and venous drainage pattern are associated with the risk of future hemorrhage from an AVM. These include evidence of previous hemorrhage (including clinically silent intralesional microbleeds), presence of an intranidal aneurysm, and draining vein stenosis.

Spontaneous regression of sporadic brain AVMs is rare and unpredictable, occurring in approximately 1% of cases. Most "obliterated" AVMs follow a hemorrhagic episode, often with venous stasis, thrombosis, and elevated intracranial pressure. Rare nonhemorrhagic cases of spontaneous AVM regression have been reported.

SPETZLER-MARTIN AVM GRADING SCALE

Size
- Small (< 3 cm) = 1
- Medium (3-6 cm) = 2
- Large (> 6 cm) = 3

Eloquence of Adjacent Brain
- Noneloquent = 0
- Eloquent = 1

Venous Drainage
- Superficial only = 0
- Deep component = 1

TREATMENT OPTIONS. Embolization, surgery, stereotactic radiosurgery, or a combination of treatments are all

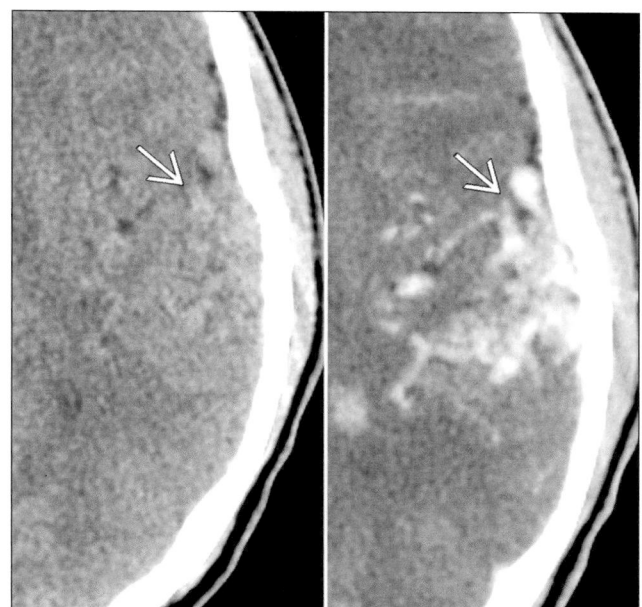

7-3. (Left) NECT shows serpentine hyperdensities ➽*. (Right) CECT shows strong uniform enhancement* ➽*. Wedge-shaped configuration is typical for AVM. Roughly 85% of AVMs are supratentorial.*

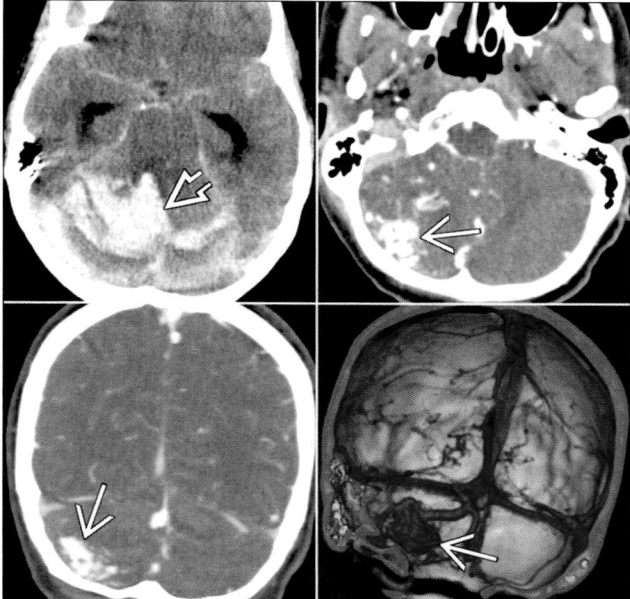

7-4. NECT scan (upper left) and CTA images in a patient with spontaneous cerebellar hemorrhage ➽ *demonstrate an underlying AVM* ➽*. Approximately 15% of AVMs are infratentorial.*

current options in treating AVMs. Best treatment varies from case to case.

Imaging

The imaging diagnosis of an uncomplicated AVM is relatively straightforward. However, the presence of hemorrhage or thrombosis can complicate its appearance. Acute hemorrhage may obliterate any typical findings of an AVM. Residua of previous hemorrhagic episodes such as dystrophic calcification, gliosis, and blood in different stages of degradation may also complicate its appearance.

GENERAL FEATURES. AVMs are complex networks of abnormal vascular channels consisting of three distinct components: (1) feeding arteries, (2) a central nidus, and (3) draining veins (7-1).

CT FINDINGS. AVMs generally resemble a "bag of worms" formed by a tightly packed tangle of vessels with little or no mass effect on adjacent brain. NECT scans typically show numerous well-delineated, slightly hyperdense serpentine vessels (7-3). Calcification is common. Enhancement of all three AVM components (feeding arteries, nidus, draining veins) is typically intense and uniform on CECT scans (7-4).

MR FINDINGS. Findings vary with vascular hemodynamics, the presence (and age) of associated hemorrhage, and secondary changes in the surrounding brain.

Because most AVMs are high-flow lesions, spins rapidly pass through the lesion and do not receive a refocusing

pulse. This produces the appearance of a tightly packed mass or a "honeycomb" of "flow voids" on both T1- and T2 scans (7-5).

Any brain parenchyma within an AVM is typically gliotic and hyperintense on T2WI and FLAIR. Contrast enhancement of AVMs is variable, depending on flow rate and direction. Draining veins typically enhance strongly and uniformly (7-6).

Hemorrhagic residua are common. T2* sequences often show foci of "blooming" both within and around AVMs.

ANGIOGRAPHY. The **feeding arteries** that supply an AVM are often enlarged and tortuous (7-5E). Flow-related angiopathy may be present, ranging from simple dilation to endothelial thickening, stenosis, and occasionally even thrombosis and occlusion. A flow-induced **"pedicle" aneurysm** is seen in 10-15% of cases.

The **nidus**, the core of the AVM, is a tightly packed tangle of abnormal arteries and veins without an intervening capillary bed. Up to 50% contain at least one aneurysmally dilated vessel (**"intranidal aneurysm"**). The nidus contains little or no brain parenchyma and hence causes no significant mass effect on the adjacent brain. Displacement of angiographic midline markers (e.g., the anterior cerebral arteries and internal cerebral veins) is therefore usually absent unless an acute hematoma is present.

As there is no intervening capillary bed between the arterial feeders and draining veins of an AVM, direct arteriovenous shunting within the nidus occurs (7-5F). **Drain-**

7-5A. Axial T1WI in a 32-year-old man with headache shows a classic wedge-shaped left parietal AVM with multiple serpentine "flow voids" ➡. A few linear foci of T1 shortening ⏩ represent thrombosed vessels within the nidus. 7-5B. T2WI in the same patient nicely demonstrates the wedge of "flow voids" ➡. The broad base toward the cortex with apex pointing toward the lateral ventricle is a typical configuration for brain AVMs.

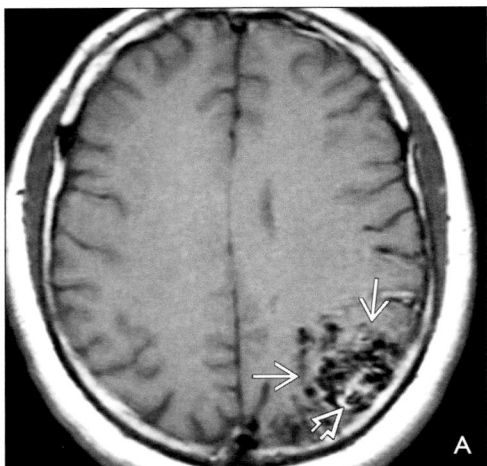
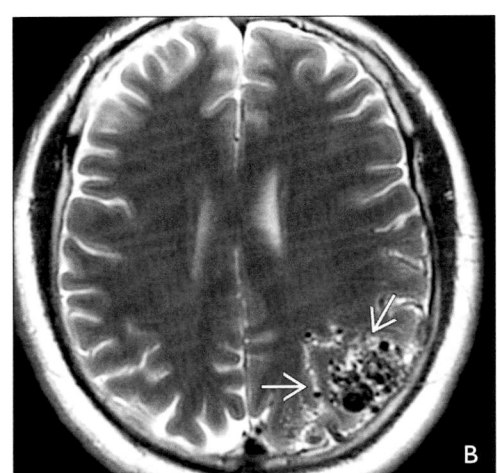

7-5C. FLAIR scan demonstrates minimal hyperintensity within and around the AVM ➡, suggesting small foci of gliotic brain. 7-5D. T1 C+ scan shows some linear and serpentine areas of enhancement ➡ that are mostly in draining veins.

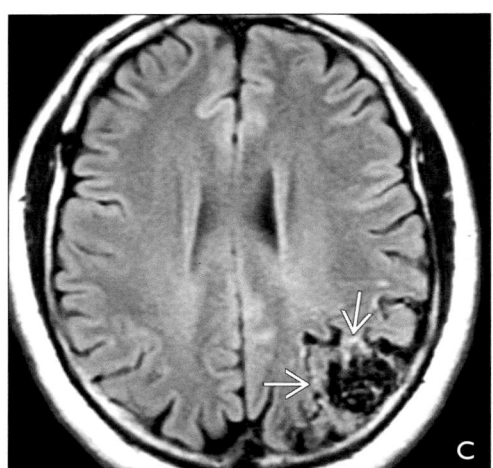
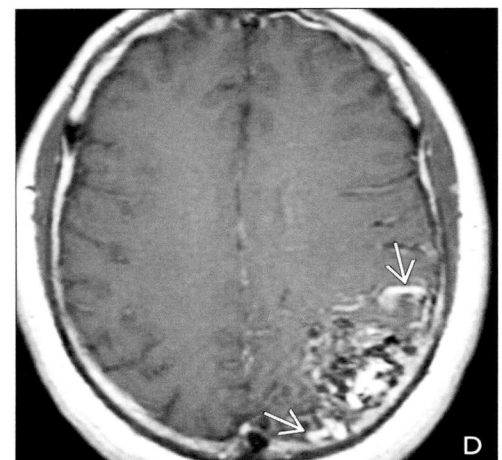

7-5E. Lateral DSA shows enlarged MCA, ACA feeding vessels ➡ with a tangle of smaller vessels in the wedge-shaped nidus ⏩. Faint opacification of the superior sagittal sinus ➚ represents arteriovenous shunting of contrast. 7-5F. Late arterial phase of the DSA shows the nidus ⏩ and "early draining" veins ➚ emptying into the SSS ➚. No deep venous drainage was identified. Spetzler-Martin grade 3 AVM.

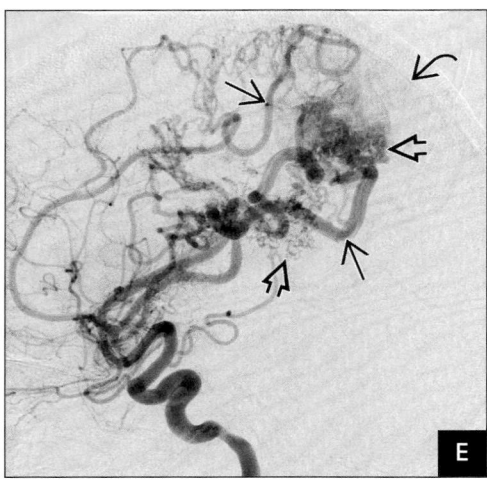
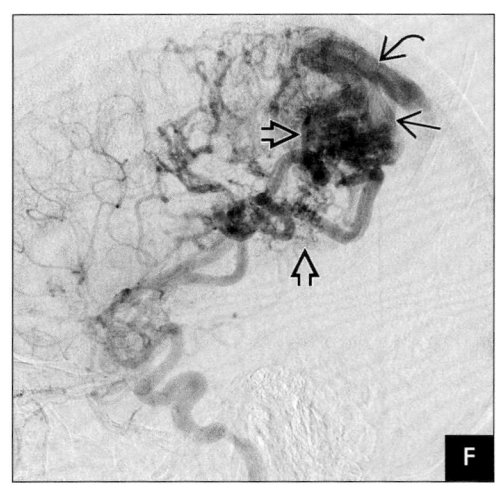

ing veins typically opacify in the mid- to late-arterial phase ("early draining" veins). Veins draining AVMs are typically enlarged, tortuous, and may become so prominent that they form varices and exert local mass effect on the adjacent cortex **(7-6)**. Stenosis of one or more "outlet" draining veins may elevate intranidal pressure and contribute to AVM hemorrhage.

CTA, especially with 3D surface rendering, may be helpful in delineating the feeding arteries and draining veins of an AVM **(7-4)**. 4D-hybrid MRA is helpful in depicting intranidal flow patterns, but DSA is still required to depict small feeding vessels.

The internal angioarchitecture of an AVM is optimally delineated by high-resolution DSA. Superselective injection of all feeding arteries delineates the nidus and helps define the presence of an intranidal aneurysm. Three-dimensional reconstructions with shaded surface display of all three AVM components may be very helpful in surgical planning or endovascular treatment.

Differential Diagnosis

Imaging findings of most uncomplicated AVMs are quite typical. However, occasionally a highly vascular neoplasm such as **glioblastoma multiforme** (GBM) displays such striking neoangiogenesis that it can mimic an AVM. Most GBMs, even extremely vascular lesions, enhance intensely and contain significant amounts of neoplasm interposed between the enlarged vessels. Occasionally, **densely calcified neoplasms** such as oligodendroglioma can mimic the "flow voids" of an AVM.

If an AVM hemorrhages spontaneously, the clot may obscure its underlying angioarchitecture **(7-7)**. A **thrombosed ("obliterated"** or **"cryptic")** AVM may not demonstrate enlarged arteries or nidus at all. Angiography may be negative or demonstrate only mass effect with "stagnating vessels" and subtle early venous drainage. These lesions may be indistinguishable from other vascular malformations (such as **cavernous malformation**) or hemorrhagic neoplasms.

Cerebral proliferative angiopathy is a large, diffuse malformation that has innumerable small feeding vessels,

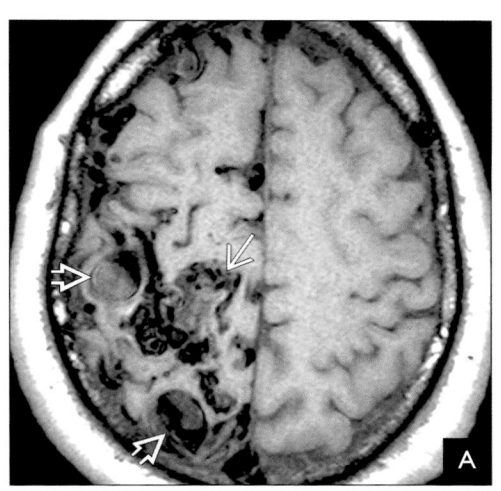

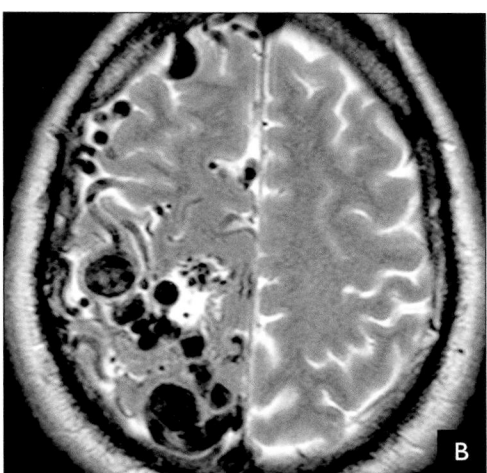

7-6A. T1WI shows extensive serpentine "flow voids" ➡ with multiple venous varices ⮀.
7-6B. T2WI shows that most of the large "flow voids" are enlarged draining veins and venous varices.

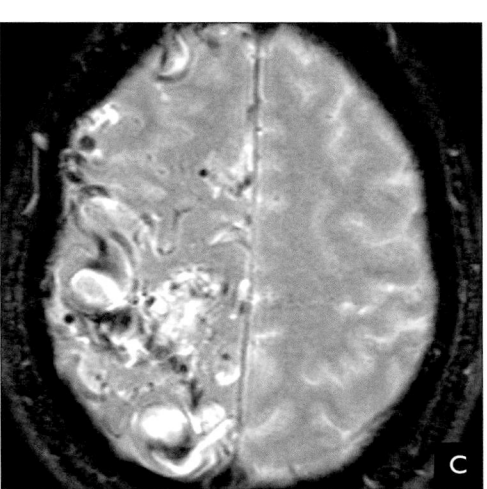

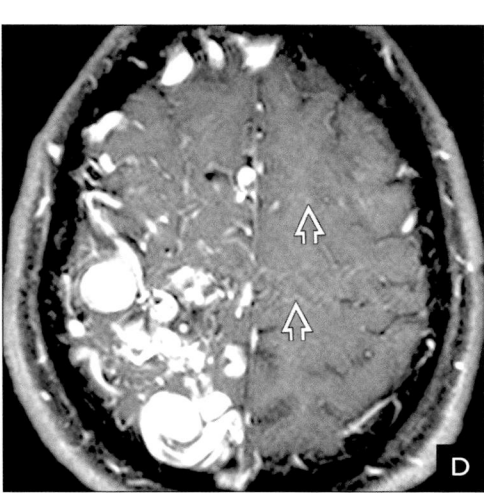

7-6C. T2* GRE shows no gross evidence of hemorrhage.
7-6D. T1 C+ FS scan shows that the serpentine "flow voids" enhance strongly, uniformly. Note phase artifact ⮀ propagating across the image.

no definable nidus, and normal brain interposed between the proliferating vascular channels (see below).

Cerebral Proliferative Angiopathy

Terminology

Cerebral proliferative angiopathy (CPA) is a rare entity characterized by diffuse angiogenesis and progressive hypervascular shunting. It is unclear whether CPA is a completely different disorder or an unusual subtype of AVM.

Pathology

Grossly, CPAs are large lesions that can occupy most of a lobe or even an entire cerebral hemisphere. Their histopathologic features and angioarchitecture are unlike those of classic BAVMs: CPAs have normal brain parenchyma interspersed between the proliferative vascular channels.

Clinical Issues

The clinical profile and natural history of CPA differ from those of classic brain AVMs. CPA generally behaves less aggressively. Most patients present with seizure (45%), severe headache (40%), or progressive neurologic deficits. Only 12% present with a hemorrhagic event. Mean age at symptom onset is 22 years. There is a 2:1 female predominance.

Patients may have laboratory evidence of ongoing angiogenesis with elevated CSF levels of VEGF and bFGF. Bevacizumab, an antiangiogenesis monoclonal antibody that binds to VEGF, has been used in a few patients with inconclusive results.

Imaging

A CPA is seen on MR as a large (usually more than six centimeters), diffusely dispersed network of innumerable dilated vascular spaces intermingled with normal brain parenchyma. Dense enhancement following contrast is typical.

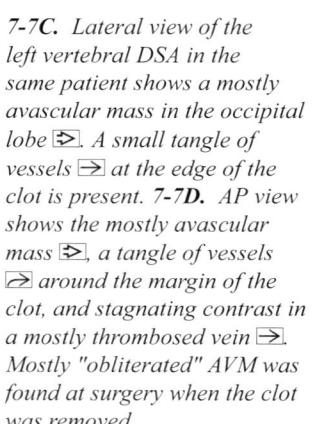

7-7A. A 55-year-old man presented with sudden onset severe headaches and visual problems. NECT scan shows a focal left occipital hemorrhage ⟹. Acute subdural blood is present along the falx and over the left hemisphere ⟹. 7-7B. Coronal CTA in the same patient shows the clot ⟹ and an unusual-appearing enhancing vessel ⟹ at the edge of the hematoma. All of the major dural sinuses are patent.

7-7C. Lateral view of the left vertebral DSA in the same patient shows a mostly avascular mass in the occipital lobe ⟹. A small tangle of vessels ⟹ at the edge of the clot is present. 7-7D. AP view shows the mostly avascular mass ⟹, a tangle of vessels ⟹ around the margin of the clot, and stagnating contrast in a mostly thrombosed vein ⟹. Mostly "obliterated" AVM was found at surgery when the clot was removed.

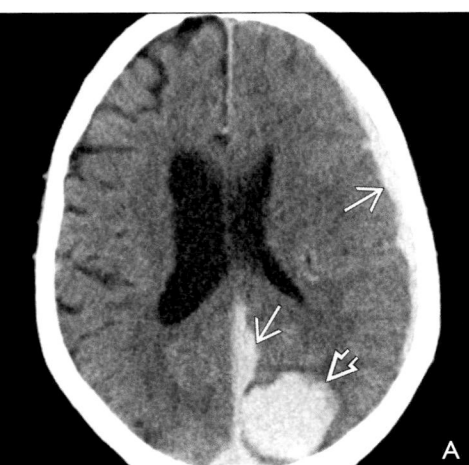

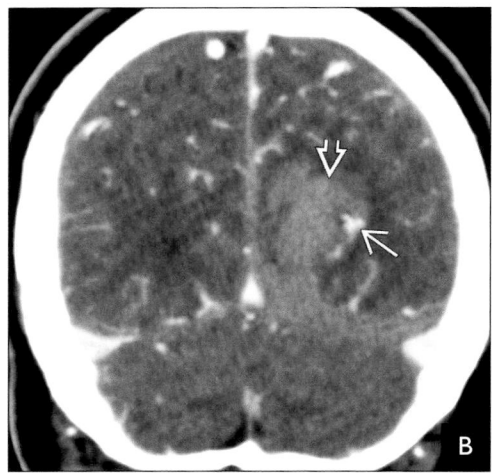

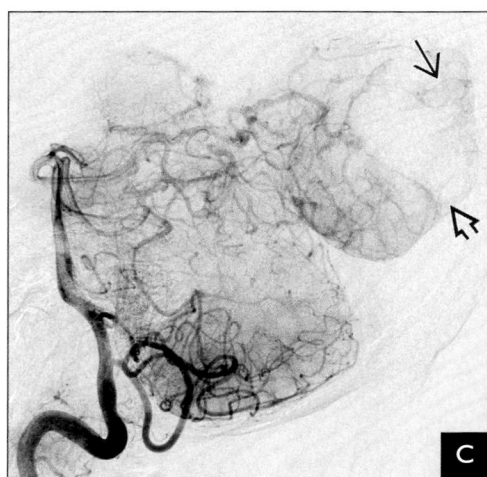

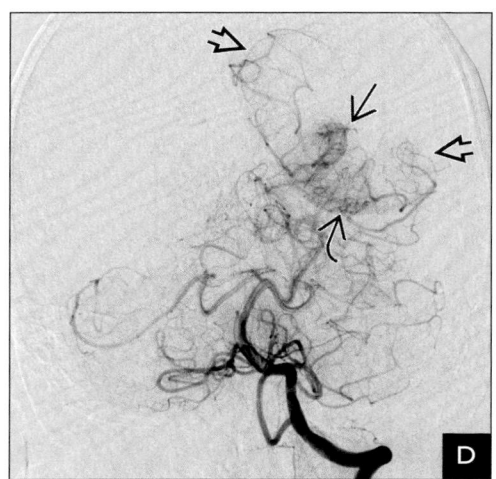

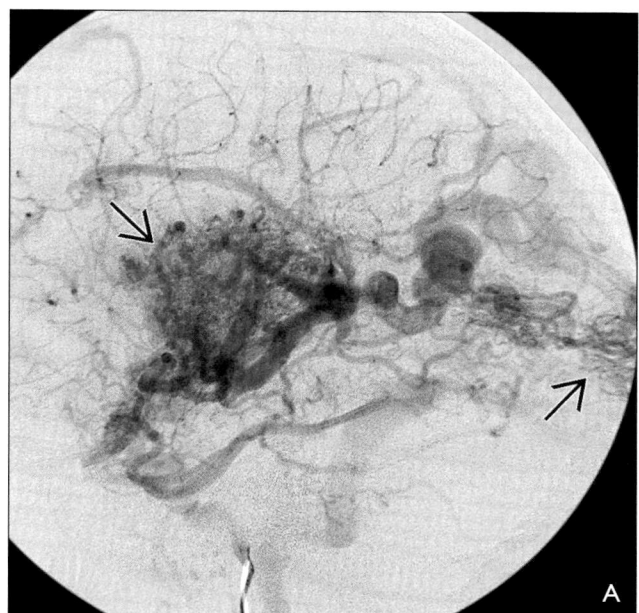

7-8A. DSA of selective internal carotid angiogram in a patient with cerebral proliferative angiopathy shows innumerable dilated vascular spaces ⇾ with no dominant feeding arteries.

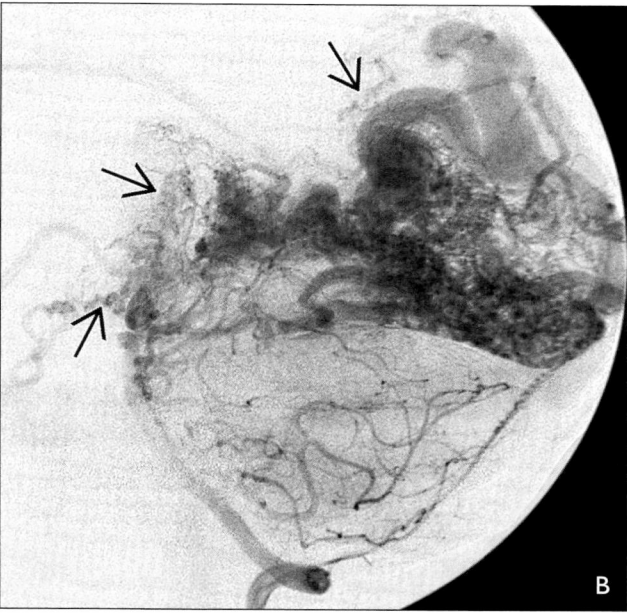

7-8B. Selective vertebral angiogram in the same patient shows additional small feeding vessels supplying the lesion ⇾. Despite its size, there are unopacified spaces within the lesion. (Courtesy P. Lasjaunias, MD.)

pCT and pMR show prolonged mean transit time and hypoperfusion abnormalities ("steal" phenomena) that extend far beyond the morphologic abnormalities.

DSA shows absence of a well-circumscribed nidus **(7-8)**. Instead, a multitude of small caliber nondominant feeding arteries are present. Recruitment of numerous "en passage" transdural feeders is common. The draining veins are only moderately enlarged relative to the striking extent of the vascular abnormality. Despite their large size, flow-related aneurysms are not a feature of CPA.

Differential Diagnosis

The major differential diagnosis of CPA is classic **brain AVM**. The absence of a dominant circumscribed nidus and the presence of brain parenchyma interspersed between the abnormal vascular channels are distinguishing features of CPA.

BRAIN ARTERIOVENOUS MALFORMATION

Etiology and Pathology
- Congenital lesion with dysregulated angiogenesis
- Solitary > > multiple (2%)
  - Multiple almost always syndromic
  - HHT, segmental arteriovenous metameric syndromes
- 85% supratentorial, 15% posterior fossa

Clinical Issues
- Most common *symptomatic* CVM
- Prevalence = 0.02-0.14% of population
- Hemorrhage risk = 2-4% per year, cumulative
- Peak age at presentation = 20-40 years
  - 25% symptomatic by age 15
  - Almost always symptomatic by age 50

Imaging
- General features
  - Arteriovenous shunting
  - No intervening capillaries
  - 3 components: Feeding arteries, nidus, draining veins
- NECT
  - Slightly hyperdense "bag of worms"
  - Tightly packed
  - Little/no mass effect
- CECT
  - Strong serpentine enhancement
- MR
  - "Honeycomb" of "flow voids"
  - No normal brain inside

Differential Diagnosis
- Highly vascular neoplasm (e.g., glioblastoma multiforme)
- Cerebral proliferative angiopathy

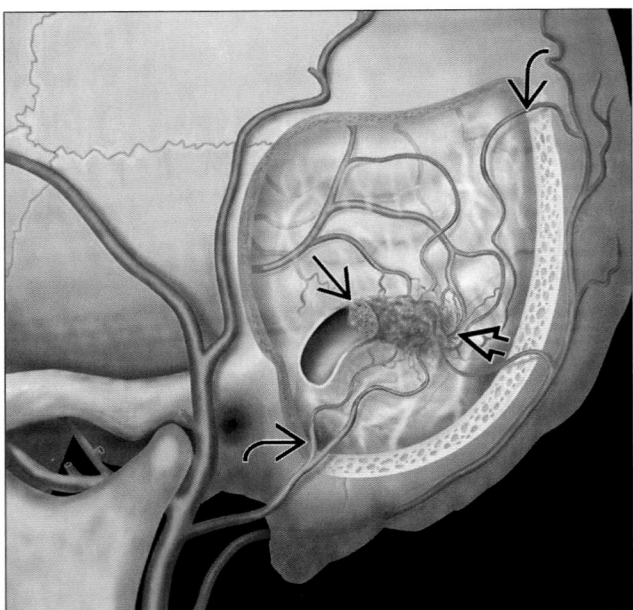

7-9. Graphic depicts dAVF with thrombosed transverse sinus ➔ with multiple tiny arteriovenous in the dural wall ➔. Lesion is mostly supplied by transosseous feeders ➔ from the external carotid artery.

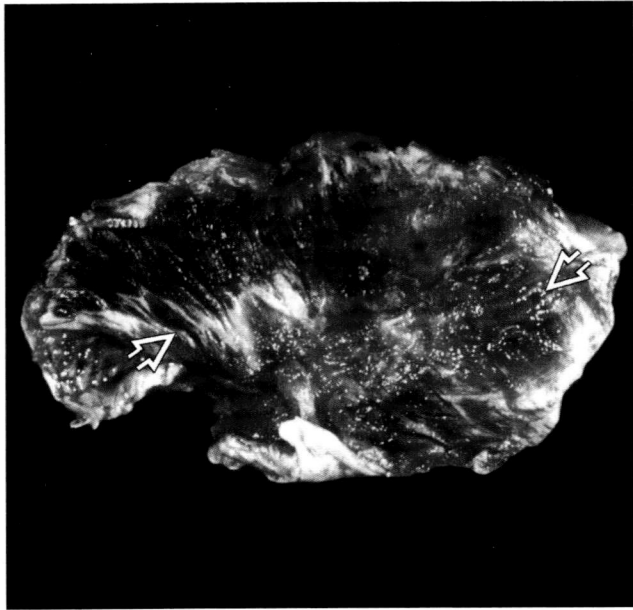

7-10. Mass-like surgical specimen from a resected dAVF in the transverse sinus wall shows innumerable crack-like vessels ➔. (Courtesy R. Hewlett, MD.)

Dural AV Fistula

Dural arteriovenous fistula (dAVF) is the second major type of cerebrovascular malformation that exhibits arteriovenous shunting. Much less common than AVMs, they exhibit a spectrum of biological behavior that ranges from relatively benign to catastrophic intracranial hemorrhage. In this section we consider typical dAVFs.

A special type of dAVF, carotid-cavernous fistula (CCF), has its own classification schema, distinctive clinical findings, and unique imaging features that differ from dAVFs elsewhere. CCF is discussed separately below.

Terminology

A dAVF, also known as a dural arteriovenous shunt, is a network of tiny, crack-like vessels that shunt blood between meningeal arteries and small venules within the wall of a dural venous sinus.

Etiology

Unlike parenchymal AVMs, adult dAVFs are usually acquired (not congenital). While the precise etiology is controversial, local hypoperfusion in a thrombosed dural venous sinus that results in elevated intrasinus pressure is the most commonly cited mechanism. Upregulated angiogenesis within the dural sinus wall occurs after thrombosis and is considered the most likely etiology. Budding/proliferation of microvascular networks connects to a plexus of thin-walled venous channels, creating microfistulas.

Pathology

LOCATION. While dAVFs can involve any dural venous sinus, the most common locations in adults are the transverse, sigmoid, and cavernous sinuses. The superior sagittal sinus is a more common site in children.

SIZE AND NUMBER. Multiple lesions in anatomically separated dural sinuses are uncommon, accounting for slightly under 8% of dAVFs. Multiple dAVFs can be synchronous (simultaneous multiplicity) or metachronous (sequential development of multiplicity).

Size varies from tiny single vessel shunts to massive complex lesions with multiple feeders and arteriovenous shunts in the sinus wall.

GROSS PATHOLOGY. Multiple enlarged dural feeders converge in the wall of a thrombosed dural venous sinus (7-9). A network of innumerable microfistulas connect these vessels directly to arterialized draining veins. These crack-like vessels may form a focal mass within the occluded sinus (7-10).

MICROSCOPIC FEATURES. Vessels within a dAVF often exhibit irregular intimal thickening with variable loss of the internal elastic lamina.

STAGING, GRADING, AND CLASSIFICATION. The most common classification of dAVFs is based on angiographic patterns of venous drainage.

Clinical Issues

EPIDEMIOLOGY. dAVFs account for 10-15% of all intracranial vascular malformations with arteriovenous shunting. AVMs are approximately 10 times as common as dAVFs.

DEMOGRAPHICS. Most dAVFs are found in adults. The peak age is 40-60 years, roughly 20 years older than the peak age for AVMs. There is no gender predilection.

PRESENTATION. Clinical presentation varies with location and venous drainage pattern. Uncomplicated dAVFs in the transverse/sigmoid sinus region typically present with either bruit and/or tinnitus. dAVFs in the cavernous sinus cause pulsatile proptosis, chemosis, retroorbital pain, bruit, and ophthalmoplegia. "Malignant" dAVFs, lesions with cortical venous drainage, may cause seizures and progressive dementia in addition to focal neurologic deficits.

Patients who present with intracranial hemorrhage or nonhemorrhagic neurologic deficits also have a higher risk of new adverse events than those with an asymptomatic fistula.

NATURAL HISTORY. The natural history of a dAVF remains poorly understood. Some lesions demonstrate angiographic progression whereas others remain relatively stable. Progression of a dAVF from low to high grade occurs but is relatively uncommon.

Prognosis depends on location and venous drainage pattern. Almost 98% of lesions without cortical venous drainage will follow a benign clinical course. Hemorrhage is rare in such cases (approximately 1.5% per year). In contrast, "malignant" dAVFs often have an aggressive clinical course, with hemorrhage (annual risk approximately 7.5% per year) and neurologic symptoms as common complications.

Multiple dAVFs are associated with angiographic progression and poor clinical prognosis, requiring an aggressive treatment and management strategy.

TREATMENT OPTIONS. A spectrum of treatments exists; the treatment goal is preventing the occurrence of intracranial hemorrhage or nonhemorrhagic neurologic

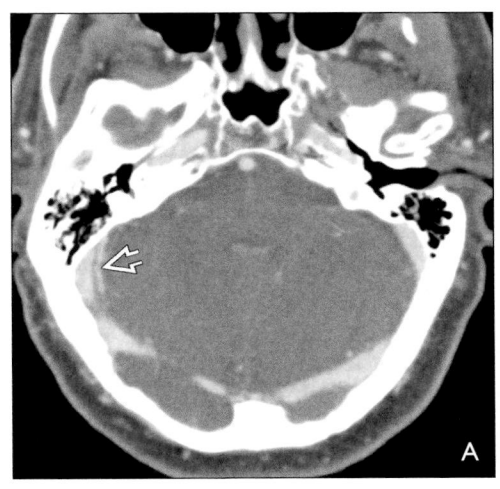

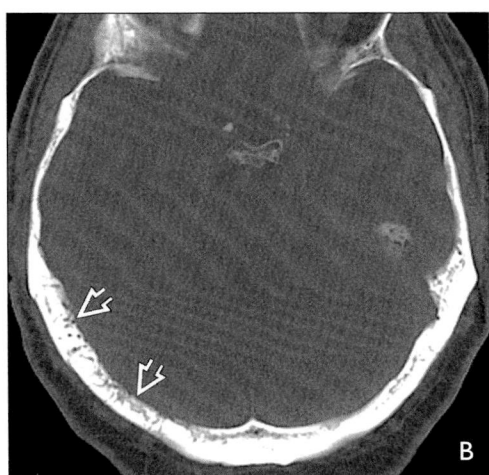

7-11A. CTA source image in a patient with right-sided tinnitus shows no obvious abnormality, although the right sigmoid sinus ➡ looks peculiar. 7-11B. Bone CT in the same patient shows multiple enlarged transosseous vascular channels ➡ in the squama of the right occipital bone.

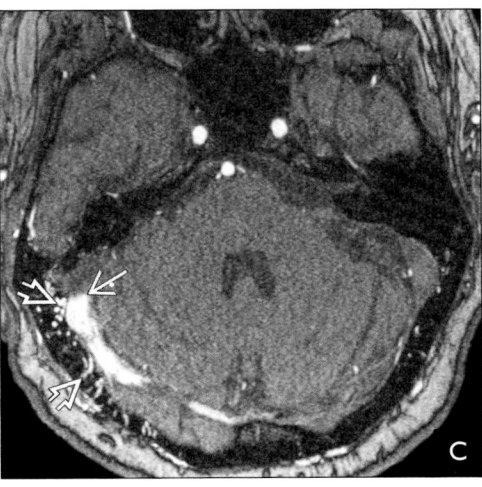

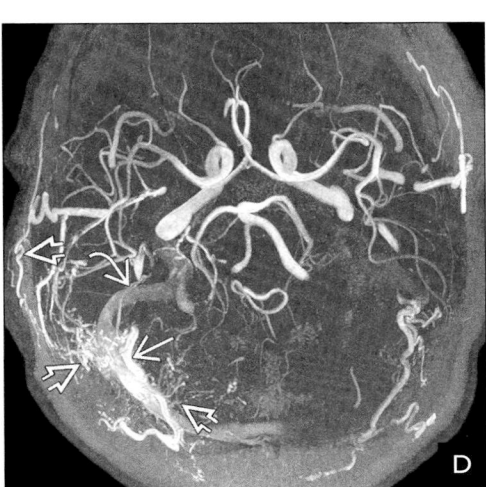

7-11C. Contrast-enhanced MRA source image shows dural sinus thrombosis ➡, multiple enhancing vascular channels ➡ characteristic of posterior fossa dAVF. 7-11D. MRA in the same patient shows innumerable tiny feeding arteries ➡ supplying a dAVF at the transverse-sigmoid sinus junction. The sinus has partially recanalized ➡, and the distal sigmoid sinus ➡ and jugular bulb are partially opacified.

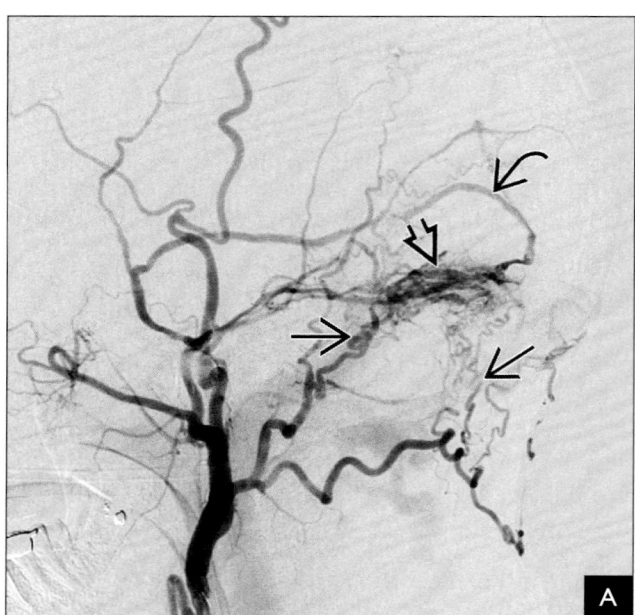

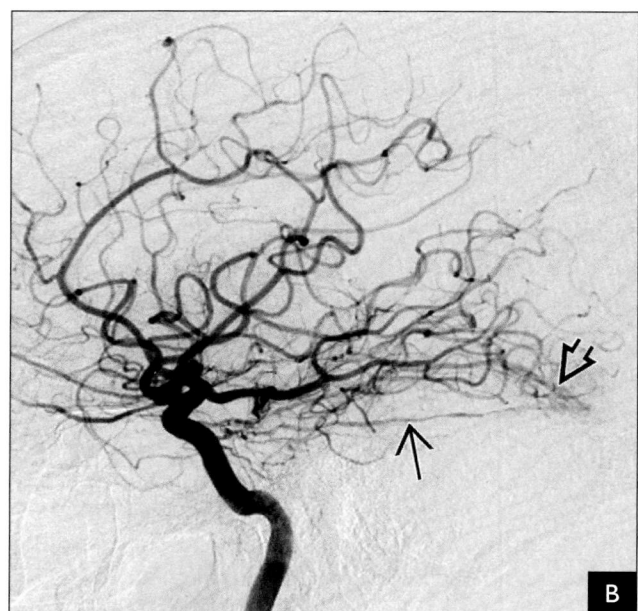

7-12A. DSA of the external carotid artery in a patient with tinnitus, dAVF in the occluded transverse sinus ⊃ supplied by the middle meningeal artery ↗, transosseous branches ⇒ from the ECA.

7-12B. Selective internal carotid angiogram in the same patient shows an enlarged meningohypophyseal trunk ⇒ that also supplies part of the dAVF ⊃.

deficits. Clinical observation may be appropriate in some patients who have minimal or no symptoms and dAVFs that demonstrate no cortical venous reflux.

In symptomatic patients, endovascular treatment with embolization of arterial feeders using particulate or liquid agents with or without coil embolization of the recipient venous pouch/sinus may be performed. Surgical resection of the involved dural sinus wall or stereotactic radiosurgery are other options.

Imaging

GENERAL FEATURES. Most dAVFs are found in the posterior fossa and skull base. While they can involve any dural venous sinus, the most common site is the transverse/sigmoid sinus junction. Between one-third and one-half of all dAVFs are found here. Less common sites are the cavernous sinus and superior petrosal sinus. dAVFs involving the superior sagittal sinus are relatively uncommon.

Cross-sectional imaging alone may be insufficient to demonstrate a dAVF. CTA, MRA, and DSA may be required both to identify a dAVF and to delineate its detailed angioarchitecture.

CT FINDINGS. CT findings vary from none to striking. Hemorrhage is uncommon in the absence of cortical venous drainage or dysplastic venous dilatation. An enlarged dural sinus or draining vein can sometimes be identified on NECT scans. Carotid-cavernous fistulas may demonstrate an enlarged superior ophthalmic vein. Dilated transcalvarial channels from enlarged tran-

sosseous feeding arteries can occasionally be seen on bone CT images and should be sought for in all patients with pulsatile tinnitus **(7-11A)**, **(7-11B)**.

Contrast-enhanced scans may demonstrate enlarged feeding arteries and draining veins. The involved dural venous sinus is often thrombosed or stenotic.

MR FINDINGS. As with CT, MR findings on standard sequences vary from normal to striking. The presence of dilated cortical veins without an identifiable nidus adjacent to normal-appearing brain may suggest the presence of a dAVF. The most common finding of a dAVF itself is a thrombosed dural venous sinus containing vascular-appearing "flow voids" **(7-11C)**, **(7-11D)**. Thrombus is typically isointense with brain on T1- and T2 scans and "blooms" on T2* sequences. Chronically thrombosed sinuses may enhance.

Parenchymal hyperintensity on T2WI and FLAIR indicates venous congestion or ischemia, usually secondary to retrograde cortical venous drainage.

ANGIOGRAPHY. While CTA/CTV with 3D shaded surface display may be useful in depicting arterial supply and venous drainage patterns, the best imaging tool for detailed delineation is DSA. Indeed, DSA with superselective catheterization of dural and transosseous feeders is usually required to identify arterial feeders, define the exact fistula site, delineate venous drainage, and identify feeding artery or remote aneurysms (found in 20% of cases).

As most dAVFs arise adjacent to the skull base, multiple enlarged dural and transosseous branches arising from the external carotid artery are usually present **(7-12A)**. Dural branches may also arise from the internal carotid and vertebral arteries **(7-13)**. An enlarged tentorial branch of the meningohypophyseal trunk commonly contributes to dAVFs at the transverse/sigmoid sinus junction **(7-12B)**.

The presence of dural sinus thrombosis, flow reversal with drainage into cortical (leptomeningeal) veins, and tortuous engorged pial veins (a "pseudophlebitic" pattern) should be identified. High-flow venopathy associated with a dAVF may result in progressive stenosis, occlusion, and subsequent hemorrhage. Dysplastic venous "pouches" may cause focal mass effect. Risk of associated intracranial hemorrhage rises significantly with the presence of leptomeningeal drainage and dysplastic venous dilatations.

Angiographic classification of dAVFs helps stratify risk of dAVF rupture and predict the clinical course of these lesions. The Cognard and Borden classifications are the most commonly used systems.

CLASSIFICATION OF dAVFs

Cognard Classification
- **Grade 1**: In sinus wall; normal antegrade venous drainage (low risk; benign clinical course)
- **Grade 2A**: In sinus; reflux to sinus, not cortical veins
- **Grade 2B**: Reflux (retrograde drainage) into cortical veins (10-20% hemorrhage)
- **Grade 3**: Direct cortical venous drainage; no venous ectasia (40% hemorrhage)
- **Grade 4**: Direct cortical venous drainage + venous ectasia (65% hemorrhage)
- **Grade 5**: Spinal perimedullary venous drainage

Borden Classification
- **Type I**: Dural arterial supply with antegrade drainage into venous sinus
  - **Type Ia**: Simple dAVF with single meningeal arterial supply
  - **Type Ib**: Complex dAVF with multiple meningeal arteries
- **Type II**: Dural supply + ↑ intrasinus pressure → antegrade sinus, retrograde cortical venous drainage
- **Type III**: Dural arteries drain into cortical veins

In either classification, *the presence of cortical venous drainage (CVD) puts a dAVF into a higher risk cate-*

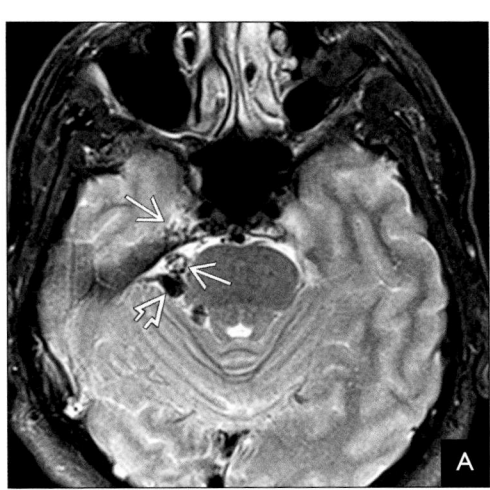

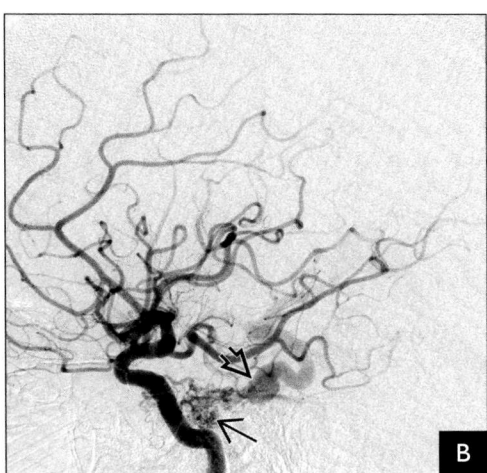

7-13A. T2WI in a 48-year-old man with right-sided trigeminal neuralgia shows a tangle of vessels ➥ in the Meckel cave and cerebellopontine angle cistern associated with a large "flow void" ➥. 7-13B. DSA of right ICA angiogram shows that the tangle of vessels ➥ is supplied by enlarged dural branches of the ICA and fistulizes directly into an enlarged "early draining" vein ➥.

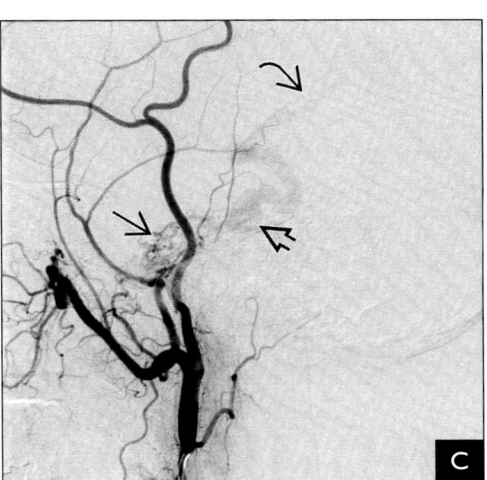

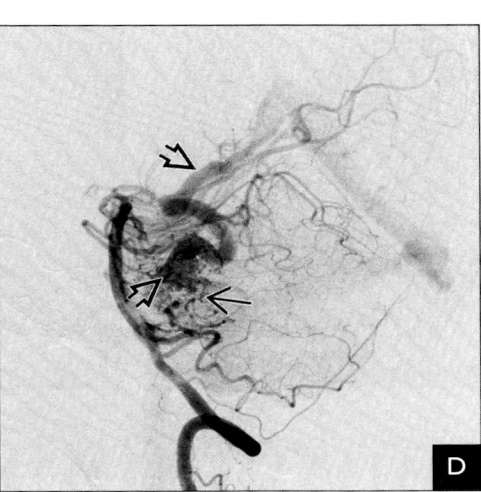

7-13C. Selective ECA angiogram shows that more enlarged feeders arise from the middle meningeal artery ➥ with early opacification of the large draining vein ➥. The prominent vein empties into a lateral mesencephalic vein that connects to the deep galenic venous system ➥. 7-13D. DSA shows that the ipsilateral vertebral artery has a number of enlarged parenchymal (pial) branches ➥ that also supply the malformation, opacify the large draining vein ➥. Mixed pial-dural AVM.

gory. Subdividing lesions with CVD into symptomatic and asymptomatic types may help improve risk stratification. dAVFs are dynamic lesions and may spontaneously regress or progress. The risk of a low-grade lesion converting to a high-grade type is relatively low, but change in symptoms should prompt imaging reevaluation.

Differential Diagnosis

The most common mimic of dAVF is a **thrombosed dural venous sinus** with prominent collateral venous drainage. Here, no enlarged arterial feeders are present, and no microfistulas can be identified in the dural sinus wall.

A **pseudolesion of the jugular bulb**, caused by slow or asymmetric flow, may create inhomogeneous signal within the jugular foramen. No thrombus is seen on T2*, and neither abnormal arterial feeders nor enlarged venous collaterals are present.

A **pial AVM** or **fistula** is rare and represents a direct arteriovenous shunt between a brain parenchymal ("pial") artery and a dilated cortical draining vein. These occur along the brain surface or within the brain itself, not within a dural venous sinus (see below).

Carotid-Cavernous Fistula

Terminology

Carotid-cavernous fistulas (CCFs) are a special type of arteriovenous shunt that develops within the cavernous sinus (7-14), (7-15). CCFs are divided into two subgroups, direct and indirect fistulas.

"Direct" CCFs are typically *high-flow* lesions that result from rupture of the cavernous internal carotid artery (ICA) directly into the cavernous sinus (CS), with or without a preexisting ICA aneurysm. **"Indirect" CCFs** are usually *slow-flow, low-pressure* lesions that represent an arteriovenous fistula between dural branches of the cavernous ICA and the cavernous sinus.

Etiology

CCFs are almost always acquired lesions and can be traumatic or nontraumatic in origin. Most *direct* CCFs are traumatic, usually secondary to central skull base fractures. Either stretch injury to the ICA or direct puncture from a bony fracture fragment may occur. A single-hole laceration/transection of the cavernous ICA with direct fistulization into the CS is the typical finding. Spontaneous (i.e., nontraumatic) rupture of a preexisting cavernous ICA aneurysm is a less common etiology.

Indirect CCFs are nontraumatic lesions and are thought to be degenerative in origin. In contrast to dAVFs elsewhere, indirect CCFs rarely occur as sequelae of dural sinus thrombosis. Most indirect CCFs are found in the dural wall of the cavernous sinus and supplied via intracavernous branches of the ICA and deep (maxillary) branches of the ECA.

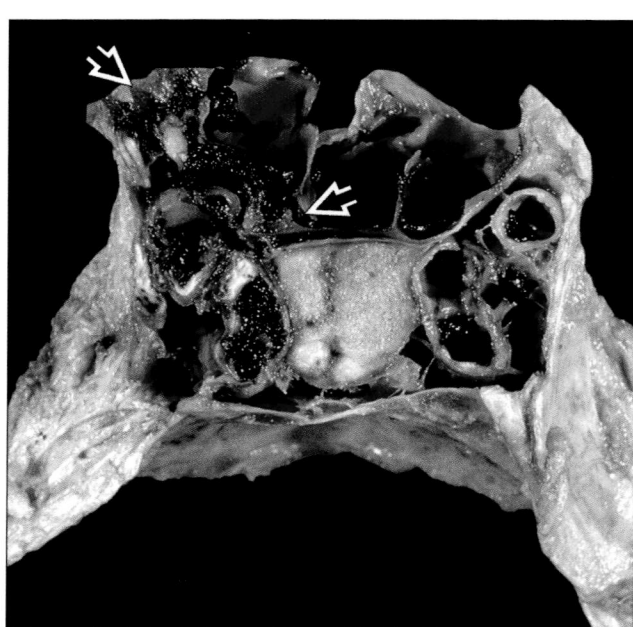

7-14. Coronal graphic depicts a carotid-cavernous fistula (CCF). The right cavernous sinus ⊳ is enlarged by numerous dilated arterial and venous channels.

7-15. Autopsy case of direct CCF with dissection of the cavernous sinus (CS) and adjacent structures shows that the right CS is enlarged ⊳ by numerous dilated vascular channels. (Courtesy B. Horten, MD.)

Pathology

GROSS PATHOLOGY. In a direct CCF, arterialized flow causes dilatation of the CS with venous hypertension and retrograde flow into the superior and inferior ophthalmic veins. Indirect CCFs demonstrate enlarged crack-like vessels within the CS that resemble those seen in typical dAVFs elsewhere.

STAGING, GRADING, AND CLASSIFICATION. CCFs are a subtype of dAVF. A specific classification for CCFs, the Barrow classification, is based on the arterial supply.

BARROW CLASSIFICATION OF CAROTID-CAVERNOUS FISTULAS

Type A: Direct ICA-cavernous sinus high-flow shunt
Type B: Dural ICA branches-cavernous sinus shunt
Type C: Dural ECA-cavernous sinus shunt
Type D: Both ICA/ECA dural branches shunt to CS

Clinical Issues

Clinical presentation, natural history, demographics, and epidemiology vary with whether the CCF is traumatic or spontaneous.

EPIDEMIOLOGY. An indirect CCF is the second most common site of intracranial dAVF, following the transverse/sigmoid sinus junction. Direct high-flow CCFs are much less common.

DEMOGRAPHICS. As direct CCFs typically occur with trauma, they are found in both genders and at all ages. Indirect CCFs are most frequent in women 40-60 years of age.

PRESENTATION. Direct CCFs may present within hours to days or even weeks following trauma. Bruit, pulsatile exophthalmos, orbital edema, decreasing vision, glaucoma, and headache are typical **(7-16)**. In severe cases, vision loss may be rapid and severe. Cranial neuropathy may occur but is less common. In rare cases, rupture of an intracavernous ICA aneurysm may cause life-threatening epistaxis.

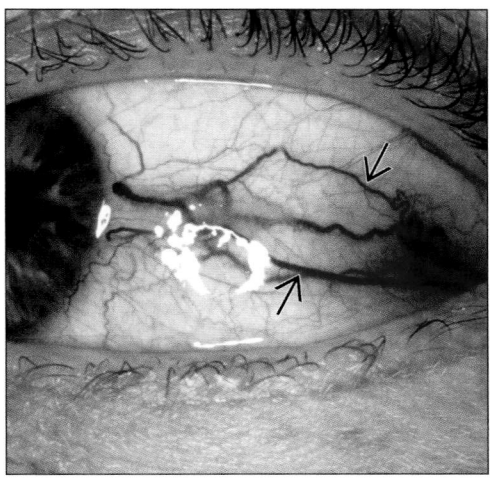

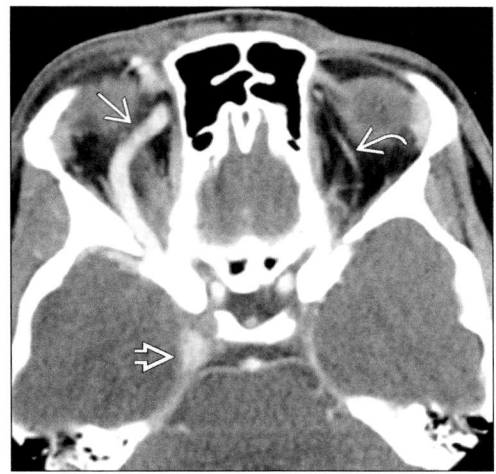

7-16. Clinical photograph of a patient with a CCF shows numerous enlarged scleral vessels ➡. 7-17. CECT scan shows classic findings of CCF. The right cavernous sinus is enlarged ➡, and the ipsilateral superior ophthalmic vein ➡ is more than 4 times the size of the left superior ophthalmic vein ➡.

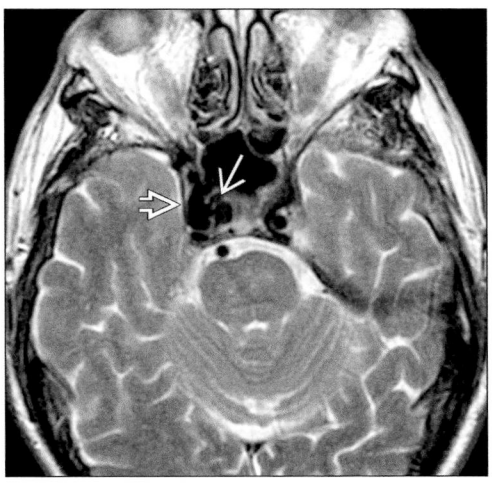

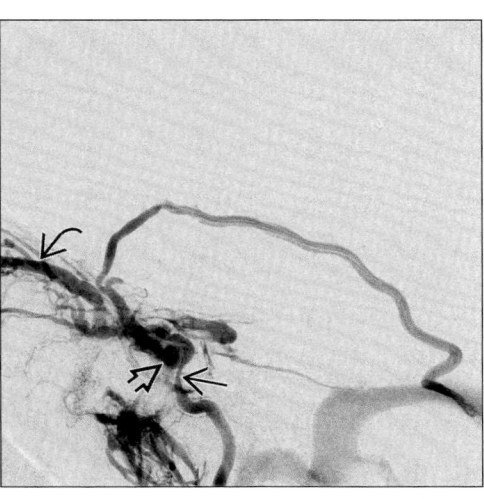

7-18. T2WI shows typical MR findings of CCF with an enlarged right cavernous sinus ➡ containing numerous abnormal "flow voids" ➡. 7-19. Lateral DSA in a case of direct CCF in a 21-year-old woman with multiple skull base fractures shows that the ICA narrows ➡ before terminating in a large venous pouch ➡. High-pressure venous reflux into the superior and inferior ophthalmic veins ➡ and the sphenoparietal sinus is present.

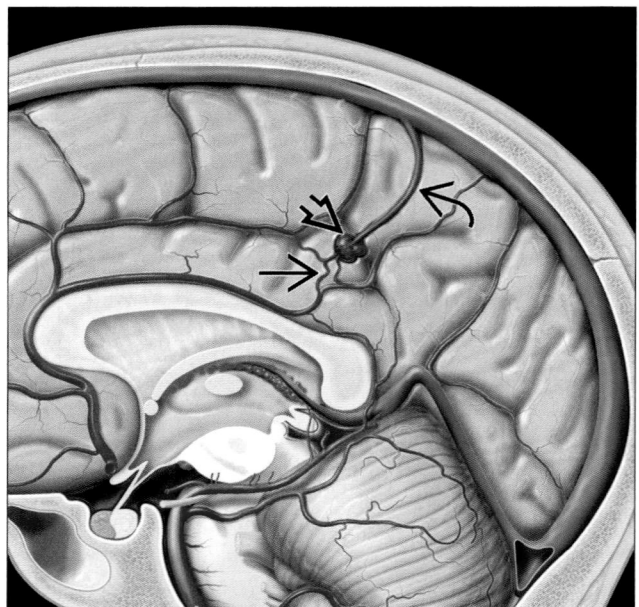

7-20. *Pial AVF with slightly enlarged ACA branches* ⊟ *connecting to a venous varix* ⊟, *dilated cortical draining vein* ⊟.

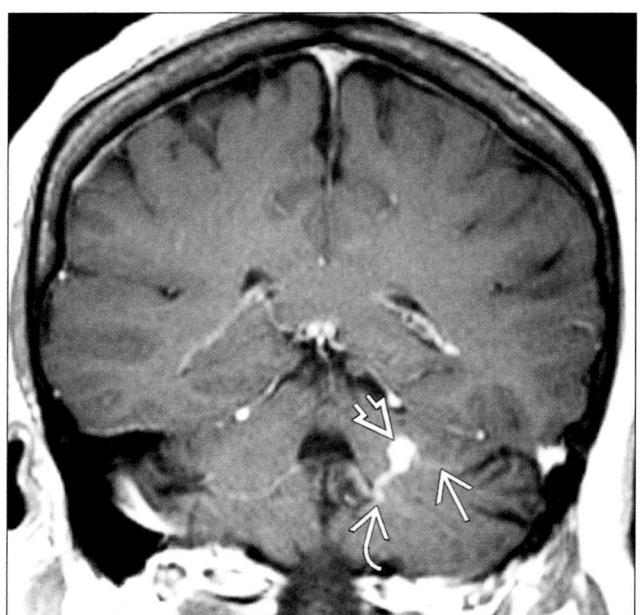

7-21. *Coronal T1 C+ scan shows a pial AVF in the posterior fossa. A small cerebellar artery* ⊟ *connects directly to a venous pouch* ⊟, *which in turn drains into a subependymal vein* ⊟ *near the fourth ventricle.*

Indirect CCFs typically cause painless proptosis with variable vision changes.

NATURAL HISTORY. In severe cases with torrential ICA-CS shunting, hemispheric ischemia may result. If retrograde intracranial venous drainage is present, catastrophic subarachnoid hemorrhage from ruptured ectatic cortical veins can occur.

TREATMENT OPTIONS. The primary goal in treating a direct CCF is fistula closure, typically by transarterial-transfistula detachable balloon embolization. Transvenous embolization via the internal jugular vein and inferior petrosal sinus is another option. If the ICA is torn, covered stent placement may be effective. Less commonly, trapping the fistula and sacrificing the parent ICA with coils or balloons may be considered. This is an option only if the patient passes balloon "test" occlusion or has sufficient collateral circulation to compensate for lack of antegrade ICA flow.

Indirect CCFs may be treated conservatively or with superselective embolization.

Imaging

GENERAL FEATURES. The general imaging features of CCF reflect the presence of AV shunting within the cavernous sinus. Depending on the degree of the shunt, findings can vary from subtle to striking.

CT FINDINGS. NECT scans may demonstrate mild or striking proptosis, a prominent CS with enlarged superior ophthalmic vein (SOV), and enlarged extraocular mus-

cles. "Dirty" fat secondary to edema and venous engorgement may be present. Occasionally, subarachnoid hemorrhage from trauma or ruptured cortical veins can be identified.

CECT scans often nicely demonstrate an enlarged SOV and CS **(7-17)**. Inferior drainage into a prominent pterygoid venous plexus and posterior drainage into the clival venous plexus are sometimes present.

MR FINDINGS. T1 scans may show a prominent "bulging" CS and SOV as well as "dirty" orbital fat. T2-weighted images may show asymmetric flow-related signal loss in the affected veins. Too many "flow voids" in the CS is a common finding with CCFs **(7-18)**.

Strong, uniform enhancement of the CS and SOV is typical. Enlarged, tortuous intracranial veins may occur with high-flow, high-pressure shunts.

Rare cases of high-flow, aggressive direct CCFs with prominent pontomesencephalic and perimedullary venous drainage causing progressive myelopathy have been reported.

ANGIOGRAPHY. DSA is required for definitive diagnosis and treatment. Complete delineation of the arterial supply and venous drainage pattern is the goal. *Direct* CCFs typically demonstrate rapid flow with very early opacification of the CS **(7-19)**. Selective ICA injection with very rapid image acquisition is often necessary to localize the fistula site precisely. A single-hole fistula is usually present, typically between the C4 and C5 ICA segments.

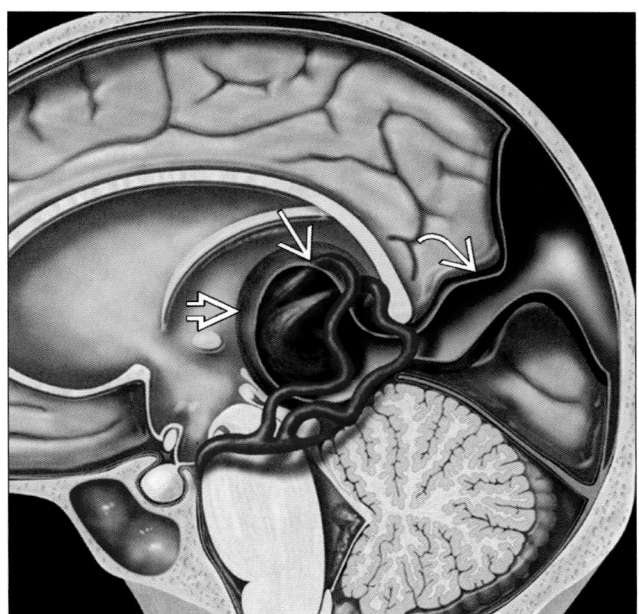

7-22. Graphic illustrates vein of Galen malformation. Enlarged choroid arteries ➡ *drain directly into dilated median prosencephalic vein (MPV)* ➡ *, falcine sinus* ➡ *. Torcular herophili (venous sinus confluence) is massively enlarged.*

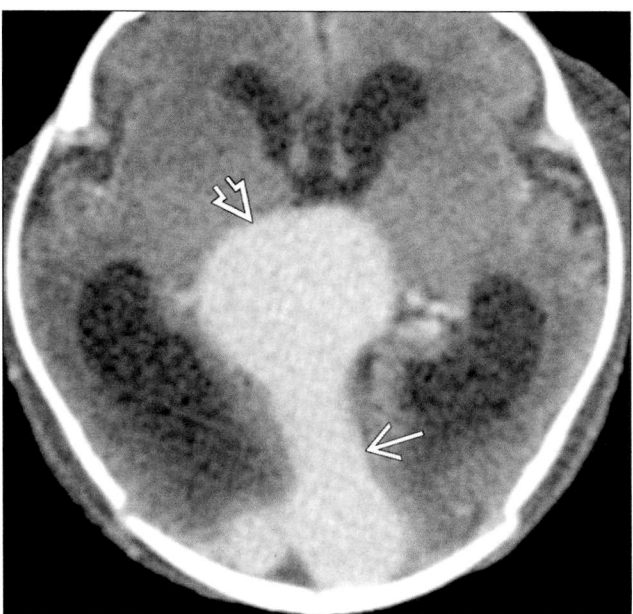

7-23. CECT scan in a newborn demonstrates a massive VGAM ➡ *draining into an enlarged falcine sinus* ➡ *, causing obstructive hydrocephalus.*

Occasionally, injection into the vertebrobasilar system with manual compression of the ipsilateral carotid artery is necessary to determine the fistula site. Venous drainage via the superior and inferior ophthalmic veins; contralateral CS; clival, pterygoid, and sphenoparietal sinuses; and intracranial cortical veins should be delineated.

Indirect CCFs often have multiple dural feeders from cavernous branches of the ICA (meningohypophyseal and inferolateral trunks) as well as deep branches of the ECA (middle meningeal and distal maxillary branches). Anastomoses between ICA and ECA feeders, such as the artery of the foramen rotundum, are common and must be delineated completely prior to embolization.

ULTRASOUND. The normal flow in the SOV is from extra- to intracranial (i.e., from orbit into CS). Flow reversal (intra- to extracranial) within an enlarged SOV can be demonstrated noninvasively using Doppler US.

Differential Diagnosis

The major differential diagnosis with CCFs is **cavernous sinus thrombosis** (CST). Both CCF and CST may cause proptosis, intraorbital edema, enlarged extraocular muscles, and the appearance of "dirty fat." In CST, the CS may appear enlarged, but prominent filling defects are present on T1 C+ MR.

Pial AV Fistula

A pial arteriovenous fistula (pAVF) is a rare vascular malformation that usually consists of a single dilated pial artery connecting directly to an enlarged cortical drain-

ing vein **(7-20)**. No intervening capillary bed or nidus is present.

Unlike dural AVFs, 80% of pAVFs are supratentorial. They typically lie on or just within the brain surface or adjacent to the ventricular ependyma **(7-21)**. pAVFs are supplied by branches of the anterior, middle, or posterior cerebral arteries and are usually associated with a venous varix.

Vein of Galen Aneurysmal Malformation

Different types of vascular malformations share a dilated vein of Galen as a common feature, but only one of these is a true vein of Galen aneurysmal malformation (VGAM). A VGAM is the most common extracardiac cause of high-output cardiac failure in newborns.

Terminology

VGAM is essentially a direct arteriovenous fistula between deep choroidal arteries and a persistent embryonic precursor of the vein of Galen **(7-22)**. The arteriovenous shunt causes flow-related aneurysmal dilatation of this primitive vein, forming a large midline venous pouch that lies behind the third ventricle.

Etiology

GENERAL CONCEPTS. In normal fetal development, arterial supply to the choroid plexus drains via a single transient midline vein, the median prosencephalic vein

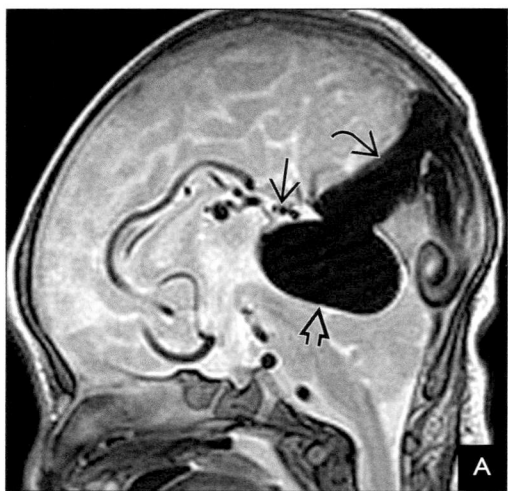

7-24A. Sagittal T2WI shows prominent arteries ⇒ supplying an enlarged median prosencephalic vein ⇒. Note enlarged falcine sinus ⇒.

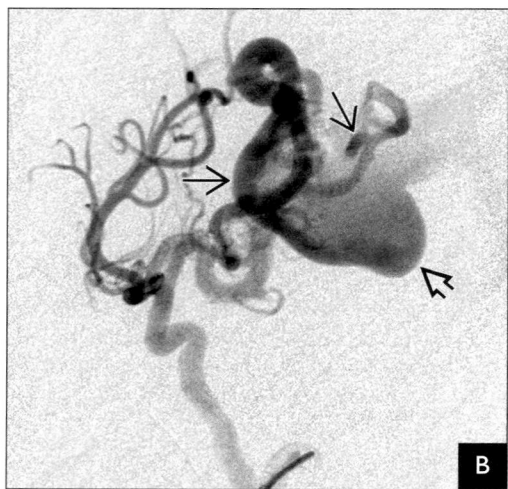

7-24B. DSA in the same patient shows that the VGAM ⇒ is supplied by multiple direct arterial fistulas ⇒.

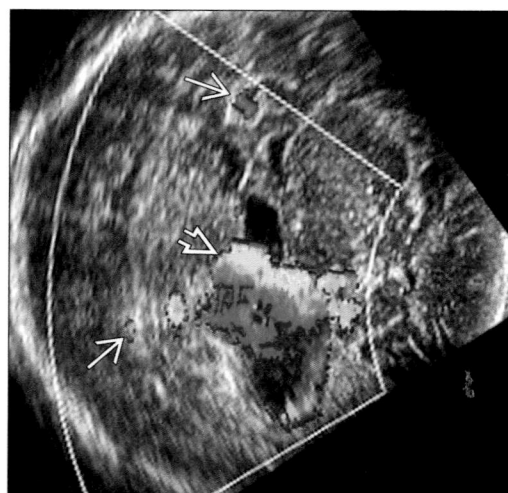

7-25. Neonatal transcranial US shows a large VGAM ⇒ posterior to the 3rd ventricle. Prominent vessels with arterial flow ⇒ supply the lesion.

(MPV) of Markowski. Normally, the developing internal cerebral veins annex drainage of the fetal choroid plexus, and the MPV regresses. In a VGAM, a high-flow fistula prevents formation of the definitive vein of Galen.

GENETICS. VGAMs are sporadic lesions with no known genetic predisposition.

Pathology

GROSS PATHOLOGY. Enlarged arteries drain directly into a dilated MPV. "Aneurysmal" dilatation of the persistent MPV forms a large venous pouch behind the third ventricle that often drains into a markedly enlarged superior sagittal sinus via an embryonic falcine sinus **(7-22)**. The ventricles are often markedly dilated. The brain is frequently atrophic. Ischemic changes are common.

MICROSCOPIC FEATURES. The wall of the venous pouch may become significantly thickened and dysplastic.

Clinical Issues

EPIDEMIOLOGY. VGAMs are rare, representing less than 1% of all cerebral vascular malformations. However, they account for 30% of symptomatic vascular malformations in children.

DEMOGRAPHICS. Neonatal VGAMs are more common than those presenting in infancy or childhood. Adult presentation is rare. There is a definite male predominance (M:F = 2:1).

PRESENTATION. Signs and symptoms vary with age of onset. In neonates, high-output congestive heart failure and a loud cranial bruit are typical. Older infants may present with macrocrania and hydrocephalus, with or without heart failure.

VGAMs in older children are often associated with developmental delay and seizures. VGAMs in young adults typically present with headache with or without hemorrhage and hydrocephalus.

NATURAL HISTORY. Prognosis is related to size of the arteriovenous shunt. Large VGAMs cause cerebral ischemia and dystrophic changes in the fetal brain. Left untreated, neonates with VGAMs typically die from progressive brain damage and intractable heart failure.

TREATMENT OPTIONS. Anatomic cure of the VGAM is not the main goal of treatment; rather, the ultimate goal is sufficient control of the malformation to allow normal brain maturation and development. Staged arterial embolization, ideally at four or five months of age, is the preferred treatment. The transvenous approach carries significant morbidity and mortality and is generally contraindicated.

Imaging

GENERAL FEATURES. A large, rounded venous pouch drains into a persistent falcine sinus or prominent straight sinus. The venous sinus confluence is often markedly enlarged.

CT FINDINGS. NECT scans show an enlarged, well-delineated, mildly hyperdense mass at the tentorial apex, usually compressing the third ventricle and causing severe obstructive hydrocephalus. Variable encephalomalacia, hemorrhage, and/or dystrophic calcification in the brain parenchyma is often present. CECT scans show strong uniform enhancement (7-23).

MR FINDINGS. Rapid but turbulent flow in the VGAM causes inhomogeneous signal loss and phase artifact (signal misregistration in the phase-encoding direction). Enlarged arterial feeders are usually seen as serpentine "flow voids" adjacent to the lesion (7-24A). Thrombus of varying ages may be present lining the VGAM.

ANGIOGRAPHY. Two forms of VGAM are recognized based on their specific angioarchitecture. The most common is the **"choroidal"** form. Here multiple branches from the pericallosal, choroidal, and thalamoperforating arteries drain directly into an enlarged, aneurysmally dilated midline venous sac (7-24B). In the rare **"mural"** form, a single or a few enlarged branches from collicular or posterior choroidal arteries drain into the sinus wall.

In more than 50% of all VGAMs, the straight sinus is hypoplastic or absent and venous drainage is into a persistent embryonic **"falcine sinus."** The falcine sinus is easily identified as it angles posterosuperiorly toward the superior sagittal sinus.

ULTRASOUND. Many VGAMs are now diagnosed antenatally. A hypoechoic to mildly echogenic midline mass behind the third ventricle is typical. Color Doppler shows bidirectional turbulent flow within the VGAM (7-25).

Differential Diagnosis

Typical imaging findings in a neonate with high-output CHF are virtually pathognomonic of VGAM. A thalamic arteriovenous malformation (AVM) with deep venous drainage may cause secondary enlargement of the vein of Galen. **Vein of Galen aneurysmal dilatation associated with an AVM** rarely presents in the neonatal period. A high-flow **giant childhood dural arteriovenous fistula** may present in infancy and clinically resemble a VGAM. Involvement of the dural venous sinuses rather than the vein of Galen or MPV is typical.

CVMs without Arteriovenous Shunting

Developmental Venous Anomaly

With the advent of contrast-enhanced MR, developmental venous anomalies have become the most frequently diagnosed intracranial vascular malformation. Once thought to be rare lesions with substantial risk of hemorrhage, the vast majority of venous "angiomas" are now recognized as asymptomatic and incidental imaging findings. Neurologic complications of these common lesions are rare.

Terminology

Developmental venous anomaly (DVA), also called **venous "angioma"** or "venous malformation," is an umbrella-shaped congenital cerebral vascular malformation composed of angiogenically mature venous elements. Dilated, thin-walled venous channels lie within (and are separated by) normal brain parenchyma.

Very rarely, a dilated or tortuous venous pouch without discernible arterial or venous tributaries occurs. In these unusual cases, the term **venous varix** is appropriate.

Etiology

GENERAL CONCEPTS. The precise etiology of DVAs is unknown. Some investigators posit arrested medullary vein development between 8 and 11 gestational weeks. Others believe DVAs represent an extreme variant of otherwise normal venous drainage. Unlike many other cerebrovascular malformations, DVAs do not express growth factors.

GENETICS.

Solitary DVA. Whereas genetic linkage studies have implicated a region on chromosome 9p in hereditary cutaneomucosal venous malformations, no genetic predisposition for the formation of isolated, sporadic brain DVAs has been identified.

An association of DVA and solitary (but not familial) cerebral cavernous malformations (CCMs) has been recently reported, suggesting that these vascular malformations probably have a different developmental mechanism. Solitary DVAs lack the *KRIT1* gene associated with familial CCMs.

Multiple DVAs. Multiple cerebral venous malformations have been reported in **blue rubber bleb nevus syn-**

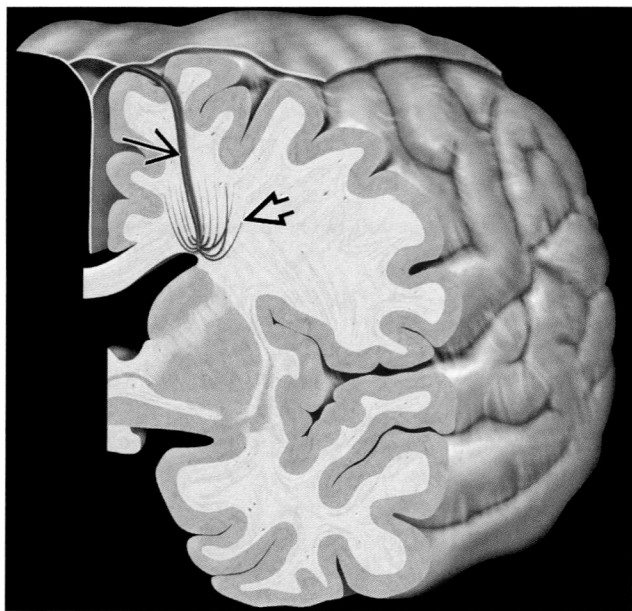

7-26. Graphic depicts DVA with enlarged medullary veins ⊳ draining into a single transmantle collector vein →.

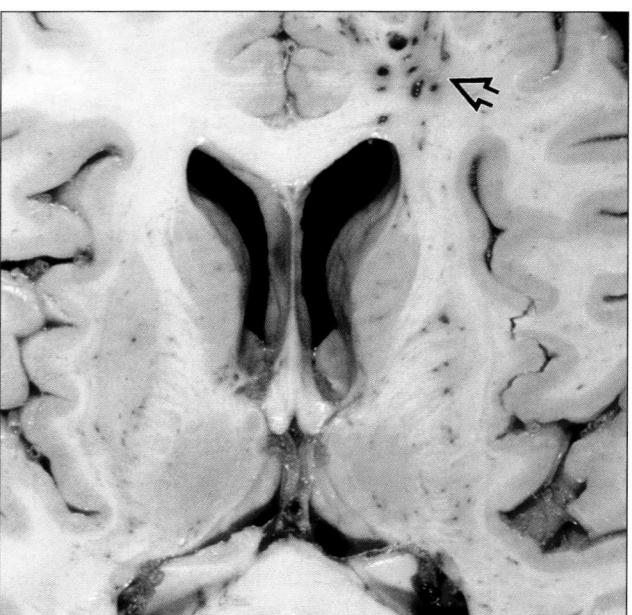

7-27. Autopsy case shows left frontal DVA as dilated medullary veins ⊳ interspersed with normal brain. (Courtesy R. Hewlett, MD.)

drome (BRBNS), with a proposed but not proven link to chromosome 9.

Pathology

LOCATION, SIZE, AND NUMBER. DVAs are found in the deep white matter (WM), adjacent to the frontal horn of the lateral ventricle **(7-26)**. The second most common location is next to the fourth ventricle. Size varies from tiny, almost imperceptible lesions to giant DVAs that can involve most of the hemispheric WM.

Solitary DVAs are much more common than multiple lesions.

GROSS PATHOLOGY. A cluster of variably sized enlarged medullary (WM) veins embedded within brain parenchyma is the usual finding **(7-27)**.

MICROSCOPIC FEATURES. Thin-walled, somewhat dilated venous channels are interspersed in normal-appearing white matter. Occasionally, the vessel walls are thickened and hyalinized. Hemorrhage and calcification are uncommon unless the DVA is associated with a CCM.

Clinical Issues

EPIDEMIOLOGY. DVA is the most common intracranial vascular malformation, accounting for 60% of all cerebrovascular malformations. Estimated prevalence on contrast-enhanced MR scans ranges from 2.5-9%.

DEMOGRAPHICS. DVAs are found in patients of all ages without gender predilection.

PRESENTATION. Most DVAs are discovered incidentally at autopsy or on imaging studies. A recent meta-analysis showed that 98% of all DVAs are asymptomatic. Two percent present with hemorrhage or infarct, probably caused by stenosis or spontaneous thrombosis of the outlet collector vein.

DVAs are occasionally associated with cortical dysplasia. In such cases, the cortical malformation may cause seizures.

DVAs may coexist with other vascular lesions that cause symptomatic intracranial hemorrhage. The most common "histologically mixed" cerebrovascular malformation is a cavernous-venous malformation. Occasionally a "triad" malformation that consists of cavernous, venous, and capillary components is identified.

Most DVAs are solitary unless they are associated with a vascular neurocutaneous syndrome such as **blue rubber bleb nevus syndrome**. DVAs may coexist with a **sinus pericranii**. Sinus pericranii is typically the cutaneous sign of an underlying venous anomaly. DVAs are also associated with **periorbital lymphatic/lymphaticovenous malformations**.

NATURAL HISTORY. Most DVAs remain asymptomatic. Longitudinal studies have demonstrated that incidentally discovered DVAs had zero symptomatic hemorrhages or infarcts in nearly 500 person-years of follow-up.

Approximately 6% of DVAs present with symptomatic hemorrhage. Most are mixed with a lesion that has an intrinsic tendency to hemorrhage (such as cavernous malformation).

TREATMENT OPTIONS. No treatment is required or recommended for solitary DVAs (they are "leave me alone!" lesions). If a DVA is histologically mixed, treatment is determined by the coexisting lesion. Preoperative identification of such mixed malformations is important as ligating the collector vein or removing its tributaries may result in venous infarction.

Imaging

GENERAL FEATURES. DVAs are composed of radially arranged medullary veins that converge on a transcortical or subependymal large collector vein. The classic appearance is that of a "Medusa head" or "upside-down umbrella."

CT FINDINGS. NECT scans are usually normal unless the DVA is very large and a prominent draining vein is present. CECT scans show numerous linear and/or punctate enhancing foci that converge on a well-delineated tubular collector vein (7-28). In atypical DVAs, perfusion CT may show a venous congestion pattern with increased CBV, CBF, and MTT in the adjacent brain parenchyma.

MR FINDINGS. If the DVA is small, it may be undetectable unless contrast-enhanced scans are obtained. T1 C+ sequences show a stellate collection of linear enhancing structures converging on the transparenchymal or subependymal collector vein (7-29), (7-30A), (7-31). The collector vein may show variable high-velocity signal loss. Because flow in the venous radicles of a DVA is typically slow, blood deoxygenates and T2* scans (GRE, SWI) show striking linear hypointensities (7-30B).

If a DVA is mixed with a cavernous malformation, blood products in various stages of degradation may be present and "bloom" on T2* sequences (7-32).

ANGIOGRAPHY. The arterial phase is normal. The venous phase shows the typical hair-like collection ("Medusa head") of dilated medullary veins within the white matter (7-33). A faint, prolonged "blush" or capillary "stain" may be present in some cases. A transitional form of venous-arteriovenous malformation with enlarged feeders and AV shunting ("early draining" vein) occurs but is uncommon. Rarely, a true venous varix may occur with a DVA.

Differential Diagnosis

Mixed vascular malformation in which the DVA provides prominent venous drainage is common. Large ("giant") **capillary telangiectasias** usually have a dominant central collector vein and may therefore resemble a DVA.

Highly vascular neoplasms such as **glioblastoma multiforme** may have arteriovenous shunting into enlarged white matter and cortical veins. **Collateral venous drainage with enlarged medullary veins** in Sturge-Weber syndrome and dural venous sinus occlusion may occasionally mimic a DVA.

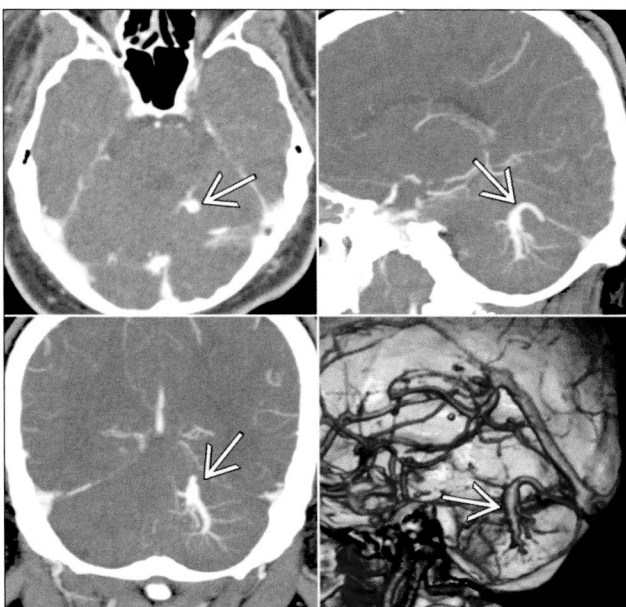

7-28. CECT, CTA depict classic DVA in the left cerebellar hemisphere ⇥.

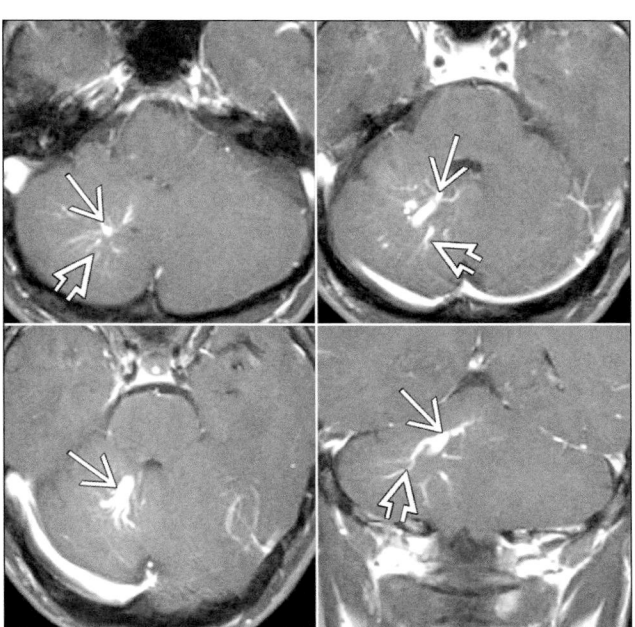

7-29. T1 C+ MR scans show classic findings of DVA with enlarged WM veins ⇥ *draining into a large collector vein* ⇥. *This was an incidental finding in an asymptomatic patient.*

7-30A. T1 C+ scan shows a classic DVA with enlarged WM veins ⬌ and a collector vein ➡ draining into the anterior aspect of the superior sagittal sinus. *7-30B.* SWI scan shows the DVA ⬌ and collector vein ➡ as hypointense structures clearly different in configuration from the normal cortical veins. A focal hemorrhage ➘ adjacent to the left frontal horn is secondary to a small cavernous malformation. DVAs are often histologically mixed lesions.

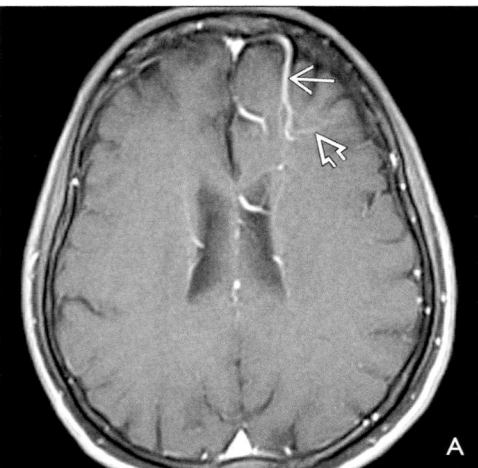
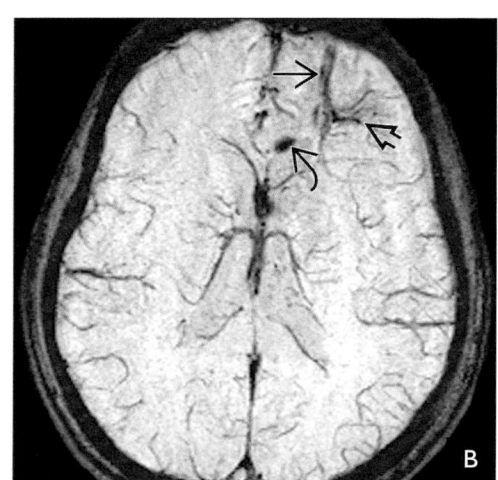

7-31A. Coronal T1 C+ scan shows multiple enlarged medullary veins ⬌ draining into the collecto" vein ➡. Normal brain parenchyma is interspersed between the venous radicles. *7-31B.* Coronal autopsy specimen shows an incidental finding of a DVA ➘. Note the normal brain in between the enlarged medullary veins and the absence of hemorrhage. (Courtesy P. Burger, MD.)

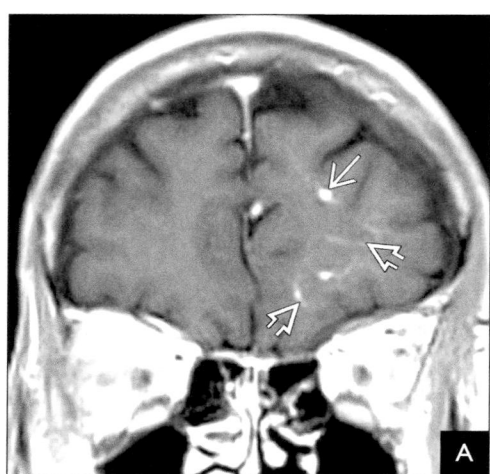
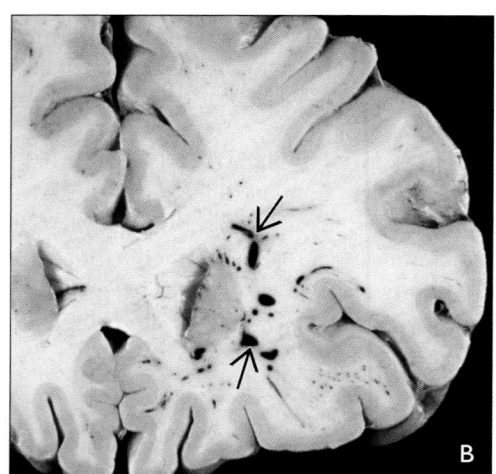

7-32A. T1 C+ FS MR in a 55-year-old man with sudden onset of right CNs VI, VII palsies shows a classic DVA ⬌ adjacent to the fourth ventricle. *7-32B.* T2* SWI shows the hypointense DVA ⬌. In addition, a small focal hematoma ➡ from a cavernous malformation in the floor of the fourth ventricle is identified; the hematoma is probably responsible for the patient's symptoms.

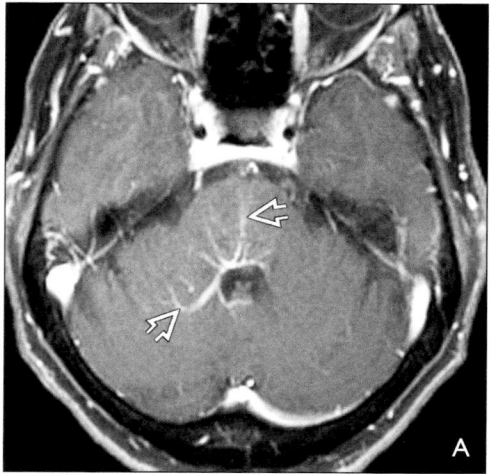
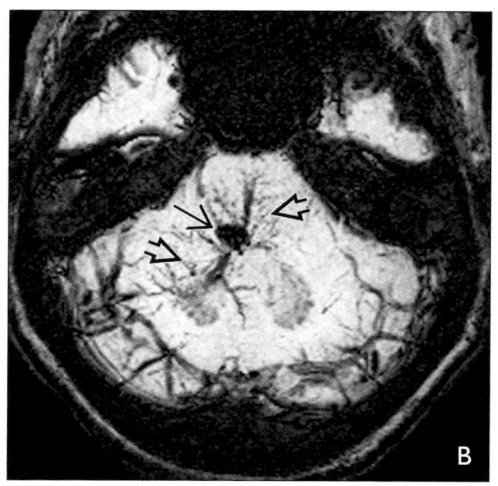

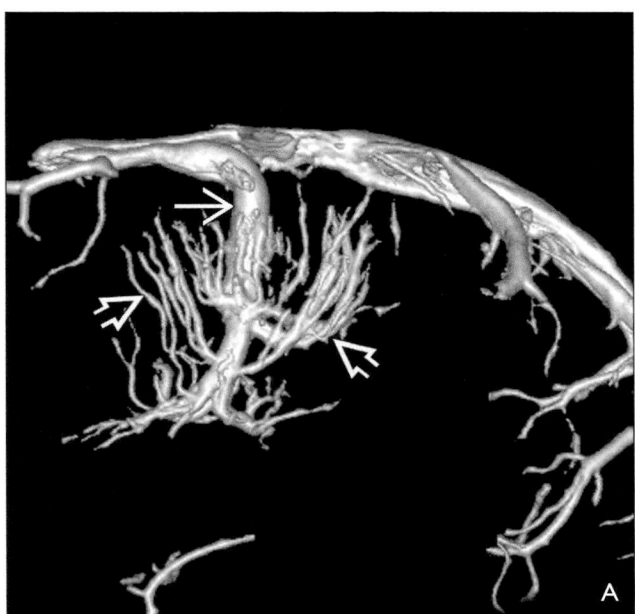

7-33A. 3D SSD demonstrates a classic DVA with enlarged medullary veins ⇉ draining into the collector vein ⇉. The appearance resembles a "Medusa head," "upside-down willow tree" or "umbrella." (Courtesy P. Lasjaunias, MD.)

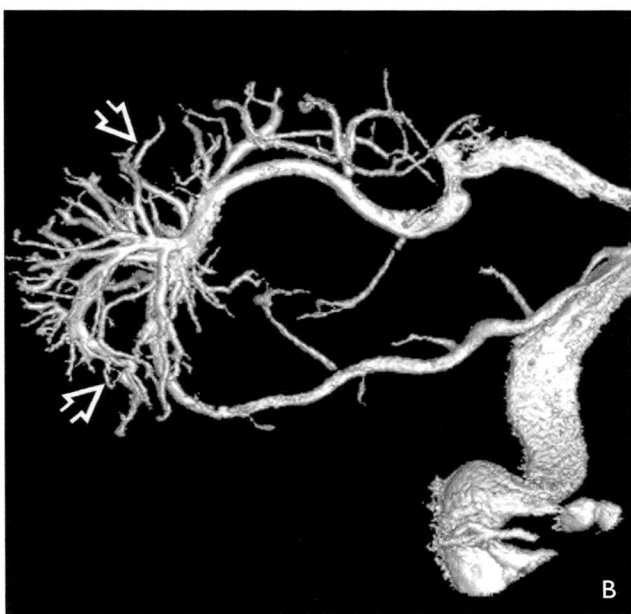

7-33B. 3D SSD in another case shows an extensive DVA with "Medusa head" ⇉ draining into the internal cerebral vein. (Courtesy P. Lasjaunias, MD.)

DEVELOPMENTAL VENOUS ANOMALY

Terminology
- DVA; also known as venous "angioma"

Etiology
- Extreme variant of normal venous drainage?
- Arrested medullary vein development?
- Chromosome 9 mutation?

Pathology
- Solitary > > multiple; small > large
- WM adjacent to ventricle (lateral > fourth)
- Enlarged WM veins interspersed with normal brain

Clinical Issues
- Epidemiology and demographics
  - Most common cerebrovascular malformation (60%)
  - Prevalence on T1 C+ MR = 2-9%
  - All ages, no gender predilection
- Natural history
  - Usually benign, nonprogressive

Imaging
- "Medusa head" of dilated veins
- Converge on large collector vein

Differential Diagnosis
- Histologically mixed malformation (usually venous + cavernous)
- Giant capillary telangiectasia
- Collateral venous drainage
  - Sturge-Weber syndrome
  - Dural sinus occlusion with shunting to deep veins

Sinus Pericranii

Terminology

Sinus pericranii (SP) is a large transcalvarial communication between the intra- and extracranial venous drainage systems. Some investigators consider SP the cutaneous manifestation of an intracranial developmental venous anomaly (DVA) as the two lesions are often—but not invariably—associated.

Etiology

GENERAL CONCEPTS. SPs can be congenital or acquired, post-traumatic or spontaneous. A congenital origin of most SPs is likely, given their frequent association with DVAs and congenital mucocutaneous malformations such as blue rubber bleb nevus syndrome **(BRBNS)**. Other possible etiologies include incomplete sutural fusion over prominent abundant diploic or emissary veins.

Scalp laceration and skull fracture that disrupts emissary veins at the outer table of the calvaria may result in development of an acquired SP.

Pathology

A bluish sac beneath or just above the periosteum of the calvaria is typical. The dilated, blood-filled sac connects through an enlarged emissary vein with the intracranial circulation **(7-34)**. The frontal lobe is the most common site, followed by the parietal and occipital lobes. SPs in the middle and posterior cranial fossae are rare.

SP may be associated with single or multiple intracranial DVAs.

Clinical Issues

EPIDEMIOLOGY. SPs are rare lesions, found in less than 10% of patients who present for treatment of craniofacial vascular malformations and 4% of patients with palpable scalp/cranial vault lesions.

DEMOGRAPHICS. Although SPs can occur at any age, most are found in children or young adults. There is no gender predilection.

PRESENTATION. A nontender, nonpulsatile somewhat bluish compressible scalp mass that increases with Valsalva maneuver and reduces in the upright position is typical. A history of "forgotten trauma" is not uncommon. Other than their cosmetic effect, most SPs are asymptomatic. SP with multiple DVAs is associated with blue rubber bleb nevus syndrome.

NATURAL HISTORY. If left alone, most SPs behave benignly and remain stable in size. There is a very small lifetime risk of air embolism or hemorrhage from direct trauma to the SP.

TREATMENT OPTIONS. Patients with SP may be referred to dermatologists because of discoloration in the scalp or forehead. Surgical removal of the extracranial component with cranioplasty is occasionally performed for cosmetic purposes. Surgery without adequate imaging may result in potentially lethal complications including hemorrhage, venous infarction (if the SP is associated with a DVA), and air embolism.

Imaging

GENERAL FEATURES. A vascular or subperiosteal scalp mass overlies a well-defined bone defect. The mass communicates directly with the intracranial venous system through the bony defect.

CT FINDINGS. An SP is iso- or hyperdense on NECT and shows strong uniform enhancement after contrast administration (7-35). The underlying calvarial defect varies in

7-34. Coronal graphic depicts a classic sinus pericranii (SP) with an expanded venous pouch under the scalp ➥ connecting to the intracranial venous system ➦ through a transcalvarial channel ➡. Some SPs are associated with a developmental venous anomaly ➘. 7-35. Sagittal CTV shows a small sinus pericranii ➡ connecting to the superior sagittal sinus through an adjacent skull defect ➦.

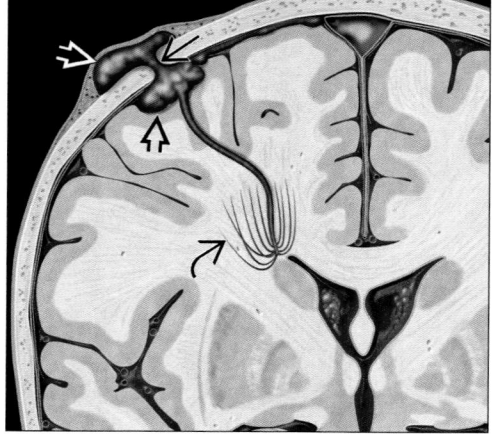

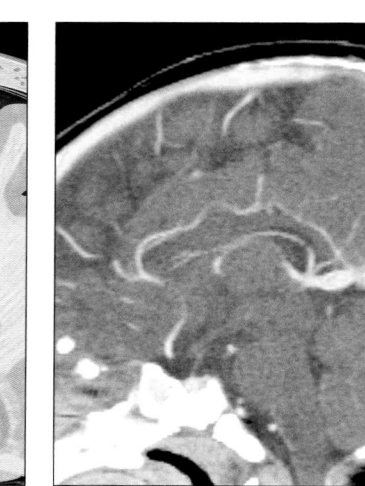

7-36. Coronal contrast-enhanced SPGR scan shows a classic sinus pericranii ➡ that connects to the superior sagittal sinus ➚ via a small transcalvarial venous channel ➥. 7-37. Late venous phase DSA shows angiographic findings of sinus pericranii with enlarged venous pouches ➡ connecting directly to the superior sagittal sinus ➚ through a transcalvarial channel ➥.

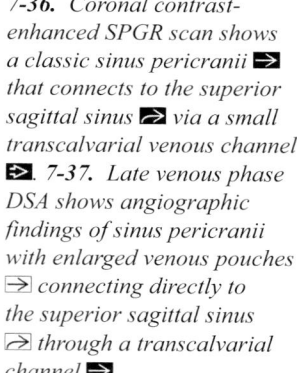

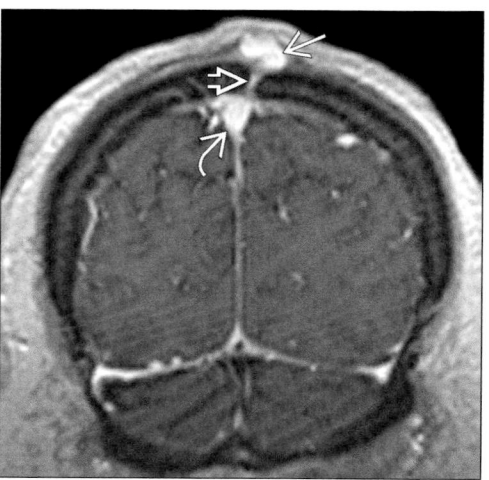

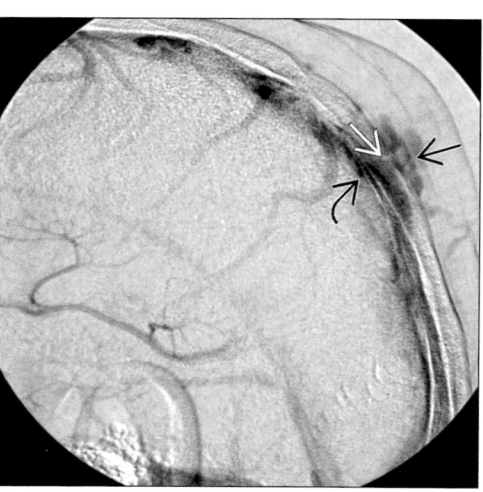

size but is typically well-demarcated. Occasionally an SP may contain calcifications (phleboliths) or thrombi.

MR FINDINGS. Most SPs are isointense on T1WI and hyperintense to brain on T2WI. "Puddling" of contrast within the SP on T1 C+ is typical **(7-36)** unless the lesion is unusually large and flow is rapid. MRV is helpful in delineating both the intra- and extracranial components.

ANGIOGRAPHY. The arterial and capillary phases are normal. Most SPs are visualized only on the very late venous phase **(7-37)**. They are seen as well-defined rounded pools of contrast that slowly accumulate within and adjacent to the skull defect containing the transcalvarial vein. Flow is variable and often bidirectional. In "closed" SPs, blood flows from and back into the adjacent dural venous sinus. "Drainer" SPs have unidirectional drainage into the venous pouch and adjacent pericranial scalp veins.

ULTRASOUND. Color Doppler may delineate the extracranial component and define flow direction. US does not define the intracranial component of an SP.

Differential Diagnosis

The imaging findings of SP are diagnostic. Other scalp and calvarial masses of infancy and childhood include **cephalocele**, **dermoid cyst**, **hemangioma**, **histiocytosis**, and **metastasis (neuroblastoma)**. In middle-aged and older adults, the most common scalp mass is a **sebaceous (trichilemmal) cyst**.

Cerebral Cavernous Malformation

Cerebral cavernous malformations (CCMs) are a distinct type of intracranial vascular malformation characterized by repeated "intralesional" hemorrhages into thin-walled, angiogenically immature, blood-filled locules called "caverns." CCMs are discrete, well-marginated lesions that do not contain normal brain parenchyma. Most are surrounded by a complete hemosiderin rim **(7-38)**.

Prior to the advent of CT and MR, cavernous malformations were sometimes called "occult" vascular malformations ("occult" to angiography as they are extremely low-flow lesions that do not exhibit arteriovenous shunting). These lesions are now easily identified on MR and hence are no longer "occult" to imaging. Cavernous malformations exhibit a wide range of dynamic behaviors. They are a relatively common cause of spontaneous nontraumatic intracranial hemorrhage in young and middle-aged adults, although they can occur at any age.

Terminology

CCMs are also known as cavernous "angiomas" or "cavernomas." They are benign malformative vascular hamartomas. CCMs are sometimes erroneously referred to as "cavernous hemangiomas." Hemangiomas are benign vascular neoplasms, not malformations.

Etiology

GENERAL CONCEPTS. CCMs are angiogenically immature lesions with endothelial proliferation and increased neoangiogenesis.

CCMs can be inherited or acquired. Acquired CCMs are rare and usually associated with prior radiation therapy (XRT). Approximately 3.5% of children who have whole brain XRT develop multiple CCMs, with a mean latency interval of approximately three years (3-102 months).

GENETICS. CCMs can be solitary and sporadic or multiple. At least half of all cases are familial, inherited as an autosomal dominant disease with variable penetrance.

Three genes have been identified in familial CCMs: *CCM1 (KRIT1)*, *CCM2 (OSM)*, and *CCM3 (PDCD10)*. Mutations in these genes account for 70-80% of all cases.

CCM1 is a pivotal inhibitor of sprouting angiogenesis and is necessary to keep vascular endothelium quiescent. Biallelic loss of a CCM gene allowing uncontrolled sprouting angiogenesis may explain the chaotic vascular architecture and dynamic progression of CCMs.

ASSOCIATED ABNORMALITIES. CCMs are the most common component in mixed vascular malformations. Cavernous-venous and cavernous-capillary are the two most frequent combinations.

Pathology

LOCATION AND SIZE. CCMs can occur anywhere in the CNS and range in size from tiny, near-microscopic lesions to giant malformations that can occupy an entire lobe or most of the cerebral hemisphere.

GROSS PATHOLOGY. A discrete raspberry-like collection of reddish-purple blood-filled "caverns" is the usual appearance **(7-39)**. Most CCMs are surrounded by a complete hemosiderin rim.

MICROSCOPIC FEATURES. CCMs consist of tightly packed epithelium-lined vascular channels ("caverns") in a collagenous stroma. The caverns typically lack elastic tissue and are usually thin-walled but may become thickened and hyalinized. Some channels are partly or completely thrombosed and contain hemorrhage in different stages of evolution. A gliotic, hemosiderin-stained rim surrounds the lesion.

CCMs do not contain brain parenchyma, but the surrounding brain often shows reactive changes and hemosiderin deposition. Dystrophic calcifications are common within CCMs.

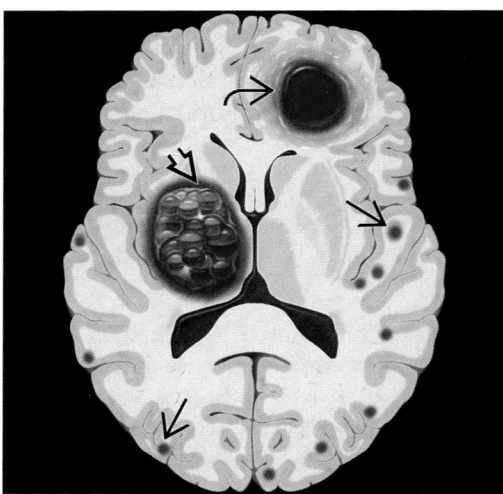

7-38. Subacute ⇗, *classic "popcorn ball"* ⇘ *appearances of CCMs. Microhemorrhages are seen as multifocal "blooming black dots"* ⇗.

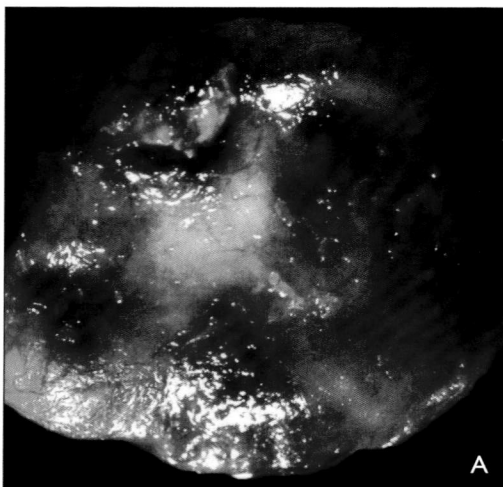

7-39A. Resected surgical specimen of CCM shows the typical well-circumscribed, lobulated, berry-like appearance.

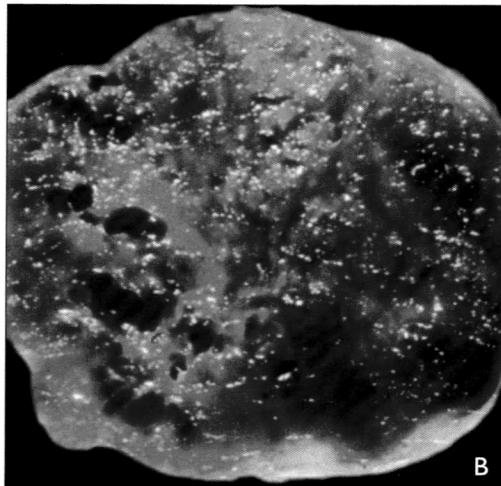

7-39B. Cut section shows multiple locules of blood in various stages of evolution.

STAGING, GRADING, AND CLASSIFICATION. The most commonly used classification of CCMs, the Zabramski classification, is based on imaging appearance, not histological findings (see box).

Clinical Issues

EPIDEMIOLOGY. CCMs are the third most common cerebral vascular malformation (after DVA and capillary telangiectasia) and are found in approximately 0.5% of the population. Two-thirds occur as a solitary, sporadic lesion; approximately one-third are multiple.

DEMOGRAPHICS. CCMs may occur at any age; they cause 10% of spontaneous brain hemorrhages in children. The imaging prevalence of CCMs increases with advancing age. Peak presentation is 40-60 years (younger in the familial multiple cavernous malformation syndrome). There is no gender predilection.

Multiple CCM syndrome is more common in Hispanic-Americans of Mexican descent. Over 90% of individuals with a positive family history have a *KRIT1* mutation and will develop one or more CCMs.

PRESENTATION. Half of all patients with CCMs present with seizures. Headache and focal neurologic deficits are also common. Small lesions, especially microhemorrhages, may be asymptomatic.

NATURAL HISTORY. CCMs have a broad range of dynamic behavior, and the clinical course of individual lesions is both highly variable and unpredictable. Repeated spontaneous intralesional hemorrhages are typical. There is a distinct propensity for lesion growth in all patients. Patients with multiple CCM syndrome typically continue to develop de novo lesions throughout their lives.

Hemorrhage risk with solitary lesions is estimated at 0.25-0.75% per year, cumulative, and is greater for women. In the familial multiple CCM form, hemorrhage risk is much higher, approaching 1-5% cumulative risk per year.

TREATMENT OPTIONS. The management of deep-seated CCMs in critical locations is controversial. At present, total surgical removal via microsurgical resection is the treatment of choice for symptomatic lesions with recurrent hemorrhages. Stereotactic radiosurgery has been used with some success in patients with brainstem CCMs that are not amenable to microsurgery.

Imaging

GENERAL FEATURES. CCMs occur throughout the CNS. The brain parenchyma is the most common site. A well-circumscribed mixed density/signal intensity mass surrounded by a complete hemosiderin rim ("popcorn ball") is the classic finding. CCMs can vary from microscopic to giant (more than six centimeters) lesions. In rare circumstances, a CCM (often mixed with venous malformations) may occupy an entire lobe of the brain.

CT FINDINGS. NECT scans are often normal as many CCMs are too small to be detected. If the lesion is large enough, it may appear hyperdense with scattered intralesional calcifications (7-40A). Most CCMs are well-delineated and do not exhibit mass effect unless there is recent hemorrhage (7-40B).

MR FINDINGS. Findings are variable, depending on the stage of evolution and pulse sequence utilized. CCMs have been divided into four types based on imaging appearance (Zabramski classification).

The classic CCM (Zabramski type 2) is a discrete reticulated or "popcorn ball" lesion caused by blood products contained within variably sized "caverns" or "locules." Fluid-fluid levels of differing signal intensities are common (7-40C). The mixed signal core is surrounded by a complete hemosiderin rim on T2WI that "blooms" on T2* sequences. CCMs with subacute hemorrhage (Zabramski type 1) are hyperintense on T1WI and mixed hyper-/hypointense on T2WI (7-41).

T2* scans (GRE, SWI) should always be performed to look for additional lesions. Punctate microhemorrhages are seen as multifocal "blooming black dots" (Zabramski type 4) in many cases with familial CCM (7-42).

Enhancement following contrast administration varies from none (the usual finding) to mild or moderate (7-43). If a CCM coexists with a DVA, the venous "angioma" may show strong enhancement. If such a histologically "mixed" vascular malformation is resected, the venous drainage must be preserved to avoid postoperative venous infarction.

ZABRAMSKI CLASSIFICATION OF CCMs
Type 1: Subacute hemorrhage
• Hyperintense on T1, hyper-/hypointense on T2
Type 2: Different age hemorrhages
• Classic = "popcorn ball"
  ○ Mixed signal with hyper/hypo on both T1 and T2
• Look for blood-filled locules with fluid-fluid levels
Type 3: Chronic hemorrhage
Type 4: Punctate microhemorrhages
• "Blooming black dots" on T2* (GRE, SWI)

ANGIOGRAPHY. CCMs have no identifiable feeding arteries or draining veins. DSA, CTA, and MRA are usually negative unless the CCM is mixed with another vascular malformation (most commonly a DVA). If acute hemorrhage has occurred, an avascular mass effect may be present. Rarely, venous pooling with contrast accumulation in one or more of the "caverns" can be identified.

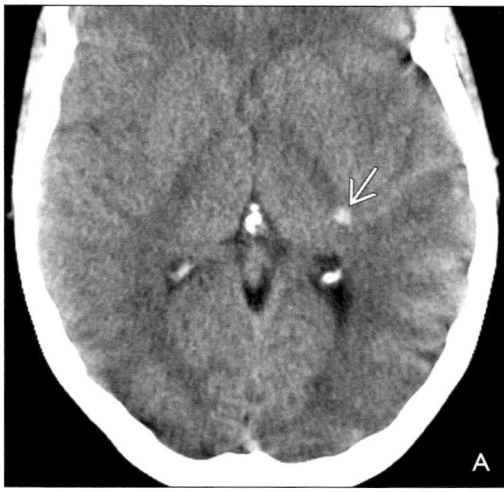
7-40A. NECT in a patient with family history of CCM shows punctate hyperdense lesion in the posterior limb of the left internal capsule ➡.

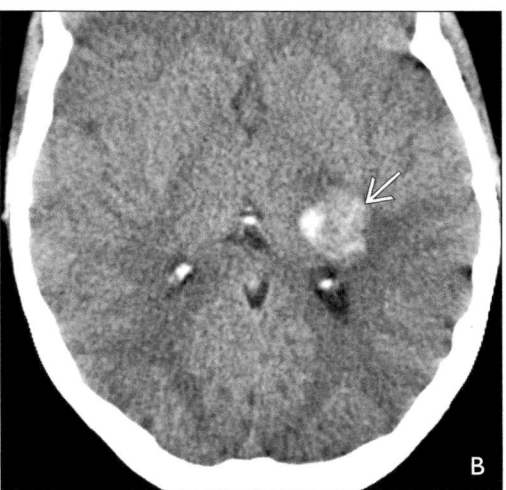
7-40B. NECT scan obtained 6 years later when the patient developed acute right hemiparesis shows that the lesion ➡ has markedly enlarged.

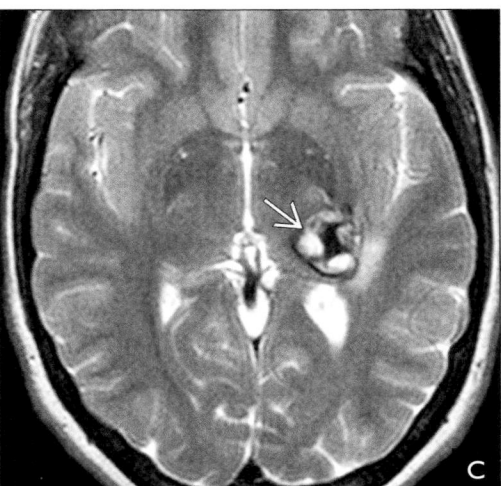
7-40C. T2WI shows classic "popcorn ball" appearance with locules of blood in different stages of evolution surrounded by hemosiderin rim ➡.

Differential Diagnosis

The most common differential diagnosis is a **mixed vascular malformation** in which a CCM is the dominant component. Occasionally, a **hemorrhagic** or **densely calcified neoplasm** (such as a glioblastoma or oligodendroglioma, respectively) can mimic a CCM.

Multifocal "black dots" on T2* scans can be seen in a number of lesions besides type 4 CCMs. Chronic hypertensive encephalopathy, amyloid angiopathy, axonal stretch injury, and cortical contusions may have similar appearances.

Hemangiomas are true benign vasoformative neoplasms and should not be mistaken for CCMs. Most are found in the skin and soft tissues of the head and neck. Hemangiomas within the CNS are rare and most commonly found in dural venous sinuses and cranial meninges, not the brain parenchyma.

CEREBRAL CAVERNOUS MALFORMATIONS

Etiology
- *CCM1*, *CCM2*, or *CCM3* mutations in familial CCM
- Negative inhibition of sprouting angiogenesis lost

Pathology
- Occur throughout CNS
- Solitary (2/3), multiple (1/3, familial)
- Multiple thin-walled blood-filled locules ("caverns")
- No normal brain inside; hemosiderin rim outside

Clinical Issues
- Third most common CVM
- Can present at any age; peak = 40-60 years
- Course variable, unpredictable
  - Repeated intralesional hemorrhages typical
  - Hemorrhage risk = 0.25-0.75% per lesion per year
  - Patients with familial CCM develop de novo lesions

Imaging
- NECT: Hyperdense ± scattered Ca++
- MR: Appearance varies
  - "Popcorn ball" with fluid-fluid levels, hemosiderin rim
  - Multifocal "blooming black dots"
- DSA usually negative

7-41A. Zabramski type 1 CCM is illustrated. (Left) T1WI shows that the lesion is hyperintense and surrounded by a hypointense hemosiderin rim ➡. (Right) T2 GRE scan shows "blooming" hypointensity both around ➡ and within the lesion. 7-41B. Microscopic section from the resected specimen in the same case shows a blood-filled cavity ➡ surrounded by thin endothelium-lined vascular channels ➡. (Courtesy R. Hewlett, MD.)*

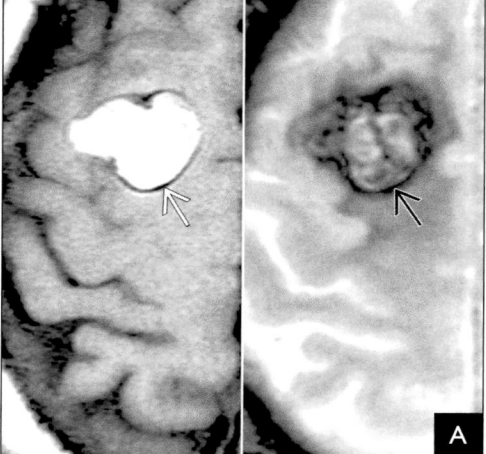

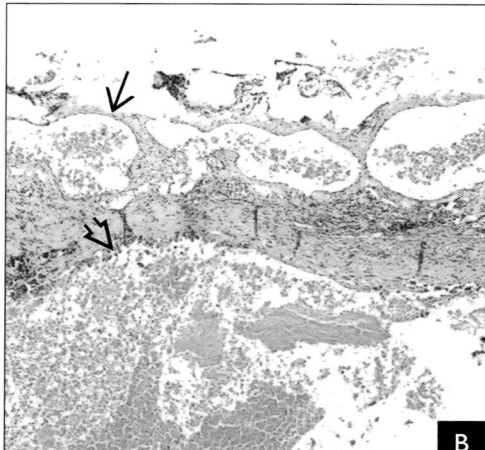

7-42A. T2WI in a patient with multiple cerebral cavernous malformations shows a large left frontal lesion with a fluid-fluid level ➡. Multiple other hypointense lesions are present ➡. 7-42B. T2 SWI shows innumerable "blooming black dots" characteristic of Zabramski type 4 CCM (punctate microhemorrhages). T2* scans are much more sensitive than FSE T2WI in depicting field inhomogeneities.*

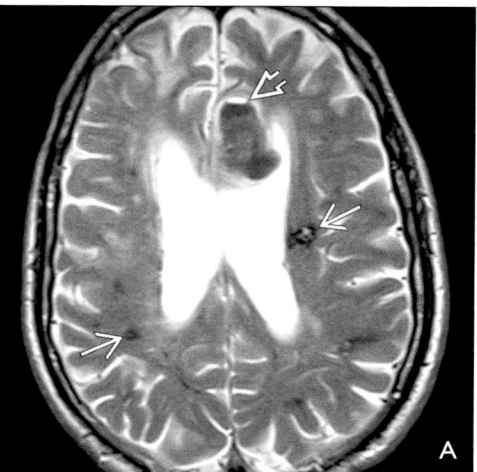

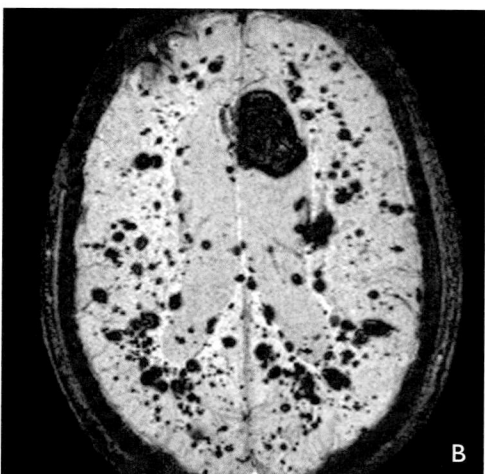

Capillary Telangiectasia

Terminology

A brain capillary telangiectasia (BCT) is a collection of enlarged, thin-walled vessels resembling capillaries. The vessels are surrounded and separated by normal brain parenchyma.

Etiology

GENERAL CONCEPTS. While their exact pathogenesis is unknown, capillary telangiectasias are probably congenital lesions. BCTs have been reported with hereditary hemorrhagic telangiectasia (HHT), but most lesions occur in the scalp and mucous membranes, not the brain parenchyma.

Cranial irradiation may cause vascular endothelial damage and induce development of multiple cavernous or telangiectatic-like lesions in the brain parenchyma. Patients with radiation-induced capillary telangiectasias typically present with seizures several years after whole brain XRT. Mean age of onset is 11-12 years, and mean latency period is nearly nine years.

GENETICS. No known genetic mutations have been identified.

Pathology

LOCATION AND SIZE. BCTs can occur anywhere in the CNS. The pons, cerebellum, and spinal cord are the most common sites (7-44). Solitary lesions are much more common than multiple BCTs. Although "giant" capillary telangiectasias do occur, the vast majority of BCTs are small, typically less than one centimeter in diameter.

GROSS PATHOLOGY. Most BCTs are often invisible to gross inspection. Only 5-10% of BCTs are larger than one centimeter in diameter. Occasionally lesions up to two centimeters occur. These can be seen as areas of poorly delineated pink or brownish discoloration in the parenchyma (7-45).

MICROSCOPIC FEATURES. A cluster of dilated, somewhat ectatic but otherwise normal-appearing capillaries interspersed within the brain parenchyma is characteris-

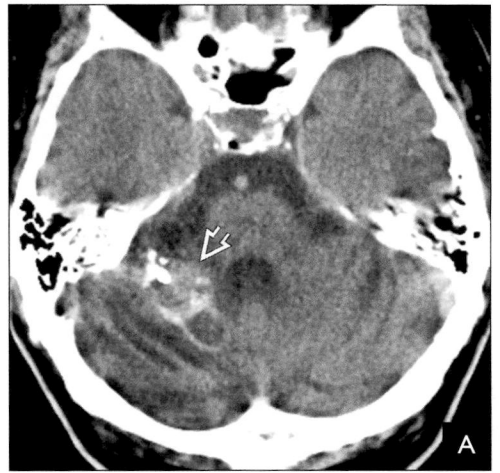

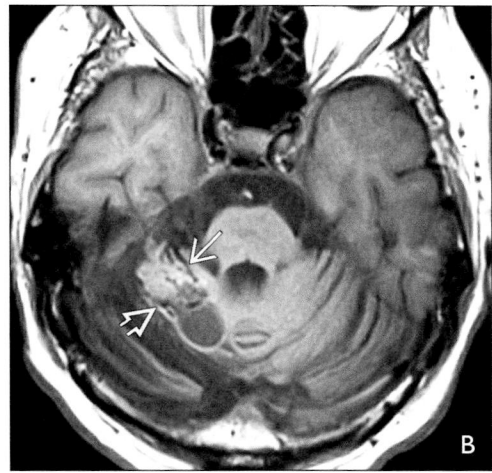

7-43A. NECT scan shows a partially calcified mixed-density mass ➡ *associated with moderately severe atrophic changes in the right cerebellar hemisphere. 7-43B. T1WI shows that the lesion* ➡ *is very heterogeneous with mixed cystic and solid components, different signal intensities, and prominent "flow voids"* ➡.

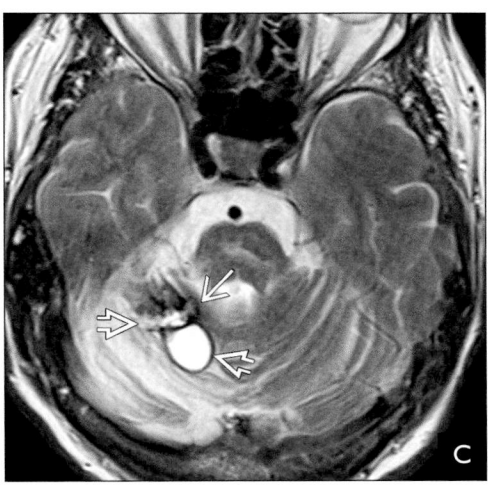

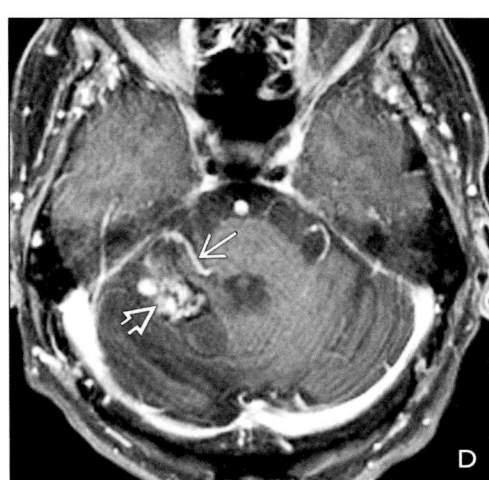

7-43C. T2WI shows prominent hypointense hemosiderin staining ➡ *surrounding hyperintense fluid-containing cavities* ➡. *7-43D. T1 C+ FS scan shows that part of the solid-appearing component demonstrates lobulated enhancement* ➡. *A prominent draining vein also enhances* ➡. *Most CCMs show minimal or no enhancement, so this is considered a variant case.*

tic **(7-46)**. Unless mixed with other malformations (such as cavernous angioma), BCTs do not hemorrhage and do not calcify. Gliosis and hemosiderin deposition are absent.

Clinical Issues

EPIDEMIOLOGY. Capillary telangiectasias are the second most common cerebral vascular malformation, representing between 10-20% of all brain vascular malformations. Skin and mucosal capillary telangiectasias are even more common than brain telangiectasias.

DEMOGRAPHICS. BCTs may occur at any age, but peak presentation is between 30-40 years. There is no gender predilection.

PRESENTATION. Most BCTs are asymptomatic and discovered incidentally. A few cases with headache, vertigo, and tinnitus have been reported.

NATURAL HISTORY. BCTs are quiescent lesions that do not hemorrhage. Very rare cases of aggressive clinical behavior have been reported.

TREATMENT OPTIONS. Isolated BCTs do not require treatment. Treatment of mixed lesions is dictated by the associated lesion.

Imaging

GENERAL FEATURES. Because normal brain is interspersed between the dilated capillaries of a BCT, no mass effect is present. Unless they are histologically mixed with other CVMs (such as a cavernous malformation), BCTs lack edema, do not incite surrounding gliosis, and neither hemorrhage nor calcify.

CT FINDINGS. Both NECT and CECT scans are usually normal.

MR FINDINGS. BCTs are inconspicuous on conventional pre-contrast MR images. T1 scans are typically normal **(7-47A)**. Large BCTs may show faint stippled hyperintensity on T2WI or FLAIR **(7-47B)**, **(7-47C)**, but small lesions are generally invisible.

T2* (GRE, SWI) is the best sequence for demonstrating a BCT. As blood flow within the dilated capillaries is quite sluggish, oxyhemoglobin is converted to deoxyhemoglo-

7-44. Graphic depicts pontine capillary telangiectasia ➡ with tiny dilated capillaries interspersed with normal brain. 7-45. Autopsy specimen shows a large pontine capillary telangiectasia ➡. Note the transverse pontine fibers ➡ passing through the lesion. (Courtesy B. Horten, MD.)

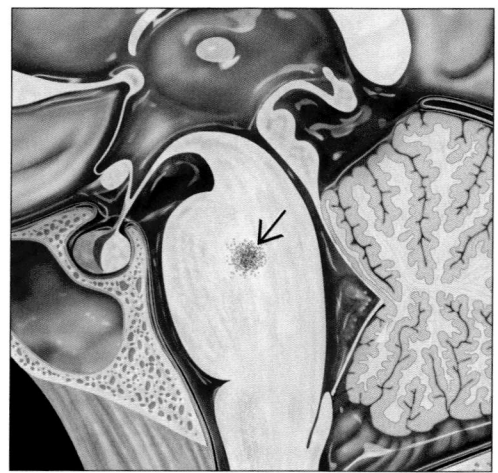

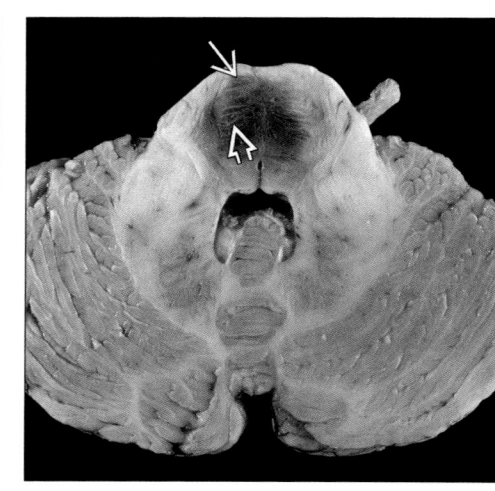

7-46A. Close-up gross photograph of a capillary telangiectasia shows innumerable enlarged pink foci ➡ in the subcortical WM produced by enlarged capillaries. 7-46B. High-power photomicrograph in the same case nicely demonstrates the blood-filled, thin-walled enlarged capillaries that are the hallmark of capillary telangiectasia. Note the normal blue-staining WM between the vessels (Luxol fast blue stain). (Courtesy P. Burger, MD.)

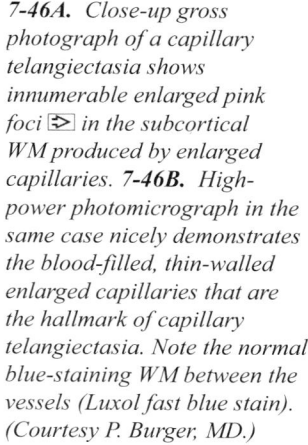

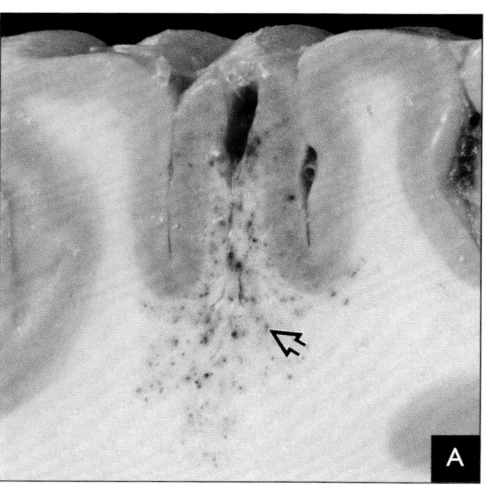

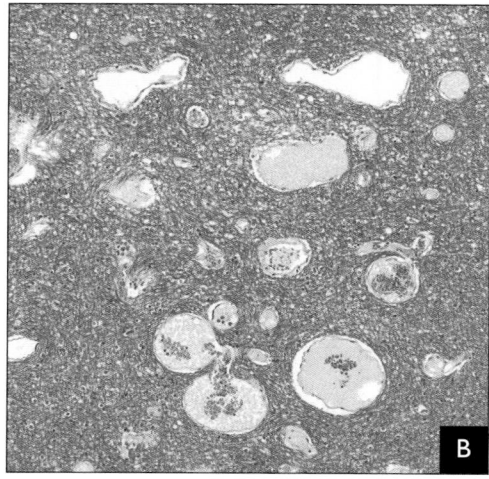

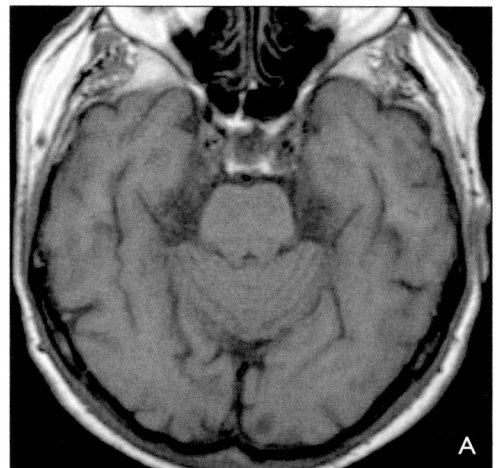

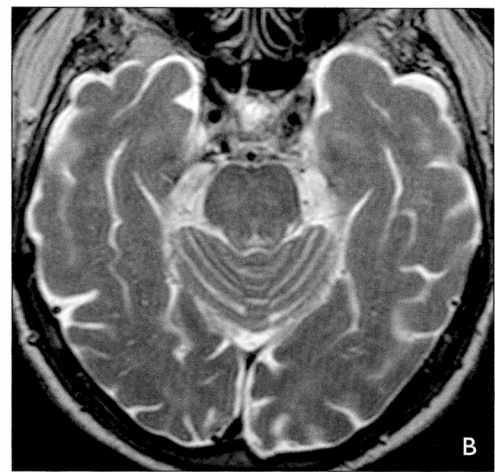

7-47A. *Series of images demonstrates classic findings of pontine capillary telangiectasia. Axial T1WI is normal.* *7-47B.* *Axial T2WI in the same patient likewise shows no abnormality.*

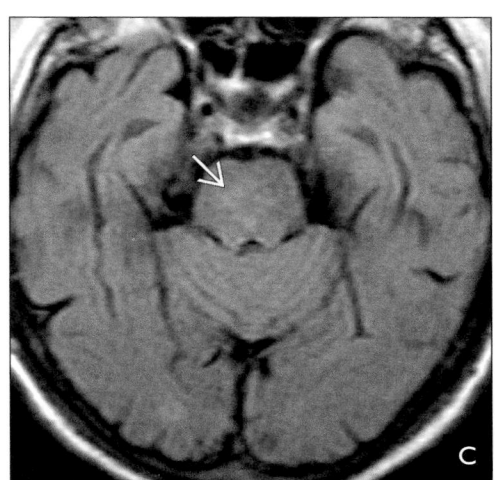

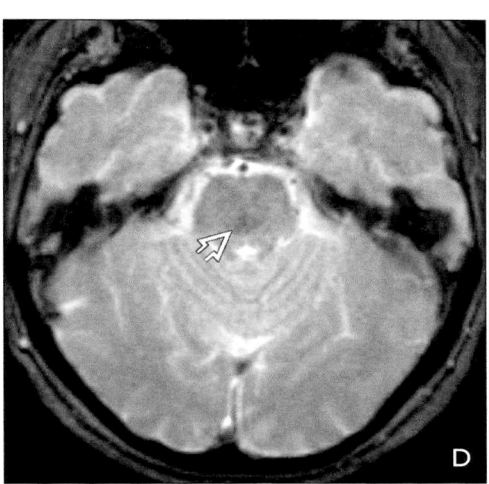

7-47C. *FLAIR scan shows faint patchy hyperintensity* ➡ *in the pons.* *7-47D.* *T2* GRE scan shows susceptibility effect with grayish hypointensity* ➡ *in the mid pons.*

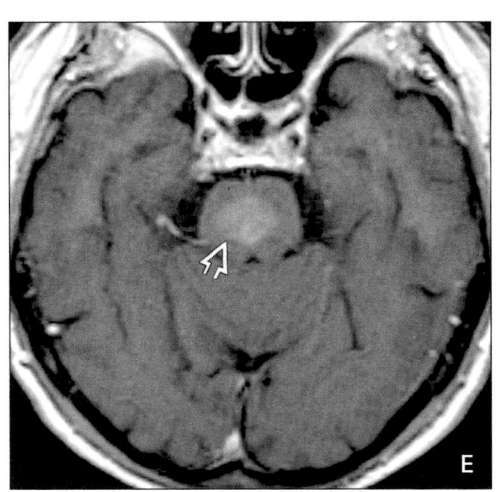

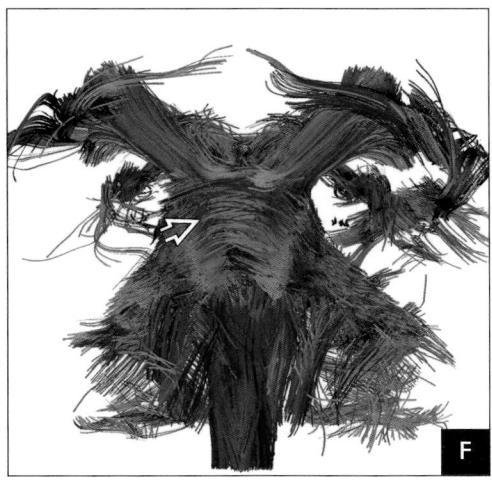

7-47E. *T1 C+ scan shows the brush-like faint enhancement* ➡ *that is characteristic of capillary telangiectasia.* *7-47F.* *DTI fiber tracking is normal. The transverse pontine fibers* ➡ *cross undisturbed through the lesion. (Courtesy P. Rodriguez, MD.)*

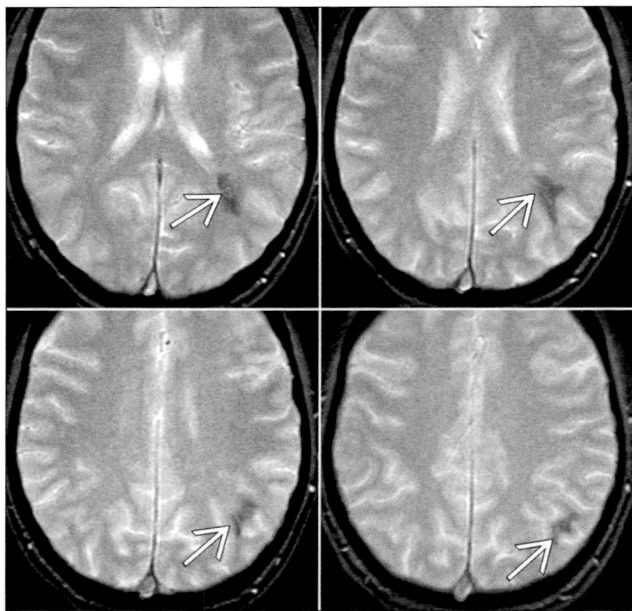

7-48. Series of T2* GRE scans shows a focal wedge-shaped subcortical hypointensity ➡ in the left parietal lobe.

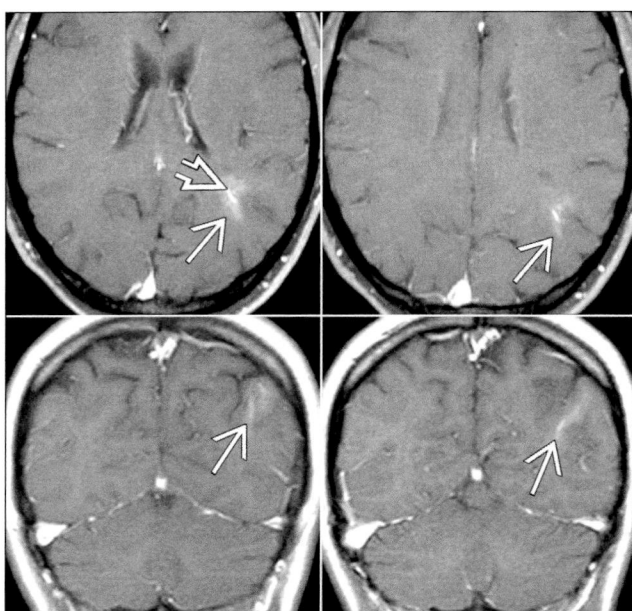

7-49. (Top) Axial and (bottom) coronal T1 C+ scans show that the lesion ➡ enhances in a brush-like fashion. A prominent central draining vein is present ➤. Imaging findings are characteristic of capillary telangiectasia (compare Figure 7-46).

bin and is visible as an area of poorly delineated grayish hypointensity **(7-47D), (7-48)**.

BCTs typically show faint stippled or poorly delineated brush-like enhancement on T1 C+ **(7-47E), (7-49)**. Larger lesions may demonstrate a linear focus of strong enhancement within the lesion, representing a draining collector vein.

As BCTs are interspersed with normal white matter tracts, DTI shows no displacement or disruption and no alteration of fractional anisotropy **(7-47F)**.

Differential Diagnosis

Because they show mild enhancement on T1 C+, BCTs are often mistaken for **neoplasms**. Yet they do not exhibit mass effect or surrounding edema. The combination of signal intensity loss on T2* and focal brush-like enhancement in a lesion that is otherwise unremarkable on standard sequences easily distinguishes BCT from primary or metastatic neoplasm.

Developmental venous anomaly and **cavernous malformation** can be histologically mixed with BCTs. **Capillary hemangiomas** are true vasoformative neoplasms, cause mass effect, and are typically found in the dura and venous sinuses, not the brain parenchyma.

Radiation-induced vascular malformations can occur and are seen as multifocal "blooming black dots" on T2* (GRE, SWI) sequences **(7-50)**. Most are cavernous malformations with microhemorrhages, not capillary telangiectasias.

CAPILLARY TELANGIECTASIAS

Pathology
- Cluster of thin-walled, dilated capillaries
  - Normal brain interspersed between vascular channels
- Can be found throughout CNS
  - Pons, cerebellum, spinal cord most common sites

Clinical Issues
- 10-20% of all cerebrovascular malformations
- All ages; peak = 30-40 years
- Rarely symptomatic
  - Most discovered incidentally at imaging

Imaging
- NECT, CECT usually normal
- MR
  - T1/T2 usually normal
  - T2* key sequence (dark gray hypointensity)
  - Brush-like enhancement on T1 C+

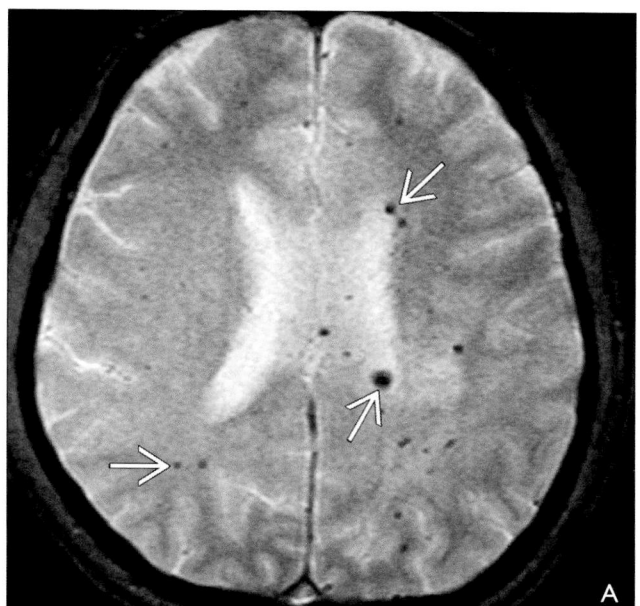

7-50A. A patient with a history of whole brain radiation 5 years earlier for a WHO grade III anaplastic astrocytoma developed seizures. T2* GRE scan shows multiple "blooming" hypointensities ➡.

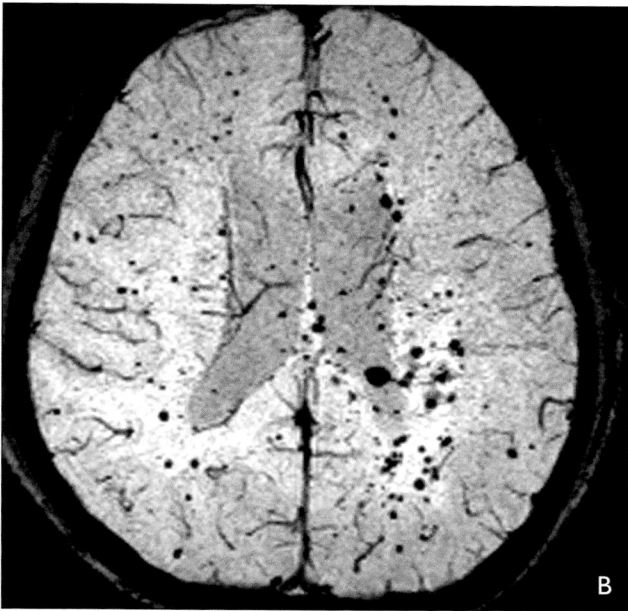

7-50B. T2* SWI scan in the same patient shows innumerable punctate microhemorrhages. Findings are consistent with radiation-induced capillary telangiectasias.

Selected References

CVMs with Arteriovenous Shunting

Arteriovenous Malformation

- Davies JM et al: Classification schemes for arteriovenous malformations. Neurosurg Clin N Am. 23(1):43-53, 2012
- Fontanella M et al: Brain arteriovenous malformations are associated with interleukin-1 cluster gene polymorphisms. Neurosurgery. 70(1):12-7, 2012
- Illies T et al: Classification of cerebral arteriovenous malformations and intranidal flow patterns by color-encoded 4D-hybrid-MRA. AJNR Am J Neuroradiol. Epub ahead of print, 2012
- Laakso A et al: Arteriovenous malformations: epidemiology and clinical presentation. Neurosurg Clin N Am. 23(1):1-6, 2012
- Meijer-Jorna LB et al: Congenital vascular malformations--cerebral lesions differ from extracranial lesions by their immune expression of the glucose transporter protein GLUT1. Clin Neuropathol. 31(3):135-41, 2012
- Geibprasert S et al: Radiologic assessment of brain arteriovenous malformations: what clinicians need to know. Radiographics. 30(2):483-501, 2010
- Lawton MT et al: A supplementary grading scale for selecting patients with brain arteriovenous malformations for surgery. Neurosurgery. 66(4):702-13; discussion 713, 2010

Cerebral Proliferative Angiopathy

- Marks MP et al: Cerebral proliferative angiopathy. J Neurointerv Surg. 4(5):e25, 2012
- Lasjaunias PL et al: Cerebral proliferative angiopathy: clinical and angiographic description of an entity different from cerebral AVMs. Stroke. 39(3):878-85, 2008

Dural AV Fistula

- Gandhi D et al: Intracranial dural arteriovenous fistulas: classification, imaging findings, and treatment. AJNR Am J Neuroradiol. 33(6):1007-13, 2012
- Gomez J et al: Classification schemes of cranial dural arteriovenous fistulas. Neurosurg Clin N Am. 23(1):55-62, 2012
- Gross BA et al: Cerebral dural arteriovenous fistulas and aneurysms. Neurosurg Focus. 32(5):E2, 2012
- Ha SY et al: Clinical and angiographic characteristics of multiple dural arteriovenous shunts. AJNR Am J Neuroradiol. Epub ahead of print, 2012
- Geibprasert S et al: Dural arteriovenous shunts: a new classification of craniospinal epidural venous anatomical bases and clinical correlations. Stroke. 39(10):2783-94, 2008

Carotid-Cavernous Fistula

- Grumann AJ et al: Ophthalmologic outcome of direct and indirect carotid cavernous fistulas. Int Ophthalmol. 32(2):153-9, 2012
- Miller NR: Dural carotid-cavernous fistulas: epidemiology, clinical presentation, and management. Neurosurg Clin N Am. 23(1):179-92, 2012
- Yoshida K et al: Transvenous embolization of dural carotid cavernous fistulas: a series of 44 consecutive patients. AJNR Am J Neuroradiol. 31(4):651-5, 2010

Pial AV Fistula

- Paramasivam S et al: Development, clinical presentation and endovascular management of congenital intracranial pial arteriovenous fistulas. J Neurointerv Surg. Epub ahead of print, 2012

Vein of Galen Aneurysmal Malformation

- Recinos PF et al: Vein of Galen malformations: epidemiology, clinical presentations, management. Neurosurg Clin N Am. 23(1):165-77, 2012
- Berenstein A et al: Endovascular management of arteriovenous malformations and other intracranial arteriovenous shunts in neonates, infants, and children. Childs Nerv Syst. 26(10):1345-58, 2010
- Alvarez H et al: Vein of galen aneurysmal malformations. Neuroimaging Clin N Am. 17(2):189-206, 2007

CVMs without Arteriovenous Shunting

Developmental Venous Anomaly

- Roccatagliata L et al: Developmental venous anomalies with capillary stain: a subgroup of symptomatic DVAs? Neuroradiology. 54(5):475-80, 2012
- Teo M et al: Developmental venous anomalies - two cases with venous thrombosis. Br J Neurosurg. Epub ahead of print, 2012
- Petersen TA et al: Familial versus sporadic cavernous malformations: differences in developmental venous anomaly association and lesion phenotype. AJNR Am J Neuroradiol. 31(2):377-82, 2010
- Ruiz DS et al: Cerebral developmental venous anomalies: current concepts. Ann Neurol. 66(3):271-83, 2009

Sinus Pericranii

- Akram H et al: Sinus pericranii: an overview and literature review of a rare cranial venous anomaly (a review of the existing literature with case examples). Neurosurg Rev. 35(1):15-26; discussion 26, 2012
- Macit B et al: Cerebrofacial venous anomalies, sinus pericranii, ocular abnormalities and developmental delay. Interv Neuroradiol. 18(2):153-7, 2012
- Vanaman MJ et al: Pediatric and inherited neurovascular diseases. Neurosurg Clin N Am. 21(3):427-41, 2010
- Park SC et al: Sinus pericranii in children: report of 16 patients and preoperative evaluation of surgical risk. J Neurosurg Pediatr. 4(6):536-42, 2009
- Gandolfo C et al: Sinus pericranii: diagnostic and therapeutic considerations in 15 patients. Neuroradiology. 49(6):505-14, 2007

Cerebral Cavernous Malformation

- Al-Holou WN et al: Natural history and imaging prevalence of cavernous malformations in children and young adults. J Neurosurg Pediatr. 9(2):198-205, 2012
- Al-Shahi Salman R et al: Untreated clinical course of cerebral cavernous malformations: a prospective, population-based cohort study. Lancet Neurol. 11(3):217-24, 2012
- Cavalcanti DD et al: Cerebral cavernous malformations: from genes to proteins to disease. J Neurosurg. 116(1):122-32, 2012
- Haasdijk RA et al: Cerebral cavernous malformations: from molecular pathogenesis to genetic counselling and clinical management. Eur J Hum Genet. 20(2):134-40, 2012
- Wüstehube J et al: Cerebral cavernous malformation protein CCM1 inhibits sprouting angiogenesis by activating DELTA-NOTCH signaling. Proc Natl Acad Sci U S A. 107(28):12640-5, 2010

Capillary Telangiectasia

- El-Koussy M et al: Susceptibility-weighted MR imaging for diagnosis of capillary telangiectasia of the brain. AJNR Am J Neuroradiol. 33(4):715-20, 2012
- Sayama CM et al: Capillary telangiectasias: clinical, radiographic, and histopathological features. Clinical article. J Neurosurg. 113(4):709-14, 2010
- Leblanc GG et al: Biology of vascular malformations of the brain. Stroke. 40(12):e694-702, 2009
- Nimjee SM et al: Review of the literature on de novo formation of cavernous malformations of the central nervous system after radiation therapy . Neurosurg Focus. 21(1):e4, 2006
- Yoshida Y et al: Capillary telangiectasia of the brain stem diagnosed by susceptibility-weighted imaging. J Comput Assist Tomogr. 30(6):980-2, 2006

8

Arterial Anatomy and Strokes

"Stroke" is a generic term that describes a clinical event characterized by sudden onset of a neurologic deficit. However, *not all strokes are the same!* Stroke syndromes have significant clinical and pathophysiological heterogeneity that is reflected in their underlying gross pathologic and imaging appearances. Arterial ischemia/infarction—the major focus of this chapter—is by far the most common cause of stroke, accounting for 80% of all cases.

The remaining 20% of strokes are mostly hemorrhagic, divided between primary "spontaneous" intracranial hemorrhage (sICH), nontraumatic subarachnoid hemorrhage (SAH), and venous occlusions. Both sICH and SAH were discussed extensively in preceding chapters, and venous occlusions will be discussed in the following chapter.

We begin by briefly reviewing the normal intracranial arteries. With this solid anatomic foundation, we then turn our attention to the etiology, pathology, and imaging manifestations of arterial strokes.

Normal Arterial Anatomy and Vascular Distributions

Clinicians frequently discuss the intracranial vasculature in two parts, the "anterior circulation" and the "posterior circulation." The **anterior circulation** consists of the intradural internal carotid artery (ICA) and its branches plus its two terminations, the anterior cerebral artery (ACA) and middle cerebral artery (MCA). Both the anterior communicating arteries (ACoAs) and the posterior communicating arteries (PCoAs) are also considered part of the anterior circulation.

The **posterior circulation** is composed of the vertebrobasilar trunk and its branches, including its terminal bifurcation into the two posterior cerebral arteries (PCAs).

We begin our discussion with the anterior circulation. We briefly consider the internal carotid artery and its segments, branches, important variants, and anomalies and then delineate the anatomy of the circle of Willis. The three major cerebral arteries (i.e., anterior, middle, posterior) are next discussed, along with their branches, variants, and vascular distributions. We conclude this section with the normal anatomy of the vertebrobasilar system.

Intracranial Internal Carotid Artery

The intracranial ICAs follow a complex course with six straight vertical or horizontal segments that are connected by three curved genua. The ICAs are divided into numbered segments. By convention, the extracranial ICA—which normally has *no* named branches in the neck—is designated as the **C1 (cervical) segment**. The cervical ICA is discussed in detail along with the other extracranial cephalocervical arteries (Chapter 10).

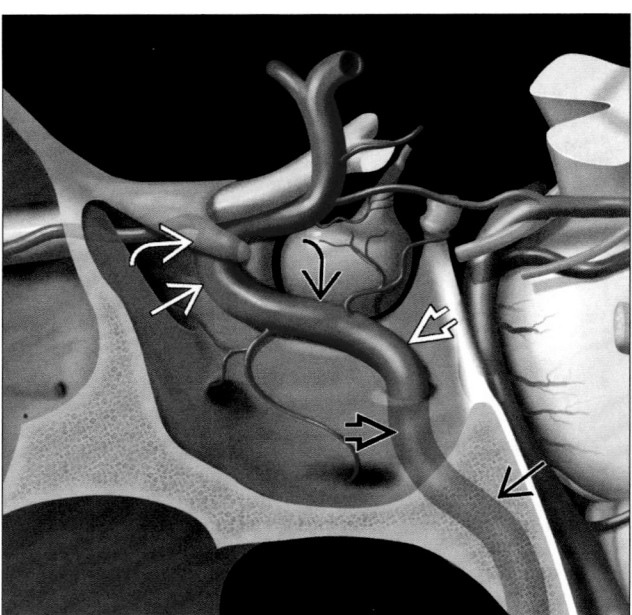

8-1. Intracranial ICA, branches. The C2 (petrous) segment ⇲ is long and L-shaped. C3 ⇲ is a short segment between C2 and the cavernous ICA (C4) ⇲. C5 ⇲ is the last extradural segment. Posterior ⇲, anterior ⇲ genua of C4 are shown.

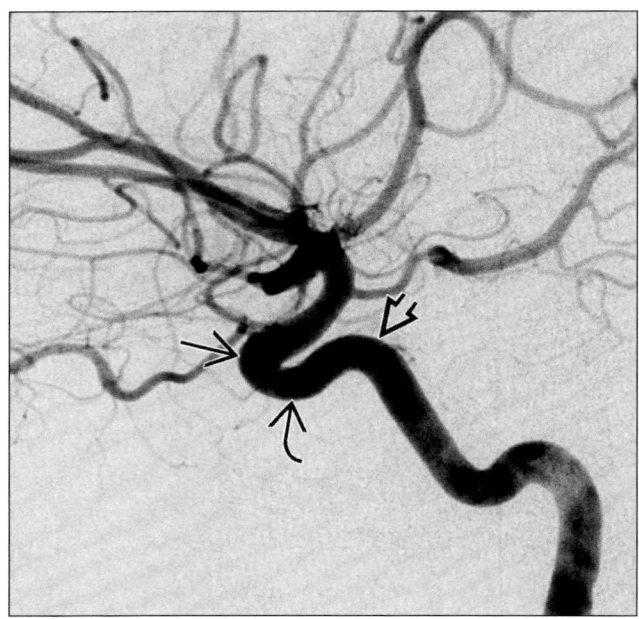

8-2. Lateral DSA shows all ICA segments. The C4 (cavernous) segment ⇲ has both a posterior ⇲ and an anterior ⇲ genu. Together, they form the angio-DSA carotid "siphon."

Normal Anatomy

C2 (Petrous) ICA Segment. The C2 (petrous) segment is contained within the carotid canal of the temporal bone and is L-shaped **(8-1)**. As it enters the skull at the exocranial opening of the carotid canal, the ICA lies just in front of the internal jugular vein. At this point, the ICA goes from being relatively mobile (in the neck) to relatively fixed (in the bone), where it is more vulnerable to traumatic shearing forces and dissection injury.

The C2 ICA has a short vertical segment, then a genu or "knee" where it turns anteromedially in front of the cochlea, and a longer horizontal segment. The ICA exits the carotid canal at the petrous apex.

The C2 segment has two small but important branches. The **vidian artery**, also known as the artery of the pterygoid canal, anastomoses with branches of the external carotid artery (ECA). The **caroticotympanic artery** is a small ICA branch that supplies the middle ear.

C3 (Lacerum) ICA Segment. The C3 (lacerum) segment is a short segment that lies just above the foramen lacerum and extends from the petrous apex to the cavernous sinus (CS). The C3 segment is covered by the **trigeminal ganglion** of CN V and has no branches.

C4 (Cavernous) ICA Segment. The C4 (cavernous) segment is one of the most important and complex of all the ICA segments. The C4 ICA has three subsegments connected by two genua **(8-2)**. In order, these are (1) a short posterior ascending (vertical) segment, (2) the posterior genu, (3) a longer horizontal segment, (4) an ante-

rior genu, and (5) an anterior vertical ascending (subclinoid) segment. As the cavernous ICA courses anteriorly, it also courses medially. Therefore, on anteroposterior or coronal views, the posterior genu is lateral to the anterior genu.

The **abducens nerve** (CN VI) is inferolateral to the ICA and is the only cranial nerve that lies *inside* the CS itself (the others are in the lateral dural wall).

The C4 ICA segment has two important branches **(8-1)**. The **meningohypophyseal trunk** arises from the posterior genu, supplying the pituitary gland, tentorium, and clival dura. The **inferolateral trunk** (ILT) arises from the lateral aspect of the intracavernous ICA and supplies cranial nerves and CS dura. Via branches that pass through the adjacent basilar foramina, the ILT anastomoses freely with branches from the ECA that arise in the pterygopalatine fossa. This important connection between the external and internal carotid circulations may provide a source of collateral blood flow in the case of ICA occlusion.

C5 (Clinoid) ICA Segment. The C5 (clinoid) segment is a short interdural segment that lies between the proximal and distal dural rings of the CS. The C5 segment terminates as the ICA exits the CS and enters the cranial cavity adjacent to the anterior clinoid process. The C5 segment has no important branches unless the ophthalmic artery originates within the CS and not in the proximal intracranial (C6) segment.

C6 (Ophthalmic) ICA Segment. The C6 (ophthalmic) segment is the first ICA segment that lies wholly within the subarachnoid space. This segment extends from the distal dural ring to just below the PCoA origin.

The C6 segment has two important branches. The **ophthalmic artery** (OA) arises from the anterosuperior aspect of the ICA, then passes anteriorly through the optic canal together with CN II. The OA has extensive anastomoses with ECA branches in and around the orbit and lacrimal gland. The **superior hypophyseal artery** arises from the posterior aspect of the C6 ICA segment and supplies the anterior pituitary lobe (adenohypophysis) and infundibular stalk as well as the optic chiasm.

C7 (COMMUNICATING) ICA SEGMENT. The C7 (communicating) segment is the last ICA segment and extends from just below the PCoA origin to the terminal ICA bifurcation into the ACA and MCA. As it courses posterosuperiorly, the ICA passes between the optic and oculomotor nerves.

The most distal ICA segment has two important branches. The **PCoA** joins the anterior to the posterior circulation. A number of perforating arteries arise from

the PCoA to supply the basal brain structures including the hypothalamus.

The **anterior choroidal artery** (AChA) arises one or two millimeters above the PCoA and initially courses posteromedially, then turns laterally in the suprasellar cistern to enter the choroidal fissure of the temporal horn. The AChA territory is reciprocal with that of the posterolateral and posteromedial choroidal arteries (both are branches of the PCA) but usually includes the medial temporal lobe, basal ganglia, and infralenticular limb of the internal capsule.

Variants and Anomalies

Three important ICA vascular anomalies must be recognized on imaging studies: An aberrant ICA (AbICA), a persistent stapedial artery, and an embryonic carotid-basilar anastomosis.

ABERRANT ICA. An AbICA is a congenital vascular anomaly that enters the posterior middle ear cavity from below and hugs the cochlear promontory as it crosses the middle ear cavity (**8-3**). The ICA finally resumes its nor-

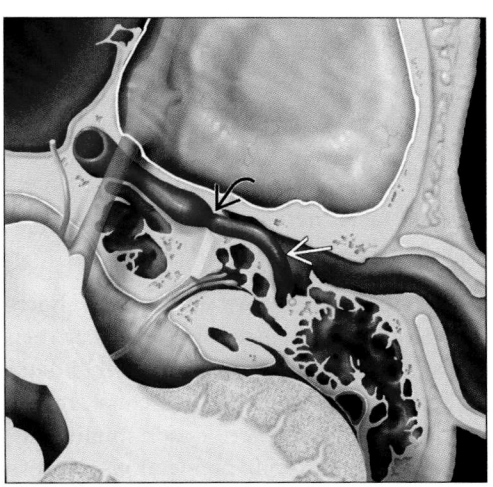
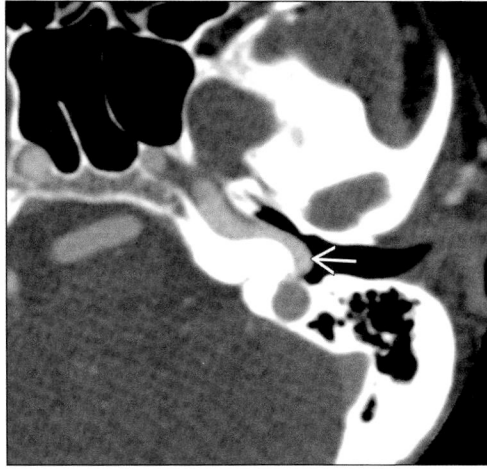

8-3. Axial graphic illustrates a classic aberrant ICA ➡ arising along the posterior cochlear promontory and crossing along the middle ear to rejoin the horizontal petrous ICA. A stenosis ➡ is often present at the reconnection site. 8-4. Axial CTA source image through the middle ear shows an AbICA ➡ looping over the cochlear promontory.

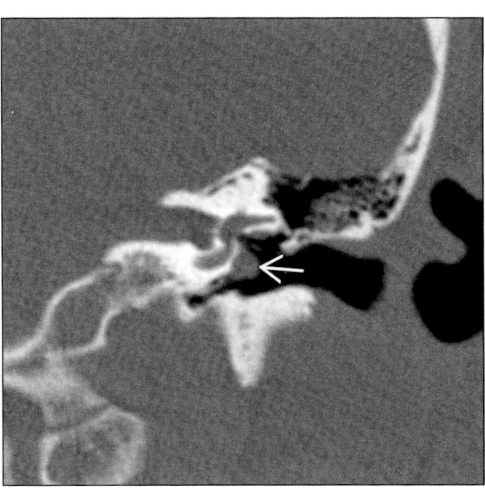
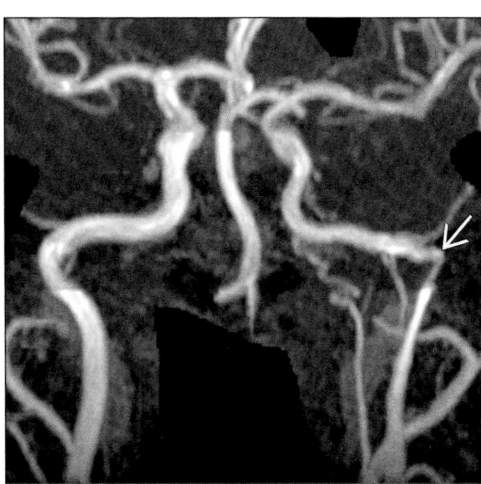

8-5. Coronal temporal bone CT at the oval window level shows an AbICA ➡ as a well-delineated soft tissue "mass" located on the cochlear promontory, mimicking a glomus tympanicum paraganglioma. 8-6. Coronal MRA shows a normal right ICA. An aberrant left ICA passes more laterally with a characteristic, sharply angled shape that resembles a "7" ➡.

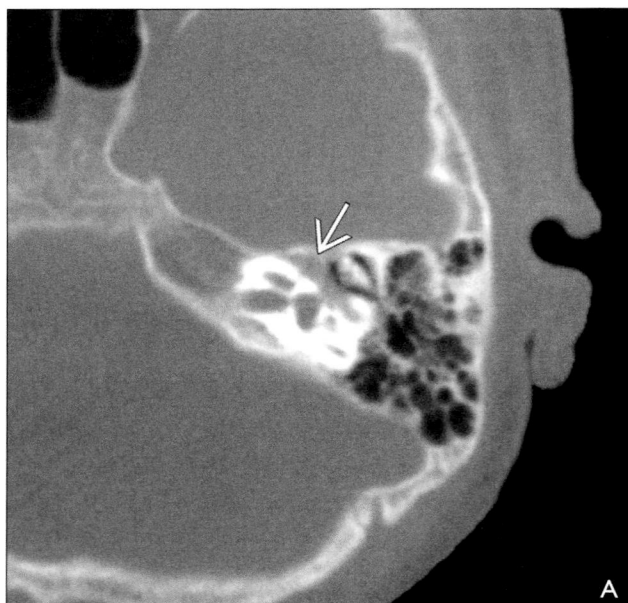

8-7A. *Characteristic findings of a persistent stapedial artery (PSA) are illustrated. Axial temporal bone CT shows an enlarged anterior tympanic segment of the facial nerve canal* ➤.

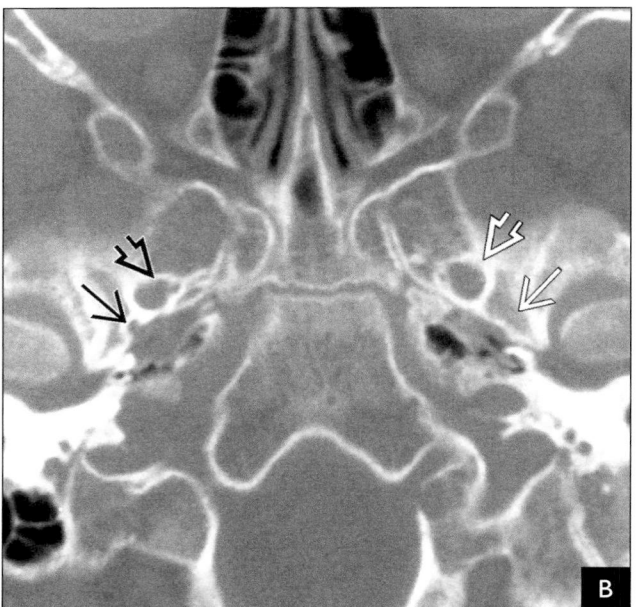

8-7B. *Bone CT in the same patient shows normal left foramen ovale* ➤, *absence of left foramen spinosum (FS)* ➤. *The right foramen ovale* ➤, *FS* ➤ *are normal. Absent FS and enlarged anterior CN VII segment are pathognomonic for PSA.*

mal, expected course as it joins the posterior lateral margin of the horizontal petrous ICA.

Patients with an AbICA typically present with pulsatile tinnitus. An AbICA is identified on otoscopic examination as a vascular-appearing retrotympanic mass lying in the anteroinferior mesotympanum. An AbICA mimics the clinical appearance of paraganglioma (glomus tympanicum, glomus jugulare). Biopsy may result in stroke or fatal hemorrhage, so this anomaly *must* be recognized by the radiologist *and* communicated to the referring clinician.

The appearance of an AbICA on CT is pathognomonic. Axial bone CT shows a tubular lesion that crosses the middle ear cavity from posterior to anterior **(8-4)**. Coronal images show a round, well-delineated soft tissue density lying on the cochlear promontory **(8-5)**.

Angiography (DSA, CTA, MRA) shows that the AbICA has a more posterolateral course than normal. A distinct angulation that resembles a "7" is often present, together with a change in contour and caliber ("pinched" appearance) before the segment resumes its normal course **(8-6)**.

PERSISTENT STAPEDIAL ARTERY. A persistent stapedial artery (PSA) is a rare congenital vascular anomaly in which the embryonic stapedial artery persists postnatally. Most PSA cases are discovered incidentally at imaging or at surgery.

A PSA arises from the C2 (petrous) ICA at the genu between the vertical and horizontal segments. The PSA passes through the stapes footplate and doubles the size

of the anterior (tympanic) facial nerve segment **(8-7A)**. Intracranially, the PSA becomes the middle meningeal artery (MMA).

Pathognomonic imaging findings are (1) the absence of the foramen spinosum (because the MMA arises from the PSA, not the ECA) **(8-7B)** and (2) an enlarged tympanic segment of the facial nerve. A PSA is often—but not invariably—associated with an AbICA.

EMBRYONIC CAROTID-BASILAR ANASTOMOSES. Early in embryonic development, connections form between the primitive carotid artery and the two longitudinal neural arteries (the fetal precursors of the basilar artery). With the exception of the posterior communicating artery, all these primitive arterial connections regress and then disappear when the definitive cerebral circulation forms. If they fail to regress, a postnatal **persistent** ("primitive" or "embryonic") **carotid-basilar anastomosis** (PCBA) remains.

There are four types of PCBA. Each is recognized and named according to its anatomic relationship with specific cranial or spinal nerves. From superior to inferior, these are a persistent trigeminal artery (CN V), persistent otic artery (CN VIII), persistent hypoglossal artery (CN XII), and proatlantal intersegmental artery (C1-3) **(8-8)**.

Persistent trigeminal artery. A persistent trigeminal artery (PTA) is the most common of the persistent embryonic carotid-basilar anastomoses and is identified in 0.1-0.2% of cases. Two types of PTA are recognized. In Saltzman type 1, the PTA supplies the distal basilar

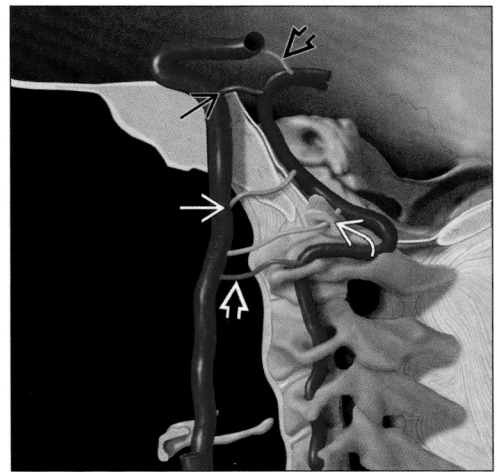

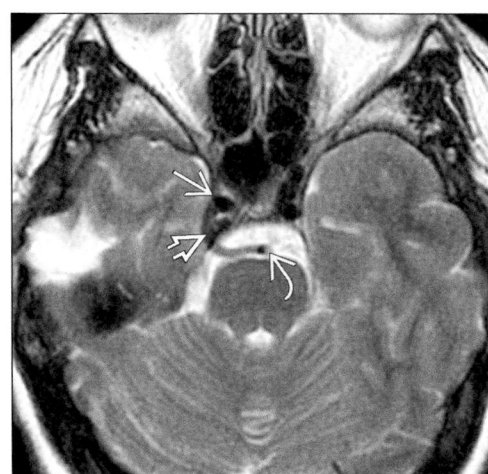

8-8. Graphic shows anastomoses between the ICA, VA. PCoA ⊟ is a normal connection. The PTA ➡ connects the cavernous ICA, BA. The POA ➡ connects the petrous ICA to the BA through the IAC. The PHA ➡ connects the cervical ICA, VA through the hypoglossal canal. The proatlantal artery ⊟ connects the cervical ICA, VA. 8-9. Axial T2WI shows a large PTA ⊟ passing posterolaterally around the sella turcica to connect the cavernous ICA ➡ to the BA ➡.

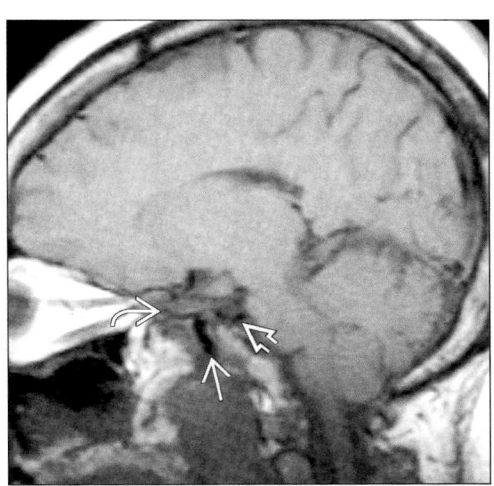

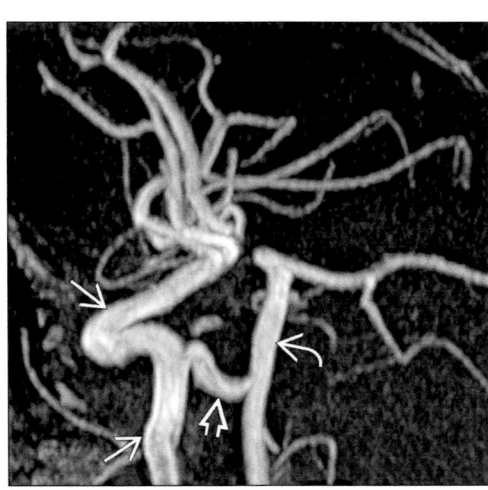

8-10. Sagittal T1-weighted MR shows the classic "Neptune's trident" appearance of a PTA. The "trident" is formed by the ascending ➡ and horizontal ➡ segments of the cavernous ICA and the PTA ⊟. 8-11. Sagittal MRA shows the complete "Neptune's trident" with the PTA ⊟ connecting the ICA ➡ to the BA ➡.

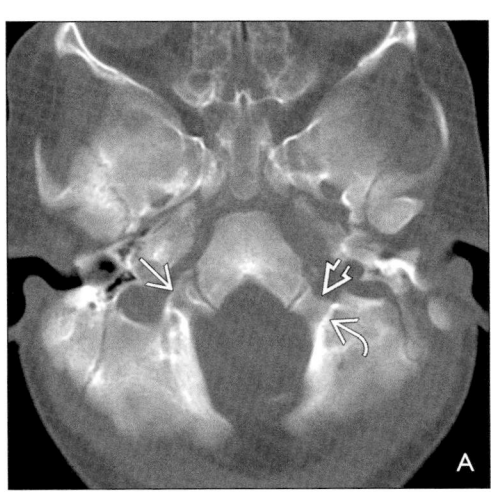

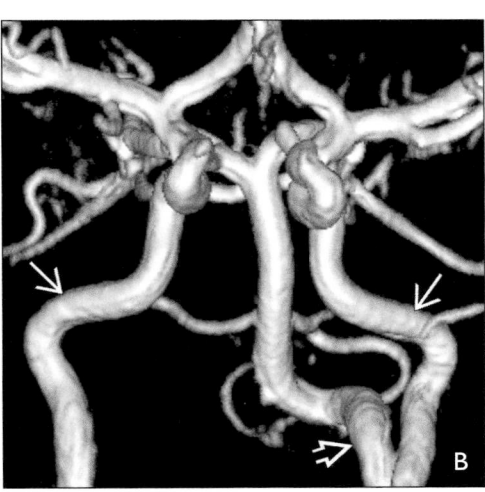

8-12A. Axial bone CT shows a normal right hypoglossal canal ➡. The left hypoglossal canal ⊟ is almost twice its size. The cortical margins of the enlarged hypoglossal canal ➡ appear intact. 8-12B. Coronal 3D MIP MRA in the same patient shows normal right and left carotid arteries ➡. The entire posterior circulation is supplied by a persistent hypoglossal artery ⊟, which accompanies the left CN XII through the enlarged hypoglossal canal.

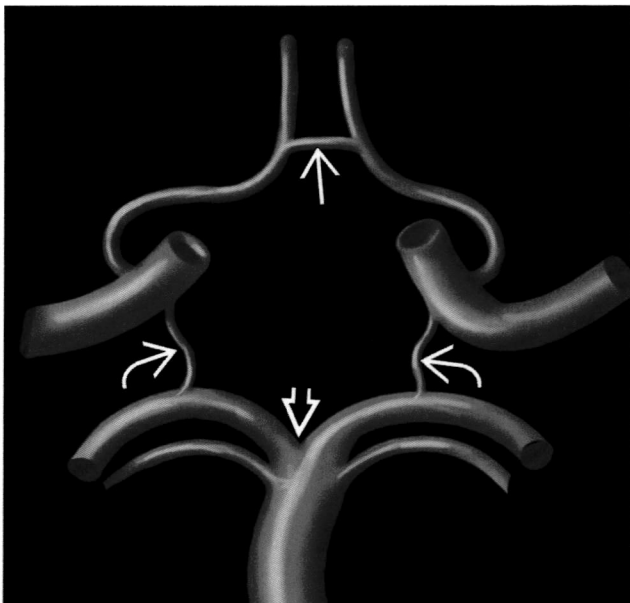

8-13. Graphic depicts the circle of Willis with the ACoA ➡ and PCoAs ➡ connecting the anterior (carotid) circulation to the posterior (vertebrobasilar) circulation ➡.

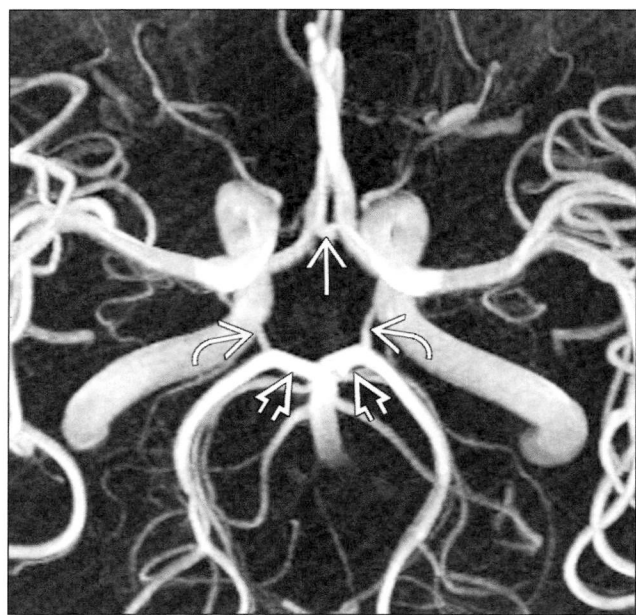

8-14. Submentovertex view of normal MRA shows the ACoA ➡, small PCoAs ➡, basilar bifurcation with large P1 PCA segments ➡ forming a "balanced" circle of Willis.

artery (BA), PCoAs are usually absent, and the proximal BA is hypoplastic. In Saltzman type 2, the PTA fills the superior cerebellar arteries while the PCAs are supplied via patent PCoAs.

As they pass posteriorly, PTAs can course either lateral or medial to the sella turcica. In the latter instance, the PTA courses posteromedially, compressing the pituitary gland and penetrating the dorsum sellae before it anastomoses with the BA. This variant is important to recognize prior to transsphenoidal surgery for pituitary adenoma.

Imaging findings of a PTA show a large vessel that connects the cavernous ICA with the BA. In 60% of cases, the PTA courses posteromedially, running through the dorsum sellae to join the BA **(8-9)**. In 40% of cases, the PTA runs posterolaterally along the trigeminal nerve, curving around (not through) the dorsum sellae.

Sagittal MR scans and MRA show a "Neptune's trident" configuration **(8-10)**, **(8-11)**. Nearly one-quarter of all PTAs have associated vascular abnormalities such as saccular aneurysm, moyamoya, aortic coarctation, and arterial fenestrations.

Persistent otic artery. Postnatally, the incidence of PCBAs is inversely related to their order of disappearance. The primitive otic artery is the first of the fetal carotid-basilar anastomoses to regress and is therefore the rarest of these uncommon anomalies. Only a few cases of persistent otic artery (POA) have been convincingly demonstrated.

Persistent hypoglossal artery. A persistent hypoglossal artery (PHA) is the second most common type of PCBA, with an estimated prevalence of 0.03-0.09%. A PHA arises from the posterior aspect of the cervical ICA, generally at the C1-2 level, and courses along CN XII through the hypoglossal canal to anastomose with the basilar artery **(8-8)**. The ipsilateral vertebral and posterior communicating arteries are hypoplastic. The posterior ICA arises from the PHA in 50% of cases.

A PHA has the highest incidence of associated aneurysms of any PCBA.

Imaging shows a large vessel that arises posteriorly from the distal cervical ICA and curves posteromedially through an enlarged hypoglossal canal to join the intracranial BA just above the foramen magnum **(8-12)**.

Proatlantal (intersegmental) artery. A proatlantal artery, also called a proatlantal intersegmental artery (PIA), is the most caudal of the PCBAs **(8-8)**. Two types are recognized: A type 1 PIA arises from the cervical ICA at the C2-3 (or lower) level, then runs posterosuperiorly and joins the suboccipital VA before coursing upward through the foramen magnum. A type 2 PIA follows a similar course but arises from the external carotid artery.

Circle of Willis

The circle of Willis (COW) is the great arterial anastomotic ring that surrounds the basal brain structures and connects the anterior and posterior circulations with each other. In the event of arterial occlusion, the COW is the most important source of potential collateral blood flow to the occluded territory.

Normal Anatomy

The COW has 10 components: Two ICAs, two proximal or horizontal (A1) anterior cerebral artery (ACA) segments, the anterior communicating artery (ACoA), two posterior communicating arteries (PCoAs), the basilar artery (BA), and two proximal or horizontal (P1) segments of the posterior cerebral arteries (PCAs) **(8-13)**, **(8-14)**. The middle cerebral artery (MCA) is *not* part of the COW.

Vascular Territory

Important perforating branches arise from all parts of the COW and supply most of the basilar brain structures. Those that arise from the ACoA and PCoA are discussed below. Perforating branches from the ACAs, MCAs, PCAs, and BA are also described along with the anatomy of their parent arteries.

The ACoA has perforating arteries that pass superiorly to supply the anterior hypothalamus and optic chiasm,

corpus callosum genu, cingulate gyrus, and pillars of the fornix. Occasionally a large, dominant perforating artery arises from the ACoA and is called the median artery of the corpus callosum. The PCoA gives origin to several perforating branches (anterior thalamoperforating arteries) that supply the thalamus.

Variants and Anomalies

COW *variants* are the rule, not the exception. One or more components of the COW is hypoplastic or absent in the majority of cases. A1 and P1 variants are described below. A hypoplastic or absent PCoA is the most common COW variant and occurs in one-quarter to one-third of all cases. An absent, duplicated, or multichanneled ACoA is seen in 10-15% of cases. Anatomic variants in the COW may cause significant flow asymmetries between the right and left ICAs or decreased volume in the BA on MRA and pMR studies; they should not be misinterpreted as vascular disease.

In contrast to normal variants, which are common, true COW *anomalies* are rare. When present, they are associated with a high prevalence of saccular aneurysms.

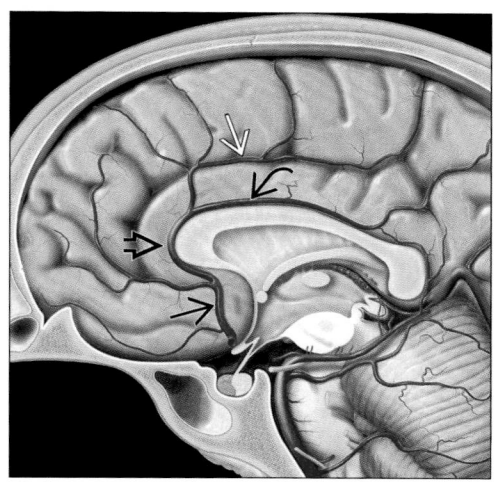

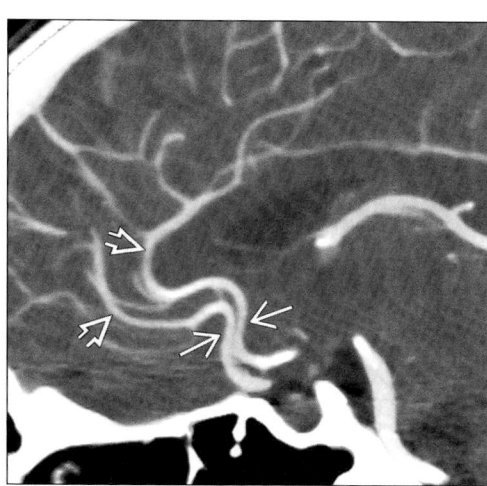

8-15. *Graphic shows the relationship of the ACA to the underlying brain. A2 segment ⇨ ascends in front of the third ventricle. A3 ⇨ curves around corpus callosum genu. Pericallosal ⇨, callosomarginal arteries ⇨ are the major terminal ACA branches.* **8-16.** *Sagittal midline MIP of CTA shows A2 segments of both ACAs ⇨ ascending in the interhemispheric fissure in front of the third ventricle, A3 segments ⇨ curving around the corpus callosum genu.*

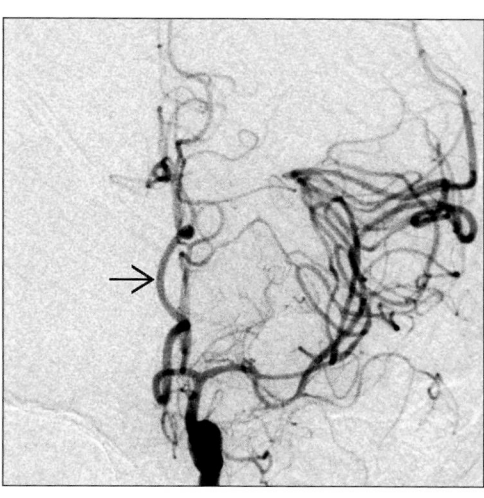

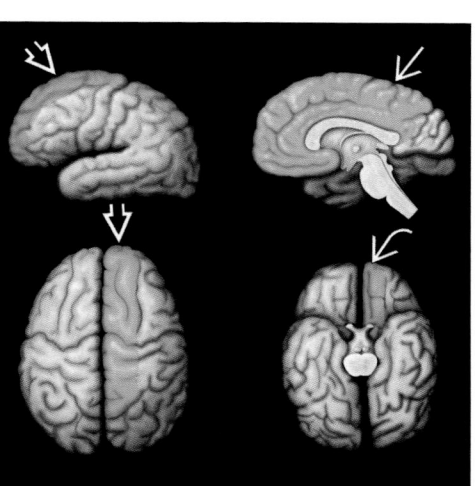

8-17. *AP view of a normal left internal carotid DSA shows the ACA ⇨ "wandering" gently from side to side across the midline in the interhemispheric fissure.* **8-18.** *ACA vascular territory (green) includes the anterior two-thirds of the medial surface of the hemisphere ⇨, a thin strip of cortex over the top of the hemisphere vertex ⇨, and a small wedge along the inferomedial frontal lobe ⇨.*

Anterior Cerebral Artery

The anterior cerebral artery (ACA) is the smaller, more medial terminal branch of the supraclinoid ICA. The ACA runs mostly in the interhemispheric fissure and has three defined segments **(8-15)**.

Normal Anatomy

A1 (HORIZONTAL) ACA SEGMENT. The first ACA segment, also termed the horizontal or A1 segment, extends medially over the optic chiasm and nerves to the midline where it is joined to the contralateral ACA by the anterior communicating artery (ACoA). Two important groups of branches arise from the A1 segment. The **medial lenticulostriate arteries** pass superiorly through the anterior perforated substance to supply the medial basal ganglia. The **recurrent artery of Heubner** arises from the distal A1 or proximal A2 ACA segment and curves backward above the horizontal ACA, then joins the medial lenticulostriate arteries to supply the inferomedial basal ganglia and anterior limb of the internal capsule.

A2 (VERTICAL) SEGMENT. The A2 or vertical ACA segment courses superiorly in the interhemispheric fissure, extending from the A1-ACoA junction to the corpus callosum rostrum **(8-16)**, **(8-17)**. The A2 segment has two cortical branches, the orbitofrontal and frontopolar arteries, that supply the undersurface and inferomedial aspect of the frontal lobe.

A3 (CALLOSAL) SEGMENT. The A3 ACA segment curves anteriorly around the corpus callosum genu, then divides into the two terminal ACA branches, the pericallosal and callosomarginal arteries. The pericallosal artery is the larger of the two terminal branches, running posteriorly between the dorsal surface of the corpus callosum and cingulate gyrus. The callosomarginal artery courses over the cingulate gyrus within the cingulate sulcus **(8-15)**.

Vascular Territory

The cortical ACA branches supply the anterior two-thirds of the *medial* hemispheres and corpus callosum, the inferomedial surface of the frontal lobe, and the anterior two-thirds of the cerebral convexity adjacent to the interhemispheric fissure **(8-18)**.

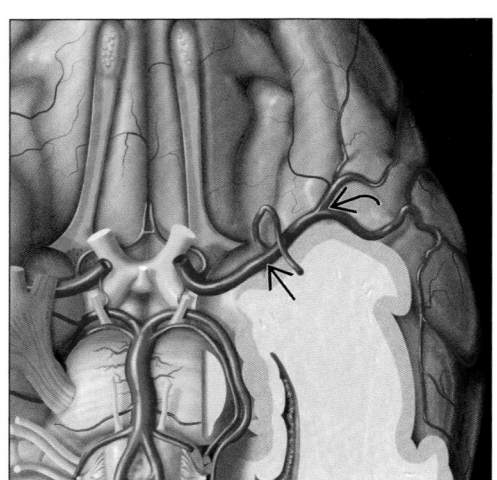

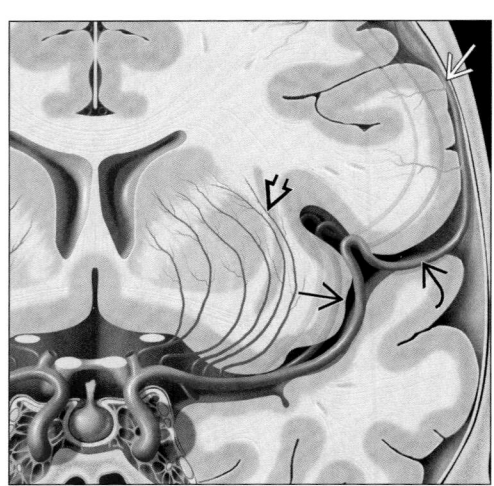

8-19. Submentovertex graphic depicts the MCA and its relationship to adjacent structures. Note the horizontal (M1) segment ➡ and the genu with bifurcation ➡ into M2 branches. 8-20. Coronal graphic shows the lateral lenticulostriate arteries ➡, M2 segments over the insula ➡, M3 segments ➡ running laterally in the sylvian fissure, M4 (cortical) branches ➡ coursing over the lateral surface of the hemisphere.

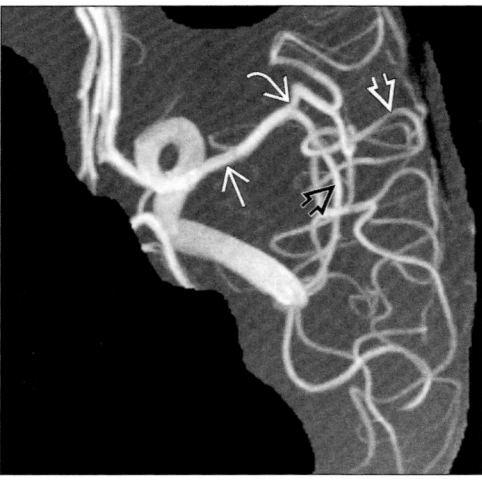

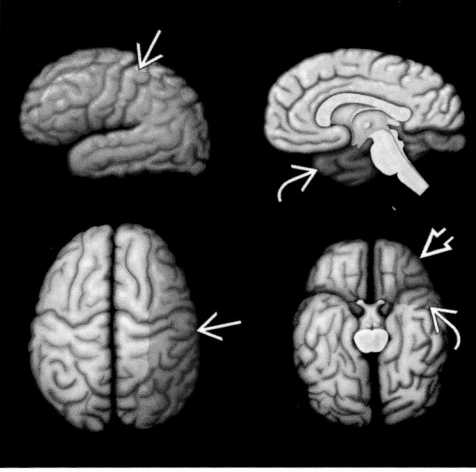

8-21. Submentovertex view of MRA shows M1 ➡, genu and bifurcation ➡, M2 segments coursing over insula ➡, M3 segments ➡ turning laterally to exit the sylvian fissure and course over the lateral surface of the hemisphere. 8-22. Vascular MCA territory (red) supplies most of the lateral surface of the hemisphere ➡, the anterior tip of the temporal lobe ➡, and the inferolateral frontal lobe ➡.

The penetrating ACA branches (mainly the medial lenticulostriate arteries) supply the medial basal ganglia, corpus callosum genu, and anterior limb of the internal capsule.

Variants and Anomalies

A rare variant is a **persistent primitive olfactory artery** (PPOA), which is a true ACA anomaly rather than a persistent carotid-basilar anastomosis (PCBA). In PPOA, a hypoplastic proximal ACA takes a very long anterior and inferomedial course along the ipsilateral olfactory tract just above the cribriform plate. It then makes a tight posterosuperior "hairpin" turn to continue as the normal distal ACA. PPOAs are frequently associated with saccular aneurysm, usually at the "hairpin" turn.

Two uncommon but important ACA anomalies are an infraoptic A1 and an azygous ACA. An **infraoptic A1** occurs when the horizontal segment passes below (not above) the optic nerve. An infraoptic A1 is associated with a high prevalence (40%) of aneurysms. A single midline or **azygous ACA** is seen with the holoprosencephaly spectrum.

Middle Cerebral Artery

The middle cerebral artery (MCA) is the larger, more lateral terminal branch of the supraclinoid ICA. The MCA has four defined segments.

Normal Anatomy

M1 (Horizontal) Segment. The M1 MCA segment extends laterally from the ICA bifurcation toward the sylvian (lateral cerebral) fissure. The MCA typically bi- or trifurcates just before it enters the sylvian fissure (8-19).

The most important branches that arise from the M1 segment are the lateral lenticulostriate group of arteries and the anterior temporal artery. The **lateral lenticulostriate arteries** supply the lateral putamen, caudate nucleus, and external capsule (8-20). The **anterior temporal artery** supplies the tip of the temporal lobe.

M2 (Insular) Segments. The post-bifurcation MCA trunks turn posterosuperiorly in the sylvian fissure, following a gentle curve (the genu or "knee" of the MCA). Several branches—the M2 or insular MCA segments—arise from the post-bifurcation trunks and sweep upward over the surface of the insula (8-20).

M3 (Opercular) Segments. The MCA branches loop at or near the top of the sylvian fissure, then course laterally under the parts ("opercula") of the frontal, parietal, and temporal lobes that hang over and enclose the sylvian fissure. These are the M3 or opercular segments (8-21).

M4 (Cortical) Segments. The MCA branches become the M4 segments when they exit the sylvian fissure and ramify over the lateral surface of the cerebral hemisphere (8-22). There is considerable variation in the cortical MCA branching patterns.

Vascular Territory

The MCA has the largest vascular territory of any of the major cerebral arteries. The MCA supplies most of the *lateral* surface of the cerebral hemisphere with the exception of a thin strip at the vertex (supplied by the ACA) and the occipital and posteroinferior parietal lobes (supplied by the PCA) (8-22). Its penetrating branches supply most of the lateral basal brain structures.

Variants and Anomalies

There is wide variability in the branching pattern of the cortical MCA vessels but few true anomalies. In contrast to the ACA/ACoA complex, MCA hypoplasia and aplasia are rare.

Duplicate origin of the MCA is rare. Here two MCA branches arise separately from the terminal segment of the ICA and then fuse to form an arterial ring. Fenestrated and accessory MCAs have been described.

Posterior Cerebral Artery

The two posterior cerebral arteries (PCAs) are the major terminal branches of the distal basilar artery. Each PCA has four defined segments (8-23).

Normal Anatomy

P1 (Precommunicating) Segment. The P1 PCA segment extends laterally from the BA bifurcation to the junction with the posterior communicating artery (PCoA). The P1 segment lies above the oculomotor nerve (CN III) and has perforating branches (the **posterior thalamoperforating arteries**) that course posterosuperiorly in the interpeduncular fossa to enter the undersurface of the midbrain.

P2 (Ambient) Segment. The P2 segment extends from the P1-PCoA junction, running in the ambient (perimesencephalic) cistern as it sweeps posterolaterally around the midbrain. The P2 segment lies above the tentorium and the cisternal segment of the trochlear nerve (CN IV). Two major cortical branches—the **anterior and posterior temporal arteries**—arise from the P2 PCA segment and pass laterally toward the inferior surface of the temporal lobe (8-23).

Several smaller but important branches also arise from the P2 PCA segment. **Thalamogeniculate arteries** and **peduncular perforating arteries** arise from the prox-

178 *Nontraumatic Hemorrhage and Vascular Lesions*

imal P2 and pass directly superiorly into the midbrain **(8-24)**.

The **medial posterior choroidal artery** (PChA) and the **lateral PChA** also arise from the P2 segment. The medial PChA curves around the brainstem and courses supero-medially to enter the tela choroidea and roof of the third ventricle. The lateral PChA enters the lateral ventricle and travels with the choroid plexus, curving around the pulvinar of the thalamus. The lateral PChA shares a reciprocal relationship with the AChA, a branch from the ICA.

P3 (Quadrigeminal) Segment. The P3 PCA is a short segment that lies entirely within the quadrigeminal cistern. It begins behind the midbrain and ends where the PCA enters the calcarine fissure of the occipital lobe **(8-25)**.

P4 (Calcarine) Segment. The P4 segment terminates within the calcarine fissure, where it divides into two terminal PCA trunks **(8-25)**. The medial trunk gives off the medial occipital artery, **parietooccipital artery**, cal-

carine artery, and **posterior splenial arteries** whereas the lateral trunk gives rise to the **lateral occipital artery**.

Vascular Territory

The PCA supplies most of the *inferior* surface of the cerebral hemisphere, with the exception of the temporal tip and frontal lobe. It also supplies the occipital lobe, posterior one-third of the medial hemisphere and corpus callosum, and most of the choroid plexus **(8-26)**. Penetrating PCA branches are the major vascular supply to the midbrain and posterior thalami.

Variants and Anomalies

A common normal variant is the **"fetal" origin of the PCA.** Here the proximal PCA arises from the internal carotid artery instead of from the basilar bifurcation. "Fetal" PCA origin is seen in 10-30% of cases. This variant is easily recognized on CTA, MRA, and DSA.

Vascular transit time in the PCA territory decreases with increasing contribution of the anterior circulation relative to that of the posterior circulation. If a large PCoA or "fetal" PCA is present on one side, this can produce

8-23. Submentovertex graphic shows the PCA segments and their relationship to the midbrain. P1 ➡, P2 ➡, P3 ➡ segments are shown. P4 segments (cortical branches) ➡ ramify over the occipital and inferior temporal lobes.
8-24. Lateral graphic depicts the PCA ➡ above and the superior cerebellar artery ➡ below the oculomotor nerve ➡. Perforating ➡, choroidal ➡, and cortical ➡ PCA branches are also shown.

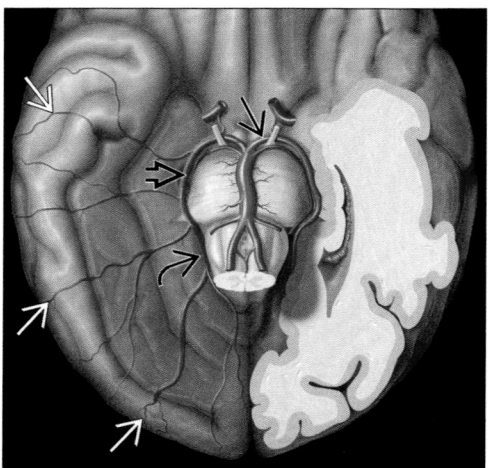
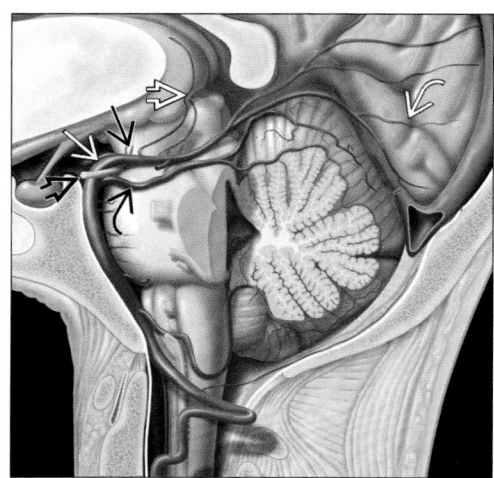

8-25. Submentovertex MRA shows the posterosubmentovertex sweep of the P2 PCAs ➡ and the medial course of the P3 segments ➡ as they pass behind the midbrain. Calcarine and P4 cortical branches ➡ are shown. 8-26. The PCA territory (purple) includes the occipital lobe and posterior third of the medial ➡ and the posterolateral surfaces of the hemisphere ➡, as well as almost the entire inferior surface of the temporal lobe ➡.

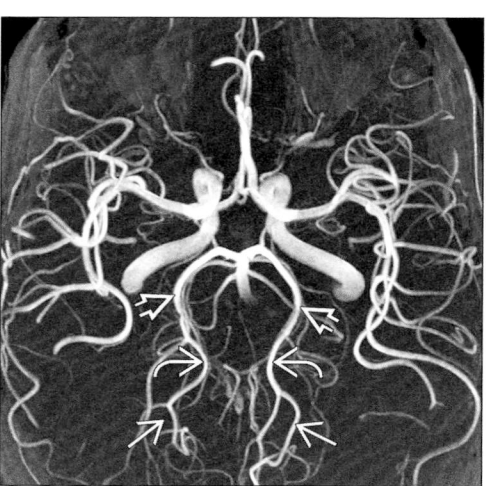
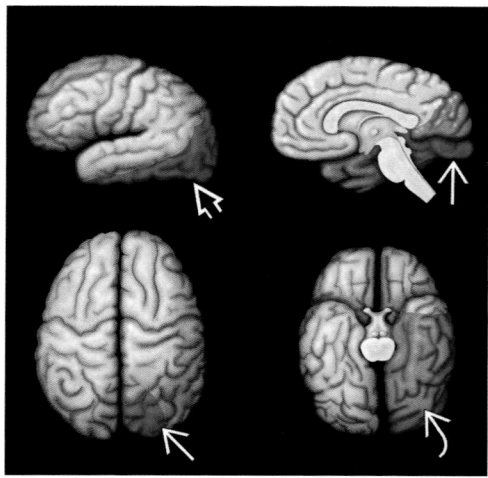

substantial left-right asymmetry on perfusion imaging. Knowledge of this common normal variant is essential as such asymmetry can mimic cerebrovascular pathology.

A rare but important PCA variant is an **artery of Percheron** (AOP). Here a single dominant thalamoperforating artery arises from the P1 segment and supplies the rostral midbrain and bilateral medial thalami **(8-74)**.

With the exception of persistent carotid-basilar anastomoses (see above), true PCA anomalies are uncommon. Early bifurcation, duplication, and fenestration of the precommunicating (P1) PCA segment have been described.

Vertebrobasilar System

The vertebrobasilar system consists of the two vertebral arteries (VAs), the basilar artery (BA), and their branches. Four VA segments are identified. Only one—the V4 segment—is intracranial.

Normal Anatomy

V1 (EXTRAOSSEOUS) SEGMENT. Each VA arises from the ipsilateral subclavian artery and courses posterosuperiorly to enter the C6 transverse foramen. Unnamed **segmental branches** arise from V1 to supply the cervical musculature and lower cervical spinal cord.

V2 (FORAMINAL) SEGMENT. The V2 segment courses superiorly through the C6-C3 transverse foramina until it reaches C2, where it first turns superolaterally through the "inverted L" of the transverse foramen and then turns upward to pass through the C1 transverse foramen **(8-27)**. An **anterior meningeal artery** and additional unnamed segmental branches arise from V2.

V3 (EXTRASPINAL) SEGMENT. The V3 segment begins after the VA exits the C1 transverse foramen. It lies on top of the C1 ring, curving posteromedially around the atlantooccipital joint before making a sharp anterosuperior turn to pierce the dura at the foramen magnum. The only major V3 branch is the **posterior meningeal artery**.

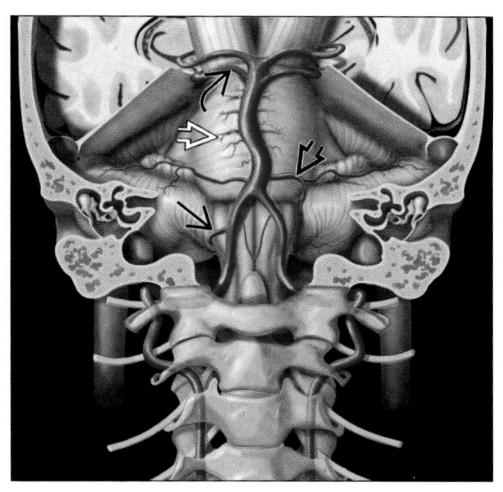
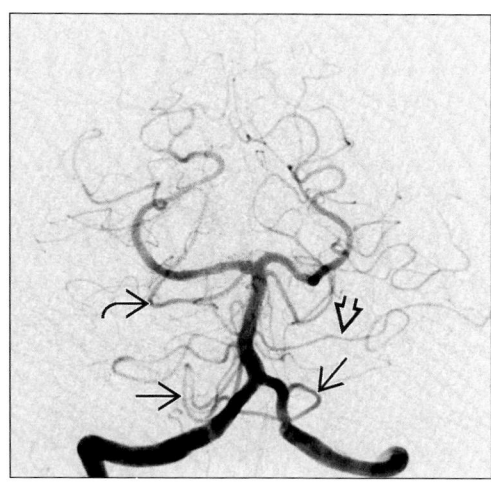

8-27. AP graphic depicts the vertebrobasilar system. PICAs ⇉ arise from the VAs before the basilar junction and curve posteriorly around the medulla. AICAs ⇉ course laterally to the CPAs. Two or more SCAs ⇉ arise from the BA just below the tentorium. Perforating BA branches ⇉ supply most of the pons. 8-28. AP DSA shows PICAs ⇉, AICAs ⇉, SCAs ⇉. The SCAs, PICAs both curve posterolaterally around the midbrain.

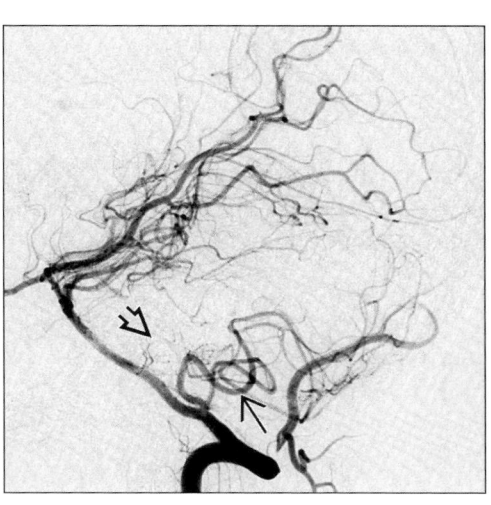
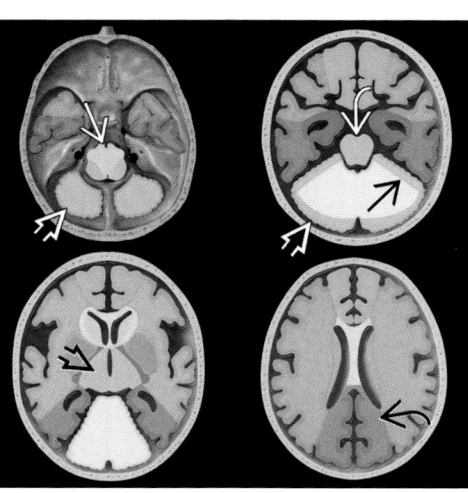

8-29. Lateral DSA shows large PICAs ⇉, small AICAs ⇉. 8-30. Graphic shows the posterior circulation vascular territories of PICAs (tan ⇉), AICAs (blue-green ⇉), SCAs (yellow), medullary perforating branches of the VA ⇉, and pontine perforating branches of the BA ⇉. Thalamic perforating branches ⇉ arise from the top of the BA, PCoAs. PCA territory is shown in purple ⇉.

V4 (INTRADURAL) SEGMENT. Once the VA becomes intradural, it courses superomedially behind the clivus and in front of the medulla. It gives off small **anterior and posterior spinal arteries** and **medullary perforating branches**. The **posterior inferior cerebellar artery (PICA)** arises from the distal VA, curves around/over the tonsil, and gives off the perforating medullary, choroid, tonsillar, and inferior cerebellar branches **(8-27), (8-28)**.

BASILAR ARTERY. The two VAs unite at or near the pontomedullary junction to form the BA. The BA courses superiorly in the prepontine cistern, lying between the clivus in front and the pons behind. It terminates in the interpeduncular fossa by dividing into the two **posterior cerebral arteries**.

Numerous small but critical **basilar perforating arteries** arise from the entire dorsal surface of the BA to supply the pons and midbrain.

The first major named BA branch is the **anterior inferior cerebellar artery (AICA) (8-29)**. The AICA arises from the proximal BA and courses ventromedially to CNs VII and VIII, frequently looping into the internal auditory meatus. It supplies both nerves as well as a relatively thin strip of the cerebellar hemisphere that lies directly behind the petrous temporal bone.

One or more (usually two to four) **superior cerebellar arteries** (SCAs) originate from each side of the distal BA, course laterally below CN III, then curve posterolaterally around the midbrain just below the tentorium **(8-28)**. SCA branches ramify over the surface of the superior cerebellum and upper vermis, curving into the great horizontal fissure.

Vascular Territory

The vertebrobasilar system normally supplies all of the posterior fossa structures as well as the midbrain, posterior thalami, occipital lobes, most of the inferior and posterolateral surfaces of the temporal lobe, and upper cervical spinal cord **(8-30)**.

Variants and Anomalies

The vertebrobasilar system has several normal variants. The two vertebral arteries vary in size, with the left VA dominant in 50% of cases, both equal size in 25%, and the right VA dominant in 25%. The left VA originates directly from the aortic arch (instead of the left subclavian artery) in 5% of cases. A small vertebral artery that ends in the PICA without connecting to the BA is another common normal variant.

The BA commonly varies in course and branching patterns. The BA and VAs can be fenestrated or partially duplicated.

Arterial Infarcts

We first focus on the pathology and imaging of major arterial ischemia-infarction, starting with acute lesions. Subacute and chronic infarcts are then discussed, followed by a brief consideration of lacunar infarcts. Lastly, we discuss watershed and hypotensive infarcts.

Acute Cerebral Ischemia-Infarction

As the clinical diagnosis of acute "stroke" is inaccurate in 15-20% of cases, imaging has become an essential component of rapid stroke triage. When and how to image patients with suspected acute stroke varies from institution to institution. Protocols are based on elapsed time since symptom onset, availability of emergent imaging with appropriate software reconstructions, clinician and radiologist preferences, and availability of neurointervention.

Because imaging has become so critical to patient management, we will focus in detail on hyperacute/acute stroke imaging. There are four "must know" questions in acute stroke triage that need to be answered rapidly and accurately: (1) Is intracranial hemorrhage or a stroke "mimic" present? (2) Is a large vessel occluded? (3) Is part of the brain irreversibly injured (i.e., is there a core of critically ischemic, irreversibly infarcted tissue)? (4) Is there a *clinically relevant* "penumbra" of ischemic but potentially salvageable tissue?

THE FOUR "MUST KNOW" ACUTE STROKE QUESTIONS

Is there intracranial hemorrhage (or a stroke "mimic")?

Is a large vessel occluded?

Is part of the brain irreversibly injured?

Is an ischemic "penumbra" present?

Terminology

Stroke—a generic term meaning sudden onset of a neurologic event—is also referred to as a cerebrovascular accident (CVA) or "brain attack."

The distinction between cerebral ischemia and cerebral infarction is subtle but important. In cerebral *ischemia*, the affected tissue remains viable although blood flow is inadequate to sustain normal cellular function. In cerebral *infarction*, frank cell death occurs with loss of neurons, glia, or both.

Timing is important in patient triage. *Hyperacute* stroke designates events within the first six hours following symptom onset. In hyperacute stroke, cell death has not yet occurred, so the combined term *acute cerebral ischemia-infarction* is often used. *Acute* strokes are those 6-48 hours from onset.

Etiology

Etiology varies with stroke subtype. Key stroke outcomes such as death, disability, and recurrence risk differ according to stroke mechanism.

STROKE SUBTYPES. Several systems have been used to classify major arterial stroke subtypes. One of the newest and simplest is the ASCO phenotypic system, which divides strokes into four subtypes: **A**therosclerotic, **s**mall vessel disease, **c**ardioembolic, and **o**ther. While all etiological classification systems (including Trial of Org 10172 in Acute Stroke Treatment [TOAST]) provide a similar distribution, the increased stroke risk in TIA patients with determined versus undetermined etiology is most evident using the ASCO classification.

Atherosclerotic (ASVD) strokes are the most common type of acute arterial ischemia/infarction, representing approximately 40-45% of cases. Most macroscopic large artery infarcts are embolic, arising from thrombi that develop at the site of an "at risk" ASVD plaque. The most common site of ASVD in the craniocervical vasculature is the carotid bifurcation (see Chapter 10), followed by the cavernous ICA segment. The most frequently occluded intracranial vessel is the middle cerebral artery (MCA).

Small vessel disease represents 15-30% of all strokes. Small artery occlusions, also called lacunar infarcts, are defined as lesions measuring less than 15 mm in diameter. Many are clinically silent although a strategically located lesion (e.g., in the internal capsule) can cause significant neurologic impairment. Lacunar infarcts can be embolic, atheromatous, or thrombotic. Most involve penetrating arteries in the basal ganglia/thalami, internal capsule, pons, and deep cerebral white matter.

Cardioembolic disease accounts for another 15-25% of major strokes. Common risk factors include myocardial infarction, arrhythmia (most often atrial fibrillation), and valvular heart disease.

Other is a heterogeneous group that combines strokes with miscellaneous but known etiologies together with strokes of undetermined etiology.

PATHOPHYSIOLOGY. An estimated two million neurons are lost each minute when a major vessel such as the MCA is suddenly occluded. Cerebral blood flow (CBF) falls precipitously. The center of the affected brain parenchyma—the densely **ischemic core**—typically has a CBF < 6-8 cm³/100 g/min. Oxygen is rapidly depleted, cellular energy production fails, and ion homeostasis is lost.

Neuronal death with irreversible loss of function occurs in the core of an acute stroke. A relatively less **ischemic penumbra** surrounding the central core is present in about half of all patients. CBF in the penumbra is significantly reduced, falling from a normal of 60 cm³/100 g/min to 10-20 cm³/100 g/min. This ischemic but not-yet-doomed-to-infarct tissue represents physiologically "at risk" but potentially salvageable tissue.

There is a well-defined histologic "hierarchy of sensitivity" to ischemic damage among the different cell types that constitute the neuropil. Neurons are the most vulnerable. They are followed (in descending order of susceptibility) by astrocytes, oligodendroglia, microglia, and endothelial cells.

There is also a geographic "hierarchy of sensitivity" to ischemic damage among the neurons themselves. Neurons in the CA1 area of the hippocampus, neocortex layers III, V, and VI, and the neostriatum are more vulnerable than other regions (e.g., the brainstem).

PREDISPOSING FACTORS AND GENETICS. Ischemic stroke is a multifactorial disease. Hypertension, diabetes, smoking, metabolic syndrome, and elevated triglycerides are significant known predisposing factors. However, all these factors together account for just part of stroke risk.

Approximately 30% of overall stroke risk is generally attributed to various genetic factors. Apart from a few single-gene disorders such as CADASIL or Fabry disease, however, no single locus with a consistent and robust association with ischemic stroke has been identified.

Pathology

LOCATION. The MCA is the most common site of large artery thromboembolic occlusion (8-31), followed by the PCA and vertebrobasilar circulation. The ACA is the least commonly occluded major intracranial vessel.

SIZE AND NUMBER. Acute infarcts can be solitary or multiple and vary in size from tiny lacunar to large territorial lesions that can involve much of the cerebral hemisphere.

GROSS PATHOLOGY. An acutely thrombosed artery is filled with soft purplish clot that may involve the entire vessel or just a short segment (8-32A). Extension into secondary branches with or without distal emboli into smaller, more peripheral vessels is common.

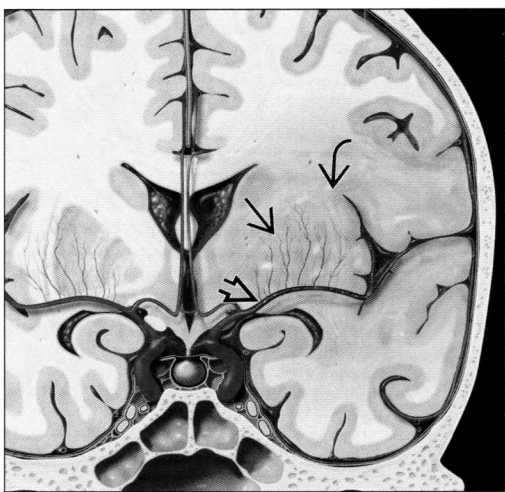

8-31. *Graphic shows proximal M1 occlusion* ⊇*. Acute ischemia is seen as subtle loss of gray-white interfaces* ⊇ *and "blurred" basal ganglia* ⊇*.*

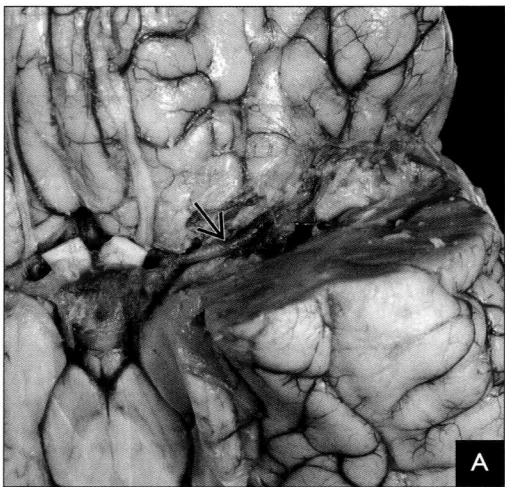

8-32A. *Autopsy specimen shows acute thrombus in the proximal MCA* ⊇*.*

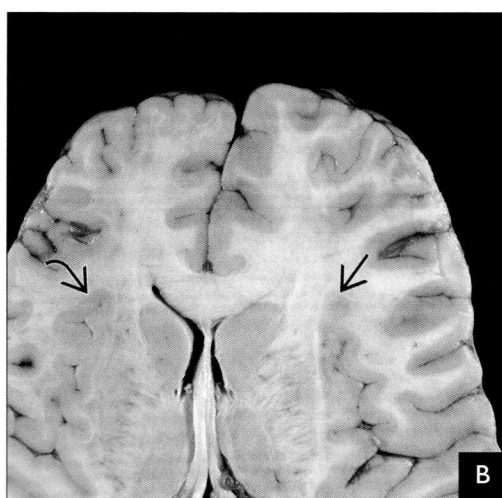

8-32B. *The same case shows swollen, "blurred" insular cortex* ⊇ *compared to the opposite normal side* ⊇*. (Courtesy R. Hewlett, MD.)*

Gross changes are minimal or absent in the first six to eight hours, after which edema in the affected vascular territory causes the brain to appear pale and swollen. The gray-white matter (GM-WM) boundaries become less distinct and more "blurred." As the gyri expand, the adjacent sulci are compressed, and the sulcal-cisternal CSF space is effaced (8-32B).

MICROSCOPIC FEATURES. Frank cerebral infarction is characterized by irreversible damage to all cells within the infarcted zone. Microscopically, neurons appear histologically normal in the first 8-12 hours. Within 12-24 hours, acutely ischemic neurons classically appear "red and dead" with hypereosinophilic cytoplasm, early karyolysis, and pyknotic nuclei. Acute infarcts are pale and often vacuolized, especially near the junction with intact brain. Astrocytic swelling without cell death predominates in the penumbral zone.

Clinical Issues

EPIDEMIOLOGY AND DEMOGRAPHICS. Stroke is the third leading cause of death in many industrialized countries and is the major worldwide cause of adult neurological disability. The age-adjusted incidence rate is about 180 per 100,000 per year.

Strokes affect patients of all ages—including newborns and neonates—although most occur in middle-aged or older adults. Children with strokes often have an underlying disorder such as right-to-left cardiac shunt, sickle cell disease, or inherited hypercoagulable syndrome. Strokes in young adults are often caused by dissection (spontaneous or traumatic) or drug abuse.

PRESENTATION. Stroke symptoms vary widely, depending on the vascular territory affected as well as the presence and adequacy of collateral flow. Sudden onset of a focal neurologic deficit such as facial droop, slurred speech, paresis, or decreased consciousness is the most common presentation.

PUBLIC AWARENESS. There have been numerous significant efforts to educate the general public about new therapeutic interventions for strokes and the urgency of dealing with a "brain attack."

Examples include a campaign by the National Stroke Association and the Stroke Awareness Foundation to publicize the many *warning signs of a stroke.* The program urges friends and family to recognize the symptoms of acute stroke and "act **FAST**."

Despite many such intense and widespread educational initiatives, the percentage of treated patients with acute stroke remains low (2-4%).

NATURAL HISTORY. Stroke outcome varies widely. Between 20-25% of strokes are considered "major" occlusions and cause 80% of adverse outcomes. Six months after stroke, 20-30% of all patients are dead, and a similar number are severely disabled.

Prognosis in individual patients depends on a number of contributing factors, i.e., which vessel is occluded, the presence or absence of robust collateral blood flow, and whether there is a significant ischemic penumbra. Nearly half of all strokes have inadequate collateral blood flow and no significant penumbra. Most patients with major vessel occlusions—even those with a significant ischemic penumbra—will do poorly unless blood flow can be restored and the brain reperfused.

Uncontrolled brain swelling with herniation and death can result from so-called malignant MCA infarction. In such cases, emergent craniectomy may be the only treatment option.

TREATMENT OPTIONS. Speed is essential, with the goal of a "door to needle" time (i.e., from arrival in the emergency department to intervention) under 60 minutes.

Stroke treatment options and inclusion/exclusion criteria are continually evolving. The single most important factor in successful intervention is patient selection, with the two most important considerations being (1) time from

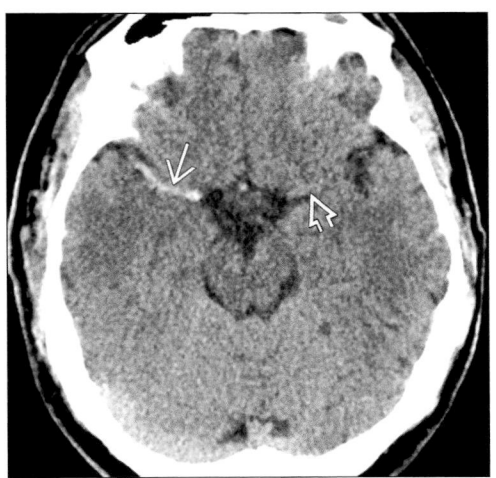

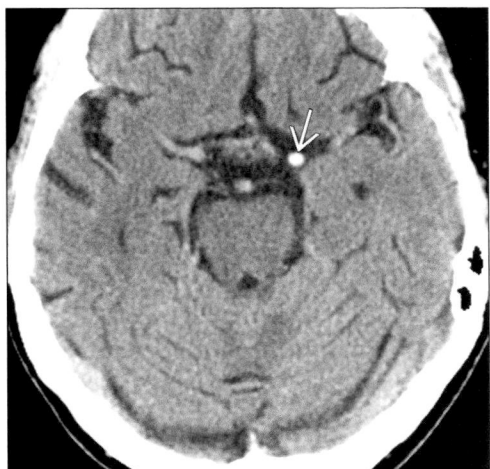

8-33. NECT scan shows a classic "hyperdense MCA" sign with acute thrombus in the right MCA ➡. Compare its striking hyperdensity with the normal, mild hyperdensity of the left MCA ➡. 8-34. NECT scan demonstrates hyperattenuating ("dense") artery sign indicating thrombus in the left internal carotid artery ➡.

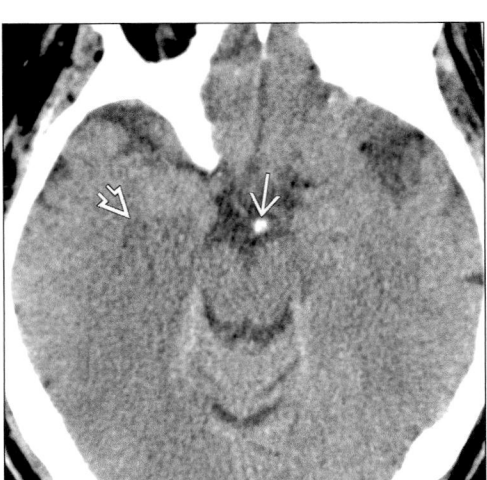

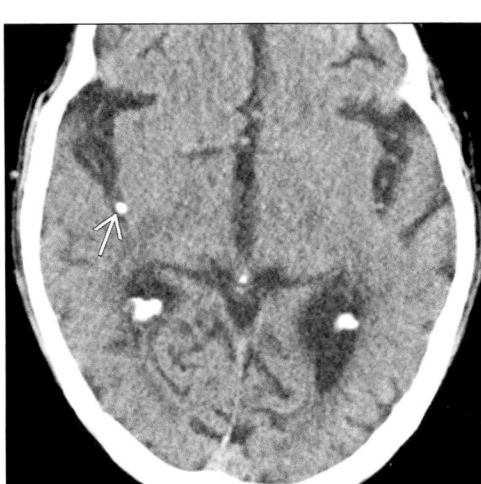

8-35. NECT scan shows "dense" artery sign ➡ in acute thrombosis of the basilar trunk. Note the hypodensity of the right occipital, inferomedial temporal lobes ➡. 8-36. NECT scan shows a calcified embolus ➡ in the angular branch of the right MCA.

symptom onset and (2) imaging findings on the screening NECT scan.

The clinically accepted therapeutic window for *intravenous* recombinant tissue plasminogen activator (rTPA) is less than three hours from ictus (the "golden hours"). *Intraarterial* thrombolysis is typically restricted to less than six hours. Exceptions to this general rule include basilar artery thrombosis and patients outside the six-hour window who have a persistent significant perfusion-diffusion mismatch.

Generally accepted imaging criteria for intraarterial thrombolysis include involvement of less than one-third of the MCA territory and absence of parenchymal hemorrhage (see below).

Intraarterial rTPA and other "clot-busting" drugs such as desmoteplase have improved outcome in selected cases. Endovascular mechanical thrombectomy offers an alternative, potentially synergistic method to thrombolysis. Its advantages include delivering site-specific therapy and tailored thrombolytic dosage. Early studies have shown improved recanalization rates and 90-day out-comes. Mechanical thrombectomy may also be suitable in patients beyond the therapeutic window or in whom thrombolytic therapy is contraindicated.

Imaging

"BRAIN ATTACK" PROTOCOLS. The primary goals of emergent stroke imaging are (1) to distinguish "bland" or ischemic stroke from intracranial hemorrhage and (2) to select/triage patients for possible reperfusion therapies.

Most protocols begin with emergent NECT to answer the *first* "must know" question in stroke imaging: Is intracranial hemorrhage or a stroke "mimic" (such as subdural hematoma or neoplasm) present? If a typical hypertensive hemorrhage is identified on the screening NECT scan in a patient with known systemic hypertension, no further imaging is generally required.

Once intracranial hemorrhage is excluded, the *second* critical issue is determining whether a major cerebral vessel is occluded. CT angiography (CTA) can be obtained immediately following the NECT scan and is the noninvasive procedure of choice for depicting potentially treat-

8-37A. Classic dense MCA sign. 8-37B. More cephalad scan in the same patient shows a hyperdense "dot" sign ➡️ *in the sylvian fissure due to thrombus extension into the proximal M2 segments. Note the "insular ribbon" sign* ➡️ *with effacement of the CSF in the sylvian fissure. Parenchymal hypodensity* ➡️ *extends to the cortical surface.*

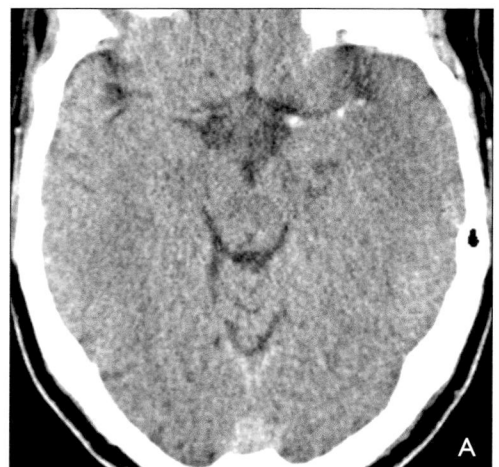
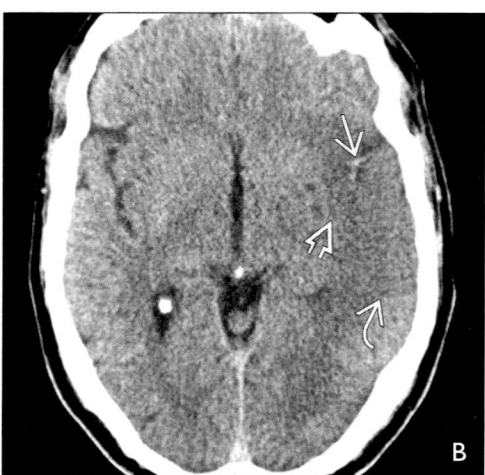

8-37C. CTA in the same patient shows an abrupt "cut-off" with a meniscus of contrast ➡️ *in the proximal left MCA. Contrast in the distal M2 and M3 segments* ➡️ *is caused by slow retrograde collateral flow from pial branches of the ACA across the watershed to M4 (cortical) branches* ➡️*. 8-37D. Left carotid DSA, AP view, in the same patient shows abrupt "cut-off" of the left M1 MCA segment* ➡️*.*

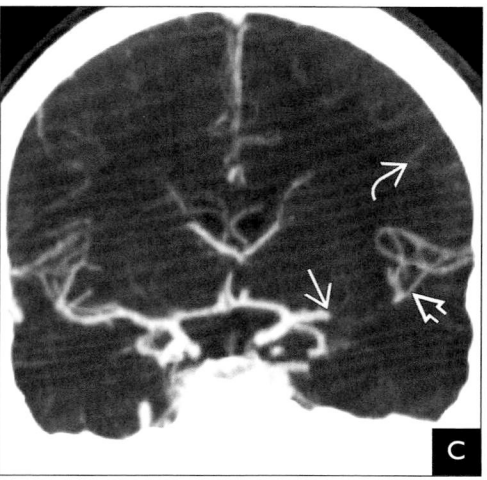
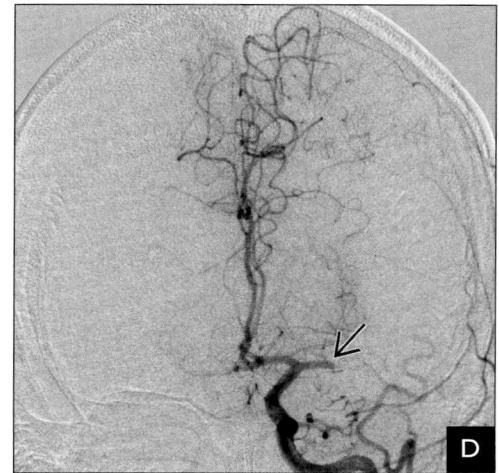

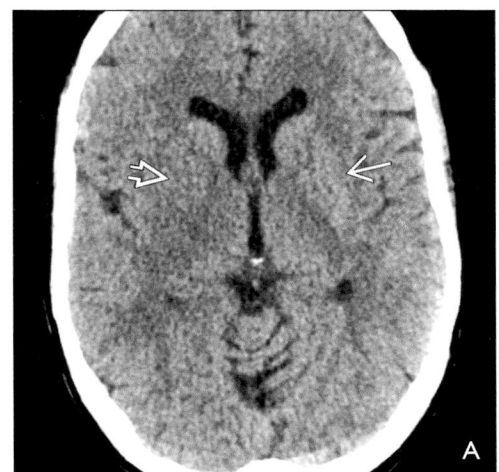

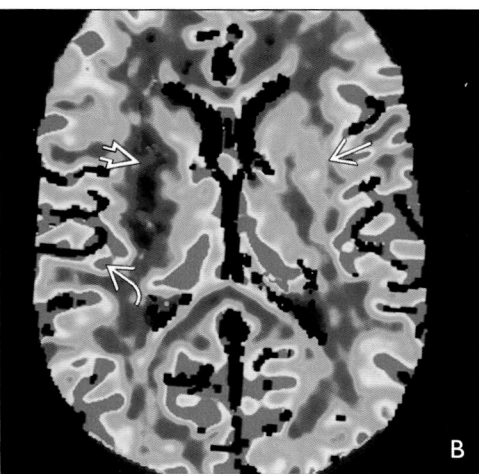

8-38A. NECT scan 3 hours after stroke onset shows hypodensity of the right basal ganglia ⇒ compared to the normal left side ⇒ ("disappearing basal ganglia" sign). 8-38B. pCT was performed. CBV shows markedly reduced blood volume in the right basal ganglia ⇒ compared to the normal left side ⇒. CBV in the cortex ⇒ overlying the basal ganglia infarct appears relatively normal.

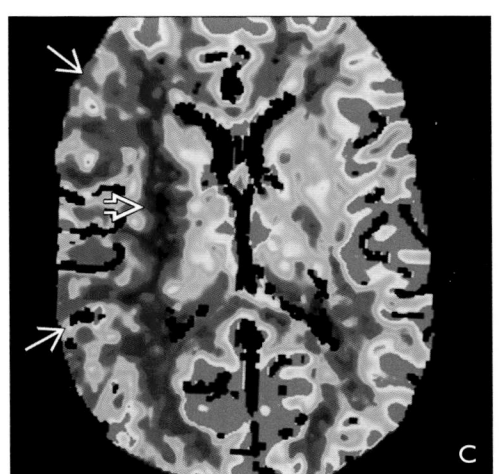

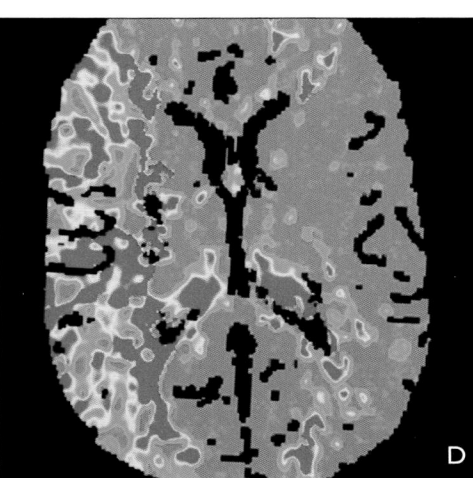

8-38C. CBF in the same patient shows markedly reduced blood flow to the entire right MCA distribution ⇒ with the most profound deficit in the right basal ganglia ⇒. The CBV/CBF "mismatch" in the cortex represents a large ischemic penumbra surrounding the densely ischemic basal ganglia. 8-38D. MTT shows that blood flow to the right MCA distribution is slow with markedly prolonged transit time.

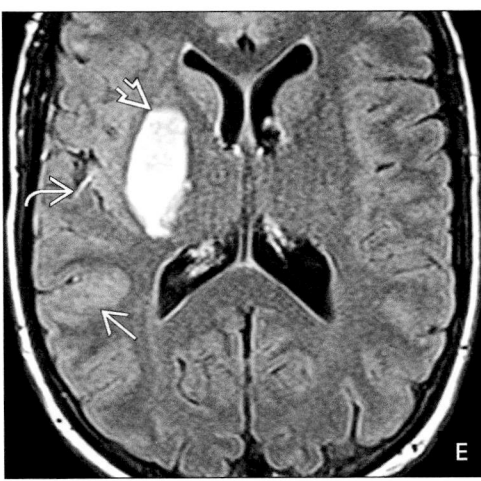

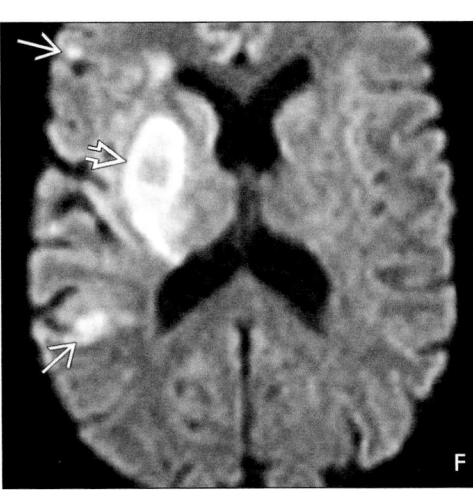

8-38E. Intraarterial thrombolytics were administered because of the large ischemic penumbra. MR obtained 24 hours later shows very hyperintense basal ganglia ⇒ with mildly swollen, hyperintense gyri in the MCA distribution ⇒. Note the hyperintense vessel ⇒ indicating slow flow. 8-38F. DWI in the same patient shows acute restriction in the right basal ganglia ⇒ with scattered foci of cortical ischemia ⇒.

able major vessel occlusions. MR angiography (MRA) is more susceptible to motion artifact, which is accentuated in uncooperative patients. DSA is typically reserved for patients undergoing intraarterial thrombolysis or mechanical thrombectomy.

The *third* and *fourth* questions can be answered with either CT or MR perfusion (pCT, pMR) studies. Both can depict what part of the brain is irreversibly damaged (i.e., the unsalvageable core infarct) and determine if there is a clinically relevant ischemic penumbra (potentially salvageable brain).

CT FINDINGS. A complete multimodal acute stroke CT protocol includes nonenhanced CT, CTA, and perfusion CT. With multidetector CT, the protocol can be completed within 15 minutes as a single examination with separate contrast material boluses.

NECT. Initial NECT scans—even those obtained in the first six hours—are abnormal in 50-60% of acute ischemic strokes if viewed with narrow window width.

The most specific but least sensitive sign is a hyperattenuating vessel filled with acute thrombus **(8-33)**. A **"dense MCA" sign** is seen in 30% of cases with documented M1 occlusion **(8-37A)**. Less common sites for a hyperdense vessel sign are the intracranial internal carotid artery **(8-34)**, basilar artery **(8-35)**, and MCA branches in the sylvian fissure ("dot" sign) **(8-37B)**. Uncommon but important NECT findings that indicate vascular occlusion include a calcified embolus, most likely from an "at-risk" ulcerated atherosclerotic plaque in the cervical or cavernous ICA **(8-36)**.

Blurring and indistinctness of gray-white matter (GM-WM) interfaces can be seen in 50-70% of cases within the first three hours following occlusion **(8-37B)**. Loss of the insular cortex (**"insular ribbon" sign**) and decreased density of the basal ganglia (**"disappearing basal ganglia" sign**) are the most common findings **(8-38A)**.

Wedge-shaped parenchymal hypodensity with indistinct GM-WM borders and **cortical sulcal effacement** develops in large territorial occlusions **(8-37B)**. If more than one-third of the MCA territory is initially involved, the likelihood of a "malignant" MCA infarct with severe

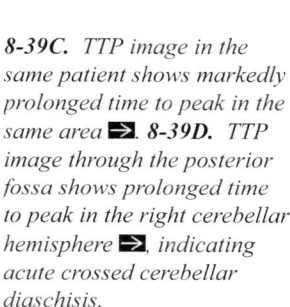

8-39A. *Axial NECT scan 5 hours after sudden onset of right hemiparesis shows left "insular ribbon" sign with hypodensity affecting the insular cortex* ➡ *and lateral aspect of the putamen* ➡ *("disappearing basal ganglia" sign). Compare to the normal right insular cortex, external capsule, putamen* ➡. *8-39B. CT perfusion with cerebral blood flow image shows markedly reduced CBF in the left MCA distribution* ➡.

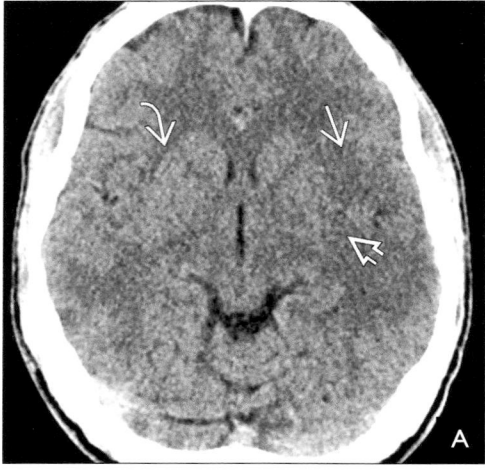

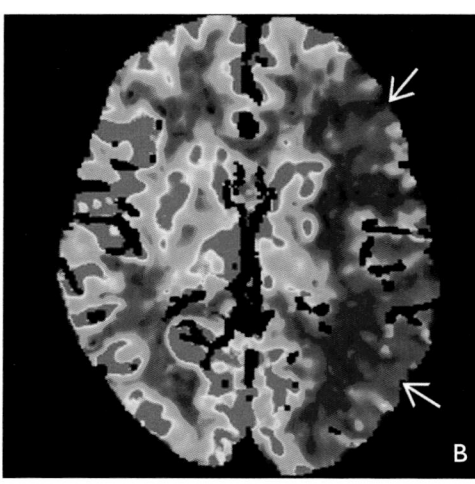

8-39C. *TTP image in the same patient shows markedly prolonged time to peak in the same area* ➡. *8-39D. TTP image through the posterior fossa shows prolonged time to peak in the right cerebellar hemisphere* ➡, *indicating acute crossed cerebellar diaschisis.*

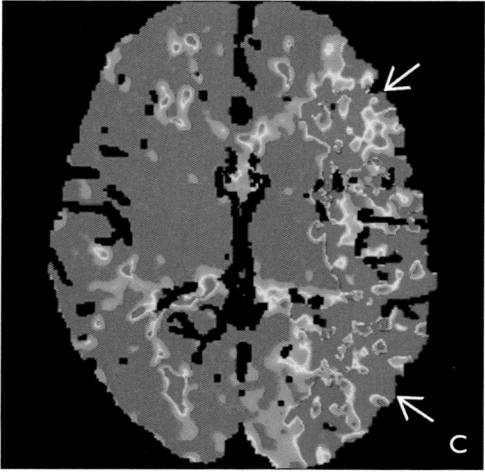

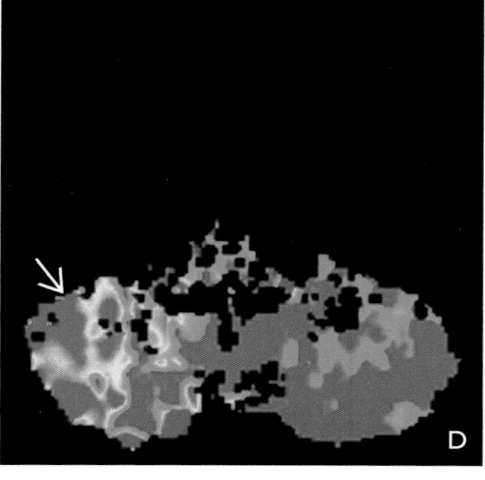

brain swelling rises, as does the risk of hemorrhagic transformation with attempted revascularization.

CECT. Standard CECT scans are rarely performed as part of most "brain attack" protocols. CECT may show enhancing vessels if slow antegrade flow or retrograde filling via collaterals over the vascular watershed zone is present. Cortical gyriform enhancement is rare in early arterial occlusion.

CTA. Multidetector row CT angiography of both the intra- and extracranial circulation is used to visualize the craniocervical vasculature from the aortic arch to the cortex. Because most strokes are embolic—from carotid atherosclerotic vascular disease (ASVD) or a cardiac source—some investigators suggest including the heart (the "triple rule-out for acute ischemic stroke").

CTA quickly answers the *second* "must know" stroke question (8-37C), i.e., is a major vessel occlusion present? CTA also localizes and defines the extent of the intravascular thrombus, assesses collateral blood flow, and characterizes atherosclerotic disease. CTA source images have been used to provide estimates of core infarct size but overestimate in 25% of cases.

pCT. The *third* and *fourth* "must know" questions can be answered with CT perfusion. pCT depicts the effect of vessel occlusion on the brain parenchyma itself. pCT can also be used to predict potential benefit after thrombolysis. Findings on pCT correlate well with those of DWI and pMR (8-38), (8-39).

Perfusion CT is obtained by monitoring the first pass of an iodinated contrast bolus through the cerebral circulation. As contrast passes through the brain, it causes transient hyperattenuation that is directly proportional to the amount of contrast in the vessels and blood in the brain.

pCT has three major parameters: Cerebral blood volume (**CBV**), cerebral blood flow (**CBF**), and mean transit time (**MTT**). CBV is defined as the volume of flowing blood in a given volume of brain. CBF is the volume of flowing blood moving through a given volume of brain in a specified amount of time. MTT is the average time it takes blood to transit through a given volume of brain.

All three pCT parameters can be depicted either visually—on a color scale—or numerically, using selected regions of interest. Color-coded perfusion maps can be visually assessed quickly and accurately.

The standard color scale is graduated from shades of red and yellow to blue and violet. With CBV and CBF, perfusion is portrayed in red/yellow/green (highest) to blue/purple/black (lowest). In normal brain, there is bilaterally symmetric perfusion in the cerebral hemispheres with higher CBF and CBV in gray matter (cortex, basal ganglia) compared to white matter. Well-perfused gray matter appears red/yellow, white matter appears blue, and ischemic brain is blue/purple. Totally nonperfused areas (i.e., the ventricles and densely ischemic central core of a major infarct) are black (8-39A), (8-39B).

Of the three standard parameters, MTT shows the most prominent regional abnormalities. Here the color scales are reversed to emphasize the abnormally prolonged transit time in the ischemic brain. With MTT, the slower the transit time, the closer to the red end of the scale. Brain with normal transit time appears blue. Parameters similar to MTT that are often used in pCT include time to peak (TTP) and time to drain (TTD).

The densely ischemic **infarct core**—the irreversibly injured brain—shows matched reduction in *both* CBV and CBF. The infarct core is seen as a dark blue/purple or black area that contrasts with the normally perfused red/yellow brain (8-38B), (8-38C). Prolonged MTT is seen as a red area, in contrast to the blue brain, in which transit time is normal (8-38D).

An **ischemic penumbra** with potentially salvageable tissue is seen as a "mismatch" between markedly reduced CBV in the infarcted core (8-38B) and a surrounding area (penumbra) characterized by decreased CBF with normal CBV (8-38C). Thus the potentially salvageable brain tissue is equivalent to CBF minus CBV. Prolonged MTT over 145% that extends beyond the core infarct area (so-called CBV/MTT mismatch) also characterizes the ischemic penumbra (8-38D).

An important ancillary finding in patients with large MCA infarcts is reduced perfusion in the opposite cerebellar hemisphere. Between 15-20% of large MCA infarcts cause hypoperfusion with reduced CBF in the contralateral cerebellum, a phenomenon called **"crossed cerebellar diaschisis"** (see below) (8-39C), (8-39D).

MR FINDINGS. While CT/CTA/pCT is often preferred because of accessibility and speed, "expedited" stroke protocols with only FLAIR, T2*, and DWI can be used. MR is superior to CT in detecting small vessel and brainstem ischemia.

T1WI. T1WI is usually normal within the first three to six hours. Subtle gyral swelling and hypointensity begin to develop within 12-24 hours and are seen as blurring of the GM-WM interfaces. With large vessel occlusions, loss of the expected "flow void" in the affected artery can sometimes be identified.

T2/FLAIR. Only 30-50% of acute strokes show cortical swelling and hyperintensity on FLAIR scans within the first four hours. Nearly all strokes are FLAIR positive by seven hours following symptom onset. T2 scans become positive slightly later, generally within 12-24 hours. Intraarterial hyperintensity on FLAIR is an early sign of stroke and indicates slow flow (not thrombosis), either from delayed antegrade flow or—more commonly—retrograde collateral filling across the cortical watershed **(8-40A)**, **(8-40B)**, **(8-41A)**. FLAIR-DWI "mismatch" (negative FLAIR, positive DWI) has been suggested as a quick indicator of viable ischemic penumbra and eligibility for thrombolysis.

T2* GRE. Intraarterial thrombus can sometimes be detected as "blooming" hypointensity on T2* (GRE, SWI) studies **(8-41B)**. Also look carefully for the presence of multifocal parenchymal microbleeds in older patients. In this age group, "blooming black dots" are most commonly caused by chronic hypertension or amyloid angiopathy. The presence of cerebral microbleeds may be an independent risk factor for subsequent anticoagulation-related hemorrhage.

T1 C+. Post-contrast T1 scans show intravascular enhancement. Parenchymal enhancement is uncommon in acute/hyperacute ischemia **(8-41E)**, **(8-41F)**.

DWI and DTI. Cellular swelling begins to develop within minutes following an ischemic insult. ADC values decrease, producing high signal intensity on DWI images **(8-40C)**, **(8-41C)**. While most investigators posit cytotoxic edema as the basis for decreased ADC, part of the decrease is due to reduced water diffusibility caused by decreased levels of astrocytic aquaporin-4 (AQP4). Aquaporins are transmembrane proteins—water channels—that facilitate bidirectional selective water transport in and out of the cell.

Around 95% of hyperacute infarcts show diffusion restriction on DWI, with hyperintensity on DWI and corresponding hypointensity on ADC **(8-38F)**, **(8-41C)**. DTI is even more sensitive than DWI, especially for pontine and medullary lesions.

A negative DWI does not exclude the diagnosis of stroke. Between 2-7% of patients with a final diagnosis of stroke are initially DWI negative. Very small (lacunar) infarcts, brainstem lesions, clot lysis with recanalization, and moderately reduced or fluctuating hypoperfusion that is not severe enough to restrict water movement have all been cited as possible reasons for DWI-negative acute strokes.

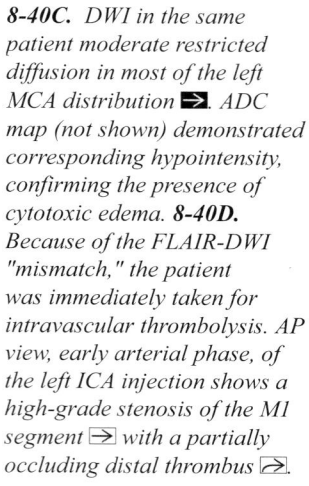

8-40A. Expedited MR with only FLAIR, GRE, and DWI was obtained in a 54-year-old woman 2 hours and 45 minutes following symptom onset. Axial FLAIR shows intravascular hyperintensity ➡ in the left MCA (compare to the normal "flow void" on the right) suggesting slow flow. 8-40B. No parenchymal abnormalities were identified in the vascular distribution of the left MCA. The only definite abnormality is hyperintensity in the posterior division branches of the left MCA ➡.

8-40C. DWI in the same patient moderate restricted diffusion in most of the left MCA distribution ➡. ADC map (not shown) demonstrated corresponding hypointensity, confirming the presence of cytotoxic edema. 8-40D. Because of the FLAIR-DWI "mismatch," the patient was immediately taken for intravascular thrombolysis. AP view, early arterial phase, of the left ICA injection shows a high-grade stenosis of the M1 segment ➡ with a partially occluding distal thrombus ➡.

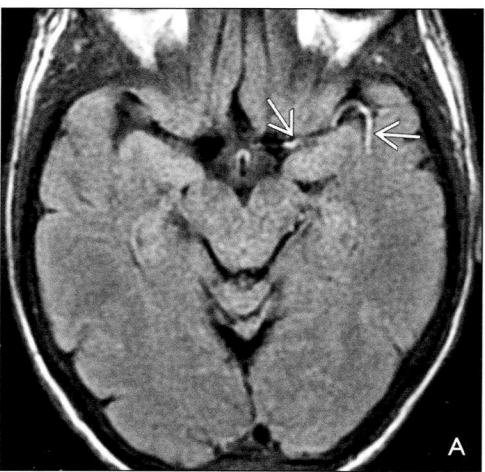

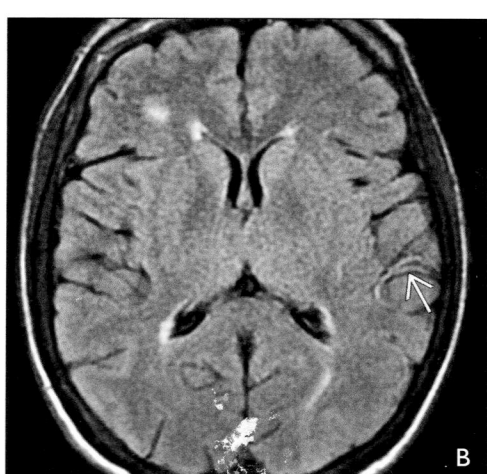

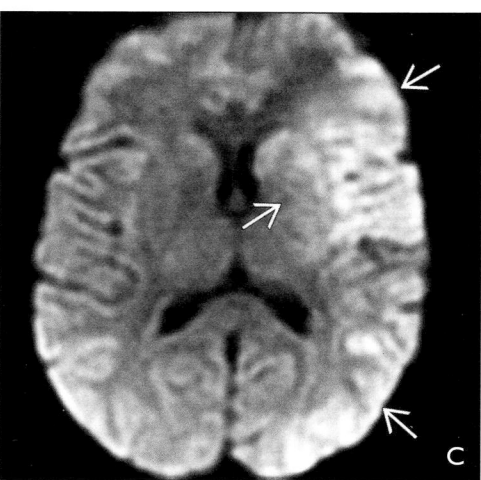

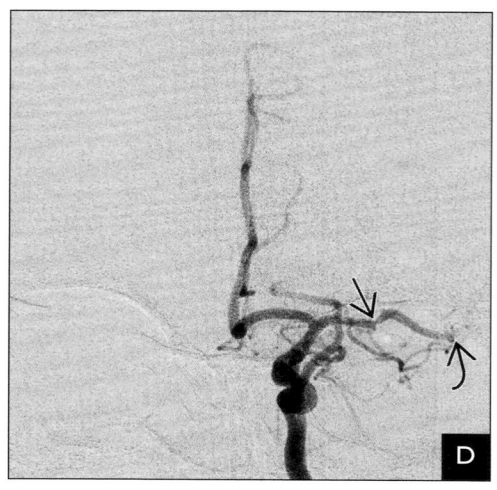

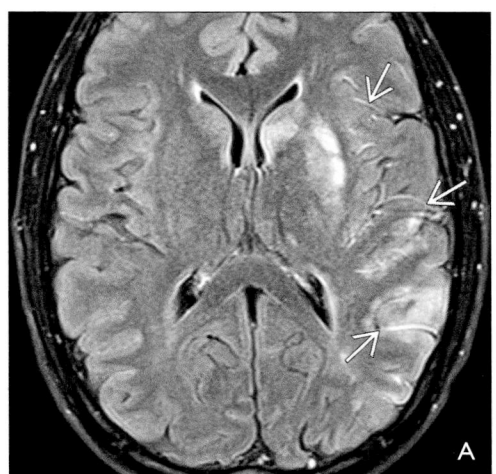
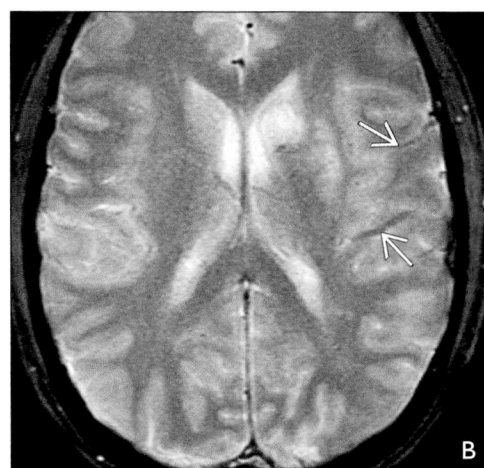

8-41A. *Acute stroke in a 47-year-old man shows patchy hyperintensity in the left caudate nucleus, lateral putamen, and parietal cortex. Note multiple linear foci of intravascular hyperintensity* ➡, *consistent with slow flow in the MCA distribution.* **8-41B.** *T2* GRE scan shows several linear hypointensities* ➡ *in the affected MCA branches, consistent with hemoglobin deoxygenation caused by slow, stagnating arterial blood flow.*

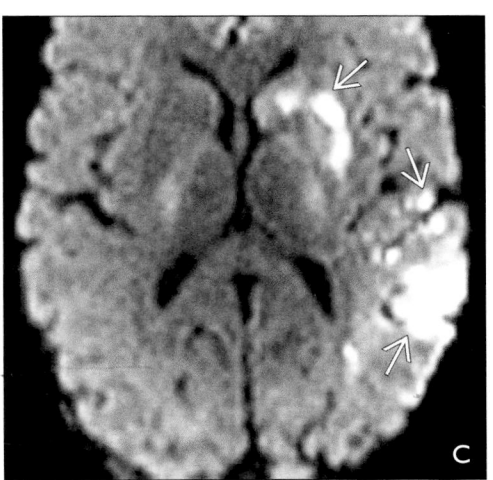
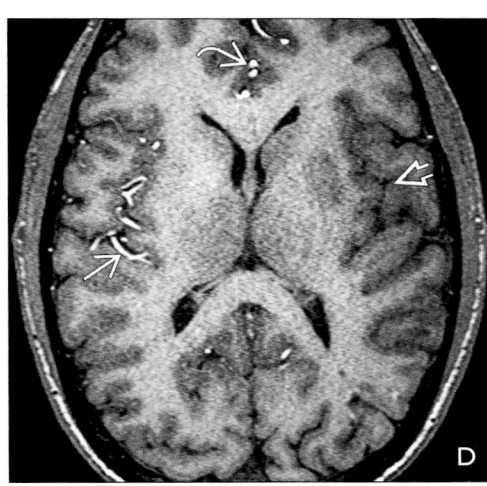

8-41C. *DWI in the same patient shows multiple patchy foci of diffusion restriction* ➡, *consistent with acute cerebral infarct.* **8-41D.** *Axial source image from 2D TOF MRA shows normal signal intensity in the right MCA* ➡ *and both ACA branches* ➡ *but no flow in the left MCA vessels* ➡.

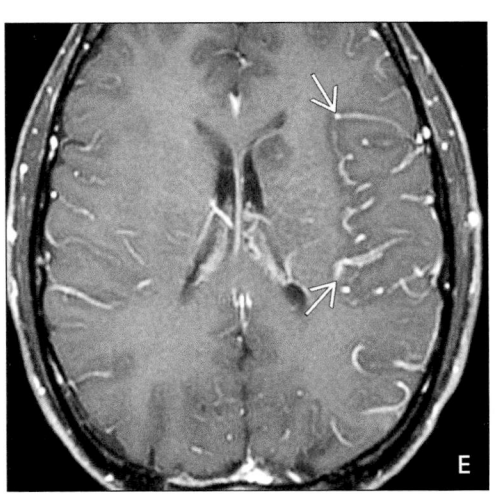
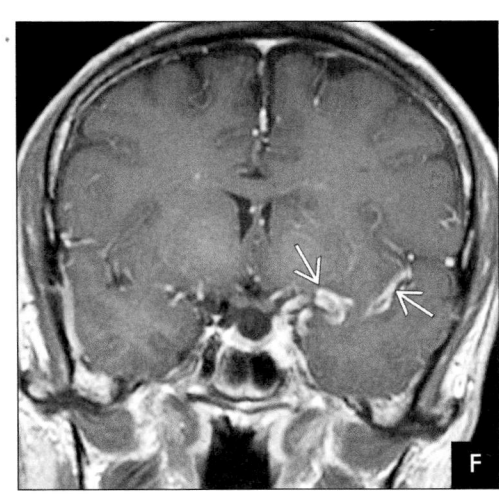

8-41E. *Axial T1 C+ FS scan shows striking intravascular enhancement in the left MCA branches* ➡, *consistent with slow flow in patent (nonthrombosed) vessels.* **8-41F.** *Coronal T1 C+ scan shows prominent intravascular enhancement in the left MCA* ➡.

8-42A. *Series of DSA images demonstrates classic angiographic findings of acute thromboembolic occlusion. Left internal carotid angiogram, early arterial phase, AP view, shows abrupt "cut-off" of the MCA ⮕. **8-42B.** Lateral view, early arterial phase, shows normal filling of both ACAs ⮕ and the ipsilateral PCA ⮕ via a large PCoA. The MCA distribution is not opacified, leaving a large "bare area" ⮕ of devascularized brain.*

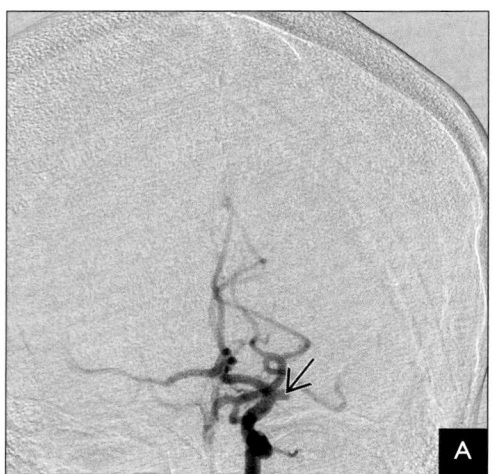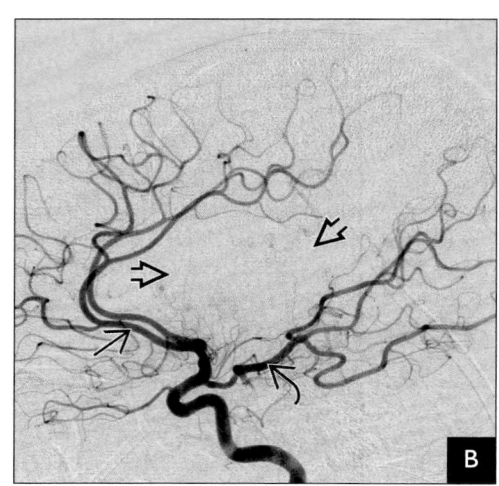

8-42C. *Later image shows that the large "bare area" remains unopacified. Cortical branches are seen high over the left parietal convexity with early retrograde filling of the distal MCA branches ⮕ via pial collaterals from the ACA and PCA. Collateral flow is also seen from the posterior temporal PCA branches ⮕ into the MCA territory. **8-42D.** Later image shows slow retrograde filling ⮕ into the MCA territory from ACA and PCA collaterals.*

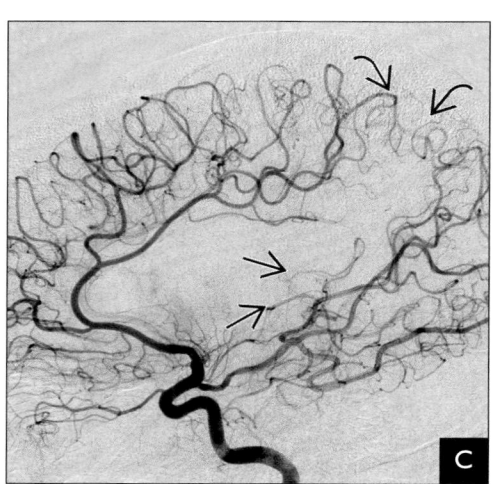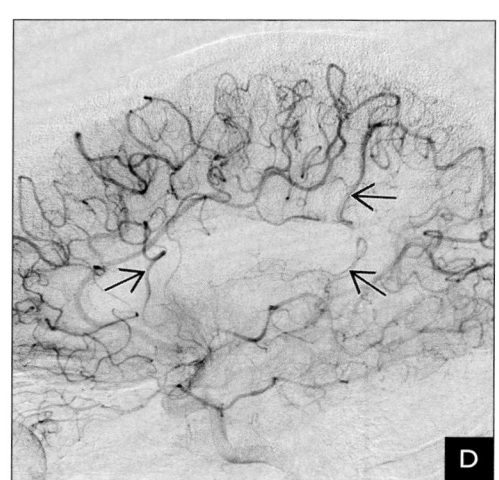

8-42E. *Capillary phase image shows a diffuse brain "blush" ⮕ in the ACA/PCA territories; contrast with the "bare area" that would normally be supplied by the MCA. Some MCA branches ⮕ are filling slowly via retrograde flow from ACA/PCA pial collaterals. **8-42F.** Venous phase shows persisting contrast ⮕ in some MCA branches that have filled in retrograde fashion via pial collaterals and are slowly emptying. Note "blush" ⮕ at the border of the "bare area" caused by "luxury perfusion."*

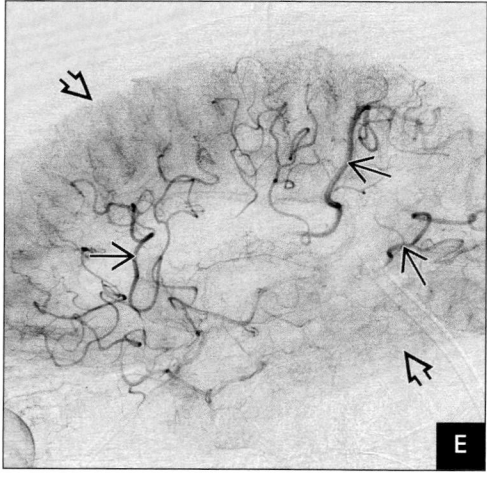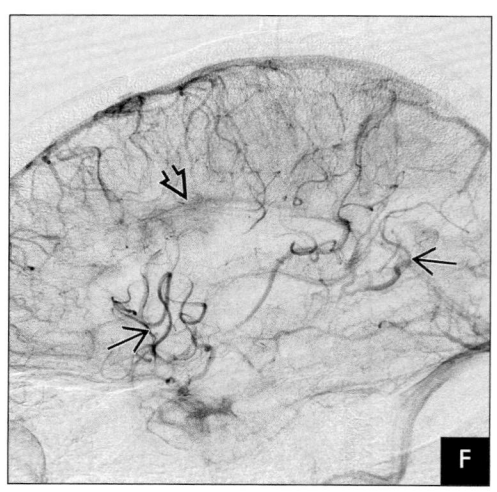

pMR. Restriction on DWI generally reflects the densely ischemic core of the infarct while pMR depicts the surrounding "at-risk" penumbra. A **DWI-PWI mismatch** is one of the criteria used in determining suitability for intraarterial thrombolysis.

ANGIOGRAPHY. As the diagnosis of acute cerebral ischemia-infarction with large vessel occlusion is already established using CTA or MRA **(8-41D)**, DSA is generally obtained only as a prelude to intraarterial thrombolysis or mechanical thrombectomy. Clot location and length can be precisely determined and collateral circulation delineated.

Major vessel occlusion is identified on DSA as interruption of the intraarterial contrast column. Frequent findings include an abrupt vessel "cut-off" **(8-37D)**, **(8-42A)**, "meniscus" sign, tapered or "rat-tail" narrowing **(8-40D)**, or "tram-track" appearance with a trickle of contrast around the intraluminal thrombus.

Other common angiographic findings include a "bare" or "naked" area of nonperfused brain **(8-42B)**, **(8-42C)**, slow antegrade filling with delayed washout of distal branches (seen as intraarterial contrast persisting into the capillary or venous phase), and pial collaterals with retrograde filling across the cortical watershed **(8-42D)**, **(8-42E)**, **(8-42F)**.

Less common signs are hyperemia with a vascular "blush" around the infarcted zone (so-called luxury perfusion) **(8-42F)** and "early draining" veins (arteriovenous shunting with contrast appearing in veins draining the infarct while the remainder of the circulation is still in the late arterial or early capillary phase).

Mass effect is rare in hyperacute stroke but very common in the acute/late acute stages.

ULTRASOUND. Carotid artery intima-media thickness as measured by Doppler US has been identified as a marker for large artery disease, which in turn is correlated with increased stroke risk.

Differential Diagnosis

The clinical differential diagnosis of acute stroke is broad. In contrast, the imaging differential diagnosis is relatively limited. Normal circulating blood is always slightly hyperdense compared to brain on NECT. A "hyperdense vessel" sign can be simulated by **elevated hematocrit** (all the vessels appear dense, not just the arteries), arterial wall **microcalcifications**, and **hypodense brain** parenchyma (e.g., diffuse cerebral edema).

The differential diagnosis of decreased perfusion on pCT includes **chronic infarct, severe microvascular ischemia,** and **extra- or intracranial stenosis** with decreased or delayed perfusion. Vascular stenoses can mimic or overestimate areas of ischemic penumbra, so

pCT should always be interpreted together with NECT and CTA.

Stroke "mimics" with restricted SWI include **infection** (does not follow defined arterial territories) and **status epilepticus** (affects cortex, spares underlying WM).

ACUTE STROKE: IMAGING

NECT
- Hyperdense vessel ± "dot" sign
- "Blurred," effaced GM-WM borders
  - "Insular ribbon" sign
  - "Disappearing" basal ganglia
- Wedge-shaped hypodensity
  - Involves both cortex, WM

CECT
- ± enhancing vessels (slow flow, collaterals)

CTA
- Site, length of thrombus
- ASVD
  - Extracranial: Aorta, carotid bifurcation
  - Intracranial: Cavernous ICA, COW + branches

pCT
- Infarct core (irreversibly damaged brain)
  - Matched perfusion (CBV, CBF both ↓)
  - ↑ MTT
- Ischemic penumbra
  - Perfusion "mismatch" (↓ CBF but normal CBV)

T1WI
- Usually normal in first 4-6 hours
- ± loss of expected "flow void"

T2WI
- Usually normal in first 4-6 hours

FLAIR (use narrow windows)
- 50% positive in first 4-6 hours
  - Cortical swelling, gyral hyperintensity
  - Intraarterial hyperintensity (usually slow flow, not thrombus)

T2* (GRE, SWI)
- Thrombus may "bloom"
- Microbleeds (chronic HTN, amyloid): ↑ risk of hemorrhage with anticoagulation

DWI and DTI
- > 95% restriction within minutes
  - Hyperintense on DWI
  - Hypointense on ADC map
- "Diffusion-negative" acute strokes
  - Small (lacunar) infarcts
  - Brainstem lesions
  - Rapid clot lysis/recanalization
  - Transient/fluctuating hypoperfusion

pMR
- DWI-PWI "mismatch" estimates penumbra

DSA
- Vessel "cut-off," "meniscus" sign, tapered/"rat-tail" narrowing
- "Bare" area of unperfused brain
- Slow antegrade or retrograde filling
- Delayed intraarterial contrast washout
- Luxury perfusion
  - "Blush" around "bare area"
  - "Early draining" veins

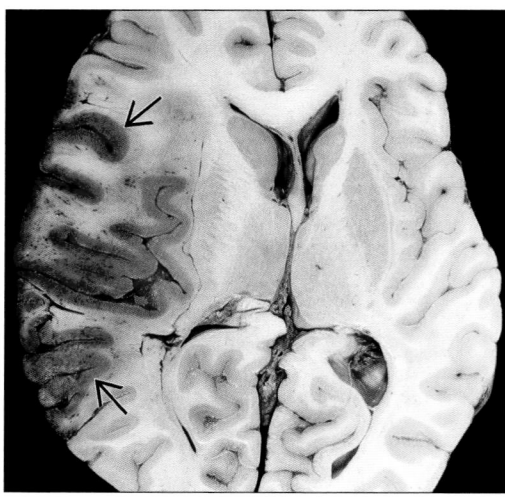

8-43. *Subacute stroke with mass effect, gyriform hemorrhagic transformation* ➡. *(Courtesy R. Hewlett, MD.)*

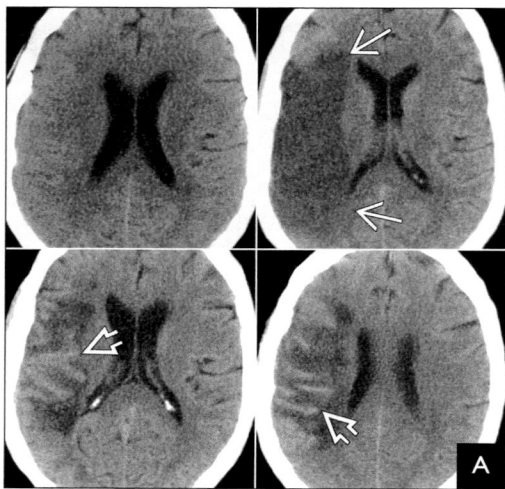

8-44A. *(Top left) NECT at 2 h shows mild sulcal effacement. At 48 h, wedge-shaped hypodensity* ➡ *involves GM, WM. (Bottom) HT* ➡ *at 1 week.*

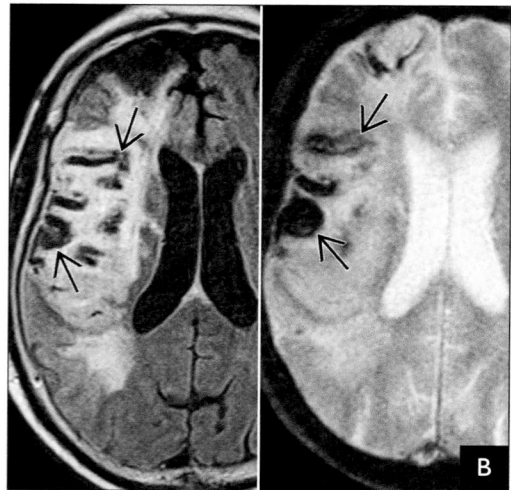

8-44B. *FLAIR (left) and GRE (right) in the same case show hemorrhagic transformation* ➡ *in this example of subacute stroke.*

Subacute Cerebral Infarcts

Terminology

Strokes evolve pathophysiologically with corresponding changes reflected on imaging studies. Although there are no firm divisions that demarcate the various stages of stroke evolution, most neurologists designate infarcts as acute, subacute, and chronic.

"Subacute" cerebral ischemia/infarction generally refers to strokes that are between 48 hours and two weeks following the initial ischemic event (8-43).

Pathology

Edema and **increasing mass effect** caused by cytotoxic edema become maximal within three to four days following stroke onset. Frank tissue necrosis with progressive influx of microglia and macrophages around vessels ensues with reactive astrocytosis around the perimeter of the stroke. Brain softening and then cavitation proceeds over the next two weeks.

Most thromboembolic strokes are initially "bland," i.e., nonhemorrhagic. **Hemorrhagic transformation** (HT) of a previously ischemic infarct occurs in 20-25% of cases between two days and a week after ictus. Ischemia-damaged vascular endothelium becomes "leaky," and blood-brain barrier permeability increases. When reperfusion is established—either spontaneously or following treatment with tissue plasminogen activator—exudation of red blood cells through the damaged blood vessel walls causes parenchymal hemorrhages. Petechial hemorrhages are more common than lobar bleeds and are most common in the basal ganglia and cortex.

Clinical Issues

HT itself generally does not cause clinical deterioration. HT is actually related to favorable outcome, probably reflecting early vessel recanalization and better tissue reperfusion.

Imaging

GENERAL FEATURES. There are significant variations within the subacute time period. Early subacute strokes have significant mass effect and often exhibit HT whereas edema and mass effect have mostly subsided by the late subacute period.

CT FINDINGS. On NECT, the wedge-shaped area of decreased attenuation seen on initial scans becomes more sharply defined. Mass effect initially increases, then begins to decrease by 7-10 days following stroke onset. HT develops in 15-20% of cases and is seen as gyriform cortical or basal ganglia hyperdensity (8-44A).

CECT follows a "2-2-2" rule. Patchy or gyriform enhancement appears as early as two days after stroke onset, peaks at two weeks, and generally disappears by two months.

MR FINDINGS. Signal intensity in subacute stroke varies depending on (1) time since ictus and (2) the presence or absence of hemorrhagic transformation.

T1WI. Nonhemorrhagic subacute infarcts are hypointense on T1WI and demonstrate moderate mass effect with sulcal effacement. Strokes with HT are initially isointense with cortex and then become hyperintense **(8-45A)**.

T2WI. Subacute infarcts are initially hyperintense compared to nonischemic brain. Signal intensity decreases with time, reaching isointensity at one to two weeks (the T2 "fogging effect") **(8-46)**. Early wallerian degeneration can sometimes be identified as a well-delineated hyperintense band that extends inferiorly from the infarcted cortex along the corticospinal tract.

FLAIR. Subacute infarcts are hyperintense on FLAIR **(8-44B)**. By one week after ictus, "final" infarct volume corresponds to the FLAIR-defined abnormality.

T2* (GRE, SWI). Petechial or gyriform "blooming" foci are present if HT has occurred in the infarcted cortex **(8-44B)**. Basal ganglia hemorrhages can be confluent or petechial.

T1 C+. The intravascular enhancement often seen in the first 48 hours following thromboembolic occlusion disappears within three or four days and is replaced by leptomeningeal enhancement caused by persisting pial collateral blood flow. Patchy or gyriform parenchymal enhancement can occur as early as two or three days after infarction and may persist for two to three months **(8-45B)**.

DWI. Restricted diffusion with hyperintensity on DWI and hypointensity on ADC persists for the first several days following stroke onset, then gradually reverses to become hypointense on DWI and hyperintense with T2 "shine-through" on ADC.

Differential Diagnosis

The major differential diagnosis of subacute cerebral infarction is **neoplasm**. Most tumors do not restrict on DWI and do not regress with time. Evolution of imaging findings in stroke occurs much more rapidly. **Infections** (e.g., encephalitis and cerebritis) can appear similar to subacute strokes but do not follow defined vascular distributions.

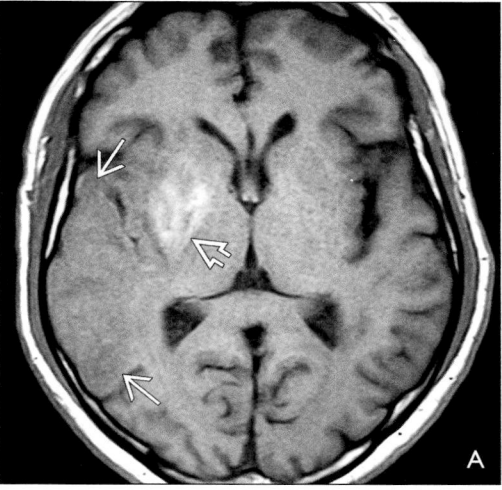

8-45A. Axial T1WI at 2 weeks after stroke onset shows hemorrhagic BG transformation ⇒, persisting gyral swelling with sulcal effacement ⇒.

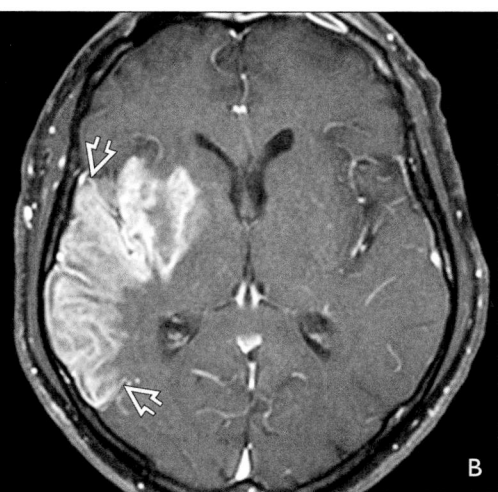

8-45B. T1 C+ FS scan in the same patient shows intense enhancement ⇒ characteristic of subacute infarction.

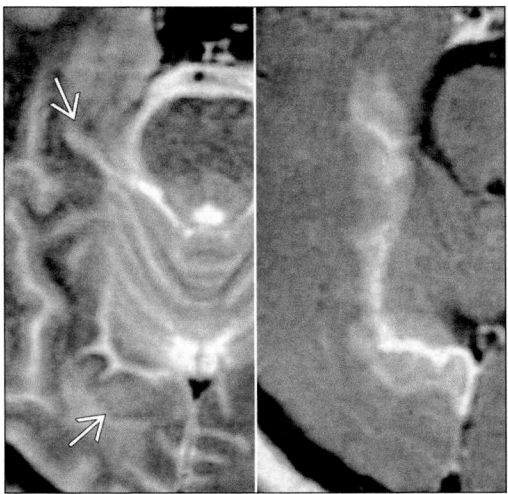

8-46. T2 "fogging effect" ⇒ (left) indicates R PCA infarct is almost isointense, but it enhances strongly on T1 C+ (right). Subacute stroke.

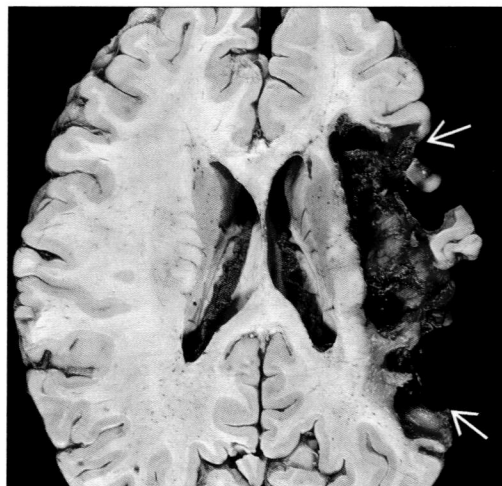

8-47. Autopsy specimen shows encephalomalacia from an old left MCA infarct ➡. (Courtesy R. Hewlett, MD.)

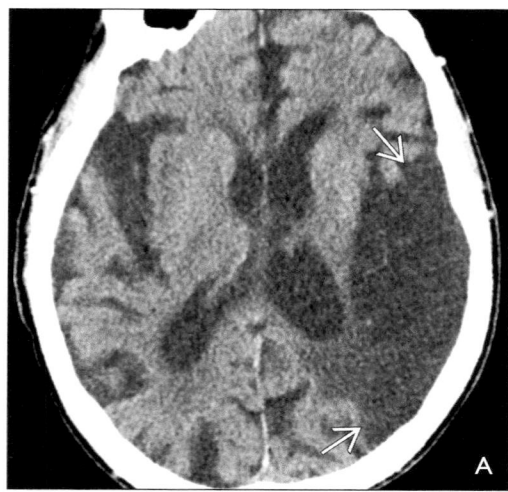

8-48A. NECT in a patient with remote stroke shows encephalomalacia in the left MCA distribution ➡. Basal ganglia were spared.

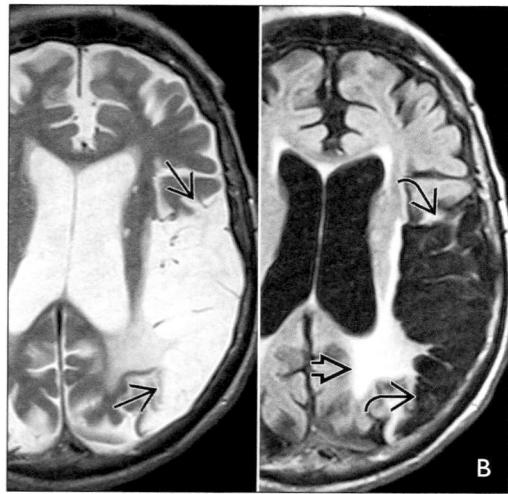

8-48B. (L) T2WI shows hyperintensity ➡ in the same distribution. (R) FLAIR shows the difference between encephalomalacia ➘, gliosis ➦.

Chronic Cerebral Infarcts

Terminology

Chronic cerebral infarcts are the end result of ischemic territorial strokes and are also called post-infarction encephalomalacia.

Pathology

The pathologic hallmark of chronic cerebral infarcts is volume loss with gliosis in an anatomic vascular distribution. A cavitated, encephalomalacic brain with strands of residual glial tissue and traversing blood vessels is the usual gross appearance of an old infarct (8-47).

Imaging

NECT scans show a sharply delineated wedge-shaped hypodense area that involves both gray (GM) and white (WM) matter and conforms to the vascular territory of a cerebral artery. The adjacent sulci and ipsilateral ventricle enlarge secondary to volume loss in the affected hemisphere (8-48A).

Wallerian degeneration with an ipsilateral small, shrunken cerebral peduncle is often present with large MCA infarcts. Look for atrophy of the contralateral cerebellum secondary to crossed cerebellar diaschisis. Dystrophic calcification is unusual, even with old hemorrhagic strokes.

Chronic infarcts older than two to three months typically do not enhance on CECT.

MR scans show cystic encephalomalacia with CSF-equivalent signal intensity on all sequences. Marginal gliosis or spongiosis around the old cavitated stroke is hyperintense on FLAIR (8-48B). DWI shows increased diffusivity (hyperintense on ADC).

Differential Diagnosis

The major differential diagnosis of chronic cerebral infarction is a **porencephalic cyst**. Porencephalic cysts typically involve the full thickness of brain, extending from the ventricle to the subpial surface of the cortex. **Post-traumatic encephalomalacia** usually shows other areas of damage and is not restricted to a vascular territory. **Postsurgical changes** also demonstrate other postoperative findings such as skull/scalp defects.

Multiple Embolic Infarcts

Cardiac and Atheromatous Emboli

PATHOETIOLOGY. Simultaneous small infarcts in multiple different vascular distributions are characteristic of embolic cerebral infarcts (8-49), (8-50). The heart is the most common source; cardiac emboli can be septic or aseptic. Peripheral signs of emboli such as splinter hemorrhages are sometimes present. Echocardiography may demonstrate valvular vegetations, intracardiac filling defect, or atrial or ventricular septal defect.

Ipsilateral hemispheric emboli are most commonly due to atheromatous internal carotid artery plaques (8-52). Many are clinically silent but convey a high risk for subsequent overt stroke.

IMAGING. In contrast to large artery territorial strokes, embolic infarcts tend to involve terminal cortical branches. The GM-WM interface is most commonly affected.

NECT scans show low-attenuation foci, often in a wedge-shaped distribution. Atherosclerotic emboli occasionally demonstrate calcification. Septic emboli are often hemorrhagic (8-51A). CECT scans may demonstrate multiple punctate or ring-enhancing lesions.

MR scans show multifocal peripheral T2/FLAIR hyperintensities. Hemorrhagic emboli cause "blooming" on T2* sequences. The most sensitive sequence is DWI.

Small peripheral foci of diffusion restriction in several different vascular distributions are typical of multiple embolic infarcts (8-51B). T1 C+ imaging shows multiple punctate enhancing foci. Septic emboli often demonstrate ring enhancement, resembling numerous microabscesses.

DIFFERENTIAL DIAGNOSIS. The major differential diagnosis of multiple embolic infarcts is **hypotensive cerebral infarction** (see below). Hypotensive infarcts are usually caused by hemodynamic compromise and tend to involve the deep internal watershed zones. **Parenchymal metastases** have a predilection for the GM-WM interface, as do embolic infarcts, but generally do not restrict on DWI.

Fat Emboli

Fat embolism syndrome (FES) is an uncommon disorder that presents as hypoxia, neurologic symptoms, and/or a petechial rash in the setting of severely displaced lower extremity long bone fractures. The term "cerebral fat emboli" (CFE) refers to the neurologic manifestations of FES.

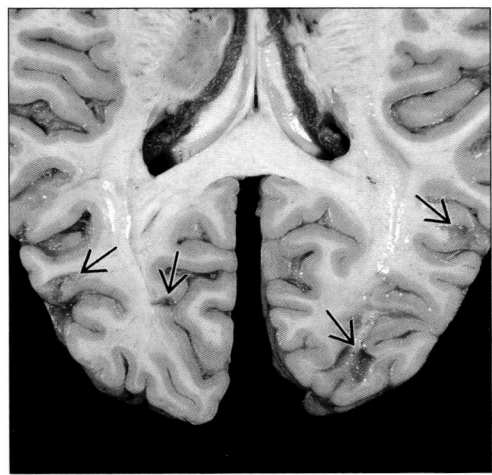

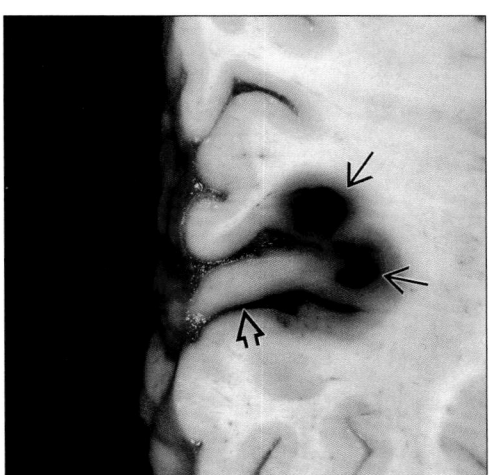

8-49. *Autopsy specimen shows multiple old healed infarcts at the gray-white matter junctions* ➡️. *(Courtesy R. Hewlett, MD.)* 8-50. *Close-up view of an autopsy specimen from a patient with infective endocarditis and septicemia shows hemorrhagic septic infarcts at the GM-WM junction* ➡️. *Focal subarachnoid hemorrhage is present in the adjacent sulci* ➡️. *(Courtesy R. Hewlett, MD.)*

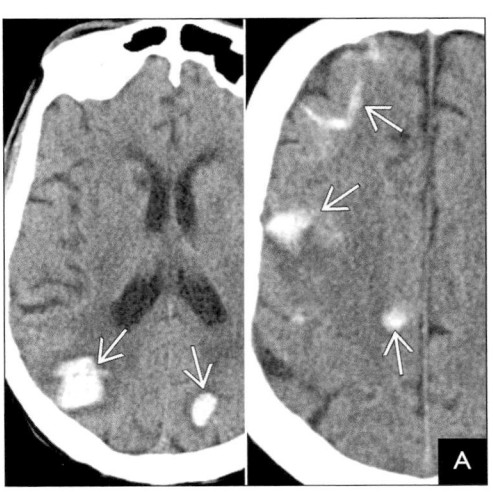

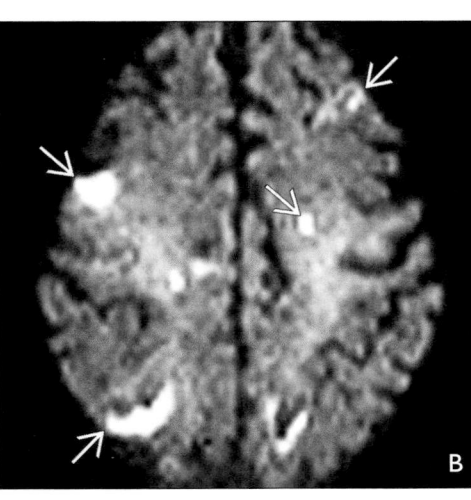

8-51A. *(Left) NECT scan in a patient with infected mitral valve, decreasing mental status shows 2 hemorrhagic foci* ➡️ *at the GM-WM junctions of both occipital lobes. (Right) Scan through the corona radiata shows additional hemorrhagic foci* ➡️. *Findings suggest multiple septic emboli.* 8-51B. *DWI shows multiple foci of restricted diffusion* ➡️ *at the GM-WM junctions of both hemispheres. Multiple embolic septic infarcts.*

8-52A. *Axial FLAIR scan in an 82-year-old man with sudden onset of left upper extremity weakness and numbness shows several scattered hyperintensities in the right parietal cortex* ➔. **8-52B.** *DWI in the same patient shows multiple small peripheral foci of diffusion restriction* ➔. *The left hemisphere appears completely normal.*

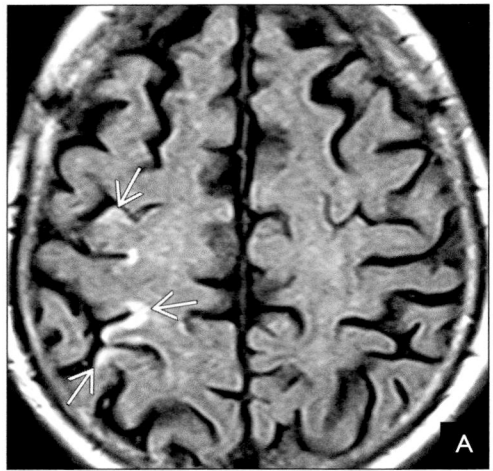
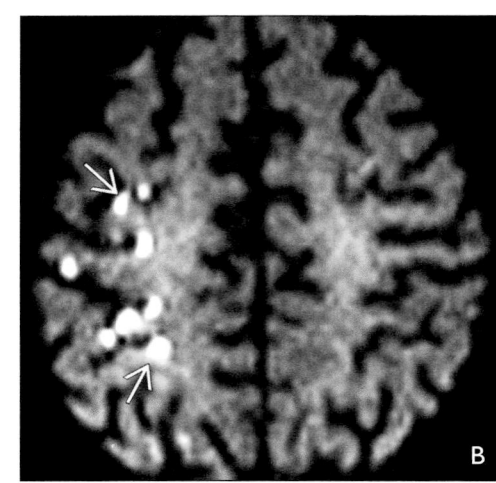

8-52C. *CTA source image in the same patient shows a densely calcified* ➔ *atherosclerotic plaque at the right carotid bifurcation. Lucency within the plaque* ➔ *suggests that it is an "at-risk" plaque.* **8-52D.** *Sagittal reconstruction shows that the calcified* ➔, *lucent* ➔ *atherosclerotic plaque causes a high-grade stenosis* ➔ *in the proximal right internal carotid artery. The multiple cortical infarcts seen on the MR were probably caused by artery-to-artery emboli.*

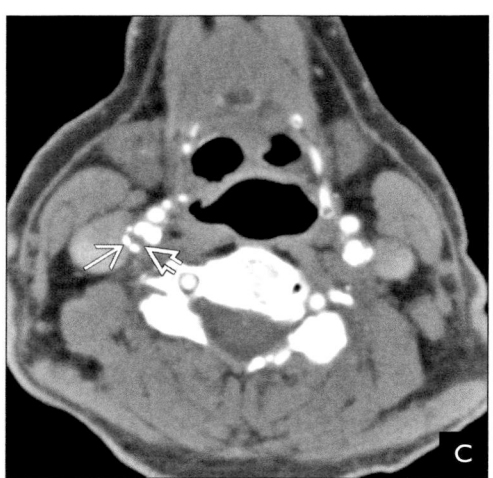
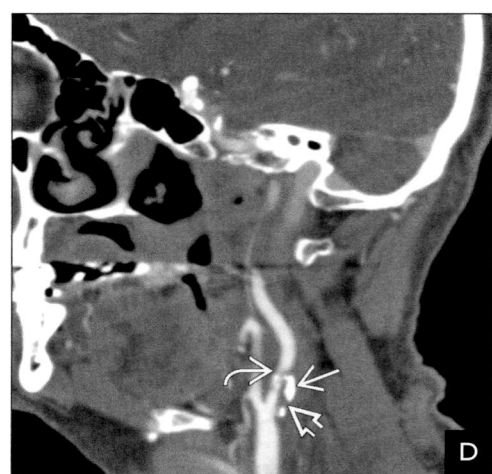

8-52E. *Axial NECT scan 3 days later shows well-demarcated focal cortical/subcortical hypodensities* ➔, *consistent with embolic infarction.* **8-52F.** *More cephalad axial NECT scan shows additional hypodensities* ➔ *corresponding to the FLAIR abnormalities that were identified on the prior MR scan. Unilateral embolic infarcts are most commonly secondary to atherosclerotic disease in the ipsilateral carotid artery.*

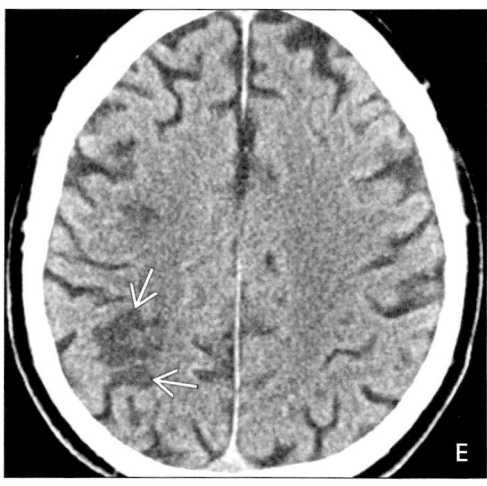
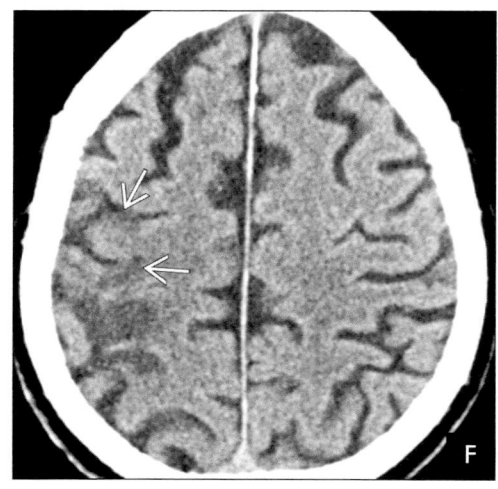

PATHOETIOLOGY. Two mechanisms have been proposed to explain the effects of FES: (1) small vessel occlusions from fat particles and (2) inflammatory changes in surrounding tissue initiated by breakdown of fat into free fatty acids and other metabolic by-products.

The pathologic hallmark of CFE is arteriolar fat emboli with perivascular microhemorrhages.

EPIDEMIOLOGY AND CLINICAL ISSUES. The overall incidence of FES in patients with long bone fractures—most commonly the femoral neck—is 0.17%. FES also occurs with elective orthopedic procedures (e.g., total hip arthroplasty), anesthesia, and systemic illness (e.g., pancreatitis).

CFE occurs in up to 80% of patients with FES. Signs and symptoms vary in severity and include headache, seizure, altered mental status, paralysis, and coma. Onset is from two hours up to two days after trauma or surgery, with a mean of 29 hours.

IMAGING. Imaging findings reflect the *effect* of the fat emboli (i.e., multifocal tiny strokes and microhemor-

rhages) on brain tissue, not the fat itself. NECT scans are therefore usually normal.

MR shows numerous (average = 50) punctate or confluent hyperintensities in the basal ganglia, periventricular WM, and GM-WM junctions on T2/FLAIR **(8-53A)**. DWI shows innumerable tiny punctate foci of diffusion restriction in multiple vascular distributions, the "star field" pattern **(8-53B)**. Solitary or multiple small hypointense "blooming" foci can be identified in up to one-third of all FES cases on T2* GRE **(8-53C)**. SWI discloses innumerable (> 200) tiny "black dots" in the majority of patients **(8-53D)**.

DIFFERENTIAL DIAGNOSIS. The major differential diagnosis of cerebral fat embolism syndrome is **multiple embolic infarcts**. Multiple cardiac or atheromatous embolic infarcts rarely produce the dozens or even hundreds of lesions seen with CFE. Lesions tend to involve the basal ganglia and corticomedullary junctions more than the white matter.

Multifocal "blooming" hypointensities on T2* can be seen with severe **diffuse axonal injury (DAI)** or **diffuse**

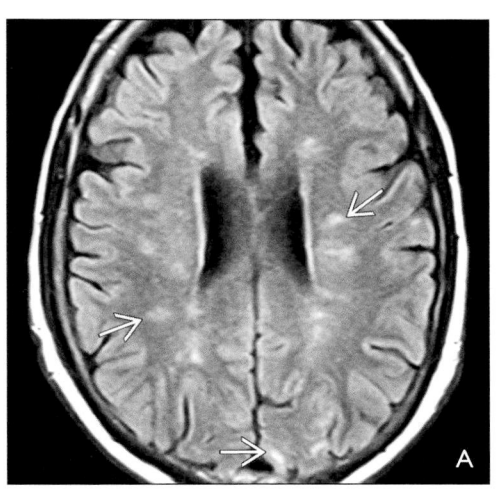
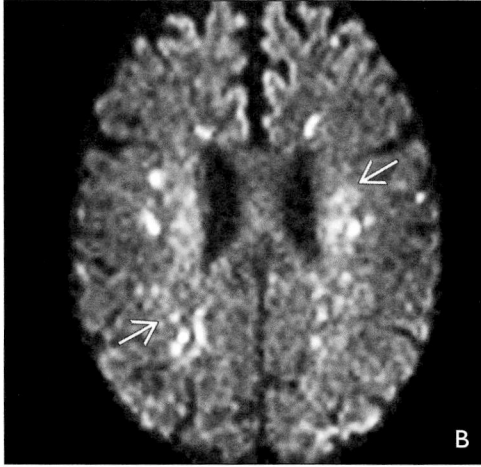

8-53A. Axial FLAIR scan in a 68-year-old man who became confused and then comatose the day after a total hip replacement shows multifocal hyperintensities ➡ *in the subcortical and deep cerebral white matter. 8-53B. DWI shows innumerable tiny foci of diffusion restriction in the deep cerebral white matter* ➡*, the "star field" pattern characteristic of cerebral fat embolism syndrome.*

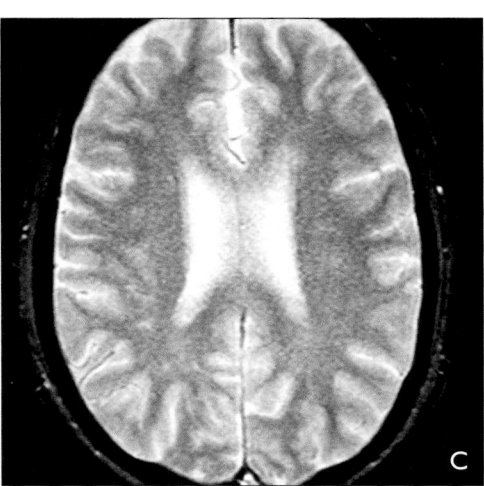
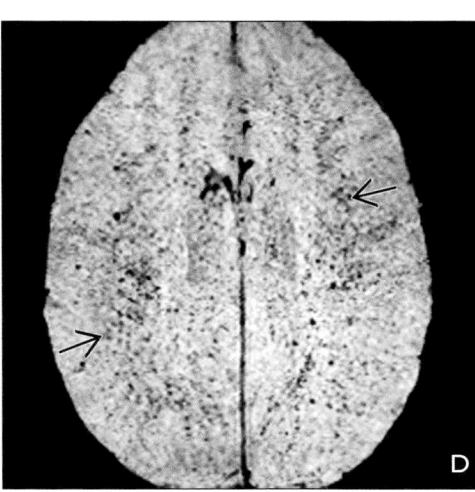

8-53C. T2 GRE scan in the same patient appears normal. 8-53D. SWI scan in the same patient shows hundreds of "blooming" hypointensities* ➡ *scattered throughout the cerebral white matter. In the setting of total hip arthroplasty, these represent microhemorrhages caused by cerebral fat embolism.*

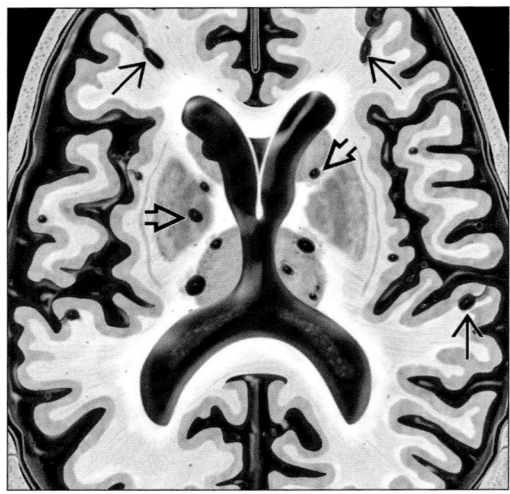

8-54. *Graphic shows lacunar infarctions in thalami, basal ganglia ⊵. Note also prominent perivascular (Virchow-Robin) spaces ⊵.*

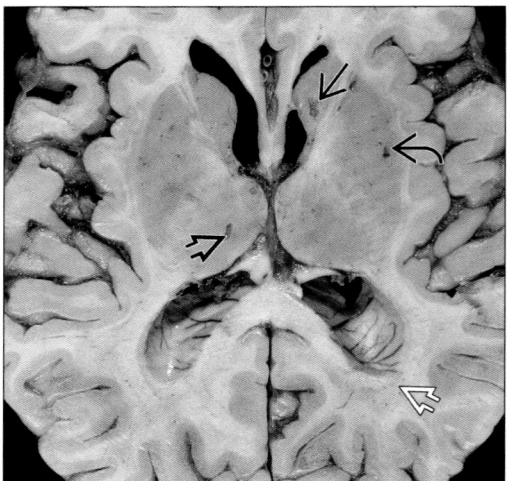

8-55. *Autopsy shows old lacunar infarcts in the caudate ⊵, putamen ⊵, thalamus ⊵, periatrial WM rarefaction ⊵. (Courtesy R. Hewlett, MD.)*

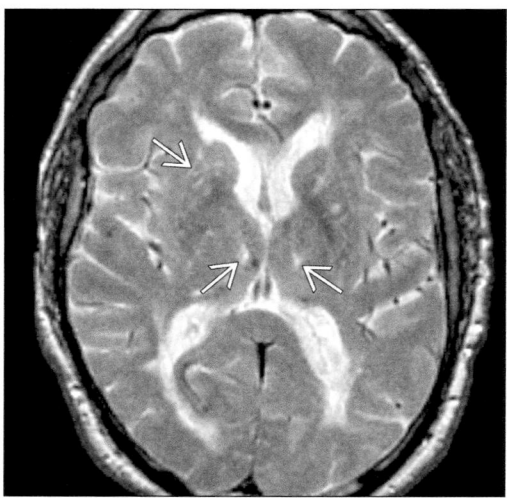

8-56. *Axial T2WI shows multiple lacunae ⊵ in the basal ganglia and thalami.*

vascular injury (DVI). As patients with CFE often have polytrauma, the distinction may be difficult on the basis of imaging studies alone. DAI and DVI tend to cause linear as well as punctate microbleeds.

Lacunar Infarcts

Terminology

The terms "lacuna," "lacunar infarct," and "lacunar stroke" are often used interchangeably. **Lacunae** are 3-15 mm CSF-filled cavities or "holes" that most often occur in the basal ganglia or cerebral white matter **(8-54)**. They are often observed coincidentally on imaging studies in older patients but are not clearly associated with discrete neurological symptoms, i.e., they are subclinical strokes. Lacunae are sometimes called "silent" strokes, a misnomer as subtle neuropsychological impairment is common in these patients.

Lacunar stroke means a clinically evident stroke syndrome attributed to a small subcortical or brainstem lesion that may or may not be evident on brain imaging. The term "état lacunaire" or **lacunar state** designates multiple lacunar infarcts.

Epidemiology and Etiology

Approximately 25% of all ischemic strokes are lacuna-type infarcts. Lacunae are considered macroscopic markers of cerebral small vessel ("microvascular") disease. They are typically caused by lipohyalinosis and atherosclerotic occlusion of perforating branches that arise from the circle of Willis and peripheral cortical arteries. These perforators are very small end arteries with few collaterals. Embolic lacunar infarcts are relatively uncommon.

Pathology

LOCATION. Lacunar infarcts are most common in the basal ganglia (putamen, globus pallidus, caudate nucleus), thalami, internal capsule, deep cerebral white matter, and pons **(8-55)**.

SIZE AND NUMBER. Lacunae are, by definition, 15 mm or less in diameter. Multiple lesions are common. Between 13-15% of patients have multiple simultaneous acute lacunar infarcts.

GROSS AND MICROSCOPIC APPEARANCE. Grossly, lacunae appear as small, pale, irregular but relatively well-delineated cystic cavities. Brown-staining siderotic discoloration can be seen in old hemorrhagic lacunae. Microscopically, ischemic lacunar infarcts demonstrate tissue rarefaction with neuronal loss, peripheral macrophage infiltration, and gliosis.

Clinical Issues

Independent risk factors for lacunar infarcts include age, hypertension, and diabetes.

Outcome of lacunar stroke is highly variable. Although most lacunae are asymptomatic, "little strokes" can mean "big trouble." A single subclinical stroke—often a lacuna—is associated with increased likelihood of having additional "little strokes" as well as developing overt clinical stroke and/or dementia. Nearly 20% of patients over 65 with white matter hyperintensities (WMHs) on T2/FLAIR MR will develop new lacunae within three years.

Between 20-30% of patients with lacunar stroke experience neurologic deterioration hours or even days after the initial event. The pathophysiology of "progressive lacunar stroke" is incompletely understood, and no treatment has been proven to prevent or halt progression.

Imaging

Imaging findings vary with whether the lacuna is acute or chronic. Acute lacunae may be invisible on NECT scans; old lacunae appear as well-defined CSF-like "holes" in the brain parenchyma.

Cavitation and lesion shrinkage are seen in more than 95% of deep symptomatic lacunar infarcts on follow-up imaging. Old lacunar infarcts are hypointense on T1- and hyperintense on T2WI **(8-56)**. The fluid in the cavity suppresses on FLAIR while the gliotic periphery remains hyperintense **(8-57)**. Multifocal white matter disease, seen as WMHs, is also common in patients with frank lacunar infarcts.

Most lacunae are nonhemorrhagic. However, parenchymal microbleeds—multifocal "blooming black dots" on T2* (GRE, SWI)—are common comorbidities in patients with lacunar infarcts and chronic hypertension.

Acute lacunar infarcts restrict on DWI, but acute DWI significantly overestimates final infarct size. Acute/early subacute lacunae may enhance on T1 C+.

Differential Diagnosis

The major differential diagnosis of lacunar infarct is **prominent perivascular spaces** (PVSs). Also known as

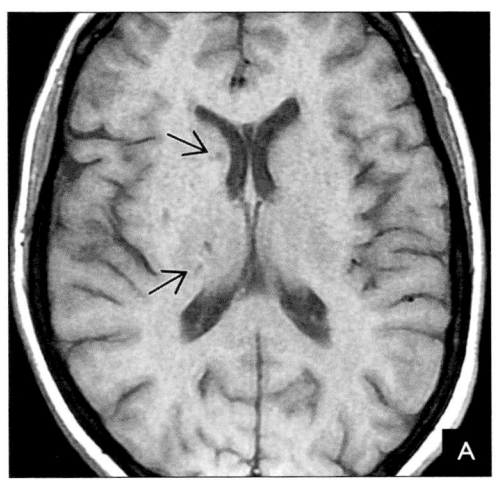

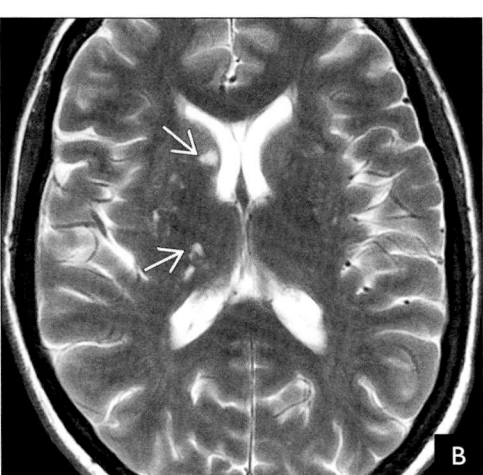

8-57A. Axial T1WI in a 43-year-old woman with a long history of drug abuse shows multiple hypointensities in the basal ganglia, thalami, and deep cerebral white matter ➔. *8-57B. Axial T2WI in the same patient demonstrates the characteristic hyperintensity and irregular shape of typical lacunar infarcts* ➔.

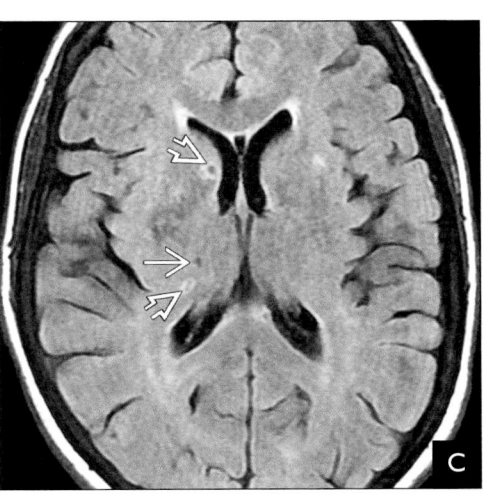

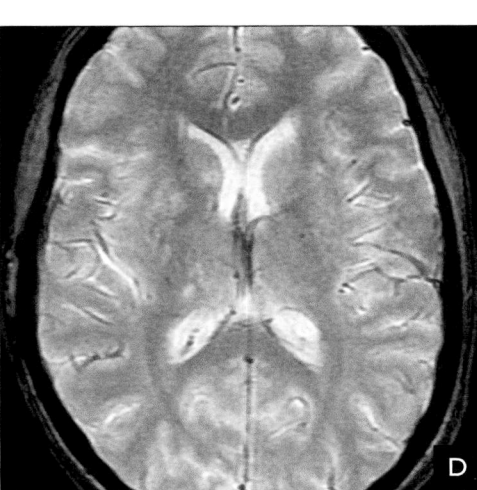

8-57C. FLAIR scan in the same patient shows that older lacunae suppress completely ➔ *whereas more recent lesions have a hyperintense rim of gliotic tissue surrounding a hypointense center* ➔ *that is not yet completely CSF-like. 8-57D. T2* GRE scan shows no evidence of hemorrhage.*

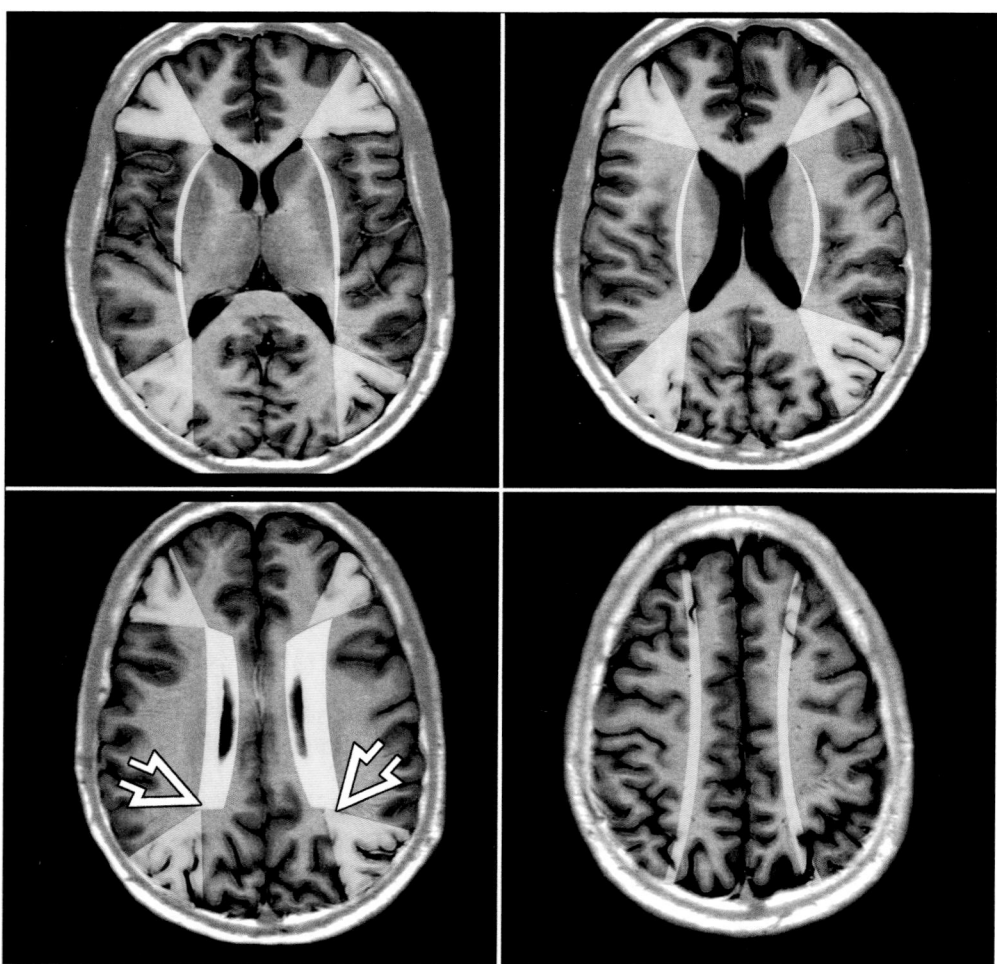

8-58. *T1-weighted images show 2 vascular watershed (WS) zones with external (cortical) WS zones in turquoise. Wedge-shaped areas between the ACAs, MCAs, PCAs represent "border zones" between the 3 major terminal vascular distributions. Curved blue lines (lower right) represent subcortical WS. The triple "border zones"* ⇒ *represent confluence of all 3 major vessels. Yellow lines indicate the internal (deep WM) WS zone between perforating arteries, major territorial vessels.*

Virchow-Robin spaces, prominent PVSs are pia-lined, interstitial fluid-filled spaces. Prominent PVSs can be found in virtually all locations and in patients of all ages, though they tend to increase in size and frequency with age. The most common locations for PVSs are the inferior third of the basal ganglia (clustered around the anterior commissure), subcortical white matter (including the external capsule), and the midbrain (see Chapter 28).

PVSs are sharply marginated and ovoid, linear, or round; lacunae tend to be more irregularly shaped. PVSs faithfully follow CSF signal intensity on all MR sequences and suppress completely on FLAIR. The adjacent brain is typically normal although a thin rim of FLAIR hyperintensity around the PVSs is present in 25% of cases.

Watershed or **"border zone" infarcts** grossly resemble lacunar infarcts on imaging studies. However, "border zone" infarcts occur in specific locations—along the cortical and subcortical white matter watershed zones—whereas lacunae are more randomly scattered

lesions that primarily affect the basal ganglia, thalami, and deep periventricular white matter.

The WMHs associated with **microvascular disease** (primarily lipohyalinosis and arteriolosclerosis) are less well-defined and usually more patchy or confluent than the small (< 15 mm) lesions that represent true lacunar infarcts. WMHs tend to cluster around the occipital horns and periventricular white matter, not the basal ganglia and thalami.

A few scattered T2/FLAIR hyperintensities are common in the **normal aging brain**. A general guideline is "one white spot per decade" until the age of 50, after which the number and size of WMHs increase at accelerated rates.

Watershed ("Border Zone") Infarcts

Terminology and Epidemiology

Watershed (WS) infarcts, also known as "border zone" infarcts, are ischemic lesions that occur in the junction between two nonanastamosing distal arterial distributions. WS infarcts are more common than generally recognized, constituting 10-12% of all brain infarcts.

Anatomy of the Cerebral "Border Zones"

Watershed zones are defined as the "border" or junction where two or more major arterial territories meet. Two distinct types of vascular border zones are recognized: An external (cortical) WS zone and an internal (deep) WS zone **(8-58)**.

The two major **external WS zones** lie in the frontal cortex (between the ACA and MCA) and parietooccipital cortex (between the MCA and PCA). A strip of paramedian subcortical white matter near the vertex of the cerebral hemispheres is also considered part of the external WS.

The **internal WS zones** represent the junctions between penetrating branches (e.g., lenticulostriate arteries, medullary white matter perforating arteries, and anterior choroidal branches) and the major cerebral vessels (MCA, ACA, and PCA) **(8-59)**.

Etiology

Two distinct hypotheses—hemodynamic compromise and microembolism—have been proposed as the etiology of hemispheric watershed infarcts. Both are likely contributing factors.

Terminal vascular distributions normally have lower perfusion pressure than main arterial trunks. Maximal vulnerability to hypoperfusion is greatest where two distal arterial fields meet together. *Hypotension with or without severe arterial stenosis or occlusion can result in hemodynamic compromise.* Flow in the affected WS zone can be critically lowered, resulting in ischemia or frank infarction. The most susceptible "border zone" is the "triple watershed" where the ACA, MCA, and PCA all converge.

External WS infarcts are the more common type. Most external WS infarcts are *embolic.* Anterior cortical WS embolic infarcts often occur in concert with internal carotid atherosclerosis. External WS infarcts in all three "border zones" are less common and usually reflect *global hypoperfusion.*

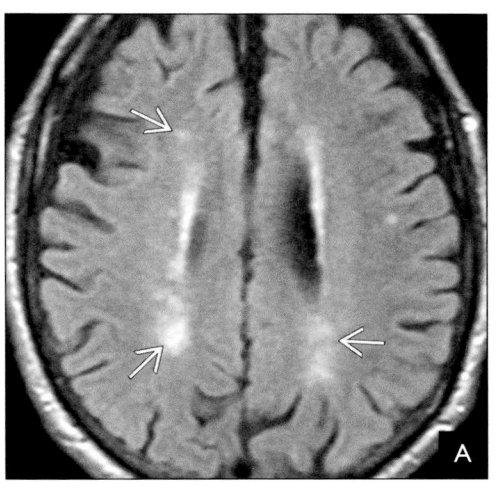

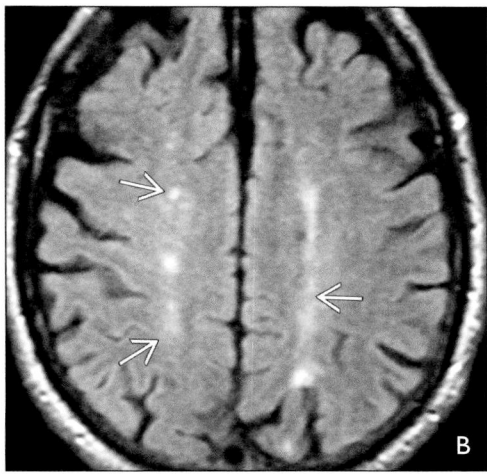

8-59A. *Nearly symmetric confluent and punctate deep white matter hyperintensities* ➡ *are seen above and behind the lateral ventricles in this middle-aged woman with left hemisphere TIAs.* **8-59B.** *FLAIR scan just above the previous image shows distinct bilateral rosary-like white matter hyperintensities* ➡.

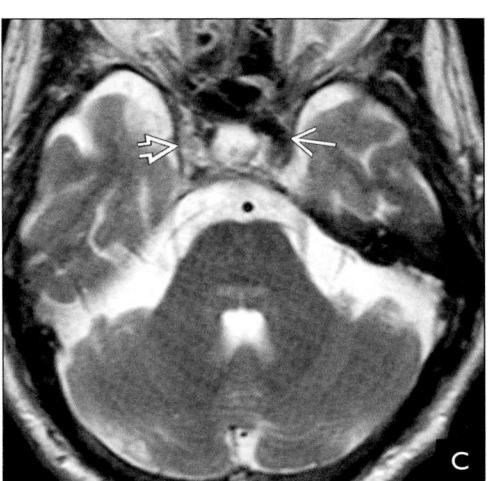

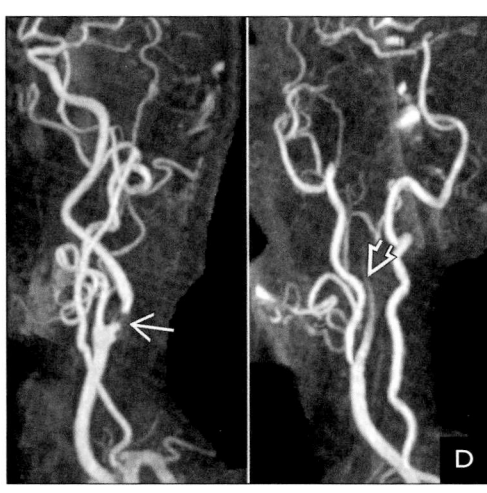

8-59C. *T2WI shows an absent "flow void" in the right cavernous ICA* ➡. *The left ICA appears normal* ➡, *yet this is the symptomatic side.* **8-59D.** *2D TOF MRA image findings explain the patient's symptoms. (L) Left ICA demonstrates a "flow gap"* ➡ *characteristic of high-grade carotid stenosis. (R) Right ICA is occluded, with "rat tail" narrowing* ➡. *Classic bilateral deep internal watershed zone hypoperfusion ischemia.*

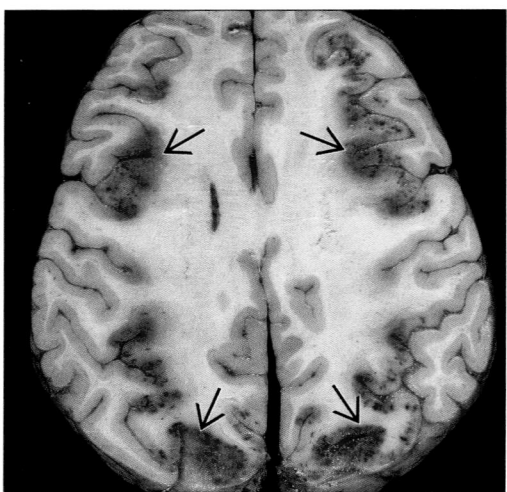

8-60. *Autopsy case shows classic external (cortical) watershed infarcts* ⇨.

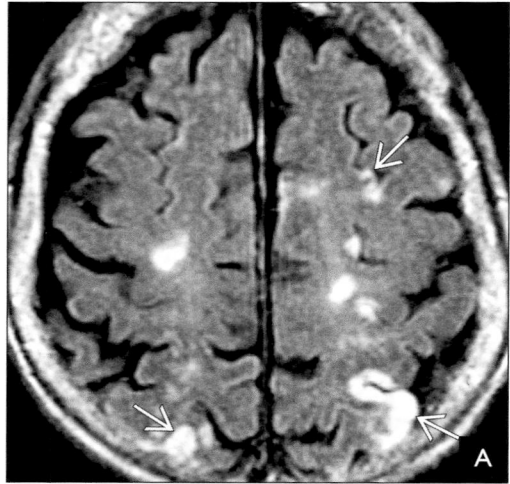

8-61A. *Axial FLAIR scan demonstrates typical findings of bilateral external (cortical) watershed infarcts* ⇨.

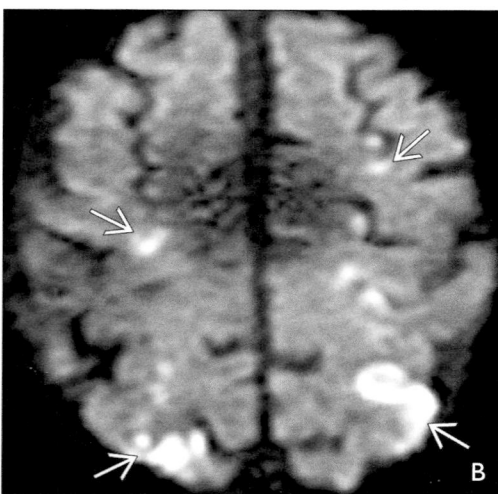

8-61B. *DWI shows multiple cortical punctate, gyriform foci of restricted diffusion* ⇨. *Hypotension with transient global hypoperfusion.*

Internal WS infarcts are rarely embolic. They represent 35-40% of all WS infarcts and are most often caused by *regional hypoperfusion* secondary to hemodynamic compromise (e.g., ipsilateral carotid stenosis).

Pathology

LOCATION. Distribution territories of the ACA, MCA, and PCA all vary considerably from individual to individual. WS infarcts likewise demonstrate moderate variability in location.

External (cortical) WS infarcts show a bimodal spatial distribution. Anteriorly, they center in the posterior frontal lobe near the junction of the frontal sulcus with the precentral sulcus. Posterior WS infarcts center in the superior parietal lobule posterolateral to the postcentral sulcus. The prevalence of WS infarcts decreases between these two areas. WS infarcts spare the medial cortex **(8-60)**.

Internal WS infarcts tend to "line up" in the white matter, parallel to and slightly above the lateral ventricles **(8-59)**. Cerebellar WS infarcts occur at the borders between the posterior inferior, anterior inferior, and superior cerebellar arteries.

SIZE AND NUMBER. WS infarcts vary in size from tiny lesions to large wedge-shaped ischemic areas. Multiple lesions are common and can be uni- or bilateral. Bilateral lesions are often related to global reduction in perfusion pressure, usually an acute hypotensive event.

Imaging

Imaging findings vary with WS infarct type. The main goals of neuroimaging in patients with WS infarcts are (1) to determine if hemodynamic impairment (i.e., vascular stenosis) is present and, if present, (2) to assess its severity.

EXTERNAL (CORTICAL) WS INFARCTS. Cortical (external) WS infarcts are wedge- or gyriform-shaped **(8-61)**.

INTERNAL WS INFARCTS. Internal "border zone" infarcts can be confluent or partial. Confluent infarcts are large, cigar-shaped lesions that lie alongside or just above the lateral ventricles. Partial infarcts are more discrete, rosary-like lesions. They resemble a line of beads extending from front to back in the deep white matter **(8-59A)**, **(8-59B)**.

Stenosis or occlusion of the ipsilateral internal carotid artery or MCA is common with unilateral lesions **(8-59C)**, **(8-59D)**. The presence and degree of hemodynamic impairment can be determined using a number of methods, including pCT, pMR, SPECT, and PET.

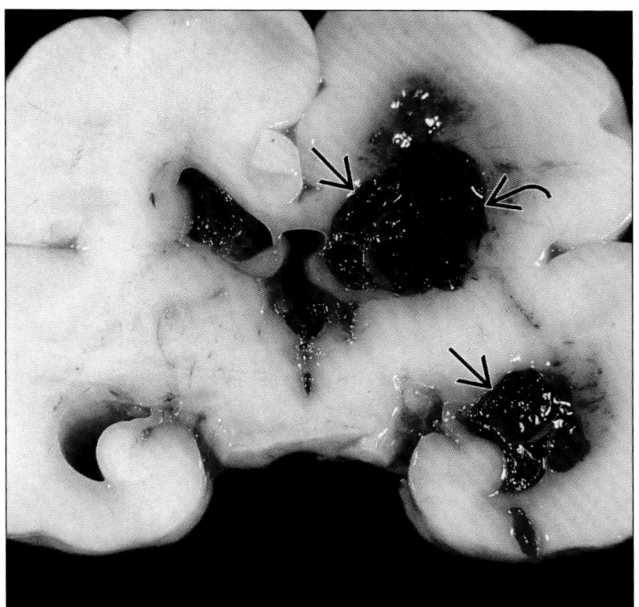

8-62. *Coronal autopsy specimen from a premature neonate shows grade III germinal matrix hemorrhage ⇗ with extension into an adjacent lateral ventricle ⇥.*

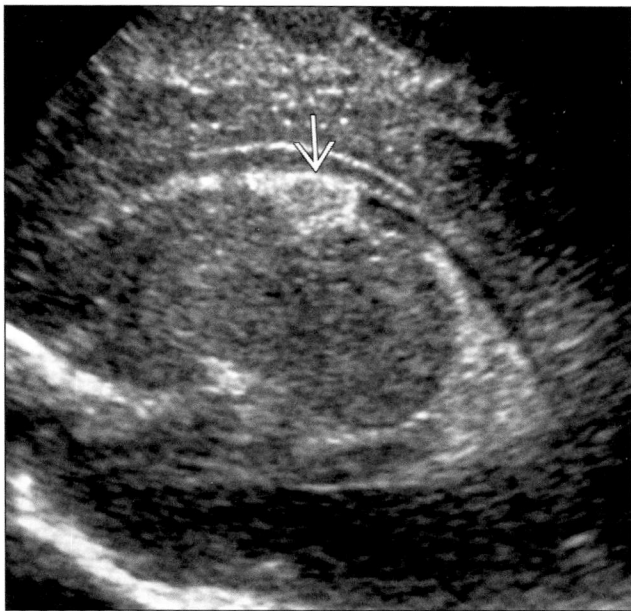

8-63. *Sagittal ultrasound in a premature infant demonstrates gray matter hemorrhage, seen as an echogenic focus in the caudothalamic notch ➥.*

Differential Diagnosis

The major differential diagnosis of WS infarction is **lacunar infarcts**. Lacunar infarcts typically involve the basal ganglia, thalami, and pons and appear randomly scattered. Multiple **embolic infarcts** can also closely resemble WS infarcts. Emboli are often bilateral and multiterritorial but can also occur at vascular "border zones."

Posterior reversible encephalopathy syndrome (PRES) typically occurs in the setting of acute hypertension. The cortex/subcortical white matter in the PCA distribution is most commonly affected, although PRES can also involve "border zones" and the basal ganglia. PRES rarely restricts on DWI (vasogenic edema) whereas "border zone" infarcts with cytotoxic edema show acute restriction.

WATERSHED ("BORDER ZONE") INFARCTS

Anatomy and Etiology
- 2 types of vascular "border zones"
  - External (cortical): Between ACA, MCA, PCA
  - Internal (deep WM): Between perforating branches, major arteries
- Etiology
  - Emboli (cortical more common)
  - Regional hypoperfusion (deep WM common)
  - Global hypoperfusion (all 3 cortical WS zones)

Imaging
- External: Wedge or gyriform
- Internal: Rosary-like line of WMHs

Hypoxic-Ischemic Injury

Hypoxic-ischemic brain injury is one of the most devastating of all brain insults. Death or severe lifelong neurologic deficits with profound functional impairment are common.

Cerebral ischemia is simply diminished blood flow. Ischemia can be focal or global. **Focal ischemia** refers to decreased or absent perfusion in a particular vascular territory, usually secondary to arterial stenosis or occlusion. Ischemia may or may not proceed to frank infarction, i.e., tissue death. **Global ischemia** occurs when overall cerebral perfusion drops below the level required to maintain normal brain function (e.g., with cardiac arrest).

Hypoxia or **hypoxemia** refers to reduced blood oxygenation. In contrast to ischemia, cerebral hypoxia is almost always global. In the initial stages of hypoxia, cardiac output and cerebral blood flow (CBF) may be maintained normally but blood oxygenation is deficient (e.g., carbon monoxide poisoning). Prolonged systemic hypoxemia results in cardiac hypoxia, which in turn diminishes output. Depressed cardiac output eventually causes global brain hypoperfusion and ischemia.

The term **global hypoxic-ischemic injury** (HII) is used to describe the pathologic and imaging findings of CNS hypoxia with or without *global* (not focal) brain ischemia. In practice, both factors often act in concert. In asphyxia, brain injury is a consequence of ischemia superimposed on hypoxia. Pure hypoxia in the absence

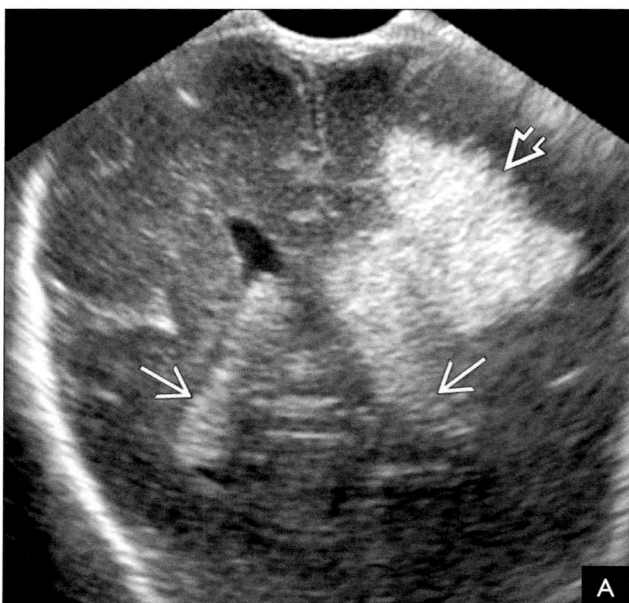

8-64A. *Oblique transfontanelle ultrasound in a 26-week premature infant shows periventricular hemorrhagic infarction (PVHI)* ⧩ *with extension into the lateral ventricles* ➥.

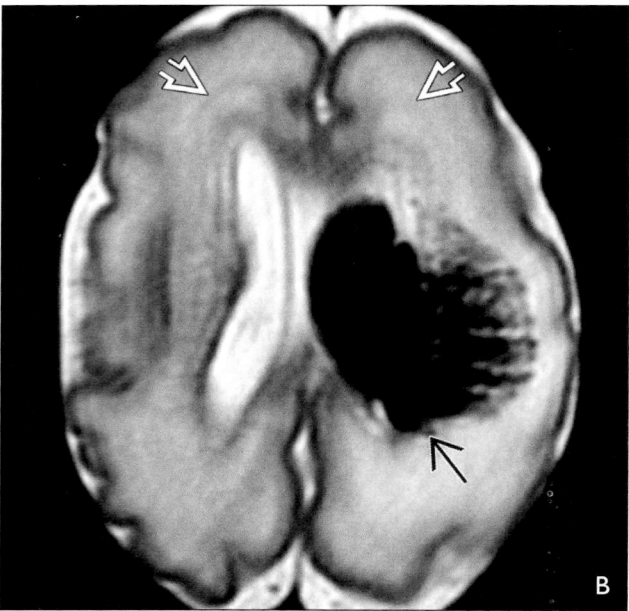

8-64B. *T2WI in the same patient shows PVHI* ➥ *and a faint dark line of neurons* ⧩ *migrating outward from the germinal matrix.*

of ischemia generally does not cause frank brain necrosis unless the hypoxic state is prolonged.

Focal ischemic disorders were discussed earlier in this chapter. Here we briefly delineate the manifestations of global brain HII. Imaging findings in HII are highly variable. The effect of HII on the mature brain of older children and adults differs significantly from its impact on the developing brain. Other factors such as insult duration and severity as well as timing of studies relative to onset also affect the imaging appearance of global cerebral HII.

Perinatal HII

Imaging findings in perinatal HII vary with insult severity, duration, and gestational age. The prenatal brain is developmentally immature, so imaging findings in these premature infants differ from findings in those born at or near term.

The spectrum of brain injury in preterm infants is surprisingly broad and includes not just HII but white matter injury of prematurity, germinal matrix hemorrhage, periventricular hemorrhagic infarction, intraventricular hemorrhage, and cerebellar injury.

HII IN PRETERM INFANTS. By definition, preterm infants are those born before 37 weeks of gestation. HII is more common in preterm neonates than in term infants. HII in preterm neonates causes approximately 50% of all cases of cerebral palsy (CP). Approximately 5% of infants < 32 weeks gestational age and 15-20% of infants born under 28 weeks develop CP.

The type of injury that may result from severe HII changes as the brain matures. Increased metabolic demand in concert with maturity of glutamate receptors changes the pattern of vulnerability to hypoxic-ischemic injury. **Severe HII** in preterm neonates preferentially affects the early myelinating and metabolically active thalami and brainstem, with relative sparing of the basal ganglia and cortex.

Imaging findings of **severe HII** in preterm infants caused by profound hypotension or circulatory arrest are variable. Increased echogenicity in the thalami at 48-72 hours is common on transcranial ultrasound. MR shows that the thalami, vermis, dorsal brainstem, lentiform nuclei, and perirolandic gyri are frequently involved. DWI abnormalities can be detected within 24 hours, although T2 prolongation and T1 shortening do not occur until a few days later.

Less profound HII causes germinal matrix hemorrhage (GMH) and intraventricular hemorrhage (IVH) and/or deep periventricular WM injury **(8-62)**. The prevalence of IVH in preterm neonates is inversely related to gestational age and birth weight. The prevalence in preterm neonates under 2,000 grams is approximately 25%.

The germinal matrix is a highly vascular structure that lies along the walls of the fetal lateral ventricles and external granular layer of the cerebellum. The germinal matrix is most prominent in the latter half of the first trimester and the second trimester. It gradually regresses during the third trimester and by 34 gestational weeks has almost completely involuted. The last area to involute—the ganglionic eminence—is located in the posterior aspect of the caudothalamic notch and is the site of most germinal matrix hemorrhages.

Peri- and intraventricular hemorrhages (including GMHs) are generally evaluated with cranial US **(8-63)**, **(8-64A)** and are divided into four grades that reflect (1) hemorrhage location (e.g., GM, ventricles) and (2) degree of ventriculomegaly (see box).

GRADING PERI- AND INTRAVENTRICULAR HEMORRHAGE IN PREMATURE INFANTS

Grade I
- Subependymal GMH (typically caudothalamic groove)
- No/minimal intraventricular extension

Grade II
- GMH + IVH (no/minimal ventriculomegaly)

Grade III
- GMH + IVH + ventriculomegaly

Grade IV
- Periventricular parenchymal hemorrhagic infarction
- Probably secondary to venous infarct
- *Not true GMH!*

White matter injury of prematurity (WMIP) was formerly called **periventricular leukomalacia** (PVL), even though it also affects gray matter. PVL basically represents end-stage WMIP. A more accurate but less commonly used description of WMIP is **encephalopathy of prematurity**.

White matter injury is common in premature infants. Prevalence is inversely related to gestational age at birth. WMIP is most likely related to the selective vulnerability of late oligodendrocyte precursor cells to lactic acidosis resulting from compromised vascular autoregulation.

White matter (WM) injury is most common adjacent to the foramen of Monro and lateral ventricle trigones; it can be noncavitary (more common) or cavitary. Frank WM necrosis may progress to cavitation and porencephalic cysts. Eventually the cysts collapse, leaving reduced gliotic white matter in the periventricular regions as the end-stage result.

The first findings on US are periventricular hyperechoic "flares" **(8-65)**. Frank periventricular cysts do not develop until three to six weeks. By six months, the cysts resolve, the ventricles enlarge, and end-stage PVL ensues.

MR initially shows periventricular T1 hypointensities and T2 hyperintensity **(8-66)**. Hemorrhage—present in nearly two-thirds of early-stage PVLs—is profoundly hypointense on T2WI **(8-64B)** and "blooms" on T2*. Because premature infants normally have higher lactate and lower NAA peaks than term infants, MRS may be difficult to interpret.

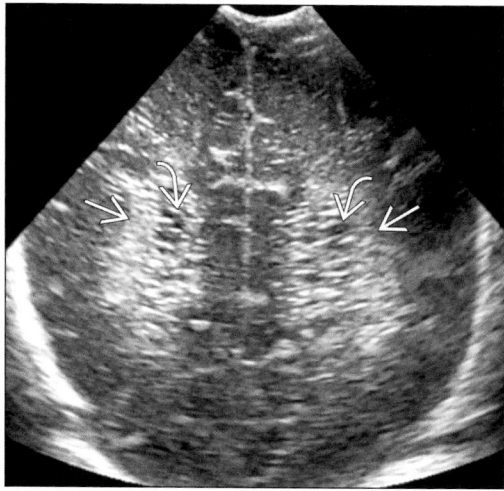

8-65. *US in a 34-week GA infant at 17 postnatal days shows WMIP with diffuse WM echogenicity* ➡️*, early cavitation* ➡️*.*

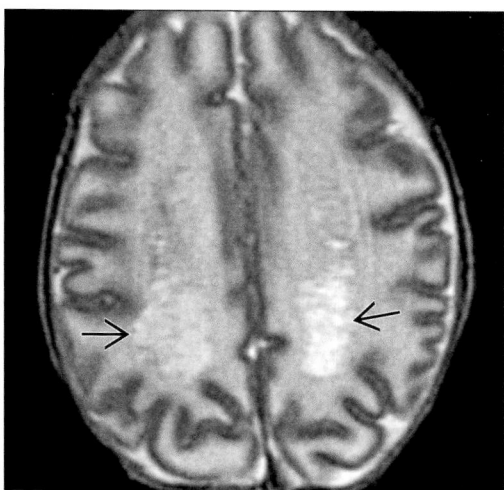

8-66. *T2WI in the same patient shows the cavitating cysts of WMIP* ➡️*.*

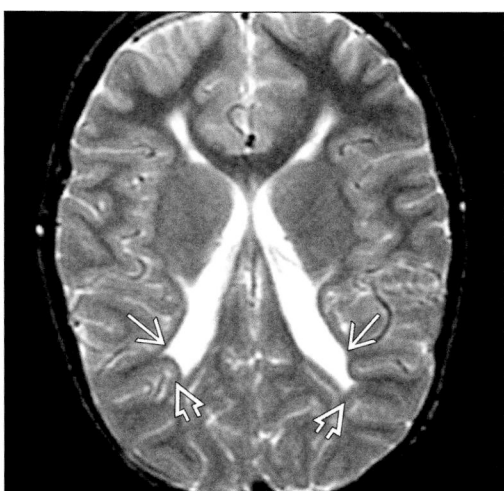

8-67. *T2WI shows end-stage WMIP with PVL, "scalloped" ventricles* ➡️*, severe WM loss. The cortex almost touches the lateral ventricles* ➡️*.*

End-stage PVL shows reduced WM volume with peritrigonal hyperintensity on T2WI. The body and splenium of the corpus callosum are thinned. In some areas, the cortex nearly touches the lateral ventricles, which are enlarged and have irregular ("scalloped") margins **(8-67)**.

HII IN PRETERM INFANTS

Clinical Issues
- < 37 weeks gestational age
- HII causes 50% of all cerebral palsy (CP) cases
  - 5% < 32 weeks develop CP
  - 15-20% < 28 weeks develop CP

Imaging
- Severe HII affects mostly thalami
- Less severe HII causes GMH, IVH
- White matter injury of prematurity
  - Oligodendrocyte precursor cells especially vulnerable
  - Periventricular, especially near trigones
  - 2/3 have coexisting hemorrhages
  - Early on US: Periventricular hyperechoic "flares"
  - Subacute: ± cysts, then resolve → gliosis
  - Late: WM ↓, enlarged ventricles with scalloped margins

HII IN TERM INFANTS. Term infants are those of 37 weeks or greater gestational age. Imaging findings of asphyxia in term infants vary with severity. Although ultrasound is often used as the initial imaging procedure, MR with DWI is the most sensitive modality for assessing neonatal HII.

Severe HII with profound perinatal hypotension or cardiocirculatory arrest in term infants preferentially affects actively myelinating brain and areas in which NMDA receptors are most highly concentrated. The deep gray matter (posterior putamina, ventrolateral thalami), hippocampi, and dorsal brainstem are most severely affected **(8-68)**. Severe HII in term infants may also cause parasagittal WS zone infarcts, especially in the perirolandic cortex.

Standard T1- and T2WI on day one are often normal. Between two and three days later, T1 basal ganglia and thalamic hyperintensity with absent or decreased signal intensity in the normally myelinated posterior limb of the internal capsule can be seen.

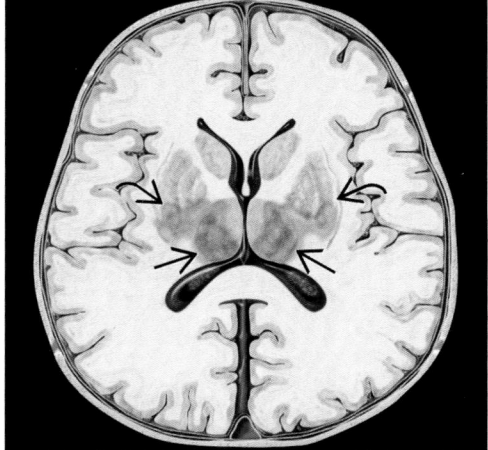
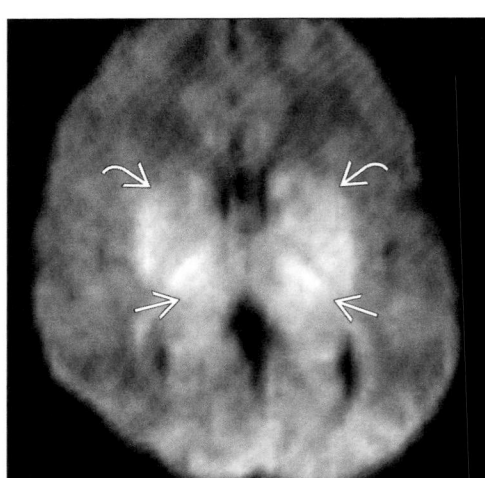

8-68. Graphic depicts severe HII in a term infant with preferential involvement of the posterior putamina ⇗, ventrolateral thalami ⇘. 8-69. DWI in a term infant with severe HII shows diffusion restriction in the basal ganglia ⇗ and ventrolateral thalami ⇘.

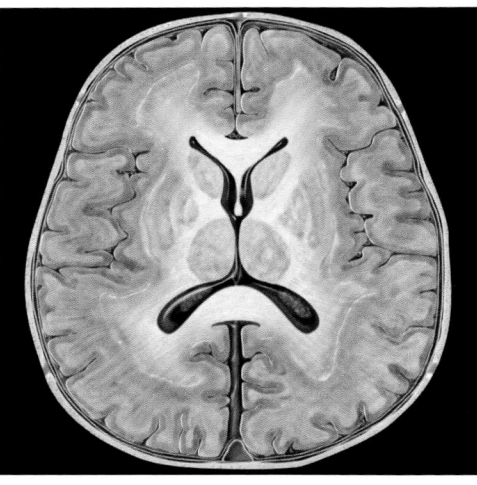
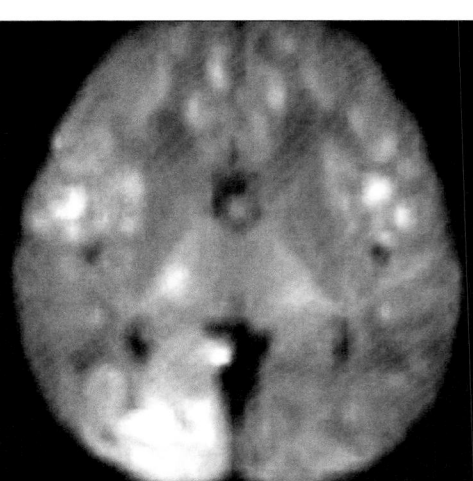

8-70. Less severe HII generally spares the deep basal ganglia but involves the cortex and subcortical WM, especially in the watershed "border zones." 8-71. DWI in a term infant with moderate HII shows relative sparing of the basal ganglia with multiple foci of restricted diffusion in the cortex and subcortical WM.

DWI is the most sensitive sequence in the first 24 hours, showing restricted diffusion and reduced ADC in the basal ganglia and thalami **(8-69)**. Abnormalities peak at three to five days and then "pseudonormalize" by the end of the first postnatal week.

MRS shows elevated Lac:NAA ratio and a glutamine-glutamate peak resonating at 2.3 ppm. MRS must be interpreted with care as lactate is present in the CSF of normal infants, phenobarbital (often used for sedation) resonates at 1.15 ppm (close to lactate at 1.3 ppm), and NAA varies with brain maturity.

Atrophy of the injured structures eventually ensues. **Ulegyria**—shrunken cortex with flattened, mushroom-shaped gyri, usually in the parietooccipital area—and cystic encephalomalacia are end-stage findings **(8-72)**.

Less severe HII with only partial asphyxia generally spares the brainstem, cerebellum, and deep gray nuclei. Prolonged partial asphyxia causes hypoperfusion in the watershed ("border") zones **(8-70)**. The parasagittal cortex and subcortical WM are most severely affected. T1 and T2 scans are initially normal, but wedge-shaped areas of diffusion restriction in the watershed zones can be seen on DWI **(8-71)**. Late findings include multicystic "border zone" cystic infarcts.

HII in Postnatal Infants and Young Children. Mild to moderate anoxic events in older infants and young children generally cause watershed zone injury, with wedge-shaped hypodensities and areas of restricted diffusion in the cortical (external) "border zones" between the major cerebral artery territories.

Severe asphyxia (usually from drowning, choking, or nonaccidental trauma) in children younger than one year of age damages the basal ganglia, lateral thalami, dorsal midbrain, and cortex.

In infants between one and two years of age, the basal ganglia, hippocampi, and anterior frontal/parietooccipital cortex are involved whereas the thalami and perirolandic cortex are relatively spared. On NECT, the cortex appears hypointense relative to the white matter (the "reversal" sign). In severe HII, diffuse cerebral edema makes the difference between the extremely hypoattenuated hemispheres and normally perfused cerebellum and brainstem especially striking ("white cerebellum" sign).

MR shows diffusion restriction in the affected areas.

HII in Older Children and Adults

Mild to moderate global HII typically results in watershed zone infarcts (see above).

Severe HII in older children and adults selectively affects the deep gray nuclei, cortex, hippocampi, and cerebellum.

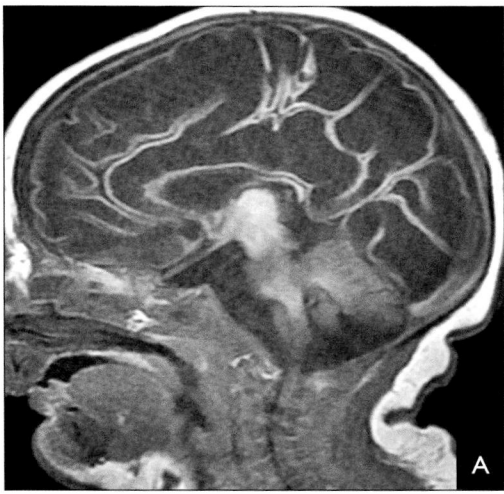

8-72A. Sagittal T1WI shows end-stage cystic encephalomalacia in a term infant imaged 5 weeks after profound birth asphyxia.

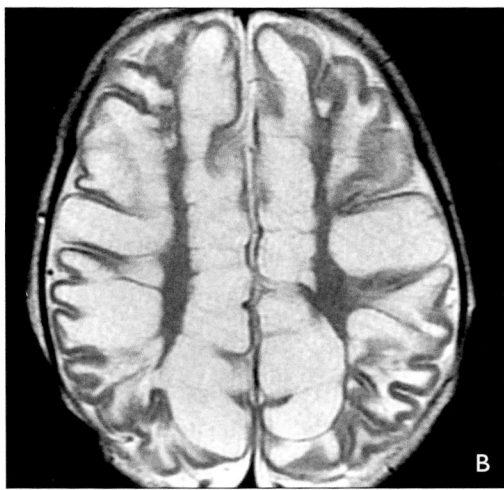

8-72B. Axial T2WI shows diffuse cystic encephalomalacia with thinned cortex.

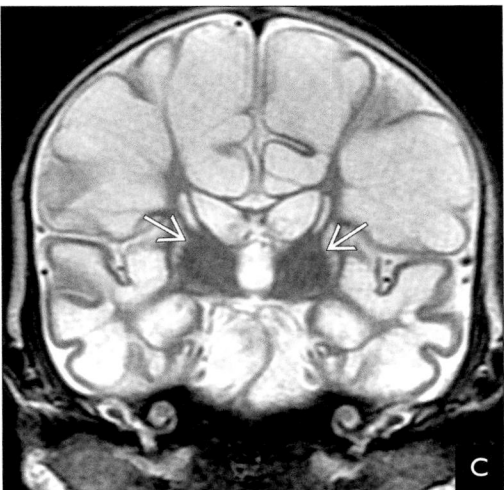

8-72C. Coronal T2WI shows diffuse cystic encephalomalacia, severely damaged WM, and small, shrunken basal ganglia ➡️

NECT shows diffuse cerebral edema with loss of normal gray-white matter differentiation and "disappearing" basal ganglia.

MR shows hyperintensity in the globi pallidi and cerebellum on T2/FLAIR. DWI demonstrates restricted diffusion in the cerebellum, basal ganglia, and cortex but typically "pseudonormalizes" within one week. In some cases of severe HII—especially those associated with carbon monoxide poisoning—delayed WM injury develops up to two to three weeks following the initial insult.

In chronic HII, T1WI may show gyriform shortening (caused by **cortical laminar necrosis**, not hemorrhage or calcification).

HII IN TERM/POSTTERM INFANTS, CHILDREN, AND ADULTS

Term Infants
- ≥ 36 weeks gestational age
- Severe
  - Deep gray nuclei, ventrolateral thalami
  - Posterior limb internal capsule, dorsal brainstem
  - Hippocampi, parasagittal watershed
  - Chronic may show ulegyria
- Less severe
  - Cortical watershed zones
  - Spares brainstem, cerebellum, deep gray nuclei

Postnatal Infants and Young Children
- Severe
  - Basal ganglia, lateral thalami, dorsal midbrain, cortex
- Mild-moderate = cortical watershed zones

Older Children and Adults
- Severe
  - Deep gray nuclei, cortex, hippocampi, cerebellum
- Mild-moderate = cortical watershed zones
  - Gyriform T1 shortening (cortical laminar necrosis)

8-73A. A 56-year-old man with > 70% stenosis of his left cervical ICA underwent carotid endarterectomy. A few hours after surgery, he became acutely confused and developed right-sided weakness. CTA source image shows markedly increased vasculature in the left hemisphere ⊳. *8-73B.* CTA with CBF appears relatively normal, but blood flow on the left (2a, 2b ROIs) is increased compared to the right side.

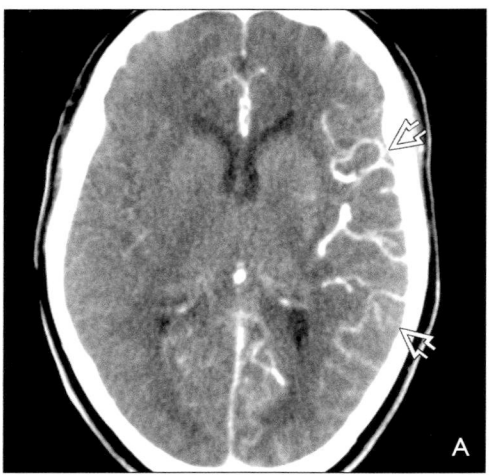

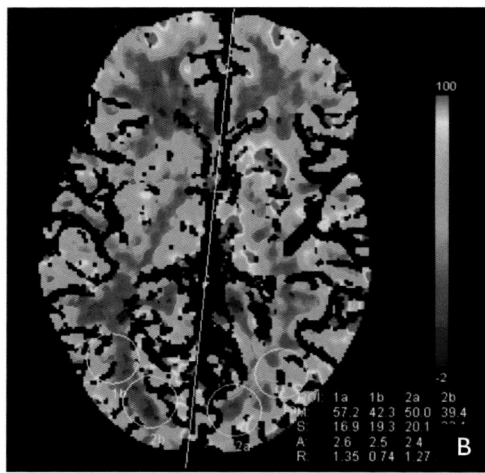

8-73C. TTP study is even more striking. The abnormal side is NOT the right MCA distribution (green) but is the left side (blue) where the TTP is markedly shortened. *8-73D.* T2WI shows gyral swelling, sulcal effacement, and hyperintensity in the left temporal and parietooccipital cortex/subcortical white matter ⊳, basal ganglia ⊳. DWI (not shown) was normal. Post-carotid endarterectomy hyperperfusion syndrome.

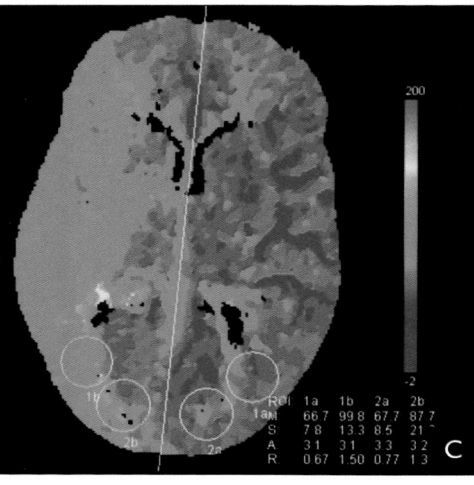

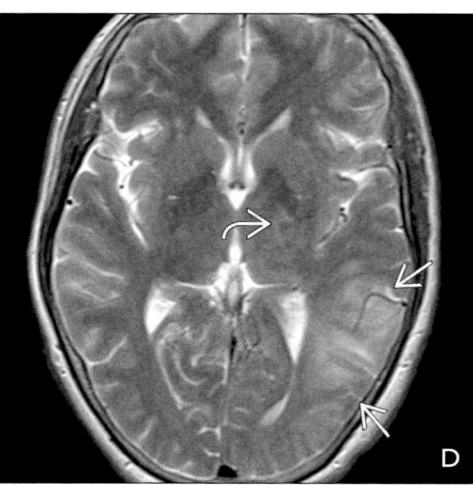

Miscellaneous Strokes

Cerebral Hyperperfusion Syndrome

Terminology

Cerebral hyperperfusion syndrome (CHS) is a rare but potentially devastating disorder. CHS is sometimes called luxury perfusion or post-carotid endarterectomy hyperperfusion and is defined as a major increase in cerebral blood flow well above normal metabolic demands.

Etiology

CHS most often occurs as a complication of carotid reperfusion procedures (i.e., endarterectomy, angioplasty, stenting, or thrombolysis). Less common causes include status epilepticus, MELAS, and hypercapnia.

Critical carotid stenosis with chronic cerebral ischemia causes endothelial dysfunction and impaired arterial autoregulation. Loss of normal vasoconstriction results in chronic dilatation of the brain "resistance" vessels. When normal perfusion is restored, this can result in rapidly increased CBF in the previously underperfused hemisphere.

Comorbid clinical risk factors include age, hypertension (especially post procedure), bilateral lesions, hemodynamically significant disease in the contralateral carotid artery, poor collateral blood flow, and diminished cerebral vascular reserve.

Clinical Issues

EPIDEMIOLOGY AND PRESENTATION. Symptomatic CHS occurs in 1-3% of carotid reperfusion procedures, although 5-10% of patients develop mild, generally asymptomatic CHS. Patients typically present within a few hours following carotid endarterectomy (CEA), usually with unilateral headache, face or eye pain, cognitive impairment, and variable neurologic deficits.

TREATMENT OPTIONS. Preventive measures include minimal intraprocedural cerebral ischemia, rigorous postoperative blood pressure monitoring and control, and adequate postoperative sedation.

Imaging

CT FINDINGS. NECT scans may show only mild gyral swelling. CTA/pCT show congested, dilated vessels with elevated blood flow and decreased MTT/TTP **(8-73A)**, **(8-73B)**, **(8-73C)**.

MR FINDINGS. T2/FLAIR scans show gyral swelling, hyperintensity, and sulcal effacement in the internal carotid distribution **(8-73D)**. T1 C+ scans may be normal or show mildly increased intravascular enhancement.

DWI is typically negative, as the edema is vasogenic rather than cytotoxic. pMR shows elevated CBF and CBV with decreased (shortened) MTT.

Differential Diagnosis

The major differential diagnosis of post-CEA CHS is **acute cerebral ischemia-infarction**. Here the MTT is prolonged (not decreased), and DWI typically shows restricted diffusion.

Acute hypertensive encephalopathy (PRES) is a dysautoregulatory disorder with a predilection for the posterior circulation. Lesions are typically bilateral, not unilateral as with post-CEA CHS.

Status epilepticus can also result in hyperperfusion. The cortex is usually more selectively involved than the white matter. The stroke-like episodes in **MELAS** are related to vasogenic edema, hyperperfusion, and neuronal damage. Cortical hyperintensity on T2/FLAIR can resemble CHS, but MRS in "normal-appearing" brain shows a characteristically elevated lactate peak.

CEREBRAL HYPERPERFUSION SYNDROME

Terminology
- CBF ↑ ↑; above normal metabolic demands

Etiology
- Common = carotid reperfusion procedure
- Less common = status epilepticus, MELAS

Clinical Issues
- 1-3% of CEA patients
- Unilateral headache, eye pain

Imaging
- Gyral swelling
- ↑ intravascular enhancement
- DWI negative (vasogenic, not cytotoxic, edema)
- pCT, pMR: Abnormally rapid blood flow
  ○ ↑ CBF, ↓ MTT

Differential Diagnosis
- Acute cerebral ischemia-infarction
- PRES

Strokes in Unusual Vascular Distributions

The vast majority of arterial strokes are easily recognizable, as they conform to the expected vascular territories of major cerebral arteries such as the ACA/MCA/PCA and posterior inferior cerebellar artery. Two unusual but important arterial occlusions are the artery of Percheron infarcts and the top of the basilar syndrome. Each is briefly discussed here.

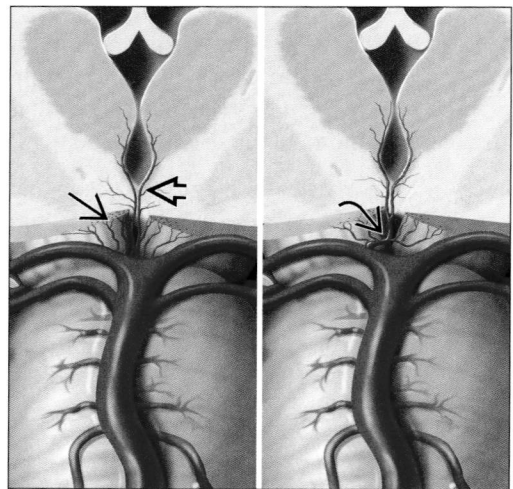

8-74. *(L) Normal basilar artery with small perforating arteries supplying midbrain* ⊇*, medial thalami* ⊇*. (R) AOP has single dominant trunk* ⊇*.*

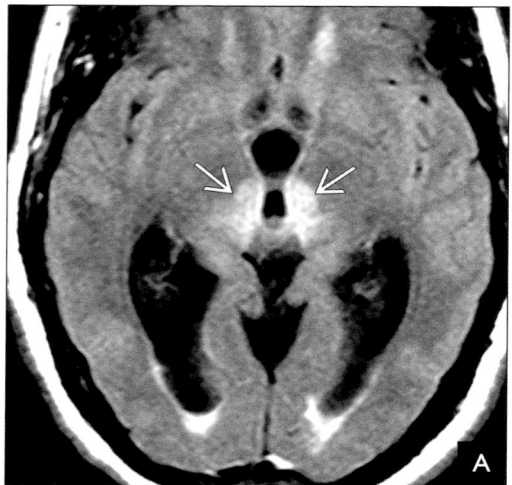

8-75A. *FLAIR scan in a patient with artery of Percheron infarct shows both medial thalami infarcts* ➡*.*

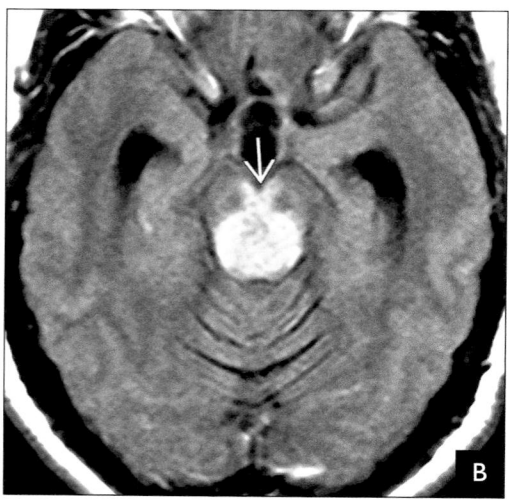

8-75B. *FLAIR in the same patient shows midbrain, peduncular "V" hyperintensity* ➡*.*

Artery of Percheron Infarction

The artery of Percheron (AOP) is a vascular variant in which a single large midbrain perforating artery arises from the P1 PCA segment to supply the midbrain and medial thalami **(8-74)**. AOP occlusion can cause obtundation, oculomotor and pupillary deficits, vertical gaze palsy, ptosis, and lid retraction.

NECT scans in early acute AOP occlusion are usually normal. Hypodense areas in both thalami extending into the central midbrain may develop later.

MR with DWI is the procedure of choice. T2/FLAIR scans show round or ovoid hyperintensities in the medial thalami, just lateral to the third ventricle **(8-75A)**. In slightly more than half of all cases, a V-shaped hyperintensity involves the medial surfaces of the cerebral peduncles and rostral midbrain **(8-75B)**. DWI shows diffusion restriction in the affected areas.

The major differential diagnosis of AOP occlusion is **"top of the basilar" infarct**. "Top of the basilar" infarcts are much more extensive, involving part or all of the rostral midbrain, occipital lobes, superior vermis, and thalami.

Deep cerebral (galenic) venous occlusions involve the basal ganglia, posterior limb of internal capsules, and typically the entire thalami. T2* (GRE, SWI) scans demonstrate "blooming" clots in the internal cerebral vein, vein of Galen, and straight sinus (see Chapter 9).

"Top of the Basilar" Infarction

"Top of the basilar" infarct is a clinically recognizable syndrome characterized by visual, oculomotor, and behavioral abnormalities caused by thrombosis of the distal basilar artery. Thrombus typically occludes both P1 PCA segments **(8-76)** and distal perforators that supply the rostral midbrain and thalami. Depending on the inferior extent of the clot, pontine perforators and one or more superior cerebellar artery territories may also be affected.

NECT scans show a "dense basilar artery" sign **(8-76)**. MR findings vary depending on thrombus extent and vascular supply to the distal PCAs. If "fetal" type PCAs or large PCoAs are present, much or all of the PCA territory may be spared. T2/FLAIR hyperintensity in the midbrain, thalami, upper pons, and superior cerebellar hemispheres is common, as is restriction on DWI **(8-77)**, **(8-78)**, **(8-79)**.

The differential diagnoses of "top of the basilar" infarct are **artery of Percheron infarction** (see above) and **deep cerebral venous occlusion** (see Chapter 9).

Selected References

Normal Arterial Anatomy and Vascular Distributions

Intracranial Internal Carotid Artery

- Teo M et al: Persistent hypoglossal artery - an increased risk for intracranial aneurysms? Br J Neurosurg. Epub ahead of print, 2012
- Uchino A et al: Persistent trigeminal artery and its variants on MR angiography. Surg Radiol Anat. 34(3):271-6, 2012
- Vasović L et al: Trigeminal artery: a review of normal and pathological features. Childs Nerv Syst. 28(1):33-46, 2012
- Komatsu F et al: Endoscopic anatomy of persistent trigeminal artery: a cadaveric study. Minim Invasive Neurosurg. 54(5-6):223-7, 2011
- Merrow AC: Persistent hypoglossal artery. Pediatr Radiol. 40 Suppl 1:S162, 2010

- Vasović L et al: Otic artery: a review of normal and pathological features. Med Sci Monit. 16(5):RA101-9, 2010
- Vasović L et al: Proatlantal intersegmental artery: a review of normal and pathological features. Childs Nerv Syst. 25(4):411-21, 2009
- Pasco A et al: Persistent carotid-vertebrobasilar anastomoses: how and why differentiating them? J Neuroradiol. 31(5):391-6, 2004
- Uchino A et al: MR angiography of anomalous branches of the internal carotid artery. AJR Am J Roentgenol. 181(5):1409-14, 2003

Circle of Willis

- Lazzaro MA et al: The role of circle of Willis anomalies in cerebral aneurysm rupture. J Neurointerv Surg. 4(1):22-6, 2012
- Rai AT et al: Cerebrovascular geometry in the anterior circulation: an analysis of diameter, length and the vessel taper. J Neurointerv Surg. Epub ahead of print, 2012
- Hendrikse J et al: Distribution of cerebral blood flow in the circle of Willis. Radiology. 235(1):184-9, 2005

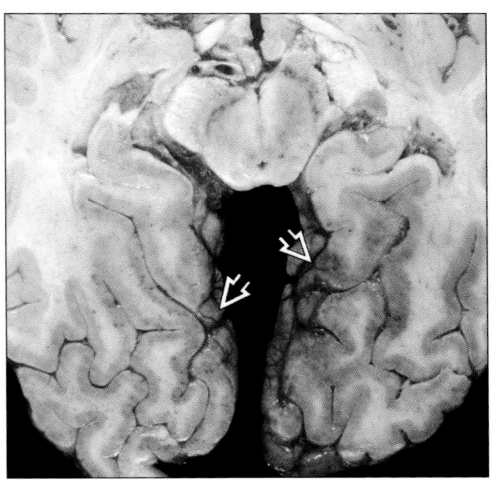
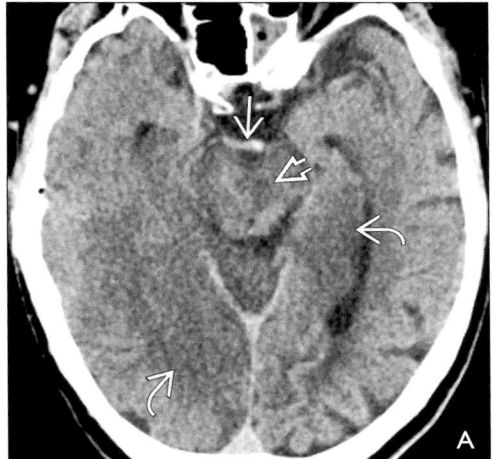
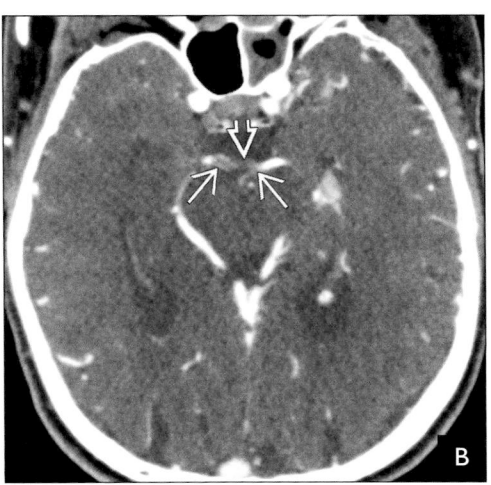
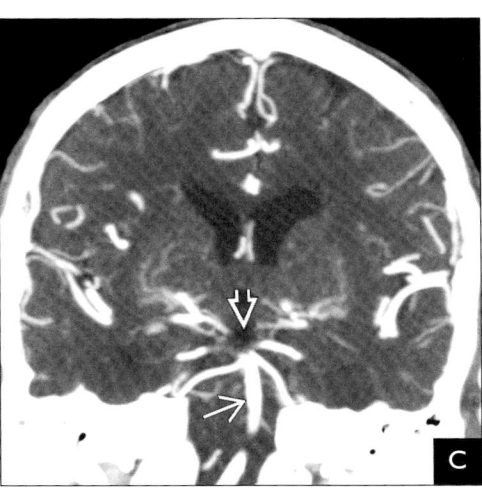

8-76. Gross autopsy specimen of a "top of the basilar" thrombosis shows bilateral occipital lobe infarcts. (Courtesy R. Hewlett, MD.) 8-77A. NECT scan in an 81-year-old man with decreased mental status following cardiac catheterization was obtained 12 hours after symptom onset. Note hyperdense BA and right P1 PCA, hypodensity in midbrain as well as in both medial temporal, occipital lobes.

8-77B. CTA source image shows thrombus with nonopacification of the basilar bifurcation, both proximal P1 PCA segments. 8-77C. Coronal MIP CTA shows that most of the proximal BA is normally opacified, but the distal BA and basilar bifurcation, proximal PCAs and SCAs are unopacified. Classic "top of the basilar" thrombosis.

8-78A. *More extensive BA thrombosis is illustrated by a series of images in a 63-year-old man. NECT scan through the midbrain shows dense BA* ➡, *hypodense midbrain* ➥, *right medial occipital lobe hypodensity* ➡. **8-78B.** *More cephalad scan shows hypodensity in the left thalamus* ➥, *corpus callosum* ➥, *both occipital lobes* ➡.

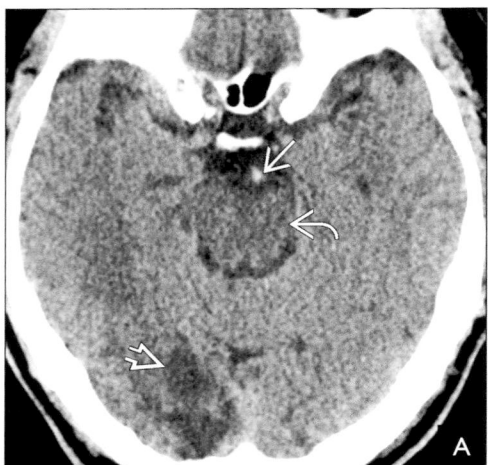
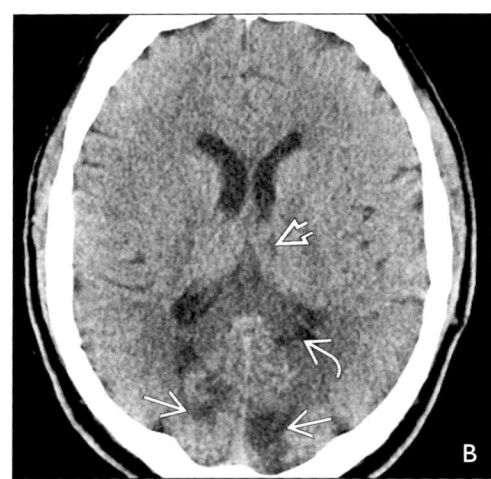

8-78C. *Sagittal CTA shows basilar artery thrombus* ➡ *with nonopacified distal basilar artery. Multiple patchy hypodensities are present in the pons* ➡ *and occipital lobe* ➥. **8-78D.** *Coronal CTA shows extensive thrombus in the BA* ➡.

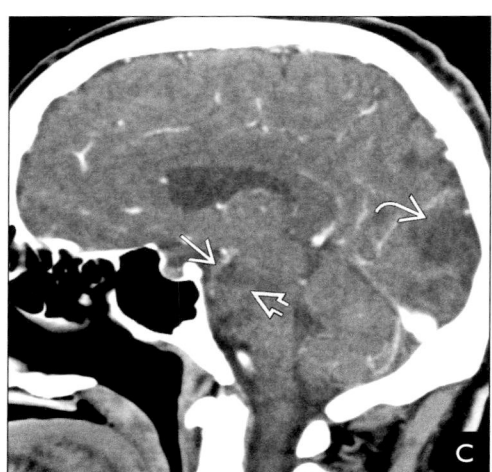
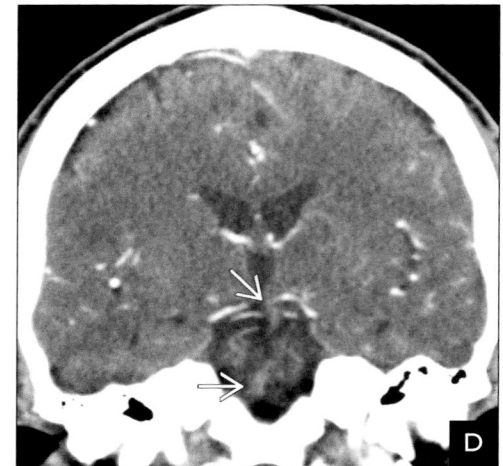

8-78E. *DWI in the same patient shows a bilateral midbrain perforating artery* ➥, *occipital infarcts* ➡. **8-78F.** *More cephalad DWI in the same patient shows infarcts in the left thalamus* ➥, *corpus callosum splenium* ➥. *Both areas are supplied by perforating branches of the distal basilar artery.*

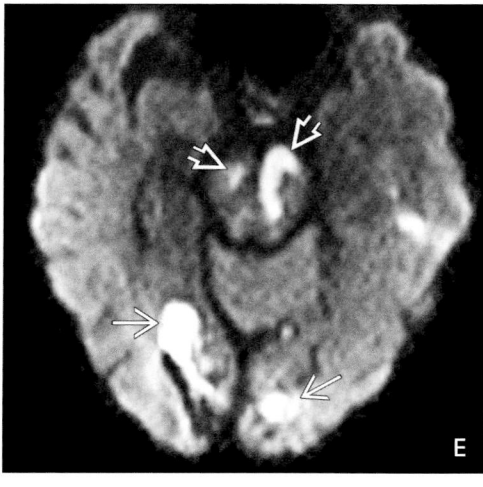
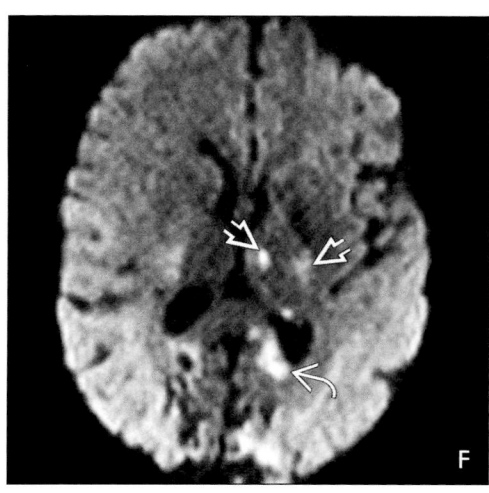

Anterior Cerebral Artery

- Horie N et al: New variant of persistent primitive olfactory artery associated with a ruptured aneurysm. J Neurosurg. 117(1):26-8, 2012
- Komiyama M: Persistent primitive olfactory artery. Surg Radiol Anat. 34(1):97-8, 2012
- Zunon-Kipré Y et al: Microsurgical anatomy of distal medial striate artery (recurrent artery of Heubner). Surg Radiol Anat. 34(1):15-20, 2012
- Kim MS et al: Diagnosis of persistent primitive olfactory artery using computed tomography angiography. J Korean Neurosurg Soc. 49(5):290-1, 2011

Middle Cerebral Artery

- Kahilogullari G et al: The branching pattern of the middle cerebral artery: is the intermediate trunk real or not? An anatomical study correlating with simple angiography. J Neurosurg. 116(5):1024-34, 2012
- Uchino A et al: Duplicate origin and fenestration of the middle cerebral artery on MR angiography. Surg Radiol Anat. 34(5):401-4, 2012
- Lame A et al: Anatomic variants of accessory medial cerebral artery. Neurosurgery. 66(6):E1217; author reply E1217, 2010

Posterior Cerebral Artery

- Wentland AL et al: Fetal origin of the posterior cerebral artery produces left-right asymmetry on perfusion imaging. AJNR Am J Neuroradiol. 31(3):448-53, 2010
- Caruso G et al: Anomalies of the P1 segment of the posterior cerebral artery: early bifurcation or duplication, fenestration, common trunk with the superior cerebellar artery. Acta Neurochir (Wien). 109(1-2):66-71, 1991

Arterial Infarcts

Acute Cerebral Ischemia-Infarction

- Amort M et al: Etiological classifications of transient ischemic attacks: subtype classification by TOAST, CCS and ASCO - a pilot study. Cerebrovasc Dis. 33(6):508-516, 2012
- Bevan S et al: Genetics of common polygenic ischaemic stroke: current understanding and future challenges. Stroke Res Treat. 2011:179061, 2011
- Doubal FN et al: Characteristics of patients with minor ischaemic strokes and negative MRI: a cross-sectional study. J Neurol Neurosurg Psychiatry. 82(5):540-2, 2011
- Fornage M et al: Genome-wide association studies of cerebral white matter lesion burden: the CHARGE consortium. Ann Neurol. 69(6):928-39, 2011
- Thomalla G et al: DWI-FLAIR mismatch for the identification of patients with acute ischaemic stroke within 4·5 h of symptom onset (PRE-FLAIR): a multicentre observational study. Lancet Neurol. 10(11):978-86, 2011
- Lui YW et al: Evaluation of CT perfusion in the setting of cerebral ischemia: patterns and pitfalls. AJNR Am J Neuroradiol. 31(9):1552-63, 2010
- Marnane M et al: Stroke subtype classification to mechanism-specific and undetermined categories by TOAST, A-S-C-O,

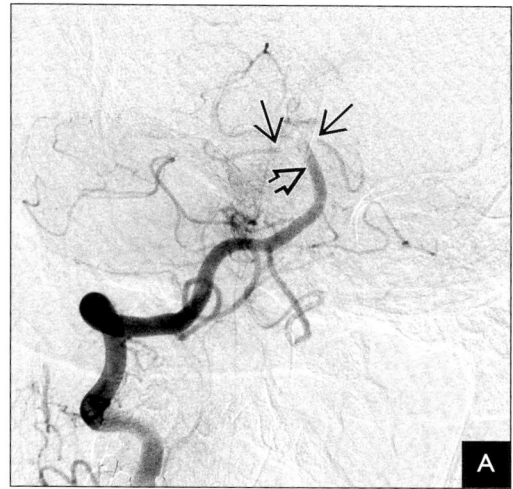

8-79A. Basilar thrombosis in a 40 yo man. DSA shows clot in distal BA ▷ that extends into the proximal superior cerebellar arteries →.

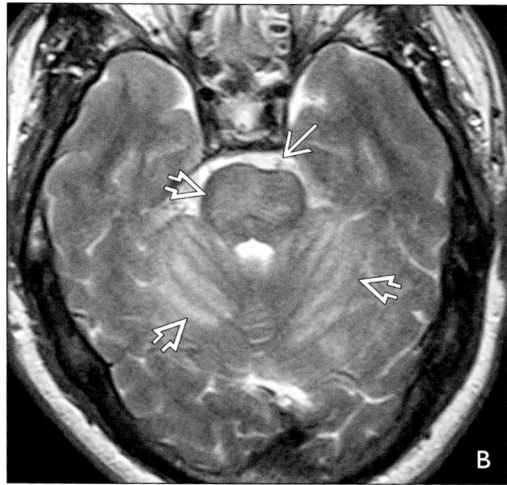

8-79B. T2WI in the same case shows absent "flow void" in basilar artery →, pontine and cerebellar hyperintensity ⇒.

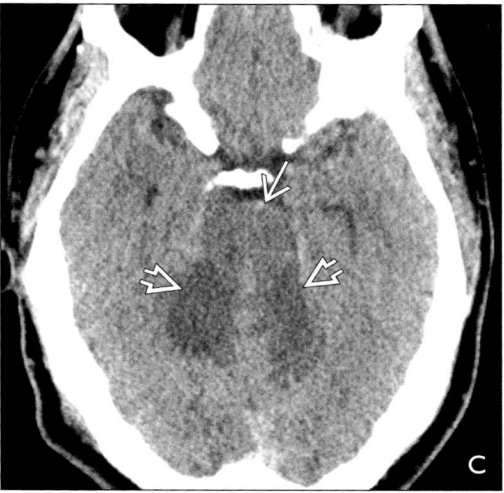

8-79C. Despite thrombolysis, the patient became "locked in." NECT scan 24 hours later shows BA thrombus →, pontine, cerebellar infarcts ⇒.

- and causative classification system: direct comparison in the North Dublin population stroke study. Stroke. 41(8):1579-86, 2010
- Zenonos G et al: Diffusion weighted imaging: what are we really seeing? Neurosurgery. 67(6):N26-9, 2010
- de Lucas EM et al: CT protocol for acute stroke: tips and tricks for general radiologists. Radiographics. 28(6):1673-87, 2008
- González RG: Imaging-guided acute ischemic stroke therapy: From "time is brain" to "physiology is brain". AJNR Am J Neuroradiol. 27(4):728-35, 2006

Subacute Cerebral Infarcts

- Alawneh JA et al: Infarction of 'non-core-non-penumbral' tissue after stroke: multivariate modelling of clinical impact. Brain. 134(Pt 6):1765-76, 2011

Multiple Embolic Infarcts

- Rafik R et al: [A rare cause of cerebral ischemic stroke: cerebral fat embolism.] Rev Neurol (Paris). 168(3):298-9, 2012
- Ryoo S et al: Branch occlusive disease: clinical and magnetic resonance angiography findings. Neurology. 78(12):888-96, 2012
- Shinohara Y et al: Changes in susceptibility signs on serial T2*-weighted single-shot echoplanar gradient-echo images in acute embolic infarction: comparison with recanalization status on 3D time-of-flight magnetic resonance angiography. Neuroradiology. 54(5):427-34, 2012
- Chin BM et al: Cerebral fat embolism: Imaging characteristics of an enigmatic entity. Presented at the 49th Annual Scientific Meeting of the American Society of Neuroradiology. Seattle, June 2011

Lacunar Infarcts

- Brundel M et al: Cerebral microinfarcts: a systematic review of neuropathological studies. J Cereb Blood Flow Metab. 32(3):425-36, 2012
- Del Bene A et al: Progressive lacunar stroke: Review of mechanisms, prognostic features, and putative treatments. Int J Stroke. 7(4):321-9, 2012
- Lee JH et al: Acute simultaneous multiple lacunar infarcts: a severe disease entity in small artery disease. Eur Neurol. 67(5):303-11, 2012
- Loos CM et al: Cavitation of deep lacunar infarcts in patients with first-ever lacunar stroke: A 2-year follow-up study with MR. Stroke. 43(8):2245-7, 2012
- Koch S et al: Imaging evolution of acute lacunar infarction: Leukoariosis or lacune? Neurology. 77(11):1091-5, 2011
- Potter GM et al: Wide variation in definition, detection, and description of lacunar lesions on imaging. Stroke. 42(2):359-66, 2011
- Bradac GB et al: Lacunes and other holes: diagnosis, pathogenesis, therapy. Neuroradiol J. 21(1): 35-52, 2008

Watershed ("Border Zone") Infarcts

- D'Amore C et al: Border-zone and watershed infarctions. Front Neurol Neurosci. 30:181-4, 2012
- Mangla R et al: Border zone infarcts: pathophysiologic and imaging characteristics. Radiographics. 31(5):1201-14, 2011
- Li HF et al: Clinical and neuroradiological features of internal watershed infarction and the occlusive diseases of carotid artery system. Neurol Res. 32(10):1090-6, 2010

Hypoxic-Ischemic Injury

- Busl KM et al: Hypoxic-ischemic brain injury: pathophysiology, neuropathology and mechanisms. NeuroRehabilitation. 26(1):5-13, 2010
- Huang BY et al: Hypoxic-ischemic brain injury: imaging findings from birth to adulthood. Radiographics. 28(2):417-39; quiz 617, 2008

Miscellaneous Strokes

Cerebral Hyperperfusion Syndrome

- De Rango P: Cerebral hyperperfusion syndrome: the dark side of carotid endarterectomy. Eur J Vasc Endovasc Surg. 43(4):377, 2012
- Lieb M et al: Cerebral hyperperfusion syndrome after carotid intervention: a review. Cardiol Rev. 20(2):84-9, 2012
- Pennekamp CW et al: Prediction of cerebral hyperperfusion after carotid endarterectomy with transcranial Doppler. Eur J Vasc Endovasc Surg. 43(4):371-6, 2012
- Noorani A et al: Cerebral hemodynamic changes following carotid endarterectomy: 'cerebral hyperperfusion syndrome'. Expert Rev Neurother. 10(2):217-23, 2010

Strokes in Unusual Vascular Distributions

- Lazzaro NA et al: Artery of percheron infarction: imaging patterns and clinical spectrum. AJNR Am J Neuroradiol. 31(7):1283-9, 2010

9

Venous Anatomy and Occlusions

Dural venous sinus and cerebral vein occlusions are relatively rare, accounting for only 1% of all strokes. They are notoriously difficult to diagnose clinically and are frequently overlooked on imaging studies as attention is focused on the arterial side of the cerebral circulation.

The risk of venous "strokes" is increased by a number of different predisposing conditions. Dehydration, pregnancy, trauma, infection, collagen-vascular disease, coagulopathies, and a spectrum of inherited disorders all enhance the likelihood of developing sinovenous occlusion.

Familiarity with both normal venous anatomy and drainage patterns is essential for understanding the imaging appearance of sinovenous occlusive disease. Therefore, in this chapter, we first briefly review the normal gross and imaging anatomy of the cerebral venous system. Because about half of all venous occlusions result in parenchymal infarcts, we also discuss their drainage territories.

Once we have laid the anatomic foundation for understanding the cranial venous system, we turn to the fascinating topic of sinovenous occlusive disease—venous "strokes"—and their mimics.

Normal Venous Anatomy and Drainage Patterns

The intracranial venous system is unlike its systemic counterparts. Brain veins and sinuses lack valves and can have bidirectional flow. In the body, veins typically accompany arteries, and their vascular territories are relatively comparable. Not so in the brain. The dural sinuses and the cerebral veins travel separately, so their drainage territories do not mirror arterial distributions. Therefore, a venous "stroke" looks and behaves quite differently from a major arterial occlusion.

The intracranial venous system has two major components, the **dural venous sinuses** and the **cerebral veins**. We begin our discussion with the dural sinuses and then turn our attention to the cerebral veins. We conclude by delineating the drainage territories of the major dural sinuses and cerebral veins.

Dural Venous Sinuses

The dural venous sinuses are subdivided into an anteroinferior group and a posterosuperior group. The posterosuperior group is the more prominent and consists of the superior sagittal sinus (SSS), inferior sagittal sinus (ISS), straight sinus (SS), sinus confluence (torcular herophili), transverse sinuses (TSs), sigmoid sinuses, and jugular bulbs.

The anteroinferior group consists of the cavernous sinus (CS), superior and inferior petrosal sinuses (SPSs, IPSs), clival venous plexus (CVP), and sphenoparietal sinus (SphPS).

General Considerations

Dural sinuses and venous plexuses are endothelium-lined channels that are contained between the outer (periosteal) and inner (meningeal) dural layers. Dural sinuses and

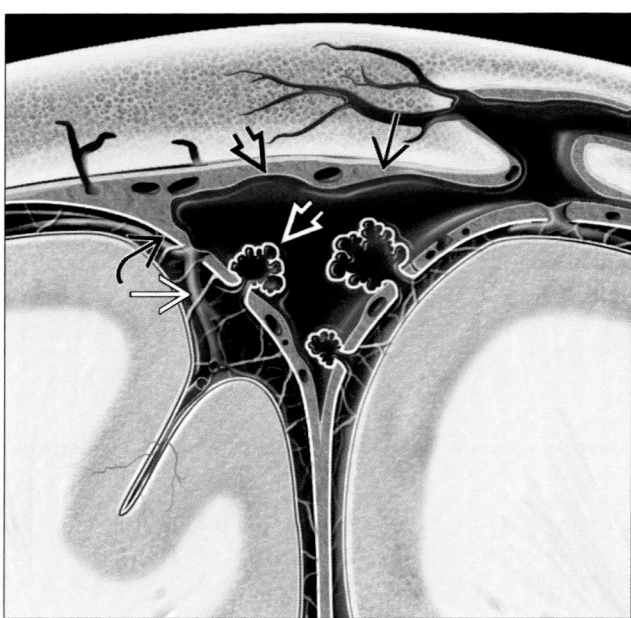

9-1. Coronal graphic shows the SSS ▷ between the outer ⟶ and inner ⟶ dural layers. CSF-containing projections (arachnoid granulations) ⟹ extend from the subarachnoid space into the SSS. Cortical veins ⟹ also enter the SSS.

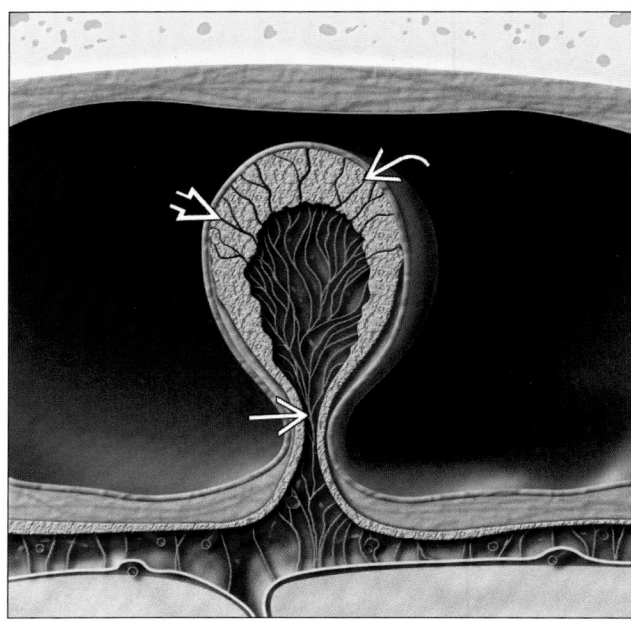

9-2. Graphic depicts an arachnoid granulation (AG) projecting into a venous sinus. CSF ⟹ extends from the SAS into the AG and is covered by a cap of arachnoid cells ⟹. Channels in the cap ⟹ drain CSF into the sinus.

plexuses—especially the cavernous sinus and clival plexus—are often fenestrated and multichanneled. At least one intrasinus septation or fibrous band is present in 30% of autopsy cases.

The dural sinuses frequently contain **arachnoid granulations** (AGs), also known as pacchionian granulations. AGs are CSF-containing projections that extend from the subarachnoid space (SAS) into dural venous sinuses **(9-1)**. A central core of CSF extends from the SAS into the granulation, which in turn is covered by an apical cap of arachnoid cells. Multiple small channels extend through the full thickness of the cap to the sinus endothelium and drain CSF into the venous circulation **(9-2)**.

While AGs can occur in all dural venous sinuses, the most common locations are the transverse and superior sagittal sinus. The cavernous sinus is a relatively uncommon site.

Superior Sagittal Sinus

The SSS is a large, curvilinear sinus that parallels the inner calvarial vault. It originates from ascending frontal veins anteriorly and runs in the midline at the junction of the falx cerebri with the calvaria **(9-3)**. The SSS increases in diameter as it courses posteriorly, collecting a number of unnamed, small, superficial cortical veins and the larger anastomotic vein of Trolard. A number of so-called venous lakes in the diploic space of the calvaria also drain into the SSS.

On coronal imaging, the SSS appears as a triangular vascular channel contained between the dural leaves of the falx cerebri. On sagittal DSA/CTA/MRA, the SSS

is seen as a sickle-shaped structure that hugs the inner table of the skull. Filling defects—AGs and fibrous septa—within the SSS are common findings on imaging studies.

Normal SSS variants include absence of its anterior segment and off-midline position. When its anterior segment is hypoplastic or absent, the SSS begins more posteriorly near the coronal suture where it receives prominent frontal veins. The SSS usually remains in the midline throughout its course. As it descends toward its termination in the venous sinus confluence, however, it may gradually course off midline.

Inferior Sagittal Sinus

Compared to the SSS, the ISS is a much smaller and more inconstant channel that lies in the bottom of the falx cerebri. The ISS lies above the corpus callosum and cingulate gyrus, collecting small tributaries as it curves posteriorly along the inferior "free" margin of the falx. The ISS terminates at the falcotentorial junction where it joins with the great cerebral vein of Galen (VofG) to form the straight sinus.

The ISS is often small or inapparent and is inconsistently visualized on imaging studies.

Straight Sinus

The SS is formed by the junction of the ISS and VofG. It runs posteroinferiorly from its origin at the falcotentorial apex. Along its course, the SS receives numerous small tributaries from the falx cerebri, tentorium cerebelli, and

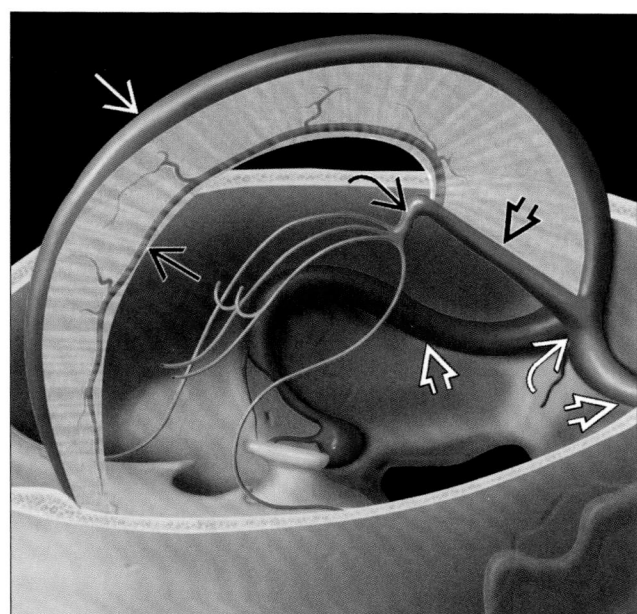

9-3. *The falx cerebri extends posteriorly from the crista galli to the falcotentorial junction and contains the SSS ➡ and the ISS ➥. The vein of Galen ➥, straight sinus ➥, sinus confluence ➥, and TSs ➥ are also illustrated.*

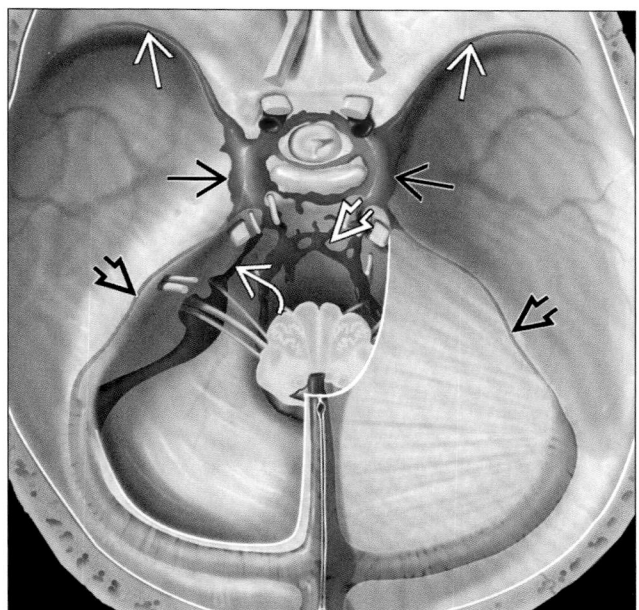

9-4. *Graphic shows the numerous interconnections among the cavernous sinuses ➥, clival venous plexus ➥, sphenoparietal sinuses ➥, and the superior ➥ and inferior ➥ petrosal sinuses.*

adjacent brain. The SS terminates by joining the superior sagittal and transverse sinuses to form the **venous sinus confluence** (torcular herophili). The venous sinus confluence is often asymmetric, with septations and intersinus channels connecting the transverse sinuses.

SS variants are relatively uncommon. A **persistent falcine sinus** is an unusual variant that is identified on 2% of normal CTAs. Here a midline venous structure—the persistent falcine sinus—connects the ISS or vein of Galen directly with the SSS. Two-thirds of patients with a persistent falcine sinus have absent/rudimentary straight sinuses.

Transverse Sinuses

The TSs, also known as lateral sinuses, are contained between attachments of the tentorium cerebelli to the inner table of the skull. The TSs curve laterally from the torcular to the posterior border of the petrous temporal bone, where they turn inferiorly and become the sigmoid sinuses.

Anatomic variations in the TSs are almost the rule rather than the exception. The two TSs are frequently asymmetric, with the right side typically larger than the left. Hypoplastic and even atretic segments are common, as are filling defects caused by arachnoid granulations and fibrous septa.

Sigmoid Sinuses and Jugular Bulbs

The sigmoid sinuses are basically the inferior continuations of the two TSs. They follow a gentle S-shaped curve, descending behind the petrous temporal bone to terminate by becoming the internal jugular veins. Side-to-side asymmetry of the sigmoid sinuses is common and normal.

The jugular bulbs are focal venous dilatations at the skull base between the sigmoid sinuses and extracranial internal jugular veins (IJVs). The IJVs and transverse/sigmoid sinuses are often asymmetric, and there is concomitant variation in size of the jugular bulbs and their osseous foramina. Jugular bulb pseudolesions with flow asymmetry are common and should not be mistaken for "real" masses (e.g., schwannoma or paraganglioma). Bone CT shows that the jugular spine and cortex around the jugular foramen are intact, not eroded or remodeled.

Cavernous Sinus

The CSs are irregularly shaped, heavily trabeculated/compartmentalized venous sinuses that lie along the sides of the sella turcica, extending from the superior orbital fissures anteriorly to the clivus and petrous apex posteriorly **(9-4)**.

Formed by a prominent lateral and much thinner—often almost inapparent—medial dural wall, the CSs contain the two cavernous internal carotid arteries (ICAs) and abducens (CN VI) nerves. CNs III, IV, V_1, and V_2 are actually *within* the lateral dural wall, not inside the CS proper **(9-5)**.

The major tributaries draining into the CSs are the superior/inferior ophthalmic veins and the sphenoparietal sinuses **(9-4)**. The two CSs communicate extensively

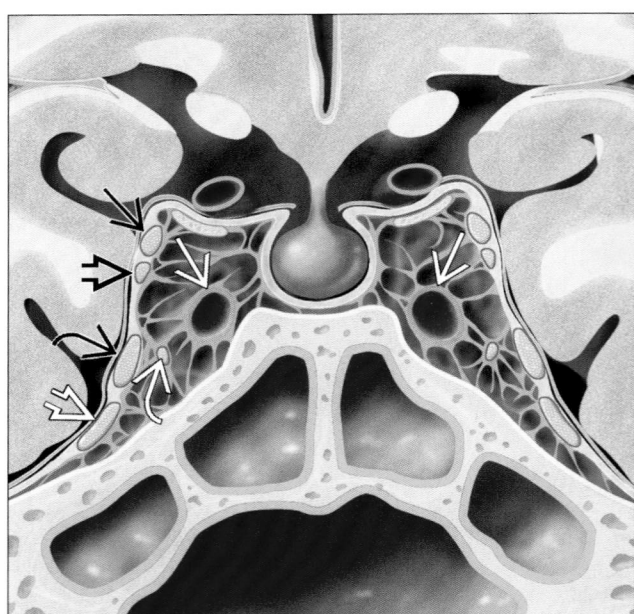

9-5. Coronal graphic shows the cavernous sinuses (CSs) and their contents. The CSs are fenestrated, septated, and multichanneled. The ICAs ⇨ and CN VI ⇨ are inside the CSs. CN III ⇨, IV ⇨, V₁ ⇨, and V₂ ⇨ lie in the lateral dural wall.

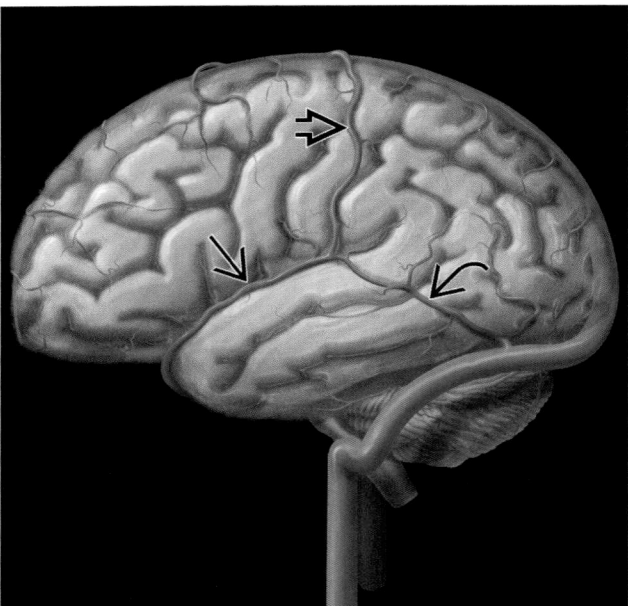

9-6. Lateral graphic depicts the superficial cortical veins. The 3 named anastomotic veins—Trolard ⇨, Labbé ⇨, and the superficial middle cerebral vein ⇨—are depicted. One or two of the superficial cortical veins are usually dominant.

with each other via intercavernous venous plexuses. The CSs drain inferiorly through the foramen ovale into the pterygoid venous plexuses and posteriorly into the clival venous plexus as well as the superior and inferior petrosal sinuses.

While the intercavernous septations and compartments are quite variable, the size and configuration of the CSs are relatively constant on imaging studies. The lateral walls normally appear straight or concave (not convex), and the venous blood enhances quite uniformly.

Superior and Inferior Petrosal Sinuses

The superior petrosal sinus (SPS) courses posterolaterally along the top of the petrous temporal bone, extending from the CS to the sigmoid sinus. The inferior petrosal sinus (IPS) courses just above the petrooccipital fissure from the inferior aspect of the clival venous plexus to the jugular bulb (9-4).

Clival Venous Plexus

The clival venous plexus (CVP) is a network of interconnected venous channels that extends along the clivus from the dorsum sellae superiorly to the foramen magnum (9-4). The CVP connects the cavernous and petrosal sinuses with each other and with the suboccipital veins around the foramen magnum.

Sphenoparietal Sinus

The sphenoparietal sinus (SphPS) courses around the lesser sphenoid wing at the rim of the middle cranial fossa. The SphPS receives superficial veins from the

anterior temporal lobe and drains into the cavernous or inferior petrosal sinus.

Cerebral Veins

The cerebral veins are subdivided into three groups: (1) superficial ("cortical" or "external") veins, (2) deep cerebral ("internal") veins, and (3) brainstem/posterior fossa veins.

Superficial Cortical Veins

The superficial cortical veins consist of a superior group, a middle group, and an inferior group.

SUPERIOR CORTICAL VEINS. Between 8 and 12 unnamed superficial veins course over the upper surfaces of the cerebral hemispheres, generally following convexity sulci. They cross the subarachnoid space and pierce the arachnoid and inner dura before draining into the SSS. In many cases, a dominant superior cortical vein, the **vein of Trolard**, courses upward from the sylvian fissure to join the SSS (9-6).

On lateral CTV, MRV, or venous phase DSA, the superior cortical veins are arranged in a spoke-like pattern, coursing centripetally toward the SSS and entering it at right angles.

MIDDLE CORTICAL VEINS. The most prominent vein in this group is the **superficial middle cerebral vein** (SMCV). The SMCV begins over the sylvian fissure and collects numerous small tributaries from the temporal, frontal, and parietal opercula that overhang the lateral cerebral fissure.

On lateral CTV, MRV, or venous phase DSA, the SMCV courses anteroinferiorly, paralleling the sylvian fissure, and curves around the temporal tip to terminate in the CS or sphenoparietal sinus.

INFERIOR CORTICAL VEINS. These veins drain most of the inferior frontal lobes and temporal poles. The **deep middle cerebral vein** (DMCV) collects tributaries from the insula, basal ganglia, and parahippocampal gyrus, then anastomoses with the **basal vein of Rosenthal** (BVR). The BVR courses posterosuperiorly in the ambient cistern, curving around the midbrain to drain into the VofG.

A prominent posterior anastomotic vein, the **vein of Labbé**, courses inferolaterally over the temporal lobe to drain into the transverse sinus **(9-6)**.

All three named superficial anastomotic veins—the vein of Trolard, vein of Labbé, and SMCV—vary in size, maintaining a reciprocal relationship with each other. If one or two are dominant, the third anastomotic vein is usually hypoplastic or absent.

Deep Cerebral Veins

The deep cerebral ("internal") veins are themselves subdivided into three groups: (1) medullary veins, (2) subependymal veins, and (3) deep paramedian veins **(9-7)**.

MEDULLARY VEINS. Innumerable small, unnamed veins originate between one and two centimeters below the cortex and course straight through the white matter toward the ventricles where they terminate in the subependymal veins **(9-8)**. These veins are generally inapparent on imaging studies throughout most of their course until they converge near the ventricles. DSA and contrast-enhanced MR may show faint linear stripes of contrast parallel to the ventricles **(9-9)**. T2* susceptibility-weighted imaging (SWI) best depicts the medullary veins because the deoxygenated blood is paramagnetic **(9-10)**.

SUBEPENDYMAL VEINS. The subependymal veins course under the ventricular ependyma, collecting blood from the basal ganglia and deep white matter (via the medullary veins) **(9-8)**. The most important named

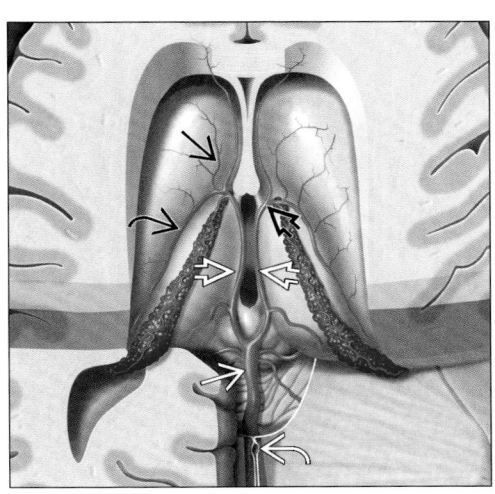
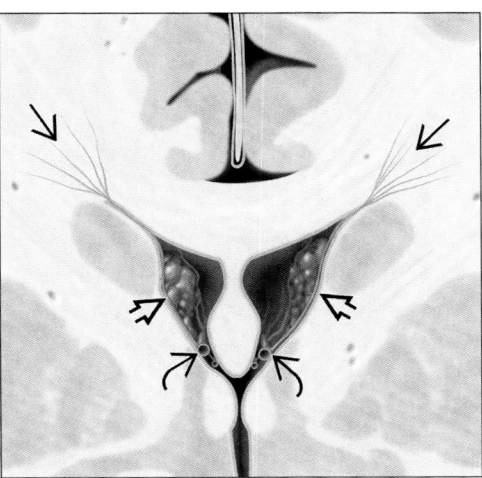
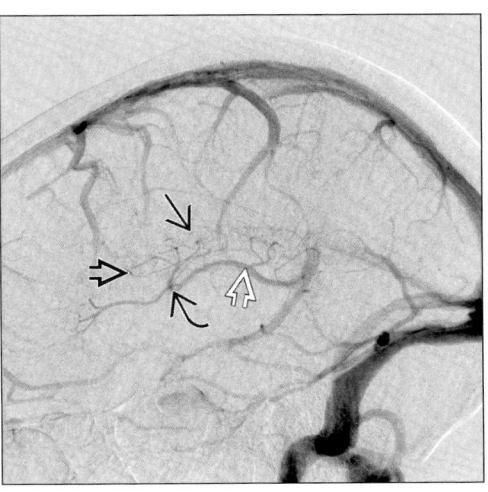
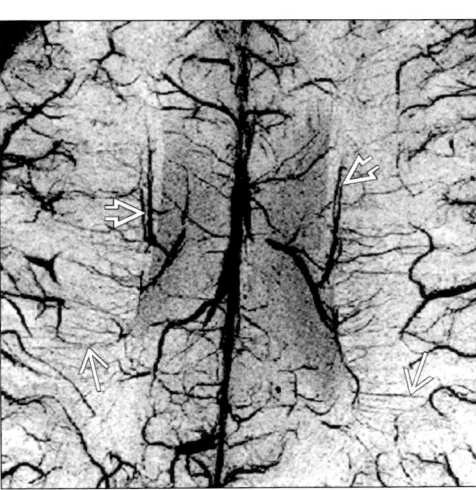

9-7. Deep cerebral and subependymal venous drainage is seen from the top down. Caudate ➡ and terminal veins ↗ form the thalamostriate veins ⊳, which drain into the internal cerebral veins ⊳, vein of Galen ➡, and straight sinus ➡. *9-8.* Coronal graphic through the coronal ventricles depicts the medullary (deep white matter) veins ➡ converging at the ventricular margins to drain into the subependymal ⊳ and thalamostriate ↗ veins. From there, they drain into the ICVs.

9-9. Venous phase DSA shows tiny medullary veins ➡ draining into subependymal veins, seen here as "dots" on end ⊳. The septal and thalamostriate veins converge near the foramen of Monro ➡ to form the internal cerebral vein ⊳. *9-10.* Close-up axial view of 3.0 T T2* SWI scan shows deoxyhemoglobin in innumerable small medullary veins ➡ that course through the white matter to converge at right angles with the ventricles and drain into the subependymal veins ⊳.

subependymal veins are the septal veins and the thalamostriate veins. The **septal veins** curve around the frontal horns of the lateral ventricles, then course posteriorly along the septi pellucidi. The **thalamostriate veins** receive tributaries from the caudate nuclei and thalami, curving medially to unite with the septal veins near the foramen of Monro to form the two internal cerebral veins **(9-8)**.

DEEP PARAMEDIAN VEINS. The **internal cerebral veins** (ICVs) and **vein of Galen** (VofG) provide drainage for most of the deep brain structures. The ICVs are paired paramedian veins that course posteriorly in the cavum velum interpositum, the thin invagination of subarachnoid space that lies between the third ventricle and the fornices. The ICVs terminate in the rostral quadrigeminal cistern by uniting with each other and the BVRs to form the VofG **(9-8)**.

The vein of Galen (great cerebral vein) curves posterosuperiorly under the corpus callosum splenium, uniting with the inferior sagittal sinus to form the straight sinus.

Brainstem/Posterior Fossa Veins

The veins that drain the midbrain and posterior fossa structures are likewise divided into three groups: (1) a superior ("galenic") group, (2) an anterior (petrosal) group, and (3) a posterior group.

SUPERIOR (GALENIC) GROUP. As the name implies, these veins drain superiorly into the vein of Galen. Major named veins in this group are the precentral cerebellar vein, the superior vermian vein, and the anterior pontomesencephalic vein **(9-11)**.

The **precentral cerebellar vein** (PCV) is a single midline vein that lies between the lingula and the central lobule of the vermis. It terminates behind the inferior colliculi by draining into the VofG. The **superior vermian vein** runs over the top of the vermis, joining the PCV and draining into the VofG **(9-11)**.

The **anterior pontomesencephalic vein** (APMV) is actually an interconnected venous plexus, not a single dominant vein. The APMV covers the cerebral peduncles and extends over the anterior surface of the pons **(9-12)**, **(9-13)**.

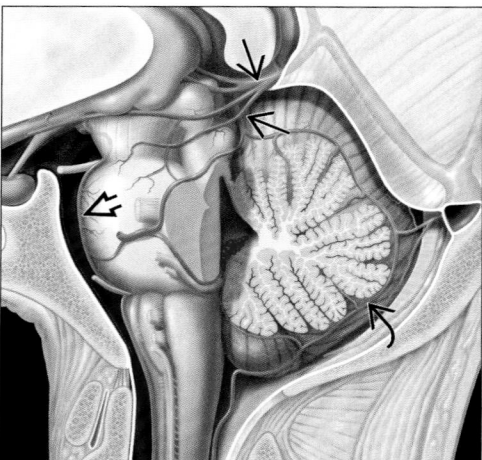
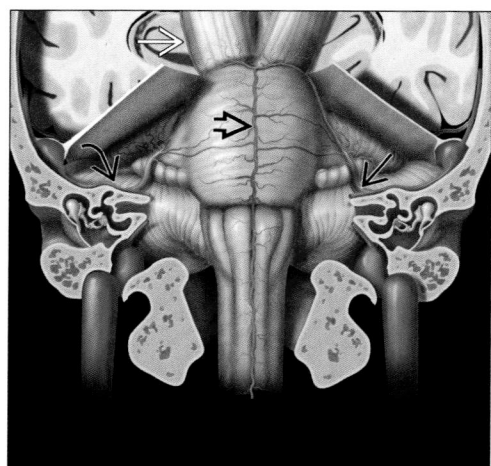

9-11. Sagittal graphic through the vermis shows the superior (galenic) group of veins ➡, the anterior group with the pontomesencephalic vein ➡, and the posterior group ➡. 9-12. Coronal graphic shows the anterior pontomesencephalic ➡ and the petrosal ➡ venous plexuses draining the pons, anterior cerebellum, and cerebellopontine angle cistern. Note anastomoses with the superior petrosal sinuses ➡ and mesencephalic veins ➡.

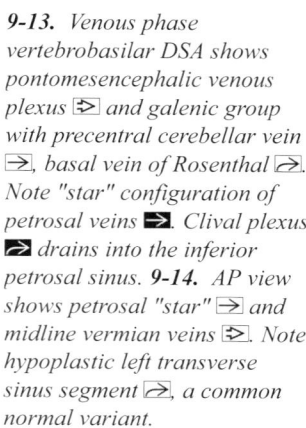
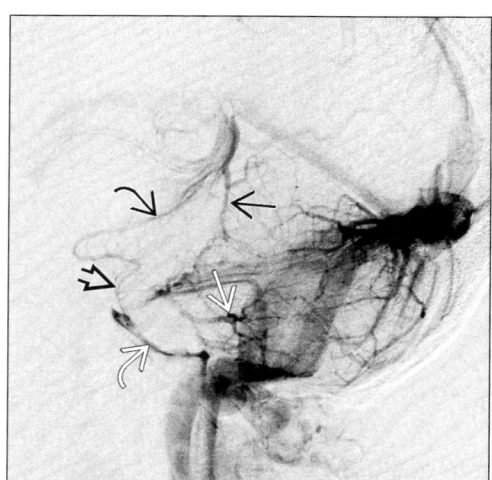
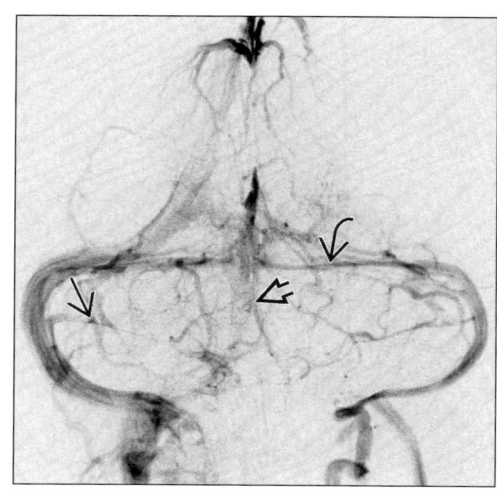

9-13. Venous phase vertebrobasilar DSA shows pontomesencephalic venous plexus ➡ and galenic group with precentral cerebellar vein ➡, basal vein of Rosenthal ➡. Note "star" configuration of petrosal veins ➡. Clival plexus ➡ drains into the inferior petrosal sinus. 9-14. AP view shows petrosal "star" ➡ and midline vermian veins ➡. Note hypoplastic left transverse sinus segment ➡, a common normal variant.

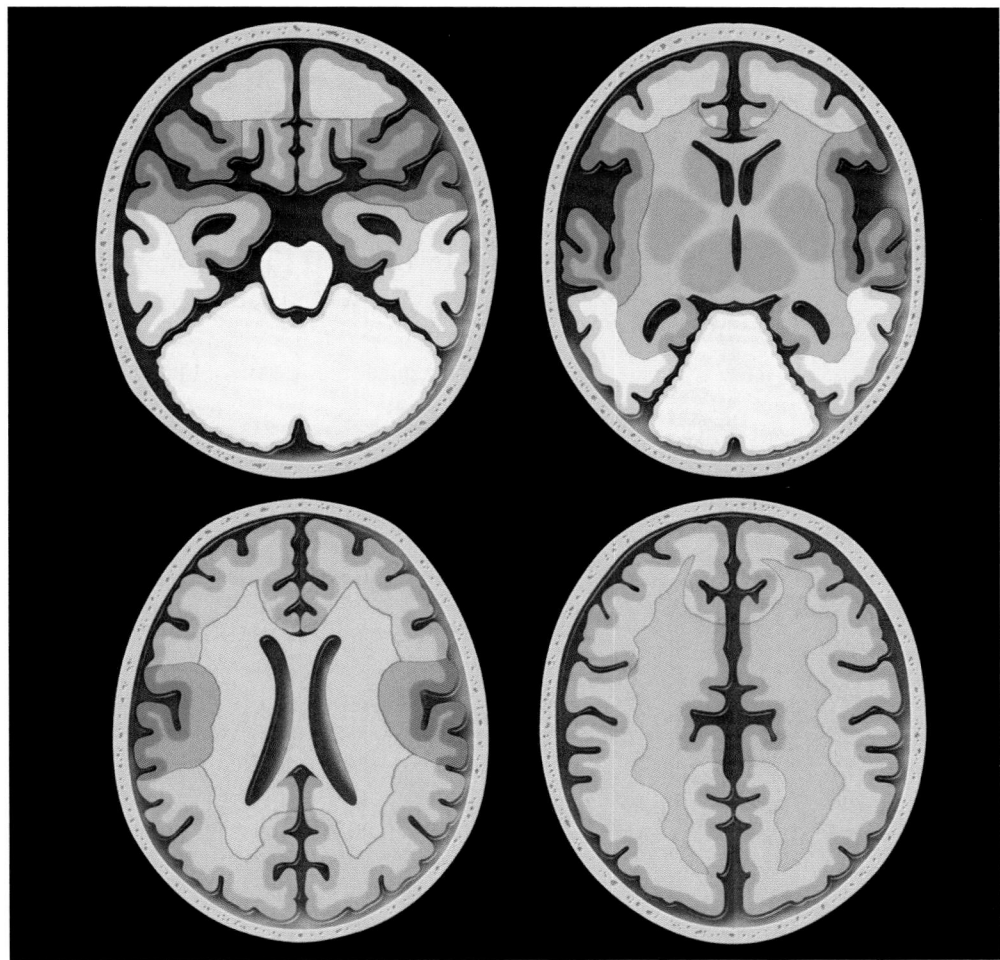

9-15. *Superficial parts of the brain (cortex, subcortical white matter) are drained by cortical veins and superior sagittal sinus (shown in green). Central core brain structures (basal ganglia, most white matter, ventricles) are drained by the deep venous system (ICVs, vein of Galen, straight sinus) (red). The veins of Labbé and the transverse sinuses drain the posterior temporal, inferior parietal lobes (yellow). The sphenoparietal, cavernous sinuses drain the area around the sylvian fissures (purple).*

ANTERIOR (PETROSAL) GROUP. The **petrosal vein** (PV) is a large venous trunk that lies in the cerebellopontine angle cistern, collecting numerous tributaries from the cerebellum, pons, and medulla. The PV and its tributaries form a prominent star-shaped vascular collection seen on AP DSA or coronal CTV **(9-14)**.

POSTERIOR (TENTORIAL) GROUP. The most prominent veins in this group are the **inferior vermian veins**, paired paramedian structures that curve under the vermis and drain the inferior surface of the cerebellum.

Venous Drainage Territories

The cerebral venous drainage territories are both less familiar and somewhat more variable than the major arterial distributions. These drainage patterns follow four basic patterns: A peripheral (brain surface) pattern, a deep (central) pattern, an inferolateral (perisylvian) pattern, and a posterolateral (temporoparietal) pattern **(9-15)**. Accurately diagnosing and delineating venous occlu-

sions depends on understanding these specific venous drainage territories.

Peripheral (Surface) Brain Drainage

Brain surface drainage generally follows a radial pattern. Most of the mid- and upper surfaces of the cerebral hemispheres together with their subjacent white matter drain centrifugally (outward) via cortical veins into the SSS.

Deep (Central) Brain Drainage

The basal ganglia, thalami, and most of the hemispheric white matter all drain centripetally (inward) into the deep cerebral veins. The internal cerebral veins, vein of Galen, and straight sinus together drain virtually the entire central core of the brain.

The most medial aspects of the temporal lobes, primarily the uncus and the anteromedial hippocampus, also drain into the galenic system via the deep middle cerebral veins and basal veins of Rosenthal.

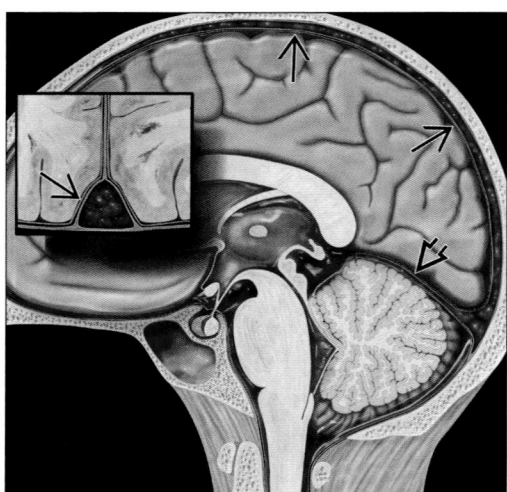

9-16. *Sagittal graphic shows SSS ⇥, SS ⇥ thrombosis. Insert shows pathologic basis of "empty delta" sign.*

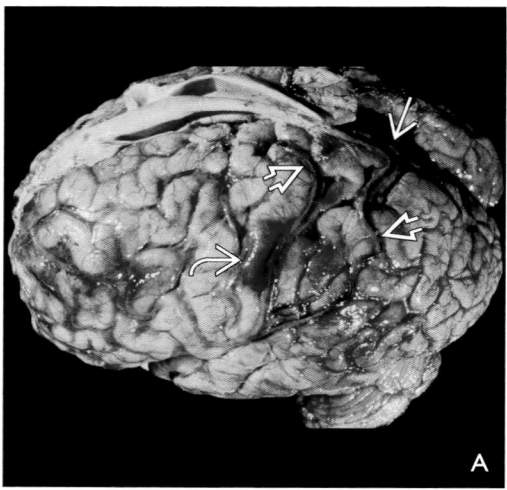

9-17A. *Autopsy case of acute SSS ⇥, cortical vein ⇥ thrombosis, venous infarcts ⇥.*

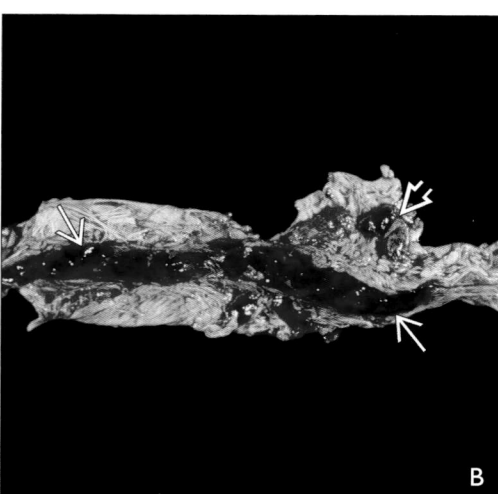

9-17B. *Gross photograph from the same case shows "currant jelly" clot in the SSS ⇥, cortical veins ⇥. (Courtesy E. T. Hedley-Whyte, MD.)*

Inferolateral (Perisylvian) Drainage

Parenchyma surrounding the sylvian (lateral cerebral) fissure consists of the frontal, parietal, and temporal opercula plus the insula. This perisylvian part of the brain drains via the superficial middle cerebral vein into the sphenoparietal sinus and cavernous sinus.

Posterolateral (Temporoparietal) Drainage

The posterior temporal lobes and inferolateral aspects of the parietal lobes drain via the superior petrosal sinuses and anastomotic vein of Labbé into the transverse sinuses.

Cerebral Venous Thrombosis

Dural venous sinus, superficial (cortical) vein, and deep vein occlusions are collectively termed cerebral venous thrombosis (CVT). CVT is an elusive diagnosis with a great diversity of causes and clinical presentations; it is also easily overlooked on imaging studies. Normal dura and circulating blood are mildly hyperdense compared to brain on NECT scans, so the subtle increased attenuation of venous thrombi can be difficult to detect. Venous sinuses lie directly adjacent to the skull, so clots can also be obscured by attenuation artifacts.

Venous infarcts can be relatively innocuous or lethal. They can mimic neoplasm, encephalitis, and numerous other nonvascular pathologies.

In this section, we consider several different types of CVT. We begin with the most common intracranial venous occlusion, dural sinus thrombosis. We next discuss superficial vein thrombosis and follow with deep cerebral occlusions.

We conclude the discussion with a consideration of cavernous sinus (CS) thrombosis/thrombophlebitis. Because of its anatomic proximity to the nose and paranasal sinuses, the CS is especially vulnerable to retrograde infection. The combination of infection and thrombosis means the clinical presentation and imaging findings of CS thrombosis have some special features not shared with other venous occlusions.

Dural Sinus Thrombosis

Terminology

Cerebral dural sinus thrombosis is defined as thrombotic occlusion of one or more intracranial venous sinuses **(9-16).** DST can occur either in isolation or in combination with cortical and/or deep venous occlusions.

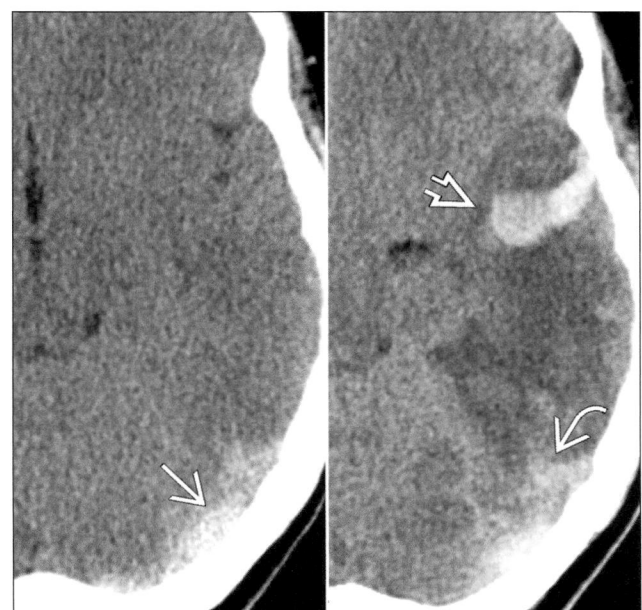

9-18. A 23-year-old woman with "migraine headache." First NECT scan (left) was called normal. Note hyperdense thrombus in left TS ➡. CT 1 day later (right) shows vein of Labbé ➡ thrombosis and large hemorrhagic infarct ➡.

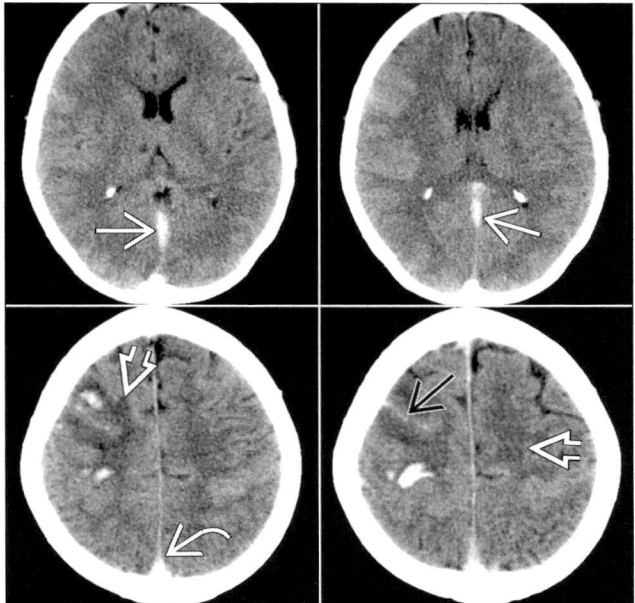

9-19. NECT in another patient shows hyperdense thrombus in the SS ➡ and SSS ➡ with bilateral edema ➡, hematomas, and convexal SAH ➡.

Etiology

A wide variety of both inherited and acquired conditions are associated with increased risk of all CVTs. A predisposing comorbidity can be identified in the majority of cases, and many affected patients have more than one predisposing factor.

The most common acquired causes of CVT are oral contraceptive use and pregnancy/puerperium. Other conditions include—but are not limited to—trauma, infection, inflammation, hypercoagulable states, elevated hemoglobin levels, dehydration, collagen-vascular disorders (such as antiphospholipid syndrome), vasculitis (such as Behçet syndrome), drugs, and Crohn disease.

Between 20-35% of all patients with CVT have an inherited or acquired prothrombotic condition. Predisposing genetic factors are common and include antithrombin III, protein C, and protein S deficiency, as well as resistance to activated protein C caused by factor V Leiden gene mutation.

Pathology

When thrombus forms in a dural sinus, venous outflow is restricted. This results in venous congestion, elevated venous pressure, and hydrostatic displacement of fluid from capillaries into the extracellular spaces of the brain. The result is blood-brain barrier breakdown with vasogenic edema. If a frank venous infarct develops, cytotoxic edema ensues.

CEREBRAL VENOUS THROMBOSIS: CAUSES

Common
- Oral contraceptives
- Prothrombotic conditions
  - Deficiency of proteins C, S, or antithrombin III
  - Resistance to activated protein C (V Leiden)
  - Prothrombin gene mutations
  - Antiphospholipid, anticardiolipin antibodies
  - Hyperhomocysteinemia
- Puerperium, pregnancy
- Metabolic (dehydration, thyrotoxicosis, etc.)

Less Common
- Infection
  - Mastoiditis, sinusitis
  - Meningitis
- Trauma
- Neoplasm-related

Rare but Important
- Collagen-vascular disorders (e.g., APLA syndrome)
- Hematologic disorders (e.g., polycythemia)
- Inflammatory bowel disease
- Vasculitis (e.g., Behçet)

LOCATION. The transverse sinus is the most commonly thrombosed dural venous sinus, followed by the SSS.

GROSS PATHOLOGY. In acute DST, the affected dural sinus appears distended by a soft, purplish clot that can be isolated to the sinus or may extend into adjacent cortical veins (9-17). In chronic DST, firm proliferative fibrous tissue fills the sinus and thickens the dura-arachnoid.

The spectrum of associated brain injury in DST varies from venous congestion to ischemia to petechial hemorrhages and frank hemorrhagic infarcts.

9-20. Axial source image from a CTV shows the classic "empty delta" sign ➡ formed by enhancing dura surrounding nonenhancing thrombus in the superior axial sinus.

9-21. Coronal T1 C+ scan in a patient with SSS ➡ and bilateral TS ➡ occlusions demonstrates the "empty delta" sign. Note prominent sulcal enhancement ➡, caused by collateral venous drainage. Original—incorrect—diagnosis was meningitis.

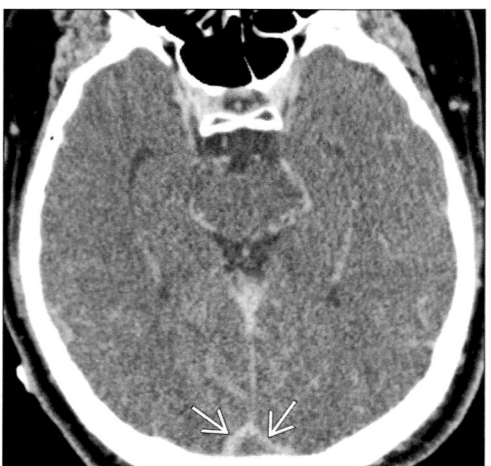
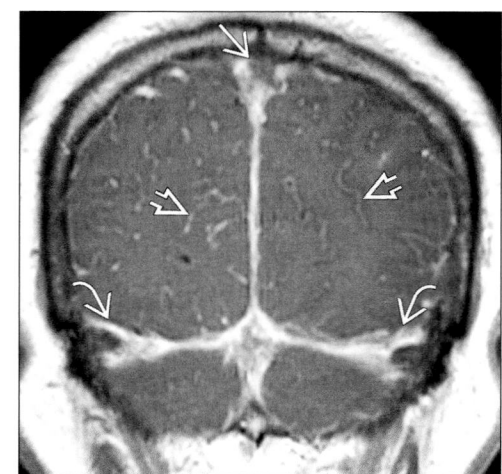

9-22A. Axial NECT scan in a 29-year-old pregnant woman with headaches, papilledema shows hyperdense right TS ➡ compared to the left sigmoid sinus ➡. 9-22B. Sagittal T1WI in the same patient shows a normal "flow void" in the straight sinus ➡. The SSS shows an absent "flow void" and—except for the CSF-filled arachnoid granulations ➡—appears filled with clot ➡ that is almost isointense with brain.

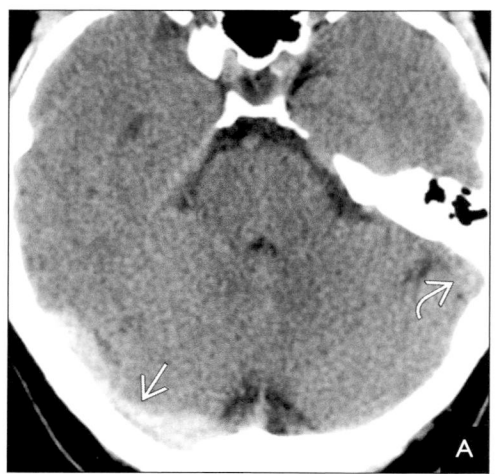
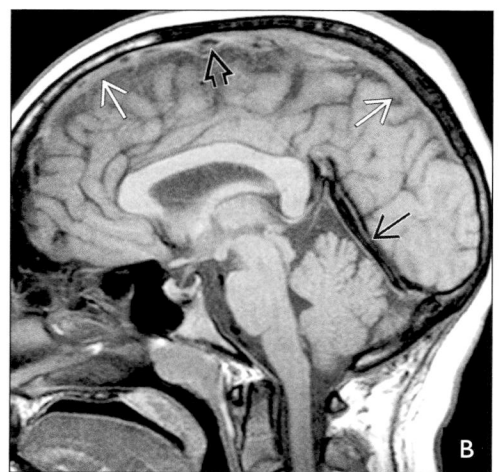

9-22C. Axial T1WI in the same patient shows an enlarged right TS that appears filled with isointense clot ➡. Compare to the normal "flow void" in the left vein of Labbé ➡ and transverse sinus ➡. 9-22D. Axial T2WI in the same patient shows that the thrombosed right TS ➡ appears very hypointense and mimics the "flow voids" of the patent left TS ➡ and vein of Labbé ➡.

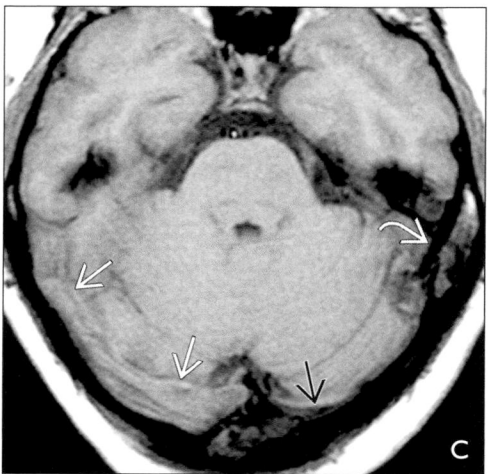
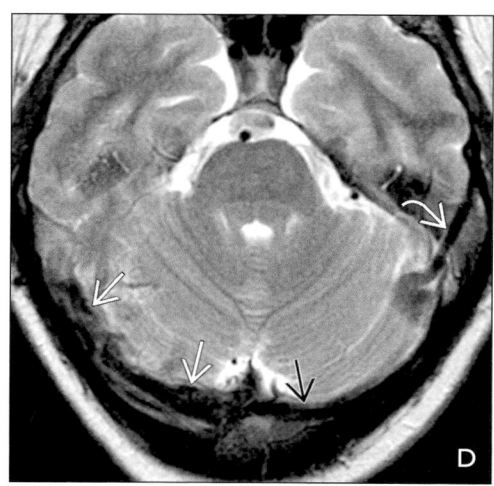

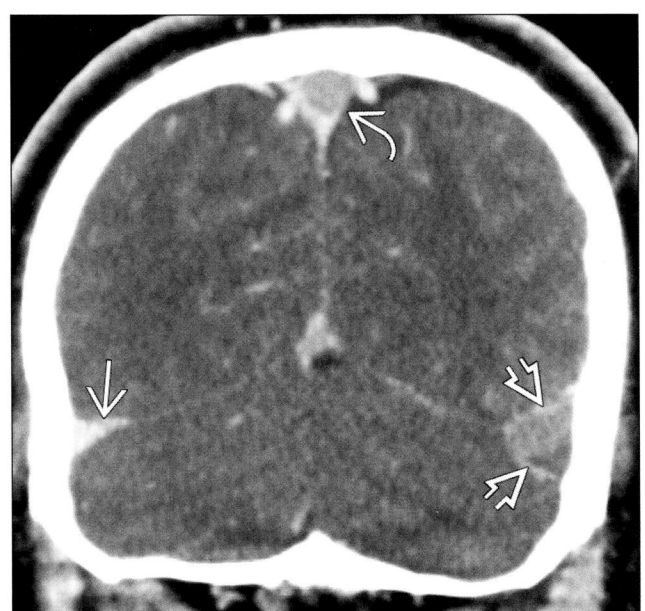

9-23. Coronal CTV shows normal right TS ⬈ and thrombus with "empty delta" sign in the enlarged, distended left TS ⬈ and SSS ⬈.

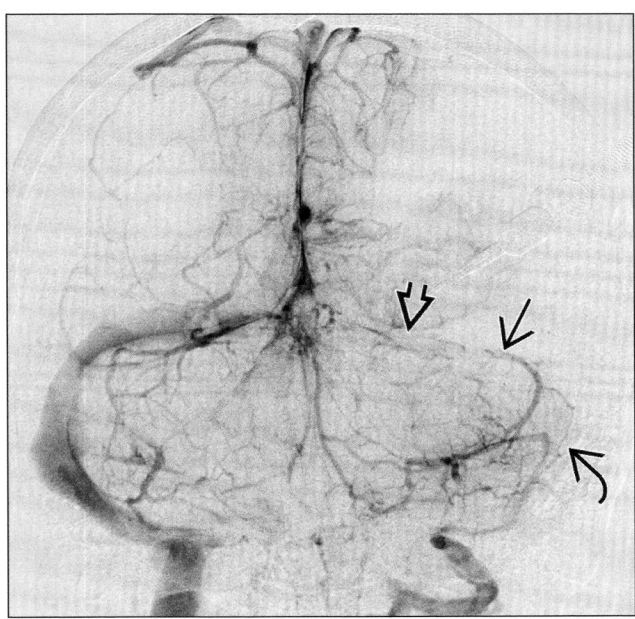

9-24. AP view, venous phase, of vertebrobasilar DSA in a patient with occlusion of the left TS ⬈ and sigmoid sinus ⬈. Note clot in adjacent tentorial vein ⬈.

Clinical Issues

EPIDEMIOLOGY. Cerebral venous occlusions represent between 0.5-1% of all acute strokes. Although CVT can occur at any age (from neonates to the elderly), it is most commonly seen in young individuals. Nearly 80% of patients are younger than 50 years of age. The estimated annual incidence is five cases per million adults.

DEMOGRAPHICS. Dural sinus thrombosis predominantly affects women (F:M = 3:1). A gender-specific risk factor (oral contraceptives, pregnancy, puerperium, and hormone replacement therapy) is present in nearly two-thirds of all women with CVT. Because of these gender-specific risk factors, mean age at presentation is nearly a decade younger in women compared to men (34 years vs. 42 years).

PRESENTATION. The clinical manifestations of CVT are varied, often nonspecific, and may be subtle—especially in neonates, children, and the elderly. Headache occurs in nearly 90% of cases and is usually nonfocal, often slowly increasing in severity over several days to weeks. Nearly 25% of patients present without focal neurologic findings, making the clinical diagnosis even more difficult.

NATURAL HISTORY. The natural history of CVTs varies widely, as does outcome. Some DSTs recanalize spontaneously without sequelae, whereas others form an arteriovenous fistula in the dural sinus wall.

Delay in diagnosis also affects outcome. The time between symptom onset and correct diagnosis averages seven days in large series. Diagnostic delay is associated with increased death and disability rates.

Following cerebral vein and/or dural sinus thrombosis, there is a small but measurable increased risk of further venous thromboembolic events, especially in male patients and those with polycythemia/thrombocythemia.

TREATMENT OPTIONS. Prompt recognition of DST has a great impact on clinical outcome. Patients with mild or minimal symptoms may require no intervention. In severe cases, mechanical thrombectomy with or without heparin infusion may succeed in reopening an occluded sinus.

DURAL SINUS THROMBOSIS:
PATHOLOGY AND CLINICAL ISSUES

Pathology
- TS > SSS > SS > CS

Clinical Issues
- Epidemiology, demographics
  - 1% of all strokes
  - Any age (newborn to elderly patients)
  - Generally younger patients (80% < 50 years)
  - F >> M (F:M = 3:1)
- Presentation
  - Headache (70%)
  - Nausea, vomiting
  - Impaired consciousness

Imaging

Keys to the early neuroradiologic diagnosis of DST are (1) a high index of suspicion, (2) careful evaluation of

9-25A. *Late acute DST in a 25-year-old man with several days of diarrhea and progressively worsening headache. NECT scan had demonstrated no definite abnormality. Axial T1WI shows mild hyperintensity in the right TS* ➡. **9-25B.** *Axial T2WI shows that the thrombus in the right TS* ➡ *is beginning to appear mildly hyperintense, unlike the very hypointense clot seen on T2WI in acute DST. Note small T2 hyperintensity in the left TS* ➡.

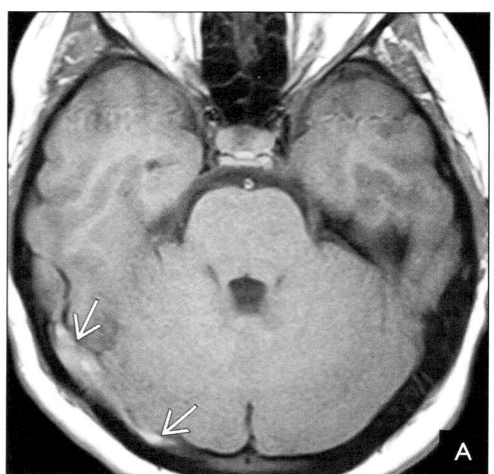

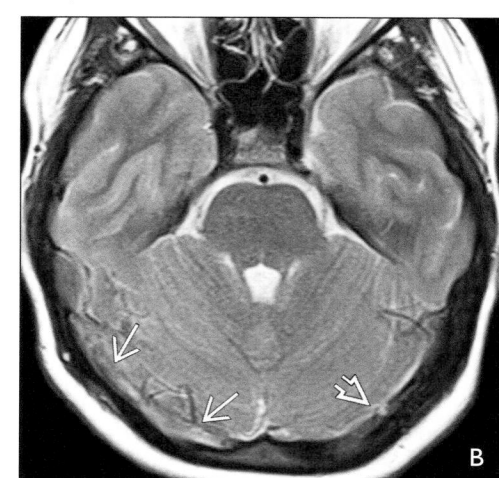

9-25C. *Axial FLAIR scan in the same patient shows that the right TS thrombus* ➡ *is mildly hyperintense. Contrast this with the normal "flow void" in the left TS* ➡. **9-25D.** *Axial T2* GRE in the same patient shows "blooming" thrombus* ➡ *in the right TS and tentorial venous tributaries* ➡.

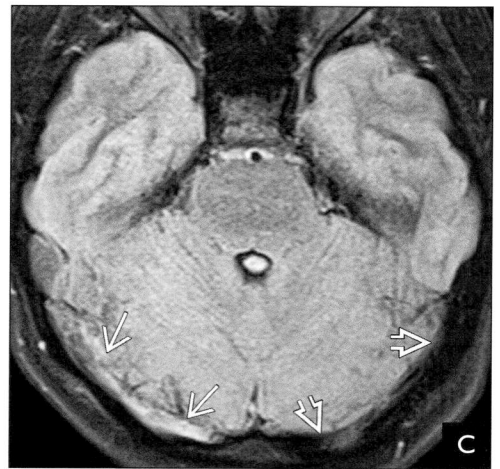

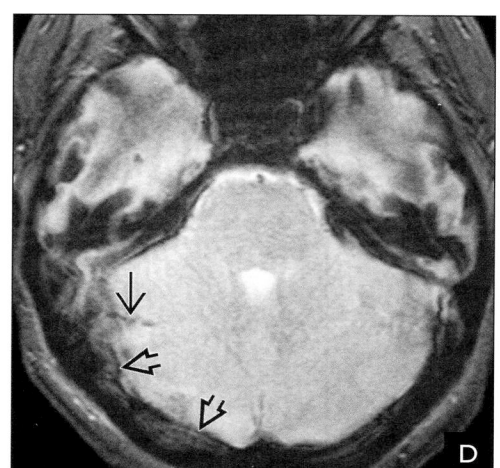

9-25E. *Axial T1 C+ FS scan shows the nonenhancing thrombus in the right TS* ➡ *surrounded by the intensely enhancing dura. The left TS shows an ovoid filling defect with CSF intensity* ➡ *containing a linear central enhancing vein* ➡. *Findings are characteristic of an arachnoid granulation.* **9-25F.** *Axial MIP of 3D TOF MRV shows nonfilling of the right transverse and sigmoid sinuses. The 2 ovoid filling defects* ➡ *in the left TS are arachnoid granulations.*

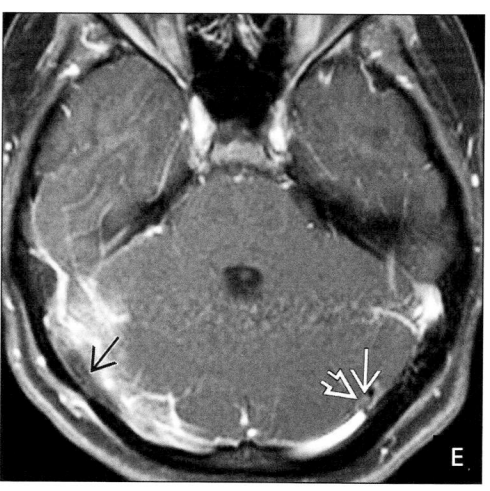

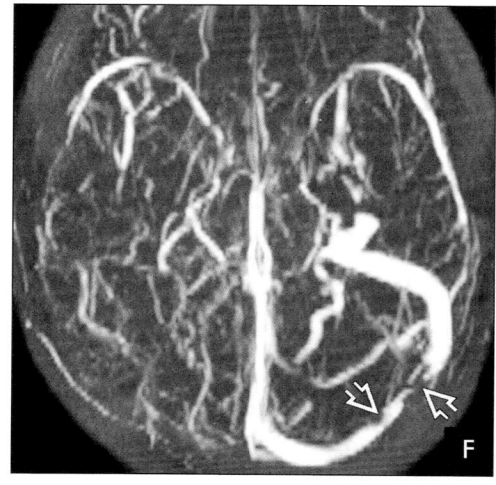

dural sinus density/signal intensity and configuration, and (3) knowledge of normal venous drainage patterns.

CT FINDINGS. *NECT may be normal early, so a normal NECT scan does **not** exclude the diagnosis of CVT!* Early signs on NECT are often subtle. Slight hyperdensity compared to the carotid arteries is seen in 50-60% of cases and may be the only hint of sinus or venous occlusion **(9-18)**. When present, a hyperattenuating vein ("cord" sign) or dural venous sinus ("dense triangle" sign) is both a sensitive and specific sign of cerebral venous occlusive disease. Parenchymal edema with or without petechial hemorrhage in the territory drained by the thrombosed sinus is a helpful but indirect sign of DST **(9-19)**.

In 70% of cases, CECT scans show an **"empty delta" sign** caused by enhancing dura surrounding nonenhancing thrombus **(9-20)**, **(9-21)**. "Shaggy," enlarged, or irregular veins suggest collateral venous drainage.

CTA/CTV has fewer artifacts than MRV and is therefore the best noninvasive method for delineating dural sinus filling defects. CTA/CTV readily demonstrates the classic "empty delta" sign of sinovenous thrombosis **(9-23)**.

MR FINDINGS. The imaging appearance of DST varies significantly with clot age, as with parenchymal hematomas. Acute, subacute, and chronic occlusions all have different findings on MR.

Acute DST. An acutely thrombosed sinus often appears moderately enlarged and displays abnormally convex—not straight or concave—margins. The "flow void" of rapidly moving blood typically seen in large venous sinuses disappears, replaced by loose but nevertheless solid blood clot. Acute DST appears *isointense* with the underlying cortex on **T1WI (9-22)**.

As hemoglobin in blood clots rapidly desaturates to deoxyhemoglobin, it becomes very *hypointense* relative to brain on **T2WI (9-22D)**. Therefore the acute T2 "dark" DVT mimics normal intrasinus "flow void." If venous congestion and edema develop secondary to obstructed outflow, they cause gyral swelling and parenchymal hyperintensity on T2/FLAIR.

Similar to parenchymal hematomas, acute venous clots *"bloom"* on **T2* (GRE, SWI)**. SWI shows the profoundly hypointense clot and dilated cortical veins.

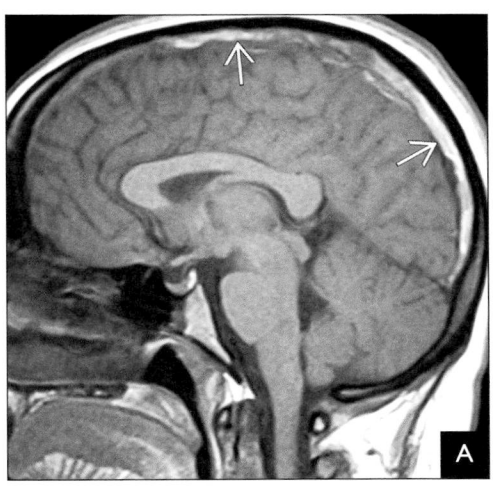

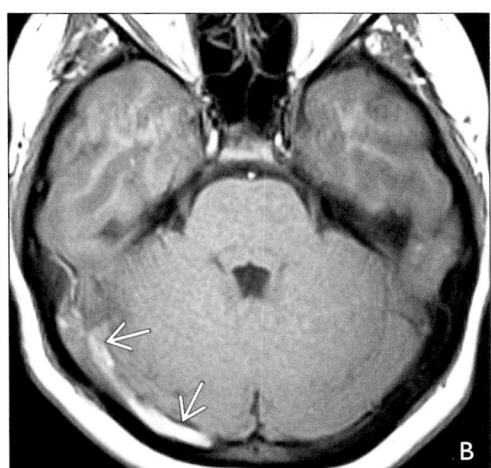

9-26A. Sagittal T1WI was obtained 5 days later in the same patient. It shows typical evolution of signal intensity from late acute to subacute thrombus. Note striking hyperintensity in the SSS ➡️. 9-26B. Axial T1WI shows the striking hyperintensity of the subacute clot in the right TS ➡️. Compare this to the mild hyperintensity seen in the late acute phase depicted on the previous page.

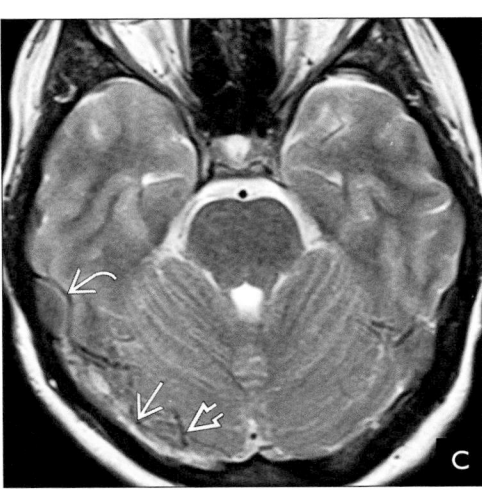

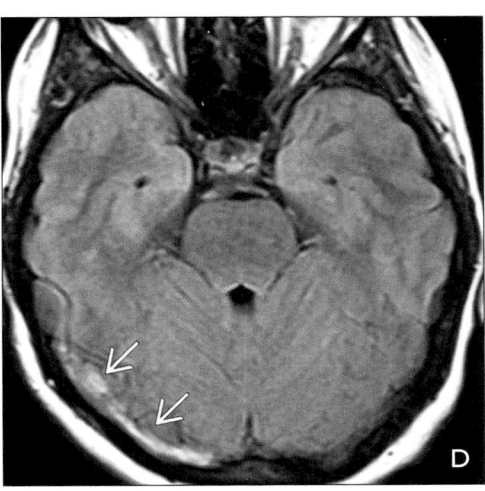

9-26C. Axial T2WI shows the classic hyperintensity of subacute thrombus ➡️ in the right TS. Note normal "flow voids" in the patent adjacent vein of Labbé ➡️ and tentorial tributary veins ➡️. 9-26D. Axial FLAIR in the same patient shows the hyperintense subacute thrombus ➡️. The adjacent cerebellum and posterior temporal lobe appear normal, without evidence of venous ischemia or infarction.

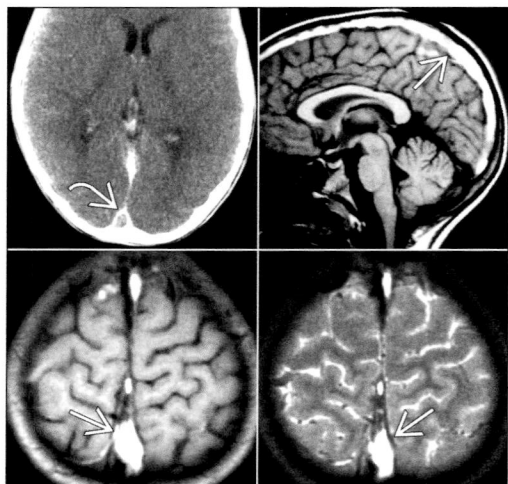

9-27. *Late subacute SSS thrombosis shows "empty delta" sign ➔ and hyperintense thrombus ➔.*

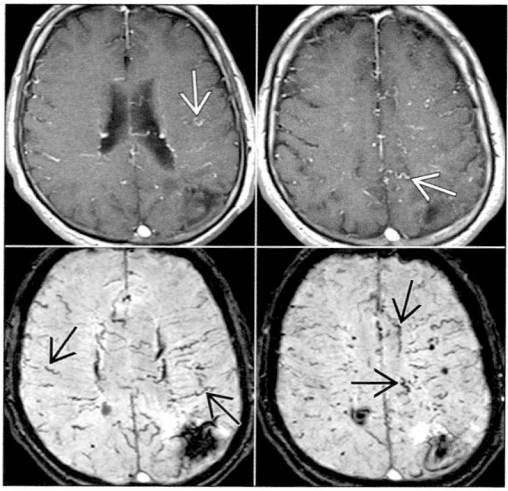

9-28. *Chronic SSS occlusion shows prominent "squiggly" parenchymal veins on T1 C+ ➔ and "flow voids" on SWI ➔.*

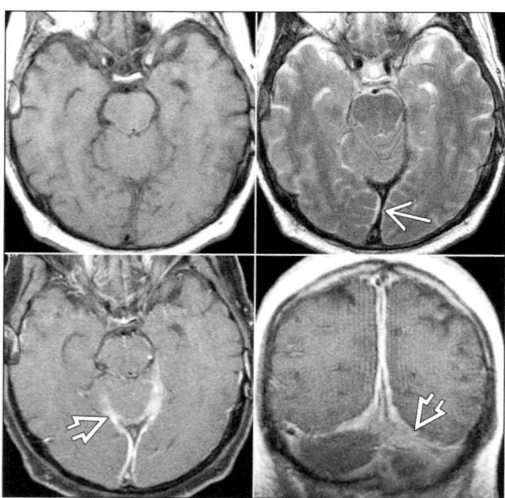

9-29. *Chronic SSS thrombosis shows hypointense ➔ thick enhancing dura ➔. (Courtesy M. Castillo, MD.)*

The appearance may nonetheless be confusing as normal-flowing but deoxygenated venous blood also appears hypointense.

Extensive DST often results in collateral venous drainage through the medullary (white matter) veins into the deep subependymal veins. The medullary veins enlarge and contain desaturated hemoglobin; thus, they are seen on T2* sequences as prominent linear hypointensities entering the subependymal veins at right angles.

T1 C+ scans also demonstrate an "*empty delta" sign*, similar to the appearance on CECT and CTA/CTV. Intrasinus thrombi usually appear as elongated *cigar-shaped* nonenhancing filling defects. If ischemia or infarction occurs secondary to the DVT, **DWI** usually shows *restriction* in the affected territory.

Coronal 2D TOF **MRV** may demonstrate *absent flow*, especially if the thrombus is in the SSS. As the TSs often have hypoplastic segments, a "flow gap" must be interpreted with caution (see below).

Late acute DST. As the intrasinus thrombus organizes, the clot begins to exhibit T1 shortening and becomes progressively hyperintense. With T2 prolongation, the thrombosed sinus gradually progresses from appearing very hypointense to isointense with brain on both T2WI and FLAIR **(9-25)**. The clot "blooms" on T2* and continues to exhibit an "empty delta" sign on T1 C+.

Subacute DST. Subacute thrombus is hyperintense on both T1 and T2/FLAIR and "blooms" on T2* sequences **(9-26)**, **(9-27)**.

Chronic DST. Chronic thrombus eventually returns to isointensity with brain on T1WI and usually remains mildly to moderately hyperintense on T2WI. Longstanding CVST often develops significant collateral drainage through the medullary veins. This is seen on T1- and T2-weighted images as tortuous, "squiggly" intraparenchymal "flow voids" that enhance on T1 C+ scans, sometimes becoming so prominent that they mimic an arteriovenous malformation **(9-28)**.

Chronic organizing thrombus develops significant neovascularity and enhances strongly on T1 C+, demonstrating a "frayed" or "shaggy" appearance.

Dura-arachnoid thickening with intense enhancement is common in longstanding chronic DST. In some cases, the dural thickening becomes so pronounced that it appears very hypointense on T2WI **(9-29)**. Any residual clot may be reduced to thin, almost inapparent hyperintensity within the thick, markedly hypointense dura-arachnoid.

ANGIOGRAPHY. DSA has been almost completely superseded by MR and CTA in the imaging diagnosis of

DST, although it is still obtained prior to thrombolysis or mechanical thrombectomy.

Typical findings of DST on DSA are those of an occluded (nonfilling) sinus **(9-24)**. Slow flow (or clot) in the adjacent cortical veins is common. Delayed emptying often makes the cortical veins appear as if they are "hanging in space."

Dural arteriovenous fistulas (dAVFs) are strongly associated with DST. Thrombosis—especially of the transverse and/or sigmoid sinus—may be the precipitating factor in development of acquired dAVFs (see Chapter 7).

Differential Diagnosis

The two major differential diagnoses of DST are pseudoocclusion caused by a **hypoplastic** or **absent sinus segment** and a **giant arachnoid granulation** (see Venous Occlusion Mimics below).

DURAL SINUS THROMBOSIS: IMAGING

Imaging
- CT
  - NECT: Can be normal or subtle with dense dural sinus ± vein
  - CECT: "Empty delta" sign (enhanced dura around nonenhancing thrombus)
- MR signal varies with clot age
  - Acute: T1 iso-, T2 hypointense, T2* "blooms," T1 C+ shows "empty delta"
  - Late acute: T1 mildly hyper-, T2/FLAIR isointense, T2* "blooms"
  - Subacute: T1 hyper-, T2/FLAIR hyperintense, T2* "blooms"
  - Chronic: T1 iso-, T2/FLAIR moderately hyperintense , T2* shows "squiggly" parenchymal "flow voids," T1 C+ shows thick, enhancing dura
  - Longstanding: T1 iso-, T2 hypointense very thick dura

Differential Diagnosis
- Pseudoocclusion
  - Hypoplastic/absent TS segment
  - Giant arachnoid granulations
- Other
  - Blood layered along tentorium (acute subdural hematoma)
  - Elevated hematocrit (all vessels abnormally dense)

Superficial Cerebral Vein Thrombosis

Superficial cerebral vein thrombosis (SCVT) can occur with or without DST. When it occurs without accompanying DST, SCVT is termed isolated cortical vein thrombosis.

Superficial Vein Thrombosis *With* DST

Two general types of SCVT with DST are recognized: DST that involves one or more small cortical draining veins and DST that affects one of the great anastomotic veins (Trolard or Labbé).

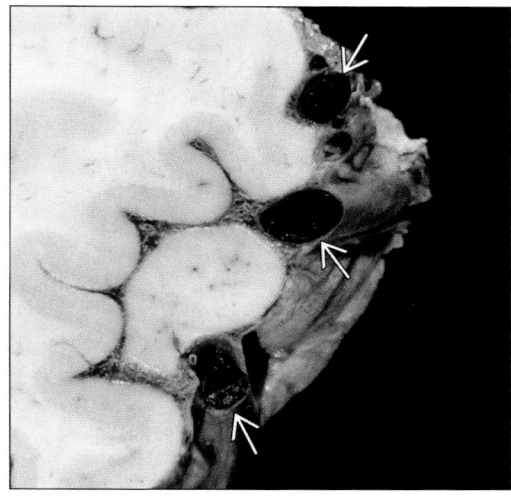

9-30. *Autopsy case shows thrombus in several cortical veins* ➡, *the pathologic basis for the "cord" sign. (Courtesy E. T. Hedley-Whyte, MD.)*

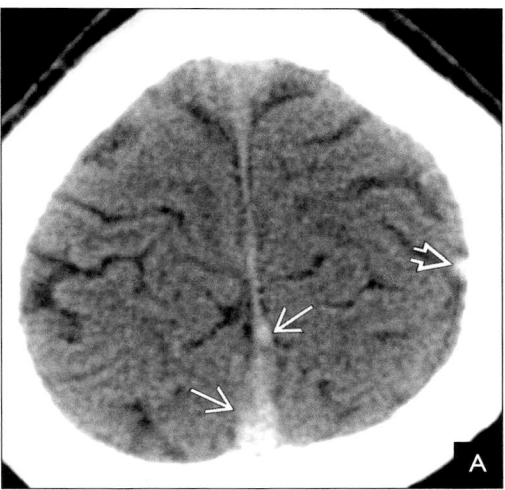

9-31A. *NECT scan shows obvious SSS thrombus* ➡ *with a hyperdense "cord" sign* ➡.

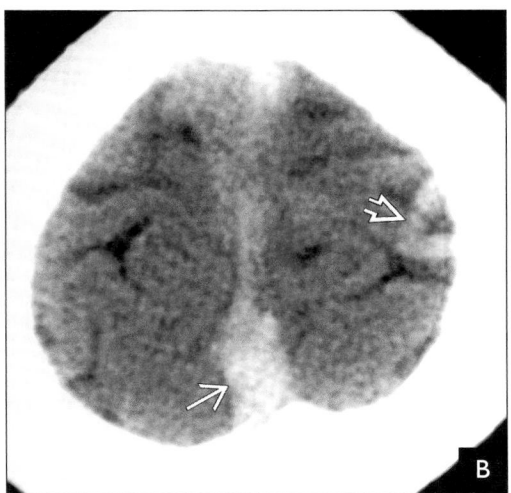

9-31B. *NECT in the same patient shows SSS thrombus* ➡ *and clot in cortical veins* ➡.

9-32A. Axial T2WI shows an expanded SSS ➥ filled with hypointense thrombus. Clot is also present in the left vein of Labbé ➥; however, the clot is essentially invisible on this sequence as it mimics a normal "flow void." *9-32B.* Axial T2* GRE in the same patient shows that "blooming" clot in the SSS ➥ extends into the thrombosed vein of Labbé ➥. No subarachnoid or parenchymal hemorrhage was identified.

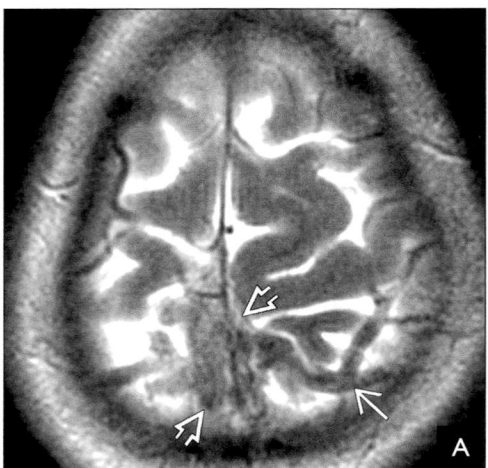
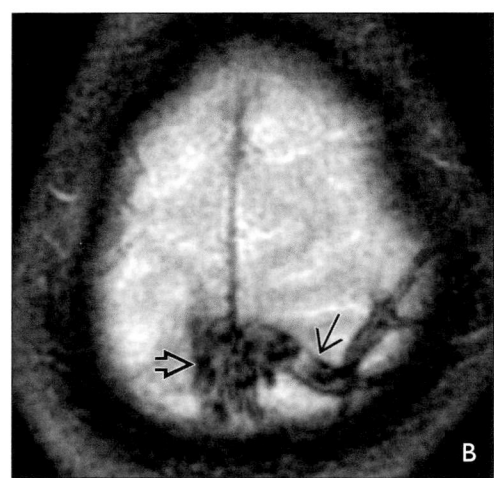

9-33A. A 46-year-old man with a family history of brain tumors presented in the ED with headache followed by a first-time seizure. NECT scan shows a hypodense lesion ➥ involving both the cortex and subcortical white matter of the right parietal convexity. Note patchy petechial hemorrhage ➥ within the lesion. *9-33B.* MR scan with SWI in the same patient shows isolated thrombosis of the right vein of Trolard ➥. The superior sagittal sinus ➥ is normal.

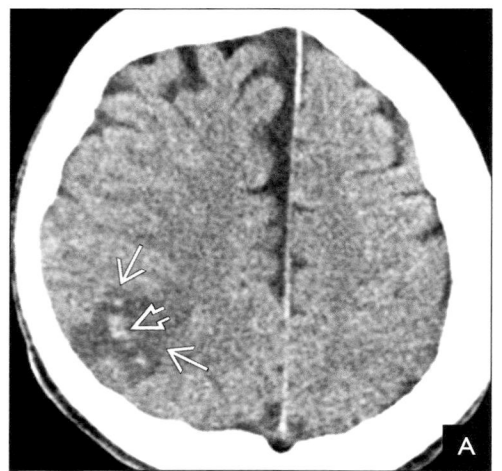
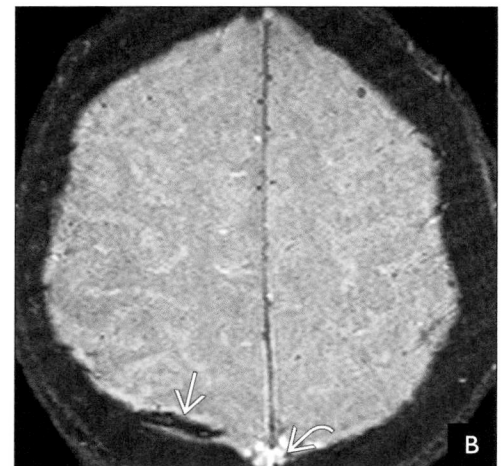

9-34. Autopsy case of TS thrombosis ➥ that occluded a dominant vein of Labbé shows extensive hemorrhagic venous infarction of the temporal, parietal, and occipital lobes ➥. (Courtesy R. Hewlett, MD.) *9-35.* Sagittal T1WI scan 3 days after a patient presented with severe headache shows late acute thrombus in the left TS ➥. Clot also occluded the dominant vein of Labbé, causing massive hemorrhage in the inferolateral temporal lobe ➥.

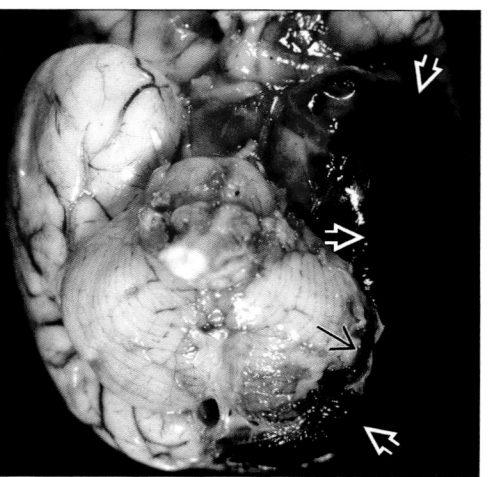
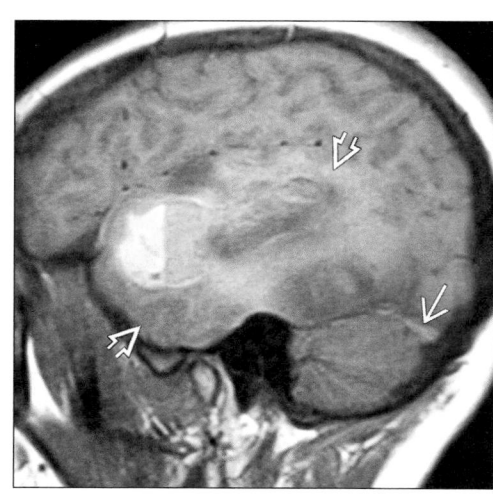

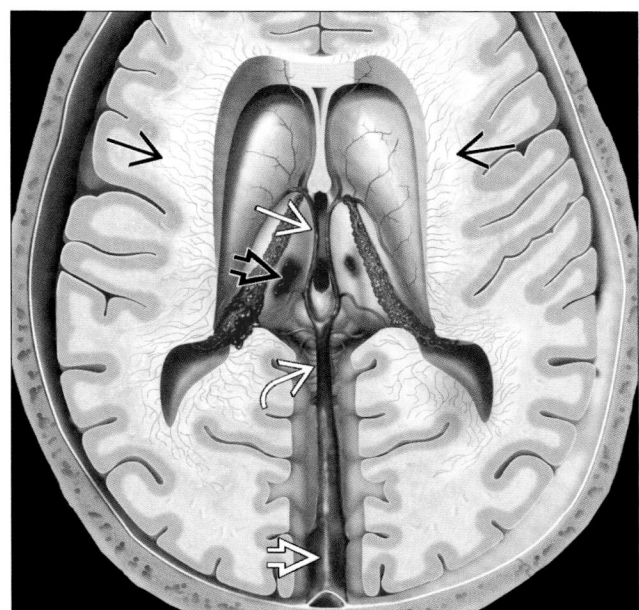

9-36. Axial graphic depicts deep venous occlusion with thrombosis of both ICVs ➡, VofG ➡, and SS ➡ with hemorrhage in both thalami ➡. Note venous congestion with edema, and engorgement of WM medullary veins ➡.

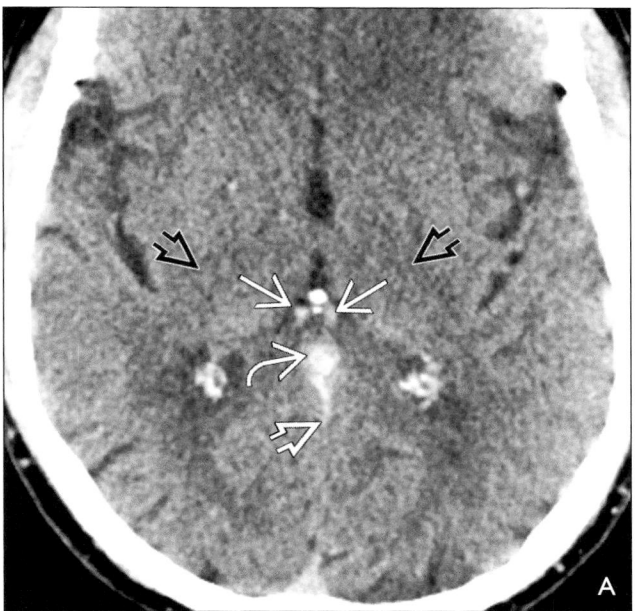

9-37A. NECT scan in a 79-year-old aphasic man imaged for "brain attack" shows hyperdensity in both ICVs ➡, VofG ➡, and SS ➡. Note hypodensity in both anterior thalami ➡ with indistinct gray-white matter interfaces.

Imaging findings of SCVT with accompanying DST are similar to those of dural sinus thrombosis alone. In addition to clot in the sinus, thrombus extends into one or more cortical veins **(9-30)**, **(9-31)**, **(9-32)**. SSS occlusion with SCVT affects the superolateral surfaces of the hemispheres, with variable amounts of edema and petechial hemorrhage involving the cortex and subcortical white matter. If the anastomotic vein of Trolard is dominant, its occlusion may result in lobar hemorrhage **(9-33)**.

Transverse sinus occlusion that extends into a dominant vein of Labbé often causes extensive posterior temporal and anterior parietal hemorrhage **(9-34)**, **(9-35)**.

Superficial Vein Thrombosis *Without* DST

SCVT in the absence of dural sinus thrombosis is rare, representing only 5% of all sinovenous occlusions. The clinical outcome of isolated SCVT is generally good.

Isolated SCVT usually presents with a nonspecific headache. Approximately 10% of patients report a "thunderclap" headache that clinically mimics aneurysmal subarachnoid hemorrhage. Symptoms such as focal neurologic deficits, seizures, and impaired consciousness are less common than with dural sinus or deep vein thrombosis.

The imaging diagnosis of isolated SCVT can be problematic. NECT is usually negative although a few cases may demonstrate focal convexal subarachnoid hemorrhage or a solitary "cord" sign that represents a hyperdense thrombosed vein. CTA/CTV is typically normal. DSA may demonstrate intraluminal thrombus and delayed venous drainage.

The MR diagnosis is difficult to establish using only standard T1- and T2-weighted sequences. MRV shows that the major dural sinuses are patent. Acute thrombi are isointense with brain on T1WI and hypointense on T2WI, making them difficult to distinguish from normal "flow voids." Focal parenchymal T2 hyperintensity in the cortical-subcortical is often present but is a nonspecific finding.

FLAIR may demonstrate focal convexal subarachnoid hemorrhage, seen as effacement of the normal hypointense sulcal CSF. Cortical-subcortical hyperintensities consistent with vasogenic edema are common associated findings.

Intraluminal thrombus can be seen as a linear hyperintensity on DWI. Venous ischemia may result in transient diffusion restriction.

T2* (GRE, SWI) sequences are key to the noninvasive diagnosis of isolated SCVT. With a sensitivity of more than 95%, they are by far the best imaging sequences for detecting solitary thrombosed cortical veins. A well-delineated tubular hypointensity with "blooming" of hemoglobin degradation products within the clot is observed at all stages of evolution, persisting for weeks or months. Patchy or petechial hemorrhages in the underlying cortex and subcortical white matter are common, as is associated convexal subarachnoid hemorrhage.

9-37B. *CTA/CTV in the same patient as shown on the previous page demonstrates normal arterial enhancement with lack of opacification of both ICVs ➡ and VofG/SS ➡. The SSS ➡ appears normal.*
9-37C. *Sagittal reconstruction confirms presence of thrombus with lack of opacification in the ICVs ➡, VofG ➡, and SS ➡. The SSS ➡ is normal.*

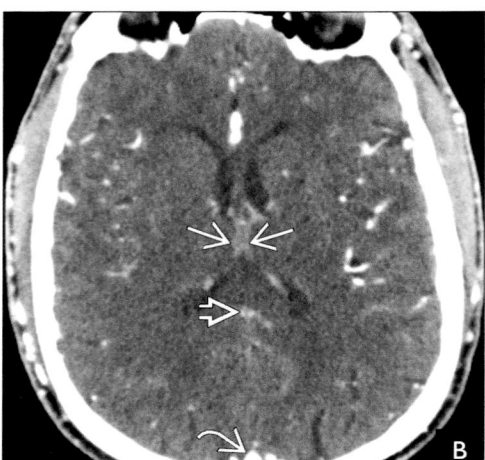
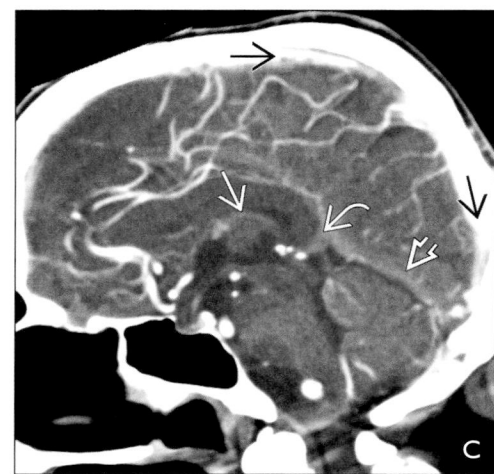

9-38A. *Sagittal T1WI in the same patient shows lack of normal "flow voids" with isointense clot present in the ICVs ➡, VofG ➡, and SS ➡.*
9-38B. *Axial T2* GRE scan shows clot with "blooming" hypointensity in the ICVs ➡, VofG ➡, and SS ➡. Note hypointensity caused by venous congestion with slow flow in the medial thalamic ➡ and deep WM medullary veins ➡.*

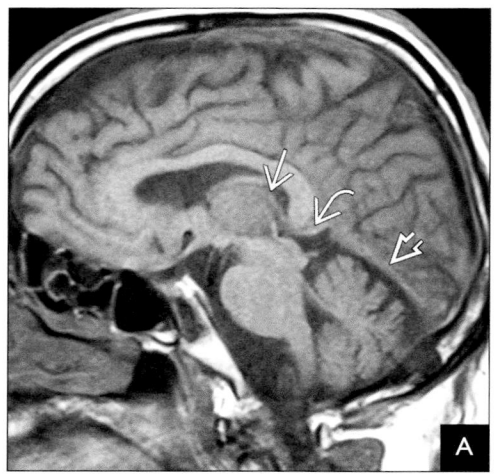
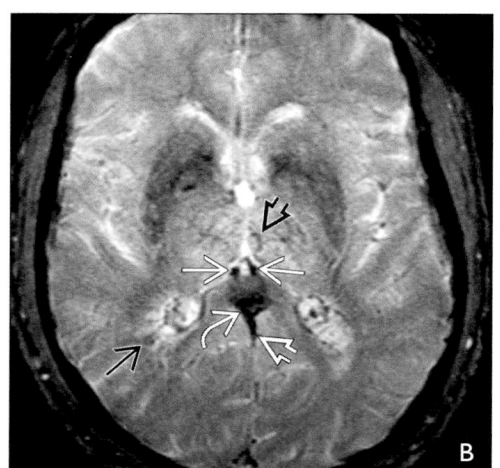

9-38C. *T2* GRE shows hypointensity from slow flow with deoxyhemoglobin in engorged subependymal ➡ and deep WM medullary veins ➡.* **9-38D.** *NECT scan 2 days later shows extensive confluent hypodensity ➡ in the entire central brain with a hemorrhagic focus in the left thalamus ➡. The hypodensity represents infarction in the deep venous drainage territory (compare with Figure 9-15). The patient died shortly afterward.*

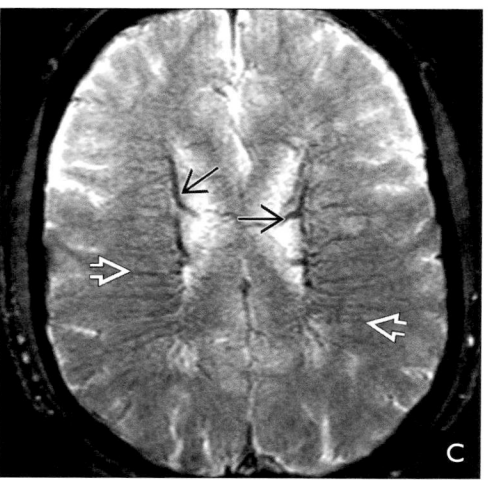
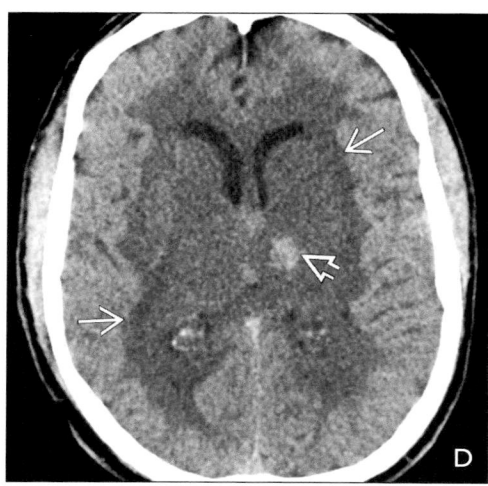

Deep Cerebral Venous Thrombosis

Deep cerebral venous thrombosis (DCVT) is a potentially life-threatening disorder with a combined mortality/disability rate of 25%.

Etiology and Pathology

The deep cerebral venous system (the ICVs and basal vein of Rosenthal, together with their tributaries, the vein of Galen, and straight sinus) is involved in approximately 15% of all patients with cerebral venoocclusive disease.

DCVT can occur either alone or in combination with other sinovenous occlusions. Isolated DCVT is present in 25-30% of cases. DCVT is almost always bilateral and results in symmetric venous congestion/infarction of the basal ganglia and thalami **(9-36)**.

Clinical Issues

The initial symptoms of DCVT are variable and nonspecific, making clinical diagnosis difficult. Most patients present with headache (80%) followed by rapid neuro-

logical deterioration and impaired consciousness (70%). Focal neurological findings are frequently absent.

Imaging

Early imaging findings on NECT may be subtle. Hyperdense ICVs and SS make the study resemble a contrast-enhanced scan **(9-37A)**. Hypodense "fading" or "disappearing" thalami with effacement of the border between the deep gray nuclei and internal capsule are important but nonspecific findings of DVT.

MR is the imaging modality of choice **(9-38)**. Acute thrombus is isointense on T1WI and hypointense on T2WI (pseudo-"flow void"). Venous congestion causes hyperintensity with swelling of the thalami and basal ganglia on T2/FLAIR in 70% of cases.

The most sensitive sequence is T2* GRE, on which acute clots show distinct "blooming." Venous congestion in the medullary and subependymal veins also appears hypointense because of slow flow and hemoglobin deoxygenation.

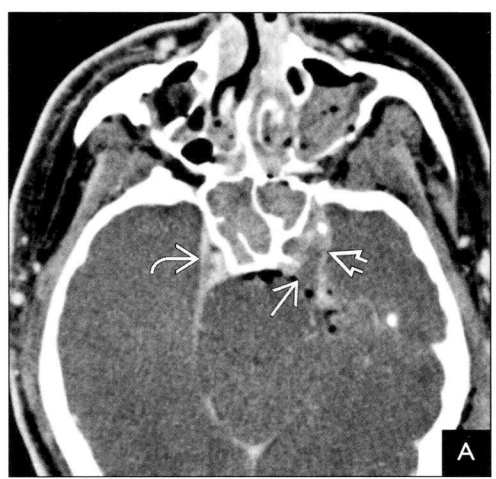

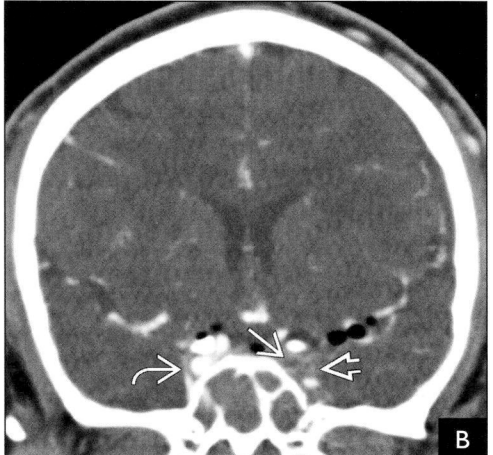

9-39A. CECT source image from CTA in a 28-year-old man with polytrauma shows filling defects in the left cavernous sinus ➱. The affected CS has a lightly convex lateral margin ➱ compared to the normal right CS ➱. 9-39B. Coronal CTA in the same patient shows occlusion of the left cavernous ICA ➱. The left CS remains unopacified because it is filled with thrombus ➱. Compare this to the normal right CS ➱.

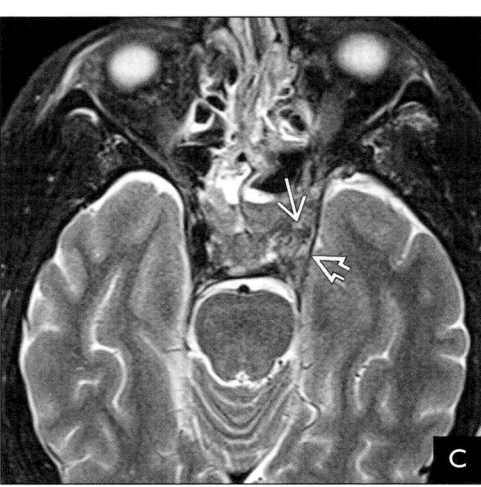

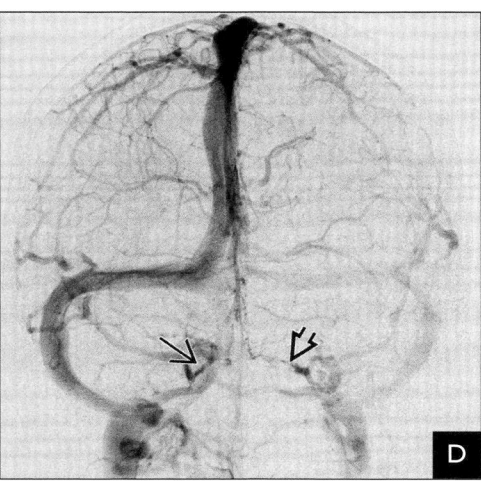

9-39C. Axial T2WI in the same patient shows left ICA occlusion, seen here as an absent "flow void" ➱. The left CS is filled with clot ➱ that appears mostly isointense with adjacent brain. 9-39D. Venous phase of right ICA angiogram demonstrates the difficulty in diagnosing CST on DSA. The right cavernous sinus ➱ is opacified, draining inferiorly into the pterygoid venous plexus. Left CS is not visualized, and subtle thrombus ➱ is present, seen here as a filling defect.

CTA/CTV and DSA demonstrate absent opacification in the deep venous drainage system **(9-37B)**, **(9-37C)**. MRV shows absence of flow in the deep drainage system.

Differential Diagnosis

The differential diagnosis of DCVT includes arterial occlusion, neoplasm, and toxic-metabolic disorders.

The artery of Percheron (AOP) is a single dominant thalamoperforating artery that arises from the basilar bifurcation or proximal posterior cerebral artery to supply both medial thalami and the midbrain. **Arterial strokes** caused by AOP thrombosis or "top of the basilar" occlusion often affect both thalami, but the arterial lesions are generally not as extensive as those of DCVT.

Bithalamic gliomas usually originate from the pons and/or midbrain with cephalad extension into the thalami and internal capsules. The ICVs can appear displaced upward but remain patent.

Carbon monoxide poisoning typically affects the globi pallidi while sparing the thalami.

SUPERFICIAL AND DEEP VEIN THROMBOSIS
Superficial Thrombosis With DST
• DST extends into adjacent veins
• Edema, hemorrhage in cortex, adjacent WM
• Can be extensive if vein of Trolard or Labbé occluded
Superficial Thrombosis Without DST
• Rare (5% of all CVTs)
• May cause convexal subarachnoid hemorrhage
• May see "cord" sign
• T2* (GRE, SWI) key to diagnosis
∘ "Blooming" thrombus in vein(s)
Deep Vein Thrombosis
• Uncommon (15% of CVTs)
• Usually both ICVs ± VofG, SS involved
• Hyperdense ICVs
• Bithalamic edema ± hemorrhage
• Can mimic neoplasm (bithalamic glioma)

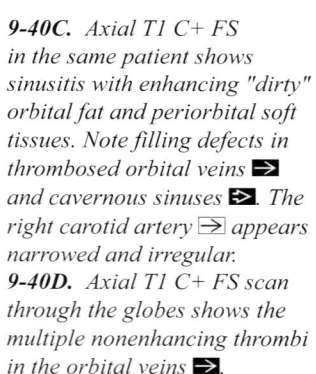

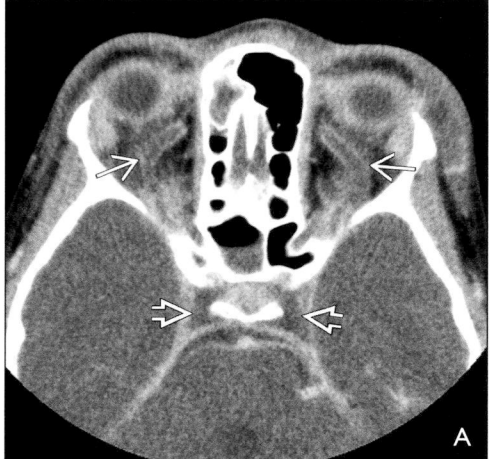

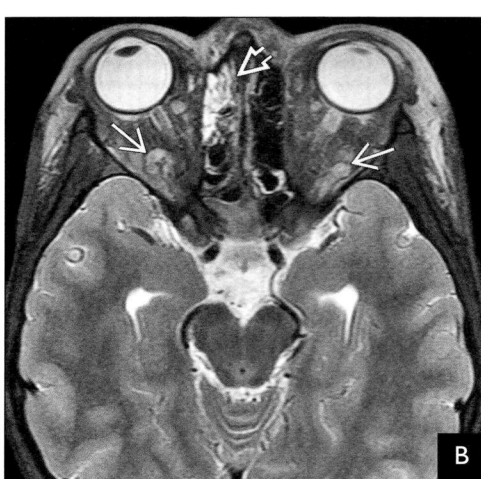

9-40A. A 5-year-old boy with sinus infection, fever, headache, and periorbital swelling presented to the ED. CECT scan shows proptosis with periorbital edema and ethmoid sinusitis with air-fluid level in the sphenoid sinus. The cavernous sinuses ⊳ and both superior ophthalmic veins → are filled with nonenhancing thrombus. 9-40B. Axial T2WI in the same patient shows the ethmoid sinusitis ⊳ and multiple enlarged intraorbital veins →.

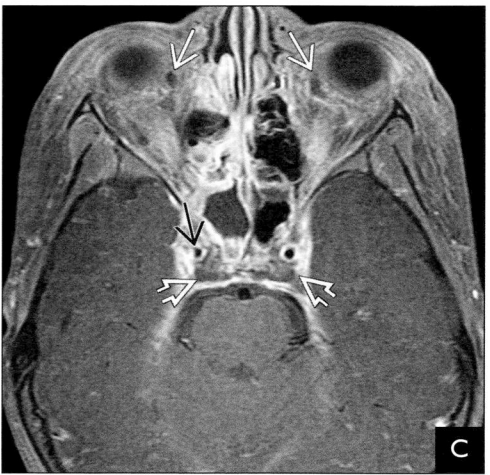

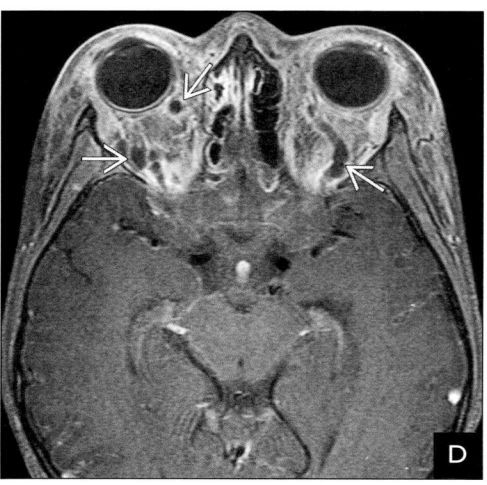

9-40C. Axial T1 C+ FS in the same patient shows sinusitis with enhancing "dirty" orbital fat and periorbital soft tissues. Note filling defects in thrombosed orbital veins → and cavernous sinuses ⊳. The right carotid artery → appears narrowed and irregular. 9-40D. Axial T1 C+ FS scan through the globes shows the multiple nonenhancing thrombi in the orbital veins →.

Cavernous Sinus Thrombosis/ Thrombophlebitis

Cavernous sinus thrombophlebitis is a rare but potentially lethal condition with significant morbidity and high mortality.

Terminology

Cavernous sinus thrombosis/thrombophlebitis (CST) is a blood clot in the cavernous sinus (CS), with or without accompanying infection (thrombophlebitis or thrombosis, respectively) **(9-39)**.

Etiology and Pathology

The CS is composed of numerous heavily trabeculated venous spaces that have numerous valveless communications with veins in the orbit, face, and neck. Infection can thus spread relatively easily through these venous conduits into the CS.

CST usually occurs as a complication of sinusitis or other midface infection. *S. aureus* is the most frequent pathogen. Other less common agents include anaerobes and angioinvasive fungal infections.

Otomastoiditis, odontogenic disease, trauma, and neoplasm are less frequent causes of CST.

Clinical Issues

EPIDEMIOLOGY. CS thrombosis without trauma, infection, or multiple other dural venous sinus occlusions is extremely rare.

PRESENTATION. Headache—especially in the CN V_1 and V_2 distributions—and fever are usually the earliest symptoms. Eye signs including orbital pain, edema, chemosis, proptosis, ophthalmoplegia, and visual loss are common.

NATURAL HISTORY. Bidirectional, bilateral spread into and out of the CS is typical. Untreated CST can be fatal. Even with antibiotics, the mortality rate of CS thrombophlebitis is 25-30%.

Imaging

CT FINDINGS. NECT scans with uncomplicated CS thrombosis may appear normal. CS thrombophlebitis causes proptosis, "dirty" orbital fat, periorbital edema, sinusitis, and lateral bulging of the CS walls. CECT scans demonstrate multiple irregular filling defects in the CS and superior ophthalmic veins **(9-40A)**. The lateral CS margins are convex (not flat or concave).

MR FINDINGS. MR scans show enlarged CSs with convex lateral margins. Acute thrombus is isointense with brain on T1WI and demonstrates variable signal intensity on T2WI. Nonenhancing filling defects within the

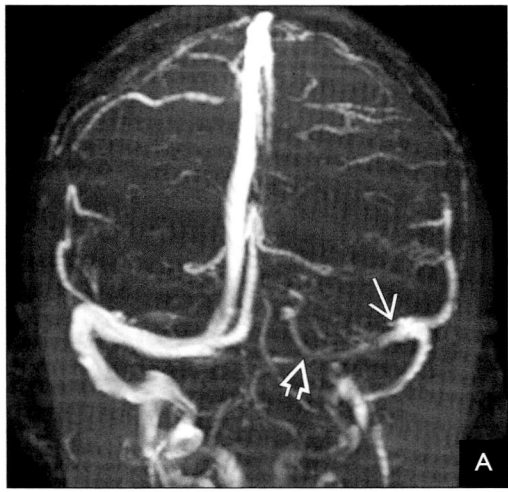

9-41A. MR venogram in a 22-year-old woman shows a dominant right TS. The left TS shows a "missing" segment ➡, possible filling defect ➡.

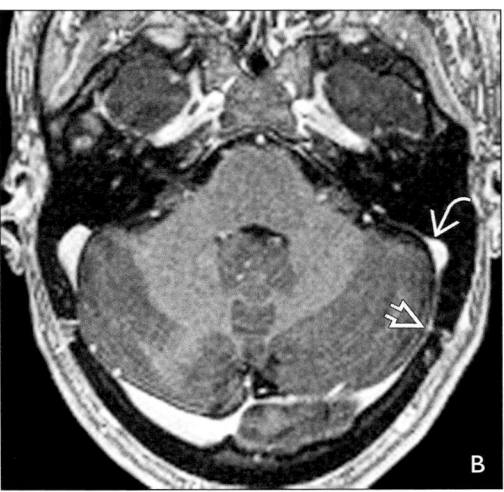

9-41B. Axial MP-RAGE shows hypoplastic but patent left TS ➡, small sigmoid sinus ➡.

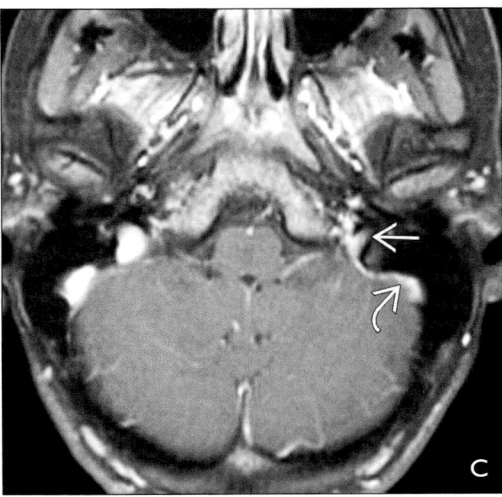

9-41C. T1 C+ FS scan shows that the left sigmoid sinus ➡ and jugular bulb ➡ are hypoplastic. "Missing" left TS is a normal variant (hypoplasia).

enhancing dural walls of the CS and thrombosed orbital veins on T1 C+ is the definitive imaging findings in CST **(9-40B), (9-40C), (9-40D)**.

ANGIOGRAPHY. The angiographic appearance of the normal CS varies from prominent and striking to minimal or none. Indeed, all of the skull base dural sinuses (superior and inferior petrosal sinuses, cavernous sinus, sphenoparietal sinuses, and clival venous plexus) are variably and inconstantly visualized on the venous phase of DSA. Nonvisualization of the CS on DSA can be a normal finding and does not indicate the presence of CS thrombosis.

In rare cases of CST, inflammation of the intracavernous carotid artery can lead to stenosis, thrombosis, or pseudoaneurysm formation.

Differential Diagnosis

The differential diagnosis of CST includes CS neoplasm, carotid-cavernous fistula, and inflammatory disorders. CS **neoplasms** such as lymphoma, meningioma, and metastases enhance uniformly and cause signifi-

cantly more mass effect than CST. **Carotid-cavernous fistula** causes "flow voids" and flow reversal from the CS into enlarged, intensely enhancing orbital veins. **Inflammatory diseases** such as sarcoid, granulomatosis with polyangiitis (formerly known as Wegener granulomatosis), and idiopathic inflammatory pseudotumor all enhance quite strongly and uniformly.

Venous Occlusion Mimics

We conclude this chapter on venous anatomy and occlusions with a brief discussion of conditions that can mimic—or obscure—venous thrombosis.

Sinus Variants

The major differential diagnosis of CVT is a **congenital anatomic variation**. The right transverse sinus is usually the dominant venous sinus and is often signifi-

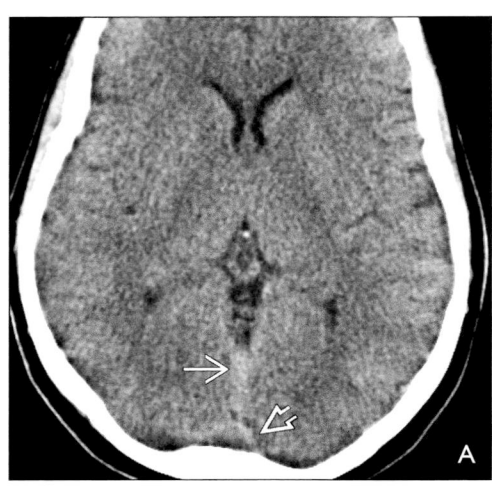
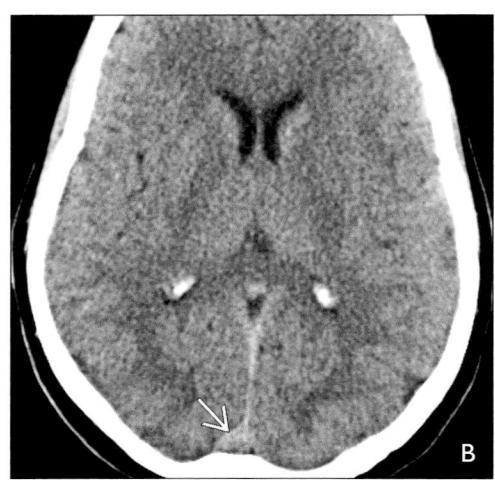

9-42A. *Axial NECT scan in a 28-year-old woman with severe headache shows mildly hyperdense straight sinus ➡ with an "empty delta"-appearing filling defect ⇲ in the sinus confluence (torcular herophili).* **9-42B.** *More cephalad NECT scan in the same patient shows that the sinus confluence ➡ appears normal.*

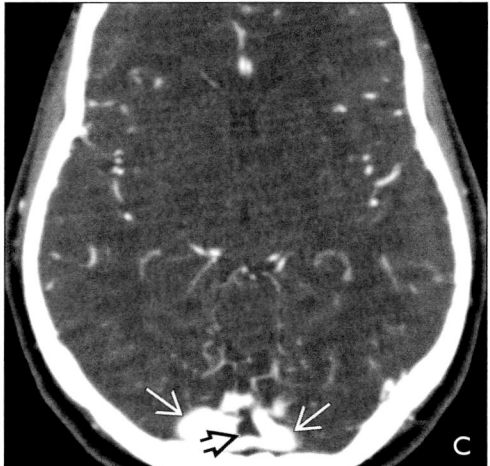
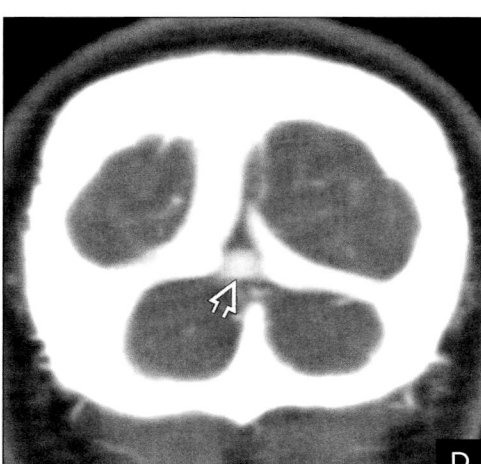

9-42C. *Because of the concern for DST, CTV was obtained. Several unusually prominent, intensely enhancing structures ➡ surround a central nonenhancing area ⇲ that could represent thrombus.* **9-42D.** *Coronal view of the CTV shows a horizontally oriented intersinus venous channel ➡ that connects a smaller left TS with the dominant right TS. Torcular anatomic variant mimics DST.*

cantly larger than the left side. A **hypoplastic transverse sinus** segment is present in one-quarter to one-third of all imaged cases and is *especially* common in the nondominant sinus (usually the left TS). In such instances, the ipsilateral jugular bulb is typically small **(9-41)**. Correlation with bone CT can also be helpful in demonstrating a small bony jugular foramen or sigmoid sinus groove. A hypoplastic transverse or sigmoid sinus is also often—but not invariably—associated with alternative venous outflow pathways such as a persistent occipital sinus or prominent mastoid emissary veins.

Variations in the torcular herophili (sinus confluence) are also common. A **high-splitting**, **segmented**, or **multichanneled sinus confluence** can have a central nonopacified area that mimics DST **(9-42)**.

The absence of occluded draining veins, enlarged venous collateral channels, or abnormally thick dural enhancement supports the diagnosis of TS sinus hypoplasia or anatomic variant vs. true CVST.

Flow Artifacts

A **"flow gap"** on 2D TOF MRV can result from a number of factors including slow intravascular or in-plane flow or complex blood flow patterns. Flow parallel to the plane of acquisition (in-plane flow) can cause signal loss on MR venography and is most prominent in vertically oriented structures such as the distal sigmoid sinus. Use of inferior saturation pulses with axial 2D TOF MRV can saturate flow in parts of the curving SSS but can be avoided by imaging in the coronal plane.

Arachnoid Granulations and Septations

Another important differential diagnosis of dural sinus thrombosis is **giant arachnoid granulation** (AG). Giant AGs are round or ovoid short-segment filling defects that exhibit CSF-like attenuation on NECT and do not enhance on CECT scans.

The MR appearance of AGs is more problematic than the associated CT findings. Giant AGs frequently do

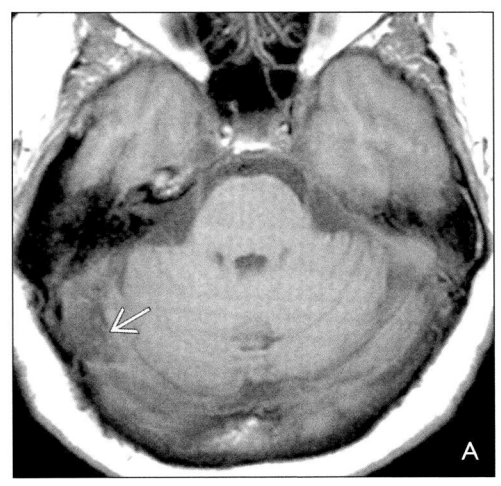

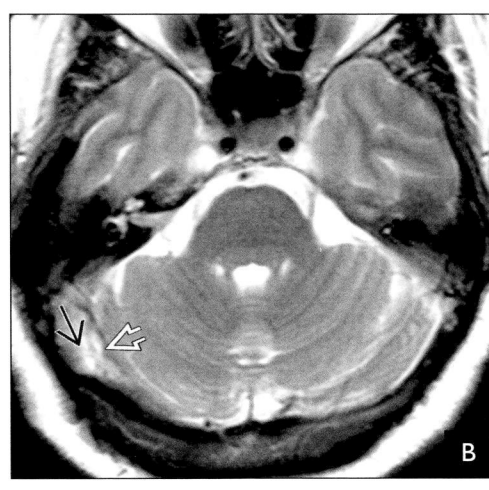

9-43A. *Axial T1WI in a patient with headaches shows a mass* ➡ *at the right transverse-sigmoid sinus junction that is hyperintense to CSF and mildly hypointense compared to the adjacent brain.* **9-43B.** *Axial T2WI shows that the ovoid mass* ⇨ *is slightly less hyperintense compared to CSF. Several internal septations* ➯ *are present within the lesion.*

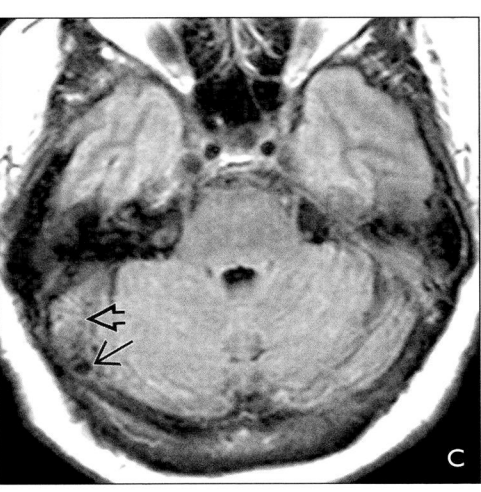

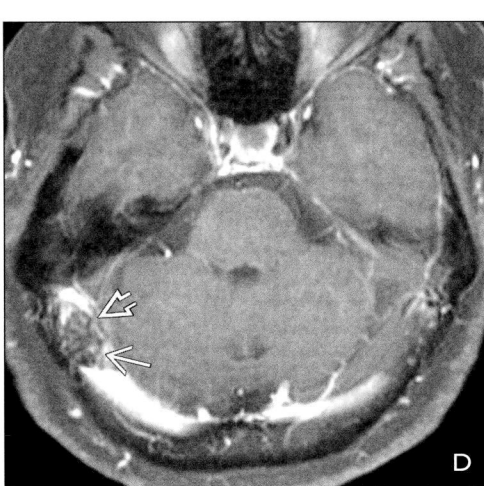

9-43C. *Parts of the lesion suppress on FLAIR* ➯, *while other parts* ⇨ *remain isointense with brain.* **9-43D.** *Axial T1 C+ FS scan shows the ovoid-shaped filling defect* ➡ *within the dominant right transverse sinus. Note enhancement of the internal septations. The nonenhancing linear area* ⇨ *that appears to enter the mass is a small vein. The majority of giant arachnoid granulations do not precisely parallel CSF signal intensity on all MR sequences!*

not follow CSF signal intensity on all sequences. CSF-incongruent signal intensity is seen on at least one sequence (most often FLAIR) in 80% of MR scans. Giant AGs do not fill the entire sinus as most thrombi do and—unlike clots—often demonstrate central linear enhancement **(9-43)**.

Septations or **trabeculations** are fibrotic bands that appear as linear filling defects in the sinuses. One to five septa are found in 30% of transverse sinuses, most commonly the right TS.

Other Venous Occlusion Mimics

Several less common entities can mimic dural sinus or cerebral vein occlusion. These include elevated hematocrit, unmyelinated brain, diffuse cerebral edema, and subdural hematoma.

High Hematocrit

The most common cause of a false-positive diagnosis of DST on NECT scan is an elevated hematocrit (i.e., patients with polycythemia vera or longstanding right-to-left cardiac shunts) **(9-44)**. This causes the appearance of a

hyperdense sinus relative to the brain parenchyma. However, the intracranial arteries in patients with high hematocrits are also similarly hyperdense.

Unmyelinated Brain

Infants and young children often have *higher* hematocrits compared to adults while the density of their unmyelinated brains is relatively *lower.* The combination of high-attenuation blood vessels and low-attenuation brain makes all vascular structures (including the dural sinuses and cortical veins) appear relatively hyperdense to dural sinus **(9-45)**.

Diffuse Cerebral Edema

Diffuse cerebral edema with decreased attenuation of the cerebral hemispheres makes the dura and all the intracranial vessels—both veins *and* arteries—appear relatively hyperdense compared to the low-density brain.

Subdural Hematoma

An acute subdural hematoma (aSDH) that layers along the straight sinus and medial tentorium can cause hyperdensity that may mimic DST on NECT scans. The dense

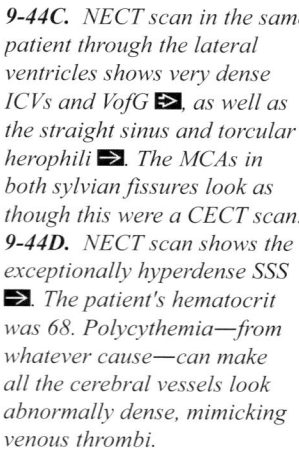

9-44A. Axial NECT (yes, this is a nonenhanced scan...) in a patient with longstanding right-to-left cardiac shunt shows hyperdensity in the transverse sinuses and sinus confluence ➡. Also note that the cranial arteries ➡ appear equally hyperdense. *9-44B.* More cephalad NECT scan shows unusually dense straight sinus and torcular herophili ➡. Again note the hyperdensity in all visualized cranial vessels—both veins and arteries.

9-44C. NECT scan in the same patient through the lateral ventricles shows very dense ICVs and VofG ➡, as well as the straight sinus and torcular herophili ➡. The MCAs in both sylvian fissures look as though this were a CECT scan. *9-44D.* NECT scan shows the exceptionally hyperdense SSS ➡. The patient's hematocrit was 68. Polycythemia—from whatever cause—can make all the cerebral vessels look abnormally dense, mimicking venous thrombi.

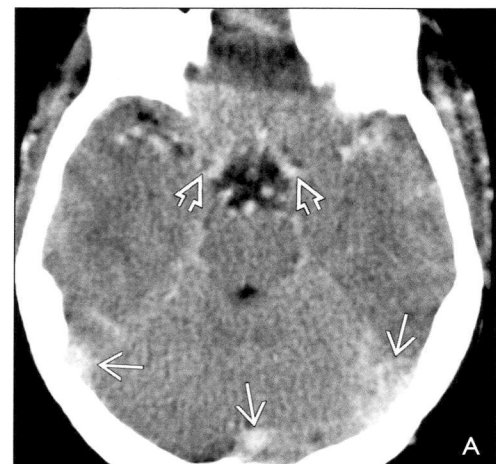
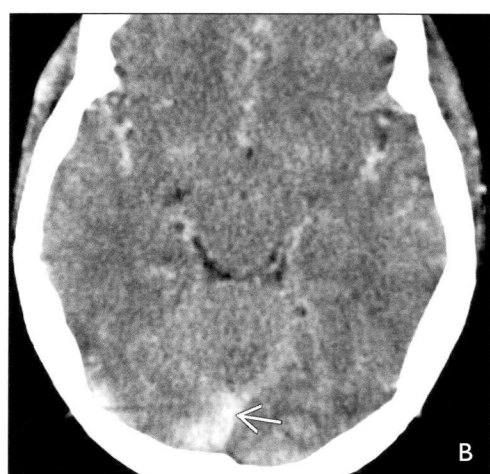
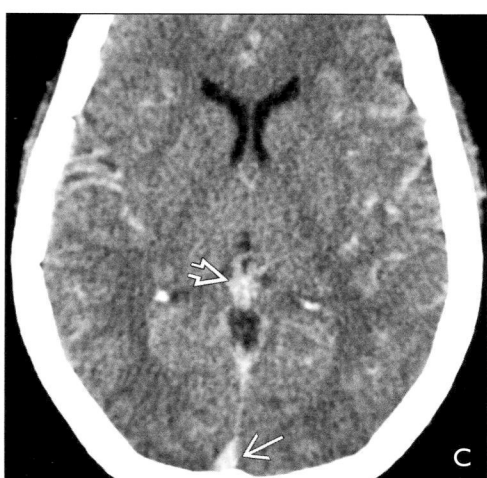
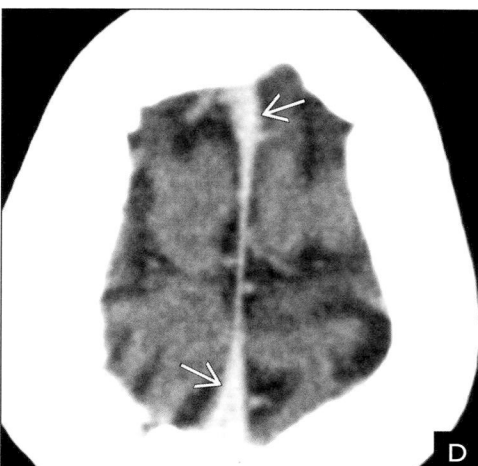

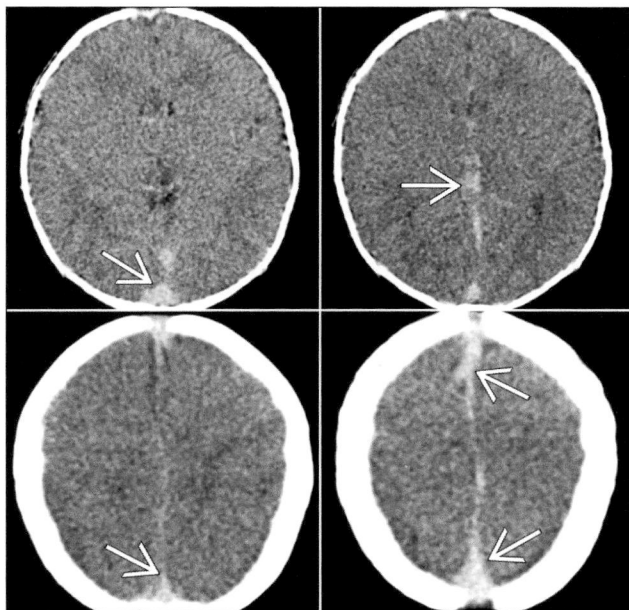

9-45. *NECT scan in a normal newborn infant. The combination of the unmyelinated hypodense brain and the physiologically elevated hematocrit makes the deep veins and dural sinuses* ⇉ *appear hyperdense, mimicking thrombosis.*

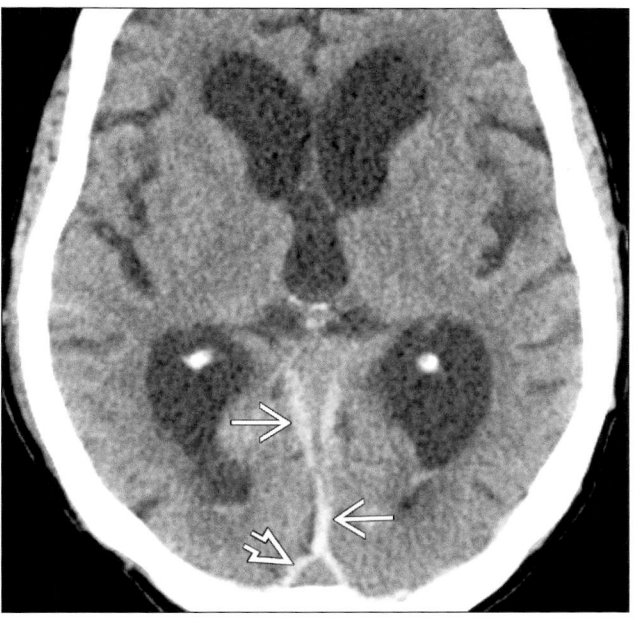

9-46. *Axial NECT scan shows subdural hemorrhage layered along the straight sinus and tentorium* ⇉, *mimicking the appearance of an "empty delta" sign* ⇉ *(which is seen on CECT—not NECT—scans).*

thrombus surrounds the relatively less dense flowing blood in the SSS and sinus confluence, mimicking an "empty delta" sign **(9-46)**. Remember: The "empty delta" sign is seen on contrast-enhanced scans, not nonenhanced scans!

CEREBRAL VENOUS OCCLUSION MIMICS

Common
- Anatomic variant
  - Hypoplastic sinus segment (TS most common)
  - Segmented, multichanneled sinus (sinus confluence)
- Flow artifacts
- Arachnoid granulations, septations

Less Common
- High-density blood (elevated hematocrit)
  - Physiologic (infants, high altitude)
  - Polycythemia vera
  - Longstanding right-to-left cardiac shunts
- Low-density brain
  - Physiologic (unmyelinated brain)
  - Pathologic (diffuse cerebral edema)
- Subdural hematoma
  - Layers along dura, sinuses
  - Looks like "empty delta" sign (NECT, not CECT)

Selected References

Normal Venous Anatomy and Drainage Patterns

- Miller E et al: Color Doppler US of normal cerebral venous sinuses in neonates: a comparison with MR venography. Pediatr Radiol. 42(9):1070-9, 2012

Dural Venous Sinuses

- Yiğit H et al: Time-resolved MR angiography of the intracranial venous system: an alternative MR venography technique. Eur Radiol. 22(5):980-9, 2012
- Chen F et al: Arachnoid granulations of middle cranial fossa: a population study between cadaveric dissection and in vivo computed tomography examination. Surg Radiol Anat. 33(3):215-21, 2011
- Strydom MA et al: The anatomical basis of venographic filling defects of the transverse sinus. Clin Anat. 23(2):153-9, 2010
- Trimble CR et al: "Giant" arachnoid granulations just like CSF? : NOT!! AJNR Am J Neuroradiol. 31(9):1724-8, 2010

Cerebral Veins

- Brockmann C et al: Variations of the superior sagittal sinus and bridging veins in human dissections and computed tomography venography. Clin Imaging. 36(2):85-9, 2012
- Nowinski WL: Proposition of a new classification of the cerebral veins based on their termination. Surg Radiol Anat. 34(2):107-14, 2012

Cerebral Venous Thrombosis

- Ageno W et al: Venous ischemic syndromes. Front Neurol Neurosci. 30:191-4, 2012

Dural Sinus Thrombosis

- Gameiro J et al: Prognosis of cerebral vein thrombosis presenting as isolated headache: early vs. late diagnosis. Cephalalgia. 32(5):407-12, 2012
- Yiğit H et al: Time-resolved MR angiography of the intracranial venous system: an alternative MR venography technique. Eur Radiol. 22(5):980-9, 2012
- Provenzale JM et al: Dural sinus thrombosis: sources of error in image interpretation. AJR Am J Roentgenol. 196(1):23-31, 2011
- Saposnik G et al: Diagnosis and management of cerebral venous thrombosis: a statement for healthcare professionals from the American Heart Association/American Stroke Association. Stroke. 42(4):1158-92, 2011
- Dlamini N et al: Cerebral venous sinus (sinovenous) thrombosis in children. Neurosurg Clin N Am. 21(3):511-27, 2010

- Kozic D et al: Overlooked early CT signs of cerebral venous thrombosis with lethal outcome. Acta Neurol Belg. 110(4):345-8, 2010
- Miranda B et al: Venous thromboembolic events after cerebral vein thrombosis. Stroke. 41(9):1901-6, 2010
- Nagai M et al: Role of coagulation factors in cerebral venous sinus and cerebral microvascular thrombosis. Neurosurgery. 66(3):560-5; discussion 565-6, 2010
- Trimble CR et al: "Giant" arachnoid granulations just like CSF? : NOT!! AJNR Am J Neuroradiol. 31(9):1724-8, 2010
- Coutinho JM et al: Cerebral venous and sinus thrombosis in women. Stroke. 40(7):2356-61, 2009
- Ferro JM et al: Delay in the diagnosis of cerebral vein and dural sinus thrombosis: influence on outcome. Stroke. 40(9):3133-8, 2009

Superficial Cerebral Vein Thrombosis

- Rathakrishnan R et al: The clinico-radiological spectrum of isolated cortical vein thrombosis. J Clin Neurosci. 18(10):1408-11, 2011

Deep Cerebral Venous Thrombosis

- Lin HC et al: Cord sign facilitates the early diagnosis of deep cerebral vein thrombosis. Am J Emerg Med. 30(1):252, 2012
- Linn J et al: Noncontrast CT in deep cerebral venous thrombosis and sinus thrombosis: comparison of its diagnostic value for both entities. AJNR Am J Neuroradiol. 30(4):728-35, 2009
- Pfefferkorn T et al: Clinical features, course and outcome in deep cerebral venous system thrombosis: an analysis of 32 cases. J Neurol. 256(11):1839-45, 2009

Cavernous Sinus Thrombosis/ Thrombophlebitis

- Desa V et al: Cavernous sinus thrombosis: current therapy. J Oral Maxillofac Surg. 70(9):2085-91, 2012
- Gamaletsou MN et al: Rhino-orbital-cerebral mucormycosis. Curr Infect Dis Rep. 14(4):423-34, 2012
- Nguyen CT et al: Cavernous sinus thrombosis secondary to sinusitis: a rare and life-threatening complication. Pediatr Radiol. 39(6):633, 2009

Venous Occlusion Mimics

- Provenzale JM et al: Dural sinus thrombosis: sources of error in image interpretation. AJR Am J Roentgenol. 196(1):23-31, 2011
- Leach JL et al: Imaging of cerebral venous thrombosis: current techniques, spectrum of findings, and diagnostic pitfalls. Radiographics. 26 Suppl 1:S19-41; discussion S42-3, 2006

Sinus Variants

- Manara R et al: Transverse dural sinuses: incidence of anatomical variants and flow artefacts with 2D time-of-flight MR venography at 1 Tesla. Radiol Med. 115(2):326-38, 2010

- Widjaja E et al: Intracranial MR venography in children: normal anatomy and variations. AJNR Am J Neuroradiol. 25(9):1557-62, 2004

Flow Artifacts

- Provenzale JM et al: Dural sinus thrombosis: sources of error in image interpretation. AJR Am J Roentgenol. 196(1):23-31, 2011

Arachnoid Granulations and Septations

- Strydom MA et al: The anatomical basis of venographic filling defects of the transverse sinus. Clin Anat. 23(2):153-9, 2010
- Trimble CR et al: "Giant" arachnoid granulations just like CSF? : NOT!! AJNR Am J Neuroradiol. 31(9):1724-8, 2010

10

Vasculopathy

The generic term "vasculopathy" literally means blood vessel pathology—of any kind, in any vessel (artery, capillary, or vein).

Because diseases such as atherosclerosis are so prevalent, evaluating the craniocervical vessels for vasculopathy is one of the major indications for neuroimaging. Large vessel atherosclerotic vascular disease (ASVD) is the single most prevalent vasculopathy in the head and neck whereas carotid stenosis or embolization from ASVD plaques are the most common causes of ischemic strokes.

With the advent and widespread availability of multidetector CT angiography, high-resolution noninvasive imaging of the cervical and intracranial vasculature has become common. Digital subtraction angiography (DSA) is now rarely used for diagnostic purposes and is generally performed only as part of a planned endovascular intervention.

In this chapter, we discuss diseases of the craniocervical arteries, first laying a foundation with normal gross and imaging anatomy of the aortic arch and great vessels. We then address the topic of atherosclerosis, starting with a general discussion of atherogenesis. Extracranial ASVD and carotid stenosis are followed by a brief overview of intracranial large and medium artery ASVD.

So-called microvascular ASVD is probably even more common than large vessel disease and its clinical burden vastly underestimated. The section on atherosclerosis concludes with a consideration of arteriolosclerosis.

The broad spectrum of nonatheromatous vasculopathy is then addressed. Finally, we devote the last section of this chapter to non-ASVD diseases of the cerebral macro- and microvasculature. While arteriolosclerosis is by far the most common cause of small vessel vascular disease, nonatherogenic microvasculopathies such as amyloid angiopathy can have devastating clinical consequences.

Normal Anatomy of the Extracranial Arteries

Aortic Arch and Great Vessels

The aorta has four major segments: The ascending aorta, transverse aorta (mostly consisting of the aortic arch), aortic isthmus, and descending aorta.

Aortic Arch

The aortic arch (AA) lies in the superior mediastinum, beginning at the level of the second right sternocostal articulation. It then curves backward and to the left over the pulmonary hilum. The AA thus has two curvatures, one that is convex upward and another that is convex forward and curving to the left.

The AA is anatomically related to a number of important structures (10-1). Cervical sympathetic branches and the left CN X (vagus nerve) lie in front of the AA. The trachea, left recurrent laryngeal nerve, esophagus, thoracic duct, and vertebral column lie behind the arch. The great vessels lie above the AA, as does the left bra-

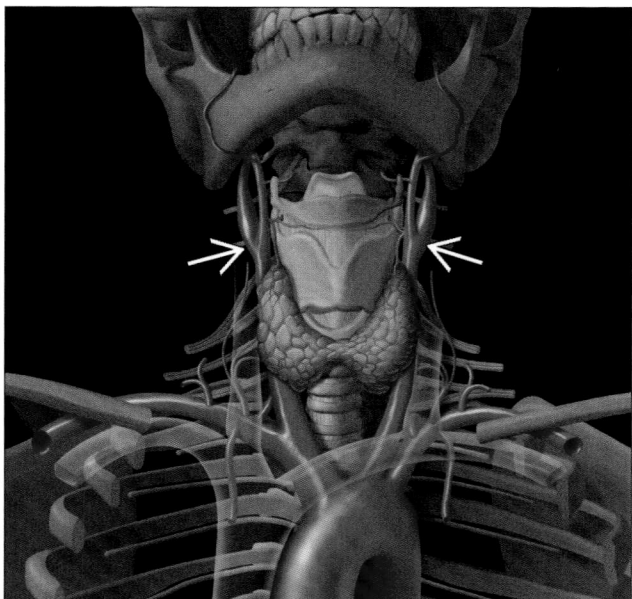

10-1. AP graphic shows normal aortic arch, its relationship to adjacent structures. Right CCA arises from brachiocephalic trunk whereas left CCA originates from arch. CCA bifurcations ➜ are around C3-4 level with the ICAs initially lateral to ECAs.

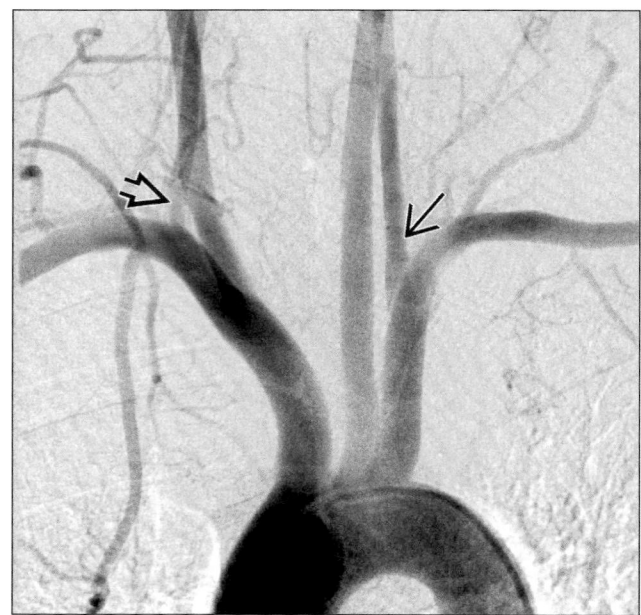

10-2. DSA shows normal aortic arch, branches. The left VA ➔ arises from the proximal left SCA and is usually dominant. The right VA ➔ arises from the SCA distal to its origin from the brachiocephalic trunk.

chiocephalic vein. The pulmonary bifurcation, ligamentum arteriosum, and left recurrent laryngeal nerve all lie below the arch.

Great Vessels

Three major vessels arise from the AA. From right to left, these are the brachiocephalic trunk, the left common carotid artery, and the left subclavian artery (10-2). Collectively, these are known as the "great vessels."

BRACHIOCEPHALIC TRUNK. The brachiocephalic trunk (BCT), also called the innominate artery, is the first and largest branch of the AA. It ascends anterior to the trachea. Near the sternoclavicular joint, the BCT bifurcates into the **right subclavian artery** (SCA) and **right common carotid artery** (CCA).

Major branches of the right SCA are the **right internal thoracic (mammary) artery**, **right vertebral artery** (right VA), **right thyrocervical trunk**, and **right costocervical trunk**. The right CCA bifurcates into its two terminal branches, the **right internal carotid artery** (ICA) and **right external carotid artery** (ECA).

LEFT COMMON CAROTID ARTERY. The left CCA arises from the apex of the AA just distal to the BCT origin. The left CCA ascends to the left of the trachea, then bifurcates into the left ECA and left ICA near the upper border of the thyroid cartilage. The left CCA lies anteromedial to the internal jugular vein.

LEFT SUBCLAVIAN ARTERY. The left SCA arises from the AA a few millimeters distal to the left CCA origin.

The left SCA ascends into the neck, passing lateral to the medial border of the anterior scalene.

Major branches of the left SCA are the **left internal thoracic (mammary) artery**, **left vertebral artery** (left VA), **left thyrocervical trunk**, and **left costocervical trunk**.

Vascular Territory

The AA and great vessels supply the neck, skull, scalp, and the entire brain.

Normal Variants

The "classic" AA with three "great vessels" originating separately from the arch is seen in 80% of cases. In 10-25% of cases, the left CCA shares a common V-shaped origin with the BCT (commonly referred to as a "bovine arch," a misnomer as this configuration bears no resemblance to the AA branching pattern seen in ruminants). The left CCA arises from the proximal BCT in another 5-7% of cases. The left CCA and left SCA share a common origin (a "left brachiocephalic trunk") in 1-2%. The left VA originates directly from the AA—not the left SCA—in 0.5-1% of cases. (10-3).

Three thoracic aorta "lumps and bumps" are normal anatomic variants that should not be mistaken for pathology. The **aortic isthmus** is a narrowed segment just distal to the left SCA and proximal to the site of the fetal ductus arteriosis. An **aortic spindle** is a circumferential bulge in the aorta just beyond the ductus. Both the aortic isthmus and spindle typically disappear after two postnatal

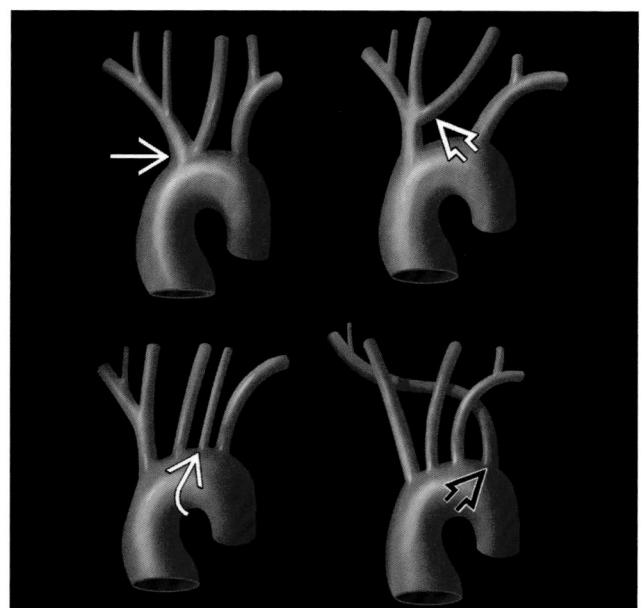

10-3. Four arch variants are depicted: Brachiocephalic trunk (BCT) and R ICA arising from V-shaped common origin ➡️, L ICA arising from BCT ⏩, L VA arising directly from arch ➡️, aberrant R SCA arising from arch as fourth "great vessel" ⏵.

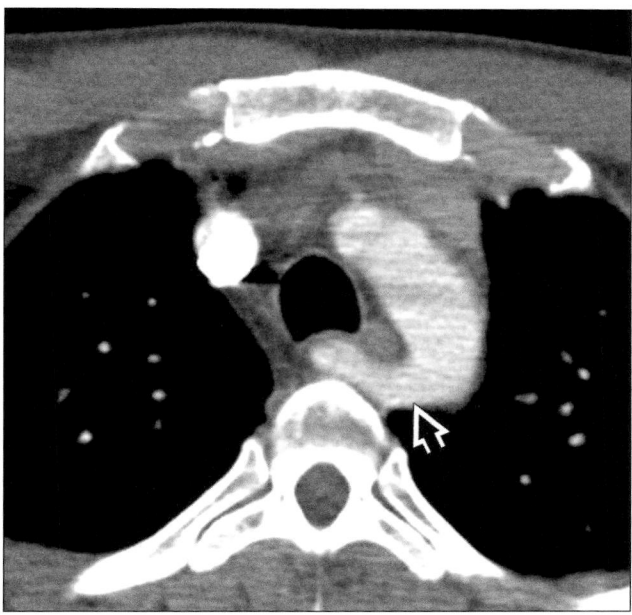

10-4. Axial CTA source image shows aberrant right SCA ⏩ arising as the last vessel from the aortic arch.

months but can persist into adulthood. A **ductus diverticulum** is a focal bulge along the anteromedial aspect of the aortic isthmus and is seen in 10% of adults.

Anomalies

Only the four most common AA anomalies are briefly discussed here. The most common congenital arch anomaly—seen in 0.5-1.0% of cases—is a **left AA with an aberrant right SCA**. Here the right SCA is the last—not the first—branch to arise from the AA **(10-4)**. Occasionally the aberrant right SCA arises from a dilated, diverticulum-like structure (Kommerell diverticulum). An aberrant right SCA is not associated with congenital heart disease.

Other important anomalies include a **right AA with mirror image branching**, which is strongly associated with cyanotic congenital heart disease (98% prevalence). Two anomalies that are rarely associated with congenital heart disease include a **right AA with aberrant left SCA** and a **double aortic arch** (DAA). In a DAA, each arch gives rise to a ventral carotid and a dorsal subclavian artery (symmetric "four-artery" sign).

Cervical Carotid Arteries

The common carotid arteries (CCAs) provide the major blood supply to the face and cerebral hemispheres. The CCAs course superiorly, anteromedial to the internal jugular veins. They terminate at about the C3-C4 or C4-C5 level by dividing into the internal and external carotid arteries (ICAs, ECAs) **(10-1)**.

Internal Carotid Artery

The cervical internal carotid artery is entirely extracranial and is designated as the C1 segment. In 90% of cases, the cervical ICA arises from the CCA posterolateral to the external carotid artery.

The C1 ICA has two parts, the carotid bulb and the ascending segment. The **carotid bulb** is the most proximal aspect of the cervical ICA and is seen as a prominent focal dilatation with a cross-sectional area nearly twice as large as that of the distal ICA.

Slipstreams from the CCA strike the CCA bifurcation and divide, with approximately 30% of the flow passing into the ECA. The majority of the flow enters the anterior part of the proximal ICA and continues cephalad. A smaller slipstream actually reverses direction in the bulb, temporarily slowing and stagnating before reestablishing normal antegrade laminar flow with the central slipstream.

The **ascending ICA segment** courses cephalad in the carotid space, a fascially defined tubular sheath that contains all three layers of the deep cervical fascia. The cervical ICA has no normal branches in the neck.

External Carotid Artery

Each ECA has eight major branches **(10-5)**.

The first ECA branch is usually the **superior thyroid artery**, which may also arise from the CCA bifurcation. The superior thyroid artery arises anteriorly from the ECA and courses inferiorly to supply the superior

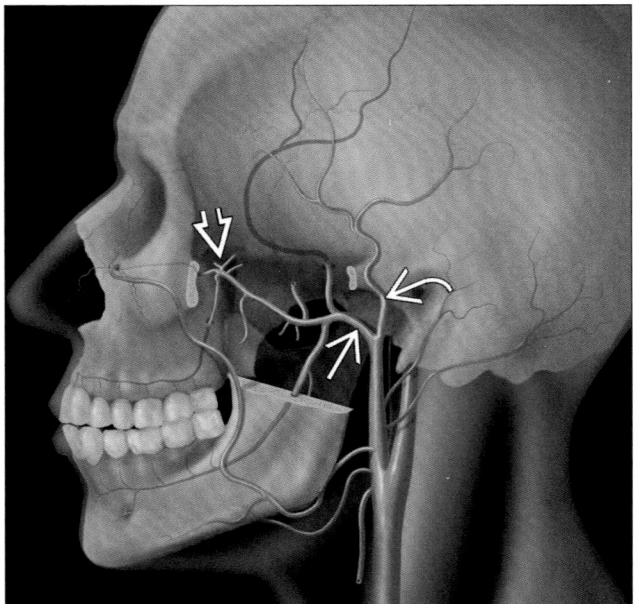

10-5. Graphic shows that the 2 terminal ECA branches are the superficial temporal ➡ and maxillary ➡ arteries. The maxillary artery divides into its distal branches within the pterygopalatine fossa ➡.

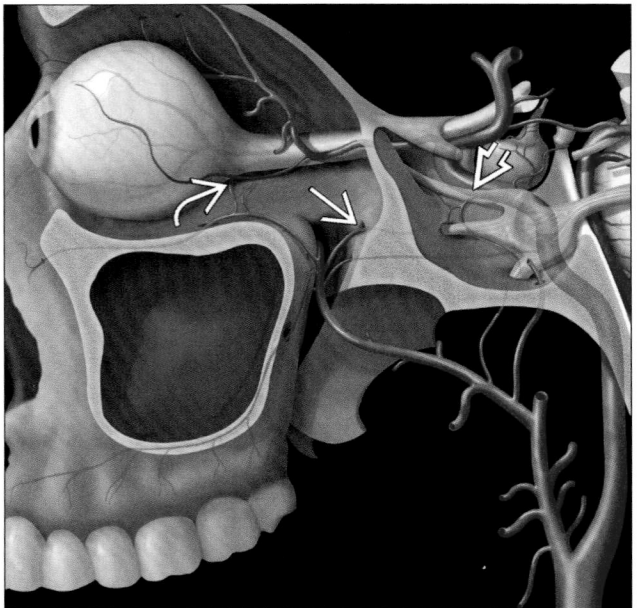

10-6. Graphic shows numerous anastomoses between the ECA and cavernous ICA, including via the artery of the foramen rotundum ➡, lateral mainstem artery ➡, and ophthalmic artery ➡.

thyroid and larynx. The **ascending pharyngeal artery** arises posteriorly from the ECA (or CCA bifurcation) and courses superiorly between the ECA and ICA to supply the naso- and oropharynx, middle ear, dura, and CNs IX-XI.

The **lingual artery** is the third ECA branch. It loops anteroinferiorly, then courses superiorly to supply the tongue, oral cavity, and submandibular gland. The **facial artery** arises just above the lingual artery, curving around the mandible before it passes anterosuperiorly to supply the face, palate, lips, and cheek.

The next two branches arise from the posterior surface of the ECA. The **occipital artery** courses posterosuperiorly between the skull base and C1 to supply the scalp, upper cervical musculature, and posterior fossa meninges. The **posterior auricular artery** is a smaller branch that also arises from the posterior ECA above the occipital artery. It courses superiorly to supply the ear and scalp.

The superficial temporal artery and maxillary artery are the two terminal branches of the ECA. The **superficial temporal artery** runs superiorly behind the mandibular condyle and loops over the zygoma to supply the scalp.

The **maxillary artery** is the larger of the two terminal ECA branches. Its first major branch is the *middle meningeal artery* (MMA), which runs superiorly and enters the calvaria through the foramen spinosum to supply the cranial meninges. The maxillary artery courses anteromedially in the masticator space and then loops into the pterygopalatine fossa, where it divides into several terminal branches that supply the deep face and nose.

Numerous anastomotic channels exist between all extracranial branches of the ECAs (except the superior thyroid and lingual arteries) and intracranial branches of the ICAs or musculospinal branches of the VAs **(10-6)**. These anastomoses (summarized in the box below) both provide an important pathway for collateral blood flow and pose a potential risk for intracranial embolization during neurointerventional procedures.

ECA-ICA-VA ANASTOMOSES

Ascending Pharyngeal Artery
- Tympanic branch → petrous ICA
- Several rami → cavernous ICA
- Odontoid arch/musculospinal branches → VA

Facial Artery
- OA → intracranial ICA

Occipital Artery
- Transosseous perforators to VA
- To muscular branches of VAs

Posterior Auricular Artery
- Stylomastoid branch to petrous ICA

Superficial Temporal Artery
- Transosseous perforators → anterior falx artery → OA

Maxillary Artery
- Vidian artery → petrous ICA
- MMA → inferolateral trunk → cavernous ICA
- Artery of foramen rotundum → inferolateral trunk → cavernous ICA
- Middle/recurrent meningeal arteries → OA → intracranial ICA
- Deep temporal → OA → intracranial ICA

Atherosclerosis

Over 90% of large cerebral infarcts are caused by thromboemboli secondary to atherosclerosis and its complications. ASVD is by far the most common cause of mortality and severe long-term disability in industrialized countries, so it is difficult to overemphasize its importance.

We begin our discussion with an overview of the etiology, biology, and pathology of atherogenesis. We then focus on extracranial ASVD before concluding with a brief discussion of the clinical and imaging manifestations of intracranial ASVD, including its microvascular manifestations.

Atherogenesis and Atherosclerosis

Terminology

The term "atherosclerosis" was originally coined to describe progressive "hardening" or "sclerosis" of blood vessels. The term "atheroma" (Greek for porridge) designates the material deposited on or within vessel walls. "Plaque" is used to describe a focal atheroma together with its epiphenomena such as ulceration, platelet aggregation, and hemorrhage.

Atherogenesis is the degenerative process that results in atherosclerosis. **Atherosclerosis** is the most common pathologic process affecting large elastic arteries (e.g., the aorta) and medium-sized muscular arteries (e.g., the carotid and vertebral arteries). **Arteriolosclerosis** describes the effects of atherogenesis on smaller arteries (and is treated separately at the end of this section). **Atherosclerotic vascular disease (ASVD)** is the generic term describing atherosclerosis in any artery, of any size, in any area of the body.

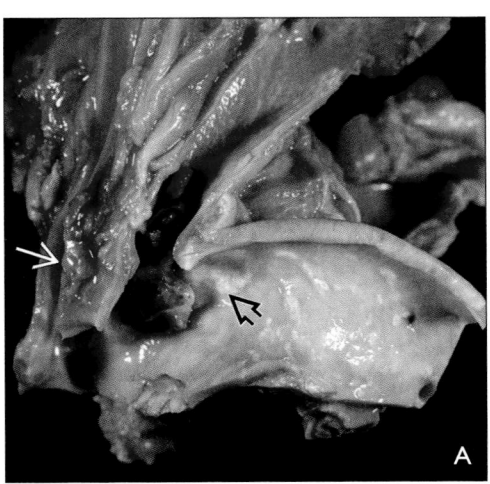

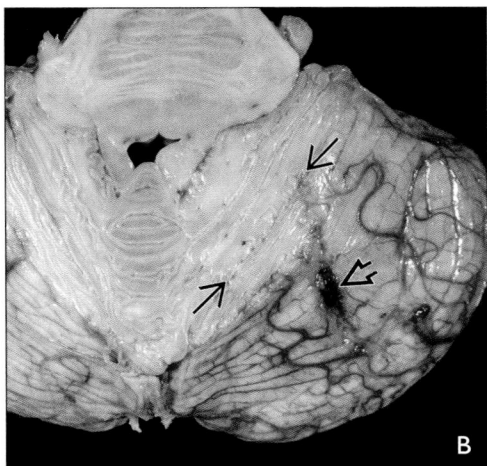

10-7A. Autopsy specimen demonstrates extensive calcification and ASVD of the aortic arch ⊳ and proximal great vessels ➡. *10-7B.* Section through the cerebellum, pons in the same case shows old hemorrhagic ⊳ and subacute embolic infarcts ➡ in the left cerebellar hemisphere.

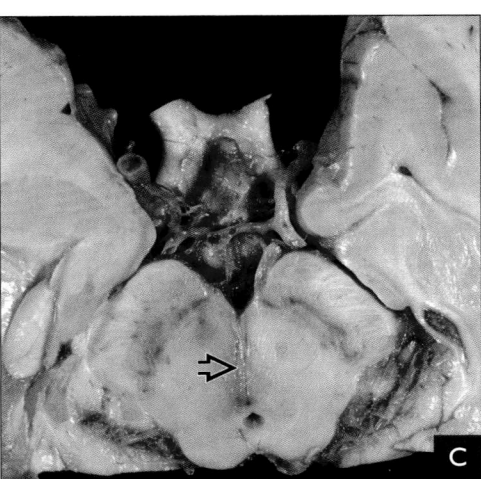

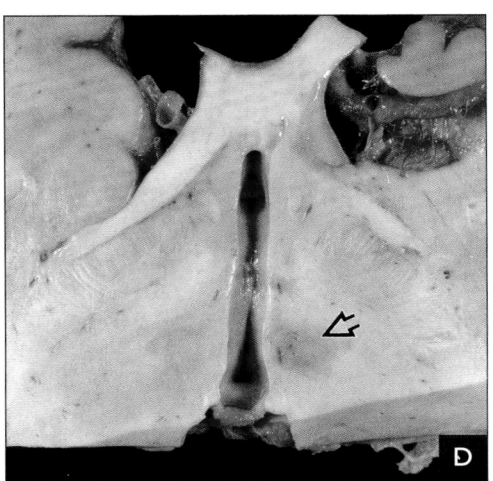

10-7C. Section through the midbrain in the same case shows an old midline penetrating artery infarction ⊳, possibly secondary to an artery of Percheron occlusion. *10-7D.* More cephalad section through the inferior third ventricle shows a subacute inferomedial thalamic infarct ⊳, consistent with artery of Percheron occlusion. (Courtesy R. Hewlett, MD.)

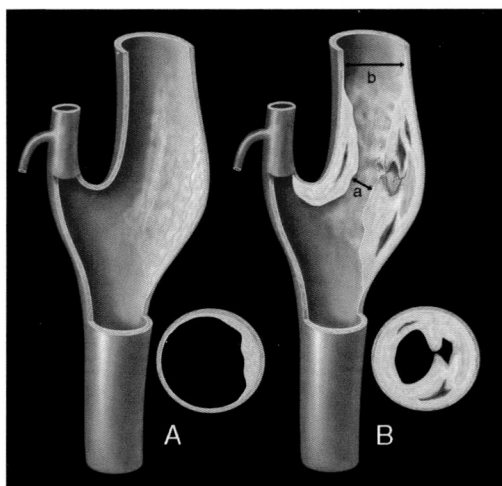

10-8. *(A) Mild ASVD with "fatty streaks." (B) Severe ASVD; % stenosis = (b-a)/b x 100; b = normal lumen, a = residual lumen diameter.*

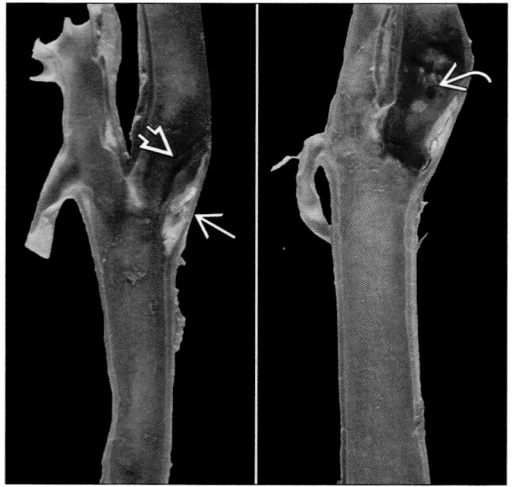

10-9. *(Left) Stable ASVD with fatty plaque* ➽, *intact intima* ➽. *(Right) Initially "at risk" plaque now shows ulceration* ➽, *disrupted intima.*

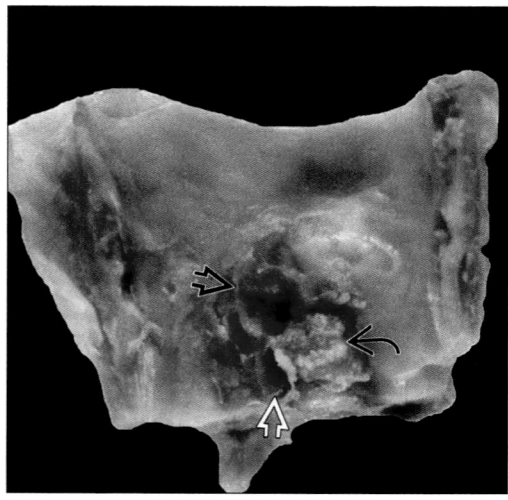

10-10. Carotid endarterectomy specimen shows ulcerated intima ➽, *calcification* ➚, *intraplaque hemorrhage* ➚. *(Courtesy J. Townsend, MD.)*

Etiology

GENERAL CONCEPTS. Atherosclerosis is a complex, slowly developing process that begins in the early teenage years and progresses over decades. Its causes are multi-factorial but appear to be a combination of lipid retention, oxidation, and modification, which in turn incites chronic inflammation. Plasma lipids, connective tissue fibers, and inflammatory cells accumulate at susceptible sites in arterial walls, forming focal atherosclerotic plaques.

Active inflammatory, innate immune, and adaptive immune mechanisms all play a key role in ASVD development. Chronic exposure to low-density lipoproteins (LDLs) modified by oxidation activates endothelial cells, inducing expression of adhesion molecules, matrix metalloproteinases, and inflammatory genes. Monocyte accumulation and macrophage differentiation are also induced as part of the inflammatory process.

Neoangiogenesis is closely associated with plaque progression and is likely the primary source of intraplaque hemorrhage. Angiogenic factors cause vasa vasorum proliferation, formation of immature vessels, and loss of capillary basement membranes. Red blood cells leak into the plaque, inducing further inflammation and increasing the risk of plaque ulceration and rupture.

GENETICS. The process of ASVD plaque development is the same regardless of race/ethnicity, gender, or geographic location. However, the *rate* at which plaques develop is faster in patients with genetic predisposition and acquired risk factors such as hypertension, smoking, type 2 diabetes, and obesity.

No single predisposing mutation for ASVD has yet been identified. To date, most investigators conclude that ASVD probably reflects the interaction of multiple intrinsic (genetic) and extrinsic (environmental) factors. A genome-wide association approach has identified multiple foci that influence the risk of systemic ASVD, especially in the setting of incidental coronary heart disease.

Pathology

LOCATION. The entire vasculature is exposed to similar environmental and genetic influences. In theory, ASVD lesions should occur randomly, with every artery—from large elastic arteries to arterioles—equally at risk of developing ASVD. Instead, ASVD occurs preferentially at highly predictable locations. In the extracranial vasculature, the most common sites are the proximal internal carotid arteries and common carotid bifurcations, followed by the aortic arch and great vessel origins **(10-7)**.

The proximal ICA exhibits an anatomic feature unlike that found in any other vessel, i.e., the **carotid bulb**. This focal post-bifurcation enlargement—together with

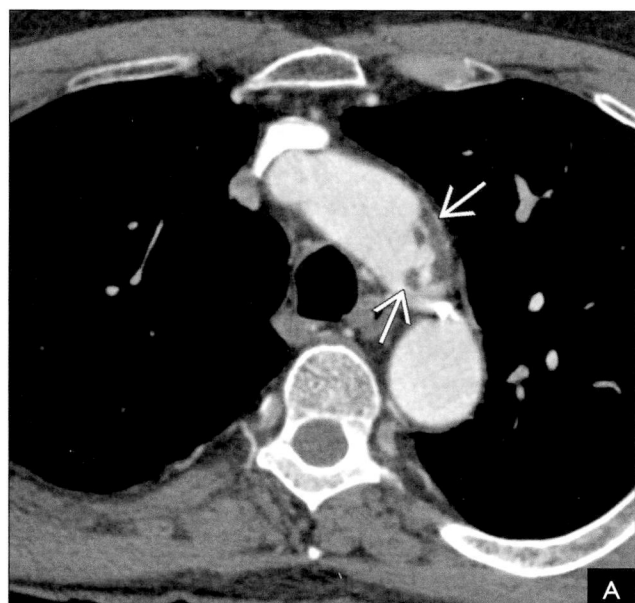

10-11A. *Axial CTA source image shows irregular, ulcerated atherosclerotic plaque* ➔ *along the aortic arch, proximal descending thoracic aorta.*

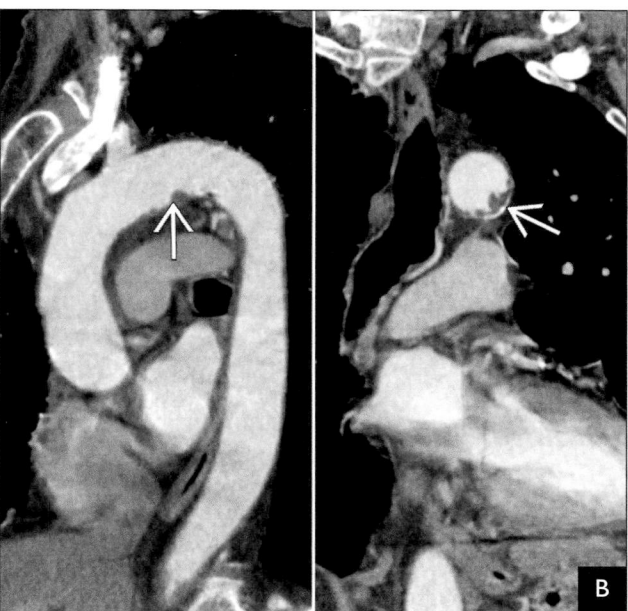

10-11B. *(Left) "Candy cane" and (right) coronal views in the same case show the plaque* ➔ *along the lesser curvature of the aortic arch. (Courtesy G. Oliveira, MD.)*

the CCA branching angle—promotes both flow separation and recirculation/stasis in the bulb. The unusual flow patterns generated by this unique geometry result in increased particle residence time and low, oscillating wall shear stresses in the outer wall of the carotid bulb. This may account for the unusually high prevalence of atheromas at this particular location.

SIZE AND NUMBER. ASVD plaques vary in size from small, almost microscopic lipid deposits to large, raised, fungating, ulcerating lesions that can extend over several centimeters and dramatically narrow the parent vessel lumen. Most plaques are 0.3-1.5 cm in diameter. With ASVD, multiple lesions in multiple locations are the rule.

GROSS PATHOLOGY. ASVD plaques develop in stages **(10-8)**. The first detectable lesion is lipid deposition in the intima, seen as yellowish "fatty streaks." Other than "fatty streaks" and slightly eccentric but smooth intimal thickening, visible changes at this early stage are minimal.

MICROSCOPIC FEATURES. ASVD plaques are classified histopathologically as "stable," "vulnerable," or "ulcerated."

Stable plaques. Uncomplicated **stable plaques**—the basic lesions of atherosclerosis—consist of cellular material (smooth muscle cells, monocytes, and macrophages), lipid (both intra- and extracellular deposits), and an overlying fibrous cap (composed of collagen, elastic fibers, and proteoglycans). The intima covering a stable plaque is thickened, but its exterior surface remains intact, with-

out disruption or ulceration. No intraplaque hemorrhage is present **(10-9)**.

Vulnerable plaques. As a necrotic core of lipid-laden foam cells, cellular debris, and cholesterol gradually accumulates under the elevated fibrous cap, the cap thins and becomes prone to rupture (**"vulnerable" plaque**) **(10-9)**.

Proliferating small blood vessels also develop around the periphery of the necrotic core. **Neovascularization** can lead to **subintimal hemorrhage** with rapid expansion, which increases pressure inside the plaque, promotes increasing lipid deposition, and enlarges the necrotic core, further weakening the overlying fibrous cap.

Ulcerated plaques. Plaque **ulceration** occurs when the fibrous cap weakens and ruptures through the intima, releasing necrotic debris **(10-10)**. Slowly swirling blood within the ulcerated denuded endothelium first allows platelets and fibrin to aggregate. An intermittent Bernoulli effect then pulls the aggregates into the rapidly flowing main artery slipstream, causing arterioarterial embolization to distal intracranial vessels.

Clinical Issues

EPIDEMIOLOGY AND DEMOGRAPHICS. Although atherogenesis actually begins in the mid-teens, most patients with symptomatic lesions are middle-aged or elderly. However, atherosclerosis is increasingly common in younger patients, contributing to the rising prevalence of strokes in patients younger than 45 years.

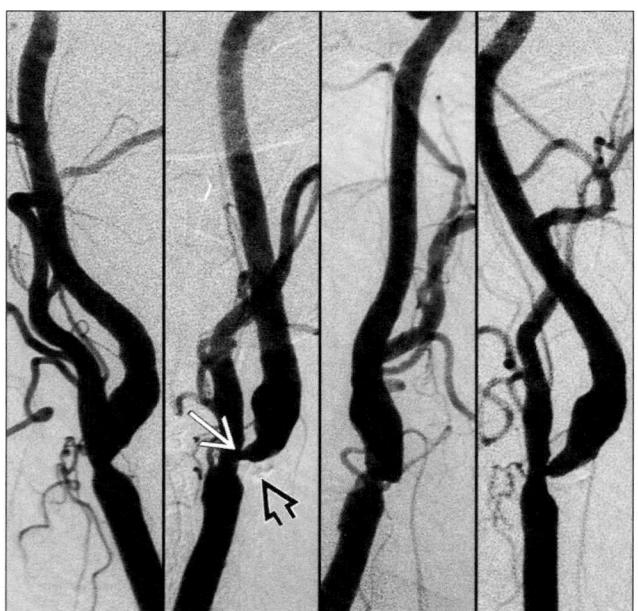

10-12. Four-view DSA shows the importance of multiple projections to profile maximum proximal ICA stenosis ➡, *calcified plaque* ▷.

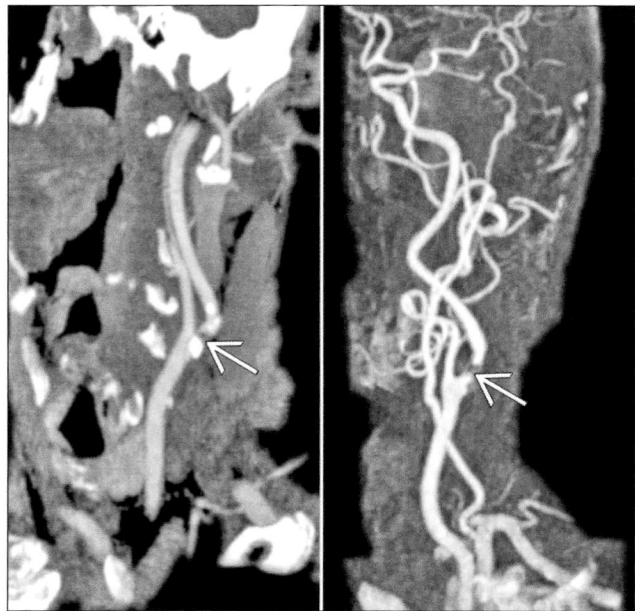

10-13. (Left) DSA shows critical ICA stenosis ➡. *(Right) MRA in the same case shows a "flow gap"* ➡ *characteristic of a high-grade flow-limiting lesion.*

There is a moderate male predominance. Although all ethnicities are affected, African-Americans are at highest risk for ASVD.

PRESENTATION. The clinical presentation of craniocervical ASVD is highly variable. As ASVD is generally a slowly progressive disorder, many lesions remain asymptomatic until they cause hemodynamically significant stenosis or thromboembolic disease. A carotid bruit may be the first clinically detectable sign of ICA stenosis. Transient ischemic attacks (TIAs) and "silent strokes" are common precursors of large territorial infarcts.

NATURAL HISTORY. The natural history of ASVD is also highly variable. ICA occlusion poses an especially high risk for eventual stroke, with over 70% of these patients eventually experiencing ischemic cerebral infarction.

TREATMENT OPTIONS. Treatment options include prevention, medical therapy (lipid-lowering regimens), and surgery or endovascular therapy (see below).

Extracranial Atherosclerosis

Extracranial ASVD is the single largest risk factor for stroke. That risk starts with the aortic arch.

Because DSA carries a small but definite risk, noninvasive imaging modalities are preferable screening procedures to evaluate patients for extracranial atherosclerosis and its complications. The major noninvasive options are CTA, high-resolution MRA, and ultrasound (US). Each technique has its advocates, advantages, disadvantages, cost considerations, and special "use case" scenar-

ios. Many investigators recommend duplex US as the initial screening test in patients with recent TIAs or minor ischemic stroke, followed by CTA for those with positive results.

An in-depth analysis and comparison of the many available vascular imaging modalities is beyond the scope of this book. We focus instead on ASVD in major anatomic sites, using examples of each technique as appropriate to demonstrate the relevant pathology.

Aortic Arch and Great Vessels

The aortic arch is an underrecognized source of intracranial ischemic strokes. Complete imaging evaluation of patients with thromboembolic infarcts in the brain should include investigation of the aortic arch.

ETIOLOGY. Aortic ASVD is more common in the descending thoracic aorta than in the ascending aorta or arch **(10-11)**. However, late diastolic retrograde flow from complex plaques in the proximal descending aorta distal to the left subclavian artery origin can reach all supraaortic arteries. Retrograde flow extends to the left SCA orifice in nearly 60% of cases, the left CCA in 25%, and the brachiocephalic trunk in 10-15%.

Aortic emboli involve the left brain in 80% of cases and show a distinct predilection for the vertebrobasilar circulation. This striking geographic distribution is consistent with thromboemboli arising from ulcerated plaques in the descending aorta that are then swept by retrograde flow into left-sided arch vessels.

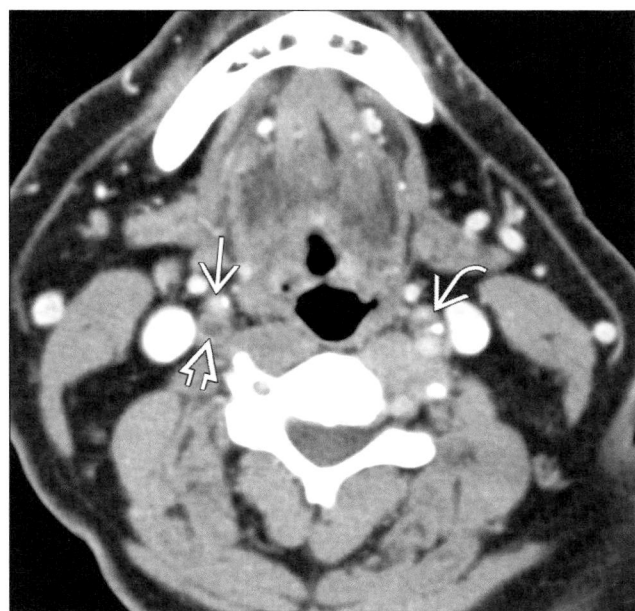

10-14. *CECT in a 60-year-old man with stroke shows a very faint dot of enhancement* ➡ *in the right proximal ICA. High-grade stenosis is caused by a "soft" ASVD plaque with hypodense lipid* ⮕. *The left ICA* ➡ *is irregular, stenotic.*

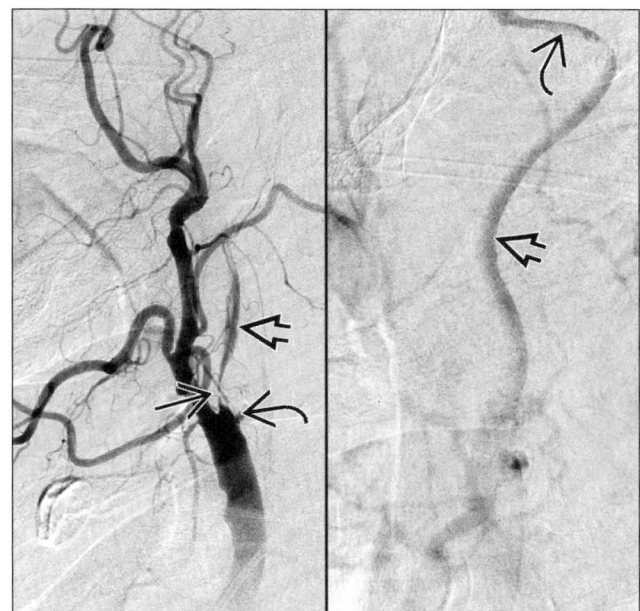

10-15. *(Left) DSA shows ulcerated plaque* ⮔ *causing high-grade, near-total stenosis* ➔ *with a "string" sign* ⮕. *(Right) Late phase shows the distal cervical ICA* ⮕. *Filling defects* ⮔ *are caused by thrombus.*

EPIDEMIOLOGY. Arch atherosclerosis is a documented independent risk factor for stroke, found on imaging studies in 10-20% of patients with acute ischemic infarcts and 25% of fatal strokes at autopsy. Ulcerated aortic plaques are present at autopsy in 60% of patients who died from cerebral infarction of unknown etiology. Aortic ASVD constitutes the only probable source of retinal emboli or cerebral infarction in nearly 25% of patients with "cryptogenic stroke," i.e., no likely cardiac or carotid source can be identified.

IMAGING. The aortic arch and proximal descending aorta should be visualized together with the extra- and intracranial vasculature. Some investigators now advocate a comprehensive "triple rule-out" CTA for acute ischemic stroke that also includes the heart and coronary arteries. Intravenous contrast is necessary to define the presence of mural thrombus, determine plaque extent, and evaluate the aortic wall for complications such as ulceration, aneurysm, and dissection.

The most common general imaging finding in aortic ASVD is irregular mural thickening with calcifications. Imaging features of aortic ASVD that are strongly correlated with stroke include atheromas located proximal to the left subclavian ostium, plaques at least four millimeters in diameter that protrude into the aortic lumen, and the presence of mobile/oscillating thrombi.

Carotid Bifurcation/Internal Carotid Arteries

Between 20-30% of all ischemic infarcts are caused by carotid artery stenosis **(10-12)**. Therefore, determining the degree of carotid stenosis on imaging studies is now both routine and required.

Three studies have shown the benefits of endarterectomy in patients with definable carotid stenosis: The North American Symptomatic Carotid Endarterectomy Trial (NASCET), the European Carotid Surgery Trial (ECST), and the Asymptomatic Carotid Atherosclerosis Group (ACAS).

Although these studies used DSA as the gold standard for determining percent stenosis, recent studies have demonstrated a linear relationship between direct millimeter carotid stenosis measures on CTA and derived percent stenosis as defined by NASCET. These studies have demonstrated the efficacy of carotid endarterectomy, angioplasty, or stenting in symptomatic patients with ICA stenosis of 70% or greater.

Carotid stenosis is classified as moderate (50-69%), severe (70-93%), and "preocclusive" or critical (94-99%) **(10-13), (10-15)**. Patients with critical stenosis are at high risk for embolic stroke as long as the ICA lumen is patent.

In addition to stenosis degree, several recent studies have demonstrated the importance of also assessing the morphologic features of ASVD plaques. Rupture of an "at risk" plaque with a large necrotic core under a thin fibrous cap is responsible for the majority of acute thrombi. As distal embolization from proximal ASVD-related clots is a common cause of cerebral ischemia/infarction, *identifying rupture-prone "vulnerable" plaques is at least as important as determining stenosis!*

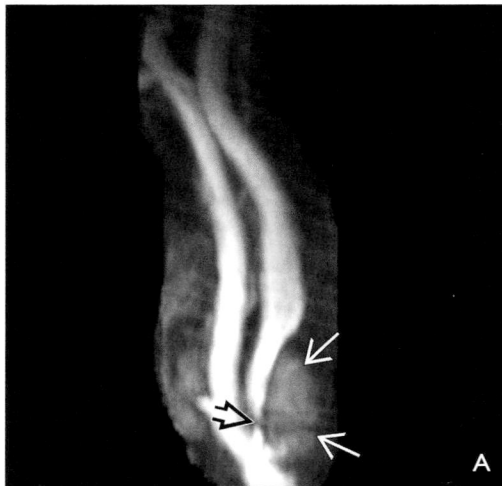

10-16A. Oblique 3.0 T MRA shows very high-grade stenosis of the right carotid artery with a "flow gap" ⊳ *caused by a large ASVD plaque* ⊳*.*

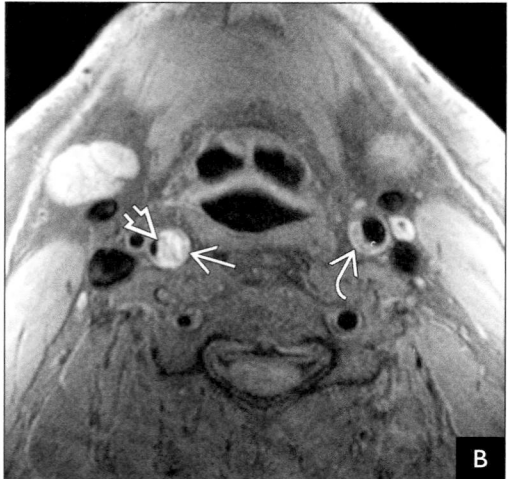

10-16B. MP-RAGE shows intraplaque hemorrhage ⊳ *with tiny residual lumen* ⊳ *in the right ICA, subintimal hemorrhage* ⊳ *in the left ICA.*

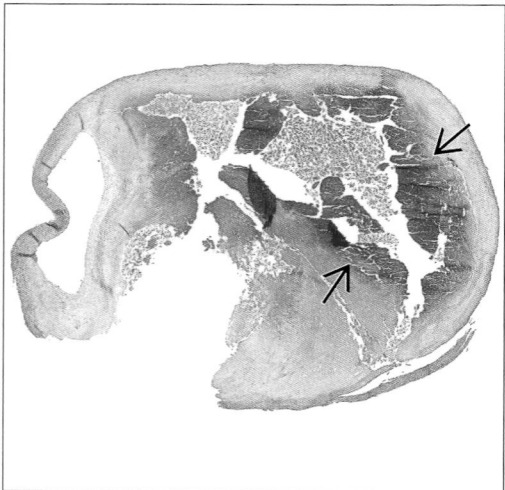

10-17. R ICA endarterectomy specimen shows that plaque hyperintensity is due to acute hemorrhage ⊳*, not lipid. (Courtesy S. McNally, MD.)*

CT Findings. The most common imaging findings in extracranial ASVD are mural calcifications, luminal irregularities, varying degrees of vessel stenosis, occlusion, and thrombosis (10-13). Elongation, ectasia, and vessel tortuosity can occur with or without other changes of ASVD.

NECT scans easily show vessel wall calcifications. Smooth plaques and extensive coalescent calcifications are associated with *decreased* risk of plaque rupture. Large atherosclerotic plaques may demonstrate one or more subintimal low-density foci. These represent the lipid-rich core of a "soft" plaque (10-14). High-density subintimal foci indicate intraplaque hemorrhage. Both findings carry increased risk of plaque rupture and concomitant distal embolization.

CECT and CTA source images display the carotid lumen in cross section. Nonstenotic smooth luminal narrowing is the most common finding in ASVD. Ulcerations—seen as irregularly shaped contrast-filled outpouchings from the lumen—are detected with 95% sensitivity and 99% specificity. Occlusion and intraluminal thrombi are also readily demonstrated.

CTA is as accurate as DSA in determining ICA stenosis. Although some carotid stenoses are irregularly shaped and noncircular, measurement of the narrowest stenosis is a reasonably reliable predictor of cross-sectional area. Differentiating total from near occlusion is essential, as patients with occlusion are usually treated medically whereas patients with high-grade lesions are eligible for emergent surgery or endovascular treatment.

In addition to calculating percent stenosis (10-8), plaque morphologic characteristics should be described in detail as decision-making is not based solely on stenosis degree. By itself, stenosis does not define complete stroke risk in symptomatic patients with < 70% stenosis or across all levels of stenoses in asymptomatic patients.

MR Findings. High-resolution MR imaging can be used to characterize carotid plaques, allowing identification of individual plaque components including lipids, hemorrhage, fibrous tissue, and calcification. Intraplaque hemorrhage has been identified as an independent risk factor for ischemic stroke at *all* degrees of stenosis, including symptomatic patients with low-grade lesions (< 50%). Therefore accurate characterization of plaque morphology is important for patient management.

High signal intensity on T1-weighted fat-suppressed scans, MRA source images, or MP-RAGE sequences represents hemorrhage into complicated "vulnerable" atherosclerotic plaques, not lipid accumulation (10-16), (10-17). Unlike intraparenchymal brain bleeds, plaque hemorrhages may remain hyperintense up to 18 months. Vulner-

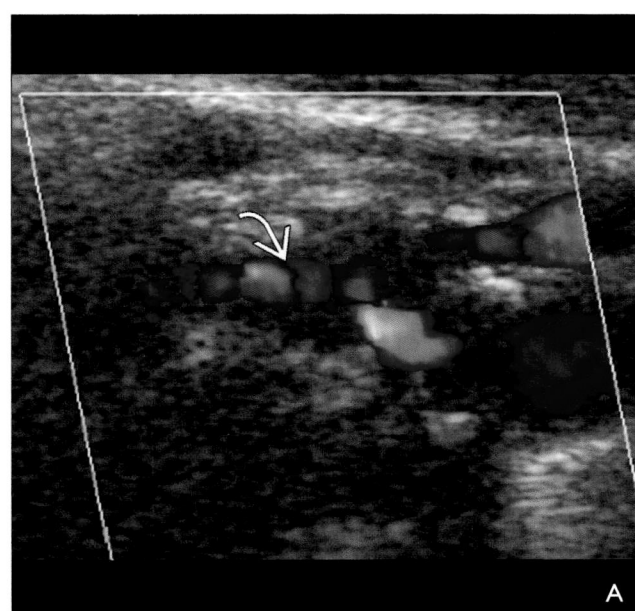

10-18A. Longitudinal color Doppler ultrasound shows high-grade ICA stenosis. The arterial lumen is significantly narrowed with "aliasing" flow artifact ➹ due to increased flow velocity.

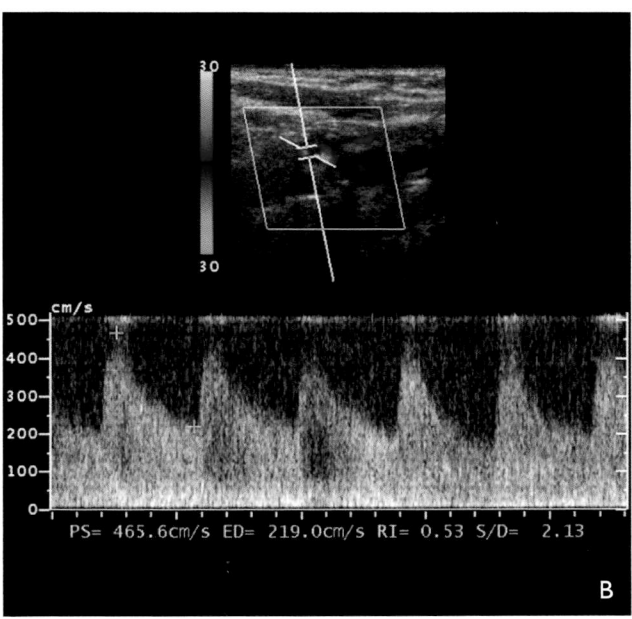

10-18B. Spectral Doppler analysis in the same case shows findings of stenosis. Both PSV and EDV are markedly increased, consistent with stenosis > 70%. (Courtesy S. S. M. Ho, MBBs.)

able plaques are usually hyperintense on T2WI whereas stable plaques are isointense on both T1- and T2WI.

T1 C+ FS scans may show enhancement around plaque margins, consistent with neovascularity in a vulnerable "at risk" plaque.

Contrast-enhanced or unenhanced 2D TOF MRA is 80-85% sensitive and 95% specific for the detection of ICA > 70% ICA stenosis. Signal loss with a "flow gap" occurs if the stenosis is > 95%. Compared to CTA and DSA, MRA tends to overestimate the degree of stenosis.

DSA. Although DSA is generally considered the gold standard of vascular imaging—especially for documenting carotid stenosis/occlusion prior to surgical or endovascular intervention—it is no longer generally used as an initial screening procedure. DSA is occasionally utilized for the detailed assessment of collateral circulation patterns.

Plaque ulceration is seen on DSA as surface irregularity in the opacified vessel lumen (10-15). The reported sensitivity of detecting plaque ulceration on DSA varies between 50-85%. Surface irregularity on DSA is associated with increased stroke risk at all degrees of stenosis.

Carotid stenosis can be identified and calculated on DSA. At least two or more views are required to profile the maximal stenosis (10-12). The NASCET calculation for percent stenosis is the normal lumen diameter minus the minimal residual lumen diameter divided by the normal lumen diameter multiplied by 100 (10-8). A 2 mm residual lumen with a 10 mm diameter represents an 80% stenosis.

"Tandem lesions" are stenoses distal to a more proximal lesion and are seen in approximately 2% of patients with hemodynamically significant cervical ICA stenosis. The most common site for a "tandem lesion" is the cavernous ICA.

Carotid thrombosis is seen as an intraluminal filling defect in the contrast column (10-15). Carotid occlusion is seen as contrast ending blindly in a blunted, rounded, or pointed pouch in the proximal ICA.

High-grade stenosis causes very slow antegrade flow with delayed contrast washout. A **"string" sign** is present when only a "trickle" ("string") of antegrade flow is detected at DSA or color Doppler (10-15). The string sign—also called carotid pseudoocclusion or preocclusion—represents > 95% stenosis. Such patients are at especially high short-term risk for stroke. Examining the late venous phase of the DSA is critical to document subtle arterial patency, as this will determine if emergent endarterectomy or stenting is a treatment option.

ULTRASOUND. US imaging includes grayscale US, color Doppler with color velocity imaging, power Doppler, and spectral Doppler analysis (10-18).

Grayscale ultrasound. Grayscale US shows a fatty or "soft" plaque as hypoechoic while a fibrous plaque is mildly echogenic. Calcified plaque is highly echogenic with distal shadowing. An ulcerated plaque appears as a

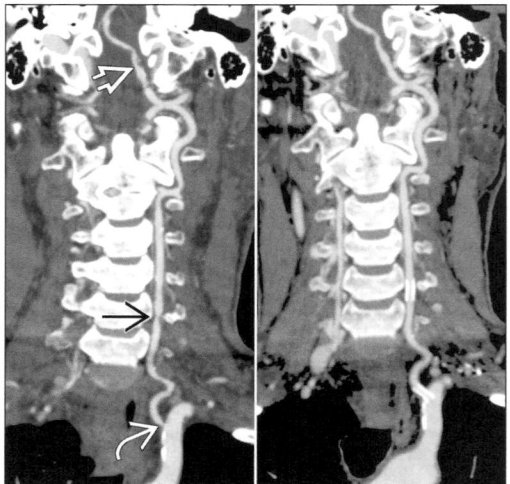

10-19. *(L) Severe VA origin* ➙*, moderate mid-cervical stenosis* ⇢*. Intracranial ASVD* ⇥*. (R) Post-stent CTA. (Courtesy C. Baccin, MD.)*

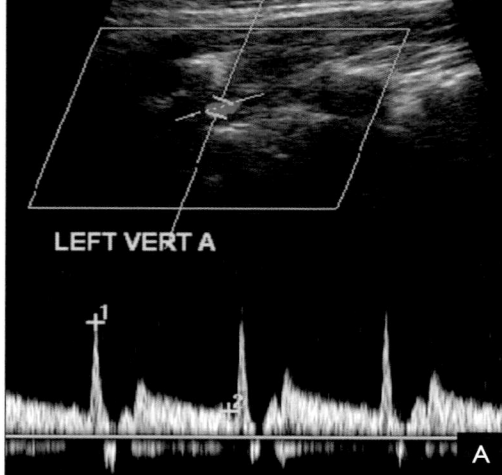

10-20A. *Longitudinal color Doppler US shows mild subclavian steal with arm resting.*

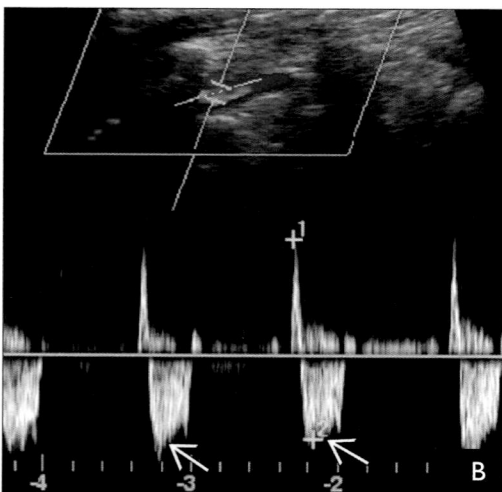

10-20B. *Steal is aggravated after arm exercise. Doppler waveform alternates with increasing retrograde flow* ➙*. (S. S. M. Ho, MBBs.)*

focal crypt with sharp or overhanging edges. Occluded vessels show absent flow with echogenic material filling the vessel lumen.

Color Doppler. Stenosis < 50% shows relatively uniform intraluminal color hues at and distal to the stenosis. Stenosis > 50% shows mildly disturbed intraluminal color hues at and distal to the stenosis.

Stenosis > 70% shows color scale shift or "aliasing" caused by elevated velocity at the stenosis together with significant poststenotic turbulence. Occluded vessels show absent color flow while high-grade near-occlusions may show a thin "trickle" of color.

Power Doppler. Power Doppler is useful in detecting low-velocity flow at and distal to preocclusive stenoses. Power Doppler is especially helpful in differentiating patent, preocclusive (high-grade) stenosis from occlusion.

Spectral Doppler. Spectral Doppler is useful for estimating the degree of stenosis from velocity parameters. Peak systolic velocity (PSV) is the most common, recommended measurement. Other useful measurements include the systolic velocity ratio (SVR), which is ICA stenosis/normal CCA, and end diastolic velocity (EDV). PSV and EDV rise with increasing stenosis.

High-grade, near-occlusive stenoses demonstrate variable velocity. High flow resistance may actually decrease the PSV, so diagnosis is based on color Doppler appearance and damped waveforms distal to the stenosis.

VELOCITY PARAMETERS

In < 50% stenosis
- PSV < 125 cm/s; EDV < 40 cm/s; SVR < 2.0

In 50-69% stenosis
- PSV = 125-229 cm/s; EDV = 40-99 cm/s; SVR = 2.0-3.9

In ≥ 70% stenosis
- PSV > 230 cm/s; EDV > 100 cm/s; SVR ≥ 4.0

Vertebral Arteries

ASVD in the extracranial vertebral arteries accounts for up to 20% of all posterior circulation ischemic strokes. Because the risk of selective VA catheterization in the presence of vasculopathy is 0.5-4%, noninvasive imaging with CTA or MRA is preferable. However, the VA's tortuous course, great variability in normal caliber, thick bony covering, and presence of adjacent veins all create special challenges for the radiologist. The right VA is adequately visualized from its origin to the basilar confluence in only 75% of patients, and the left VA is well seen in approximately 70%.

Although mid- and distal cervical segment lesions occur, extracranial ASVD is most common at or near the VA origin **(10-19)**. Calcification and stenosis are the most common findings. CTA, MRA, color Doppler sonography, and DSA can all provide diagnostic images.

A special type of VA pathology is called **subclavian steal**. Here the SCA or brachiocephalic trunk is severely stenotic or occluded *proximal* to the vertebral artery origin. Flow reversal in the affected VA occurs as blood is recruited (i.e., "stolen") from the opposite vertebral artery, crosses the basilar artery (BA) junction, and flows in retrograde fashion down the VA into the subclavian artery to supply the shoulder and arm distal to the stenosis/occlusion.

Subclavian steal can be complete or partial, symptomatic or occult, and is often an incidental finding. Symptomatic patients present with posterior circulation symptoms secondary to vertebrobasilar insufficiency and brainstem ischemia. Episodic dizziness, diplopia, dysarthria, nausea, and visual disturbances are typical and are aggravated by exercise of the affected arm and shoulder. Significant blood pressure differential (> 20 mmHg) between arms is usually associated with symptomatic subclavian steal.

Noninvasive imaging of subclavian steal can be problematic. Because superior saturation bands are applied in 2D TOF MRA, reversed flow direction in a vertebral artery can mimic occlusion. Standard TOF MRA alone may not be adequate to differentiate *reversed* flow from *absent* flow, so confirmation and quantification with additional imaging—either bolus-timed or direction-encoded phase-contrast MRA, color Doppler US, or DSA—is required **(10-20)**.

DSA shows a severely stenotic or occluded VA with collateral filling from the contralateral VA through the BA junction and/or multiple enlarged, unnamed muscular branches **(10-21)**.

On the basis of hemodynamic changes in the VA, three degrees of subclavian steal are recognized on US. In occult steal, symptoms are absent, hemodynamic changes are minimal, and the only finding may be systolic deceleration. In moderate or partial steal, power Doppler spectrum shows alternating or partially reversed flow. In complete steal, VA flow is completely reversed. Dynamic tests with exercise are recommended for confirmation and treatment considerations.

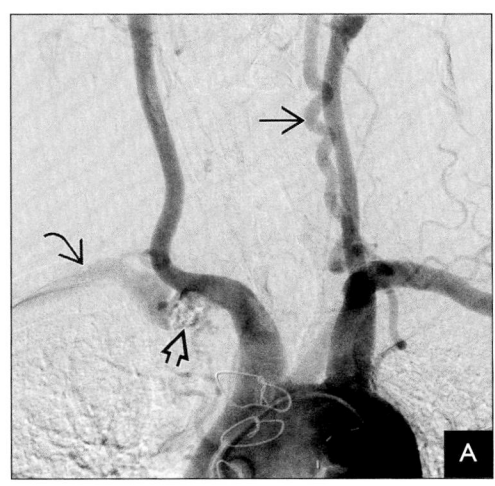

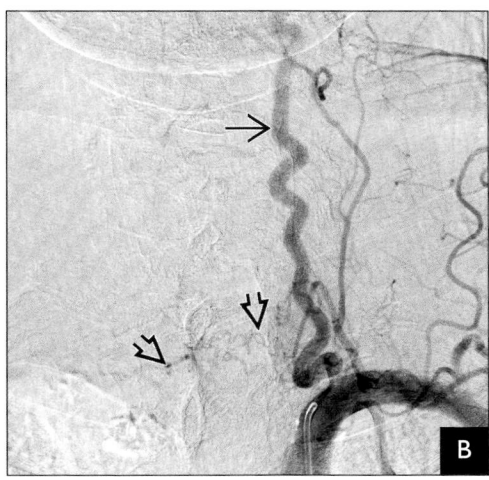

10-21A. *Middle-aged man with systemic ASVD and history of cardiac bypass surgery experienced episodic dizziness. LAO view of aortic arch DSA shows a large calcification at the right SCA origin ⊵ with minimal contrast in the distal SCA ⊿. The right vertebral artery is unopacified. The left VA is enlarged and tortuous ⊐.* **10-21B.** *Selective left SCA angiogram shows the prominent VA ⊐, enlarged muscular branches ⊵ collateralizing to the right SCA vascular distribution.*

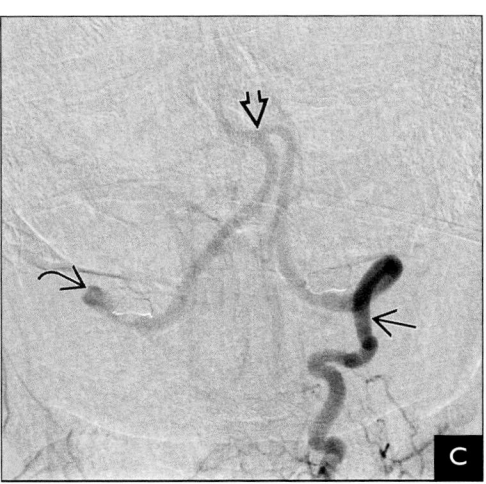

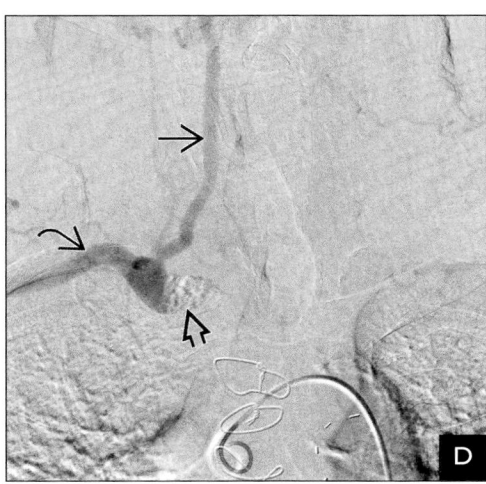

10-21C. *AP view of the left SCA injection shows that blood flows up the left VA ⊐, across the basilar junction ⊵, and down the right VA ⊿. There is transient filling of the proximal basilar artery, but most of the posterior fossa circulation remains unopacified.* **10-21D.** *Delayed image from the aortic arch injection shows retrograde filling of the right VA ⊐ and SCA ⊿ distal to the calcification ⊵ and high-grade stenosis. Classic subclavian steal.*

10-22. *Autopsy case shows the distribution of intracranial ASVD. Most severe disease is in the vertebrobasilar system* ➡️*, ICAs* ➡️*, and proximal MCAs* ➡️*. (Courtesy R. Hewlett, MD.)* **10-23.** *Autopsy case of vertebrobasilar dolichoectasia (VBD) shows yellow atheromatous plaques* ➡️ *in an extremely tortuous basilar artery. Note the mild ectasia of both middle cerebral arteries* ➡️*. (Courtesy R. Hewlett, MD.)*

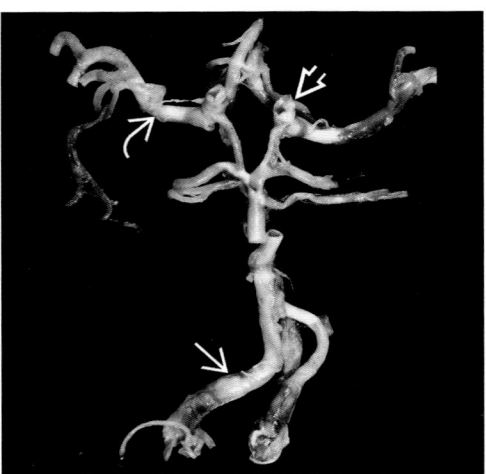
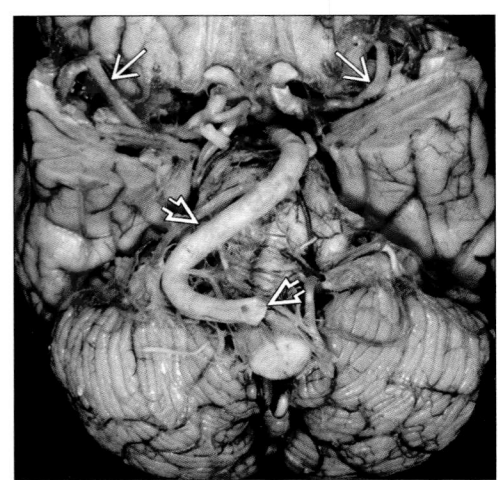

10-24A. *Sagittal T1WI in an elderly man without hypertension or dementia shows an extremely elongated "flow void" of the basilar artery* ➡️*. The dolichoectatic artery indents and elevates the third ventricle* ➡️*, which appears compressed and draped over the basilar bifurcation.* **10-24B.** *Coronal T1 C+ scan in the same case shows slow flow with enhancement in the ectatic basilar artery* ➡️*. Note that the third ventricle is elevated, compressed* ➡️ *by the VBD.*

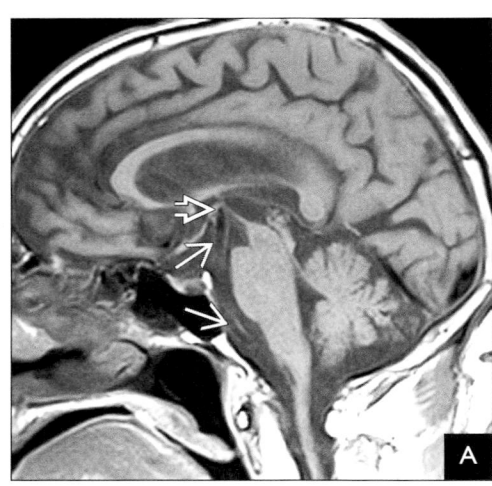
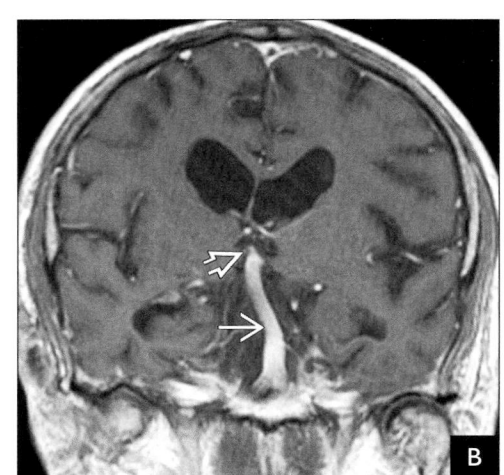

10-25. *Autopsy case demonstrates ASVD fusiform ectasias of the ICAs* ➡️ *and MCAs* ➡️*. The posterior (vertebrobasilar) circulation is relatively spared* ➡️*. (Courtesy R. Hewlett, MD.)* **10-26.** *Autopsy case shows extreme ectasia of the horizontal MCA segment* ➡️*. (Courtesy R. Hewlett, MD.)*

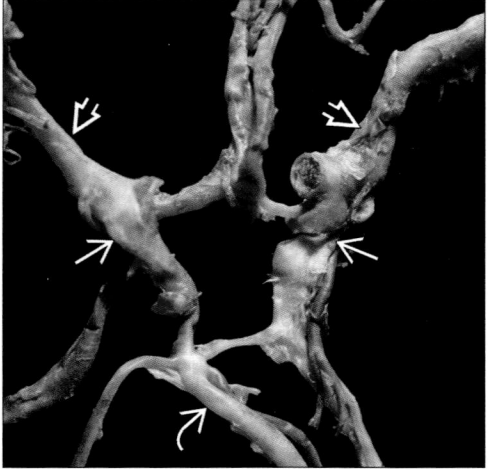
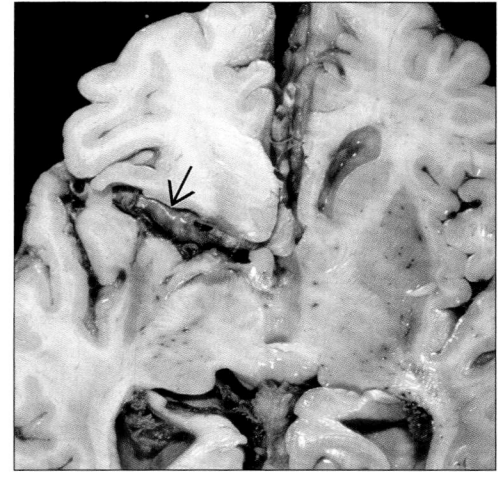

Differential Diagnosis

The major differential diagnoses of extracranial ASVD include dissection, dissecting aneurysm, vasospasm, and fibromuscular dysplasia. All usually spare the carotid bulb.

Dissection (either traumatic or spontaneous) is more common in young/middle-aged patients and occurs in the *middle* of extracranial vessels. Extracranial dissections typically terminate at the exocranial opening of the carotid canal. Most are smooth or display minimal irregularities whereas calcifications and ulcerations—common in carotid plaques—are absent.

Mid-segment vessel narrowing with a focal mass-like outpouching of the lumen is typical of **dissecting aneurysm**. **Vasospasm** is more common in the intracranial vessels. When it involves the cervical carotid or vertebral arteries, it also typically spares the proximal segments.

Fibromuscular dysplasia (FMD) spares the carotid bulb and usually affects the middle or distal aspects of the extracranial carotid and vertebral arteries. A "string of beads" appearance is typical. Long-segment tubular narrowing is less common and may reflect coexisting dissection.

Less common mimics of extracranial ASVD include congenital hypoplasia and small vessel size secondary to reduced distal run off. Congenital **internal carotid artery hypoplasia**, featuring a small ipsilateral bony carotid canal, is rare. A congenital **hypoplastic vertebral artery** is common and considered a normal variant. Here the VA often terminates in the posterior inferior cerebellar artery (PICA) and the contralateral VA is typically large. If both PCAs have a so-called fetal origin from the ICAs and the P1 PCA segments are absent, the entire vertebrobasilar system may appear relatively hypoplastic.

Diminished distal flow—"run off"—occurs when intracranial pressure becomes markedly elevated or if there is severe vasospasm of the intracranial vessels. The lumen of the affected cervical vessel diminishes in proportion to the reduced run off.

Intracranial Atherosclerosis

One of the most serious and disabling manifestations of ASVD is stroke. Most acute ischemic strokes are thromboembolic, most often secondary to cardiac sources or plaques in the cervical ICA.

Many clinicians focus on extracranial carotid artery disease, considering intracranial ASVD (IASVD) a relatively infrequent cause of stroke. However, recent studies have demonstrated that intracranial ASVD accounts for

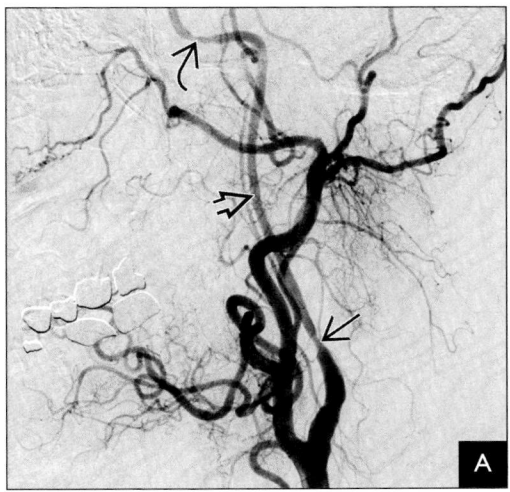

10-27A. Lateral DSA shows high-grade narrowing of the cervical ICA ➔, small distal ICA ➔ (from reduced flow), "tandem" stenosis ➔.

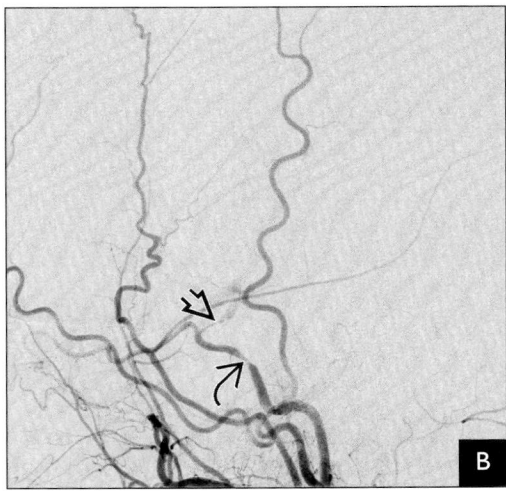

10-27B. Intracranial view shows the high-grade cavernous ICA stenosis ➔ together with near-complete occlusion of the supraclinoid ICA ➔.

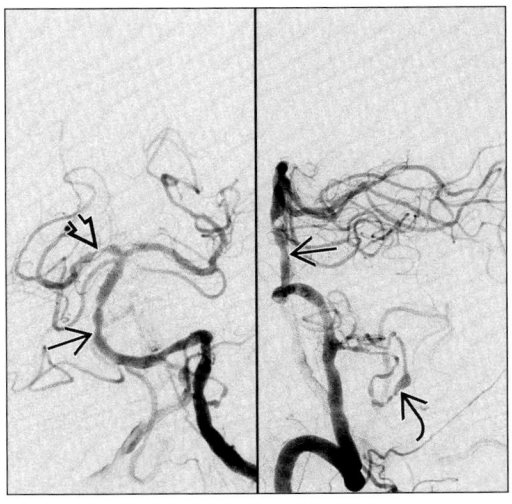

10-28. (Left) AP, (right) lateral DSA show extensive changes of ASVD in the vertebrobasilar artery ➔, proximal right PCA ➔, PICA ➔.

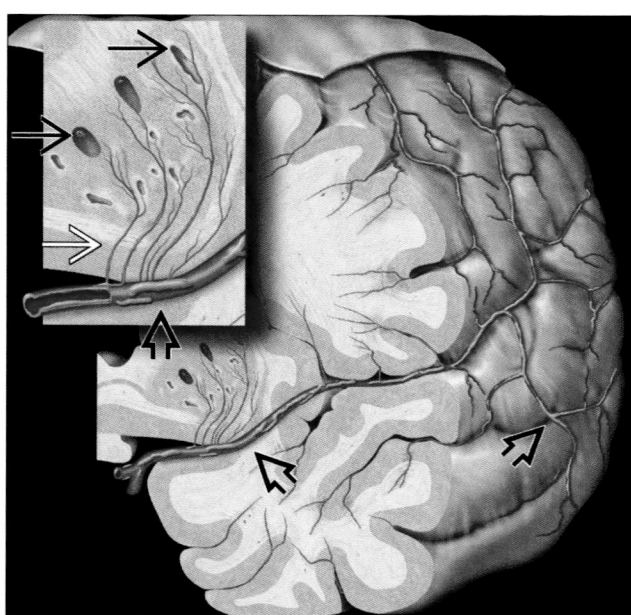

10-29. Coronal graphic shows atherosclerotic plaques ⊵ involving the major intracranial arteries and their branches. Inset shows penetrating (lenticulostriate) arteries ⊳ and lacunar infarcts ⊵.

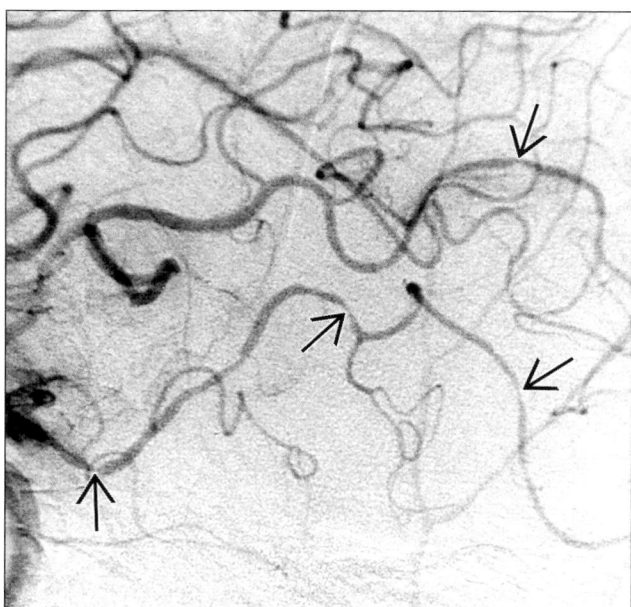

10-30. Magnified lateral DSA shows severe intracranial ASVD with numerous foci of irregular narrowing and dilatation in distal MCA branches ⊳ mimicking vasculitis.

5-10% of all ischemic strokes. Nearly half of all patients with fatal cerebral infarction have at least one intracranial plaque-associated luminal stenosis at autopsy (10-22).

With an expanding variety of treatment options now available, accurate delineation of intracranial ASVD is imperative for individualized patient care. In this section, we briefly review the manifestations of intracranial ASVD ranging from asymptomatic vascular ectasias to fusiform aneurysms and life-threatening but potentially treatable stenoocclusive disease.

Ectasia

Generalized nonfocal vessel elongation is called "ectasia," "dolichoectasia," "arteriectasis," or "dilative arteriopathy." Elongated, tortuous vessels are common manifestations of advanced atherosclerosis throughout the body and also occur in both the cervical and intracranial arteries. When ectasia occurs in the posterior circulation, it is termed "vertebrobasilar dolichoectasia" (VBD) (10-23).

Many—if not most—ectatic intracranial vessels are asymptomatic and discovered incidentally at autopsy or on imaging studies. These vascular enlargements are most common in middle-aged and elderly patients (10-24).

Ectasias can involve any part of the intracranial circulation but are most common in the vertebrobasilar arteries and supraclinoid ICA (10-25). Multifocal disease is common. Ectasias may extend from the basilar and internal carotid arteries into the proximal M1 or P1 segments (10-26). Imaging findings of uncomplicated ectasias are

one or more elongated arteries that do not demonstrate focal aneurysmal dilatation.

Atherosclerotic Fusiform Aneurysm

Atherosclerotic fusiform aneurysms (FAs) are focal arterial enlargements that are usually superimposed on an ectatic artery. ASVD FAs are most common in the vertebrobasilar circulation. When they occur in the anterior circulation, they can produce a rare but dramatic manifestation called a giant "serpentine" aneurysm. ASVD FAs are discussed in detail in Chapter 6.

Intracranial Stenoocclusive Disease

The advent of effective endovascular techniques to treat intracranial stenoocclusive disease has made detection and accurate delineation of IASVD as important as identifying and characterizing extracranial ASVD.

EPIDEMIOLOGY. Atherosclerosis that causes large artery intracranial occlusive disease (LAICOD) is now a well-defined yet relatively neglected and poorly understood stroke subtype. Recent studies have shown that the overall prevalence of IASVD in patients with concurrent extracranial disease varies between 20% and 50%, and 12% of patients have diffuse (multifocal) intracranial ASVD.

Between 8-10% of all strokes in North America are related to LAICOD. The prevalence of intracranial ASVD is especially high in blacks, Hispanics, and Asians, in whom some studies have demonstrated a preponderance of intracranial stenosis relative to extracranial carotid stenosis. Insulin resistance and metabolic syndrome are significant risk factors for intracranial vs. extracranial ASVD.

CLINICAL ISSUES. Overall, symptomatic patients with moderate to severe stenosis (i.e., 70-99%) in the intracranial circulation have a 25% two-year risk for recurrent stroke.

Clinical course varies significantly with stenosis sublocation. The vessel-specific mean overall annual mortality is 6.8% for middle cerebral artery stenosis, 11.6% for vertebrobasilar stenosis, and 12.4% for intracranial ICA stenosis.

Symptomatic IASVD generally has a poor prognosis as conservative (i.e., medical) management frequently fails. Stroke recurrence rates in patients with IASVD treated with either warfarin or aspirin are unacceptably high. Among patients with symptomatic IASVD who fail antithrombotic therapy, the subsequent rates of stroke or vascular death are even higher, up to 45% per year.

The availability of endovascular techniques such as intracranial angioplasty has opened new treatment avenues for LAICOD. A variety of balloon-expandable, drug-eluting, and self-expanding stents are also now available as options.

IMAGING. Imaging findings generally resemble those of extracranial ASVD. Mural calcifications are common and are frequently identified on NECT scans. Calcification in the carotid siphon (cavernous and supraclinoid ICA) is related to overall ASVD burden. Patterns vary from scattered stippled foci to thick continuous linear ("railroad track") deposits. The degree of carotid siphon calcification correlates with the prevalence of lacunar infarcts but is not associated with large thromboembolic territorial strokes.

Angiography best depicts IASVD (10-27), (10-28). While CTA accurately depicts > 50% stenoses of large intracranial arterial segments (cavernous and supraclinoid ICA, proximal MCA), lesser degrees of stenosis and ASVD in smaller second- or third-order branches are best depicted on DSA. Compared with CTA and DSA, MRA less accurately depicts intracranial atherosclerosis—especially in second- and third-order branches or when the residual vessel lumen is less than one millimeter.

Solitary or multifocal stenoses alternating with areas of post-stenotic dilatation are typical of IASVD (10-29). When atherosclerosis affects distal branches of the major intracranial vessels, the appearance can mimic that of vasculitis (see below) (10-30).

Imaging the *intracranial* circulation in patients with a hemodynamically significant *extracranial* stenosis is imperative. A **"tandem" stenosis**—defined as any lesion with an *intra*cranial stenosis > 50% in the same vascular distribution distal to a primary *extra*cranial stenosis—is present in 20% of patients (10-27). Cumulative stroke and/or death rate is higher than with either stenosis alone.

DIFFERENTIAL DIAGNOSIS. The major differential diagnoses of intracranial ASVD are vasculitis, vasospasm, and dissection. **Vasculitis** occurs at all ages but is more common in middle-aged patients. Vasculitis and ASVD appear virtually identical on angiography. Remember: The most common cause of a vasculitis-like pattern in an older patient isn't vasculitis, it's ASVD!

Vasospasm spares the cavernous ICA and is usually more diffuse than ASVD. A history of trauma, subarachnoid hemorrhage, or drug abuse (typically with sympathomimetics) is common. **Intracranial dissection**—especially in the anterior circulation—is rare and usually occurs in young patients.

Arteriolosclerosis

Terminology

Arteriolosclerosis is also known as **small vessel disease** or—less specifically—cerebral microvascular disease. Arteriolosclerosis is a microangiopathy that typically affects small arteries (i.e., arterioles), especially in the subcortical and deep cerebral white matter (WM).

The term **leukoariosis** is sometimes used by neurologists to designate the confluent WM lesions associated with arteriolosclerosis, i.e., small vessel vascular disease. This is one of the most grossly visible markers that aging and vascular risk factors inflict on the brain.

Etiology and Pathology

Aging, chronic hypertension (HTN), hypercholesterolemia, and diabetes mellitus (DM) are the most common factors that predispose to cerebral microvascular disease. Genetic risk factors include the *APOE*E4* genotype.

Gross pathologic features of cerebral arteriolosclerosis include generalized volume loss, multiple lacunar infarcts, and deep white matter spongiosis. Stenosis or occlusion of small vessels by arteriolosclerosis and lipohyalinosis probably results in WM microinfarctions.

The microscopic correlates of the deep periventricular white matter lesions identified on imaging studies have a spectrum of findings. Degenerated myelin (myelin "pallor"), axonal loss with increased extracellular fluid, lipofibrohyalinosis with small vessel occlusion, gliosis, spongiosis, and enlarged perivascular spaces can all be present in varying degrees.

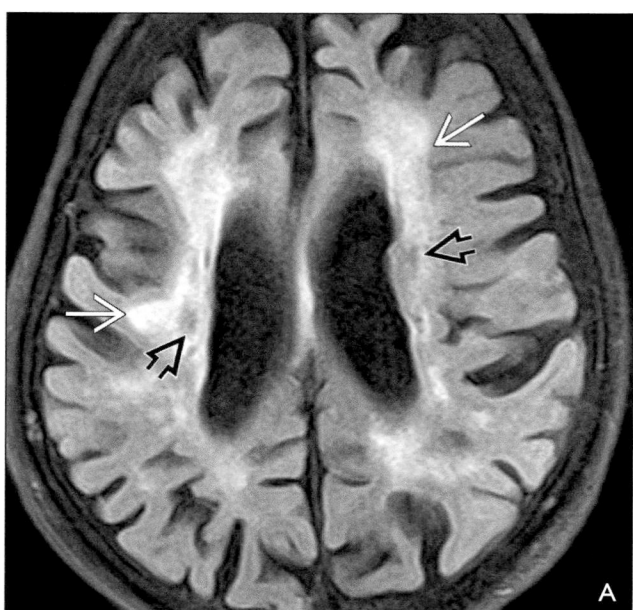

10-31A. Axial FLAIR scan in an elderly demented patient with chronic hypertension and small vessel vascular disease shows volume loss, confluent periventricular WM hyperintensities ➡, and multiple lacunar infarcts ⊳.

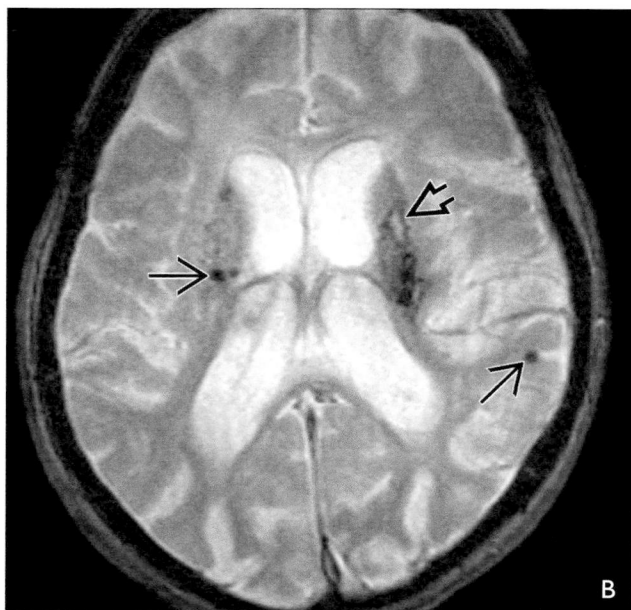

10-31B. T2* GRE scan in the same patient shows multifocal hypointensities characteristic of cerebral microbleeds ➡, old hypertensive basal ganglia hemorrhage ⊳.

Clinical Issues

The clinical manifestations of cerebral small vessel vascular disease vary widely and range from normal or minimal cognitive impairment (MCI) to severe dementia. Although there is relatively poor correlation between the degree of WM changes on imaging studies and cognitive performance, the severity of small vessel disease at autopsy correlates significantly with the degree of cognitive impairment.

Imaging

Imaging studies typically reflect white matter rarefaction and spongiosis associated with varying degrees of generalized volume loss.

CT. Patchy and/or confluent WM hypodensities that spare the cortex are typical findings on NECT. Periventricular lesions have a broad or confluent base with the ventricular surface and are especially prominent around the atria of the lateral ventricles. Lesions are almost always nonenhancing on CECT.

MR. Patchy or confluent periventricular and subcortical white matter hypointensities are seen on T1WI. The lesions are hyperintense on T2WI and are especially prominent on FLAIR (10-31A). T2* (GRE, SWI) sequences often demonstrate multifocal "blooming" hypointensities, especially in the presence of chronic hypertension (10-31B).

Chronic arteriolosclerosis does not enhance on T1 C+ and does not demonstrate restricted diffusion on DWI.

ULTRASOUND. Carotid intimal-medial thickness and arterial stiffness are emerging as markers of arterial aging and may serve as surrogate risk markers for vascular cognitive impairment.

Differential Diagnosis

The most important differential diagnosis is **normal age-related hyperintensities**. There is significant overlap between imaging findings in cognitively normal individuals and patients with MCI. Scattered periventricular WM lesions are almost universal after age 65. Between 2-6% of normal elderly patients demonstrate extensive/confluent WM lesions. "Silent" lacunar infarcts are seen in one-third of asymptomatic healthy elderly patients.

Other significant differential considerations include **enlarged perivascular (Virchow-Robin) spaces** (PVSs). Prominent PVSs can be seen in patients of all ages and in virtually all locations, although they do increase with age. The most common site is the inferior one-third of the basal ganglia around the anterior commissure. PVSs contain interstitial fluid but behave like CSF, i.e., they suppress completely on FLAIR. Perilesional hyperintensity is seen in 25% of cases.

Demyelinating disease typically causes ovoid or triangular periventricular lesions that commonly involve the callososeptal interfaces, which are rarely involved by arteriolosclerosis.

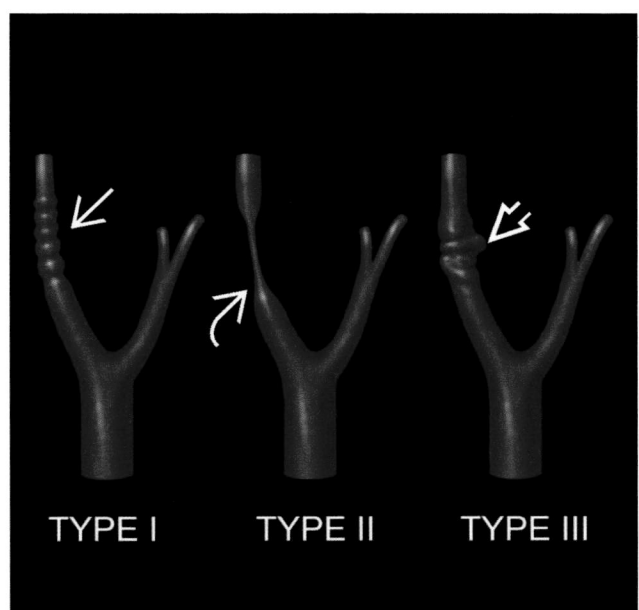

10-32. Graphic of the carotid bifurcation shows the principal subtypes of FMD. Type 1 appears as alternating areas of constriction and dilatation ➘, type 2 as tubular stenosis ➚, and type 3 as focal corrugations ± diverticulum ➘.

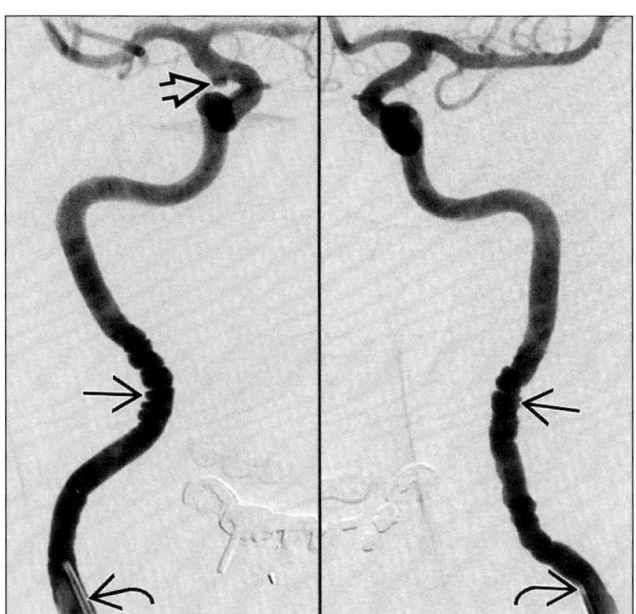

10-33. AP DSA shows type 1 FMD in both ICAs with sparing of the bulbs ➚, "string of beads" in mid-cervical segments ➘, small unruptured saccular aneurysm ➘ of the right supraclinoid ICA.

Subcortical arteriosclerotic encephalopathy (SAE) is associated with Binswanger-type vascular dementia and is a clinical (not an imaging) diagnosis.

Nonatheromatous Vascular Diseases

While ASVD is by far the most common disease to affect the craniocervical vasculature, a number of other nonatheromatous disorders can affect the brain, causing stroke or stroke-like symptoms. In this section, we briefly discuss some of the most important entities, including fibromuscular dysplasia, vasculitis, and non-ASVD non-inflammatory vasculopathies such as cerebral amyloid disease.

Fibromuscular Dysplasia

Terminology

Fibromuscular dysplasia (FMD) is an uncommon segmental nonatherosclerotic, noninflammatory disease of unknown etiology that affects medium and large arteries in many areas of the body.

Etiology

The exact pathoetiology of FMD remains unknown. It is more common in first-degree relatives of patients with the disease, but most patients have no family history of FMD.

Pathology

LOCATION. Although virtually any artery in any location can be affected, FMD affects some arteries far more than others. The renal arteries are affected in 75% of cases; about 35% of these are bilateral.

The cervicocephalic vessels are involved in up to 70% of cases. The ICA is the most common site; VA FMD is seen in 20% of cases. Approximately half of all cervicocephalic FMD cases involve more than one artery (usually either both ICAs or one ICA and a VA). Intracranial FMD is very rare.

FMD carries an increased risk of developing intracranial saccular aneurysms. Intracranial saccular aneurysms are present in approximately 7-10% of patients with cervical FMD.

SIZE AND NUMBER. Size varies from small focal lesions with minimal beading to extensive disease involving most of the vessel one to two centimeters distal to its origin. Multiple arterial systems are involved in 25-30% of cases. When multisystem disease is present, the renal arteries are almost always involved.

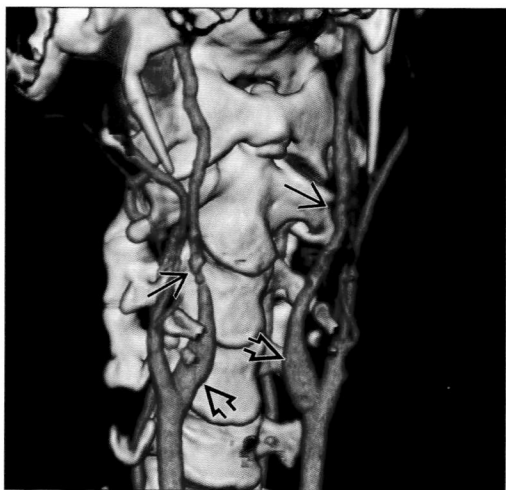

10-34. *Oblique CTA shows type 1 FMD with "string of beads" appearance in both carotid arteries ➡. Note the sparing of carotid bulbs ▷.*

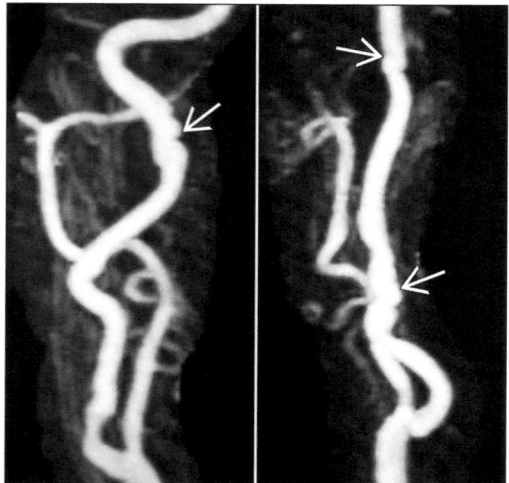

10-35. *TOF MRA shows FMD ➡ with "string of beads" appearance in both cervical carotid arteries.*

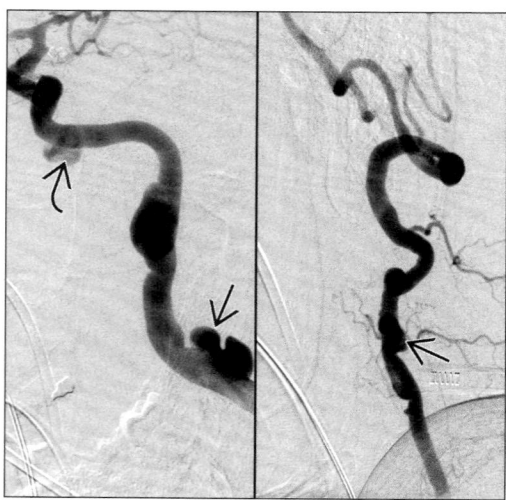

10-36. *(L) DSA of internal carotid, (R) vertebral arteries with type 3 FMD shows diverticulum-like outpouchings ➡, saccular aneurysm ➘.*

STAGING, GRADING, AND CLASSIFICATION. FMD is classified histologically into three categories according to which arterial wall layer is affected (media, intima, or adventitia) **(10-32)**. By far the most common type (type 1) is medial fibroplasia, accounting for approximately 85% of all FMD cases. Here the media has alternating thin and very thick areas formed by concentric rings of fibrous proliferations and smooth muscle hyperplasia. Inflammatory cells are absent.

Intimal fibroplasia (type 2) accounts for less than 10% of FMD cases. Focal band-like and smooth long-segment narrowings both occur. Histologically, the intima is markedly thickened by circumferential or eccentric collagen deposition, and the internal elastic lamina is fragmented. Lipid and inflammatory components are absent.

Adventitial (periarterial) fibroplasia (type 3) is the least common type of FMD, accounting for less than 5% of cases. Dense collagen replaces the delicate fibrous tissue of the adventitia and may infiltrate the adjacent periarterial tissues.

Clinical Issues

EPIDEMIOLOGY. Once thought to be a relatively rare vasculopathy, FMD is identified in 0.5% of all patients screened with CTA for ischemic neurologic symptoms.

FMD primarily affects individuals between the ages of 20 and 60 years, but it may also occur in infants, children, and the elderly. Gender disparity in FMD is striking with a 9:1 female predominance.

PRESENTATION. Sudden onset of high blood pressure in a young woman is a typical presentation of renal FMD. Carotid or vertebral FMD typically presents at an older age, generally around 50 years. Cervical FMD can present with transient ischemia attack, bruit, stroke, or dissection (often with Horner syndrome, i.e., ptosis, pupil constriction, facial anhidrosis).

NATURAL HISTORY AND TREATMENT. The natural history of FMD is unclear as many cases are now discovered incidentally on imaging studies.

To date, no prospective randomized trials have compared the efficacy of different treatment options. "Watch and wait" for patients with renal FMD without hypertension and with normal renal function is common, as is antiplatelet therapy for asymptomatic individuals with cervical FMD. Percutaneous balloon angioplasty is recommended for patients with recent-onset or resistant hypertension, TIA, or stroke. Surgery is generally used only to treat aneurysms.

Imaging

TECHNICAL CONSIDERATIONS. In the past, DSA was considered the gold standard for the diagnosis of FMD. However, CTA accurately depicts FMD in the cervicocephalic arteries and also allows visualization of the intracranial vessels to detect the presence of associated aneurysms. TOF MRA is problematic because artifacts caused by patient motion or in-plane flow and susceptibility gradients can mimic the appearance of FMD. Duplex sonography and color Doppler can depict FMD only when the lesion is located proximally.

Because multisystem disease is common, patients with newly diagnosed carotid and/or vertebral FMD should also have their renal arteries examined.

IMAGING. Imaging findings vary with FMD subtype. Between 80-90% of patients demonstrate findings typical for medial fibroplasia (type 1 FMD). An irregular "corrugated" or "string of beads" appearance with alternating areas of constriction and dilatation that are wider than the original lumen is the typical appearance **(10-33)**, **(10-34)**, **(10-35)**. In type 2 (intimal fibroplasia), a smooth, long-segment tubular narrowing is present. In type 3 (adventitial) FMD, asymmetric diverticulum-like outpouchings from one side of the artery are present **(10-36)**.

All three cervical FMD subtypes spare the carotid bifurcations and great vessel origins, involve the middle segments, and are most common at the C1-C2 level. Complications of cervicocephalic FMD include dissection, intracranial aneurysm with or without subarachnoid hemorrhage **(10-33)**, **(10-36)**, and arteriovenous fistulas.

Differential Diagnosis

The major differential diagnosis of FMD is **atherosclerosis**. FMD is most common in young women, a group that is generally at low risk for ASVD. FMD involves the middle to distal portions of the affected arteries, not the origins.

The smooth, tapered "tubular" narrowing of intimal FMD can be difficult to distinguish from **spontaneous dissection**, which also occurs as a complication of FMD. Other **nonatherosclerotic vasculopathies** such as Takayasu arteritis and giant cell arteritis can mimic tubular (i.e., intimal) FMD.

Dissection

Craniocervical arterial dissection (CAD) is an uncommon but important cause of ischemic stroke in young and middle-aged adults. Timely therapy can reduce the immediate stroke risk and mitigate long-term sequelae of craniocervical dissections, so imaging diagnosis is crucial to patient management.

Terminology

A **dissection** is a vessel wall tear permitting blood to penetrate into and delaminate ("dissect") wall layers **(10-37)**. A dissecting aneurysm is a dissection characterized by an outpouching that extends beyond the vessel wall. Most occur with subadventitial dissections and are more accurately designated as pseudoaneurysms (i.e., they lack all normal vessel wall components).

Etiology

CAD can be extra- or intracranial.

Almost 60% of *extracranial* dissections are "spontaneous," i.e., nontraumatic. The remainder result from blunt or penetrating injury. Most nontraumatic dissections occur secondary to an underlying vasculopathy such as FMD, Marfan syndrome, or other connective tissue disorder (e.g., Ehlers-Danlos type 4). Less common predisposing conditions include hypertension, migraine headaches, vigorous physical activity, hyperhomocysteinemia, and recent pharyngeal infection.

Intracranial dissections are usually traumatic. Iatrogenic dissections (typically secondary to endovascular procedures) are becoming increasingly common.

Pathology

LOCATION. Dissections typically occur in the most mobile segment of a vessel, often starting or ending where the vessel transitions from a relatively free position to a position fixed by an encasing bony canal. The extracranial ICA is the most common overall site in the head and neck. Extracranial ICA dissections spare the carotid bulb and often extend up to—but only occasionally into—the skull base **(10-38)**. Vertebral dissections are most common between the skull base and C1 and between C1 and C2.

Intracranial dissections are rare, accounting for just 1-2% of all cervicocephalic dissections. The most common site is the vertebral artery. Dissections in the anterior circulation are even less common. They almost always involve the supraclinoid ICA, with or without extension into the proximal MCA.

SIZE AND NUMBER. Dissections can be limited to a focal intimal tear and small subintimal hematoma. Most are solitary, long-segment lesions that extend for several centimeters. Approximately 20% involve two or more vessels. Multiple dissections are more common if an underlying vasculopathy such as Marfan, Ehlers-Danlos type 4, or FMD is present.

GROSS PATHOLOGY. An intimal tear permits dissection of blood into the vessel wall, resulting in a medial or subendothelial hematoma. The hematoma nar-

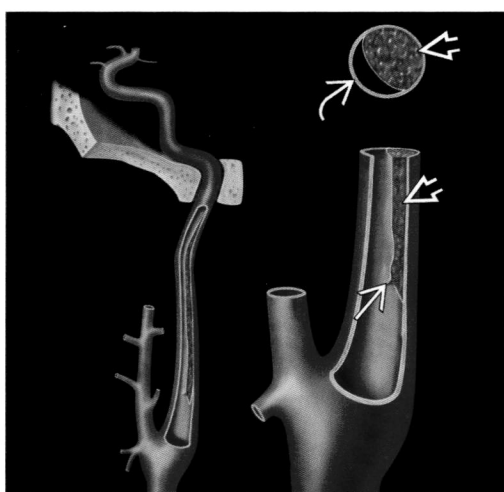

10-37. *Extracranial ICA dissection shows intimal tear ➡, subintimal thrombus ➡ compressing the residual lumen ➡. The bulb is spared.*

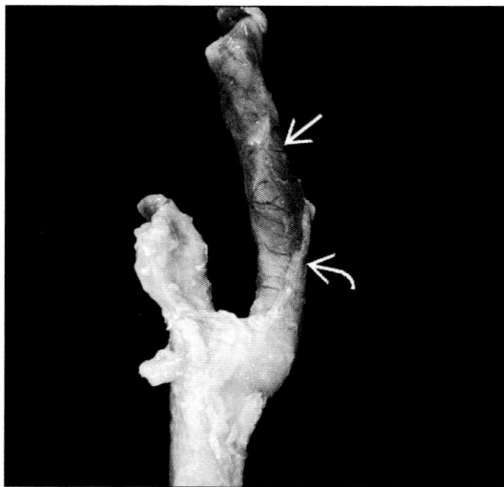

10-38. *Extracranial ICA dissection shows extensive mural thrombus ➡. Dissection begins ➡ distal to the bulb. (Courtesy R. Hewlett, MD.)*

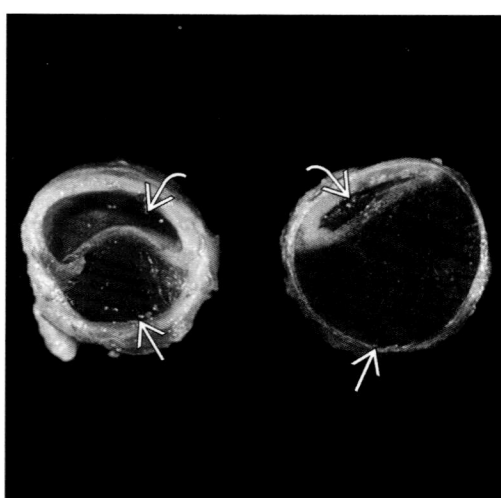

10-39. *Two axial sections show carotid dissection with subintimal hematoma ➡, compressed residual lumen ➡. (Courtesy R. Hewlett, MD.)*

rows and may occlude the parent vessel lumen (10-39). Occasionally dissections—especially in the vertebral artery—extend through the adventitia and present with subarachnoid hemorrhage.

Clinical Issues

EPIDEMIOLOGY AND DEMOGRAPHICS. The annual incidence of ICA dissection is 2.5-3 cases per 100,000. The incidence of VA dissection is approximately half that of the ICA.

Although dissections occur at all ages, most are found in young and middle-aged adults. Peak age is 40 years. Carotid dissections are more common in men whereas vertebral dissections are more common in women.

CAD accounts for approximately 2% of all ischemic strokes. In young and middle-aged patients with no or minimal ASVD risk factors, dissections may account for 10-25% of all ischemic strokes.

PRESENTATION. Neck pain and headache are the most common symptoms. One or more lower cranial nerve palsies including postganglionic Horner syndrome may occur. Pulsatile tinnitus is a less frequent presentation.

NATURAL HISTORY. The natural history of most extracranial CADs is benign. Approximately 90% of stenoses resolve, and 60% of all occlusions recanalize. The risk of recurrent dissection is low; 2% in the first month, then 1% per year thereafter (usually in another vessel).

Persistent headache, pulsatile tinnitus, postganglionic Horner syndrome, and ischemic stroke are uncommon but well-recognized complications of CAD.

Intracranial CAD is much more problematic. Stroke is more common, and spontaneous recanalization is less frequent.

TREATMENT OPTIONS. Anticoagulation is the recommended treatment for extracranial arterial dissection. Six months of antiplatelet therapy in asymptomatic patients with stable imaging findings is common. Intravenous heparin with oral warfarin is an option, as is endovascular stenting. The treatment of intracranial CAD is controversial.

Imaging

Both lumen-opacifying procedures (e.g., CTA, conventional DSA, MRA) and cross-sectional techniques that visualize the vessel wall itself (e.g., CT, MR) should be used to delineate the full extent of disease.

GENERAL FEATURES. Dissections can present as stenosis, occlusion, or aneurysmal dilatation.

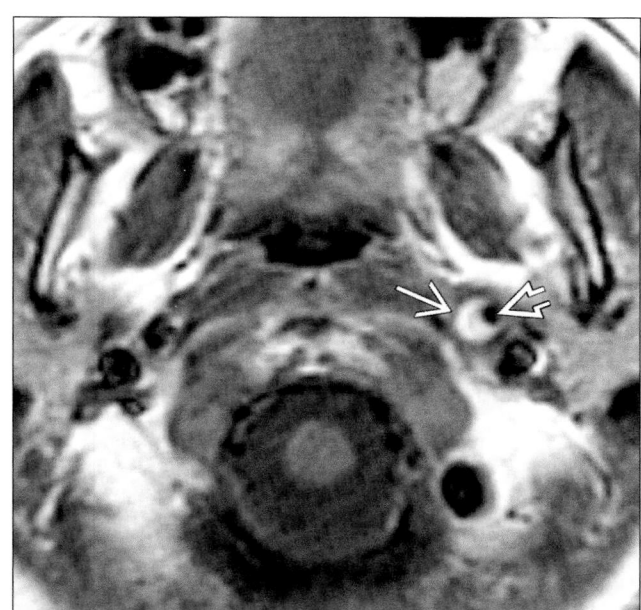

10-40. Axial T1WI shows the classic findings of extracranial carotid dissection with subacute subintimal hematoma. Note the crescent-shaped hyperintensity ➡ surrounding the narrowed "flow void" ⧉ of the mid-cervical ICA.

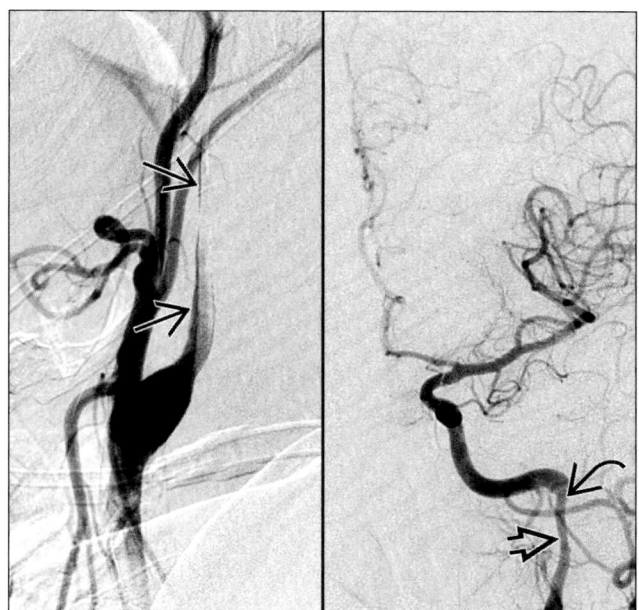

10-41. DSA in 2 cases of cervical ICA dissection. (Left) Classic "rat-tail" narrowing ⤳ of the mid carotid with sparing of the bulb. (Right) Upper ICA dissection ⧈ terminates at the exocranial opening of the bony carotid canal ⤳.

CT FINDINGS. NECT may show crescent-shaped thickening caused by the wall hematoma. Approximately 20% of vertebral artery dissections cause posterior fossa subarachnoid hemorrhage.

CECT may show narrowing of the dissected vessel with or without aneurysmal dilatation.

MR FINDINGS. T1WI with fat saturation is the best sequence for demonstrating CAD. A hyperintense crescent of subacute blood adjacent to a narrowed "flow void" in the patent lumen is typical (10-40). T2WI may show laminated layers of thrombus that "blooms" on T2* (10-42).

At least half of all patients with cervicocephalic dissections have cerebral or cerebellar infarcts, best depicted on DWI. Multiple ipsilateral foci of diffusion restriction are typical findings.

ANGIOGRAPHY. Extracranial ICA dissections typically spare the carotid bulb, beginning two to three centimeters distal to the bifurcation and terminating at the exocranial opening of the carotid canal (10-41). Vertebral dissections are most common around the skull base and upper cervical spine.

CTA shows an eccentrically narrowed lumen surrounded by a crescent-shaped mural thickening. A dissection flap can sometimes be identified. Pseudoaneurysms are common. An opacified double lumen ("true" plus "false" lumen) occurs in less than 10% of cases.

The most common finding on DSA is a smooth or slightly irregular, tapered mid-cervical narrowing. CAD with occlusion shows a flame-shaped "rat-tail" termination (10-41). Occasionally a subtle intimal tear or flap, a double lumen, narrowed or occluded true lumen, or pseudoaneurysm can be identified. If the dissection is subadventitial and does not narrow the vessel lumen, DSA can appear entirely normal; the paravascular hematoma must be detected on cross-sectional imaging.

Intracranial dissections are more difficult to diagnose than their extracranial counterparts (10-43), (10-44). They are significantly smaller and findings are often subtle.

Differential Diagnosis

The major differential diagnosis of *extracranial* arterial dissection is type 2 (intimal) **fibromuscular dysplasia**. A common complication of FMD is dissection, so the two conditions are interrelated and may be indistinguishable on imaging studies alone. Although multiple dissections do occur, they are much less common than multifocal FMD; careful evaluation of the other cervicocephalic vessels for typical changes of FMD may be helpful.

Atherosclerosis is more common than dissection in older patients. ASVD typically involves the great vessel origins and carotid bulb, sites that are almost always spared by dissection. As ASVD is a systemic disorder, multiple vessels in multiple vascular distributions are usually affected. Dissection, on the other hand, is solitary unless an underlying vasculopathy such as Marfan or Ehlers-Danlos syndrome is present (10-42).

10-42A. *T1WI in a 28-year-old woman with Marfan syndrome and a 4-day history of neck pain shows dissection of both cervical internal carotid arteries* ➡️*, both vertebral arteries* ⮞*. Mural thrombus surrounds tiny residual "flow voids" in all 4 vessels.* **10-42B.** *T2* GRE in the same patient demonstrates that the mural thrombus around the distal cervical ICAs "blooms"* ⮞*.*

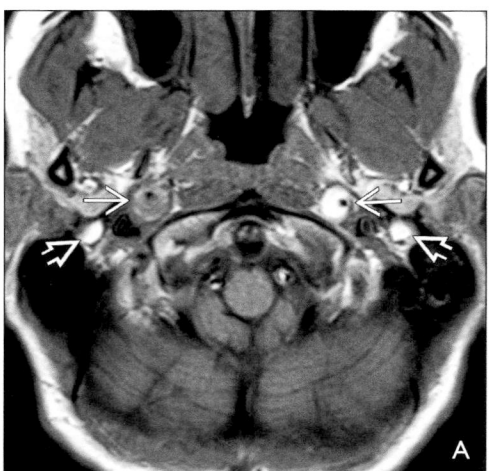

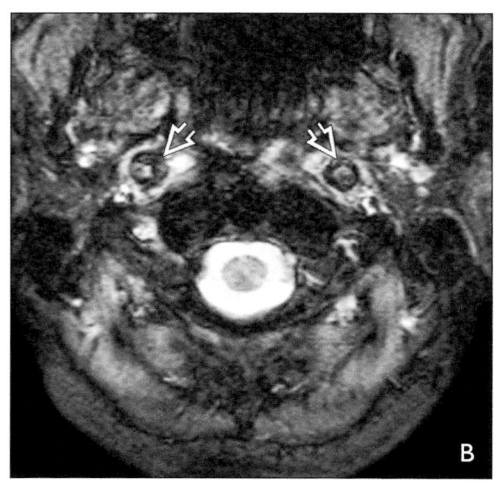

10-42C. *More cephalad T1WI through the skull base shows that the dissections of both ICAs extend into the petrous carotid canals* ➡️*.* **10-42D.** *(L) Coronal MRA shows dissections in all 4 cervicocephalic vessels* ➡️*, including petrous intracranial ICA segments* ⮞*. (R) Oblique view shows that left ICA dissection* ➡️ *spares the carotid bulb* ⮞*. Note the cervical carotid pseudoaneurysm* ➡️*.*

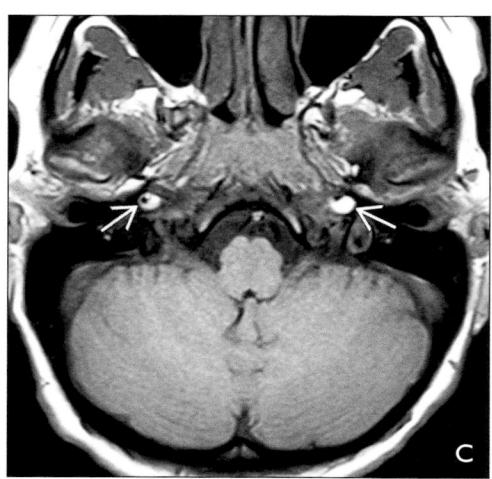

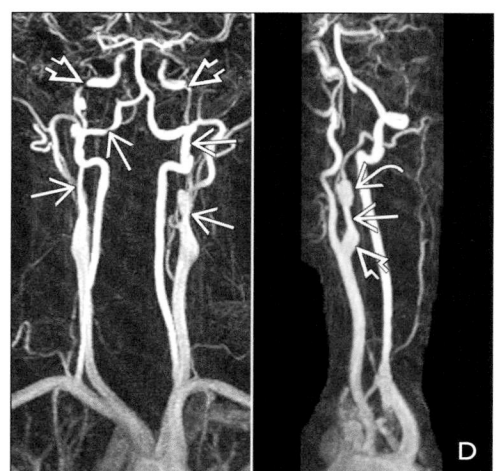

10-42E. *(L) AP and (R) lateral MRAs of right carotid, vertebral arteries show long tapered narrowing of mid-cervical ICA* ➡️*, another pseudoaneurysm* ⮞*. High-grade stenosis of the VA is present between C1 and the skull base* ⮞*.* **10-42F.** *Contrast-enhanced TOF MRA of the intracranial circulation shows stenosis of the ascending right ICA segment* ➡️ *while the left ICA appears occluded* ⮞*. The intracranial vertebral arteries and basilar junction* ⮞ *appear normal.*

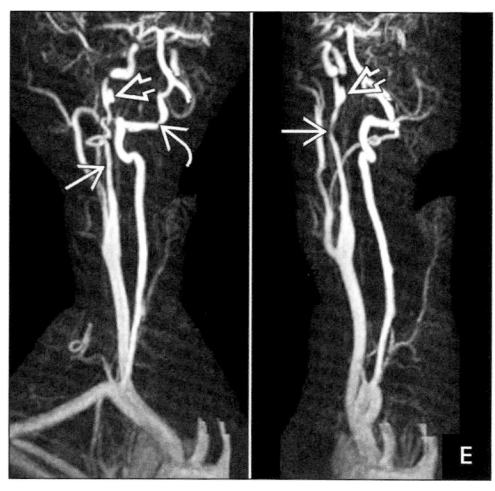

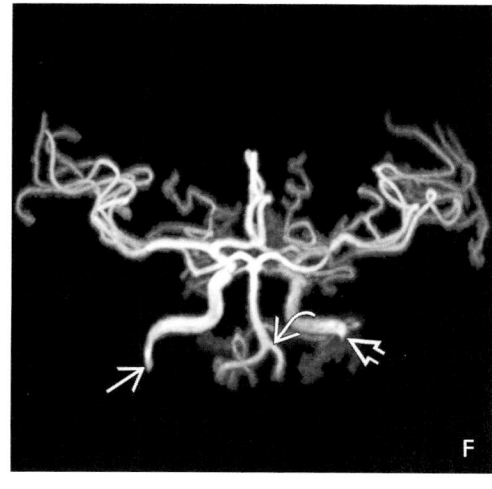

Arterial **thrombosis** without an underlying dissection can cause tapered "rat-tail" narrowing or occlusion. Imaging findings of isolated thrombosis are difficult to distinguish from those of dissection complicated by a secondary superimposed thrombosis.

Vasospasm or reduced distal flow can cause diffuse narrowing of the extracranial vessels. Catheter-induced vasospasm during angiography typically resolves quickly.

Vasospasm and atherosclerosis are the major differential diagnostic considerations for *intracranial* dissections. Both affect multiple vessels in several vascular distributions whereas intracranial CAD almost always is limited to the supraclinoid ICA and proximal MCA.

Vasoconstriction Syndromes

Vasospasm with multifocal intracranial foci of arterial constriction and dilation is a common, well-recognized complication of aneurysmal subarachnoid hemorrhage (aSAH) and is the most common cause of severe vasoconstriction. aSAH-induced vasospasm is discussed in detail in Chapter 6. Vasospasm and vasospasm-like arterial constrictions can occur in the absence of aSAH, trauma, or infection. Two conditions—reversible cerebral vasoconstriction syndrome and postpartum angiopathy—are less well-known cerebral vasoconstriction syndromes that can produce identical imaging findings.

Reversible cerebral vasoconstriction syndrome (RCVS, also known as Call-Fleming syndrome) is associated with nonaneurysmal subarachnoid hemorrhage, pregnancy, and exposure to certain drugs.

The typical patient is a middle-aged woman with recurrent, sudden, severe ("thunderclap") headaches. RCVS often causes convexal subarachnoid hemorrhage and may be complicated by ischemic stroke. The diagnosis requires demonstration of multifocal segmental arterial constrictions that resolve, then recur **(10-45)**. The major differential diagnosis of RCVS is vasospasm related to aSAH and CNS vasculitis.

Postpartum cerebral angiopathy (PPCA) is a rare but important neurological complication of pregnancy.

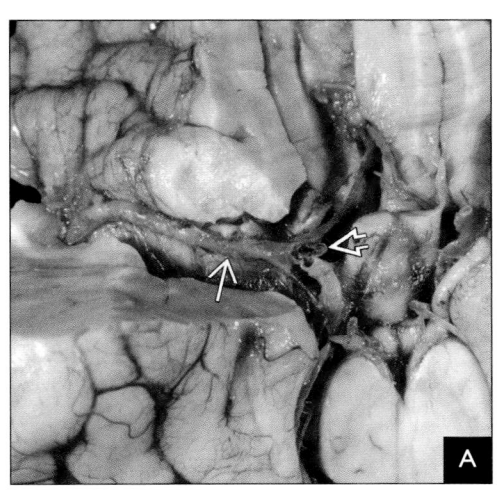

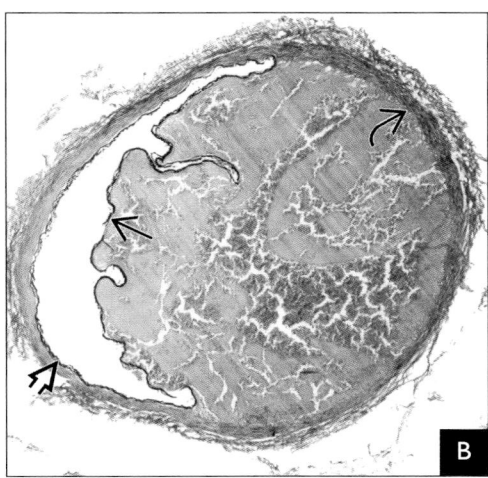

10-43A. Autopsy case shows intracranial dissection extending from the supraclinoid ICA ⊡ into the horizontal (M1) MCA segment ⊡. *10-43B.* Low-power photomicrograph of the MCA seen in cross section shows organizing hematoma between the intima and internal elastic lamina ⊡ and the muscular layer ⊡ of the vessel wall. The lumen ⊡ is patent but severely narrowed. (Courtesy R. Hewlett, MD.)

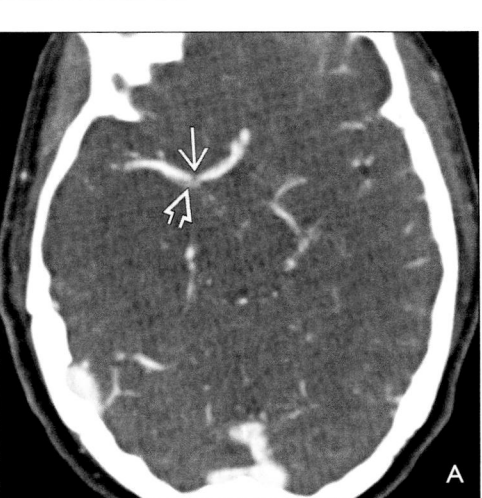

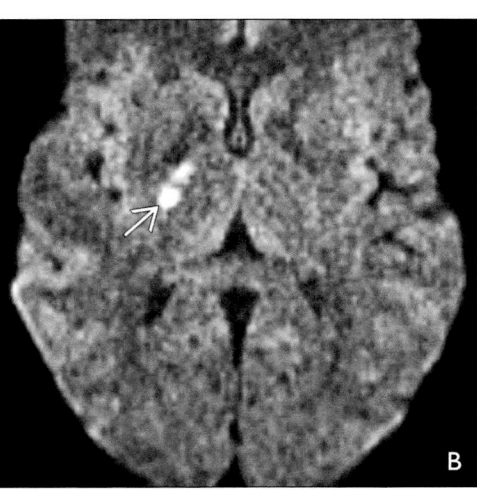

10-44A. CTA in a patient with supraclinoid ICA dissection shows hyperdense clot ⊡ surrounding a very narrow distal ICA ⊡. *10-44B.* DWI in the same patient shows a focal acute infarct in the posterior limb of the right internal capsule ⊡ caused by embolization from the supraclinoid ICA dissection.

Patients often have a history of migraines and generally present with sudden severe ("thunderclap") headache and variable hypertension. Multiple foci of segmental narrowing in the intracranial circulation is the typical finding on imaging studies (10-46). The vasoconstriction generally resolves with time or intraarterial nimodipine. Atypical cases of PPCA may cause frank cerebral infarction.

CEREBRAL VASOCONSTRICTION SYNDROMES

Vasospasm
• Most often secondary to aSAH

Reversible Cerebral Vasoconstriction Syndrome
• Terminology: RCVS or Call-Fleming syndrome
• Middle-aged woman with "thunderclap" headache
• Waxing, waning multifocal segmental narrowings

Postpartum Cerebral Angiopathy
• HTN, headache (may be "thunderclap")
• Multifocal segmental stenoses

Vasculitis and Vasculitides

Terminology

The generic terms "vasculitis" and "angiitis" denote inflammation of blood vessels affecting arteries, veins, or both. The plural "vasculitides" is a more generic term that is often used interchangeably. "Arteritis" is more specific and refers solely to inflammatory processes that involve arteries.

Classification

Classifying vasculitis is difficult and controversial. The two most widely used classifications are the 1990 American College of Rheumatology (ACR) criteria and the 2007 Chapel Hill Consensus Conference (CHCC) criteria.

The ACR identified seven widely accepted types of vasculitis: Giant cell arteritis, Takayasu arteritis, Wegener granulomatosis, Churg-Strauss syndrome, polyarteritis nodosa, Henoch-Schönlein purpura, and hypersensitivity vasculitis. This system was developed prior to the

10-45A. AP vertebral DSA in a 41-year-old woman with "thunderclap" headache shows multiple areas of vasoconstriction ⇨ and dilatation. 10-45B. Repeat vertebral DSA 2 weeks later shows almost complete resolution. Reversible cerebral vasoconstriction syndrome.

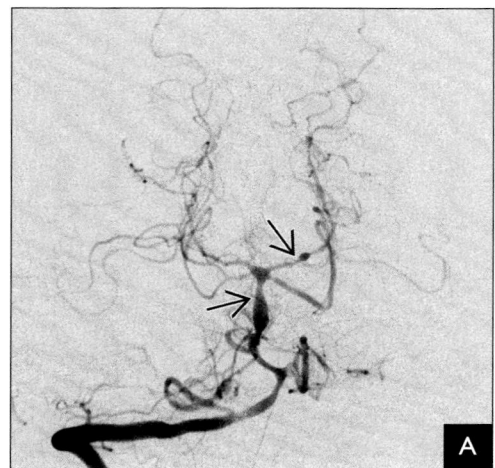

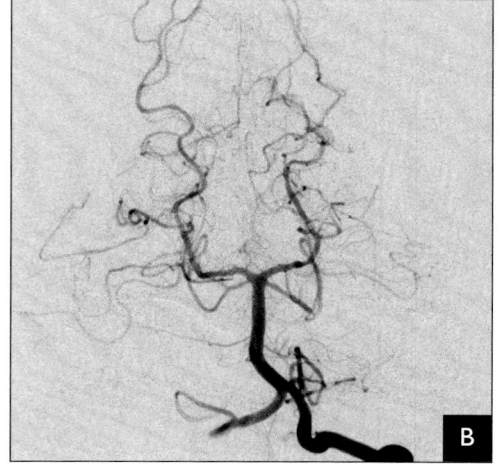

10-46A. Common carotid angiogram, lateral view, in a 28-year-old postpartum woman shows multifocal "beaded" areas of alternating stenoses and dilatations ⇨, characteristic of vasculitis. 10-46B. Vertebral angiogram, AP view, in the same patient shows multiple "beaded" foci ⇨ in the posterior circulation as well. Postpartum angiopathy.

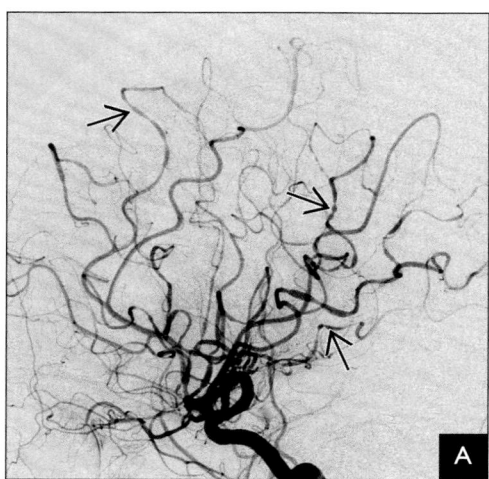

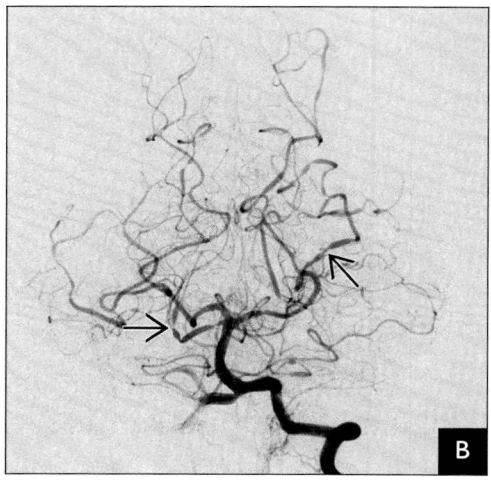

recognition of antineutrophil cytoplasmic autoantibodies (ANCAs), which now play a key role in the differential diagnosis of patients with small vessel vasculitis.

The CHCC further differentiated immune-complex-mediated vasculitides and cryoglobulinemic vasculitis, recognized ANCA-associated vasculitis (AAV), and distinguished microscopic polyangiitis from polyarteritis nodosa (PAN).

Etiology

Vasculitis can be caused by infection, collagen-vascular disease, immune complex deposition, drug abuse, and even neoplasms (e.g., lymphomatoid granulomatosis). The general pathologic features of many vasculitides are quite similar (10-47). As a result, the definitive diagnosis depends primarily on hematologic and immunohistochemical characteristics. Other "surrogate" clinical markers such as glomerulonephritis and granulomatous inflammation of the airways have recently been added to help distinguish among the various vasculitides.

Pathology

While the vasculitides are a heterogeneous group of CNS disorders, they are characterized histopathologically by two cardinal features: Inflammation and necrosis in blood vessel walls (10-48). Infarcts in multiple vascular distributions are common (10-49).

Imaging

As imaging in most vasculitides is similar regardless of etiology, this discussion will focus on the general features of vasculitis as it affects the brain.

CT FINDINGS. NECT scans are relatively insensitive and are often normal. In a few cases, the first imaging manifestation of vasculitis is subarachnoid hemorrhage (especially convexal SAH).

Multifocal hypodensities in the basal ganglia and subcortical white matter that demonstrate patchy enhancement on CECT are common.

MR FINDINGS. Involvement of the cortex/subcortical white matter together with the basal ganglia (BG) is strongly suggestive of vasculitis. T1 scans can be normal or show multifocal cortical/subcortical and BG hypointensities. T2/FLAIR scans demonstrate hyperintensities in the same areas (10-50A). T2* (GRE, SWI) may show parenchymal microhemorrhages and/or SAH in some cases.

Patchy enhancement with punctate and linear lesions is common on T1 C+ scans. Acute lesions with cerebral ischemia show multiple foci of diffusion restriction in

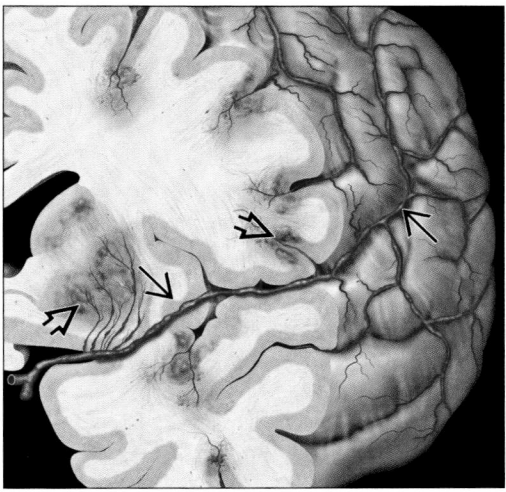

10-47. Graphic shows vasculitis ⇨ with multifocal infarcts, scattered hemorrhages ⊳ in the basal ganglia and at the gray-white matter junction.

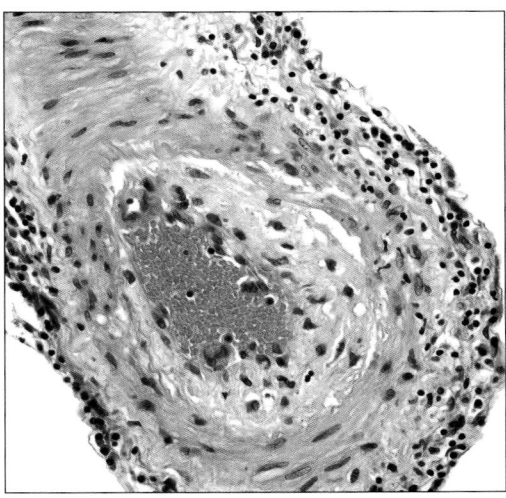

10-48. Photomicrograph shows thick vessel wall with inflammation and necrosis, the cardinal features of vasculitis. (Courtesy R. Hewlett, MD.)

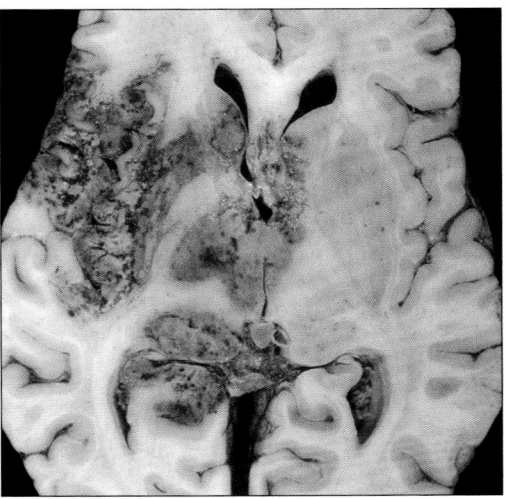

10-49. Autopsy specimen shows vasculitis with multifocal cortical, basal ganglia lesions characterized by necrosis, petechial hemorrhages.

the cortex, subcortical white matter, and basal ganglia **(10-50B)**.

ANGIOGRAPHY. DSA is more sensitive than either CTA or MRA. Findings include multifocal irregularities, stenoses, and vascular occlusions **(10-50C)**. Pseudoaneurysm formation and branch occlusions occur but are less common. Although the circle of Willis and horizontal segments of the ACA, MCA, and PCA can be affected, the distal branches of these vessels are most frequently involved **(10-50D)**.

Differential Diagnosis

The major differential diagnosis of vasculitis is **atherosclerotic vascular disease** (ASVD). ASVD typically occurs in older patients and involves larger intracranial arteries (e.g., the carotid siphon, vertebral and basilar arteries). However, ASVD can affect second- and third-order branches and thus mimic vasculitis.

Vasospasm can also mimic vasculitis. However, vasospasm most commonly affects the major cerebral vessels. A history of trauma or subarachnoid hemorrhage is common but not invariably present. **Reversible cerebral vasoconstriction syndrome** and **postpartum angiopathy** can be indistinguishable from vasculitis.

Other Macro- and Microvasculopathies

A broad spectrum of both inherited and acquired noninflammatory, nonatherosclerotic diseases can involve the intracranial vasculature. In this section, we briefly review a few of the more important miscellaneous vasculopathies that affect both large and small cerebral vessels.

Sickle Cell Disease

Sickle cell disease (SCD) is one of the best characterized human monogenic disorders and the most common worldwide cause of childhood stroke. African-American and African-Brazilian children are among the most affected children outside of continental Africa.

ETIOLOGY AND PATHOLOGY. SCD is an inherited, autosomal recessive chronic hemolytic anemia caused by a point mutation in the β-globin gene cluster. The forma-

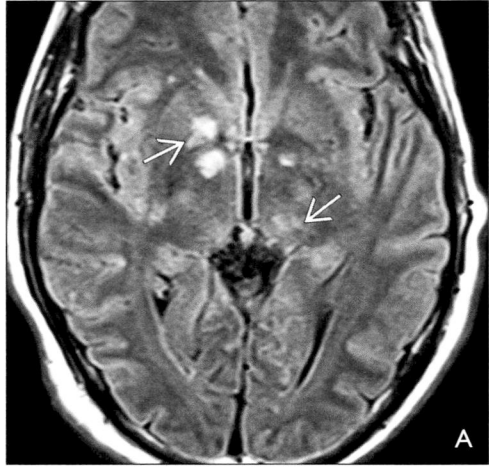
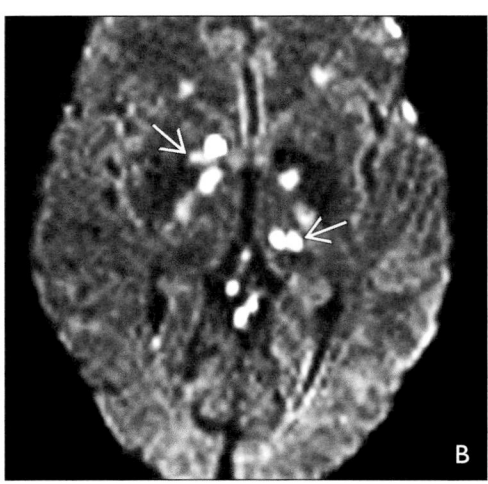

10-50A. Axial FLAIR scan in a patient with a history of recent streptococcal meningitis shows several hyperintense foci in the basal ganglia and thalami ➡. 10-50B. DWI in the same patient shows multiple foci of restricted diffusion ➡ in the basal ganglia. Other images (not shown) demonstrated peripheral lesions in the cortex and subcortical white matter. Findings suggest infarcts secondary to meningitic vasculitis.

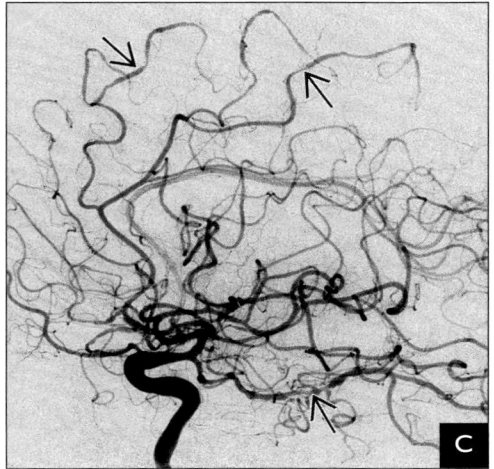
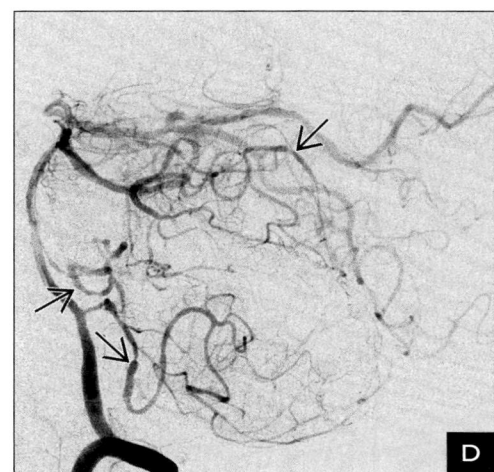

10-50C. Right internal carotid artery angiogram, lateral view, arterial phase, shows multifocal segmental areas of arterial narrowing and dilatation ➡, classic findings of vasculitis. 10-50D. Vertebral angiogram in the same patient shows additional foci of segmental constrictions alternating with dilatations ➡.

tion of Hgb S induces a change in shape ("sickling") and rigidity of red blood cells, which then stagnate in and damage the endothelium of small vessels. Progressive fibrosis, narrowing, and eventually occlusion result. The brain microvasculature assumes an inflammatory, procoagulant state that probably contributes to the high incidence of ischemic stroke in patients with SCD.

CLINICAL ISSUES. The most common CNS complication of SCD is stroke. Other neurologic manifestations of SCD include decreased cognitive function ("silent stroke") and headache. Most patients experience repeated ischemic events with worsening motor and intellectual deficits.

Approximately 75% of SCD-related strokes are ischemic, and 25% are hemorrhagic. Stroke risk is highest between the ages of two and five years.

IMAGING. A diffusely thickened calvaria with expanded diploic space secondary to increased hematopoiesis is a frequent finding, as is reconversion of "yellow" to "red" (hematopoietic) marrow **(10-51A)**.

Generalized volume loss with sulcal and ventricular enlargement together with multiple hypodensities in the cortex and cerebral white matter is common on NECT scans. CECT scans may show punctate enhancing foci in the basal ganglia (BG) and deep white matter from enlarged "moyamoya" type collaterals.

MR scans often demonstrate subcortical and white matter hyperintensities along the deep watershed zone on T2/FLAIR **(10-51B)**. A moyamoya-like pattern with supraclinoid ICA stenosis may develop with especially severe SCD **(10-52)**. In such cases, an "ivy" sign with serpentine hyperintensities in the cerebral sulci from leptomeningeal collaterals can be seen on FLAIR.

Moyamoya Disease

TERMINOLOGY. Moyamoya disease (MMD) is an idiopathic progressive arteriopathy characterized by stenosis of the distal (supraclinoid) ICAs and formation of an abnormal vascular network at the base of the brain **(10-53)**. Multiple enlarged "telangiectatic" lenticulostriate, thalamoperforating, leptomeningeal, dural, and pial arteries develop as compensatory circulation. These "moyamoya

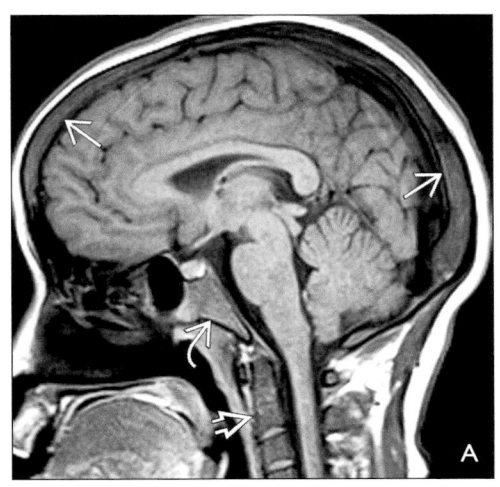
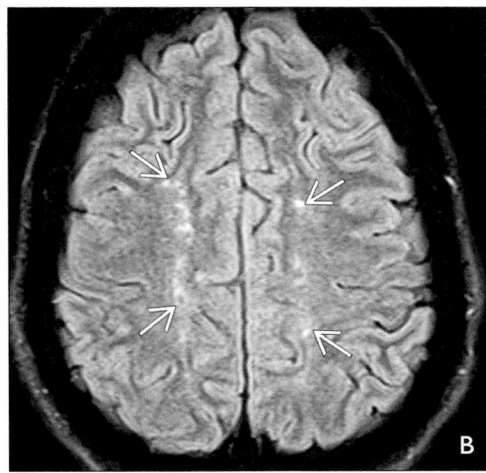

10-51A. Sagittal T1WI in a 29-year-old woman with sickle cell disease (SCD) shows thick calvaria with hypointense hematopoietic marrow ➡. The clivus ➡ and cervical vertebral bodies ➡ are also hypointense. The intervertebral discs appear "brighter" than the vertebral bodies. 10-51B. FLAIR scan in the same patient shows punctate hyperintensities in both watershed zones ➡, a common finding in SCD.

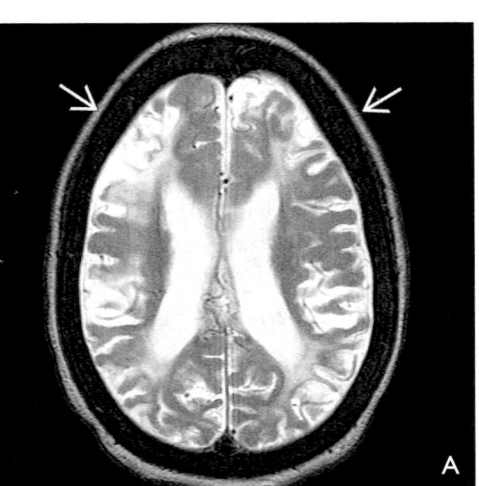
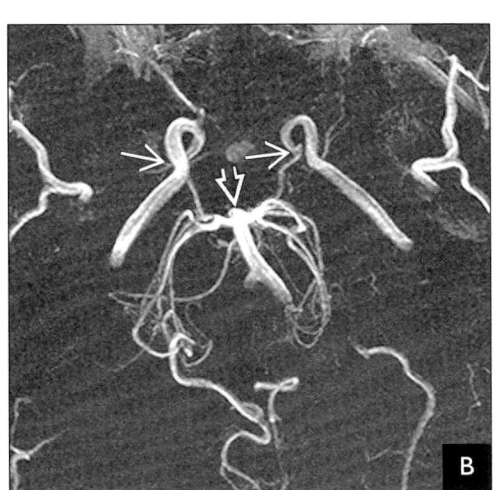

10-52A. Axial T2WI in an 11-year-old child with sickle cell disease shows markedly thickened calvaria with hypointense marrow ➡, atrophy with multiple cortical and deep WM infarcts. 10-52B. Submentovertex MIP of the MRA in the same patient shows occlusion of both supraclinoid ICAs ➡. The vertebrobasilar circulation ➡ appears relatively normal.

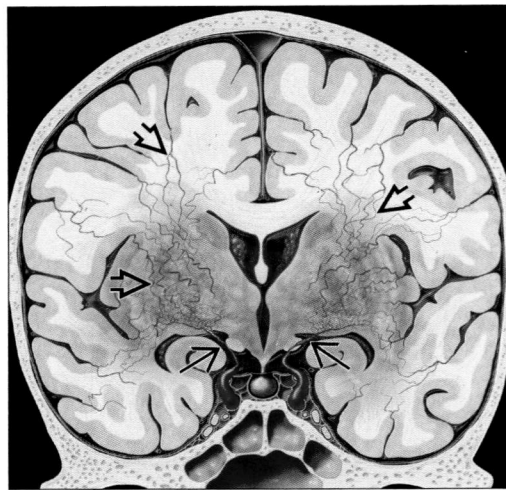

10-53. Graphic of MMD shows severely narrowed supraclinoid ICAs ⟶, striking "puff of smoke" from extensive basal ganglia, WM collaterals ▷.

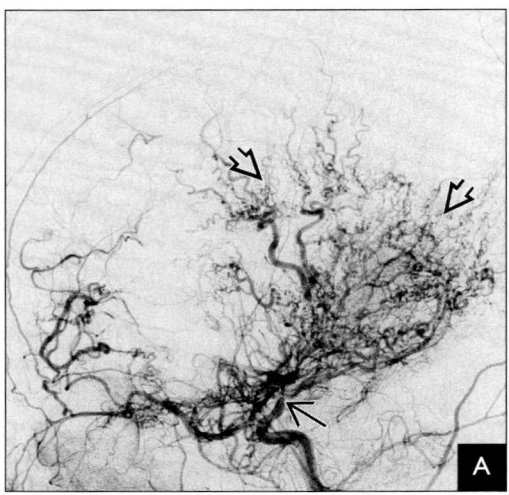

10-54A. MMD in a 3-year-old shows near-total supraclinoid ICA stenosis ⟶ with innumerable tortuous enlarged moyamoya-like collaterals ▷.

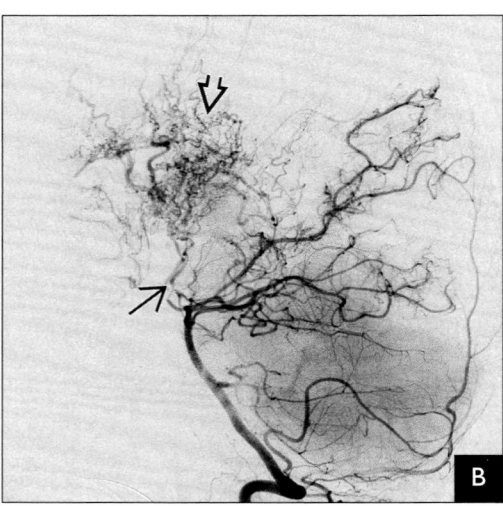

10-54B. Vertebral angiogram in the same patient shows moyamoya-like collaterals ▷ from enlarged thalamoperforating arteries ⟶.

collaterals" can become so extensive that they resemble the "puff of smoke" from a cigarette, the Japanese term for which the disease is named **(10-54)**.

ETIOLOGY. The pathophysiology of MMD has been extensively investigated but remains poorly understood. Genetic, acquired, and environmental factors have all been implicated. Aberrant expression of IgG and S100 A4 proteins in the walls of MMD vessels has been demonstrated, but its significance is uncertain.

Approximately 5-10% of Asian MMD cases are familial. The disease is also associated with several genetically transmitted disorders including neurofibromatosis type 1, trisomy 21 (Down syndrome), and a spectrum of hemoglobinopathies such as sickle cell anemia. Collagen vascular diseases including Marfan and Ehlers-Danlos syndromes have also been associated with MMD.

Moyamoya-*like* collateral vessels can develop with any slowly progressive arteriopathy that affects the major intracranial arteries. When this pattern occurs with a known disease association, it is sometimes termed "pseudo-moyamoya" to distinguish it from "true" (i.e., idiopathic) MMD.

PATHOLOGY. The pathologic changes of MMD are very different from those of ASVD and vasculitis. The terminal ICAs show severe stenosis with concentric and eccentric fibrocellular intimal thickening without significant inflammatory cell infiltration. Subintimal lipid deposition, hemorrhage, and necrosis are absent. The internal elastic lamina is typically tortuous and stratified.

CLINICAL ISSUES. MMD is most prevalent in Japan and Korea, where its estimated incidence is 0.35-0.54 per 100,000 people. MMD is increasingly diagnosed worldwide, but its incidence in Europeans is estimated at one-tenth that of Japanese population.

Moyamoya has two peak ages of presentation. Two-thirds of cases occur in children, and at least half of these occur under the age of 10 years. Between one-quarter and one-third present in adults with peak presentation in the fifth decade.

The clinical features of MMD in children differ from those in adults. When MMD presents in childhood, the initial symptoms are usually ischemic. In adults, approximately half of all patients develop intracranial hemorrhage from rupture of the fragile moyamoya collateral vessels. The other 50% present with TIAs or cerebral infarcts.

MMD is relentlessly progressive, and long-term outcome is generally poor. Even relatively "asymptomatic" patients commonly have cognitive disturbances and silent ischemic infarcts. Cerebral revascularization surgery, primarily encephalo-duro-arterio-synangiosis in children and superficial temporal artery-MCA bypass in adults, has been performed with some success.

IMAGING. Multiple enhancing punctate "dots" (CECT) or "flow voids" (MR) in the basal ganglia are the most striking findings in MMD. T1 and T2 scans show markedly narrowed supraclinoid ICAs with multiple tortuous, serpentine "flow voids" **(10-55A)**, **(10-55B)**. The appearance of multiple tiny collateral vessels in enlarged CSF spaces has been likened to "swimming worms in a bare cistern."

An "ivy" sign with sulcal hyperintensity from slow flow in leptomeningeal collaterals is sometimes seen on FLAIR and correlates with decreased vascular reserve in the affected hemisphere.

Multiple microbleeds can be detected on T2* GRE scans in 15-40% of patients and are associated with increased risk of overt cerebral hemorrhage. Susceptibility-weighted imaging (SWI) shows increased conspicuity of deep medullary veins, an appearance dubbed the "brush" sign.

T1 C+ scans often show contrast stagnating in slow-flowing collateral vessels both in the brain parenchymal and over its surface **(10-55C)**.

Diffusion tensor imaging (DTI) demonstrates loss of microstructural integrity in normal-appearing white matter, seen as lowered FA and elevated ADC. pMR may demonstrate chronic cerebral hypoperfusion in the internal carotid artery territories, seen as increased rCBV secondary to compensatory vasodilatation and delayed TTP due to proximal vessel stenosis.

DSA, CTA, and MRA show predominantly anterior circulation disease with marked narrowing of both supraclinoid ICAs ("bottle neck" sign). The PCAs are less commonly involved. Prominent deep-seated lenticulostriate and thalamoperforator collaterals are present, forming the "puff of smoke" appearance characteristic of moyamoya. Numerous transosseous and transdural collaterals from the extracranial to intracranial circulation may develop.

DIFFERENTIAL DIAGNOSIS. The differential diagnosis of idiopathic ("true") moyamoya disease includes other slowly developing occlusive vasculopathies. **Radiation therapy, neurofibromatosis type 1 (NF1), trisomy 21, sickle cell disease,** and even **atherosclerosis** may develop multiple small moyamoya-like collateral vessels.

Classic moyamoya typically affects *both* supraclinoid ICAs while sparing the posterior circulation. A unilateral **"aplastic"** or **twig-like M1 MCA** is a rare nonprogressive congenital anomaly that should be differentiated from MMD. Degenerative stenoocclusive disease with **"segmental" high-grade stenosis** or occlusion of the M1 MCA with a network of small vessels bridging the gap

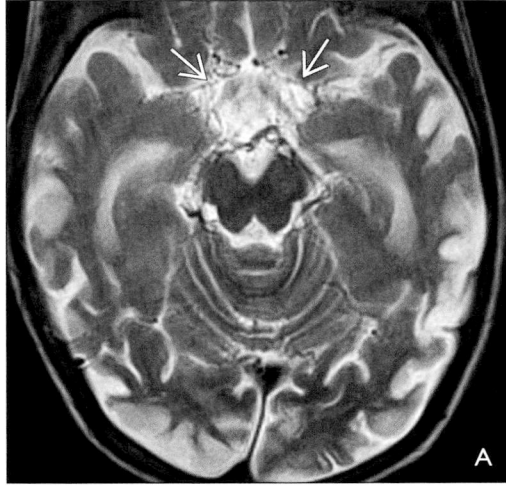

10-55A. T2WI shows severely attenuated, almost thread-like supraclinoid ICAs, MCAs ➡ with marked cortical atrophy, enlarged temporal horns.

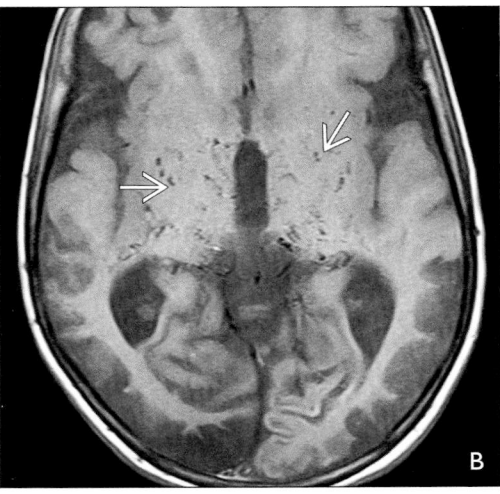

10-55B. T1WI in the same patient shows multiple "flow voids" from enlarged moyamoya collaterals in the basal ganglia, thalami ➡.

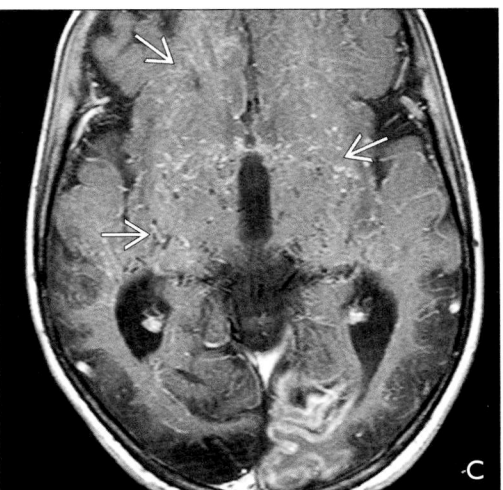

10-55C. T1 C+ shows "puff of smoke" (punctate/ serpentine enhancing vessels in basal ganglia, thalami, deep WM ➡). (Courtesy H. Els, MD.)

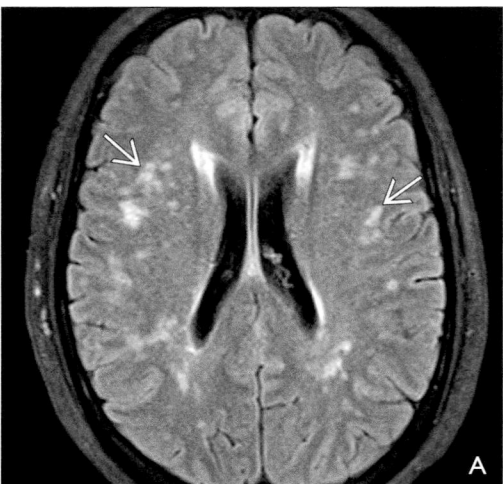

10-56A. Axial FLAIR scan in a 48 yo man with multiple stroke-like episodes shows multifocal subcortical and deep WM hyperintensities ➡.

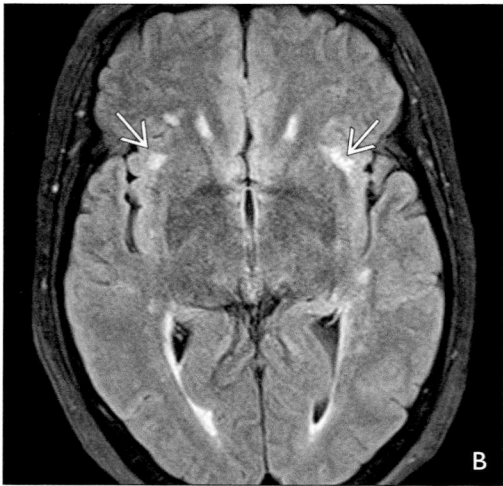

10-56B. FLAIR scan through the basal ganglia shows external capsule lesions ➡, *highly suggestive of CADASIL.*

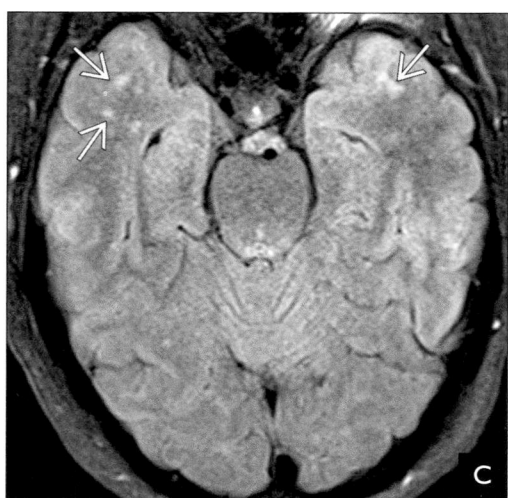

10-56C. FLAIR scan in the same patient shows anterior temporal lobe WM hyperintensities ➡. *NOTCH3 mutation confirmed CADASIL.*

between the horizontal and distal segments should also be differentiated from MMD.

MOYAMOYA DISEASE

Terminology
- Moyamoya = "puff of smoke"

Etiology, Epidemiology
- Progressive arteriopathy → stenosis supraclinoid ICAs
- Idiopathic or associated with NF1, sickle cell disease, etc.

Pathology
- Fibrocellular intimal thickening
- No inflammation, hemorrhage, lipid deposition

Clinical Issues
- Worldwide distribution, most common in Japan
- Children (70%, usually < 10 years)
  - TIAs, stroke
- Adults (30%)
  - Hemorrhage > stroke
- Relentless course
- Revascularization (encephalo-duro-arterial-synangiosis, extracranial-intracranial bypass)

Imaging
- Stenosis/occlusion of supraclinoid ICAs
- Innumerable basal collaterals
- Atrophy
- Strokes (chronic, acute)
- Hemorrhage
  - Parenchymal
  - Subarachnoid

Moyamoya-like Vascular Collaterals
- Moyamoya disease
- Radiation therapy
- Neurofibromatosis type 1 (NF1)
- Trisomy 21
- Sickle cell disease
- Slowly progressive ASVD

CADASIL

CADASIL is the acronym for **c**erebral **a**utosomal **d**ominant **a**rteriopathy with **s**ubcortical **i**nfarcts and **l**eukoencephalopathy. CADASIL is an autosomal dominant disease of the cerebral microvasculature that primarily affects smooth muscle cells in penetrating cerebral and leptomeningeal arteries.

ETIOLOGY AND PATHOLOGY. CADASIL is caused by highly stereotyped missense point mutations in the *NOTCH3* gene. Fourteen distinct familial forms of CADASIL have been identified with mutations in different *NOTCH3* exons. These mutations all cause an odd number of cysteine residues within an epidermal growth factor (EGF) repeat in the extracellular domain of *NOTCH3*.

The pathologic hallmark of CADASIL is accumulation of granular osmiophilic material in the basement membranes of small arteries and arterioles that causes severe fibrotic thickening and stenosis. Long penetrating cerebral arteries and their branches are especially affected. At autopsy, mild to moderate diffuse cerebral atrophy with multiple lacunar infarcts in the periventricular white matter, basal ganglia, thalamus, midbrain, and pons is present.

CLINICAL ISSUES. Although symptoms are restricted to the CNS, arterial changes of CADASIL are systemic. While its exact prevalence is unknown, CADASIL has been identified as the most common monogenic heritable cause of stroke and vascular dementia in adults. At initial presentation, only 35% of patients have a first-degree relative with known CADASIL.

The classic clinical presentation involves a young to middle-aged adult without identifiable vascular risk factors. The main clinical manifestations are recurrent ischemic strokes (60-85%), migraine headache (which occurs in 25-75% of cases and is often the earliest manifestation of the disease), psychiatric disturbances (20-40%), and progressive cognitive impairment (20-40%). Although symptom onset is generally in the third decade, CADASIL can present in children.

Between 5-10% of CADASIL patients develop epileptic seizures, typically late in the disease course. A small number of patients present with an acute reversible encephalopathy syndrome with fever, confusion, coma, and seizure lasting several days.

CADASIL generally follows a progressive course, causing disability and dementia in 75% of cases. CADASIL patients who have a high lesion burden on baseline MR studies are at high risk for more rapid disease progression.

IMAGING. Imaging is important in raising the possible diagnosis of CADASIL, as characteristic patterns may precede overt symptoms by more than a decade. The typical findings are multiple lacunar infarcts in the basal ganglia and high signal intensity lesions in the subcortical and periventricular white matter (WM).

NECT scans can be normal early in the disease course or show hypodense foci in the affected regions.

Bilateral, multifocal T2 and FLAIR hyperintensities in the periventricular and deep WM begin to appear by age 20. Although these findings are nonspecific, involvement of the **anterior temporal lobe** and **external capsule** has high sensitivity and specificity in differentiating CADASIL from the much more common sporadic cerebral small vessel disease (primarily arteriolosclerosis and lipohyalinosis) **(10-56)**. DTI can demonstrate ultrastructural tissue damage with reduced FA even in "normal-appearing" WM.

Lacunar infarcts in the subcortical WM, basal ganglia, thalamus, internal capsule, and brainstem are found in

75% of patients between 30-40 years of age and increase in both number and prominence with age. Mild to moderate generalized cerebral atrophy is a relatively late finding and is independently associated with the extent of cognitive decline.

Cerebral microbleeds (CMBs) are found on T2* scans in 25% of patients between 40-50 years old and are seen in nearly 50% of patients over 50. CMBs can be either the initial neurologic manifestation or a development when patients take antiplatelet agents.

DIFFERENTIAL DIAGNOSIS. The clinical diagnosis of CADASIL is often elusive, with at least one-third of all patients initially misdiagnosed with MS, dementia, or CNS vasculitis. Using electron microscopy to detect granular osmiophilic deposits in skin biopsy specimens is highly reliable, and immunostaining for NOTCH3 ECS increases both sensitivity and specificity to over 90%.

The imaging differential diagnosis of CADASIL includes sporadic subcortical arteriosclerotic encephalopathy, mitochondrial encephalomyopathy with lactic acidosis and stroke-like episodes (MELAS), vasculitis, and antiphospholipid syndromes. **Subcortical arteriosclerotic encephalopathy (SAE)** is a hypertension-associated disorder that causes WM disease and lacunar infarcts. Unlike CADASIL, the lesions generally do not involve the anterior temporal WM.

MELAS typically shows cortical and subcortical lesions and may present acutely as hyperintense gyral swelling on T2/FLAIR that resolves with clinical recovery. **Antiphospholipid syndromes** and **protein S deficiency** can both present in young and middle-aged adults. Cortical and lacunar infarcts, vasculitis-like findings on DSA, dural sinus thromboses, and WM hyperintensities on T2/FLAIR are common.

Other hereditary small vessel diseases of the cerebral vasculature can mimic CADASIL. A second known single-gene disorder that directly affects cerebral small vessels is termed **CARASIL** (**c**erebral **a**utosomal **r**ecessive **a**rteriopathy with **s**ubcortical **i**nfarcts and **l**eukoencephalopathy). Most CARASIL cases have been reported in Japanese patients.

Hereditary systemic angiopathy (HSA) is a systemic microvasculopathy associated with cerebral calcifications, retinopathy, progressive nephropathy, and hepatopathy. Other small vessel disorders—hereditary endotheliopathy, retinopathy, nephropathy, and stroke (HERNS), hereditary vascular retinopathy (HVR), and cerebroretinal vasculopathy (CRV)—may simply represent different phenotypes of the same oculocerebral disease.

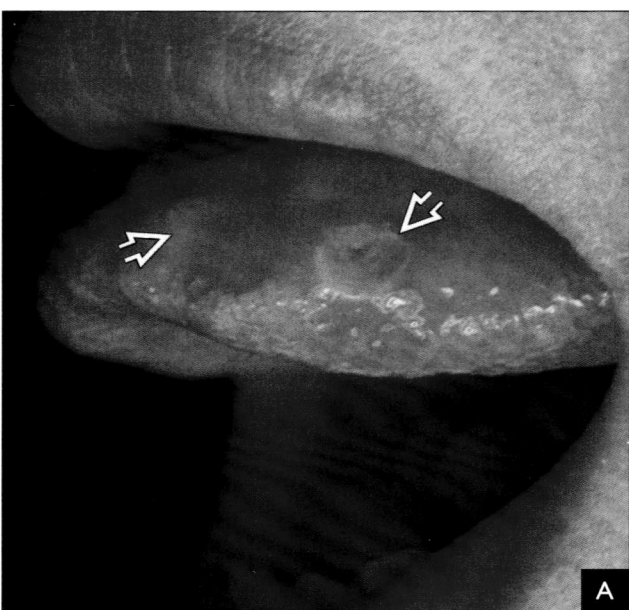

10-57A. Clinical photograph of a patient with Behçet disease shows the classic oral ulcers ➲ *involving the tongue and oral mucosa.*

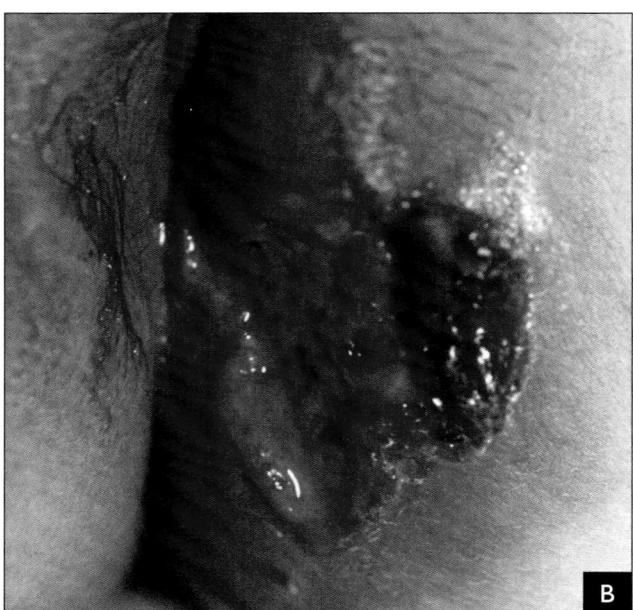

10-57B. Clinical photograph of the same patient shows aphthous genital ulcers. (Courtesy E. T. Tali, MD.)

Behçet Disease

Behçet disease (BD) is a chronic, idiopathic, relapsing-remitting, multisystem, inflammatory vascular disease that is characterized mainly by skin lesions. The CNS is involved in 20-25% of patients. When BD occurs in the CNS, it is termed neuro-Behçet disease (NBD).

ETIOLOGY AND PATHOLOGY. CNS involvement in NBD is divided into parenchymal and nonparenchymal lesions. Parenchymal NBD is mainly a meningoencephalitis, with lesions in the brainstem, hemispheres, spinal cord, or meningoencephalitic lesions.

Nonparenchymal manifestations of NBD include dural sinus thrombosis, arterial occlusion, and/or aneurysms. Dural sinus and cortical vein thrombosis with intracranial hypertension is found in 10-35% of patients. Occlusion and pseudoaneurysm formation involving the intra- and extracranial arteries has been reported in NBD but is rare compared to venous disease.

Typical histologic findings of NBD are perivascular necrosis with mild inflammatory infiltrates and oligodendroglial degeneration.

CLINICAL ISSUES. While BD is most common in the Mediterranean region, the Middle East, and East Asia (especially Japan), it has a worldwide distribution. NBD typically affects young adults and has a moderate male predominance.

The major clinical features of BD are mucocutaneous recurrent oral and genital ulcers, aphthous stomatitis,

ophthalmologic lesions such as uveitis and iridocyclitis, and multiple arthralgias (10-57). Parenchymal NBD typically presents with pyramidal symptoms while nonparenchymal disease usually causes elevated intracranial pressure secondary to dural sinus occlusion.

The clinical course of BD is typically chronic and may span up to a decade, although fulminant disease with rapid clinical deterioration has been reported. Neurologic involvement usually occurs months to years following systemic disease but is the initial presentation in 5% of patients. Overall mortality of NBD is low (5%).

IMAGING. Although any part of the CNS can be affected, brainstem involvement—especially of the cerebral peduncles—is typical and occurs in 50% of cases (10-58). The thalamus and basal ganglia are the second most common sites of involvement, followed by the cerebral hemispheric white matter. Between 10-50% of NBD cases demonstrate focal lesions in the spinal cord.

Typical MR findings are small circular, linear, crescent-shaped, or irregular foci of T2/FLAIR hyperintensity in the midbrain. Mass effect is usually minimal, but during the acute phase, large brainstem and/or basal ganglia lesions can exhibit significant mass effect, extending into the diencephalon and mimicking neoplasm.

Mild to moderate patchy enhancement following contrast administration is common; strong, uniform enhancement is rare.

DIFFERENTIAL DIAGNOSIS. The major differential diagnosis of BD includes **multiple sclerosis**, **sarcoidosis**,

neoplasm, and **systemic inflammatory disease**. Oligoclonal bands are absent in the CSF and the myelin basic protein is typically normal, helping distinguish BD from MS. Skin lesions are generally absent in sarcoid while serum ACE levels are usually (but not invariably) elevated.

Widespread brainstem involvement extending into the cerebral peduncles, thalami, basal ganglia, and periventricular WM has been reported and can mimic gliomatosis cerebri or lymphoma. Biopsy may be required to distinguish BD from neoplasm.

Systemic inflammatory diseases such as **systemic lupus erythematosus**, **antiphospholipid syndrome**, and **Sjögren disease** can resemble BD when they involve the CNS. Skin lesions are common in these disorders, but the oral and genital aphthous ulcers seen in BD are absent.

Sweet syndrome, also known as acute febrile neutrophilic dermatosis, is a multisystem inflammatory disorder that often manifests as a vasculitis presenting with painful erythematous skin plaques, fever, and leukocytosis. Neuro-Sweet and NBD can appear identical on MR imaging, with T2/FLAIR hyperintensities in the brainstem and basal ganglia. The CNS involvement in neuro-Sweet is usually transient, mimicking a relapsing and remitting encephalitis, whereas NBD usually follows a much more chronic, slowly progressive course.

Systemic Lupus Erythematosus

TERMINOLOGY. Systemic lupus erythematosus (SLE or "lupus") is a multisystem complex autoimmune disorder that affects the respiratory, cardiovascular, gastrointestinal, genitourinary, and musculoskeletal systems, as well as the CNS. Most diagnoses of lupus are established on the basis of systemic findings and laboratory abnormalities with imaging playing an important but ancillary role in diagnosis and management.

When overt CNS symptoms are present, the disorder is termed CNS lupus (CNS SLE) or neuropsychiatric systemic lupus erythematosus (NPSLE).

ETIOLOGY. SLE is an autoimmune disorder characterized by immune complex deposition, vasculitis, and vasculopathy. Multiple components of the immune system are affected, including the complement system, T sup-

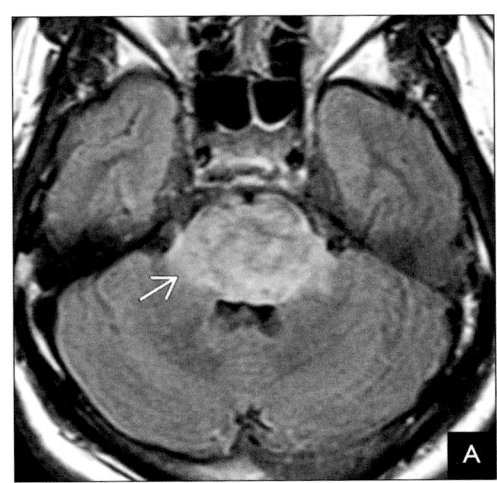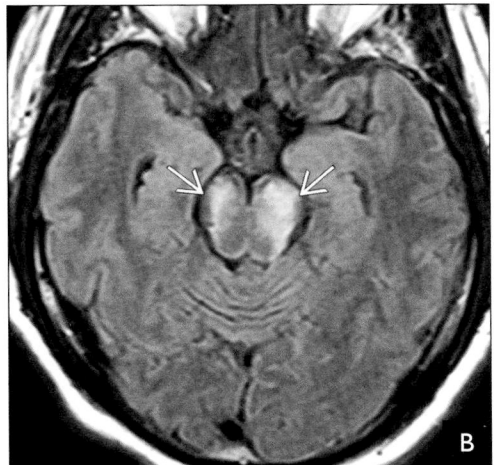

10-58A. Axial FLAIR scan in a 30-year-old man with fever, oral ulcers, and bilateral upper extremity weakness shows a heterogeneously hyperintense mass in the pons ➡. 10-58B. The lesions extend cephalad into both cerebral peduncles ➡, which also appear enlarged. Additional lesions were present in the basal ganglia (not shown).

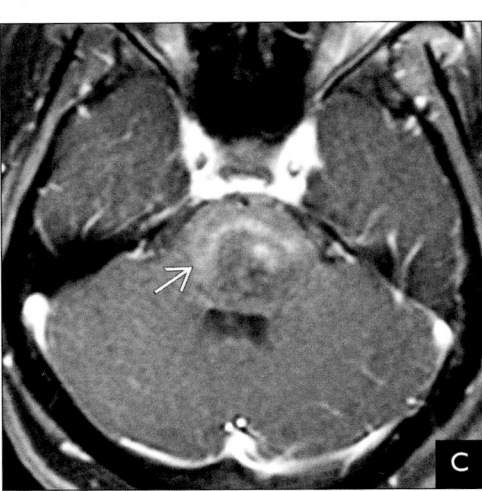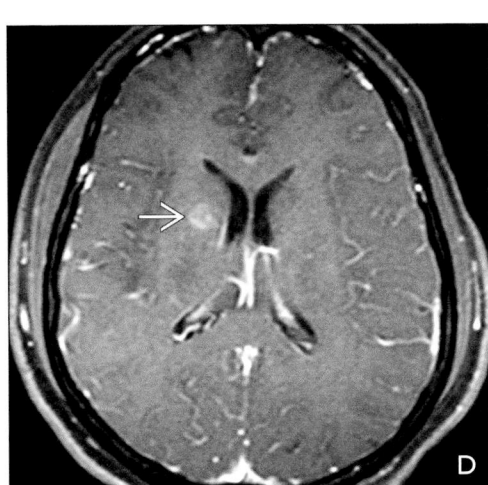

10-58C. Axial T1 C+ FS scan in the same patient shows that the pontine mass ➡ enhances moderately but heterogeneously. 10-58D. T1 C+ FS scan shows a ring-enhancing lesion in the right caudate nucleus and anterior limb of the internal capsule ➡. Biopsy-proven Behçet disease.

pressor cells, and cytokine products. Circulating autoantibodies may be produced for many years before overt clinical SLE symptoms emerge.

Activation of the complement system, together with formation and deposition of immune complexes in tissues, recruits B lymphocytes, resulting in formation of autoantibodies. Normal immune suppression fails, resulting in an unchecked autoimmune response. Immune system dysfunction also results in frequent infections and increased prevalence of lymphoreticular malignancy.

CNS lupus is generally considered an angiopathic disease, although neural autoimmune damage, demyelination, and thromboembolism may be contributing factors. Lupus-related cerebral ischemia/infarction can result from coagulopathy (secondary to antiphospholipid syndrome), accelerated atherosclerosis (often associated with corticosteroid treatment), thromboembolism (secondary to Libman-Sacks endocarditis), or a true primary lupus vasculitis.

PATHOLOGY. The most frequent gross findings in patients with NPSLE are generalized volume loss with cortical atrophy and enlarged ventricles. Focal atrophy, cerebral infarcts, and hemorrhage are also common.

Lupus angiitis/vasculitis is characterized histopathologically by marked endothelial hyperplasia and obliterative intimal fibrosis in small arteries and arterioles. Occlusive fibrin thrombi without histologic evidence of vasculitis can also occur.

CLINICAL ISSUES. SLE affects one out of every 700 white females and one out of every 245 black females. CNS SLE occurs at all ages, with peak onset between the second and fourth decades. In adults, over 90% of patients are females. In children, the F:M ratio is 2-3:1.

Lupus onset can be insidious, and early clinical diagnosis can be elusive. Diagnostic criteria for SLE have been established by the American College of Rheumatology and include malar or discoid rash, oral and/or nasal ulcers, arthritis, serositis, renal disease, and vasculitis.

CNS lupus occurs in 30-40% of cases and can be a serious, potentially life-threatening manifestation of SLE. Indeed, CNS lupus accounts for 15-20% of lupus-related deaths.

10-59A. Axial FLAIR scan in a 33-year-old woman with acute exacerbation of her CNS lupus shows confluent hyperintensity expanding the medulla ➡. 10-59B. FLAIR scan through the vertex in the same patient shows patchy cortical and subcortical hyperintensities in the left frontal and parietal lobes ➡. Mild mass effect with sulcal effacement ➡ is present. The right hemisphere appears normal.

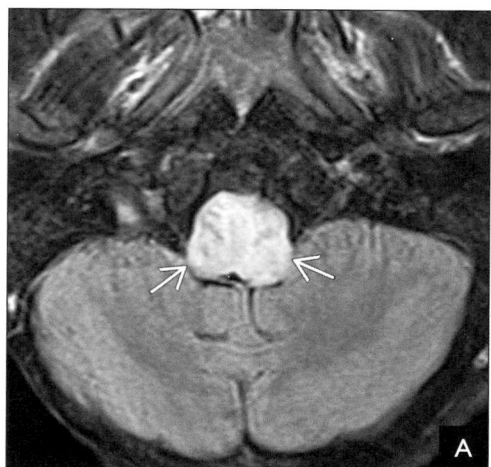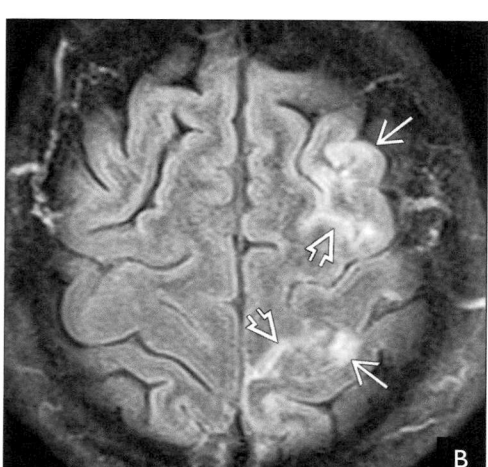

10-59C. T1 C+ FS scan in the same patient shows mild patchy enhancement in the cortex and subcortical WM of the left hemisphere ➡. 10-59D. DWI shows foci of restricted diffusion in the right frontal cortex ➡.

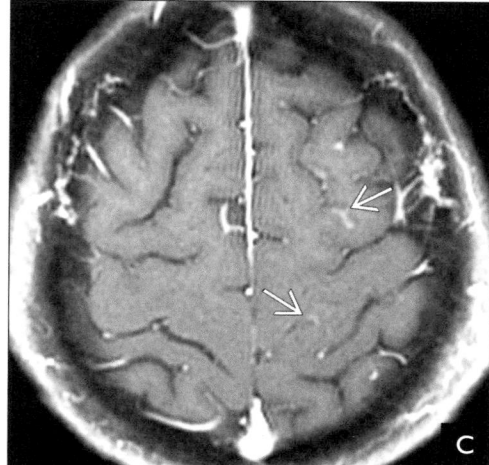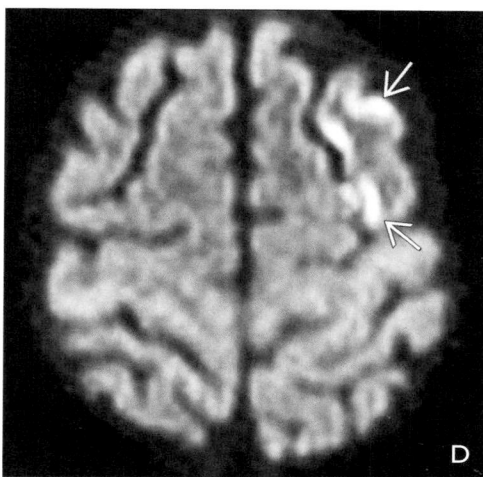

IMAGING. Imaging abnormalities occur in 25-75% of NPSLE patients and are associated with disease severity/activity, increasing age, and documented neurologic events.

Initial NECT scans are often normal or show scattered patchy cortical/subcortical hypodensities. Large territorial infarcts and dural sinus occlusions occur but are less common. Spontaneous intracranial hemorrhages can occur in SLE patients with uremia, thrombocytopenia, and hypertension.

MR findings vary from normal to striking. The most common finding, seen in 25-50% of newly diagnosed NPSLE patients, is that of multiple small subcortical and deep WM hyperintensities on T2/FLAIR **(10-59)**. Large confluent lesions that resemble acute disseminated encephalomyelitis (ADEM) occur but are generally seen only in patients with CNS symptoms **(10-60)**. Diffuse cortical, basal ganglia, and brainstem lesions—suggestive of vasculopathy or vasculitis—are also common.

Acute lesions demonstrate transient enhancement on T1 C+ studies and restricted diffusion. pMR in patients with NPSLE shows elevated CBV and CBF.

Dural venous sinus and cortical/deep venous thrombosis occur in 20-30% of NPSLE cases. Systemic hypertension is common in SLE patients. Posterior reversible encephalopathy syndrome (PRES) is a rare but treatable manifestation of CNS lupus.

DIFFERENTIAL DIAGNOSIS. The imaging differential diagnosis of NPSLE is broad and includes **arteriolosclerosis** ("small vessel disease"), **multiple sclerosis**, **Susac syndrome**, non-lupus **antiphospholipid syndromes**, **Lyme disease**, and **other vasculitides** such as primary angiitis of the CNS.

There is a significant overlap of lupus with antiphospholipid syndrome (APS): Between 25-40% of SLE patients have APS (see below). While there are no universally accepted diagnostic imaging criteria for NPSLE, the presence of multifocal infarcts and "migratory" edematous areas is suggestive of the disease.

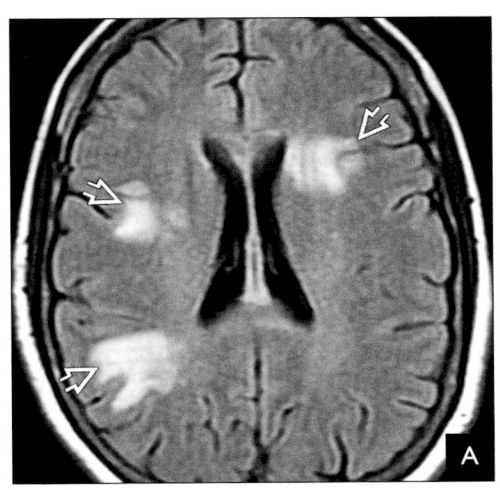

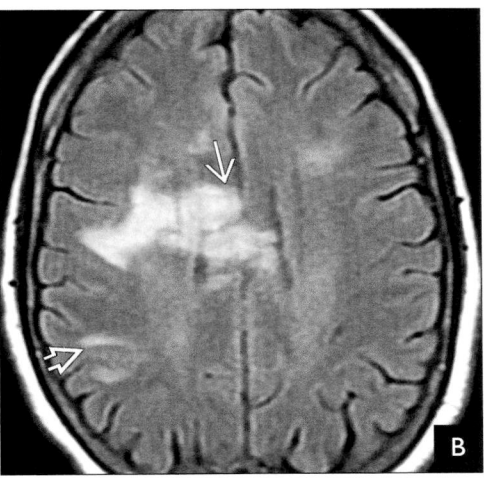

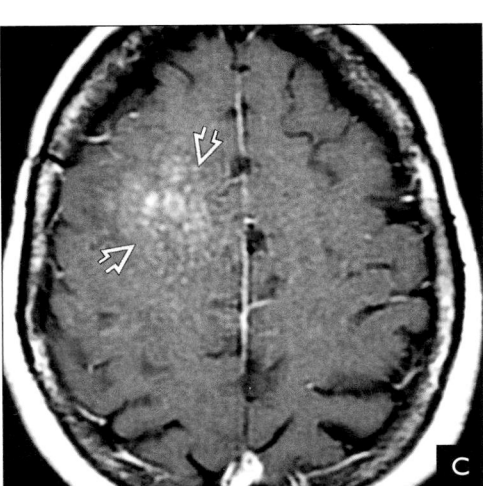

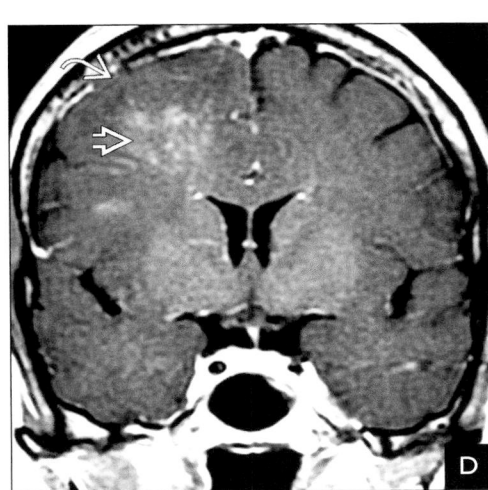

10-60A. Axial FLAIR scan in a 55-year-old woman with unusual neuropsychiatric symptoms shows patchy and confluent hyperintensities in the subcortical and deep periventricular WM ➡. *10-60B. Axial FLAIR scan in the same patient shows subcortical WM lesions* ➡ *in addition to "fluffy" confluent lesions that cross the corpus callosum* ➡ *and resemble ADEM.*

10-60C. Coronal T1 C+ scan in the same patient shows mild punctate and linear foci of enhancement in the subcortical and deep cerebral WM ➡. *10-60D. Coronal T1 C+ shows patchy and linear enhancing foci in the subcortical WM* ➡. *Note the burr hole* ➡ *from biopsy. Histopathologic examination disclosed CNS lupus vasculitis.*

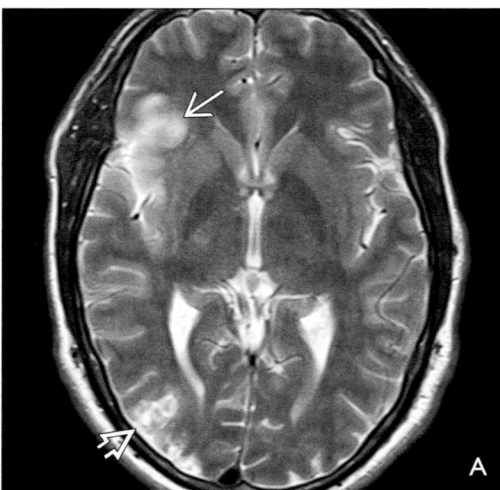

10-61A. Axial T2WI in a 36-year-old man with documented APS and multiple strokes shows acute gyral edema ➡, parietal encephalomalacia ➡.

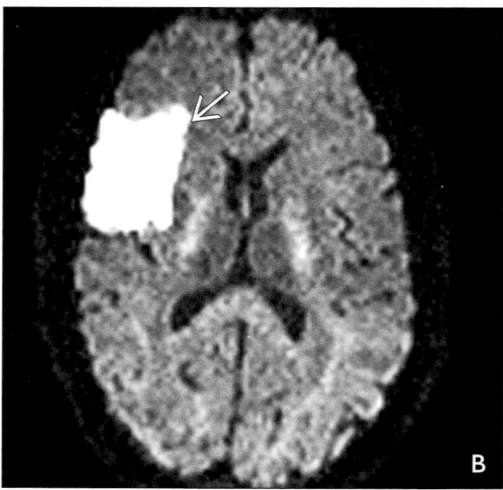

10-61B. DTI trace image in the same patient shows acute restriction in the anterior division of the right middle cerebral artery ➡.

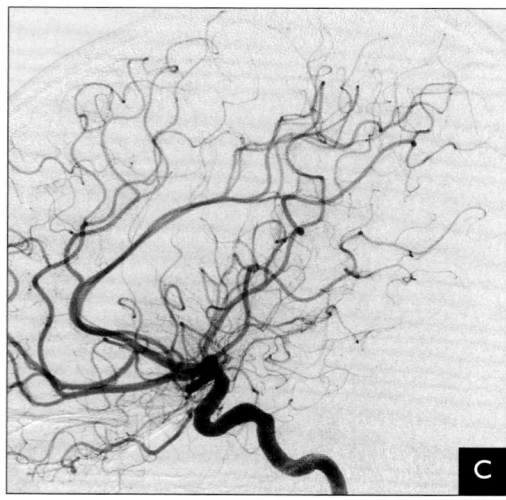

10-61C. Lateral DSA in the same patient shows no evidence of vasculitis.

Antiphospholipid Syndrome

TERMINOLOGY AND ETIOLOGY. APS is a multisystem disorder characterized by arterial or venous thrombosis, early strokes, cognitive dysfunction, and pregnancy loss. APS with widespread livedo reticularis and ischemic cerebrovascular episodes is called **Sneddon syndrome**.

CLINICAL ISSUES. The spectrum of antiphospholipid-mediated syndromes reflects end-organ injury due to microangiopathic disease and endothelial dysfunction. Variable clinical manifestations include skin disease (livedo reticularis rash, splinter hemorrhages); cardiac, pulmonary, and renal involvement; hematologic disorders; and neuropsychiatric symptoms.

The diagnosis of APS requires the presence of at least one clinical criterion (e.g., vascular thrombosis or pregnancy morbidity) and one laboratory finding, i.e., persistently positive lupus anticoagulant, antiphospholipid antibodies (e.g., anticardiolipin antibodies), or anti-β2 glycoprotein 1 antibody.

Mean age of onset is 50 years. There is a 2:1 female predominance (women with APS are often initially diagnosed because of pregnancy loss). A rare complication of APS is HELLP syndrome (**h**emolysis, **e**levated **l**iver enzymes, **l**ow **p**latelets).

CNS involvement in APS is common. Manifestations of CNS APS include cerebrovascular disease with arterial thrombotic events (early onset TIA, stroke) or venous occlusions, MS-like syndromes, seizure, headache, and cognitive dysfunction. A rare "catastrophic" antiphospholipid syndrome is characterized by multiorgan accelerated and widespread vessel occlusions and has a mortality rate approaching 50%. Catastrophic acute CNS APS can cause acute encephalopathy as well as arterial and venous infarcts.

IMAGING. Mixed-age multifocal cortical/subcortical infarcts, parietal-dominant atrophy with relative sparing of the frontal and temporal lobes, and "too many for age" deep WM hyperintensities on T2/FLAIR scans are typical findings in APS **(10-61)**. Both arterial and venous thromboses are common.

DIFFERENTIAL DIAGNOSIS. APS in the CNS can be difficult to distinguish from **multiple sclerosis**. The absence of callososeptal lesions is a helpful differential feature. **Multi-infarct ("vascular") dementia** usually lacks the parietal-dominant atrophy of APS. **SLE** commonly occurs with APS and may present with similar clinical and imaging findings.

Cerebral Amyloid Disease

TERMINOLOGY. Cerebral amyloid disease encompasses a heterogeneous group of biochemically and genetically diverse CNS disorders. Cerebral amyloid disease occurs in several forms. By far the most common is an age-related microvasculopathy termed **cerebral amyloid angiopathy** (CAA), also known as congophilic angiopathy. Amyloid deposition in neuritic plaques is also a prominent feature of **Alzheimer disease** (AD).

Uncommon manifestations of CNS amyloid disease include a focal, tumefactive mass-like lesion called an **amyloidoma.** Rarely, cerebral amyloid disease presents as an **amyloid β-related angiitis** (ABRA) with diffuse inflammatory changes that primarily affect the white matter. ABRA is also known as CAA-related inflammation.

ETIOLOGY. CAA is caused by the accumulation of aggregated Aβ in small cerebral vessels. Aβ is derived from proteolytic cleavage of amyloid precursor protein. Two amino acid species, a 42-aa length (Aβ42) and a shorter 40-aa (Aβ40) length, are associated with amyloid-related brain disease. Aβ42 is principally found in AD-associated neuritic plaques whereas the shorter, relatively more soluble Aβ40 is the major form found in CAA.

Imbalance between Aβ production and clearance is considered a key element in the formation of CNS amyloid deposits. These deposits accumulate in the abluminal portion of the muscular layer and adventitia of cerebral arterioles and capillaries, causing progressive disruption of the neurovascular unit. The geographic distribution of Aβ deposits corresponds anatomically to the perivascular drainage pathways by which interstitial fluid (ISF) and solutes are eliminated from the brain.

Aβ transport between the neuropil and cerebral circulation is blocked in CAA. Failure to clear Aβ from the brain has two major consequences: (1) intracranial hemorrhages associated with rupture of Aβ-laden vessels in CAA and (2) altered neuronal function caused by pathologic accumulation of Aβ and other soluble metabolites in AD. The most frequent vascular abnormality seen in AD is CAA.

GENETICS. Amyloid precursor protein is encoded by the *APP* gene on chromosome 21.

CAA can be primary or secondary, sporadic or familial. Sporadic CAA is much more common than familial CAA and is strongly associated with presence of the *APOE*E4* allele.

Hereditary forms of CAA are generally familial and occur as an autosomal dominant disorder with several recognized subtypes, including Dutch, Italian, Flemish/British, and Icelandic subtypes. Hereditary CAA is generally more severe and earlier in onset compared to the sporadic disease form.

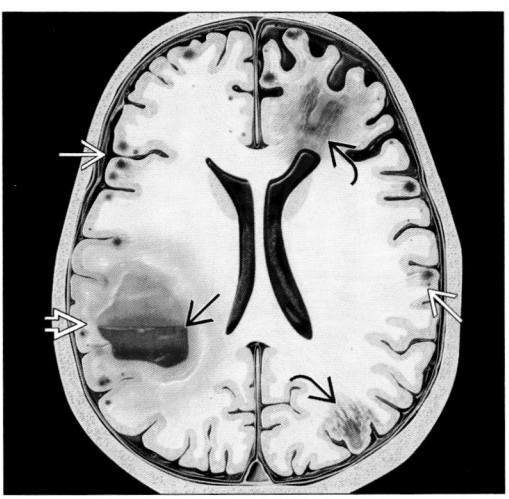

10-62. Acute hematoma ➡ *with a fluid level* ➡; *microbleeds* ➡ *and old lobar hemorrhages* ➷ *are also typical findings in cerebral amyloid disease.*

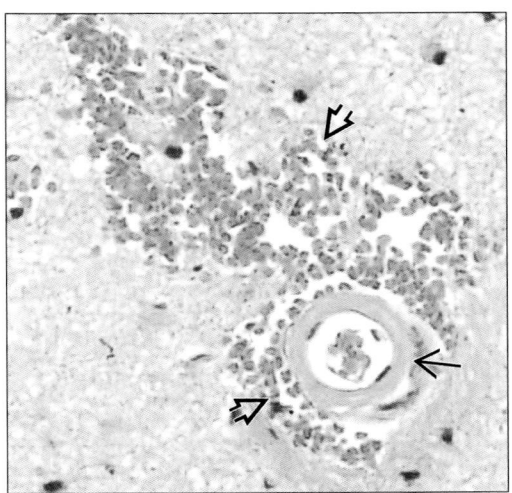

10-63. High-power H&E shows thickened arteriole ➷ *with perivascular hemorrhages* ➷, *characteristic findings of CAA.*

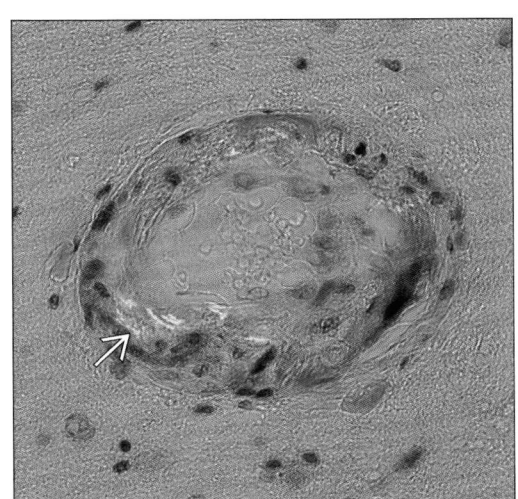

10-64. Congo red stain in polarized light shows thickened arteriole with apple-green birefringence ➡. *CAA. (Courtesy B. K. DeMasters, MD.)*

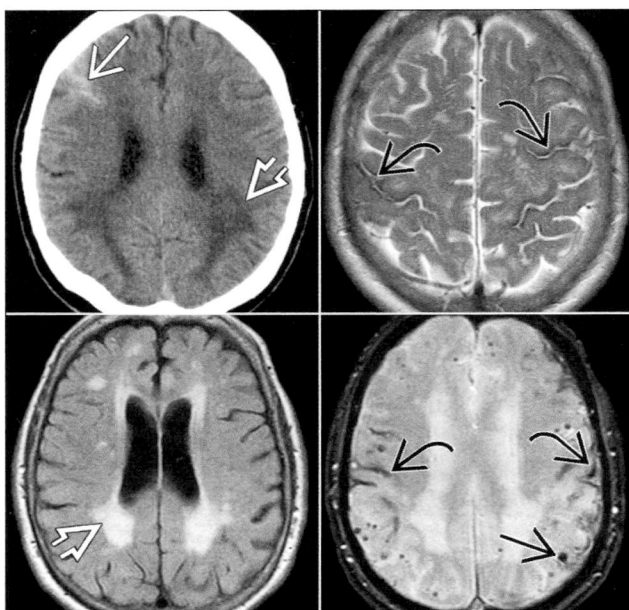

10-65. Scans in a patient with headache and CAA show convexal SAH ➔, confluent WM lesions ➔, superficial siderosis ➢, and microbleeds ➔. (Courtesy M. Castillo, MD.)

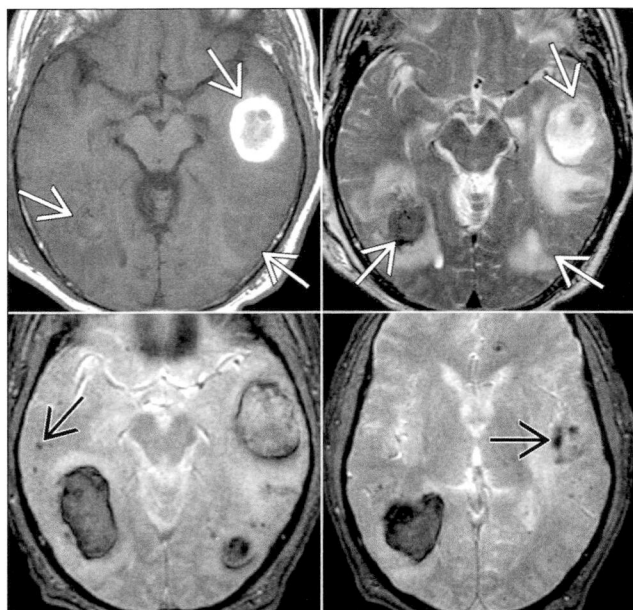

10-66. MR scans demonstrate multiple lobar hemorrhages of different ages ➔, multifocal peripheral "blooming black dots" ➔ that are classic for CAA.

Secondary CAA has been associated with hemodialysis, medullary thyroid carcinoma, and type 2 diabetes.

PATHOLOGY. CAA is characterized by progressive deposition of Aβ fibrils in the walls of small to medium-sized arteries and penetrating arterioles, with preferential involvement of the supratentorial cortex and leptomeninges. The cerebellum, brainstem, and basal ganglia are relatively spared.

Gross pathologic findings include major lobar hemorrhages (most commonly frontal or frontoparietal), cortical petechial hemorrhages, small cerebral infarcts, and white matter ischemic lesions **(10-62)**.

Microscopic features include a "smudgy" eosinophilic thickening of leptomeningeal and cortical vessels **(10-63)**. Severe cases can demonstrate vessel "splitting" (a "lumen within a lumen" appearance), fibrinoid necrosis, pseudoaneurysm formation, and thrombosis. Aβ-related angiitis demonstrates mural and perivascular inflammatory changes with necrosis, variable numbers of multinucleated giant cells, epithelioid histiocytes, eosinophils, and lymphocytes.

On Congo red stains, CAA vessels have a salmon-colored "congophilic" appearance. A characteristic yellow-green color ("birefringence") appears when the affected vessels are viewed using polarized light **(10-64)**. Immuno-histochemistry using antibodies against Aβ is positive. Amyloid-laden blood vessels are also immunoreactive for matrix metalloproteinase (MMP-19).

CLINICAL ISSUES. CAA causes 5-20% of all nontraumatic cerebral hemorrhages and is now recognized as a major cause of spontaneous intracranial hemorrhage and cognitive impairment in the elderly.

Advancing age is the strongest known risk factor for developing CAA. Sporadic CAA usually occurs in patients older than 55 years whereas the hereditary forms present one or two decades earlier. Patients with Aβ-related angiitis also tend to be younger than those with sporadic, noninflammatory CAA.

Autopsy studies show a CAA prevalence of 20-40% in nondemented and 50-60% in demented elderly populations. CAA is present in over 90% of AD patients at post-mortem examination.

The most common clinical manifestations of CAA are focal neurologic deficits (with recurrent lobar hemorrhages) and cognitive impairment (with multiple chronic microbleeds).

The clinical presentation of patients with CAA-related inflammation (e.g., ABRA) differs, usually resembling an autoimmune-mediated vasculitis or a subacute meningoencephalitis. Headache and cognitive decline are common. Occasionally ABRA patients have a more fulminant course characterized by rapidly progressive dementia, seizure, and focal neurologic deficits. Three-quarters of patients with biopsy-proven ABRA respond to corticosteroid therapy, so establishing the correct histopathologic diagnosis is crucial for patient management.

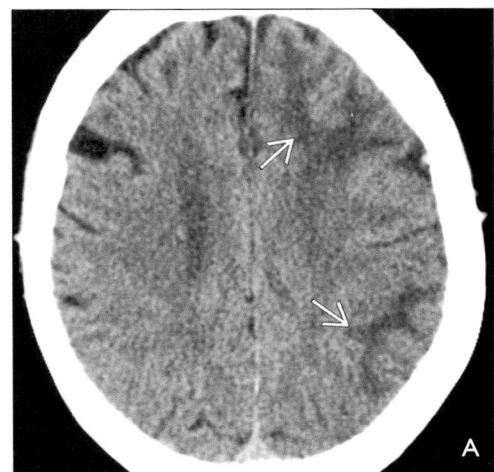
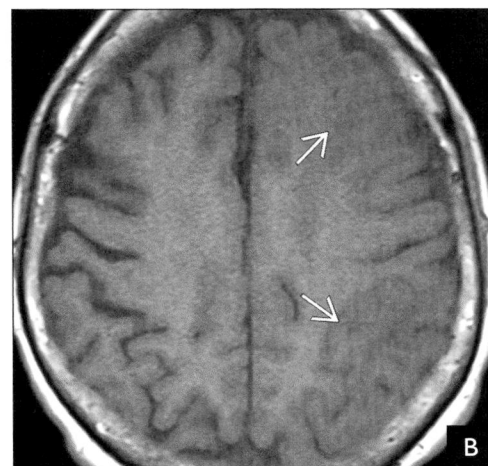

10-67A. NECT scan in an 83-year-old normotensive man with rapidly progressive dementia and right-sided weakness shows confluent subcortical WM hypointensities ➡ in the left frontal and parietal lobes. *10-67B.* T1WI in the same patient shows hypointense swollen gyri ➡ in the left hemisphere together with effacement of the adjacent sulci.

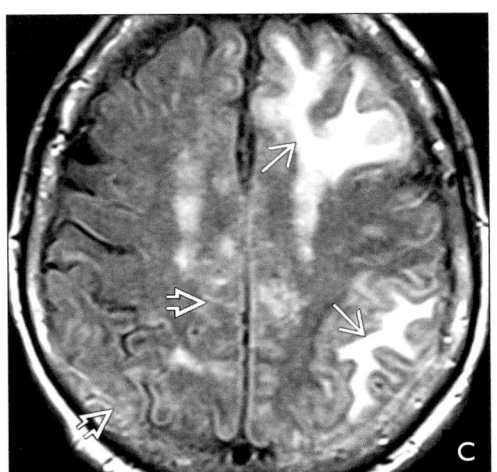
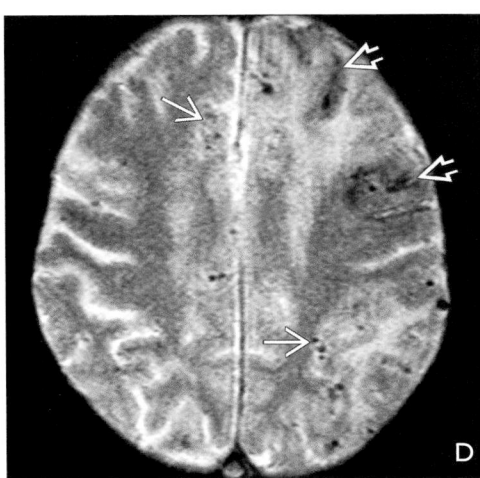

10-67C. FLAIR scan shows striking confluent WM hyperintensity in the left frontal, parietal lobes ➡ with patchy cortical and subcortical hyperintensities ➡ in the right hemisphere and along the medial surfaces of both hemispheres. *10-67D.* T2* GRE scan shows multiple "blooming" cortical/subcortical hypointensities ➡ and linear hypointensity along the left hemisphere sulci ➡, suggestive of siderosis.

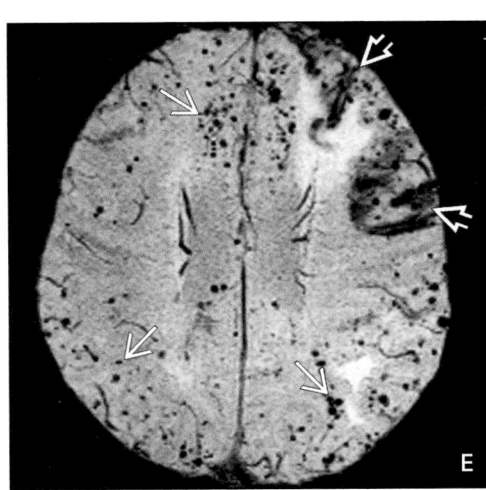
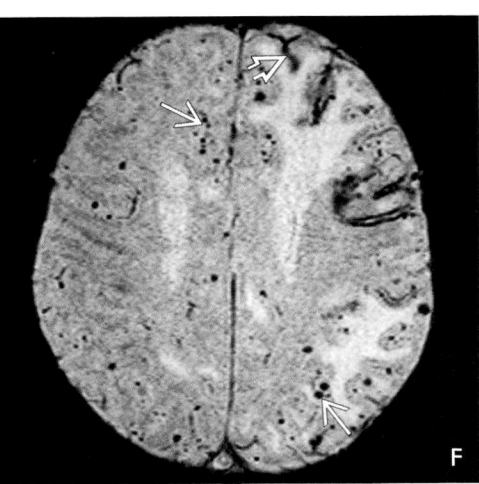

10-67E. T2* SWI scan through the upper ventricles shows innumerable peripheral "blooming black dots" in both hemispheres ➡ as well as the superficial siderosis ➡ characteristic of cerebral amyloid angiopathy. *10-67F.* T2* SWI through the corona radiata shows additional areas of siderosis ➡ and microhemorrhages ➡. Because of the clinical findings plus cerebral edema and mass effect, this case represents CAA-related inflammation (ABRA).

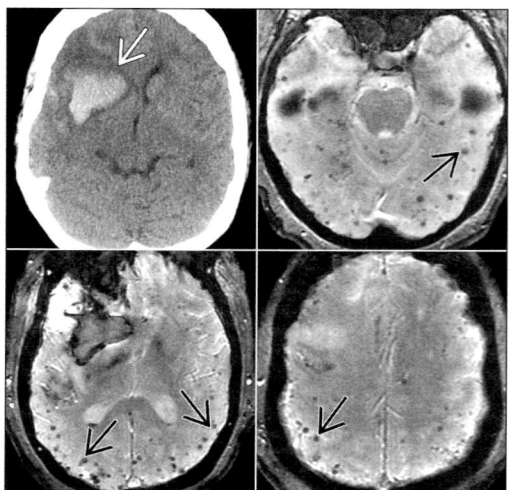

10-68. CAA shows hematoma with fluid-fluid level on NECT ➡, multiple peripheral microbleeds on GRE ➡. (Courtesy P. Hildenbrand, MD.)

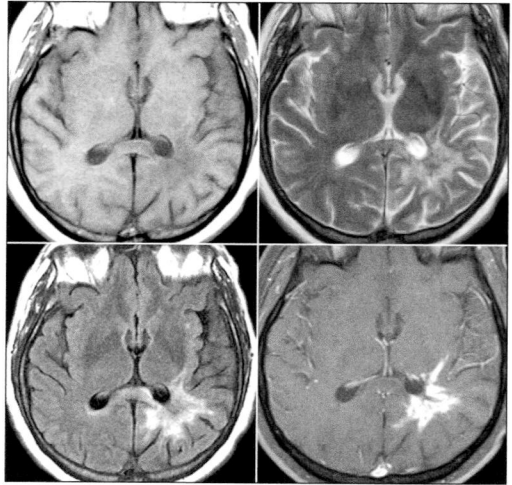

10-69. Biopsy-proven cerebral amyloidoma shows a solitary enhancing periventricular mass. No microbleeds were present on T2* imaging.

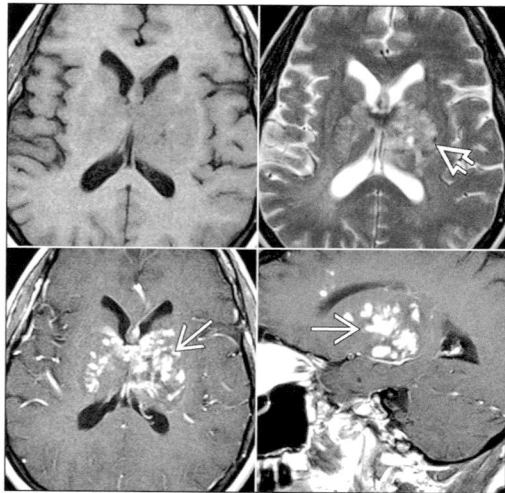

10-70. Biopsy-proven case of infiltrating cerebral amyloid disease with multifocal enhancement ➡, petechial hemorrhages ➡.

IMAGING. Imaging findings vary with the type of cerebral amyloid disease. CAA is by far the most common form; amyloidomas and ABRA are rare.

CT. NECT scans in patients with acute manifestations of CAA typically show a hyperdense lobar hematoma with varying peripheral edema. Multiple irregular confluent white matter hypointensities together with generalized volume loss are common. Enhancement on CECT is rare in cerebral amyloid disease and occurs only if a focal mass ("amyloidoma") or ABRA is present.

Occasionally, patients with CAA can present with so-called convexal subarachnoid hemorrhage (cSAH) (10-65). In cSAH, the basal cisterns appear normal, but one or more adjacent convexity sulci demonstrates curvilinear hyperdensity consistent with blood.

MR. Signal intensity of a CAA-associated lobar hematoma varies with clot age (10-66). Acute hematomas are isointense on T1WI and iso- to hypointense on T2WI.

The vast majority of patients with CAA have focal or patchy confluent WM hyperintensity on T2/FLAIR. Large asymmetric areas of confluent WM hyperintensity on T2/FLAIR with or without microhemorrhages are characteristic of ABRA (10-67). Mass effect is typically absent unless ABRA or a focal amyloid mass ("amyloidoma") is present.

In addition to residual from lobar hemorrhages, T2* (GRE, SWI) sequences demonstrate multifocal punctate "blooming black dots" in the leptomeninges, cortex, and subcortical WM (10-68). The basal ganglia and cerebellum are relatively spared.

CAA-associated hemorrhages typically do not enhance on T1 C+. Both ABRA and amyloidoma may show such striking enhancement that they mimic meningitis, encephalitis, or neoplasm (10-69), (10-70), (10-71).

Nuclear medicine. Patients with CAA have significantly decreased cerebral perfusion on 99m Tc-ECD SPECT studies.

Use of positron emission tomography (PET) amyloid imaging agents such as carbon 11-labeled Pittsburgh Compound B (11C PiB) has facilitated the in vivo evaluation of cerebral amyloid disease, with good overall agreement between 11C PiB and either very low or very high Aβ loads.

Coregistered PET and T2* MR demonstrate significantly increased 11C PiB retention at microbleed sites, indicating that microbleeds occur preferentially in regions of concentrated amyloid deposition.

DIFFERENTIAL DIAGNOSIS. The major differential diagnosis of CAA is **chronic hypertensive encephalopathy** (CHtnE). The microbleeds associated with CHtnE

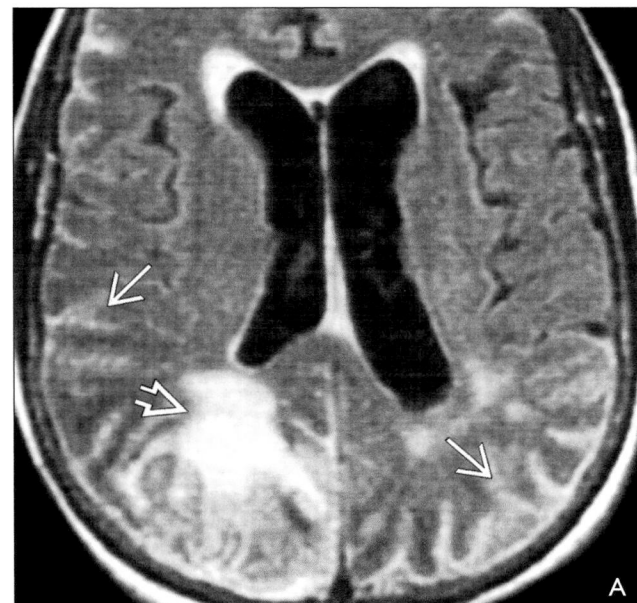

10-71A. Axial FLAIR scan in a patient with inflammatory cerebral amyloid disease shows bilateral sulcal hyperintensities ⮞ with right occipital lobe confluent hyperintensity ⮞.

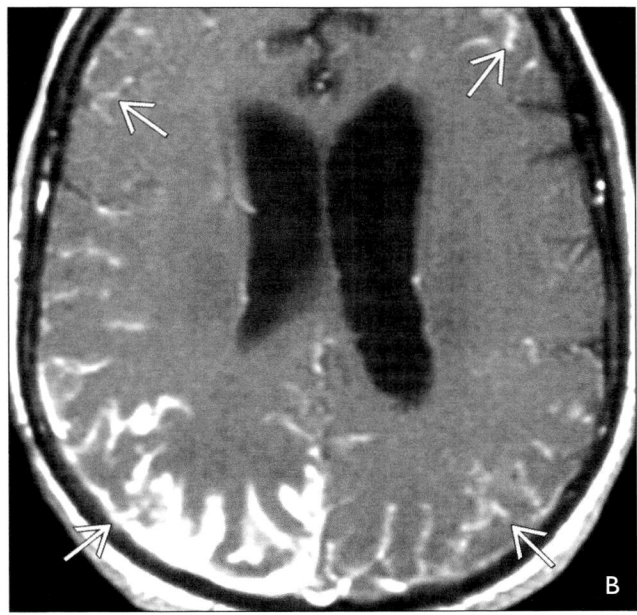

10-71B. T1 C+ in the same patient shows striking sulcal enhancement ⮞. Biopsy-proven Aβ-related angiitis (ABRA). (Courtesy D. Jacobs, MD.)

often involve the basal ganglia and cerebellum. Peripheral microbleeds occur but are less common than CAA-related microhemorrhages, which typically affect the cortex and leptomeninges.

Hemorrhagic lacunar infarcts can demonstrate "blooming" hemosiderin deposits. The basal ganglia and deep cerebral WM are the most common sites, helping distinguish these infarcts from the peripheral microbleeds of CAA.

Multiple cavernous angiomas (Zabramski type 4) typically involve the subcortical WM, basal ganglia, and cerebellum. The cortex is a less common site. "Locules" of blood with fluid-fluid levels and hemorrhages at different stages of evolution are often present in addition to multifocal "blooming black dots" on T2*.

Hemorrhagic metastases at the gray-white matter junction can resemble CAA. The multifocal microbleeds typical of CAA lack mass effect, peripheral edema, and enhancement.

Because of their mass effect, edema, and enhancement patterns, ABRA and amyloidoma are difficult to distinguish from **infection** or **neoplasm** without biopsy.

CEREBRAL AMYLOID DISEASE

Terminology and Etiology
- Most common form
  - Cerebral amyloid angiopathy (CAA)
  - Also known as congophilic angiopathy
- Less common forms
  - Amyloidoma
  - Inflammatory CAA (Aβ-related angiitis, ABRA)
- Aβ40 deposited in meningeal, cortical arterioles

Pathology
- Lobar bleeds, microhemorrhages
- "Congophilic"; birefringent

Clinical Issues
- Causes 5-20% of spontaneous ICHs in elderly
  - Normotensive
  - Dementia
- ↑ age = strongest risk factor

Imaging
- Classic = lobar hemorrhages of different ages
- Common = multifocal microbleeds
  - "Blooming" hypointensities on T2*
  - Typically cortical, meningeal (pial)
  - Posterior > anterior
  - Cerebellum, brainstem, basal ganglia generally spared
- Less common = Aβ-related inflammatory angiitis
  - T2/FLAIR parenchymal hyperintensity
  - Edema, mass effect
  - ± T2* "blooming" microbleeds
  - ± sulcal-cisternal enhancement
- Rare = intracerebral amyloidoma
  - Focal mass(es), often periventricular
  - Biopsy required to distinguish from neoplasm

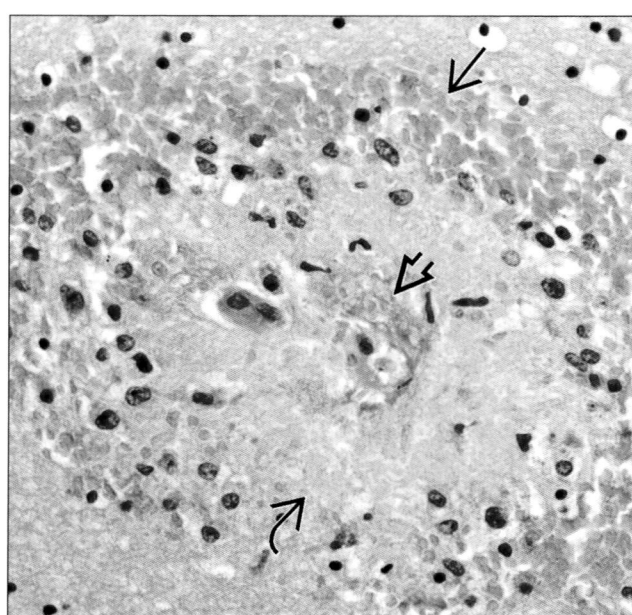

10-72. High-power H&E micropathology image of DIC shows thickened, thrombosed arteriole ➔ with perivascular necrosis ➔ surrounded by a ring of hemorrhage ➔. (Courtesy R. Hewlett, MD.)

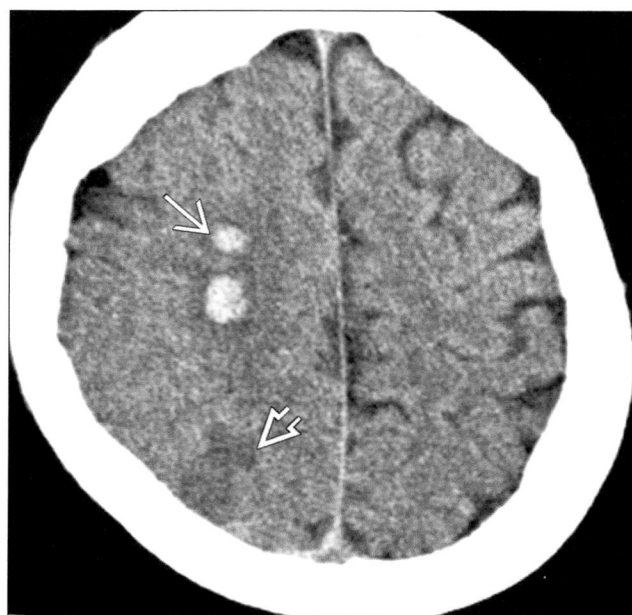

10-73. Axial NECT in a 42-year-old man with AML and DIC shows hemorrhagic foci in the subcortical WM ➔. A hypodense lesion ➔ involves the right parietal cortex and subcortical WM.

Thrombotic Microangiopathies

TERMINOLOGY. The thrombotic microangiopathies (TMAs), also known collectively as thrombotic microangiopathic syndromes, are a heterogeneous group of microvascular occlusive disorders characterized by thrombocytopenia, erythrocyte fragmentation (intravascular hemolysis), and ischemic organ damage.

The major TMAs are **disseminated intravascular coagulopathy** (DIC), **malignant hypertension** (mHTN), and **thrombotic thrombocytopenic purpura** (TTP) with or without **hemolytic-uremic syndrome** (HUS). TTP and HUS share hemolytic anemia and thrombocytopenia as common features and are therefore often grouped together as TTP/HUS (or HUS/TTP).

ETIOLOGY. Endothelial cell injury is the common denominator in the sequence of events leading to TMA development. The microangiopathic cascade begins with loss of physiologic thromboresistance and leukocyte adhesion to damaged endothelium. This is followed by complement consumption, abnormal von Willebrand factor release with decreased fragmentation by the metalloproteinase ADAMTS13, and increased vascular shear stress with mechanical injury to erythrocytes.

Multiple triggers such as infection with septicemia and segmental microvascular necrosis, drugs, toxins, cancer, chemotherapy, bone marrow transplantation, and pregnancy have all been associated with TMAs. A classic toxin-induced TMA is HUS following enterohemorrhagic *Escherichia coli* O104:H4 infection. Here

extremely powerful toxins known as verotoxins or Shiga toxins cause widespread vascular endothelial injury that in turn leads to multiorgan infarcts and hemorrhages.

TMAs are characterized hematologically by platelet aggregation, profound thrombocytopenia, microcirculatory occlusions with ischemia or infarctions, microangiopathic hemolytic anemia, and microhemorrhages in multiple organs.

PATHOLOGY. Biopsy is rarely performed in TMA.

Gross pathology demonstrates multiple widespread foci of necrosis and hemorrhage. Arteriolar and capillary wall thickening, endothelial swelling and fragmentation, subendothelial accumulation of protein and cellular debris, and multiple platelet-fibrin occlusive thrombi are characteristic histopathologic findings **(10-72)**.

CLINICAL ISSUES. TMAs are rare. The overall incidence is estimated at less than 1:1,000,000 per year. Although the TMAs share a common pathophysiology, the clinical findings vary depending on the underlying disease.

DIC is the most common TMA, causing 80% of all cases. DIC is associated with a spectrum of comorbid pathologies including infection, tumor, vascular abnormalities, obstetrical and neonatal complications, massive tissue necrosis, and drug reactions. DIC is characterized clinically by thrombosis and/or hemorrhage at multiple sites.

Malignant HTN is the second most common TMA. Patients typically present with elevated blood pressure and papilledema, often accompanied by retinal hemorrhage and exudates. Pregnant patients with mHTN are eclamptic or preeclamptic.

TTP is the least common TMA. TTP is primarily a disease of children but can also affect young adults. Approximately half of all patients develop CNS symptoms, usually seizures and/or fluctuating neurologic deficits. Fever, renal insufficiency, and a purpuric rash over the trunk and limbs are common. The classic laboratory triad consists of thrombocytopenia, elevated lactate dehydrogenase, and schistocytosis. The majority of TTP patients have ADAMTS13 deficiency.

Although their symptoms often overlap, CNS disease is more common in TTP while renal involvement predominates in HUS. HUS is defined by the triad of mechanical hemolytic anemia, thrombocytopenia, and renal impairment. Complement dysregulation—not ADAMTS13 deficiency—is characteristic of HUS.

Renal failure and stroke from intravascular coagulopathy or thrombotic microangiopathy are among the most serious complications of TMA. Treatment is mainly supportive and often includes plasma exchange, steroids,

vincristine, and/or rituximab. Antibiotics are usually avoided in *E. coli*-induced hemorrhagic enterocolitis due to the potential for augmented verotoxin release by dying and dead bacteria. Splenectomy and cyclophosphamide have been proposed as salvage therapies in severe TTP.

IMAGING. Multifocal cortical and subcortical ischemic and hemorrhagic infarcts are typical **(10-73)**. NECT scans can be normal early in the disease course. Positive findings include peripheral poorly defined irregular hypoattenuating foci or hemorrhage with relatively well-delineated hyperdensities surrounded by variable edema. Mixed patterns with both hypo- and hyperdense lesions are also common **(10-74A)**.

Signal intensity on MR varies with clot age. Multifocal cortical/subcortical hyperintensities on T2/FLAIR are common in acute TMA. The most sensitive sequence is T2* (GRE, SWI). Punctate gyral "blooming" hypointensities are typical **(10-74B)**, **(10-74C)**. DWI shows multiple foci of diffusion restriction **(10-74D)**, **(10-75)**.

HUS/TTP and mHTN can cause a PRES-like imaging pattern with posterior cortical/subcortical or brainstem

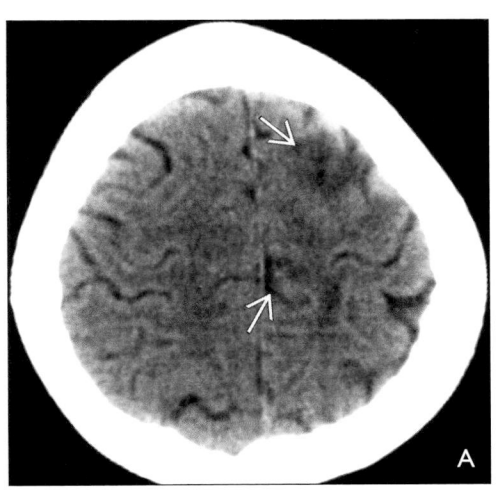

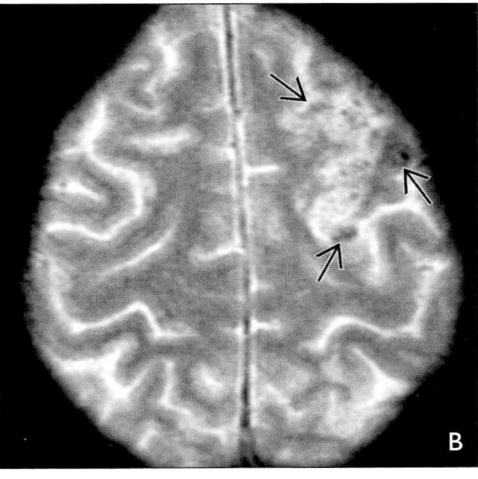

10-74A. Axial NECT scan in a 45-year-old woman with AML, mental status changes shows scattered cortical and subcortical hypodensities ➡. 10-74B. T2 GRE scan in the same patient shows multifocal, peripherally located microbleeds ➡.*

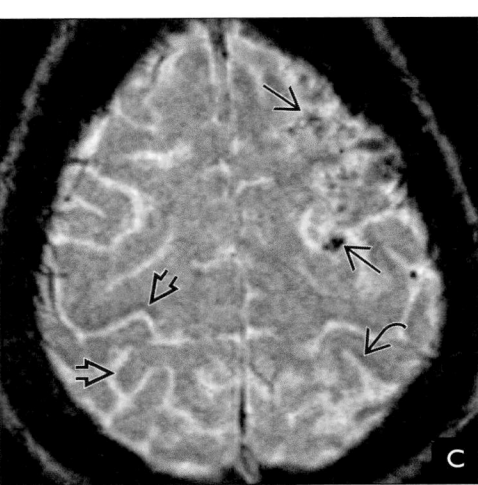

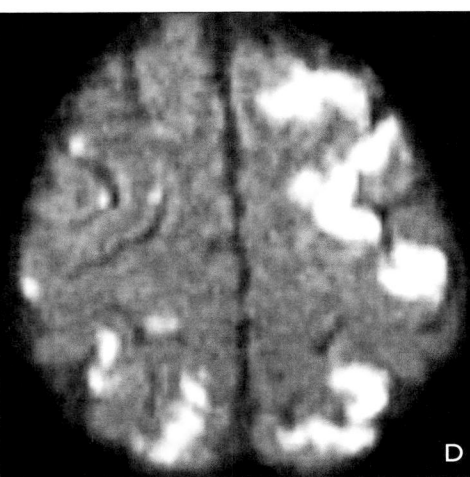

10-74C. T2 SWI scan better delineates the left frontal cortical/subcortical microbleeds ➡. In addition, subtle lesions in the right hemisphere are seen ⊳ as are additional left hemisphere lesions ➡. 10-74D. DWI in the same patient shows multiple foci of restricted diffusion in the cortex and subcortical WM of both hemispheres. Laboratory studies confirmed TTP.*

hyperintensities. DWI in these cases is typically but not invariably normal.

DIFFERENTIAL DIAGNOSIS. The major differential diagnosis of TMAs, especially HUS/TTP, is **acute hypertensive encephalopathy** (e.g., PRES). HUS/TTP can cause a PRES-like syndrome with identical imaging findings. Clinical history (nonpregnant patient) and laboratory findings should distinguish between these two entities.

Multiple cerebral infarcts, especially septic emboli, can mimic the peripheral cortical lesions of TMA. Hemorrhagic septic emboli are typically not as diffuse as TMA-associated lesions. However, **septicemia with segmental microvascular necrosis** can cause a diffuse hemorrhagic encephalopathy that may be exacerbated by DIC **(10-76)**.

Antiphospholipid antibody syndrome complicated by HELLP syndrome can mimic TMA.

Cortical venous thrombosis with or without dural sinus occlusion can cause multiple peripheral hemorrhages. The hemorrhages and infarcts in TMA are typically more diffuse, and evidence for dural sinus thrombosis is absent.

THROMBOTIC MICROANGIOPATHIES

Terminology
- Microvascular occlusive disorders with
  - Thrombocytopenia
  - Intravascular hemolysis
  - Ischemic organ damage
- Major types
  - Disseminated intravascular coagulopathy
  - Malignant hypertension
  - HUS/TTP

Etiology
- Endothelial cell injury
- Multiple triggers
  - Infection (e.g., septicemia, enterohemorrhagic *E. coli*)
  - Drugs
  - Cancer or chemotherapy
  - Pregnancy

Imaging
- Cortical/subcortical ischemic infarcts
- Multifocal microhemorrhages

Differential Diagnosis
- PRES
- Septic emboli
- Antiphospholipid antibody syndrome

10-75A. FLAIR scan in a 54-year-old woman with chronic renal failure shows confluent hyperintensities in the periventricular WM of both frontal lobes ⇨. Scattered patchy hyperintense foci are present in the deep WM of both hemispheres ⇨. 10-75B. T2* GRE scan shows a few scattered focal hypointensities in the deep cerebral WM ⇨.

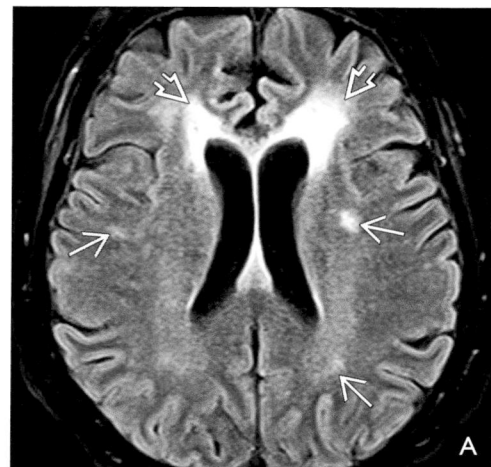
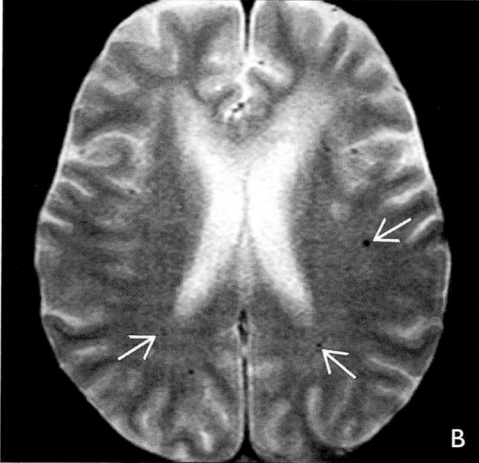

10-75C. T2* SWI scan in the same patient shows multiple "blooming black dots" in the deep cerebral WM of both hemispheres ⇨. 10-75D. More cephalad SWI scan in the same patient shows more "blooming" foci in the corona radiata ⇨. Findings are consistent with microhemorrhages in HUS/TTP.

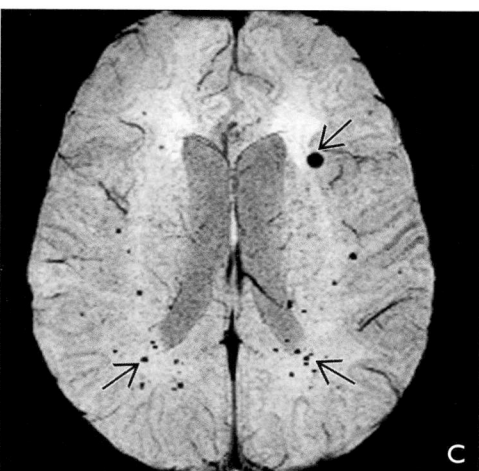
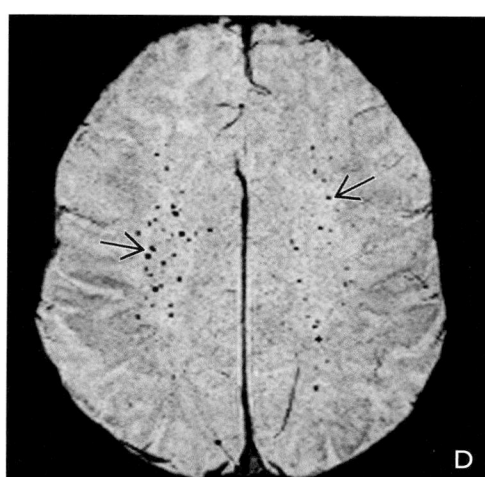

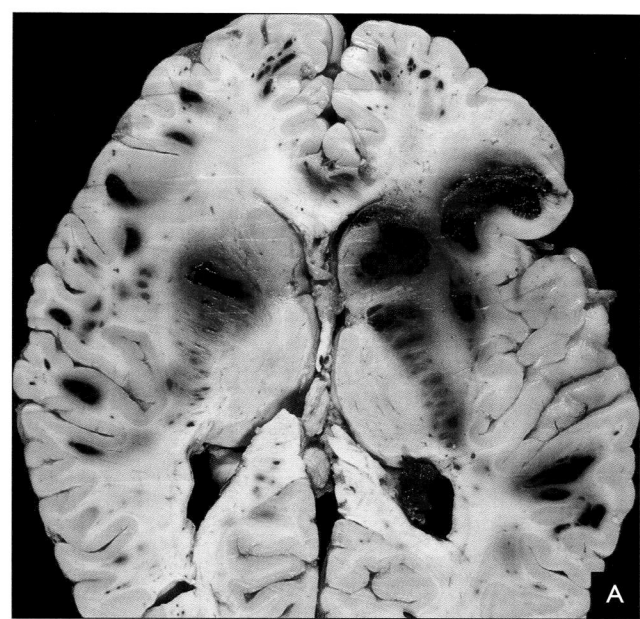

10-76A. *Autopsy from a 70 yo man with gram-negative septicemia shows multifocal petechial hemorrhages in the subcortical WM, basal ganglia. Most are small ovoid or linear lesions, but some scattered confluent hemorrhages are present.*

10-76B. *More cephalad section through the corona radiata shows extensive subcortical, deep WM lesions with almost complete sparing of the cortical GM. (Courtesy R. Hewlett, MD.)*

Selected References

Normal Anatomy of the Extracranial Arteries

Aortic Arch and Great Vessels

- Finlay A et al: Surgically relevant aortic arch mapping using computed tomography. Ann Vasc Surg. 26(4):483-90, 2012

- Ramos-Duran L et al: Developmental aortic arch anomalies in infants and children assessed with CT angiography. AJR Am J Roentgenol. 198(5):W466-74, 2012

- Restrepo CS et al: Multidetector computed tomography of congenital anomalies of the thoracic aorta. Semin Ultrasound CT MR. 33(3):191-206, 2012

- Welch CS et al: The five-vessel arch: independent origin of both vertebral arteries from the aortic arch. J Comput Assist Tomogr. 36(2):275-6, 2012

- Layton KF et al: Bovine aortic arch variant in humans: clarification of a common misnomer. AJNR Am J Neuroradiol. 27(7):1541-2, 2006

Cervical Carotid Arteries

- Kamenskiy AV et al: Three-dimensional geometry of the human carotid artery. J Biomech Eng. 134(6):064502, 2012

- Saba L et al: Imaging of the carotid artery. Atherosclerosis. 220(2):294-309, 2012

Atherosclerosis

Atherogenesis and Atherosclerosis

- Arboix A et al: [Complex aortic atheroma plaques: study of 71 patients with lacunar infarcts.] Med Clin (Barc). 138(4):160-4, 2012

- Phan TG et al: Carotid artery anatomy and geometry as risk factors for carotid atherosclerotic disease. Stroke. 43(6):1596-601, 2012

- Bressler J et al: Genetic variants identified in a European genome-wide association study that were found to predict incident coronary heart disease in the atherosclerosis risk in communities study. Am J Epidemiol. 171(1):14-23, 2010

- Insull W Jr: The pathology of atherosclerosis: plaque development and plaque responses to medical treatment. Am J Med. 122(1 Suppl):S3-S14, 2009

Extracranial Atherosclerosis

- Byrnes KR et al: The current role of carotid duplex ultrasonography in the management of carotid atherosclerosis: foundations and advances. Int J Vasc Med. 2012:187872, 2012

- van den Oord SC et al: Assessment of subclinical atherosclerosis using contrast-enhanced ultrasound. Eur Heart J Cardiovasc Imaging. Epub ahead of print, 2012

- van Gils MJ et al: Carotid atherosclerotic plaque progression and change in plaque composition over time: A 5-year follow-up study using serial CT angiography. AJNR Am J Neuroradiol. 33(7):1267-73, 2012

- Boussel L et al: Ischemic stroke: etiologic work-up with multidetector CT of heart and extra- and intracranial arteries. Radiology. 258(1):206-12, 2011

- Cheung HM et al: Late stage complicated atheroma in low-grade stenotic carotid disease: MR imaging depiction--prevalence and risk factors. Radiology. 260(3):841-7, 2011
- Qiao Y et al: Identification of intraplaque hemorrhage on MR angiography images: a comparison of contrast-enhanced mask and time-of-flight techniques. AJNR Am J Neuroradiol. 32(3):454-9, 2011
- Capmany RP et al: Complex atheromatosis of the aortic arch in cerebral infarction. Curr Cardiol Rev. 6(3):184-93, 2010
- Furtado AD et al: The triple rule-out for acute ischemic stroke: imaging the brain, carotid arteries, aorta, and heart. AJNR Am J Neuroradiol. 31(7):1290-6, 2010
- Ota H et al: Carotid intraplaque hemorrhage imaging at 3.0-T MR imaging: comparison of the diagnostic performance of three T1-weighted sequences. Radiology. 254(2):551-63, 2010
- Huang HH et al: Time-of-flight MR angiography not for diagnosing subclavian steal syndrome. Radiology. 253(3):897, author reply 897-8, 2009
- Chao A-C et al: The relationship between carotid artery diameter and percentage of stenosis. Neuroradiol J. 20(1):103-109, 2007
- Puchner S et al: CTA in the detection and quantification of vertebral artery pathologies: a correlation with color Doppler sonography. Neuroradiology. 49(8):645-50, 2007

Intracranial Atherosclerosis

- Fisher M et al: Pathogenesis of intracranial atherosclerosis. Ann Neurol. 72(1):149, 2012
- López-Cancio E et al: Biological signatures of asymptomatic extra- and intracranial atherosclerosis: The Barcelona-AsIA (Asymptomatic Intracranial Atherosclerosis) study. Stroke. 43(10):2712-9, 2012
- Siddiqui FM et al: Endovascular management of symptomatic extracranial stenosis associated with secondary intracranial tandem stenosis. A multicenter review. J Neuroimaging. 22(3):243-8, 2012
- Hong NR et al: The correlation between carotid siphon calcification and lacunar infarction. Neuroradiology. 53(9):643-9, 2011

Arteriolosclerosis

- Smallwood A et al: Cerebral subcortical small vessel disease and its relation to cognition in elderly subjects: a pathological study in the Oxford Project to Investigate Memory and Ageing (OPTIMA) cohort. Neuropathol Appl Neurobiol. 38(4):337-43, 2012
- Gorelick PB et al: Vascular contributions to cognitive impairment and dementia: a statement for healthcare professionals from the American Heart Association/American Stroke Association. Stroke. 42(9):2672-713, 2011

Nonatheromatous Vascular Diseases

Fibromuscular Dysplasia

- Olin JW et al: The United States registry for fibromuscular dysplasia: results in the first 447 patients. Circulation. 125(25):3182-90, 2012
- Olin JW et al: Diagnosis, management, and future developments of fibromuscular dysplasia. J Vasc Surg. 53(3):826-36, 2011
- Touzé E et al: Fibromuscular dysplasia of cervical and intracranial arteries. Int J Stroke. 5(4):296-305, 2010
- de Monyé C et al: MDCT detection of fibromuscular dysplasia of the internal carotid artery. AJR Am J Roentgenol. 188(4):W367-9, 2007

Dissection

- Patel RR et al: Cervical carotid artery dissection: current review of diagnosis and treatment. Cardiol Rev. 20(3):145-52, 2012
- Rodallec MH et al: Craniocervical arterial dissection: spectrum of imaging findings and differential diagnosis. Radiographics. 28(6):1711-28, 2008

Vasoconstriction Syndromes

- Fugate JE et al: Fulminant postpartum cerebral vasoconstriction syndrome. Arch Neurol. 69(1):111-7, 2012
- Marder CP et al: Multimodal imaging of reversible cerebral vasoconstriction syndrome: a series of 6 cases. AJNR Am J Neuroradiol. 33(7):1403-11, 2012
- Rozen TD: Reversible postpartum cerebral vasoconstriction syndrome. Arch Neurol. 69(6):792-3, 2012
- Tan LH et al: Reversible cerebral vasoconstriction syndrome: an important cause of acute severe headache. Emerg Med Int. 2012:303152, 2012
- Ansari SA et al: Reversible cerebral vasoconstriction syndromes presenting with subarachnoid hemorrhage: a case series. J Neurointerv Surg. 3(3):272-8, 2011

Vasculitis and Vasculitides

- Mandell DM et al: Vessel wall MRI to differentiate between reversible cerebral vasoconstriction syndrome and central nervous system vasculitis: preliminary results. Stroke. 43(3):860-2, 2012
- Salvarani C et al: Adult primary central nervous system vasculitis. Lancet. 380(9843):767-77, 2012
- Watts R et al: Development and validation of a consensus methodology for the classification of the ANCA-associated vasculitides and polyarteritis nodosa for epidemiological studies. Ann Rheum Dis. 66(2):222-7, 2007

Other Macro- and Microvasculopathies

- Charidimou A et al: Sporadic cerebral amyloid angiopathy revisited: recent insights into pathophysiology and clinical spectrum. J Neurol Neurosurg Psychiatry. 83(2):124-37, 2012
- Houkin K et al: Review of past research and current concepts on the etiology of moyamoya disease. Neurol Med Chir (Tokyo). 52(5):267-77, 2012
- Lin R et al: Clinical and immunopathological features of moyamoya disease. PLoS One. 7(4):e36386, 2012
- Radhi M et al: Thrombotic microangiopathies. ISRN Hematol. 2012:310596, 2012
- Scully M et al: Guidelines on the diagnosis and management of thrombotic thrombocytopenic purpura and other thrombotic microangiopathies. Br J Haematol. 158(3):323-335, 2012

- Seo BS et al: Clinical and radiological features of patients with aplastic or twiglike middle cerebral arteries. Neurosurgery. 70(6):1472-80; discussion 1480, 2012

- Wang PI et al: Perfusion-weighted MR imaging in cerebral lupus erythematosus. Acad Radiol. 19(8):965-70, 2012

- Wengert O et al: Cerebral amyloid angiopathy-related inflammation: a treatable cause of rapidlyprogressive dementia. J Neuropsychiatry Clin Neurosci. 24(1):E1-2, 2012

- Biffi A et al: Cerebral amyloid angiopathy: a systematic review. J Clin Neurol. 7(1):1-9, 2011

- Curiel R et al: PET/CT imaging in systemic lupus erythematosus. Ann N Y Acad Sci. 1228:71-80, 2011

- Currie S et al: Childhood moyamoya disease and moyamoya syndrome: a pictorial review. Pediatr Neurol. 44(6):401-13, 2011

- Ellchuk TN et al: Suspicious neuroimaging pattern of thrombotic microangiopathy. AJNR Am J Neuroradiol. 32(4):734-8, 2011

- Horie N et al: "Brush sign" on susceptibility-weighted MR imaging indicates the severity of moyamoya disease. AJNR Am J Neuroradiol. 32(9):1697-702, 2011

- Lee SK et al: Rapid atypical progression of neuro-Behçet's disease involving whole brainstem and bilateral thalami. J Korean Neurosurg Soc. 50(1):68-71, 2011

- Luyendijk J et al: Neuropsychiatric systemic lupus erythematosus: lessons learned from magnetic resonance imaging. Arthritis Rheum. 63(3):722-32, 2011

- Maarouf CL et al: Alzheimer's disease and non-demented high pathology control nonagenarians: comparing and contrasting the biochemistry of cognitively successful aging. PLoS One. 6(11):e27291, 2011

- Mosca L et al: NOTCH3 gene mutations in subjects clinically suspected of CADASIL. J Neurol Sci. 307(1-2):144-8, 2011

- Pandey P et al: Neurosurgical advances in the treatment of moyamoya disease. Stroke. 42(11):3304-10, 2011

- Singh JS et al: Case 176: Neuro-sweet syndrome. Radiology. 261(3):989-93, 2011

- Choi JC: Cerebral autosomal dominant arteriopathy with subcortical infarcts and leukoencephalopathy: a genetic cause of cerebral small vessel disease. J Clin Neurol. 6(1):1-9, 2010

- Fertrin KY et al: Genomic polymorphisms in sickle cell disease: implications for clinical diversity and treatment. Expert Rev Hematol. 3(4):443-58, 2010

- Mayer M et al: Antiphospholipid syndrome and central nervous system. Clin Neurol Neurosurg. 112(7):602-8, 2010

- Richard E et al: Characteristics of dyshoric capillary cerebral amyloid angiopathy. J Neuropathol Exp Neurol. 69(11):1158-67, 2010

- Steiger HJ et al: Cerebral angiopathies as a cause of ischemic stroke in children: differential diagnosis and treatment options. Dtsch Arztebl Int. 107(48):851-6, 2010

- Lalani TA et al: Imaging findings in systemic lupus erythematosus. Radiographics. 24(4):1069-86, 2004

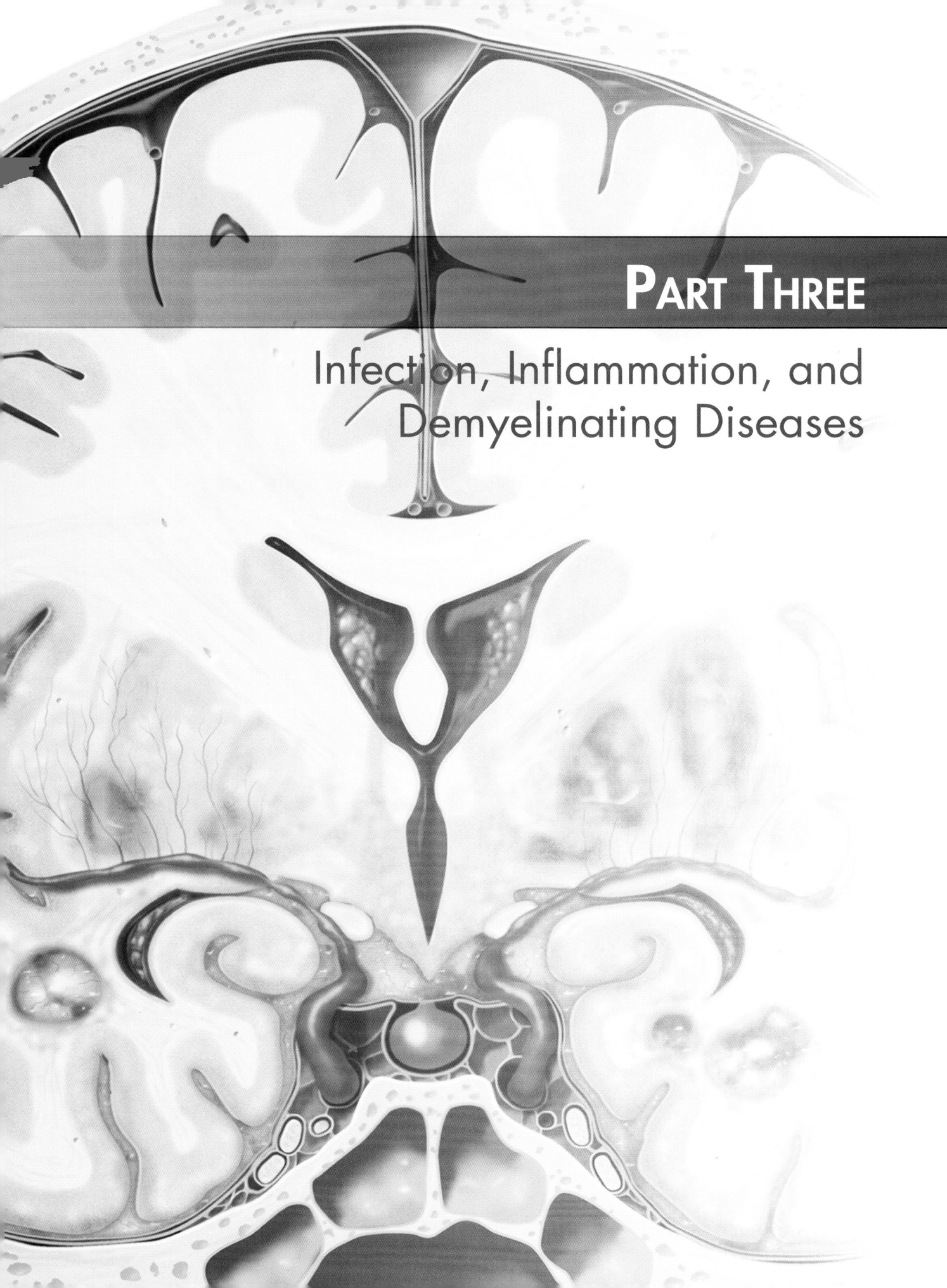

PART THREE

Infection, Inflammation, and Demyelinating Diseases

11

Approach to Infection, Inflammation, and Demyelination

The plague (both literal and figurative) of infectious diseases has been a threat to humankind for millennia. Parasitic infestations have been identified in Egyptian mummies from the Old Kingdom and still affect people today. Our ancient enemies—tuberculosis and malaria—once seemed to be under relative control. But are they? Absolutely not. One in three people in the world has been infected with *M. tuberculosis*.

In the antibiotic era, once-dreaded infections may seem a distant memory. But are they truly relegated to the medical history scrap heap? Hardly.

I once heard Dr. Joshua Lederberg, who shared the 1958 Nobel Prize in Physiology or Medicine for his discoveries concerning recombination and organization of bacterial genes, make a very telling comment. He remarked, "We are in an 'evolutionary foot race' with our closest competitors, viruses and bacteria." Guess who's winning? One doesn't need to be a genius to guess just *who* is winning ... and it isn't us humans!

Widespread use of antibiotics had its inevitable result. Adaptive evolution has rendered some organisms resistant even to the "antibiotics of last resort." Outbreaks of diverse multidrug-resistant organisms, once rare, are reported with increasing frequency. Methicillin-resistant *Staphylococcus aureus* (MRSA) and vancomycin-resistant *Enterococcus* (VRE) have achieved significant rates of colonization and infection in most intensive care units. To date, interventions aimed at reducing transmission of resistant bacteria in such high-risk settings have been relatively ineffective.

Misuse or mismanagement of first-line drugs has also resulted in the development of multidrug-resistant TB (MDR TB). MDR TB and the recent emergence of extensively drug-resistant TB (XDR TB) jeopardize the major gains achieved by several decades of TB control. The significant progress made in reducing TB-related deaths in immunocompromised patients is also threatened by these developments.

While any part of the human body can become inflamed or infected, the brain has long been considered an "immunologically protected" site because of the blood-brain barrier. Although CNS infections are considerably less common than their systemic counterparts, the brain is by no means invulnerable to onslaught from pathogenic organisms.

The role of medical imaging in the emergent evaluation of intracranial infection ideally should be supportive, not primary. But in many health care facilities worldwide, triage of acute CNS disease frequently uses brain imaging as an initial noninvasive "screening procedure." Therefore, the radiologist may be the first—not the last—to recognize the presence of possible CNS infection.

In this part, we devote chapters 12 and 13 to CNS infections. HIV/AIDS is covered in Chapter 14. The last chapter, Chapter 15, considers the surprisingly broad spectrum of noninfectious idiopathic inflammatory and demyelinating disorders that affect the CNS.

CNS Infections

Intracranial infections are caused by a broad range of pathogenic agents; well over 200 different organisms have been described as causing CNS infections of one type or another. Imaging findings are often nonspecific, so a careful history and appropriate clinical-laboratory investigations are necessary for accurate diagnosis and appropriate treatment.

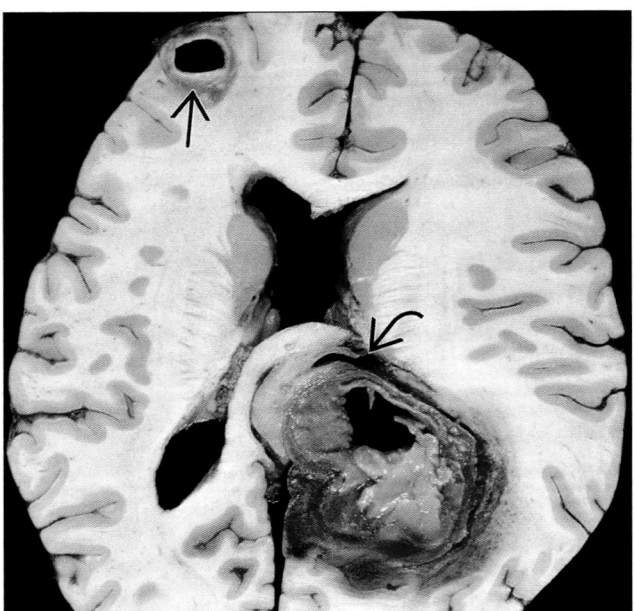

11-1. Note small, well-encapsulated frontal lobe abscess ➔ with a larger, less well-defined lesion in the contralateral hemisphere. The large abscess ruptured into the ventricle ⇗, causing pyocephalus and death. (Courtesy R. Hewlett, MD.)

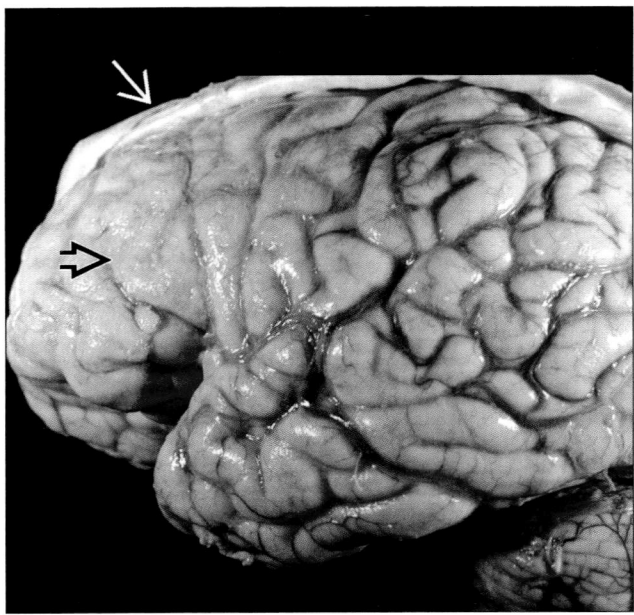

11-2. Autopsy specimen shows the dura ➔ reflected up to reveal a purulent-appearing collection in the underlying subdural space ⇒. Findings are typical for a pyogenic subdural empyema. (Courtesy R. Hewlett, MD.)

CNS infections can be classified in several ways. The most common method is to divide them into congenital/neonatal and acquired infections. Categorizing infections purely according to disease category, i.e., pyogenic, viral, granulomatous, parasitic, etc., is also very common. As imaging findings overlap considerably, this system is of little help to the radiologist.

In this text we follow a combination of classifications. We first subdivide infections into congenital and acquired disorders. Congenital infections are discussed in Chapter 12. Because this is a relatively short discussion, we combine these with acquired pyogenic and viral infections.

Our discussion of pyogenic infections begins with the meninges (meningitis). We follow with a consideration of focal brain infections (cerebritis, abscess), the often-lethal complication of ventriculitis (pyocephalus) (11-1), and pus collections in the extraaxial spaces (subdural/epidural empyemas) (11-2). We then focus on the CNS manifestations of acquired viral infections.

In Chapter 13, we consider the pathogenesis and imaging of tuberculosis, fungal infections, and parasitic and protozoal infestations. We conclude this second chapter on infections with a brief discussion of spirochetes and emerging CNS infections (e.g., the rare hemorrhagic viral fevers).

HIV/AIDS

In the more than three decades since AIDS was first identified, the disease has become a worldwide epidemic. With the development of effective combination antiretroviral therapies, HIV/AIDS has evolved from a virtual death sentence to a chronic but manageable disease—if the treatment is (1) available and (2) affordable. As treated patients with HIV/AIDS now often survive for a decade or longer, the imaging spectrum of HIV/AIDS has also evolved.

Treated HIV/AIDS as a chronic disease looks very different from HIV/AIDS in so-called high-burden regions of the world. In such places, HIV in socioeconomically disadvantaged patients often behaves as an acute, fulminant infection. Comorbid diseases such as TB, malaria, or overwhelming bacterial sepsis are common complications and may dominate the imaging presentation.

Complications of HAART treatment itself have created newly recognized disorders such as immune reconstitution inflammatory syndrome (IRIS). In Chapter 14, we consider the effect of HIV itself on the CNS (HIV encephalitis) as well as opportunistic infections, IRIS, miscellaneous manifestations of HIV/AIDS, and HIV-associated neoplasms.

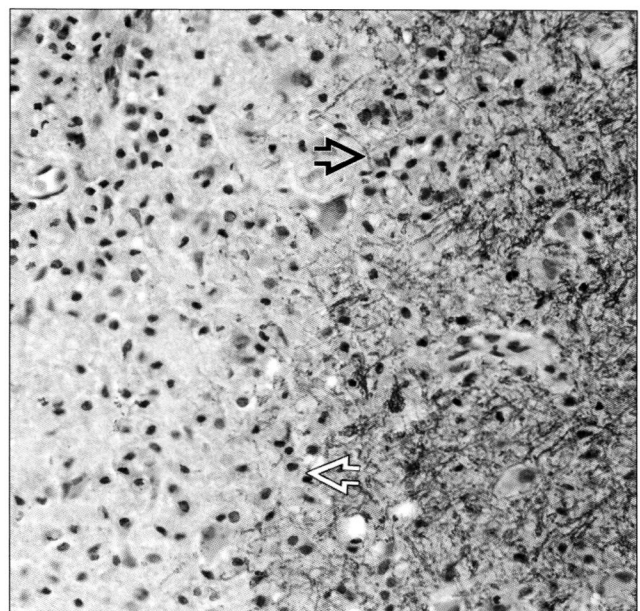

11-3. H&E/Luxol fast blue stain emphasizes the sharp interface between lesion (pale-staining tissue ⊳) and normal parenchyma (blue-staining tissue ⊳) typical of most demyelinating plaques. (Courtesy B. K. DeMasters, MD.)

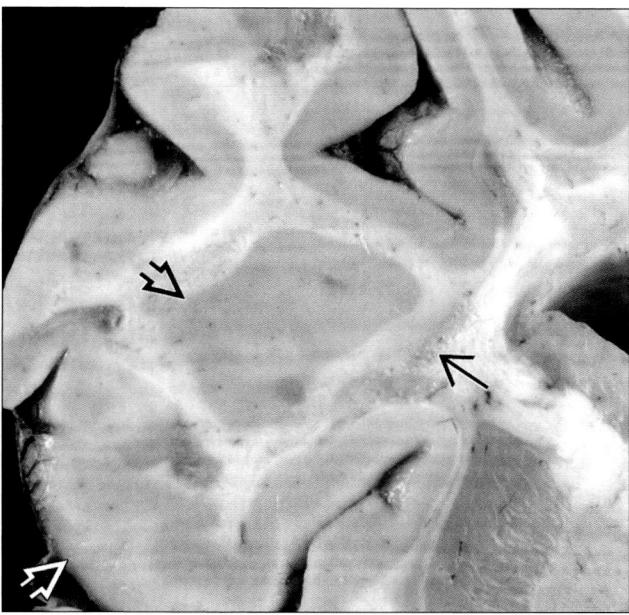

11-4. Gross autopsy with close-up view of "tumefactive" demyelinating disease ⊳ shows peripheral necrosis → with mass effect on the adjacent gyrus ⊳. (Courtesy B. K. DeMasters, MD.)

Demyelinating and Inflammatory Diseases

The final chapter in this part is devoted to demyelinating and noninfectious inflammatory diseases of the CNS.

Infection is caused by microorganisms. *Inflammation* is not synonymous with infection. Inflammation (from the Latin meaning "to ignite" or "set alight") is the response of tissues to a variety of pathogens (which may or may not be infectious microorganisms). The inflammatory "cascade" is complex and multifactorial. It involves the vascular system, immune system, and cellular responses such as microglial activation, the primary component of the brain's innate immune response.

The CNS functions as a unique microenvironment that responds differently from the body's other systems to infiltrating immune cells. The brain white matter is especially susceptible to inflammatory disease. Inflammation can be acute or chronic, manageable or life-threatening. Imaging plays a central role in the identification and follow-up of neuroinflammatory disorders.

The bulk of Chapter 15 is devoted to multiple sclerosis (11-3). Also included is a discussion of MS variants (11-4) and the surprisingly broad spectrum of idiopathic (noninfectious) inflammatory demyelinating dis-

eases (IIDDs) such as neuromyelitis optica. Susac syndrome is a retinocochleocerebral vasculopathy that is often mistaken for MS on imaging studies, so it too is discussed in the context of IIDDs.

Post-infection, post-vaccination, autoimmune-mediated demyelinating disorders are considered next. Acute disseminated encephalomyelitis (ADEM) and its most fulminant variant, acute hemorrhagic leukoencephalitis (AHLE), are delineated in detail.

We close the chapter with a discussion of neurosarcoid and inflammatory pseudotumors.

Selected References

- Huskins WC et al: Intervention to reduce transmission of resistant bacteria in intensive care. N Engl J Med. 364(15):1407-18, 2011

CNS Infections

- Gupta RK et al: Imaging of central nervous system viral diseases. J Magn Reson Imaging. 35(3):477-91, 2012
- Nickerson JP et al: Neuroimaging of pediatric intracranial infection--part 1: techniques and bacterial infections. J Neuroimaging. 22(2):e42-51, 2012
- Mullins ME: Emergent neuroimaging of intracranial infection/inflammation. Radiol Clin North Am. 49(1):47-62, 2011

HIV/AIDS

- Huis in 't Veld D et al: The immune reconstitution inflammatory syndrome related to HIV co-infections: a review. Eur J Clin Microbiol Infect Dis. 31(6):919-27, 2012
- Silva AC et al: Neuropathology of AIDS: an autopsy review of 284 cases from Brazil comparing the findings pre- and post-HAART (highly active antiretroviral therapy) and pre- and postmortem correlation. AIDS Res Treat. 2012:186850, 2012
- Valcour V et al: Pathogenesis of HIV in the central nervous system. Curr HIV/AIDS Rep. 8(1):54-61, 2011
- Smith AB et al: From the archives of the AFIP: central nervous system infections associated with human immunodeficiency virus infection: radiologic-pathologic correlation. Radiographics. 28(7):2033-58, 2008

Demyelinating and Inflammatory Diseases

- Pierson E et al: Mechanisms regulating regional localization of inflammation during CNS autoimmunity. Immunol Rev. 248(1):205-15, 2012
- Ransohoff RM et al: Innate immunity in the central nervous system. J Clin Invest. 122(4):1164-71, 2012
- Zettl UK et al: Immune-mediated CNS diseases: a review on nosological classification and clinical features. Autoimmun Rev. 11(3):167-73, 2012
- Hu W et al: The pathological spectrum of CNS inflammatory demyelinating diseases. Semin Immunopathol. 31(4):439-53, 2009

12

Congenital, Acquired Pyogenic, and Acquired Viral Infections

Infectious diseases can be conveniently divided into congenital/neonatal and acquired infections. As infections of the developing brain have different manifestations and long-term neurological consequences compared to those that affect the more mature (fully developed) brain, we begin our discussion of CNS infections with this group of disorders.

We then delineate the first major category of acquired infections, i.e., pyogenic infections. We start with meningitis, the most common of the pyogenic infections. Abscess, together with its earliest manifestations (cerebritis) is discussed next, followed by considerations of ventriculitis (a rare but potentially fatal complication of deep-seated brain abscesses) and intracranial empyemas.

We close the chapter with a discussion of the pathologic and imaging manifestations of acquired viral infections.

Congenital Infections

With two exceptions (toxoplasmosis and syphilis), most congenital infections are viral and are usually secondary to transplacental passage of the agent.

Six members of the herpesvirus family cause neurologic disease in children: Herpes simplex virus 1 and 2 (HSV1, HSV2), varicella-zoster (VZV), Epstein-Barr (EBV), Cytomegalovirus (CMV), and human herpesvirus 6 (HHV-6). Aside from CMV, herpes encephalitis, and congenital HIV, congenital infections are now relatively rare because of childhood immunization and prenatal screening.

Infections of the fetal nervous system result in a spectrum of findings that depends on both the specific agent and timing of the infection. When infections occur early in fetal development (e.g., during the first trimester), they usually result in miscarriage or malformations such as lissencephaly.

When infections occur later, encephaloclastic manifestations predominate. Microcephaly with frank brain destruction and widespread encephalomalacia are common.

We begin with a brief overview of the so-called TORCH infections. We then consider specific agents individually, beginning with the most common of the congenital infections, Cytomegalovirus.

TORCH Infections

Terminology

Congenital infections are often grouped together and simply called **TORCH** infections—the acronym for **to**xoplasmosis, **r**ubella, **C**ytomegalovirus, and **h**erpes. If

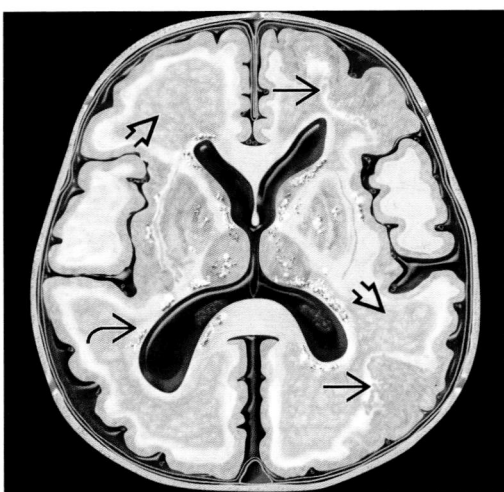

12-1. Congenital CMV is shown with periventricular parenchymal calcifications ➡, damaged white matter ⇥, dysplastic cortex ⇥.

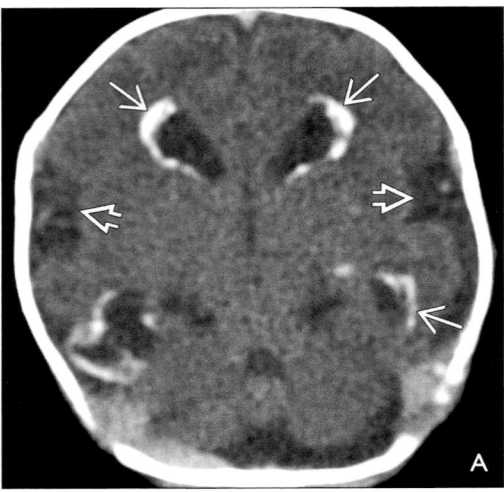

12-2A. NECT in a newborn with CMV shows microcephaly, large ventricles, shallow sylvian fissures ⇥, striking periventricular Ca++ ⇥.

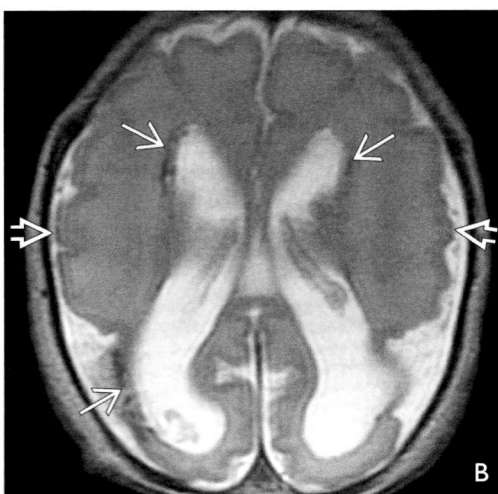

12-2B. T2WI in the same patient shows large ventricles, periventricular calcifications ➡, simplified gyral pattern ⇥.

congenital syphilis is included, the grouping is called TORCH(S) or (S)TORCH.

Etiology

In addition to the recognized "classic" TORCH infections, a host of new organisms have been identified as causing congenital and perinatal infections. These include HIV, hepatitis B, varicella, and tuberculosis.

Imaging

Toxoplasmosis, rubella, CMV, and HIV all cause parenchymal calcifications. CMV causes periventricular cysts, clefts, schizencephaly, and migrational defects. Rubella and herpes simplex virus (HSV) cause lobar destruction and encephalomalacia. Congenital syphilis is relatively rare but when it occurs, it causes basilar meningitis.

TORCH infections should be considered in newborns and infants with microcephaly, parenchymal calcifications, chorioretinitis, and intrauterine growth restriction.

Congenital Cytomegalovirus

CMV is the leading cause of nonhereditary deafness in children and is the most common cause of congenital infection in developed countries.

Terminology and Etiology

Congenital Cytomegalovirus infection is also called CMV encephalitis. CMV is a ubiquitous DNA virus that belongs to the human herpesvirus family.

Pathology

The timing of the gestational infection determines the brain insult. Early gestational CMV infection causes germinal zone necrosis with subependymal dystrophic calcifications. White matter volume loss occurs at all gestational ages and can be diffuse or multifocal. Malformations of cortical development are common (12-1).

Microscopic examination shows cytomegaly with viral inclusions in the nuclei and cytoplasm. Patchy and focal cellular necrosis, particularly of germinal matrix cells, is typical of first trimester infection. Vascular inflammation and thrombosis are also common.

Clinical Issues

EPIDEMIOLOGY. CMV is the most common of all congenital infections. Between 0.25-1% of newborn infants have CMV in their urine or saliva, as documented by PCR. Of these, only 10% develop CNS or systemic symptoms.

PRESENTATION AND NATURAL HISTORY. Infants with asymptomatic congenital CMV infections may be developmentally normal. Sensorineural hearing loss and mild developmental delay are the major long-term risks.

Newborns with systemic manifestations (e.g., hepatosplenomegaly, petechiae, and jaundice) have a slightly worse prognosis. Slightly over half of all infants with systemic manifestations also have CNS involvement. The vast majority with microcephaly, ventriculomegaly, and parenchymal calcifications have major neurodevelopmental sequelae (e.g., cerebral palsy, epilepsy, mental retardation).

TREATMENT OPTIONS. Early (before gestational week 17) maternal hyperimmunoglobulin therapy improves the outcome of fetuses from women with primary CMV infection. The use of antiviral agents is also being explored for the treatment of symptomatic congenital CMV beyond the neonatal period. Antiviral agents that specifically target CMV are ganciclovir (GCV), valganciclovir (VGVC), foscarnet (FOS), and cidofovir. VGVC is well-tolerated and may improve or help preserve auditory function in infected infants.

Imaging

GENERAL FEATURES. Imaging features of congenital CMV include microcephaly with ventriculomegaly, intracranial calcifications, white matter disease, and neuronal migration disorders. As a general rule, the earlier the infection, the more severe the findings.

CT FINDINGS. NECT scans show intracranial calcifications and ventriculomegaly in the majority of symptomatic infants. Calcifications are predominantly periventricular, with a predilection for the germinal matrix zones **(12-2A)**. Calcifications vary from numerous bilateral thick calcifications to subtle or faint punctate unilateral foci. Occasionally, calcification may be entirely absent; its lack should not preclude a diagnosis of congenital CMV.

MR FINDINGS. CMV exhibits a broad spectrum of MR abnormalities including microcephaly with ventriculomegaly, white matter volume loss, delayed myelination, and periventricular cysts. Migrational abnormalities are present in approximately 10-50% of cases. Cortical abnormalities range from minor dysgenesis with a simplified gyral pattern and "open" sylvian fissures to a near-agyric lissencephalic pattern **(12-2B)**.

T1 scans show subependymal hyperintense foci caused by the periventricular calcifications. Enlarged ventricles with germinolytic cysts in the adjacent white matter are common.

T2-weighted and FLAIR images show myelin delay or destruction and white matter volume loss with focal or

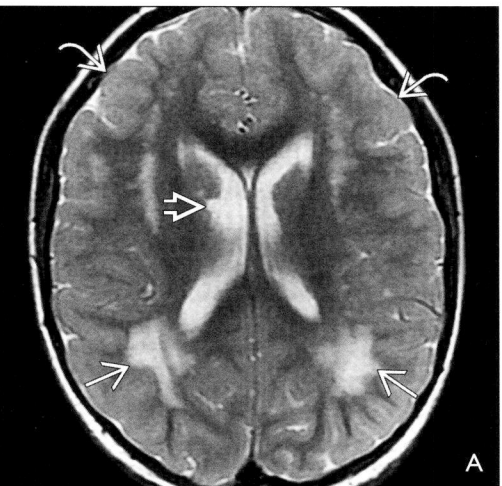

12-3A. T2WI in a 3-year-old girl with CMV shows confluent WM hyperintensities ➡, a connatal cyst ➡, malformations of cortical development ➡.

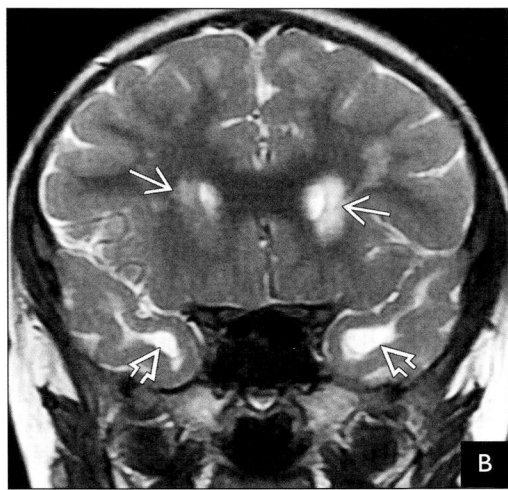

12-3B. Coronal T2WI in the same patient shows periventricular WM hyperintensities ➡, anterior temporal lobe cysts ➡.

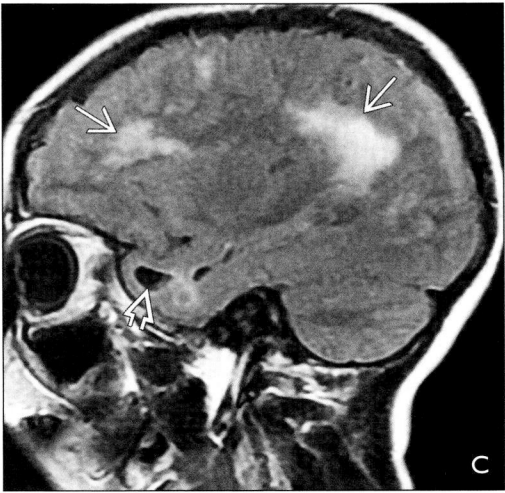

12-3C. Sagittal FLAIR shows the WM hyperintensities ➡, anterior temporal lobe cysts ➡.

confluent hyperintensities in most cases. Periventricular cysts, especially in the anterior temporal lobe, are common **(12-3)**.

ULTRASOUND. Sonography shows enlarged ventricles. Focal periventricular hyperechogenic foci that correspond to the subependymal calcifications observed on NECT scans are common. Germinolytic cysts may be present along the caudothalamic grooves. Lenticulostriate mineralizing vasculopathy occurs in 25-30% of cases and is seen as uni- or bilateral curvilinear echogenic streaks within the basal ganglia and thalami.

Fetal MR is more sensitive than US in the early detection of CMV-associated abnormalities.

Differential Diagnosis

The differential diagnosis of congenital CMV includes other TORCH infections, especially toxoplasmosis. **Toxoplasmosis** is much less common and typically causes scattered parenchymal calcifications, not the dominant subependymal pattern observed in CMV. Microcrania

and cortical dysplasia are also significantly less common in congenital toxoplasmosis.

Lymphocytic choriomeningitis (LCM) may mimic CMV on NECT scans. LCM typically causes necrotizing ependymitis and aqueductal obstruction with hydrocephalus and macrocephaly, not microcephaly.

The **pseudo-TORCH syndromes** such as Baraitser-Reardon and Aicardi-Goutières are rare autosomal recessive demyelination and degeneration disorders. Basal ganglia and brainstem calcifications are more common than the subependymal pattern characteristic of CMV.

Congenital Toxoplasmosis

Etiology and Pathology

Congenital toxoplasmosis (toxo) is caused by intrauterine infection with *Toxoplasma gondii*, a ubiquitous obligate intracellular parasite. Infected domestic cats are a major source of infection, which is usually acquired from undercooked meat or food products (usually fresh fruit and vegetables) contaminated by cat feces.

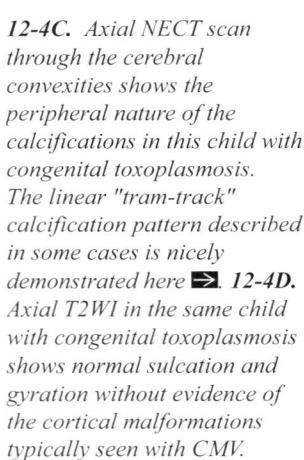

12-4A. *Axial NECT scan through the lateral ventricles in a 12-year-old retarded girl with known congenital toxoplasmosis. Punctate and linear calcifications primarily involve the cerebral cortex and subcortical white matter. Only a single periventricular calcification is present* ➡, *contrasting this case with CMV.* *12-4B.* *Axial NECT scan at the upper ventricular level in the same case shows more peripheral punctate calcifications.*

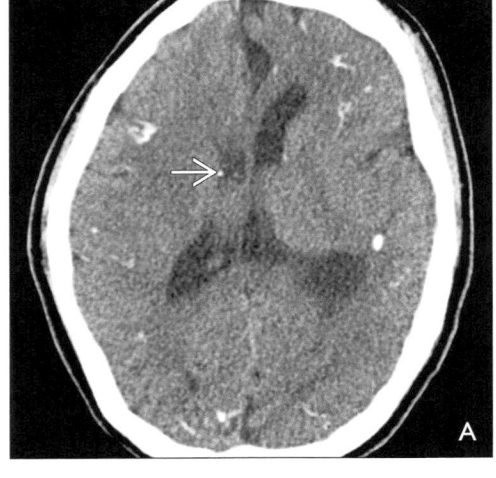

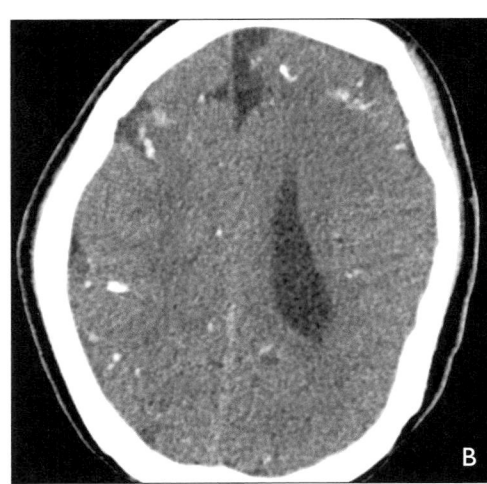

12-4C. *Axial NECT scan through the cerebral convexities shows the peripheral nature of the calcifications in this child with congenital toxoplasmosis. The linear "tram-track" calcification pattern described in some cases is nicely demonstrated here* ➡. *12-4D. Axial T2WI in the same child with congenital toxoplasmosis shows normal sulcation and gyration without evidence of the cortical malformations typically seen with CMV.*

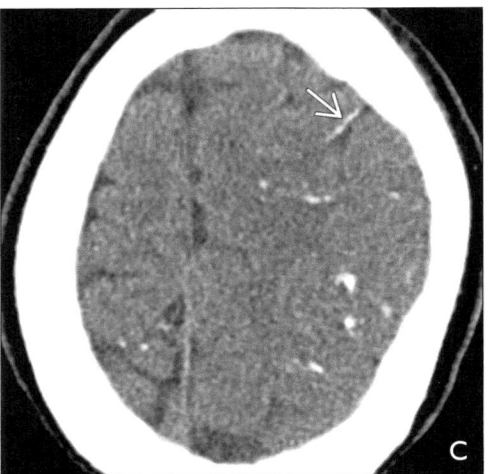

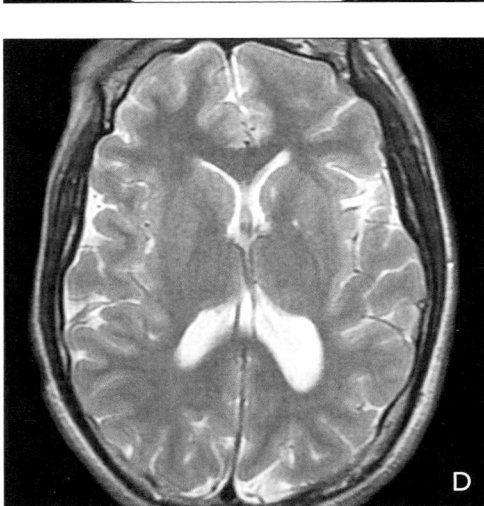

Macrocephaly with hydrocephalus and ependymitis are prominent gross features of congenital toxo. In contrast to CMV, malformations of cortical development are rare.

Clinical Issues

Toxoplasmosis is the second most common congenital infection. Approximately 5 in 1,000 pregnant women are infected with toxo. Estimates of the risk of fetal transmission vary from 10-100%.

Congenital toxo causes hepatosplenomegaly, growth retardation, chorioretinitis, and brain damage. Infants with subclinical infection at birth are at risk for delayed cognitive, motor, and visual defects.

Imaging and Differential Diagnosis

With some exceptions, imaging features of congenital toxo resemble those of CMV. NECT scans show extensive parenchymal calcifications that are predominantly cortical and subcortical (12-4). MR scans show multiple subcortical cysts and moderate to severe ventriculomegaly.

The major differential diagnosis of congenital toxo is CMV. The calcifications in toxo tend to be more peripheral while those of CMV are generally periventricular. Macrocephaly—not microcephaly—is typical. Malformations of cortical development are common in CMV but rare in toxo.

Congenital (Perinatal) HIV

The imaging presentation of congenital HIV infection is quite different from the findings in acquired HIV/AIDS. Congenital HIV resembles the other congenital viral infections and is therefore discussed here. Acquired HIV/AIDS is considered separately (see Chapter 14).

Etiology

The causative agent is the retrovirus human immunodeficiency virus type 1 (HIV). At least 90% of congenital HIV cases are vertically transmitted (mother-to-child transmission). Most infants become infected at birth or during the third trimester. Occasionally older infants are infected during breast feeding.

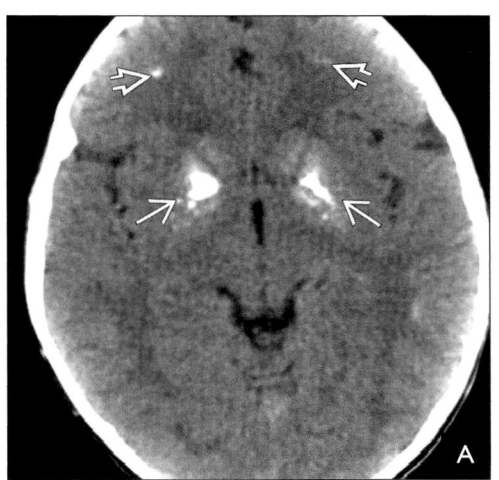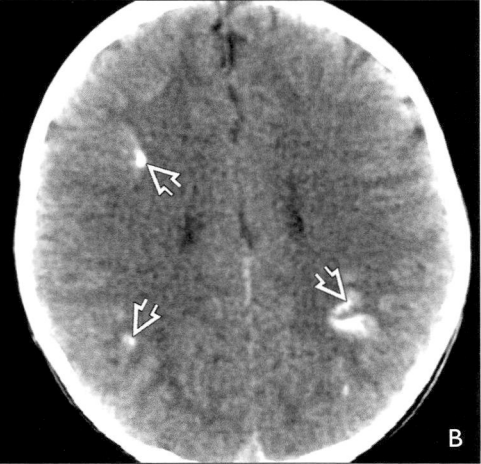

12-5A. Axial NECT scan in a 5-year-old child with congenital HIV shows bilateral symmetric calcifications in the basal ganglia ➡ and the subcortical white matter ⮞. 12-5B. Axial NECT scan in the same patient shows fairly symmetric punctate and curvilinear calcifications at the gray-white matter junctions ⮞ caused by mineralizing microangiopathy. (Courtesy V. Mathews, MD.)

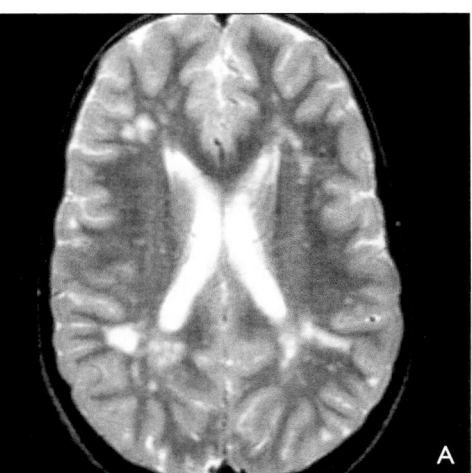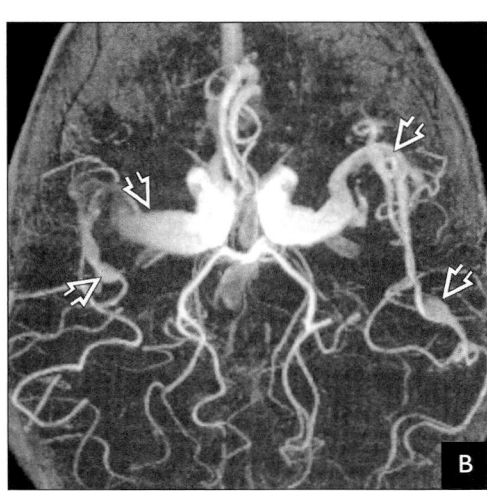

12-6A. Axial T2WI MR in an 11 year old demonstrates late manifestations of congenital HIV. Note prominent ventricles and sulci as well as multifocal white matter hyperintensities. 12-6B. Submentovertex view of an MRA obtained in the same patient shows striking fusiform arteriopathy in both middle cerebral arteries ⮞.

Pathology

The most characteristic gross finding is generalized brain volume loss with symmetric enlargement of the ventricles and subarachnoid spaces. Multiple foci of microglia, macrophages, and multinucleated giant cells containing viral particles are typical. Patchy myelin pallor and vacuolization are common. Mineralizing microangiopathy with basal ganglia calcifications and endothelial hypertrophy with gross cerebral vasculopathy are seen in some cases.

Clinical Issues

EPIDEMIOLOGY. Congenital HIV infection is diminishing as highly active antiretroviral therapy (HAART) becomes more widely available. Children account for just 2% of all HIV/AIDS patients in the USA and Europe but still represent 5-25% of cases worldwide. Congenital and acquired CMV infections are strong independent correlates of mother-to-child HIV transmission.

PRESENTATION AND NATURAL HISTORY. Symptoms generally begin around 12 postnatal weeks. Developmental delay, progressive motor dysfunction, and failure to thrive are the most common CNS symptoms. Hepatosplenomegaly and lymphadenopathy are common systemic manifestations of congenital HIV.

Approximately 20% of infected infants die. While opportunistic infections are less common in HIV-infected children compared to adults, stroke is more common.

Imaging

The most striking and consistent finding is atrophy, particularly in the frontal lobes. Bilaterally symmetric basal ganglia calcifications are common (12-5). Calcifications are sometimes identified in the hemispheric white matter and cerebellum.

Ectasia and fusiform enlargement of intracranial arteries is found in 3-5% of cases (12-6). Strokes with foci of restricted diffusion may occur as complications of the underlying vasculopathy.

Differential Diagnosis

The differential diagnosis of congenital HIV is other TORCH infections. **Cytomegalovirus** is characterized by periventricular calcifications, microcephaly, and cortical dysplasia. Other than volume loss, the brain in congenital HIV appears normal. **Toxoplasmosis** is much less common than CMV and causes scattered parenchymal calcifications, not symmetric basal ganglia lesions.

Congenital Herpes Encephalitis

Terminology

CNS involvement in herpes simplex virus (HSV) infection is called **congenital** or **neonatal HSV** when it involves neonates and herpes simplex encephalitis (HSE) in individuals beyond the first postnatal month. In this section, we discuss neonatal HSV; HSE is discussed below with other acquired viral infections.

Etiology

Approximately 75-80% of neonatal herpes encephalitis is caused by HSV type 2. The remainder is caused by HSV1. The morbidity and mortality in neonatal HSV2 encephalitis are significantly worse compared to HSV1 encephalitis.

Pathology

Neonatal HSV encephalitis is a diffuse disease, without the predilection for the temporal lobes and limbic system seen in older children and adults.

Early changes include meningoencephalitis with necrosis, hemorrhage, and microglial proliferation. Atrophy with gross cystic encephalomalacia and parenchymal calcifications is typical of late-stage HSV. Near-total loss of brain substance with hydranencephaly is seen in severe cases.

Clinical Issues

EPIDEMIOLOGY. HSV2 is one of the most prevalent sexually transmitted infections worldwide. Approximately 2% of women are infected by HSV2 during pregnancy. The majority are asymptomatic, and many infected individuals are unaware of the disease. Neonatal HSV infections are vertically transmitted, occurring in approximately one in 3,200 deliveries in the United States. Prevalence is higher in African-Americans, low-income mothers, and mothers with multiple sexual partners.

The vast majority (85%) of neonatal HSV is acquired at parturition, and 10% is contracted postnatally. Only 5% of cases are due to **in utero** transmission. The risk is increased with primary maternal infection during the third trimester and can be decreased by cesarean delivery.

PRESENTATION. Neonatal HSV infection causes three disease patterns: (1) skin, eye, and mouth disease, (2) encephalitis, and (3) disseminated disease with or without CNS disease. Approximately 50% of all infants with neonatal HSV will have CNS involvement, either isolated or as part of disseminated disease.

Lethargy, fever, poor feeding, seizures, and bulging fontanelle are common. Typical onset of symptoms sec-

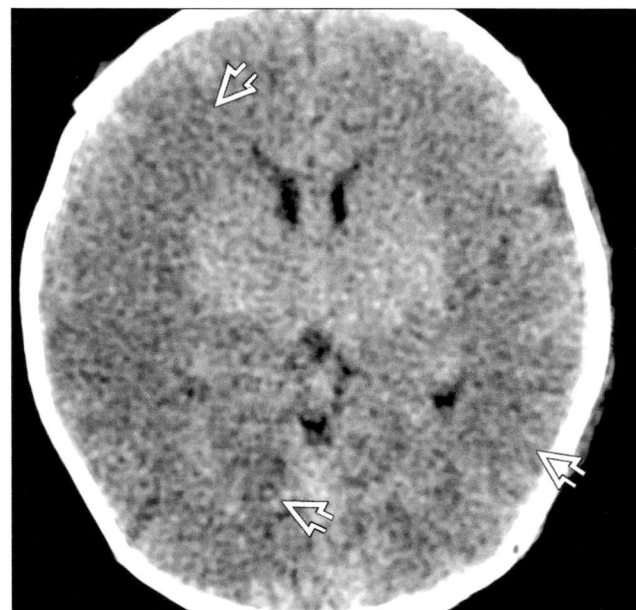

12-7. NECT in a neonate with HSV2 encephalitis shows widespread confluent hypodensity of the gray, white matter ⮕. *The basal ganglia are relatively unaffected.*

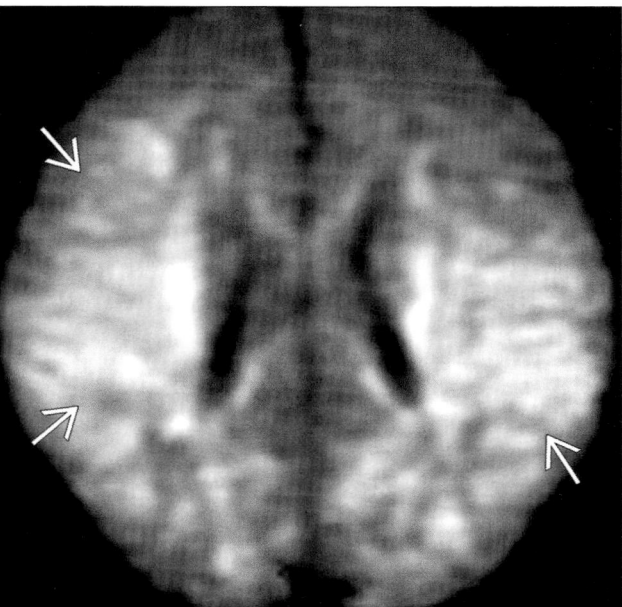

12-8. DWI in a 2-week-old infant with seizures, bulging fontanelles demonstrates extensive foci of restricted diffusion in both hemispheres ⮕. *HSV2 encephalitis.*

ondary to peripartum HSV infection is two to four weeks following delivery (peak = 16 days). The definitive diagnosis is based on PCR or viral isolation from ulcerated vesicles and/or scarifying mucocutaneous lesions.

NATURAL HISTORY. Death by one year of age occurs in approximately 50% of untreated neonates with overt CNS disease and 85% with disseminated infection. Half of surviving infants have permanent deafness, vision loss, cerebral palsy, and/or epilepsy.

TREATMENT OPTIONS. Antiviral therapy with high-dose acyclovir significantly reduces morbidity, especially in infants with disseminated disease, and should be initiated whenever perinatal HSV encephalitis is suspected.

maging

Unlike childhood or adult herpes simplex encephalitis, neonatal HSV CNS infection is much more diffuse. Both gray and white matter are affected.

CT FINDINGS. NECT scans may be normal early in the disease course, but widespread areas of hypoattenuation involving both cortex and subcortical white matter soon appear **(12-7)**. Hemorrhages may develop and are seen as multifocal punctate and curvilinear hyperdensities in the basal ganglia and cortex.

MR FINDINGS. MR is the imaging procedure of choice in suspected cases of neonatal HSV although the watery, unmyelinated neonatal brain makes it difficult to discriminate between infection and unaffected brain.

In the early stages, T1WI may be normal or demonstrate mild hypointensity in the affected areas. T2WI and FLAIR are more sensitive. Hyperintensity in the cortex, subcortical white matter, and basal ganglia is typical. Hemorrhagic foci are uncommon in early stages but may develop later and are best seen on T2* (GRE, SWI) sequences.

Foci of patchy enhancement, with or without meningeal enhancement, are common on T1 C+ scans. In later stages, T1 shortening and T2 hypointensity with "blooming" on T2* GRE secondary to hemorrhagic foci may develop **(12-9)**.

DWI is key to the diagnosis of congenital HSV encephalitis. In half of all patients, DWI demonstrates bilateral or significantly more extensive disease than seen on conventional MR **(12-8)**. Areas of restricted diffusion may be the only positive imaging findings in early cases. Late-stage disease shows severe volume loss with enlarged ventricles and multicystic encephalomalacia **(12-10)**, **(12-11)**.

ULTRASOUND. Ultrasound demonstrates linear echoes in the basal ganglia, similar to CMV.

Differential Diagnosis

The major differential diagnosis for neonatal HSV is **other TORCH infections**. Neonates with HSV are usually normal for the first few days after delivery. Brain scans are normal or minimally abnormal early in the disease course. Calcifications and migrational anomalies are absent.

12-9A. *A 4-week-old infant born to an HSV2-positive mother had several days of fever, lethargy. T1WI shows multiple bilateral cortical, basal ganglia foci of T1 shortening* ➡ *suggestive of subacute hemorrhage.* *12-9B. More cephalad scan in the same patient shows additional areas of cortical T1 shortening* ➡.

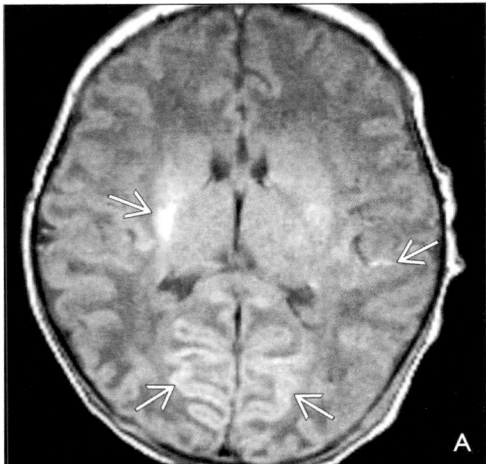
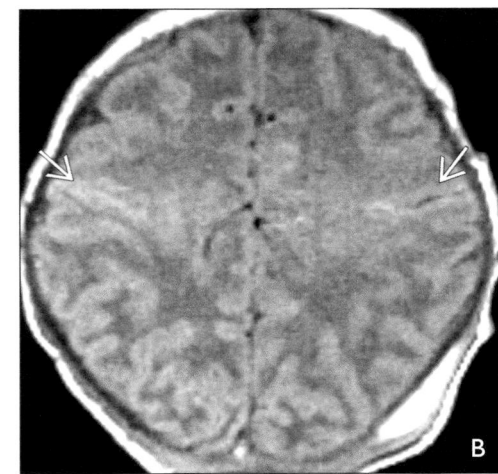

12-9C. *T2WI in the same infant obtained 1 month later shows dramatic interval changes of multicystic encephalomalacia with blood-fluid levels* ➡. *Note extensive areas of ribbon-like T2 shortening in the cortex* ➡ *secondary to hemorrhage.* *12-9D. More cephalad scan in the same patient illustrates extensive cystic encephalomalacia underlying more foci of gyral T2 shortening* ➡. *This case illustrates both early and late changes of congenital HSV.*

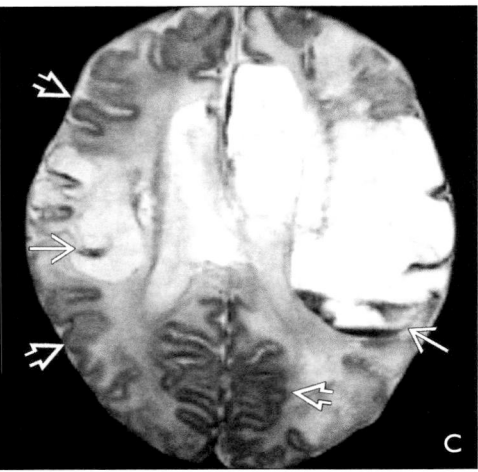
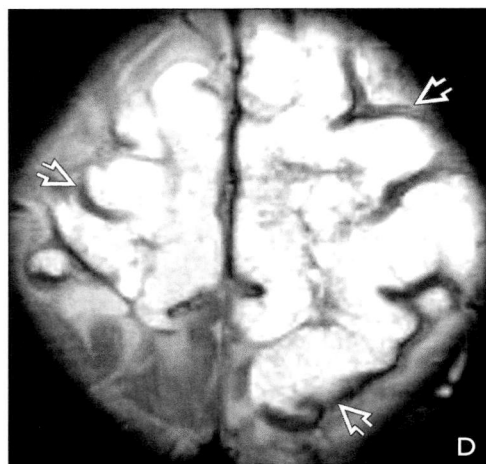

12-10. *Autopsied brain from an infant with end-stage HSV shows markedly enlarged ventricles with extensive cystic encephalomalacia in both hemispheres* ➡. *12-11. Coronal FLAIR in a microcephalic infant with a history of peripartum HSV2 shows extensive bihemispheric cystic encephalomalacia* ➡, *gliosis* ➡.

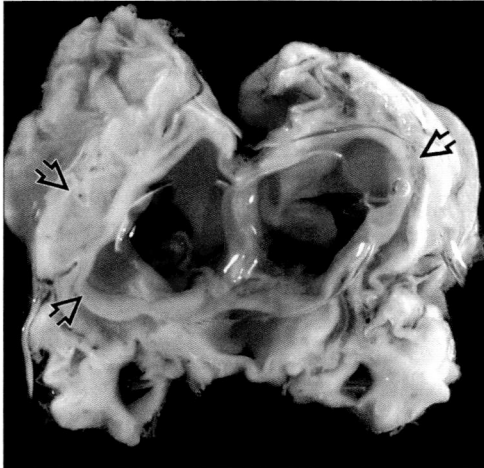
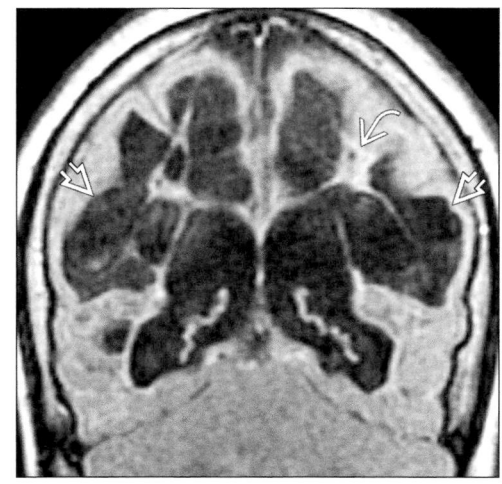

In some cases, HSV causes watershed distribution ischemic injury in areas remote from the primary herpetic lesions and may be difficult to distinguish from **hypoxic-ischemic injury** (HII). However, term infants with HII follow a different clinical course, becoming symptomatic in the intrapartum or immediate postnatal period. Profound HII preferentially affects the perirolandic cortex and sulcal depths, white matter, hippocampi, and deep gray nuclei including the ventrolateral thalami. Hemorrhage with "blooming" on T2* GRE is uncommon.

Other Congenital Infections

Rubella

Humans are the only reservoir for the rubella virus. Transmission is via virus-contaminated respiratory secretions. With the advent of measles-mumps-rubella vaccination, the worldwide prevalence of congenital rubella syndrome (CRS) has declined dramatically. Approximately 100,000 infants are born with CRS, mostly in countries with low national vaccination rates.

Early in utero infection results in miscarriage, fetal death, or congenital malformations in surviving infants. Late infection causes generalized brain volume loss, dystrophic calcifications, and regions of demyelination and/or gliosis.

The clinical spectrum of CRS includes ophthalmic, auditory, cardiac, and craniofacial defects. Imaging findings are nonspecific, varying from parenchymal calcifications on NECT scans to multiple foci of T2/FLAIR hyperintensity and volume loss with mildly enlarged ventricles and sulci (12-12).

Congenital Syphilis

Congenital syphilis (CS) is caused by transplacental passage of the *Treponema pallidum* spirochete from untreated mothers with syphilis. The prevalence of CS is low in most of the developed world although there has been a mild resurgence of the disease reported in several European countries.

Up to 60% of infants infected with CS are asymptomatic at birth. Symptoms typically develop later in infancy, are often subtle and nonspecific, and include seizures, stroke, and signs of increased intracranial pressure.

The most common imaging findings in CS are hydrocephalus and meningitis with leptomeningeal enhancement.

Lymphocytic Choriomeningitis

Congenital lymphocytic choriomeningitis (LCM) is a rare congenital infection caused by an arenavirus carried by feral hamsters and house mice. Its incidence during pregnancy is unknown.

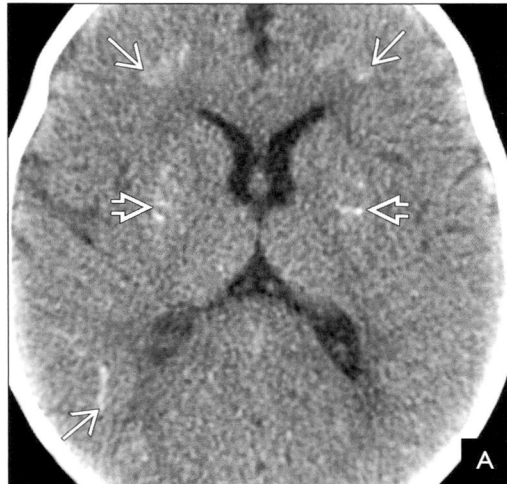

12-12A. NECT scan in an 18-month-old boy with congenital rubella shows subtle subcortical ➜, basal ganglia calcifications ➡.

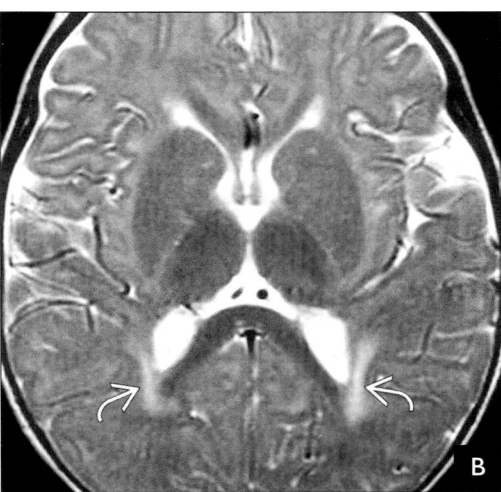

12-12B. T2WI in the same patient shows striking delayed myelination, symmetric periventricular hyperintensities ➜.

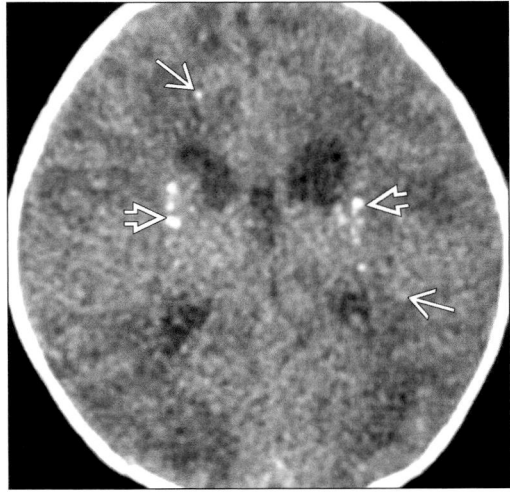

12-13. NECT in an infant with congenital lymphocytic choriomeningitis shows scattered parenchymal ➜, basal ganglia calcifications ➡.

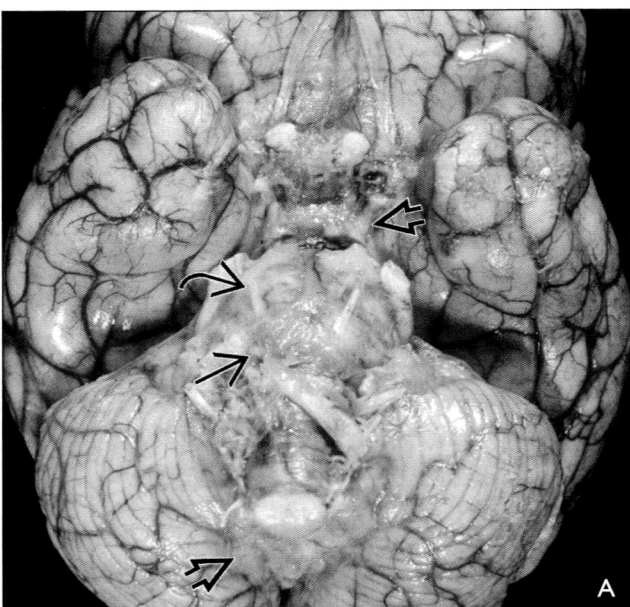

12-14A. Autopsied brain shows typical changes of severe meningitis with dense purulent exudate covering the pons ⮕, coating the cranial nerves ⮕, and filling all the basal cisterns ⮕.

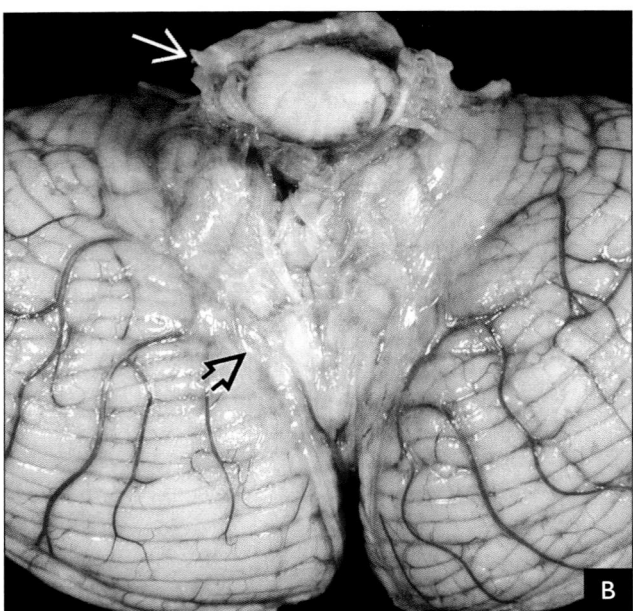

12-14B. The exudate coats the medulla ⮕ and completely fills the cisterna magna ⮕. (Courtesy R. Hewlett, MD.)

LCM causes a necrotizing ependymitis with aqueductal obstruction and hydrocephalus. The imaging appearance of LCM is virtually identical to that of CMV and toxo with scattered basal ganglia calcifications on NECT (12-13).

TORCH(S) INFECTIONS

Terminology
- Acronym for
  - **TO**xoplasmosis
  - **R**ubella
  - **C**ytomegalovirus
  - **H**erpes
  - **S**yphilis
- Others
  - HIV
  - Rubella
  - Lymphocytic choriomeningitis

Pathology
- Timing of infection during fetal development determines pathology of insult
- Timing more important than specific agent involved
  - Early insult → brain malformations
  - Late insult → encephaloclastic, destructive changes

General Imaging Findings
- Calcifications
  - Periventricular (especially CMV)
  - Parenchymal (especially toxo)
- Microcephaly, ventriculomegaly
- Migrational defects
  - Polymicrogyria
  - Schizencephaly
- Volume loss
- White matter hyperintensities
- Germinolytic cysts

Acquired Pyogenic Infections

Meningitis

Terminology

Meningitis is an acute or chronic inflammatory infiltrate of meninges and CSF. **Pachymeningitis** involves the dura-arachnoid; **leptomeningitis** affects the pia and subarachnoid spaces.

Etiology

Meningitis can be acquired in several different ways. *Hematogenous spread* from remote systemic infection is the most common route. Direct *geographic extension* from sinusitis, otitis, or mastoiditis is the second most common method of spread. *Penetrating injuries* and *skull fractures* (especially of the skull base) are rare but important causes of meningitis.

Many different infectious agents can cause meningitis. Most cases are caused by acute pyogenic (bacterial) infection. Meningitis can also be acute lymphocytic (viral) or chronic (tubercular or granulomatous).

The most common responsible agent varies with age, geography, and immune status. Group B β-hemolytic streptococcal meningitis is the leading cause of newborn

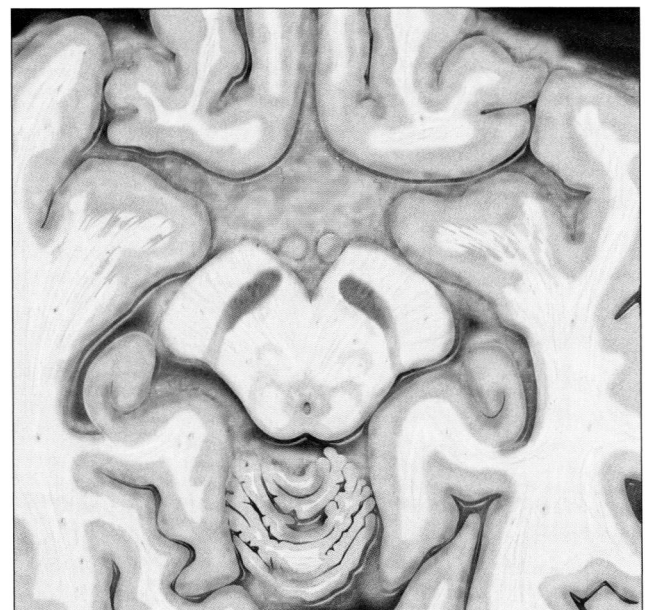

12-15. Graphic of meningitis shows diffuse purulent exudate that involves the leptomeninges and fills the basal cisterns and sulci. The underlying brain is mildly hyperemic.

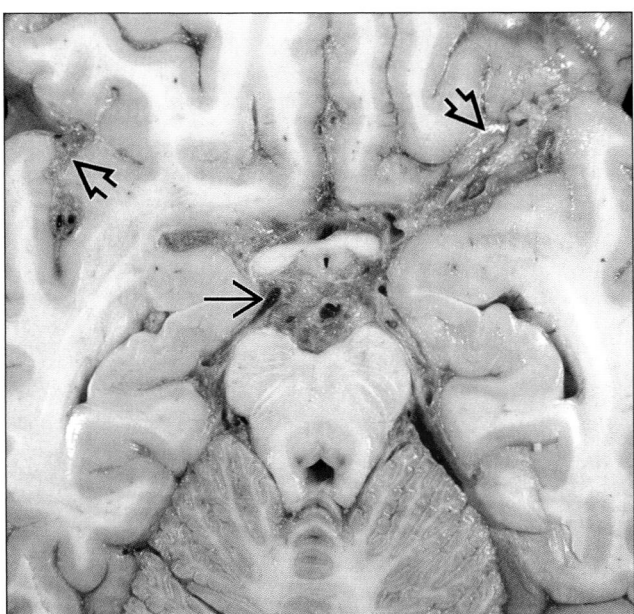

12-16. Axial autopsy section shows meningitis with exudate completely filling the suprasellar cistern ⊇ and sylvian fissures ⊋. (Courtesy R. Hewlett, MD.)

meningitis in developed countries while enteric, gram-negative organisms (typically *Escherichia coli*, less commonly *Enterobacter* or *Citrobacter*) cause the majority of cases in developing countries.

Vaccination has significantly decreased the incidence of *Haemophilus influenzae* meningitis, so the most common cause of childhood bacterial meningitis is now *Neisseria meningitidis*. Adult meningitis is typically caused by *Streptococcus pneumoniae* or *N. meningitidis*. *Listeria monocytogenes*, *S. pneumoniae*, and *N. meningitidis* affect elderly patients. Tuberculous meningitis is common in developing countries and in immunocompromised patients (e.g., HIV/AIDS, solid organ transplant recipients).

Pathology

LOCATION. The basal cisterns and subarachnoid spaces are the CSF spaces most commonly involved by meningitis (12-14), (12-15), (12-16), followed by the cerebral convexity sulci.

GROSS PATHOLOGY. Cloudy CSF initially fills the subarachnoid spaces, followed by development of a variably dense purulent exudate that covers the pial surfaces. Vessels within the exudate may show inflammatory changes and necrosis.

MICROSCOPIC FEATURES. The meningeal exudate contains the inciting organisms, inflammatory cells, fibrin, and cellular debris. The underlying brain parenchyma is often edematous, with subpial astrocytic and microglial proliferation.

Meningoencephalitis shows inflammatory changes in the pia, and the perivascular spaces may act as a conduit for extension from the pia into the underlying brain parenchyma.

Clinical Issues

EPIDEMIOLOGY AND DEMOGRAPHICS. Pyogenic meningitis is the most common cause of acute febrile encephalopathy and reaches all social strata. The overall prevalence of meningitis is estimated at 3:100,000 in industrialized countries. In the United States, meningitis is diagnosed in 62:100,000 emergency department visits.

PRESENTATION. Presentation depends on patient age. In adults, headache, fever, nuchal rigidity, and altered mental status are common symptoms. Fever, lethargy, and irritability are common in infants. Children with *N. meningitidis* infection may develop a purpuric rash. Seizures occur in 30% of patients.

CSF shows leukocytosis (mainly polymorphonuclear cells), elevated protein, and decreased glucose.

NATURAL HISTORY. Despite rapid recognition and effective therapy, meningitis still has significant morbidity and mortality rates. Death rates from 15-25% have been reported in disadvantaged children with poor living conditions.

Complications are both common and numerous. **Extraventricular obstructive hydrocephalus** is one of the earliest and most common complications. The choroid plexus can become infected, causing choroid plexitis and then **ventriculitis**. Infection can also extend from the pia along the perivascular spaces into the brain parenchyma itself, causing **cerebritis** and then **abscess**.

Sub- and epidural **empyemas** or sterile **effusions** may develop. **Cerebrovascular complications** of meningitis include vasculitis, thrombosis, and occlusion of both arteries and veins.

TREATMENT OPTIONS. Specific antibiotic therapy should be based on culture and sensitivity.

Imaging

GENERAL FEATURES. Imaging should be used in conjunction with—and not as a substitute for—appropriate clinical and laboratory evaluation. Imaging studies are best used to confirm the diagnosis and assess possible complications. While CT is commonly employed as a screening examination in cases of suspected meningitis, both primary and acute manifestations of meningitis as well as secondary complications are best depicted on MR.

CT FINDINGS. Initial NECT scans may be normal or show only mild ventricular enlargement **(12-17A)**. "Blurred" ventricular margins indicate acute obstructive hydrocephalus with accumulation of extracellular fluid in the deep white matter. Bone CT should be carefully evaluated for sinusitis and otomastoiditis.

As the cellular inflammatory exudate develops, it replaces the normally clear CSF. The cisterns and sulci appear effaced as they become almost isodense with brain **(12-18A)**.

CECT shows intense enhancement of the inflammatory exudate as it covers the brain surfaces, extending into and filling the sulci **(12-17B)**, **(12-18B)**, **(12-19)**.

MR FINDINGS. The purulent exudates of acute meningitis are isointense with underlying brain on T1WI, giving the appearance of "dirty" CSF. The exudates are isointense with CSF on T2WI and do not suppress on FLAIR **(12-20A)**. Hyperintensity in the subarachnoid cisterns and superficial sulci on FLAIR is a typical but nonspecific finding of meningitis.

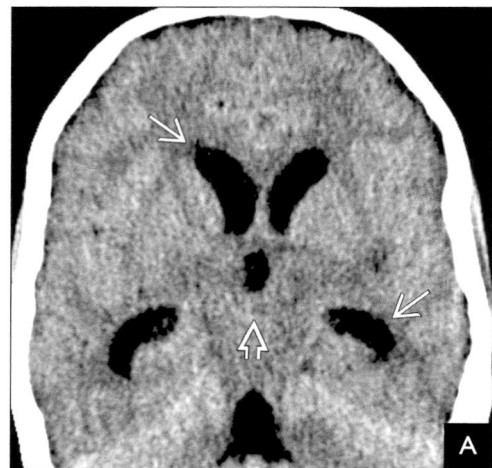
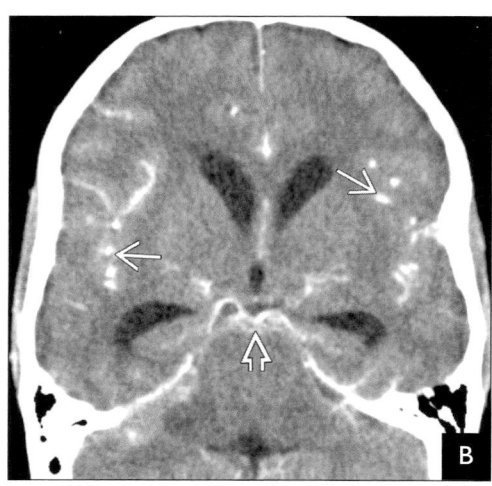

12-17A. NECT scan shows typical changes of meningitis with enlarged ventricles, slightly "blurred" margins ➡, effaced suprasellar and interpeduncular cisterns ➡. 12-17B. CECT scan in the same patient shows enhancing exudate filling the sylvian fissures ➡, coating the surface of the pons and interpeduncular cistern ➡.

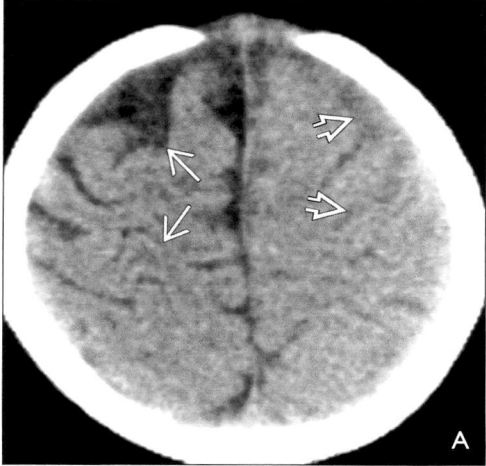
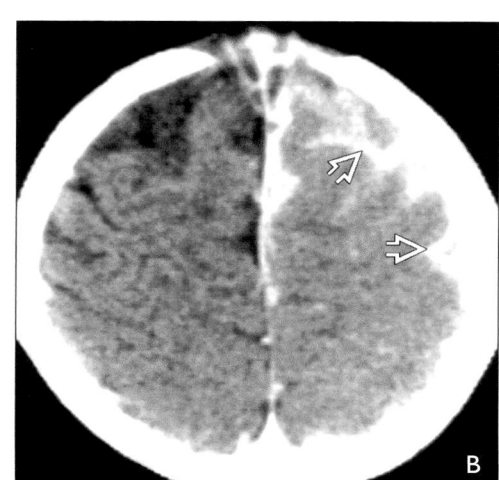

12-18A. NECT scan in a child with meningitis shows relatively normal-appearing CSF-filled sulci over the right cerebral hemisphere ➡. In contrast, sulci over the left convexity are effaced ➡ and filled with pus, appearing almost isointense with the underlying cortex. 12-18B. CECT scan in the same patient shows intense enhancement of the left-sided exudate that covers the brain surface and completely fills the sulci ➡.

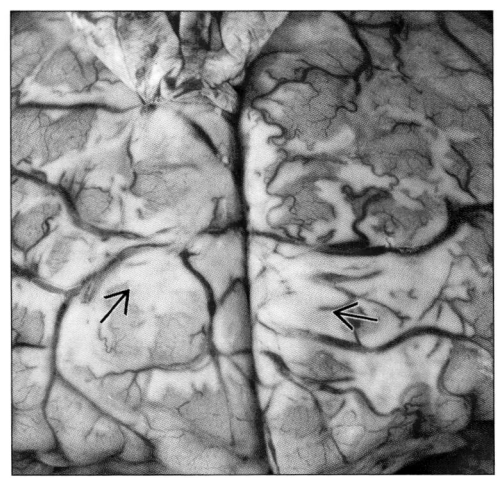

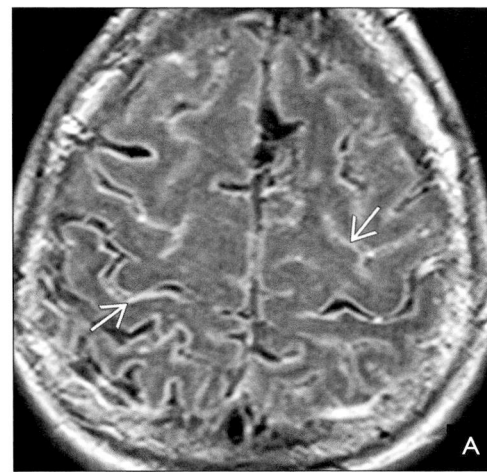

12-19. *Close-up view of autopsied brain displays purulent exudate filling the subarachnoid spaces and obliterating the convexity sulci ➡. (Courtesy R. Hewlett, MD.)* *12-20A.* *FLAIR scan in a patient with pyogenic meningitis shows hyperintensity covering the pial surfaces of all the convexity gyri ➡.*

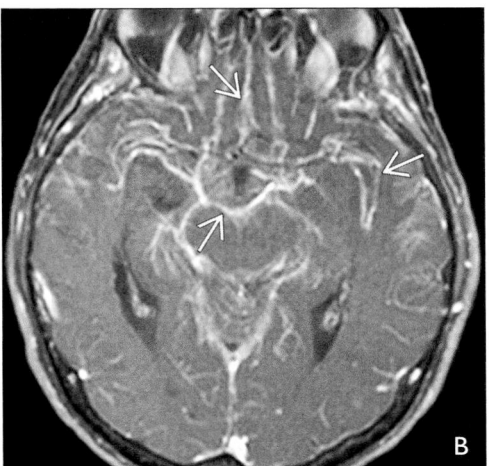

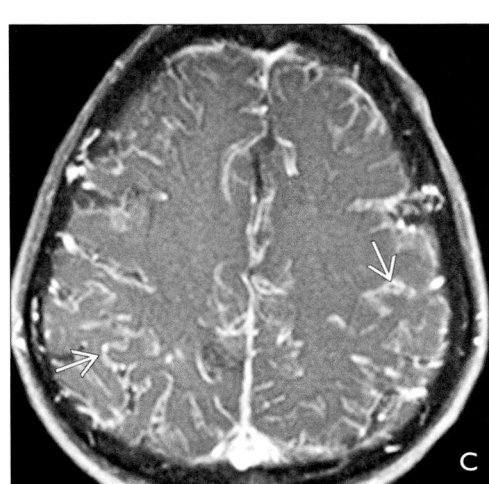

12-20B. *T1 C+ FS scan in the same patient shows diffuse, intense enhancement of the basal cisterns, sulci ➡. 12-20C.* *Scan through the corona radiata in the same patient shows that the enhancement covers the pial surfaces of the gyri and fills the convexity sulci ➡. Classic findings of pyogenic meningitis.*

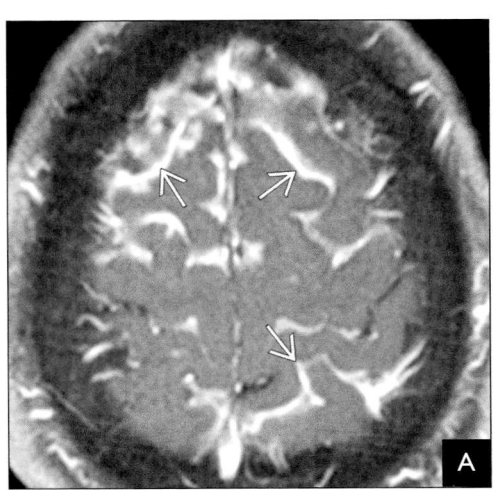

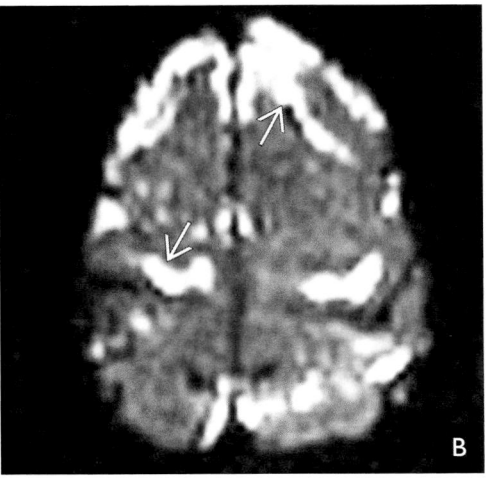

12-21A. *T1 C+ FS scan in a case of especially severe pyogenic meningitis shows diffuse, intensely enhancing exudate completely filling all the convexity sulci ➡. 12-21B.* *DWI in the same patient shows that the pus in the sulci restricts strongly ➡.*

DWI is especially helpful in meningitis, as the purulent subarachnoid space exudates usually show restriction (12-21B). Meningitis enhances intensely and uniformly on T1 C+ (12-20B), (12-20C), (12-21A). A curvilinear pattern that follows the gyri and sulci (the "pial-cisternal" pattern) is more common than dura-arachnoid enhancement. Delayed contrast-enhanced FLAIR scans may be a helpful addition in detecting subtle cases.

ANGIOGRAPHY. Irregular foci of constriction and dilatation characteristic of vasculitis can sometimes be identified on CTA or DSA.

COMPLICATIONS OF MENINGITIS. Other than hydrocephalus, complications from meningitis are relatively uncommon. Post-meningitis reactive **effusions**—sterile CSF-like fluid pockets—develop in 5-10% of children treated for acute bacterial meningitis. Effusions are generally benign lesions that regress spontaneously over a few days and do not require treatment.

Effusions can occur either in the subdural (most common) or subarachnoid spaces. The frontal, parietal, and temporal convexities are the most common sites. NECT shows bilateral crescentic extraaxial collections that are iso- to slightly hyperdense compared to normal CSF.

Effusions are iso- to slightly hyperintense to CSF on T1WI and isointense on T2WI. They are often slightly hyperintense relative to CSF on FLAIR (12-22A). Effusions usually do not enhance on T1 C+ but occasionally demonstrate enhancement along the medial (cerebral) surfaces of the lesions. Effusions do not restrict on DWI, differentiating them from subdural empyemas (12-22B).

Less common complications include pyocephalus (ventriculitis), empyema (12-23), cerebritis and/or abscess, and ischemia. All are discussed separately below.

Differential Diagnosis

The major differential diagnosis of infectious meningitis is neoplastic or **"carcinomatous" meningitis**, which can appear identical on imaging so clinical information is essential. Remember: Sulcal/cisternal FLAIR hyperintensity is a nonspecific finding and can be seen with a number of different entities (see box).

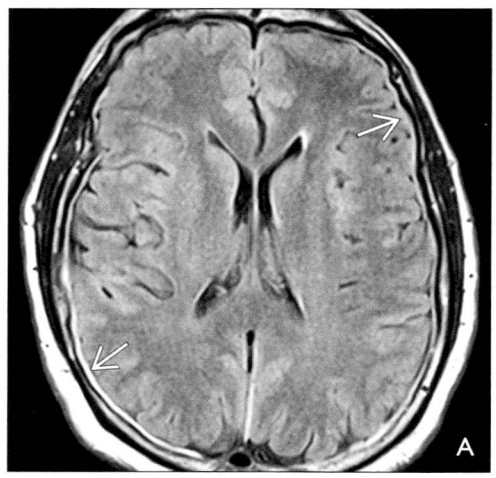
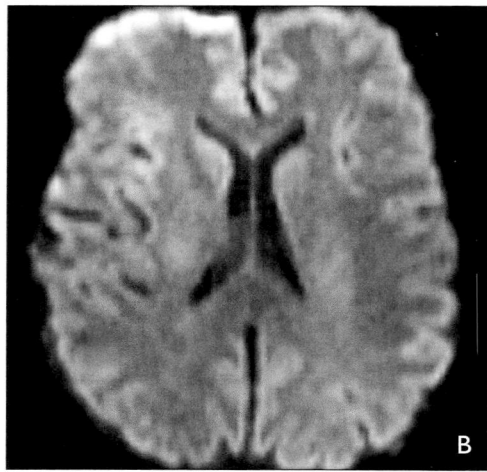

12-22A. Axial FLAIR scan in a 60-year-old man with headaches, history of recent staphylococcus meningitis shows a thin hyperintense subdural fluid collection ➔. The collection did not enhance on T1 C+ (not shown). 12-22B. DWI in the same patient shows no diffusion restriction. Subdural effusion. (Courtesy P. Hildenbrand, MD.)

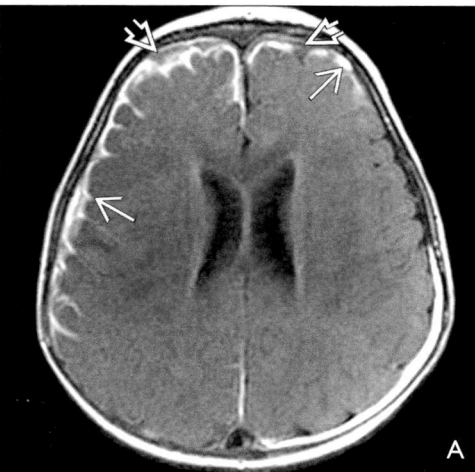
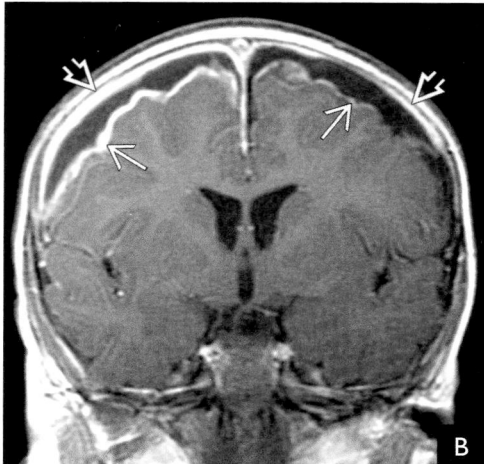

12-23A. Axial T1 C+ scan in a child with pyogenic meningitis shows pia-subarachnoid space enhancement that follows the surfaces of the brain, extending into the sulci ➔. A small bifrontal fluid collection ⊳ is present. 12-23B. Coronal T1 C+ scan shows that the meningitis extends over the brain surface ➔. The fluid collections are encased by a thickened membrane ⊳ under the calvaria. Subdural empyemas complicating meningitis.

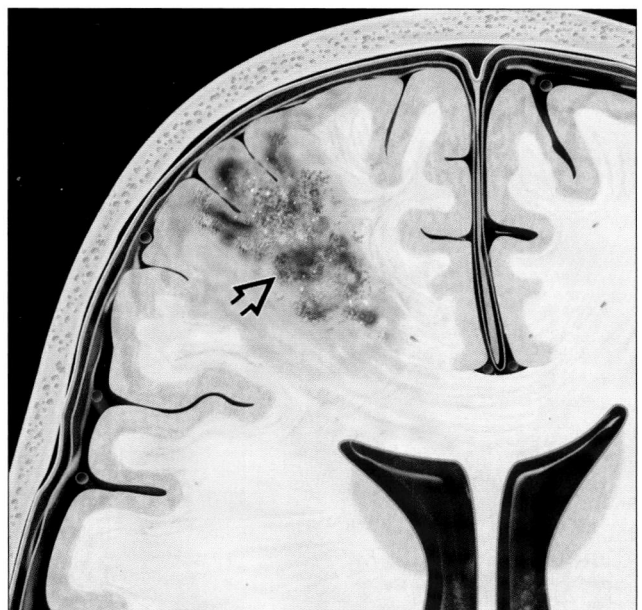

12-24. *Axial graphic shows early cerebritis (the initial phase of abscess formation) in the right frontal lobe. There is a focal unencapsulated mass of petechial hemorrhage, inflammatory cells, and edema* 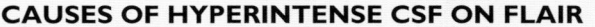.

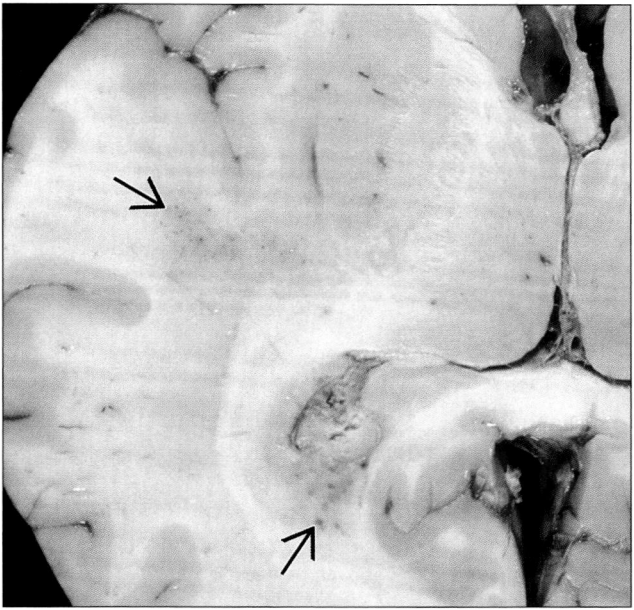

12-25. *Autopsy specimen from a patient with sepsis, seizures shows 2 small foci of early cerebritis with unencapsulated edema, petechial hemorrhages* ➡. *(Courtesy R. Hewlett, MD.)*

CAUSES OF HYPERINTENSE CSF ON FLAIR

Common
- Blood
  - Subarachnoid hemorrhage
- Infection
  - Meningitis
- Artifact
  - Susceptibility
  - Flow
- Tumor
  - CSF metastases

Less Common
- High inspired oxygen
  - 4-5x signal with 100% O_2
- Prominent vessels
  - Stroke (pial collaterals)
  - "Ivy" sign (moyamoya)
  - Pial angioma (Sturge-Weber)

Rare but Important
- Fat (ruptured dermoid)
- Gadolinium in CSF
  - Renal failure
  - Blood-brain barrier leakage

Abscess

Terminology

A cerebral abscess is a localized infection of the brain parenchyma.

Etiology

Most abscesses are caused by hematogenous spread from an extracranial location (e.g., lung or urinary tract infection, endocarditis). Abscesses may also result from penetrating injury or direct geographic extension from sinonasal and otomastoid infection. These typically begin as extraaxial infections such as empyema (see below) or meningitis (see above) and then spread into the brain itself.

Abscesses are most often bacterial but they can also be fungal, parasitic, or (rarely) granulomatous. Although myriad organisms can cause abscess formation, the most common agents in immunocompetent adults are *Streptococcus* species, *Staphylococcus aureus*, and pneumococci. *Citrobacter* is a common agent in neonates. In 20-30% of abscesses, cultures are sterile and no specific organism is identified.

Proinflammatory molecules such as tumor necrosis factor-α (TNF-α) and interleukin-1-β (IL1-β) induce various cell adhesion molecules (CAMs) that facilitate extravasation of peripheral immune cells and promote abscess development.

Bacterial abscesses are relatively uncommon in immunocompromised patients. *Klebsiella* is common in diabetics, and fungal infections by *Aspergillus* and *Nocardia* are common in transplant recipients. In patients with HIV/AIDS, toxoplasmosis and tuberculosis are the most common opportunistic infections.

Pathology

Four general stages are recognized in the evolution of a cerebral abscess: (1) early cerebritis, (2) late cerebritis, (3) early capsule, and (4) late capsule. Each has its own

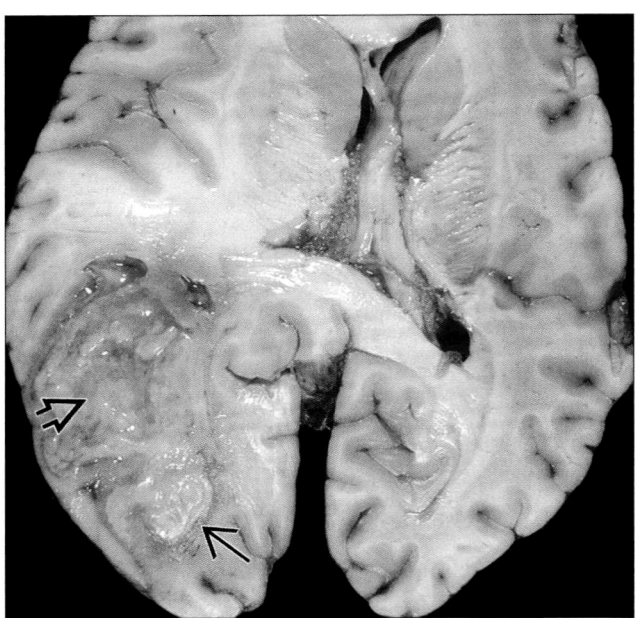

12-26. Autopsy case demonstrates typical pathologic findings of late cerebritis with significant mass effect, edema. The coalescing lesion shows some central necrosis ⊵ and an ill-defined rim of petechial hemorrhage ⊵.

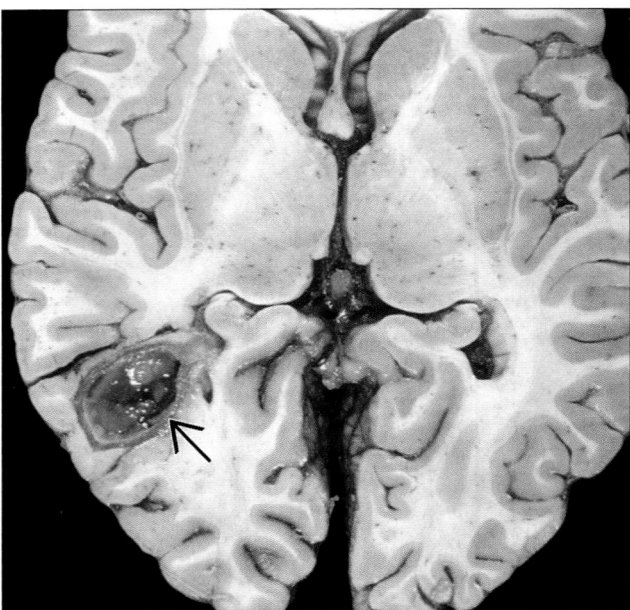

12-27. Another autopsy case shows typical findings of a cerebral abscess at the early capsule stage. The liquefied necrotic core of the lesion is surrounded by a well-developed capsule ⊵. (Courtesy R. Hewlett, MD.)

distinctive pathologic appearance, which in turn determines the imaging findings.

EARLY CEREBRITIS. In the early cerebritis stage of abscess formation, infection is focal but not yet localized (12-24). An unencapsulated, edematous, hyperemic mass of leukocytes and bacteria is intermixed with patchy necrotic foci and petechial hemorrhages (12-25). Early cerebritis typically begins three to five days after the initial infection.

LATE CEREBRITIS. The next stage of abscess formation is late cerebritis, which begins at four or five days after infection and lasts between 10 days and two weeks. Necrotic foci coalesce, forming a confluent core. The necrotic center is surrounded by a poorly organized rim of inflammatory cells, macrophages, granulation tissue, and fibroblasts. Capillary proliferation and surrounding vasogenic edema become more prominent (12-26).

EARLY CAPSULE. The early capsule stage starts around two weeks and may last for a month or two. The necrotic core liquefies, and proliferating granulation tissue around the rim gradually forms a well-delineated collagenous capsule (12-27). Vasogenic edema begins to decrease.

LATE CAPSULE. With treatment, the central cavity gradually involutes and shrinks, collagen deposition further thickens the wall, and the surrounding vasogenic edema disappears. This late capsule stage begins several weeks following infection and may last for several months. Eventually, only a small nonenhancing gliotic nodule of collagen and fibroblasts remains.

Clinical Issues

EPIDEMIOLOGY. Brain abscesses are rare. Only 2,500 cases are reported annually in the USA.

DEMOGRAPHICS. Brain abscesses occur at all ages but are most common in patients between the third and fourth decades. Almost 25% occur in children under the age of 15 years. The M:F ratio is 2:1 in adults and 3:1 in children.

PRESENTATION. Headache, seizure, and focal neurologic deficits are the typical presenting symptoms. Fever is common but not universal. CSF cultures may be normal early in the infection.

PROGNOSIS. Brain abscesses are potentially fatal but treatable lesions. Rapid diagnosis, stereotactic surgery, and appropriate medical treatment have reduced mortality to 2-4%.

Imaging

GENERAL FEATURES. Imaging findings evolve with time and are related to the stage of abscess development. MR is more sensitive than CT and is the procedure of choice.

EARLY CEREBRITIS. Very early cerebritis may be invisible on CT. A poorly marginated cortical/subcortical hypodense mass is the most common finding (12-28A). Early cerebritis often shows little or no enhancement on CECT.

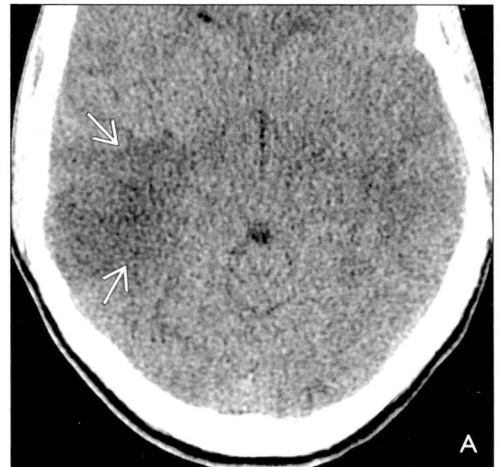

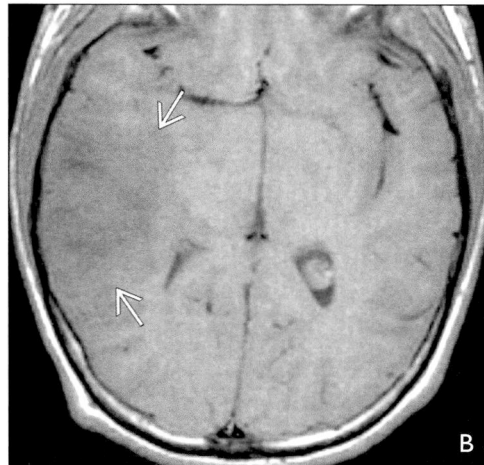

12-28A. A 16-year-old male with a 2-day history of headache, nausea, vomiting, and disorientation following an upper respiratory infection. NECT shows an ill-defined hypodensity ➔ with mild mass effect in the right posterosuperior temporal lobe. Because the lesion involved both the cortex and subcortical WM, the initial imaging diagnosis was territorial infarction. 12-28B. MR was obtained. T1WI shows an ill-defined hypointense mass ➔ in the posterior temporal lobe.

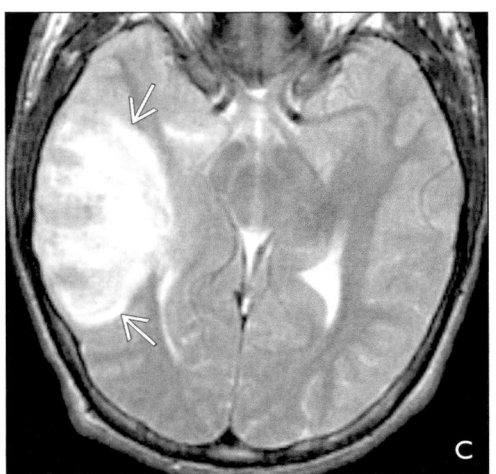

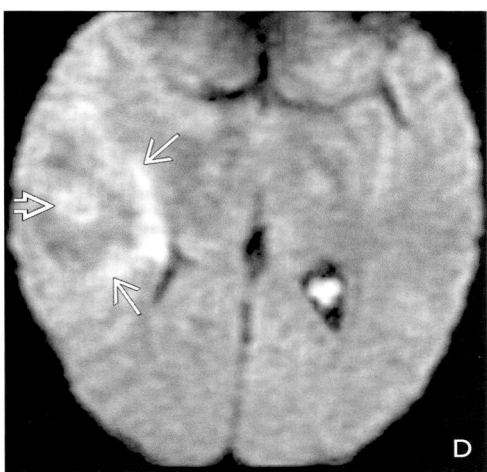

12-28C. T2WI in the same patient shows a mixed iso- and hyperintense mass ➔. 12-28D. DWI shows mild restricted diffusion at the periphery ➔ and center ➔ of the lesion, not what would be expected for a late acute cerebral infarct.

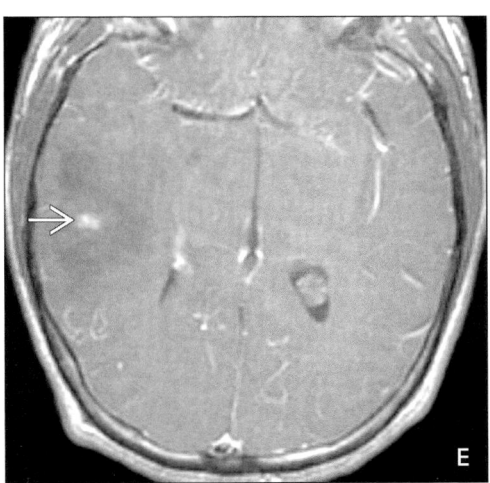

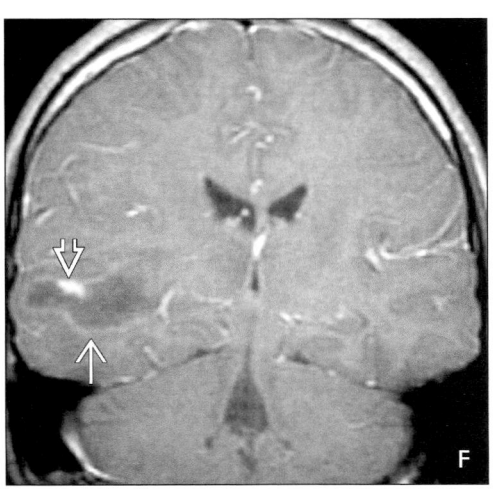

12-28E. T1 C+ scan shows a tiny enhancing focus ➔ in the center of the largely nonenhancing mass. The enhancement corresponds to the center of the diffusion restriction noted on DWI image. 12-28F. Slightly delayed coronal T1 C+ scan shows the enhancing focus ➔ as well as a faint rim of peripheral enhancement around the lesion ➔. Typical imaging findings of early cerebritis.

12-29A. *Axial T1WI in a 12-year-old boy with a 5-day history of a flu-like illness and increasing headache shows a predominantly hypointense mass* ⇨ *with an incomplete, slightly hyperintense rim* ➡. *12-29B. T2WI shows a "double rim" sign with hypointense outer* ⇨, *hyperintense inner rim* ➡.

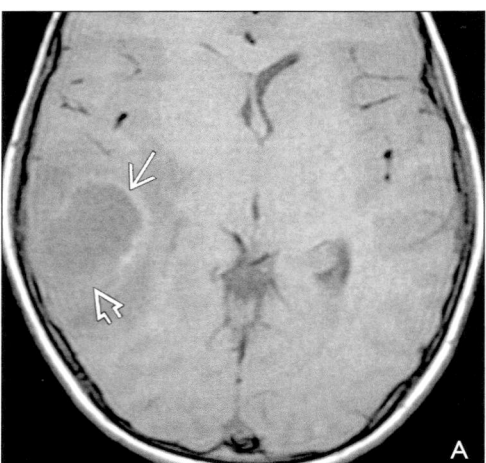

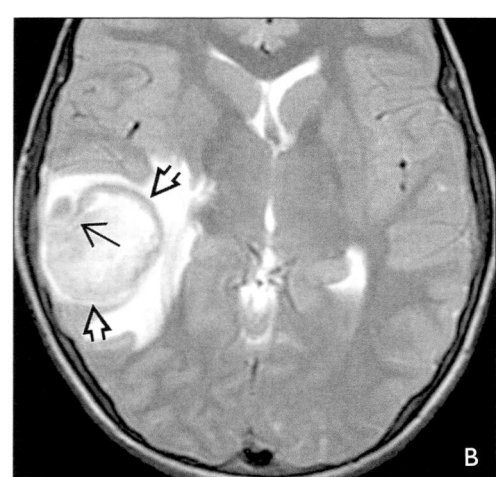

12-29C. *The rim* ⇨ *is hyperintense on FLAIR. Moderate peripheral edema is present.* *12-29D. T1 C+ FS scan shows rim enhancement* ⇨ *around the nonenhancing center of the mass.*

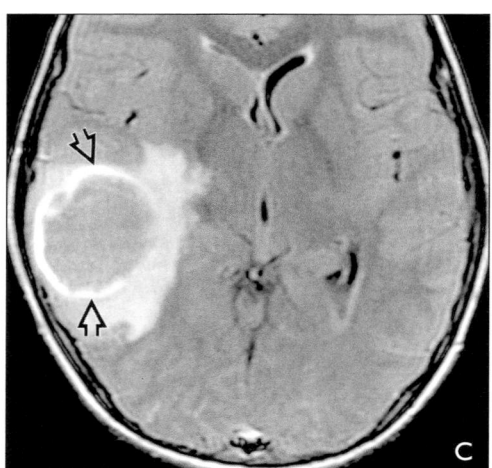

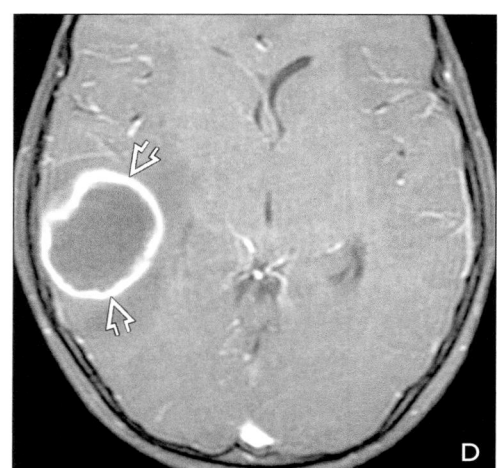

12-29E. *DWI shows that the center of the lesion restricts strongly* ➡. *12-29F. MRS of the cavity TR 2,000 TE 35. Amino acids (valine, leucine, isoleucine) at 0.9 ppm* ➡, *acetate at 1.9 ppm* ➡, *lactate at 1.3 ppm* ➈, *and succinate at 2.4 ppm (double straight arrows). Imaging findings are those of an abscess at the late cerebritis/early capsule stage.*

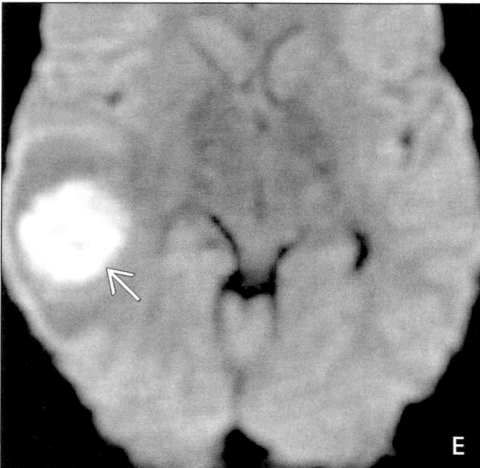

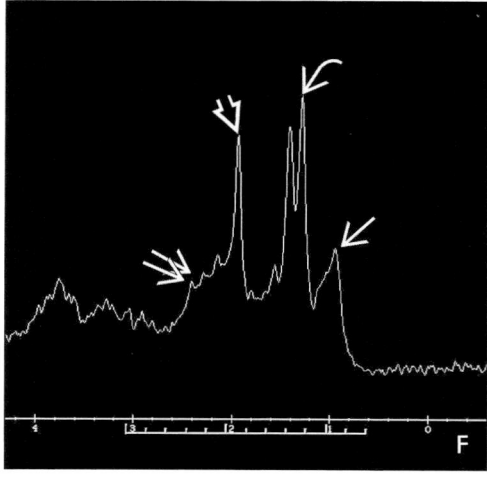

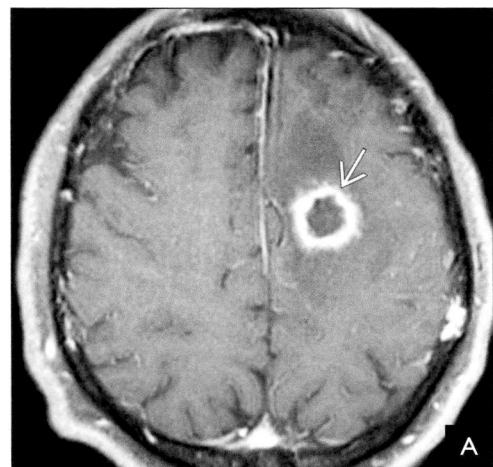

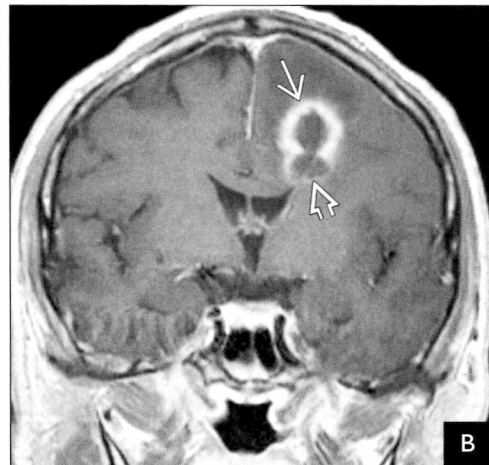

12-30A. Axial T1 C+ FS scan in a 65-year-old man with a dental abscess and 2-week history of headache shows a left posterior frontal ring-enhancing mass ➡. 12-30B. Coronal T1 C+ FS scan shows that the abscess wall ➡ is thinnest on its deepest side ➡, next to the lateral ventricle. Note edema, mass effect on the ventricle.

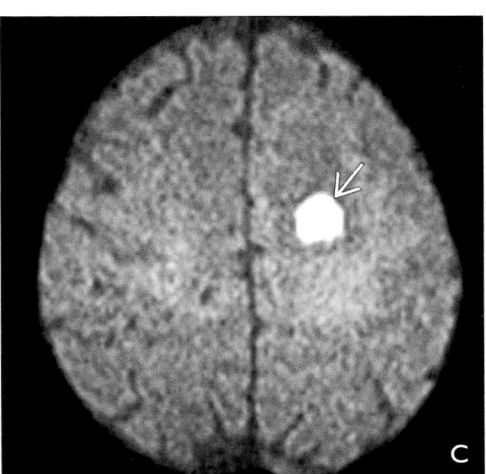

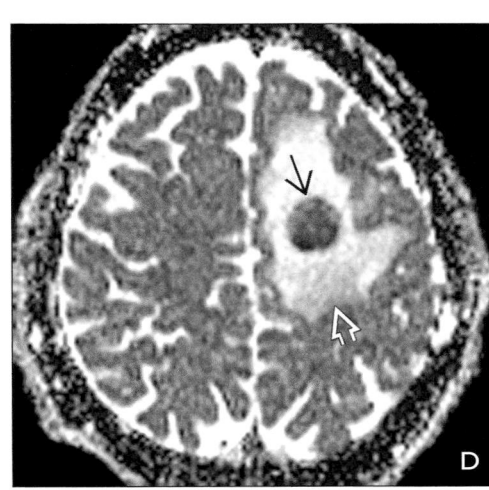

12-30C. The mass restricts strongly on DWI ➡. 12-30D. ADC shows that the mass ➡ is very hypointense compared to normal brain parenchyma, confirming that the hyperintensity seen on DWI is true diffusion restriction. The hyperintensity ➡ surrounding the mass is edema.

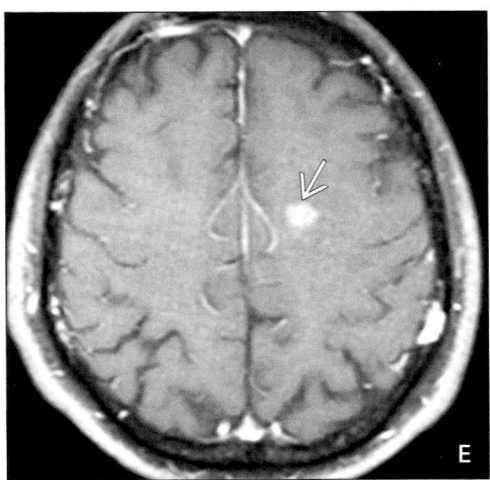

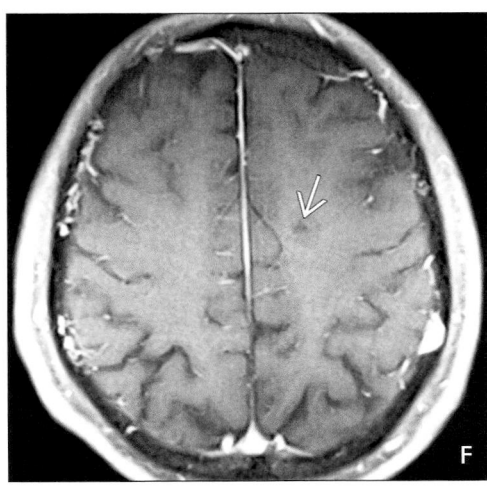

12-30E. The patient was treated with intravenous antibiotics for 6 weeks. Follow-up scan at the end of treatment shows a small residual enhancing nodule ➡ with almost complete resolution of the surrounding edema. 12-30F. Follow-up T1 C+ FS scan 1 year later shows that only a small hypointense nonenhancing focus remains ➡.

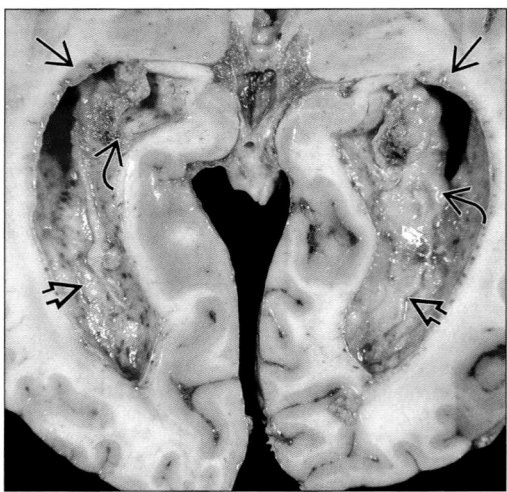

12-31. Autopsy case of IVRBA shows ependymal infection ⤵, choroid plexitis ⤵, pus adhering to ventricular walls ⤵. (Courtesy R. Hewlett, MD.)

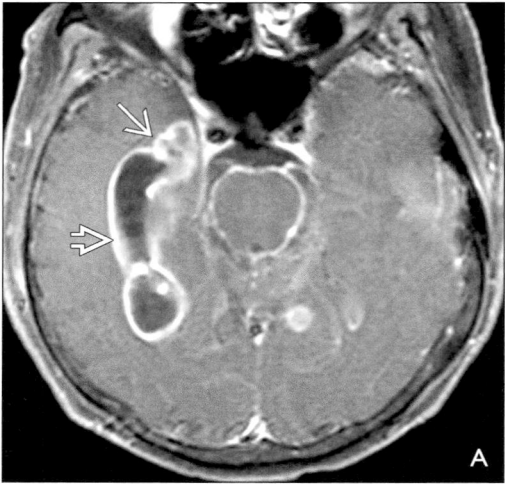

12-32A. Axial T1 C+ FS scan shows meningitis, abscess ➡ with intraventricular rupture ⤵.

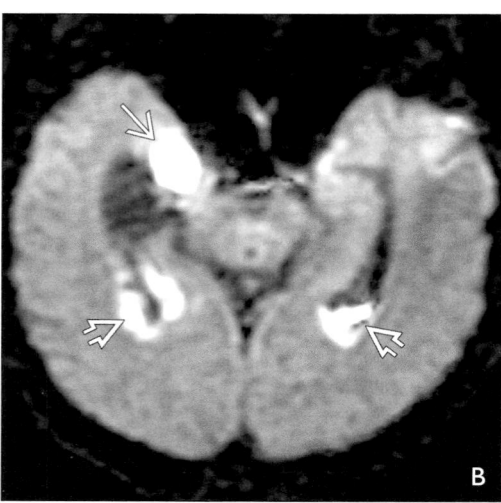

12-32B. DWI in the same patient shows that the abscess ➡ and ventriculitis ⤵ restrict.

Early cerebritis is hypo- to isointense on T1WI and hyperintense on T2/FLAIR. T2* GRE may show punctate "blooming" hemorrhagic foci. Patchy enhancement may or may not be present. DWI shows diffusion restriction **(12-28)**.

LATE CEREBRITIS. A better-delineated central hypodense mass with surrounding edema is seen on NECT. CECT typically shows irregular rim enhancement.

Late cerebritis has a hypointense center and an iso- to mildly hyperintense rim on T1WI. The central core of the cerebritis is hyperintense on T2WI while the rim is relatively hypointense. Intense but somewhat irregular rim enhancement is present on T1 C+ images. Late cerebritis restricts strongly on DWI. MRS shows cytosolic amino acids (0.9 ppm), lactate (1.3 ppm), and acetate (1.9 ppm) in the necrotic core **(12-29)**. The abscess wall demonstrates low rCBV on pMR.

EARLY CAPSULE. Abscesses in the early capsule stage are well-delineated round or ovoid masses with liquefied, hyperintense cores on T2/FLAIR. The rim of the abscess is usually thin, complete, smooth, and hypointense on T2WI. A "double rim" sign demonstrating two concentric rims, the outer hypointense and the inner hyperintense relative to cavity contents, is seen in 75% of cases **(12-29B)**. Abscess rims become significantly more hypointense on T2* SWI scans. The necrotic center of encapsulated abscesses restricts strongly on DWI **(12-30)**.

T1 C+ sequences show a thin enhancing rim. The rim of encapsulated abscesses is thinnest on its deepest (ventricular) side **(12-30B)**. "Daughter" abscesses (satellite lesions) are present in 10-15%.

LATE CAPSULE. As the cavity collapses, the capsule thickens even as the overall mass diminishes in size and gradually disappears. Contrast enhancement in the resolving abscess may persist for months, long after clinical symptoms have resolved **(12-30E)**.

Differential Diagnosis

The differential diagnosis of abscess varies with its stage of development. Early cerebritis is so poorly defined that it can be difficult to characterize and can mimic many lesions, including **cerebral ischemia** or neoplasm.

Once a ring develops around the necrotic center, the differential diagnosis is basically that of a generic ring-enhancing mass. While there are many ring-enhancing lesions in the CNS, the most common differential diagnosis is infection vs. **neoplasm (glioblastoma or metastasis)**. Tumors have increased rCBV in their "rind," usually do not restrict (or if they do, not as strongly as abscess), and do not demonstrate cytosolic amino acids on MRS.

Less common entities that can appear as a ring-enhancing mass include **demyelinating disease**, in which the ring is usually incomplete and "open" toward the cortex. Resolving hematomas can exhibit a vascular, ring-enhancing pattern.

Ventriculitis

Primary intraventricular abscess is rare. A collection of purulent material in the ventricle is more likely due to intraventricular *rupture* of a brain abscess (IVRBA), a catastrophic complication. Recognition and prompt intervention are necessary to treat this highly lethal condition.

Terminology

Ventriculitis is also called **ependymitis**, **pyocephalus**, and (less commonly) ventricular empyema.

Etiology

Infection of the ventricular ependyma most often occurs when a pyogenic abscess ruptures through its thin, medial capsule into the adjacent ventricle. Risk of IVRBA increases if an abscess is deep-seated, multiloculated, and/or close to the ventricular wall. A reduction of one millimeter between the ventricle and brain abscess increases the rupture rate by 10%.

Ventriculitis can also occur as a complication of meningitis, usually via spread of infection through the choroid plexus (choroid plexitis) into the CSF.

Patients who require external ventricular drainage (EVD) are also at risk for development of device-related ependymal infections. The infection rate of external ventriculostomy catheters is high, with reported incidences ranging from 5-20%. The most common pathogens are *Staphylococcus*, *Streptococcus*, and *Enterobacter*. Nosocomial ventriculitis and ventriculomeningitis are potentially life-threatening complications of EVD.

Pathology

Autopsy examination shows that the ependyma, subependymal region, and choroid plexus are congested and covered with pus **(12-31)**. Hemorrhagic ependymitis may be present. Hydrocephalus with pus obstructing the aqueduct is common.

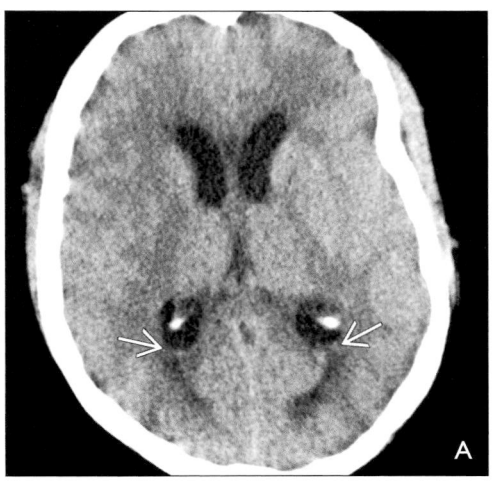
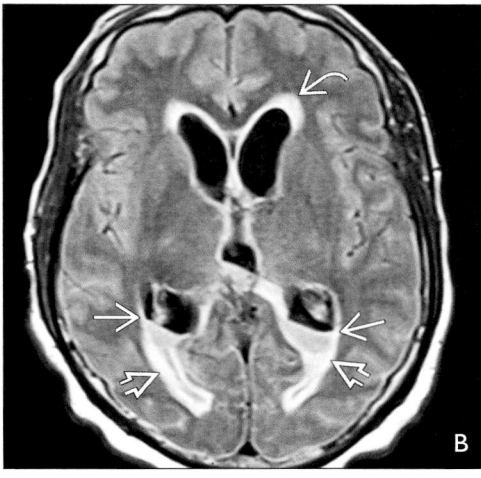

12-33A. Axial NECT in a 28-year-old female drug abuser with severe headache shows enlarged ventricles with indistinct ("blurred") margins, possible fluid-debris levels in both occipital horns ➡. 12-33B. FLAIR scan in the same patient shows transependymal CSF migration ➡, thickened hyperintense ependyma ➡ with distinct fluid-debris levels ➡.

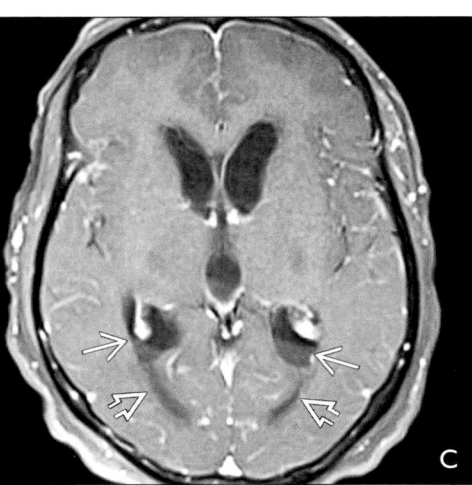
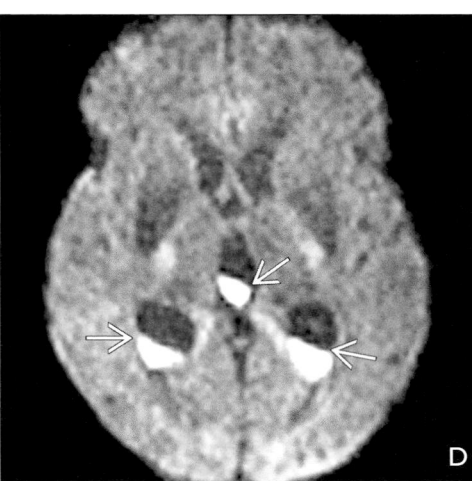

12-33C. Axial T1 C+ FS in the same patient shows debris-fluid levels ➡ in the lateral and third ventricles but no enhancement of the thickened ventricular ependyma ➡. 12-33D. DWI shows intense restriction of the intraventricular debris ➡. Stereotactic-guided ventriculostomy and drainage was performed. Klebsiella was cultured from the ventricular CSF. The patient expired despite high-dose intravenous antibiotics.

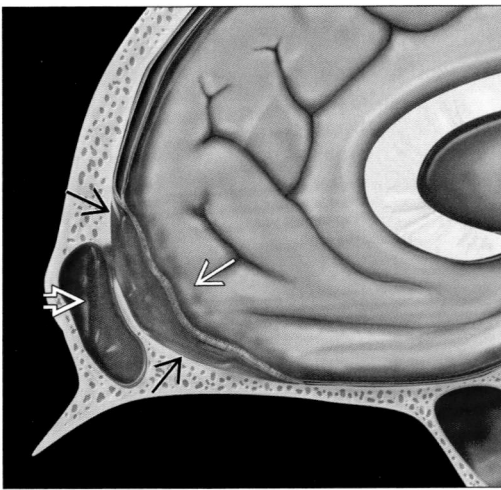

12-34. Purulent frontal sinusitis ⇨ *with extension into epidural space causes epidural empyema* ⇾, *frontal lobe cerebritis* ⇨.

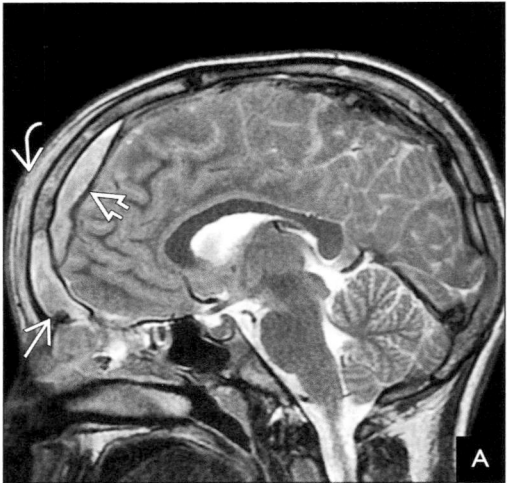

12-35A. Sagittal T2WI in a child with frontal sinusitis ⇨ *causing scalp cellulitis* ⇾, *epidural empyema* ⇨.

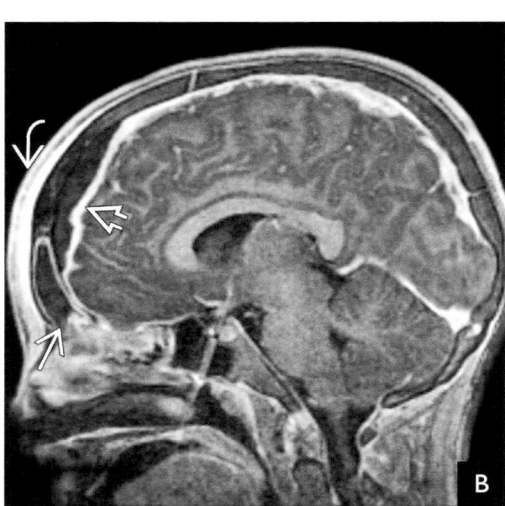

12-35B. T1 C+ scan (same case) shows the frontal sinusitis ⇾, *cellulitis* ⇾, *enhancing thickened dura* ⇨ *behind the epidural empyema.*

Clinical Issues

EPIDEMIOLOGY AND DEMOGRAPHICS. The incidence of IVRBA varies. Recent studies estimate that intraventricular rupture occurs in up to 35% of brain abscesses. Males are more commonly affected than females.

PRESENTATION. Clinical features of IVRBA can be indistinguishable from those of brain abscesses without intraventricular rupture. In general, headaches are more severe and are accompanied by signs of meningeal irritation. Rapid deterioration of clinical status is typical.

NATURAL HISTORY AND TREATMENT OPTIONS. Image-guided stereotactic aspiration is the simplest, safest method to obtain pus for culture and to decompress the abscess cavity. The combination of third-generation cephalosporins and metronidazole is the mainstay of initial empirical antimicrobial treatment. The choice of definitive antibiotics depends on culture results.

Despite aggressive medical and surgical management, many patients do poorly and succumb to the disease. Overall mortality is 25-85%. Only 40% of patients survive with good functional outcome.

Imaging

Ventriculomegaly with a debris level in the dependent part of the occipital horns together with periventricular hypodensity is the classic finding on NECT scans **(12-33A)**. The ventricular walls enhance on CECT.

MR should be the first-line imaging modality in cases of suspected IVRBA. Irregular ventricular debris that appears hyperintense to CSF on T1WI and hypointense on T2WI with layering in the dependent occipital horns is typical.

Enhancement varies from none to striking **(12-32A)**, **(12-33C)**. Some degree of ependymal enhancement can be identified in 60% of cases.

The most sensitive sequences are FLAIR and DWI. A "halo" of periventricular hyperintensity is usually present on both T2WI and FLAIR scans **(12-33B)**. DWI shows diffusion restriction of the layered debris **(12-32B)**, **(12-33D)**.

Differential Diagnosis

The differential diagnosis of IVRBA is limited. Sudden deterioration of a patient with a known cerebral abscess together with intraventricular debris and pus on MR is almost certainly IVRBA.

Ependymal enhancement *without* intraventricular debris and pus is a nonspecific finding on imaging studies. Mild, thin, linear enhancement of the periventricular and ependymal veins is normal, especially around the frontal horns, septi pellucidi, and atria of the lateral ventricles.

Primary malignant CNS neoplasms such as **glioblastoma multiforme** and **primary CNS lymphoma** can spread along the ventricular ependyma, giving it a thick or nodular "lumpy-bumpy" appearance. **Germinoma** and **metastasis** from an extracranial primary neoplasm can both cause irregular ependymal thickening and enhancement.

Empyemas

Extraaxial infections of the CNS are rare but potentially life-threatening conditions. Early diagnosis and prompt treatment are essential to maximize neurologic recovery.

Terminology

Empyemas are pus collections that can occur in either the subdural or epidural space.

Etiology

The pathophysiological basis of empyemas varies with patient age. Empyemas in infants and young children are most commonly secondary to bacterial meningitis.

In older children and adults, over two-thirds of empyemas occur as extension of infection from paranasal sinus disease. Infection can erode directly through the thin posterior wall of the frontal sinus, which is half the thickness of the anterior wall **(12-34)**. Infection may also spread indirectly in retrograde fashion through valveless bridging emissary veins.

Approximately 20% of empyemas in older children and adults are secondary to otomastoiditis. Rare causes of empyemas include penetrating head trauma, neurosurgical procedures, or hematogenous spread of pathogens from a distant extracranial site.

The most common organisms are staphylococci and streptococci.

Pathology

LOCATION. Subdural empyemas (SDEs) are much more common than epidural empyemas (EDEs). In approximately 15% of cases, pus involves both the epi- and subdural spaces.

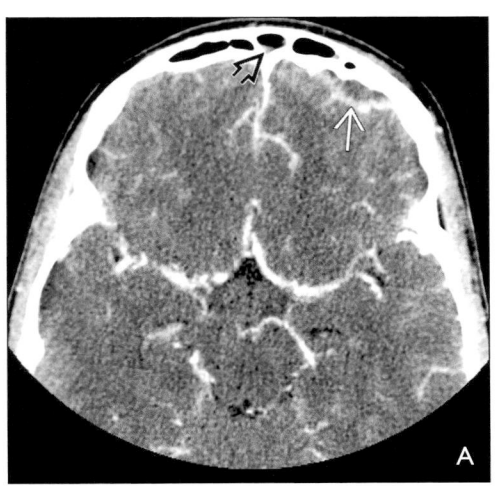

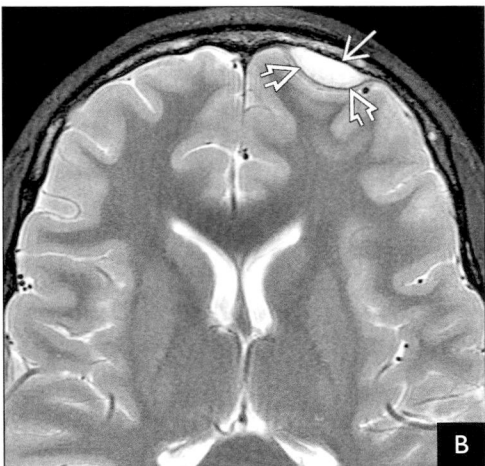

12-36A. *CECT scan was obtained in a 14-year-old male who developed severe left frontal headache after 2 weeks of sinusitis. A biconvex lentiform fluid collection with enhancing rim ➡ was identified. Note frontal sinusitis ⬒. **12-36B.** Axial T2WI in the same case shows a lentiform hyperintense left frontal fluid collection ➡. The inwardly displaced dura is seen as a thin black line ➡, confirming that the collection is indeed in the epidural space.*

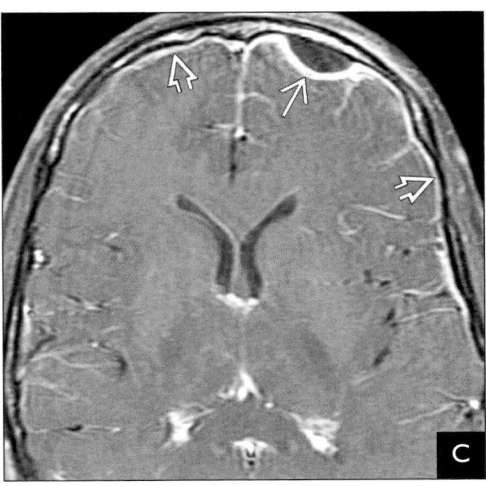

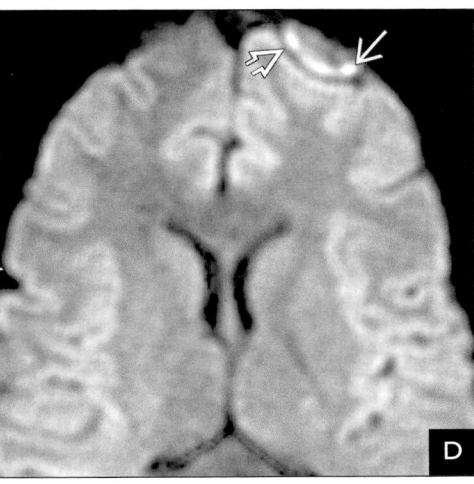

12-36C. *Axial T1 C+ FS scan in the same patient shows that the displaced dura and underlying arachnoid ➡ enhance intensely and uniformly. Note reactive dural thickening extending over the left hemisphere and across the midline ⬒. **12-36D.** Axial DWI that shows only a small crescent of the collection ➡ that lies immediately outside the displaced dura ➡ restricts. Note lack of underlying cerebritis. Epidural empyema was drained under stereotactic guidance.*

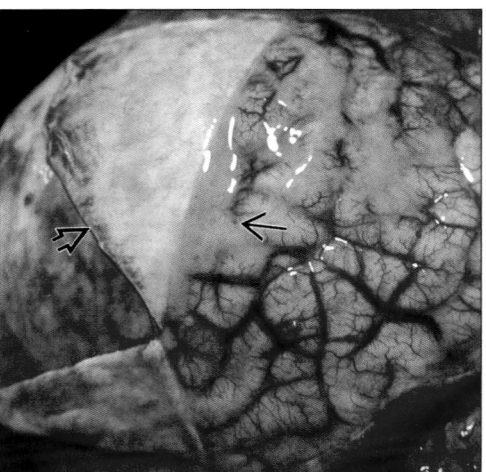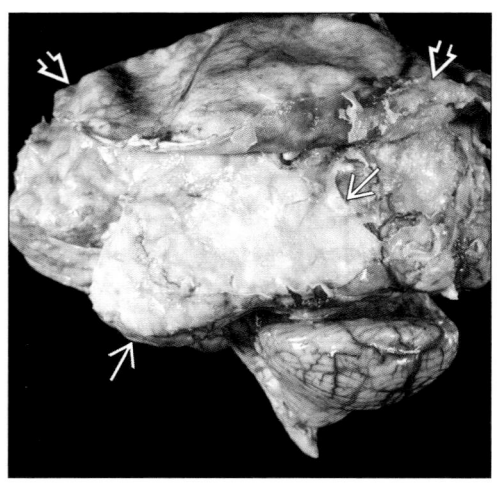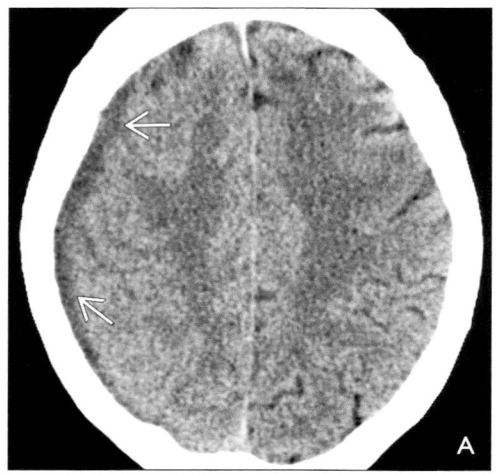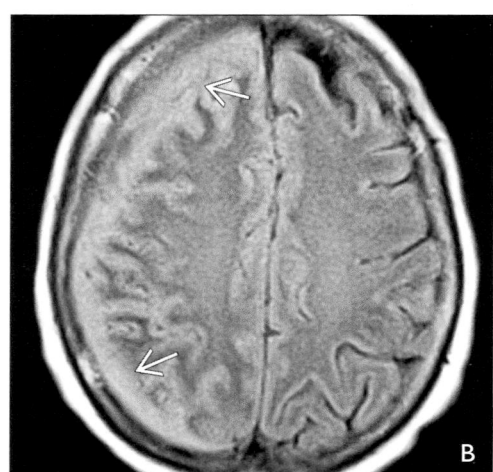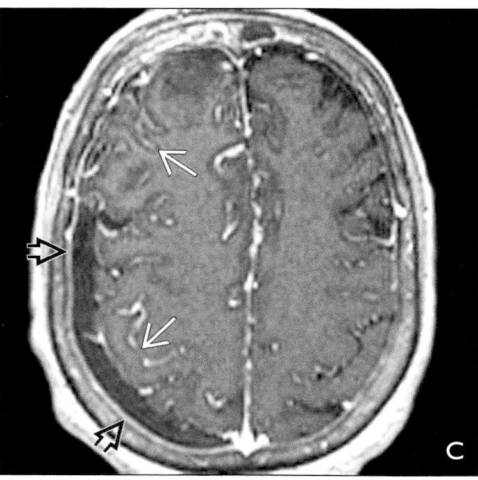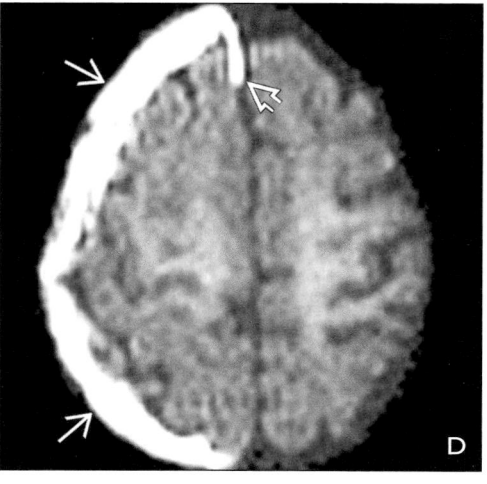

12-37. Autopsy case demonstrates findings of acute SDE. The dura ⊳ has been reflected back, revealing a cloudy fluid collection ⇒ in the subdural space. (Courtesy R. Hewlett, MD.) *12-38.* Lateral view of a more chronic subdural empyema shows that the thick yellowish collection ⇒ extends over the entire frontal and temporal lobes. The overlying dura ⊳ has been reflected superiorly to display the collection. (Courtesy R. Hewlett, MD.)

12-39A. A 51-year-old man with acute sinusitis developed severe headache and decreasing mental status. NECT scan shows a curvilinear hypodense collection ⇒ that covers the right hemisphere and compresses the underlying brain. The fluid collection is slightly hyperdense compared to CSF in the left hemispheric sulci. *12-39B.* FLAIR scan in the same case shows that the fluid collection ⇒ does not suppress. The underlying sulci are hyperintense, suggesting possible meningitis.

12-39C. Axial contrast-enhanced SPGR for stereotactic aspiration shows that the outer margin of the collection enhances ⊳. Curvilinear enhancement in the surface sulci ⇒ is consistent with meningitis. *12-39D.* Axial DWI shows that the collection ⇒ restricts strongly and uniformly. Note interhemispheric extension ⊳ does not cross the midline. Subdural empyema was drained at craniotomy and S. pneumoniae was cultured from the fluid collection.

SIZE AND NUMBER. Empyemas vary in size and extent. They range from small, focal epidural collections (12-34) to extensive subdural infections that spread over most of the cerebral hemisphere and extend into the interhemispheric fissure (12-37), (12-38). Loculated and/or multiple unilateral collections are more common than separate bilateral empyemas.

GROSS AND MICROSCOPIC FEATURES. The most common gross appearance of an empyema is an encapsulated, thick, yellowish, purulent collection lying between the dura and the arachnoid. Early empyemas may be unencapsulated collections of cloudy, more fluid-like material (12-37).

Microscopic features are those of nonspecific inflammatory infiltrate with varying amounts of granulation tissue.

Clinical Issues

EPIDEMIOLOGY. SDEs and EDEs are rare in the developed world due to the early and judicious use of antibiotics. The incidence of extraaxial CNS infections is higher in patients with limited access to medical care.

DEMOGRAPHICS. Extraaxial CNS infections can occur at any age but tend to occur at a significantly earlier age than brain abscesses. Males are more often affected than females. An adolescent male with significant headache and fever should elicit a high index of suspicion for sinusitis complications and prompt immediate imaging evaluation.

PRESENTATION. Most patients have fever and headaches preceded by symptoms of sinusitis or otomastoiditis. Meningismus is common. "Pott puffy tumor"—localized swelling of the forehead— is considered a specific sign for subperiosteal abscess of the frontal bone. A "Pott puffy tumor" is seen in up to one-third of patients with frontal SDE. Orbital cellulitis is a less common but significant sign of empyema.

NATURAL HISTORY AND TREATMENT OPTIONS. The interval between initial infection (usually sinusitis) and onset of the empyema is typically one to three weeks. EDEs have a better prognosis than SDEs. Once established, untreated empyemas can spread quite rapidly, extending from the extraaxial spaces into the subjacent

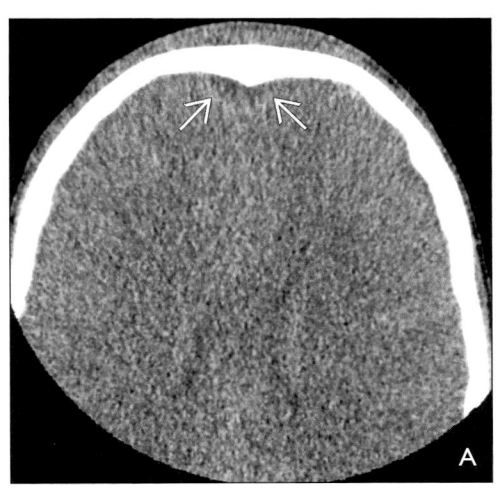
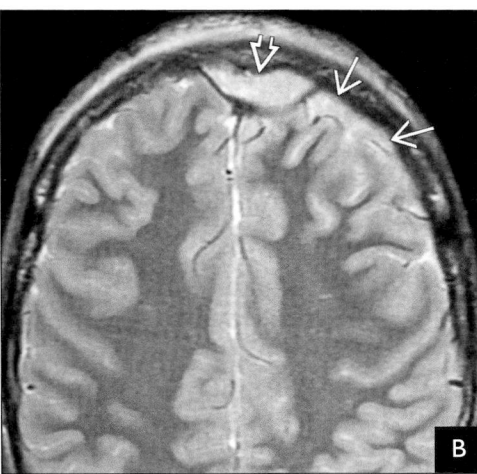

12-40A. *Axial sinus CT with soft tissue windows in a child with severe headache, forehead swelling, and acute frontal sinusitis (not shown) demonstrates an ill-defined lens-shaped midline hypodensity ➡ behind the inner table of the calvaria.* *12-40B.* *T2WI demonstrates both an EDE ➡ and an SDE ➡.*

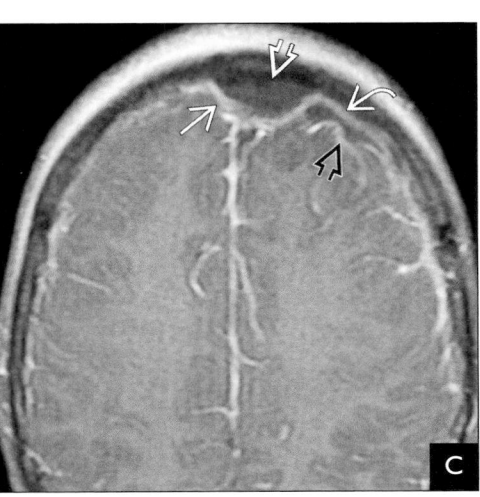
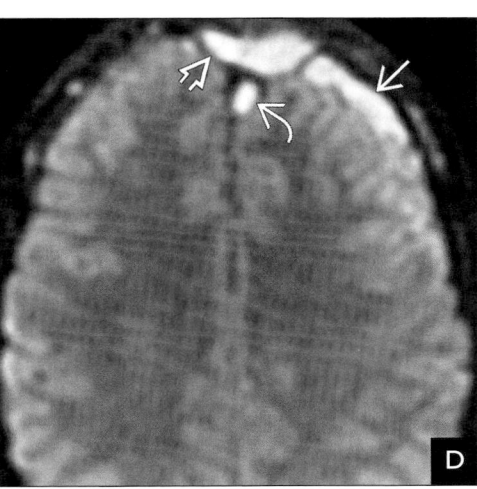

12-40C. *T1 C+ FS scan shows that the EDE ➡ crosses the midline, displacing the thickened dura posteriorly ➡. The SDE is seen positioned between the thickened dura on the outside ➡ and the enhancing arachnoid ➡ on the inside.* *12-40D.* *DWI shows that both the EDE ➡ and the SDE ➡ restrict strongly and equally. Note the small subdural empyema in the interhemispheric fissure ➡. Combined EDEs and SDEs occur in 15% of cases.*

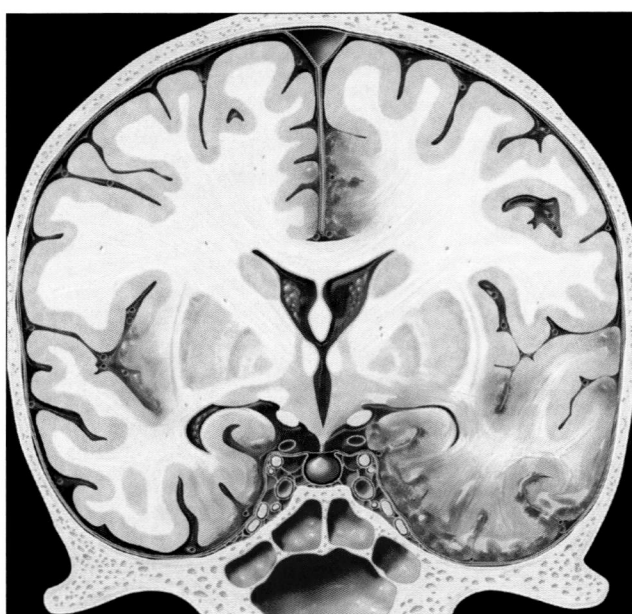

12-41. *Coronal graphic shows the classic features of herpes encephalitis with bilateral but asymmetric involvement of the limbic system. There is inflammation involving the temporal lobes, cingulate gyri, and insular cortices.*

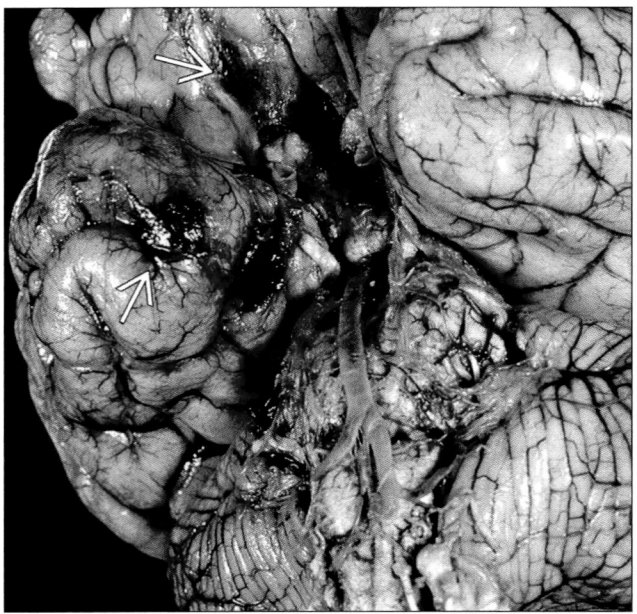

12-42. *Autopsied brain from a patient with HSE shows characteristic hemorrhagic lesions in the anteromedial temporal lobes, subfrontal regions ➡. (Courtesy R. Hewlett, MD.)*

brain. Besides cerebritis and abscess formation, the other major complication of empyema is cortical vein thrombosis with venous ischemia.

Surgical drainage and rapid initiation of empiric intravenous antibiotic therapy (initially vancomycin and a third-generation cephalosporin) has been shown to reduce mortality. Mortality of treated empyemas is still significant, ranging from 10-15%.

Imaging

Imaging is essential to the early diagnosis of empyema. NECT scans may be normal or show a hypodense extraaxial collection **(12-39A)**, **(12-40A)** that demonstrates peripheral enhancement on CECT **(12-36A)**. Bone CT should be evaluated for signs of sinusitis and otomastoiditis.

MR is the procedure of choice for evaluating potential empyemas. T1 scans show an extraaxial collection that is mildly hyperintense relative to CSF. SDEs are typically crescentic and lie over the cerebral hemisphere. The extracerebral space is widened and the underlying sulci are compressed by the collection. SDEs often extend into the interhemispheric fissure but do not cross the midline.

EDEs are biconvex and usually more focal than SDEs. The inwardly displaced dura can sometimes be identified as a thin hypointense line between the epidural collection and the underlying brain. In contrast to SDEs, frontal EDEs may cross the midline, confirming their epidural location **(12-35A)**, **(12-36B)** **(12-40C)**.

Empyemas are iso- to hyperintense compared to CSF on T2WI **(12-40B)** and are hyperintense on FLAIR **(12-39B)**. Hyperintensity in the underlying brain parenchyma may be caused by cerebritis or ischemia (either venous or arterial).

SDEs typically demonstrate striking diffusion restriction on DWI **(12-39D)**, **(12-40D)**. EDEs are variable but usually have at least some restricting component **(12-36D)**.

Empyemas show variable enhancement depending on the amount of granulomatous tissue and inflammation present. The encapsulating membranes, especially on the outer margin, enhance moderately strongly **(12-35B)**, **(12-36C)**, **(12-39C)**, **(12-40C)**.

Differential Diagnosis

The major differential diagnosis of extraaxial empyema is a nonpurulent extraaxial collection, especially subdural effusion and subdural hygroma.

A **chronic subdural hematoma** (cSDH) is often hypodense on NECT scan and hyperintense on T2/FLAIR. Residual blood in the extraaxial collection "blooms" on T2* (GRE, SWI). The membranes that encapsulate a cSDH enhance. In contrast to subdural empyemas, cSDHs typically do not restrict on DWI.

A **subdural hygroma** is a sterile, nonenhancing, nonrestricting CSF collection that occurs with a tear in the arachnoid that allows escape of CSF into the subdural space. A **subdural effusion** is usually post-meningitic, is typically bilateral, and does not restrict on DWI.

EMPYEMAS

Etiology
- Infants, young children
  - Meningitis
- Older children, adults
  - Sinusitis, otomastoiditis

Pathology
- SDEs > > EDEs
- EDE focal
  - Usually adjacent to sinus, mastoid
- SDE can spread diffusely
  - Over hemispheres
  - Along tentorium/falx

Clinical Issues
- M:F = 2:1
- Typical case: Child with headache, fever
- "Pott puffy tumor" common with frontal SDE
- SDEs can spread rapidly, are surgical emergencies!

Imaging
- Bone CT: Look for sinus, ear infection
- EDE is focal, biconvex, can cross midline
- SDE is crescentic, covers hemisphere, may extend into interhemispheric fissure
- SDEs restrict strongly on DWI; EDEs variable

Differential Diagnosis
- Chronic subdural hematoma
- Subdural hygroma
- Subdural effusion

Acquired Viral Infections

Herpes Simplex Encephalitis

Several members of the herpesvirus family are neurotropic viruses that may cause significant neurologic disease. HSV1 typically involves the skin and facial mucosa while HSV2 is associated with genital infection. HHV-7 is increasingly recognized as a major cause of morbidity and mortality in lung transplant recipients, whereas Epstein-Barr virus (EBV) and HHV-8 have proven oncogenic potential.

Congenital HSV2 and CMV were both considered above, as their manifestations in newborn infants differ from those of acquired herpesvirus infections. HSV1 and HHV-6 are discussed here. Varicella-zoster and EBV are discussed below as "Miscellaneous Encephalitides."

Terminology

Recall that CNS involvement in herpes simplex virus infection is called congenital or neonatal HSV when it involves neonates but is designated herpes simplex encephalitis (HSE) in all individuals beyond the first post-

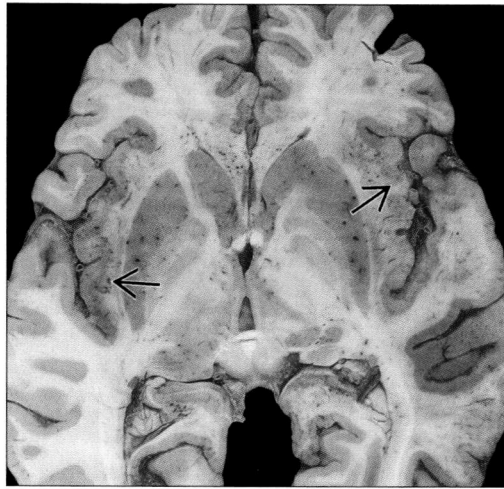

12-43. Axial autopsy section in HSE shows petechial hemorrhages in the insular cortex of both temporal lobes ➡. (Courtesy R. Hewlett, MD.)

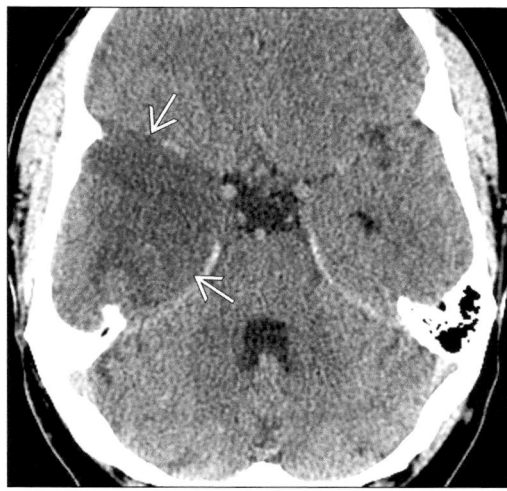

12-44. NECT in a 52-year-old man with HSE shows hypodensity, mild mass effect in right anteromedial temporal lobe ➡.

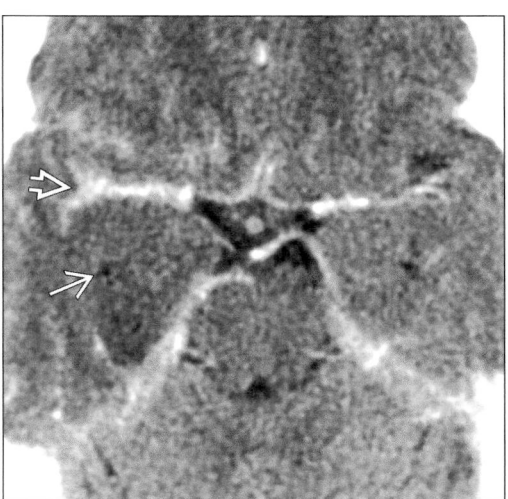

12-45. CECT scan in a patient with declining mental status shows right temporal lobe edema ➡, minimal enhancement ➡. PCR positive for HSV1.

12-46A. A 68-year-old man presented to the emergency department with viral prodrome, confusion. Initial NECT scan (not shown) was negative. MR was obtained emergently. Some motion artifact is present, but FLAIR scan shows hyperintensity in both insular cortices ➡. *12-46B.* DWI shows marked diffusion restriction in both insular cortices ➡. Somewhat less striking hyperintensity is seen in both anterior temporal lobes ➡.

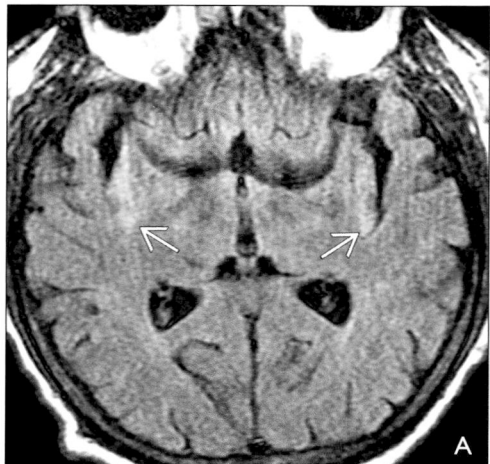

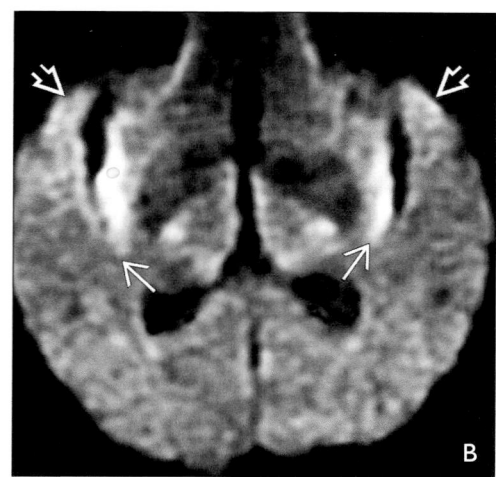

12-46C. More cephalad DWI in the same patient shows symmetric restricted diffusion in both cingulate gyri ➡. Because of the strong suspicion for HSE, the patient was placed on antiviral agents. PCR was positive for HSV1. *12-46D.* Despite treatment, the patient did poorly. Repeat NECT scan 2 weeks later shows confluent hemorrhages in both anteromedial temporal lobes ➡.

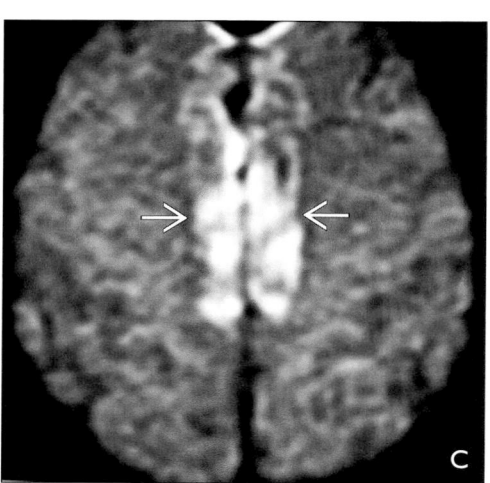

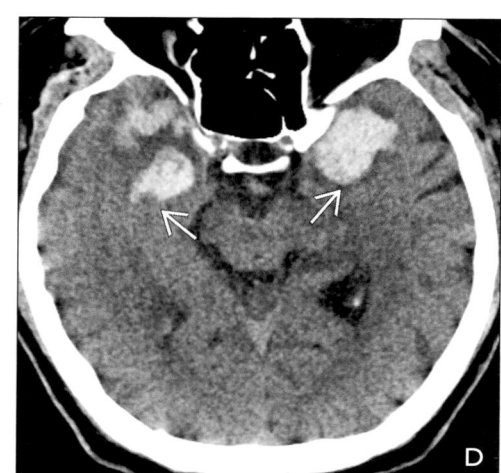

12-46E. Hemorrhagic necrosis is also seen in the right insular cortex ➡, although the left insula is spared. Note blood-fluid level in the occipital horn of the right lateral ventricle ➡. *12-46F.* More cephalad scan shows hemorrhagic necrosis in the right cingulate gyrus ➡. Bilateral but asymmetric involvement is typical of HSE.

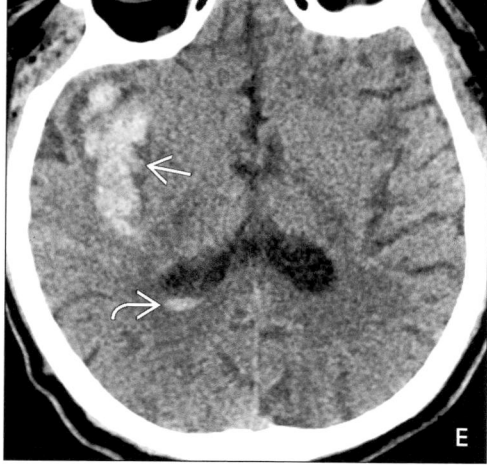

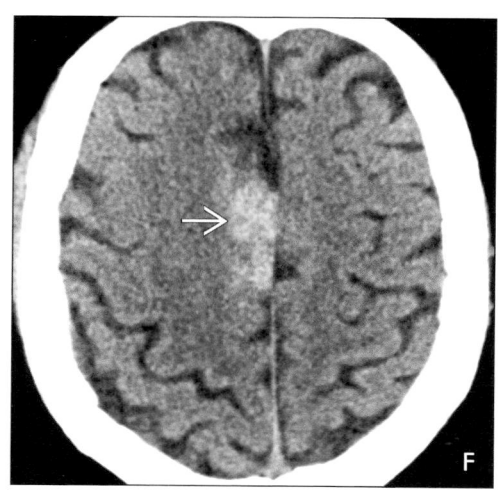

natal month. HSE is also sometimes called herpes simplex virus encephalitis.

Etiology

Over 95% of HSE is caused by HSV1, an obligate intracellular pathogen. The virus initially gains entry into cells in the nasopharyngeal mucosa, invades sensory lingual branches of the trigeminal nerve, then passes in retrograde fashion into the trigeminal ganglion. It establishes a lifelong latent infection within sensory neurons of the trigeminal ganglion, where it can remain dormant indefinitely.

Viral gene expression is largely silent until viral reactivation occurs. Reactivation of latent herpesvirus infection can occur spontaneously or may be triggered by trauma, stress, immunosuppression, or hormonal fluctuations.

Pathology

LOCATION. HSE has a striking affinity for the limbic system **(12-41)**. The anterior and medial temporal lobes, insular cortex, subfrontal area, and cingulate gyri are most frequently affected **(12-42)**. Bilateral but asymmetric disease is typical **(12-43)**. Extratemporal, extralimbic involvement occurs but is more common in children compared to adults. When it occurs, extralimbic HSE most often involves the parietal cortex. Brainstem-predominant infection is uncommon. The basal ganglia are usually spared.

GROSS PATHOLOGY. HSE is a fulminant, hemorrhagic, necrotizing encephalitis. Massive tissue necrosis accompanied by numerous petechial hemorrhages and severe edema is typical. Inflammation and tissue destruction are predominantly cortical but may extend into the subcortical white matter. Advanced cases demonstrate gross temporal lobe rarefaction and cavitation.

MICROSCOPIC FEATURES. Perivascular lymphocytic cuffing with diffuse neutrophil infiltration into the necrotic parenchyma is typical. Large "owl's-eye" viral inclusions in neurons, astrocytes, and oligodendrocytes are seen in the acute and subacute phases. Tissue destruction with neuronophagia and apoptosis is striking.

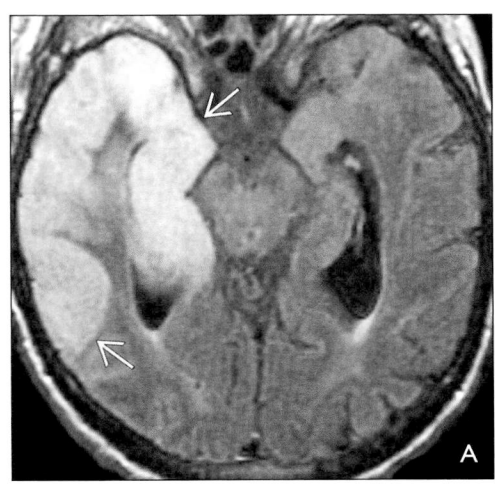
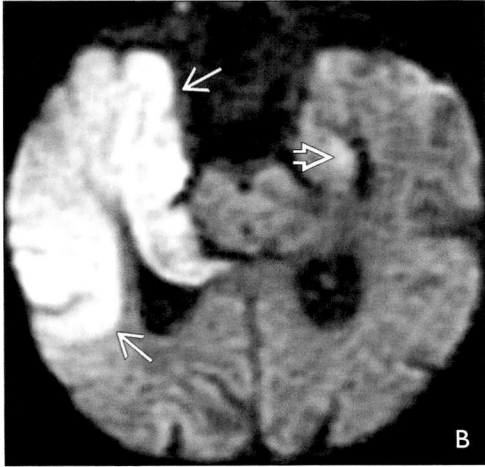

12-47A. Axial FLAIR scan in a 37-year-old man with PCR-proven HSE shows striking hyperintensity, cortical swelling of the right temporal lobe. The left side appears normal. 12-47B. DWI in the same patient shows striking restricted diffusion in the cortex of the right temporal lobe. A subtle area of diffusion restriction is noted in the left medial temporal lobe.

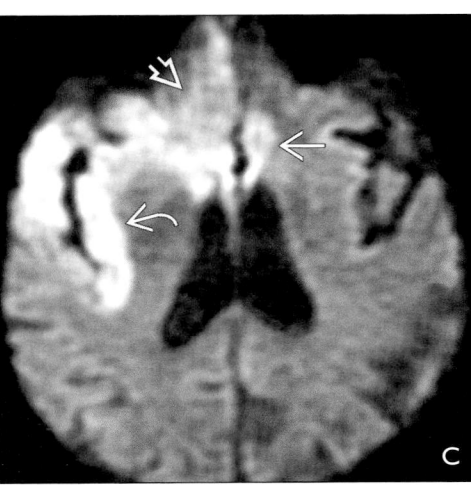
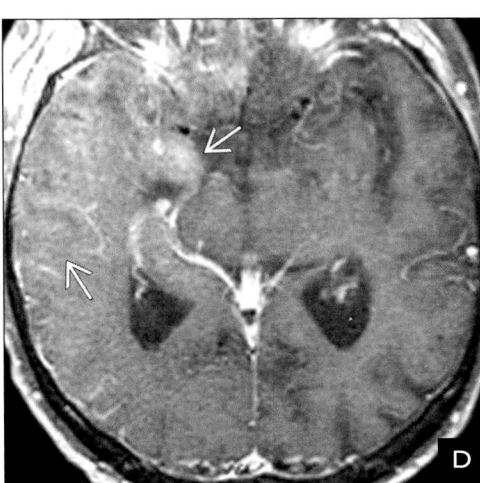

12-47C. More cephalad DWI in the same patient shows restricted diffusion in the right insular cortex, right subfrontal region, and cingulate gyrus, as well as subtle involvement of the left cingulate gyrus. 12-47D. T1 C+ FS scan shows patchy enhancement in the right temporal lobe cortex. In this case, involvement of the left limbic system is subtle and can be identified only on DWI.

12-48A. Axial T1WI in a 37-year-old man with confusion and altered mental status 3 weeks after hematopoietic stem cell transplant appears normal. *12-48B.* T2WI in the same patient shows subtle hyperintensity in the amygdala and hippocampus of the left medial temporal lobe ➡.

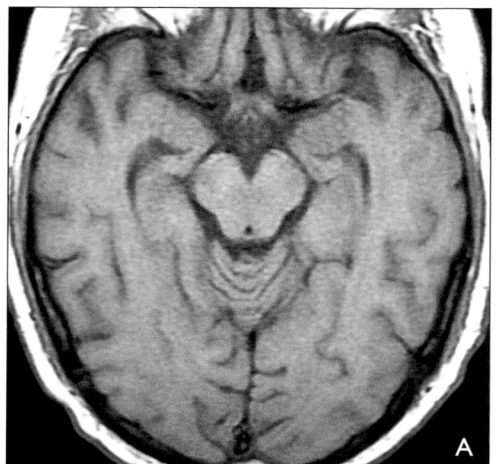
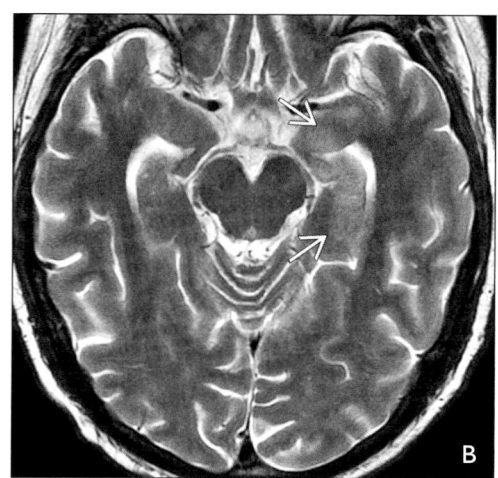

12-48C. The hyperintensity in the left mesial temporal lobe is much better appreciated on FLAIR scan ➡. *12-48D.* T2* GRE scan shows no evidence of hemorrhage.

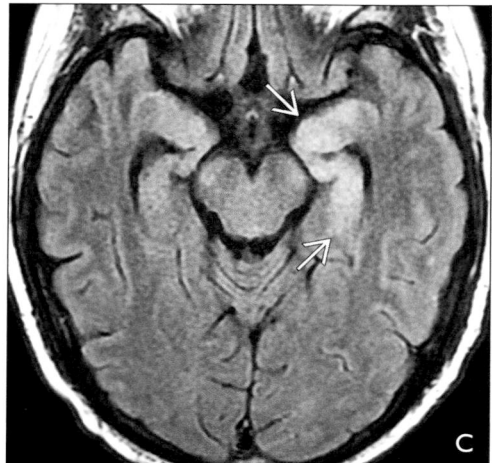
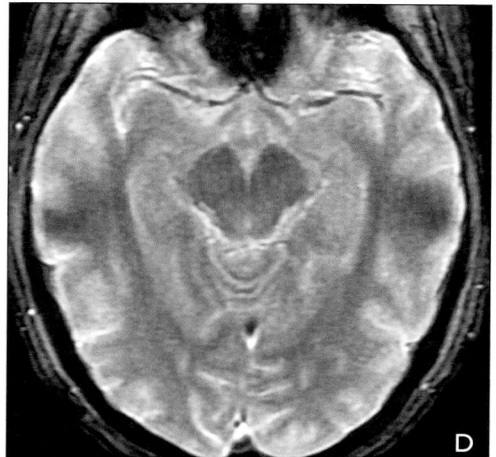

12-48E. DWI demonstrates restricted diffusion in the left temporal lobe ➡. The right temporal lobe appears normal. *12-48F.* T1 C+ scan shows no evidence of enhancement. HHV-6 encephalopathy was subsequently documented. Exclusive involvement of the mesial temporal lobe without evidence for abnormalities outside the hippocampus and amygdala helps differentiate HHV-6 encephalopathy from HSE.

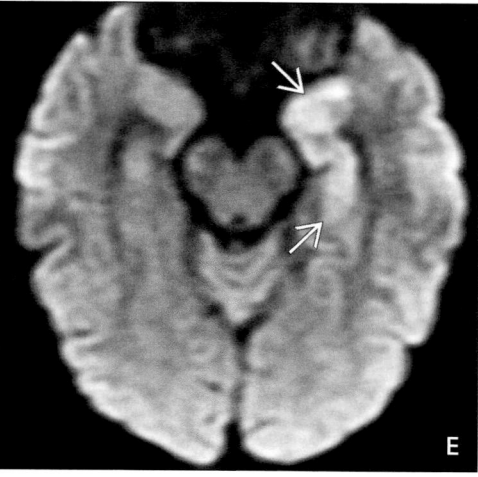
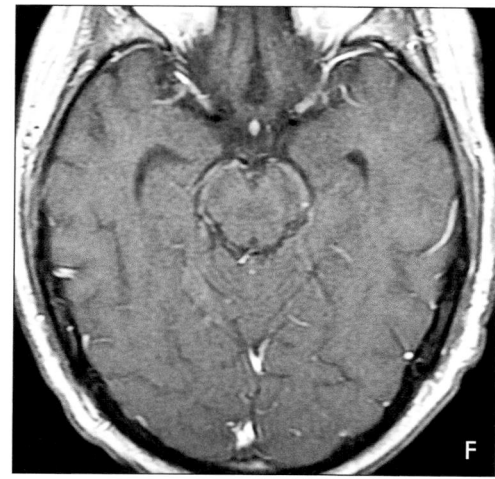

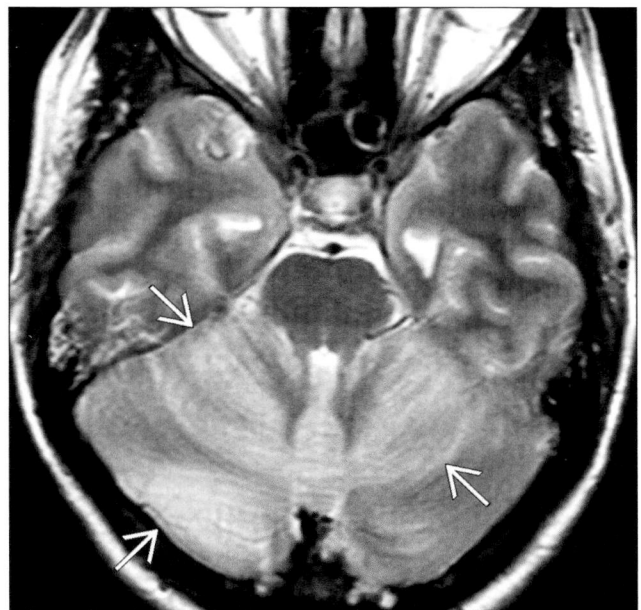

12-49. T2WI in a 9-year-old girl with a 2-week history of ear infection, headaches, confusion, and ataxia shows acute cerebellitis. Note edema and mass effect, seen as hyperintensity in both cerebellar hemispheres ➥. PCR was positive for VZV.

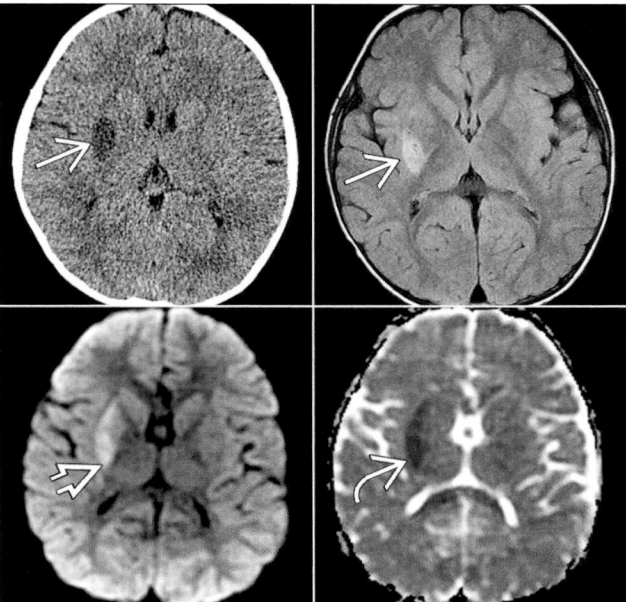

12-50. VZV vasculitis with basal ganglia infarct in a 4-year-old girl. NECT and FLAIR scans show putaminal infarct ➥ that restricts as shown on DWI ➥ and ADC ➥.

Clinical Issues

EPIDEMIOLOGY. HSV1 is the most common worldwide cause of sporadic (i.e., nonepidemic) viral encephalitis. Overall prevalence is 1-3:1,000,000.

DEMOGRAPHICS. HSE may occur at any age. It follows a bimodal age distribution, with one-third of all cases occurring between the ages of six months and three years and one-half seen in patients older than 50. There is no gender predilection.

PRESENTATION. A viral prodrome followed by fever, headache, seizures, behavioral changes, and altered mental status is typical.

NATURAL HISTORY. HSE is a devastating infection with mortality rates ranging from 50-70%. Rapid clinical deterioration with coma and death is typical. Nearly two-thirds of survivors have significant neurological deficits despite antiviral therapy.

TREATMENT OPTIONS. Antiviral therapy with intravenous acyclovir should be started immediately if HSE is suspected. Definitive diagnosis requires PCR confirmation. CSF PCR is 96-98% sensitive.

Imaging

CT FINDINGS. NECT is often normal early in the disease course. Hypodensity with mild mass effect in one or both temporal lobes and the insula may be present **(12-44)**. CECT is usually negative, although patchy or gyriform enhancement may develop after 24-48 hours **(12-45)**.

MR FINDINGS. MR is the imaging procedure of choice **(12-46)**. T1 scans show gyral swelling with indistinct gray-white interfaces. T2 scans demonstrate cortical/subcortical hyperintensity with relative sparing of the underlying white matter. FLAIR is the most sensitive sequence and may be positive before signal changes are apparent on either T1- or T2WI. Bilateral but asymmetric involvement of the temporal lobes and insula is characteristic of HSE but is not always present.

T2* (GRE, SWI) may demonstrate petechial hemorrhages after 24-48 hours. Gyriform T1 shortening, volume loss, and confluent curvilinear "blooming" foci on T2* are seen in the subacute and chronic phases of HSE.

HSE shows restricted diffusion early in the disease course, sometimes preceding visible FLAIR abnormalities. Enhancement varies from none (early) to intense gyriform enhancement several days later **(12-47)**.

Differential Diagnosis

The major differential diagnoses for HSE are neoplasm, acute cerebral ischemia, status epilepticus, other encephalitides (especially HHV-6), and paraneoplastic limbic encephalitis. Infiltrating neoplasms such as **gliomatosis cerebri** and **diffuse low-grade astrocytoma** usually involve white matter or white matter plus cortex.

Acute cerebral ischemia-infarction occurs in a typical vascular distribution, involving both the cortex and white matter. Onset is typically sudden compared to HSE, and a history of fever or a viral prodrome with flu-like illness is lacking. Especially in immunocompro-

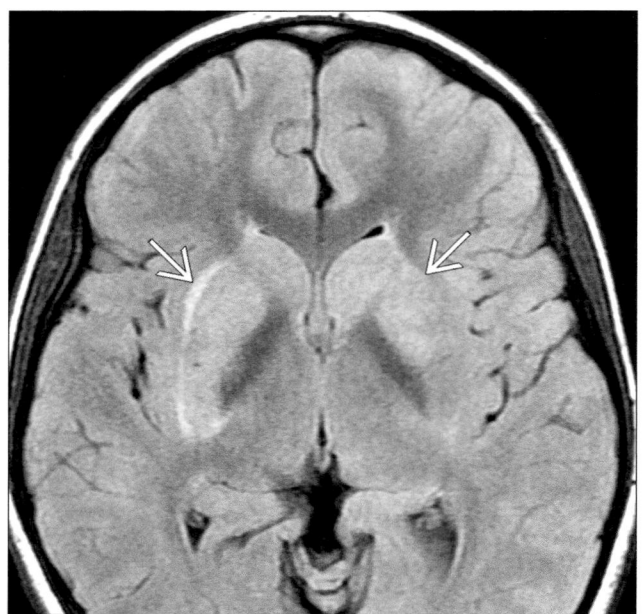

12-51. Axial FLAIR scan in a 13-year-old girl with fever and headache shows bilateral hyperintensities in the basal ganglia ➡. PCR was positive for EBV.

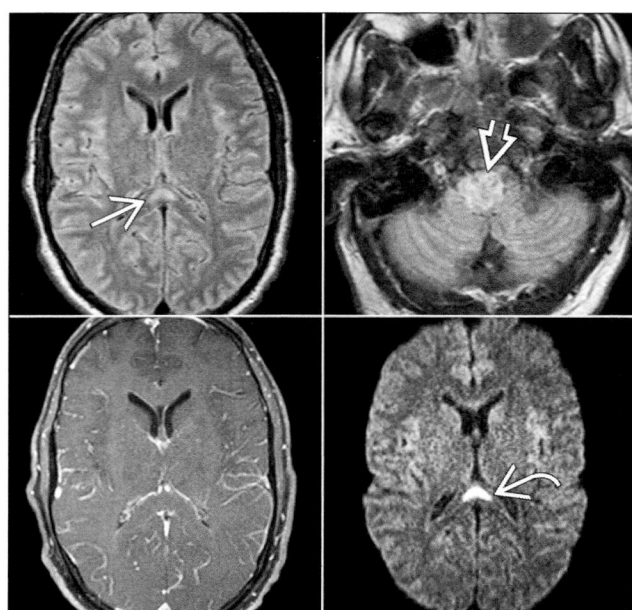

12-52. EBV encephalitis in a 29 yo man with headache, fever, diplopia, somnolence. FLAIR scans show sulcal hyperintensities, focal lesions in CC splenium ➡, medulla ➡. The WM lesions do not enhance, but the splenium lesion restricts on DWI ➡.

mised patients, late acute/subacute HSE itself can have a "pseudo-ischemic" appearance caused by widespread dead or dying neurons.

Status epilepticus is usually unilateral and typically involves just the cortex. Postictal edema is transient but generally more widespread, often involving most or all of the hemispheric cortex.

HHV-6 encephalitis usually involves just the medial temporal lobes but, if extrahippocampal lesions are present, it may be difficult to distinguish from HSE solely on the basis of imaging findings. Other viral encephalitides typically lack the frontotemporal limbic preferential distribution seen in HSE.

Limbic encephalitis has a more protracted, subacute onset (weeks to months), but imaging findings may be virtually indistinguishable from those of HSE. History of an extracranial primary carcinoma (often lung) and neuronal antibodies in the serum and CSF are helpful differentiating features.

HHV-6 Encephalopathy

Etiology

More than 90% of the general population is seropositive for HHV-6 by two years of age. Most primary infections are asymptomatic, after which the virus remains latent.

Clinical Issues

HHV-6 can become pathogenic in immunocompromised patients, especially those with hematopoietic stem cell or solid organ transplantation. The median interval between transplantation and onset of neurologic symptoms is three weeks. Patients typically present with altered mental status, short-term memory loss, and seizures.

Imaging

NECT scans are typically normal. MR shows predominant or exclusive involvement of one or both medial temporal lobes (hippocampus and amygdala) **(12-48)**. Extrahippocampal disease is much less common than with HSE. Transient hyperintensity of the mesial temporal lobes on T2WI and FLAIR with restriction on DWI is typical. T2* (GRE, SWI) scans show no evidence of hemorrhage.

Differential Diagnosis

The major differential diagnosis is **herpes simplex encephalitis** (HSE). The disease course of HSE is more fulminant. Extratemporal involvement and hemorrhagic necrosis are common in HSE but rare in HHV-6 encephalopathy. In contrast to HSE, in HHV-6, MR imaging abnormalities tend to resolve with time.

Postictal hippocampal hyperemia is transient, and extrahippocampal involvement is absent.

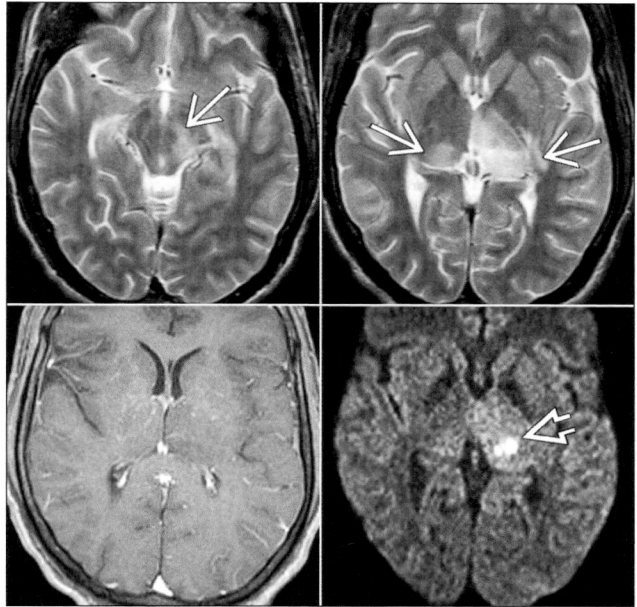

12-53. Typical findings of WNV encephalitis include bilateral but asymmetric nonenhancing lesions in the basal ganglia and midbrain 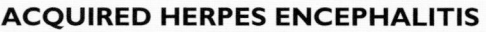. *DWI may demonstrate restriction* ➡.

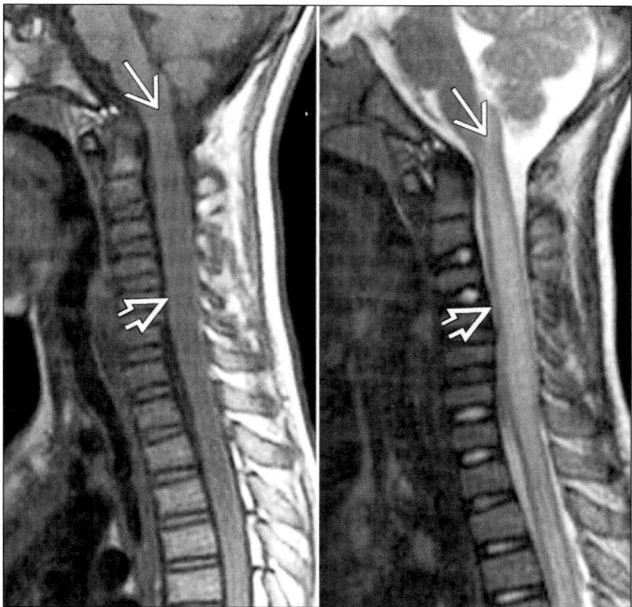

12-54. Sagittal T1 (left) and T2 (right) scans show findings of rabies encephalomyelitis. Note involvement of the medulla ➡ *and cervicothoracic spinal cord* ➡. *(Courtesy R. Ramakantan, MD.)*

ACQUIRED HERPES ENCEPHALITIS

Etiology of Herpes Simplex Encephalitis (HSE)
- > 95% of HSE caused by HSV1
  - Reactivation of latent virus in trigeminal ganglion
  - Trauma, stress, immunosuppression can trigger

Pathology
- HSE: Striking affinity for limbic system
  - Temporal lobes, insular cortex, subfrontal, cingulate gyri
- Hemorrhagic, necrotizing encephalitis

Clinical Issues
- HSE is most common cause of nonepidemic viral encephalitis
- Bimodal age distribution (6 months to 3 years, > 50 years)
- High mortality, morbidity

Imaging
- Bilateral but asymmetric temporal lobe, insular cortex lesions
  - FLAIR most sensitive
  - Restricts on DWI

Differential Diagnosis of HSE
- Neoplasm (gliomatosis cerebri)
- Stroke (vascular distribution, both GM, WM)
- Postictal hyperemia
- Other encephalitis (limbic, HHV-6)

HHV-6 Encephalitis
- Patients often immunocompromised
  - Hematopoietic stem cell, solid organ transplants
- Bilateral medial temporal lobes
  - Extratemporal involvement less common than in HSE
- Differential diagnosis
  - HSE, limbic encephalitis
  - Postictal hyperemia

Miscellaneous Acute Encephalitides

Viral encephalitis is a medical emergency. Prognosis depends on both the specific pathogen and host immunologic status. Timely, accurate diagnosis and prompt therapy can improve survival and reduce the likelihood of brain injury.

Many viruses can cause encephalitis. Over 100 different viruses in more than a dozen families have been implicated in CNS infection. HSV1, Epstein-Barr virus, mumps, measles, and enteroviruses are responsible for most cases of encephalitis in immunocompetent patients.

Viral infection of the CNS is almost always part of generalized systemic disease. Most viruses infect the brain via hematogenous spread. Others—such as some of the herpesviruses and rabies virus—are neurotropic and spread directly from infected mucosa or conjunctiva along nerve roots into the CNS.

CSF or serum analysis with pathogen identification by PCR amplification establishes the definitive diagnosis. Nevertheless, imaging is essential to early diagnosis and treatment.

The most common nonepidemic viral encephalitis, herpes encephalitis, was discussed earlier. In this section we consider additional examples of viral CNS infections. We begin with two other members of the herpesvirus family—varicella-zoster virus and Epstein-Barr virus. We then turn our attention to selected sporadic and epidemic encephalitides.

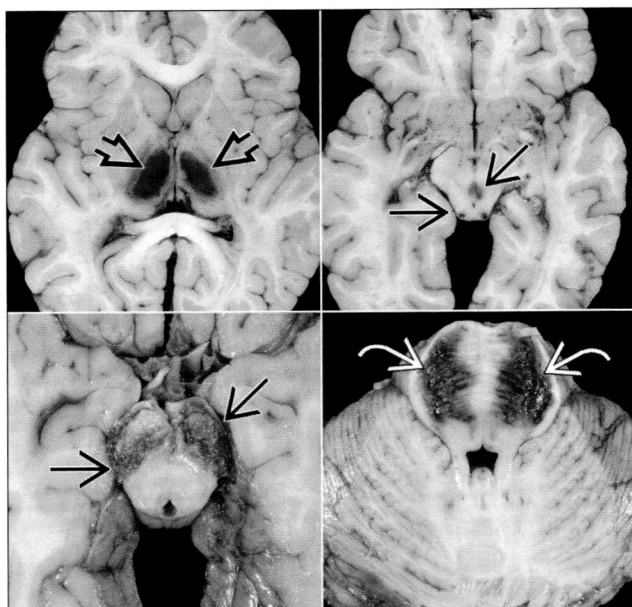

12-55. Series of autopsy photographs demonstrates the characteristic findings of acute necrotizing encephalopathy with bilaterally symmetric hemorrhagic necrosis in the thalami ⇒, midbrain ⇒, and pons ➜. (Courtesy R. Hewlett, MD.)

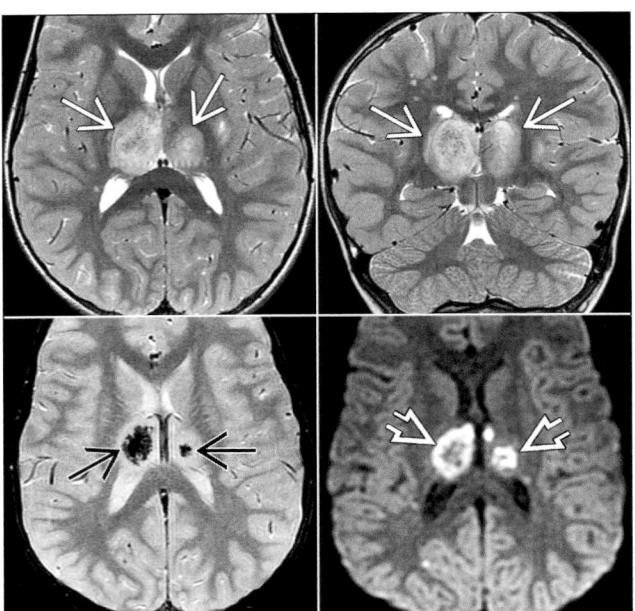

12-56. ANE in a 4-year-old obtunded girl with influenza A shows bithalamic hyperintense lesions on T2WI ➜ with hemorrhage on T2 ⇒. Note diffusion restriction ➜. (Courtesy C. D. Phillips, MD.)*

Varicella-Zoster Encephalitis

The incidence of varicella-zoster (VZV) infection has decreased significantly since the introduction of a live attenuated VZV vaccine in 1995. Yet despite widespread vaccination rates, VZV continues to cause CNS disease. VZV, which causes chickenpox (varicella) and shingles (zoster), also causes Bell palsy, Ramsay-Hunt syndrome, meningitis, encephalitis, myelitis, Reye syndrome, and postherpetic neuralgia.

VZV encephalitis has a wide age range with a median age at diagnosis of 46 years. Between 25-30% of patients are under 18 years of age.

Symptoms generally begin 10 days after chickenpox rash or varicella vaccination. Note, however, that many patients with CNS VZV disease present without the characteristic accompanying zoster rash.

Meningitis is the most frequent overall manifestation (50% of cases) and the most common clinical presentation in immunocompetent patients (90%). Encephalitis is the second most common CNS presentation (42%) but the most common manifestation in immunodeficient patients (67%). The most common presentation in children is acute cerebellar ataxia. Acute disseminated encephalomyelitis (ADEM) is rare (8%).

Cerebellitis with diffuse cerebellar swelling and hyperintensity on T2/FLAIR scan is common (12-49). Children may develop multifocal leukoencephalopathy with patchy foci of T2/FLAIR hyperintensity. VZV vasculopathy with stroke causes multifocal cortical, basal ganglia, and deep white matter hyperintensities (12-50). Enhancement on T1 C+ FS scans is variable in VZV encephalitis and, when it occurs, it is typically patchy and mild. Restriction on DWI is common.

Epstein-Barr Encephalitis

Epstein-Barr virus (EBV) causes infectious mononucleosis. Uncontrolled proliferation of EBV-infected B cells results in post-transplant lymphoproliferative disease (PTLD). EBV is found in more than 90% of PTLD cases occurring within the first post-transplant year.

Mononucleosis is usually a benign, self-limiting disease. Neurologic complications occur in less than 7% of cases, but occasionally CNS disease can be the sole manifestation of EBV infection. Seizures, polyradiculomyelitis, transverse myelitis, encephalitis, cerebellitis, meningitis, and cranial nerve palsies have all been described as complications of EBV.

EBV has a predilection for deep gray nuclei. Bilateral diffuse T2/FLAIR hyperintensities in the basal ganglia and thalami are common (12-51). Patchy white matter hyperintensities are seen in some cases. EBV can also cause a transient, reversible lesion of the corpus callosum splenium that demonstrates restriction on DWI (12-52).

The differential diagnosis of EBV includes ADEM and other viral infections, especially West Nile virus.

West Nile Virus Encephalitis

West Nile virus (WNV) is a mosquito-borne Flavivirus that causes periodic epidemics of febrile illness and sporadic encephalitis in Africa, the Mediterranean basin, Europe, and southwest Asia. The first outbreak in the western hemisphere occurred in New York in 1999. Since then, WNV has spread across North America and into parts of Central and South America. WNV is now the most common cause of epidemic meningoencephalitis in North America.

WNV cycles between mosquito vectors and bird hosts; humans are incidental hosts. Transmission increases in warmer months; in the northern hemispheres, peak activity is from July through October. Nearly 80% of human WNV infections are clinically silent. Mild, self-limited fever is seen in 20%. Less than 1% of patients develop neuro-invasive disease. Immunosuppressed patients and the elderly are at higher risk.

WNV CNS infection can result in meningitis, encephalitis, and acute flaccid paralysis/poliomyelitis. The definitive diagnosis is made by PCR.

Bilateral hyperintensities on T2/FLAIR in the basal ganglia, thalami, and brainstem are typical **(12-53)**. WNV

may cause a transient corpus callosum splenium lesion. Lesions restrict on DWI but rarely enhance.

Rabies Encephalitis

Rabies encephalitis is caused by a neurotropic RNA virus of the Rhabdoviridae family and is a significant public health problem in developing countries.

Nearly 55,000 deaths due to rabies encephalitis occur annually, 99% of them in Asia and Africa. The dog is the major vector and viral reservoir, although other mammals (e.g., bats, wolves, raccoons, skunks, and mongooses) may act as major hosts. The virus is abundant in the saliva of the infected animal and is deposited in bite wounds.

The virus replicates in muscle tissues at the wound, then infects motor neurons, and accesses the CNS by retrograde axoplasmic flow.

Human rabies encephalitis is a rapidly fulminant disease that is invariably fatal once clinical symptoms become evident. The history and clinical presentation are highly suggestive, but the definitive diagnosis requires labora-

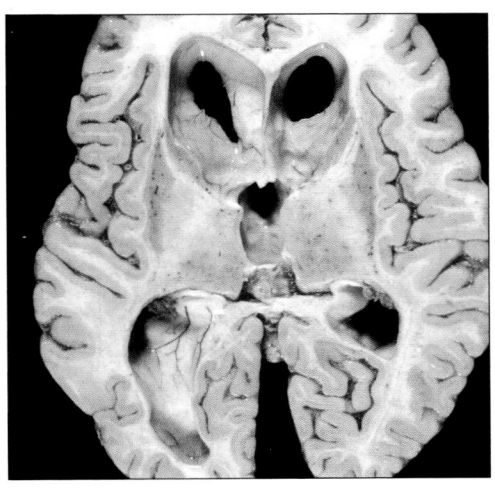

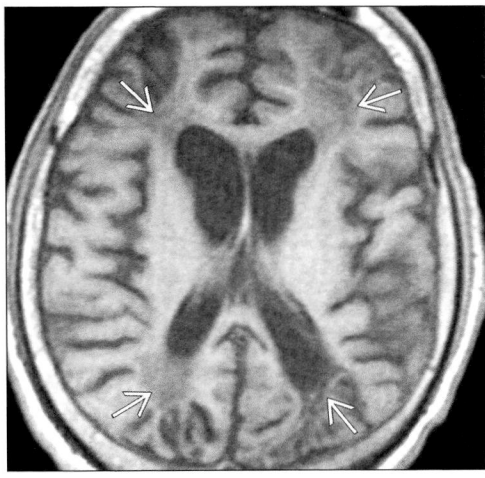

12-57. Autopsy of SSPE shows grossly enlarged ventricles and sulci with striking volume loss in the basal ganglia and cerebral white matter. In the occipital poles, the white matter is so thin the ventricles almost contact the cortical gray matter. 12-58. Axial T1WI in a 16-year-old male with deteriorating school performance and behavioral changes shows gross atrophy with bifrontal and bioccipital hypointensities ➡. CSF was positive for measles antibodies.

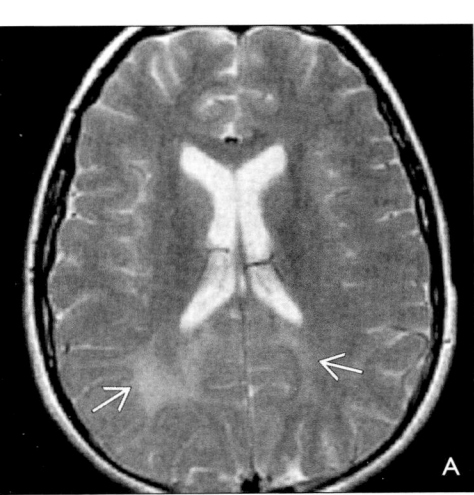

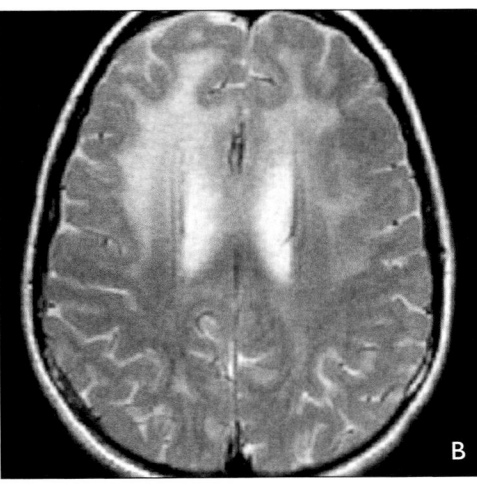

12-59A. Axial T2WI in a 13 year old with unexplained cognitive decline and progressive motor impairment shows bilateral but asymmetric white matter hyperintensities in both occipital lobes ➡. The frontal white matter appears normal. The ventricles are mildly enlarged for the patient's age. 12-59B. Six months later, the white matter hyperintensity has spread to involve both the frontal and parietal lobes. CSF was positive for measles antibodies.

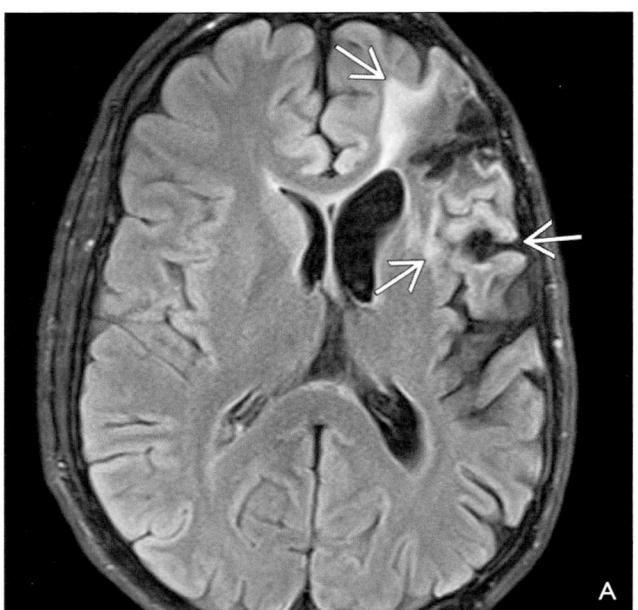

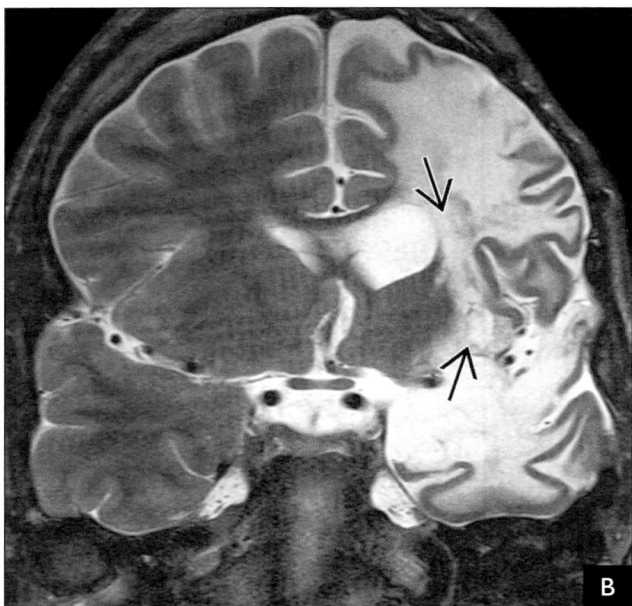

12-60A. Axial FLAIR in a 23 yo with medically refractory epilepsy secondary to RE shows left frontotemporal lobe volume loss with left lateral ventricle, sulcal enlargement. Note hyperintensity in the WM, basal ganglia, insula, cortex ➡.

12-60B. Coronal T2WI in the same patient confirms the frontotemporal atrophy and shows the insular volume loss ➔ especially well. Rasmussen encephalitis.

tory confirmation of rabies antigen or rabies antibodies or isolation of the virus from biological samples.

Rabies virus has a predilection for the brainstem, thalami, and hippocampi. MR shows poorly delineated hyperintensities in the dorsal medulla and upper spinal cord **(12-54)**, pontine tegmentum, periaqueductal gray matter, midbrain, medial thalami/hypothalami, and hippocampi. Hemorrhage and enhancement are generally absent, helping differentiate rabies from Japanese encephalitis and other viral encephalitides.

Influenza-associated Encephalopathy

Influenza-associated encephalitis or encephalopathy (IAE) is characterized by high fever, convulsions, severe brain edema, and high mortality. It usually affects children younger than five years. Onset of neurologic deterioration occurs a few days to a week after the first signs of influenza infection. Many viruses have been reported as causing IAE, most recently H3N2 and influenza A (H1N1, also known as swine flu).

Imaging studies are abnormal in the majority of cases. Symmetric bilateral thalamic lesions, hemispheric edema, and reversible lesions in the corpus callosum splenium and white matter are common. Findings resembling posterior reversible encephalopathy syndrome (PRES) have also been reported.

Acute Necrotizing Encephalopathy

Acute necrotizing encephalopathy (ANE) is a more severe, life-threatening form of IAE characterized by high fever, seizures, and rapid clinical deterioration

within two or three days after symptom onset. The disease is often fatal. Most cases occur in children or young adults.

ANE causes symmetric, often hemorrhagic, brain necrosis. The thalami, midbrain tegmentum, and pons are most severely affected **(12-55)**. Periventricular white matter, cerebellar, and spinal cord involvement has been reported in some cases.

CT may be normal early in the disease course. Bilaterally symmetric hyperintensity in the thalami is seen on T2/FLAIR **(12-56)**. The midbrain, pons, cerebellum, and deep cerebral white matter are frequently involved. T2* (GRE, SWI) shows "blooming" foci of petechial hemorrhage, most often in the thalami. Restriction on DWI has been described in some cases.

Miscellaneous Viral Encephalitides

A host of other viral encephalitides have been identified. While some (such as rotavirus encephalitis) are widespread, others (e.g., Japanese encephalitis, LaCrosse encephalitis, Nipah virus encephalitis) currently have a more restricted geographic distribution.

OTHER ACUTE VIRAL ENCEPHALITIDES

Varicella-Zoster Encephalitis
- After chickenpox or vaccination
- Cerebellitis, leukoencephalopathy, vasculopathy

Epstein-Barr Virus Encephalitis
- Rare mononucleosis complication
- Bilateral basal ganglia, WM/splenium

West Nile Virus Encephalitis
- Most common epidemic meningoencephalitis in North America
- Bilateral basal ganglia, thalami, brainstem

Rabies Encephalitis
- Developing > > developed countries
- Brainstem, thalami, spinal cord

Influenza-associated Encephalopathy (IAE)
- HINI (influenza A or "swine flu")
- Bilateral thalami, corpus callosum splenium

Acute Necrotizing Encephalopathy
- More fulminant form of IAE (often fatal)

Rotavirus Encephalitis
- Common GI pathogen in children
- Cerebellitis, corpus callosum splenium

Japanese Encephalitis
- Most common human endemic encephalitis
  ○ Korea, Japan, India, Southeast Asia
- Bilateral thalami, basal ganglia, substantia nigra, hippocampi
- High morbidity, mortality

LaCrosse Encephalitis
- School-aged children (midwest USA)
- Mimics HSE but more benign

Chronic Encephalitides

Some viruses cause acute, fulminating CNS infection. Others have a more insidious onset, producing a "slow" chronic infection. Some—such as the measles virus—can cause both. In this section, we briefly consider two chronic encephalitides: The measles reactivation syndrome called subacute sclerosing panencephalitis and Rasmussen encephalitis.

Other chronic encephalitides such as progressive multifocal leukoencephalopathy and variant Creutzfeldt-Jakob disease are considered in detail in subsequent chapters but briefly summarized in the box below.

Subacute Sclerosing Panencephalitis

Subacute sclerosing panencephalitis (SSPE) is a rare progressive encephalitis that occurs years after measles virus infection. A few cases in immunocompromised patients occur following immunization. The measles virus infects neurons and remains latent for years. Why and how reactivation occurs is not fully understood.

Measles virus disproportionately affects children in regions with low measles vaccination rates. Almost all patients are children or adolescents; adult-onset SSPE occurs but is rare. There is a 2:1 male predominance. SSPE is rare in developed countries where vaccination rates are high.

On average, clinical manifestations appear six years after measles virus infection. Symptom onset is often insidious, with behavioral and cognitive deterioration, myoclonic seizures, and progressive motor impairment. Elevated measles antibody titers in CSF establish the diagnosis.

SSPE shows relentless progression **(12-57)**. More than 95% of patients die within five years, most within one to six months after symptom onset. To date, there is no effective treatment.

Imaging may be normal in the early stages of the disease, so normal MR does not exclude SSPE. Inflammatory infiltrates in cortical gray matter are the major pathologic findings in early SSPE; gray matter reduction in the frontotemporal cortex may occur before other lesions become apparent **(12-58)**. Other abnormal findings eventually develop, with bilateral but asymmetric cortical and subcortical white matter, periventricular, and basal ganglia hyperintensity on T2/FLAIR sequences **(12-59)**.

Diffuse atrophy with ventricular and sulcal enlargement ensues as the disease progresses **(12-57)**. MRS shows decreased NAA and choline with elevated myoinositol and glutamine/glutamate.

Rasmussen Encephalitis

Rasmussen encephalitis (RE) is also called chronic focal (localized) encephalitis. RE is a rare progressive chronic encephalitis characterized by drug-resistant epilepsy, progressive hemiparesis, and mental impairment.

The exact etiology of RE is unknown. Viral infection or autoimmune disease involving glutamate receptors with glutamine toxicity have been suggested as possible etiologies. Biopsy findings are nonspecific, with leptomeningeal and perivascular lymphocytic infiltrates, microglial nodules, neuronal loss, and gliosis.

Patients are clinically normal until seizures begin, usually between the ages of 14 months and 14 years. Peak onset is between three and six years. Neurologic deficits are progressive, and the seizures often become medically refractory. Treatment options have included immunomodulatory therapy, focal cortical resection, and functional hemispherectomy.

Initial imaging studies are usually normal. With time, hyperintensity on T2/FLAIR develops in the cortex and subcortical white matter of the affected hemisphere **(12-60)**. The disease is characterized by unilateral progressive cortical atrophy. Basal ganglia atrophy is seen in the majority of cases. MRS findings are nonspecific with decreased NAA and increased Cho. Myoinositol may be mildly elevated.

CHRONIC ENCEPHALITIDES

Subacute Sclerosing Panencephalitis (SSPE)
- Measles virus reactivation
- Occurs years after initial infection
- Almost always fatal
- White matter hyperintensity
- Progressive atrophy

Rasmussen Encephalitis
- Etiology unknown (viral, autoimmune)
- Medically refractory epilepsy
- Unilateral
- WM hyperintensity, volume loss

Progressive Multifocal Leukoencephalopathy
- JC polyomavirus reactivation
- Immunocompromised patients
  - HIV/AIDS
  - Chemotherapy
  - Immunomodulating agents
- Progressive demyelination
  - Bilateral but asymmetric WM disease
- Usually no enhancement (acute may show peripheral)
- Diagnosis confirmed with CSF PCR

Variant Creutzfeldt-Jakob Disease
- Prion-mediated spongiform leukoencephalopathy
- Hyperintense BG, cortex on FLAIR
- Restricts on DWI

Selected References

Congenital Infections

TORCH Infections

- Nickerson JP et al: Neuroimaging of pediatric intracranial infection--part 2: TORCH, viral, fungal, and parasitic infections. J Neuroimaging. 22(2):e52-63, 2012
- Shet A: Congenital and perinatal infections: throwing new light with an old TORCH. Indian J Pediatr. 78(1):88-95, 2011

Congenital Cytomegalovirus

- Alcendor DJ et al: Infection and upregulation of proinflammatory cytokines in human brain vascular pericytes by human cytomegalovirus. J Neuroinflammation. 9:95, 2012
- Del Rosal T et al: Treatment of symptomatic congenital cytomegalovirus infection beyond the neonatal period. J Clin Virol. 55(1):72-4, 2012
- Gabrielli L et al: Congenital cytomegalovirus infection: patterns of fetal brain damage. Clin Microbiol Infect. 18(10):E419-E427, 2012
- Manara R et al: Brain magnetic resonance findings in symptomatic congenital cytomegalovirus infection. Pediatr Radiol. 41(8):962-70, 2011
- Fink KR et al: Neuroimaging of pediatric central nervous system cytomegalovirus infection. Radiographics. 30(7):1779-96, 2010

Congenital Toxoplasmosis

- Robert-Gangneux F et al: Epidemiology of and diagnostic strategies for toxoplasmosis. Clin Microbiol Rev. 25(2):264-96, 2012

Congenital (Perinatal) HIV

- Khamduang W et al: The interrelated transmission of HIV-1 and cytomegalovirus during gestation and delivery in the offspring of HIV-infected mothers. J Acquir Immune Defic Syndr. 58(2):188-92, 2011

Congenital Herpes Encephalitis

- Berardi A et al: Neonatal herpes simplex virus. J Matern Fetal Neonatal Med. 24 Suppl 1:88-90, 2011
- Lanari M et al: Neuroimaging examination of newborns in vertically acquired infections. J Matern Fetal Neonatal Med. 24 Suppl 1:117-9, 2011
- James SH et al: Antiviral therapy for herpesvirus central nervous system infections: neonatal herpes simplex virus infection, herpes simplex encephalitis, and congenital cytomegalovirus infection. Antiviral Res. 83(3):207-13, 2009
- Vossough A et al: Imaging findings of neonatal herpes simplex virus type 2 encephalitis. Neuroradiology. 50(4):355-66, 2008

Other Congenital Infections

- Karthikeyan K et al: Congenital rubella syndrome: a continuing conundrum. Lancet. 379(9830):2022, 2012
- Rodríguez-Cerdeira C et al: Congenital syphilis in the 21st century. Actas Dermosifiliogr. 103(8):679-693, 2012
- Bonthius DJ et al: Lymphocytic choriomeningitis virus infection of the developing brain: critical role of host age. Ann Neurol. 62(4):356-74, 2007

Acquired Pyogenic Infections

Meningitis

- Modi A et al: The etiological diagnosis and outcome in patients of acute febrile encephalopathy: A prospective observational study at tertiary care center. Neurol India. 60(2):168-73, 2012
- Nickerson JP et al: Neuroimaging of pediatric intracranial infection--part 1: techniques and bacterial infections. J Neuroimaging. 22(2):e42-51, 2012
- Takhar SS et al: U.S. emergency department visits for meningitis, 1993-2008. Acad Emerg Med. 19(6):632-9, 2012
- Hughes DC et al: Role of imaging in the diagnosis of acute bacterial meningitis and its complications. Postgrad Med J. 86(1018):478-85, 2010

Abscess

- Nathoo N et al: Taming an old enemy: a profile of intracranial suppuration. World Neurosurg. 77(3-4):484-90, 2012
- Toh CH et al: Differentiation of pyogenic brain abscesses from necrotic glioblastomas with use of susceptibility-weighted imaging. AJNR Am J Neuroradiol. 33(8):1534-8, 2012
- Piatt JH Jr: Intracranial suppuration complicating sinusitis among children: an epidemiological and clinical study. J Neurosurg Pediatr. 7(6):567-74, 2011
- Shachor-Meyouhas Y et al: Brain abscess in children - epidemiology, predisposing factors and management in the modern medicine era. Acta Paediatr. 99(8):1163-7, 2010
- Erdoğan E et al: Pyogenic brain abscess. Neurosurg Focus. 24(6):E2, 2008

Ventriculitis

- Gadgil N et al: Intraventricular brain abscess. J Clin Neurosci. 19(9):1314-6, 2012
- Nathoo N et al: Taming an old enemy: a profile of intracranial suppuration. World Neurosurg. 77(3-4):484-90, 2012
- Beer R et al: Management of nosocomial external ventricular drain-related ventriculomeningitis. Neurocrit Care. 10(3):363-7, 2009
- Lee TH et al: Clinical features and predictive factors of intraventricular rupture in patients who have bacterial brain abscesses. J Neurol Neurosurg Psychiatry. 78(3):303-9, 2007
- Fujikawa A et al: Comparison of MRI sequences to detect ventriculitis. AJR Am J Roentgenol. 187(4):1048-53, 2006

Empyemas

- Blumfield E et al: Pott's puffy tumor, intracranial, and orbital complications as the initial presentation of sinusitis in healthy adolescents, a case series. Emerg Radiol. 18(3):203-10, 2011

- Gupta S et al: Neurosurgical management of extraaxial central nervous system infections in children. J Neurosurg Pediatr. 7(5):441-51, 2011

- Hicks CW et al: Identifying and managing intracranial complications of sinusitis in children: a retrospective series. Pediatr Infect Dis J. 30(3):222-6, 2011

- Wong AM et al: Diffusion-weighted MR imaging of subdural empyemas in children. AJNR Am J Neuroradiol. 25(6):1016-21, 2004

Acquired Viral Infections

Herpes Simplex Encephalitis

- Egdell R et al: Herpes simplex virus encephalitis. BMJ. 344:e3630, 2012

- Sabah M et al: Herpes simplex encephalitis. BMJ. 344:e3166, 2012

- Sureka J et al: Clinico-radiological spectrum of bilateral temporal lobe hyperintensity:a retrospective review. Br J Radiol. 85(1017):e782-92, 2012

- Ward KN et al: Herpes simplex serious neurological disease in young children: incidence and long-term outcome. Arch Dis Child. 97(2):162-5, 2012

- De Tiège X et al: The spectrum of herpes simplex encephalitis in children. Eur J Paediatr Neurol. 12(2):72-81, 2008

HHV-6 Encephalopathy

- Noguchi T et al: CT and MRI findings of human herpesvirus 6-associated encephalopathy: comparison with findings of herpes simplex virus encephalitis. AJR Am J Roentgenol. 194(3):754-60, 2010

- Sauter A et al: Spectrum of imaging findings in immunocompromised patients with HHV-6 infection. AJR Am J Roentgenol. 193(5):W373-80, 2009

Miscellaneous Acute Encephalitides

- Pahud BA et al: Varicella zoster disease of the central nervous system: epidemiological, clinical, and laboratory features 10 years after the introduction of the varicella vaccine. J Infect Dis. 203(3):316-23, 2011

- Bartynski WS et al: Influenza A encephalopathy, cerebral vasculopathy, and posterior reversible encephalopathy syndrome: combined occurrence in a 3-year-old child. AJNR Am J Neuroradiol. 31(8):1443-6, 2010

- Ormitti F et al: Acute necrotizing encephalopathy in a child during the 2009 influenza A(H1N1) pandemia: MR imaging in diagnosis and follow-up. AJNR Am J Neuroradiol. 31(3):396-400, 2010

- Rao AS et al: Case report: magnetic resonance imaging in rabies encephalitis. Indian J Radiol Imaging. 19(4):301-4, 2009

Chronic Encephalitides

- Cece H et al: Epidemiological findings and clinical and magnetic resonance presentations in subacute sclerosing panencephalitis. J Int Med Res. 39(2):594-602, 2011

- Irislimane M et al: Serial MR imaging of adult-onset Rasmussen's encephalitis. Can J Neurol Sci. 38(1):141-2, 2011

- Ng WF et al: A 7-year-old boy dying of acute encephalopathy. Brain Pathol. 20(1):261-4, 2010

- Aydin K et al: Reduced gray matter volume in the frontotemporal cortex of patients with early subacute sclerosing panencephalitis. AJNR Am J Neuroradiol. 30(2):271-5, 2009

13

Tuberculosis, Fungal, Parasitic, and Other Infections

Overview

Infectious diseases are increasingly worldwide phenomena, with what once seemed exclusively local indigenous diseases rapidly spreading around the globe. New pathogens have emerged, as viruses such as HIV—almost unheard-of 30 years ago—have become global health concerns. The rise in food and waterborne pathogens is unmistakable. Immigration and widespread travel have resulted in formerly exotic "tropical diseases" such as neurocysticercosis and other parasitic infections becoming commonplace.

In this chapter we continue the delineation of acquired infections that we began in Chapter 12 with pyogenic and viral CNS infections. We first turn our attention to mycobacterial infections, focusing primarily on tuberculosis. We follow with an in-depth discussion of fungal and parasitic infections. We close the chapter with a brief consideration of miscellaneous and emerging CNS infections to remind us that the "hot zone" is right outside our windows, no matter where we live!

Mycobacterial Infections

Mycobacteria are small, rod-shaped acid-fast bacilli with more than 125 recognized species. They are divided into three main groups, each with a different signature disease: (1) *Mycobacterium tuberculosis (*tuberculosis), (2) nontuberculous mycobacteria ("atypical" mycobacterial spectrum infections), and (3) *M. leprae* (leprosy). Each group has different pathologic features, clinical manifestations, and imaging findings.

Of the three groups, the so-called *M. tuberculosis* complex is responsible for the vast majority of human mycobacterial infections. It causes more than 98% of CNS tuberculosis (TB) and is therefore the major focus of our discussion. We follow with a brief review of nontuberculous mycobacterial infection and its rare manifestations in the head and neck. Leprosy causes peripheral neuropathy but virtually never affects the CNS and is not considered further.

Tuberculosis

Etiology

Most TB is caused by *M. tuberculosis*. Less common species that are also considered part of the *M. tuberculosis* complex include *M. africanum*, *M. microti*, *M. canetti,* and *M. bovis*.

Human-to-human transmission is typical. Animal-to-human transmission via *M. bovis*, a common pathogen in the past, is now rarely encountered.

Neurotuberculosis is secondary to hematogenous spread from extracranial infection, most frequently in the lungs. The GI and GU tracts, musculoskeletal system, and lymph nodes are less common sources.

Pathology

CNS TB has several distinct pathological manifestations. Acute/subacute TB **meningitis** (TBM) constitutes 70-80% of cases. An inflammatory reaction ("exudate") with a variable admixture of exudative, proliferative, and necrotizing components in the subarachnoid cisterns is the typical finding (13-1). Rarely, TBM presents as an isolated pachymeningitis with focal or diffuse dura-arachnoid thickening.

The second most common manifestation of neurotuberculosis is a focal parenchymal infection with central caseating necrosis (TB granuloma or **tuberculoma**).

The least common manifestation of CNS TB is "abscess," which contains macrophages and liquefied necrotic debris. (As it usually does not contain pus with neutrophils, most TB "abscesses" are more correctly called pseudoabscesses.) TB **pseudoabscesses** are rare in immunocompetent patients but are found in 20% of patients coinfected with TB and HIV.

LOCATION. TB meningitis has a striking predilection for the basal cisterns although exudates in the superficial convexity sulci do occur.

Tuberculomas are space-occupying masses of granulomatous tissue. The majority occur in the cerebral hemispheres, especially the frontal and parietal lobes and basal ganglia. Occasionally, CNS TB presents as a focal dural (13-11), intraventricular (choroid plexus), or isolated calvarial lesion.

TB abscesses can be found anywhere in the brain, from the hemispheres to the midbrain to the cerebellum.

SIZE AND NUMBER. Tuberculomas vary in size. The majority are small (less than 2.5 cm), and the "miliary" nodules are often just a few millimeters in diameter. "Giant" tuberculomas can reach four to six centimeters.

Tuberculomas also vary in number, ranging from a solitary lesion to innumerable small "miliary" lesions.

GROSS PATHOLOGY. TBM is seen as a dense, diffuse, glutinous exudate that accumulates in the basal cisterns, coating the brain surfaces and cranial nerves

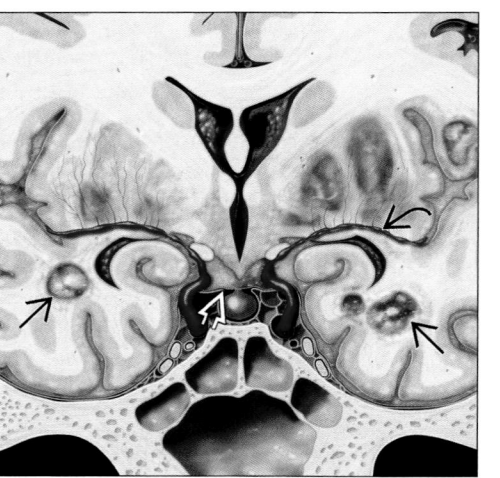

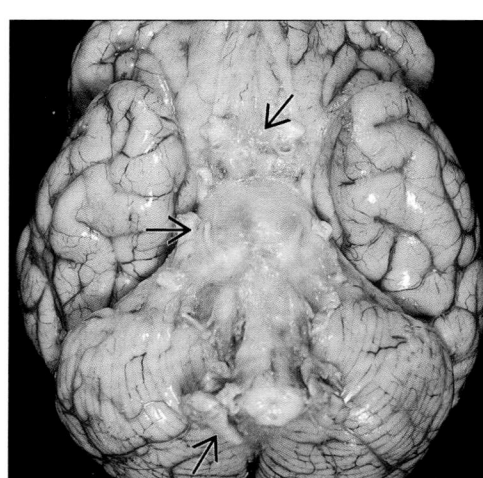

13-1. Coronal graphic shows basilar TB meningitis ➡ and tuberculomas ➡, which often coexist. Note the vessel irregularity ➡ and early basal ganglia ischemia related to arteritis. 13-2. Autopsy case shows typical findings of TB meningitis with dense exudates extending throughout the basal cisterns ➡. Gross appearance is indistinguishable from that of pyogenic meningitis. (Courtesy R. Hewlett, MD.)

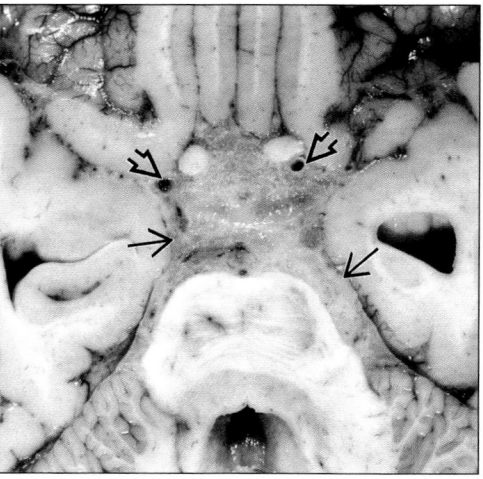

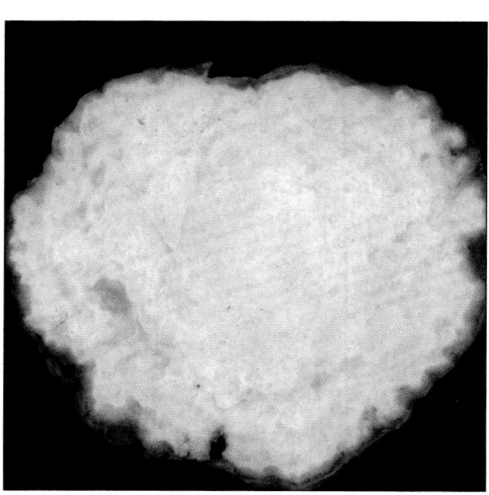

13-3. Axial section through the suprasellar cistern in another autopsied case of TBM shows thick exudate ➡ filling the suprasellar cistern and coating the pons. Note the extremely small diameter of the supraclinoid ICAs ➡ due to TB vasculitis. (Courtesy R. Hewlett, MD.) 13-4. Surgically resected TB gumma shows the solid "cheesy" appearance of a caseating granuloma. (Courtesy R. Hewlett, MD.)

(13-2). The suprasellar/chiasmatic region, ambient cisterns, and interpeduncular fossa are most commonly involved (13-3).

Tuberculomas have a creamy, cheese-like, necrotic center surrounded by a grayish granulomatous rim (13-4).

MICROSCOPIC FEATURES. Edema, perivascular infiltrates, and microglial reaction are common in brain tissue immediately under the tuberculous exudate.

The inflammatory exudate encases major vessels and their perforating branches, invading vessel walls and causing a true panarteritis (sometimes called "endarteritis obliterans"). Vessel occlusion with secondary infarcts are identified in 40% of autopsied cases of TBM, most commonly in the basal ganglia and internal capsule. Large territorial infarcts are less common.

Tuberculomas demonstrate central caseating necrosis with surrounding multinucleated giant cells (generally Langerhans type), epithelioid histiocytes, plasma cells, and lymphocytes. Acid-fast bacilli may be difficult to identify.

TB pseudoabscesses consist of vascular granulation tissue with acid-fast bacilli, liquefied necrotic debris, and macrophages.

Clinical Issues

EPIDEMIOLOGY. TB is endemic in many developing countries and is reemerging in developed countries because of widespread immigration and HIV/AIDS. Worldwide, 8-10 million new cases are reported each year. The highest prevalence is in Southeast Asia, which accounts for one-third of all cases.

CNS infections account for only 2-5% of all TB infections but are among the most devastating of its many manifestations. One of the most common "brain tumors" in endemic countries is tuberculoma, which accounts for 10-30% of all brain parenchymal masses.

CNS TB occurs in both immunocompetent and immunocompromised patients. Among people with latent TB infection, HIV is the strongest known risk factor for progression to active TB. In TB and HIV/AIDS coinfection, each disease also greatly amplifies the lethality of the other.

DEMOGRAPHICS. CNS TB occurs at all ages, but 60-70% of cases occur during the first two decades. There is no gender predilection.

PRESENTATION. The most common manifestation of active CNS TB is meningitis. Presentation varies from fever and headache with mild meningismus to confusion, lethargy, seizures, and coma. Symptoms of increased intracranial pressure are common.

Cranial neuropathies, especially involving CNs II, III, IV, VI, and VII, are common.

DIAGNOSIS. CSF shows low glucose, elevated protein, and lymphocytic pleocytosis. Acid-fast bacilli can sometimes be identified visually in CSF smears, but the definitive diagnosis depends on positive PCR or growth and identification of *M. tuberculosis* in cultures.

NATURAL HISTORY AND TREATMENT. Prognosis is variable and depends on the patient's immune status as well as treatment. Untreated TB can be fatal in four to eight weeks. Even with treatment, one-third of patients deteriorate within six weeks. Overall mortality is 25-30% and is even higher in drug-resistant TB.

Multidrug-resistant TB (MDR TB) is resistant to at least two of the first-line anti-TB drugs, isoniazid and rifampin. **Extensively drug-resistant TB (XDR TB)** is defined as TB that is resistant to isoniazid and rifampin, any fluoroquinolone, and at least one of three injectable second-line drugs (i.e., amikacin, kanamycin, or capreomycin).

Common complications of CNS TB include hydrocephalus (70%) and stroke (up to 40%). The majority of survivors have long-term morbidity with seizures, mental retardation, neurologic deficits, and even paralysis.

CNS TB: ETIOLOGY, PATHOLOGY, AND CLINICAL ISSUES

Etiology
- *Mycobacterium tuberculosis* complex
  - Vast majority caused by *M. tuberculosis*
  - Other mycobacteria (e.g., *M. bovis*) rare
- Human-to-human transmission
- Hematogenous spread from extracranial site
  - Lung > GI, GU
  - Other: Bone, lymph nodes

Pathology
- TB meningitis (70-80%)
  - Exudative, proliferative, necrotizing inflammatory reaction
  - Basal cisterns > convexity sulci
- Tuberculoma (TB granuloma) (20-30%)
  - Caseating necrosis
  - Cerebral hemispheres, basal ganglia
- Pseudoabscess (rare)

Epidemiology and Demographics
- 8-10 million new cases annually
- All ages, but 60-70% in children < 20 years
- CNS TB in 2-5% of cases
- 10-30% of brain parenchymal masses in endemic areas

Presentation and Diagnosis
- Fever, headache, meningismus, signs of ↑ ICP
- PCR best, most rapid definitive diagnosis

Prognosis
- Overall mortality (25-30%)
- Worse with MDR or XDR TB

Imaging

GENERAL FEATURES. Early diagnosis and treatment is necessary to reduce the significant morbidity and mortality associated with CNS TB. As CT scans may be normal in the earliest stages of TBM, contrast-enhanced MR is the imaging procedure of choice.

CT FINDINGS.

TB meningitis. Nonspecific hydrocephalus is the most frequent finding on NECT. "Blurred" ventricular margins indicate extracellular fluid accumulation in the subependymal WM. As the disease progresses, iso- to mildly hyperdense basilar and sulcal exudates replace and efface the normal hypodense CSF (13-5A). CECT usually shows intense enhancement of the basilar meninges and subarachnoid spaces (13-5B).

Patients who deteriorate during treatment often develop new hydrocephalus, infarcts, exudates, or tuberculomas.

Tuberculoma. NECT scans show one or more iso- to slightly hyperdense round, lobulated, or crenated masses with variable perilesional edema. Calcification can be seen in healed granulomas (13-6). CECT scans demonstrate punctate, solid, or ring-like enhancement (13-7).

Pseudoabscess. TB pseudoabscesses are hypodense on NECT with significant mass effect and surrounding edema. Ring enhancement is seen on CECT (13-5B).

MR FINDINGS.

TB meningitis. Basilar exudates are isointense with brain on T1WI, giving the appearance of "dirty" CSF (13-8). FLAIR scans show increased signal intensity in the sulci and cisterns. Marked linear or nodular meningeal enhancement is seen on T1 C+ FS sequences. Focal or diffuse dura-arachnoid enhancement (pachymeningitis) with or without involvement of the underlying subarachnoid spaces may occur but is uncommon (13-12).

Tuberculous exudates often extend into the brain parenchyma along the perivascular spaces, causing a meningoencephalitis.

Vascular complications are common complications of TBM. The "flow voids" of major arteries may appear reduced. Parenchyma adjacent to meningeal inflam-

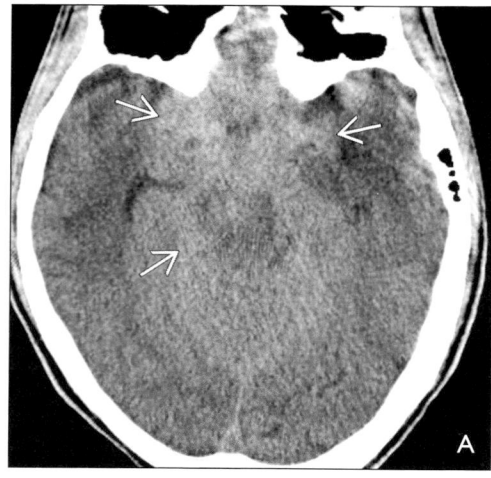
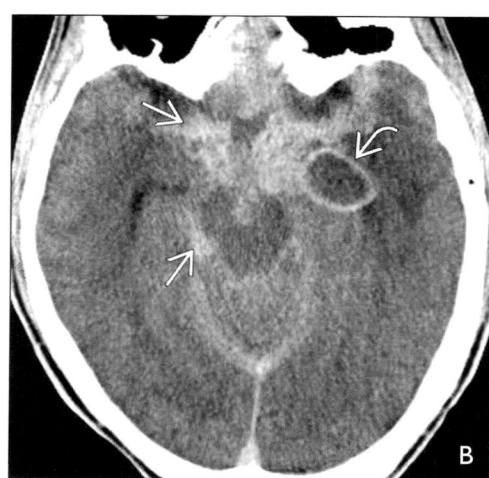

13-5A. NECT scan in TBM shows complete effacement of all basal cisterns by a mildly hyperdense exudate ➡. 13-5B. CECT scan in the same patient shows that the exudate enhances moderately ➡. The left medial temporal lobe ring-enhancing mass ➡ with surrounding edema could represent either a tuberculoma or TB pseudoabscess. (Courtesy A. T. Maydell, MD, S. Andronikou, MD.)

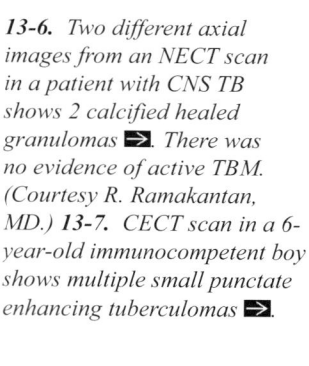
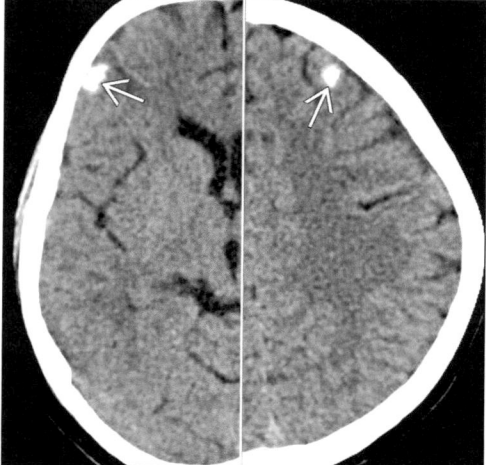
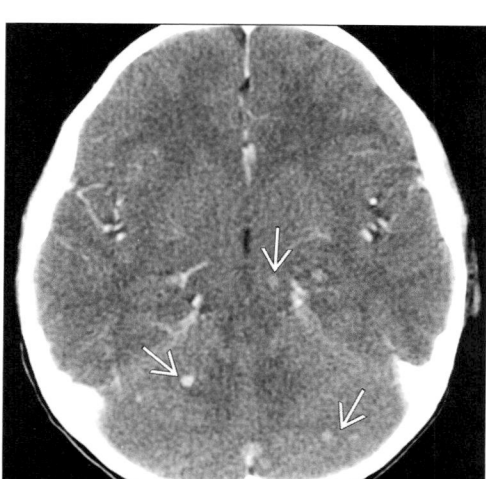

13-6. Two different axial images from an NECT scan in a patient with CNS TB shows 2 calcified healed granulomas ➡. There was no evidence of active TBM. (Courtesy R. Ramakantan, MD.) 13-7. CECT scan in a 6-year-old immunocompetent boy shows multiple small punctate enhancing tuberculomas ➡.

mation may demonstrate necrosis. Penetrating artery infarcts with enhancement and restricted diffusion are common **(13-8)**.

Tuberculoma. Most TB granulomas are solid caseating lesions that appear hypo- or isointense with brain on T1WI and hypointense on T2WI **(13-9A)**. Liquefied areas may be T2 hyperintense with a hypointense rim **(13-10A)**.

Enhancement is variable, ranging from small punctate foci to multiple rim-enhancing lesions. Mild to moderate round or lobulated ring-like enhancement around a nonenhancing center is the most typical pattern **(13-9B)**, **(13-10B)**. pMR shows elevated rCBV in the cellular, hypervascular, enhancing rim.

Solid caseating tuberculomas do not restrict on DWI although liquefied foci may restrict.

MRS can be very helpful in characterizing tuberculomas and distinguishing them from neoplasm or pyogenic abscess. A prominent decrease in NAA:Cr with a modest decrease in NAA:Cho is typical. A large lipid peak with absence of other metabolites such as amino acids and succinate is seen in 85-90% of cases **(13-10C)**.

Pseudoabscess. Unlike tuberculomas, TB pseudoabscesses are usually hyperintense to brain on T2/FLAIR and restrict on DWI. A ring-enhancing multiloculated lesion or multiple separate lesions is the typical finding on T1 C+ images. MRS shows lipid and lactate peaks without evidence of cytosolic amino acids.

Differential Diagnosis

The major differential diagnosis of *TBM* is **pyogenic or carcinomatous meningitis**, as their imaging findings can be indistinguishable. **Carcinomatous meningitis** is usually seen in older patients with a known systemic or primary CNS neoplasm.

Neurosarcoidosis can also mimic TBM. Infiltration of the pituitary gland, infundibulum, and hypothalamus is common.

The major differential diagnosis of multiple parenchymal *tuberculomas* is **neurocysticercosis** (NCC). NCC usually shows multiple lesions in different stages of evolution. Tuberculomas can also resemble pyogenic **abscesses** or **neoplasms**. Abscesses restrict on DWI. Tuberculomas have a large lipid peak on MRS and lack the elevated Cho typical of neoplasm.

TB *pseudoabscesses* appear identical to pyogenic abscesses on standard imaging studies. Both show restricted diffusion. MRS of TB pseudoabscesses shows no evidence of cytosolic amino acids, the spectral hallmark of pyogenic lesions.

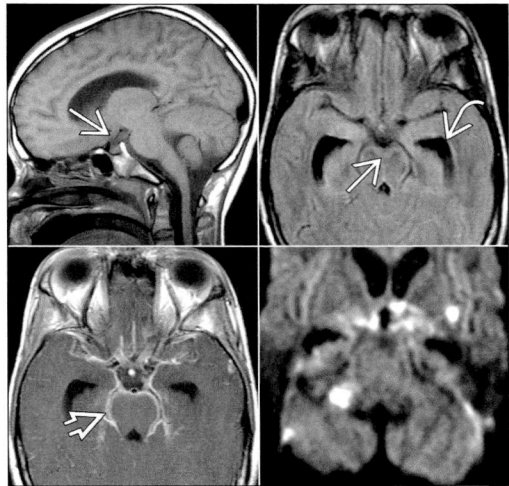

13-8. TBM with "dirty" CSF ➡, *hydrocephalus* ➡, *basilar meningeal enhancement* ➡, *restricted diffusion. (Courtesy S. Andronikou, MD.)*

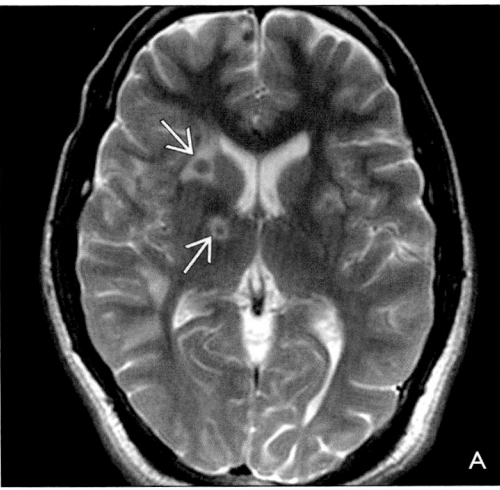

13-9A. T2WI shows multifocal tuberculomas as hypointense foci surrounded by edema ➡.

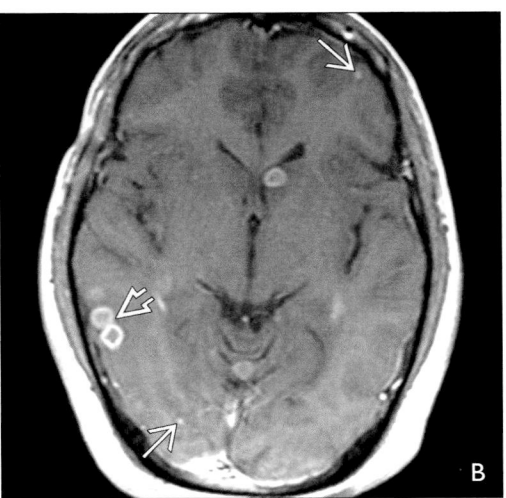

13-9B. T1C+ scan in the same case illustrates additional lesions with punctate ➡, *ring enhancement* ➡. *(Courtesy R. Ramakantan, MD).*

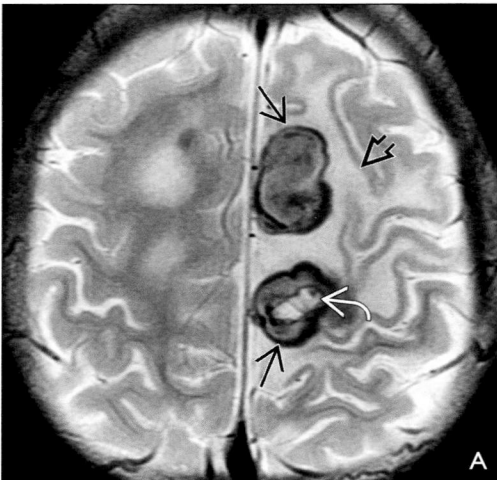

13-10A. *Axial T2WI shows hypointense caseating tuberculomas* →, *edema* ⇨. *Central liquefaction is hyperintense* ↩.

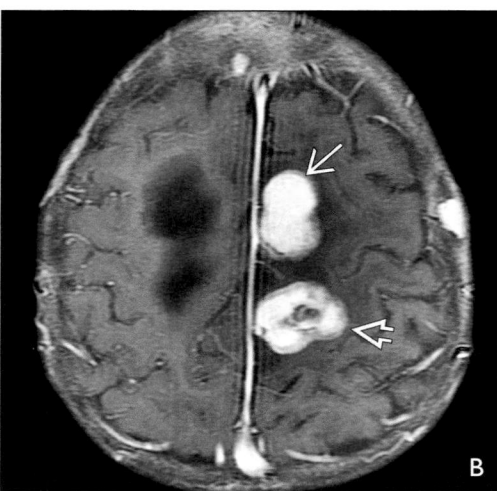

13-10B. *T1C+FS shows both solid* →, *thick rim enhancement* ⇨.

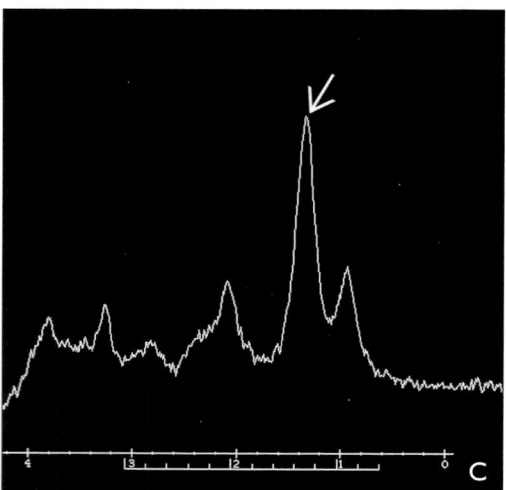

13-10C. *MRS with TE = 35 msec shows decreased NAA, prominent lipid lactate peak* →.

CNS TUBERCULOSIS: IMAGING

General Features
- Best procedure = contrast-enhanced MR
- Findings vary with pathology
  - TB meningitis
  - Tuberculoma
  - Abscess
- Combination of findings (usually TBM, tuberculoma)

CT Findings
- TB meningitis
  - Can be normal in early stages!
  - Nonspecific hydrocephalus common
  - "Blurred" ventricular margins
  - Effaced basilar cisterns, sulci
  - Iso-/mildly hyperdense exudates
  - Thick, intense pia-subarachnoid space enhancement
  - Can cause pachymeningopathy with diffuse dura-arachnoid enhancement
  - Look for secondary parenchymal infarcts
- Tuberculoma
  - Iso-/hyperdense parenchymal mass(es)
  - Round, lobulated > irregular margins
  - Variable edema
  - Punctate, solid, or ring enhancement
  - May cause focal enhancing dural mass
  - Chronic, healed may calcify
- Abscess
  - Hypodense mass
  - Perilesional edema usually marked
  - Ring enhancement

MR Findings
- TB meningitis
  - Can be normal
  - "Dirty" CSF on T1WI
  - Hyperintense on FLAIR
  - Linear, nodular pia-subarachnoid space enhancement
  - May extend via perivascular spaces into brain
  - Vasculitis, secondary infarcts common
  - Penetrating arteries > large territorial infarcts
- Tuberculoma
  - Hypo-/isointense with brain on T1WI
  - Most are hypointense on T2WI
  - Rim enhancement
  - Rare = dural-based enhancing mass
  - Large lipid peak on MRS
- Abscess
  - T2/FLAIR hyperintense
  - Striking perilesional edema
  - Rim, multiloculated enhancement

Differential Diagnosis
- TBM
  - Pyogenic, carcinomatous meningitis
  - Neurosarcoid
- Tuberculoma
  - Neurocysticercosis
  - Primary or metastatic neoplasm
  - Pyogenic abscess
  - Dural-based mass can mimic meningioma

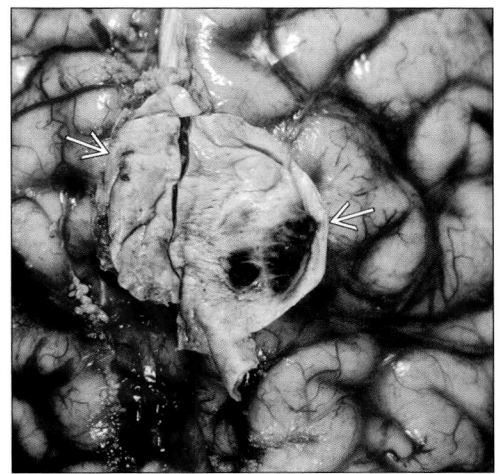

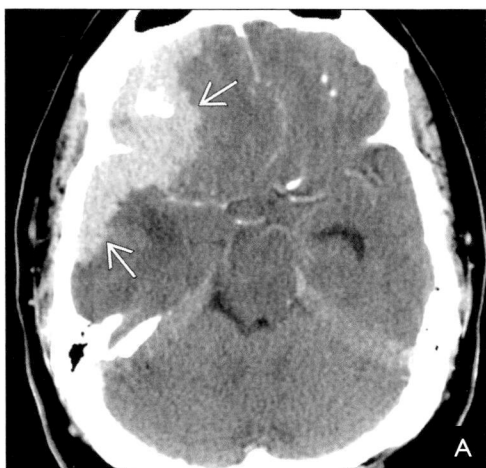

13-11. Gross autopsy case shows TB as a focal dural mass ➡. Appearance is indistinguishable from that of meningioma. 13-12A. CECT scan in a case of proven dura-based TB inflammatory pseudotumor shows extensive "en plaque" enhancing right frontotemporal mass ➡.

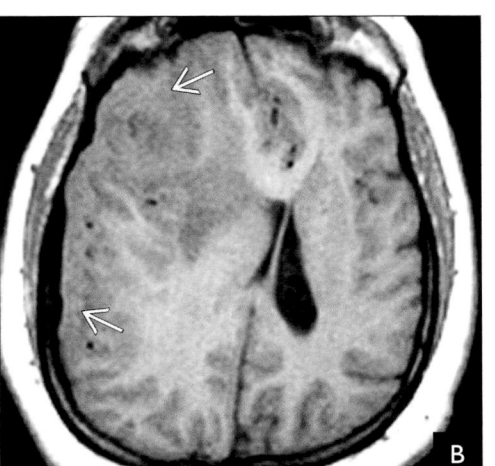

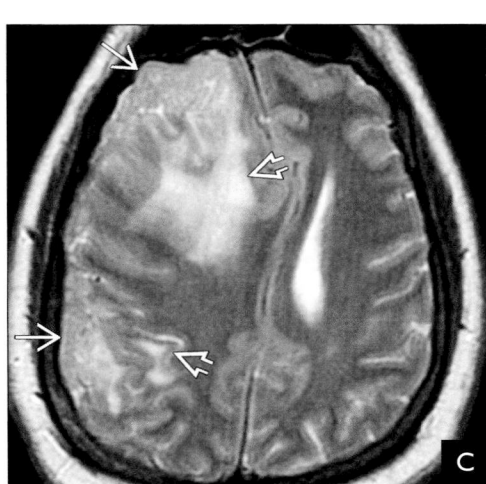

13-12B. T1WI in the same patient shows that the mass ➡ is isointense with the underlying cortex. 13-12C. T2WI shows that the mass ➡ is moderately hyperintense compared to the underlying brain and is associated with significant edema ➡ in the underlying brain parenchyma.

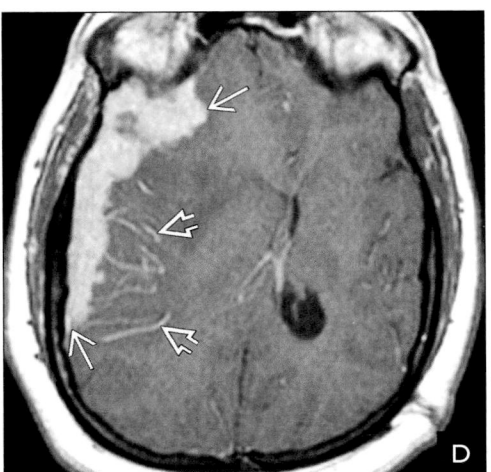

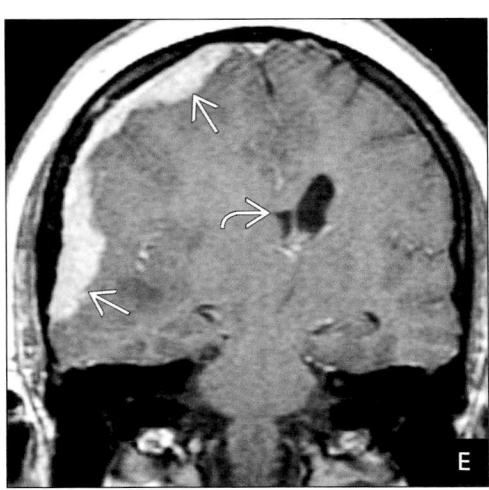

13-12D. T1 C+ scan demonstrates that the dura-based mass ➡ enhances intensely and uniformly. Note contrast stasis (intravascular enhancement) in the underlying middle cerebral artery branches ➡. 13-12E. Coronal T1 C+ scan shows the enhancing dura-based pseudotumor ➡ causing significant mass effect, evidenced by subfalcine herniation of the lateral ventricles ➡. (Courtesy A. Sillag, MD.)

Nontuberculous Mycobacterial Infections

Nontuberculous mycobacteria (NTM) are ubiquitous organisms that are widely distributed in water and soil. Human disease is usually caused by environmental exposure, not human-to-human spread.

Compared to *M. tuberculosis*, NTM infections are uncommon. Most are caused by two closely related "atypical" mycobacteria, *M. avium* and *M. intracellulare*, which are collectively called *M. avium-intracellulare complex* (MAIC). Less common NTM include *M. abscessus*, *M. fortuitum*, and *M. kansasii*.

The most common manifestation of MAIC infection is pulmonary disease, which usually occurs in adults with intact systemic immunity. Disseminated systemic infections are primarily seen in immunocompromised patients.

Three disease patterns are seen in the head and neck: (1) chronic cervical lymphadenitis, (2) immune reconstitu-tion inflammatory syndrome (IRIS), and (3) CNS disease **(13-13)**.

Nontuberculous Cervical Lymphadenitis

CLINICAL ISSUES. Subacute or chronic neck infection is by far the most common manifestation of MAIC in the head and neck. Children younger than five years and immunocompromised adults are typically affected. Most patients are afebrile and present with a painless, slowly enlarging submandibular or preauricular mass. Chest radiographs show no evidence of pulmonary TB.

IMAGING. NECT scans demonstrate one or more enlarged, isodense, solid or cystic-appearing level I and II lymph node(s). Unilateral disease is more common than bilateral disease. Inflammatory changes in the surrounding tissues are minimal or absent.

Rim enhancement is common on CECT **(13-14)**. Occasionally, fistulization to the skin occurs.

MR shows hyperintense, cystic-appearing lymph node(s) with minimal surrounding inflammation on fat-saturated T2-weighted images **(13-15A)**. T1 C+ FS illustrates

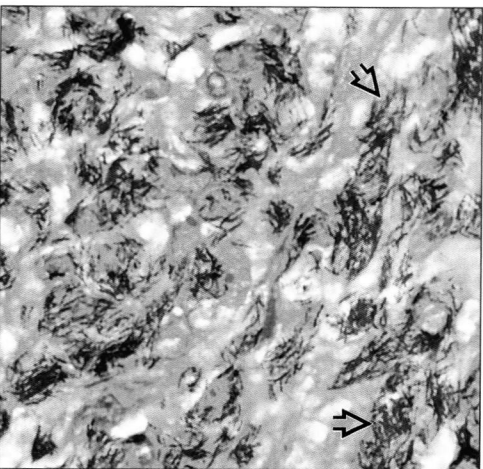

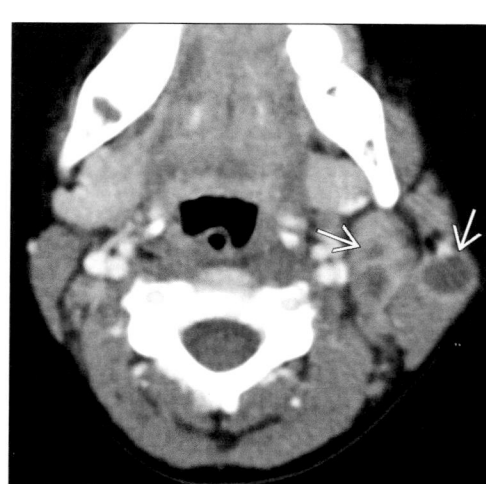

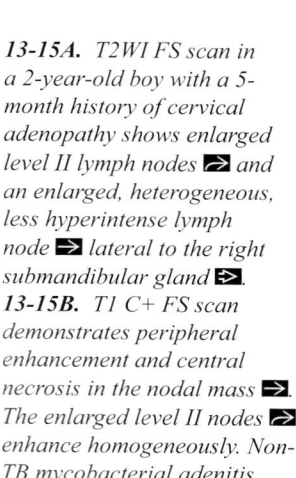

13-13. Biopsy specimen of a CNS mycobacterial spindle cell pseudotumor from a patient with AIDS demonstrates large numbers of acid-fast bacilli ⧖ that fill epithelioid histiocytes. Granulomas, multinucleated giant cells are absent. (Courtesy B. K. DeMasters, MD.) 13-14. Axial CECT scan in a 2-year-old girl with a painless left neck mass shows multiple ring-enhancing lymph nodes ➡ with low-attenuation centers. Non-TB mycobacterial adenitis.

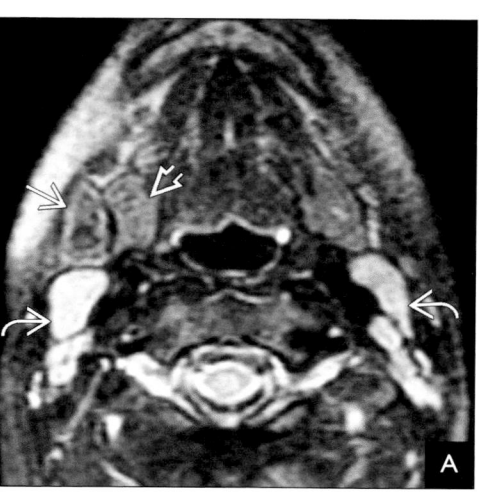

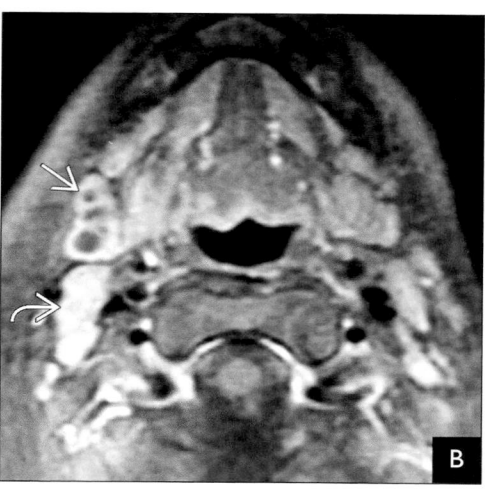

13-15A. T2WI FS scan in a 2-year-old boy with a 5-month history of cervical adenopathy shows enlarged level II lymph nodes ➚ and an enlarged, heterogeneous, less hyperintense lymph node ➘ lateral to the right submandibular gland ⧖. 13-15B. T1 C+ FS scan demonstrates peripheral enhancement and central necrosis in the nodal mass ➡. The enlarged level II nodes ➚ enhance homogeneously. Non-TB mycobacterial adenitis.

marked peripheral enhancement around the nonenhancing necrotic centers (13-15B).

DIFFERENTIAL DIAGNOSIS. The major differential diagnosis of nontuberculous cervical lymphadenitis is **suppurative lymphadenopathy**. Patients present with fever and painful mass(es). Cellulitis with stranding of fat and adjacent structures is common.

Tuberculosis causes 95% of cervical lymphadenitis cases in adults but only 8% in children. Half of all cases occur in immunocompromised patients. Imaging studies demonstrate multiple enlarged posterior triangle and internal jugular nodes. Bilateral lesions are typical. Co-existing pulmonary disease is common.

Less common mimics are cat scratch disease and second branchial cleft cysts. **Cat scratch disease** presents one to two weeks following the incident and is seen as reactive adenopathy in regional nodes draining the lesion. **Second branchial cleft cyst** can mimic a cystic lymph node but is located between the submandibular gland and sternocleidomastoid muscle.

MAIC-associated IRIS

Atypical microbacterial IRIS outside the CNS is common, usually occurring as pulmonary disease and/or lymphadenitis, but MAIC-associated CNS IRIS is very rare. Reported findings are perivascular granulomatous inflammation with multiple enhancing parenchymal lesions on T1 C+ scans.

CNS Disease

In comparison to CNS TB, MAIC infections are uncommon. MAIC causes a localized mass-like inflammatory lesion called a mycobacterial spindle cell pseudotumor. The most common sites are the lymph nodes, lungs, and skin.

Most reported cases in the head and neck are found in the nose and orbit. Intracranial lesions are exceptionally rare; almost all are found in patients with HIV/AIDS.

At biopsy, mycobacterial pseudotumors contain sheets of epithelioid histiocytes with mixed inflammatory cell infiltrate and little necrosis. Innumerable acid-fast intracellular organisms can be demonstrated but granulomas and multinucleated giant cells are absent (13-13).

Imaging studies show an enhancing, dural-based mass that mimics meningioma or neurosarcoidosis.

> **NONTUBERCULOUS MYCOBACTERIAL INFECTION**
>
> **Etiology and Clinical Issues**
> - Non-TB mycobacteria (NTM)
>   - "Atypical" mycobacteria
>   - Most common = *M. avium, M. intracellulare*
>   - Collectively termed *M. avium-intracellulare complex* (MAIC)
> - Pulmonary disease (immunocompetent)
> - Disseminated systemic disease (immunocompromised)
> - Head and neck disease less common; CNS rare
>
> **Nontuberculous Cervical Lymphadenitis**
> - Subacute/chronic lymphadenopathy
> - Immunocompetent children < 5 years
> - Typical presentation: Painless submandibular, preauricular mass
> - Imaging shows enlarged, ring-enhanced node(s)
>
> **Immune Reconstitution Inflammatory Syndrome**
> - HIV(+) patient with disseminated MAIC placed on HAART
> - Usually involves lungs, lymph nodes
> - CNS disease very rare
>   - Disseminated enhancing parenchymal lesions
>
> **CNS Disease due to NTM**
> - Clinical issues
>   - CNS MAIC < < < CNS TB
>   - Immunocompromised adults
> - Pathology
>   - Mass-like (mycobacterial spindle cell pseudotumor)
>   - Histiocytes, inflammatory cells, intracytoplasmic acid-fast bacilli
>   - Lymph nodes, lungs, skin > > nose and orbit > CNS
> - Imaging
>   - Focal dural-based mass
>   - Can mimic meningioma, neurosarcoid

Fungal Infections

Fungi are ubiquitous organisms with a widespread distribution. Although CNS fungal infections are uncommon, their prevalence is rising as the number of immunocompromised patients increases worldwide.

Terminology

CNS fungal infections are also called cerebral mycosis. A focal "fungus ball" is also called a mycetoma or fungal granuloma.

Etiology

FUNGAL PATHOGENS. A number of fungal pathogens can cause CNS infections. The most common are *Coccidioides immitis, Aspergillus fumigatus, Cryptococcus*

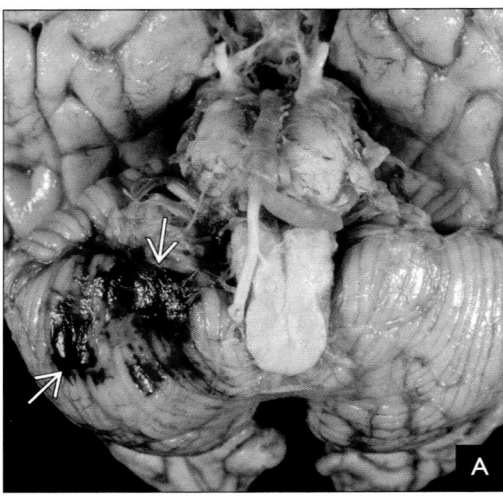

13-16A. Autopsy case demonstrates multiple hemorrhagic infarcts ➡ typical of fungal infection.

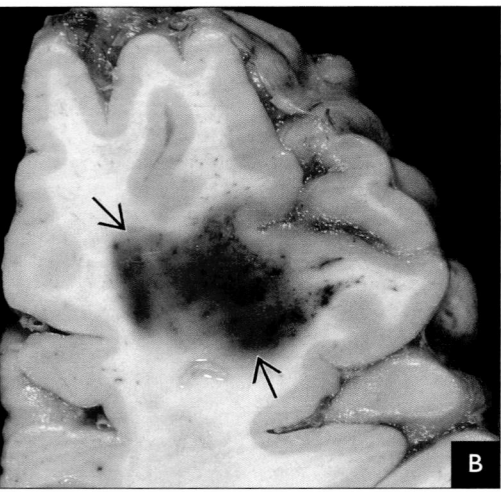

13-16B. Axial section through the cerebral hemisphere in the same case shows a hemorrhagic subcortical infarct ➡. (Courtesy R. Hewlett, MD.)

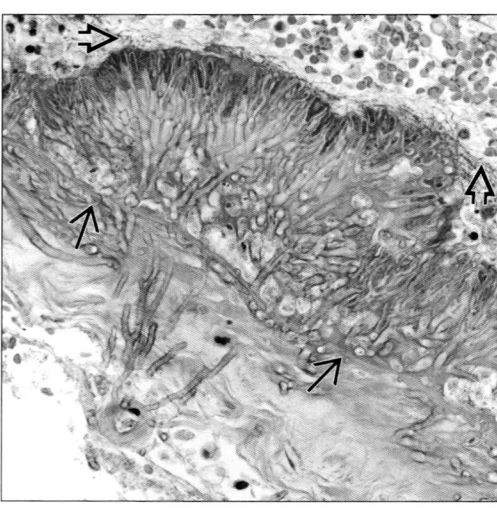

13-17. Corona-like arrays of Aspergillus ➡ penetrate the wall of a leptomeningeal blood vessel ➡. (Courtesy B. K. DeMasters, MD.)

neoformans, Histoplasma capsulatum, Candida albicans, and *Blastomyces dermatitidis.* Members of the Zygomycetes class (especially the *Mucor* genus) can also become pathogenic.

The specific agents vary with immune status. Candidiasis, mucormycosis, and cryptococcal infections are usually opportunistic infections. They occur in patients with predisposing factors such as diabetes, hematological malignancies, and immunosuppression. Coccidioidomycosis and aspergillosis affect both immunocompetent and immunocompromised patients.

ENVIRONMENTAL EXPOSURE. Aside from *C. albicans* (a normal constituent of human gut flora), most fungal infections are initially acquired by inhaling fungal spores in contaminated dust and soil.

Coccidioidomycosis occurs in areas with low rainfall and high summer temperatures (e.g., Mexico, southwestern United States, some parts of South America) whereas histoplasmosis and blastomycosis occur in watershed areas with moist air and damp, rotting wood (e.g., Africa, around major lakes and river valleys in North America).

SYSTEMIC AND CNS INFECTIONS. Sufficiently large numbers of inhaled spores can produce pulmonary infection. In immunocompetent patients, fungi such as *Blastomycosis* and *Histoplasma* are usually confined to the lungs where they cause focal granulomatous disease.

Hematogenous spread from the lungs to the CNS is the most common route of infection. Fungal sinonasal infections may invade the skull base and cavernous sinus directly. Sinonasal disease with intracranial extension (rhinocerebral disease) is the most common pattern of *Aspergillus* and *Mucor* CNS infection.

Disseminated fungal disease usually occurs only in immunocompromised patients.

Pathology

CNS mycoses have four basic pathologic manifestations: Diffuse meningeal disease (most common), solitary or multiple focal parenchymal lesions (common), disseminated nonfocal parenchymal disease (rare), and focal dura-based masses (rarest).

LOCATION. The meninges are the most common site, followed by the brain parenchyma and spinal cord.

SIZE AND NUMBER. Parenchymal mycetomas vary in size from tiny (a few millimeters) to one or two centimeters. Large lesions are rare although multiple lesions are common.

GROSS PATHOLOGY. The most common gross finding is basilar meningitis with congested meninges. Parenchymal fungal infections can be either focal or disseminated.

Fungal abscesses are encapsulated lesions with a soft tan or thick mucoid-appearing center, an irregular reddish margin, and surrounding edema. Disseminated disease is less common and causes a fungal cerebritis with diffusely swollen brain.

Hemorrhagic infarcts, typically in the basal ganglia or at the gray-white matter junction, are common with angioinvasive fungi (13-16). On rare occasions, fungal infections can produce dura-based masses that closely resemble meningioma.

MICROSCOPIC FEATURES. Microscopic features of CNS fungal infections vary with the specific agent (13-17). *Blastomyces*, *Histoplasma*, *Cryptococcus*, and *Candida* are yeasts. *Aspergillus* has branching septated hyphae whereas *Mucor* has broad nonseptated hyphae. *Candida* has pseudohyphae. *Coccidioides* has sporangia that contain endospores.

Fungal abscesses exhibit central coagulative necrosis with moderate amounts of acute (polymorphonuclear leukocytic) or chronic (lymphohistiocytic) inflammation mixed with variable numbers of fungal organisms.

Abscesses are surrounded by a rim of granulation tissue, perivascular hemorrhage, and thrombosed vessels. Fungal granulomas are less common and are characterized by the presence of multinucleated giant cells.

Extraaxial fungal infections are characterized predominantly by spindle cell proliferations.

Clinical Issues

EPIDEMIOLOGY. Epidemiology varies with the specific fungus. Many infections are both common and asymptomatic (e.g., approximately 25% of the entire population in the USA and Canada are infected with *Histoplasma*).

Candidiasis is the most common nosocomial fungal infection worldwide. *Aspergillosis* accounts for 20-30% of fungal brain abscesses and is the most common cerebral complication following bone marrow transplantation. *Mucor* is ubiquitous but generally infects only immunocompromised patients.

DEMOGRAPHICS. Immunocompetent patients have a bimodal age distribution with fungal infections disproportionately represented in children and older individu-

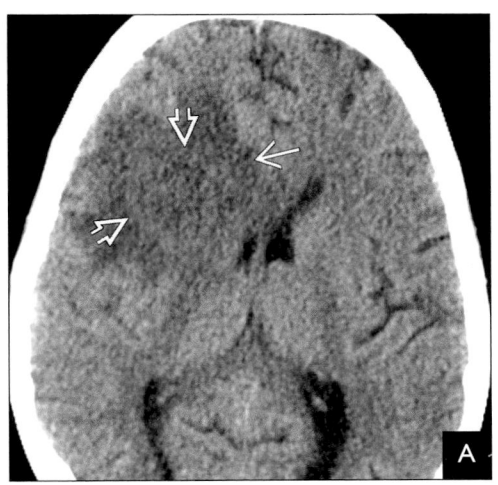
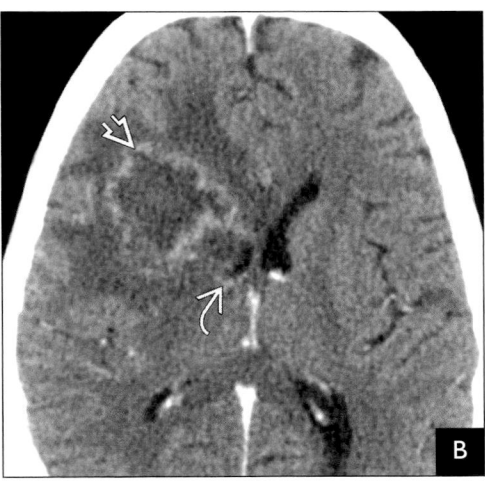

13-18A. *Axial NECT scan in an immunocompetent patient shows a hypodense mass with a faint rim of hyperdensity* ➡ *surrounded by significant edema* ➡. *13-18B. CECT scan in the same patient shows an irregular, crenelated enhancing rim* ➡ *with edema, adjacent ventriculitis* ➡. *Aspergilloma was found at surgery.*

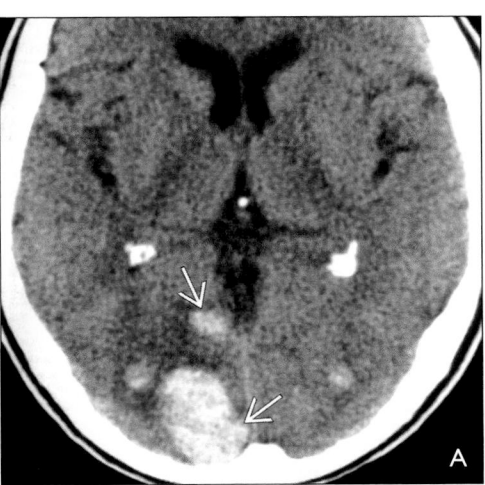
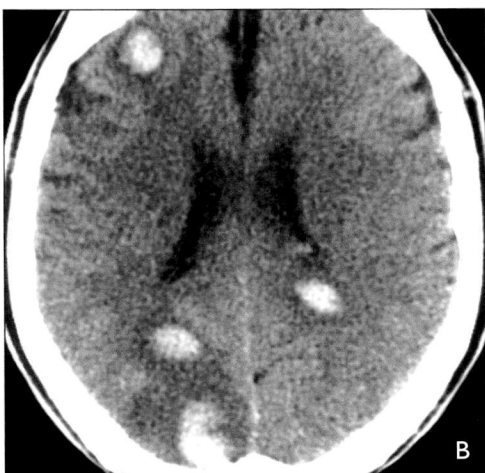

13-19A. *NECT scan shows multifocal parenchymal hemorrhages* ➡ *in both occipital lobes caused by angioinvasive fungal infection. 13-19B. More cephalad NECT scan in the same patient shows that additional hemorrhagic lesions are scattered throughout both hemispheres. Hemorrhagic mycetomas from angioinvasive aspergillosis were documented at surgery.*

als. There is a slight male predominance. Immunocompromised patients of all ages and both sexes are at risk.

PRESENTATION. Nonspecific symptoms such as weight loss, fever, malaise, and fatigue are common. Many patients initially have symptoms of pulmonary infection. CNS involvement is presaged by headache, meningismus, mental status changes, and/or seizure.

DIAGNOSIS. Imaging and laboratory findings are likewise often nonspecific. While microscopic features are helpful in diagnosis, cultures are necessary to document the species and type of fungal infection.

The diagnosis of aggressive fungal infections can be especially difficult in immunocompromised patients. There are no available serological or PCR-based diagnostic tests for some fungi (e.g., *Mucor*). Biopsy remains the only reliable method to diagnose these infections.

NATURAL HISTORY. Prognosis depends on the patient's underlying disease as well as prompt, accurate diagnosis and initiation of appropriate antifungal therapy.

FUNGAL DISEASES OF THE CNS

Etiology and the Environment
- General features
  - Most are ubiquitous, worldwide
  - Most from spores in soil (exception = *Candida*)
- Normal or both normal/immunocompromised
  - Histoplasmosis, blastomycosis
  - Aspergillosis, coccidioidomycosis
- Usually immunocompromised
  - Candidiasis, cryptococcosis, mucormycosis

Pathology
- 4 basic manifestations
  - Diffuse meningeal disease
  - Solitary/multiple focal parenchymal masses
  - Diffuse/disseminated nonfocal parenchymal disease
  - Focal dura-based mass(es)
- Angioinvasive fungi (*Mucor*, *Aspergillus*) can cause hemorrhagic infarcts

Clinical Issues
- Risk factors
  - Congenital/acquired immunocompromised states
  - Diabetes
- Age
  - Bimodal (children, older individuals) but can affect any age

---

13-20A. Sagittal T1 C+ scan in a 30-year-old man with cocci meningitis/ventriculitis shows obstructive hydrocephalus with marked enlargement of the fourth ventricle ➡️. Thick enhancing exudate ➡️ entirely fills the suprasellar and prepontine cisterns, the cisterna magna and extends inferiorly around the cervical spinal cord. 13-20B. Axial T1 C+ scan in the same patient shows extensive enhancement in the basal and ambient cisterns ➡️. Note ependymitis ➡️.

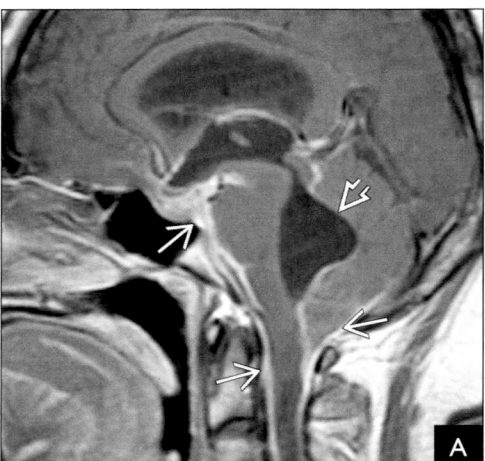

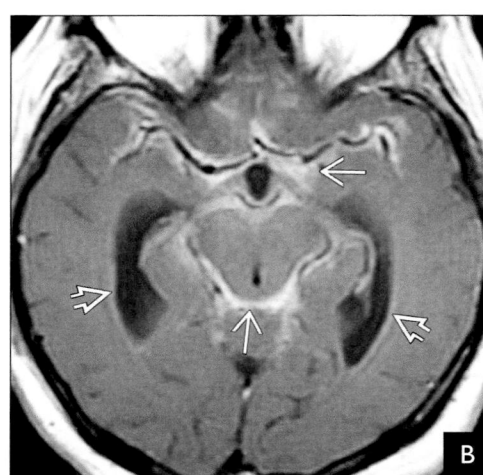

13-21A. T1WI in an immunocompromised patient with disseminated fungal infection shows diffuse brain atrophy, multifocal confluent hypointensities in the cortex and subcortical white matter ➡️. A focal cystic-appearing mass is present in the right basal ganglia ➡️. 13-21B. FLAIR scan shows diffuse hyperintensity throughout most of the cortex, subcortical white matter, and basal ganglia ➡️. Fungal cerebritis with focal basal ganglia mycetoma ➡️.

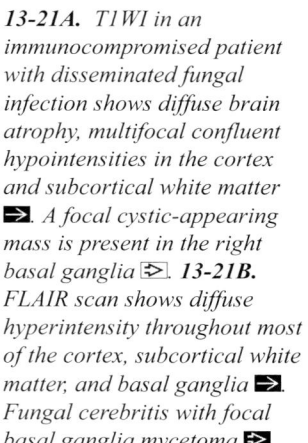

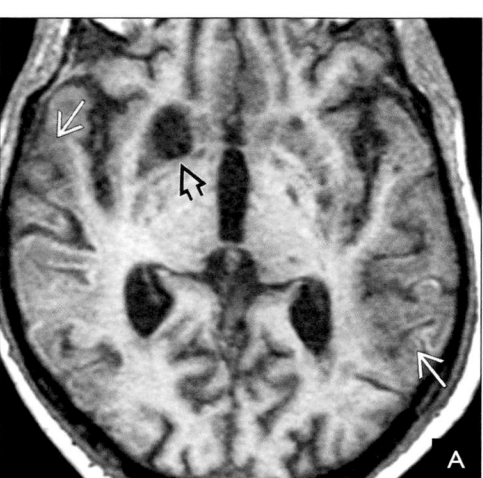

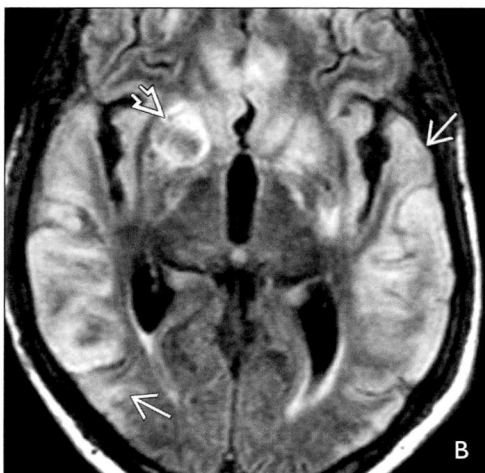

maging

GENERAL FEATURES. Findings vary with the patient's immune status. Well-formed fungal abscesses are seen in immunocompetent patients. Imaging early in the course of a rapidly progressive infection in an immunocompromised patient may show diffuse cerebral edema more characteristic of encephalitis than fungal abscess.

CT FINDINGS. Findings on NECT include hypodense parenchymal lesions caused by focal granulomas or ischemia **(13-18)**. Hydrocephalus is common in patients with fungal meningitis. Patients with coccidioidal meningitis may demonstrate thickened, mildly hyperdense basal meninges.

Disseminated parenchymal infection causes diffuse cerebral edema. Multifocal parenchymal hemorrhages are common in patients with angioinvasive fungal species **(13-19)**, **(13-25)**.

Mycetoma in the paranasal sinuses is usually seen as a single opacified hyperdense sinus that contains fine round to linear calcifications. Fungal sinusitis occasionally becomes invasive, crossing the mucosa to involve blood vessels, bone, orbit, cavernous sinuses, and intracranial cavities. Focal or widespread bone erosion with adjacent soft tissue infiltration can mimic neoplasm. Bone CT with reconstructions in all three standard planes is helpful to assess skull base involvement, and T1 C+ FS MR is the best modality to delineate disease spread beyond the nose and sinuses **(13-26)**.

Diffuse meningeal disease demonstrates pia-subarachnoid space enhancement on CECT. Multiple punctate or ring-enhancing parenchymal lesions are typical findings of parenchymal mycetomas.

MR FINDINGS. Fungal meningitis appears as "dirty" CSF on T1WI. Parenchymal lesions are typically hypointense on T1WI but demonstrate T1 shortening if subacute hemorrhage is present **(13-23)**. Irregular walls with nonenhancing projections into the cavity are typical.

T2/FLAIR scans in patients with fungal cerebritis show bilateral but asymmetric cortical/subcortical and basal ganglia hyperintensity **(13-21)**. Focal lesions (mycetomas) show high signal foci that typically have a periph-

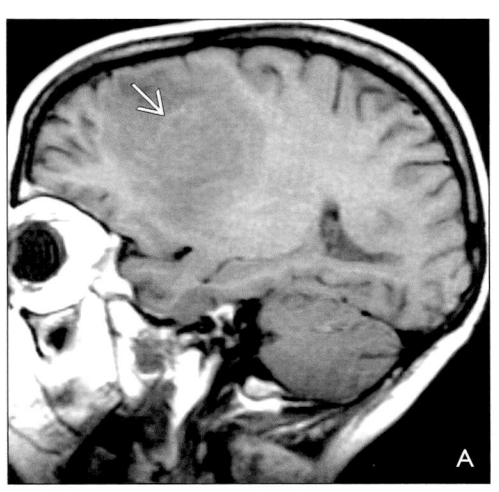

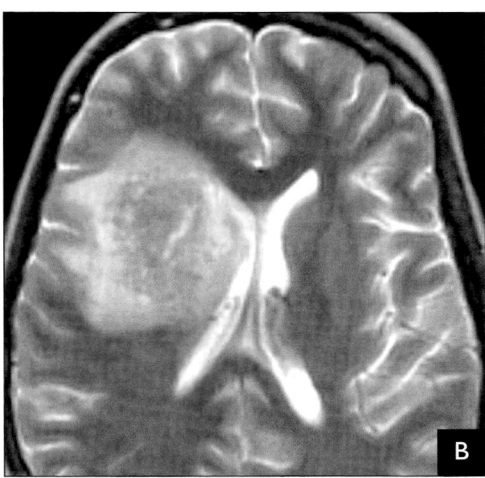

13-22A. Sagittal T1WI in the same case as Figure 13-18 shows hypointense edema surrounding a mildly hyperintense rim ➡. *13-22B. Axial T2WI shows that the lesion is mostly hypointense relative to cortex.*

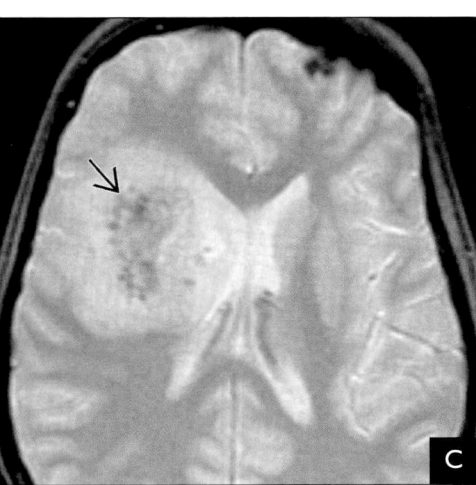

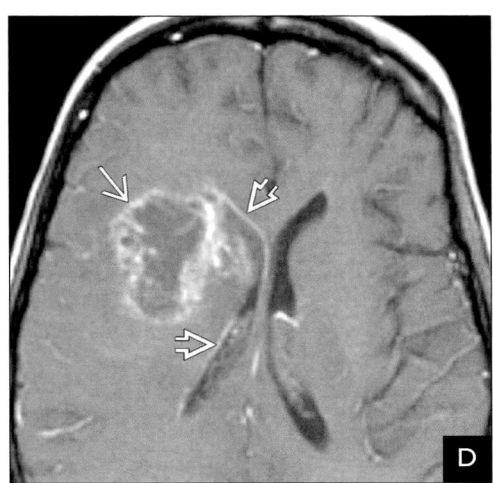

13-22C. T2* GRE shows multiple punctate "blooming" foci ➔ *within the mass, consistent with petechial hemorrhages. 13-22D. Axial T1 C+ shows the irregular, crenelated enhancing rim* ➡ *that surrounds the central nonenhancing lesion core. Note extension into the lateral ventricle with diffuse ependymal enhancement* ➡. *Aspergilloma was found at surgery and confirmed by histopathology.*

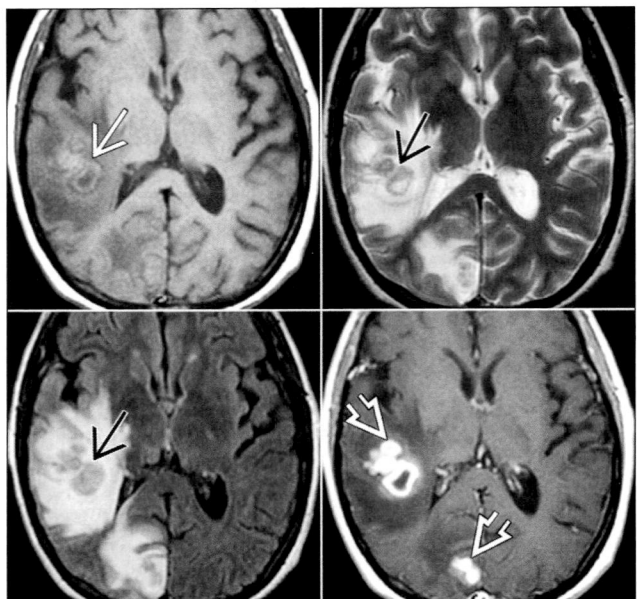

13-23. Multiple Nocardia abscesses in a 35-year-old woman. Note the distinct hyperintense rims on T1WI ➡️ and the hypointensity on T2/FLAIR scans ➡️, solid and rim enhancement ➡️.

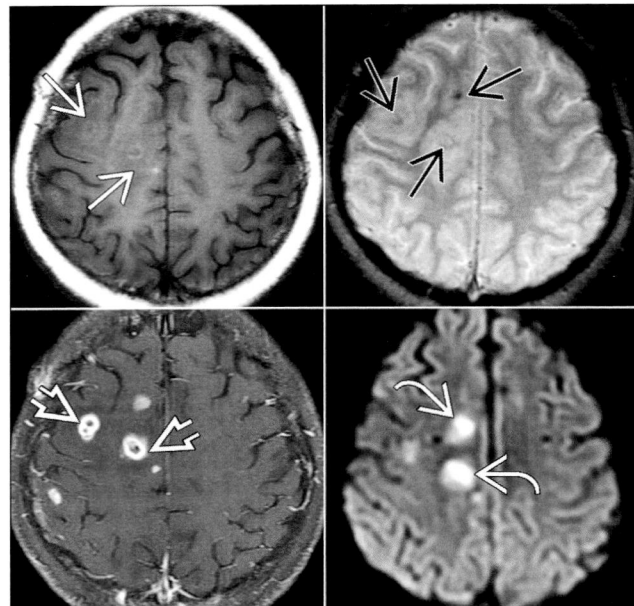

13-24. Aspergillus abscesses in an immunosuppressed patient. Axial T1WI shows punctate and ring-like hyperintense foci ➡️ with "blooming" on T2 ➡️. Nodular and rim enhancement is seen on T1 C+ FS ➡️. Most of the lesions restrict on DWI ➡️.*

eral hypointense rim, surrounded by vasogenic edema. T2* scans may show "blooming" foci caused by hemorrhages or calcification (13-24). Focal paranasal sinus and parenchymal mycetomas usually restrict on DWI (13-26D).

T1 C+ FS scans usually show diffuse, thick, enhancing basilar leptomeninges (13-20). Angioinvasive fungi may erode the skull base, cause plaque-like dural thickening, and occlude one or both carotid arteries (13-27), (13-28). Parenchymal lesions show punctate, ring-like, or irregular enhancement (13-22), (13-24).

MRS shows mildly elevated Cho and decreased NAA. A lactate peak is seen in 90% of cases, while lipid and amino acids are identified in approximately 50%. Multiple peaks resonating between 3.6 and 3.8 ppm are common and probably represent trehalose.

Differential Diagnosis

Imaging findings of fungal meningitis are nonspecific and resemble those of pyogenic, tubercular, and carcinomatous meningitis.

Fungal abscesses can sometimes be differentiated from **pyogenic abscesses** by their more irregularly shaped walls and internal nonenhancing projections, together with resonance between 3.6 and 3.8 ppm on MRS. **TB** can have crenelated margins and appear similar to fungal abscesses on standard imaging studies. Gross hemorrhage is more common with fungal than either pyogenic or tubercular abscesses.

Other mimics of fungal abscesses are primary **neoplasm** (e.g., glioblastoma with central necrosis) or metastases.

FUNGAL INFECTIONS: IMAGING

CT
- Meningitis
  - Iso-/hyperdense meninges
- Abscess
  - Hypodense center
  - Hyperdense rim
  - Variable hemorrhage (angioinvasive infections)
- Sinonasal disease
  - Hyperdense (mycetoma)
  - May demonstrate Ca++
  - ± bone destruction
  - ± intracranial extension

MR
- Meningitis
  - "Dirty" CSF
  - Isointense with brain on T1WI
  - Hyperintense on T2/FLAIR
- Abscess
  - Hypointense center, hyperintense rim on T1WI
  - Hyperintense center, hypointense rim on T2WI
  - Hemorrhagic "blooming" foci on T2* common
  - Restriction on DWI
  - Strong enhancement on T1 C+
  - MRS lactate in 90%, lipids and amino acids in 50%; multiple peaks at 3.6-3.8 ppm

Differential Diagnosis
- Pyogenic, granulomatous meningitis
- Pyogenic abscess
- Neoplasm (primary, metastatic)

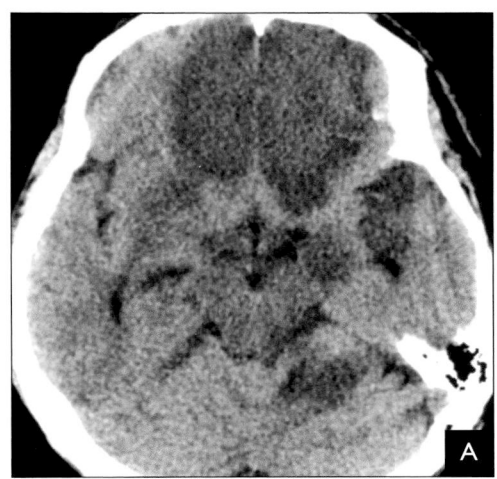

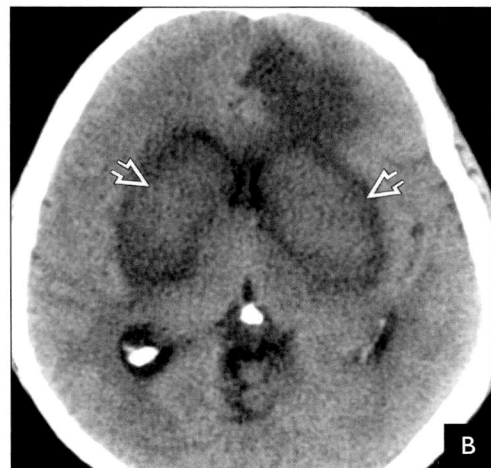

13-25A. NECT scan of angioinvasive aspergillosis shows hypodense infarcts in the cerebellum, midbrain, frontal and temporal lobes. 13-25B. Axial NECT scan in the same patient shows that the basal ganglia infarcts exhibit some hemorrhagic transformation ➡.

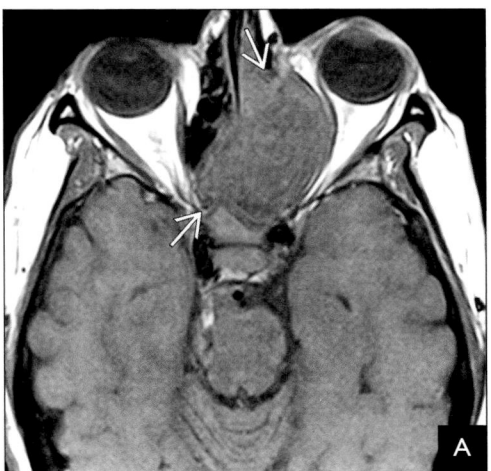

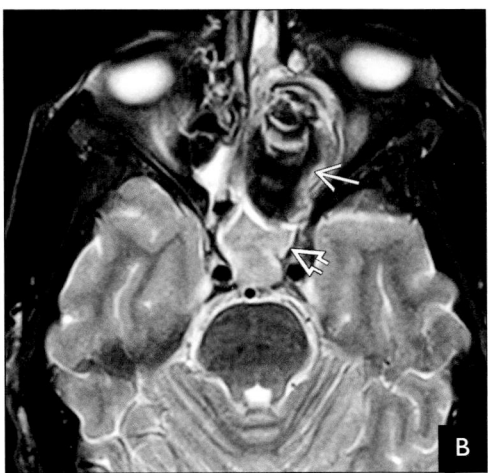

13-26A. Series of images demonstrates a focal sinonasal mycetoma. Axial T1WI shows an expansile, destructive isointense mass ➡ in the nose and ethmoid sinus. The lesion invades the left orbit and extends posteriorly, obstructing the sphenoid sinus. 13-26B. The lesion is somewhat mixed signal intensity on T2WI FS but mostly appears profoundly hypointense ➡. Note obstructive changes in the sphenoid sinus ➡.

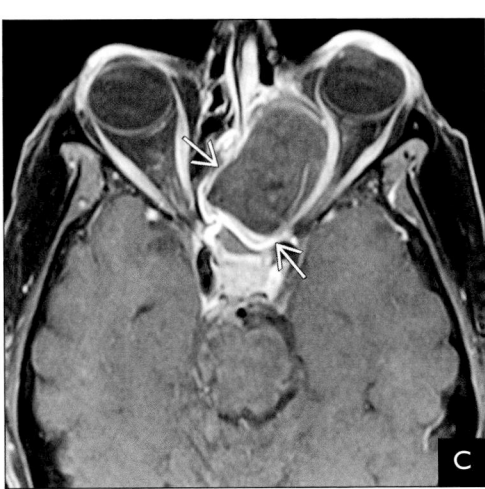

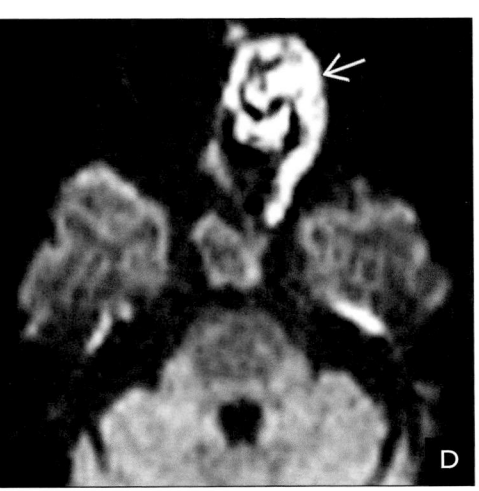

13-26C. T1 C+ FS scan shows peripheral enhancement around the margins of the mass ➡. 13-26D. The mass shows diffusion restriction ➡.

13-27. *Close-up view of autopsied cavernous sinus with invasive fungal sinusitis occluding the left cavernous internal carotid artery ➡. (Courtesy R. Hewlett, MD.)* **13-28A.** *Bone CT in a patient with poorly controlled diabetes, invasive mucormycosis. Note bone invasion, destruction at orbital apex, sphenoid sinus ➡.*

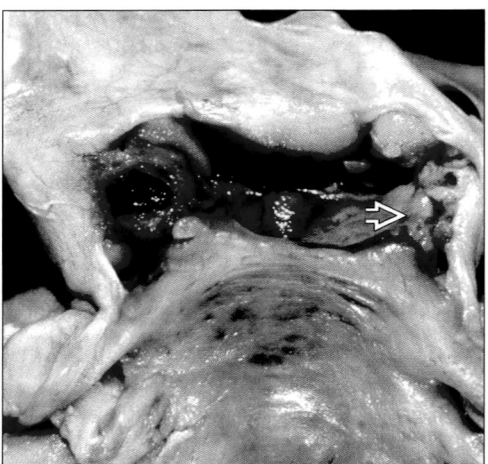
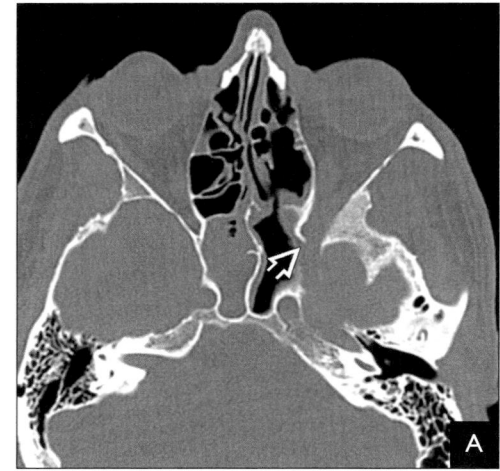

13-28B. *Axial T2WI FS shows normal right cavernous ICA "flow void" ➡ with left cavernous sinus mass, occluded ICA ➡. **13-28C.** T1 C+ FS scan in the same patient shows the left cavernous sinus invasion ➡, occluded carotid artery ➡.*

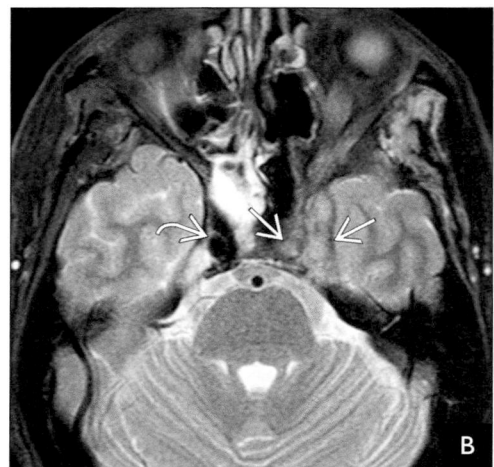
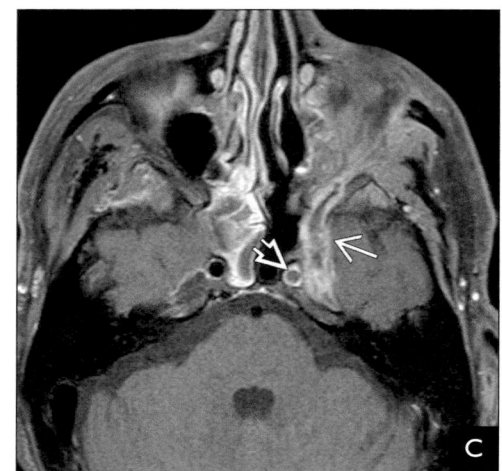

13-28D. *T1 C+ FS scan through the top of the cavernous sinus shows the invaded enhancing left side ➡ with absent "flow void" ➡ (compare to the normal right side ➡). **13-28E.** Coronal T1 C+ FS shows the normal right cavernous ICA ➡, the occluded left ICA ➡, and the cavernous sinus infiltration ➡. Invasive sinonasal mucormycosis in a diabetic patient is a potentially lethal lesion. This patient died from a massive left MCA stroke shortly after the scan.*

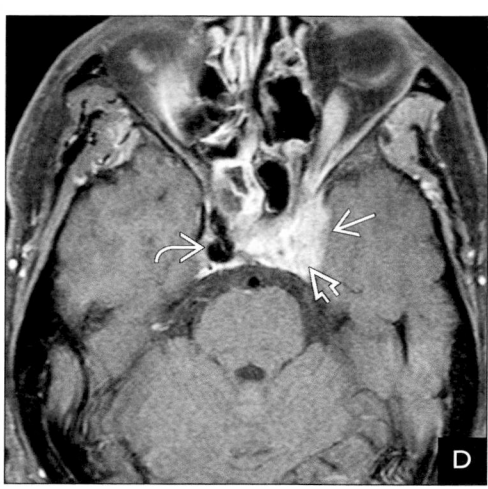
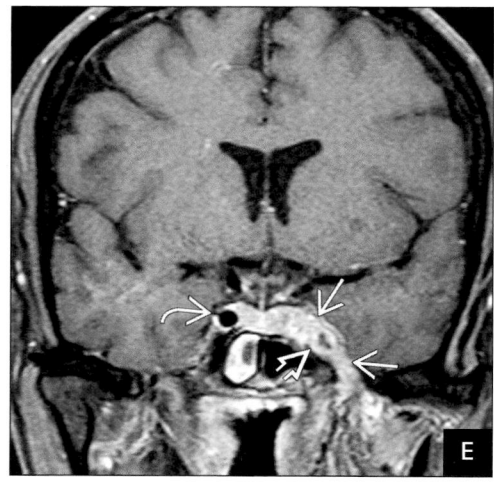

Parasitic Infections

Once considered endemic only in countries with poor sanitation and adverse economic conditions, widespread travel and immigration has made parasitic diseases a global health concern.

With the exception of neurocysticercosis, CNS parasitic disease is rare. When they infest the brain, parasites can cause very bizarre-looking masses that can mimic neoplasm.

Neurocysticercosis

Cysticercosis is the most common parasitic infection in the world, and CNS lesions eventually develop in 60-90% of patients with cysticercosis.

Terminology

When cysticercosis infects the CNS, it is termed neurocysticercosis (NCC). A "cysticercus" cyst in the brain is actually the secondary larval form of the parasite. The "scolex" is the head-like part of a tapeworm, bearing hooks and suckers. In the larval form, the scolex is invaginated into one end of the cyst, which is called the "bladder."

Etiology

Most NCC cases are caused by encysted larvae of the pork tapeworm *Taenia solium* and are acquired through fecal-oral contamination. Humans become infected by ingesting *T. solium* eggs. When the eggs enter the intestine, they hatch and release their primary larvae (oncospheres) that disseminate via the bloodstream to virtually any organ in the body.

Pathology

LOCATION. *T. solium* larvae are most common in the CNS, eyes, muscles, and subcutaneous tissue. The intracranial subarachnoid spaces are the most common CNS site, followed by the brain parenchyma and ventricles (fourth > third > lateral ventricles) **(13-29)**. NCC cysts in the depths of sulci may incite an intense inflammatory response, effectively "sealing" the sulcus over the cysts and making them appear intraaxial.

SIZE AND NUMBER. Most parenchymal NCC cysts are relatively small, from a few millimeters to around one centimeter in diameter. Occasionally, multiple large NCC cysts up to several centimeters can form in the subarachnoid space (the "racemose" form of NCC that resembles a bunch of grapes).

Numbers vary from solitary lesions (20-50% of cases) to multiple small cysts.

GROSS PATHOLOGY. Four stages of NCC development and regression are recognized. Patients may have multiple lesions at different stages of evolution.

In the **vesicular stage**, viable larvae (the cysticerci) appear as translucent, thin-walled, fluid-filled cysts with an eccentrically located, whitish, invaginated scolex **(13-30), (13-31)**.

In the **colloidal vesicular stage**, the larvae begin to degenerate. The cyst fluid becomes thick and turbid. A striking inflammatory response is incited and characterized by a collection of multinucleated giant cells, macrophages, and neutrophils. A fibrous capsule develops, and perilesional edema becomes prominent.

The **granular nodular stage** represents progressive involution with collapse and retraction of the cyst into a granulomatous nodule that will eventually calcify. Edema persists, but pericystic gliosis is the most common pathologic finding at this stage. In the **nodular calcified stage**, the entire lesion becomes a fibrocalcified nodule **(13-32)**. No host immune response is present.

MICROSCOPIC FEATURES. The cyst wall has three distinct layers—namely the outer cuticular, middle cellular ("pseudoepithelial"), and inner fibrillary or reticular layer. Viable larvae have a rostellum with hooklets and muscular suckers.

Clinical Issues

EPIDEMIOLOGY. In countries where cysticercosis is endemic, calcified NCC granulomas are found in 10-20% of the entire population. Of these, approximately 5% (400,000 out of 75 million) will become symptomatic.

DEMOGRAPHICS. NCC occurs at all ages, but peak symptomatic presentation is between 15 and 40 years. There is no gender or race predilection.

PRESENTATION. NCC is a clinically pleomorphic disease with a range of manifestations. Signs and symptoms depend on number and location of larvae, developmental stage, infection duration, and presence or absence of host immune response.

Seizures/epilepsy are the most common symptoms (80%) and are a result of inflammation around degeneration cysts. Headache (35-40%) and focal neurologic deficit (15%) are also common. Between 10-12% of patients exhibit signs of elevated intracranial pressure. Other manifestations such as cerebrovascular disorders occur in less than 10% of symptomatic NCC patients.

NATURAL HISTORY. Many patients remain asymptomatic for years. The average time from infestation until symptoms develop is two to five years. The time to progress through all four stages varies from one to nine years with a mean of five years.

TREATMENT OPTIONS. Oral albendazole with or without steroids, excision/drainage of parenchymal lesions, and endoscopic resection of intraventricular lesions are treatment options.

NEUROCYSTICERCOSIS: ETIOLOGY AND EPIDEMIOLOGY

Etiology
- Pork tapeworm (*T. solium*)
- Fecal-oral transmission
- Ingested eggs hatch in intestine
- Release, disseminate oncospheres
- Larvae encyst in brain

Epidemiology
- Most common parasitic infection worldwide
- CNS lesions develop in 60-90% of infected individuals

Imaging

GENERAL FEATURES. Imaging findings depend on several factors: (1) lifecycle stage of *T. solium* at presentation, (2) host inflammatory response, (3) number and location of parasites, and (4) associated complications such as hydrocephalus and vascular disease.

Vesicular stage. NECT shows a smooth thin-walled cyst that is isodense to CSF. There is no surrounding edema and no enhancement on CECT.

MR shows that the cyst is isointense with CSF on T1 and T2/FLAIR. The scolex is discrete, nodular, and hyperintense. Enhancement is typically absent. Disseminated or "miliary" NCC has a striking "salt and pepper brain" appearance (13-33), (13-34) with notable lack of perilesional edema.

Colloidal vesicular stage. Cyst fluid is hyperdense relative to CSF on NECT and demonstrates a ring-enhancing capsule on CECT. Moderate to marked edema surrounds the degenerating dying larvae.

13-29. NCC. Convexity cysts have a scolex ➔ and surrounding inflammation. Inflammation around the largest cyst "seals" the sulcus ➔ and makes it appear parenchymal. "Racemose" cysts ⬧ without scolices are seen in the basal cisterns. 13-30. NCC in vesicular stage has a clear fluid-filled cyst ➔ and a white eccentrically positioned scolex ⬧. Note the second granular nodular lesion ➔. (Courtesy R. Hewlett, MD.)

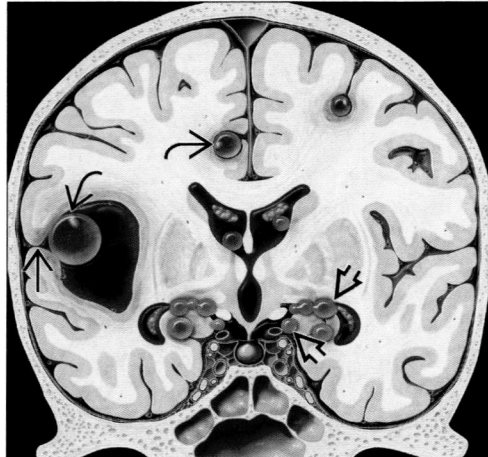
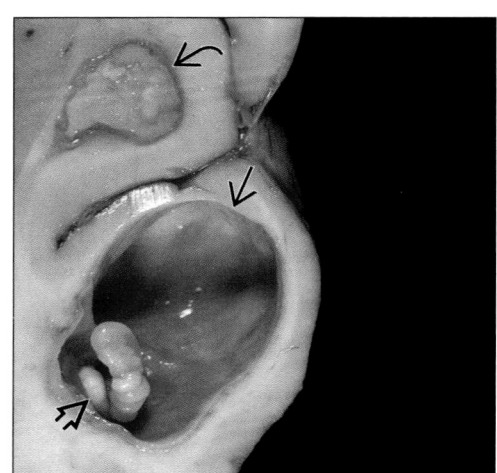

13-31. Low-power photomicrograph of cysticercus shows the invaginated scolex ➔ lying within the thin-walled cyst ⬧, also known as the bladder. (Courtesy B. K. DeMasters, MD.) 13-32. Close-up view shows a nodular calcified NCC cyst ➔. Note the lack of inflammation and lack of mass effect. (Courtesy R. Hewlett, MD.)

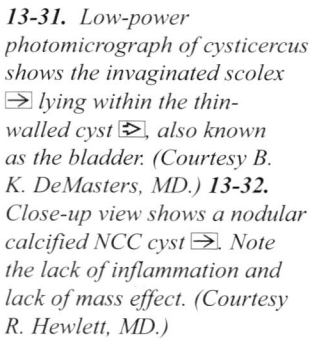
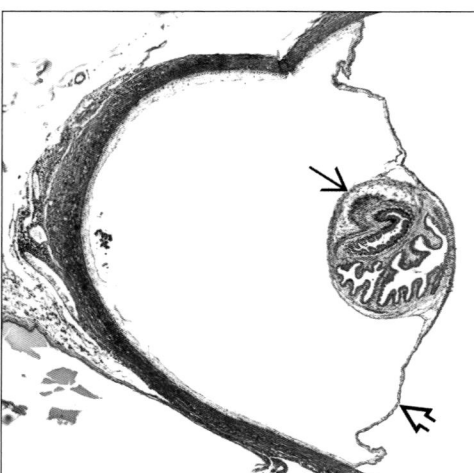
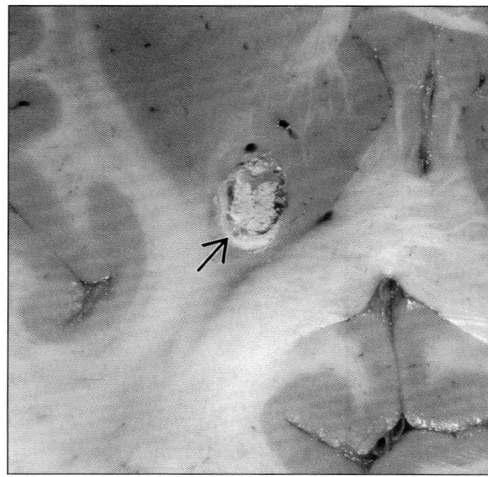

MR shows that the cyst fluid is mildly hyperintense to CSF on T1WI and that the scolex appears hyperintense on FLAIR **(13-35)**. Moderate to marked surrounding edema is present **(13-36B)**. No restriction is seen on DWI. Enhancement of the cyst wall is typically intense and often slightly "shaggy" **(13-36D)**, **(13-37)**. MRS shows a succinate peak resonating at 2.4 ppm as well as a lactate peak and a small acetate peak.

Granular nodular stage. NECT shows mild residual edema. CECT demonstrates an involuting, mildly to moderately enhancing nodule.

The cyst wall appears thickened and retracted, and the perilesional edema diminishes substantially, eventually disappearing. Nodular or faint ring-like enhancement is typical at this stage **(13-36D)**.

Nodular calcified stage. A small calcified nodule without surrounding edema or enhancement is seen on CT **(13-36A)**. Shrunken, calcified lesions are seen as hypointensities on T1- and T2-weighted images. Perilesional edema is absent. "Blooming" on T2* GRE is seen and may show multifocal "blooming black dots" if mul-

tiple calcified nodules are present **(13-36C)**. Quiescent lesions do not enhance on T1 C+.

SPECIAL FEATURES. "Racemose" NCC shows multilobulated, variably sized, grape-like lesions in the basal cisterns. Most cysts lack an identifiable scolex. Arachnoiditis with fibrosis and scarring demonstrates rim enhancement around the cysts and along the brain surfaces **(13-38)**. Obstructive hydrocephalus is common.

NCC-associated vasculitis with stroke is a rare but important complication of "racemose" NCC that can mimic tuberculosis. Most infarcts involve small perforating vessels although large territorial infarcts have been reported.

Intraventricular NCC may be difficult to detect on CT. FLAIR and CISS are the most sensitive sequences for detecting intraventricular cysts on MR.

Differential Diagnosis

The differential diagnosis of NCC depends on lesion type and location. Subarachnoid/cisternal NCC can resemble **TB meningitis**. In contrast to NCC, the thick purulent

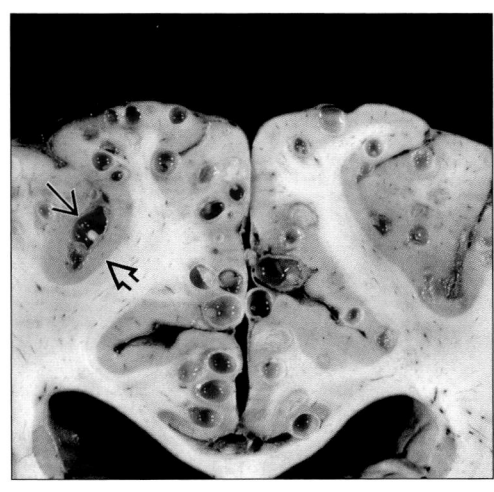
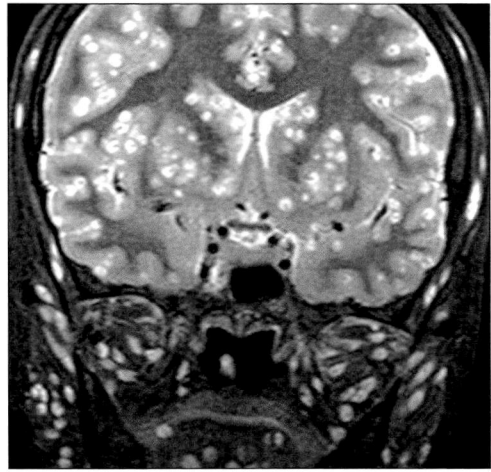

13-33. Disseminated NCC with innumerable cysts, mostly in the subarachnoid space. Note that cyst with scolex in the depth of a frontal sulcus ➡ is surrounded by cortex ➡, making what is actually a subarachnoid cyst appear intraparenchymal. 13-34. T2WI shows disseminated vesicular NCC with "salt and pepper brain" appearance. Innumerable tiny hyperintense cysticerci with scolices (seen as small black "dots" inside the cysts) are present. Perilesional edema is absent.

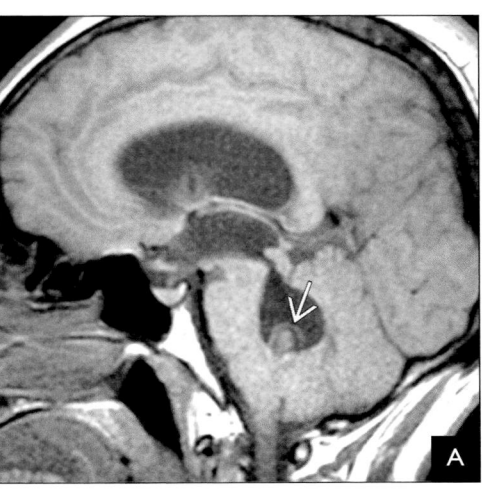
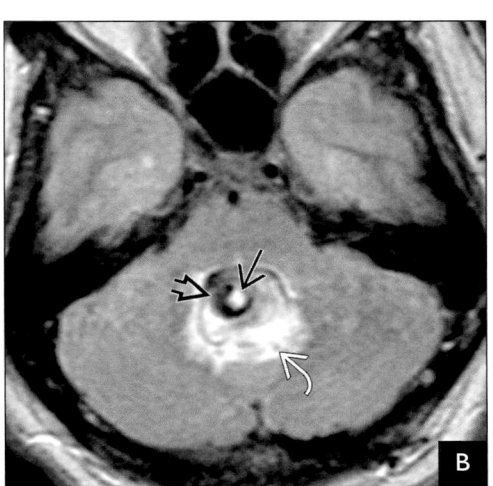

13-35A. Sagittal T1WI shows hydrocephalus, NCC cyst in the fourth ventricle ➡. 13-35B. Axial FLAIR scan in the same patient shows that the cyst fluid suppresses ➡ while the scolex ➡ is hyperintense. Extracellular fluid has accumulated around the margins of the obstructed fourth ventricle ➡.

A

B

basilar exudates typical of TB are solid and lack the cystic features of "racemose" NCC. **Carcinomatous meningitis** and **neurosarcoid** are also rarely cystic.

Abscess and **multifocal septic emboli** can resemble parenchymal NCC cysts but demonstrate a hypointense rim on T2WI and restrict strongly on DWI. A succinate peak on MRS helps distinguish a degenerating NCC cyst from abscess.

A giant parenchymal colloidal-vesicular NCC cyst with ring enhancement can mimic **neoplasm**, **tuberculoma**, or **toxoplasmosis**.

The differential diagnosis of intraventricular NCC cyst includes **colloid cyst** (solid), **ependymal cyst** (cystic but lacks a scolex), and **choroid plexus cyst.**

NEUROCYSTICERCOSIS: PATHOLOGY AND IMAGING

Pathology
- Location, size, and number
  - Subarachnoid spaces > parenchyma > ventricles
  - Usually < 1 cm but can be giant
  - Solitary (20-50%); if multiple, can be innumerable
- 4 stages of development, healing, regression
  - Vesicular (viable larva): Cyst + scolex
  - Colloidal vesicular (dying larva): Intense inflammation, edema
  - Granular nodular (healing): Cyst involutes, edema diminishes
  - Nodular calcifying (healed): Quiescent fibrocalcified nodule

Imaging
- Varies with stage
  - Vesicular: Cyst with "dot" (scolex), no edema, no enhancement
  - Colloidal vesicular: Ring enhancement, edema striking
  - Granular nodular: Faint rim enhancement, edema decreased
  - Nodular calcified: CT Ca++, MR "black dots"
- Common to have lesions in different stages

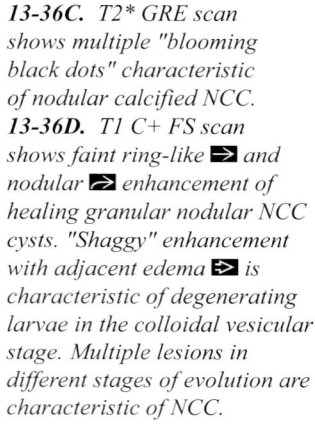

13-36A. *NECT scan in a patient with NCC shows multiple nodular calcified lesions ➡. A few demonstrate adjacent edema ➤. 13-36B. FLAIR scan shows a few hypointense foci ➡ caused by quiescent NCC in the nodular calcified stage. Several foci of perilesional edema are apparent around lesions in the colloidal vesicular stage ➤, while minimal residual edema surrounds lesions in the granular nodular stage ➡.*

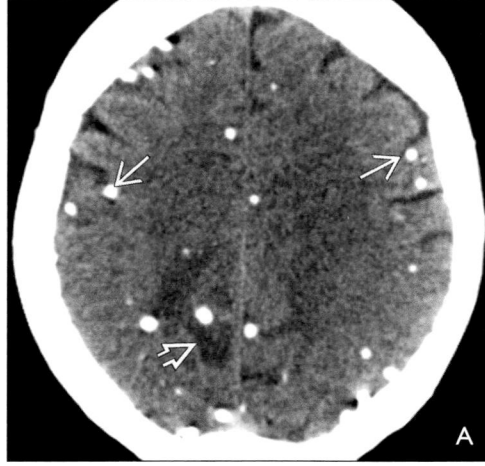

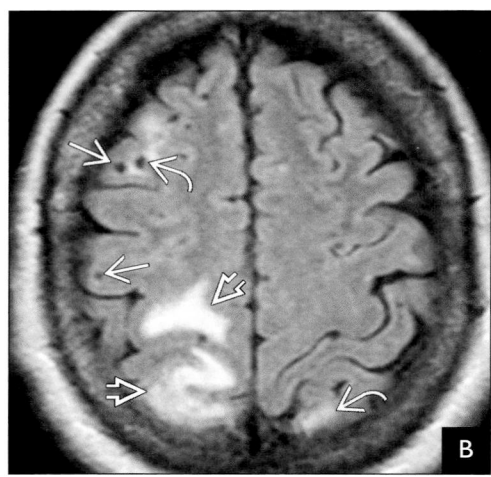

13-36C. *T2* GRE scan shows multiple "blooming black dots" characteristic of nodular calcified NCC. 13-36D. T1 C+ FS scan shows faint ring-like ➡ and nodular ➤ enhancement of healing granular nodular NCC cysts. "Shaggy" enhancement with adjacent edema ➤ is characteristic of degenerating larvae in the colloidal vesicular stage. Multiple lesions in different stages of evolution are characteristic of NCC.*

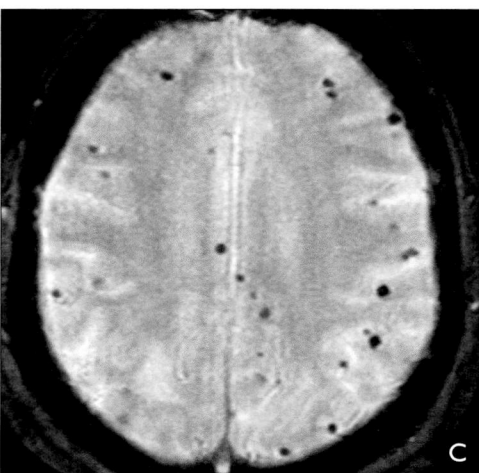

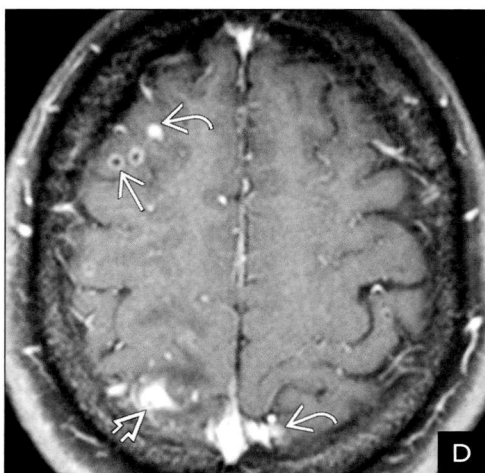

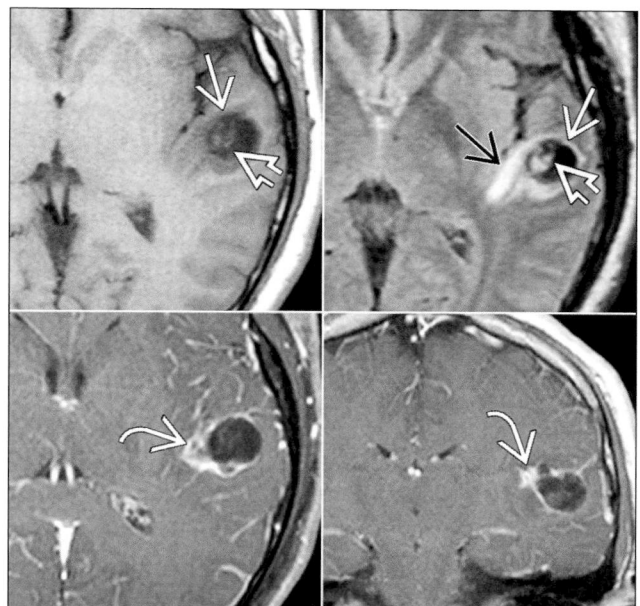

13-37. Solitary degenerating colloidal vesicular NCC cyst ➡ with scolex ➡ demonstrates perilesional edema ➡, "shaggy" enhancement ➡.

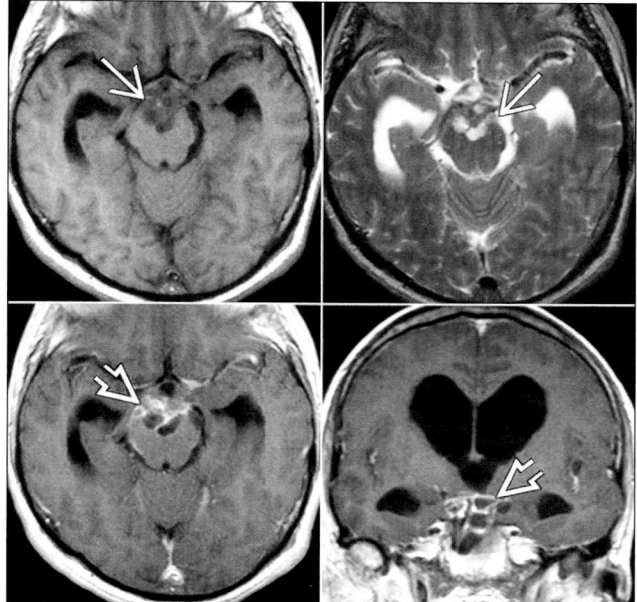

13-38. "Racemose" NCC. Multiple small cysts without visible scolices fill the suprasellar cistern ➡. Note hydrocephalus, meningeal reaction with moderate rim enhancement around the "bunch of grapes" cysts ➡. (Courtesy P. Rodriguez, MD.)

Echinococcosis

Terminology and Etiology

Infection by *Echinococcus* is called echinococcosis.

Two species of *Echinococcus* tapeworms, *E. granulosis* (EG) and *E. multilocularis/alveolaris* (EM/EA), are responsible for most human CNS infections. EG infestation is also called **hydatid disease** or hydatid cyst (HC). Infection with EM/EA is also known as **alveolar echinococcosis**.

Epidemiology

After NCC, echinococcosis is the second most common parasitic infection that involves the CNS. Humans—most often children—become accidental intermediate hosts by ingesting eggs in soil contaminated by excrement from a definitive host. Approximately 1-2% of patients with EG and 3-5% of patients with EM/EA develop CNS disease.

EG usually affects children whereas EM/EA is more common in adults.

Pathology

The gross appearances of EG and EM/EA differ. EG typically produces a well-delineated cyst **(13-39)**. EM/EA has numerous irregular small cysts and appears as an infiltrative, invasive, neoplasm-like lesion in both liver and brain.

Hydatid cysts can be uni- or multilocular with "daughter cysts." The wall of a hydatid cyst has three layers: An outer dense fibrous pericyst, a middle laminated membranous ectocyst, and an inner germinal layer (the endocyst). It is the germinal layer that can produce "daughter cysts."

Imaging

The most common imaging appearance of HC is that of a large, unilocular, thin-walled cyst without calcification, edema, or enhancement on CT **(13-40)**. Occasionally, a single large cyst will contain multiple "daughter cysts" **(13-41)**.

MR shows that cyst fluid is isointense with CSF on T1- and T2-weighted images. Sometimes a detached germinal membrane and hydatid "sand" can be seen in the dependent portion of the cyst **(13-42)**.

EA consists of numerous irregular cysts that—unlike HC—are not sharply demarcated from surrounding brain and usually enhance following contrast administration. Irregular peripheral or ring-like, heterogeneous, nodular, and cauliflower-like patterns have been reported **(13-43)**.

Differential Diagnosis

The differential diagnosis of a supratentorial intraaxial cystic mass is extensive and includes cystic neoplasms, abscess, parasitic cysts, and neuroglial cysts. Of these, the most difficult to distinguish from HCs are neuroglial cysts and porencephalic cysts. **Neuroglial cysts** are rarely as large as HCs. **Porencephalic cysts** are literally "holes in the brain" adjacent to—and usually connected with—an enlarged ventricle.

13-39A. Autopsy case shows brain after the removal of a huge unilocular hydatid cyst. Note the well-demarcated border ➔ between the cyst cavity and the brain. There is no surrounding edema, and the mass effect relative to the size of the cyst is minimal. 13-39B. Photograph of the external cyst wall ➔ with cut view of the cyst ⧨ shows the typical thin wall of a classic hydatid cyst. (Courtesy R. Hewlett, MD.)

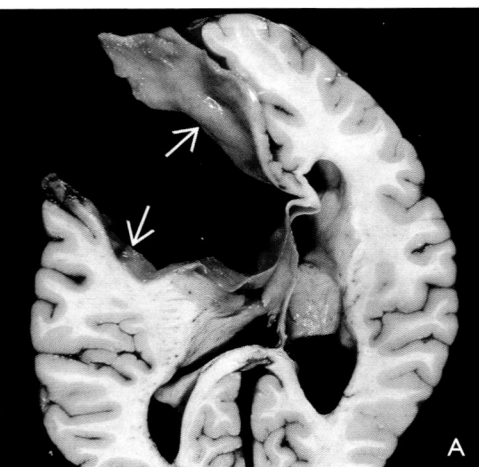

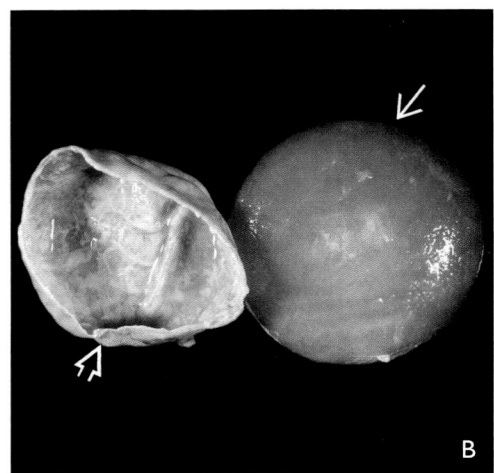

13-40A. Axial T1WI shows a unilocular hydatid cyst ➔. Mass effect relative to the overall cyst size is only moderate. 13-40B. T2WI in the same patient nicely demonstrates the typical three-layered cyst wall ⧨. (Courtesy R. Hewlett, MD.)

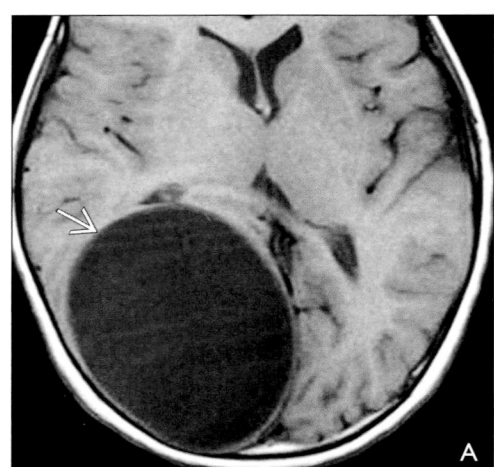

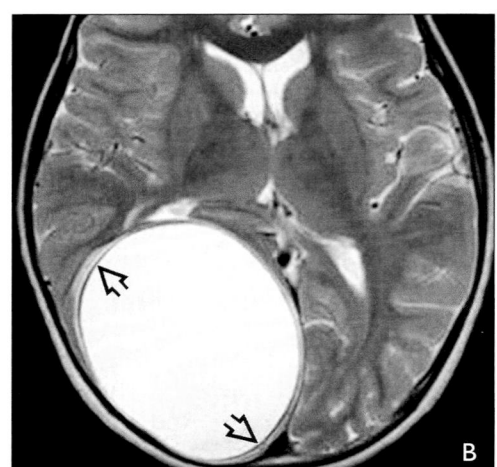

13-41. CECT scan shows a multiloculated hydatid cyst that contains multiple "daughter cysts." (Courtesy S. Nagi, MD.) 13-42. Series of axial MR scans with T1WI, FLAIR, DWI, and ADC (clockwise from top left corner) shows a hydatid cyst ➔ with detached germinal membrane ⧨ and hydatid "sand" in the dependent part of the cyst ➔. Surrounding edema, mass effect is minimal.

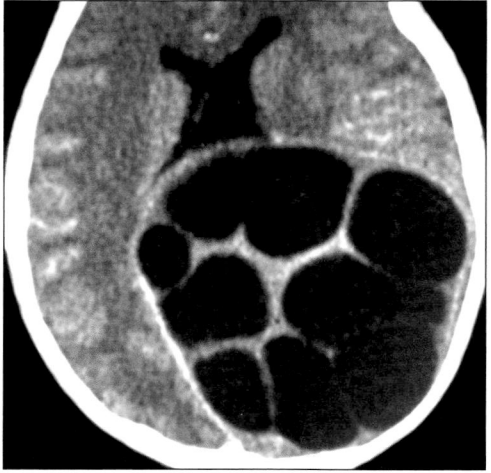

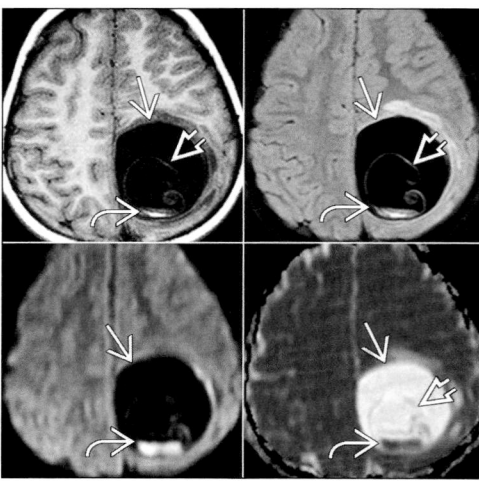

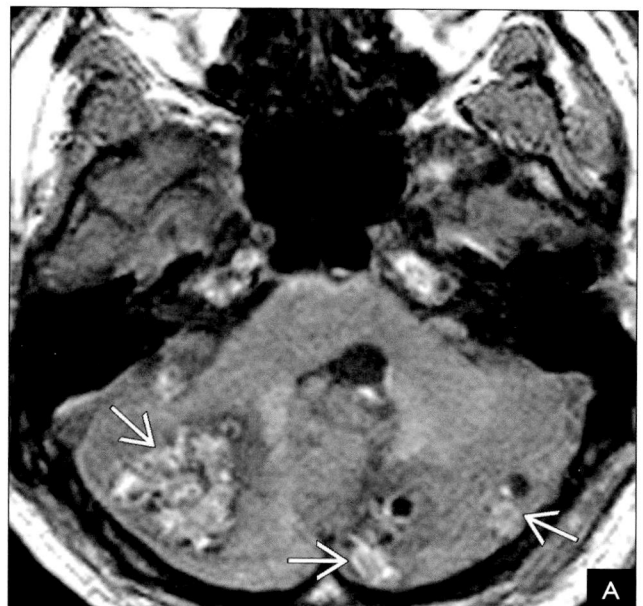

13-43A. T1 C+ scan in a 20-year-old man with alveolar echinococcosis shows cauliflower-like clusters of multiple small, irregular, ring-enhancing cysts ➡.

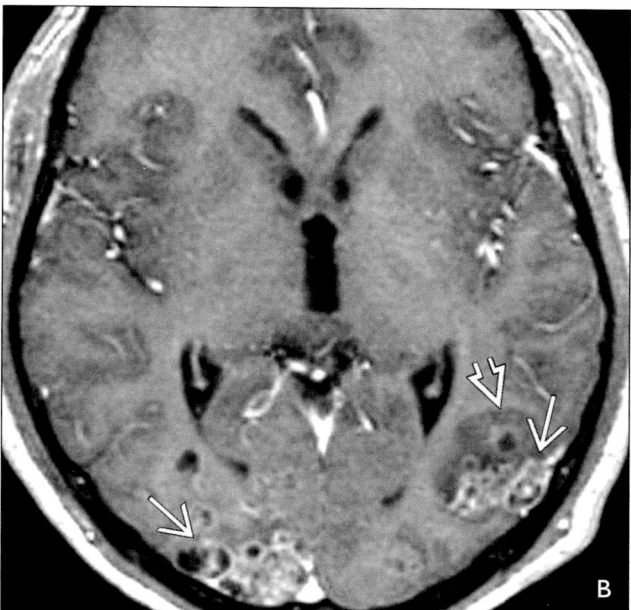

13-43B. More cephalad T1 C+ scan shows additional collections of enhancing cysts ➡, edema ➡. FLAIR scans (not shown) demonstrated edema around all of the clusters. (Courtesy M. Thurnher, MD.)

Amebiasis

Terminology and Etiology

Amoebae are free-living organisms that are distributed worldwide. Species of the *Acanthamoeba* (Ac) genus are found in soil and dust, fresh or brackish water, and a variety of other locations ranging from hot tubs and hydrotherapy pools to air conditioning units, contact lens solutions, and dental irrigation units. *Balamuthia mandrillaris* is a soil-dwelling organism. *Naegleria fowleri* is found in both soil and fresh water. *Entamoeba histolytica* occurs in food or water contaminated with feces.

Up to 10% of the population worldwide is infected with EH, but CNS disease is rare.

Pathology

Two basic types of CNS amebic infection occur: Primary amebic meningoencephalitis (PAM) and granulomatous amebic encephalitis (GAE). Amebic abscess occurs but is relatively uncommon in Western and industrialized countries.

Gross autopsies of PAM show a necrotizing, hemorrhagic meningitis and angiitis with focal lesions in the orbitofrontal and temporal lobes, brainstem, and upper spinal cord **(13-44)**, **(13-45)**. Numerous trophozoites are present, but no cysts are seen because of disease acuity.

GAE demonstrates granulomatous inflammation with multinucleated giant cells, trophozoites, and cysts. An amebic abscess has pus with trophozoites at the edge of the lesion.

Clinical Issues

Primary amebic meningoencephalitis is an acute, rapidly progressive, necrotizing hemorrhagic meningoencephalitis caused by *N. fowleri*. Healthy children and immunocompetent young adults swimming in warm fresh water during the summer are the typical victims, presenting with fever, headache, and altered mental status. *N. fowleri* invades the olfactory mucosa and enters the brain along the olfactory nerves. PAM is almost always fatal. Death within 48-72 hours is typical.

Granulomatous encephalitis is a subacute to chronic condition usually caused by one of six *Acanthamoeba* species or *B. mandrillaris*. GAE shows no seasonal predilection. GAE is generally associated with immunodeficiency (e.g., HIV/AIDS, organ transplantation) and chronic debilitating conditions such as malnutrition and diabetes. Presentation ranges from headache and chronic low-grade fever to fulminant infection (with BM). Focal symptoms are present for an average of two or three months.

Amebic abscess in the CNS is rare even in endemic areas and is usually caused by *E. histolytica*. Most patients have intestinal or liver infection. Amebic abscess is not related to immunodeficiency. Patients develop headache, altered mental status, and meningeal symptoms.

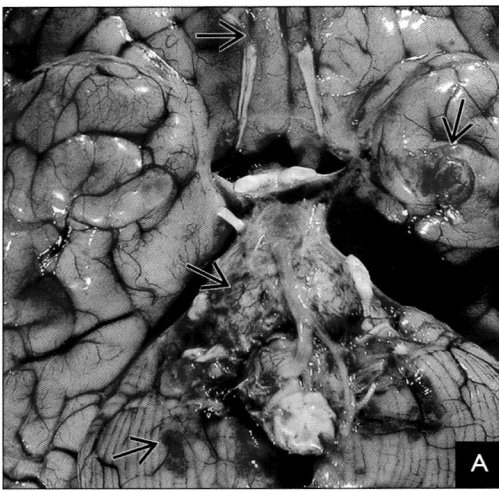

13-44A. Gross pathology from a patient with amebic meningoencephalitis shows multiple basilar hemorrhagic exudates ➡.

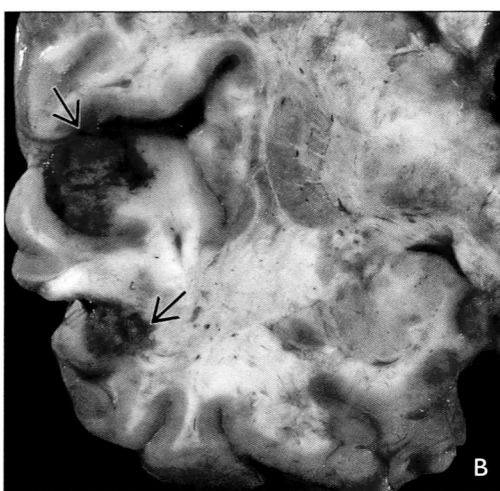

13-44B. Coronal cut section in the same case shows numerous focal parenchymal hemorrhages ➡.

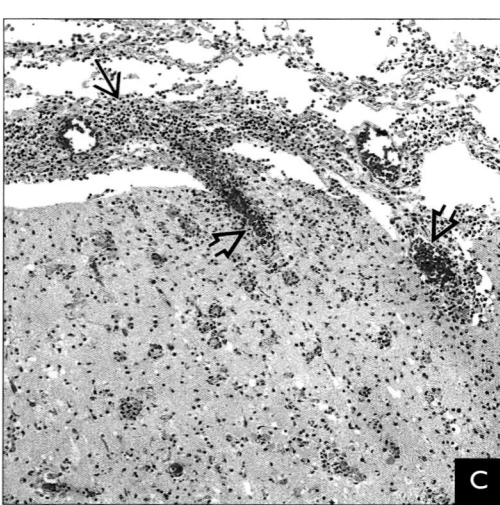

13-44C. Histology shows meningitis ➡, hemorrhage/inflammatory cells in Virchow-Robin spaces ➡. (Courtesy B. K. DeMasters, MD.)

Imaging

A broad spectrum of imaging findings in amebic meningoencephalitis has been described, including meningeal exudates, multifocal hemorrhagic parenchymal lesions (13-46), and pseudotumoral lesions with necrosis (13-47).

PAM demonstrates findings of leptomeningitis with sulcal obliteration and enhancement, especially along the perimesencephalic cisterns. Multifocal parenchymal lesions with involvement of posterior fossa structures, diencephalon, and thalamus are typical. Necrotizing angiitis with hemorrhages and frank infarction is seen in some cases.

GAE demonstrates a multifocal pattern with discrete lesions at the corticomedullary junction and/or a pseudotumoral pattern with a solitary mass-like lesion (13-48).

Amebic abscesses are usually located in the basal ganglia or at the gray-white matter junction. Solitary or multiple irregularly shaped ring-enhancing hemorrhagic lesions are the typical imaging finding (13-47).

Differential Diagnosis

The imaging features of amebiasis are nonspecific. Amebic abscesses and meningoencephalitis can mimic disease caused by other pyogenic, parasitic, and granulomatous infections. Multifocal parenchymal and pseudotumoral lesions can mimic neoplasm.

Malaria

Terminology and Etiology

Cerebral malaria (CM) is caused by infection with the protozoan parasite *Plasmodium* and is transmitted by infected *Anopheles* mosquitoes. Four species cause human disease: *P. falciparum*, *P. vivax*, *P. ovale*, and *P. malariae*. Of these, *P. falciparum* has the most severe morbidity and mortality and causes 95% of all CM cases.

The lifecycle of a malaria parasite involves the female *Anopheles* mosquito and a human host. Sporozoites are inoculated into humans during the mosquitoes' "blood meal." The sporozoites invade and replicate asexually in liver cells, maturing into schizonts that rupture and release merozoites. The merozoites infect red blood cells (RBCs). Merozoites can develop into trophozoites, which undergo asexual reproduction in the blood, or into gametocytes, which reproduce sexually in deep tissue capillaries. Gametocytes are ingested by mosquitoes, and the cycle is repeated over and over again (13-49).

Pathology

Grossly the brain appears swollen, and its external surface is often a characteristic dusky dark red. Deposition

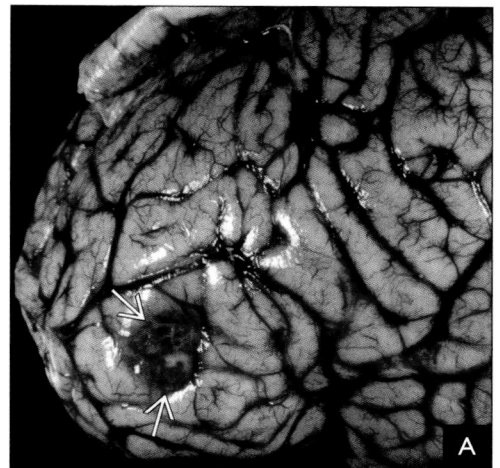
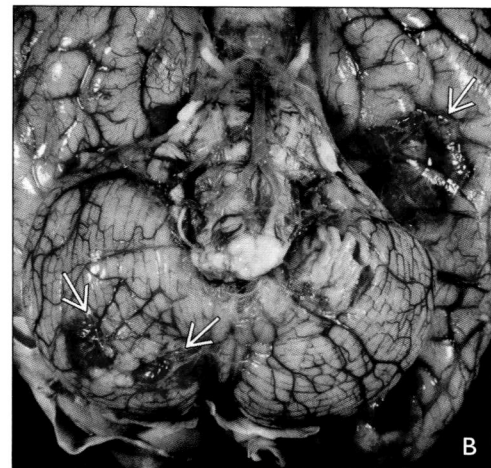

13-45A. Lateral view of autopsied brain from a patient with amebic encephalitis shows focal parenchymal hemorrhage ➡. *13-45B.* Submentovertex view in the same case shows superficial cerebellar and temporal lobe hemorrhages ➡. (Courtesy R. Hewlett, MD.)

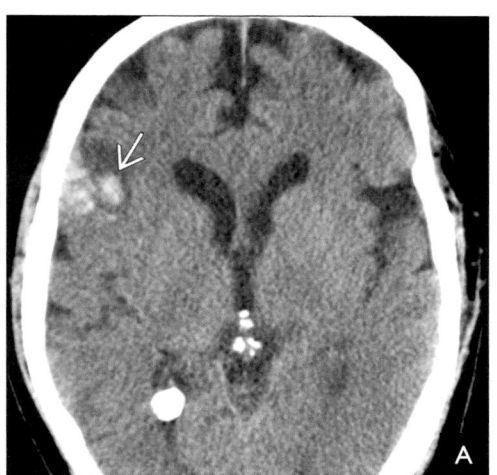
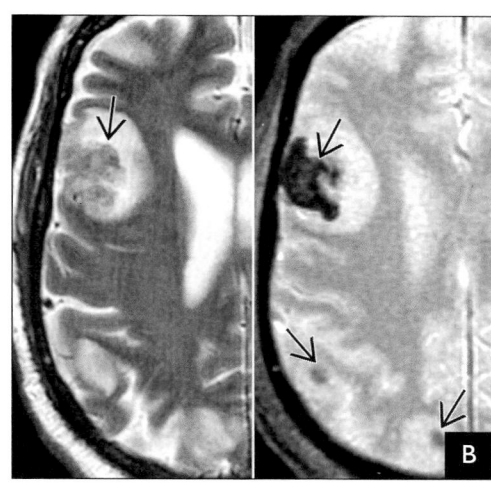

13-46A. Axial NECT scan in a patient with seizure following a recent trip to central Africa during which he waded briefly in fresh water. Note patchy hemorrhage in the right posterior frontal lobe ➡. *13-46B.* (Left) T2WI and (right) T2* GRE in the same patient show multiple parenchymal hemorrhages ➡ with "blooming." Biopsy disclosed amebic granuloma.

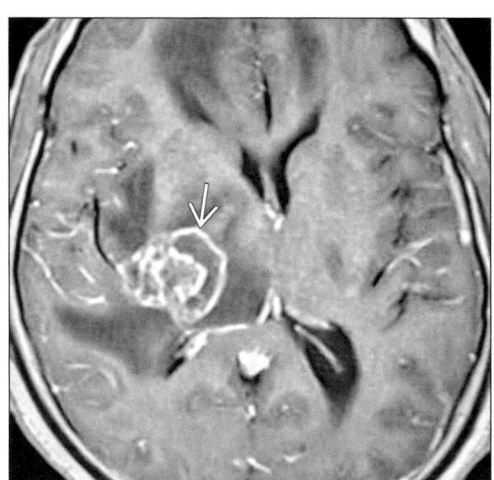
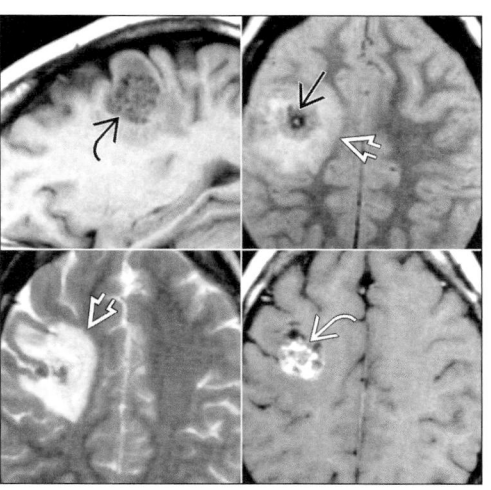

13-47. Axial T1 C+ scan shows a solitary inhomogeneously enhancing right thalamic mass ➡. Biopsy disclosed "tumefactive" amebic granuloma. *13-48.* Series of MR scans in another patient with fever, seizure shows a solitary inhomogeneous conglomerate-appearing mass ➡ with central hemorrhage ➡, perilesional edema ➡, and mixed nodular/ring enhancement ➡. Granulomatous amebic encephalitis. (Both cases courtesy R. Hewlett, MD.)

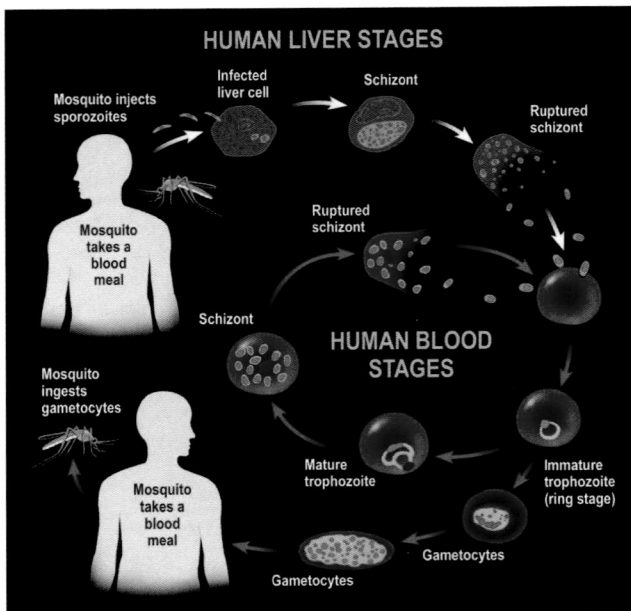

13-49. *Sporozoites inoculated into blood infect the liver cells. When mature, they rupture the cells, releasing merozoites that infect RBCs. Merozoites develop into trophozoites or gametocytes, which are then ingested by uninfected mosquitoes.*

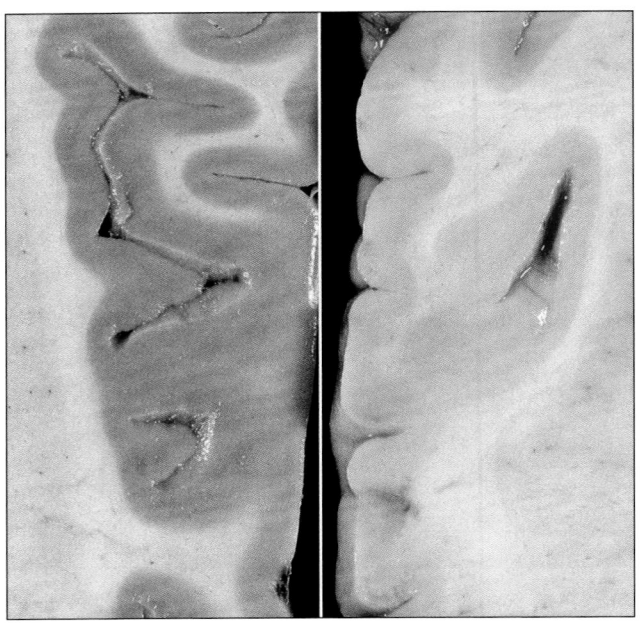

13-50. *Classic "slate gray" edematous cortex of cerebral malaria (left) compared to normal brain (right). (Courtesy R. Hewlett, MD.)*

of malaria pigment can give the cortex a slate gray color **(13-50)**. Petechial hemorrhages are often seen in the subcortical white matter, corpus callosum, cerebellum, and brainstem.

The major microscopic feature is sequestration of parasitized red blood cells in the cerebral microvasculature **(13-51)**. Perivascular ring and punctate microhemorrhages are common. Diagnostic black malarial pigment ("hemozoin bodies") within sequestered, hemoglobin-depleted "ghost" RBCs is common. Malaria parasites remain intravascular, so encephalitic inflammatory changes are absent.

Clinical Issues

EPIDEMIOLOGY AND DEMOGRAPHICS. Falciparum malaria is a leading cause of poor health, neurodisability, and death in tropical countries. Approximately 40% of the world's population is at risk. Between 250 and 500 million new cases of malaria develop every year. The majority of cases occur in sub-Saharan Africa where children under five years of age are most affected. Peak prevalence is between one and three years.

Severe malaria develops in 1% of symptomatic malaria infections. Of these, cerebral malaria is the most severe manifestation. The incidence of cerebral malaria is 1,120 per 100,000 per year in endemic areas. Malaria causes approximately one million deaths each year.

Malaria is generally restricted to tropical and subtropical areas with altitudes under 1,500 meters and to travelers or immigrants coming from endemic areas. A few

isolated cases of "airport malaria" have been reported. For such cases, falciparum malaria occurred in individuals who never traveled outside the country but became infected by imported anopheline mosquitoes at or around an international airport.

PRESENTATION AND NATURAL HISTORY. The incubation period from infection to symptom development is one to three weeks. Shaking chills followed by cyclical high fever and profuse sweating is typical and corresponds temporally to RBC lysis after schizonts mature. *P. falciparum*, *P. ovale*, and *P. vivax* are characterized by fever every 48 hours whereas *P. malariae* cycles every 72 hours.

Prognosis is variable. Individuals with sickle cell trait generally have milder disease. In other cases, headache, altered sensorium, and seizures develop and can be followed within one to two days by impaired consciousness, coma, and death. Mortality in cerebral malaria is 15-20% even with appropriate therapy. While many surviving patients recover completely, between 10-25% of affected children have long-term neurologic deficits.

P. falciparum relapse is rare. *P. vivax* and *P. ovale* can relapse, as dormant liver stages allow the parasite to survive during colder periods. Active forms can arise months to years later.

Imaging

Imaging findings on NECT vary from normal to striking. The most typical finding is focal infarcts in the cortex, basal ganglia, and thalami. Gross hemorrhage can occur but is rare. Diffuse cerebral edema can occur in severe CM.

MR shows focal hyperintensities in the basal ganglia, thalami, and white matter on T2/FLAIR **(13-52)**. Confluent hyperintensities can occur in severe cases although large territorial infarcts are rare.

T2* scans demonstrate multifocal "blooming" petechial hemorrhages in the basal ganglia and cerebral white matter. These linear and punctate hypointensities are especially striking on susceptibility-weighted imaging (SWI) **(13-53)**, **(13-54)**. Malarial lesions generally do not enhance on T1 C+.

Differential Diagnosis

CM is a clinical diagnosis and should be considered in any patient with a febrile illness and impaired consciousness who lives in—or has recently traveled to—endemic malaria areas!

Differential diagnosis varies with patient age. The major imaging differential diagnosis of CM in adults is **multiple cerebral emboli/infarction**, which more commonly involves the gray-white matter junction or cortex. Multifocal WM petechial hemorrhages on T2* are nonspecific and can be seen in **fat emboli** syndrome, **acute hemorrhagic leukoencephalitis**, **diffuse vascular injury**, and **thrombotic microangiopathies** such as disseminated intravascular coagulopathy.

The major differential diagnosis of CM in children is **acute necrotizing encephalopathy** and **infantile bilateral striatal necrosis**. These are generally influenza-associated diseases and follow flu-like respiratory infection or rotavirus gastroenteritis.

Other Parasitic Infections

Schistosomiasis, paragonimiasis, sparganosis, trichinosis, and trypanosomiasis can occasionally involve the CNS. Although these parasitic infestations can occur at any age, they most commonly affect children and young adults.

Brain involvement is relatively uncommon. When it does occur, these parasites are associated with significant mortality and morbidity. Because imaging often resembles

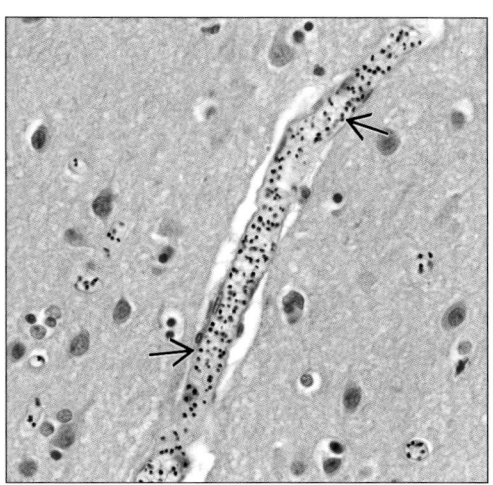

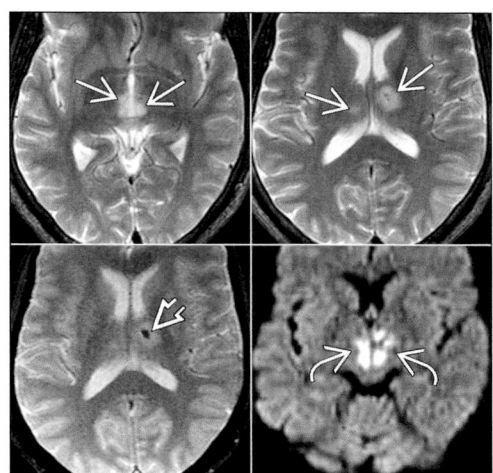

13-51. In cerebral malaria, parasites convert metabolized hemoglobin to hemozoin ("malarial pigment"), seen here as tiny black "dots" in sequestered red blood cells ➡. *(Courtesy B. K. DeMasters, MD.)* *13-52. Scans in a patient with malaria show T2 basal ganglia hyperintensities* ➡ *that "bloom" on T2* GRE* ➡, *restrict on DWI* ➡. *(Courtesy R. Ramakantan, MD.)*

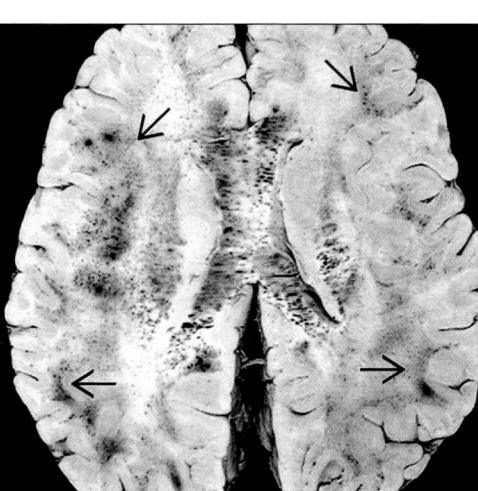

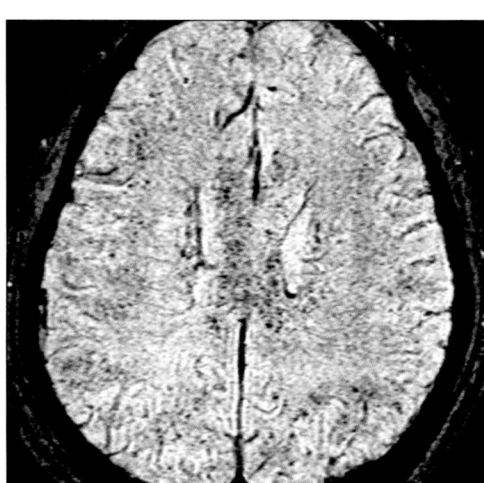

13-53. CM shows innumerable petechial WM hemorrhages ➡ *in the subcortical, deep white matter. (Courtesy L. Chimelli: A morphological approach to the diagnosis of protozoal infections of the CNS. Patholog Res Int. 2011 July 14. Open source.)* *13-54. T2* SWI in a patient with cerebral malaria shows innumerable punctate "blooming" microhemorrhages throughout the WM. (Courtesy K. Tong, MD.)*

neoplasm, a history of travel to—or residence in—an endemic area is key to the diagnosis.

Schistosomiasis

Schistosomiasis, also known as bilharziasis, is a trematode (fluke) infection that affects more than 200 million people worldwide.

Several *Schistosoma* species cause human disease. *Schistosoma haematobium* is endemic in Africa, especially the Nile River basin. *S. mansoni* is also endemic in Africa (the mid-continent and lake region), South America, and the Caribbean **(13-56)**. *S. japonicum* is endemic in China, and *S. mekongi* is endemic in Southeast Asia.

Schistosoma species have a complex lifecycle. Ova in human urine and feces hatch in fresh water and enter snails as their intermediate host. Snails release motile larvae (cercariae) that infect humans wading or swimming in infested water. The larvae penetrate skin and migrate to the liver or lungs where they mature. Adult worms migrate to venous plexuses in the intestines (*S. mansoni, S. japonicum*) or bladder (*S. hematobium*).

The mature worms release eggs, which can be shed in urine or feces. Eggs can also disseminate to ectopic sites, including the brain. Focal meningeal and firm parenchymal masses are the typical gross pathologic findings. On microscopic examination, schistosome eggs show no spine (*S. japonicum*) or a terminal (*S. haematobium*) or lateral (*S. mansoni*) spine.

Typical imaging findings of neuroschistosomiasis are single or multiple conglomerated heterogeneous lesion(s) with edema and mass effect. A central linear enhancement surrounded by multiple punctate nodules (an "arborized" appearance) on T1 C+ MR **(13-55)** has been described as characteristic.

Paragonimiasis

Paragonimiasis is another snail-borne trematode infection. Humans become infected by eating undercooked fresh water crabs or crayfish contaminated by *Paragonimus westermani*, a lung fluke endemic in Asia and Central and South America. Worms penetrate the skull base foramina and meninges, then directly invade the brain

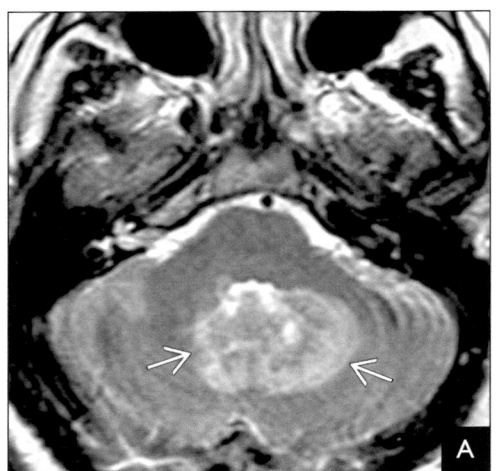
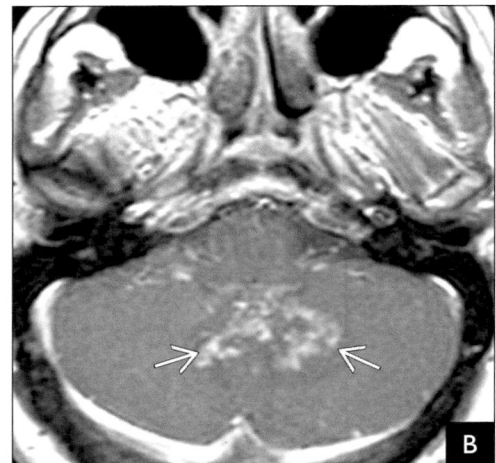

13-55A. Axial T2WI in a 34-year-old man with schistosomiasis shows a mixed hypo- and hyperintense lesion ➡ involving the vermis and both cerebellar hemispheres. 13-55B. Axial T1 C+ scan shows a patchy "arborization" pattern of enhancement ➡.

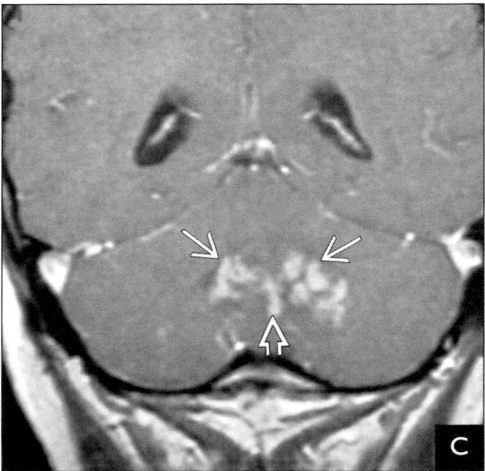
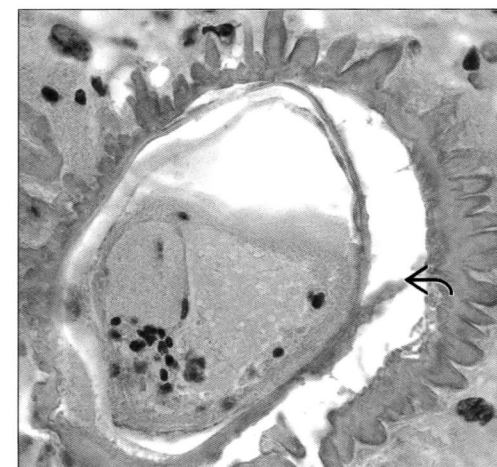

13-55C. Coronal T1 C+ shows patchy enhancement ➡ around a central linear focus ➡, suggesting an "arborization" pattern. 13-56. Microscopic view from the biopsied lesion shows the encysted S. mansoni with the classic lateral spine ➡. (Courtesy D. Kremens, MD, S. Galetta, MD.)

where they elicit a granulomatous inflammatory reaction. Adolescent males are most commonly affected.

Imaging shows a heterogeneous mass with multiple conglomerated ring-enhancing lesions surrounded by edema (13-57). Intralesional hemorrhage is common.

Sparganosis

Sparganosis is a rare parasitic infection caused by the larval cestode of *Spirometra mansoni*. Nearly half of all reported cases are due to ingestion of raw or undercooked frogs or snakes. Sparganosis is endemic in Southeast Asia, China, Japan, and Korea.

Imaging studies show an irregularly shaped mass, usually in the cerebral white matter, surrounded by edema. The most common imaging finding is the "tunnel" sign, a hollow tube ("tunnel") several centimeters long created by the burrowing worm. The "tunnel" is surrounded by an enhancing rim of reactive inflammatory granulomatous tissue. The second most common feature of cerebral sparganosis is a conglomerate mass of ring- or bead-like enhancing lesions (13-58).

Sparganosis is typically characterized by the simultaneous presence of new and old lesions. Lesions in different stages of evolution from acute infection to cortical atrophy with white matter volume loss and calcifications around degenerated/dead worms are typical of this particular parasitic infestation.

Differential Diagnosis

Most parasitic infections share several common features. They usually present as mass-like lesions with edema and multiple "conglomerate" ring-enhancing foci. **Metastasis** and **glioblastoma multiforme** are two common neoplasms that can appear very similar to parasitic masses. **Inflammatory granulomas** (e.g., TB granulomas) can also mimic parasitic granulomas and are often endemic in the same geographic areas.

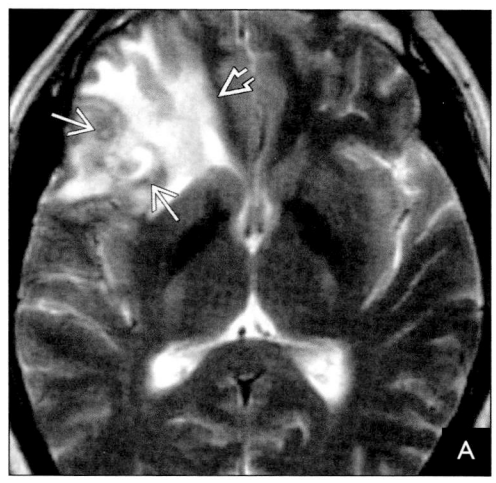

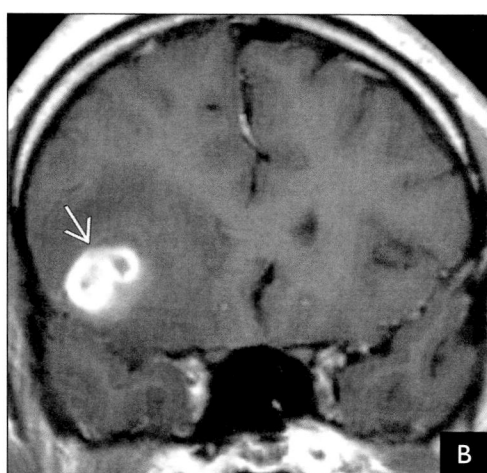

13-57A. *Axial T2WI in a young man from Southeast Asia shows a heterogeneous right frontal lobe mass with intralesional hypointensities ⇨ suggesting hemorrhage. Moderate perilesional edema ⇨ is present.* **13-57B.** *Coronal T1 C+ shows conglomerate ring-enhancing lesions ⇨. Paragonimiasis granuloma was found at surgery.*

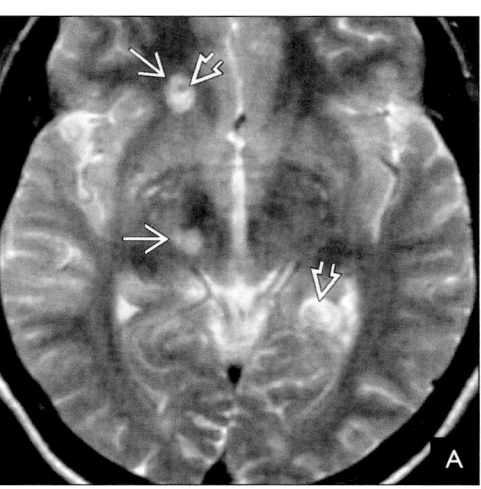

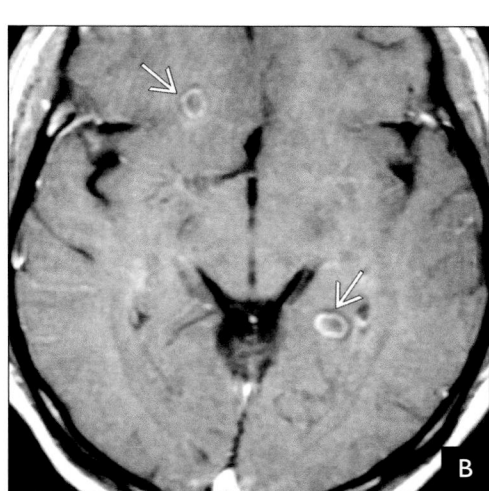

13-58A. *Axial T2WI in a patient with known sparganosis shows multiple ring-like hyperintensities ⇨ with central hypointense foci ⇨.* **13-58B.** *Axial T1 C+ scan in the same patient shows nonspecific ring enhancement ⇨. No "tunnel" sign was present. (Courtesy M. Castillo, MD.)*

Miscellaneous and Emerging CNS Infections

Spirochete Infections of the CNS

Two spirochete species can cause significant CNS disease: *Borrelia* (e.g., Lyme disease, relapsing fever borreliosis) and *Treponema* (neurosyphilis).

Lyme Disease

TERMINOLOGY. Lyme disease (LD) is also known as Lyme borreliosis. LD with neurologic disease is called Lyme neuroborreliosis (LNB) or neuro-Lyme disease. **Relapsing fever borreliosis** is a multisystem disease that infects a variety of tissues including the CNS (rare).

Lyme disease is a multisystem inflammatory disease caused by *B. burgdorferi* in the United States and *B.*

garinii or *B. afzelii* in Europe. LD is a zoonosis maintained in animals such as field mice and white-tailed deer. LD is transmitted to humans by bite of *Ixodes* ticks and requires 24-48 hours of tick attachment.

Relapsing fever (RF) borreliosis is caused by arthropod-borne spirochetes of the genus *Borrelia*. The major agents vary worldwide. In North America, RF is generally caused by *B. hermsii* and *B. turicatae* and is transmitted by tick bites. Rodents are the reservoir organism.

ETIOLOGY. The precise mechanism of CNS involvement is unclear. Direct brain infection/invasion, antigen-driven autoimmune-mediated mechanisms, and vasculitis-like processes have been postulated.

CLINICAL ISSUES.

Epidemiology and demographics. LD is now the most common vector-borne disease in the United States with 20,000 new cases reported each year. Prevalence varies significantly with geography. Between 90-95% of cases in the United States occur in the Mid-Atlantic states, Michigan, and Minnesota. Occurrence peaks during the early summer, especially May and June.

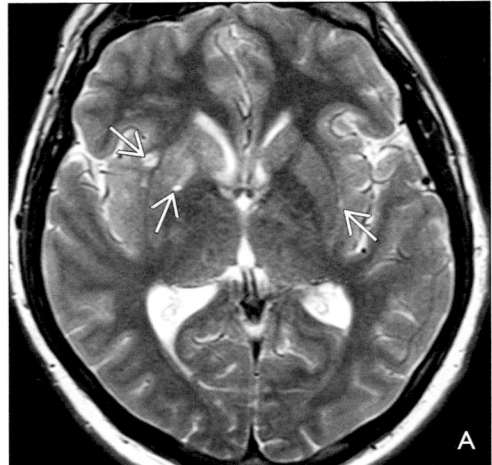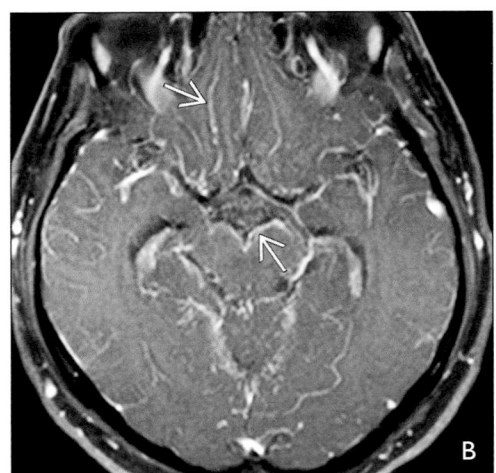

13-59A. T2WI in a 37-year-old man with ataxia, ophthalmoplegia, and documented Lyme meningoencephalitis shows multifocal hyperintensities in the basal ganglia, white matter ➡️. *13-59B. T1 C+ FS scan in the same patient shows diffuse pial enhancement* ➡️ *consistent with meningitis.*

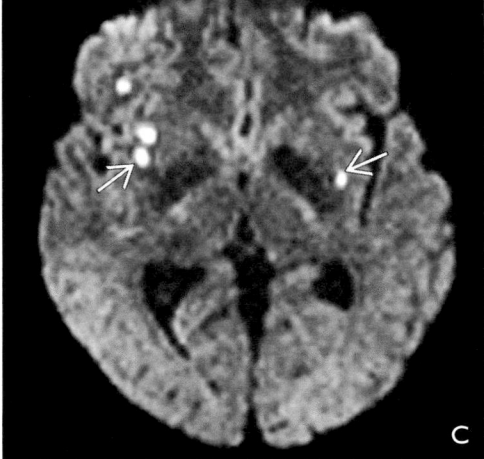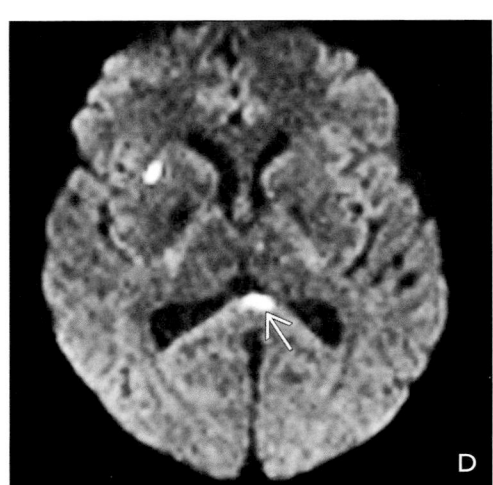

13-59C. DWI shows multiple foci of restricted diffusion ➡️. *13-59D. More cephalad scan shows additional foci of restricted diffusion, including one in the corpus callosum splenium* ➡️.

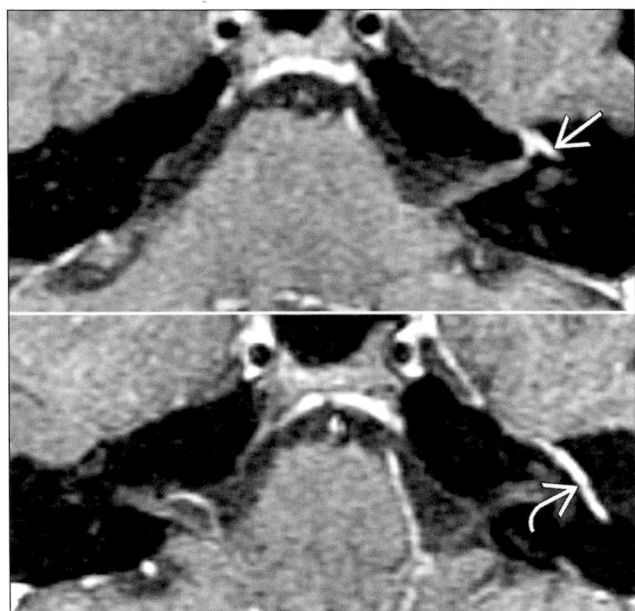

13-60. Two axial images in a patient with Lyme disease and a left Bell palsy show enhancement of the geniculate ➡ and horizontal ➡ facial nerve segments. (Courtesy P. Hildenbrand, MD.)

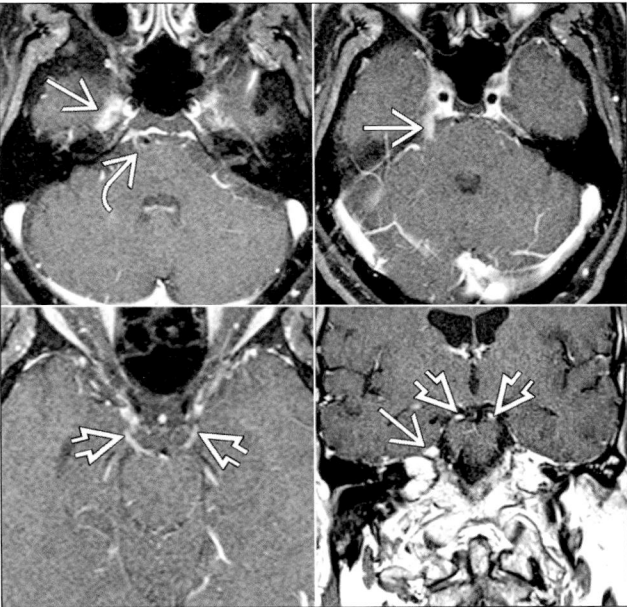

13-61. T1 C+ FS scans in a patient with Lyme disease and multiple cranial nerve palsies show enhancement of the right fifth ➡ and sixth ➡ CNs as well as both oculomotor nerves ➡. (Courtesy P. Hildenbrand, MD.)

LD occurs at all ages, but peak presentation is between 16 and 60 years. Thirty percent of cases occur in children.

Presentation. North American LD occurs in stages. Stage 1 occurs between 2 and 30 days after the initial tick bite and is characterized by erythema migrans—a characteristic round, outwardly expanding, target-like ("bull's-eye") rash—and "summer flu" symptoms such as fever, headache, and malaise. Migrating myalgias and pain in large joints may develop ("Lyme arthritis").

Stage 2 occurs one to four months after infection and presents with neurologic and cardiac symptoms. Neurologic symptoms develop in approximately 10-15% of cases, while cardiac involvement occurs in 8%. Stage 3 can occur several years following the initial infection and manifests as arthritic and chronic neurologic symptoms.

The classic triad of North American LNB consists of aseptic meningitis, cranial neuritis, and radiculoneuritis. Uni- or bilateral facial palsy is common and helps differentiate LNB from other disorders. Erythema migrans, "Lyme arthritis," and carditis are also common.

The most common symptom in children is headache, followed by facial nerve palsy and meningismus.

The most common presentation of European LNB is the triad of Bannwarth syndrome: Lymphocytic meningitis, cranial neuropathy, and painful radiculitis. Erythema migrans, "Lyme arthritis," and carditis are all uncommon manifestations of European LD.

Natural history. The diagnosis and treatment of chronic Lyme disease is controversial. To date, there is no systematic evidence that *B. burgdorferi* can be identified in patients with chronic symptoms following treated LD. Multiple prospective trials have demonstrated that prolonged courses of antibiotics neither prevent nor alleviate post-Lyme syndromes and may result in severe adverse events.

PATHOLOGY. Findings of meningitis and radiculitis predominate. Microscopic features include nonspecific perivascular T-lymphocytic cuffing and plasma cell infiltrates with axonal degeneration. Lymphocytes and plasma cells accumulate in autonomic ganglia of the peripheral nervous system. Spirochetes can be identified in the leptomeninges, nerve roots, and dorsal root ganglia, but not in the CNS parenchyma.

IMAGING. NECT and CECT scans are usually normal.

The most common MR finding is multiple small (two to eight millimeters) subcortical and periventricular white matter hyperintensities on T2/FLAIR (13-59). These are identified in approximately half of all patients with LNB. Large "tumefactive" lesions are uncommon.

Cranial nerve involvement is common in North American LNB. CN VII is the most frequently involved (13-60), followed by CNs V and III. Unilateral disease is more common than bilateral disease although multiple nerves can be affected (13-61). Uniform enhancement on T1 C+ FS is the typical finding.

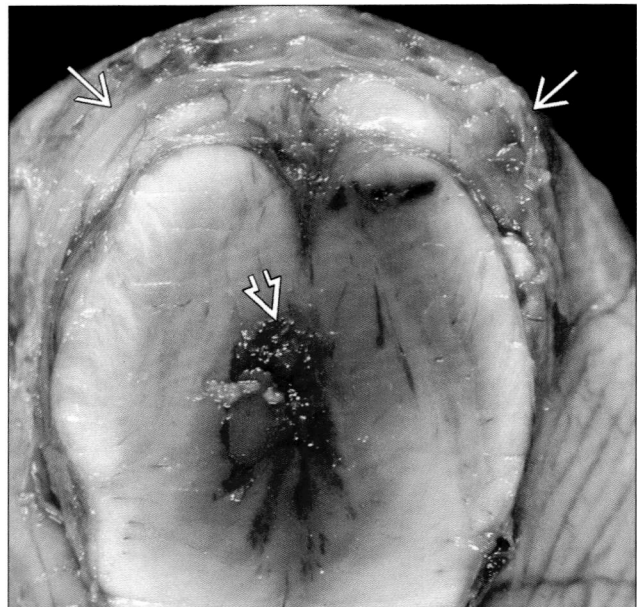

13-62. Close-up view of autopsied brain demonstrates the typical findings of meningovascular syphilis. Exudate covers the pons ➡. A syphilitic gumma ⬎ is also present. (Courtesy R. Hewlett, MD.)

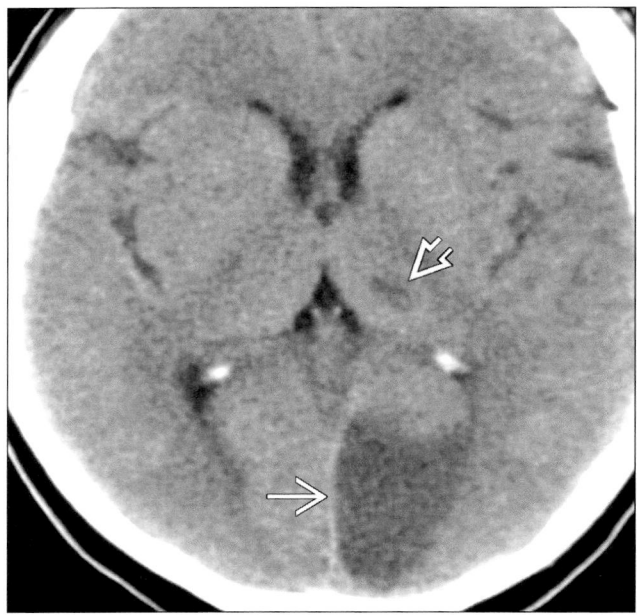

13-63. NECT scan in a patient with meningovascular syphilis shows left occipital ➡, thalamic infarcts ➡. DSA (not shown) disclosed vasculitis-like findings. (Courtesy P. Hildenbrand, MD.)

Spinal cord involvement by *B. burgdorferi* is very rare but is more common in European LD. Diffuse or multifocal hyperintense lesions on T2WI with patchy cord and linear nerve root enhancement is common in *B. garinii* radiculomyelopathy.

Enhancement of LNB white matter lesions varies from none to moderate. Occasionally "horseshoe" or incomplete ring enhancement occurs and can mimic demyelinating disease.

In European LNB, enhancement of cauda equina and lower spinal cord nerve roots is more common than cranial nerve enhancement.

DIFFERENTIAL DIAGNOSIS. The major differential diagnosis of LNB is demyelinating disease. **Multiple sclerosis** (MS) frequently involves the periventricular white matter. Callososeptal involvement is more common in MS compared to LNB. Cranial nerve enhancement—especially CN VII—is less common than with LNB.

Susac syndrome typically involves the middle layers of the corpus callosum and is often accompanied by sensorineural hearing loss (rare in LNB) and visual symptoms.

Vasculitis involves the basal ganglia more than LNB does and rarely affects the cranial nerves.

Neurosyphilis

TERMINOLOGY AND ETIOLOGY. Syphilis is a chronic systemic infectious disease caused by the spirochete *Tre-*

ponema pallidum. Syphilis is usually transmitted via sexual contact although some cases of vertical transmission from mother to fetus have been reported. Neurosyphilis (NS) is also called neurolues. A focal syphilitic granuloma is called a gumma.

EPIDEMIOLOGY AND DEMOGRAPHICS. Once expected to be eradicated with the use of penicillin, syphilis has become dramatically more prevalent since 2000, primarily because of HIV/AIDS. Syphilis and HIV have emerged as important copathogens with reciprocal augmentation in both transmission and disease progression. HIV-positive patients tend to experience more aggressive symptomatology and are at greater risk of developing neurologic disease.

The M:F ratio is 2:1. Most patients are between 18 and 64 years with a mean age of slightly over 50 years. Congenital syphilitic gummatous lesions are exceptionally rare.

CLINICAL ISSUES. Between 5-10% of patients with untreated syphilis develop NS. *T. pallidum* disseminates to the CNS within days after exposure, although symptomatic NS can occur up to 25 years after the initial chancre. Peak occurrence is 15 years after primary infection.

NS has been divided into five major but overlapping clinicopathologic categories, i.e., asymptomatic, meningeal, meningovascular, parenchymatous, and gummatous. Neuropsychiatric disturbances are the most common presentation. Clinical manifestations can occur during any stage of the infection.

Early NS generally presents as meningovascular disease. Late NS is associated with chronic syphilis in the brain and spinal cord but rarely presents with classic tabes dorsalis or general paresis. Neuropsychiatric disturbances, primarily cognitive impairment and personality change, are common.

CSF VDRL tests are specific but not especially sensitive tests for NS. CSF VDRL is positive in just over 60% of cases. *T. pallidum* hemagglutination assay is positive in 80-85%.

PATHOLOGY. Brain syphilitic gumma is a completely curable disease, so appropriate diagnosis is essential for patient treatment. Syphilitic gummata consist of a dense inflammatory infiltrate with large numbers of lymphocytes and plasma cells surrounding a central caseous necrotic core. Vascular proliferation, endarteritis with intimal thickening, and perivascular inflammation are characteristic findings. The definitive histologic diagnosis is obtained using fluorescent isothiocyanate-labeled monoclonal antibodies or PCR.

Gummata probably arise from excessive response of the cell-mediated immune system. Nearly two-thirds are located along brain surfaces, especially over the cerebral convexities. Direct extension from syphilitic meningovascular pial inflammation into the adjacent brain along the penetrating perivascular spaces is the probable mechanism (13-62). Dural thickening and inflammation adjacent to cerebral gummata are common.

IMAGING. Meningovascular syphilis may cause a vasculopathy with lacunar or territorial infarcts that are indistinguishable from thromboembolic strokes (13-63).

Syphilitic gummata are hypo- or mixed-density lesions on NECT that enhance intensely on CECT. A ring-like or diffuse enhancement pattern is typical.

MR shows the gummata are hypointense on T1 and heterogeneously hyperintense on T2WI. Marked enhancement on T1 C+ is seen, and a dural "tail" is present in one-third of cases (13-64).

DIFFERENTIAL DIAGNOSIS. Syphilitic gummata are most commonly misdiagnosed as **primary** or **metastatic neoplasms.** HIV/AIDS patients who have positive blood/

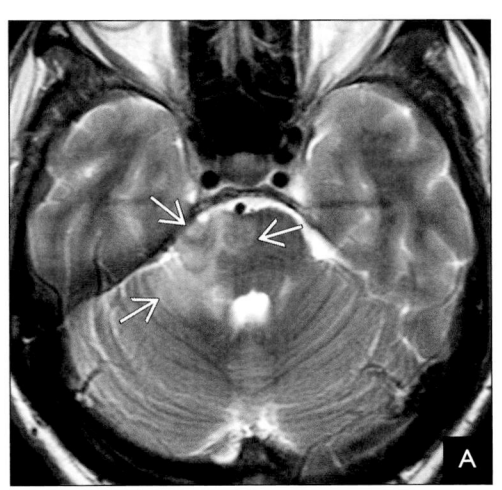
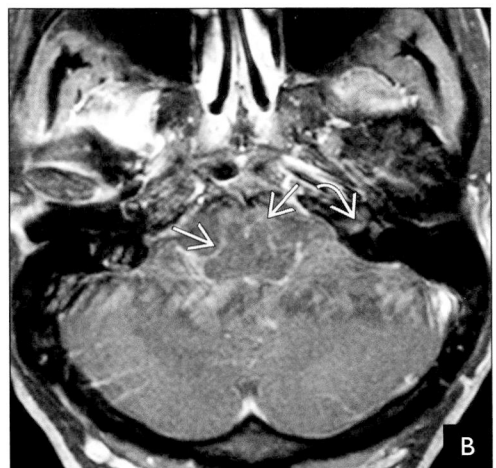

13-64A. Axial T2WI in a 47-year-old HIV-positive man with trigeminal neuralgia shows a mixed iso-/hyperintense mass involving the pons, cerebellum, and trigeminal nerve ➡. 13-64B. Axial T1 C+ FS demonstrates pial enhancement surrounding the medulla ➡ and extending into the left internal auditory canal ➡.

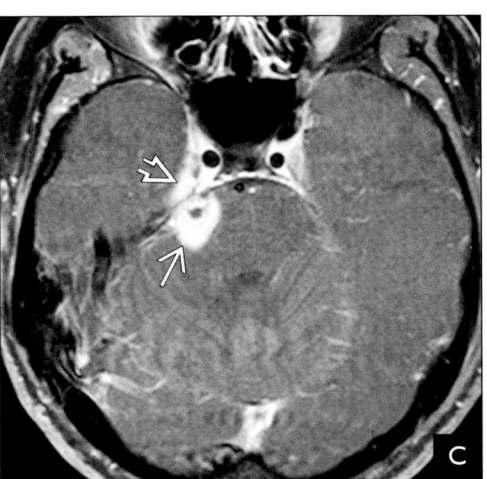
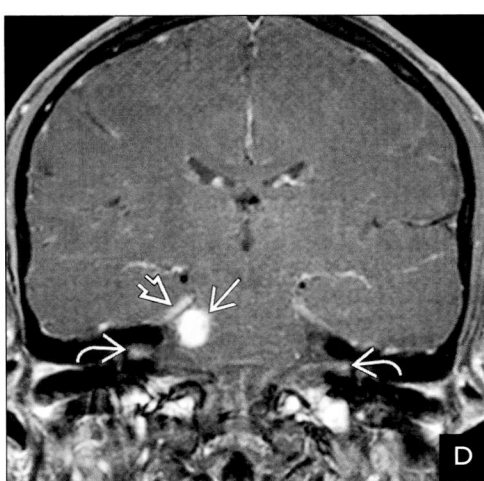

13-64C. More cephalad T1 C+ FS scan in the same patient shows intense enhancement in the pons and cerebellum ➡ with extension into Meckel cave ➡ and thickening of the adjacent dura. 13-64D. Coronal T1 C+ scan demonstrates the syphilitic gumma ➡, adjacent dural thickening ➡, and enhancement in both internal auditory canals ➡. The patient's CD4 count at the time of imaging was 200. Biopsy-proven meningovascular syphilis.

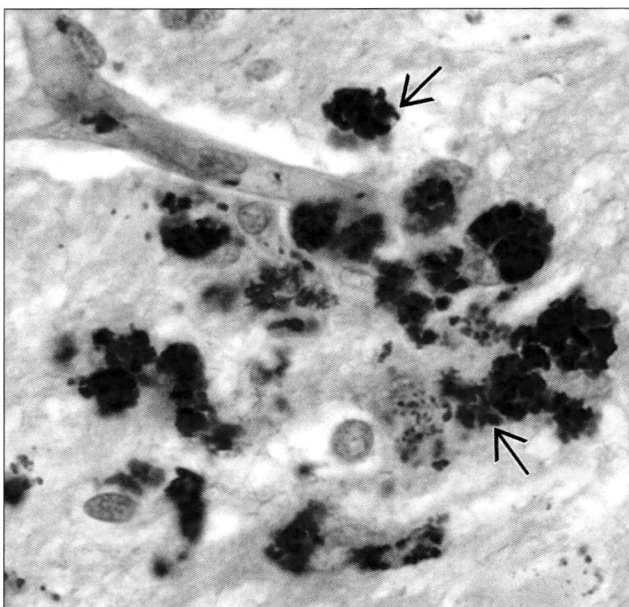

13-65. *Clumped intracytoplasmic bacilli are intensely PAS positive ➡. Individual organisms are difficult to identify. (Courtesy B. K. DeMasters, MD.)*

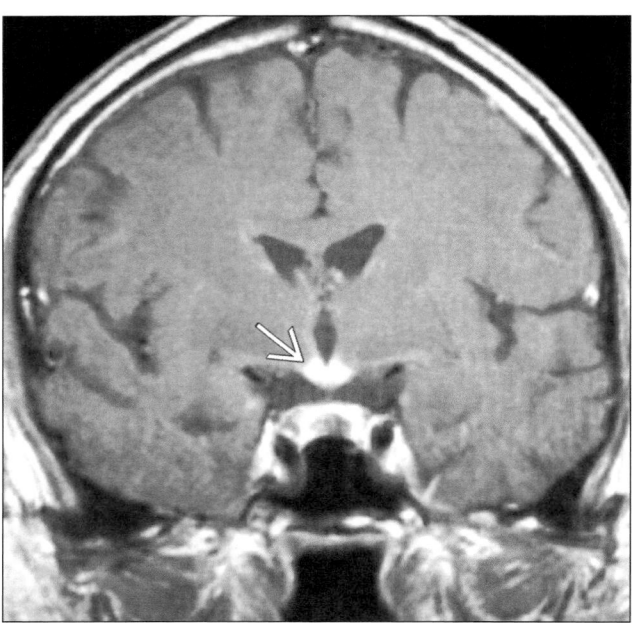

13-66. *Coronal T1 C+ scan shows hypothalamic enhancement ➡ in a patient with documented CNS Whipple disease. (Courtesy B. K. DeMasters, MD.)*

CSF syphilis titers and a cerebral mass lesion with characteristic imaging findings might warrant an empiric trial of intravenous penicillin G with follow-up imaging.

Miscellaneous and Emerging CNS Infections

We briefly discuss several unusual infections in this section. Some of these rare infections are potentially curable if recognized early in the disease course. Others are emerging infections—mostly viruses—about which much is still unknown and for which no cures currently exist.

Emerging infections are diseases that are literally emerging to infect humans. Some of these are zoonoses (i.e., diseases transmitted from animals to humans) while others are insect-borne. Most rarely affect the CNS, but when they do, the results can be disastrous. Examples of the latter include the hemorrhagic viral fevers such as Korean hemorrhagic fever, Rift Valley fever, hantavirus, dengue, and Ebola.

CNS Whipple Disease

TERMINOLOGY AND ETIOLOGY. Whipple disease is a chronic multisystem disorder caused by the bacterium *Tropheryma whippelii.*

EPIDEMIOLOGY AND DEMOGRAPHICS. CNS Whipple disease is a subset of an already-rare disease with a prevalence of one case per 10,000 carriers of the bacterium.

There is no known association with HIV/AIDS or other immunodeficiency syndromes.

PATHOLOGY. The diagnosis of Whipple disease is established by immunohistochemistry (positive antibodies to *T. whippelii*) or PCR. PCR is highly sensitive and specific and can be performed on small bowel, lymph node, or brain biopsy specimens. Between 70-80% of cases have positive CSF PCR.

Histologic features include loose aggregates of histiocytes, lymphocytes, and plasma cells with little or no granulomatous inflammation. Gray-tinged foamy macrophages on H&E contain sickle-shaped PAS-positive intracytoplasmic granules that represent clumps of bacilli **(13-65)**.

CLINICAL ISSUES. Whipple disease can occur at any age but is most common in middle-aged white men. Mean age at onset is 50 years.

Clinical symptoms vary. Systemic symptoms include diarrhea, malabsorption, weight loss, migratory polyarthralgias, fever, and night sweats. Lymphadenopathy is common.

Approximately 5% of Whipple disease patients initially present with symptoms of brain involvement; additional patients develop CNS symptoms later in the disease course.

Encephalopathy with nonspecific cognitive changes, including dementia, altered consciousness, and psychiatric disturbances, is the most frequent presentation.

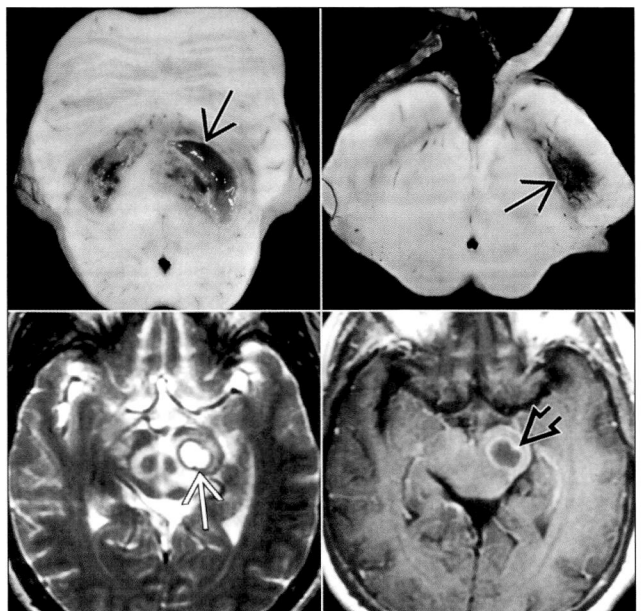

13-67. Listeriosis shows classic findings of midbrain abscess ➡. T2WI (left), T1 C+ (right) a few days before death show focal hyperintense mass in the left cerebral peduncle with hypointense rim ➡, perilesional edema, ring enhancement ➡.

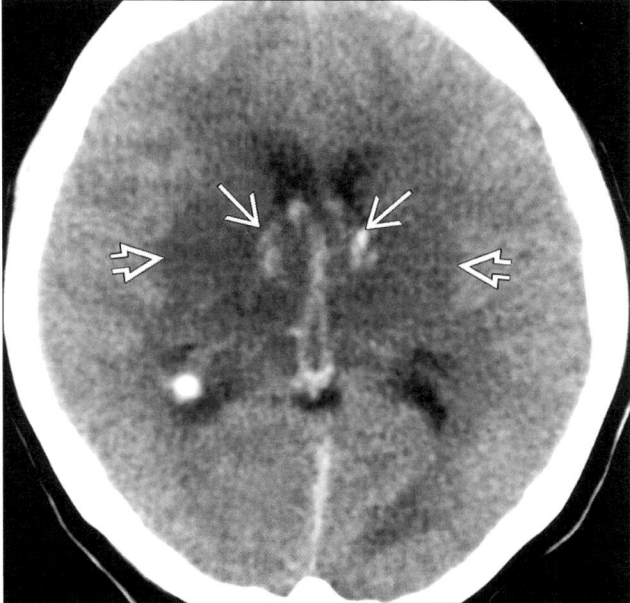

13-68. NECT scan in a patient with dengue fever shows bilateral basal ganglia, thalamic hypodensities ➡ with focal petechial hemorrhages ➡.

Ophthalmoplegia and supranuclear palsy are common. Hypothalamic dysfunction occurs in about one-third of all patients, and cranial nerve palsies are present in 25%.

Without treatment, Whipple disease is invariably fatal. Some patients improve dramatically or stabilize with appropriate antibiotic therapy. Even with antibiotics, however, many patients relapse. The prognosis in patients with CNS Whipple disease is especially grim. Approximately one-quarter die within four years, and another 25% survive with major neurologic deficits.

IMAGING. Imaging findings in CNS Whipple disease are nonspecific. Lesions tend to cluster in the thalami, hypothalamus, quadrigeminal plate, periaqueductal gray matter, and medial temporal lobes **(13-66)**. Multifocal disease is much more common than solitary lesions.

Midline or bilaterally symmetric hyperintense lesions on T2/FLAIR that display mild enhancement on T1 C+ are typical. Corticospinal tract hyperintensity occurs in some patients and may resemble amyotrophic lateral sclerosis. Whipple disease usually does not restrict on DWI.

DIFFERENTIAL DIAGNOSIS. The differential diagnosis of CNS Whipple disease includes granulomatous processes such as **neurosarcoid** and **tuberculosis**. Mesial temporal lesions may simulate **herpes encephalitis** or **autoimmune/limbic encephalitis**. Most CNS Whipple disease lesions have minimal or no mass effect, so neoplasm such as **lymphoma** or **diffusely infiltrating astrocytoma** is a less likely consideration.

Listeriosis

Listeriosis is an emerging food borne zoonotic infection caused by *Listeria monocytogenes*, a gram-positive facultative intracellular bacterium that dwells in soil, vegetation, or animal reservoirs. There are six species of *Listeria*, only one of which—*L. monocytogenes*—is pathogenic in humans.

Listeria causes gastroenteritis, mother-to-fetus infection, septicemia, and CNS infection in immunocompromised individuals, pregnant women, and newborns. Cases in immunocompetent people are rare.

CNS listeriosis shows a specific tropism for the meninges and brainstem. Symptoms include fever, headache, cranial nerve palsies, vertigo, and somnolence. Once symptoms of CNS disease develop, the mortality rate is 25-30%.

Imaging findings are generally nonspecific. CNS listeriosis can occur as meningitis, encephalitis, cerebritis, or abscess. In the appropriate clinical setting, a focal midbrain, pons, or medulla T2/FLAIR hyperintense, ring-enhancing mass with significant perilesional edema should suggest the possibility of *L. monocytogenes* abscess **(13-67)**.

Hemorrhagic Viral Fevers

The Centers for Disease Control and Prevention (CDC) has identified six biological agents as "category A" (easily disseminated or transmitted from person to person, resulting in high mortality rate and potential for major public health risk): Anthrax, smallpox, botulism, tularemia, viral hemorrhagic fever, and plague. Of these, the **viral hemorrhagic fevers** are the most likely to affect the CNS.

Filoviruses such as Ebola and Marburg are single-stranded negative-sense RNA viruses that cause acute hemorrhagic fever with high mortality rates. Most of these patients do not survive long enough to develop CNS symptoms, and most are never imaged. Currently there are no licensed vaccines or therapeutics to counter human filovirus infections. Confirmed cases of Ebola hemorrhagic fever have been reported in Africa. No confirmed case has ever been reported in the United States or Europe.

Hemorrhagic fevers with known CNS complications include dengue hemorrhagic fever/dengue shock syndrome and hantavirus with renal syndrome.

Dengue infection is caused by a flavivirus with four serotypes, two of which (serotypes 2 and 3) are the principal agents with CNS involvement. In endemic areas, dengue has become the most frequent cause of encephalitis, surpassing even Herpes simplex virus. Dengue is the most important flavivirus with respect to global disease incidence and the potential for spread beyond nonendemic regions **(13-68)**.

Symptomatic CNS involvement occurs in 5-20% of patients with confirmed acute dengue virus infection and dengue hemorrhagic fever. Imaging studies show multiple hemorrhagic foci. Frank infarcts and pituitary apoplexy have been reported in some cases.

Many patients with **hantavirus** or **Korean hemorrhagic fever** renal syndromes develop CNS symptoms such as acute psychiatric disorders, epilepsy, and meningismus. Autopsy studies demonstrate pituitary hemorrhage in 37%, pituitary necrosis in 5%, and brainstem hemorrhage in nearly 70%. In the few reported cases, MR showed pituitary hemorrhage and reversible splenium lesion in the corpus callosum.

elected References

Mycobacterial Infections

Tuberculosis

- Chou PS et al: Central nervous system tuberculosis: a forgotten diagnosis. Neurologist. 18(4):219-22, 2012
- Leeds IL et al: Site of extrapulmonary tuberculosis is associated with HIV infection. Clin Infect Dis. 55(1):75-81, 2012
- Li H et al: Central nervous system tuberculoma. J Clin Neurosci. 19(5):691-5, 2012
- Gupta RK et al: Central nervous system tuberculosis. Neuroimaging Clin N Am. 21(4):795-814, vii-viii, 2011
- Omar N et al: Diffusion-weighted magnetic resonance imaging of borderzone necrosis in paediatric tuberculous meningitis. J Med Imaging Radiat Oncol. 55(6):563-70, 2011
- Androulaki A et al: Inflammatory pseudotumor associated with Mycobacterium tuberculosis infection. Int J Infect Dis. 12(6):607-10, 2008
- du Plessis J et al: CT features of tuberculous intracranial abscesses in children. Pediatr Radiol. 37(2):167-72, 2007
- Bernaerts A et al: Tuberculosis of the central nervous system: overview of neuroradiological findings. Eur Radiol. 13(8):1876-90, 2003

Nontuberculous Mycobacterial Infections

- Arkun K et al: Atypical mycobacterial brain abscess presenting as a spindle cell lesion in an immunocompetent patient. Clin Neuropathol. 31(3):155-8, 2012
- Morrison A et al: Mycobacterial spindle cell pseudotumor of the brain: a case report and review of the literature. Am J Surg Pathol. 23(10):1294-9, 1999

Fungal Infections

- DeMasters BK: Fungal infections. In Burger P et al: Diagnostic Pathology: Neuropathology. Salt Lake City: Amirsys Publishing. II.2:50-61, 2012
- Chow FC et al: Cerebrovascular disease in central nervous system infections. Semin Neurol. 31(3):286-306, 2011
- Luthra G et al: Comparative evaluation of fungal, tubercular, and pyogenic brain abscesses with conventional and diffusion MR imaging and proton MR spectroscopy. AJNR Am J Neuroradiol. 28(7):1332-8, 2007
- Mueller-Mang C et al: Fungal versus bacterial brain abscesses: is diffusion-weighted MR imaging a useful tool in the differential diagnosis? Neuroradiology. 49(8):651-7, 2007
- Gaviani P et al: Diffusion-weighted imaging of fungal cerebral infection. AJNR Am J Neuroradiol. 26(5):1115-21, 2005

Parasitic Infections

- Abdel Razek AA et al: Parasitic diseases of the central nervous system. Neuroimaging Clin N Am. 21(4):815-41, viii, 2011

Neurocysticercosis

- Abdel Razek AA et al: Parasitic diseases of the central nervous system. Neuroimaging Clin N Am. 21(4):815-41, viii, 2011
- Carabin H et al: Clinical manifestations associated with neurocysticercosis: a systematic review. PLoS Negl Trop Dis. 5(5):e1152, 2011
- Kimura-Hayama ET et al: Neurocysticercosis: radiologic-pathologic correlation. Radiographics. 30(6):1705-19, 2010

Echinococcosis

- Abdel Razek AA et al: Parasitic diseases of the central nervous system. Neuroimaging Clin N Am. 21(4):815-41, viii, 2011
- Shahlaie K et al: Parasitic central nervous system infections: echinococcus and schistosoma. Rev Neurol Dis. 2(4):176-85, 2005

Amebiasis

- Abdel Razek AA et al: Parasitic diseases of the central nervous system. Neuroimaging Clin N Am. 21(4):815-41, viii, 2011

Malaria

- Wilson CS: Malaria. In Foucar K et al: Diagnostic Pathology: Blood and Bone Marrow. Salt Lake City: Amirsys Publishing. 7.52-59, 2012
- Chimelli L: A morphological approach to the diagnosis of protozoal infections of the central nervous system. Patholog Res Int. 2011:290853, 2011
- Idro R et al: Cerebral malaria: mechanisms of brain injury and strategies for improved neurocognitive outcome. Pediatr Res. 68(4):267-74, 2010
- Singh P et al: Amebic meningoencephalitis: spectrum of imaging findings. AJNR Am J Neuroradiol. 27(6):1217-21, 2006

Other Parasitic Infections

- Kleinschmidt-DeMasters BK: Other parasitic infections. In Burger P et al: Diagnostic Pathology: Neuropathology. Salt Lake City: Amirsys Publishing. II.2.78-83, 2012
- Abdel Razek AA et al: Parasitic diseases of the central nervous system. Neuroimaging Clin N Am. 21(4):815-41, viii, 2011
- Song T et al: CT and MR characteristics of cerebral sparganosis. AJNR Am J Neuroradiol. 28(9):1700-5, 2007
- Shahlaie K et al: Parasitic central nervous system infections: echinococcus and schistosoma. Rev Neurol Dis. 2(4):176-85, 2005

Miscellaneous and Emerging CNS Infections

Spirochete Infections of the CNS

- Kayal AK et al: Clinical spectrum of neurosyphilis in North East India. Neurol India. 59(3):344-50, 2011

- Lantos PM: Chronic Lyme disease: the controversies and the science. Expert Rev Anti Infect Ther. 9(7):787-97, 2011

- Makhani N et al: A twist on Lyme: the challenge of diagnosing European Lyme neuroborreliosis. J Clin Microbiol. 49(1):455-7, 2011

- Ghanem KG: Review: Neurosyphilis: an historical perspective and review. CNS Neurosci Ther. 16(5):e157-68, 2010

- Liu H et al: Induction of distinct neurologic disease manifestations during relapsing fever requires T lymphocytes. J Immunol. 184(10):5859-64, 2010

- Agarwal R et al: Neuro-lyme disease: MR imaging findings. Radiology. 253(1):167-73, 2009

- Fargen KM et al: Cerebral syphilitic gummata: a case presentation and analysis of 156 reported cases. Neurosurgery. 64(3):568-75; discussioin 575-6, 2009

- Hildenbrand P et al: Lyme neuroborreliosis: manifestations of a rapidly emerging zoonosis. AJNR Am J Neuroradiol. 30(6):1079-87, 2009

- Günther G et al: Tick-borne encephalopathies: epidemiology, diagnosis, treatment and prevention. CNS Drugs. 19(12):1009-32, 2005

Miscellaneous and Emerging CNS Infections

- Kleinschmidt-DeMasters BK: Whipple disease. In Burger P et al: Diagnostic Pathology: Neuropathology. Salt Lake City: Amirsys Publishing. II.2.16-19, 2012

- Wildemberg LE et al: Dengue hemorrhagic fever: a condition associated with multiple risk factors for pituitary apoplexy. Endocr Pract. Epub ahead of print, 2012

- Bui-Mansfield LT et al: Imaging of hemorrhagic fever with renal syndrome: a potential bioterrorism agent of military significance. Mil Med. 176(11):1327-34, 2011

- Iagodova ES: [Affection of central nervous system in hemorrhagic fever with renal syndrome.] Klin Med (Mosk). 89(2):60-2, 2011

- Ramadan M et al: Listeria rhomboencephalitis. N Z Med J. 124(1344):98-102, 2011

- Soares CN et al: Review of the etiologies of viral meningitis and encephalitis in a dengue endemic region. J Neurol Sci. 303(1-2):75-9, 2011

- Baek SH et al: Reversible splenium lesion of the corpus callosum in hemorrhagic fever with renal failure syndrome. J Korean Med Sci. 25(8):1244-6, 2010

- Black DF et al: MR imaging of central nervous system Whipple disease: a 15-year review. AJNR Am J Neuroradiol. 31(8):1493-7, 2010

- Oevermann A et al: Rhombencephalitis caused by Listeria monocytogenes in humans and ruminants: a zoonosis on the rise? Interdiscip Perspect Infect Dis. 2010:632513, 2010

- Hautala T et al: Central nervous system-related symptoms and findings are common in acute Puumala hantavirus infection. Ann Med. 42(5):344-51, 2010

- Drnda A et al: Listeria meningoencephalitis in an immunocompetent person. Med Arh. 63(2):112-3, 2009

- Hayashi T et al: Critical roles of NK and CD8+ T cells in central nervous system listeriosis. J Immunol. 182(10):6360-8, 2009

- Matlani M et al: Dengue encephalitis: an entity now common in dengue-prone regions. Trop Doct. 39(2):115-6, 2009

14

HIV/AIDS

In this chapter we explore the "many faces" of HIV/AIDS as it affects the central nervous system. We start by placing the disease in its epidemiological and demographic context, then turn our attention to the pathology and imaging spectrum of CNS HIV/AIDS.

We next discuss the manifestation of HIV itself in the brain, i.e., HIV encephalitis. We follow with a consideration of unusual but important associated findings such as HIV vasculopathy, HIV-associated bone marrow changes, and benign salivary gland lymphoepithelial lesions.

We then consider the broad spectrum of opportunistic infections that complicate HIV/AIDS and what happens when an HIV-positive patient is also coinfected with TB, another sexually transmitted disease, or malaria.

New insights about treated AIDS and the phenomenon of immune reconstitution inflammatory syndrome (IRIS) are then presented. We conclude the chapter by discussing neoplasms that occur in the setting of HIV/AIDS (the so-called AIDS-defining malignancies).

Overview

Introduction

It has been more than 30 years since a new syndrome associated with profound suppression of cell-mediated immunity was first identified. The causative agent, a retrovirus, was given the appropriate name of human immunodeficiency virus (HIV), and the syndrome it caused was named acquired immunodeficiency syndrome (AIDS).

It required nearly a decade to develop highly active multidrug multiclass treatment regimens for HIV/AIDS. Highly active antiretroviral therapy (HAART), also called combination antiretroviral therapy (cART), has resulted in a dramatic decline in mortality for treated patients. Overall AIDS-related deaths have dropped by nearly 20% in the last five years.

In wealthy industrialized countries in which widespread access to HAART is readily available, HIV/AIDS has evolved from a virtual death sentence to a chronic but manageable disease. Survival in these countries has increased from a mean of 10.5 years to 22.5 years in a single decade. That's the good news. The bad news? Progress is fragile and unevenly distributed. In many less-developed "high burden" parts of the world, HIV incidence is still rising in epidemic numbers. The personal and socioeconomic consequences of the HIV/AIDS epidemic have been devastating.

Epidemiology

Summaries of the global AIDS epidemic indicate that in 2010 (the most recent year for which data are available), the number of people living with HIV totalled 34 million. Of these, nearly 70% were in sub-Saharan Africa, and 3.4 million were children under the age of 15 years. Women

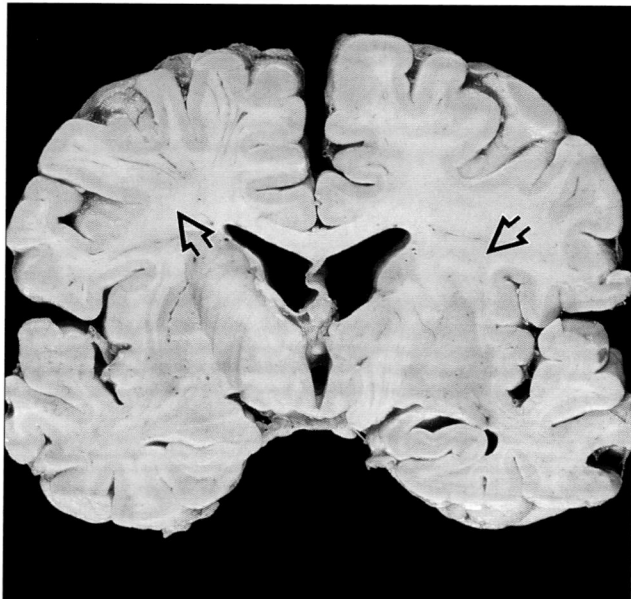

14-1. Coronal autopsy of HIVE shows generalized volume loss with enlargement of the lateral ventricles, sylvian fissures. "Hazy," poorly defined abnormalities are present in the WM ⊳ but spare the subcortical U-fibers. (B. K. DeMasters, MD.)

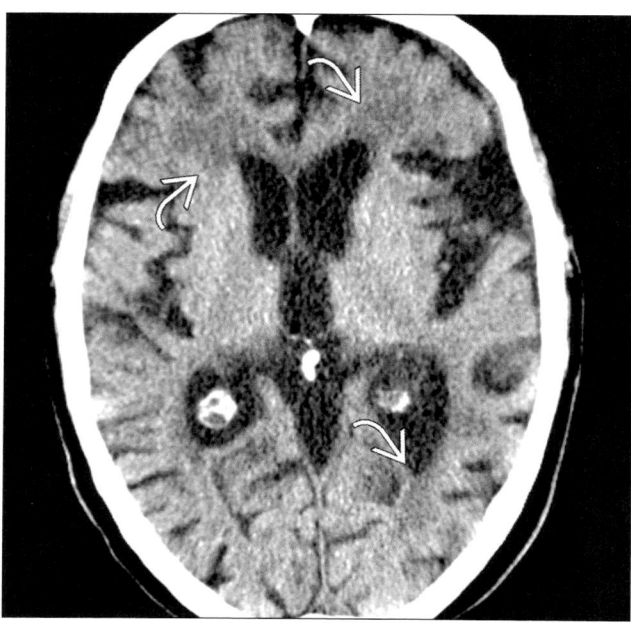

14-2. Axial NECT scan in a 38-year-old man with longstanding HIV/AIDS shows gross cerebral atrophy and multifocal hypodensities ⇨ in the subcortical white matter.

now account for almost 52% of adult cases globally. A total of 2.7 million new HIV infections occur annually—97% in low- and middle-income countries—while 1.8 million infected individuals die each year from HIV/AIDS and its complications.

The vast majority of HIV/AIDS patients now live in low- to middle-income regions while most of the patients with access to HAART live in high-income countries. Access to antiretroviral therapy in less-developed countries has increased only slightly and reaches just 35% of all patients who need treatment in those countries. Although the number of new infections has been significantly reduced since their peak in 1999, this number continues to outpace the number of people placed on HAART.

This disparity means that socioeconomic determinants of health affect both the prevalence and manifestations of HIV/AIDS. The same disease can have vastly different consequences—and therefore imaging appearances—in different parts of the world. Coinfection and comorbidity from other diseases further complicate imaging diagnosis and patient management.

Demographics

HIV is transmitted through unprotected sexual intercourse (anal or vaginal), transfusion of contaminated blood, and sharing of contaminated needles, as well as between mother and infant during pregnancy, childbirth, and breastfeeding.

HIV prevalence varies widely with geography, race/ethnicity, and gender. Sub-Saharan Africa accounts for nearly 70% of the global prevalence of HIV, disproportionately affecting women and young people. As a result of improved therapeutics and monitoring, HIV infections are also a growing concern in the elderly.

The most recently available data indicate that gay and bisexual men remain the population most heavily affected by HIV in the United States. New infection rates have been relatively stable since 2006 but are disproportionately higher in African-American males compared to African-American females as well as higher in white males compared to white females.

Individuals with sexually transmitted diseases (including chlamydia, gonorrhea, syphilis, herpes, and human papillomavirus) are more likely than uninfected persons to acquire HIV infection. Approximately 10% of patients with hepatitis C are coinfected with HIV.

HIV Infection

HIV is a neurovirulent infection that has both direct and indirect effects on the CNS. Neurologic complications can arise from the HIV infection itself, from opportunistic infections or neoplasms, and from treatment-related metabolic derangements.

In this section we consider the effects of the HIV virus itself on the brain. Extracranial manifestations of HIV/AIDS may also be identified on brain imaging studies, so we discuss these as well.

HIV Encephalitis

Between 75-90% of HIV/AIDS patients have demonstrable HIV-induced brain injury at autopsy (14-1). While many patients remain asymptomatic for variable periods, brain infection is the initial presenting symptomatology in 5-10% of cases. Approximately 25% of treated HIV/AIDS patients develop moderate cognitive impairment despite good virologic response to therapy.

Terminology

HIV encephalitis (HIVE) and HIV leukoencephalopathy (HIVL) are the direct result of HIV infection of the brain. Opportunistic infections are absent early although coinfections or multiple infections are common later in the disease course.

HIV-associated neurocognitive disorders (HANDs) are the most frequent neurological manifestations of HIVE and HIVL. The term "acquired immunodeficiency dementia complex" refers specifically to HIV-associated dementia.

Etiology

HIV is a pathogenic neurotropic human RNA retrovirus. **HIV-1** is responsible for most cases of HIV/AIDS. **HIV-2** infection is predominantly a disease of heterosexuals and is found primarily in West Africa. Unless otherwise noted in this discussion, "HIV" or "HIV infection" refers to HIV-1 infection.

HIV initially infects Langerhans (dendritic) cells in the skin and mucous membranes. Its envelope protein gp120 binds to CD4 receptors in these dendritic cells, which then migrate to lymphoid tissues and infect CD4-positive T cells. The virus proliferates in and then destroys the infected T cells. A burst of viremia develops within days and leads to widespread tissue dissemination.

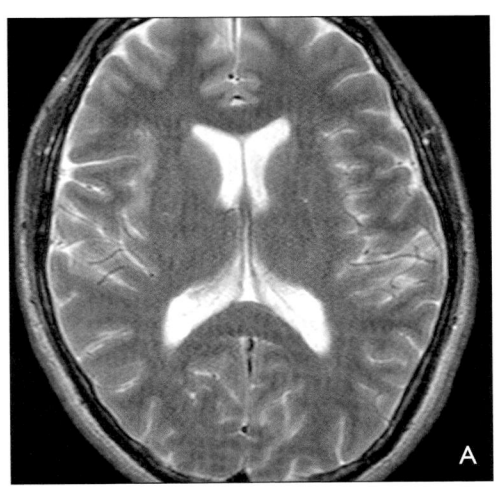

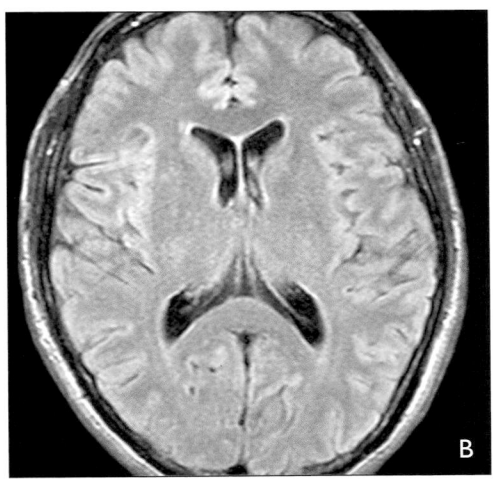

*14-3A. Axial T2WI in a 45-year-old man with early dementia shows minimal enlargement of the lateral ventricles and sulci. **14-3B.** Axial FLAIR shows no evidence of white matter hyperintensities.*

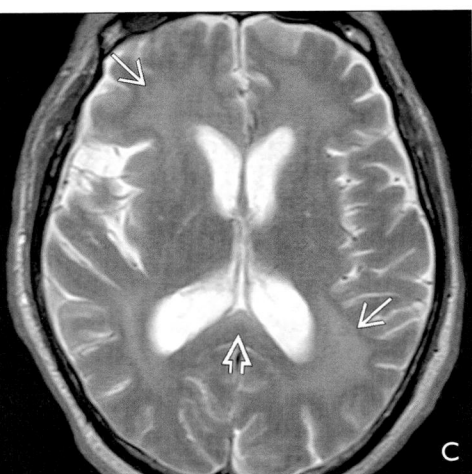

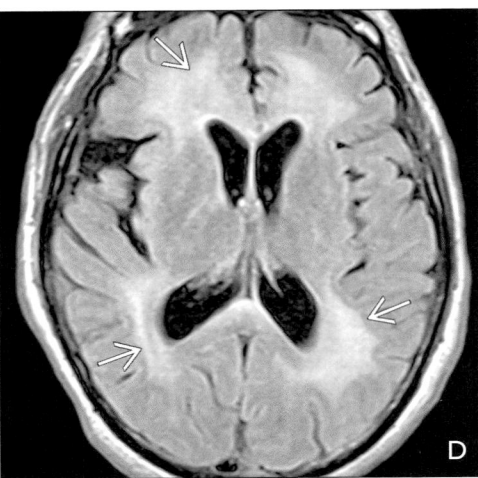

14-3C. Four years later, the same patient has developed severe HIV-associated dementia. Axial T2WI shows significantly increased volume loss, reflected by the enlarged lateral ventricles and sulci. Symmetric confluent hyperintensities have developed in the cerebral white matter ➡ and corpus callosum splenium ⇨. 14-3D. Axial FLAIR scan shows the dramatic interval white matter changes of severe HIV encephalitis ➡. Note sparing of the subcortical U-fibers even at this late stage.

The two major targets of viral infection are lymphoid tissue—especially T cells—and the CNS. HIV-infected monocytes and lymphocytes migrate across the intact blood-brain barrier, penetrating the brain within 24-48 hours after initial exposure.

Although HIV-1 does not directly infect neurons, it persists in brain perivascular macrophages and microglia. Some non-CNS peripheral reservoirs of virus also persist and may play an active role in ongoing brain injury, even with adequate treatment.

Pathology

GROSS PATHOLOGY. Brain pathology in HIV/AIDS varies with patient age and disease acuity. In early stages, the brain appears grossly normal. Advanced HIVE results in generalized brain volume loss ("atrophy") with enlarged ventricles and subarachnoid spaces.

MICROSCOPIC FEATURES. HIVE is characterized by gliosis, microglial clusters, perivascular macrophage accumulation, and multinucleated giant cells. The mult-

inucleated giant cells contain viral antigens and are immunoreactive for the envelope protein gp120.

Immune activation (encephalitis) is often disproportionate to the amount of HIV virus present in the brain. Disseminated patchy foci of white and gray matter damage with myelin pallor and diffuse myelin loss are prominent features. HIV infects astrocytes but does not directly infect neurons. However, neurons can be injured indirectly by viral proteins and neurotoxins.

HIVL is characterized by ill-defined, diffuse myelin pallor with poorly demarcated areas of myelin loss. Lesions are most prominent in the deep periventricular white matter (WM) and corona radiata.

Clinical Issues

EPIDEMIOLOGY. Almost 60% of all AIDS patients eventually develop overt neurologic manifestations. Although HAART has significantly improved survival, approximately 15-25% of treated patients develop moderate cognitive impairment or full-blown AIDS dementia complex. In countries with widespread access to HAART,

14-4A. Axial T2WI in a 43-year-old patient with HIV/ AIDS and mild early cognitive impairment shows diffuse, confluent, bilaterally symmetric hyperintensity in the cerebral white matter ➡. Note sparing of the subcortical U-fibers. 14-4B. Axial FLAIR scan in the same patient shows the "hazy" confluent white matter hyperintensity ➡ characteristic of HIVE. No atrophy is present, and—with the exception of a single focal left parietal lesion ➡—the subcortical WM is spared.

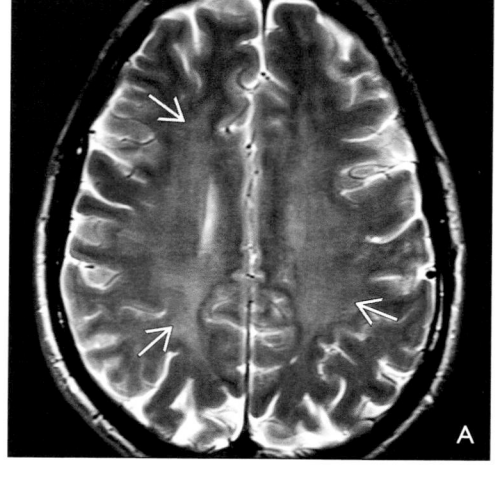
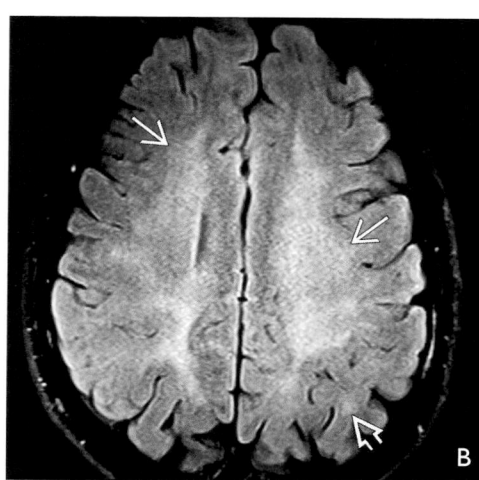

14-4C. Axial T1 C+ FS in the same patient shows no parenchymal or meningeal enhancement. 14-4D. Axial DWI shows no evidence of restricted diffusion. The slight hyperintensity in the hemispheric white matter is not true diffusion restriction; rather, it is secondary to T2 "shine-through."

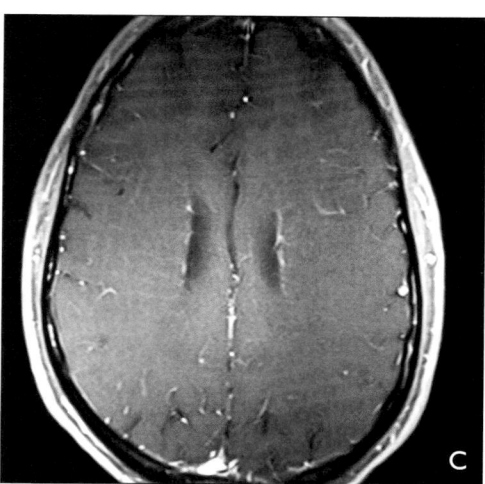
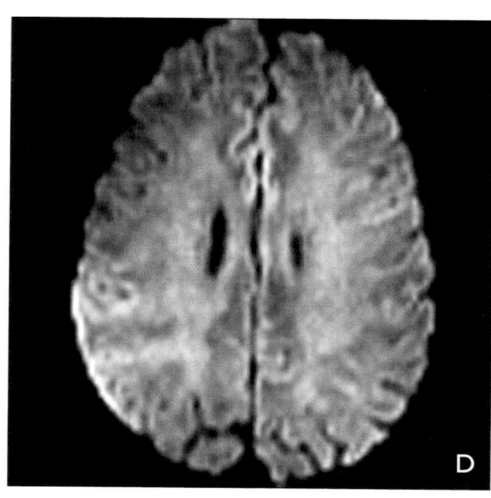

AIDS dementia complex has become the most common neurologic complication of HIV infection.

DEMOGRAPHICS. Both adult and pediatric HIV-positive patients can develop HIVE. From one-third to two-thirds of adult AIDS patients and 30-50% of pediatric cases are affected. The gender distribution of HIVE reflects that of HIV and varies with geographic region.

Age is consistently identified as a risk factor for HIV-related cognitive impairment. There is growing evidence that abnormal brain proteins accumulate in HIV-infected brains. Excess hyperphosphorylated tau, amyloid, and α-synuclein have all been identified and may contribute to the development of accelerated neurodegenerative syndromes and AIDS dementia complex.

PRESENTATION. Some patients develop symptoms of an acute retroviral syndrome (ARVS) during the initial viremia. ARVS develops two to four weeks after infection and consists of sore throat, fever, lymphadenopathy, nausea, rashes, and variable neurologic changes.

HANDs develop as intermediate- and long-term complications. Early brain infection with HIV is often asymptomatic, and cognitive and functional performances are both initially normal. Full-blown HIV-associated dementia causes advanced cognitive impairment and marked impact on daily function.

NATURAL HISTORY. Nearly half of HIV-infected patients in the United States demonstrate sub-par performance on neuropsychological tests. Slowly progressive impairment of fine motor control, verbal fluency, and short-term memory is characteristic. Severe deterioration and subcortical dementia with near vegetative state may develop in the final stages.

The latency period for HIV-2 infection is generally longer and the viral loads lower than with HIV-1. Immunodeficiency therefore evolves more slowly. Patients with HIV-2 infection do develop the same spectrum of opportunistic infections found in HIV-1.

TREATMENT OPTIONS. HAART has decreased morbidity and mortality in HIV/AIDS. It does not prevent development of HIVE but does decrease its overall severity.

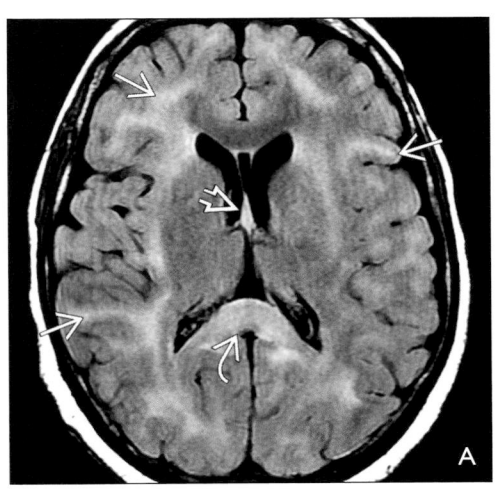

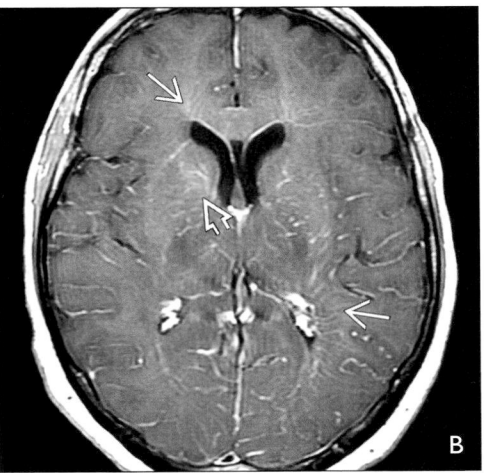

14-5A. FLAIR scan in a 33-year-old woman with fulminant onset of HIVE shows bilateral confluent hyperintensity ➡️ throughout the subcortical and deep WM, including the corpus callosum splenium ➡️ and fornix ➡️. 14-5B. T1 C+ scan shows multifocal linear and punctate enhancing foci, presumably around penetrating arteries ➡️ and deep WM veins ➡️.

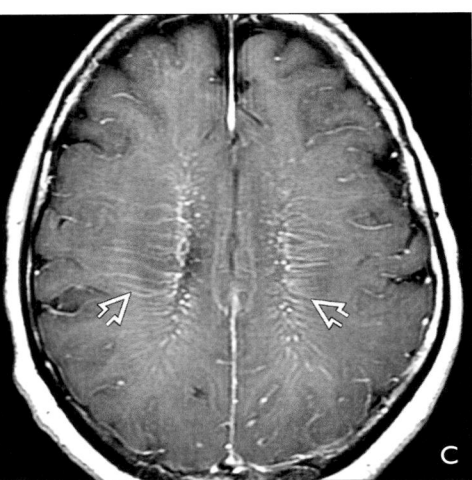

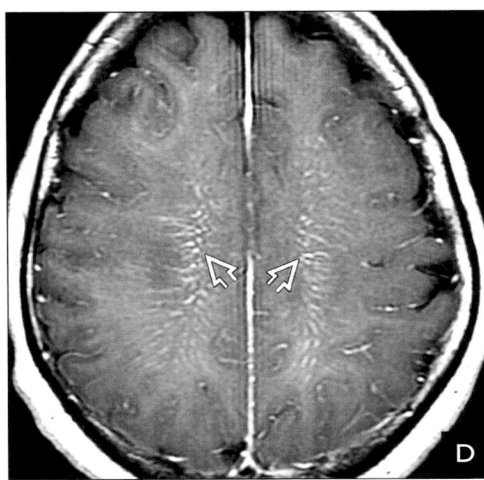

14-5C. More cephalad T1WI C+ scan in the same patient shows striking enhancement around the deep medullary veins of both hemispheres ➡️. 14-5D. T1 C+ scan through the corona radiata shows striking linear and punctate enhancement ➡️ suggesting acute inflammatory changes around the medullary veins. Findings probably represent acute demyelination in fulminant HIVE.

HIV ENCEPHALITIS

Terminology
- HIV encephalitis (HIVE)
  - Direct results of HIV brain infection
  - HIV-associated neurocognitive disorders (HAND)
  - Most serious is AIDS dementia complex

Etiology
- HIV is neurotropic retrovirus
  - Most human infections caused by HIV-1
  - HIV-2 primarily in West Africa
- HIV-infected monocytes, T cells cross blood-brain barrier in 24-48 hours

Clinical Issues
- Epidemiology
  - 60% of AIDS patients develop neurologic disease
  - 15-25% of HAART-treated patients develop AIDS dementia complex
- Presentation
  - Acute retroviral syndrome rare
  - More common = slow progressive impairment

Imaging

GENERAL FEATURES. HIVE does not cause mass effect. Even in the post-HAART era, the most common finding remains generalized progressive volume loss that is disproportionate to the patient's age. Cortical thinning and bilateral white matter lesions are the most common parenchymal abnormalities.

CT FINDINGS. NECT scans may be normal in the early stages. Mild to moderate atrophy with patchy or confluent white matter hypodensity develops as the disease progresses (14-2). HIVE does not enhance on CECT.

MR FINDINGS. Generalized volume loss with enlarged ventricles and sulci is best appreciated on T1WI or thin-section inversion recovery sequences. Reduced gray matter volume in the medial and superior frontal gyri has been identified as a possible early imaging marker for HIVE. White matter signal intensity is generally normal or near-normal on T1WI.

T2/FLAIR initially shows bilateral, patchy, relatively symmetric white matter hyperintensities. With time, confluent "hazy," ill-defined hyperintensity in the subcortical and deep cerebral white matter develops, and volume loss ensues (14-3). HIVE usually does not enhance on T1 C+ and usually shows no restriction on DWI (14-4). In fulminant cases, perivenular enhancement may indicate acute demyelination (14-5).

Advanced imaging modalities may show early changes of HIVE not readily apparent on standard MR. MRS demonstrates neuronal damage as decreased NAA. mI, a marker of glial activation, is often elevated. Other reported early changes in HIVE include increased choline to creatine (Cho:Cr) ratios bilaterally in the frontal gray and white matter, in the left parietal white matter, and in total Cho:Cr ratio.

DTI shows that patients with AIDS-related dementia exhibit significantly elevated mean and radial diffusivity in the parietal white matter compared to nondemented patients with HIVE. Radial diffusivity is affected to a much greater extent than axial diffusivity, suggesting that demyelination is the prominent disease process in white matter.

Differential Diagnosis

The major differential diagnosis of HIVE is **progressive multifocal leukoencephalopathy** (PML). PML has patchy white matter lesions that can be unilateral or bilateral and appear as strikingly asymmetric hyperintensities on T2/FLAIR. Both the hemispheric and posterior fossa white matter are commonly affected. PML often involves the subcortical U-fibers, which are usually spared in HIVE.

Coinfections with other infectious agents are common in HIVE and may complicate the imaging appearance. **Cytomegalovirus** (CMV) can also cause a diffuse white matter encephalitis and ependymitis. **Toxoplasmosis** causes multifocal punctate and "target" or ring-enhancing lesions that are more prominent in the basal ganglia. **Herpes encephalitis** and **HHV-6 encephalitis** both involve the temporal lobes, especially the cortex.

HIV ENCEPHALITIS: IMAGING

NECT
- Normal or atrophy ± WM hypodensity

MR
- Volume loss with ↑ sulci, ventricles
- T2/FLAIR "hazy" WM symmetric hyperintensity
  - Spares subcortical U-fibers
- No mass effect
- Usually no enhancement
  - Possible exception = acute fulminant HIVE

Differential Diagnosis
- Progressive multifocal leukoencephalopathy (PML)
  - Coinfection with HIVE common
  - Usually asymmetric
  - Often involves U-fibers
- Opportunistic infections
  - Coinfection with HIVE common
  - CMV causes encephalitis, ependymitis
  - Toxoplasmosis: Multiple enhancing rings
  - Herpes, HHV-6 usually involve temporal lobes

Other Manifestations of HIV/AIDS

Vasculopathy

Cardiovascular disease has long been recognized as a consequence of HIV infection. While the etiology and pathogenesis of the cardiovascular disease are unknown, HIV affects every aspect of the cardiac axis, causing a

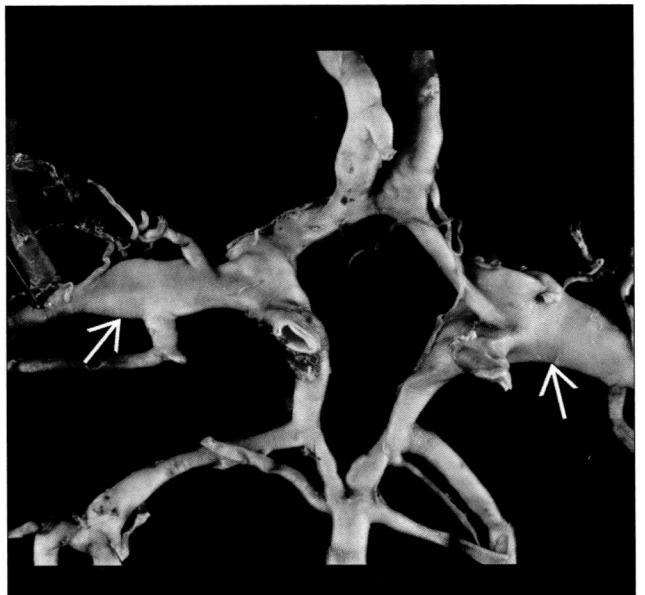

14-6. *Autopsy case in a hemophiliac child with AIDS and HIV vasculopathy shows striking fusiform dilatation of both middle cerebral arteries* ➔ *as well as all components of the circle of Willis. (Courtesy L. Rourke, MD.)*

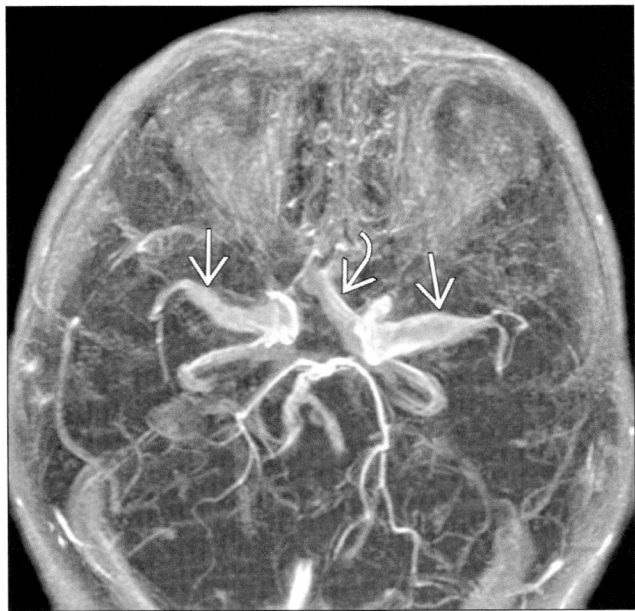

14-7. *Submentovertex 2D TOF MRA in another child with HIV/AIDS and HIV vasculopathy shows marked fusiform enlargement of both middle cerebral arteries* ➔ *and less dramatic enlargement of the left ACA* ➔.

spectrum of disease ranging from cardiomyopathy and myocarditis to peripheral vascular disease. HIV-associated vasculopathy is an increasingly recognized clinical entity, causing high morbidity and increasing mortality.

Stroke is an uncommon but growing cause of mortality and morbidity in HIV/AIDS patients. Autopsy series have found a 4-29% prevalence of cerebral infarction in patients with documented HIV/AIDS. Many of these strokes are due to non-HIV CNS coinfection, lymphoma, cardioembolic sources, or primary vasculitis. Approximately 5-6% are true HIV-associated vasculopathy with small vessel intimal thickening, mineralization, and perivascular inflammatory infiltrates.

HIV vasculopathy (HIV-V) and varicella-zoster virus (VZV) vasculitis are uncommon but increasingly important causes of stroke in the HIV/AIDS population.

HIV VASCULOPATHY. Striking nonatherosclerotic fusiform ectasias of the major intracranial arteries occur, usually in children with congenital HIV/AIDS **(14-6)**, **(14-7)**. HIV-V is generally associated with large hemispheric strokes.

VZV VASCULOPATHY. CNS varicella-zoster virus vasculopathy affects both large and small cerebral vessels. Large vessel disease is most common in immunocompetent individuals whereas small vessel disease usually develops in immunocompromised patients. Overt neurological disease often occurs months after zoster and sometimes presents without any history of zoster rash.

The diagnosis can be confirmed by finding anti-VZV antibody in CSF.

HIV/AIDS patients with VZV-V are generally younger than those with HIV-V. In contrast those associated with HIV-V, most strokes associated with VZV-V are small, deep-seated, subcortical infarcts. Large cortical hemispheric strokes are relatively rare.

HIV/AIDS Bone Marrow Changes

The calvaria and skull base, as well as part of the facial bones and upper cervical spine, are visible on sagittal T1-weighted brain MRs **(14-8)**. The cranium and mandible alone account for approximately 13% of active (red) marrow in adult humans. Add the cervical spine plus facial bones, and these structures together represent 15-20% of all bone marrow activity; therefore, carefully examining all the bones visible on brain MRs may provide important information regarding hematopoietic status.

Bone marrow abnormalities are common in HIV/AIDS patients and have been implicated in the brain injury underlying cognitive deterioration and dementia. Anemia before AIDS onset is strongly predictive of HIV-associated dementia (HAD). Escalation in monocyte trafficking from bone marrow into the brain in late-stage infection may represent a critical determinant of HAD neuropathogenesis.

PATHOLOGY. Pathologic processes alter the composition of bone marrow, causing a relative increase in cellular hematopoietic tissue and a corresponding replacement of adipose tissue. Extracellular hemosiderin, hypercellularity, and increased numbers of monocytes and macrophages all contribute significantly to marrow hypercellularity.

The most common skeletal abnormalities in HIV/AIDS patients are myelodysplasia (69% of biopsy specimens), evidence of reticuloendothelial iron blockade (65%), hypercellularity (53%), megaloblastic hematopoiesis (38%), lymphocytic aggregates (36%), plasmacytosis (25%), fibrosis (20%), and granulomas (13%). Most of the marrow abnormalities associated with HIV infection are related directly to the infection itself or its complications, not to therapeutic intervention.

IMAGING. Subtle changes in bone marrow may be difficult to detect on conventional MR images. Imaging findings that suggest marrow abnormalities are nonspecific. The prolonged T1 relaxation times alter signal intensity of hematopoietic bone marrow. Fatty T1 hyperintense "yellow" marrow is replaced with T1 hypointense tissue **(14-9)**. The calvaria and clivus appear mottled or "gray." The affected vertebral bodies appear hypointense relative to the intervertebral discs (the "bright disc" sign).

Hypercellular bone marrow in HIV/AIDS patients may demonstrate reduced mean diffusivity on quantitative imaging before any grossly visible changes become apparent.

Benign Lymphoepithelial Lesions

Salivary gland disease is an important manifestation of HIV infection. Most lesions represent either benign non-neoplastic lymphoepithelial cysts or reactive lymphoid hyperplasia.

Benign lymphoepithelial lesions of the salivary glands include a spectrum of disorders ranging from the lymphoepithelial sialadenitis (LESA) of Sjögren syndrome to lymphoepithelial cysts (LEC) to both HIV-related and -unrelated cystic lymphoid hyperplasia (CLH). LESA, LEC, and CLH share a common microscopic appearance characterized by epimyoepithelial islands and/or epithelium-lined cysts in a lymphoid stroma. However, they differ greatly regarding their etiology, clinical presentation, and management.

Benign lymphoepithelial lesions of HIV (BLL-HIV) are nonneoplastic cystic masses that enlarge salivary glands.

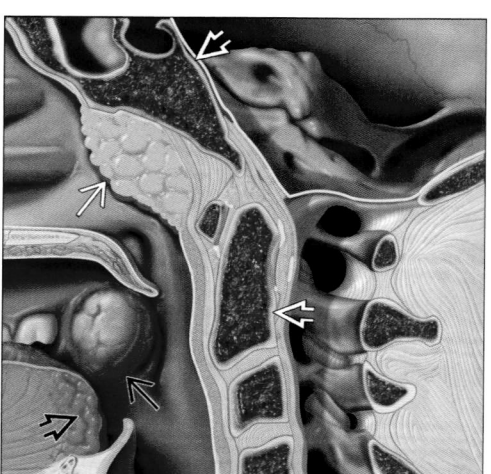

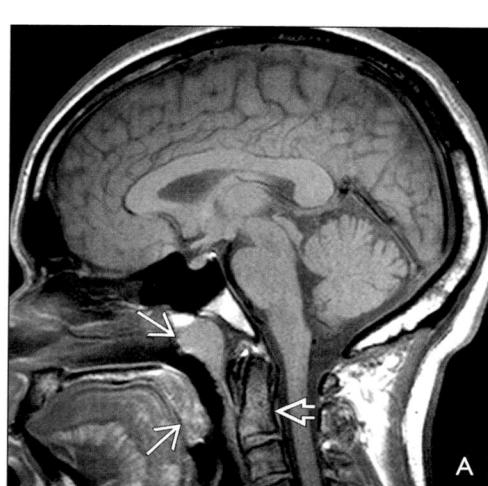

14-8. Graphic depicts other head and neck manifestations of HIV/AIDS. Note prominent lymphoid tissue (adenoids ➡, tonsils ➡, Waldeyer ring ⇒), reconversion of yellow to red (hematopoietic) marrow in the cervical spine, skull ➡. 14-9A. Sagittal T1WI in a 43-year-old man who has been HIV-positive for 20 years and treated with HAART shows unusually prominent lymphatic tissue ➡, "dark" vertebral bodies ➡ indicating reconversion of yellow to red marrow.

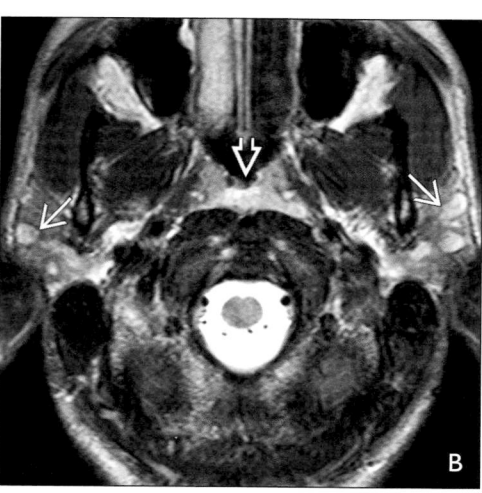

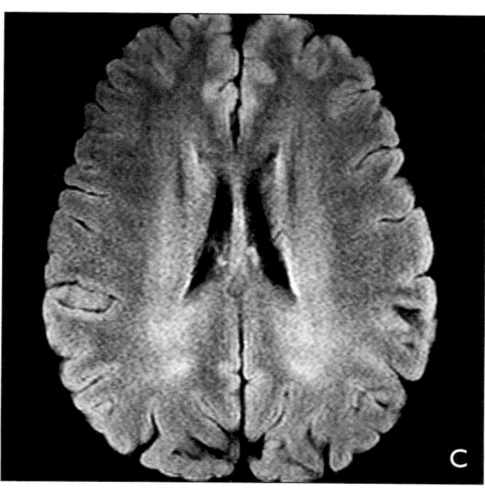

14-9B. Axial T2WI through the foramen magnum shows hyperintense lymphoepithelial cysts in both parotid glands ➡, prominent adenoids ➡. 14-9C. FLAIR scan in the same patient shows the "hazy" hyperintensity in the periventricular WM characteristic of HIVE. Little volume loss is present, and the patient exhibited only mild cognitive impairment.

Bilateral lesions are common. The parotid glands are most frequently affected **(14-10)**.

NECT scans show multiple bilateral well-circumscribed cysts within enlarged parotid glands. A thin enhancing rim is present on CECT scans **(14-11)**. The cysts are homogeneously hyperintense on T2WI and demonstrate rim enhancement on T1 C+ **(14-9)**, **(14-12)**.

Lymphoid Hyperplasia

Lymphoid hyperplasia is common in patients with HIV/AIDS. Immunohistochemistry, fluorescent in situ hybridization (FISH), and transmission electron microscopy have all identified HIV in lymph nodes, tonsils, and adenoidal tissue. Histologic evaluation of adenoids and tonsils excised from HIV/AIDS patients demonstrates a spectrum of changes including florid follicular hyperplasia, follicle lysis, attenuated mantle zone, and the presence of multinucleated giant cells.

Affected patients can be asymptomatic or present with a nasopharyngeal mass, nasal stuffiness or bleeding, hearing loss, or cervical lymphadenopathy.

Lymphoid hyperplasia of Waldeyer ring is the most common finding observed on brain MR **(14-10)**, **(14-11)**. Unusually prominent tonsils and adenoids in a patient over 25-30 years of age should raise suspicion of HIV infection.

The differential diagnosis of benign reactive lymphoid hyperplasia in HIV/AIDS patients is lymphoma.

Opportunistic Infections

With the advent of HAART, the prevalence of CNS opportunistic infections has decreased five- to ten-fold. Nevertheless, these infections and HIV coinfections such as tuberculosis continue to create substantial morbidity.

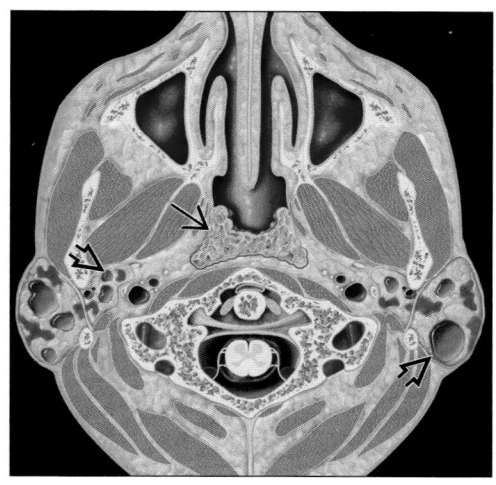
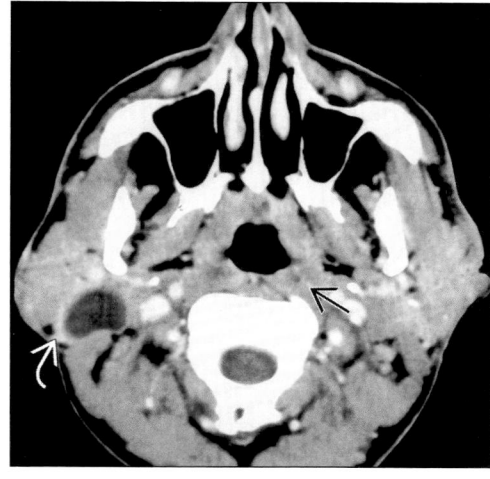

14-10. Axial graphic shows typical lymphoid and lymphoepithelial lesions of HIV/AIDS. Note the hyperplastic tonsils ➔, multiple cysts in the superficial and deep lobes of both parotid glands ➔. **14-11.** Axial CECT scan in a 33-year-old man with HIV/AIDS shows a large right parotid cyst with enhancing rim ➔ and enlarged Waldeyer ring ➔.

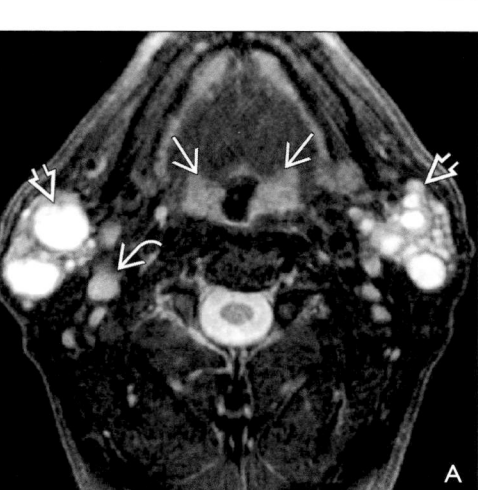
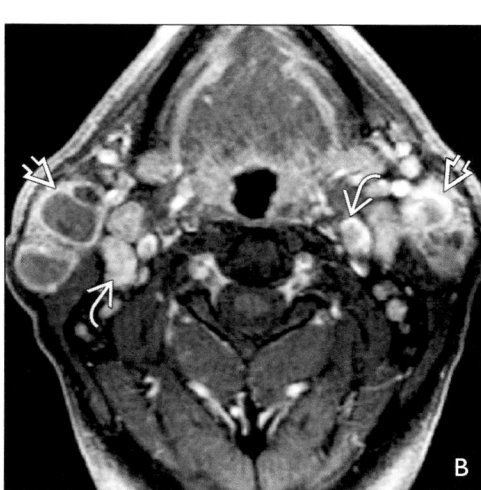

14-12A. Axial T2WI in a 31-year-old HIV-positive man shows hyperplastic Waldeyer ring ➔, prominent deep cervical lymph nodes ➔, and multiple variably sized cysts ➔ in both parotid glands. **14-12B.** Axial T1 C+ FS scan in the same patient shows rim-enhancing cysts in both parotid glands ➔, enlarged deep cervical lymph nodes ➔.

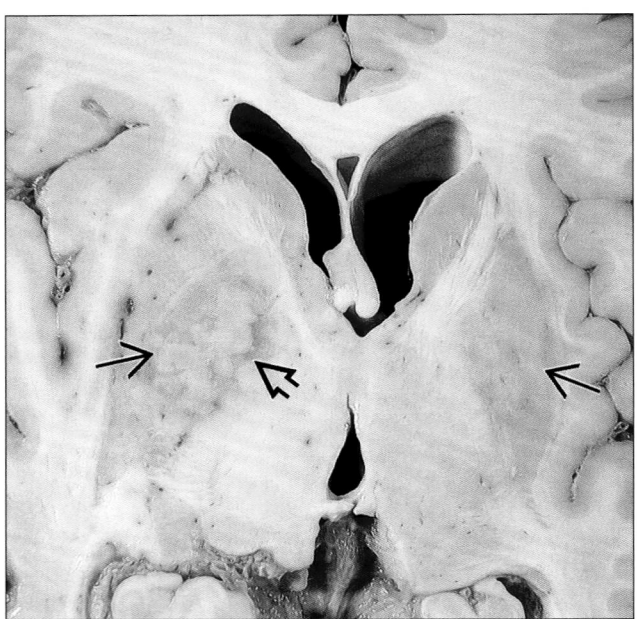

14-13. Axial gross pathology from an HIV-positive patient shows ill-defined toxoplasmosis abscesses in both basal ganglia ➔. *Note hemorrhage* ➢ *surrounding central necrosis in the right lesion. (Courtesy R. Hewlett, MD.)*

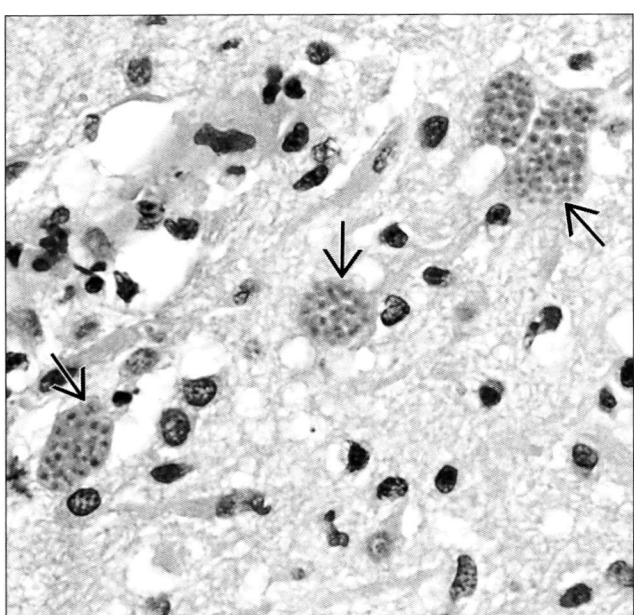

14-14. H&E photomicrograph of toxoplasmosis shows multiple encysted organisms ➔. *(Courtesy B. K. DeMasters, MD.)*

Toxoplasmosis

Toxoplasmosis is the most common opportunistic infection and overall cause of a mass lesion in patients with HIV/AIDS.

Terminology and Etiology

Toxoplasmosis (toxo) is caused by the ubiquitous intracellular parasite *Toxoplasma gondii*. Between 20-70% of the population is seropositive for *T. gondii*, so infection in HIV/AIDS patients generally represents reactivation of latent infection.

T. gondii is an obligate intracellular parasite. Although any mammal can be a carrier and act as an intermediate host, cats are the definitive host. Humans become infected when the organism is accidentally ingested. The parasites rapidly multiply as tachyzoites. When the tachyzoites invade the CNS, they become bradyzoites and form parenchymal cysts.

Pathology

LOCATION, SIZE, AND NUMBER. CNS toxo most commonly involves the basal ganglia, thalami, corticomedullary junctions, and cerebellum **(14-13)**. Multifocal lesions are more common than solitary ones; only 15-20% of toxo lesions are solitary masses. Most lesions are small, averaging two to three centimeters in diameter.

GROSS AND MICROSCOPIC FEATURES. The macroscopic appearance of CNS toxo in patients with HIV/AIDS is that of poorly circumscribed necrotizing abscesses with a hyperemic border and soft yellowish contents.

Microscopic features include coagulative necrosis, encysted toxo organisms, numerous free tachyzoites, and minimal host inflammatory response **(14-14)**.

Clinical Issues

DEMOGRAPHICS. Toxo prevalence varies widely. In countries in which HAART is widely available, its prevalence has diminished four-fold over the past decade, decreasing from 25% to 3-10%. The overall prevalence of toxo in resource-poor regions is much higher. In Africa, 35-50% of all HIV/AIDS patients develop CNS toxoplasmosis. Immunocompromised patients are most likely to develop toxo when their CD4 counts fall below 200.

PRESENTATION. Most HIV/AIDS patients with toxo present with focal neurologic findings superimposed on symptoms of global encephalopathy such as headache, confusion, and lethargy. Mild hemiparesis is the most common focal abnormality. Chorea is relatively rare.

NATURAL HISTORY AND PROGNOSIS. CNS toxo is fatal if left untreated, yet early institution of therapy can be curative. Treated patients usually improve significantly within two to four weeks. In resource-poor socioeconomic environments, median survival is only 28 months.

maging

CT FINDINGS. The most common finding on NECT scan is multiple ill-defined hypodense lesions in the basal ganglia or thalamus with moderate to marked peripheral edema.

Enhancement on CECT is closely correlated to CD4 count. In patients with counts under 50, enhancement is absent or faint. Enhancement becomes more pronounced as the CD4 count rises. Multiple punctate and ring-enhancing masses are the most common finding.

MR FINDINGS. T1WI shows a hypointense mass that occasionally demonstrates mild peripheral hyperintensity caused by coagulative necrosis or hemorrhage.

Alternating concentric zones of hyper- and hypointensity with marked perilesional edema are seen on T2WI **(14-15A)**. The central T2 hyperintensity corresponds histologically to necrotizing abscess. As a toxo abscess organizes, intensity diminishes and eventually the lesion becomes isointense relative to white matter. Perilesional hyperintensity represents edema with demyelination.

One or more nodular and ring-enhancing masses are typical on T1 C+ **(14-15B)**, **(14-15C)**, **(14-15D)**. A ring-shaped zone of peripheral enhancement with a small eccentric mural nodule represents the "eccentric target" sign. The enhancing nodule is a collection of concentrically thickened vessels while the rim enhancement is caused by an inflamed vascular zone that borders the necrotic abscess cavity.

Disseminated toxoplasmosis encephalitis, also called microglial nodule encephalitis, produces multifocal T2 hyperintensities in the basal ganglia and subcortical white matter. Enhancement may be absent or minimal despite fulminant disease.

MRS findings are nonspecific and often show a lipid-lactate peak. Toxo shows reduced rCBV on SPECT and pMR scans **(14-16)**.

Differential Diagnosis

The major differential diagnosis is **primary CNS lymphoma** (PCNSL). AIDS-related CNS toxo has positive findings on serology in 80% of cases, and CSF PCR

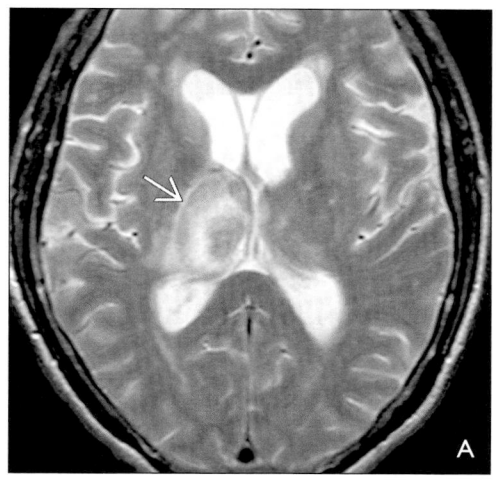

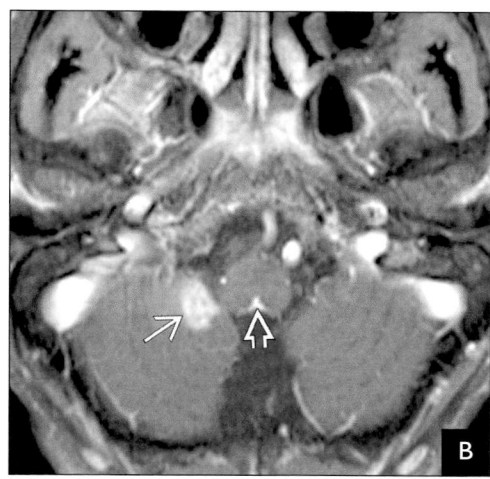

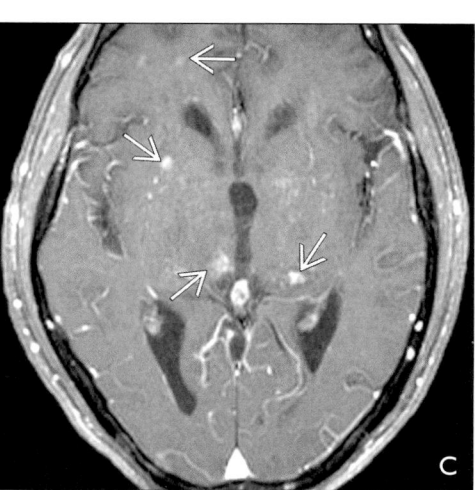

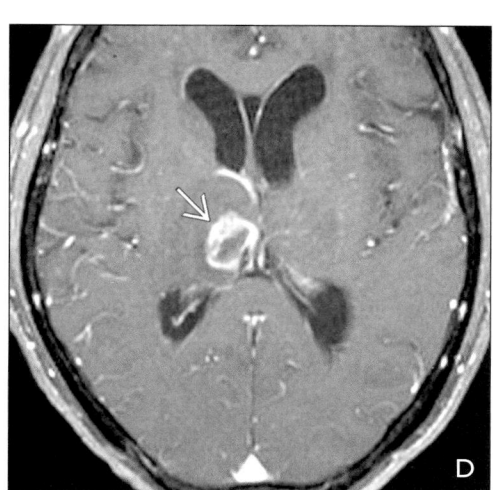

14-15A. Axial T2WI in a 60-year-old HIV-positive man with markedly elevated toxo titers was obtained when he stopped taking HAART and became comatose. Generalized volume loss is present. Note focal lesion in the right thalamus ➡ has three alternating concentric zones: A central hypointense zone, a middle hyperintense ring, and an outer isointense rim. 14-15B. Axial T1 C+ MR in the same patient shows focal enhancing lesions in the right cerebellum ➡ and dorsal medulla ➡.

14-15C. Axial T1 C+ FS through the third ventricle shows multiple punctate enhancing lesions ➡. 14-15D. Axial T1 C+ FS shows that the hyperintense layer seen on the T2WI enhances ➡ whereas the center and periphery of the lesion remain unenhanced. Multifocal toxoplasmosis.

14-16A. T2WI in an HIV-positive patient with toxoplasmosis shows multiple hyperintense lesions in both basal ganglia ➡, as well as a larger confluent lesion ⮞ around the occipital horn of the right lateral ventricle. 14-16B. FLAIR scan in the same patient shows multiple small, mostly hyperintense WM lesions ➡. A large "tumefactive" lesion ⮞ with a hypointense rim, hyperintense center, and striking peripheral edema is present.

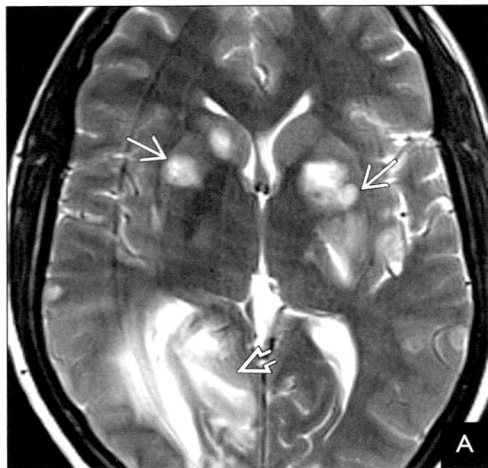
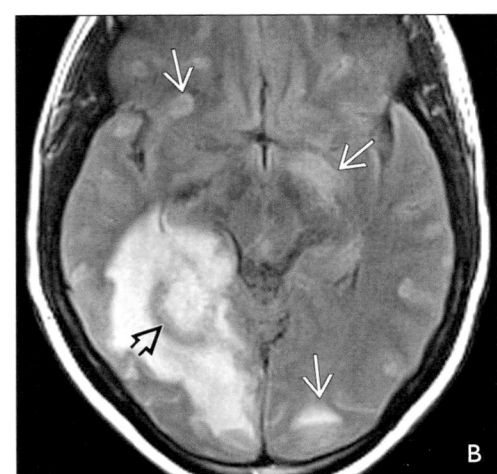

14-16C. More cephalad FLAIR scan in the same patient shows large, heterogeneously hyperintense lesions but numerous smaller foci scattered throughout the brain in the cortex and subcortical WM ➡. 14-16D. T1 C+ FS scan shows that the "tumefactive" lesion enhances strongly but heterogeneously ⮞. Several other enhancing lesions are present ➡.

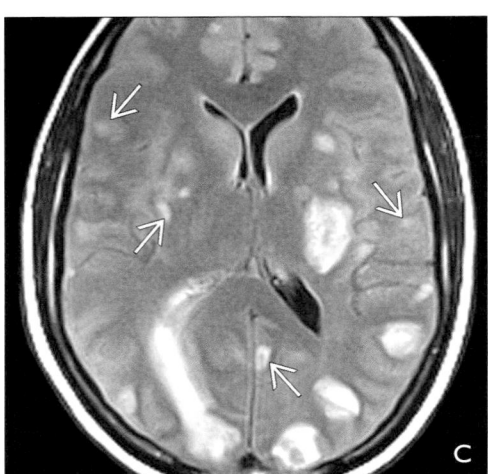
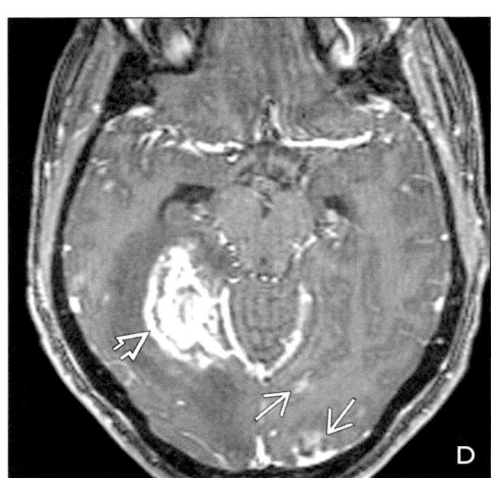

14-16E. More cephalad T1 C+ FS scan in the same patient demonstrates additional enhancing lesions ➡ including a "target" lesion in the left basal ganglia ⮞. 14-16F. pMR scan in the same patient shows that the "tumefactive" lesion has markedly reduced rCBV ➡, consistent with toxoplasmosis rather than lymphoma.

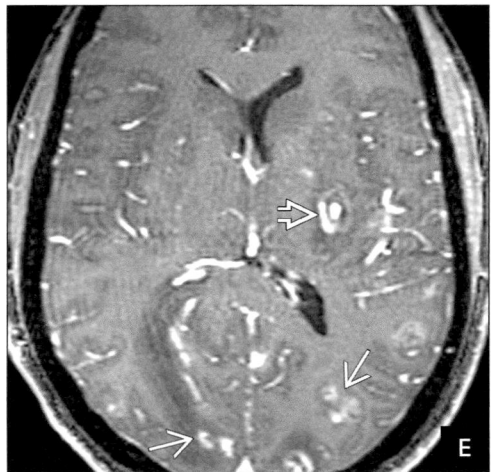
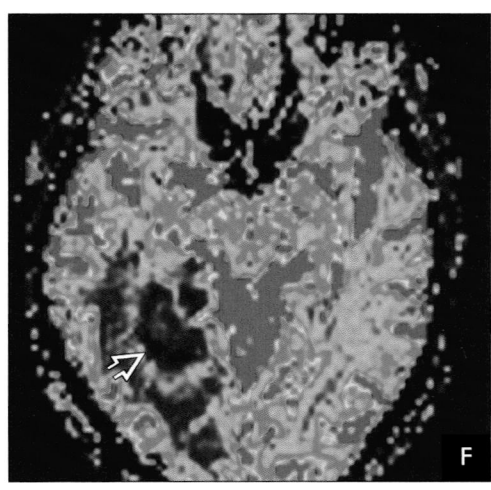

is definitive. Solitary lesions are uncommon. Approximately 70% of isolated CNS masses in HIV/AIDS patients are PCNSL.

Cryptococcosis

Fungal infections can be life-threatening in immunocompromised patients, especially those with HIV/AIDS. While many different fungi can cause CNS infection, the most common fungi to affect patients with HIV/AIDS are *Candida albicans*, *Aspergillus* species, and *Cryptococcus neoformans* (crypto). Cryptococcosis in immunocompetent patients was briefly discussed in Chapter 13. Here we focus on its appearance in immunocompromised patients.

Etiology and Epidemiology

Cryptococcus neoformans is excreted in mammal and bird feces and is found in soil and dust. Crypto is a ubiquitous fungus with worldwide distribution. The lungs are usually the primary infection site. CNS infection occurs when organisms circulating in the blood are deposited in the subarachnoid cisterns and perivascular spaces.

Crypto is the third most common CNS infectious agent in HIV/AIDS patients, after HIV and *T. gondii*. Prior to HAART, crypto CNS infections occurred in 10% of HIV patients, but it is now relatively rare in developed countries. Crypto usually occurs when CD4 counts drop below 50-100 cells/μL.

Pathology

CNS cryptococcal infection takes three main forms: Meningitis, gelatinous pseudocysts (14-17), and focal mass lesions called cryptococcomas. Cryptococcomas and meningitis are the most common forms in immunocompetent patients whereas meningitis and gelatinous pseudocysts are the most common forms in HIV/AIDS patients.

In crypto meningitis or meningoencephalitis, the meninges become thickened and cloudy. Gelatinous mucoid-like cryptococcal capsular polysaccharides and budding yeast accumulate within dilated perivascular spaces (14-18). Multiple gelatinous pseudocysts occur in the basal ganglia, midbrain, dentate nuclei, and subcortical white matter (14-19).

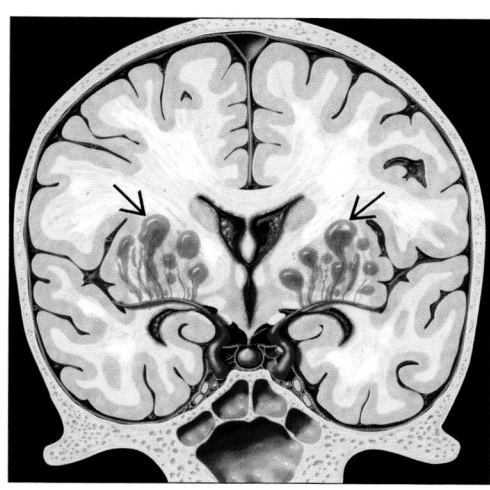

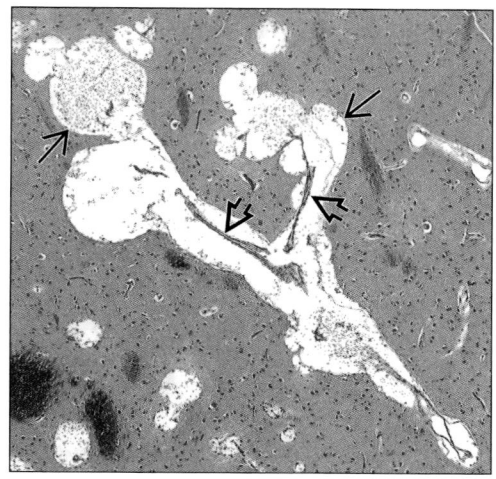

14-17. Coronal graphic shows multiple dilated perivascular spaces ➡ filled with gelatinous mucoid-appearing material characteristic of cryptococcal infection in HIV/AIDS patients.
14-18. Photomicrograph shows a branching vessel cut in longitudinal section ➡ surrounded by enlarged perivascular spaces stuffed full of cryptococcal gelatinous pseudocysts ➡. (Courtesy B. K. DeMasters, MD.)

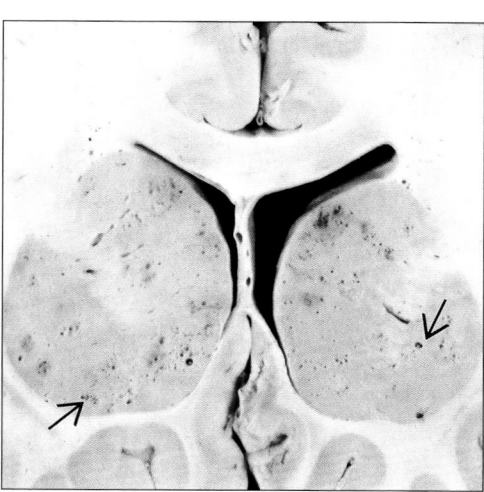

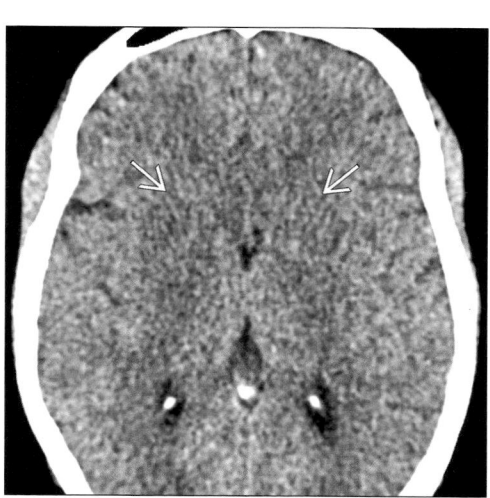

14-19. Coronal view shows multiple tiny cryptococcal cysts in the perivascular spaces of the basal ganglia ➡. (Courtesy B. K. DeMasters, MD.) 14-20. Axial NECT scan in an HIV-positive patient shows hypodense basal ganglia ➡. (Courtesy N. Omar, MD.)

Clinical Issues

Crypto in patients with HIV/AIDS typically presents as meningitis or meningoencephalitis. Common symptoms are headache, seizure, and blurred vision. Focal neurologic deficits are uncommon.

Imaging

NECT scans often show hypodensity in the basal ganglia **(14-20)**. Enhancement varies with immune status. CECT scans in immunocompromised patients typically show no enhancement.

Cryptococcal gelatinous pseudocysts are hypointense to brain on T1WI and very hyperintense on T2WI **(14-21)**. The lesions generally follow CSF signal intensity and suppress on FLAIR **(14-22)**. Perilesional edema is generally absent. Lack of enhancement on T1 C+ is typical although mild pial enhancement is sometimes observed.

Differential Diagnosis

Enlarged perivascular spaces (PVSs) are a common normal finding in virtually all patients and are seen at all ages. They can occur in clusters and typically follow CSF signal intensity. Enlarged PVSs do not enhance. In HIV/AIDS patients with CD4 counts under 20, symmetrically enlarged PVSs should be considered cryptococcal infection and treated as such.

Toxoplasmosis usually has multifocal ring- or "target"-like enhancing lesions with significant surrounding edema. **Tuberculosis** usually demonstrates strong enhancement in the basal meninges. Tuberculomas are generally hypointense on T2WI. **Primary CNS lymphoma** in HIV/AIDS patients often shows hemorrhage, necrosis, and ring enhancement. Solitary lesions are more common than multifocal involvement.

Progressive Multifocal Leukoencephalopathy

Terminology

Progressive multifocal leukoencephalopathy (PML) is an opportunistic infection caused by the JC virus (JCV), a member of the Papovaviridae family. The virus was

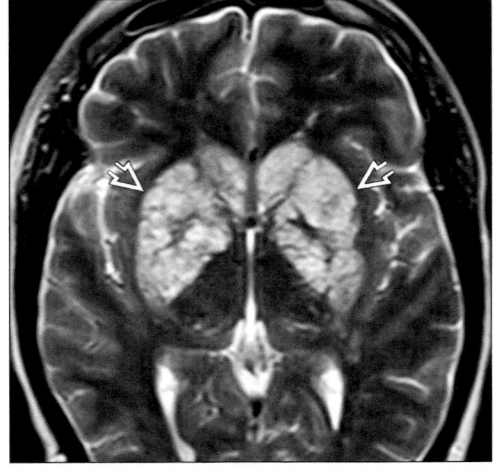

14-21. T2WI in the same patient as Figure 14-20 demonstrates that the lentiform nuclei and the heads of both caudate nuclei are grossly expanded by innumerable hyperintense cysts ⇨ characteristic of cryptococcal gelatinous pseudocysts. (Courtesy N. Omar, MD.)
14-22A. Axial T2WI in a 55-year-old man with HIV/AIDS shows enlarged perivascular spaces in both cerebral peduncles ⇨ and in the left anterior perforated substance ⇨.

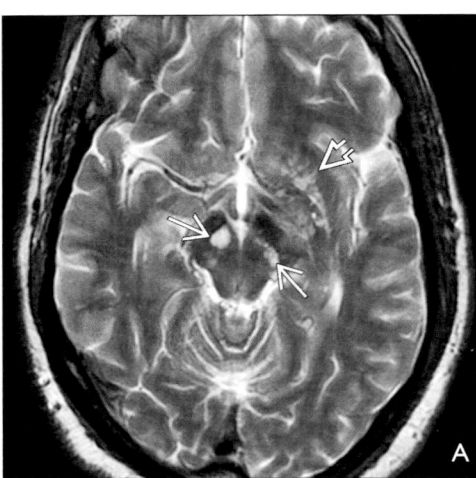

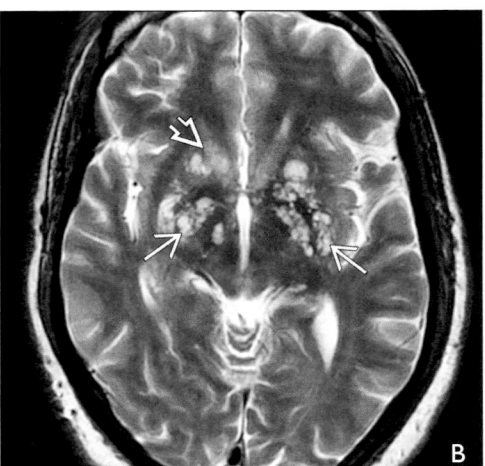

14-22B. Axial T2WI in the same patient shows multiple gelatinous pseudocysts in both lenticular nuclei ⇨ as well as the head of the right caudate nucleus ⇨. 14-22C. FLAIR scan in the same patient shows that the pseudocysts suppress. Note "hazy" hyperintensity in the cerebral white matter ⇨ consistent with HIVE. (Courtesy T. Markel, MD.)

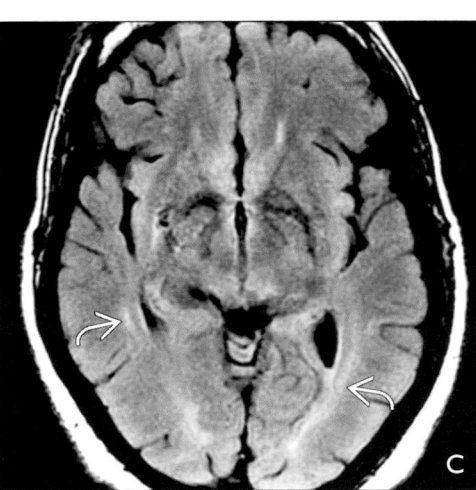

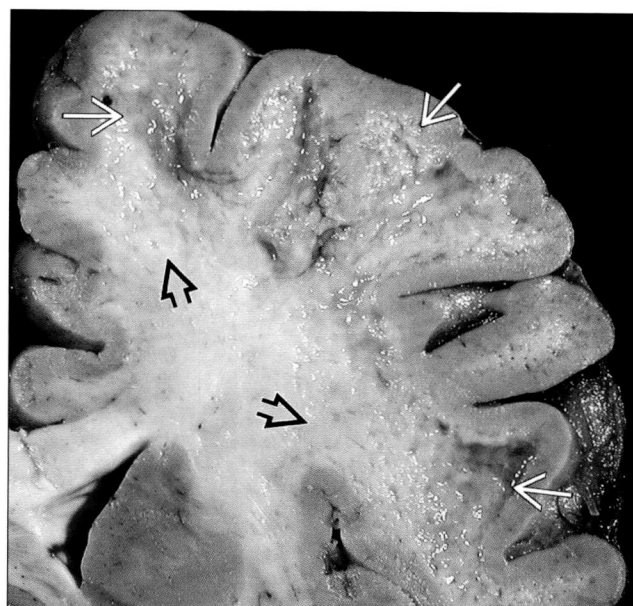

14-23. Close-up coronal view of autopsied brain from a patient with severe advanced PML shows coalescent, spongy-appearing, demyelinated foci along the cortical gray-white matter junction ➘ extending into the subcortical and deep WM ⊃.

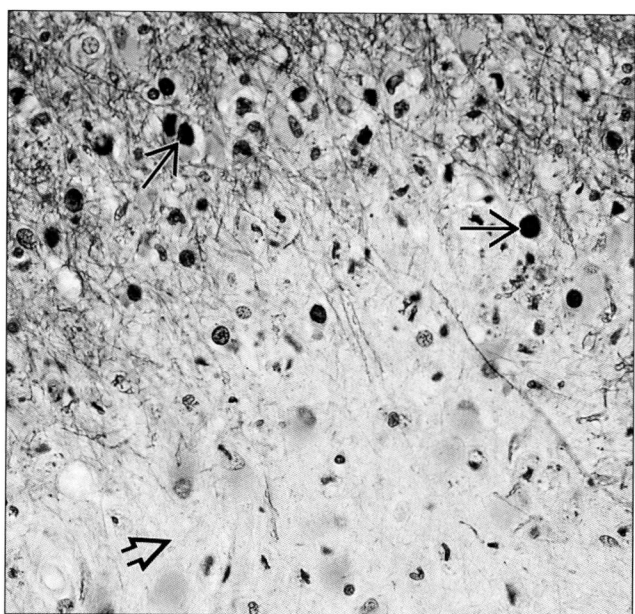

14-24. Dark infected oligodendrocytes ➔ are concentrated at the edge of the pink-appearing demyelinated foci ⊃ in this classic microscopic image of PML. (Both cases courtesy B. K. DeMasters, MD.)

named "JC" after it was first isolated from autopsied brain tissue from a patient named John Cunningham.

Over the past two decades, the spectrum of JCV CNS infection has expanded beyond "classic" PML. Some investigators have suggested distinguishing between classic PML (cPML) and inflammatory PML (iPML). Other neurotropic forms of JCV infection include JCV encephalopathy (JCE), JC meningitis (JCM), and JCV infection of the cerebellar granular layer (JCV granule cell neuronopathy).

Etiology

JCV is a ubiquitous virus that circulates widely in the environment, primarily in sewage. More than 85% of the adult population worldwide has antibodies against JCV. Asymptomatic infection is probably acquired in childhood or adolescence and remains latent until the virus is reactivated.

In some immunocompromised patients, the reactivated JCV becomes neurotropic and infects oligodendrocytes, causing a progressive demyelinating encephalopathy, i.e., PML.

Three phases in the development of PML have been identified. The first phase is the primary but clinically inapparent infection. In the second phase, the virus persists as a latent peripheral infection, primarily in the kidneys, bone marrow, and lymphoid tissue. The third phase is that of reactivation and dissemination with hematogenous spread to the CNS.

HIV-induced immunodeficiency is now the most common predisposing factor for symptomatic JCV infection and is responsible for 80% of all cases. PML also occurs in the setting of collagen vascular disease, immunosuppression for solid organ or bone marrow transplantation, chemotherapy with rituximab for hematologic malignancies, and treatment with the immunosuppressive agent natalizumab for multiple sclerosis or Crohn disease.

The expanding spectrum of PML now also includes patients *without* severe depletion of cellular immunity. This generally occurs in conditions with less overt immunodeficiency such as idiopathic CD4 lymphocytopenia, systemic lupus erythematosus, cirrhosis, psoriasis, and even pregnancy. Cases of PML in the absence of *any* documented immunodeficiency have also been reported.

Pathology

LOCATION. Activated JC virus almost exclusively affects oligodendrocytes, causing multifocal asymmetric demyelination with a predilection for the frontal and parietooccipital WM.

SIZE AND NUMBER. Initial PML lesions are small, generally measuring a few millimeters in diameter. As the disease progresses, small foci coalesce into confluent lesions that can occupy large volumes of white matter.

GROSS PATHOLOGY. Early lesions appear as small yellow-tan round to ovoid foci at the gray-white matter junction. The cortex remains normal. With lesion coalescence, large spongy-appearing depressions in the cere-

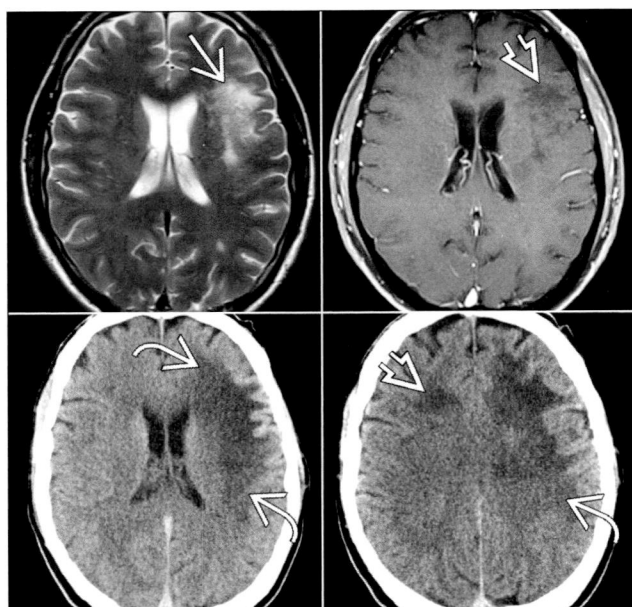

14-25. cPML in a 32-year-old HIV-positive man. Confluent left frontal T2 hyperintensity ➡ *spares cortex, does not enhance* ⟱. *NECT 6 weeks later shows the left frontal lesion has increased in size* ⟱, *and a new right frontal hypodensity is present* ⟱.

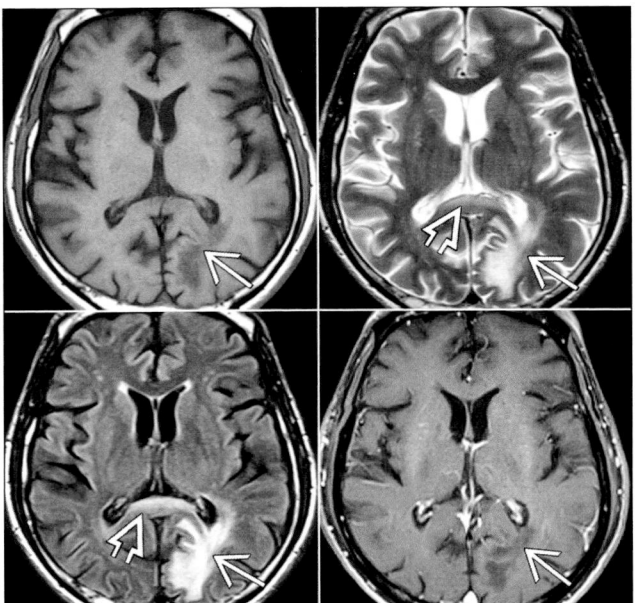

14-26. MR in a clinically deteriorating 46-year-old HIV-positive patient with a CD4 count < 10 shows a confluent nonenhancing left occipital lesion ➡ *that crosses the corpus callosum* ⟱. *CSF was PCR-positive for JCV.*

bral and cerebellar white matter appear **(14-23)**. Unlike ischemic infarcts, PML lesions are rarely completely cavitated.

MICROSCOPIC FEATURES. Demyelination ranges from myelin pallor to severe loss. Pale-staining demyelinating foci are bordered by large infected oligodendrocytes with violaceous nuclear inclusions **(14-24)**. With the exception of cerebellar granular neurons, neuronal infection is rare.

Clinical Issues

EPIDEMIOLOGY. In the pre-HAART era, PML affected between 3-7% of HIV-positive patients and caused 18% of all CNS-related AIDS deaths. The increasingly widespread use of HAART has significantly reduced the prevalence of PML in patients with HIV/AIDS. The incidence has dropped from 0.7 to 0.07 per 100 person-years in the decade since the institution of HAART.

The incidence of natalizumab-associated PML is estimated at 1:1,000. Risk increases with duration of exposure.

PRESENTATION AND NATURAL HISTORY. Until recently, PML was the only known manifestation of CNS JCV infection. Newly recognized presentations include PML-associated immune reconstitution inflammatory syndrome (IRIS, see below). Rare presentations include JCE, JCM, and an oligodendrocyte-sparing cerebellar syndrome associated with isolated infection of cerebellar granule cell neurons ("JCV granule cell neuronopathy").

The most common symptoms of PML are altered mental status, headache, lethargy, motor deficits, aphasia, and gait difficulties. In approximately 25% of patients, PML is the initial manifestation of AIDS and can appear early in the disease course while CD4 counts are above 200 cells/μL.

PML in untreated HIV/AIDS patients is often fatal with death in 6-8 months. HAART may stabilize the disease and improve overall survival, but PML is still the second most common cause of all AIDS-related deaths, second only to lymphoma.

PML in natalizumab-treated MS carries a high morbidity and mortality rate. Drug withdrawal and plasma exchange therapy have been used with some success to increase survival in these patients.

The diagnosis of PML is usually suggested by imaging findings in HIV/AIDS patients and confirmed by CSF that is PCR-positive for JCV.

Imaging

GENERAL FEATURES. Imaging plays a key role in the diagnosis and follow-up of JCV infections. cPML can appear as solitary or multifocal widespread lesions. Any area of the brain can be affected, although the supratentorial lobar white matter is the most commonly affected site. The posterior fossa white matter—especially the middle cerebellar peduncles—is the second most common location. In occasional cases, a solitary lesion in the subcortical U-fibers is present.

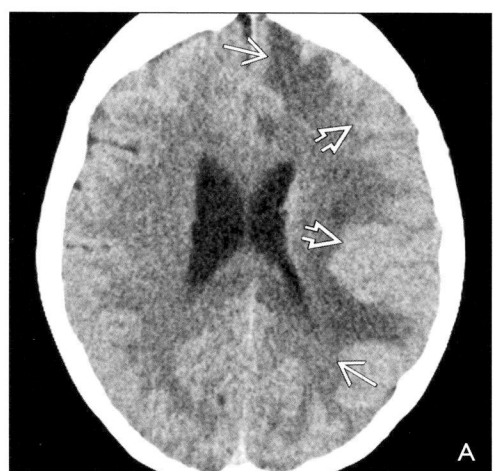

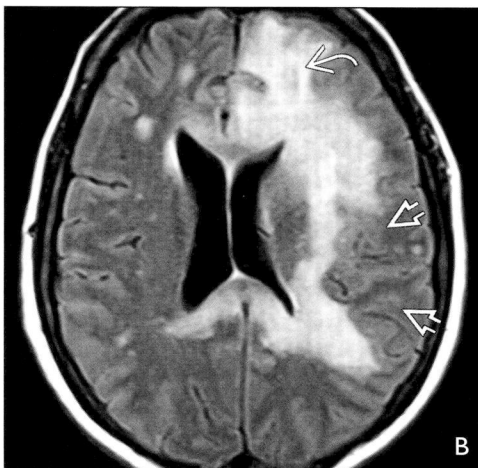

14-27A. *A 54-year-old woman on chemotherapy for AML developed headaches and visual problems. Axial NECT scan shows an extensive hypodense lesion that occupies most of the left hemisphere white matter* ➡. *Note cortical swelling* ⬈, *mass effect on the left lateral ventricle.* *14-27B.* *FLAIR shows confluent white matter hyperintensity crossing the corpus callosum as well as sulcal obliteration and cortical hyperintensity* ⬈. *Note focal ring-like lesion* ➡ *in the left frontal lobe.*

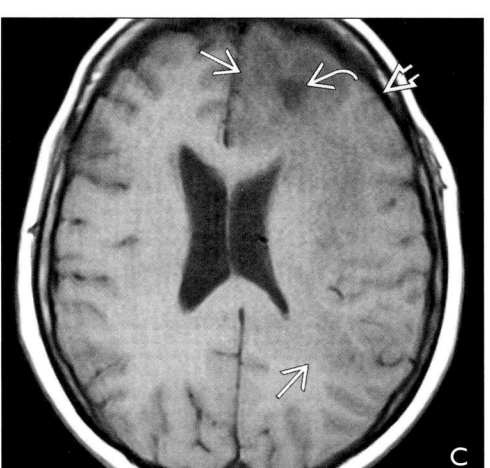

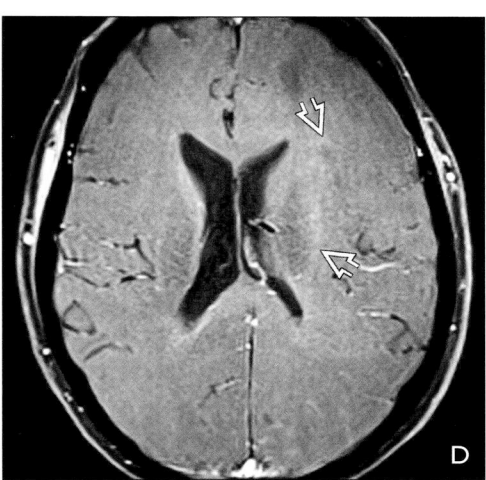

14-27C. *Axial T1WI shows ill-defined white matter hypointensity* ➡ *with effacement of the left superficial sulci* ⬈ *and a focal hypointense left frontal mass* ⬈. *14-27D.* *T1 C+ FS shows faint but definite enhancement around the advancing margins of several lesions* ⬈.

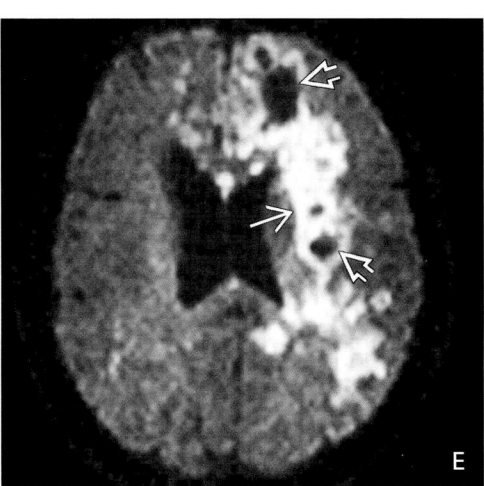

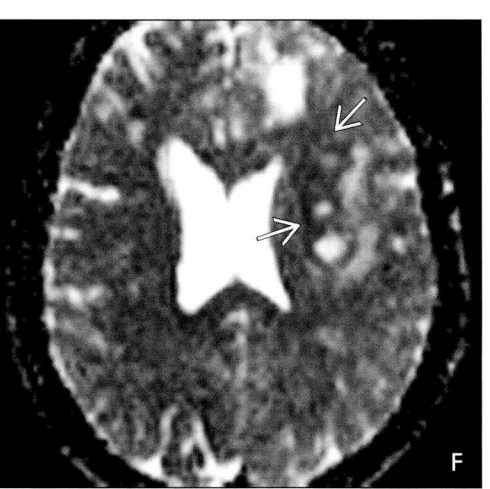

14-27E. *DWI shows restricted diffusion in many new white matter lesions* ➡ *whereas the centers of several older lesions* ⬈—*including the ring-like area in the left frontal lobe—do not restrict.* *14-27F.* *ADC shows restriction in the active margins of inflammation* ➡. *The patient's CSF PCR was positive for JC virus. With the mass effect and subtle enhancement, this was thought to represent the inflammatory PML (iPML) variant.*

Extent varies from small scattered subcortical foci to large bilateral but asymmetric confluent WM lesions. In the early acute stage of infection, some mass effect with focal gyral expansion can be present. At later stages, encephaloclastic changes with atrophy and volume loss predominate.

CT Findings. More than 90% of cPML cases show hypodense areas in the subcortical and deep periventricular WM on NECT **(14-25)**; 70% are multifocal. PML lesions generally do not enhance on CECT.

MR Findings.

Classic PML (cPML). Multifocal, bilateral but asymmetric, irregularly shaped hypointensities on T1WI are typical. The lesions are heterogeneously hyperintense on T2WI **(14-26)** and frequently extend into the subcortical U-fibers all the way to the undersurface of the cortex, which remains intact even in advanced disease **(14-27)**. Smaller, almost microcyst-like, very hyperintense foci within and around the slightly less hyperintense confluent lesions represent the characteristic spongy lesions seen in more advanced PML.

PML generally does not enhance on T1 C+ scans although faint peripheral rim-like enhancement occurs in 5% of all cases **(14-28)**. The exception is hyperacute PML in the setting of IRIS (see below) and in MS patients on natalizumab. In these cases, striking foci with irregular rim enhancement are frequently—but not invariably—present. Corticosteroids significantly decrease the prevalence and intensity of enhancement.

Appearance on DWI varies according to disease stage. In newly active lesions, DWI restricts strongly. Slightly older lesions show a central core with low signal intensity and high mean diffusivity (MD) surrounded by a rim of higher signal intensity and lower MD. Chronic "burned out" lesions show increased diffusion due to disorganized cellular architecture **(14-28)**.

DTI shows reduced fractional anisotropy consistent with disorganized white matter structure. As cPML lesions are comparatively avascular, pMR demonstrates reduced rCBV compared to unaffected white matter.

Findings on MRS are nonspecific, with decreased NAA reflecting neuronal loss. Increased choline, consistent

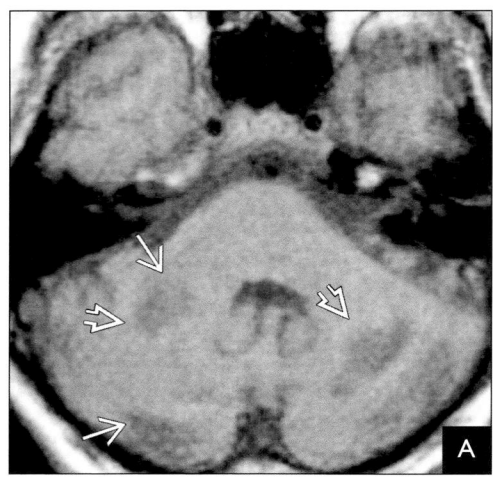

14-28A. *Axial T1WI MR in a 42-year-old HIV-positive woman with cerebellar cPML and gait difficulties shows several hypointense lesions in the cerebellum* ➡. *Note faint hyperintensity along the margins of the more anterior cerebellar lesions* ➡. ***14-28B.*** *Axial T2WI in the same patient shows the characteristic involvement of both middle cerebellar peduncles* ➡.

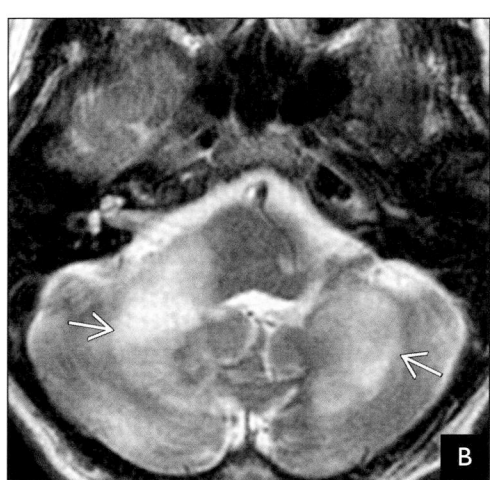

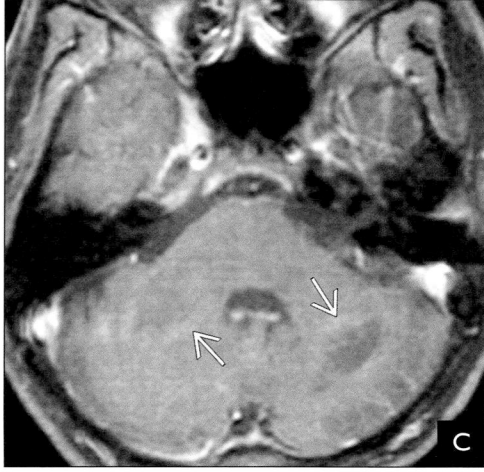

14-28C. *Axial T1 C+ FS scan shows very faint rim enhancement around the lesions* ➡. ***14-28D.*** *DWI in the same patient shows lesions in 3 different stages. The right posterior cerebellar lesion* ➡ *shows no restriction, the right middle cerebellar peduncle lesion* ➡ *restricts strongly and uniformly, and the left cerebellar lesion shows restriction around the lesion's rim* ➡.

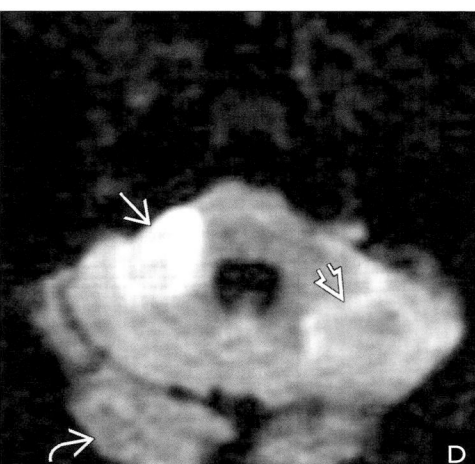

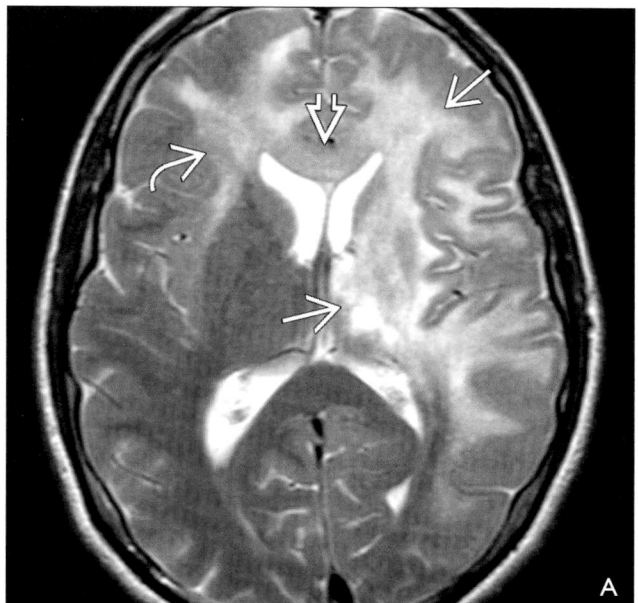

14-29A. A 27 yo HIV(+) man developed acute confusion, right-sided weakness. Axial T2WI shows confluent heterogeneous hyperintensity in left cerebral WM, basal ganglia ➡ that crosses the corpus callosum ➡ to involve the right frontal lobe ➡.

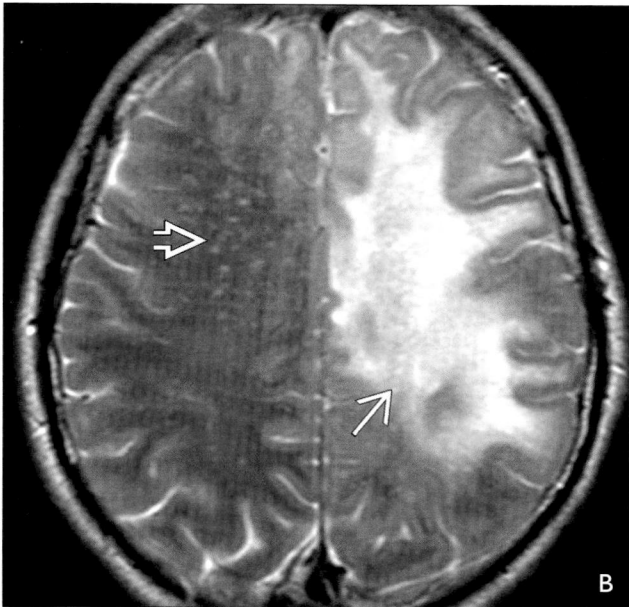

14-29B. More superior image shows the inhomogeneously hyperintense nature of the lesion ➡. Tiny hyperintense microcysts are present in the right frontal white matter ➡. Acute inflammatory PML.

with myelin destruction, and a lipid-lactate peak from necrosis are often present. Myoinositol is variable but may be elevated, consistent with inflammatory change.

Inflammatory PML (iPML). Imaging findings in iPML are identical to those of cPML except that the lesions demonstrate peripheral enhancement and/or mass effect **(14-29)**. Acute iPML may have relatively increased vascularity and rCBV caused by the inflammatory angiogenic effect. In some patients, lesions may demonstrate features of iPML early and then evolve to cPML later in the disease course.

Miscellaneous JCV infections. JCV meningitis has no distinguishing features from other meningitides, demonstrating nonspecific sulcal-cisternal hyperintensity on FLAIR and enhancement on T1 C+ FS scans.

JCE initially affects the hemispheric gray matter, then extends into the subcortical white matter. JCV infection of the cerebellar granular layer is seen as cerebellar atrophy with T2 hyperintensity in the affected folia.

Differential Diagnosis

The major differential diagnosis of cPML is **HIV encephalitis**. HIVE demonstrates more symmetric WM disease while sparing the subcortical U-fibers. **Immune reconstitution inflammatory syndrome (IRIS)** is usually more acute and demonstrates strong but irregular ring-like enhancement.

Other opportunistic infections in immunocompromised patients such as toxoplasmosis and CMV should be considered. Toxoplasmosis is more mass-like while CMV typically causes ependymitis/ventriculitis, retinitis, and polyradiculopathy.

PROGRESSIVE MULTIFOCAL LEUKOENCEPHALOPATHY (PML)

Etiology
- Caused by JC virus
  - Ubiquitous; > 85% of adults have JCV antibodies
  - Acquired in childhood, latent until reactivated
- Most common predisposing condition = HIV (80%)
- Less common = collagen vascular, immunosuppression, MS treated with natalizumab (20%)
- Rare = systemic lupus erythematosus, pregnancy

Pathology
- Activated virus almost exclusively affects oligodendrocytes
- Multifocal demyelination

Clinical Issues
- Epidemiology
  - PML in pre-HAART = 3-7% of HIV(+) patients
  - Prevalence ↓↓
- Major CNS JCV syndrome = classic PML
- Others = inflammatory PML (iPML), JC encephalitis/meningitis, cerebellar granule layer

Imaging
- Multifocal WM lesions
  - Bilateral but asymmetric
  - Involve subcortical U-fibers
  - Spare cortex
- Usually no mass, no enhancement (unless iPML)

Differential Diagnosis
- HIVE (doesn't involve U-fibers)
- IRIS (PML-IRIS most common)
- Other opportunistic infections (e.g., CMV)

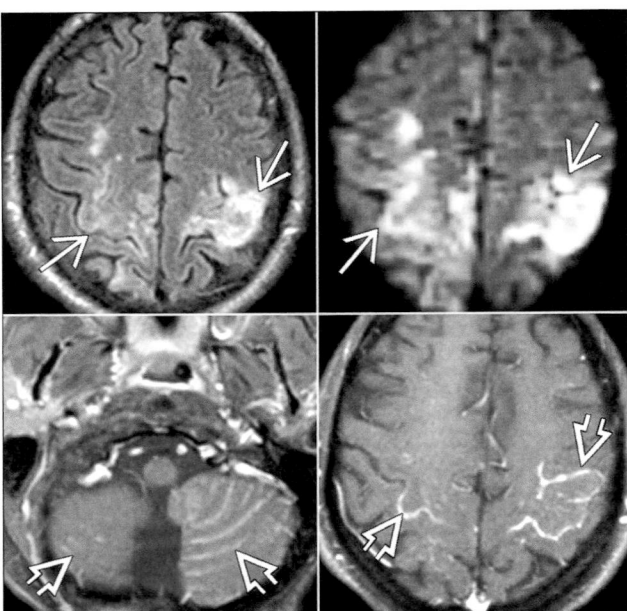

14-30. *CMV meningoencephalitis in a 32-year-old HIV-positive man. FLAIR shows hyperintensity in both parietal lobes, corresponding restriction on DWI* ➡. *T1 C+ scans show enhancement in the posterior fossa, convexity sulci* ➡.

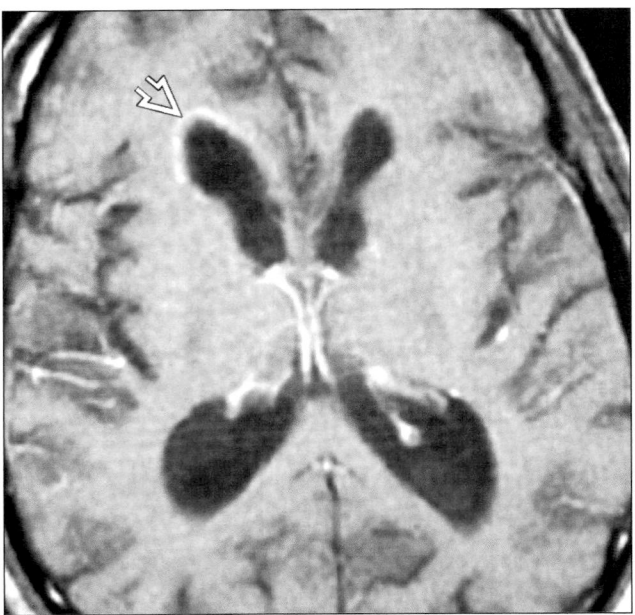

14-31. *T1 C+ scan in a patient with HIV encephalitis shows generalized volume loss. Note striking ependymal enhancement* ➡, *atypical for HIV encephalitis. CMV ventriculitis.*

Other Opportunistic Infections

A number of other infectious/inflammatory processes can cause or exacerbate preexisting CNS disease in patients with HIV/AIDS. These include Cytomegalovirus, sexually transmitted diseases (especially neurosyphilis), tuberculosis, fungal infections, malaria, and bacterial abscesses. In this section we focus on acquired Cytomegalovirus infection (congenital CMV was discussed in Chapter 12), the "deadly intersection" between HIV/AIDS and TB coinfection, and the "triple collision" when HIV, TB, and malaria all overlap.

Cytomegalovirus

Cytomegalovirus (CMV) is a member of the herpesvirus family. While it is a ubiquitous virus, CMV typically remains latent until reactivated. Several risk factors predispose patients to the development of overt CMV CNS disease: T-cell depletion syndromes, anti-thymocyte globulin, allogenic stem cell transplants, and HIV/AIDS. All cause severe, protracted T-cell immunodeficiency.

CNS CMV is a late-onset disease in immunocompromised patients. With increasing use of HAART, less than 2% of HIV/AIDS patients develop overt symptoms of CMV infection. Patients with CD4 counts under 50 cells/μL are most at risk.

Mortality in CNS CMV is high despite therapy with a combination of antiviral drugs. Ganciclovir-resistant CMV has developed, making prophylactic therapy difficult in high-risk patients.

In contrast to congenital CMV in which the virus causes parenchymal calcifications, acquired CMV most commonly manifests as meningoencephalitis and ventriculitis/ependymitis. While the imaging findings of meningoencephalitis resemble those of other infections **(14-30)**, enhancement along the ventricular ependyma in an immunocompromised patient is highly suggestive of CMV **(14-31)**.

Retinitis and myelitis with radiculitis are the two most frequent extracranial presentations.

Tuberculosis

TB is one of the most devastating coinfections in immunocompromised patients and is the main cause of morbidity and mortality in HIV-infected patients worldwide. The emergence of multidrug-resistant and extensively drug-resistant TB (MDR TB and XDR TB) has occurred almost entirely in patients coinfected with HIV.

More than one-third of all HIV/AIDS patients worldwide are coinfected with TB, and this deadly combination is disproportionately prevalent in highly endemic, resource-limited regions such as sub-Saharan Africa.

HIV is the most powerful known risk factor for reactivation of latent TB to active disease. HIV patients who are coinfected with TB have a 100 times greater risk of developing active TB compared to non-HIV patients. Conversely, the host immune response to TB enhances HIV replication and accelerates disease progression.

In turn, TB coinfection exacerbates the severity and accelerates the progress of HIV. In such patients, AIDS can behave as an acute fulminating illness with meningitis, bacterial abscesses, sepsis, coma, and death **(14-32)**. Mortality approaches 100%, and median survival is measured in days to a few weeks.

TB is treated *first* in HIV-related infection both to preserve the effectiveness of HAART and to prevent the development of TB-IRIS (see below).

The typical imaging findings in HIV-associated CNS TB may differ slightly from those in immunocompetent patients, looking like TB "gone wild" with multiple parenchymal granulomas and pseudoabscesses **(14-33)**.

Immunocompromised patients with CD4 counts under 200 cells/µL mount a significantly attenuated immunological response. While meningitis is the most common manifestation of HIV-associated CNS TB, enhancement of meningeal inflammation, tuberculomas, and pseudoabscesses is often mild or absent even though greater numbers of acid-fast bacilli are present.

Malaria

Seroprevalence of HIV-1 is high in patients with severe malaria. HIV coinfected patients generally have a higher parasite burden, more complications, and a significantly higher case mortality rate. In-hospital parasitemia, renal impairment, and clinical deterioration are common in these coinfected patients, so early identification of both infections is important for management.

HIV, TB, and malaria are three pandemics that overlap in resource-poor tropical countries. The least deadly condition is HIV infection without the other two comorbid disorders. The most deadly combinations are HIV-TB and HIV-TB-malaria.

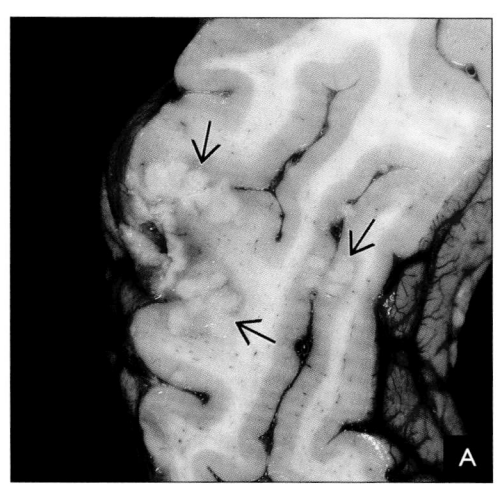

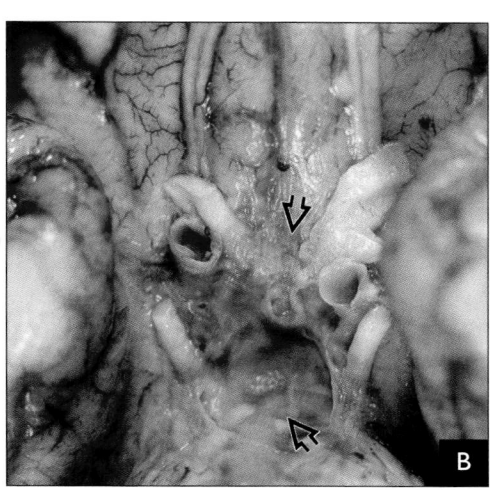

14-32A. Series of autopsy images, all from the same patient, shows the "cascade" of catastrophes caused by HIV-TB coinfection. Several of many multiple old healed granulomas ➡ from prior CNS TB are shown in this axial section obtained through the temporal lobe. 14-32B. The patient became HIV positive, which reactivated his latent TB, causing severe tuberculous meningitis ➡ as seen on this view of the basilar cisterns.

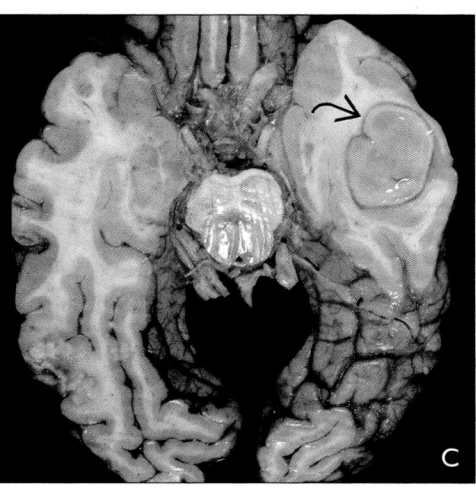

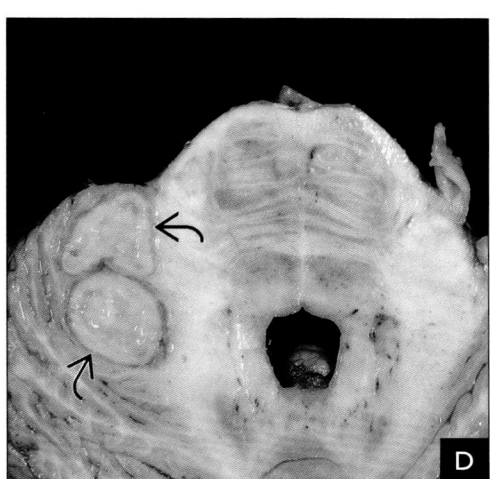

14-32C. With his immune system severely weakened, the patient became septic and developed several acute pyogenic abscesses. Note that the abscess in the temporal lobe ➡ is relatively poorly encapsulated. 14-32D. Two other abscesses are shown in the cerebellum ➡. The ultimate cause of death was acute overwhelming sepsis. (Courtesy R. Hewlett, MD.)

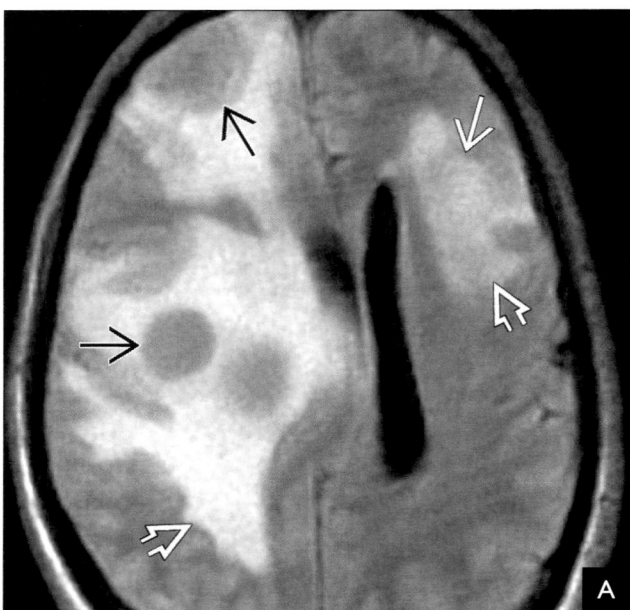

14-33A. *An HIV-positive patient with CD4 count < 50 with rapidly progressive left-sided weakness, decreased mental status. Axial FLAIR shows several hypointense* ⇥ *and 1 hyperintense* ⇥ *lesion with marked mass effect, significant edema* ⇥.

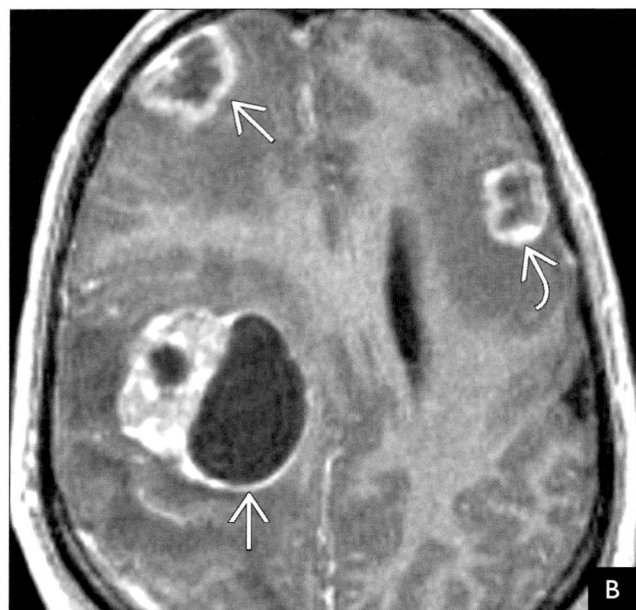

14-33B. *Axial T1 C+ scan in the same patient shows multiple rim-enhancing masses. This severely immunocompromised patient had both granulomas* ⇥ *and a pseudoabscess* ⇥ *in the setting of fulminant reactivated TB. (Courtesy S. Candy, MD.)*

MISCELLANEOUS OPPORTUNISTIC INFECTIONS

Cytomegalovirus (CMV)
- Herpesvirus family
- Develops in 2% of HIV/AIDS patients
- CD4 count usually < 50
- Imaging
  - Meningitis
  - Ventriculitis/ependymitis

Tuberculosis
- 1/3 of HIV/AIDS patients coinfected
- HIV most powerful known risk factor for reactivating latent TB
  - 100x risk for non-AIDS patients
- TB enhances HIV replication, accelerates disease
  - May present as acute, fulminant, fatal infection
  - TB "gone wild"

Malaria
- HIV coinfection worsens outcome
- "Triple combination" of HIV-TB-malaria more deadly than HIV-malaria

---

Immune Reconstitution Inflammatory Syndrome

Terminology

CNS immune reconstitution inflammatory syndrome (IRIS) is a recently recognized T-cell-mediated encephalitis that occurs in the setting of treated HIV or autoimmune disease (e.g., multiple sclerosis). CNS IRIS is also called neuro-IRIS.

Etiology

Most investigators consider neuro-IRIS a dysregulated immune response and pathogen-driven disease whose clinical expression depends on host susceptibility, the intensity and quality of the immune response, and the specific characteristics of the "provoking pathogen" itself.

IRIS occurs when restored immunity causes an exaggerated immune response to infectious or noninfectious antigens. IRIS develops in two distinct scenarios, "unmasking" IRIS and "paradoxical" IRIS. Both differ in clinical expression, disease management, and prognosis although their imaging manifestations are similar.

"Unmasking" IRIS occurs when antiretroviral therapy reveals a subclinical, previously undiagnosed opportunistic infection. Immune restoration leads to an immune response against a living pathogen. Here brain parenchyma is damaged by both the replicating pathogen and the incited immune response.

"Paradoxical" IRIS occurs when a patient who has been successfully treated for a recent opportunistic infection unexpectedly deteriorates after initiation of antiretroviral therapy. Here there is no newly acquired or reactivated infection. The recovering immune response targets persistent pathogen-derived antigens or self-antigens and causes tissue damage.

Several different underlying pathogens have been identified with IRIS. The most common are JC virus (PML-IRIS), tuberculosis (TB-IRIS), and fungal infections, especially *Cryptococcus* (crypto-IRIS). Some parasitic infections—such as toxoplasmosis—are relatively common in HIV/AIDS patients but rarely associated with IRIS.

Not all neurotropic viruses cause IRIS. HIV itself rarely causes neuro-IRIS. Herpes viruses (e.g., HSV, VZV, CMV) are all rarely reported causes of neuro-IRIS.

An unusual type of IRIS occurs in MS patients treated with natalizumab who subsequently develop PML. Natalizumab-related PML is managed by discontinuation of the drug and instituting plasmapheresis/immunoadsorption (PLEX/IA). Neurologic deficits and imaging studies in some patients worsen during subsequent immune reconstitution, causing **natalizumab-associated PML-IRIS**. Two types are recognized: Patients with early PML-IRIS (develops *before* institution of PLEX/IA) and patients with late PML-IRIS (IRIS develops *after* treatment with PLEX/IA). Neurologic outcome is generally worse in early PML-IRIS with a mortality rate approaching 25%.

Pathology

There are no specific histologic features or biomarkers for neuro-IRIS; rather, the diagnosis is established on the basis of clinical manifestations, exclusion of other disorders, and imaging or histopathologic evidence of inflammatory reaction.

Clinical Issues

EPIDEMIOLOGY. Between 15-35% of AIDS patients beginning HAART develop IRIS. Of these, approximately 1% develop neuro-IRIS. The two most important risk factors are a low CD4 count and a short time interval between treatment of the underlying infection and the commencement of antiretroviral therapy. The highest risk is in patients with a count less than 50 cells/μL.

Epidemiology varies according to the specific "provoking pathogen." The most common cause of neuro-IRIS is JC virus. Latent virus is reactivated when patients become immunodeficient. The reactivated virus infects oligodendrocytes, causing the lytic demyelination characteristic of progressive multifocal leukoencephalopathy

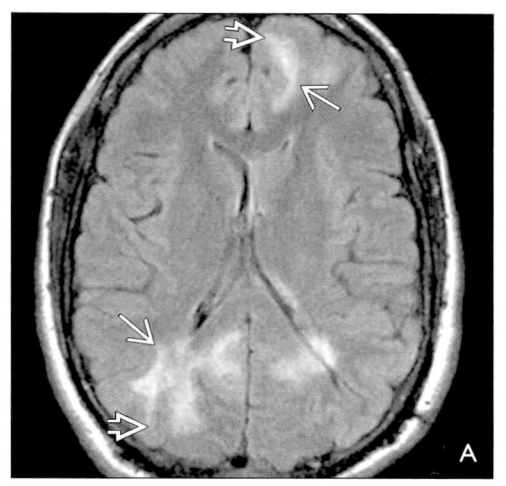
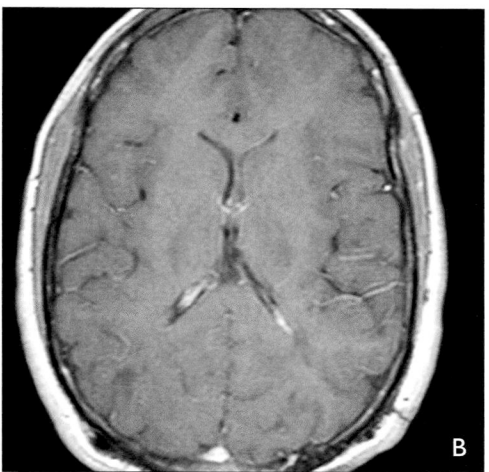

14-34A. Initial FLAIR MR in an HIV-positive male obtained prior to beginning HAART shows bilateral but asymmetric white matter hyperintensities ➡. Note lesions extending into the subcortical U-fibers ⋙, suggesting PML. 14-34B. Axial T1 C+ scan in the same patient shows no enhancement.

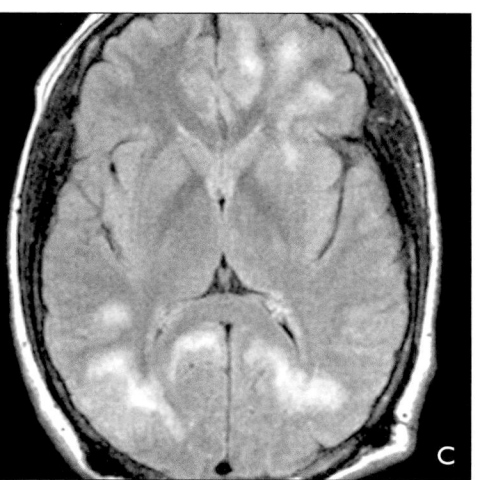
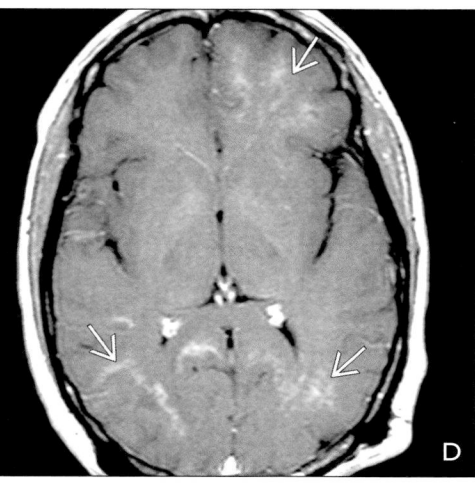

14-34C. The patient deteriorated 3 weeks following institution of combination antiretroviral therapy despite rising CD4 counts and significantly decreased viral load. Repeat FLAIR scan shows significant interval increase in the white matter disease. 14-34D. T1 C+ scan shows interval appearance of multifocal, wild-looking, irregular enhancement ➡. CSF was PCR-positive for JCV. PML-IRIS. (Courtesy T. Hutchins, MD.)

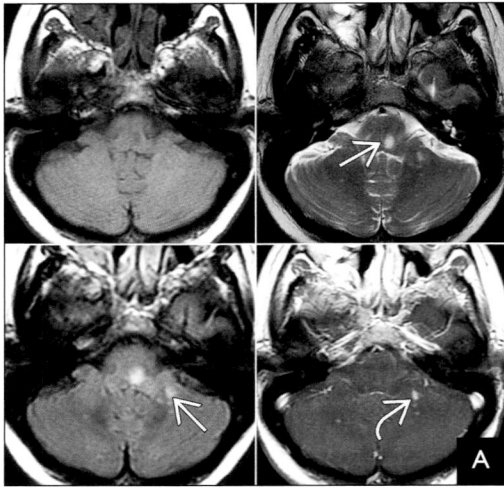

14-35A. *Natalizumab-associated PML-IRIS in MS. Baseline imaging shows posterior fossa lesions* ➡ *with a solitary focus of punctate enhancement* ➘.

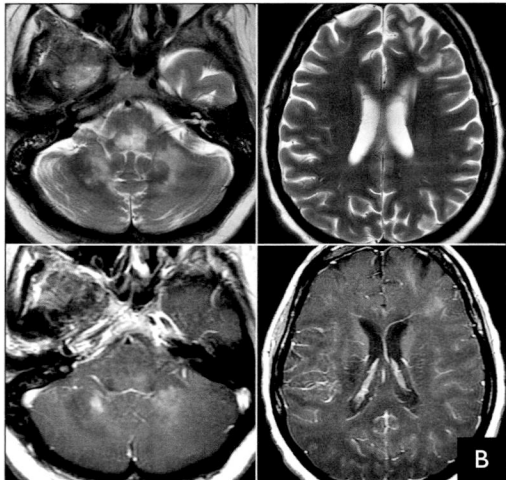

14-35B. *Three months later, symptoms had progressed. Existing lesions have enlarged, and new lesions have appeared.*

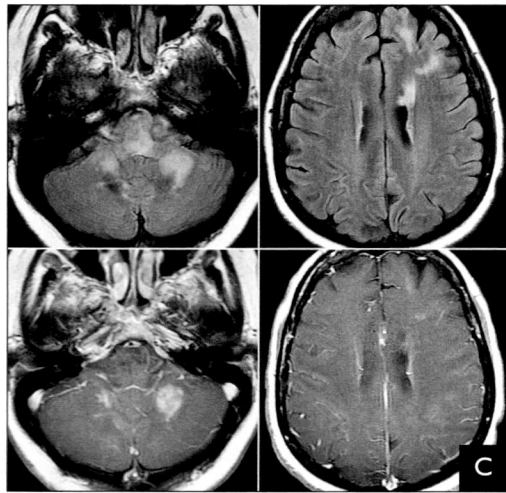

14-35C. *Following PLEX/IA treatment, the disease stabilized.*

(PML). Nearly 17% of patients with preexisting PML worsen after beginning HAART and are considered to have "unmasking" **PML-IRIS.**

TB-IRIS occurs in 15% of patients who are coinfected with TB if antiretroviral therapy is initiated before the TB is adequately treated. Pulmonary involvement and lymphadenitis are the most common manifestations. Almost 20% of TB-IRIS patients develop neurological involvement characterized by meningitis, tuberculomas, and radiculomyelopathies. TB-IRIS occurs as both "unmasking" and "paradoxical" IRIS.

"Paradoxical" **crypto-IRIS** affects 20% of HIV-infected patients in whom antiretroviral therapy was initiated after treatment of neuromeningeal cryptococcosis. The major manifestation of crypto neuro-IRIS is aseptic recurrent meningitis. Parenchymal cryptococcomas are rare.

Despite the high prevalence of parasitic infestations in resource-poor countries, only a few cases of parasite-associated neuro-IRIS have been reported. All have been caused by *T. gondii.*

Natalizumab-associated IRIS is rare. To date, approximately 50 cases have been reported. Most are PML-IRIS.

PRESENTATION. Neuro-IRIS is a polymorphic condition with heterogeneous clinical manifestations. The most common presentation is clinical deterioration of a newly treated HIV-positive patient despite rising CD4 counts and diminishing viral loads.

NATURAL HISTORY AND TREATMENT OPTIONS. Given that a low CD4 T-cell count is a major risk factor for developing IRIS, starting HAART at a count of $> 350/\mu L$ will prevent most cases.

Systemic IRIS is usually mild and self-limited. Prognosis in neuro-IRIS is variable. Corticosteroids and cytokine neutralization therapy have been used for treatment of neuro-IRIS with mixed results and are controversial.

Patients with neuro-IRIS may die within days to weeks. Mortality from PML-IRIS exceeds 40% while that of crypto-IRIS is about 20%. TB-IRIS mortality is slightly lower (13%).

Imaging

Imaging manifestations of neuro-IRIS vary depending on the "provoking pathogen" but typically reflect the generic imaging features of inflammatory disease. Bizarre-looking parenchymal masses and progressively enlarging, enhancing lesions **(14-34)** are typical of PML-IRIS but occur in slightly less than half of all cases **(14-35).**

TB-IRIS patients can develop florid TB pseudoabscesses (TB "gone wild") and/or rapidly increasing enhancement

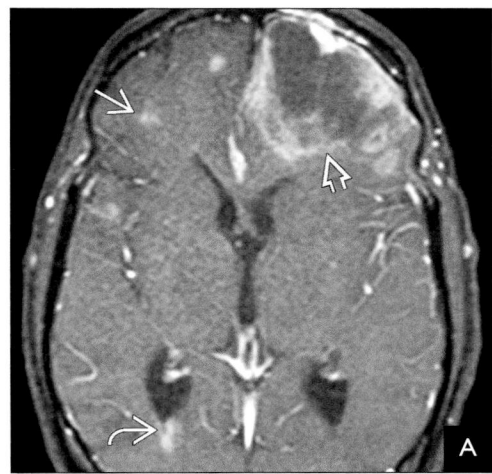

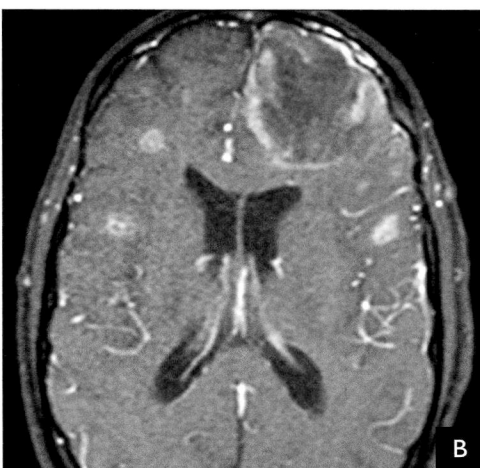

14-36A. *A 38-year-old HIV-positive man with a remote history of cardiac Chagas disease experienced acute worsening 2 weeks following initiation of HAART. T1 C+ FS scan shows multiple ring-like* ⧩ *and nodular enhancing lesions* ➡, *ventriculitis* ↗. ***14-36B.*** *More cephalad scan shows additional lesions.*

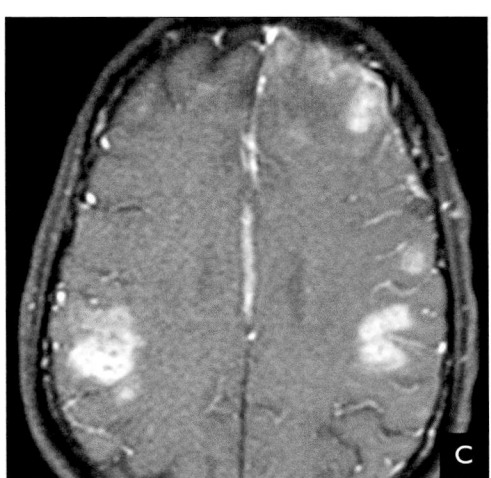

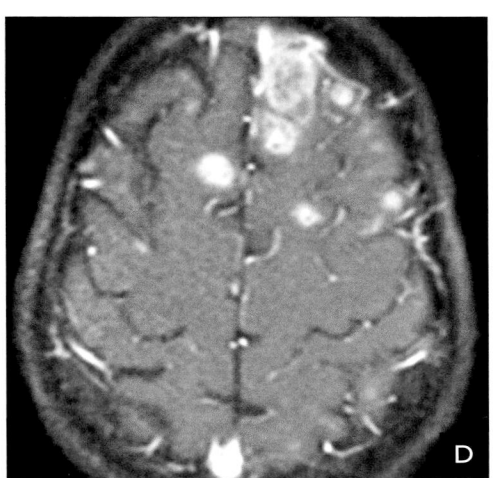

14-36C. *Multiple heterogeneously enhancing lesions are seen at the gray-white matter interfaces of both hemispheres.* ***14-36D.*** *Axial T1 C+ FS scan through the vertex shows many more lesions.*

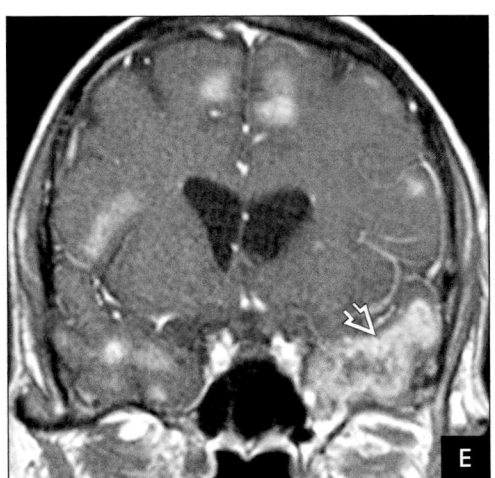

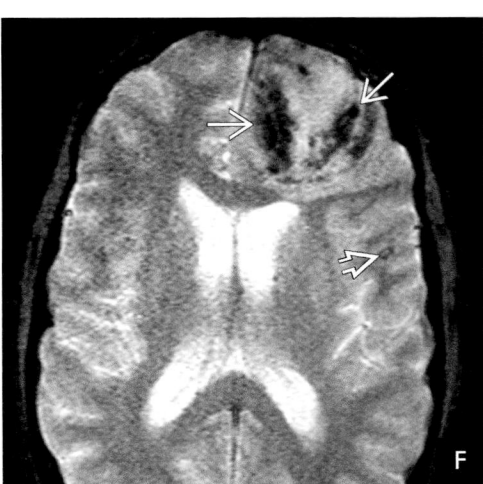

14-36E. *Coronal T1 C+ scan shows multiple enhancing foci at the gray-white matter interfaces, as well as a large necrotic-looking left temporal lobe mass* ⧩. ***14-36F.*** *T2* GRE scan shows multiple large* ➡ *and small* ⧩ *hemorrhages. Parasite-IRIS from reactivation of latent Chagas disease.*

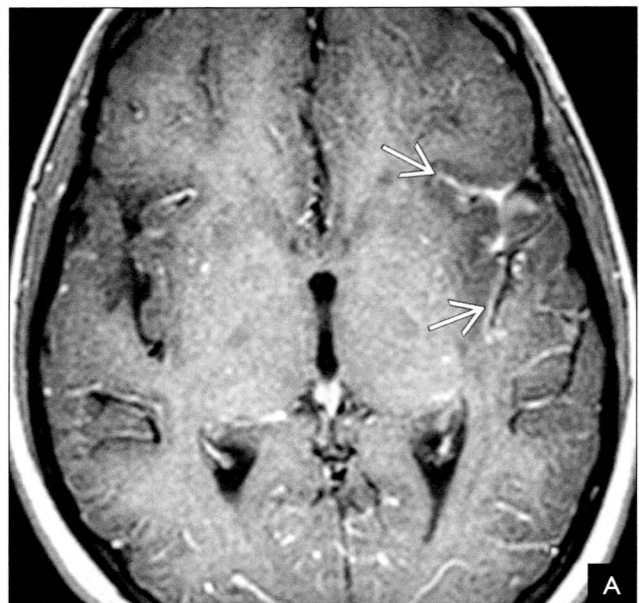

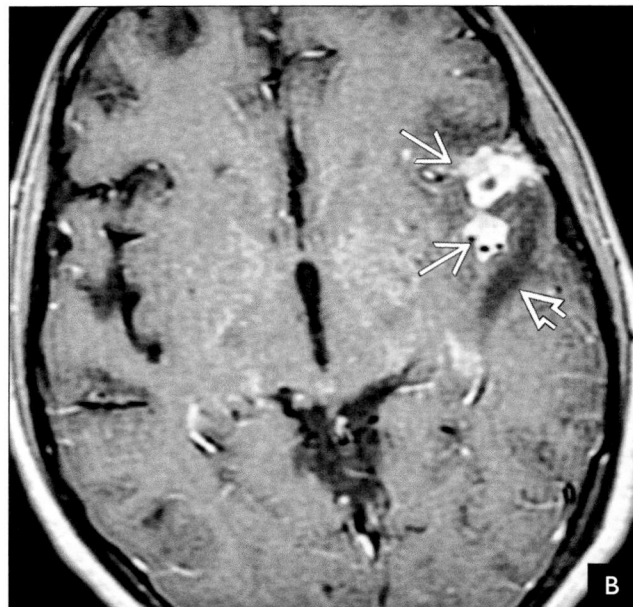

14-37A. Axial T1 C+ scan in an HIV-positive patient with tuberculous meningitis shows meningeal enhancement in the left sylvian fissure ➡.

14-37B. The patient was placed on HAART and subsequently developed significant worsening of symptoms. The meningeal enhancement ➡ has increased significantly and is now nodular and mass-like. Note significant edema ➡. TB-IRIS.

in the basilar meninges **(14-37)**. Less common types of IRIS include fungal-IRIS and parasite-IRIS **(14-36)**.

Differential Diagnosis

IRIS can have varying presentations and different degrees of severity, making clinical diagnosis difficult. Neuro-IRIS should be considered in any immunocompromised patient with unexpected neurologic deterioration within a few weeks or months after immune restoration. Natalizumab-treated MS patients who experience paradoxical worsening may have PML or PML-IRIS.

The major imaging differential diagnosis of neuro-IRIS is **non-IRIS-associated opportunistic infection**. Contrast enhancement in combination with mass effect is more typical of IRIS but may be absent early in the disease course. The distinction is important, as IRIS requires control of the inflammatory response (currently steroids) whereas non-IRIS opportunistic infections need immune restoration. Brain biopsy may be required to detect the typical perivascular and parenchymal inflammatory changes of IRIS.

AIDS-defining neoplasms, particularly **lymphoma**, may mimic IRIS with findings of necrosis and irregular ring enhancement. Dermatological manifestations of IRIS can be simulated by Kaposi sarcoma.

IMMUNE RECONSTITUTION INFLAMMATORY SYNDROME (IRIS)

Terminology and Etiology
- Neuro-IRIS
  - "Unmasking" IRIS (HAART "unmasks" existing subclinical opportunistic infection)
  - "Paradoxical" IRIS (treated infection worsens after HAART)
- Pathogens associated with neuro-IRIS
  - JC virus (PML-IRIS) most common
  - Tuberculosis (TB-IRIS) next most common
  - Fungi (crypto-IRIS)
  - Drugs (natalizumab-associated PML-IRIS)
  - Parasites (rare, except for toxo-IRIS)
  - Neurotropic viruses (e.g., HIV, herpesviruses) rarely cause IRIS

Epidemiology
- 15-35% of AIDS patients starting HAART develop IRIS
- Of these, 1% develop neuro-IRIS
- CD4 count < 50 cells/μL = ↑↑ risk of IRIS

Imaging
- Varies with "provoking pathogen"
- Rapidly increasing mass effect common
- Variable enhancement, often bizarre and "wild"

Differential Diagnosis
- Non-IRIS-associated opportunistic infections
- AIDS-defining malignancies
  - Especially lymphoma

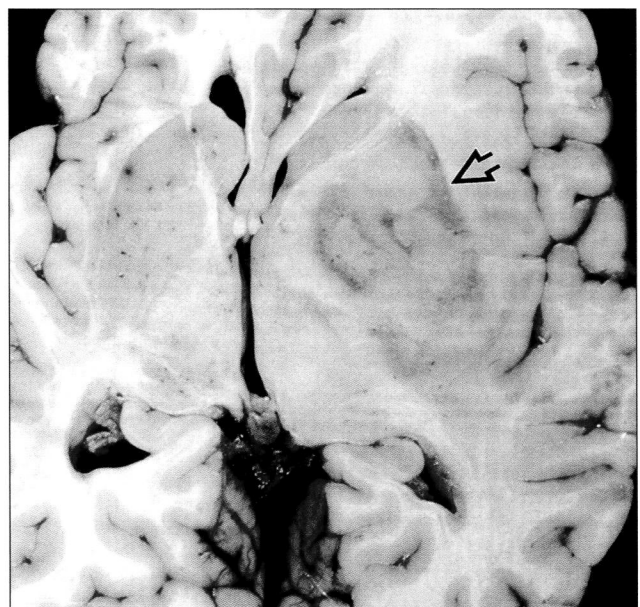

14-38. Autopsy case of AIDS-related PCNSL shows a solitary mass in the basal ganglia with central necrosis and peripheral hemorrhage ➡. (Courtesy R. Hewlett, MD.)

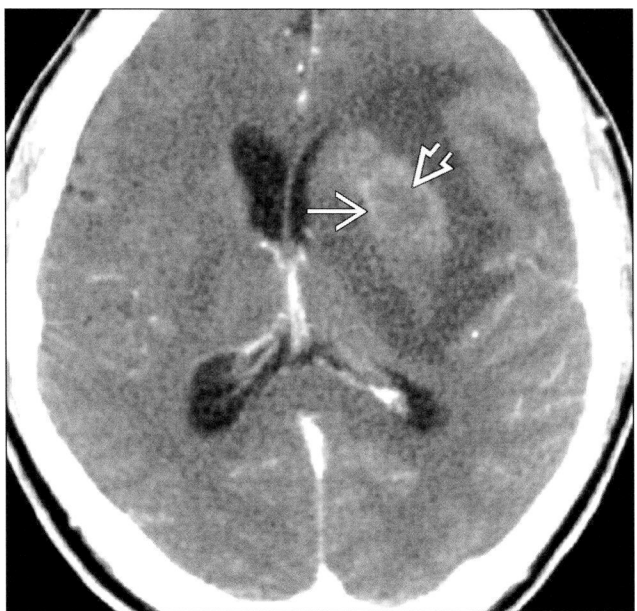

14-39. Axial CECT scan in a different HIV-positive patient shows a solitary mass in the left basal ganglia with central necrosis ➡ and mild rim enhancement ➡. Perilesional edema is marked. Biopsy disclosed PCNSL.

Neoplasms in HIV/AIDS

AIDS-defining malignancies include certain non-Hodgkin lymphomas, Kaposi sarcoma (KS), and cervical cancer. With the exception of cervical cancer, HIV-associated malignancies in the United States peaked in the mid-1990s and have since declined. With primary central nervous system lymphoma (PCNSL), malignancy risk is linked to the patient's immune status and increases with CD4 counts less than 50-100 cells/μL. In some cases, i.e., with cervical intraepithelial neoplasia (CIN), HAART is associated with disease regression.

We now briefly discuss the AIDS-defining malignancies that can affect the scalp, skull, and brain: PCNSL and KS.

HIV-associated Lymphomas

HIV-associated lymphomas are typically the diffuse large B-cell non-Hodgkin type. Epstein-Barr virus (EBV) infection is most often associated with infectious mononucleosis. An estimated 1% of all lymphoproliferative, epithelial, and mesenchymal neoplasms are linked to EBV infection. EBV plays an especially prominent role in the development of lymphoma in patients with HIV or transplant-related immunosuppression.

PCNSLs are the second most common cerebral mass lesion in AIDS (exceeded only by toxoplasmosis) and

develop in 2-6% of patients. PCNSLs cause approximately 70% of all solitary brain parenchymal lesions in HIV/AIDS patients.

PCNSLs present as single or (less commonly) multiple masses. More than 90% are supratentorial, with preferential location in the basal ganglia and deep white matter abutting the lateral ventricle. PCNSLs often cross the corpus callosum. Central necrosis and hemorrhage are common in AIDS-related lymphomas (14-38), which is reflected in the imaging findings (14-39), (14-40).

The major differential diagnosis is **toxoplasmosis**. Toxoplasmosis is more commonly multiple, and lesions often exhibit the "eccentric target" sign, i.e., an eccentrically located nodule within a ring-enhancing mass. pMR is helpful in distinguishing PCNSL from toxoplasmosis; lymphoma typically has increased rCBV whereas toxoplasmosis does not. PET and SPECT are also helpful imaging adjuncts, as lymphoma is "hot" but toxo is "not."

Kaposi Sarcoma

Kaposi sarcoma (KS) is the most common sarcoma in immunosuppressed patients. The next most frequent non-KS sarcoma is leiomyosarcoma, followed by angiosarcoma and fibrohistiocytic tumors.

Kaposi sarcoma develops from a combination of factors: HHV-8 infection (also known as Kaposi sarcoma-associated herpesvirus), altered immunity, and an inflammatory or angiogenic milieu. EBV infection is common in patients with HIV-associated leiomyosarcomas.

There has been a marked decline in the incidence of AIDS-related KS since the advent of antiretroviral therapy. Transplant-related KS often resolves after reduction of immunosuppression, highlighting the role of cellular immune response in the control of HHV-8 infection.

KS is the most common neoplasm in untreated AIDS patients. Overall, the most common site is the skin **(14-41)**, followed by mucous membranes, lymph nodes, and viscera. Classic KS is an indolent tumor with purplish or dark brown plaques and nodules, usually on the extremities. AIDS-associated KS is much more aggressive. Lesions most commonly occur on the face, genitals, and mucous membranes **(14-42)**.

Cranial KS is unusual and much less common than CNS lymphoma. When it occurs, cranial KS is typically seen as a localized scalp thickening **(14-43)** or an infiltrating soft tissue mass in the skin of the face and neck **(14-44)**. Calvarial invasion is unusual. KS is isointense with muscle on T1WI, hyperintense on T2WI, and enhances strongly on CECT or T1 C+ MR.

AIDS-DEFINING MALIGNANCIES

HIV-associated Lymphoma
- Etiology and pathology
  - Often associated with EBV
  - Most are diffuse large B-cell NHL type
- Clinical issues
  - Second most common mass lesion in AIDS
  - Occurs in 2-6% of HIV/AIDS patients
  - 70% of solitary CNS masses in HIV(+) patients
- Imaging
  - Hemorrhage, necrosis common
  - Supratentorial (90%)
  - Basal ganglia, deep WM (often crosses corpus callosum)
  - Often ring-enhancing
  - ↑ rCBV

Kaposi Sarcoma
- Etiology and pathology
  - Associated with HHV-8
  - Most common sarcoma in immunosuppressed
- Clinical issues
  - Antiretrovirals ↓↓ prevalence
  - Skin, mucous membranes, lymph nodes, scalp
- Imaging
  - Localized scalp thickening
  - Infiltrating soft tissue mass in skin of face or neck

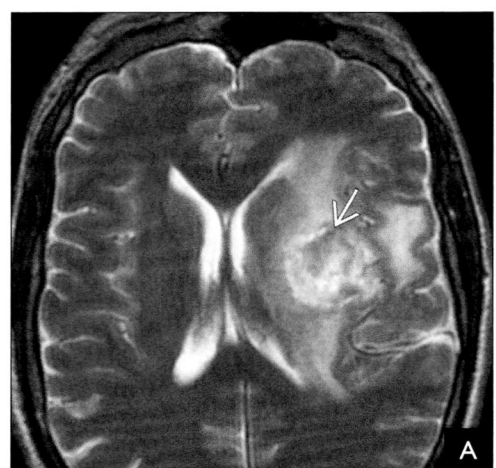
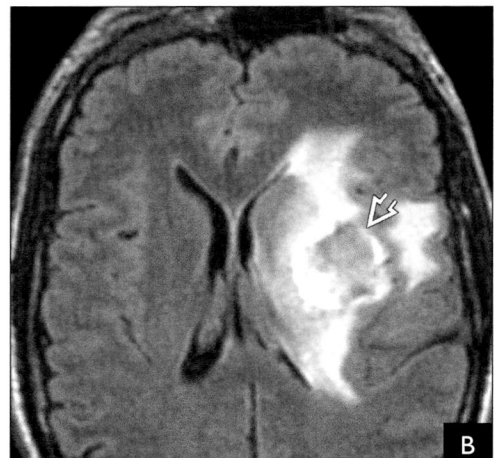

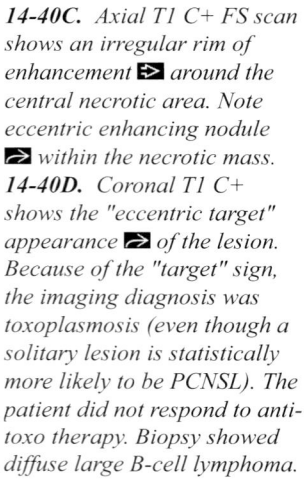

14-40A. Axial T2WI in an HIV/AIDS patient who developed right-sided weakness shows a solitary heterogeneous mass ⮕ at the junction of the left basal ganglia and deep white matter. 14-40B. The center of the lesion is isointense ⮕ with brain on FLAIR.

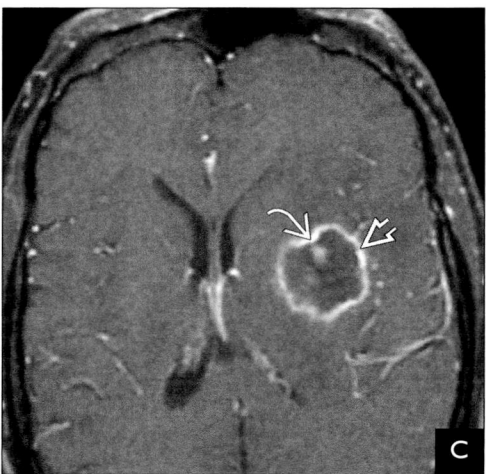
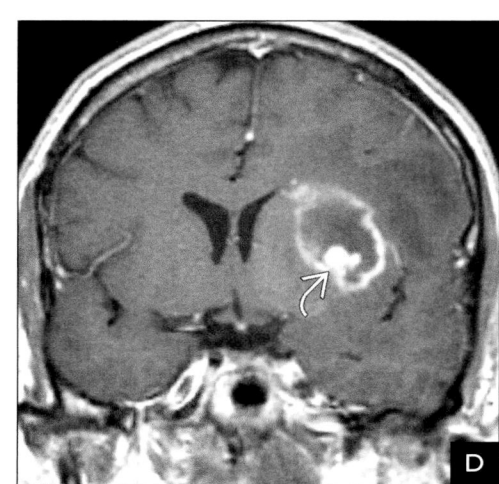

14-40C. Axial T1 C+ FS scan shows an irregular rim of enhancement ⮕ around the central necrotic area. Note eccentric enhancing nodule ⮕ within the necrotic mass. 14-40D. Coronal T1 C+ shows the "eccentric target" appearance ⮕ of the lesion. Because of the "target" sign, the imaging diagnosis was toxoplasmosis (even though a solitary lesion is statistically more likely to be PCNSL). The patient did not respond to anti-toxo therapy. Biopsy showed diffuse large B-cell lymphoma.

elected References

verview

Epidemiology

- Dean D et al: Neuro-AIDS in the developing world. Neurology. 78(7):499-500, 2012

IV Infection

HIV Encephalitis

- Becker JT et al: Factors affecting brain structure in men with HIV disease in the post- HAART era. Neuroradiology. 54(2):113-21, 2012
- Towgood KJ et al: Mapping the brain in younger and older asymptomatic HIV-1 men: frontal volume changes in the absence of other cortical or diffusion tensor abnormalities. Cortex. 48(2):230-41, 2012

- Valcour V et al: Central nervous system viral invasion and inflammation during acute HIV infection. J Infect Dis. 206(2):275-282, 2012
- Prado PT et al: Image evaluation of HIV encephalopathy: a multimodal approach using quantitative MR techniques. Neuroradiology. 53(11):899-908, 2011
- Valcour V et al: Pathogenesis of HIV in the central nervous system. Curr HIV/AIDS Rep. 8(1):54-61, 2011
- Chen Y et al: White matter abnormalities revealed by diffusion tensor imaging in non-demented and demented HIV(+) patients. Neuroimage. 47(4):1154-62, 2009

Other Manifestations of HIV/AIDS

- Gutierrez J et al: HIV/AIDS patients with HIV vasculopathy and VZV vasculitis: a case series. Clin Neuroradiol. 21(3):145-51, 2011
- Ntusi NB et al: Progressive human immunodeficiency virus-associated vasculopathy: time to revise antiretroviral therapy guidelines? Cardiovasc J Afr. 22(4):197-200, 2011
- World Health Organization: Global health sector strategy on HIV/AIDS, 2011-2015. Geneva, Switzerland: WHO Press, 2011

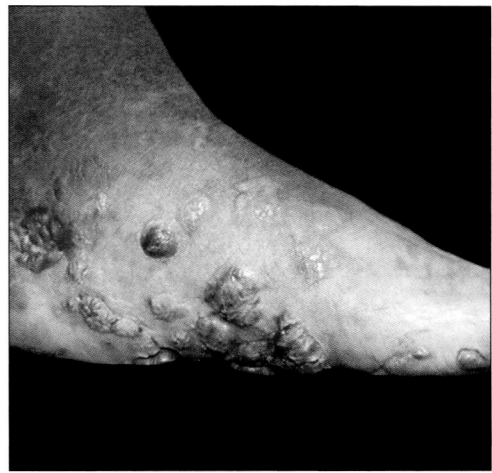

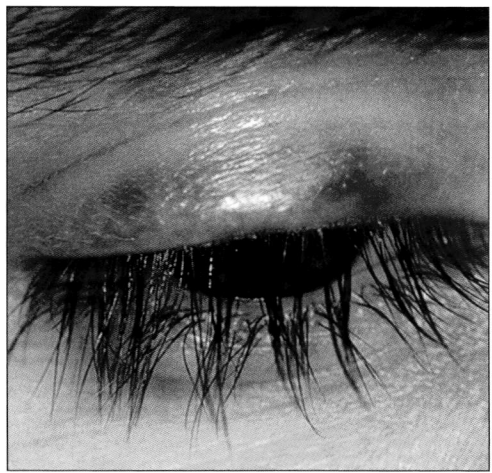

14-41. Clinical photograph shows classic Kaposi sarcoma presenting with multiple nodular skin lesions. (Courtesy T. Mentzel, MD.) 14-42. Patients with AIDS-related KS often present with lesions in unusual anatomic sites, as did this young patient with small reddish lesions on his upper eyelid. (Courtesy T. Mentzel, MD.)

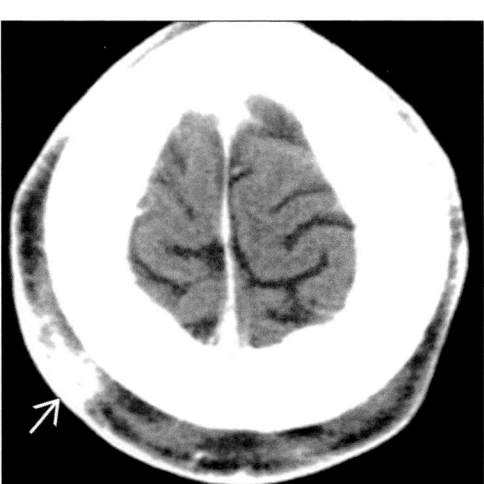

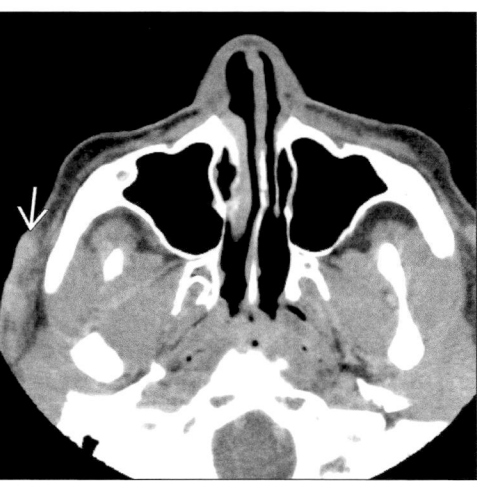

14-43. CECT scan shows Kaposi sarcoma of the scalp in this AIDS patient. Note infiltration of the skin and subcutaneous tissues ➡. 14-44. Kaposi sarcoma of the skin of the face and neck in this AIDS patient is seen as superficial nodules involving the cutis and subcutaneous tissues ➡.

- Ragin AB et al: Bone marrow diffusion measures correlate with dementia severity in HIV patients. AJNR Am J Neuroradiol. 27(3):589-92, 2006
- Gilden DH et al: The protean manifestations of varicella-zoster virus vasculopathy. J Neurovirol. 8 Suppl 2:75-9, 2002
- Connor MD et al: Cerebral infarction in adult AIDS patients: observations from the Edinburgh HIV Autopsy Cohort. Stroke. 31(9):2117-26, 2000
- Karcher DS et al: The bone marrow in human immunodeficiency virus (HIV)-related disease. Morphology and clinical correlation. Am J Clin Pathol. 95(1):63-71, 1991

Opportunistic Infections

- Tan IL et al: HIV-associated opportunistic infections of the CNS. Lancet Neurol. 11(7):605-17, 2012

Toxoplasmosis

- Robert-Gangneux F et al: Epidemiology of and diagnostic strategies for toxoplasmosis. Clin Microbiol Rev. 25(2):264-96, 2012

Progressive Multifocal Leukoencephalopathy

- Ferenczy MW et al: Molecular biology, epidemiology, and pathogenesis of progressive multifocal leukoencephalopathy, the JC virus-induced demyelinating disease of the human brain. Clin Microbiol Rev. 25(3):471-506, 2012
- Piza F et al: JC virus-associated central nervous system diseases in HIV-infected patients in Brazil: clinical presentations, associated factors with mortality and outcome. Braz J Infect Dis. 16(2):153-6, 2012
- Bag AK et al: JC virus infection of the brain. AJNR Am J Neuroradiol. 31(9):1564-76, 2010
- Smith AB et al: From the archives of the AFIP: central nervous system infections associated with human immunodeficiency virus infection: radiologic-pathologic correlation. Radiographics. 2008 Nov-Dec;28(7):2033-58. Review. Erratum in: Radiographics. 29(2):638, 2009

Other Opportunistic Infections

- Hendriksen IC et al: Diagnosis, clinical presentation, and in-hospital mortality of severe malaria in HIV-coinfected children and adults in Mozambique. Clin Infect Dis. 55(8):1144-53, 2012
- Tshikuka Mulumba JG et al: Severity of outcomes associated to types of HIV coinfection with TB and malaria in a setting where the three pandemics overlap. J Community Health. Epub ahead of print, 2012
- Daikos GL et al: Multidrug-resistant tuberculous meningitis in patients with AIDS. Int J Tuberc Lung Dis. 7(4):394-8, 2003

Immune Reconstitution Inflammatory Syndrome

- Achenbach CJ et al: Paradoxical immune reconstitution inflammatory syndrome in HIV-infected patients treated with combination antiretroviral therapy after AIDSdefining opportunistic infection. Clin Infect Dis. 54(3):424-33, 2012
- Huis in 't Veld D et al: The immune reconstitution inflammatory syndrome related to HIV co-infections: a review. Eur J Clin Microbiol Infect Dis. 31(6):919-27, 2012
- Post MJ et al: CNS-immune reconstitution inflammatory syndrome in the setting of HIV infection, part 1: Overview and discussion of progressive multifocal leukoencephalopathy-immune reconstitution inflammatory syndrome and cryptococcal-immune reconstitution inflammatory syndrome. AJNR Am J Neuroradiol. Epub ahead of print, 2012
- Post MJ et al: CNS-immune reconstitution inflammatory syndrome in the setting of HIV infection, part 2: Discussion of neuro-immune reconstitution inflammatory syndrome with and without other pathogens. AJNR Am J Neuroradiol. Epub ahead of print, 2012
- Worodria W et al: Clinical spectrum, risk factors and outcome of immune reconstitution inflammatory syndrome in patients with tuberculosis-HIV coinfection. Antivir Ther. 17(5):841-848, 2012
- Johnson T et al: Immune reconstitution inflammatory syndrome and the central nervous system. Curr Opin Neurol. 24(3):284-90, 2011
- Martin-Blondel G et al: Pathogenesis of the immune reconstitution inflammatory syndrome affecting the central nervous system in patients infected with HIV. Brain. 134(Pt 4):928-46, 2011
- Tan IL et al: Immune reconstitution inflammatory syndrome in natalizumab-associated PML. Neurology. 77(11):1061-7, 2011
- Anderson AM et al: Human immunodeficiency virus-associated cytomegalovirus infection with multiple small vessel cerebral infarcts in the setting of early immune reconstitution. J Neurovirol. 16(2):179-84, 2010
- Marais S et al: Neuroradiological features of the tuberculosis-associated immune reconstitution inflammatory syndrome. Int J Tuberc Lung Dis. 14(2):188-96, 2010

Neoplasms in HIV/AIDS

- Malfitano A et al: Human immunodeficiency virus-associated malignancies: a therapeutic update. Curr HIV Res. 10(2):123-32, 2012
- Shiels MS et al: Proportions of Kaposi sarcoma, selected non-Hodgkin lymphomas, and cervical cancer in the United States occurring in persons with AIDS, 1980-2007. JAMA. 305(14):1450-9, 2011

HIV-associated Lymphomas

- Kaplan LD: HIV-associated lymphoma. Best Pract Res Clin Haematol. 25(1):101-17, 2012

Kaposi Sarcoma

- Bhatia K et al: Sarcomas other than Kaposi sarcoma occurring in immunodeficiency: interpretations from a systematic literature review. Curr Opin Oncol. 24(5):537-46, 2012

15

Demyelinating and Inflammatory Diseases

In the previous chapters, we discussed congenital and acquired infections. Here, we focus on the surprisingly broad spectrum of noninfectious idiopathic inflammatory and demyelinating disorders that can affect the CNS.

CNS inflammatory syndromes have been classified in numerous ways: By presentation (clinically isolated vs. polysymptomatic disease), pattern (monofocal or multifocal), geography (brain vs. spinal cord vs. peripheral nervous system), disease severity (from asymptomatic to severe), and disease course (monophasic, multiphasic, relapsing-remitting, progressive, etc.).

In this chapter, we follow a simplified approach, dividing our discussion into multiple sclerosis and its mimics, post-infection/post-vaccination inflammatory disorders, and inflammatory-like disorders.

We begin with multiple sclerosis (MS), delineating its etiology and pathology, epidemiology and clinical phenotypes, imaging appearance, and differential diagnosis.

Although MS is by far the most common CNS demyelinating disorder, a number of other neuro-inflammatory demyelinating conditions can affect the CNS. Following our detailed discussion of MS, we delineate several special variants of so-called idiopathic inflammatory demyelinating lesions (IIDLs). Some—such as Balo con-

centric sclerosis and Schilder disease—may actually be MS variants, while others are most likely separate entities. We also include IIDLs with restricted topographical distribution, i.e., neuromyelitis optica (NMO) (also known as Devic disease or aquaporin-4 antibody disease). Susac syndrome—an immune-mediated microvascular endotheliopathy that can closely resemble MS—is also included here.

We then turn our attention to post-infection, post-vaccination inflammatory syndromes. We focus on two particularly important entities: Acute disseminated encephalomyelitis (ADEM) and the fulminant, highly lethal acute hemorrhagic encephalomyelitis (AHEM).

The chapter concludes by discussing three important inflammatory-like disorders of unknown or uncertain etiology: Neurosarcoidosis, idiopathic inflammatory pseudotumors, and chronic inflammatory demyelinating polyneuropathy (CIDP).

Multiple Sclerosis

Terminology

Multiple sclerosis (MS) is a progressive neurodegenerative disorder characterized histopathologically by multiple inflammatory demyelinating foci called "plaques."

Etiology

GENERAL CONCEPTS. MS is a complex, multifactorial disease whose precise pathogenesis remains unknown. Nevertheless, most investigators consider MS an autoimmune-mediated process in which environmental factors act upon genetically susceptible individuals.

Some investigators have proposed an alternative explanation, suggesting that MS is caused or exacerbated by abnormal CNS venous outflow. They have termed this purported vascular condition "chronic cerebrospinal venous insufficiency" (CCSVI). Some concepts related to MS pathoetiology are briefly summarized here.

Autoimmune-mediated demyelination. Immune-mediated events—whether inherent or environmentally triggered—are thought to cause myelin loss and oligodendrocyte death leading to axonal degeneration. Disordered T-cell homeostasis and cytokine networks have been cited as promoting inflammatory damage.

Environmental factors. Environmental factors including Epstein-Barr virus (EBV) exposure and geographic variability clearly contribute to MS risk. For example, EBV infection has been strongly associated with MS compared to age-matched controls. The relative risk of MS in EBV-negative individuals is very low.

The risk of MS also varies across race and geographic regions. MS occurs less often in non-whites compared to whites. MS frequency also increases with increasing latitude.

Chronic cerebrospinal venous insufficiency. Initial reports claimed a prevalence of 100% sensitivity and specificity for CCSVI in MS. Invasive endovascular procedures for treatment of CCSVI were performed with purported success. However, independent follow-up studies have not demonstrated a benefit for angioplasty or stenting in MS. No significant interaction between MS and CCSVI has been demonstrated for any hemodynamic parameters as determined by color Doppler ultrasonography.

GENETICS. The strongest identified genetic risk factor for MS is the human leukocyte antigen (*HLA-A*) gene in the major histocompatibility complex (MHC). Genome-wide association studies have pinpointed nearly 50 additional risk loci that play a key role in disease susceptibility. Despite recent progress, however, all the identified risk loci together account for only 50% of the inherited MS risk. Therefore, much of the genetic architecture underlying MS susceptibility remains to be determined.

15-1. Sagittal graphic illustrates multiple sclerosis plaques involving the corpus callosum, pons, and spinal cord. Note the characteristic perpendicular orientation of the lesions ⮕ at the callososeptal interface along penetrating venules. 15-2. Axial autopsy section shows typical ovoid, grayish MS plaques oriented perpendicularly and adjacent to the lateral ventricles ⮕, along medullary (deep WM) veins ⮕. (Courtesy R. Hewlett, MD.)

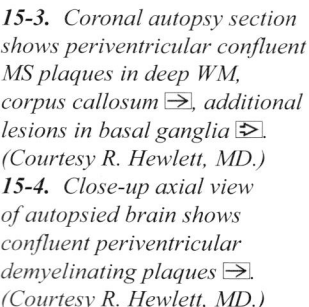
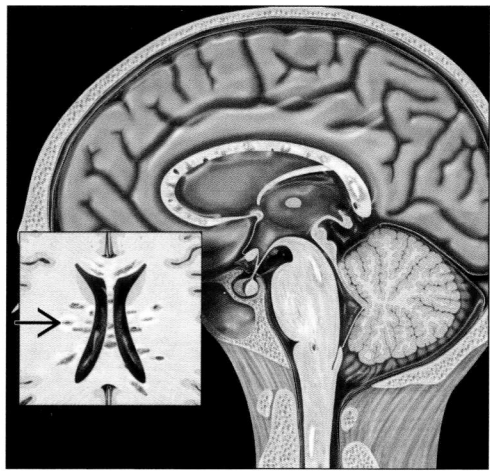
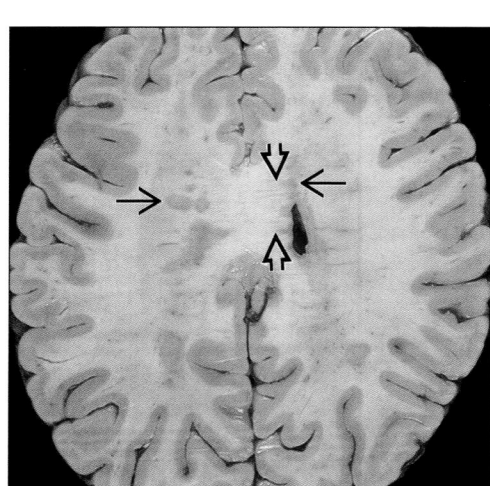

15-3. Coronal autopsy section shows periventricular confluent MS plaques in deep WM, corpus callosum ⮕, additional lesions in basal ganglia ⮕. (Courtesy R. Hewlett, MD.) 15-4. Close-up axial view of autopsied brain shows confluent periventricular demyelinating plaques ⮕. (Courtesy R. Hewlett, MD.)

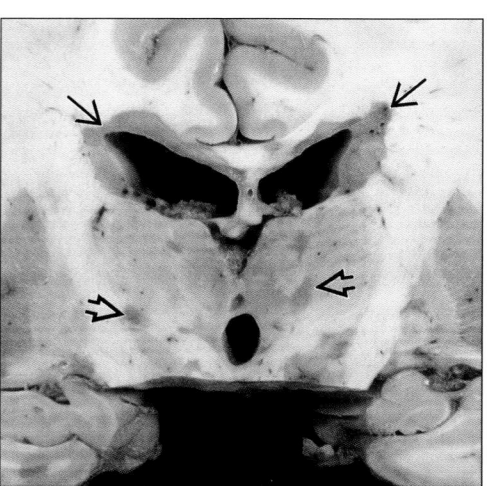
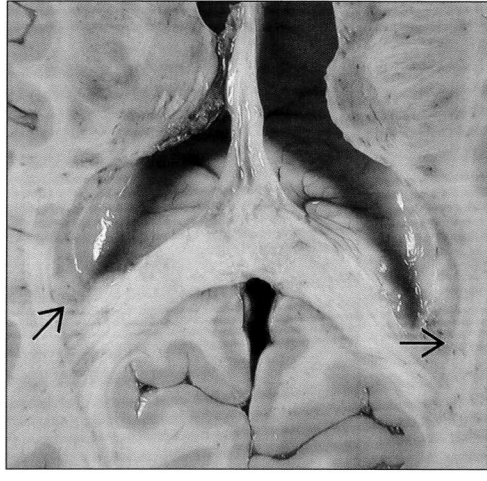

athology

LOCATION. Most MS plaques are supratentorial. Less than 10% occur in the posterior fossa although infratentorial lesions are relatively more common in children.

MS plaques in the deep cerebral white matter are linear, round, or ovoid lesions that are oriented perpendicular to the lateral ventricles **(15-1)**. Between 50-90% of all supratentorial lesions occur at or near the callososeptal interface. Centripetal perivenular extension is common, causing the appearance of "Dawson fingers" radiating outward from the lateral ventricles **(15-2)**, **(15-3)**.

Other commonly affected areas include the subcortical U-fibers, brachium pontis, brainstem, and spinal cord. Gray matter (cortex and basal ganglia) lesions are seen in 10% of cases **(15-4)**.

SIZE AND NUMBER. MS plaques vary in size. While most are small—between 5 and 10 millimeters—large lesions can reach several centimeters in diameter. MS plaques are usually multiple although 30% of giant "tumefactive" plaques initially occur as solitary lesions. These

"tumefactive" MS plaques are relatively more common in children and young adults compared to middle-aged and older patients.

GROSS PATHOLOGY. MS plaque classification is based on temporal progression. Three types are identified: Acute, chronic active, and chronic silent lesions. All occur along a continuum and evolve with time. Acute MS plaques are a tan-yellow color and have ill-defined margins with a granular texture. Chronic silent plaques have more distinctly defined borders and are grayish in color with scarred and excavated, depressed centers **(15-5)**.

MICROSCOPIC FEATURES. Low-power images of myelin stains show a sharp contrast between the "robin's-egg blue" of normally myelinated white matter and the pale-staining, almost pinkish areas of myelin loss **(15-6)**.

There is significant variability in the major histologic features of MS, i.e., inflammation, demyelination, remyelination, and axonal injury. Each is found in varying degrees in different patients as well as in the same patient at different stages of lesion evolution.

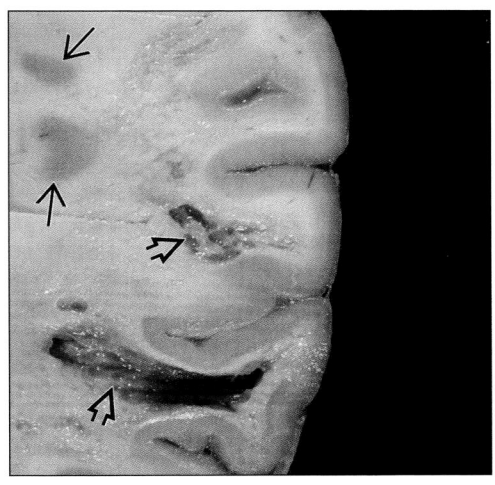
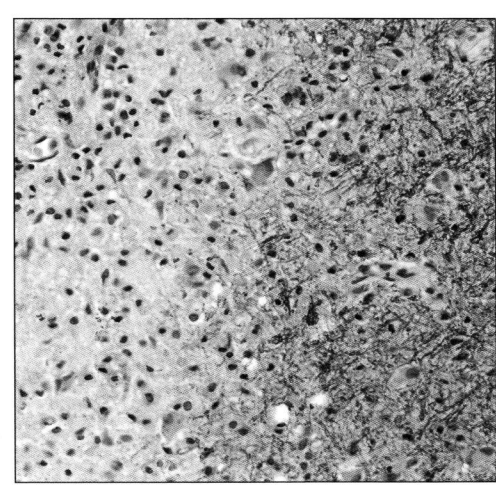

15-5. Close-up view of autopsied MS shows several cavitated, chronic inactive lesions with their well-defined margins and scarred excavated depressed centers ▷ as well as 2 grayish chronic active lesions ➡. (Courtesy R. Hewlett, MD.) 15-6. Luxol fast blue myelin stain shows relatively normal "robin's-egg blue" tissue on the right, pinkish demyelinated tissue on the left in classic MS. (Courtesy B. K. DeMasters, MD.)

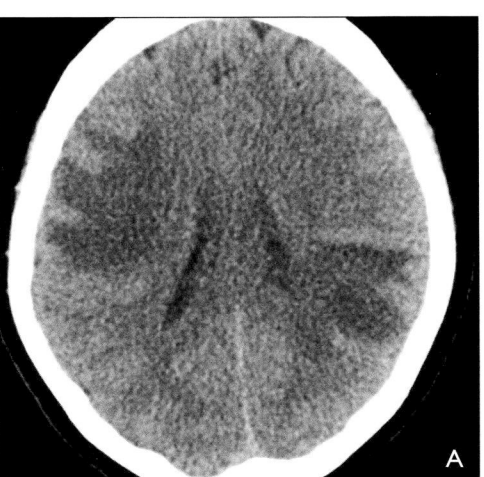
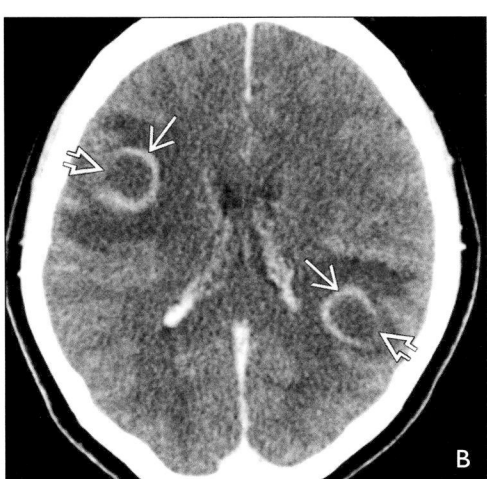

15-7A. NECT scan in a 47-year-old woman with headache, numbness, and tingling shows two areas of confluent hypodensity in the WM of both cerebral hemispheres. 15-7B. CECT shows incomplete ("horseshoe") ring enhancement ➡ surrounded by edema. The right is incomplete with the "open" end ➱ pointing toward the cortex, which appears spared. Lesions were initially called abscesses or metastases. Multiple sclerosis.

Acute MS plaques are characterized by robust inflammatory infiltration combined with features of myelin destruction. Acute lesions are often hypercellular, with large numbers of foamy macrophages and prominent perivascular T-cell lymphocytic cuffing. Normal-appearing white matter outside the plaques also frequently demonstrates immunopathologic changes including microglial activation, T-cell infiltration, and perivascular lymphocytic cuffing.

Chronic plaques range from chronic active to chronic silent lesions. Chronic active lesions have continuing inflammation around their outer borders. Chronic silent ("burned out") lesions are characterized by hypocellular regions, myelin loss, absence of active inflammation, and glial scarring.

MULTIPLE SCLEROSIS: PATHOLOGY

Location
- Supra- (90%), infratentorial (10%) (higher in children)
- Deep cerebral/periventricular WM
- Predilection for callososeptal interface
- Perivenular extension (Dawson fingers)

Size and Number
- Multiple > solitary
- Mostly small (5-10 mm)
- Giant "tumefactive" plaques can be several cm
- 30% of "tumefactive" MS lesions solitary

Gross Pathology
- Active: Yellow-tan, ill-defined margins ± edema
- Chronic active: Grayish, flat
- Chronic silent: Scarred, depressed, excavated

Microscopic Features
- Active: Hypercellular with robust inflammation, myelin destruction
- Chronic active: Inflammation around borders
- Chronic silent: Glial scarring, no active inflammation

15-8A. Sagittal T1WI in a 19-year-old woman with longstanding MS shows findings of chronic "burned out" disease. Volume loss with multiple hypointense ovoid and triangular lesions in the deep periventricular WM ➡ is present. 15-8B. Axial T1WI shows the ill-defined hyperintense rims ➡ surrounding the plaques ➡, giving the distinct "lesion-within-a-lesion" appearance.

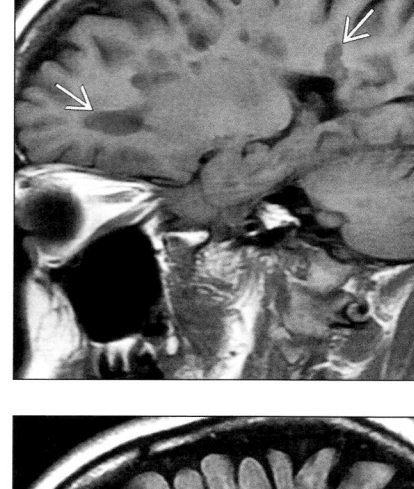
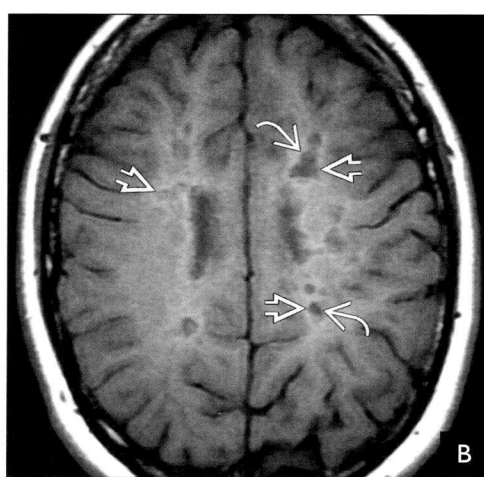

15-8C. FLAIR shows the characteristic triangle configuration of typical deep white matter MS plaques seen in the sagittal plane. The broad bases of the triangles are oriented toward the ventricular surface ➡ with the apices ➡ pointing toward the cortex. 15-8D. T2WI shows the ovoid perivenular plaques ➡ that are oriented perpendicular to the lateral ventricles as seen in the axial plane.

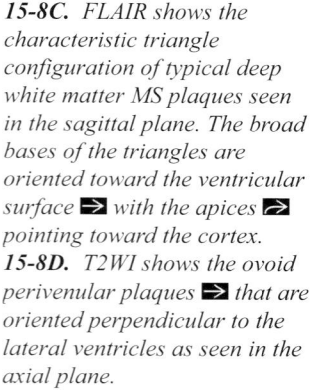
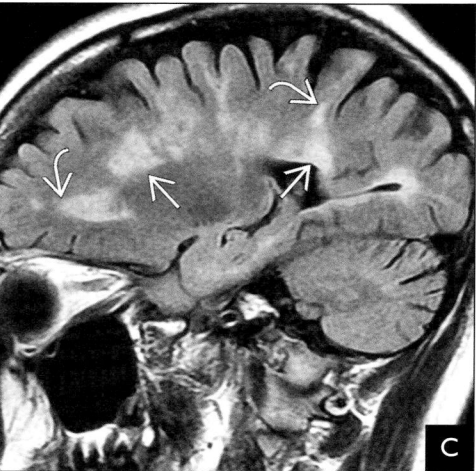
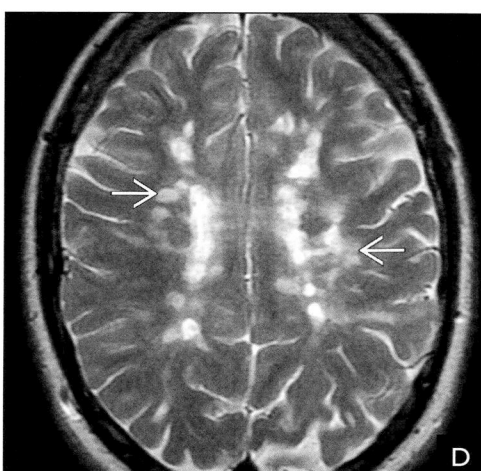

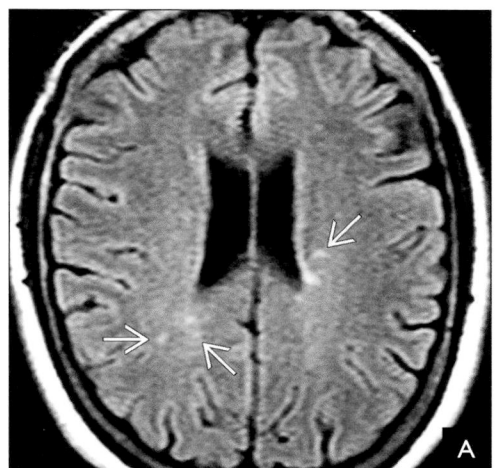

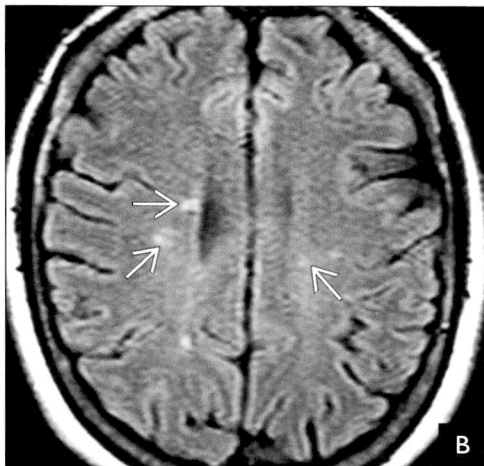

15-9A. Axial FLAIR scan in a middle-aged patient with a multi-year history of vague numbness and tingling shows a few scattered periventricular white matter hyperintensities ➡. *15-9B.* Axial FLAIR in the same patient shows additional lesions ➡. Their ovoid shape, perivenular extension, and perpendicular orientation are highly suggestive of MS.

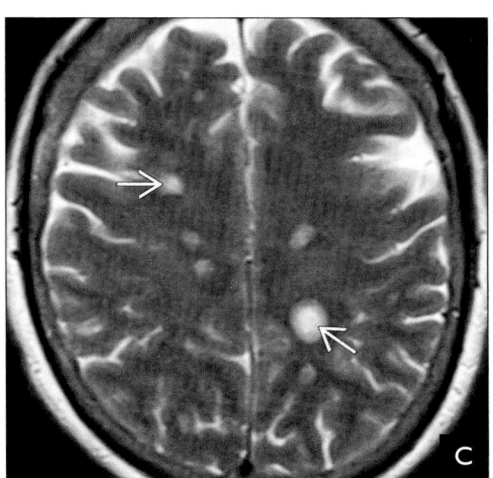

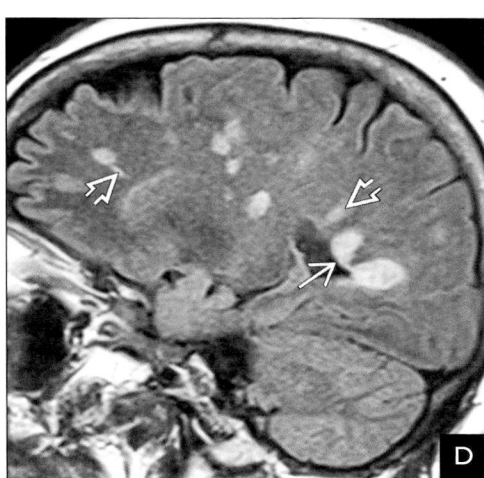

15-9C. The patient presented 2 years later with acute exacerbation of her symptoms accompanied by confusion and disorientation. Note additional white matter lesions with very hyperintense centers ➡ surrounded by slightly less hyperintense rims. *15-9D.* Sagittal FLAIR shows multiple deep WM lesions. Note triangle-shaped occipital lesions with their broad bases at the ventricular surface ➡. Several ovoid-shaped lesions ➡ surrounding medullary veins are present.

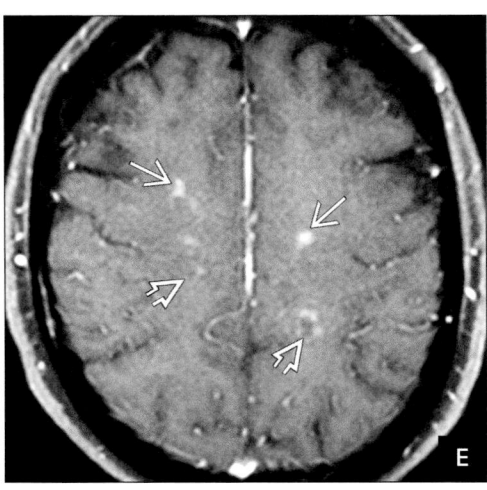

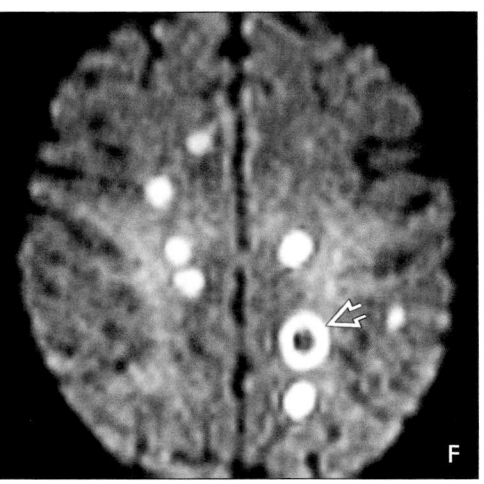

15-9E. T1 C+ FS scan shows punctate ➡ and incomplete rim enhancement ➡ in some of the lesions. *15-9F.* DWI shows multiple foci of diffusion restriction. The left parietal lesion with incomplete ("horseshoe") rim enhancement shows diffusion restriction in the periphery ➡ surrounding a nonrestricting hypointense core. The lesion was biopsied and showed typical changes of MS. The patient was later determined to have secondary progressive disease on the basis of her clinical course.

15-10A. Axial FLAIR in a 28-year-old man with 3 weeks of visual symptoms shows several hypointense white matter lesions ➡. The left hemisphere lesions demonstrate a more hypointense center surrounded by a less hypointense rim. 15-10B. T2WI shows additional lesions ➡. The large left frontal lesion has a very hyperintense center surrounded by a thin hypointense rim ⇨ and peripheral edema.

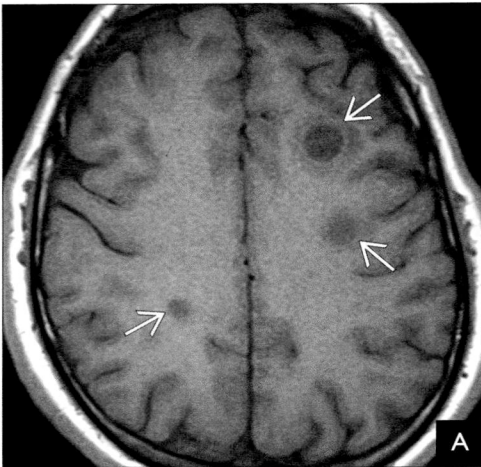

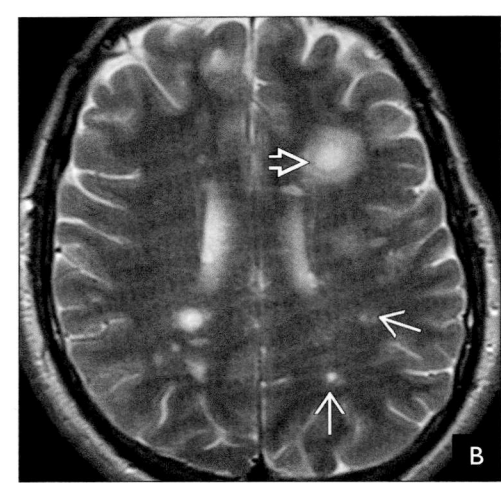

15-10C. Sagittal FLAIR shows small triangle-shaped hyperintensities at the callososeptal interface ➡. Note alternating areas of hyper- and isointensity along the undersurface of the corpus callosum ⇨, the "dot-dash" sign of early MS. 15-10D. Axial T1 C+ FS shows multiple enhancing lesions in the posterior fossa ➡, including an incomplete rim-enhancing lesion ➡ and an infiltrating lesion at the root entry zone of the left trigeminal nerve ➡.

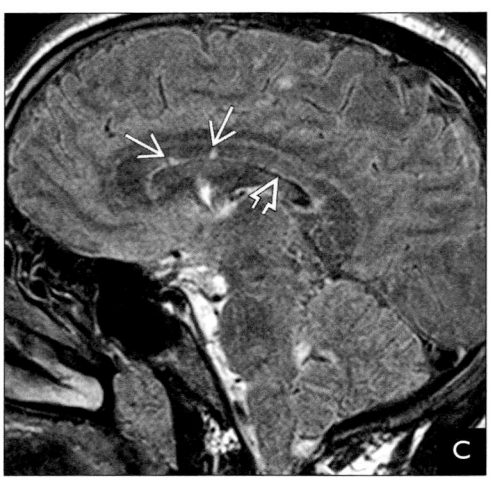

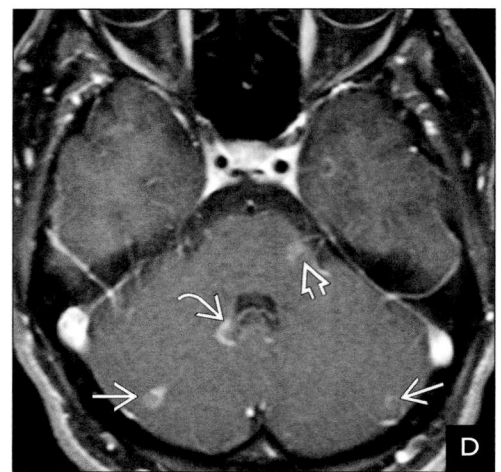

15-10E. Axial T1 C+ FS shows multiple foci of punctate and ring enhancement in the cerebral white matter. Note "target" appearance of the left frontal lesion ➡. CSF findings were consistent with a diagnosis of MS. The patient was placed on high-dose steroids. 15-10F. Repeat T1 C+ FS scan obtained 5 days later shows almost complete fading of the contrast-enhancing lesions. Steroids can dramatically reduce enhancement of MS lesions.

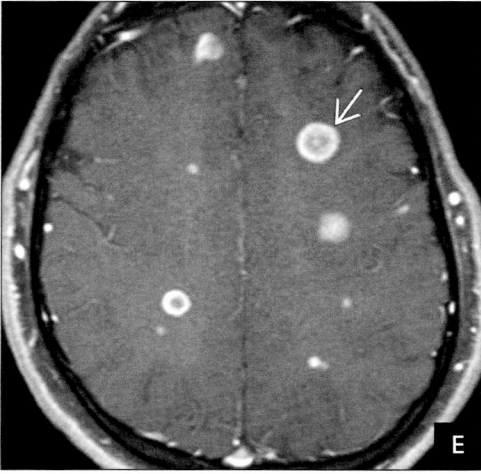

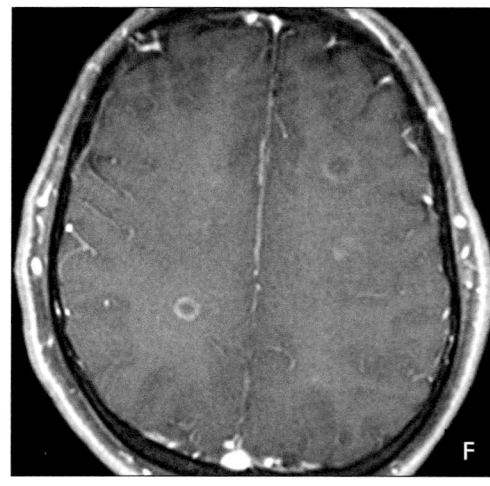

linical Issues

EPIDEMIOLOGY. MS is the most frequent primary demyelinating pathology in the CNS, affecting approximately 350,000 people in the USA and 2.5 million worldwide. It is the most common chronic nontraumatic neurological disease among young and middle-aged people in the developed world. The risk of MS is increased 15-35 times in first-order relatives of patients with clinically definite MS compared to the general population.

DEMOGRAPHICS. Onset typically occurs in young to middle-aged adults from 20-40 years of age. Although median age at initial diagnosis is approximately 30 years, up to 10% of all patients with MS become symptomatic in childhood. Between 10-25% of children initially diagnosed as having acute disseminated encephalomyelitis (ADEM) are ultimately diagnosed with MS.

The overall F:M ratio is 1.77:1, but it is higher (3-5:1) in children. Caucasians of Northern European descent living in temperate zones are the most commonly affected ethnic group. MS is significantly less common in Asians and Africans. For example, African-American men have a 40% lower MS risk than white men.

PRESENTATION. Clinical presentation varies with heterogeneous neurological manifestations, evolution, and disability. The interplay between inflammatory and neurodegenerative processes typically results in intermittent neurological disturbances followed by progressive accumulation of disabilities.

The first attack of MS (most commonly optic neuritis, transverse myelitis, or a brainstem syndrome) is known as a clinically isolated syndrome. Half of patients with optic neuritis eventually develop MS.

CLINICAL MS SUBTYPES. Four major clinical MS subtypes are recognized: Relapsing-remitting, secondary-progressive, primary-progressive, and progressive-relapsing MS. A fifth type, radiologically isolated syndrome, has recently been described.

Relapsing-remitting MS. The vast majority—about 85%—of all MS patients experience relapses alternating

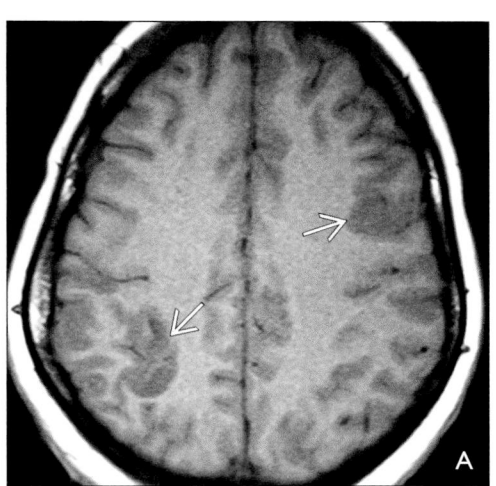

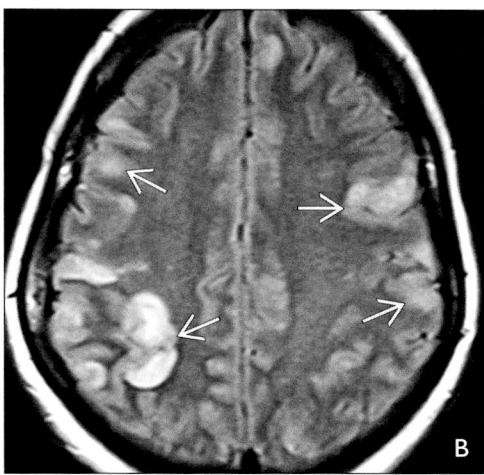

15-11A. Axial T1WI in a 32-year-old woman with psychiatric symptoms and first-time seizures shows several foci of mostly cortical hypointensity ➡. 15-11B. FLAIR scan in the same patient shows multifocal cortical and subcortical hyperintensities ➡.

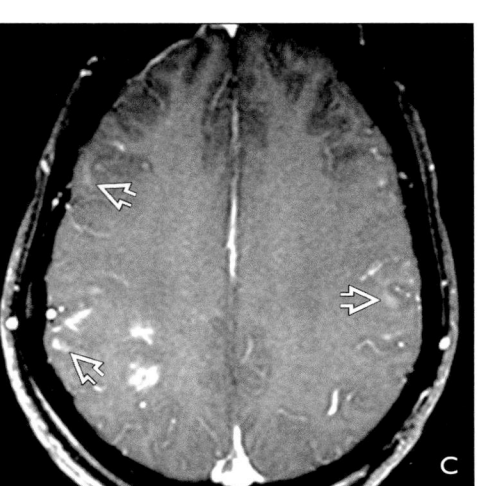

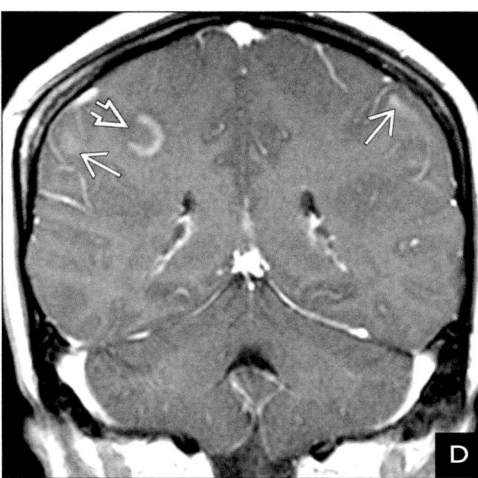

15-11C. T1 C+ FS scan shows patchy areas of cortical and subcortical enhancement ➡. 15-11D. Coronal T1 C+ scan shows an incomplete "horseshoe" ring of enhancement in the subcortical WM ➡. Other faint areas of peripheral enhancement are seen ➡. The imaging diagnosis was vasculitis, but subsequent biopsy disclosed MS.

15-12A. Series of images demonstrates "tumefactive" MS. Axial T1WI shows large heterogeneously hypointense lesions in both cerebral hemispheres ➡ with significant perilesional edema ⬦.
15-12B. T2WI shows that the lesions ➡ are very hyperintense and surrounded by a thin hypointense rim ➡ and perilesional edema ⬧.

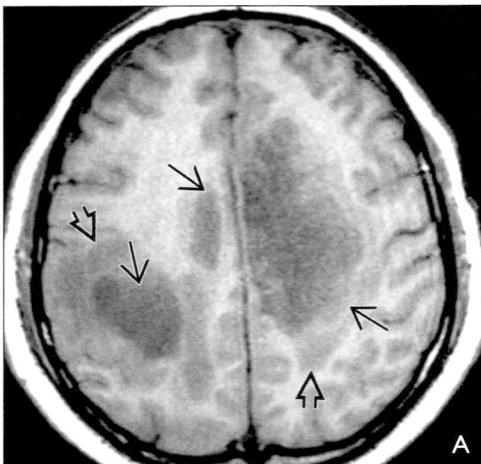

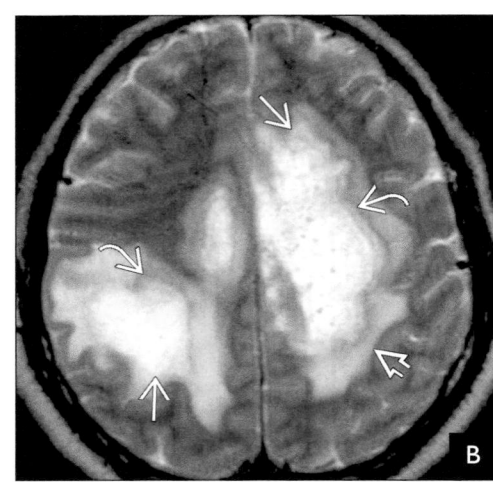

15-12C. The hypointense rims of the lesion show striking but incomplete ring enhancement ➡. *15-12D.* DWI shows that the enhancing rims restrict moderately ➡.

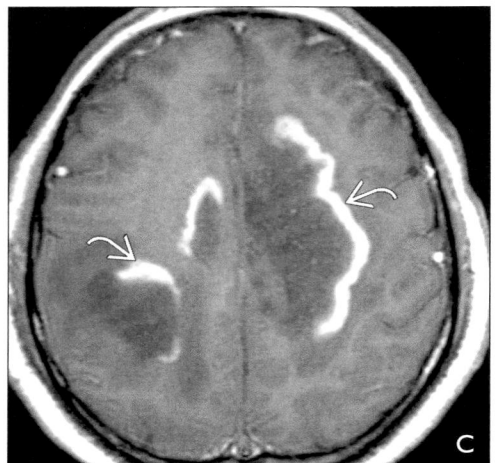

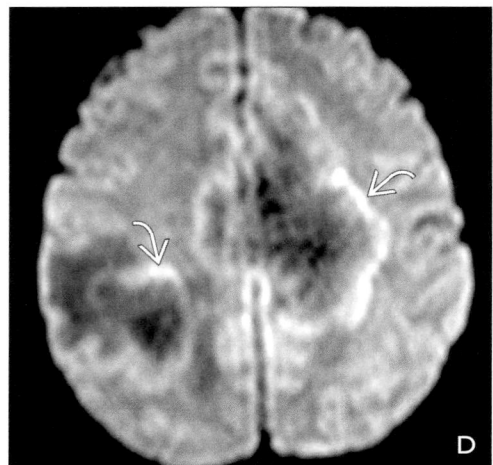

15-12E. The rims demonstrate low ADC values ➡ in this patient with biopsy-proven "tumefactive" MS. (Courtesy P. Rodriguez, MD.) *15-13.* Autopsy specimen in another case demonstrates typical findings of "tumefactive" demyelination with a horseshoe-shaped demyelinating mass ➡, the "open" end ⬦ toward the cortex. (Courtesy R. Hewlett, MD.)

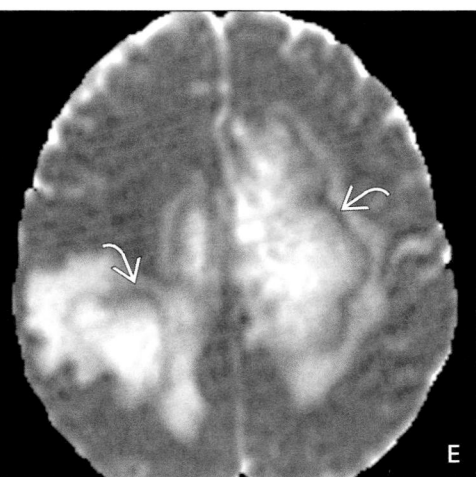

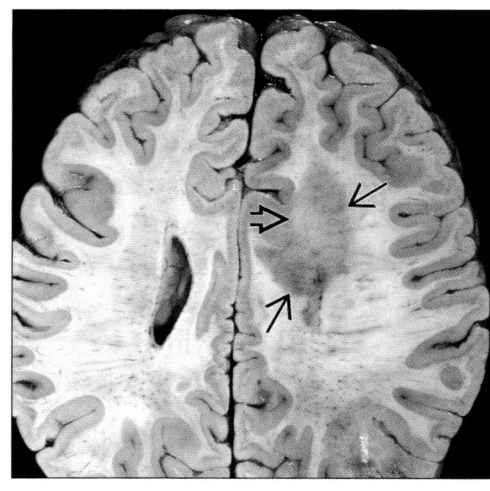

with remission phases and are classified as having relapsing-remitting MS (RR MS).

Secondary-progressive MS. Secondary-progressive MS (SP MS) is also called relapsing-progressive MS. Almost half of RR MS patients enter an SP stage within 10 years. By 25 years following initial diagnosis, 90% of RR MS cases become the SP MS subtype.

Primary-progressive MS. Primary-progressive MS (PP MS) is progressive from the outset and lacks periods of remission. Approximately 5-10% of patients have PP MS.

Progressive-relapsing MS. This rare form of MS is characterized by progressive disease with clear acute relapses interposed between episodes of variable recovery.

Radiologically isolated syndrome. Radiologically isolated syndrome (RIS) refers to MR findings suggestive of MS in persons without typical MS symptoms and with a normal neurological examination. Half of the patients with RIS are initially imaged because of headache; some have subclinical cognitive impairment similar to that seen in MS.

NATURAL HISTORY. Natural history varies. The majority of MS patients follow a protracted course with gradual deterioration and increasing disability. Approximately one-third have an initial episode followed by normal or near-normal function. Acute rapid neurologic deterioration without remission is uncommon.

Approximately two-thirds of patients with RIS show evidence of imaging progression; one-third develop neurological symptoms within five years. Cortical and cervical cord lesions are important predictors of conversion to clinically definite MS. Pregnancy seems to shorten the time to conversion from RIS in some patients.

TREATMENT OPTIONS. Treatment options are numerous and continue to evolve. Immunosuppressant and immunomodulatory regimens are typically included. While the initiation and management of immunomodulatory drugs has to be individualized, studies have shown both a significant decrease in relapse rate and a reduction of brain lesion accumulation when therapy is introduced at an early stage.

The diagnosis of CCSVI in MS and the use of venous angioplasty to treat it is highly controversial. Some investigators claim that endovascular treatment reduces relapse rates and cumulative disability in patients with RR MS, but randomized controlled studies assessing clinical efficacy have not been performed.

MULTIPLE SCLEROSIS: CLINICAL ISSUES

Epidemiology
- Most common CNS primary demyelinating disease
- Most common chronic neurologic disease in young

Demographics
- Peak onset = 20-40 years (10% in childhood)
- F:M = almost 2:1
- Risk ↑ 15-35x in first-order relatives of MS patients
- Caucasians > > Africans, Asians
- Temperate zone > > tropics

Presentation
- Optic neuritis (50% develop clinically definite MS)
- Sensory, motor disturbances

Clinical MS Subtypes
- Relapsing-remitting (85%)
- Secondary-progressive (RR often becomes SP)
- Primary-progressive (5-10%)
- Progressive-relapsing (rare)

Imaging

GENERAL FEATURES. Tissue loss with generalized brain atrophy is common. Atrophy begins early in the disease and progresses throughout its course. Enlarged ventricles and sulci with white matter volume loss and a thinned corpus callosum are typical findings.

CT FINDINGS. NECT is often normal early in the disease course, especially with mild cases. Solitary or multiple ill-defined white matter hypodensities may be present. Acute or subacute lesions may show mild to moderate punctate, patchy, or ring enhancement on CECT (15-7). Enhancement increases with delayed or double-dose scans.

MR FINDINGS. Over 95% of patients with "clinically definite" MS have positive findings on MR scans. Therefore, MR is the procedure of choice for both initial evaluation and treatment follow-up. The most recent revised McDonald criteria for MS diagnosis rely on MR imaging to demonstrate dissemination in both space and time (see below).

REVISED McDONALD CRITERIA FOR MS DIAGNOSIS

Dissemination in Space
- ≥ 1 T2 hyperintense lesion(s)
- In at least 2 of the following 4 areas
  - Periventricular
  - Juxtacortical
  - Infratentorial
  - Spinal cord

Dissemination in Time
- *Either* new T2 or Gd-enhancing lesion(s) on follow-up MR
- *Or* simultaneous presence of
  - Asymptomatic Gd-enhancing *and*
  - Nonenhancing lesions at any time

15-14A. *Sagittal T1WI in a 53-year-old man with severe longstanding MS shows a strikingly thinned corpus callosum* ➡️. *The sulci are widened, the lateral ventricle* ➡️ *is enlarged, and the midbrain appears atrophic* ➡️. **15-14B.** *Axial T1WI shows severe bifrontal volume loss, large sulci and ventricles, and numerous cavitating periventricular WM plaques* ➡️.

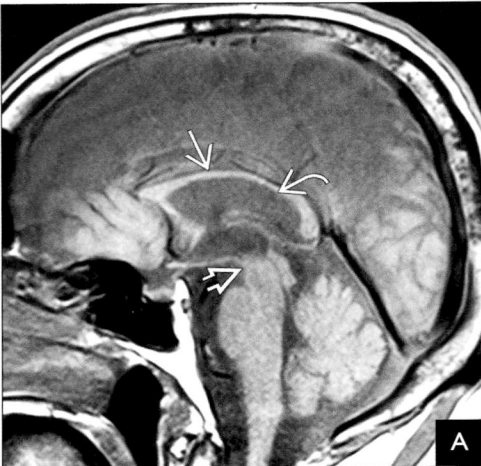
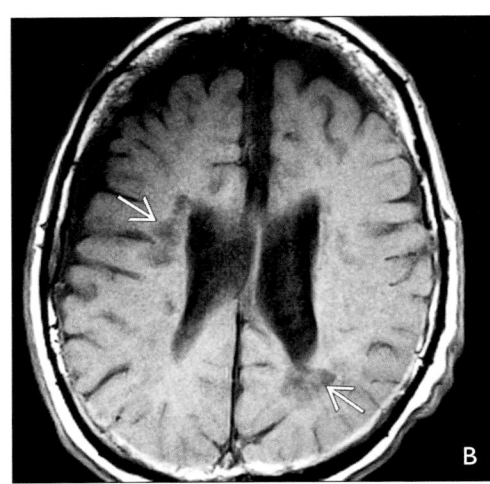

15-14C. *T2WI through the basal ganglia shows the volume loss, periventricular confluent demyelination* ➡️. *The basal ganglia* ➡️ *and thalami* ➡️ *appear profoundly hypointense.* **15-14D.** *FLAIR scan better demonstrates the extensive confluent periventricular demyelination* ➡️.

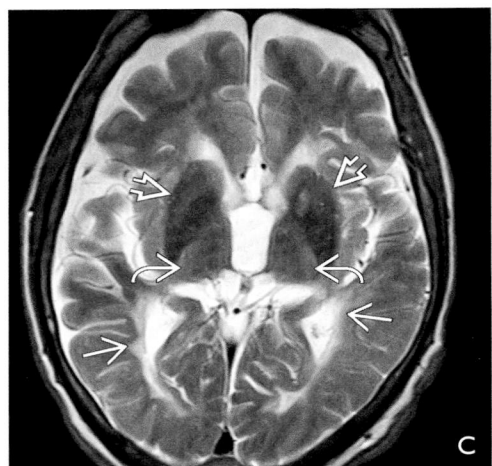
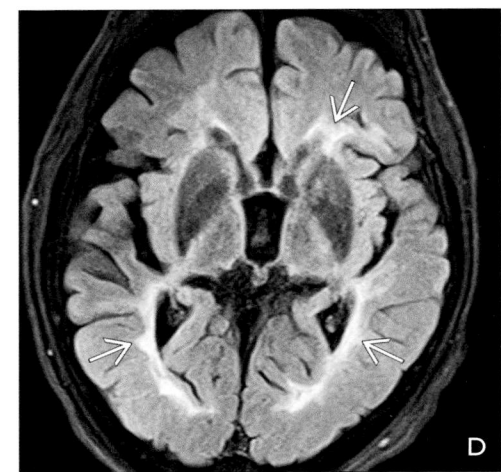

15-14E. *FLAIR scan through the upper lateral ventricles shows extensive confluent WM hyperintensity* ➡️ *with multiple cavitating foci* ➡️. **15-14F.** *Sagittal FLAIR scan shows the unusually extensive periventricular demyelination, atrophy. The frontal* ➡️ *and convexity* ➡️ *sulci, volume loss are especially prominent.*

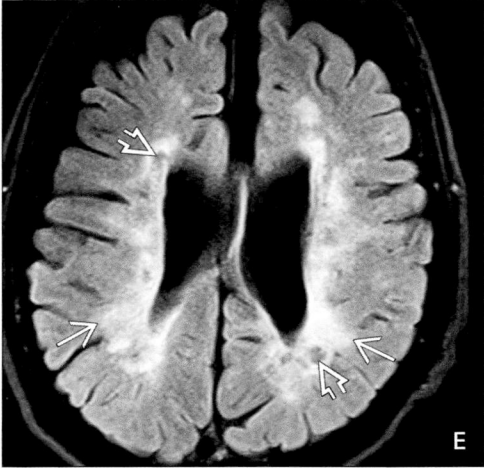
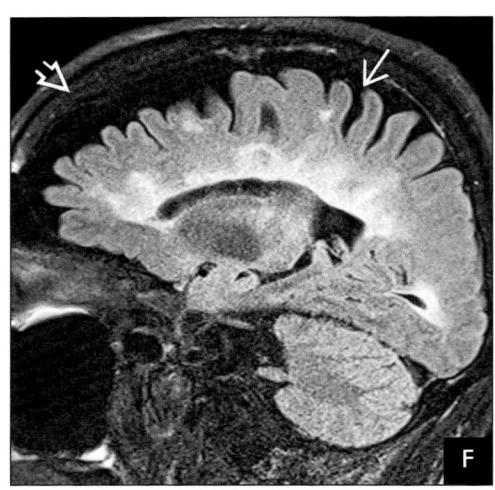

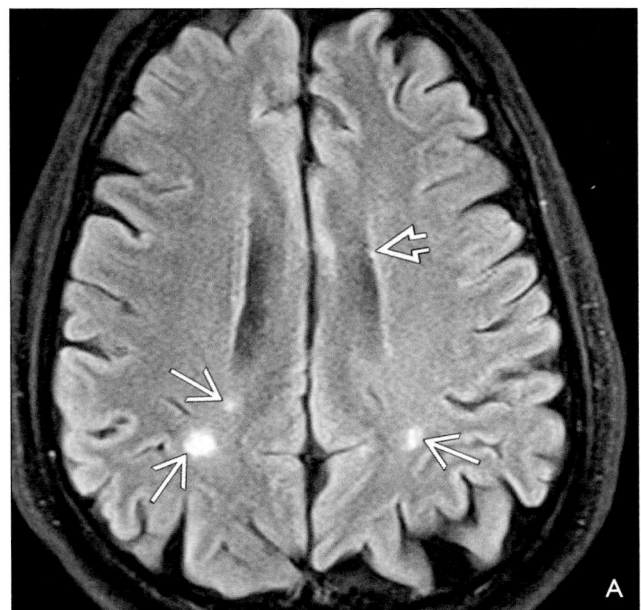

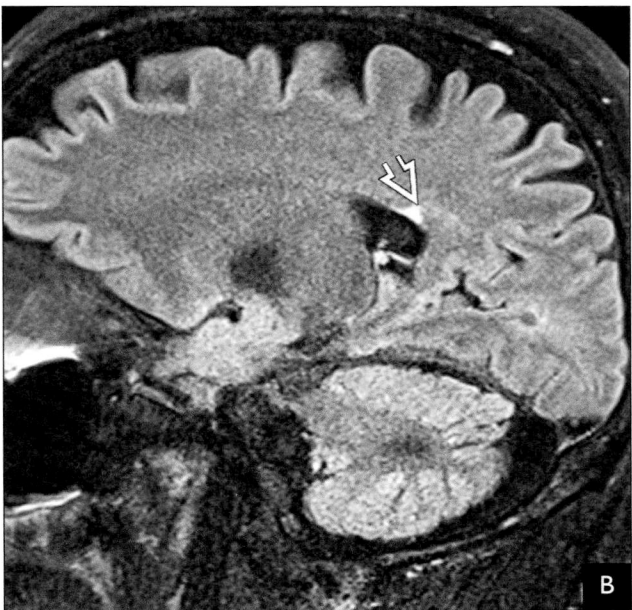

15-15A. FLAIR scan in a neurologically normal 58-year-old woman scanned for headache shows at least 3 definite ➡ and 1 probable ⇉ deep WM hyperintensities.

15-15B. Sagittal FLAIR scan shows a classic triangular lesion ⇉ suggesting MS. Radiologically isolated syndrome. CSF studies were positive for MS.

T1WI. Most MS plaques are hypo- or isointense on T1WI. The hypointensity ("black holes") correlates with axonal destruction. T1 hyperintensity is an independent predictor of atrophy, disability, and advancing disease. A faint, poorly delineated peripheral rim of mild hyperintensity secondary to lipid peroxidation and macrophage infiltration often surrounds sharply delineated hypointense "black holes." This gives many subacute and chronic lesions a characteristic "beveled" or "lesion-within-a-lesion" appearance **(15-8)**.

Chronic and severe cases typically show moderate volume loss and generalized atrophy. The corpus callosum becomes progressively thinner and is best delineated on sagittal T1WI.

T2/FLAIR. T2WI shows multiple hyperintense linear, round, or ovoid lesions surrounding the medullary veins that radiate centripetally away from the lateral ventricles. Larger lesions often demonstrate a very hyperintense center surrounded by a slightly less hyperintense peripheral area and variable amounts of perilesional edema **(15-9)**.

MS plaques often assume a distinct triangular shape with the base adjacent to the ventricle on sagittal FLAIR or T2WI images **(15-9C)**. One of the earliest findings is alternating areas of linear hyperintensity along the ependyma on sagittal FLAIR, known as the "ependymal 'dot-dash'" sign **(15-10)**.

Cortical demyelinating lesions are common and present in early MS and may even precede the appearance of classic WM plaques in some patients **(15-11)**.

Basal ganglia hypointensity is seen in 10-20% of chronic moderate to severe MS cases and is probably secondary to degenerative changes with heavy metal ion deposition **(15-14)**.

T1 C+. MS plaques demonstrate transient enhancement during the active stage of demyelination. Punctate, nodular, and rim patterns are seen **(15-10)**. A prominent incomplete rim ("horseshoe") of enhancement with the "open" nonenhancing segment facing the cortex can be present **(15-11)**, especially in large "tumefactive" lesions **(15-12)**, **(15-13)**.

Enhancement disappears within six months in more than 90% of lesions. Steroid administration significantly reduces lesion enhancement and conspicuity and may render some lesions virtually invisible **(15-10)**.

DWI. The overwhelming majority of acute plaques show normal or *increased* diffusivity, not restricted diffusion. While a few acute MS plaques can demonstrate restriction on DWI, such an appearance is atypical and should not be considered a reliable biomarker of active plaques **(15-9)**.

MRS. MRS may allow early distinction between relapsing-remitting and secondary-progressive MS. Secondary-progressive MS shows decreased NAA in normal-appearing gray matter consistent with axonal/neuronal loss or dysfunction. Myoinositol levels are elevated in acute lesions and are also increased in normal-appearing white matter. "Tumefactive" MS shows nonspecific findings (elevated choline, decreased NAA, and high lactate).

Advanced imaging techniques. Some studies using DTI have reported reduced longitudinal diffusivity in areas of axonal injury. Others have used magnetization transfer imaging (MTI) to detect subtle myelin loss in nonlesional tissue (i.e., normal-appearing white matter). While these techniques may be useful to measure treatment changes in populations and to characterize pathophysiology, they are rarely helpful in refining the diagnosis for an individual patient. When the diagnosis of MS is uncertain based on brain imaging findings, it is probably more helpful to image the spinal cord.

Differential Diagnosis

Multifocal T2/FLAIR "white spots" are nonspecific imaging findings and have a broad differential diagnosis. Hyperintensities in the correct location (callososeptal interface, periventricular) or of the correct shape (triangular) may represent "radiologically isolated" early MS **(15-15)**. It is helpful to suggest whether such lesions do or do not meet McDonald criteria.

Multifocal enhancing white matter lesions can be caused by acute disseminated encephalomyelitis (ADEM), autoimmune-mediated vasculitis, and Lyme disease. **ADEM** usually has a history of viral prodrome or recent vaccination. **Vasculitis** often preferentially involves the basal ganglia and spares the callososeptal interface. **Lyme disease** (LD) can appear identical to MS. Cranial nerve enhancement is more common in LD than in MS.

Susac syndrome (see below) is often mistaken for MS on imaging studies as both have multifocal T2/FLAIR white matter hyperintensities and both commonly affect young adult women. Lesions in Susac syndrome preferentially involve the middle of the corpus callosum, not the callososeptal interface.

"Tumefactive" MS can mimic **abscess** or **neoplasm** (**glioblastoma multiforme** [GBM] or **metastasis**). *"Tumefactive" demyelination often has an incomplete or "horseshoe" pattern of enhancement.* **Progressive multifocal leukoencephalopathy** (PML) and **immune reconstitution inflammatory syndrome** (PML-IRIS) occur in a few MS patients treated with natalizumab. Irregular, "wild" enhancement in such cases may be difficult to distinguish from acute "tumefactive" MS.

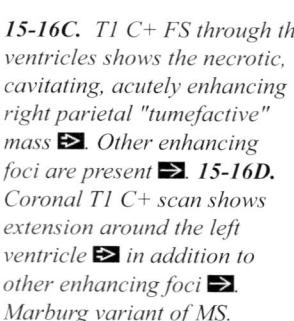

15-16A. A 26-year-old man presented with a short history of visual disturbances and left upper extremity weakness followed by rapid onset of numbness and then quadriplegia. Axial FLAIR scan shows a large heterogeneously hyperintense lesion in the right parietal white matter ➡ with a smaller lesion on the left ⮞. 15-16B. Axial T1 C+ FS in the same case shows multiple bilateral incomplete ring-enhancing lesions ⮞ in the deep and periventricular white matter.

15-16C. T1 C+ FS through the ventricles shows the necrotic, cavitating, acutely enhancing right parietal "tumefactive" mass ⮞. Other enhancing foci are present ➡. 15-16D. Coronal T1 C+ scan shows extension around the left ventricle ⮞ in addition to other enhancing foci ➡. Marburg variant of MS.

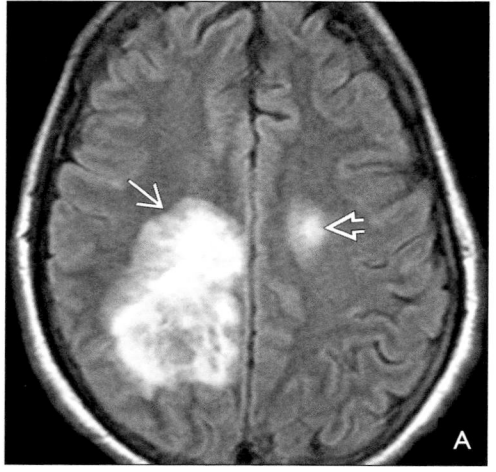

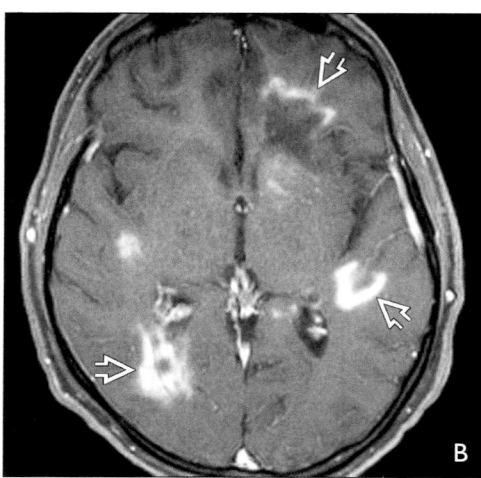

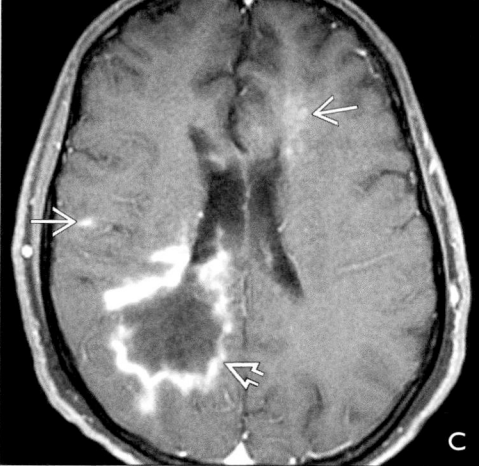

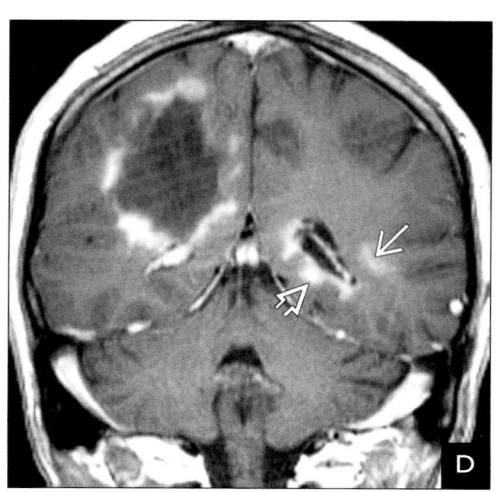

MULTIPLE SCLEROSIS: IMAGING

CT
- Patchy/confluent hypodensities
- Mild/moderate, patchy, ring enhancement

MR
- Hypointense on T1WI ± faint hyperintense rim
- Very hyperintense center on T2WI, slightly less hyperintense rim
  - Callososeptal interface
  - Triangular on sagittal
  - Ovoid, perivenular on axial
  - Subpial, intracortical lesions common
- Active plaques enhance ("tumefactive" partial rim)
- Steroids suppress enhancement

Differential Diagnosis
- Multifocal T2/FLAIR hyperintensities
  - ADEM, Lyme disease
  - Vasculitis, Susac syndrome
- Solitary "tumefactive" MS
  - Neoplasm (GBM, metastasis)
  - PML/PML-IRIS in natalizumab-treated MS

Other Neuroinflammatory Demyelinating Diseases

Several rare neuroinflammatory disorders are grouped into an umbrella category called idiopathic inflammatory demyelinating diseases (IIDDs). IIDDs are classified according to clinical symptoms and signs, lesion distribution, neuroimaging features, and CSF characteristics.

The three general categories of idiopathic inflammatory demyelinating lesions (IIDLs) are (1) fulminant or acute IIDLs (e.g., Marburg disease, Schilder disease, and Balo concentric sclerosis), (2) monosymptomatic IIDLs (e.g., isolated optic neuritis), and (3) IIDLs restricted to a particular geographic distribution (e.g., neuromyelitis optica and isolated transverse myelitis). Some of these unusual IIDLs such as Marburg disease and Balo concentric sclerosis are probably MS variants and are discussed below as such. Others—e.g., neuromyelitis optica—are now considered completely different entities.

Multiple Sclerosis Variants

In this section, we briefly delineate three unusual but important IIDDs that affect the brain and often present as an acute fulminating demyelinating disorder: Marburg disease, Schilder disease, and Balo concentric sclerosis.

Marburg Disease

TERMINOLOGY AND CLINICAL ISSUES. Marburg disease (MD) is an acute fulminant MS variant character-ized by rapid, relentless progression and an exceptionally severe clinical course. Patients are typically young adults.

MD course is generally monophasic. Striking neurologic deterioration occurs within days or weeks after onset. Death within a year—usually secondary to brainstem involvement—is common.

PATHOLOGY. MD lesions are much more destructive than typical MS plaques and are characterized histopathologically by massive macrophage infiltration, necrosis, and severe axonal injury. Multiple lesions throughout the brain and spinal cord often form large coalescent white matter plaques.

IMAGING. Imaging shows multifocal diffusely disseminated disease with focal and confluent white matter hyperintensities on T2/FLAIR. Strong patchy enhancement on T1 C+ is typical, and large, cavitating, incomplete, ring-enhancing, "tumefactive" lesions are common **(15-16).**

MARBURG DISEASE

Clinical Issues
- Rare acute fulminate MS variant
  - Rapid neurologic deterioration
  - Monophasic, relentless progression
  - Death usually within 1 year
- Usually young adults

Pathology and Imaging
- Multifocal > solitary disease
  - Characterized by coalescent WM plaques
  - Brain (including posterior fossa), spinal cord lesions
- Lesions characterized by massive inflammation, necrosis
- Imaging shows diffusely disseminated disease
  - Large cavitating lesions
  - Incomplete ("open") enhancing rim
  - Multiple other patchy enhancing foci

Schilder Disease

TERMINOLOGY AND CLINICAL ISSUES. Schilder disease (SD)—also known as myelinoclastic diffuse sclerosis—is a rare disorder characterized by one or more inflammatory demyelinating white matter plaques. SD is typically a disease of childhood and young adults. Median age at presentation is 18 years, with a slight female predominance.

Clinical features are atypical for MS and include signs of increased intracranial pressure, aphasia, and behavioral symptoms. CSF is usually normal, and there is no history to suggest acute disseminated encephalomyelitis (ADEM) (i.e., no fever, infection, or preceding vaccination). Approximately 15% of cases progress to MS.

PATHOLOGY. Solitary unilateral masses are present in two-thirds of cases. Most are large lesions, measuring several centimeters in diameter.

The histopathologic features of SD consist of WM demyelination, lymphocytic perivascular infiltrates, and microglial proliferation.

IMAGING. Imaging shows a subcortical hypodense lesion on NECT scans. MR shows a hypointense lesion on T1WI that is hyperintense on T2/FLAIR. Rim enhancement—often the incomplete or "open ring" pattern—is seen during the acute inflammatory stage **(15-17)**.

The lesion rim usually restricts on DWI during the acute phase. MRS is nonspecific, showing a decreased but present NAA peak with increased Cho:Cr ratio. Lactate and lipid-lactate complexes are common.

DIFFERENTIAL DIAGNOSIS. The differential diagnosis of SD can be difficult. **"Tumefactive" MS** can appear identical to SD on imaging studies. SD often mimics intracranial neoplasm or abscess both in clinical presen-

tation and on imaging studies. **Pyogenic abscess** generally shows strong diffusion restriction in the lesion core. Perfusion MR may be helpful in distinguishing SD from **metastasis** and **glioblastoma multiforme**.

Balo Concentric Sclerosis

TERMINOLOGY AND CLINICAL ISSUES. Balo concentric sclerosis (BCS) is a rare aggressive MS variant usually characterized by acute onset and rapid clinical deterioration. Peak presentation is between 20 and 50 years. Most reported cases occur in young adult males.

Not all cases of BCS are rapidly progressive and invariably fatal. BCS occasionally follows a relatively benign course without clinically apparent relapsing episodes.

PATHOLOGY. BCS is an inflammatory demyelinating disease related to MS. The pathologic hallmark of BCS is a peculiar pattern of concentric rings that resembles a tree trunk or onion bulb. Large demyelinated plaques with alternating rims of myelin preservation and destruction give the lesion its characteristic appearance **(15-18)**. BCS can occur as a solitary mass or, less commonly, as multiple lesions.

15-17A. Axial T2WI in a 12-year-old girl shows a solitary hyperintense left parietal mass ➥ that involves the subcortical white matter. Note relatively minimal mass effect for the size of the lesion. Perilesional edema is absent. 15-17B. Axial T1 C+ in the same patient shows incomplete or "open ring" peripheral enhancement with the nonenhancing margin just beneath the cortex.

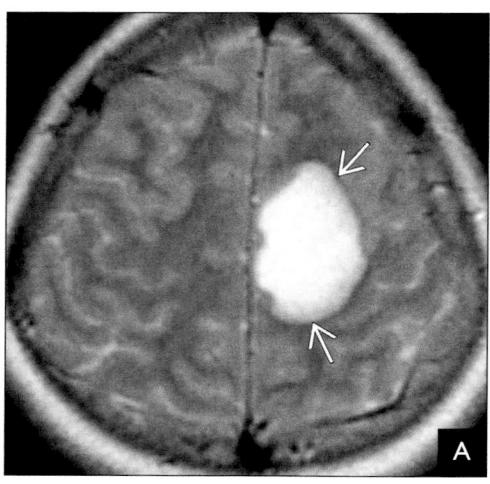
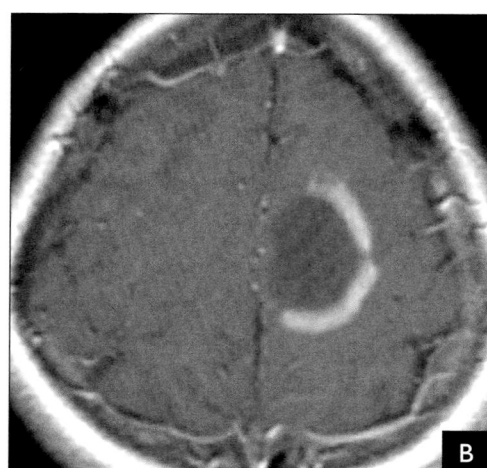

15-17C. Sagittal T1 C+ shows the incomplete or "horseshoe" pattern of enhancement especially well. Note lack of significant mass effect on the underlying lateral ventricle. 15-17D. Coronal T1 C+ again demonstrates the partial rim enhancement along the deep and lateral surfaces of the mass. Biopsy-proven Schilder disease.

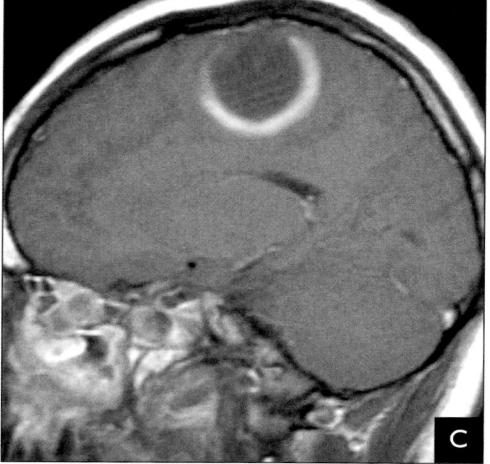
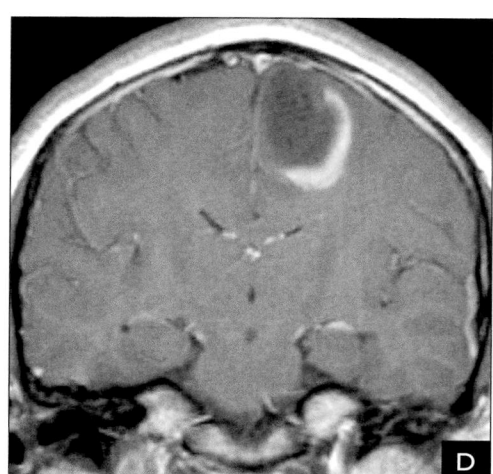

IMAGING. Imaging studies reflect the distinctive gross pathology of BCS and vary with disease stage. Acute lesions have significant surrounding edema. Two or more alternating bands of differing signal intensities are seen on T2WI and resemble a "whirlpool" of concentric rings. The actively demyelinating layers enhance on T1 C+ sequences **(15-19A)**. Other more typical MS-like plaques can also be present.

Mild to moderate diffusion restriction is seen in the outermost rings on DWI. MRS findings are nonspecific and resemble those of MS (e.g., elevated choline with decreased NAA).

Subacute or chronic BCS shows two or more alternating bands of iso- and hypointensity on T1WI. The concentric layers appear iso- and hyperintense on T2WI **(15-19B)**. Edema and mass effect are minimal, and the lesions do not enhance on T1 C+.

DIFFERENTIAL DIAGNOSIS. The concentric ring pattern ("onion bulb" or "whirlpool" appearance) is highly suggestive of the diagnosis. A somewhat similar "bull's-eye" configuration is occasionally seen in **relapsing MS**, but the classic multiple layered bands are absent. **ADEM** also lacks distinctive band-like layers.

OTHER MS VARIANTS

Schilder Disease
- Myelinoclastic diffuse sclerosis
  - Rare acute/subacute demyelinating disorder
  - Lesions may resolve; 15% progress to MS
- Young adults
  - Mean age at onset = 18 years
- Clinical features atypical for MS, ADEM
  - CSF normal
  - No history of fever, flu, vaccination
- Solitary > multifocal lesions
- Lesions look like "tumefactive" MS
- Differential diagnosis: Neoplasm, abscess

Balo Concentric Sclerosis
- Concentric rings of demyelination/myelin preservation
  - Resemble tree trunk or onion bulb
  - Solitary > multifocal
- "Whirlpool" hyperintense concentric rings on T2WI
  - Minimal mass effect, edema
- Actively demyelinating layers enhance

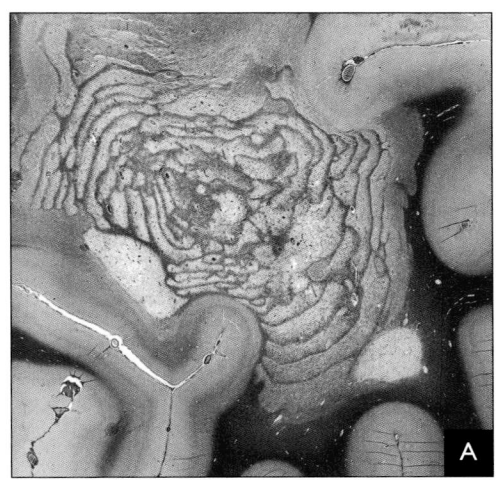

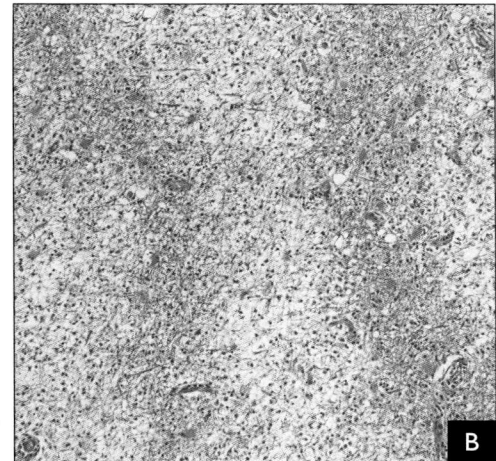

15-18A. Luxol fast blue myelin stain shows gross pathology findings of Balo concentric sclerosis. Note concentric rings of demyelinated, pale-staining areas alternating with the thinner blue layers of preserved myelin. 15-18B. High-power H&E stain in the same case shows pale pink demyelinated areas alternating with darker pink layers of preserved myelin. (Courtesy B. K. DeMasters, MD, and S. Ludwin, MD.)

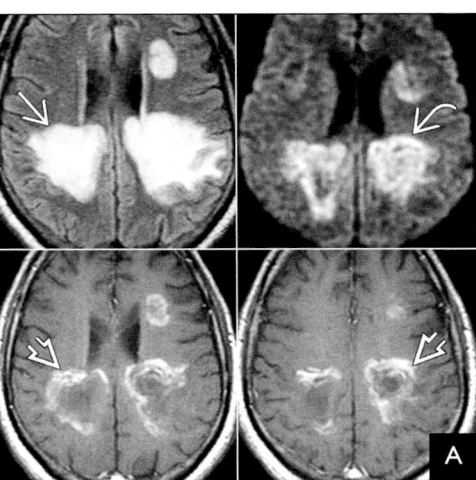

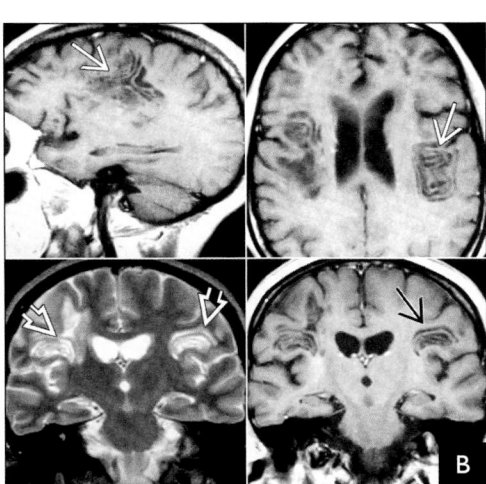

15-19A. Acute Balo concentric sclerosis is illustrated by the fluffy-appearing confluent WM lesions on FLAIR ➡. The lesions restrict on DWI ➡, show concentric laminated ("onion bulb") enhancement ➡. 15-19B. Follow-up scans after acute symptoms subsided show alternating rings of iso- and hyperintensity on T1 scans ➡ and iso-/hyperintensity on T2WI ➡. No enhancement is seen on T1 C+ ➡. (Courtesy P. Rodriguez, MD.)

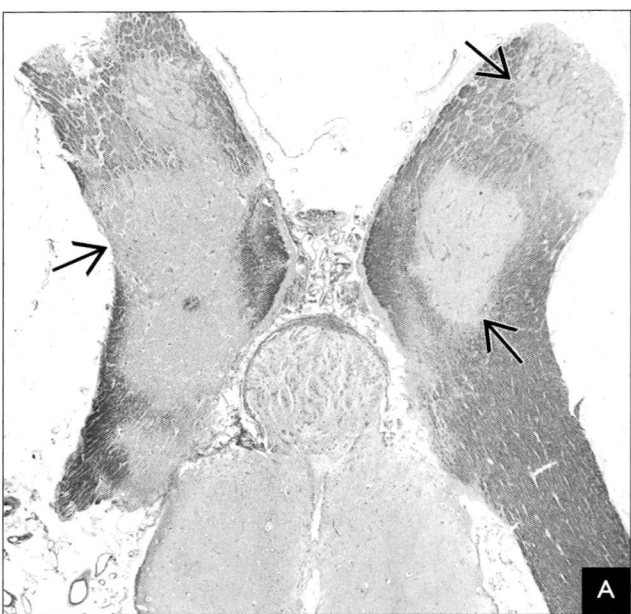

15-20A. Luxol fast blue stain of a section through the optic chiasm shows classic demyelinating foci characteristic of neuromyelitis optica ➡.

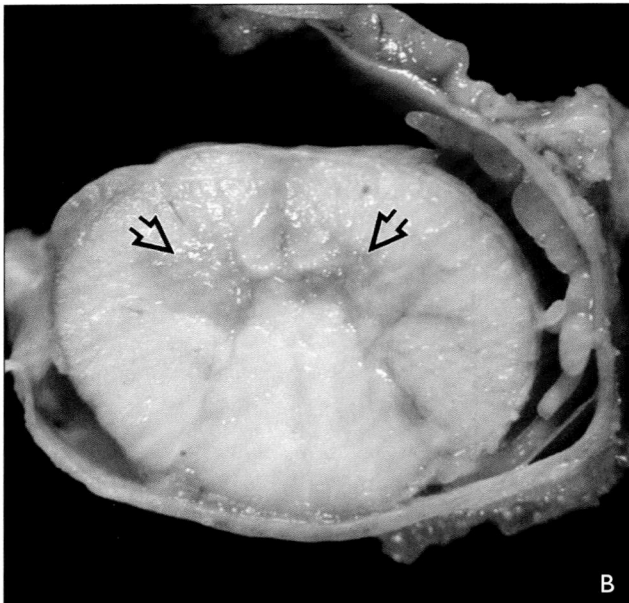

15-20B. Axially sectioned spinal cord in the same case shows cavitating central cord lesions ➡. (Courtesy R. Hewlett, MD.)

Neuromyelitis Optica

Terminology

Neuromyelitis optica (NMO)—also known as **Devic syndrome**—is classified as one of the idiopathic inflammatory demyelinating disorders with restricted topographical distribution. Several other entities are also considered part of the **NMO spectrum disorders** (see below).

NMO is a severe form of acute demyelinating disease that preferentially involves the spinal cord and optic nerves. The cerebral white matter is relatively spared.

Etiology

NMO was once considered a "special form" of MS but is now recognized as a distinct entity. NMO is a B-cell mediated disease characterized by the presence of antibodies to aquaporin-4 (AQP4). AQP4 is the most abundant water channel in the CNS and is located in the foot processes of astrocytes surrounding the blood-brain barrier.

A specific biomarker of the disease, NMO-IgG, is 90% specific and 70-75% sensitive for NMO. NMO-IgG is almost always negative in MS and other autoimmune disorders, such as Sjögren syndrome and SLE.

Pathology

LOCATION. One or both optic nerves are involved. together with the spinal cord. The cervical cord is most commonly affected, and lesions typically extend over three or more consecutive segments (15-20).

MICROSCOPIC FEATURES. Selective AQP4 loss and vasculocentric complement and immunoglobulin deposition are characteristic. Note, however, that antibody-independent AQP4 loss also occurs in other demyelinating conditions, namely Balo disease and some cases of MS.

It is the *immunohistochemical* staining pattern of NMO-IgG that is diagnostic. NMO-IgG binds to the abluminal face of microvessels at sites of immune complex deposition in NMO lesions. Actively demyelinating NMO lesions demonstrate vessel hyalinization, a finding not present in MS or ADEM.

Clinical Issues

NMO SPECTRUM DISORDERS. The spectrum of NMO disorders has recently expanded beyond standard Devic disease. The NMO spectrum now includes limited forms such as recurrent longitudinally extensive myelitis and bilateral simultaneous or recurrent optic neuritis, Asian optic-spinal MS, optic neuritis or myelitis associated with lesions in specific brain areas (e.g., hypothalamus, periventricular nucleus, and brainstem), and myelitis/optic neuritis associated with systemic autoimmune disease.

EPIDEMIOLOGY AND DEMOGRAPHICS. NMO is far less common than MS. NMO is most common in Caucasian women with a F:M ratio of nearly 3:1. Although onset varies from childhood to the elderly, mean age at initial diagnosis is 35-40 years. The yearly incidence of NMO in Caucasians is estimated at 0.4 per million person-years.

NMO SPECTRUM DISORDERS

Neuromyelitis Optica (NMO)
- Also known as Devic disease/syndrome

Other NMO Spectrum Disorders
- Recurrent longitudinally extensive myelitis
- Bilateral simultaneous/recurrent optic neuritis
- Asian optic-spinal MS
- Optic neuritis or myelitis + specific brain lesions
- Optic neuritis or myelitis + systemic autoimmune disease

Etiology and Pathology
- Aquaporin-4 antibodies
- Vasculocentric IgG deposition

PRESENTATION AND NATURAL HISTORY. NMO can be idiopathic or related to other clinical entities (e.g., viral or bacterial infections, connective tissue or endocrine disorders). It is characterized by severe uni- or bilateral optic neuritis and transverse myelitis occurring simultaneously at disease onset. Involvement of other CNS regions sometimes occurs later in the disease course.

NMO follows an unpredictable course, but prognosis is generally worse than for MS. The vast majority of cases (85-90%) are relapsing, but NMO occasionally occurs as a monophasic illness. Relapsing NMO generally results in severe residual injury that accumulates with each subsequent attack.

Almost 30% of NMO patients are initially misdiagnosed with MS. NMO-IgG seropositivity is detected in 3-5% of patients who have a clinically isolated syndrome at the time of initial presentation.

TREATMENT OPTIONS. Recent studies suggest that the therapeutic options in NMO should be immunosuppressive rather than immunomodulatory drugs. Rituximab decreases the frequency of attacks and helps mitigate disability.

Imaging

MR is the procedure of choice in evaluating patients with suspected NMO. Imaging during an acute attack shows (1) a hyperintense, enhancing cord lesion that extends over three or more contiguous vertebral segments and (2)

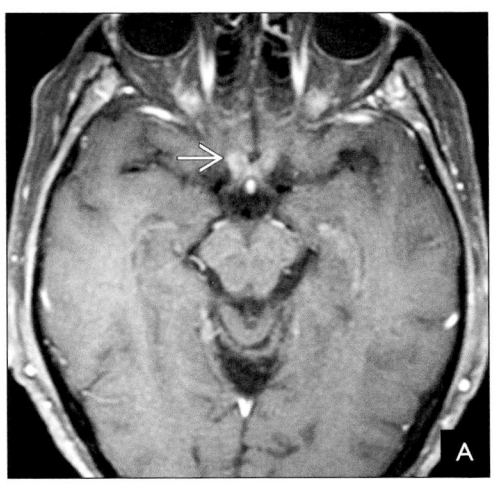
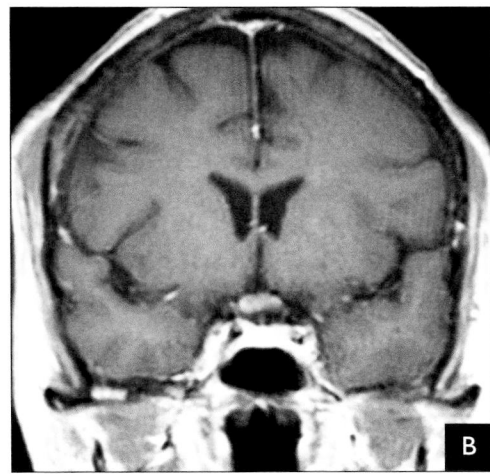

15-21A. Axial T1 C+ FS in a patient with serologically proven NMO shows optic chiasm enhancement →. 15-21B. Coronal T1 C+ scan in the same patient confirms the optic chiasm enhancement. T2/FLAIR scans (not shown) showed no evidence of other lesions.

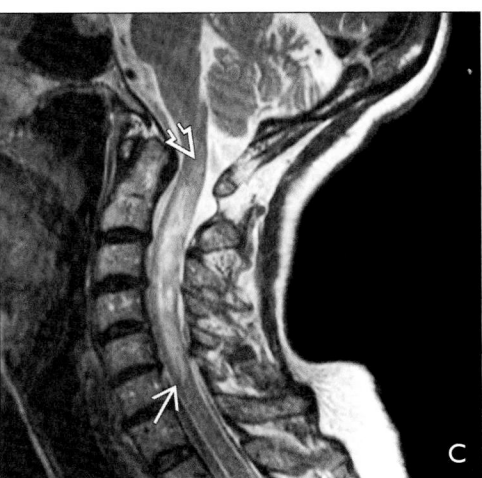
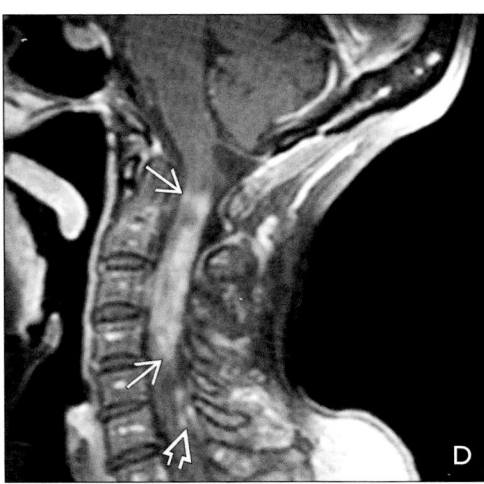

15-21C. Sagittal T2WI in the same patient shows patchy central hyperintensity extending from the lower medulla → to C5-C6 →. The cervical cord appears moderately swollen and symmetrically enlarged. 15-21D. T1 C+ scan shows confluent heterogeneous enhancement from the upper C2 to the C4-5 interspace → and a smaller patchy region at C6 →.

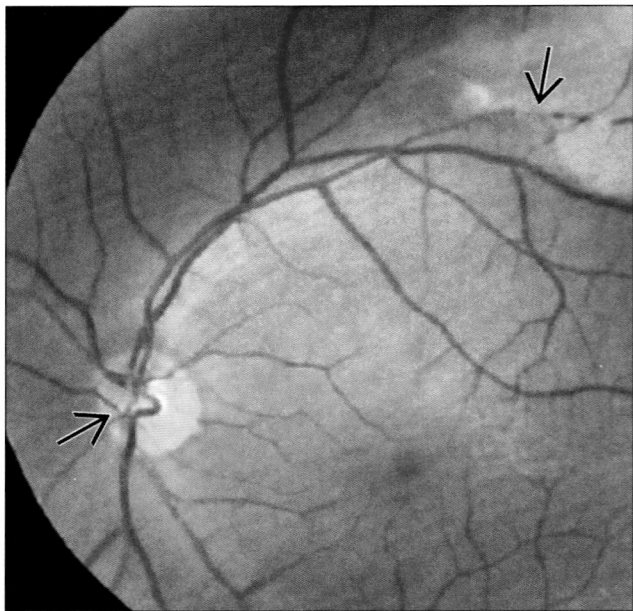

15-22. Funduscopic examination shows multiple retinal artery branch occlusions and irregularities ➔.

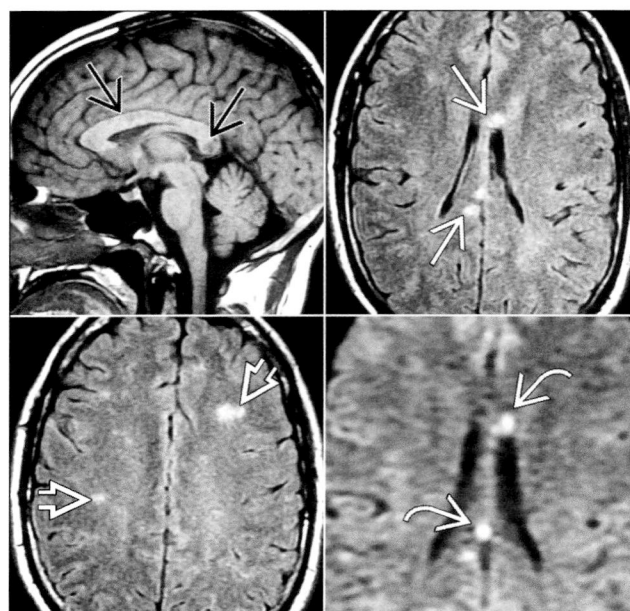

15-23. Classic findings of Susac syndrome with middle callosal "holes" on sagittal T1WI ➔, multifocal ovoid callosal ➔ and WM hyperintensities ➔ on FLAIR, diffusion restriction on DWI ➔. (Courtesy P. Rodriguez, MD.)

optic nerve hyperintensity and/or enhancement, consistent with acute optic neuritis (15-21).

Between 30-60% of NMO patients also have nonspecific T2/FLAIR hyperintensities in the cerebral white matter, so this finding does *not* exclude the diagnosis.

DWI in NMO shows higher diffusivity and lower FA compared to MS.

Differential Diagnosis

The major differential diagnosis of NMO is MS. The brain is more involved in **multiple sclerosis** while multisegmental contiguous spinal cord disease is typical of NMO. NMO must also be distinguished from cases of **isolated optic neuritis** and **transverse myelitis**, both of which are components of NMO.

REVISED NMO DIAGNOSTIC CRITERIA

Required
- Optic neuritis
- Acute myelitis
- Hyperintense, enhancing cord lesion ≥ 3 segments

Plus Two or More Supportive Criteria
- Disease-onset MR imaging nondiagnostic for MS
- Contiguous spinal cord lesions on MR ≥ 3 vertebral segments
- NMO-IgG seropositivity

Susac Syndrome

Susac syndrome is a relatively recently recognized syndrome that is often mistaken for MS on imaging studies.

Nevertheless, Susac has a distinct clinical presentation and highly suggestive imaging appearance.

Terminology

Susac syndrome (SS) is also known as retinocochleocerebral vasculopathy, RED-M (for **r**etinopathy, **e**ncephalopathy, and **d**eafness-associated **m**icroangiopathy), and SICRET (**s**mall **i**nfarcts of **c**ochlear, **r**etinal, and **e**ncephalic **t**issue).

Etiology

Most investigators have concluded SS is a multisystem immune-mediated microvascular occlusive endotheliopathy and not a true primary demyelinating disorder.

Pathology

The findings are those of a microangiopathy with microinfarcts. The infarcts can be acute or subacute and involve either the cortex or white matter or both. The microvasculature is abnormal. Intraluminal hyaline thrombi, perivascular inflammatory changes with aggregates of macrophages, and prominent activated endothelial cells are typical histologic features of SS.

Clinical Issues

EPIDEMIOLOGY. SS is a rare disorder. Its true prevalence is unknown, but the incidence is probably more common than previously thought, as many SS cases have been misdiagnosed as MS.

DEMOGRAPHICS. SS predominantly affects young adult women between 20-40 years. Mean age at presentation is 35 years. The F:M ratio is 3-5:1.

PRESENTATION. The classic clinical triad in SS consists of acute or subacute encephalopathy, sensorineural hearing loss, and branch retinal artery occlusions (15-22), although not all patients initially present with the full triad. SS encephalopathy is characterized by severe or migrainous headaches in 50% of cases. Inflamed retinal arterioles with branch retinal artery occlusions are typically present at fluorescein angiography.

Waxing and waning changes in mental status with memory impairment, confusion, and behavioral and psychiatric disturbances are common, often dominant features. Hearing loss is typically low- to mid-frequency and can be uni- or bilateral, symmetric or asymmetric. Associated vertigo, ataxia, and nystagmus are common.

Muscle and skin lesions ("livedo racemosa") have also been reported in patients with SS.

NATURAL HISTORY. The clinical course of SS is unpredictable. It is often but not invariably self-limited, resolving within two to four years. Some patients have a relapsing-remitting course, while others experience permanent neurologic deficits (most commonly deafness and impaired vision).

TREATMENT OPTIONS. The management goal is to prevent permanent neurologic damage. Early, aggressive, and sustained immunosuppressive therapy is recommended. Intravenous glucocorticoids with the addition of immune globulin or cyclophosphamide in refractory cases have produced a good response in many patients.

Imaging

CT FINDINGS. NECT and CECT scans are usually normal. Temporal bone CT is helpful to exclude other causes of sensorineural hearing loss.

MR FINDINGS. Sagittal T1WI in patients with chronic SS may show typical "punched-out" hypointense lesions in the middle layers of the corpus callosum (15-23). T2/FLAIR shows multiple periventricular and deep white matter hyperintensities in over 90% of cases (15-24). Almost 80% show corpus callosal involvement with

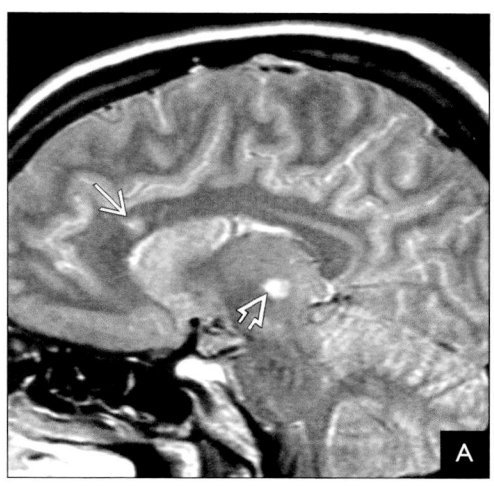

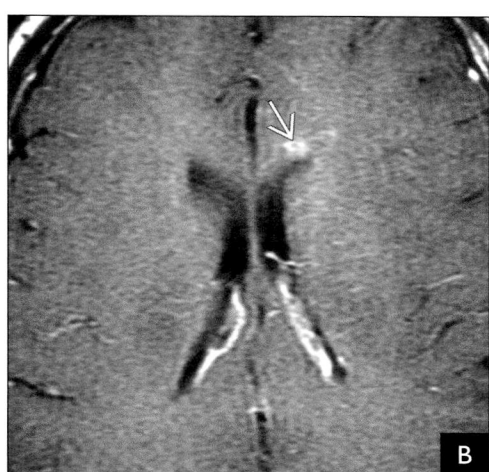

15-24A. A 27-year-old woman presented with headaches, blurred vision, dizziness, and buzzing and ringing in both ears. Sagittal T2WI shows 2 hyperintense foci, one in the middle of the corpus callosum genu ➡ and a second lesion in the thalamus ➡. 15-24B. Axial T1 C+ shows that the corpus callosum genu lesion ➡ enhances.

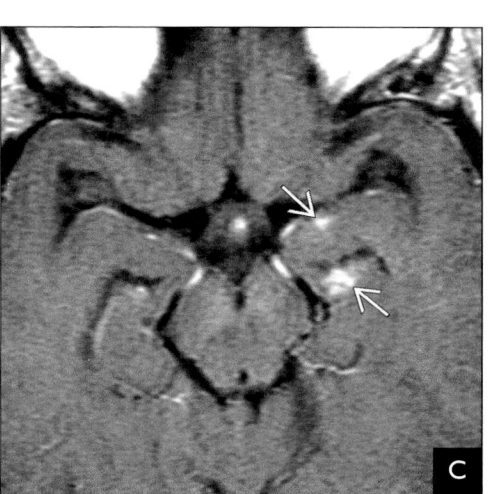

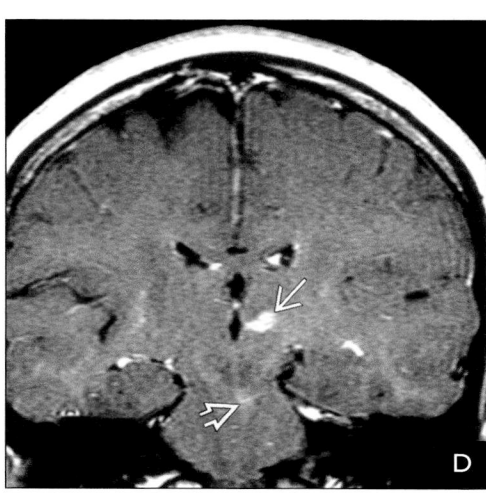

15-24C. Close-up view of axial T1 C+ through the suprasellar cistern shows 2 additional enhancing lesions ➡ in the left temporal lobe. 15-24D. Coronal T1 C+ shows that the left thalamic lesion ➡ enhances. Another small enhancing lesion is present in the mid-pons ➡. Imaging findings plus clinical history are virtually diagnostic of Susac syndrome.

15-25A. Series of FLAIR scans demonstrates progressive disease in a patient with Susac syndrome. Initial sagittal FLAIR scan shows 2 hyperintense lesions in the middle of the corpus callosum splenium ➡.

15-25B. More lateral scan demonstrates multiple punctate and ovoid hyperintensities in the subcortical and deep white matter ➡. A lesion is also present in the thalamus ⇉.

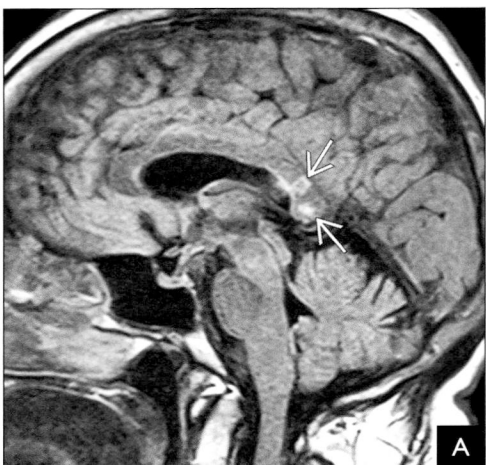
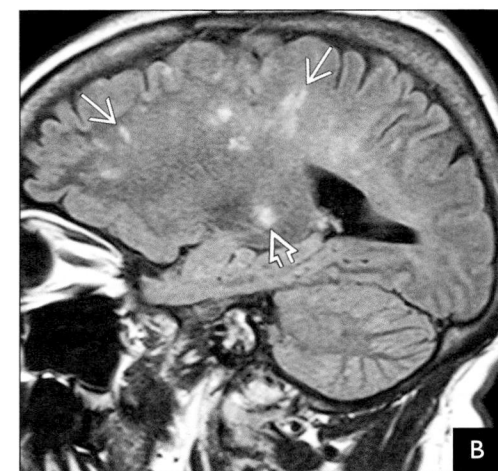

15-25C. Axial FLAIR shows multiple punctate, ovoid hyperintensities ➡. There are also confluent deep WM lesions of lesser hyperintensity in both parietal lobes ⇨. *15-25D.* The patient's symptoms continued to worsen. Nearly 18 months later, she was almost completely blind and deaf. Repeat sagittal FLAIR scan shows marked interval volume loss with thin corpus callosum and widened sulci.

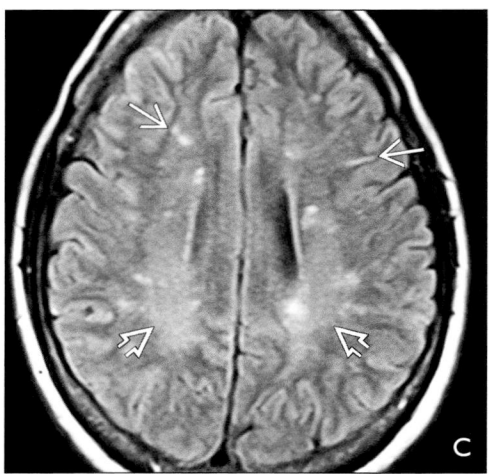
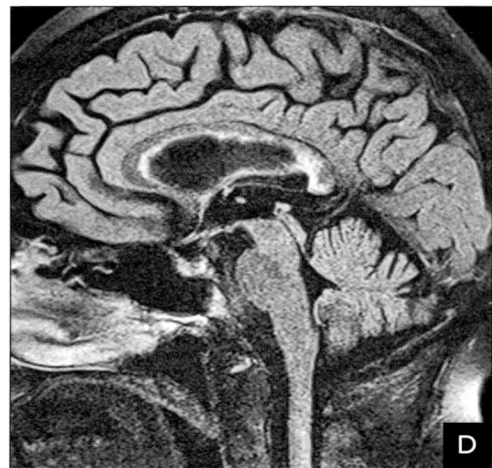

15-25E. Sagittal FLAIR scan now shows confluent deep periventricular WM lesions ➡ that involve most of the corona radiata but spare the subcortical association fibers. The lateral ventricle is significantly enlarged compared to the comparable scan from 18 months earlier. *15-25F.* Axial FLAIR scan now shows sulcal widening, enlargement of the lateral ventricles, confluent WM disease. Severe progression in Susac syndrome is uncommon but clinically devastating.

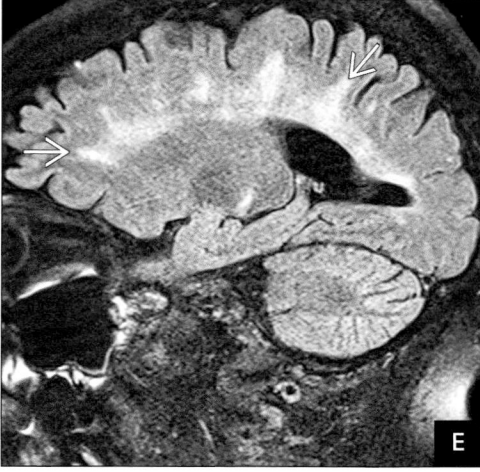
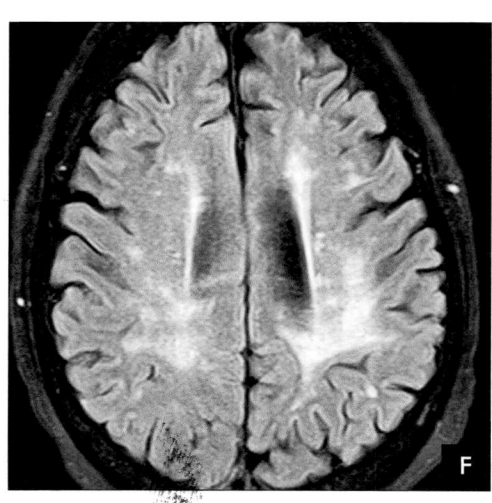

lesions that typically involve the middle of the corpus callosum and spare the undersurface **(15-25)**. Basal ganglia lesions occur in 70% of cases and brainstem lesions in nearly one-third **(15-24)**.

Acute SS lesions show punctate enhancement on T1 C+. Leptomeningeal enhancement occurs in 30% of patients. DTI shows widespread white matter disruption with focal damage to the corpus callosum genu.

Differential Diagnosis

The major imaging differential diagnoses of SS are MS, ADEM, and Lyme disease. **Multiple sclerosis** preferentially involves the undersurface of the corpus callosum, which is usually spared in SS. Auditory involvement with hearing loss is unusual in MS.

ADEM and **Lyme disease** rarely involve the middle layers of the corpus callosum. ADEM is generally monophasic, preceded by a viral prodrome or history of vaccination.

Vasculitis and **thromboembolic infarcts** are other differential considerations. Both rarely affect the corpus callosum.

SUSAC SYNDROME

Terminology
- Retinocochleocerebral vasculopathy

Etiology and Pathology
- Immune-mediated
  - Probably not true demyelinating disorder
- Occlusive microendotheliopathy
  - Perivascular inflammation with microinfarcts

Clinical Issues
- F > > M
- Clinical triad
  - Headache, encephalopathy
  - Sensorineural hearing loss
  - Vision abnormalities

Imaging
- T2/FLAIR WM hyperintensities (> 90%)
  - Involvement of corpus callosum (CC) (80%)
  - Middle of CC > > callososeptal interface
- Basal ganglia lesions (70%)
- Variable enhancement (usually punctate)

Differential Diagnosis
- Multiple sclerosis
- ADEM
- Lyme disease
- Vasculitis

Post-Infection/Post-Immunization Demyelination

Some investigators consider acute disseminated encephalomyelitis and acute hemorrhagic leukoencephalopathy part of the idiopathic inflammatory demyelinating disease spectrum. As they are associated with antecedent viral infection or immunization, we consider them separately here.

Acute Disseminated Encephalomyelitis

Terminology

Acute disseminated encephalomyelitis (ADEM) is a post-infection, post-immunization disorder that is also called **parainfectious encephalomyelitis**. Once considered a purely monophasic illness, recurrent and multiphasic forms of ADEM are now recognized.

Etiology

The immunohistopathologic features of ADEM mimic those of experimental allergic encephalitis, an induced autoimmune disease precipitated by myelin antibodies. Therefore, most investigators consider ADEM an immune-mediated CNS demyelinating disorder.

Pathology

LOCATION. As the name implies, ADEM can involve both the brain and spinal cord. White matter lesions usually predominate, but basal ganglia involvement is seen in nearly half of all cases. Spinal cord lesions are found in 10-30%.

A rare ADEM variant, acute infantile bilateral striatal necrosis, occurs one to two weeks following a respiratory illness. Viral and streptococcal infections have been implicated and cause enlarged hyperintense basal ganglia, caudate nuclei, and interna/external capsules.

SIZE AND NUMBER. Lesion size varies from a few millimeters to several centimeters ("tumefactive" ADEM) and have a punctate to flocculent configuration. Multiple lesions are more common than solitary lesions.

GROSS PATHOLOGY. Small lesions are often inapparent on gross examination. Large "tumefactive" lesions cause a gray-pink white matter discoloration and often extend all the way to the cortex-white matter junction **(15-26)**. Mass effect is minimal compared to lesion size. Gross

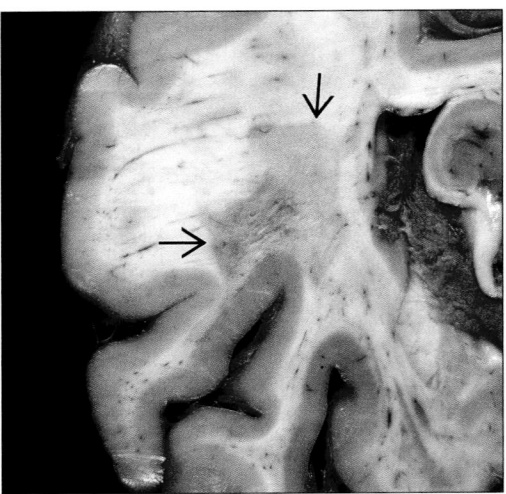

15-26. *Autopsy shows necrotizing demyelination* ➡ *characteristic of post-infection, post-vaccination disorders. (Courtesy R. Hewlett, MD.)*

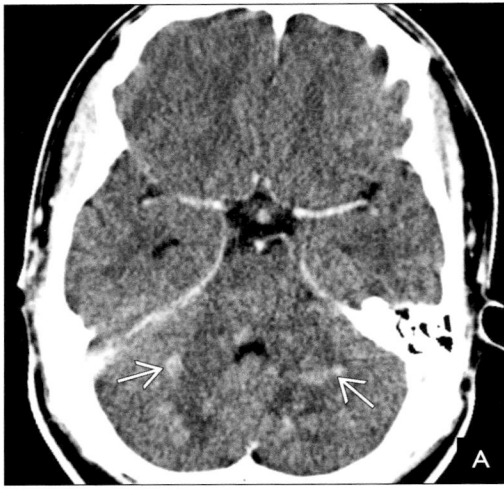

15-27A. *Axial CECT in a patient with ADEM shows multifocal enhancing lesions in the posterior fossa* ➡.

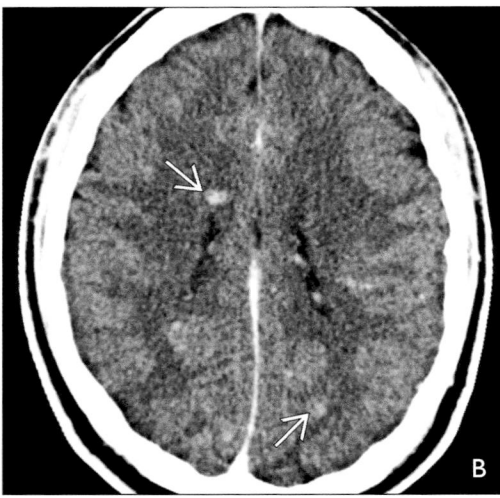

15-27B. *Axial CECT in the same patient also shows supratentorial enhancing lesions* ➡.

intralesional hemorrhage is rare and is more characteristic of acute hemorrhagic leukoencephalitis (AHLE) than ADEM.

MICROSCOPIC FEATURES. "Sleeves" of pronounced perivenular demyelination with macrophage-predominant inflammatory infiltrates are typical. The outer margins of ADEM lesions are indistinct compared to the relatively well-delineated edges of MS plaques. Viral inclusion bodies are generally absent, unlike viral encephalitis.

Clinical Issues

EPIDEMIOLOGY AND DEMOGRAPHICS. ADEM is second only to MS as the most common acquired idiopathic inflammatory demyelinating disease. Unlike MS, there is no female predominance. ADEM occurs most commonly in spring and autumn.

ADEM can occur at any age but—perhaps because of the frequency of immunizations and antigen exposure—is more common in childhood, with peak occurrence between five and eight years. The overall estimated incidence is 0.8 per 100,000 persons annually. The incidence of childhood ADEM is estimated at 2-10 cases per million children per year. Between 10-25% of children with ADEM are eventually diagnosed with MS.

PRESENTATION. Symptoms typically occur a few days to a few weeks following antigenic challenge (e.g., infection or vaccination). The majority of children with ADEM have a nonspecific febrile illness preceding onset. Viral exanthema is usually absent. Unlike MS, optic neuritis is rare.

NATURAL HISTORY. Disease course and outcome vary. **Monophasic ADEM** is the most common type. However, the disease sometimes follows an atypical course, waxing and waning over a period of several months.

Recurrent ADEM is characterized by a second episode occurring more than three months after the initial illness and involving the *same* anatomic area(s) as the original illness. **Multiphasic ADEM** is characterized by one or more subsequent events that involve a *different* anatomic area as demonstrated by a new lesion on MR or a new focal neurologic deficit.

More than half of all patients recover completely within one or two months after onset, while approximately 20% experience some residual functional impairment. Overall mortality is relatively high (10-25%).

ACUTE DISSEMINATED ENCEPHALOMYELITIS (ADEM)

Etiology and Pathology
- Post-infection, post-immunization
- Immune-mediated perivenular demyelination

Clinical Issues
- Second only to MS as acquired demyelinating disease
- No female predominance
- Occurs at all ages, but children 5-8 years most affected
- Course, outcome vary
  - Monophasic ADEM: Most common
  - Recurrent ADEM: Second episode, same site
  - Multiphasic ADEM: Multiple episodes, different sites
- Recover completely (> 50%)
- Mortality (10-25%)

Imaging

CT FINDINGS. Unless large "tumefactive" lesions are present, NECT is usually normal. CECT may show multifocal punctate or partial ring-enhancing lesions (15-27).

MR FINDINGS. T1WI is often normal or shows only "dirty" grayish foci in the white matter. Multifocal hyperintensities on T2/FLAIR are the most common findings and vary from small round/ovoid foci to flocculent "cotton ball" lesions with very hyperintense centers surrounded by slightly less hyperintense areas with "fuzzy" margins (15-28).

Bilateral but asymmetric involvement is typical. Basal ganglia and posterior fossa lesions are common.

T1 C+ scans show enhancement that varies from minimal or none to striking and intense (15-29). Punctate, linear, ring, and incomplete ring patterns all occur. Large "tumefactive" lesions with horseshoe-shaped enhancement resemble "tumefactive" MS (15-30). Unlike MS, cranial nerve enhancement is relatively common in ADEM.

Severe acute lesions may show restriction on DWI. MRS is nonspecific with low NAA and elevated lactate. The magnetization transfer ratio (MTR) in normal-appearing white matter is usually normal.

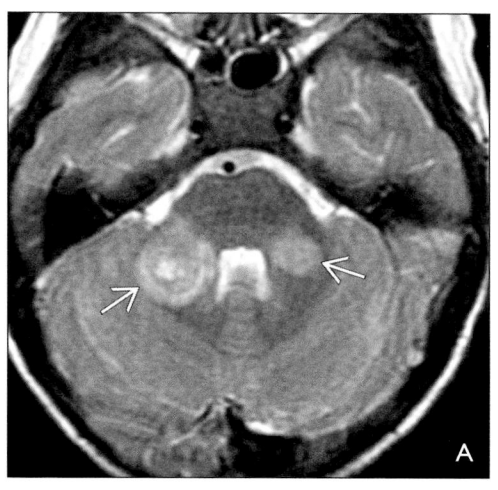
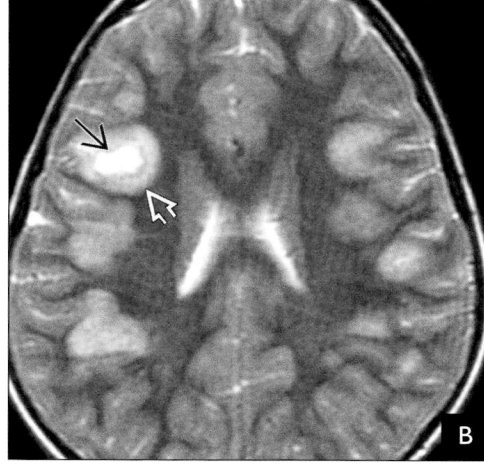

15-28A. "Flocculent" ADEM lesions are illustrated in this case. Axial T2WI shows bilateral brachium pontis lesions with a "fluffy" appearance and "fuzzy" margins ➡. *15-28B.* Axial T2WI in the same patient shows classic subcortical "fluffy" hyperintensities of ADEM. The cortex overlying the lesions appears intact. Note the right frontal lesion with a very hyperintense center ➡, slightly less hyperintense periphery ➡.

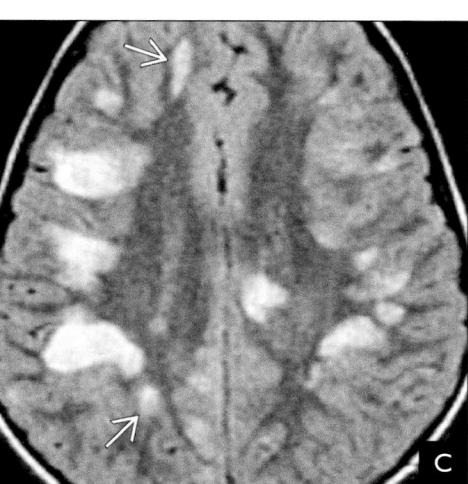
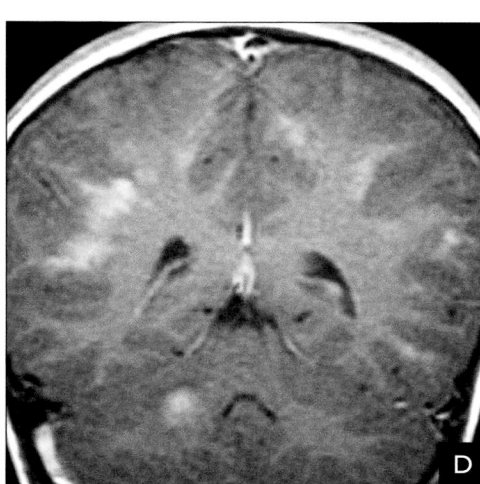

15-28C. FLAIR scan demonstrates additional subcortical hyperintensities ➡ that were not as conspicuous on the T2WI. *15-28D.* Coronal T1 C+ scan shows linear and round "fluffy" enhancement in the lesions.

Differential Diagnosis

The major differential diagnosis of ADEM is **multiple sclerosis**. ADEM may be difficult to distinguish from MS on the basis of imaging findings alone. "Tumefactive" lesions—including those with incomplete ring enhancement—occur in both disorders. ADEM is more common in children and often has a history of viral infection or immunization preceding the illness. MS more commonly involves the callbacksoseptal interface, but periventricular lesions in ADEM are common. MS typically has a relapsing-remitting course while most (but not all!) cases of ADEM are monophasic (15-31).

Other diagnostic considerations include **viral encephalitis**, autoimmune-mediated **vasculitis**, and **collagen-vascular disease**. Occasionally, **neurosarcoidosis** with parenchymal involvement and CNS **Whipple disease** can mimic ADEM.

ADEM: IMAGING

CT
 • NECT: Usually normal
 • CECT: Punctate, partial ring enhancement
 MR
 • Multifocal T2/FLAIR hyperintensities
   ∘ Bilateral but asymmetric WM lesions
   ∘ Subcortical, periventricular
   ∘ Small round/ovoid to flocculent "cotton balls"
   ∘ Basal ganglia, posterior fossa, cranial nerves often involved
 • Enhancement varies from none to striking
   ∘ Multifocal punctate, linear, partial ring
   ∘ Can be perivenular
   ∘ Large lesions ("tumefactive") rare
 Differential Diagnosis
 • MS
 • Encephalitis, vasculitis, collagen-vascular disease
 • "Tumefactive" ADEM mimics neoplasm

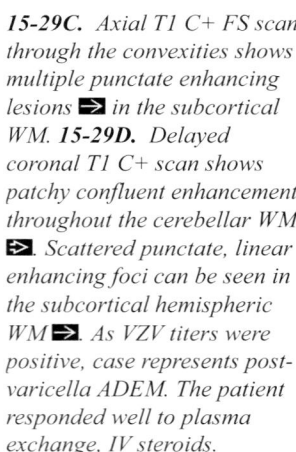

15-29A. A 37-year-old woman with a history of Bell palsy 2 years earlier presented with fever, malaise, and myalgia. Two weeks later, she complained of headache and unsteady gait, then became drowsy and eventually comatose. Axial T1 C+ FS scan shows multifocal patchy enhancement ➡ in the posterior fossa WM.
15-29B. Axial T1 C+ FS scan shows several punctate ➡, incomplete ring-enhancing lesions ➤ in both hemispheres.

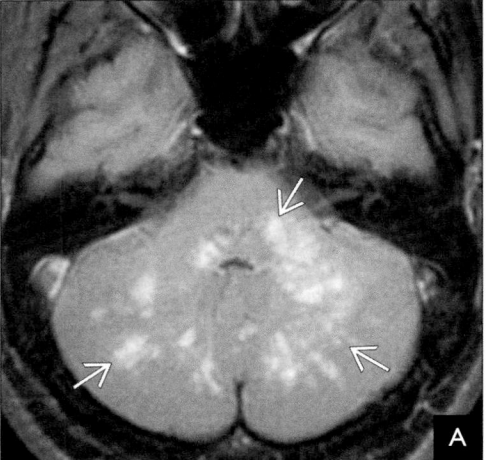

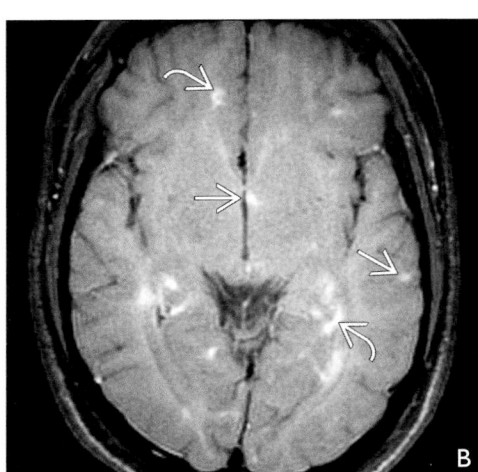

15-29C. Axial T1 C+ FS scan through the convexities shows multiple punctate enhancing lesions ➡ in the subcortical WM. 15-29D. Delayed coronal T1 C+ scan shows patchy confluent enhancement throughout the cerebellar WM ➤. Scattered punctate, linear enhancing foci can be seen in the subcortical hemispheric WM ➡. As VZV titers were positive, case represents post-varicella ADEM. The patient responded well to plasma exchange, IV steroids.

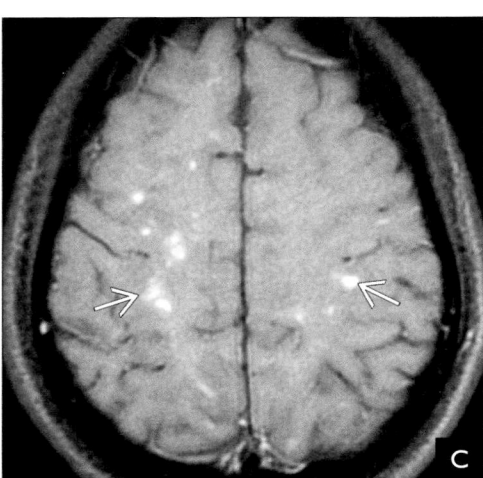

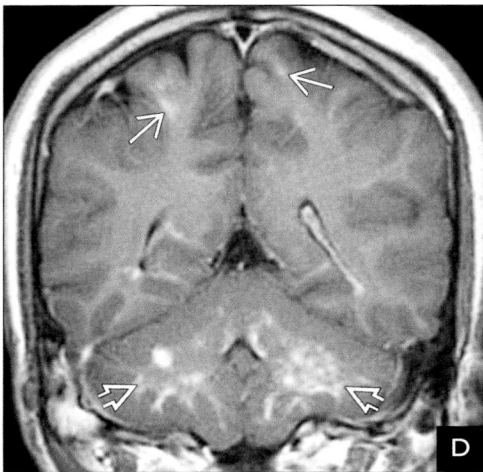

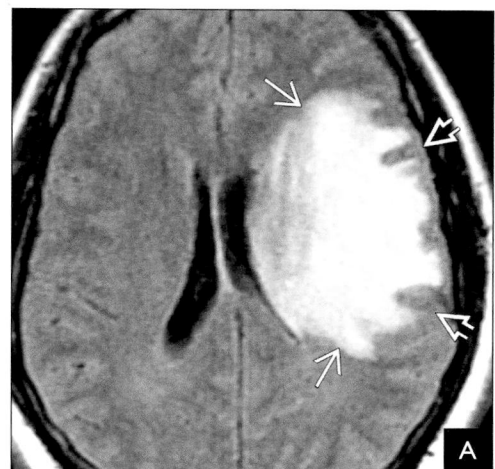

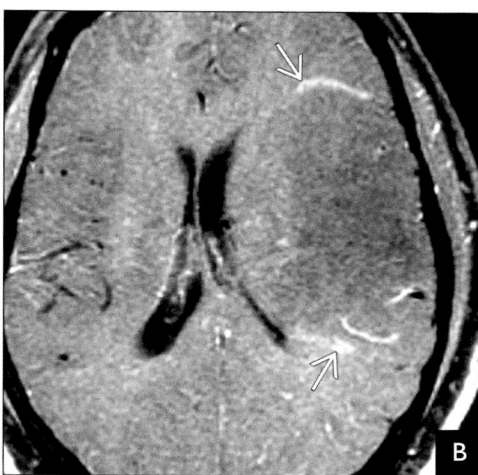

15-30A. FLAIR scan in a patient of acute "tumefactive" MS shows a large confluent hyperintense mass that exclusively involves the white matter ➡, sparing the cortex ➡. No other lesions were present. 15-30B. T1 C+ FS in the same patient shows partial rim enhancement around the mostly nonenhancing mass ➡. Biopsy disclosed acute demyelinating disease without evidence of neoplasm or infection.

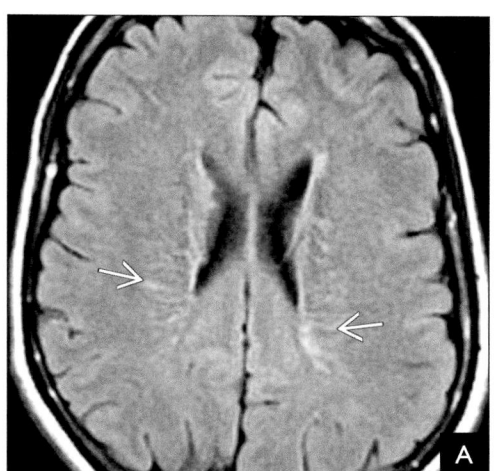

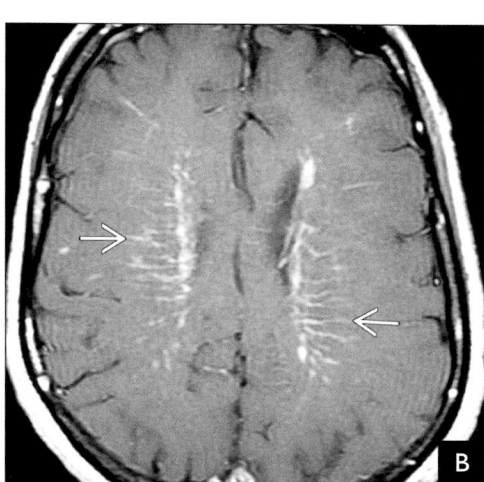

15-31A. Multiphasic ADEM is illustrated in this case of a 52-year-old woman who presented with left-sided headache, retroorbital pain, and visual loss. Axial FLAIR scan shows enlarged hyperintense perivenular spaces ➡ in the deep cerebral white matter. 15-31B. Axial T1 C+ scan in the same patient shows striking linear enhancement ➡ along the deep medullary veins and perivascular spaces.

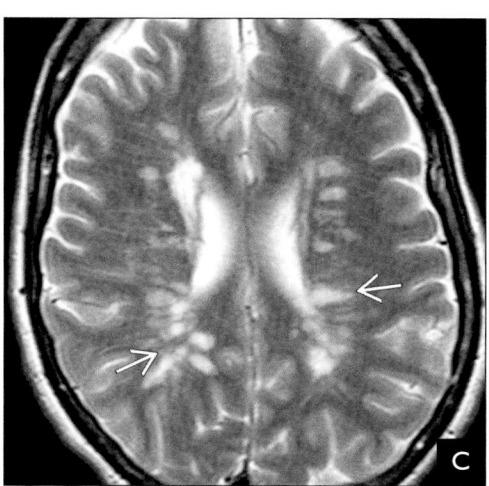

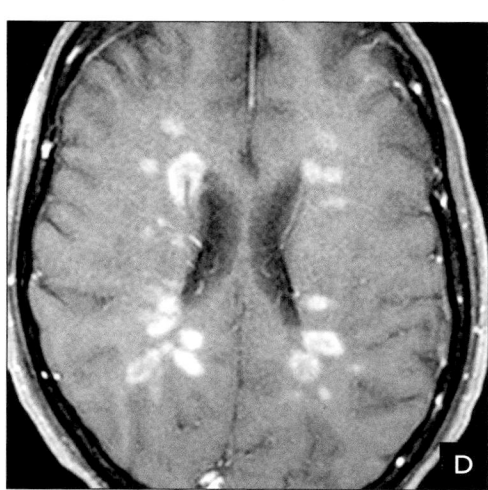

15-31C. Repeat imaging was obtained 4 months later because of worsening symptoms. Axial T2WI shows multiple ovoid and triangular hyperintensities ➡ oriented perpendicular to the lateral ventricles. These were considered characteristic for perivenular demyelination. 15-31D. Axial T1 C+ FS scan shows that the ovoid hyperintensities demonstrate ring, punctate, and linear enhancement. Biopsy disclosed demyelinating disease most consistent with ADEM.

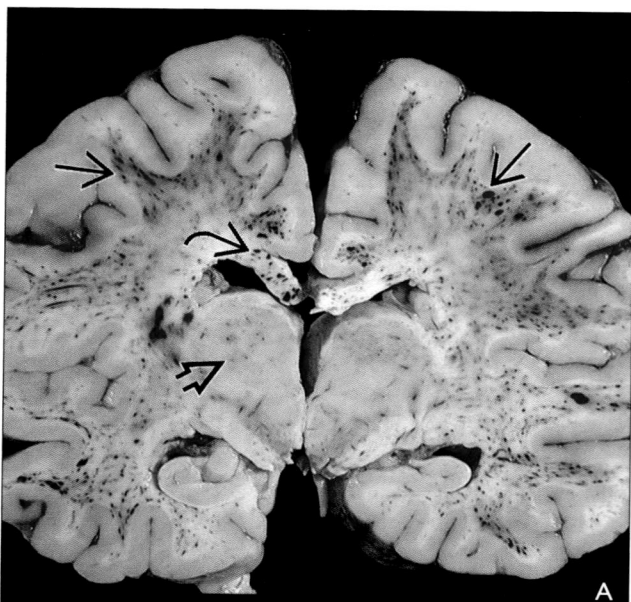

15-32A. Coronal autopsy of AHLE shows innumerable bilaterally symmetric petechial WM hemorrhages ➡ extending into subcortical U-fibers. Note lesions in corpus callosum ➡. The cortex is completely spared but not the deep gray nuclei ➡.

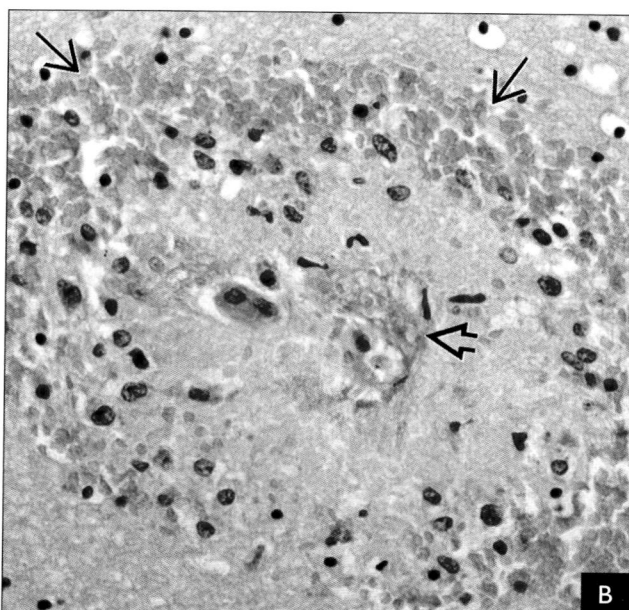

15-32B. H&E photomicrograph in the same case shows a ring of perivascular hemorrhage ➡ surrounding a thrombosed vessel ➡. (Case courtesy R. Hewlett, MD.)

Acute Hemorrhagic Leukoencephalitis

Terminology

Acute hemorrhagic leukoencephalitis (AHLE) is also known as acute hemorrhagic leukoencephalopathy, acute hemorrhagic encephalomyelitis (AHEM), and Weston Hurst disease.

Some investigators include AHLE as part of the ADEM spectrum—as a hyperacute, exceptionally severe, extremely fulminant manifestation of ADEM. Because the histologic and imaging features of AHLE differ significantly from ADEM, in this text we consider AHLE separately from ADEM.

Etiology

The precise etiology of AHLE is unclear. History of a viral prodrome or flu-like illness is common but not invariably present. Cross-reactivity between myelin basic protein moieties and various infectious agent antigens probably causes an acute autoimmune-mediated demyelination.

Pathology

LOCATION. AHLE predominantly affects the white matter but may involve both the brain and spinal cord. Both the cerebral hemispheres and posterior fossa structures are affected. Despite its name, AHLE may affect the gray matter. Basal ganglia involvement is common, but the cortical gray matter is generally (but not invariably) spared.

SIZE AND NUMBER. AHLE has two distinct manifestations: Focal macroscopic parenchymal hemorrhages and innumerable petechial microbleeds. A few cases combine features of both.

GROSS PATHOLOGY. The typical gross appearance is that of diffuse brain swelling with focal confluent and/or petechial white matter hemorrhagic necrosis (15-32A).

MICROSCOPIC FEATURES. Fibrinoid necrosis of vessel walls with perivascular demyelination, hemorrhage, and mononuclear inflammatory cell cuffing are the pathologic hallmarks of AHLE (15-32B). Diffuse, mostly neutrophilic infiltrates are typical, in contrast to the macrophage-predominant infiltrates typical of ADEM.

Clinical Issues

EPIDEMIOLOGY AND DEMOGRAPHICS. AHLE is considerably less common than ADEM. Approximately 2% of all ADEM cases are of the hyperacute hemorrhagic type that could be considered consistent with AHLE. While AHLE occurs at all ages, most patients are children and young adults.

PRESENTATION AND NATURAL HISTORY. Most AHLE cases begin with a viral illness or vaccination followed by rapid neurological deterioration. Fever and lethargy with increasing somnolence, decreased mental status, impaired consciousness, and long-tract signs are the most common clinical symptoms.

Untreated AHLE has a very poor prognosis. Rapid clinical deterioration and death usually occur within days to a week after symptom onset. Mortality is 60-80%. The disease course is fulminant and almost always fatal if untreated.

TREATMENT OPTIONS. Aggressive treatment with intravenous high-dose corticosteroids, immunoglobulin, cyclophosphamide, and plasmapheresis has been used with some success in a few cases.

Imaging

Imaging evaluation plays a key role in patients with a clinical history that suggests possible AHLE.

CT FINDINGS. NECT may be normal unless macroscopic confluent hemorrhages are present. Petechial microhemorrhages are generally invisible, but white matter edema with diffuse, relatively asymmetric hypodensity in one or both hemispheres may be present.

MR FINDINGS. T1 scans are often normal unless lobar hemorrhage is present. T2/FLAIR findings vary from subtle to striking. Multifocal scattered or confluent

hyperintensities as well as bilateral confluent hyperintensity of the cerebral white matter are typical but nonspecific findings **(15-33)**.

While large lobar confluent hemorrhages are easily identified on most standard sequences **(15-34)**, **(15-35)**, T2* scans are the key to diagnosis. SWI sequences are more sensitive than GRE, especially when only microbleeds are present **(15-33)**, **(15-36)**, **(15-37)**.

Multifocal punctate and linear "blooming" hypointensities in the corpus callosum that extend through the full thickness of the hemispheric white matter to the subcortical U-fibers are typical findings on T2*. Striking sparing of the overlying cortex is common. Additional lesions are frequently present in the basal ganglia, midbrain, pons, and cerebellum.

Enhancement on T1 C+ occurs in 50% of cases and ranges from linear perivascular space enhancement to larger patchy or confluent foci.

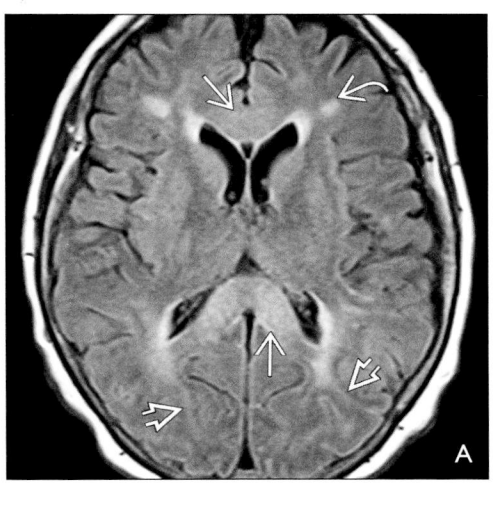

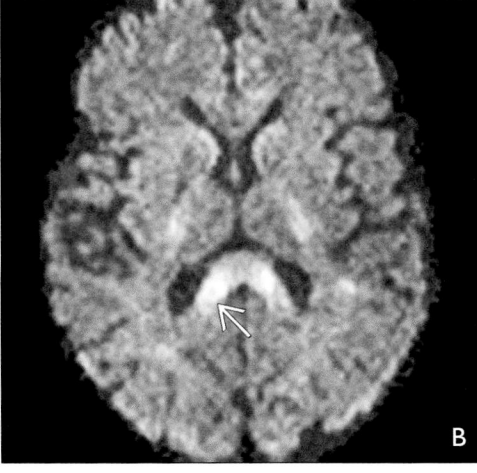

15-33A. A 69-year-old woman had a viral exanthem followed several days later by lethargy and progressive decline in mental status. Axial FLAIR shows confluent hyperintensity in both the splenium and genu of the corpus callosum ➡️*, together with bifrontal focal hemispheric white matter lesions* ➡️ *and subtle confluent hyperintensity in the occipital subcortical white matter* ➡️*. 15-33B. DWI shows restricted diffusion in the corpus callosum splenium* ➡️*.*

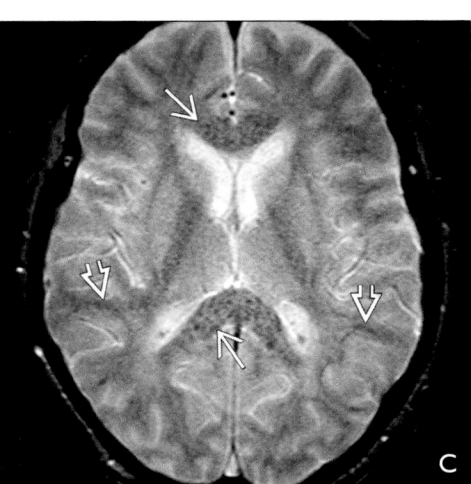

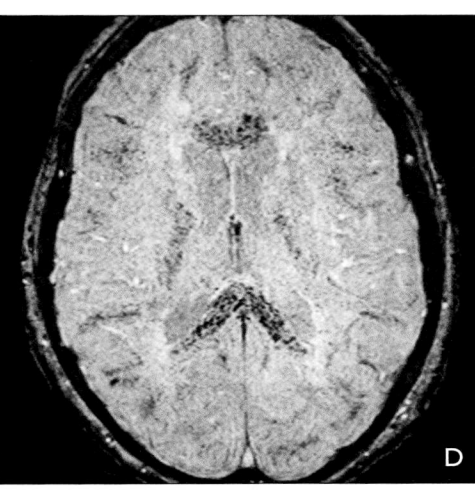

15-33C. T2 GRE scan shows punctate hypointensities in the corpus callosum* ➡️ *with subtle "blooming" in the subcortical white matter* ➡️*. 15-33D. The patient continued to deteriorate, so repeat MR with susceptibility-weighted imaging (SWI) was obtained. Innumerable bilaterally symmetric punctate and linear "blooming" hypointensities are seen throughout the WM with striking sparing of cortical gray matter. AHLE was diagnosed on imaging and confirmed with biopsy.*

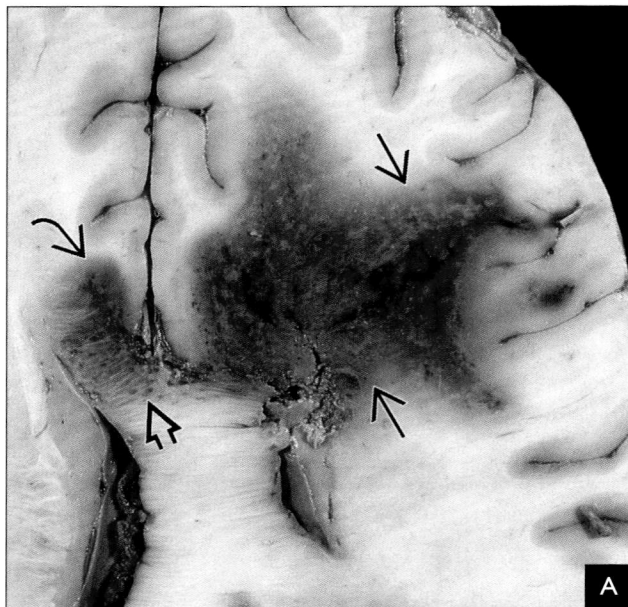

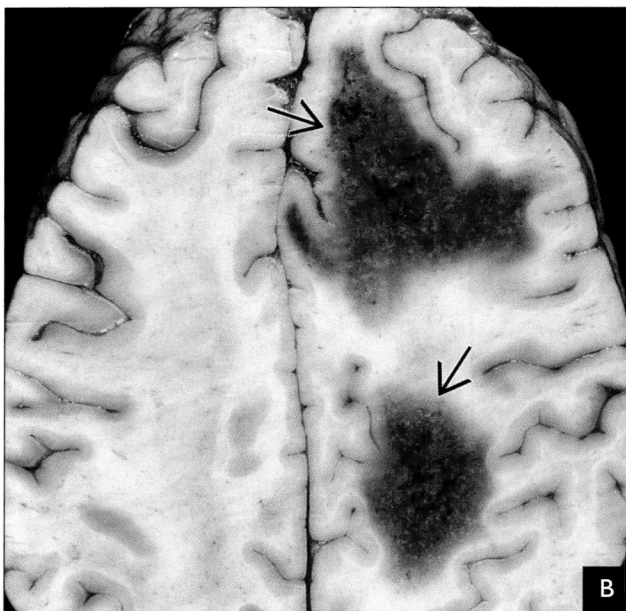

15-34A. Axial brain section in autopsied case of AHLE demonstrates a large confluent area of grossly hemorrhagic necrosis ⇒. Note that the lesion crosses the corpus callosum genu ⇒ to involve the opposite frontal lobe ⇒.

15-34B. The same case demonstrates 2 additional areas of gross hemorrhagic necrosis ⇒. Findings, clinical history of prior flu-like illness with rapidly progressive clinical course are characteristic of AHLE. (Courtesy R. Hewlett, MD.)

Differential Diagnosis

The major differential diagnosis of AHLE is **ADEM**. Both share a number of similar features. However, ADEM usually follows a much less fulminant course and does not demonstrate the characteristic lobar or perivascular hemorrhages of AHLE.

Other entities that should be considered in the differential diagnosis include fulminant multiple sclerosis, acute necrotizing encephalopathy, and macrophage activation syndrome. Acute fulminant **multiple sclerosis** (Marburg type) is not characterized by high fever or marked leukocytosis. The prominent hemorrhagic foci on MR imaging seen with AHLE are absent.

Acute necrotizing encephalopathy (ANE) is a rare but recognized complication of viral infections—such as influenza A and B, human herpesvirus 6, varicella-zoster—and mycoplasmal infection. Imaging is quite different from that of AHLE. Virtually all cases of ANE show bilateral symmetric lesions in the thalami, internal capsules, and upper brainstem tegmentum.

Macrophage activation syndrome (MAS) can have a neurological presentation and MR findings that resemble AHLE. However, a history of rheumatological disease is typical in MAS, and hyperferritinemia is a laboratory hallmark of the disease that is absent in AHLE.

The petechial microhemorrhages of AHLE can be found in a number of other unrelated disorders including diffuse vascular injury, fat emboli, thrombotic thrombo-

cytopenic purpura, sepsis, vasculitis, hemorrhagic viral fevers, malaria, and rickettsial diseases.

ACUTE HEMORRHAGIC LEUKOENCEPHALITIS (AHLE)

Terminology
- Also called acute hemorrhagic encephalomyelitis (AHEM), Weston Hurst disease

Etiology and Pathology
- Similar to ADEM (viral/post-viral autoimmune-mediated)
- May represent fulminant form of ADEM

Clinical Issues
- Rare; 2% of ADEM cases
- All ages affected, especially children/young adults
- Fever, lethargy, impaired consciousness
- Rapidly progressive, often lethal course

Imaging
- General features
  - White matter edema
  - Focal macroscopic hemorrhages or multifocal microbleeds
- CT may be normal or demonstrate hypodense white matter
- MR procedure of choice
  - Multifocal scattered or confluent lesions on T2/FLAIR
  - Corpus callosum, cerebral WM, pons, cerebellum ± basal ganglia (BG)
  - Cortical GM generally spared
  - T2* (GRE, SWI) depicts microbleeds
  - 50% show variable enhancement

Differential Diagnosis
- ADEM
- Fulminant MS (Marburg type)
- Acute necrotizing encephalopathy

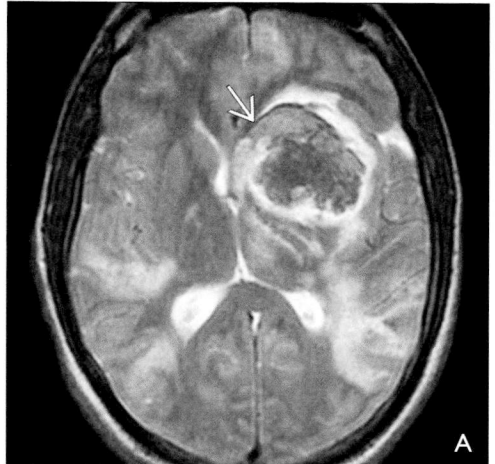

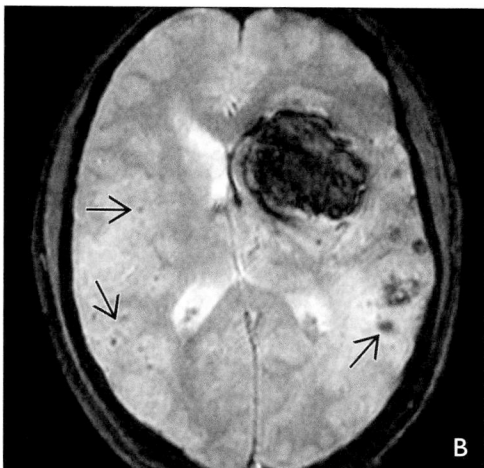

15-35A. Axial T2WI in a patient with presumed MS, rapid progression shows multifocal WM lesions, hemorrhagic left frontal mass ➡. 15-35B. T2* GRE scan shows numerous other "blooming" foci ⇒ in the WM lesions. Imaging and clinical picture are most consistent with AHLE. (Courtesy R. Ramakantan, MD.)

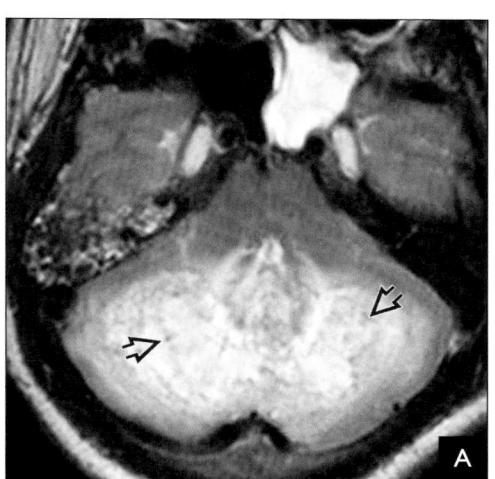

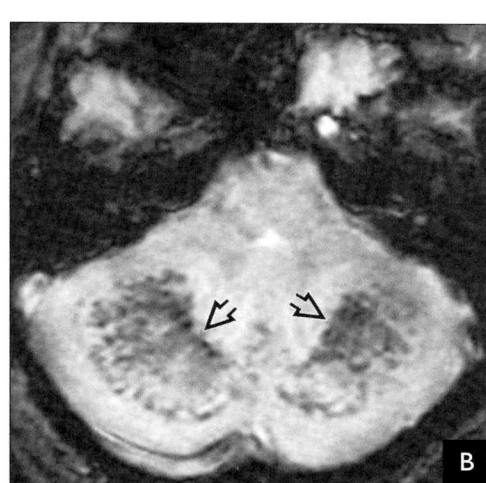

15-36A. T2WI in a patient with ataxia shows diffuse confluent cerebellar hyperintensity with multifocal hypointense areas ⇒. 15-36B. T2* GRE shows multiple petechial hemorrhages ⇒. Clinical, imaging findings most consistent with AHLE. (Courtesy R. Ramakantan, MD.)

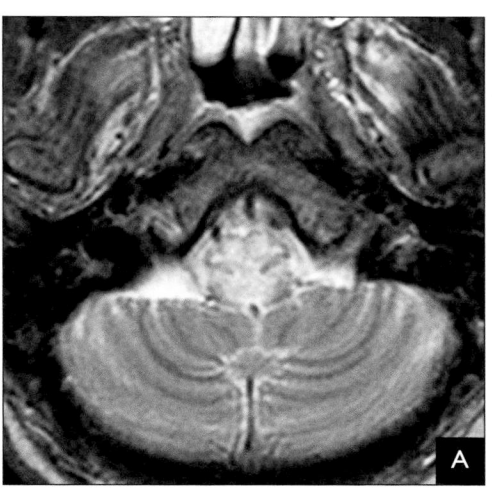

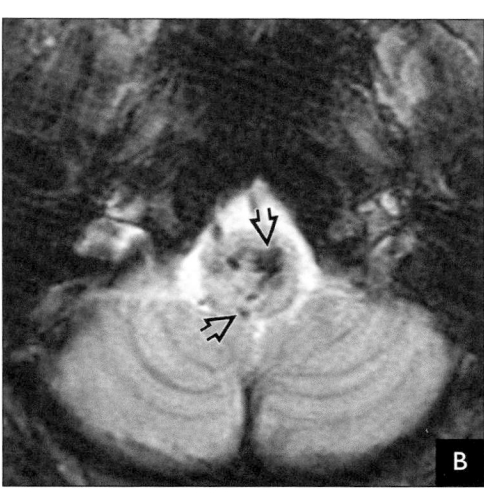

15-37A. T2WI in a 65-year-old man with rapidly progressive gait disturbance and extremity weakness shows a swollen hyperintense medulla; spine imaging showed similar findings in the upper cervical cord. 15-37B. T2* GRE scan shows multifocal "blooming" hypointensities ⇒ consistent with hemorrhagic foci. AHLE localized to the medulla and cervical spinal cord without other involved areas is uncommon.

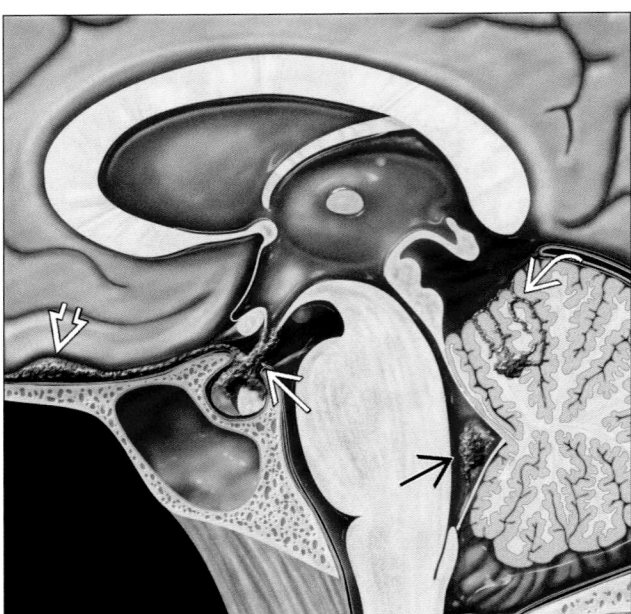

15-38. Graphic illustrates common neurosarcoid locations: (1) infundibulum, extending into the pituitary ➡, (2) plaque-like dura-arachnoid thickening ➡, and (3) synchronous lesions of the superior vermis ➡ and fourth ventricle choroid plexus ➡.

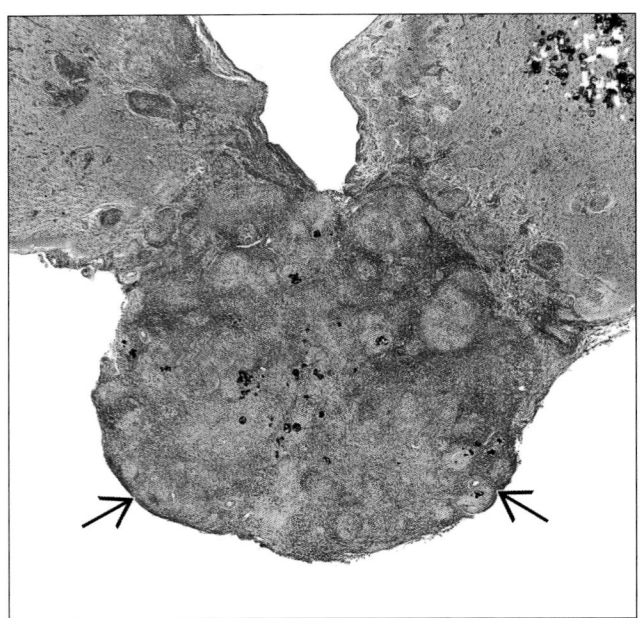

15-39. Coronal low-power photomicrograph shows sarcoidosis expanding the third ventricle floor and thickening the proximal infundibulum ➡. (Courtesy B. K. DeMasters, MD.)

Inflammatory-like Disorders

Neurosarcoidosis

Terminology

Sarcoidosis ("sarcoid") is a multisystem inflammatory disorder characterized by discrete noncaseating epithelioid granulomas. When sarcoidosis affects the CNS it is termed "neurosarcoid" (NS).

Etiology

The etiology of sarcoidosis remains unknown. Although the initiating event in its pathogenesis remains elusive, the prevailing view is that genetically susceptible individuals develop sarcoidosis following exposure to as-yet-unidentified antigens. A reactive inflammatory cascade ensues that appears to be driven primarily through CD4-positive T cells.

Pathology

LOCATION. Systemic distribution is variable as sarcoidosis affects multiple body parts, especially the lymph nodes and lungs. The hilar nodes are the overall most common site.

The CNS is involved in approximately 5% of cases, usually in combination with disease elsewhere. Only 5-10% of NS cases are confined to the CNS and occur without evidence of systemic sarcoidosis.

Sarcoid can involve any part of the nervous system or its coverings. The most common location is the leptomeninges, especially around the base of the brain. Diffuse leptomeningeal thickening with or without more focal nodular lesions is seen in about 40% of cases **(15-38)**.

The hypothalamus and infundibulum are also favored intracranial sites. NS can involve cranial nerves, eye and periorbita, bone, the ventricles and choroid plexus, and the brain parenchyma itself. Both supra- and infratentorial compartments are affected. Sarcoid can also involve the spinal leptomeninges, cord, and nerve roots.

SIZE AND NUMBER. NS lesions vary in size from tiny granulomas that infiltrate along the pia and perivascular spaces to large dura-based masses that closely resemble meningioma. Multiple lesions are more common than solitary lesions.

GROSS PATHOLOGY. The gross appearance varies widely and depends on location. Somewhat nodular diffuse basilar leptomeningeal thickening is common. Extension of the granulomas into the brain perivascular spaces is a frequent finding, as are infiltration and enlargement of the hypothalamus and infundibulum. Single or multifocal discrete firm yellow-tan granulomas are typical findings.

Fibrocollagenous tissue becomes progressively more prominent with longstanding disease and may result in dense meningeal fibrosis, seen as a pachymeningopathy with or without focal dural masses.

MICROSCOPIC FEATURES. Sarcoid granulomas are non-caseating collections with central aggregates of epithelioid histiocytes and multinucleated giant cells together with variable numbers of benign-appearing lymphocytes and plasma cells **(15-39)**. There is no histologic or immunohistochemical evidence of infection or neoplasm.

linical Issues

EPIDEMIOLOGY AND DEMOGRAPHICS. NS has a bimodal age distribution. The largest peak occurs during the third and fourth decades with a second smaller peak in patients—especially women—over the age of 50 years. There is a moderate female predominance.

Sarcoidosis is distributed worldwide although prevalence varies significantly with geography and ethnicity. African-Americans and North European whites have the highest disease incidence. In the USA, the lifetime risk in African-Americans is nearly three-fold higher than in Caucasians.

PRESENTATION. Symptoms vary with location. The most common presentation of NS is isolated or multiple cranial nerve deficits, which is seen in 50-75% of patients. Involvement of virtually every cranial nerve has been reported. Facial nerve palsy is the most frequent finding. The optic nerve is the second most commonly affected nerve, causing visual field defects, blurry vision, or optic nerve head edema.

Nonspecific symptoms of NS include headache, fatigue, seizures, encephalopathy, cognitive deficits, and psychiatric disturbances. Symptoms of pituitary/hypothalamic dysfunction such as diabetes insipidus or panhypopituitarism are seen in 10-15% of cases.

NATURAL HISTORY. NS has a variable course. It can be relatively asymptomatic and clinically indolent. Nearly two-thirds of patients experience a self-limited monophasic illness. One-third follow a chronic remitting-relapsing course with new symptoms suggesting the development of additional granulomas.

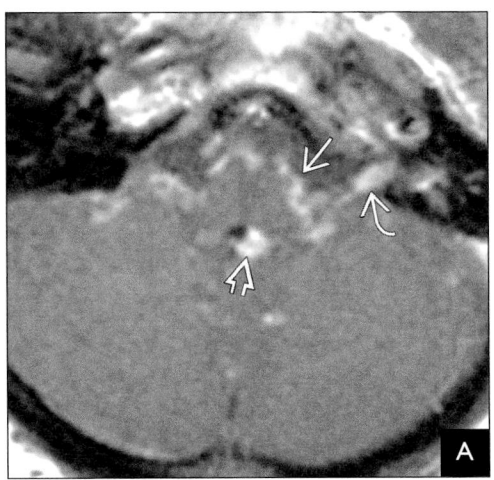

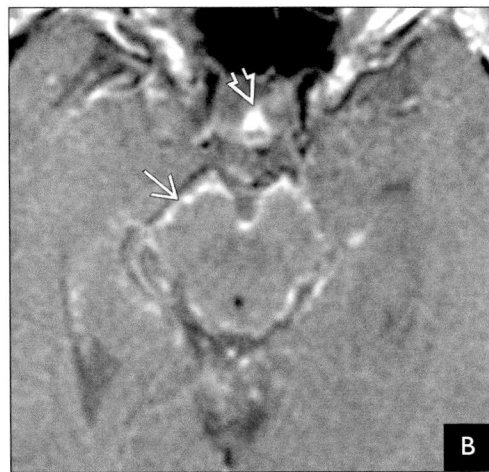

15-40A. *Axial T1 C+ scan in a patient with neurosarcoid shows linear and nodular thickening along the pial surface of the medulla* ➡, *as well as lesions in the fourth ventricle* ➡ *and CNs IX-XI* ➡. *15-40B.* *Axial T1 C+ in the same patient shows that the midbrain is almost completely covered with linear and nodular sarcoid deposits* ➡. *Note the thickened infundibular stalk* ➡.

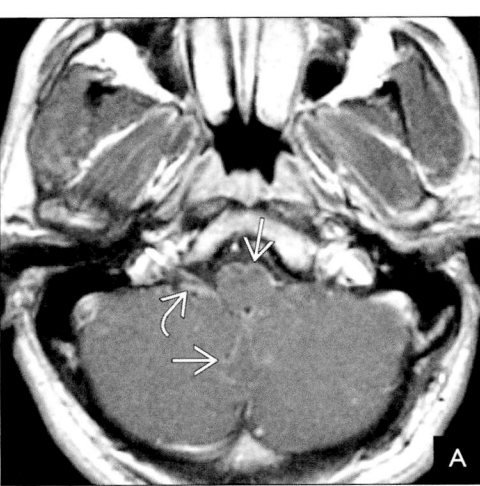

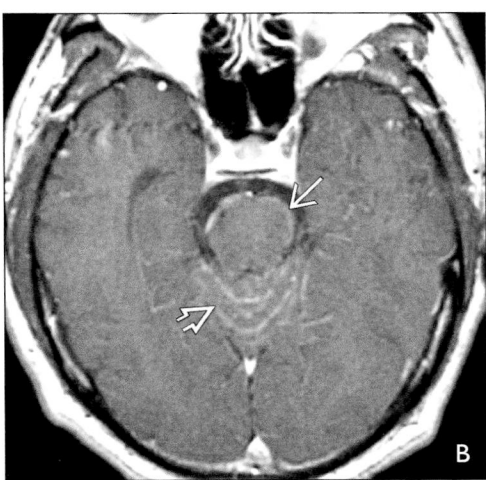

15-41A. *Axial T1 C+ scan in another case of neurosarcoid shows more subtle leptomeningeal enhancement along the surface of the medulla and tonsils* ➡ *as well as infiltration along CNs IX-XI* ➡. *15-41B.* *Axial T1 C+ scan in the same case shows linear enhancement along the upper pons* ➡ *as well as prominent nodular and linear enhancement in the vermian sulci* ➡. *Leptomeningeal enhancement is the most common imaging finding in neurosarcoid.*

TREATMENT OPTIONS. As there is no known cure for NS, the treatment goal is symptom alleviation. Most patients with NS respond to steroids. Some are relatively refractory to treatment with corticosteroids and immuno-suppressive agents.

Imaging

GENERAL FEATURES. Systemic sarcoidosis has protean manifestations and is one of the great mimickers of many other diseases. NS is no different, and findings vary widely. Specific imaging features are described below and summarized according to frequency in the accompanying box.

CT FINDINGS. Depending on the amount of fibrosis present, NS can appear slightly hyperdense relative to normal brain parenchyma on NECT scan. Leptomeningeal disease may enhance on CECT, resembling tuberculosis or pyogenic meningitis. Dura-based masses are typically modestly hyperdense and enhance strongly and uniformly on CECT.

Sarcoidosis involving the calvaria or skull base is uncommon. Well-circumscribed "punched-out" lesions with nonsclerotic margins can be seen on bone CT.

MR FINDINGS. NS is isointense with brain on T1WI and hyperintense relative to CSF. Sulci filled with leptomeningeal infiltrates appear effaced. Dura-based masses resemble meningiomas, so large lesions sometimes create a distinct CSF-vascular "cleft" between the lesion and the brain. More often, the subarachnoid space is filled, and the border between sarcoid and brain is indistinct.

Signal intensity on T2 depends on the amount of fibrocollagenous material present. Longstanding dural lesions are relatively hypointense. Parenchymal infiltration along the perivascular spaces causes a vasculitis-like reaction with edema, mass effect, and hyperintensity on T2/FLAIR.

The most common finding on T1 C+ scans is nodular or diffuse leptomeningeal thickening, found in approximately one-third to one-half of all cases (15-40), (15-41).

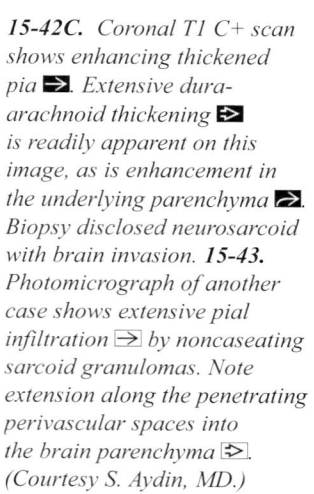

15-42A. Axial T2WI in a 44-year-old woman with worsening headaches, diplopia shows extensive edema ➡ in an enlarged left temporal lobe with early uncal, hippocampal herniation ➡. Very hypointense dural thickening is present along the entire surface of the middle cranial fossa ➡.
15-42B. Axial T1 C+ scan shows intense dura-arachnoid thickening and enhancement ➡. Note involvement of the underlying sulci ➡ with some parenchymal enhancement ➡.

15-42C. Coronal T1 C+ scan shows enhancing thickened pia ➡. Extensive dura-arachnoid thickening ➡ is readily apparent on this image, as is enhancement in the underlying parenchyma ➡. Biopsy disclosed neurosarcoid with brain invasion. 15-43. Photomicrograph of another case shows extensive pial infiltration ➡ by noncaseating sarcoid granulomas. Note extension along the penetrating perivascular spaces into the brain parenchyma ➡. (Courtesy S. Aydin, MD.)

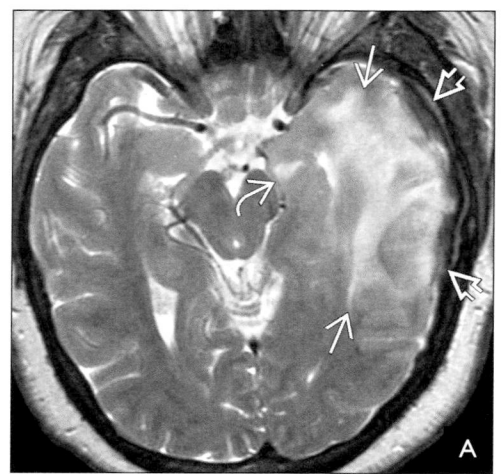

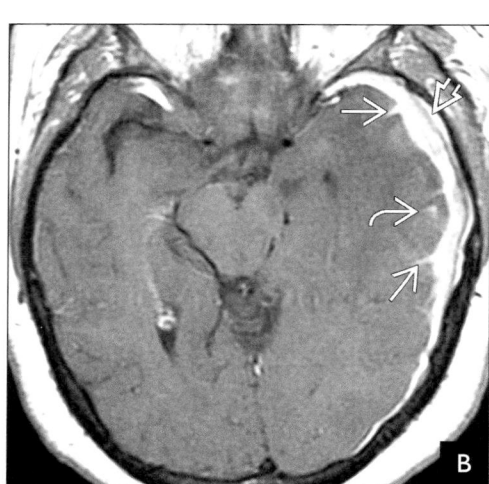

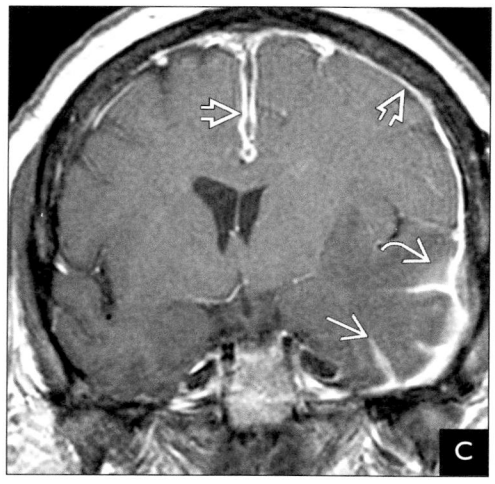

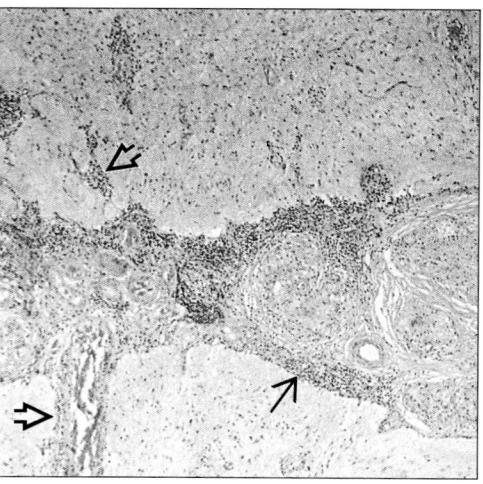

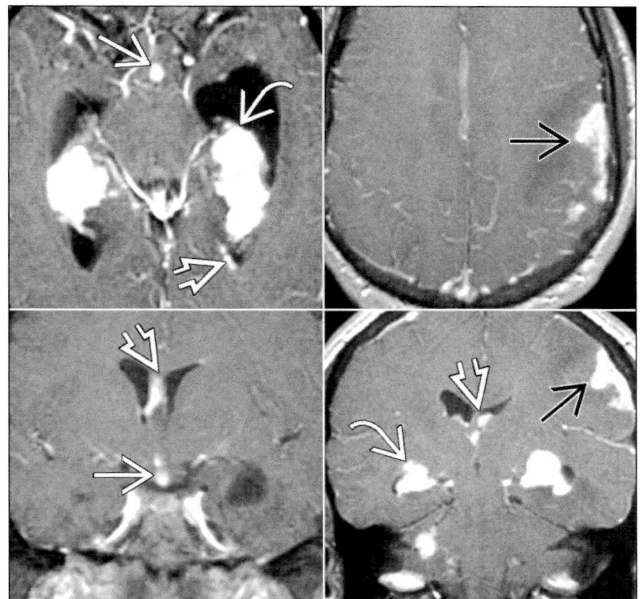

15-44. *Collage of T1 C+ scans shows NS with involvement of the infundibulum* ➡, *choroid plexus* ➡, *ependyma* ➡, *meninges* ➡.

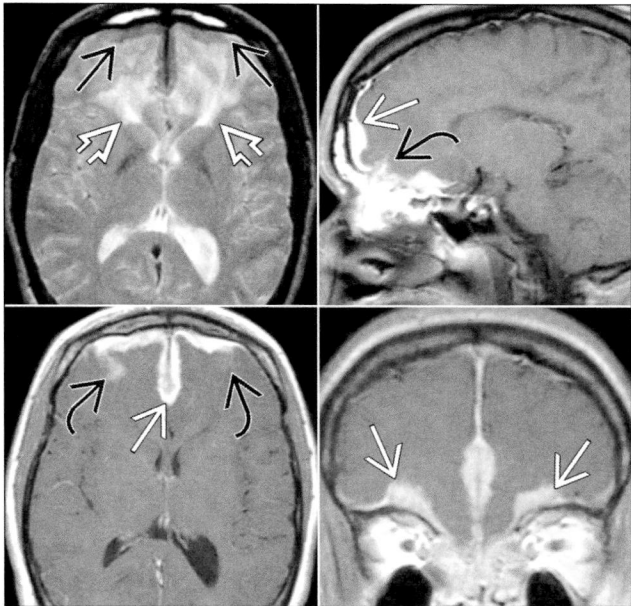

15-45. *NS with dura-arachnoid thickening is hypointense on T2WI* ➡, *enhances strongly and uniformly* ➡. *Parenchymal extension along perivascular spaces causes edema* ➡, *enhancement* ➡.

Half of NS patients eventually develop parenchymal disease **(15-42)**, **(15-43)**. Hypothalamic and infundibular thickening with intense enhancement is seen in 5-10% of cases. Multifocal nodular enhancing masses or more diffuse perivascular infiltrates may develop **(15-44)**. Solitary parenchymal or dura-based masses are less common **(15-44)**, **(15-45)**. In rare cases, coalescing granulomas form a focal expansile mass ("tumefactive" NS) **(15-46)**.

NS may cause solitary or multifocal thickened enhancing cranial nerves **(15-47)**, **(15-48)** as well as enhancing masses in the ventricles and choroid plexus **(15-44)**.

NEUROSARCOID: IMAGING

Most Common
- Linear/nodular leptomeningeal enhancement
  - Predilection for basilar cisterns
- Parenchymal enhancing lesions
  - Thick enhancing hypothalamus/pituitary stalk, gland
  - Perivascular infiltrating lesions
- Cranial nerve thickening, enhancement
  - Any nerve can be involved
  - Facial, optic nerves most common

Less Common
- Solitary or multiple dura-based masses
  - Can be diffuse, plaque-like
  - Focal, discrete mass(es)
- Diffuse/focal nonenhancing T2/FLAIR hyperintensities
- Hydrocephalus

Rare but Important
- "Tumefactive" parenchymal masses
- Choroid plexus mass(es)

Differential Diagnosis

The differential diagnosis of NS depends on lesion location. **Meningitis**—especially TB meningitis—can look very similar to NS of the basilar leptomeninges. **Carcinomatous meningitis** can also resemble leptomeningeal NS.

The differential diagnosis of dura-based NS includes **meningioma, lymphoma,** and **idiopathic inflammatory pseudotumor,** while hypothalamic/infundibular/pituitary NS may look like **histiocytosis** or lymphocytic **hypophysitis.**

Coalescent parenchymal NS looks like **primary CNS lymphoma** or **metastases** while multifocal enhancing lesions can resemble **multiple sclerosis, metastases,** and **intravascular lymphoma.** The differential diagnosis of solitary or multiple cranial NS is broad and includes infection, demyelinating disease, and neoplasm.

Idiopathic Inflammatory Pseudotumors

Idiopathic inflammatory pseudotumors (IIPs) are uncommon lesions that can be virtually indistinguishable from "real" neoplasms. IIPs are benign nonneoplastic cellular aggregates that are also known as idiopathic hypertrophic pachymeningopathy, plasma cell granuloma, and inflammatory myofibroblastic tumor.

IIPs have been described in virtually all body systems. They can affect any part of the CNS but are typically

15-46A. Series of images demonstrates "tumefactive" neurosarcoid diagnosed on preoperative imaging studies as neoplasm. Axial T1WI in a 45-year-old man with syncope, dizziness, seizures, and longstanding difficulty with short-term memory shows no definite abnormality. 15-46B. Axial T2WI in the same patient shows an infiltrating hyperintense mass in the right temporal lobe ➡.

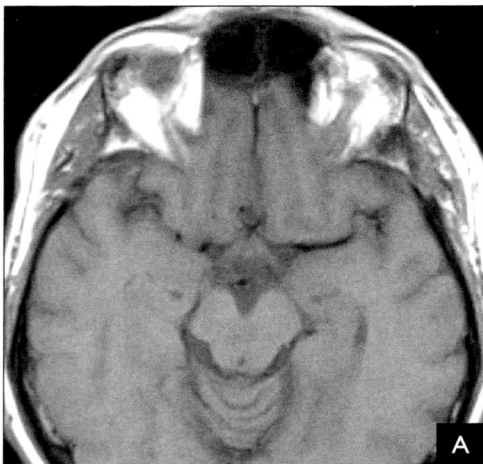
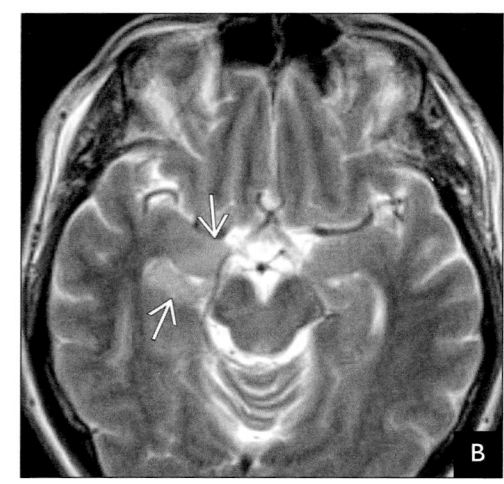

15-46C. FLAIR scan in the same patient shows that the mass ➡ involves most of the uncus and is wrapped around the temporal horn of the lateral ventricle. 15-46D. Axial T1 C+ FS scan shows mild to moderate but somewhat patchy enhancement of the mass ➡. Note that the infundibular stalk ➡ appears normal and that there is no evidence of enhancement or mass effect elsewhere.

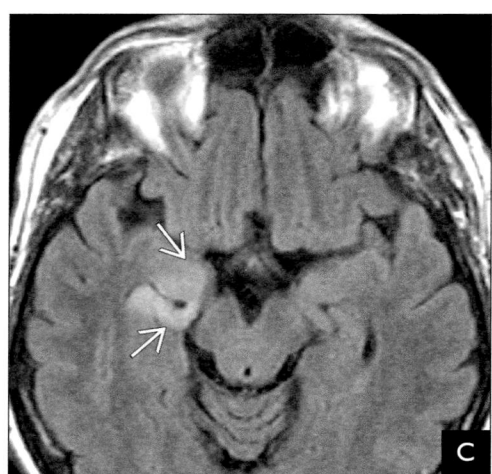
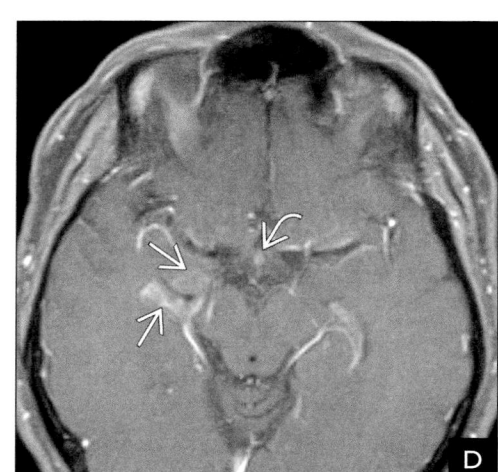

15-46E. Adjacent T1 C+ FS image shows the extensively infiltrating nature of the mass ➡. No other abnormalities are present. 15-46F. Low-power H&E photomicrograph from resected surgical specimen shows extensive parenchymal infiltration by noncaseating granulomas. Histologic diagnosis is isolated neurosarcoid.

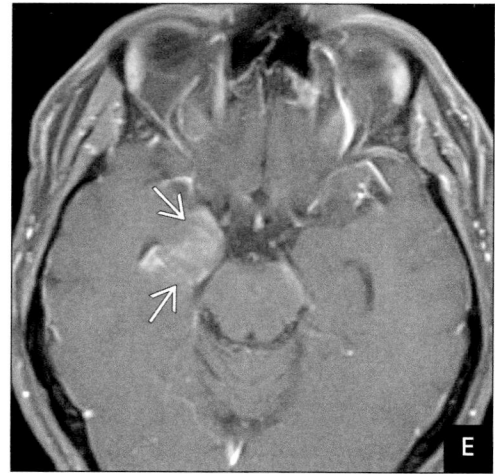
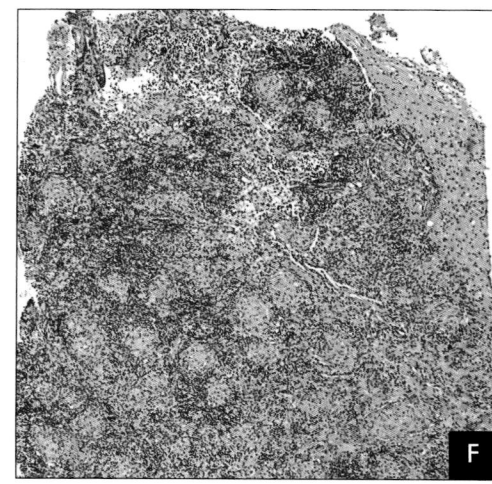

meninges-based lesions that can be isolated or invasive. Focal or mass-like dura-arachnoid thickening is the typical imaging finding.

The differential diagnosis of noninvasive IIP includes en plaque **meningioma** and benign, nonneoplastic causes of dura-arachnoid thickening. **Neurosarcoid, intracranial hypotension, prior surgery, dural sinus thrombosis, chronic subdural hematoma**, and residua of **chronic meningitis** are among the many entities that cause this nonspecific appearance on imaging studies.

Invasive IIPs behave aggressively and may simulate **malignant neoplasm** or **fungal infection**. The definitive diagnosis requires biopsy, as there are no pathognomonic imaging characteristics. IIPs are discussed in detail and extensively illustrated in Chapter 26.

Chronic Inflammatory Demyelinating Polyneuropathy

A rare type of localized autoimmune demyelinating disease, **chronic inflammatory demyelinating polyneuropathy (CIDP)**, is characterized by repeated episodes of demyelination and remyelination with "onion bulb" hypertrophy of the affected nerves. CIDP usually affects spinal and peripheral nerve roots but occasionally involves cranial nerves.

CIDP is characterized by chronic progressive or relapsing symmetric sensorimotor involvement. Clinically, CIDP is often initially diagnosed as Guillain-Barré syndrome, Bickerstaff encephalitis, or multiple sclerosis.

Diffuse thickening with striking hyperintensity on T2/STIR and mild to moderate enhancement of one or more cranial nerves is the typical imaging manifestation of intracranial CIDP **(15-49)**. Parenchymal demyelinating foci consistent with MS are commonly—but not invariably—present.

The imaging differential diagnosis of intracranial CIDP includes **neurosarcoidosis** and cranial nerve infiltration secondary to **lymphoma** or **metastases**. **Multiple sclerosis, Lyme disease**, and **acute disseminated encephalomyelitis** (ADEM) can all cause cranial nerve enhancement but do not cause the striking symmetric enlargement that characterizes CIDP.

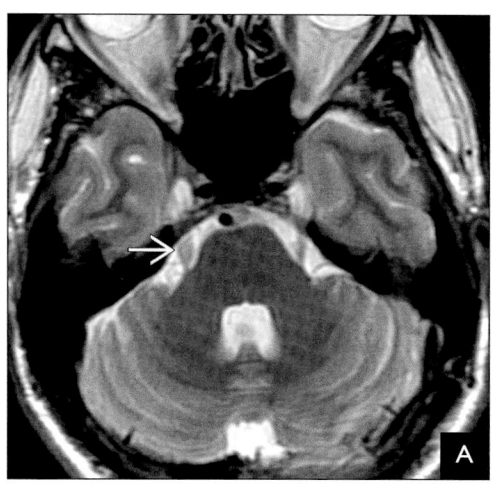

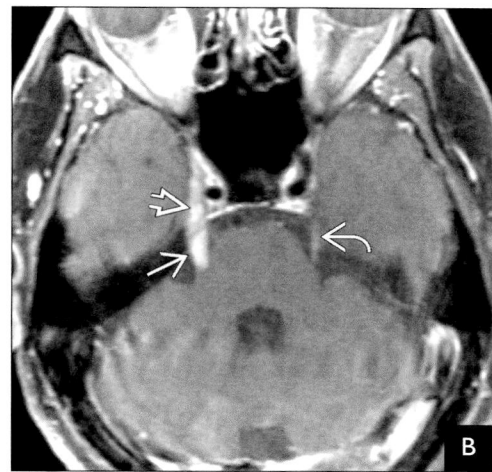

15-47A. A 50-year-old man presented with right CN V₂ facial numbness, headache, and diplopia. Serum ACE was elevated. Axial T2WI shows the right CN V appears moderately thickened ➡. 15-47B. Axial T1 C+ FS shows the thickened right CN V enhances from the root entry zone ➡ all the way into Meckel cave ➡. The left CN V also enhances slightly ➡. Patient was placed on steroids; 6 months later, nerves appeared normal. Presumed neurosarcoid. (Courtesy P. Hildenbrand, MD.)

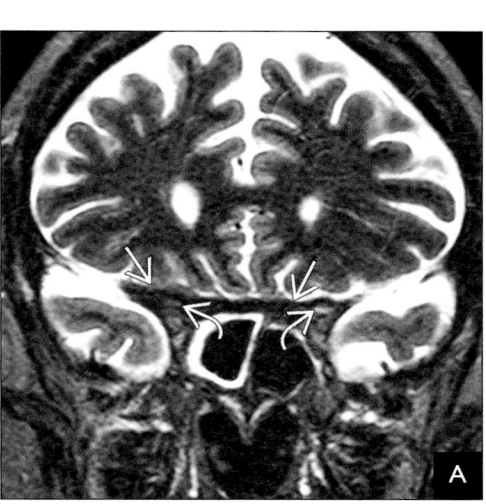

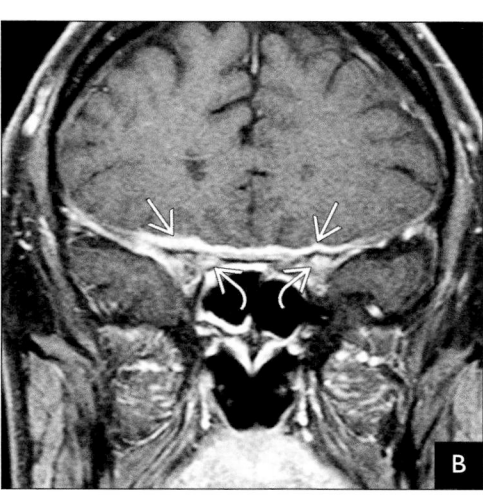

15-48A. Coronal T2WI with fat saturation in a 50-year-old man with progressive vision loss shows thickened hypointense dura ➡ extending along the planum sphenoidale, anterior clinoid processes. Both optic nerves appear compressed ➡. 15-48B. Coronal T1 C+ FS shows striking enhancement ➡. Both optic nerves show abnormal enhancement ➡. Biopsy-proven idiopathic inflammatory pseudotumor without evidence of neoplasm, infection, or noncaseating granulomas.

15-49A. Chronic inflammatory demyelinating polyneuropathy (CIDP) in a 23-year-old woman with bilateral trigeminal nerve deficits shows striking hyperintensity and fusiform enlargement of both CN Vs ➡ on this T2-weighted fat-suppressed scan. 15-49B. Image through the midbrain and upper orbits in the same patient shows hugely enlarged, markedly hyperintense ophthalmic nerves ➡.

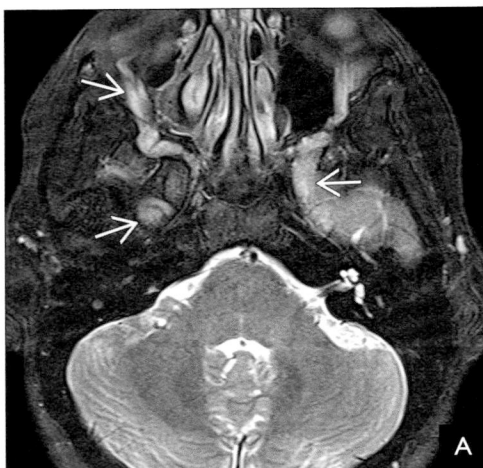
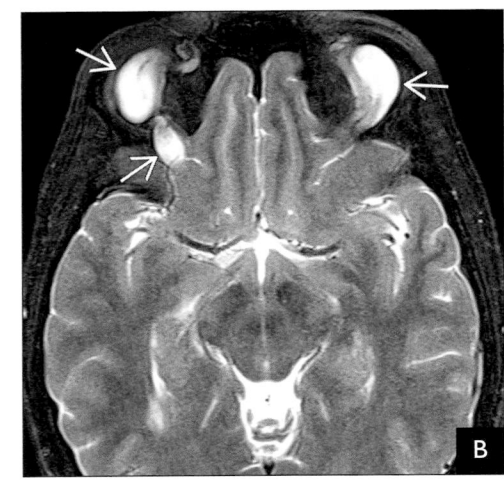

15-49C. Coronal STIR scan in the same patient shows fusiform rope-like enlargement and moderate hyperintensity of both mandibular nerves, extending from Meckel cave into the deep face ➡. 15-49D. Coronal STIR scan through the orbits shows the massively but symmetrically enlarged hyperintense ophthalmic nerves ➡.

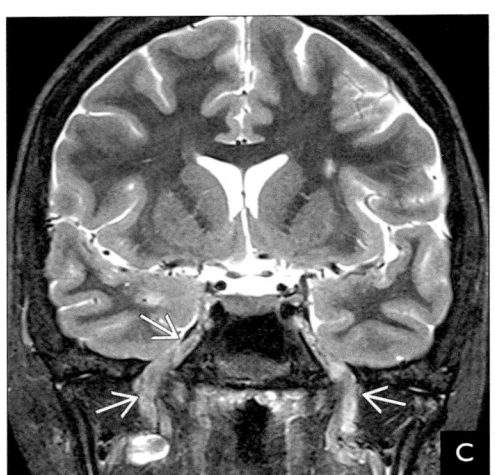
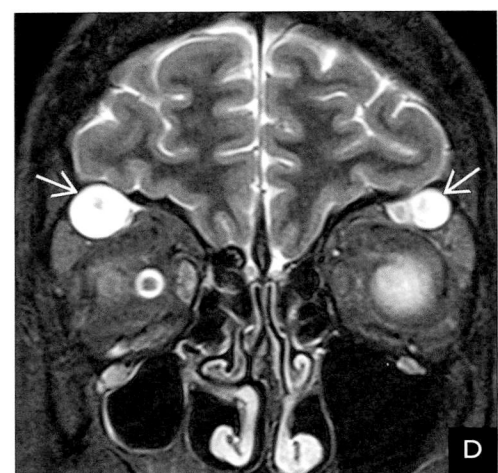

15-49E. Coronal T1 C+ FS shows that the enlarged trigeminal nerves enhance moderately ➡ but somewhat heterogeneously. 15-49F. Coronal T1 C+ FS shows mild to moderate enhancement of both ophthalmic divisions of CN V ➡. The patient had been diagnosed with MS, but no brain lesions were identified. CNS CIDP was confirmed at biopsy.

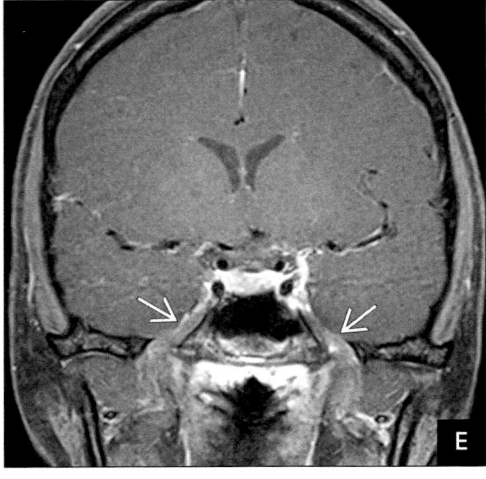
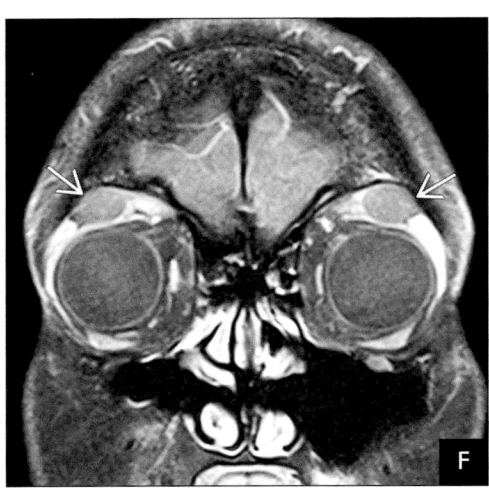

elected References

Multiple Sclerosis

- Balashov KE et al: Acute demyelinating lesions with restricted diffusion in multiple sclerosis. Mult Scler. Epub ahead of print, 2012
- Ceccarelli A et al: MRI in multiple sclerosis: a review of the current literature. Curr Opin Neurol. 25(4):402-9, 2012
- Chitnis T et al: Consensus statement: evaluation of new and existing therapeutics for pediatric multiple sclerosis. Mult Scler. 18(1):116-27, 2012
- Garaci FG et al: Brain hemodynamic changes associated with chronic cerebrospinal venous insufficiency are not specific to multiple sclerosis and do not increase its severity. Radiology. 265(1):233-9, 2012
- Granberg T et al: Radiologically isolated syndrome - incidental magnetic resonance imaging findings suggestive of multiple sclerosis, a systematic review. Mult Scler. Epub ahead of print, 2012
- Popescu BF et al: Meningeal and cortical grey matter pathology in multiple sclerosis. BMC Neurol. 12:11, 2012
- Salvi F et al: Venous angioplasty in multiple sclerosis: neurological outcome at two years in a cohort of relapsing-remitting patients. Funct Neurol. 27(1):55-9, 2012
- Tillema J et al: Non-lesional white matter changes in pediatric multiple sclerosis and monophasic demyelinating disorders. Mult Scler. Epub ahead of print, 2012
- Flynn LC et al: Current thoughts on chronic cerebrospinal venous insufficiency in multiple sclerosis. Curr Opin Ophthalmol. 22(6):463-7, 2011
- Ghezzi A et al: Chronic cerebro-spinal venous insufficiency (CCSVI) and multiple sclerosis. Neurol Sci. 32(1):17-21, 2011
- Giorgio A et al: Cortical lesions in radiologically isolated syndrome. Neurology. 77(21):1896-9, 2011
- International Multiple Sclerosis Genetics Consortium: Genetic risk and a primary role for cell-mediated immune mechanisms in multiple sclerosis. Nature. 476(7359):214-9, 2011
- Polman CH et al: Diagnostic criteria for multiple sclerosis: 2010 revisions to the McDonald criteria. Ann Neurol. 69(2):292-302, 2011
- Ratcliffe MR et al: Demyelinating disorders of the adult central nervous system: a pictorial review of MR imaging findings. Neurographics 1(1):17-30, 2011

ther Neuroinflammatory emyelinating Diseases

- Eckstein C et al: A differential diagnosis of central nervous system demyelination: beyond multiple sclerosis. J Neurol. 259(5):801-16, 2012

Multiple Sclerosis Variants

- Kraus D et al: Schilder's disease: non-invasive diagnosis and successful treatment with human immunoglobulins. Eur J Paediatr Neurol. 16(2):206-8, 2012
- Mealy MA et al: Epidemiology of neuromyelitis optica in the United States: a multicenter analysis. Arch Neurol. 69(9):1176-80, 2012
- Talab R et al: Marburg variant multiple sclerosis - a case report. Neuro Endocrinol Lett. 32(4):415-20, 2011
- Wengert O et al: Images in clinical medicine. Baló's concentric sclerosis. N Engl J Med. 365(8):742, 2011
- Wang L et al: Balo's concentric sclerosis. Lancet. 376(9736):189, 2010
- Cañellas AR et al: Idiopathic inflammatory-demyelinating diseases of the central nervous system. Neuroradiology. 49(5):393-409, 2007
- Kavanagh EC et al: Diffusion-weighted imaging findings in Balo concentric sclerosis. Br J Radiol. 79(943):e28-31, 2006
- Benavente E et al: Neuromyelitis optica-AQP4: an update. Curr Rheumatol Rep. 13(6):496-505, 2011
- Matsuoka T et al: Reappraisal of aquaporin-4 astrocytopathy in Asian neuromyelitis optica and multiple sclerosis patients. Brain Pathol. 21(5):516-32, 2011
- Wingerchuk DM et al: Revised diagnostic criteria for neuromyelitis optica. Neurology. 66(10):1485-9, 2006

Neuromyelitis Optica

- Dellavance A et al: Anti-aquaporin-4 antibodies in the context of assorted immune-mediated diseases. Eur J Neurol. 19(2):248-52, 2012
- Asgari N et al: A population-based study of neuromyelitis optica in Caucasians. Neurology. 76(18):1589-95, 2011
- Benavente E et al: Neuromyelitis Optica-AQP4: an update. Curr Rheumatol Rep. 13(6):496-505, 2011
- Matsuoka T et al: Reappraisal of aquaporin-4 astrocytopathy in Asian neuromyelitis optica and multiple sclerosis patients. Brain Pathol. 21(5):516-32, 2011
- Argyriou AA et al: Neuromyelitis optica: a distinct demyelinating disease of the central nervous system. Acta Neurol Scand. 118(4):209-17, 2008
- Wingerchuk DM et al: Revised diagnostic criteria for neuromyelitis optica. Neurology. 66(10):1485-9, 2006

Susac Syndrome

- Mateen FJ et al: Susac syndrome: clinical characteristics and treatment in 29 new cases. Eur J Neurol. 19(6):800-11, 2012
- Bienfang DC et al: Case records of the Massachusetts General Hospital. Case 24-2011. A 36-year-old man with headache, memory loss, and confusion. N Engl J Med. 365(6):549-59, 2011
- Bitra RK et al: Review of Susac syndrome. Curr Opin Ophthalmol. 22(6):472-6, 2011
- Demir MK: Case 142: Susac syndrome. Radiology. 250(2):598-602, 2009

Post-Infection/Post-Immunization Demyelination

Acute Disseminated Encephalomyelitis

- Parrish JB et al: Acuted disseminated encephalomyelitis. Adv Exp Med Biol. 724:1-14, 2012
- Zettl UK et al: Immune-mediated CNS diseases: a review on nosological classification and clinical features. Autoimmun Rev. 11(3):167-73, 2012
- Lim CC: Neuroimaging in postinfectious demyelination and nutritional disorders of the central nervous system. Neuroimaging Clin N Am. 21(4):843-58, viii, 2011

Acute Hemorrhagic Leukoencephalitis

- Kao HW et al: Value of susceptibility-weighted imaging in acute hemorrhagic leukoencephalitis. J Clin Neurosci. Epub ahead of print, 2012
- Borlot F et al: Acute hemorrhagic encephalomyelitis in childhood: Case report and literature review. J Pediatr Neurosci. 6(1):48-51, 2011
- Lann MA et al: Acute hemorrhagic leukoencephalitis: a critical entity for forensic pathologists to recognize. Am J Forensic Med Pathol. 31(1):7-11, 2010

Inflammatory-like Disorders

Neurosarcoidosis

- Saidha S et al: Etiology of sarcoidosis: does infection play a role? Yale J Biol Med. 85(1):133-41, 2012
- Terushkin V et al: Neurosarcoidosis: presentations and management. Neurologist. 16(1):2-15, 2010
- Lury KM et al: Neurosarcoidosis--review of imaging findings. Semin Roentgenol. 39(4):495-504, 2004
- Smith JK et al: Imaging manifestations of neurosarcoidosis. AJR Am J Roentgenol. 182(2):289-95, 2004

Idiopathic Inflammatory Pseudotumors

- Yavuzer D et al: Intracranial inflammatory pseudotumor: case report and review of the literature. Clin Neuropathol. 29(3):151-5, 2010

Chronic Inflammatory Demyelinating Polyneuropathy

- Kamm C et al: Autoimmune disorders affecting both the central and peripheral nervous system. Autoimmun Rev. 11(3):196-202, 2012
- Kale HA et al: Magnetic resonance imaging findings in chronic inflammatory demyelinating polyneuropathy with intracranial findings and enhancing, thickened cranial and spinal nerves. Australas Radiol. 51 Spec No, 2007
- Quan D et al: A 71-year-old male with 4 decades of symptoms referable to both central and peripheral nervous system. Brain Pathol. 15(4):369-70, 373, 2005

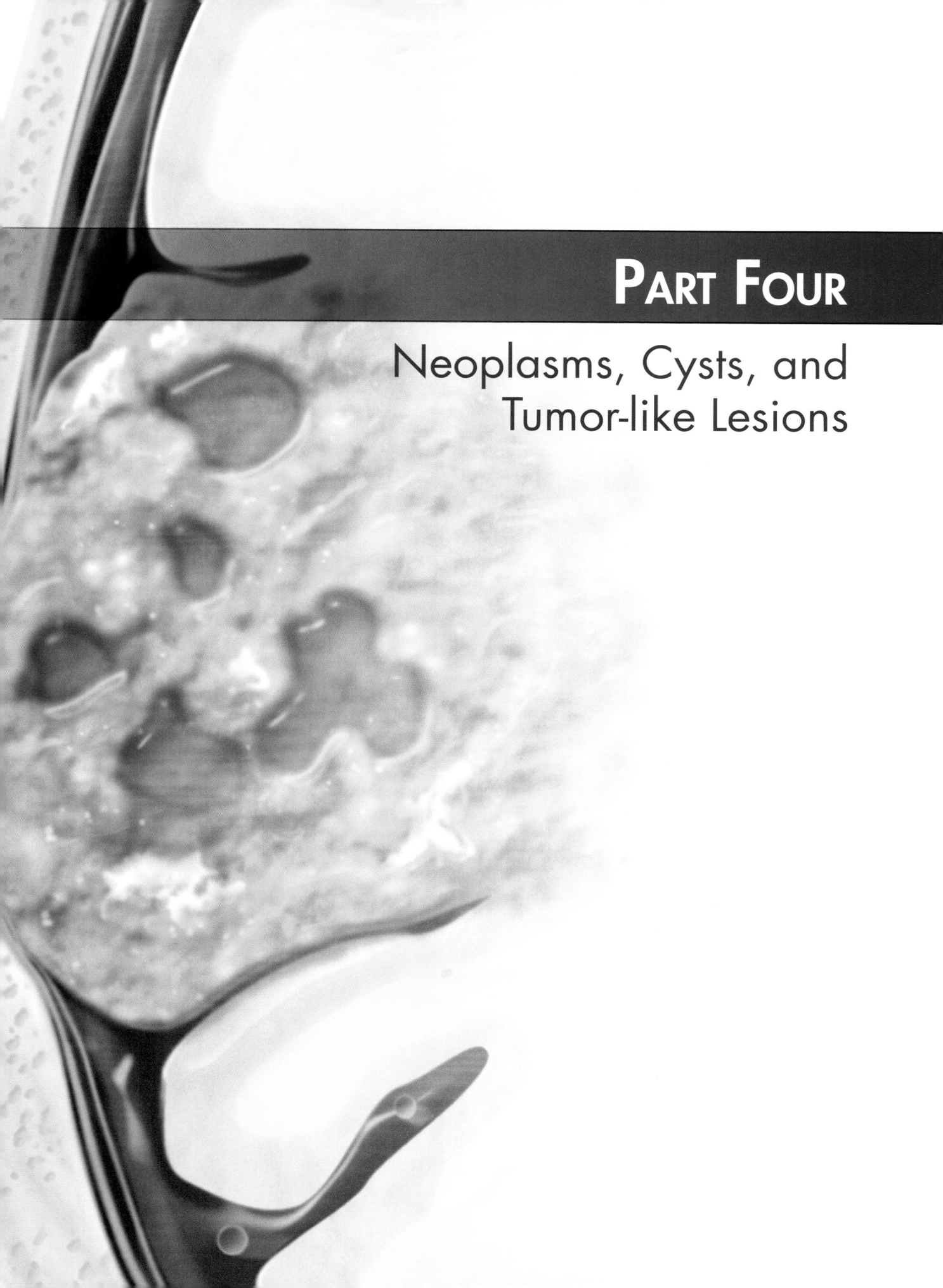

PART FOUR

Neoplasms, Cysts, and Tumor-like Lesions

16

Introduction to Neoplasms, Cysts, and Tumor-like Lesions

The most widely accepted classification of brain neoplasms is sponsored by the World Health Organization (WHO). Since 1986, a working group of world-renowned neuropathologists has convened approximately every seven years for an editorial and consensus update conference on brain tumor classification and grading. The results are then published as the *WHO Classification of Tumours of the Central Nervous System.*

The most recent edition—the fourth—was published in 2007 and is the version followed in this text. (The fifth edition is not scheduled for publication until 2014.) Between editions, updates are published in *Brain Pathology,* the official journal of the International Society of Neuropathologists.

Each edition of the WHO classification has added important new entities and redefined or clarified existing ones. The now-familiar dysembryoplastic neuroepithelial tumor (DNET) was codified in the 1993 edition. Two new tumors—chordoid glioma of the third ventricle and atypical teratoid/rhabdoid tumor—were added in 2000.

The current edition introduced the most extensive changes to date, adding eight new tumor entities and four new variants. All are included in this text. In addition, we include and briefly discuss neoplasms described since

2007 (e.g., pituitary blastoma and embryonal tumor with abundant neuropil and true rosettes [ETANTR]).

Classification and Grading of CNS Neoplasms

Brain tumors are both classified and graded. **Classifications** traditionally attempt to assign CNS neoplasms to discrete categories based on the histologic similarity of tumor cells to normal or embryonic constituents of the nervous system. The first widely accepted classification of brain tumors was formulated by Bailey and Cushing in 1926. Most subsequent systems—including the WHO—are modifications of that classification.

Classifications do form the logical basis for approaching CNS neoplasms despite their shortcomings and inconsistencies. Classifications based strictly on histologic criteria are gradually transitioning to a combination of genetic and molecular characteristics. If the genetic or molecular "signature" of a tumor has been identified, it is noted in this text.

Histological **grading** is a means of predicting the biological behavior of tumors and an important guide to therapeutic decisions. While many different grading schemas have been proposed, the WHO system is the most widely accepted and is utilized in this text. Most tumors have been assigned WHO grades and ICD-O (International Classification of Diseases for Oncology) codes, but a number of other tumors—especially those that are newly defined—remain ungraded or have been given only provisional codes.

Tumors of Neuroepithelial Tissue

Neoplasm	Grade	Neoplasm	Grade
ASTROCYTIC		**OTHER NEUROEPITHELIAL**	
Pilocytic astrocytoma	I	Astroblastoma	N/A
Pilomyxoid astrocytoma	II	Chordoid glioma of third ventricle	II
Subependymal giant cell astrocytoma	I	Angiocentric glioma (ANET)	I
Pleomorphic xanthoastrocytoma	II		
Diffuse astrocytoma	II	**NEURONAL, MIXED GLIONEURONAL**	
Anaplastic astrocytoma	III	Gangliocytoma	I
Glioblastoma multiforme	IV	Ganglioglioma	I
Gliosarcoma	IV	DIG/DIA	I
Gliomatosis cerebri	III	DNET	I
		Central neurocytoma	II
OLIGODENDROGLIAL		Extraventricular neurocytoma	II
Oligodendroglioma	II	Cerebellar liponeurocytoma	II
Anaplastic oligodendroglioma	III	Paraganglioma (spinal cord)	I
Oligoastrocytoma	II-III	Papillary glioneural tumor	I
		Rosette-forming glioneuronal tumor	I
EPENDYMAL			
Subependymoma	I	**PINEAL REGION**	
Myxopapillary ependymoma	I	Pineocytoma	I
Ependymoma	II	PPTID	II-III
Anaplastic ependymoma	III	Pineoblastoma	IV
		PTPR	II-III
CHOROID PLEXUS			
Choroid plexus papilloma	I	**EMBRYONAL**	
Atypical choroid plexus papilloma	II	Medulloblastoma	IV
Choroid plexus carcinoma	III	PNET	IV
		AT/RT	IV

Table 16-1. *AT/RT = atypical teratoid/rhabdoid tumor; DIG/DIA = desmoplastic infantile ganglioglioma or astrocytoma; DNET = dysembryoplastic neuroepithelial tumor; N/A = central nervous system tumor not assigned a grade by the World Health Organization; PNET = primitive neuroectodermal tumor; PPTID = pineal parenchymal tumor of intermediate differentiation; PTPR = papillary tumor of the pineal region. Table adapted from Louis DN et al: World Health Organization Classification of Tumours of the Central Nervous System. 4th ed. Lyon, France: IARC Press, 2007.*

General Considerations

CNS neoplasms are divided into primary and metastatic tumors, each accounting for about half of all brain tumors. Primary neoplasms are divided into six major categories. The largest by far is "tumors of neuroepithelial tissue" **(Table 16-1)**, followed by tumors of the meninges. Tumors of cranial and spinal nerves as well as lymphomas and hematopoietic neoplasms are less common but nevertheless important groupings.

In this text, we group two categories of primary CNS neoplasms by geographic location. Thus pineal region tumors and germ cell tumors (which are primarily but not exclusively found in the pineal region) are considered together. Tumors of the sellar region are likewise discussed as a group.

The current WHO classification also includes familial tumor syndromes such as neurofibromatosis types 1 and 2, tuberous sclerosis complex, von Hippel-Lindau disease, and Li-Fraumeni. We consider these in the last part of this text in connection with congenital malformations.

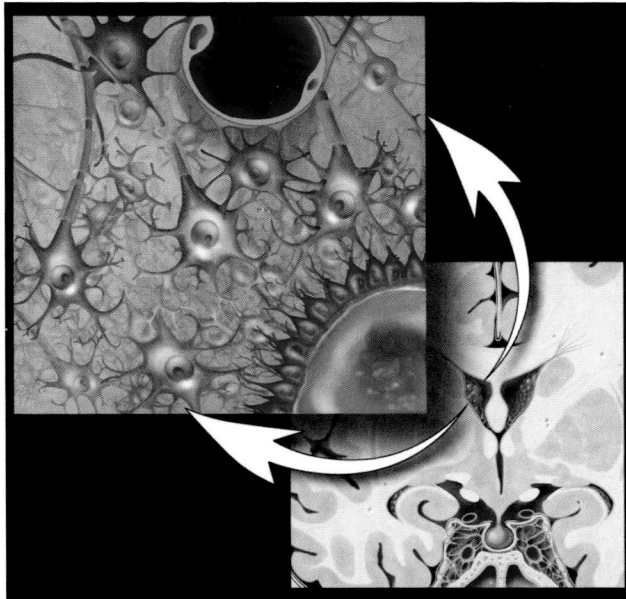

16-1. Cellular constituents of the neuropil include astrocytes, oligodendrocytes, neurons, microglia, choroid plexus, and ependymal cells. Each cell type was once thought to undergo malignant transformation, producing a corresponding neoplasm.

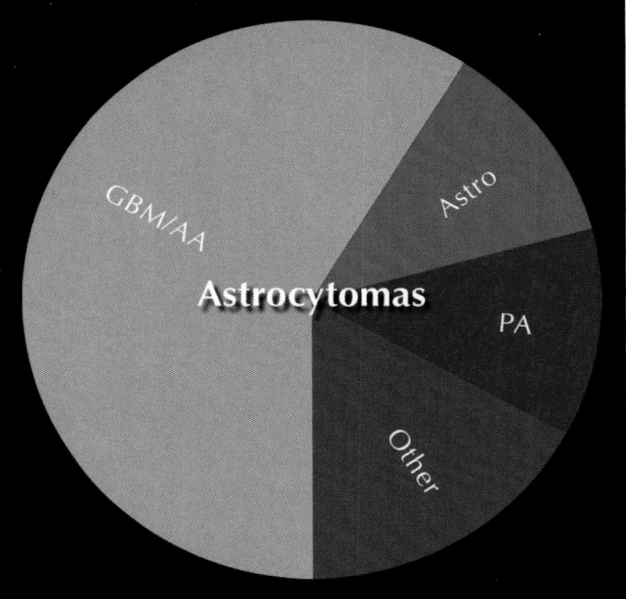

16-2. Astrocytomas are the largest group of primary brain tumors. More than half are AA (WHO grade III), GBM (grade IV). Astrocytoma (grade II), pilocytic astrocytoma (grade I) account for about 1/3 of all cases.

Tumors of Neuroepithelial Tissue

Tumors of neuroepithelial tissue is a huge category and therefore has been divided into several discrete tumor subtypes, each corresponding to a specific component of the neuropil. The primary constituents of the neuropil are neurons and glial cells, with the latter far outnumbering the former.

Glial neoplasms constitute one of the most heterogeneous groups of brain tumors. Tumors of putative glial cell origin were originally called "gliomas" (because of their supposed derivation from glue-like glial cells). The more accurate and current term is "neuroepithelial" or "neuroectodermal" tumors, reflecting tumor origin from nervous system precursor cells.

We begin our discussion of neuroepithelial tumors with a general overview of tumorigenesis, then follow with a brief consideration of each major tumor subgroup, beginning with astrocytomas.

Origin of Neuroepithelial Tumors

The neuropil contains several subtypes of glial cells: Astrocytes, oligodendrocytes, ependymal cells, and modified ependymal cells that form the choroid plexus. In the past, each subtype was thought to give rise to a specific type of "glioma." In this rather simplistic view, abnormal astrocytes were considered the source of astrocytomas, oligodendrogliomas to originate from oligodendrocytes, etc. **(16-1)**.

A paradigm shift in our understanding of cancer origins has occurred over the last few years. Many—if not most—primary neoplasms of the brain parenchyma are now thought to arise from **pluripotential neural stem cells** (NSCs). These NSCs persist in two areas of the postnatal brain: The subventricular zone—the region located under the ependyma of the brain ventricles—and the dentate gyrus of the hippocampus **(16-3)**.

Normal neurogenesis and gliogenesis continue throughout life. Brain NSCs have a high rate of proliferation and are thus prone to genetic errors. When these brainstem cells mutate, they become tumor progenitor cells (tumor stem cells) that can generate phenotypically diverse neoplasms.

Tumor stem cells have the capacity for continuous proliferation and self-renewal. They are inherently resistant to drugs and toxins, which may account for the general failure of many malignant brain tumors to respond to conventional nontargeted cancer therapies (i.e., ionizing radiation and chemotherapy).

Recent studies have shown that other factors may also contribute to the development of neuroepithelial tumors. The **brain stromal microenvironment** influences tumor formation and growth through cell-cell and cell-matrix contacts.

The molecular pathways responsible for tumor proliferation, invasion, angiogenesis, and anaplastic transformation also seem to contribute. Identification of these pathways provides important new prognostic and predic-

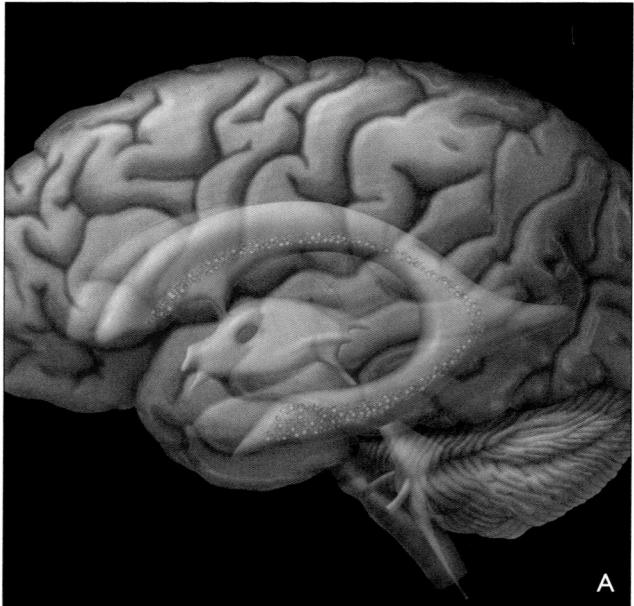

16-3A. Sagittal graphic depicts neural stem cells in yellow, shown arising from the subventricular zone just under the ependyma of the lateral ventricles.

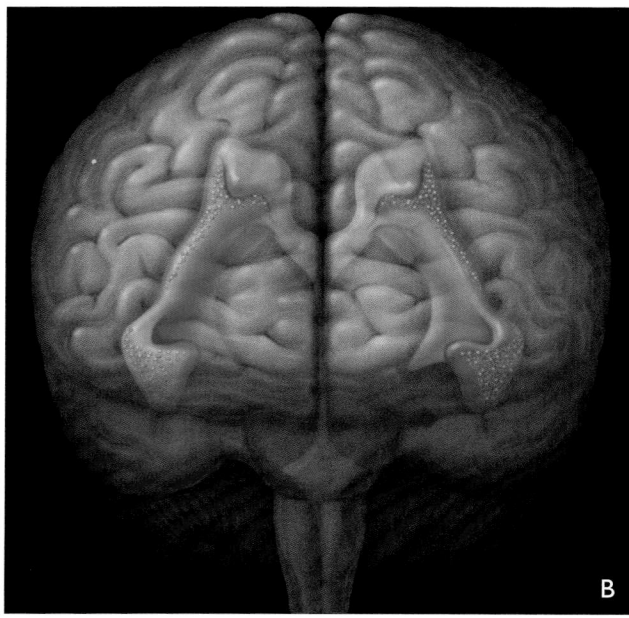

16-3B. Coronal graphic depicts neural stem cells in the subventricular zones of both lateral ventricles.

tive factors to guide treatment. For example, proangiogenic factors such as vascular endothelial growth factor (VEGF) and the methylation status of gene promotor of methylguanine-methyltransferase (MGMT) are emerging as important determinants in treating glioblastomas.

"Epigenetic" mechanisms involve heritable changes in gene expression that are not accompanied by changes in DNA sequence. For example, microRNAs are important regulators of developmental growth and differentiation. Genetically distinct microRNA expression signatures resembling those of radial glia, oligoneuronal precursors, neuronal precursors, neuroepithelial/neural crest precursors, and astrocyte precursors have been identified and, when altered, may play a key role in oncogenesis.

In the future, tumors may well be classified according to their molecular profiles and genetic signatures. Nevertheless—at least for the present—neuroepithelial tumors retain their traditional histologic classification as discussed below.

Astrocytomas

There are many histologic types and subtypes of astrocytomas. Astrocytomas can be relatively localized (and generally behave more benignly) or diffusely infiltrating with an inherent tendency to malignant degeneration.

The more localized astrocytic tumors are less common than the diffusely infiltrating astrocytomas **(16-2)**. Two of the localized tumors, pilocytic astrocytoma (PA) and subependymal giant cell astrocytoma (SEGA), are designated WHO grade I neoplasms. Neither displays a ten-

dency to malignant progression although a variant of PA, pilomyxoid astrocytoma, may behave more aggressively.

The most common astrocytomas are diffusely infiltrating neoplasms in which no distinct border between tumor and normal brain is present (even though the tumor may look discrete on imaging studies). The lowest grade of diffusely infiltrating astrocytoma is called simply "diffuse astrocytoma" and is designated WHO grade II. Anaplastic astrocytoma (AA) is WHO grade III, and glioblastoma (GBM) is a grade IV neoplasm. All diffusely infiltrating astrocytomas have an inherent tendency to malignant progression. *Note that there is no such thing as a grade I diffusely infiltrating astrocytoma.*

Patient age has a significant effect on neoplasm type and location **(16-4)**, **(16-5)**. This is especially true for astrocytomas. Astrocytomas in adults tend to be malignant (e.g., AA, GBM) and to affect the cerebral hemispheres. In contrast, PAs are tumors of children and young adults. They are common in the cerebellum and around the third ventricle but rarely occur in the hemispheres.

Nonastrocytic Glial Neoplasms

Oligodendrogliomas, ependymomas, histologically mixed glial neoplasms (most commonly oligodendroglioma mixed with astrocytoma), and choroid plexus tumors are all considered nonastrocytic glial neoplasms.

OLIGODENDROGLIAL TUMORS. Oligodendroglial tumors vary from a diffusely infiltrating but relatively well-differentiated WHO grade II neoplasm (oligodendroglioma) to anaplastic oligodendrogliomas (WHO

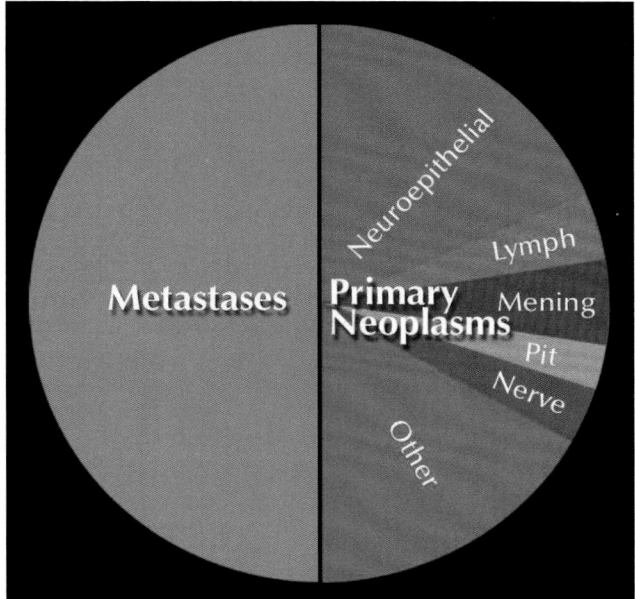

16-4. Graphic depicts the relative prevalence of brain tumors in adults. Roughly half are metastases from systemic cancers; the other half are primary neoplasms.

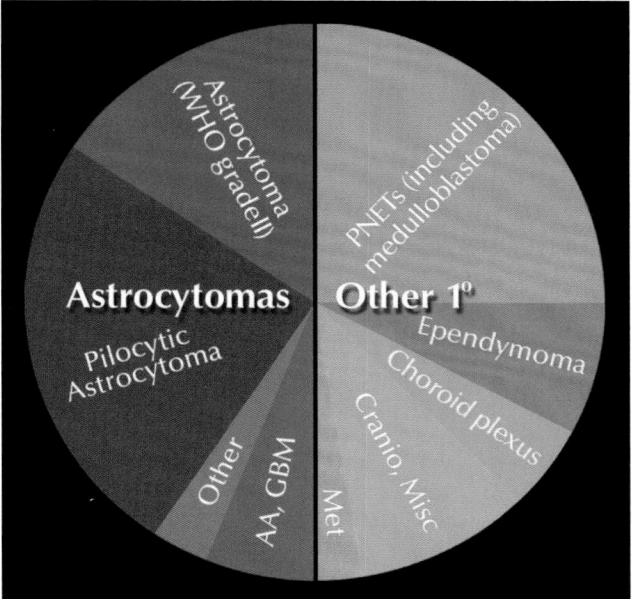

16-5. Graphic depicts the relative prevalence of brain tumors in children. Metastases, anaplastic astrocytoma, and glioblastoma multiforme are rare. Pilocytic astrocytoma and PNETs are more common compared to adults.

grade III). Oligodendrogliomas can be mixed with astrocytic or other elements. These so-called mixed gliomas are graded according to the most anaplastic element, which is usually the astrocytic component.

For treatment determination, however, molecular profiling (1p,19q deletion) is more important than the histologic characteristics of an oligodendroglioma.

EPENDYMAL TUMORS. Ependymal tumors vary from WHO grade I to III. Subependymoma, a benign-behaving neoplasm of middle-aged and older adults that occurs in the frontal horns and fourth ventricle, is a WHO grade I tumor. So is myxopapillary ependymoma, a tumor of young and middle-aged adults that is almost exclusively found at the conus, cauda equina, and filum terminale of the spinal cord.

Ependymoma, generally a slow-growing tumor of children and young adults, is a WHO grade II neoplasm that may arise anywhere along the ventricular system and in the central canal of the spinal cord. Infratentorial ependymomas, typically arising within the fourth ventricle, occur predominantly in children. Supratentorial ependymomas are more common in the cerebral hemispheres than the lateral ventricle and are usually tumors of young children. Anaplastic ependymomas are biologically more aggressive, have poorer prognosis, and are designated WHO grade III neoplasms.

Each of these ependymomas, while histologically similar, is developmentally and molecularly distinct and has specific identifiable genetic mutations.

CHOROID PLEXUS TUMORS. Choroid plexus tumors are papillary intraventricular neoplasms derived from choroid plexus epithelial cells. Almost 80% of choroid plexus tumors are found in children and are one of the most common brain tumors in children under the age of three years.

Choroid plexus tumors have classically been divided into choroid plexus papillomas (CPPs), which are WHO grade I tumors, and choroid plexus carcinomas (CPCas), designated WHO grade III. CPPs are five to ten times more common than CPCas. Both CPPs and CPCas can spread diffusely through the CSF, so the entire neuraxis should be imaged prior to surgical intervention.

The 2007 WHO classification recognizes a new intermediate grade of choroid plexus tumor. These tumors have been designated "atypical choroid plexus papillomas" (aCPPs) and are considered WHO grade II neoplasms.

OTHER NEUROEPITHELIAL TUMORS. Rare neuroepithelial neoplasms include astroblastoma, chordoid glioma of the third ventricle, and angiocentric glioma.

Neuronal and Mixed Glioneuronal Tumors

Neuroepithelial tumors with ganglion-like cells, differentiated neurocytes, or poorly differentiated neuroblastic cells are characteristic of this heterogeneous group.

Ganglion cell neoplasms (gangliocytoma, ganglioglioma), desmoplastic infantile ganglioglioma or astrocytoma (DIG/DIA), neurocytoma (central as well as the newly described extraventricular variant), dysembryoplastic neuroepithelial tumor (DNET), papillary glioneuronal tumor, rosette-forming glioneuronal tumor (of the fourth ventricle), and cerebellar liponeuroblastoma are included.

Pineal Region Tumors

Pineal region neoplasms account for less than 1% of all intracranial neoplasms and can be germ cell tumors or pineal parenchymal tumors. Pineal parenchymal tumors are less common than germ cell tumors. Germ cell neoplasms do occur in other intracranial sites but are discussed together with pineal parenchymal neoplasms.

Pineocytoma is a very slowly growing, well-delineated pineal parenchymal tumor that is usually found in adults. Pineocytomas are WHO grade I. Pineoblastoma is a highly malignant primitive embryonal tumor mostly found in children. Highly aggressive and associated with early CSF dissemination, pineoblastomas are WHO grade IV neoplasms.

A newly described tumor, pineal parenchymal tumor of intermediate differentiation (PPTID), is intermediate in malignancy and has been added to the WHO classification. PPTIDs are WHO grade II or III neoplasms. Many "aggressive" pineocytomas would probably be reclassified as PPTIDs according to the new criteria. Another recently described neoplasm, papillary tumor of the pineal region (PTPR), is a rare neuroepithelial tumor of adults. No formal WHO grade has been assigned, but PTPRs are provisionally designated WHO grade II or III neoplasms.

Embryonal Tumors

The embryonal tumor group includes medulloblastoma, CNS primitive neuroectodermal tumors (PNETs), and atypical teratoid/rhabdoid tumors (AT/RTs). All are highly malignant invasive tumors. All are WHO grade IV and are mostly tumors of young children.

Meningeal Tumors

Meningeal tumors are the second largest category of primary CNS neoplasms. They are divided into meningiomas and mesenchymal, nonmeningothelial tumors (i.e., tumors that are *not* meningiomas). Hemangiopericytomas, hemangioblastomas, and melanocytic lesions are also considered as part of the meningeal tumor grouping **(Table 16-2)**.

Meningiomas

Meningiomas arise from meningothelial (arachnoidal) cells. Most are attached to the dura but can occur in other locations (e.g., choroid plexus of the lateral ventricles).

While meningiomas have many histologic subtypes (e.g., meningothelial, fibrous, psammomatous), each with a different ICD-O code, the current WHO schema classifies them rather simply. Most meningioma subtypes are benign, have a low risk of recurrence and/or aggressive growth, and are grouped together as WHO grade I neoplasms.

Atypical meningiomas, as well as the chordoid and clear cell variants, are WHO grade II tumors. Anaplastic (malignant) meningiomas, including the papillary and rhabdoid subtypes, correspond to WHO grade III.

Both WHO grade II and III meningiomas have a greater likelihood of recurrence and/or aggressive behavior. The WHO classification also notes that meningiomas of any subtype or grade with a high proliferation index and/or brain invasion have a greater likelihood of aggressive behavior.

Mesenchymal Nonmeningothelial Tumors

Both benign and malignant nonmeningothelial mesenchymal tumors can originate in the CNS. Most correspond to tumors of soft tissue or bone. Generally, both a benign and malignant (sarcomatous) type occur. Lipomas and liposarcomas, chondromas and chondrosarcomas, osteomas and osteosarcomas are examples.

Hemangiopericytoma (HPC) is a highly cellular, very vascular mesenchymal tumor that is almost always attached to the dura. HPCs are WHO II or III neoplasms.

Hemangioblastoma (HGBL) is a WHO grade I neoplasm consisting of stromal cells and innumerable small blood vessels. It occurs both sporadically and as part of von Hippel-Lindau (VHL) syndrome.

Primary melanocytic neoplasms of the CNS are rare. They arise from leptomeningeal melanocytes and can be diffuse or circumscribed, benign or malignant.

Tumors of Cranial (and Spinal) Nerves

Schwannoma

Schwannomas are benign encapsulated nerve sheath tumors that consist of well-differentiated Schwann cells. They can be solitary or multiple. Multiple schwannomas are associated with neurofibromatosis type 2 (NF2) and schwannomatosis, a syndrome characterized by multiple schwannomas but lacking other features of NF2.

Intracranial schwannomas are almost always associated with cranial nerves (CN VIII is by far the most common) but occasionally occur as parenchymal lesions. Schwannomas do not undergo malignant degeneration and thus are designated WHO grade I neoplasms **(Table 16-3)**.

Meningeal Tumors				
Neoplasm	Grade	Neoplasm		Grade
MENINGOTHELIAL		**NONMENINGOTHELIAL MESENCHYMAL**		
Meningioma	I	Lipoma		I
Atypical meningioma	II	Liposarcoma		N/A
Anaplastic/malignant meningioma	III	Chondroma		I
		Chondrosarcoma		N/A
OTHER RELATED		Osteoma		N/A
Hemangioblastoma	I	Osteosarcoma		N/A
		Osteochondroma		N/A
PRIMARY MELANOCYTIC		Hemangioma		I
Diffuse melanocytosis	N/A	Hemangiopericytoma		II-III
Melanocytoma	N/A			
Malignant melanoma	N/A			
Meningeal melanomatosis	N/A			

Table 16-2. *N/A = central nervous system tumor not assigned a grade by the World Health Organization. Table adapted from Louis DN et al: World Health Organization Classification of Tumours of the Central Nervous System. 4th ed. Lyon, France: IARC Press, 2007.*

Neurofibroma

Neurofibromas (NFs) are diffusely infiltrating extraneural tumors that consist of Schwann cells and fibroblasts. Solitary scalp neurofibromas occur, and multiple NFs or plexiform NFs occur as part of neurofibromatosis type 1. Neurofibromas correspond histologically to WHO grade I. Plexiform neurofibromas may degenerate into malignant peripheral nerve sheath tumors (MPNSTs). MPNSTs are graded from WHO II to IV, the same three-tiered system used for soft tissue sarcomas.

Lymphomas and Hematopoietic Tumors

Primary CNS lymphoma and histiocytic tumors are the only two entities the WHO includes in this category. For our discussion, we include neoplasms such as leukemia and plasma cell tumors that usually reflect secondary involvement from systemic disease. Also included are disorders such as lymphomatoid granulomatosis, posttransplant lymphoproliferative disorder (PTLD), and nonneoplastic tumor-like histiocytic masses that may involve the CNS.

Primary CNS Lymphoma

Primary CNS lymphoma (PCNSL) is considered an extranodal malignant lymphoma that initially arises in the CNS. PCNSL must be distinguished from secondary involvement by extracranial systemic lymphoma.

Although PCNSL occurs in both immunocompetent and immunocompromised patients, the success of antiretroviral therapy in HIV/AIDS patients and improved survival in other immunocompromised patients has dramatically increased its prevalence. PCNSL now represents about 4% of all primary intracranial neoplasms.

PCNSL can occur as both focal parenchymal and intravascular tumor. PCNSL can be single or multiple and is most commonly seen in the cerebral hemispheres. More than 95% of PCNSLs are diffuse large B-cell lymphomas.

Leukemia

Leukemia is the most common form of childhood cancer. Once relatively uncommon, the prevalence of CNS involvement has risen as more effective treatment prolongs survival.

Histiocytic Tumors

Histiocytic tumors are a poorly understood heterogeneous group of tumors and tumor-like conditions. A wide variety of neoplastic and nonneoplastic histiocytic proliferations characterize these disorders. Some behave relatively benignly, and others are potentially lethal.

Germ Cell Tumors

Intracranial germ cell tumors (GCTs) are morphologic and immunophenotypic homologues of germinal neoplasms that arise in the gonads and extragonadal sites. From 80-90% occur in adolescents. Most occur in the midline (pineal region, around the third ventricle).

Germinomas are the most common intracranial GCT. Teratomas differentiate along ectodermal, endodermal, and mesodermal lines. They can be mature, immature, or

Other Tumors

Neoplasm	Grade	Neoplasm	Grade
CRANIAL & SPINAL NERVE TUMORS		**SELLAR REGION TUMORS**	
Schwannoma	I	Craniopharyngioma	I
Neurofibroma	I	Adamantinomatous	
MPNST	II-IV	Papillary	
		Granular cell tumor of neurohypophysis	I
GERM CELL TUMORS		Pituicytoma	I
Germinoma	II	Spindle cell oncocytoma of adenohypophysis	I
Embryonal carcinoma	N/A		
Yolk sac tumor	N/A	**LYMPHOMA/HEMATOPOIETIC**	
Mixed germ cell tumor	N/A	Malignant lymphoma	N/A
Teratoma	N/A	Plasmacytoma	N/A
Mature teratoma		Leukemia/granulocytic sarcoma	N/A
Immature teratoma			
Teratoma with malignant degeneration			

Table 16-3. *MPNST = malignant peripheral nerve sheath tumor; N/A = central nervous system tumor not assigned a grade by the World Health Organization. Table adapted from Louis DN et al: World Health Organization Classification of Tumours of the Central Nervous System. 4th ed. Lyon, France: IARC Press, 2007.*

occur as teratomas with malignant transformation. Other miscellaneous GCTs include the highly aggressive yolk sac tumor, embryonal carcinoma, and choriocarcinoma.

Germ cell tumors are discussed in detail with tumors of the pineal region.

Sellar Region Tumors

The sellar region is one of the most anatomically complex areas in the brain. Yet the official WHO classification of sellar region tumors includes only craniopharyngioma and rare tumors such as granular cell tumor of the neurohypophysis, pituicytoma, and spindle cell oncocytoma of the adenohypophysis.

The sellar region contains many structures besides the craniopharyngeal duct and infundibular stalk that give rise to masses seen on imaging studies. The most common of these masses—pituitary adenoma—is not part of the WHO classification but is included here, as are variants (such as pituitary hyperplasia) and nonneoplastic tumor-like masses (e.g., hypophysitis and hypothalamic hamartoma) that can mimic neoplasms.

Pituitary Adenoma

Pituitary adenomas account for the majority of sellar/suprasellar masses in adults. They are classified by size as microadenomas (≤ 10 mm) and macroadenomas (≥ 11 mm).

Craniopharyngioma

Craniopharyngioma is a benign (WHO grade I), often partially cystic neoplasm that is the most common nonneuroepithelial intracranial neoplasm in children. It shows a distinct bimodal age distribution with the cystic adamantinomatous type seen mostly in children and a smaller peak in middle-aged adults. The less common papillary type is usually solid and found almost exclusively in adults.

Miscellaneous Sellar Region Tumors

Granular cell tumor of the neurohypophysis, also called choristoma, is a rare tumor of adults that usually arises from the infundibulum. Pituicytomas are glial neoplasms of adults that also usually arise within the infundibulum. Spindle cell oncocytoma of the adenohypophysis is an oncocytic nonendocrine neoplasm. All of these rare tumors are WHO grade I. The diagnosis is usually histological, as differentiating these tumors from each other and from other adult tumors such as macroadenoma can be problematic.

Metastatic Tumors

Metastatic neoplasms represent nearly half of all CNS tumors. In Chapter 27, we consider the "many faces" of CNS metastatic disease as well as the intriguing topic of paraneoplastic syndromes.

Paraneoplastic neurologic syndromes (PNSs) are rare nervous system dysfunctions in cancer patients that are not due to metastases or local effects of a tumor. Classic PNSs with "onconeural" antibodies and several recently described nonparaneoplastic encephalitides are likewise included in Chapter 27.

ntracranial Cysts

Cysts are common findings on neuroimaging studies and, for purposes of discussion, included in this part of the text. Although our focus is primarily neoplasms, nonneoplastic CNS cysts can sometimes be confused with "real" brain tumors and are often considered in the differential diagnosis of mass lesions in specific anatomic locations.

We therefore take an anatomic- and imaging-based approach to intracranial cysts. Here the key consideration is not cyst wall histopathology (as in brain neoplasms) but anatomic location.

The four key anatomy-based questions to pose when considering the imaging diagnosis of an intracranial cyst are: (1) Is the cyst extra- or intraaxial? (2) Is it supra- or infratentorial? (3) Is it midline or off-midline? (4) If the cyst is intraaxial, is it in the brain parenchyma or inside the ventricles?

While many cysts can be found in multiple locations, each type has its own "preferred" (i.e., most common) site. The three major anatomic sublocations are the extraaxial spaces (including the scalp and skull), the brain parenchyma, and the cerebral ventricles.

xtraaxial Cysts

This is the second largest group of nonneoplastic cysts. The chapter on nonneoplastic cysts considers these first, beginning from the scalp and skull and proceeding inward to the arachnoid. The uncommon but important "neoplasm-associated cysts" that are sometimes seen around extraaxial tumors such as macroadenoma, meningioma, and vestibular schwannoma are probably a form of arachnoid cyst. Epidermoid and dermoid cysts are also included in this discussion.

ntraaxial (Parenchymal) Cysts

The most common parenchymal cysts are enlarged perivascular spaces and hippocampal sulcus remnants, followed by porencephalic (encephaloclastic) cysts. Neuroglial cysts—parenchymal cysts lined by nonneoplastic gliotic brain—are relatively uncommon.

Intraventricular Cysts

Intraventricular cysts are less common than cysts in the brain parenchyma. The most common intraventricular cysts are choroid plexus cysts, which are almost always incidental findings on imaging studies. Colloid cysts are the second most common cyst but the most important to diagnose because they can suddenly and unexpectedly obstruct the foramen of Monro. Acute obstructive hydrocephalus and even death can result.

Selected References

- Osborn AG et al: The new World Health Organization Classification of Central Nervous System Tumors: what can the neuroradiologist really say? AJNR Am J Neuroradiol. 33(5):795-802, 2012

Classification and Grading of CNS Neoplasms

Tumors of Neuroepithelial Tissue

- Faria CM et al: Epigenetic mechanisms regulating neural development and pediatric brain tumor formation. J Neurosurg Pediatr. 8(2):119-32, 2011
- Pollo B: Neuropathological diagnosis of brain tumours. Neurol Sci. 32 Suppl 2:S209-11, 2011
- Rahman M et al: The cancer stem cell hypothesis: failures and pitfalls. Neurosurgery. 68(2):531-45; discussion 545, 2011
- Vergani F et al: World Health Organization grade II gliomas and subventricular zone: anatomic, genetic, and clinical considerations. Neurosurgery. 68(5):1293-8; discussion 1298-9, 2011
- Moser JJ et al: The microRNA and messengerRNA profile of the RNA-induced silencing complex in human primary astrocyte and astrocytoma cells. PLoS One. 5(10):e13445, 2010

Meningeal Tumors

- Perry A et al: Meningiomas. In Louis DN et al: WHO Classification of Tumours of the Central Nervous System. Lyon, France: IARC Press. 163-86, 2007

Tumors of Cranial (and Spinal) Nerves

- Jones NB et al: Prognostic factors and staging for soft tissue sarcomas: an update. Surg Oncol Clin N Am. 21(2):187-200, 2012

Intracranial Cysts

- Osborn AG et al: Intracranial cysts: radiologic-pathologic correlation and imaging approach. Radiology. 239(3):650-64, 2006

17

Astrocytomas

Approximately half of all primary brain tumors arise from glial cells, probably via their neural stem cell progenitors. Nearly 75% of these "gliomas" are astrocytomas. Astrocytomas thus comprise the single largest group of all primary CNS neoplasms.

Astrocytomas form a surprisingly diverse group of neoplasms with many different histologic types and subtypes. These fascinating tumors differ widely in preferential location, peak age, clinical manifestations, morphologic features, biological behavior, and prognosis.

In this chapter, we discuss the full pathologic spectrum of astrocytic tumors, along with their clinical features and imaging findings. For purposes of discussion, astrocytomas are subdivided into two general categories: A relatively "localized," comparatively more benign-behaving group and a "diffusely infiltrating," more biologically aggressive group. This distinction is somewhat arbitrary and imperfect, as some "circumscribed" astrocytomas occasionally become more aggressive and infiltrate adjacent structures despite their low-grade histology.

Other tumors such as pleomorphic xanthoastrocytoma occupy an intermediate position but, for purposes of this discussion, are included with the localized group.

Origin of Astrocytomas

Astrocytomas were originally named for their putative origin from the stellate-shaped cells—"astrocytes"—that are the dominant component of the neuropil (vastly out-

numbering neurons). It was once assumed that astrocytes could undergo both hyperplasia (nonneoplastic "reactive astrocytosis") and neoplastic transformation.

There is increasing evidence that astrocytomas do *not* arise from neoplastic transformation of normal mature astrocytes. Instead, astrocytomas are probably derived from neural stem cells (NSCs) that have been stimulated by different oncogenes. Insufficient p53-dependent tumor suppression associated with high H-Ras oncogenic susceptibility has been suggested as the origin of most diffuse astrocytomas, the majority of which carry *TP53* mutations.

Recent studies have also shown that microRNAs are important regulators of developmental growth and differentiation. Genetically distinct microRNA signatures have been identified with a variety of different precursor cells including radial glia, oligoneuronal precursors, neuronal precursors, neuroepithelial/neural crest precursors, and astrocyte precursors. microRNA probably plays a key role in the oncogenesis of astrocytomas as well as other primary CNS malignancies.

Classification and Grading

While tumor staging is commonly used for neoplasms elsewhere in the body, CNS neoplasms are first classified (into specific tumor types) and then graded (a measure of malignancy).

To date, tumor classification has been based primarily on histologic features. However, use of molecular profiling is increasingly common and may ultimately become the basis for tumor classification as well as patient management.

CLASSIFICATION. Between 10-15% of astrocytomas grow slowly, tending to remain localized and relatively well-circumscribed. These astrocytomas generally follow a relatively indolent clinical course. Only two astrocytoma subtypes—pilocytic and subependymal giant cell astrocytomas—are considered truly benign. On occasion, even these relatively localized neoplasms behave aggressively (see below).

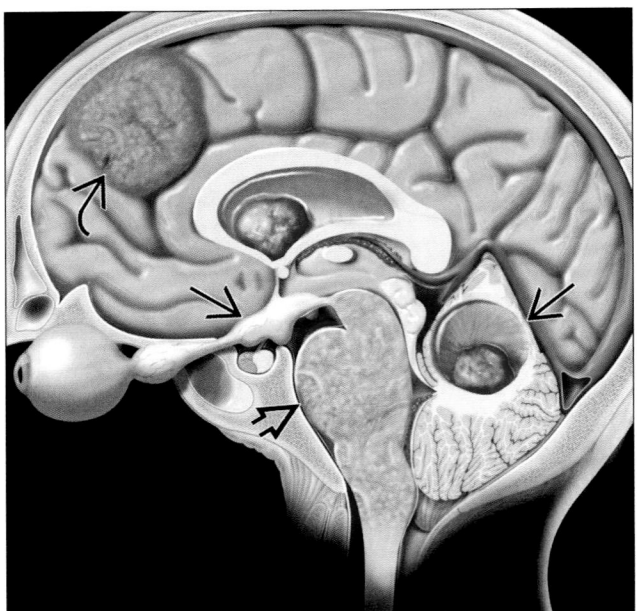

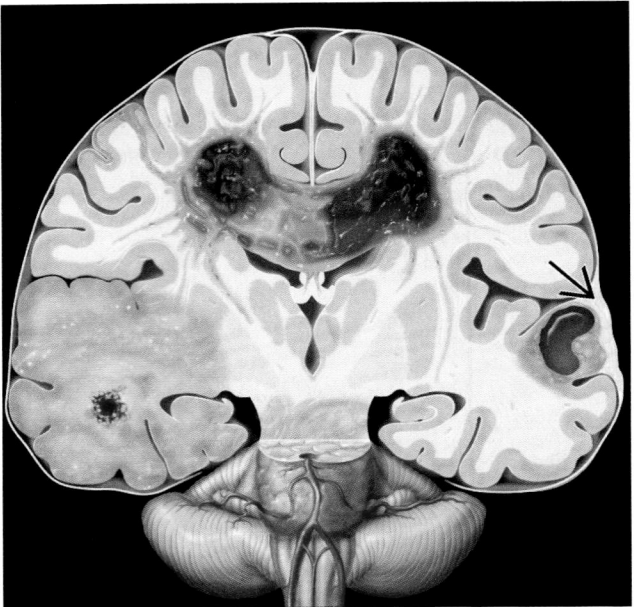

17-1. Childhood astrocytomas are illustrated. Pilocytic astrocytoma is common in the cerebellum, hypothalamus/optic nerves ➡. Pontine tumors ➡ are diffusely infiltrating WHO II-IV tumors. Hemispheric astrocytomas ➹ are uncommon.

17-2. Coronal graphic shows the classic astrocytomas of adulthood. Low-grade astrocytoma (brainstem), AA (temporal lobe), GBM (corpus callosum), and PXA with cyst, meningeal reaction ➡ are shown.

The vast majority of astrocytomas grow more rapidly and diffusely infiltrate adjacent tissues. They demonstrate relentless progression and display an inherent propensity to undergo malignant degeneration. The most malignant varieties—glioblastoma multiforme and anaplastic astrocytoma—represent well over half of all astrocytomas.

GRADING. In this text, we follow the World Health Organization (WHO) grading system of astrocytomas, designating them from grade I to grade IV. Grade I lesions have low proliferative potential, and patients have relatively prolonged survival. Surgical resection alone may be curative, so grade I astrocytomas rarely require adjuvant therapy. Two histologic subtypes of astrocytomas—pilocytic and subependymal giant cell astrocytoma—are designated WHO grade I neoplasms.

By far the largest group of astrocytomas is composed of diffusely infiltrating tumors. All diffusely infiltrating astrocytomas are *at least* WHO grade II neoplasms, and most are grades III-IV. In the WHO system, there is no such thing as a grade I diffuse astrocytoma. Because of their intrinsic tendency to undergo progressive genetic alterations and malignant transformation, mean survival of patients with grade II astrocytomas is under a decade.

Grading of diffusely infiltrative astrocytic tumors should be based on the areas with the most marked anaplasia. Tumors with cytological atypia alone are designated grade II (i.e., low-grade diffuse astrocytoma). Astrocytomas that demonstrate anaplasia and mitotic activity are grade III tumors (anaplastic astrocytoma). If microvas-

cular endothelial proliferation ("neovascularity") and necrosis are also present, the neoplasm is designated a grade IV astrocytoma (glioblastoma multiforme).

Distinguishing a grade II from a grade III astrocytoma on the basis of histological features alone can be difficult. Neuropathologists often add a measure of cellular proliferation called the MIB-1 labeling index as a surrogate estimate for subsequent biological behavior of the tumor.

Age and Location in Astrocytomas

There is a striking effect of age on both astrocytoma subtype and preferred location. Some astrocytomas (such as pilocytic astrocytoma) occur almost exclusively in children, while others (e.g., glioblastoma multiforme) are far more common in adults.

There is also a very strong anatomic preference with certain astrocytomas occurring frequently in some locations and very rarely in others. With some exceptions, most astrocytomas in children are localized tumors that primarily occur in the posterior fossa **(17-1)**. The vast majority of adult astrocytomas are diffusely infiltrating, supratentorial, and located in the cerebral hemispheres **(17-2)**.

CHILDHOOD ASTROCYTOMAS. Although brain tumors account for only 1-2% of all neoplasms, they cause 20-25% of cancers in children between one and 15 years of age. Astrocytomas account for nearly half of all intracranial neoplasms in this age group.

Newborns and infants. Astrocytomas are rare in newborns and infants. When they occur in this age group, they tend to be supratentorial, rather than the preferential infratentorial location seen in children. Congenital astrocytomas are large, bulky, highly malignant hemispheric neoplasms. **Glioblastoma multiforme** (GBM) is the most common congenital astrocytoma.

A rare variant of pilocytic astrocytoma called **pilomyxoid astrocytoma** can also present in infants, generally as a large H-shaped hypothalamic mass that extends laterally into one or both temporal lobes.

Children. The vast majority of childhood astrocytomas are either localized tumors such as **pilocytic astrocytoma** (WHO grade I) or **low-grade diffusely infiltrating astrocytoma** (WHO grade II). Less than 10% of astrocytomas in children are malignant (grades III-IV).

The only other grade I astrocytoma that commonly occurs in children is **subependymal giant cell astrocytoma** (SEGA). SEGAs virtually always occur in the setting of tuberous sclerosis. SEGAs are almost exclusively found in the lateral ventricle near the foramen of Monro, attached to the septi pellucidi.

In addition to specific tumor types, childhood astrocytomas have a particularly strong predilection for certain anatomic locations. After the age of one to two years, more than half are infratentorial; the cerebellum and the brainstem are the most common sites. Cerebellar and tectal plate astrocytomas are usually pilocytic astrocytomas, whereas most brainstem "gliomas" are diffusely infiltrating fibrillary astrocytomas (usually grades II-III).

The second most common overall astrocytoma site in children clusters around the third ventricle, hypothalamus, and optic chiasm. Most astrocytomas in this location are pilocytic, including the rare pilomyxoid variant.

The cerebral hemispheres are the least common site of astrocytomas in children. The astrocytoma most frequently seen here is the grade II diffusely infiltrating low-grade astrocytoma, which is usually a tumor of older children and young adults. Hemispheric pilocytic astrocytomas occur but are quite rare.

ASTROCYTOMAS IN YOUNG ADULTS. Diffusely infiltrating astrocytoma (WHO grade II) is the most common of all primary CNS neoplasms in patients between the ages of 18 and 30 years. Most occur in the hemispheric white matter.

Pleomorphic xanthoastrocytoma (PXA) is a WHO grade II-III neoplasm. PXAs are usually cortically based hemispheric tumors that present with epilepsy. PXAs are more common in young adults than in children.

ADULTHOOD ASTROCYTOMAS. In contrast to astrocytomas in children, astrocytomas in patients over the age of 30 years are mostly supratentorial and occur primarily in the cerebral hemispheres. Diffusely infiltrating astrocytomas are the most common tumor type.

In general, the older the patient, the higher the tumor grade. For example, pilocytic astrocytomas are rare in adults. Anaplastic astrocytoma (AA) and glioblastoma multiforme are much more common in middle-aged and older adults than low-grade (i.e., grade II) diffusely infiltrating astrocytoma.

AGE AND ASTROCYTOMAS

Newborn/Infant
- Rare
- Supratentorial > > infratentorial
- Large, bulky, malignant (GBM) hemispheric mass
- Less common = pilomyxoid astrocytoma

Children/Young Adults
- Common
- Infratentorial > supratentorial
- Pilocytic > diffusely infiltrating astrocytoma > subependymal giant cell astrocytoma (SEGA)
- Pilocytic astrocytoma
  - Cerebellum, fourth ventricle > pons, medulla
  - Optic chiasm/hypothalamus > tectum
  - Hemispheric PA rare
- Diffusely infiltrating astrocytoma
  - Low grade > high grade
  - Brainstem, cerebral hemispheres > cerebellum
- SEGA
  - Look for signs of tuberous sclerosis
  - Most at/around foramen of Monro

Middle-Aged/Older Adults
- Older the patient, the more malignant the astrocytoma
- GBM > anaplastic > > low-grade astrocytoma
- Usually involve hemispheric WM
- Posterior fossa very rare

Localized Astrocytic Tumors

In this section, we consider the relatively "localized" or circumscribed astrocytomas. Localized astrocytomas are significantly less common than diffusely infiltrating astrocytomas.

Recall that only two localized astrocytomas, **pilocytic astrocytoma** (PA) and **subependymal giant cell astrocytoma**, are designated WHO grade I neoplasms. WHO grade I tumors do not display an inherent tendency to malignant progression. Remote metastases are rare, and when they occur, they generally maintain their innocent histologic (i.e., grade I) features.

Pilomyxoid astrocytoma (PMA), considered by some neuropathologists a rare but more aggressive PA variant, is generally designated as a WHO grade II neoplasm. Because it behaves quite differently from PA, PMA is discussed separately.

Pilocytic Astrocytoma

Terminology

Pilocytic astrocytoma, sometimes termed "juvenile pilocytic astrocytoma" or "cystic cerebellar astrocytoma," is a well-circumscribed, typically slow-growing glioma of young patients.

Etiology

Most investigators believe PAs arise from an as-yet-unidentified astrocytic precursor cell, probably a neural stem cell. There is a syndromic association with neurofibromatosis type 1 (NF1) (15% of NF1 patients develop PAs). Unlike diffusely infiltrating astrocytomas, PAs have a very low prevalence of *TP53* mutations.

Pathology

LOCATION. PAs may arise anywhere in the neuraxis but have a distinct predilection for certain sites. The cerebellum is the most common location, accounting for nearly 60% of all PAs.

The second most common site is in and around the optic nerve/chiasm and hypothalamus/third ventricle, which together account for between one-quarter and one-third of all PAs. The third most common location is the pons and medulla. PAs also occur in the tectum where they may cause aqueductal stenosis.

The cerebral hemispheres are a reported but uncommon location of PA. When they occur outside the posterior fossa, optic pathway, or suprasellar region, PAs tend to be cortically based cysts with a tumor nodule that usually does not abut the pial surface.

GROSS PATHOLOGY. PAs are typically well-delineated soft grayish tumors that often form intratumoral cysts (17-3). The walls of most PA-associated cysts usually consist of compressed but otherwise normal brain

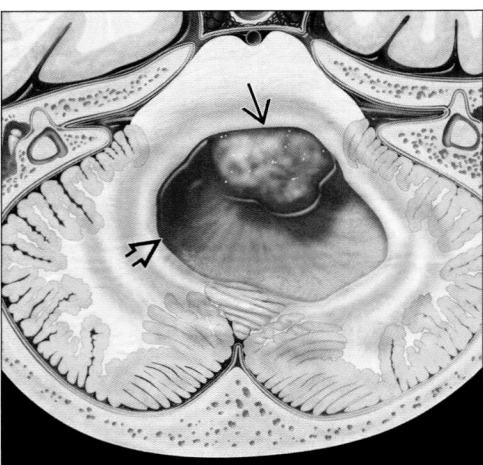
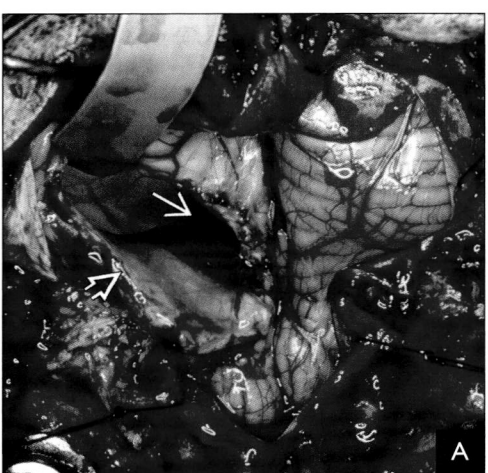
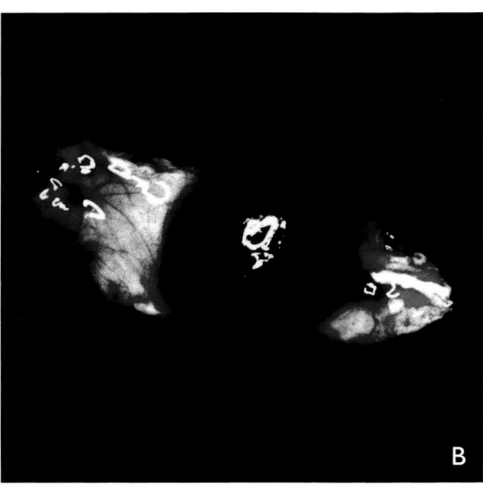
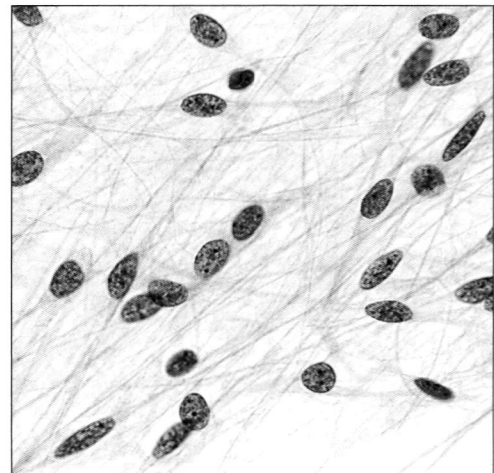

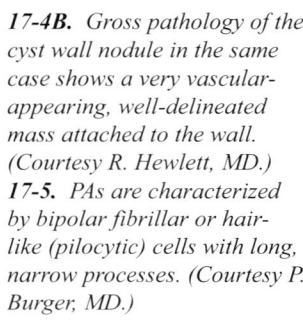

17-3. Graphic depicts typical cerebellar pilocytic astrocytoma with a vascular-appearing tumor nodule ➡, large nonneoplastic cyst ➡. The cyst wall consists of compressed but otherwise histologically normal brain parenchyma. 17-4A. Intraoperative photograph shows a cerebellar hemisphere cyst ➡ that is held open by a retractor. The cyst wall consists of compressed brain parenchyma. A reddish nodule ➡ is barely visible.

17-4B. Gross pathology of the cyst wall nodule in the same case shows a very vascular-appearing, well-delineated mass attached to the wall. (Courtesy R. Hewlett, MD.) 17-5. PAs are characterized by bipolar fibrillar or hair-like (pilocytic) cells with long, narrow processes. (Courtesy P. Burger, MD.)

parenchyma with the neoplastic element confined to the mural tumor nodule **(17-4)**. Cyst contents are typically a protein-rich xanthochromic fluid.

Macrocystic PAs are preferentially located in the cerebellum and (less commonly) the cerebral hemispheres.

More infiltrative PAs without cyst formation are more common in the optic pathways (optic pathway "glioma") and hypothalamus.

MICROSCOPIC FEATURES. The classic finding of PA is a biphasic pattern of two distinct astrocyte populations. The dominant type is composed of compact, hair-like ("pilocytic") bipolar cells with Rosenthal fibers (electron-dense glial fibrillary acidic protein [GFAP]-positive cytoplasmic inclusions) **(17-5)**. Intermixed are loosely textured, hypocellular, GFAP-negative areas that contain multipolar cells with microcysts. Immunohistochemistry with MIB-1 is typically less than 1%, indicating low proliferative potential.

Rare anaplastic PA variants do occur in children but are more common in adults. Increased cellularity and cytological atypia with > 5 mitoses per high-powered field and a high Ki-67 or MIB-1 proliferative index are features that suggest anaplastic PA. Increased L1CAM expression correlates with Ki-67 index and is also associated with recurrence risk.

STAGING, GRADING, AND CLASSIFICATION. PA is a WHO grade I tumor. Tumor dissemination occasionally occurs but is rare.

linical Issues

EPIDEMIOLOGY. PA accounts for 5-10% of all gliomas and is the most common primary brain tumor in children. PAs represent nearly 25% of all CNS neoplasms and 85% of posterior fossa astrocytomas in this age group.

DEMOGRAPHICS. More than 80% of PAs occur in patients under 20. The peak incidence is in "middle-aged" children between the ages of five and 15 years. There is no gender predilection.

PRESENTATION. Symptoms vary with location. Cerebellar PAs often present with headache, morning nausea, and vomiting, as intraventricular obstructive hydrocephalus is common. Ataxia, visual loss, and cranial nerve palsies also occur.

Optic pathway PAs typically present with visual loss. An uncommon presentation of a PA involving the hypothalamus is diencephalic syndrome, a rare but potentially lethal cause of failure to thrive despite adequate caloric intake.

Pontine and medullary PAs are uncommon but typically present with multiple cranial nerve palsies.

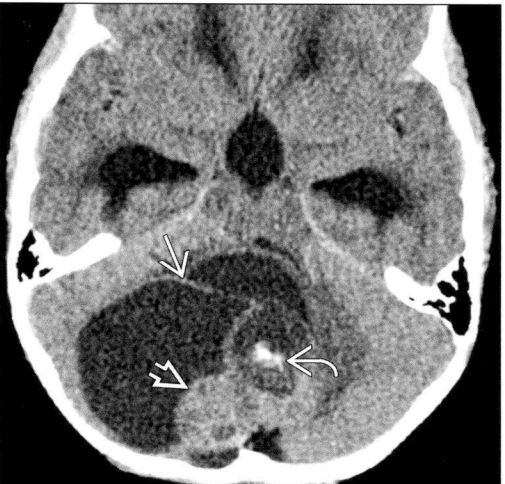

17-6. NECT scan shows a posterior fossa PA with cysts ➡, *solid tumor nodule* ➡, *Ca++* ➡, *associated obstructive hydrocephalus.*

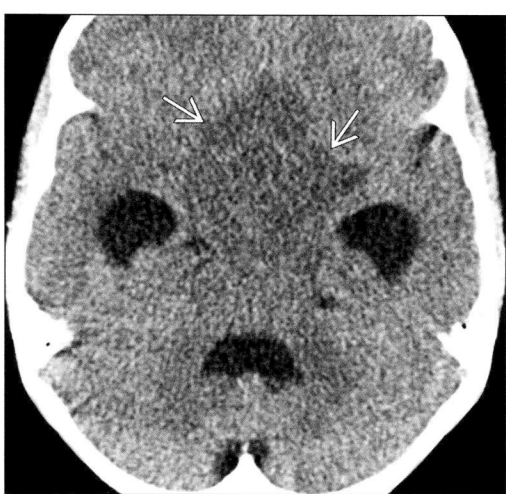

17-7. NECT scan in a visual pathway/hypothalamic PA shows a hypodense suprasellar mass with somewhat ill-defined borders ➡.

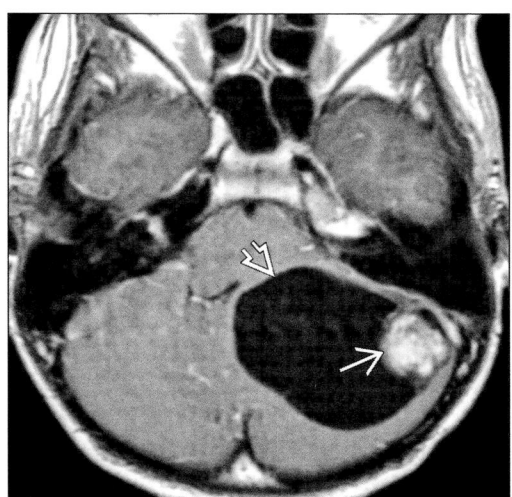

17-8. T1 C+ shows a classic PA in the cerebellum with an enhancing mural nodule ➡, *nonenhancing cyst wall* ➡, *little peritumoral edema.*

17-9A. T1WI in a 7-year-old girl with morning headaches and vomiting shows a mostly solid, slightly hypointense mass in the fourth ventricle ➜. *17-9B. The mass is heterogeneously hyperintense on T2WI* ➜.

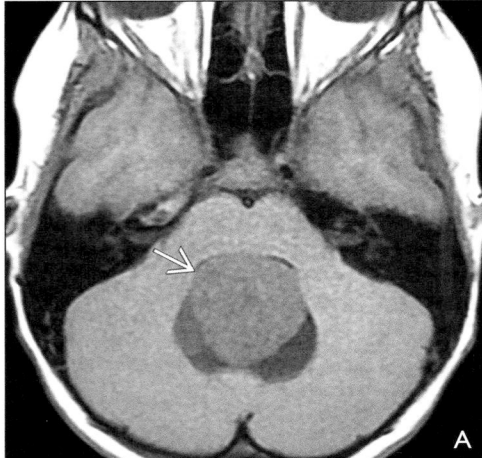

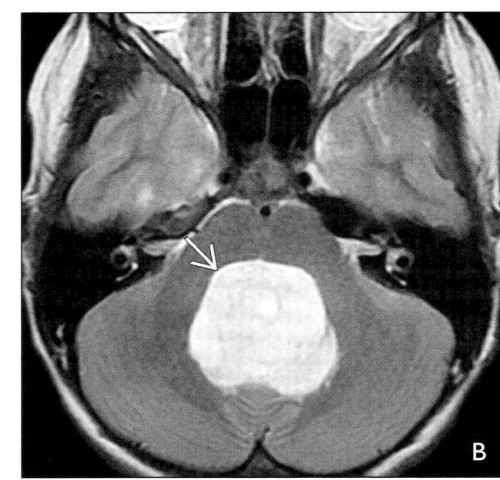

17-9C. T1 C+ FS scan in the same patient shows strong, slightly heterogeneous enhancement in the solid portion of the mass ➜ *with rim enhancement* ➤ *around a small cyst. 17-9D. The mass* ➜ *shows no evidence of restricted diffusion on DWI.*

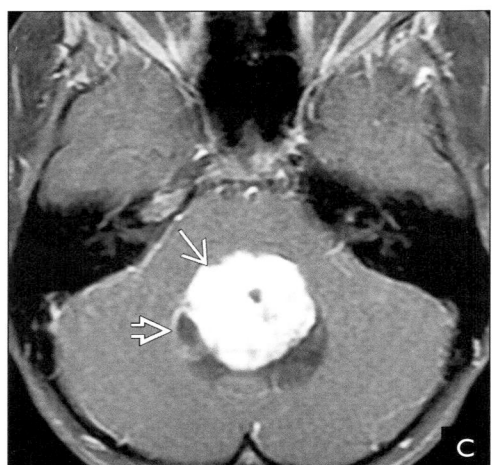

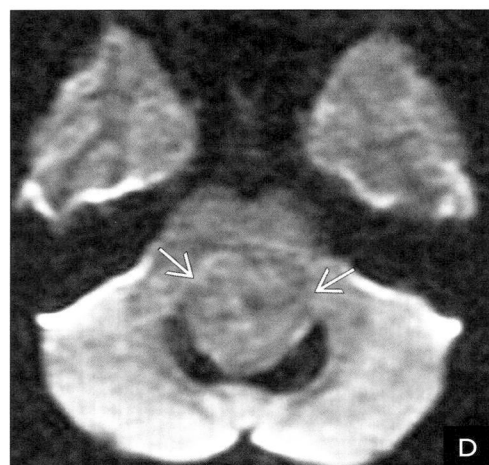

17-9E. pMR shows that the mass ➜ *has a low rCBV. 17-9F. MRS in the same case with TE = 288 msec shows a "pseudomalignant" spectrum with an elevated choline peak* ➜.

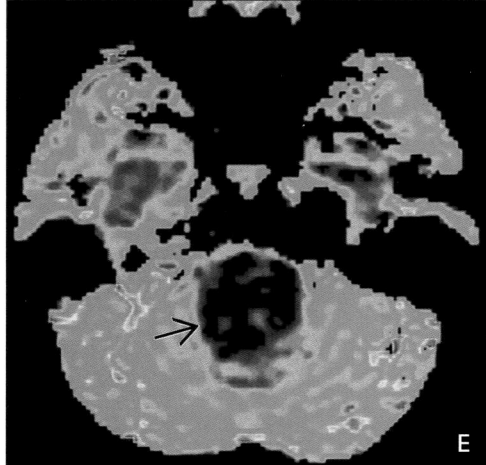

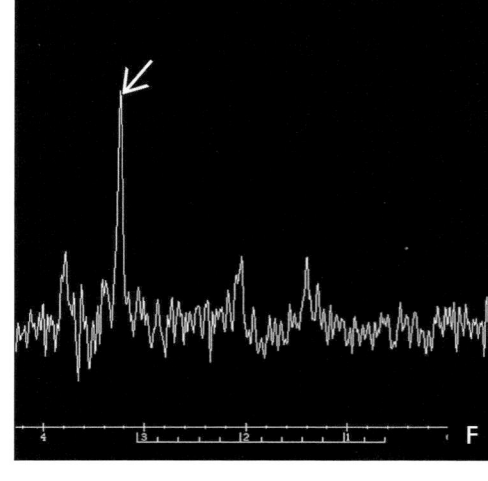

NATURAL HISTORY. PAs generally grow slowly. Ten-year survival exceeds 90%, even with partially resected tumors. Almost half of residual tumors show spontaneous regression or arrested long-term growth.

Rare cases of disseminated grade I PA have been reported. However, some cases that were initially diagnosed as "aggressive" or "atypical" PA may be pilomyxoid astrocytoma (PMA). PMAs generally have an earlier age of onset, more aggressive clinical course, and poorer prognosis than PA.

...aging

Similar to clinical presentation, imaging findings vary with PA location. The most common appearance of a posterior fossa PA is a well-delineated cerebellar cyst with a mural nodule.

PAs in and around the optic nerve, chiasm, third ventricle, and tectum tend to be solid, infiltrating, and less well-marginated. When they occur in these locations, PAs tend to expand the affected structures, which maintain their underlying anatomic configuration.

PAs in the tectum expand the collicular plate and may cause aqueductal obstruction. The rare hemispheric PA typically presents as a cortically based lesion, usually a cyst with a mural nodule.

CT FINDINGS. NECT scans show a mixed cystic/solid **(17-6)** or solid mass with focal mass effect **(17-7)** and little, if any, adjacent edema. Calcification occurs in 10-20% of cases. Hemorrhage is uncommon; if present, the tumor may be a pilomyxoid astrocytoma rather than PA.

Most PAs enhance on both CT and MR scans. The most common pattern, seen in approximately half of all cases, is a nonenhancing cyst with a strongly enhancing mural nodule **(17-8)**. A solid enhancing mass with central necrosis is seen in 40%, and 10% show solid homogeneous enhancement. If delayed scans are obtained, a contrast-fluid level may accumulate within the cyst.

MR FINDINGS. Cystic PAs are usually well-delineated and appear slightly hyperintense to CSF on both T1- and T2WI **(17-9)**. They do not suppress completely on FLAIR. The mural nodule is iso-/hypointense on T1WI and iso-/hyperintense on T2WI. Solid PAs appear iso- or

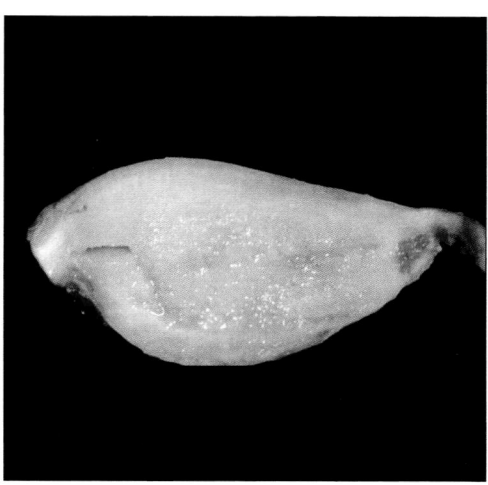

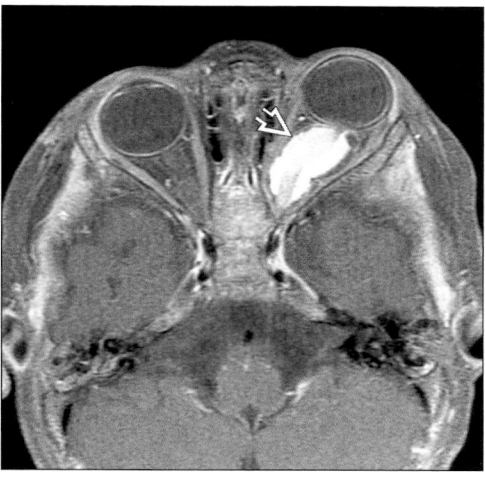

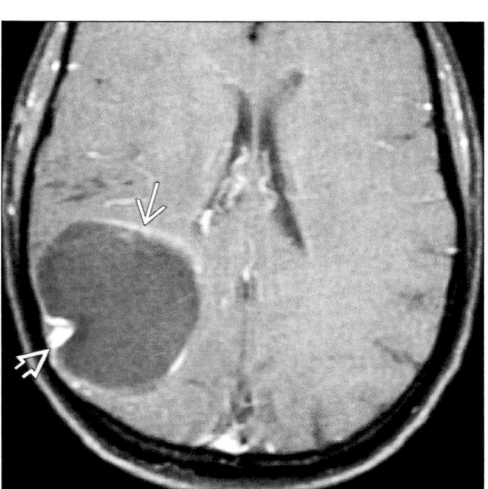

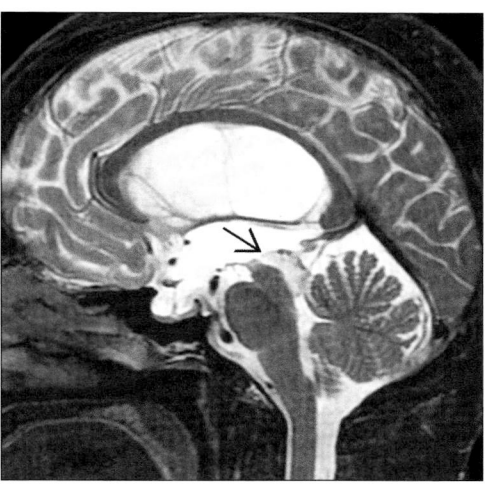

17-10. Gross pathology of an optic nerve "glioma" shows fusiform enlargement of the optic nerve. Most optic nerve gliomas are pilocytic astrocytomas. Less commonly, they are WHO grade II diffusely infiltrating astrocytomas. (Courtesy R. Hewlett, MD.) 17-11. Axial T1 C+ FS shows typical fusiform enlargement, intense enhancement of optic nerve "glioma" ➡ (pilocytic astrocytoma).

17-12. T1 C+ FS scan shows a large right parietal cystic mass with rim enhancement ➡, mural nodule ➡. Biopsy-proven pilocytic astrocytoma. 17-13. Sagittal T2WI FS in a middle-aged man with longstanding headaches shows hydrocephalus, aqueductal obstruction caused by a hyperintense tectal mass ➡. Imaging remained unchanged over 5 years. This is a presumed PA.

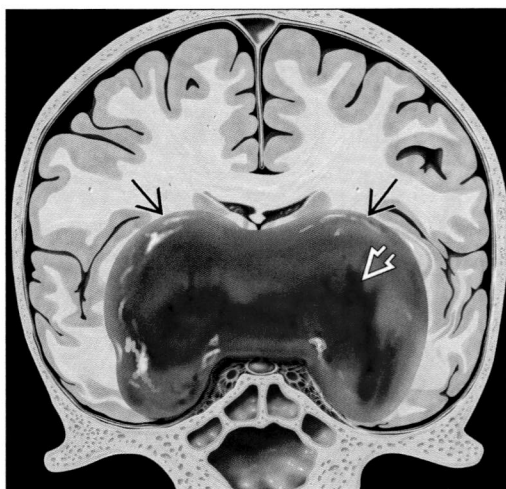

17-14. *PMA with bulky H-shaped hypothalamic/ chiasmatic region mass extending to temporal lobes. Shiny myxoid matrix* →, *hemorrhage* ⇒.

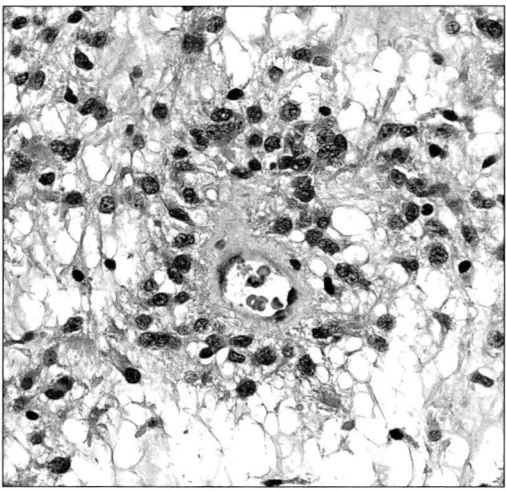

17-15. *Loose perivascular formations in a basophilic myxoid matrix are classic histologic features of PMA. (Courtesy P. Burger, MD.)*

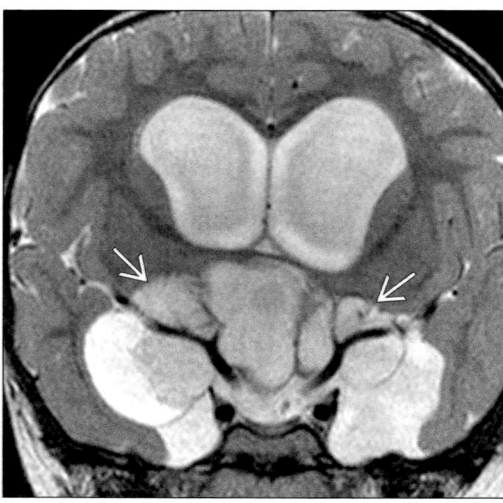

17-16. *Coronal T2WI shows a large lobulated PMA* → *that involves the hypothalamus and both medial temporal lobes.*

hypointense to parenchyma on T1WI and hyperintense on T2/FLAIR **(17-13)**. Posterior extension along the optic radiations is not uncommon with a suprasellar PA and does not denote malignancy.

PAs contain numerous capillaries with fenestrations and open endothelial tight junctions that permit the escape of large macromolecules across the blood-brain barrier. They may therefore show striking enhancement following contrast administration. Intense but heterogeneous enhancement of the nodule in a cystic PA is typical. Enhancement of the cyst wall itself varies from none to moderate. A variant pattern is a solid mass with central necrosis and a thick peripherally enhancing "rind" of tumor.

PAs in the optic nerve, optic chiasm, and hypothalamus/third ventricle show quite variable enhancement (from none to striking) **(17-10)**, **(17-11)** whereas hemispheric PAs generally present with a cyst plus an enhancing mural nodule **(17-12)**.

MRS in PAs often shows elevated Cho, low NAA, and a lactate peak—paradoxical findings that are more characteristic of malignant neoplasms than this clinically benign-behaving tumor **(17-9F)**. pMR shows low to moderate rCBV **(17-9E)**.

ANGIOGRAPHY. Solid PAs are usually avascular whereas cystic PAs may show moderately intense, prolonged vascular staining of the mural nodule. Arteriovenous shunting with "early draining" veins is uncommon.

Differential Diagnosis

The differential diagnosis of PA depends on location. Posterior fossa PAs can resemble **medulloblastoma**, especially when they are mostly solid midline tumors. Medulloblastomas typically restrict on DWI whereas PAs do not.

Ependymoma is a plastic-appearing tumor that extrudes out the foramen of Magendie and lateral recesses. The imaging appearance of **hemangioblastoma** (HGBL) can resemble PA, but HGBLs are tumors of middle-aged adults rather than children. HGBLs have significant peritumoral edema and markedly elevated rCBV.

The major differential diagnosis of hypothalamic PAs is **pilomyxoid astrocytoma**. PMAs tend to occur in younger children and infants. Hemorrhage is rare in PA but relatively common in PMA. **Demyelinating disease** and post-viral inflammation can mimic visual pathway PAs. Optic neuritis can cause enlargement and enhancement of the optic nerves and chiasm.

The differential diagnosis of a hemispheric PA with a "nodule plus cyst" appearance is **ganglioglioma**. Gangliogliomas are generally cortically based and often calcify.

Pleomorphic xanthoastrocytomas (PXA) can present with a solid "nodule plus cyst" but are tumors of young adults, not children. PXAs often incite meningeal reaction ("dural tail" sign).

ilomyxoid Astrocytoma

Pilomyxoid astrocytoma (PMA) is a newly described neoplasm that was originally considered just a "juvenile" variant of pilocytic astrocytoma (PA). Now recognized as a distinct entity, PMA has a unique histological appearance and differs from PA in its presentation as well as its clinical course.

athology

LOCATION. Although PMAs may occur anywhere along the neuraxis, they have a strong geographic predilection for the suprasellar region. Almost 60% center in the hypothalamus/optic chiasm, often extending into both temporal lobes **(17-14)**.

About 40% of PMAs occur in atypical locations, mostly the cerebral hemispheres. In contrast to PA, PMAs in the cerebellum or fourth ventricle are rare.

GROSS PATHOLOGY. PMAs are generally large, bulky, but relatively well-circumscribed masses. A glistening appearance caused by the myxoid component is common. Hemorrhage and necrosis are more common than with PA.

MICROSCOPIC FEATURES. Rosenthal fibers and the characteristic biphasic pattern of PA are absent. Instead, PMAs consist of monomorphic piloid tumor cells embedded in a striking, mucopolysaccharide-rich myxoid matrix. The neoplastic cells often display an angiocentric pattern that some investigators consider almost pathognomonic of PMA **(17-15)**. PMAs are GFAP and vimentin positive. MIB-1 is usually in the 1-2% range.

STAGING, GRADING, AND CLASSIFICATION. PMA is considered a WHO grade II neoplasm.

linical Issues

EPIDEMIOLOGY. The exact incidence of PMA is unknown but is estimated at 0.5-1% of all astrocytomas, considerably less common than PA. Between 5-10% of cases diagnosed histologically as "aggressive" PAs before 2007 may actually be PMAs.

DEMOGRAPHICS. Although PMA has a relatively wide age range, it typically occurs at an earlier mean age than PA. Suprasellar PMAs are typically tumors of infants and children younger than four years. PMAs in atypical locations are more common in adolescents and young adults.

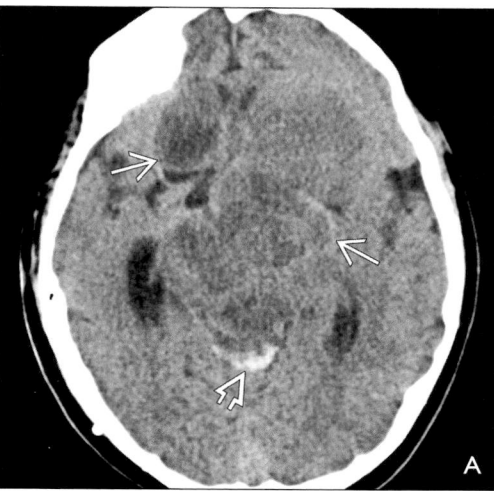

17-17A. Patient diagnosed with PA at age 2. NECT at age 10 shows a large, mixed-density suprasellar mass ➡ with possible hemorrhage ➡.

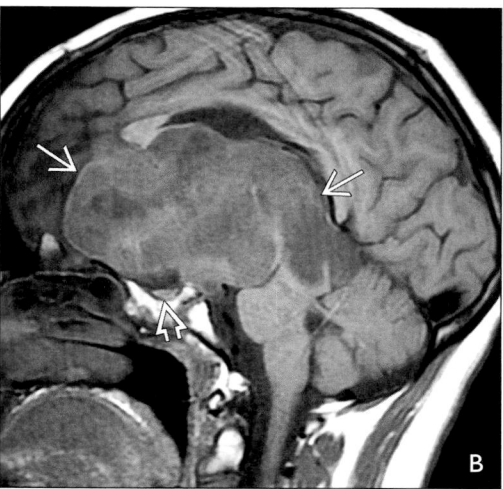

17-17B. Sagittal T1WI in the same patient shows that the enormous mass ➡ has mixed iso- and hypointense signal. The pituitary ➡ is normal.

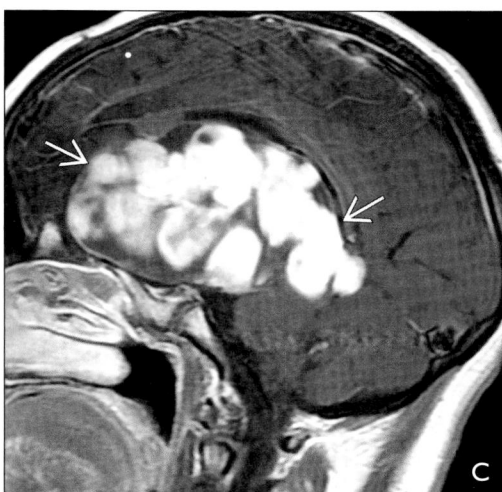

17-17C. T1 C+ in the same patient shows strong but heterogeneous enhancement ➡. Reexamination of the original pathology disclosed PMA.

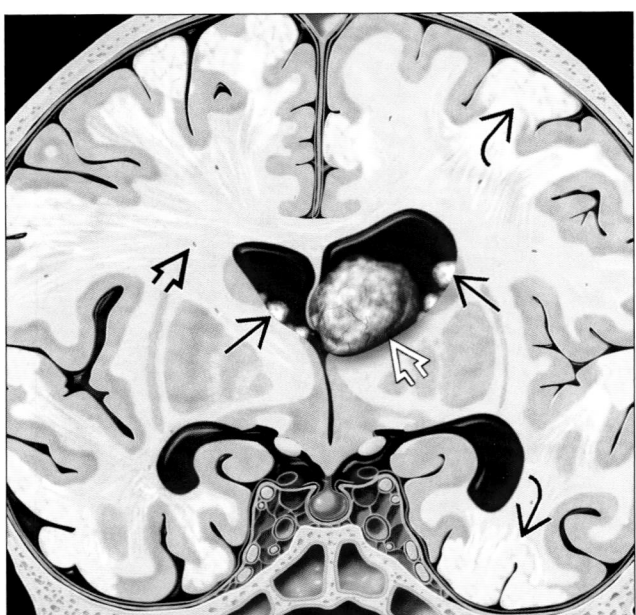

17-18. *Coronal graphic shows an SEGA ➘ in a patient with tuberous sclerosis. Note subependymal nodules ➔ and cortical tubers ➔ with "blurring" of the gray-white interface. Prominent radial glial bands ➘ are also present in the medullary WM.*

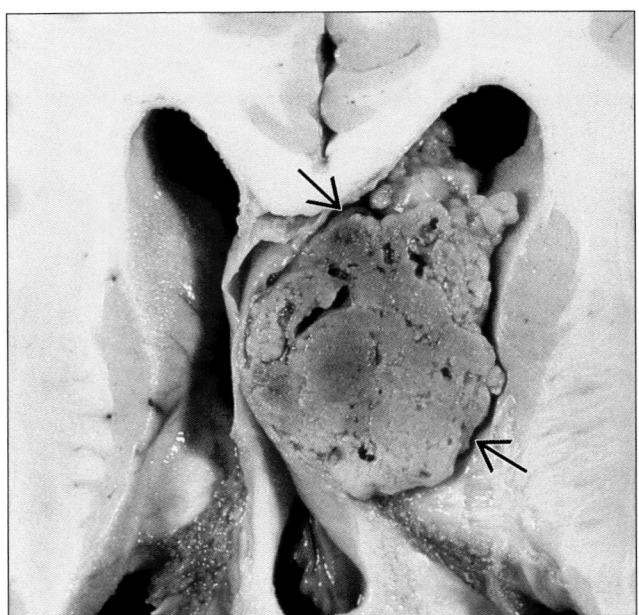

17-19. *Close-up view of an autopsy specimen from a patient with TSC shows a well-circumscribed lobulated mass ➔ in the frontal horn near the foramen of Monro. Subependymal giant cell astrocytoma.*

PRESENTATION. Clinical presentation is often insidious. Infants may present with signs of increased intracranial pressure, failure to thrive, and diencephalic syndrome. Hypothalamic dysfunction and visual disturbances are common.

NATURAL HISTORY. Patients with PMAs generally have a worse prognosis that those with PA. Post-treatment recurrence rate is higher, progression-free interval is smaller, and overall survival is shorter.

Imaging

The imaging features of PMA are similar to those of PA. Both tumors often display solid and cystic components. T2 signal intensity and ADC values are generally higher in PMA (17-16), reflecting the higher proportion of myxoid matrix in these tumors.

Approximately 20% of PMAs demonstrate evidence of intratumoral hemorrhage on T2* (GRE, SWI), which is very rare in PAs. Both tumors show strong but heterogeneous enhancement after contrast administration (17-17). CSF dissemination is common with PMA, so the entire neuraxis should be imaged.

Differential Diagnosis

The major differential diagnosis of PMA is other astrocytomas. **Pilocytic astrocytoma** tends to occur in somewhat older children (5-15 years), and the posterior fossa is the most common overall site. Intratumoral hemorrhage is rare. PAs are usually indolent tumors that may spread locally but rarely disseminate.

Low-grade diffuse astrocytoma occurs in older patients (peak age is 20-45 years), rarely hemorrhages, does not enhance, and typically affects the cerebral hemispheres rather than the hypothalamus/optic chiasm. **Glioblastoma multiforme** often hemorrhages but rarely involves the diencephalon and usually affects older patients.

FEATURES THAT DISTINGUISH PMA FROM PA

Pathology
- Piloid cells + myxoid background
- Angiocentric growth
- WHO grade II

Clinical Issues
- More common in infants, children < 4 years
- More aggressive behavior

Imaging
- Hypothalamus/optic chiasm > > cerebellum
- Large, bulky, H-shaped tumor
- Hemorrhage more common in PMA

Subependymal Giant Cell Astrocytoma

Subependymal giant cell astrocytoma (SEGA) is a localized, circumscribed, WHO grade I astrocytic tumor that occurs in patients with tuberous sclerosis complex (TSC).

Terminology

SEGA is a neuroglial tumor composed of spine to large cells that occurs near the foramen of Monro in patients with TSC.

tiology

The origin of SEGAs and their relationship to the subependymal hamartomas that are a near-constant feature of TSC is controversial. While there are histological similarities between the two lesions, mitotic figures are found only in SEGAs.

GENETICS. The *TSC1* and *TSC2* genes encode the tumor suppressor proteins hamartin and tuberin, respectively. Mutations prevent the hamartin/tuberin heterodimer from deactivating Rheb, leading to mTOR upregulation. mTOR upregulation leads to uncontrolled cell growth and protein synthesis.

athology

LOCATION. Nearly all SEGAs are located in the lateral ventricles, adjacent to the foramen of Monro **(17-18)**. A few cases of extraventricular SEGA have been reported.

SIZE AND NUMBER. SEGAs vary in size from tiny to lesions measuring several centimeters in diameter. The average tumor size is 10-15 mm.

Most SEGAs are solitary lesions. So-called double SEGAs occur in up to 20% of cases.

GROSS PATHOLOGY. SEGAs are well-circumscribed solid intraventricular masses that infrequently hemorrhage or undergo necrosis **(17-19)**. Calcification is common.

MICROSCOPIC FEATURES. SEGA tumor cells display a wide spectrum of astroglial phenotypes that may be indistinguishable from subependymal nodules (SENs). Large pyramidal cells that resemble astrocytes or ganglion cells are typical. Nuclei are large, round, and usually eccentric with open chromatin and prominent nucleoli. Mitoses are variable but generally few in number, so MIB-1 is low.

STAGING, GRADING, AND CLASSIFICATION. SEGAs are WHO grade I neoplasms.

Clinical Issues

EPIDEMIOLOGY. SEGAs arise in a relatively small proportion (10-20%) of patients with TSC but cause up to 25% of the morbidity associated with this condition.

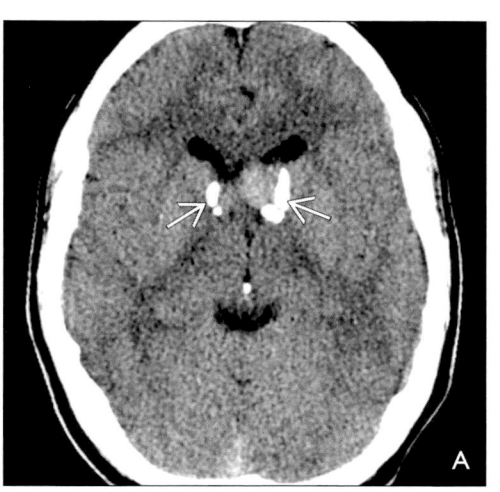

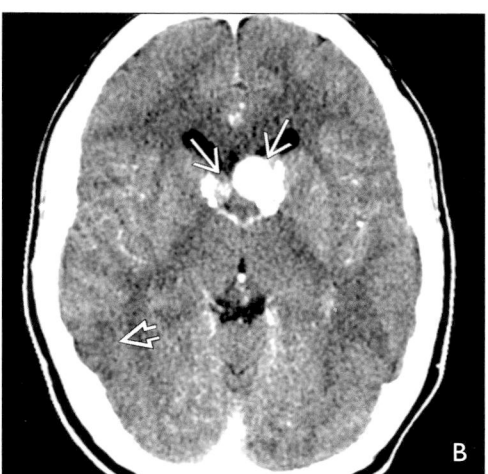

17-20A. NECT scan in a child with TSC shows slightly hyperdense calcified masses in the frontal horns of both lateral ventricles ➡. *17-20B. CECT scan in the same patient shows that the noncalcified portions of the masses enhance strongly* ➡. *Note the hypodense cortical tuber* ➡.

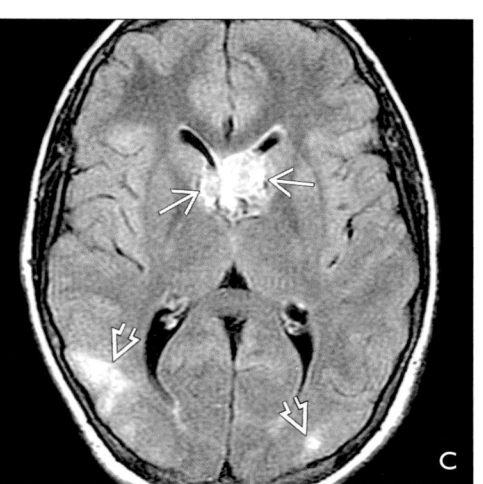

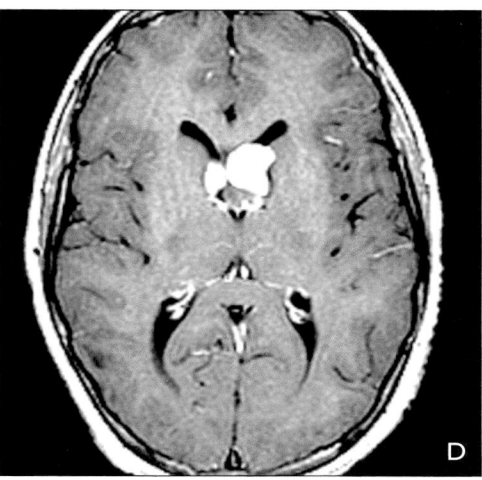

17-20C. FLAIR scan in the same patient shows that the masses ➡ *are heterogeneously hyperintense. Again note the cortical tubers* ➡. *17-20D. T1 C+ shows the intense enhancement of the masses. Subependymal giant cell astrocytomas in a tuberous sclerosis complex patient.*

DEMOGRAPHICS. SEGAs generally occur in the setting of tuberous sclerosis complex and typically develop during the first two decades of life. Mean age at diagnosis is 11 years. Sporadic SEGAs without obvious TS stigmata occur but are extremely rare.

PRESENTATION. Epilepsy in TS patients is related to cortical tubers, not SEGA. SEGAs are generally asymptomatic until they cause obstructive hydrocephalus. Headache, vomiting, and loss of consciousness are typical symptoms.

NATURAL HISTORY. Prognosis is generally good, as SEGA grows slowly and rarely invades adjacent brain. Many patients with SEGAs have small lesions that may remain relatively stable. Median growth rate generally ranges from 2.5-5.6 mm per year.

The clinical course of SEGA, however, is not invariably so benign. The main concern is obstructive hydrocephalus, which may develop suddenly and result in rapidly rising intracranial pressure.

TREATMENT OPTIONS. When imaging findings are indeterminate and a lesion near the foramen of Monro cannot be clearly identified as an SEN or SEGA, close interval follow-up imaging (initially every six months, then annually if there is no evidence of growth) is recommended. A lesion in this location should be treated as soon as it shows evidence of enlargement.

Surgical resection has been the treatment of choice as regrowth rates after complete tumor removal are very low. However, not all SEGAs can be resected completely. Other treatment options now include stereotactic radiosurgery and mTOR inhibitor therapy with everolimus.

Imaging

The most important ancillary imaging findings to identify are those of TSC (see Chapter 39). In the absence of a known family history, mental retardation, epilepsy, or cutaneous stigmata, imaging may provide the first clues to the diagnosis of TSC.

CT FINDINGS. SEGAs are hypo- to isodense, variably calcified lesions near the foramen of Monro (17-20A). Calcified SENs may be seen along the lateral ventricle margins, especially the caudothalamic grooves. Hydrocephalus is present in 15% of cases. "Blurred" lateral ventricle margins indicate severe obstructive hydrocephalus with transependymal CSF migration.

SEGAs demonstrate strong but heterogeneous enhancement (17-20B). An enhancing lesion at the foramen of Monro on CECT scan should be considered SEGA until proven otherwise.

MR FINDINGS. SEGAs are hypo- to isointense compared to cortex on T1WI and heterogeneously iso- to hyperintense on T2WI. Calcified foci are mildly hyperintense on T1WI, hypointense on T2WI, and "bloom" on T2*. Close inspection of the lateral ventricle walls may disclose unsuspected SENs.

FLAIR is especially useful for detecting subtle CNS features of TSC such as cortical tubers and white matter radial migration lines. Streaky linear hyperintensities extending through the white matter to the subjacent ventricle or wedge-shaped hyperintensities underlying expanded ("clubbed") gyri are typical (17-20C).

SEN enhancement is much more visible on MR than on CT. Between 30-80% of SENs enhance following contrast administration, so enhancement alone is insufficient to distinguish an SEN from an SEGA. Although a mass at the foramen of Monro larger than 10-12 mm in diameter is usually an SEGA (17-20D), only progressive enlargement is sufficient to differentiate an SEGA from an SEN.

Differential Diagnosis

The major differential diagnosis of SEGA in a patient with TSC is a benign nonneoplastic **subependymal nodule**. The distinction is important as the lesions evolve differently. SENs remain stable and do not need to be treated whereas SEGAs gradually enlarge and eventually require surgical treatment. Both SEGAs and SENs calcify. SEGAs arise only near the foramen of Monro whereas SENs can be located anywhere around the ventricular wall, especially along the caudothalamic groove. Although SENs are much more common than SEGAs, a partially calcified enhancing lesion at the foramen of Monro larger than five millimeters is more likely to be an SEGA than an SEN.

Other intraventricular neoplasms besides SEGA can arise in the lateral ventricle near the foramen of Monro. **Subependymoma** is a tumor of middle-aged and elderly patients whereas SEGA is a tumor of children and young adults. **Choroid plexus papilloma** (CPP) occasionally arises within the third ventricle and may extend superiorly through the foramen of Monro. CPPs are generally found in children under the age of 5 years.

Central neurocytoma is a "bubbly" tumor that arises in the lateral ventricle body, usually not next to the foramen of Monro. **Chordoid glioma** is a tumor of the third ventricle that is more common in adults.

Low-grade **diffusely infiltrating astrocytoma** can arise in the septi pellucidi or fornices, but these tumors typically neither calcify nor enhance. Imaging stigmata of TSC (such as SENs and cortical tubers) are absent.

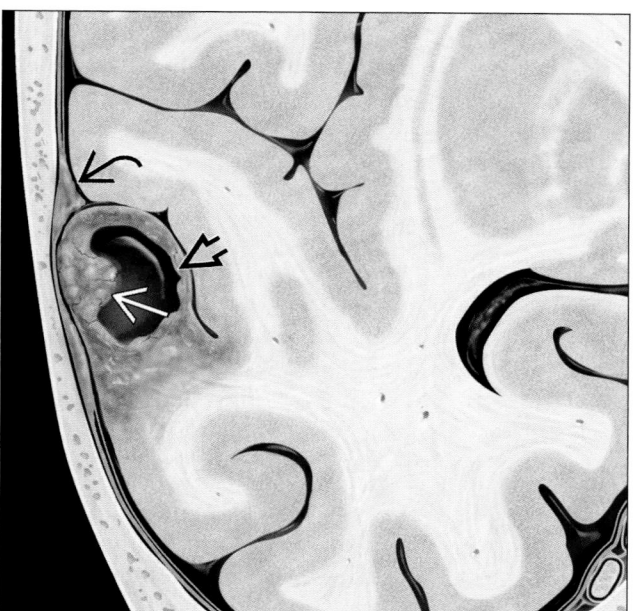

17-21. Coronal graphic depicts pleomorphic xanthoastrocytoma with cyst ⊟, nodule abutting pial surface ➡, reactive thickening of the adjacent dura-arachnoid ➢.

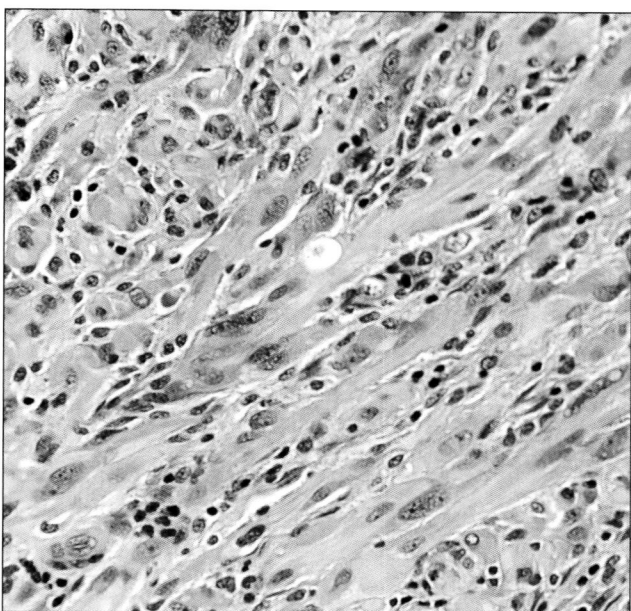

17-22. Classic histologic features of PXA include somewhat fascicular architecture and cells that appear pleomorphic but not "monstrous." The bulk of the lesion is compact, noninfiltrating. (Courtesy P. Burger, MD.)

Pleomorphic Xanthoastrocytoma

Terminology

Pleomorphic xanthoastrocytoma (PXA) is a relatively focal, superficial, seizure-associated tumor. Despite its striking cellular pleomorphism, it generally has a favorable prognosis if totally excised.

Pathology

LOCATION. Over 95% of PXAs are supratentorial hemispheric masses. Most are superficial, cortically based neoplasms that often involve the temporal (40-50%), frontal (33%), or parietal (20%) lobes. Cerebellar and spinal cord PXAs have been reported but are very rare.

SIZE AND NUMBER. PXAs are usually solitary lesions although a few multicentric lesions have been reported.

GROSS PATHOLOGY. The most common gross appearance is that of a relatively discrete solid or partially cystic mass with a mural nodule that abuts or is attached to the leptomeninges (17-21). Dural invasion is rare. The deep tumor margins may be indistinct with focal parenchymal infiltration into the adjacent subcortical white matter.

MICROSCOPIC FEATURES. The most striking features of PXA are its pleomorphism, dense reticulin network, compact architecture, and lipidization of tumor cells. Fibrillary and giant, multinucleated, neoplastic astrocytes are intermixed with large, lipid-containing, GFAP-positive cells (17-22). Almost all PXAs are GFAP positive and show S100 immunoreactivity. Neuronal markers such as synaptophysin and neurofilament protein are often present. Mitotic figures are rare or absent.

STAGING, GRADING, AND CLASSIFICATION. PXAs are WHO grade II tumors. Between 10-15% display anaplastic features including higher cellularity and increased mitoses, along with some vascular proliferation and occasional necrotic foci. The WHO grade for a "PXA with anaplastic features" has not yet been defined.

Clinical Issues

EPIDEMIOLOGY. PXA is a rare tumor, accounting for slightly less than 1% of all astrocytomas.

DEMOGRAPHICS. PXAs are generally tumors of children and young adults; almost two-thirds of patients are under the age of 18 at initial presentation.

PRESENTATION. Because of its characteristic superficial cortically based location, the most common presentation is longstanding epilepsy.

NATURAL HISTORY. Recurrence following gross total resection is uncommon. Mitotic activity and extent of resection are the only predictors of subsequent biologic behavior. Overall five-year survival is approximately 80%, and the 10-year survival rate is 70%.

Malignant transformation occurs but is uncommon. Anaplastic PXA is an aggressively growing, malignant tumor that may disseminate throughout the CNS.

Imaging

CT FINDINGS. NECT scans show a well-delineated, peripheral, cortically based mass that contacts the leptomeninges. Two imaging patterns are common. A "cyst + nodule" configuration is present in 70% of cases, and a predominantly solid mass with intratumoral cysts is seen in 30%. The overlying skull may be thinned and remodeled on bone CT. Calcifications are present in 40% of cases, but gross intratumoral hemorrhage is rare.

The mural nodule of a PXA shows moderate to intense enhancement on CECT.

MR FINDINGS. The solid component of a PXA is heterogeneously hypo- or isointense relative to cortex on T1WI **(17-23A)**. Over 90% of the tumor nodules demonstrate heterogeneous hyperintensity on T2WI and FLAIR. If calcifications or hemorrhage is present, "blooming" on T2* can be seen. The cystic portions of PXA are usually hyperintense relative to CSF on T2WI and FLAIR sequences **(17-23B)**, **(17-23C)**.

Moderate enhancement of the tumor nodule is typical following contrast administration **(17-23D)**. Over 90% of PXAs abut the pia and may incite reactive thickening of the adjacent dura. A "dural tail" sign was seen in 15-50% of cases in reported series.

Differential Diagnosis

The major differential diagnosis of PXA is **ganglioglioma**, another cortically based tumor that often causes epilepsy. Other less common tumors with a "cyst + nodule" appearance can mimic PXA, including hemispheric **pilocytic astrocytoma**. **Dysembryoplastic neuroepithelial tumor (DNET)** has a similar presentation and age range but typically has a multicystic "bubbly" appearance.

Diffuse (low-grade) fibrillary astrocytoma usually involves the white matter and does not involve the meninges. **Oligodendroglioma** can present as a slow-growing cortical-white matter junction lesion that remodels the adjacent calvaria, but the "cyst + nodule" pattern is usually absent.

17-23A. Coronal inversion recovery scan in a 19-year-old man with longstanding temporal lobe epilepsy shows a partially cystic right temporal lobe mass ➡ that remodels the adjacent calvaria ➘. 17-23B. Coronal T2WI shows that the lesion ➡ is predominantly hyperintense. The smooth remodeling of the adjacent calvaria ➘ can be especially well appreciated on this image.

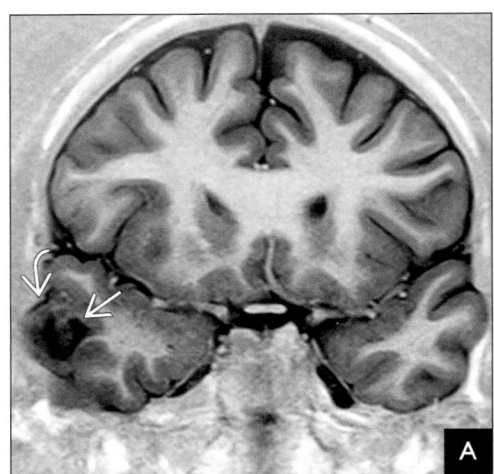
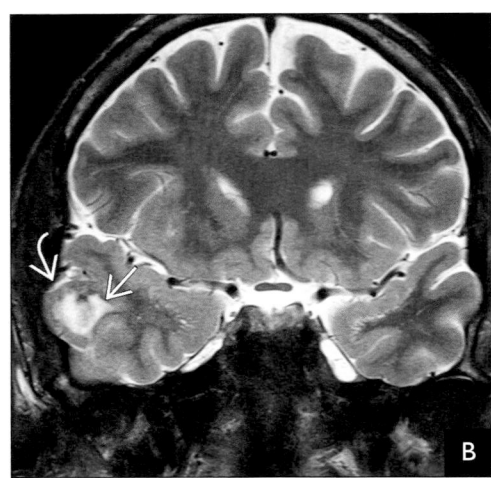

17-23C. Coronal FLAIR scan shows that the lesion is heterogeneously hyperintense ➘. 17-23D. Coronal T1 C+ scan demonstrates an enhancing nodule ➡ that abuts the dura, causing minimal thickening and enhancement ➘. WHO grade II pleomorphic xanthoastrocytoma was removed at surgery.

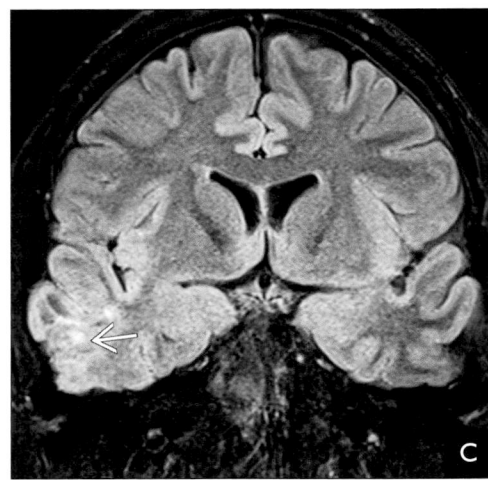
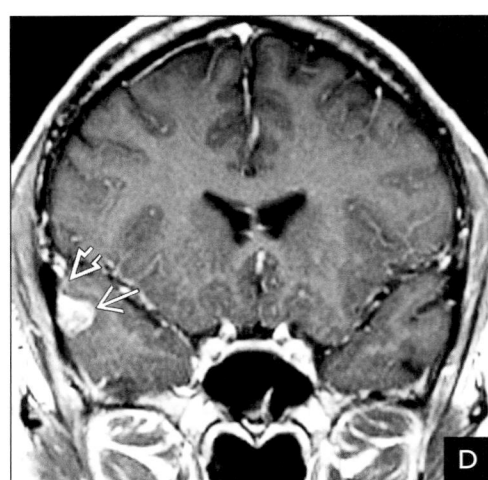

**CORTICALLY BASED TUMORS
WITH "CYST + NODULE"**

Common
- Ganglioglioma
- Metastasis

Less Common
- Pilocytic astrocytoma
- Pleomorphic xanthoastrocytoma
- Glioblastoma multiforme

Rare
- Hemangioblastoma
- Desmoplastic infantile astrocytoma/ganglioglioma
- Papillary glioneuronal tumor
- Schwannoma

Diffusely Infiltrating Astrocytomas

Low-Grade Diffuse Astrocytoma

Terminology

Low-grade diffusely infiltrating glioma with astrocytic differentiation is also known as grade II astrocytoma or low-grade astrocytoma (LGA). Most LGAs are composed of fibrillary neoplastic astrocytes. LGAs tend to grow slowly but have an intrinsic tendency for malignant progression to anaplastic astrocytoma (AA) and (ultimately) glioblastoma multiforme (GBM).

Etiology

GENERAL CONCEPTS. Astrocytomas were once thought to arise from neoplastic transformation of differentiated astrocytes. Recent evidence indicates that neural stem cells destined for astrocytic differentiation are probably the precursor cell of origin.

GENETICS. Mutations in *IDH1* are present in 85% of adolescent and adult LGAs. *P53* mutations are present in 25% of cases. In general, diffuse low-grade gliomas with complex chromosomal aberrations have a greater tendency for aggressive behavior (i.e., shorter progression-free survival) than tumors that display only simple aberrations.

Pathology

LOCATION. Nearly two-thirds of LGAs are supratentorial. The cerebral hemispheres are the most common overall site with tumors distributed approximately equally between the frontal and temporal lobes. Almost 20%

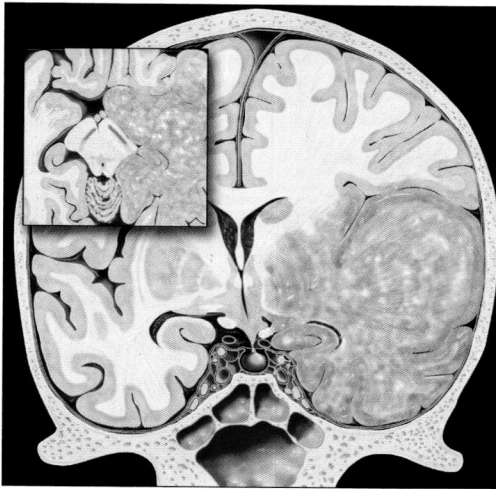

17-24. Diffusely infiltrating astrocytoma (WHO grade II). The tumor expands the temporal lobe, infiltrating cortex/subcortical WM.

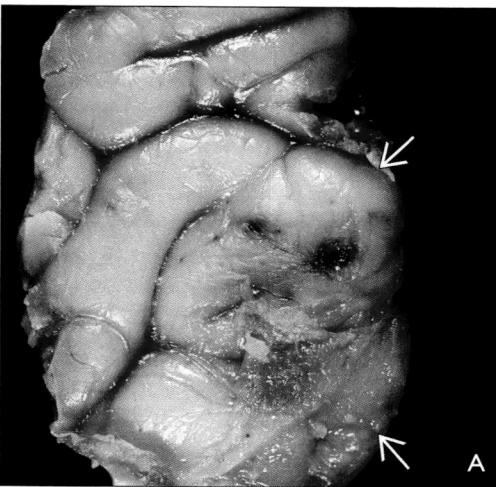

17-25A. Surgical specimen from resected diffusely infiltrating astrocytoma shows expansion of cortex ➔*, mass effect on underlying gyri.*

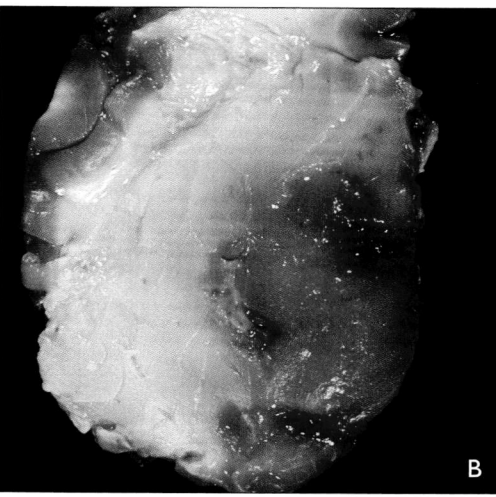

17-25B. Cut section shows tumor infiltrates cortex, subcortical WM. No discernible border between normal, abnormal brain. (R. Hewlett, MD.)

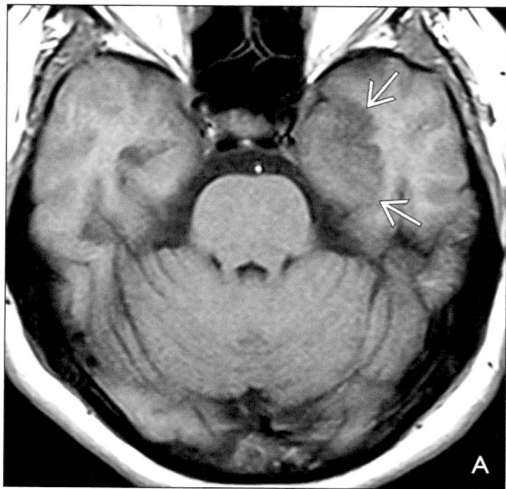

17-26A. T1WI in a 37 yo man with seizures shows homogeneously hypointense left medial temporal lobe mass ➡ in cortex, subcortical WM.

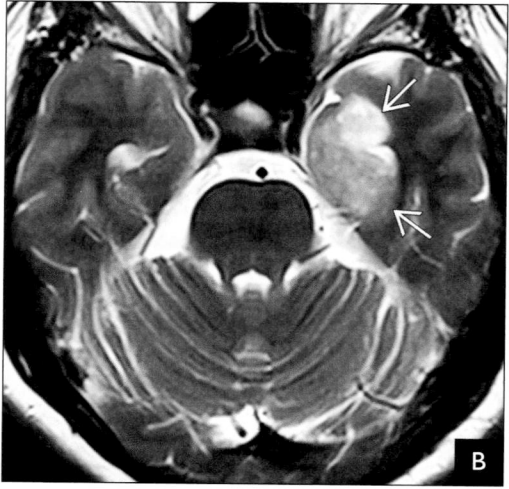

17-26B. T2WI in the same patient shows that the mass ➡ is heterogeneously hyperintense.

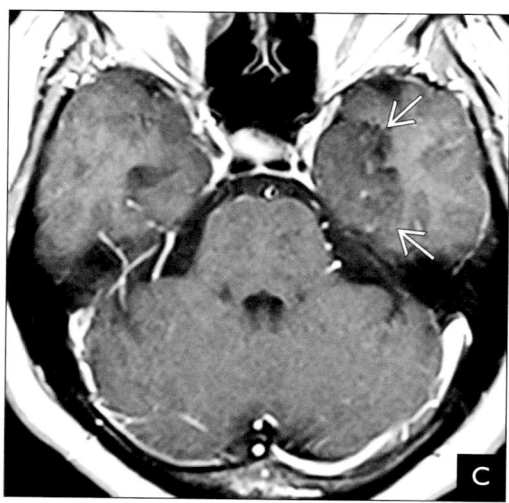

17-26C. The mass ➡ does not enhance on this T1 C+ scan. Diffusely infiltrating astrocytoma, WHO grade II, was found at surgery.

involve the deep gray nuclei, especially the thalami **(17-24)**.

Approximately one-third of LGAs are infratentorial. LGA accounts for 50% of brainstem tumors in children and typically involves the pons. The medulla is a less frequent site. The cerebellum is an uncommon location for LGA.

SIZE AND NUMBER. Frontal lobe LGAs may become rather large before producing symptoms. LGA is the most common underlying neoplasm in gliomatosis cerebri, an extensively infiltrating diffuse tumor that often involves several lobes and the deep gray nuclei. Temporal lobe lesions are often smaller at initial presentation because of their propensity to cause complex partial seizures.

GROSS PATHOLOGY. LGAs are infiltrating lesions with ill-defined borders. Enlargement and distortion of invaded structures is typical. Gray-white matter interfaces are blurred **(17-25)**. Occasional cysts and calcification may be present. Hemorrhage is rare.

MICROSCOPIC FEATURES. The most common LGA is **fibrillary astrocytoma**. An infiltrating "diffuse" hypercellular tumor with mild to moderate nuclear atypia is typical. A loosely structured, often microcystic tumor matrix or fine fibrillary background is a classic finding. Mitotic activity is rare or absent, and the MIB-1 index is low.

Immunohistochemistry in LGAs is helpful in establishing the diagnosis. IDH-1 positivity is present in almost all cases of adult and adolescent LGAs, as is Olig2 positivity. Variable GFAP reactivity is seen.

STAGING, GRADING, AND CLASSIFICATION. By definition, diffuse low-grade astrocytomas are WHO grade II neoplasms.

Clinical Issues

EPIDEMIOLOGY. LGA is less common than AA and GBM, accounting for between 10-15% of astrocytomas in adults. LGA is the second most common astrocytoma of childhood (after pilocytic astrocytoma).

DEMOGRAPHICS. Although LGAs can occur at all ages, the majority of supratentorial tumors are found in patients 20-45 years of age. Brainstem LGAs are more common in children. There is a very slight male predominance.

PRESENTATION. Presentation depends on location. Seizure is the most common presentation of hemispheric lesions.

NATURAL HISTORY. Patients with LGAs have a median survival of 6-10 years. Recurrence following surgical resection is common, and most tumors progress to a higher grade astrocytoma within 10 years. Children and patients with gross total resection as well as tumors with *IDH1* mutations have somewhat better survival.

Imaging

CT FINDINGS. NECT shows an ill-defined homogeneous mass that is usually hypointense relative to white matter. Calcification is seen in 20% of cases. Gross cystic change and hemorrhage are rare. CECT shows no enhancement.

MR FINDINGS. Moderate mass effect with adjacent cortical expansion is common. LGAs are hypointense on T1WI and hyperintense on T2/FLAIR **(17-26)**. The tumor may appear somewhat circumscribed on MR, but neoplastic cells generally infiltrate adjacent normal-appearing brain. T2* scans may show "blooming" foci if calcification is present. LGAs do not enhance following contrast administration.

DWI shows no restriction. MRS is nonspecific, with elevated choline, low NAA, and a high mI:Cr ratio. MR perfusion shows relatively low rCBV **(17-27)**. If stereotactic biopsy is performed, any foci of increased rCBV should be targeted, as they may represent areas of early malignant degeneration.

Differential Diagnosis

The major *imaging* differential diagnoses of LGA are other astrocytomas and oligodendroglioma. **Anaplastic astrocytoma**, a WHO grade III neoplasm, is generally indistinguishable from LGA on the basis of standard imaging findings alone. pCT or pMR may demonstrate elevated rCBV in AA, but the definitive diagnosis requires histologic confirmation.

Pilocytic astrocytoma is generally more circumscribed and better demarcated than LGA, often has a "cyst + nodule" configuration rather than an infiltrating appearance, and usually demonstrates moderate to strong enhancement following contrast administration.

Encephalitis with T2/FLAIR hyperintensity shows enhancement on T1 C+ and restriction on DWI.

The major *pathologic* differential diagnosis of LGA is normal brain or nonspecific gliosis. At the opposite end of the spectrum, anaplastic astrocytoma may be a consideration as features such as nuclear atypia may overlap with those of LGA. AAs usually demonstrate higher cellularity and greater cytological atypia, as well as a higher MIB-1 rate (generally more than 5%).

Oligodendroglioma is generally cortically based, more often calcifies, and frequently has enhancing foci. Histologically mixed tumors such as **oligoastrocytoma** are usually more heterogeneous appearing than LGA.

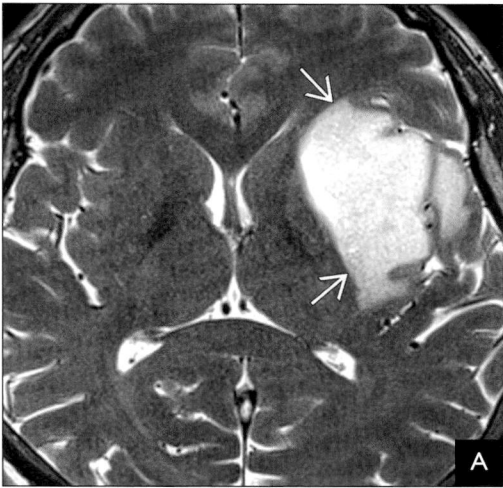

17-27A. *T2WI shows a hyperintense left insular temporal lobe mass that appears quite sharply demarcated from underlying brain* ➡.

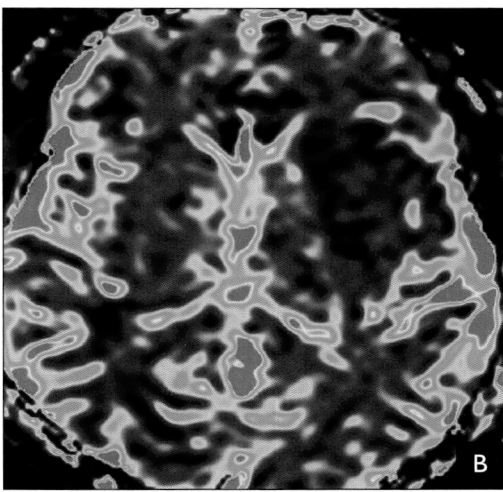

17-27B. *pMR shows no foci of increased rCBV that would suggest foci of malignant degeneration.*

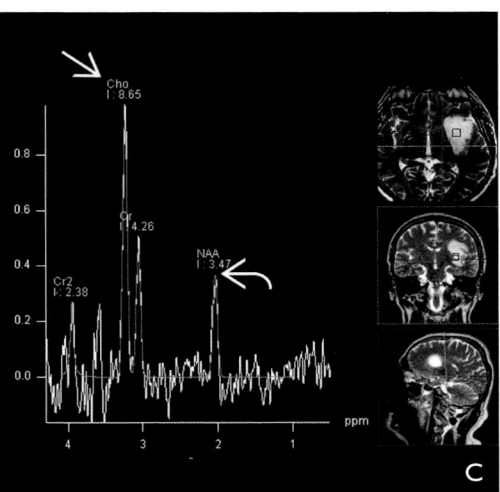

17-27C. *MRS shows elevated Cho* ➡*, low NAA* ➡*, no lactate peak. WHO grade II astrocytoma. (Courtesy M. Thurnher, MD.)*

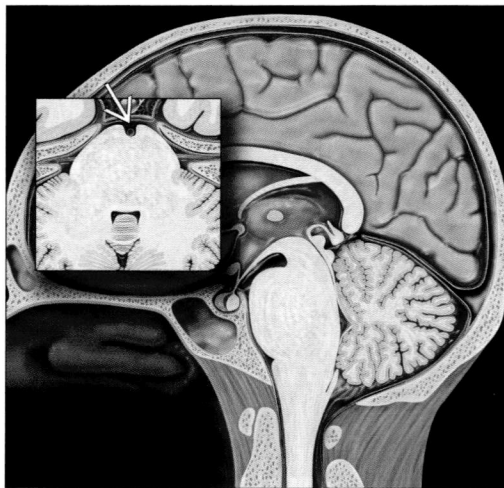

17-28. *Diffusely infiltrating pontine glioma expands pons, wrapping around basilar artery* ➡. *Most are WHO II-IV fibrillary astrocytomas.*

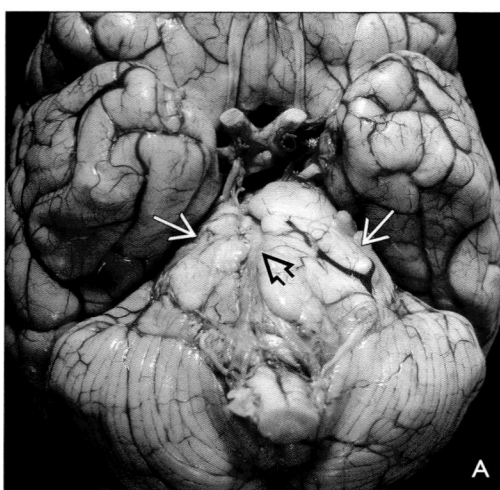

17-29A. *Autopsy specimen shows a diffuse pontine glioma expanding the pons* ➡, *almost completely encasing the basilar artery* ➡.

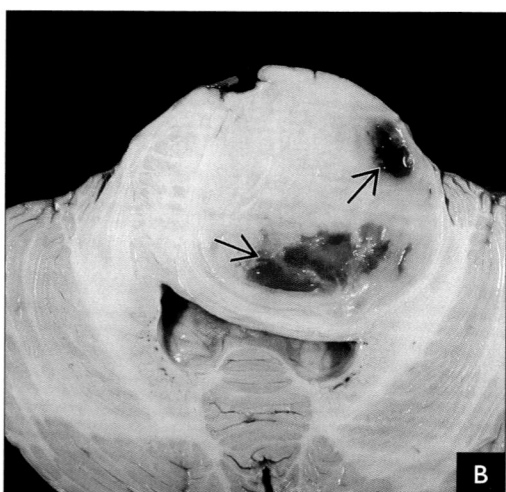

17-29B. *Cut section shows infiltrating tumor. AA (WHO III) with necrotic, hemorrhagic foci of GBM* ➡. *(Courtesy R. Hewlett, MD.)*

DIFFUSELY INFILTRATING ASTROCYTOMA

Terminology
- Also known as low-grade astrocytoma or diffuse astrocytoma

Etiology
- Neural stem cells destined for astrocytic differentiation
- *IDH1* mutations (85%), *P53* mutations (25%)

Pathology
- Supratentorial > infratentorial
- Infiltrating, ill-defined borders
- WHO grade II
- Inherent tendency to undergo malignant degeneration

Clinical Issues
- 10-15% of astrocytomas in adults
- Second most common astrocytoma in children
- Peak age = 20-45 years
- Median survival = 6-10 years

Imaging
- Hypodense on NECT; no enhancement
- Hypointense on T1, hyperintense on T2/FLAIR
- No enhancement, hemorrhage
- MRS nonspecific (↑ Cho, ↓ NAA, no lactate)
- Low rCBV
  - Foci of ↑ rCBV suspicious for malignant degeneration

Differential Diagnosis
- Anaplastic astrocytoma
- Pilocytic astrocytoma
- Oligodendroglioma
- Encephalitis

Diffuse Intrinsic Pontine Gliomas

Brainstem gliomas are uncommon tumors in adults. When they do occur, low-grade phenotypes predominate. In contrast, so-called pediatric brainstem gliomas (BSGs) are significantly more common. They constitute between 10-15% of all childhood brain tumors and are the main cause of death in this group.

Pediatric BSGs can involve the midbrain, pons, or medulla. They are much more heterogeneous than their rarer adult counterparts. All pediatric BSGs are astrocytomas, but their histologic subtypes and prognosis vary substantially. Therefore, *not all pediatric BSGs are the same—geography, tumor grade, and patient outcome are remarkably variable!*

Pathology and Clinical Issues

Pediatric BSGs are divided into two groups by histology and location. The most common pediatric BSGs are **diffuse** pontine astrocytomas (sometimes generically termed "gliomas") **(17-28)**. These BSGs are infiltrative fibrillary astrocytomas that typically involve the pons. Most begin as low-grade (WHO grade II) tumors, but foci of anaplasia (WHO grade III or even IV) are common **(17-29)**. Prognosis is generally poor.

The second group of pediatric BSGs consists of focal lesions that involve the midbrain, tectum, or lower brainstem. These **focal** tumors are generally **pilocytic astrocytomas** (WHO grade I neoplasms) or low-grade astrocytomas (LGAs) and have a much better prognosis. Dorsally exophytic focal gliomas of the cervicomedullary junction also have a better prognosis than the diffusely infiltrating pontine astrocytomas.

Imaging

Imaging features vary with tumor type and location.

Pediatric BSGs expand and diffusely infiltrate the pons, are hyperintense on T2WI, and compress but do not invade the fourth ventricle. They are often anteriorly exophytic and may almost completely engulf the basilar artery **(17-30)**. Grade II fibrillary astrocytomas do not enhance, but degeneration into higher grade tumor may produce necrosis, focal enhancement, and occasionally even intratumoral hemorrhage.

Tectal, tegmental, and dorsally exophytic gliomas are less common than the pediatric BSGs.

Tectal gliomas focally enlarge the colliculi, often obstruct the cerebral aqueduct, and rarely invade adjacent structures. Tectal gliomas are hyperintense on T2/FLAIR, generally show little or no enhancement, and are typically stable in size over many years **(17-13)**.

Focal tegmental mesencephalic gliomas resemble tectal gliomas, except they occur in the central midbrain instead of the colliculi.

Dorsally exophytic gliomas are T2/FLAIR hyperintense, nonenhancing lesions with well-circumscribed borders. Peritumoral edema is generally absent **(17-31)**.

Differential Diagnosis

The general differential diagnosis of BSG is **brainstem encephalitis**, **demyelinating disease** (MS, ADEM), **neurofibromatosis type 1** (NF1), and **osmotic demyelination**. All can cause solitary or multifocal poorly delineated hyperintensity on T2/FLAIR.

A "fat" pons can be mimicked by **intracranial hypotension**. Inferior displacement of the midbrain and pons (brain "sagging") can make these structures look abnormally large. Signal intensity is normal on T2/FLAIR, and ancillary signs of intracranial hypotension such as dural-venous engorgement, effacement of the suprasellar cistern, subdural hematoma(s), and acquired tonsillar herniation help distinguish this condition from pontine glioma.

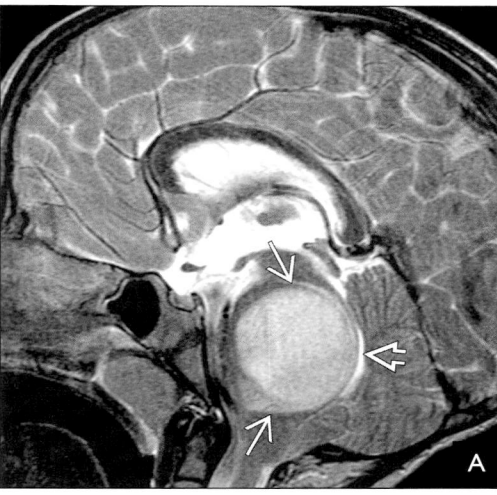

17-30A. T2WI in a child with diffuse pontine glioma shows a hyperintense mass ➡ *expanding pons, displacing fourth ventricle* ➡ *posteriorly.*

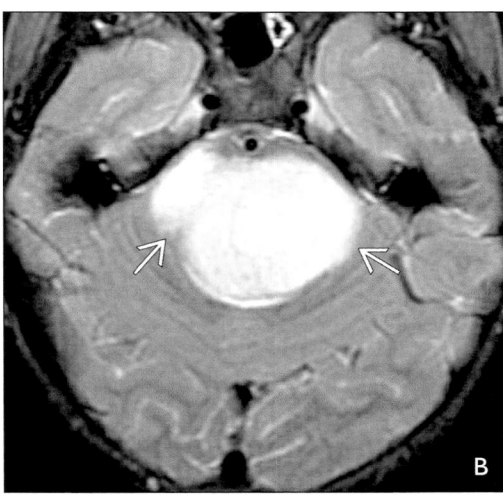

17-30B. T2 FS scan shows that the mass is hyperintense with poorly defined margins ➡. *WHO grade II diffusely infiltrating astrocytoma.*

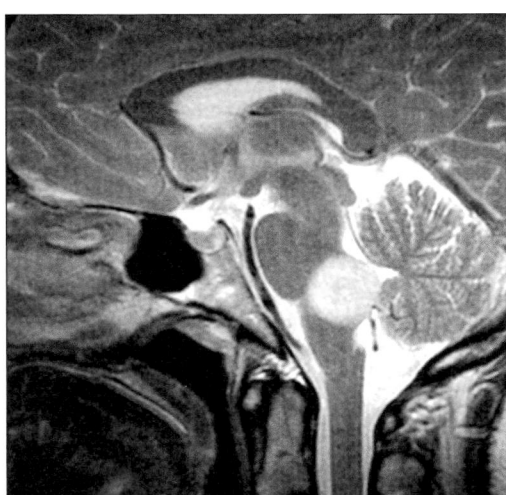

17-31. Sagittal T2WI shows a dorsally exophytic medulla mass. It is a fibrillary astrocytoma, also a WHO II tumor, but with generally better prognosis.

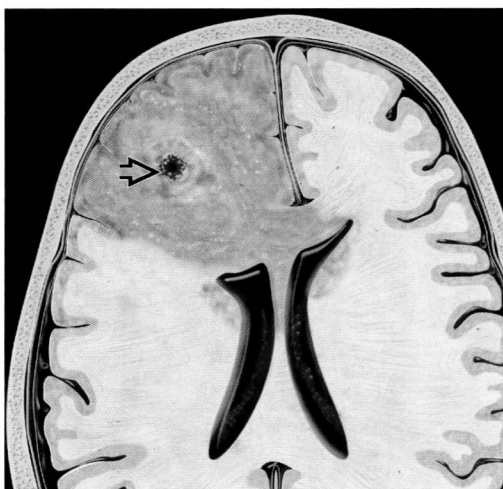

17-32. Anaplastic astrocytoma (WHO grade III) diffusely infiltrates the right frontal lobe. Focal area of degeneration into GBM is depicted ⊵.

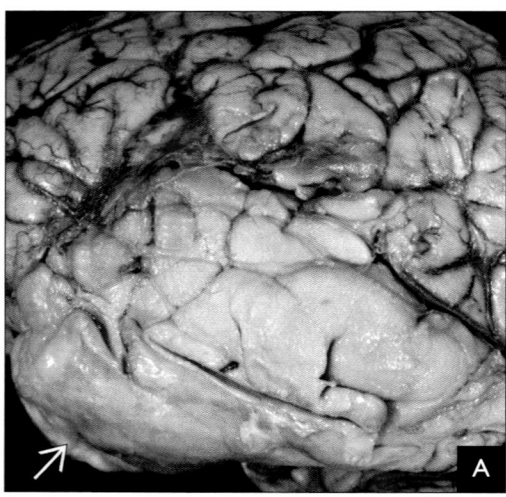

17-33A. Autopsy case of anaplastic astrocytoma shows massive expansion of the entire temporal lobe ➔.

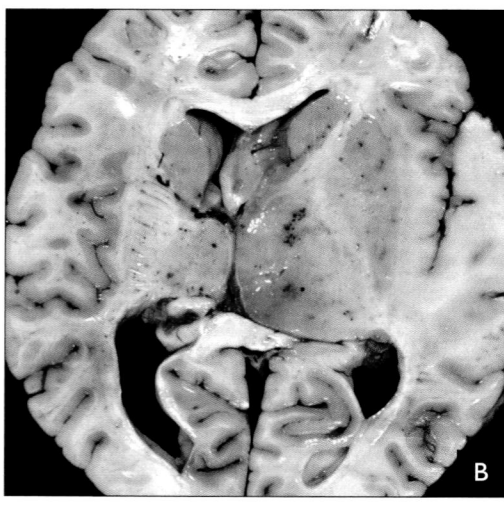

17-33B. Axial section shows that the mass is poorly marginated and infiltrates both gray and white matter. (Courtesy R. Hewlett, MD.)

DIFFUSE INTRINSIC PONTINE GLIOMAS

Epidemiology
- Rare in adults
- 10-15% of childhood brain tumors

Pathology
- Adults: Low grade > high grade
- Children
  - Pons: Diffusely infiltrating (WHO II-IV)
  - Tectum, tegmentum: Pilocytic astrocytoma

Prognosis
- Adults: Generally better prognosis
- Children
  - Diffusely infiltrating pontine = poor prognosis
  - Tectum, dorsally exophytic mesencephalic = better

Imaging
- "Fat" pons, tectum, or medulla
  - T2/FLAIR hyperintensity
  - Any enhancement suspicious for anaplasia

Differential Diagnosis
- Brainstem encephalitis
- Demyelinating disease
- Intracranial hypotension
  - Brainstem "sagging" → "fat" pons

Anaplastic Astrocytoma

Terminology

Anaplastic astrocytoma (AA) is a mitotically active, diffusely infiltrating WHO grade III astrocytoma that has an intrinsic propensity to undergo further malignant degeneration into glioblastoma multiforme (GBM).

Etiology

GENERAL CONCEPTS. AAs can either develop de novo or arise from malignant degeneration of grade II lesions. About 75% of AAs evolve from a low-grade astrocytoma (LGA) that develops multiple genetic alterations. De novo AAs probably arise from precursor stem and progenitor cells committed to astrocytic differentiation.

GENETICS. AAs display a high frequency of *P53* mutations and LOH of 17p.

Pathology

LOCATION. The most common site of AA is the cerebral hemispheres (17-32). The thalami are frequently involved, either by extension of a hemispheric lesion or as the primary tumor site. The pons is the most common site in children.

SIZE AND NUMBER. AAs vary greatly in size and are usually solitary but widely infiltrating lesions. Multifocal AAs occur but are rare.

GROSS PATHOLOGY. AAs cause gross expansion of the affected brain without frank tissue destruction, enlarging adjacent gyri and often extending into the basal ganglia. AAs vary in consistency from rubbery infiltrations to fleshy, highly cellular tumors with poorly delineated margins (17-33). Cysts and intratumoral hemorrhage are rare.

MICROSCOPIC FEATURES. AAs are characterized by moderate to markedly increased cellularity, rare to abundant mitotic activity, and variable degrees of nuclear atypia. Nuclear features may be relatively bland and overlap with grade II astrocytoma or markedly atypical, resembling GBM. Necrosis and microvascular proliferation are absent.

Ki-67 (MIB-1) is elevated, generally in the 5-15% range.

Immunohistochemistry generally shows GFAP and Olig2 positivity. Most cases likewise express IDH-1. Diffuse p53 positivity is present in a minority of cases.

STAGING, GRADING, AND CLASSIFICATION. Anaplastic astrocytomas are WHO grade III tumors, intermediate in malignancy between LGA (WHO grade II) and GBM (WHO grade IV).

Clinical Issues

EPIDEMIOLOGY. AAs represent one-third of all astrocytomas, second in frequency only to GBM.

PRESENTATION. AAs can occur at all ages, but peak presentation is between 40-50 years. There is a slight male predominance.

NATURAL HISTORY. Prognosis is generally poor, with mean survival of two or three years. Progression to GBM is very common and generally occurs within two years following initial diagnosis. Patients with IDH-1-negative AAs have an especially dismal prognosis, equivalent to that of GBM.

TREATMENT OPTIONS. Treatment is resection with adjuvant radiation therapy and chemotherapy (e.g., temozolomide [Temodar]).

Imaging

GENERAL FEATURES. An infiltrating expansile mass that predominantly involves the hemispheric white matter is typical.

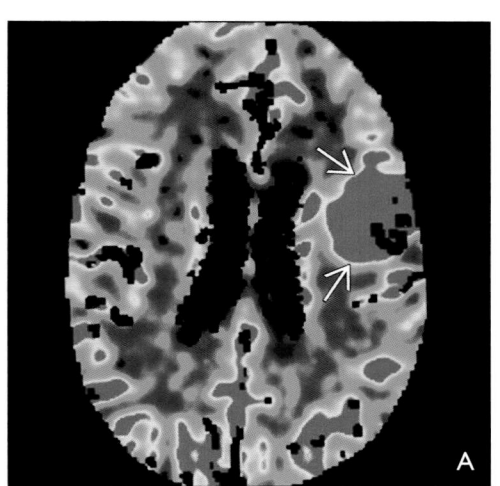
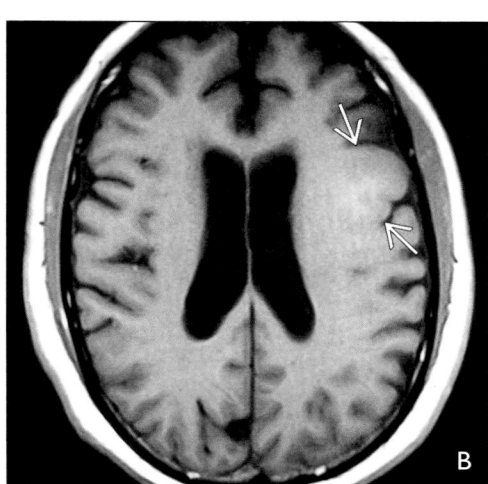

17-34A. A 72-year-old man with sudden right-sided weakness was brought to the emergency department for "brain attack." NECT scan (not shown) demonstrated a left posterior frontal mass. CT perfusion obtained as part of the emergent stroke protocol shows markedly elevated rCBV in the mass ➜. 17-34B. T1WI shows a mostly isointense expansile mass ➜ that effaces the gray-white matter interface.

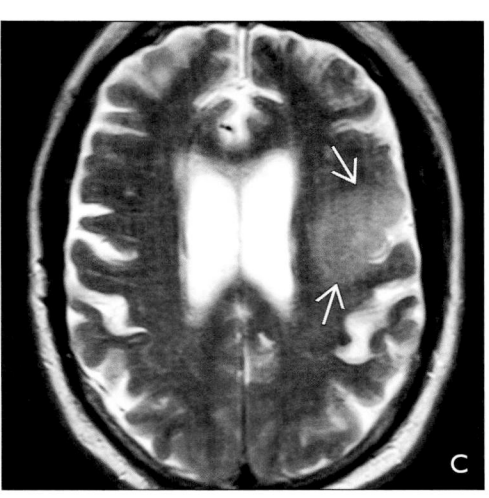
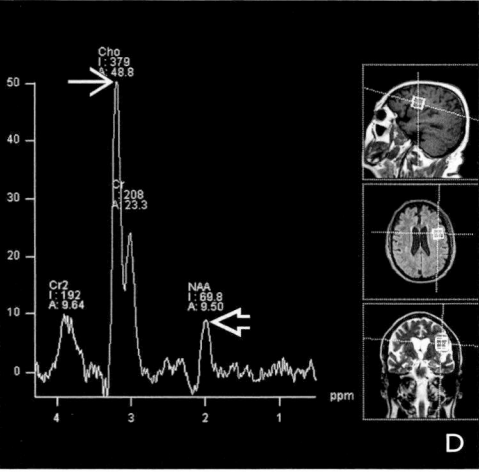

17-34C. T2WI with slight motion degradation shows that the mass ➜ is hyperintense with ill-defined margins. T1 C+ FS scan (not shown) demonstrated no enhancement. 17-34D. MRS shows markedly elevated Cho ➜, decreased NAA ➜ suggesting neoplasm. With increased rCBV despite the lack of enhancement, this tumor is most likely an anaplastic astrocytoma. Histopathology confirmed WHO grade III anaplastic astrocytoma.

CT FINDINGS. AAs are ill-defined low-density lesions on NECT. If the lesion began in an LGA, calcification may be present.

The majority of AAs do not enhance on CECT. When present, enhancement is often focal, patchy, poorly delineated, and heterogeneous.

MR FINDINGS. Most AAs are hypointense on T1WI and hyperintense on T2/FLAIR **(17-34)**. The margins may appear grossly discrete, but tumor cells invariably infiltrate adjacent brain. Hemorrhage and calcification are uncommon, so T2* "blooming" is typically absent.

Contrast enhancement varies from none to moderate. Between 50-70% of AAs show some degree of enhancement. Focal, nodular, homogeneous, patchy, or even ring-enhancing patterns may be seen.

The presence of enhancement is clinically significant. Nonenhancing AAs behave more like low-grade tumors. In contrast, preoperative enhancement is associated with increased recurrence risk and shortened survival. Enhancement may indicate a more malignant astrocytoma, with foci tending toward glioblastoma (grade IV).

AAs generally do not restrict on DWI. MRS shows elevated choline and decreased NAA. The mI:Cr ratio is generally lower than that of LGAs. DTI can be helpful in delineating early white matter tract invasion.

Perfusion MR shows increased rCBV in the most malignant parts of the tumor. Color choline maps are helpful in guiding stereotactic biopsy, improving diagnostic accuracy with decreased sampling error **(17-35)**.

Differential Diagnosis

The major differential diagnosis of AA is **other diffusely infiltrating astrocytomas**. Imaging findings of AA are often indistinguishable from those of LGA. GBMs usually have an irregular enhancing rim surrounding a necrotic nonenhancing core. Hemorrhage with spin dephasing and "blooming" on T2* is common.

Oligodendroglioma and **mixed oligoastrocytoma** may also be indistinguishable from AA. Oligodendrogliomas are usually cortically based tumors whereas AA more often diffusely infiltrates white matter.

17-35A. FLAIR scan in a 34-year-old woman shows a widely infiltrating hyperintense mass in the corpus callosum, deep periventricular WM ➡. *17-35B. T1 C+ FS scan shows a small ring-enhancing focus in the middle of the mass* ➡.

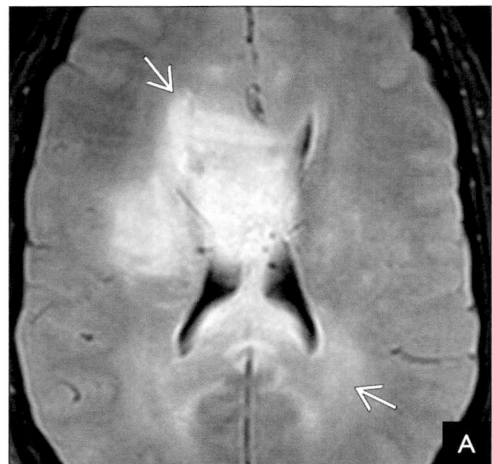
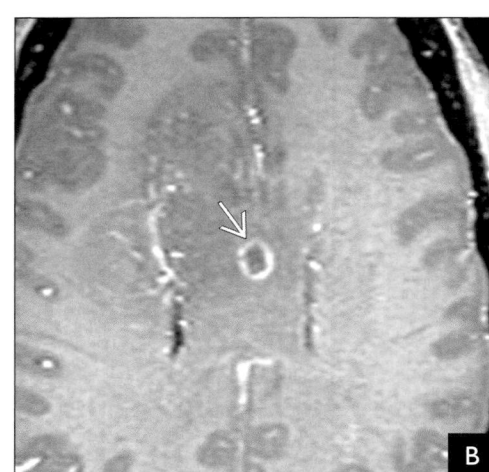

17-35C. MRS shows elevated Cho ➡, *low NAA* ➡. *17-35D. Cho:NAA map shows that choline is highest in the area of ring-like enhancement, suggesting high-grade malignant neoplasm. Histologic diagnosis was anaplastic astrocytoma (WHO grade III). (Courtesy M. Thurnher, MD.)*

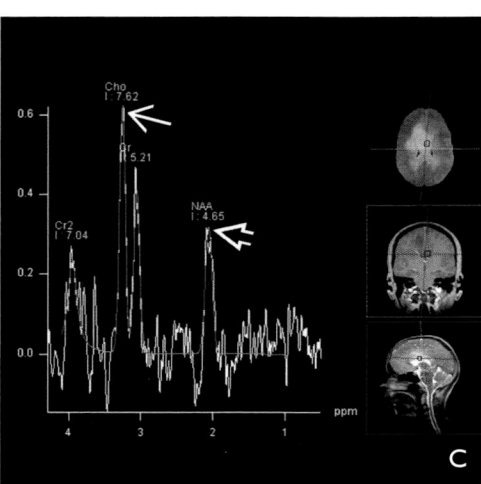
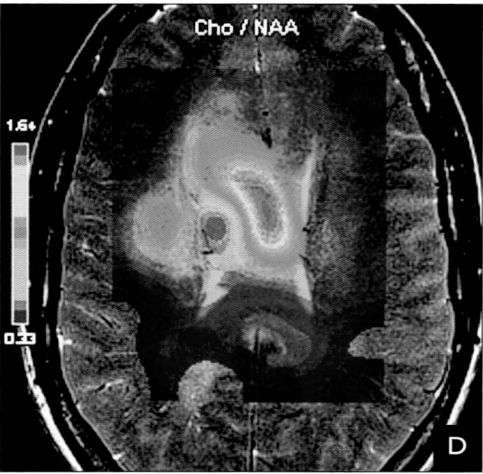

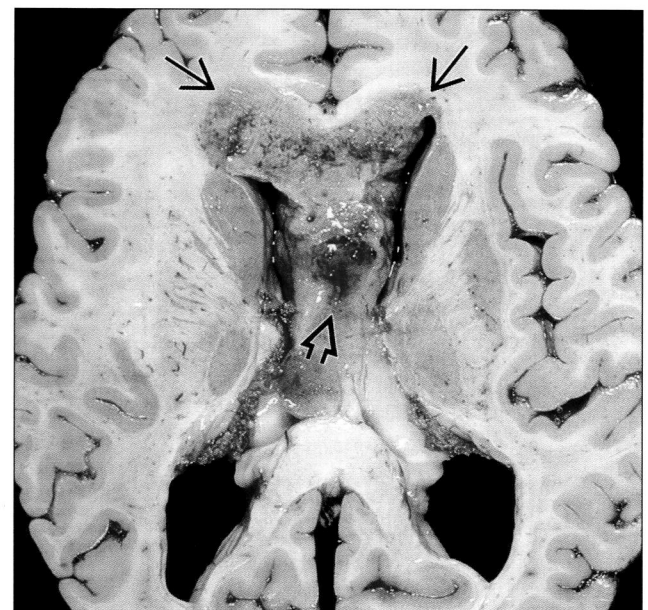

17-36. Autopsy specimen shows "butterfly" glioblastoma multiforme ⇒ crossing corpus callosum genu, extending into and enlarging fornix ⊵. (Courtesy R. Hewlett, MD.)

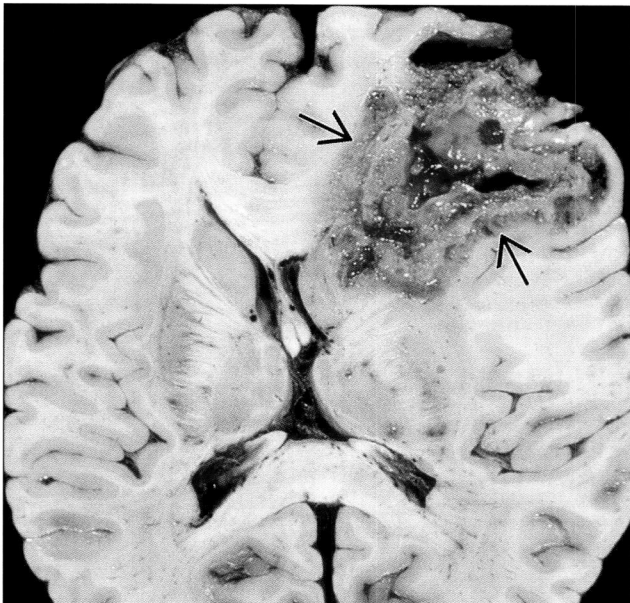

17-37. Autopsy specimen shows classic primary glioblastoma multiforme with hemorrhage, viable "rind" of tumor ⇒ surrounding a necrotic core. (Courtesy R. Hewlett, MD.)

Infection (**cerebritis** and **encephalitis**) may cause parenchymal edema and enhancement. Restriction on DWI is common. **Status epilepticus** may cause gyriform enhancement and edema in a nonvascular distribution. Seizure history is usually but not invariably present.

ANAPLASTIC ASTROCYTOMA

Etiology
- 75% evolve from low-grade astrocytoma

Pathology
- 1/3 of all astrocytomas
  - Second only to GBM
- Diffusely infiltrating
- Lacks necrosis, hemorrhage
- WHO grade III

Clinical Issues
- Peak age = 40-50 years
- Mean survival = 2-3 years
- Degenerates into GBM

Imaging
- Diffusely infiltrating T2/FLAIR hyperintense WM mass
- 50-70% enhance
  - Can be focal, nodular, patchy, or ring-like
  - Enhancement correlates with poor prognosis
- MRS, pMR helpful for guiding biopsy

Differential Diagnosis
- Other astrocytomas (LGA, GBM)
- Oligodendroglioma, oligoastrocytoma
- Cerebritis, encephalitis

Glioblastoma Multiforme

Glioblastoma multiforme is the most common primary brain tumor and the most malignant of the astrocytomas.

Terminology

Glioblastoma multiforme (GBM) is also called grade IV astrocytoma and malignant astrocytoma (the latter term is more generic, as it also refers to anaplastic astrocytoma). Two forms of GBM are currently recognized: Primary ("de novo") GBM and secondary GBM (tumor arising from a previously lower grade astrocytoma). While these two types share similar histology, they differ genetically.

Etiology

GENERAL CONCEPTS. Primary GBMs arise abruptly, usually within a few months, without a recognizable precursor lesion. These tumors probably originate from neural stem cells. In contrast, **secondary GBMs** develop more slowly, arising from malignant degeneration of a lower grade diffuse astrocytoma (WHO grade II or III).

MicroRNAs are highly conserved regulators of gene expression and play a key role in controlling glioma cell proliferation. microRNAs are important regulators of growth and differentiation in transformed neural precursor cell types. Recent studies using microRNA expression profiles have identified *five* clinically and genetically distinct subclasses of glioblastoma, each related to a different neural precursor cell type.

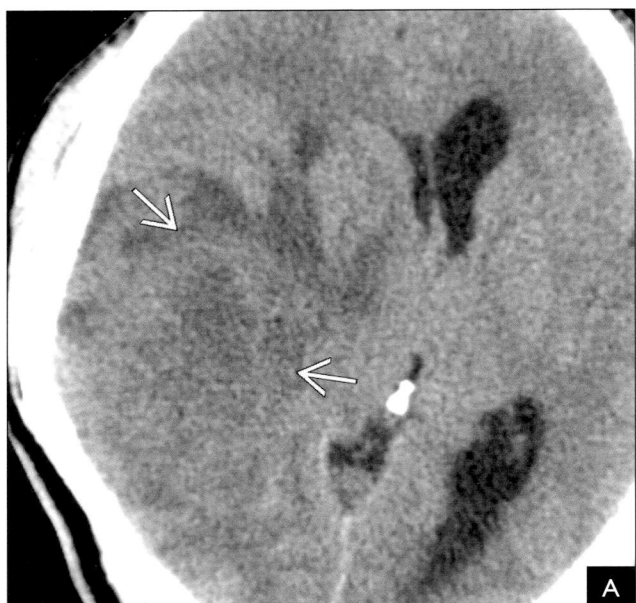

17-38A. NECT scan shows typical findings of GBM with a large, mixed iso-/hypodense mass ⇒ that compresses and displaces lateral ventricles.

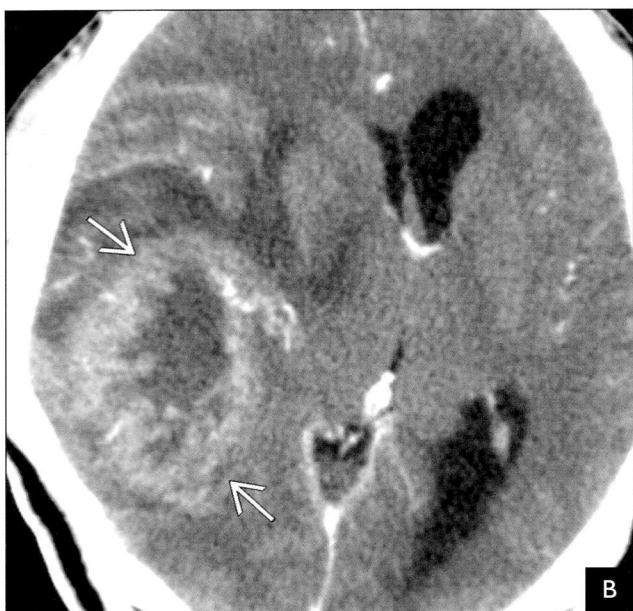

17-38B. CECT scan in the same patient shows the irregular enhancing "rind" of tissue ⇒ surrounding the nonenhancing necrotic core of the tumor.

GENETICS. The high frequency of *IDH1* and *IDH2* mutations in astrocytomas, secondary glioblastomas, and oligodendrogliomas suggests that these tumors share a common progenitor cell population. The absence of this molecular marker in primary glioblastomas suggests a different cell of origin. Both glioblastoma subtypes acquire a similar histological phenotype as a result of common genetic alterations, including the loss of tumor suppressor genes on chromosome 10q.

A number of mutations have been identified in GBMs. Only a few of the more important ones are discussed here. *EGFR* amplification occurs in 40-50% of primary GBMs (rarely in secondary tumors) while *TP53* mutations are more common in secondary GBMs (but also occur in primary lesions). *IDH1* mutation occurs in secondary GBM.

Three inherited cancer syndromes—namely **neurofibromatosis type 1** (NF1), **Li-Fraumeni**, and **Turcot syndrome**—demonstrate an enhanced propensity to develop GBM.

Pathology

LOCATION. The cerebral hemispheres are the most common site in adults. GBMs preferentially involve the subcortical and deep periventricular white matter, easily spreading across compact tracts such as the corpus callosum and corticospinal tracts **(17-36)**. The basal ganglia and thalami are other common tumor locations.

The brainstem—especially the pons—is a common site in children. GBMs of the cerebellum and spinal cord are very rare.

SIZE AND NUMBER. GBMs vary in size. Primary GBMs are generally larger, more necrotic lesions while secondary GBMs initially develop as small foci within a larger "sea" of lower grade astrocytoma.

Because GBMs spread quickly and widely along compact white matter tracts, up to 20% appear as multifocal lesions at the time of initial diagnosis. Between 2-5% of multifocal GBMs are true synchronous, independently developing tumors.

GROSS PATHOLOGY. The most frequent appearance is a reddish-gray "rind" of tumor surrounding a necrotic core **(17-37)**. Mass effect and peritumoral edema are typically marked. Increased vascularity and intratumoral hemorrhage are common. Symmetric involvement of the corpus callosum is also common, the "butterfly glioma" pattern.

MICROSCOPIC FEATURES. Necrosis and microvascular proliferation are the histologic hallmarks of GBMs, distinguishing them from anaplastic astrocytomas.

Varied tumor cells comprise GBMs; hence the "multiforme" part of GBM. Pleomorphic fibrillary astrocytes, gemistocytes, bipolar bland-appearing but mitotically active small cells (including "microglia"), and large bizarre multinucleated giant cells are all common features.

GBMs generally have a high proliferation index (MIB-1), usually exceeding 10%.

Immunohistochemistry shows GFAP and Olig2 positivity. IDH-1 is very helpful in differentiating secondary glioblastomas (positive) from primary glioblastomas (negative).

STAGING, GRADING, AND CLASSIFICATION. GBMs are all WHO grade IV neoplasms.

Clinical Issues

EPIDEMIOLOGY. GBM is the most common primary brain tumor, representing between 12-15% of all intracranial neoplasms and 60-75% of astrocytomas. Primary tumors account for 95% of all GBMs. Only 5% of GBMs are secondary tumors, arising from a preexisting lower grade astrocytoma.

DEMOGRAPHICS. GBMs can occur at any age (including in neonates and infants), but overall peak age is 45-75 years. Primary GBMs tend to occur in older adults (peaking between 60 and 75 years) while secondary GBMs occur a decade or two earlier. The M:F ratio is almost equal, although primary GBMs occur slightly more often in men and secondary tumors slightly more often in women.

PRESENTATION. Presentation varies with location, but seizure, focal neurologic deficits, and mental status changes are the most common symptoms. Headache from elevated intracranial pressure is also common. Approximately 2% of GBMs present with sudden stroke-like onset caused by acute intratumoral hemorrhage. Underlying GBM should always be a diagnostic consideration in an older normotensive patient with a spontaneous, unexplained intracranial hemorrhage.

NATURAL HISTORY. GBM is a relentless progressive disease. Mean survival in patients with a primary GBM is under one year. Younger patients with secondary GBMs may survive somewhat longer.

TREATMENT OPTIONS. Gross total surgical resection followed by concurrent radiation and chemotherapy may modestly prolong survival but with highly variable quality of life. Tumor "debulking" is generally ineffective.

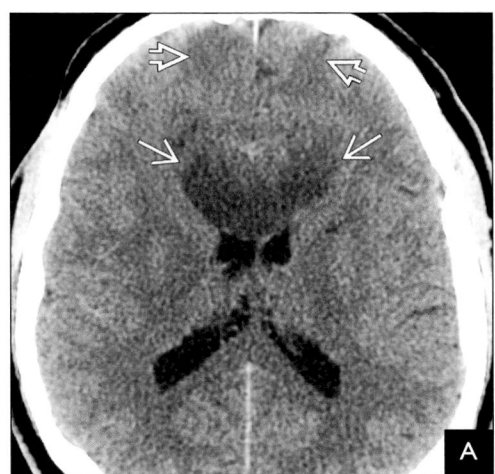

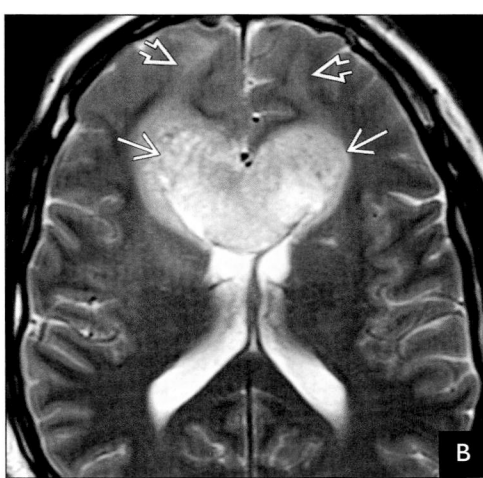

17-39A. NECT scan in a patient with a typical GBM shows an ill-defined hypodense mass expanding the corpus callosum genu ➡. Hypodense subcortical WM foci are seen in both frontal lobes ➡. 17-39B. T2WI shows that the mass ➡ is heterogeneously hyperintense on T2WI. Note edema extending into both anterior frontal lobes ➡.

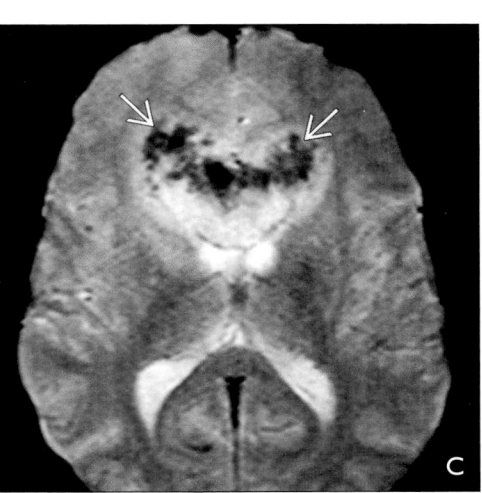

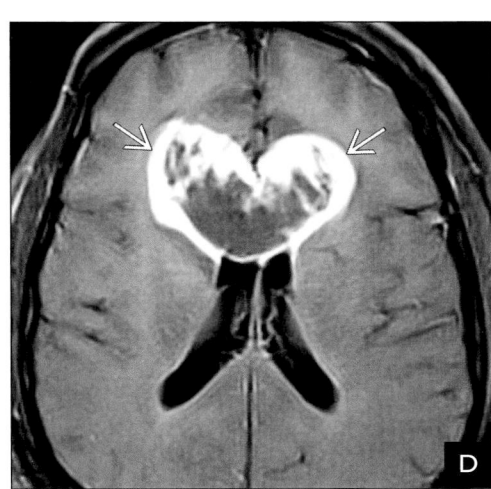

17-39C. T2 GRE shows patchy, confluent hemorrhage ➡. 17-39D. T1 C+ FS scan shows that a thick enhancing "rind" of tumor ➡ surrounds the necrotic core of the mass. No enhancement is seen in the edematous areas that were identified on T2WI, but viable neoplastic cells always extend far beyond visible enhancement or signal abnormality.*

Imaging

GENERAL FEATURES. At least 90-95% of GBMs demonstrate a thick, irregular, enhancing "rind" of tumor surrounding a necrotic core.

In rare cases, no dominant mass is present. Instead, tumor extends diffusely throughout the cerebral white matter. Confluent and patchy white matter hyperintensities on T2/FLAIR scans mimic small vessel vascular disease. An even rarer variant is "primary diffuse leptomeningeal gliomatosis." Here tumor extends diffusely around the brain surfaces, mostly between the pia and the glia limitans of the cortex.

CT FINDINGS. Most GBMs demonstrate a hypodense central mass surrounded by an iso- to moderately hyperdense rim on NECT **(17-38A)**. Hemorrhage is common but calcification rare. Marked mass effect and significant hypodense peritumoral edema are typical ancillary findings.

CECT shows strong but heterogeneous irregular rim enhancement **(17-38B)**. Prominent vessels in highly vascular GBMs are seen as linear enhancing foci adjacent to the mass.

MR FINDINGS. T1WI shows a poorly marginated mass with mixed signal intensity. Subacute hemorrhage is common. T2/FLAIR shows heterogeneous hyperintensity with indistinct tumor margins and extensive vasogenic edema **(17-39)**, **(17-40)**. Necrosis, cysts, hemorrhage at various stages of evolution, fluid/debris levels, and "flow voids" from extensive neovascularity may be seen. T2* imaging often shows foci of susceptibility artifact **(17-39)**.

T1 C+ shows strong but irregular ring enhancement surrounding a central nonenhancing core of necrotic tumor. Nodular, punctate, or patchy enhancing foci outside the main mass represent macroscopic tumor extension into adjacent structures. Microscopic foci of viable tumor cells are invariably present far beyond any demonstrable areas of enhancement or edema on standard imaging sequences.

Most GBMs do not restrict on DWI. DTI may show reduced fractional anisotropy and disrupted white matter

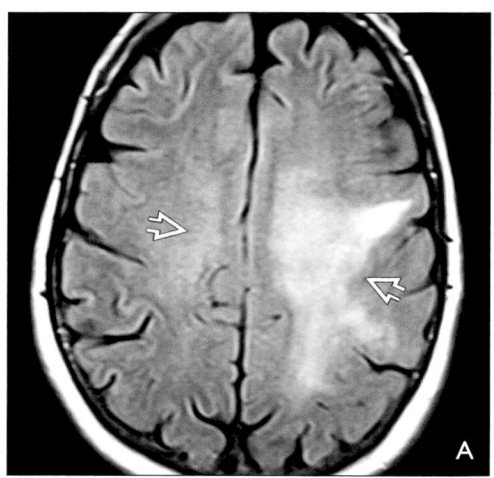
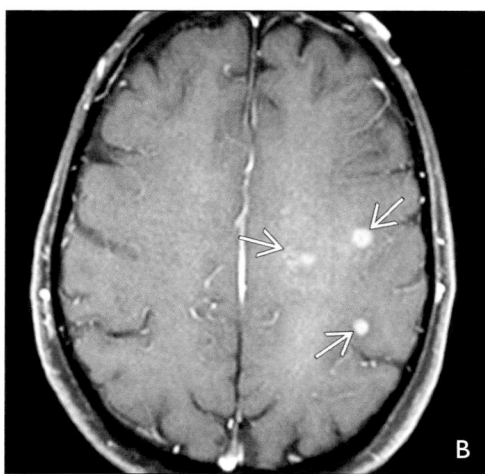

17-40A. FLAIR scan in a 68-year-old woman with confusion and right arm weakness, remote history of breast cancer shows confluent hyperintensity in the corona radiata of both hemispheres ⇨. 17-40B. T1 C+ FS scan shows multiple foci of linear and solid dot-like enhancement ➡ in the left hemisphere.

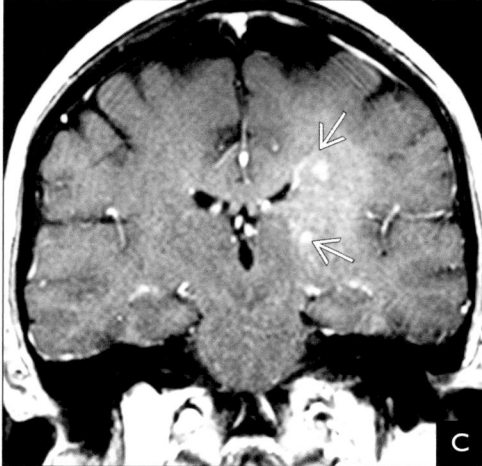
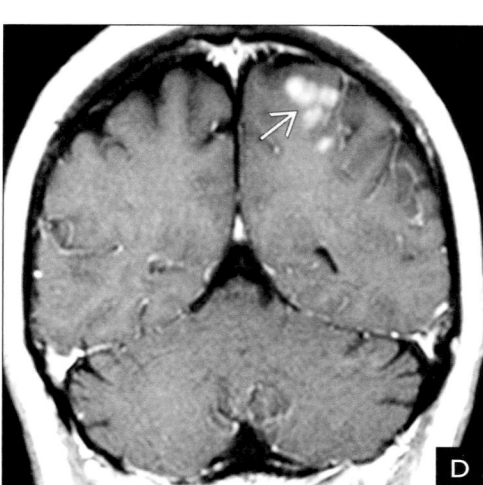

17-40C. Coronal T1 C+ scan shows the dot-like and linear foci of contrast enhancement ➡. 17-40D. More posterior T1 C+ scan shows a cluster of nodular enhancing foci ➡. Biopsy disclosed GBM. Occasionally, GBM presents as a diffusely infiltrating multifocal neoplasm without a dominant mass as in this case.

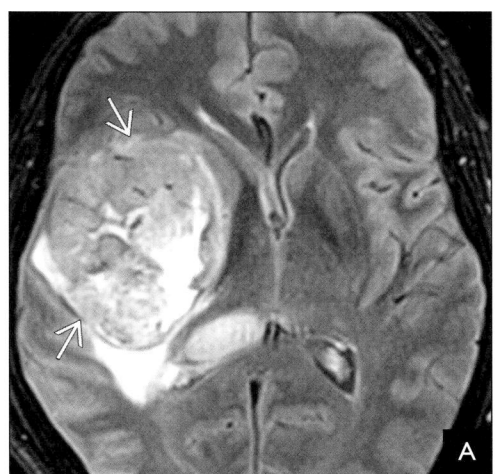

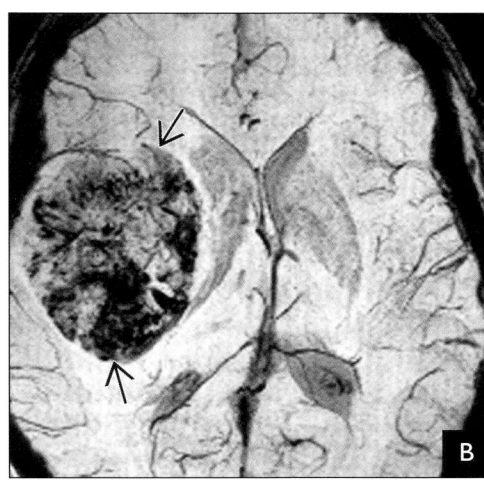

17-41A. T2WI shows a very heterogeneous-appearing mass ➜ in the right temporal lobe, basal ganglia, thalamus. 17-41B. T2* SWI scan shows extensive "blooming" foci ➡ consistent with intratumoral hemorrhage.

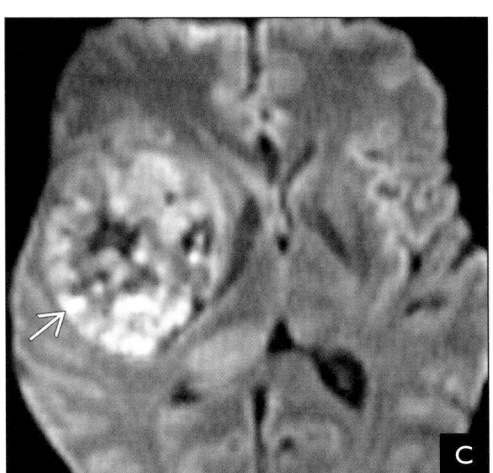

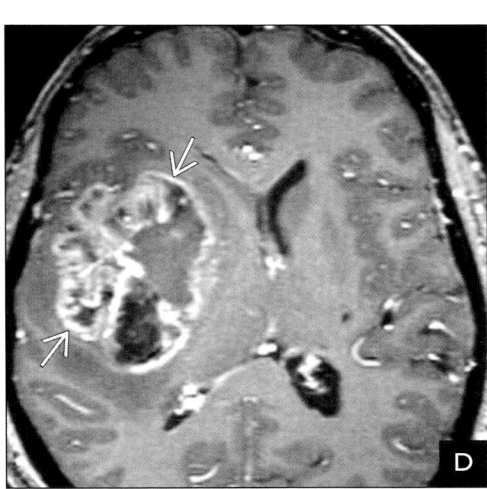

17-41C. DWI shows restricted diffusion in the areas of highest cellularity ➜. 17-41D. T1 C+ FS scan shows irregular rim and nodular enhancement around the mass ➜.

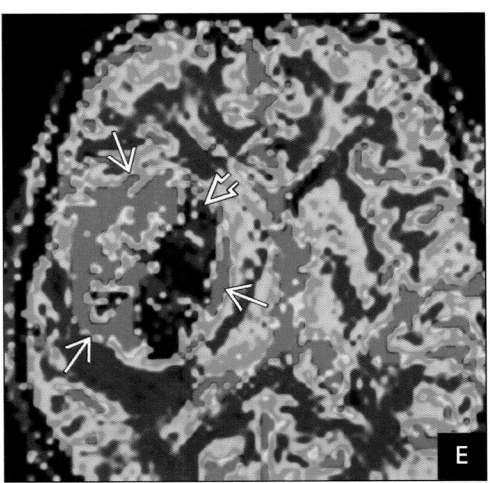

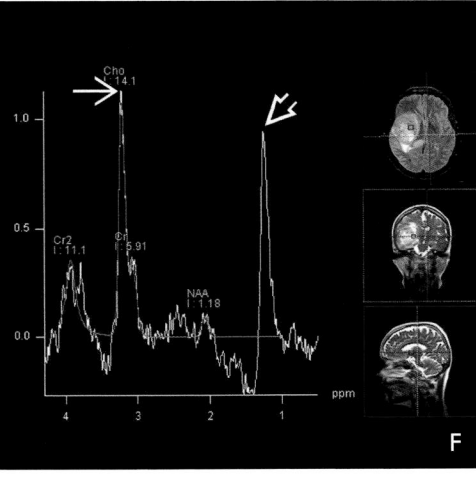

17-41E. pMR shows elevated rCBV around the rim and in the solid part of the tumor ➜, low or absent signal in the necrotic center ➜. 17-41F. MRS shows high choline ➜, low NAA, large lactate peak ➡. Glioblastoma multiforme. (Courtesy M. Thurnher, MD.)

17-42. Graphic shows many potential GBM routes of spread. Preferential tumor spread is along compact WM tracts but can be ependymal, subpial, diffuse CSF ("carcinomatous meningitis"). Dural, skull invasion and extracranial metastases occur but are rare. 17-43. Series of autopsy cases illustrates patterns of GBM dissemination. Axial section through the pons and cerebellum shows multiple discrete foci of parenchymal tumor ➔. (Courtesy E. T. Hedley-Whyte, MD.)

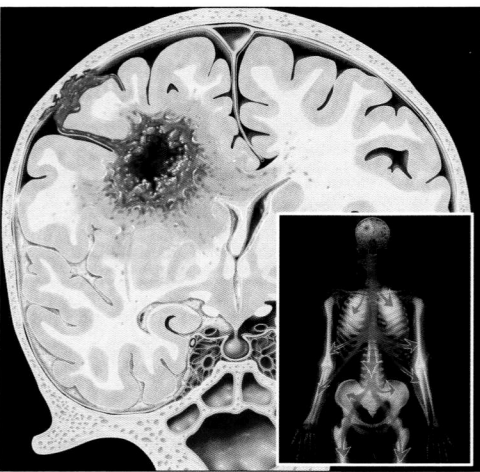 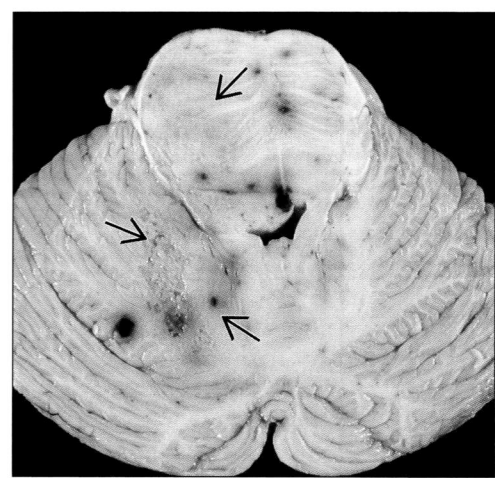

17-44. "Carcinomatous meningitis" from GBM coats the surface of the brainstem and cerebellum, basilar artery, and cranial nerves. Gross appearance is virtually indistinguishable from that of pyogenic meningitis. (Courtesy R. Hewlett, MD.) 17-45. Glioblastoma has spread around both lateral ventricles in a thick band of subependymal tumor ➔. (Courtesy R. Hewlett, MD.)

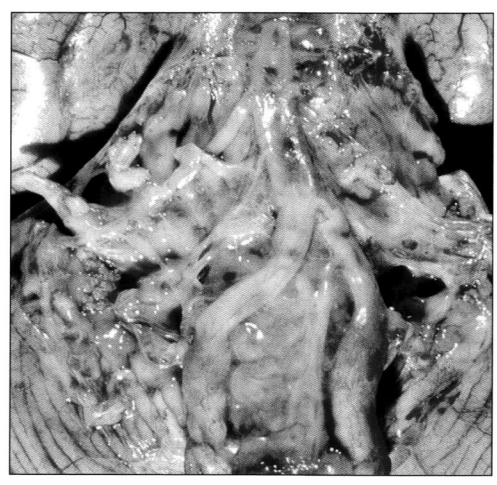 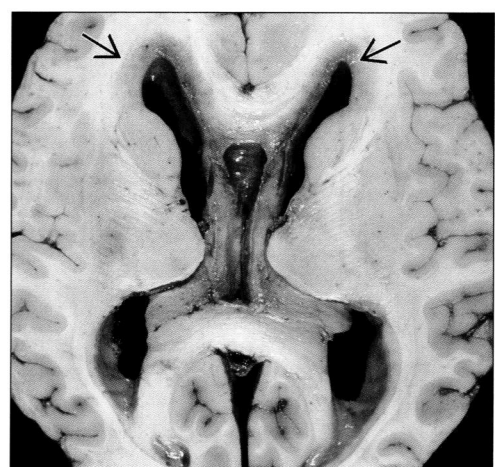

17-46A. Coronal autopsied brain shows a necrotic, hemorrhagic temporal lobe GBM. 17-46B. Lumbar (left) and thoracic (right) spine in the same case show multiple metastases in the vertebral bodies ➔. Extracranial spread of GBM is rare although documented in this case. (Courtesy E. T. Hedley-Whyte, MD.)

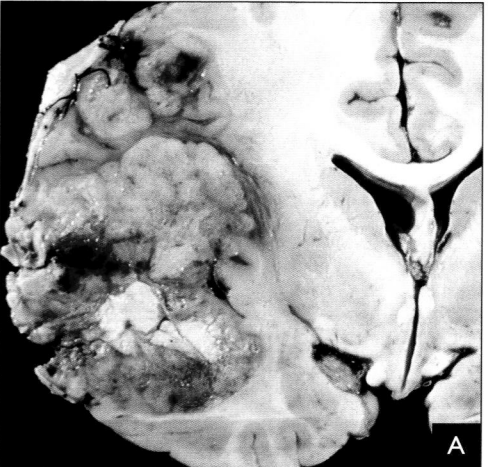 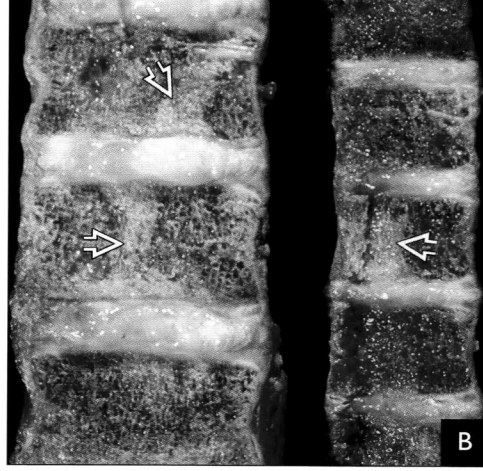

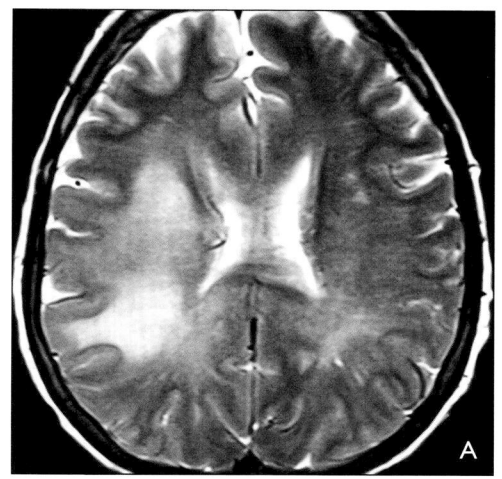

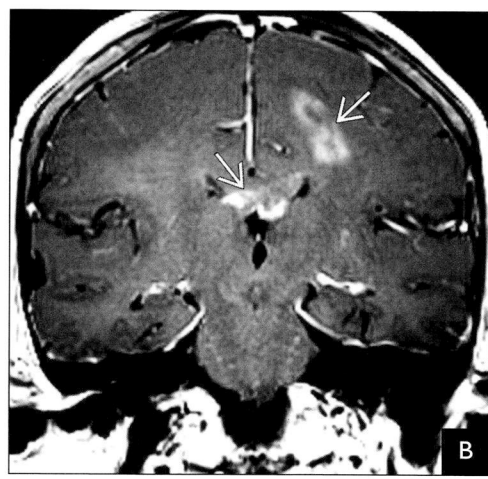

17-47A. *T2WI shows diffuse confluent and patchy WM hyperintensity in this elderly patient with increasing confusion, left-sided weakness.* ***17-47B.*** *Coronal T1 C+ in the same patient shows enhancement in the left hemispheric WM, corpus callosum* ➡. *Biopsy disclosed diffusely infiltrating GBM.*

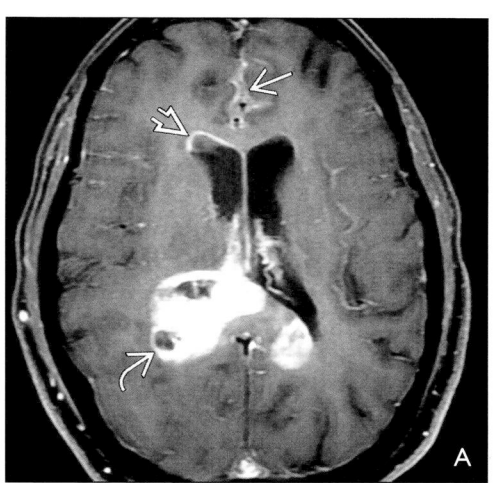

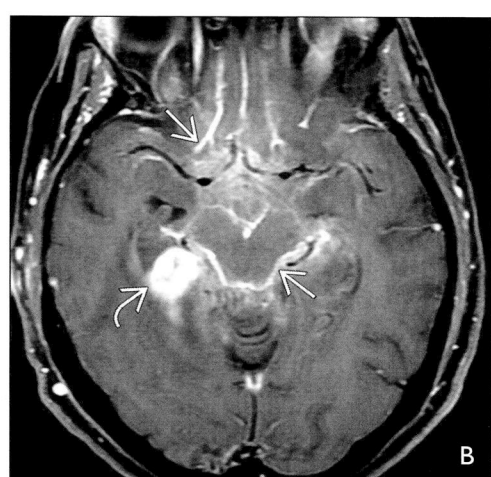

17-48A. *Series of T1 C+ FS scans demonstrates GBM* ➡ *with widespread CSF dissemination. Note ependymal* ➡, *sulcal-cisternal* ➡ *enhancement.* ***17-48B.*** *Lower T1 C+ FS scan shows the primary tumor* ➡ *together with a diffuse coating of midbrain, enhancement throughout the suprasellar cistern extending into both sylvian fissures and olfactory sulci* ➡.

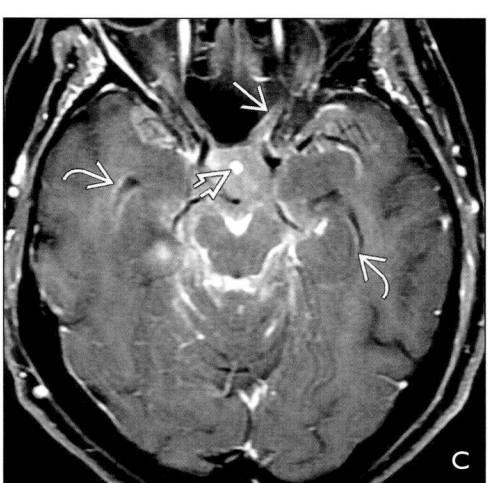

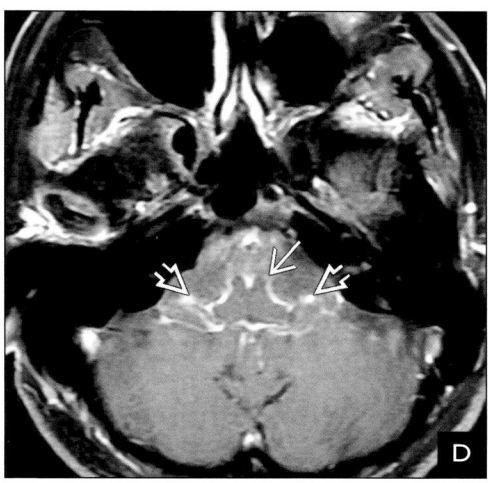

17-48C. *Enhancing tumor thickens and coats the infundibular stalk* ➡, *extends along the optic nerve sheath into the orbit* ➡, *and fills the interpeduncular cistern. Note ependymal spread around both temporal horns* ➡. ***17-48D.*** *Medulla is diffusely coated with tumor* ➡, *and enhancing tumor is seen along CNs IX-XI* ➡. *GBM can spread throughout the entire CSF space ("carcinomatous meningitis"). Numerous "drop metastases" to the lumbosacral sac were also present.*

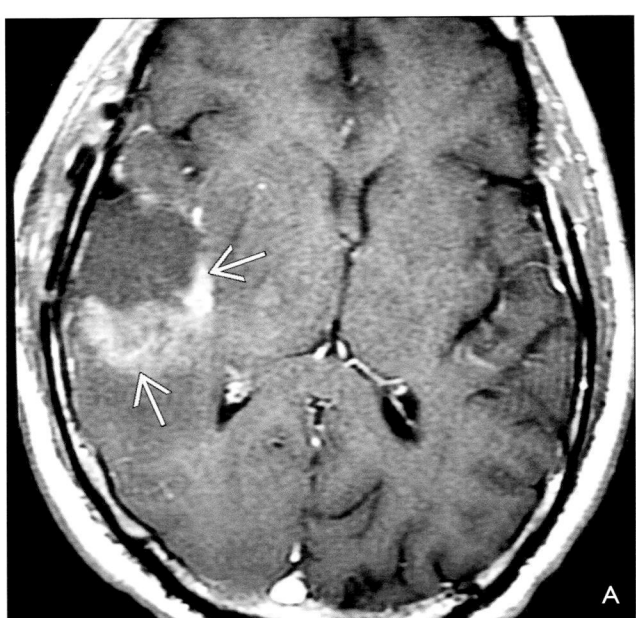

17-49A. *Immediately following resection of a right temporal lobe GBM, T1 C+ scan was obtained. Residual enhancing tumor lines the resection cavity* ➡.

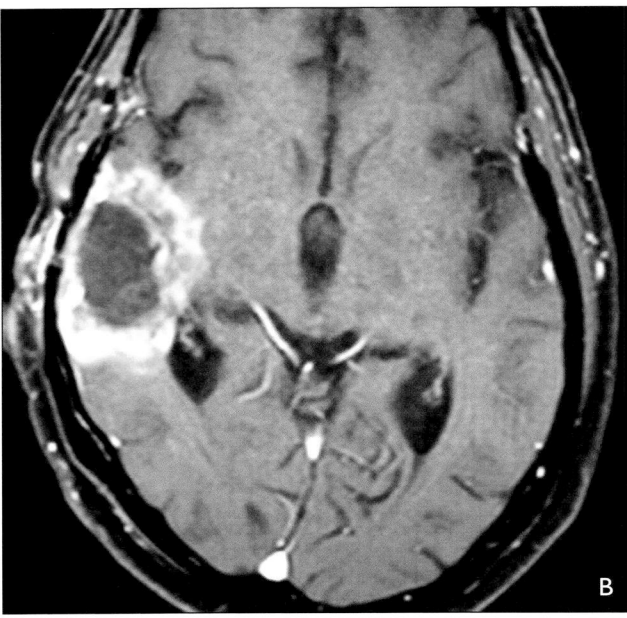

17-49B. *The patient received radiation and concurrent temozolomide. Five weeks later, thick enhancement surrounds the resection bed. Biopsy disclosed mostly necrotic tumor. The enhancement represented pseudoprogression.*

tracts from tumor invasion. MRS usually shows elevated choline, decreased NAA and mI, and a lipid/lactate peak resonating at 1.33 ppm. pMR shows elevated rCBV in the tumor "rind" and increased vascular permeability **(17-41)**.

ANGIOGRAPHY. Angiography shows a prominent capillary phase tumor "blush," enlarged/irregular-appearing vessels, and "pooling" of contrast. Arteriovenous shunting is common, seen as "early draining" veins.

PATTERNS OF GBM SPREAD. GBM is the most common primary CNS neoplasm to cause "brain-to-brain" metastases. While some primary tumors such as medulloblastoma, ependymoma, and germinoma tend to disseminate almost exclusively through CSF pathways, GBMs are notorious for their ability to spread via multiple routes **(17-42)**, **(17-43)**, **(17-44)**, **(17-45)**, **(17-46)**. Because GBM spreads so rapidly and viable tumor cells are present throughout much of the normal-appearing brain, many neuropathologists and oncologists consider glioblastoma a "whole-brain" disease.

White matter metastases. The most common route of GBM spread is throughout the white matter **(17-47)**. Tumor spreads directly into (and beyond) the peritumoral edema. Dissemination along compact white matter tracts such as the corpus callosum, fornices, anterior commissure, and corticospinal tract can result in tumor implantation in geographically remote areas such as the pons, cerebellum, medulla, and spinal cord.

CSF dissemination. GBM often seeds the CSF, filling the sulci and cisterns. Diffuse coating of cranial

nerves and the pial surface of the brain is also common. This appearance of "carcinomatous meningitis" may be indistinguishable on imaging studies from pyogenic meningitis **(17-48)**.

"Drop metastases" can extend inferiorly into the spinal canal, covering the spinal cord, thickening nerves, and causing focal mass-like deposits within the thecal sac.

Ependymal and subependymal spread. GBM spread along the ventricular ependyma also occurs but is less common than diffuse CSF dissemination. The interior of the ventricles—most often the lateral ventricles—is coated with enhancing tumor and resembles pyogenic ventriculitis on contrast-enhanced imaging **(17-48)**.

Subependymal tumor spread also occurs, producing a thick neoplastic "rind" as tumor "creeps" and crawls around the ventricular margins.

Skull-dura invasion. Direct invasion of GBM through the pia and into the dura-arachnoid is rare. In exceptional cases, tumor erodes into and sometimes even through the calvaria, extending into the subgaleal soft tissues.

Extra-CNS metastases. Hematogenous spread of GBM to systemic sites occurs but is rare. Bone marrow (especially the vertebral bodies), liver, lung, and even lymph node metastases can occur.

GBM PSEUDOPROGRESSION. Contrast-enhanced MR is currently the imaging mainstay for monitoring treatment response in patients with GBMs. Treatment decisions are guided by criteria that equate increased enhancement with progressive tumor burden, treatment failure, and poor prognosis.

However, standard imaging can neither distinguish recurrent or progressive tumor from treatment-induced parenchymal injury nor identify admixtures of tumor and parenchymal injury. **Radiation necrosis** and **pseudoprogression** are the two major types of treatment-related effects that can mimic tumor recurrence. Radiation necrosis is a delayed response, but pseudoprogression typically occurs within three months.

Following surgical resection and radiotherapy with concurrent temozolomide, lesion enlargement on the first follow-up MR is often observed **(17-49)**. Almost half of all patients show increased mass effect and new areas of enhancement compared to immediate baseline postoperative imaging. Of these, approximately 40% are secondary to pseudoprogression rather than "true" tumor progression.

Distinguishing early "true" progression from pseudoprogression is difficult. pMR with dynamic susceptibility-weighted contrast enhancement can be used to map rCBV and estimate tissue microvasculature across lesions. Early studies suggest that rCBV can quantify tumor burden relative to components of pseudoprogression and radiation necrosis.

The use of biodegradable **carmustine (Gliadel) wafers** also complicates postoperative imaging. Ring enhancement occurs within one postoperative day and peaks at one month. Restricted diffusivity may last up to one year.

ifferential Diagnosis

The major neoplasm that should be distinguished from GBM is **metastasis**. Metastases are often multiple and tend to occur peripherally at the gray-white matter junction. Even large metastases are round or ovoid, not infiltrating like GBM.

Other GBM mimics include anaplastic astrocytoma, anaplastic mixed oligodendroglioma, and primary CNS lymphoma. **Anaplastic astrocytomas** generally do not enhance, although some do and may be difficult to distinguish from GBM on imaging alone.

Anaplastic oligodendroglioma and **anaplastic oligoastrocytoma** may infiltrate white matter in a manner similar to GBM and may be difficult to diagnose without biopsy. **Primary CNS lymphoma** often involves the corpus callosum but is rarely necrotic in the absence of HIV/AIDS.

The major nonneoplastic differential diagnosis of GBM is **abscess**. Abscesses typically have thinner, more regu-

lar rims and restrict on DWI. MRS often shows succinate and cytosolic amino acids, which are rare in GBM.

"Tumefactive" demyelination in the subcortical white matter may demonstrate peripheral rim enhancement. A "horseshoe" pattern, often draped around a sulcus, is common. An incomplete rim with the open segment pointing toward the sulcus and cortex is typical for "tumefactive" demyelination.

GLIOBLASTOMA MULTIFORME

Etiology
- "Primary" GBM: De novo, probably from neural stem cells
  - 95% of GBMs
- "Secondary" GBM: Malignant progression of lower grade astrocytoma
  - 5% of GBMs

Pathology
- Most common primary CNS neoplasm
  - 60-75% of astrocytomas
- Hemispheres > > pons > > cerebellum, spinal cord
- Thick "rind" of tumor around central necrosis (95%)
  - Hemorrhage common, Ca++ rare
- Histologic hallmarks: Neovascularity, necrosis

Clinical Issues
- Any age, but peak = 45-75 years
- Relentless progression
  - Survival < 1 year

Imaging
- Thick, irregular tumor around central necrosis (95%)
- Strong but heterogeneous enhancement
- "Brain to brain" spread common
  - Hemispheric white matter, fiber tracts
  - CSF ("carcinomatous meningitis," spine "drop mets")
  - Ependymal/subependymal "creeping" tumor spread

Differential Diagnosis
- Common: Metastasis, abscess
- Less common: AA, anaplastic oligo, lymphoma
- Rare: "Tumefactive" demyelination

Gliosarcoma

Terminology

Gliosarcoma (GS) is a glioblastoma variant that contains distinct gliomatous and sarcomatous components.

Etiology

Gliosarcoma can be primary or secondary. Most GSs are primary tumors and arise de novo. Secondary GSs occur in patients with previously resected and irradiated GBMs or as radiation-induced tumors in patients without any prior history of GBM.

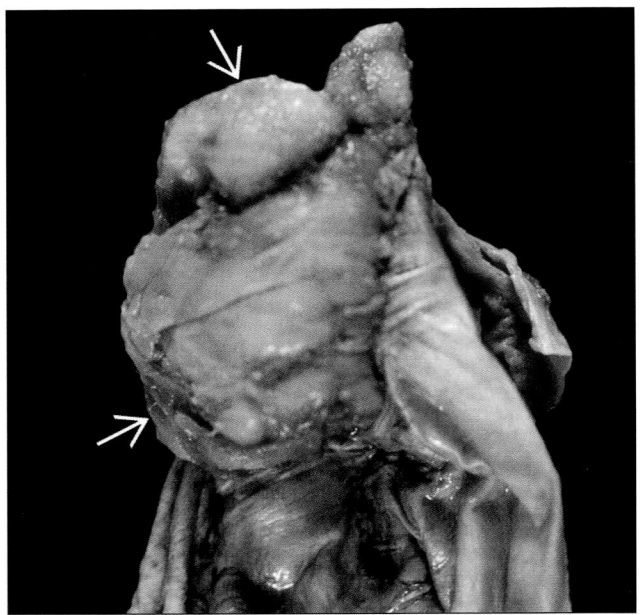

17-50. Autopsy case of gliosarcoma demonstrates a dura-based tumor nodule ➡ that appears very similar to meningioma. (Courtesy Rubinstein Collection, AFIP Archives.)

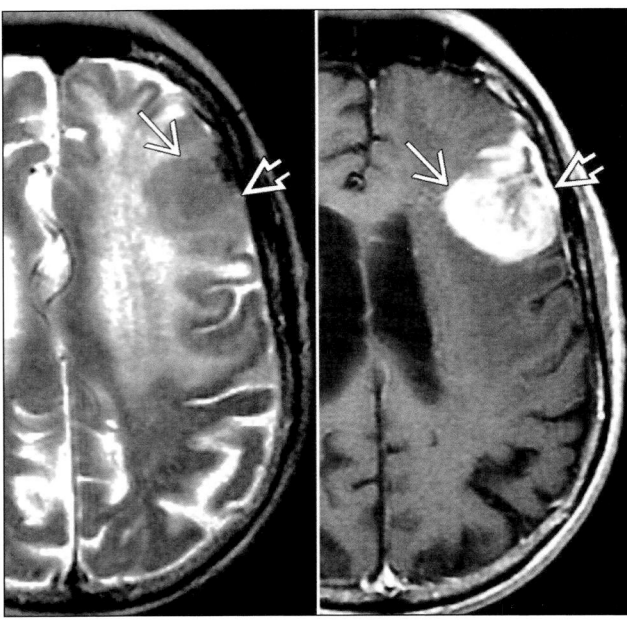

17-51. T2WI (left), T1 C+ (right) show an enhancing left frontal mass ➡ that involves brain parenchyma, invades the dura ➡. Gliosarcoma. (Courtesy L. Ginsberg, MD.)

The genetic profile of GS is similar to that of primary GBM, except for rare EGFR amplification. MGMT methylation and *IDH1* mutation are rare.

Pathology

Gliosarcoma is characterized by a biphasic tissue pattern. Areas that exhibit both neoplastic glial and metaplastic mesenchymal elements are present within the same tumor. The gliomatous element may be geographically separated from—or intermingled with—the mesenchymal component **(17-50)**.

Histologically, the glial component meets the usual criteria for GBM (see above). The mesenchymal component may display a wide variety of morphologic features with fibroblastic, cartilaginous, osseous, muscle, or adipose cell lineage.

Gliosarcomas are WHO grade IV neoplasms.

Clinical Issues

Gliosarcomas are rare, accounting for approximately 2% of all glioblastomas. Peak age is the fifth to seventh decades. Prognosis is grim with median survival of eight months for secondary GSs and 14 months for primary GSs. Local recurrence is typical. In contrast to GBM, extracranial metastases are relatively common, occurring in 15-30% of cases.

Imaging

Imaging studies show a heterogeneous-appearing, broad-based, peripheral hemispheric mass with moderate to marked surrounding edema. Irregular lesions with thick walls that demonstrate dense ring-like enhancement are seen in 80% of cases **(17-51)**.

Gliosarcomas usually abut the meninges but may not demonstrate dural attachment or obvious invasion. An enhancing dural "tail" often extends peripherally from the tumor mass.

Differential Diagnosis

The major differential diagnosis of GS is **anaplastic meningioma**. **Other sarcomas**, dural **metastases**, **lymphoma**, **plasmocytoma**, and **neurosarcoid** can all present as dura-based lesions with variable brain invasion.

Gliomatosis Cerebri

Terminology

Gliomatosis cerebri (GC) is also known as diffuse cerebral gliomatosis. While other glial neoplasms such as oligodendroglioma sometimes produce a GC-like growth pattern, most GCs exhibit astrocytic lineage and are therefore considered in this chapter.

GC is characterized by unusually widespread infiltration of the brain parenchyma. By definition, GC involves at least three lobes of the brain, frequently extending into the basal ganglia and deep cerebral white matter.

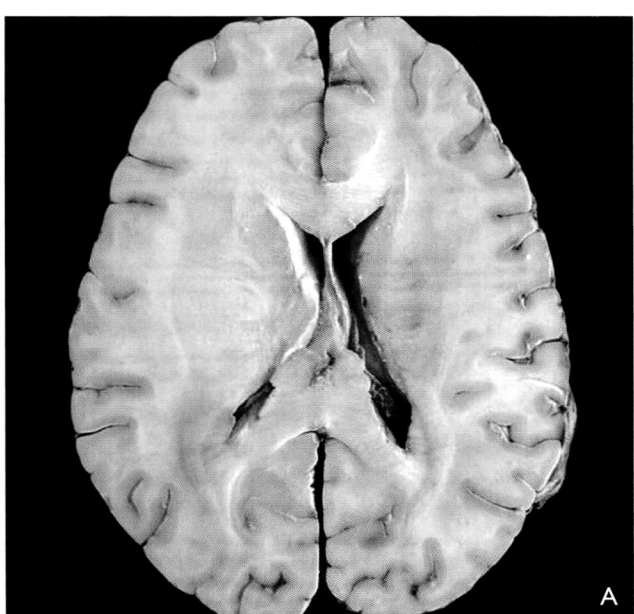

17-52A. Autopsy case of gliomatosis cerebri shows diffuse expansion and slight discoloration of the cerebral WM, infiltration of the basal ganglia.

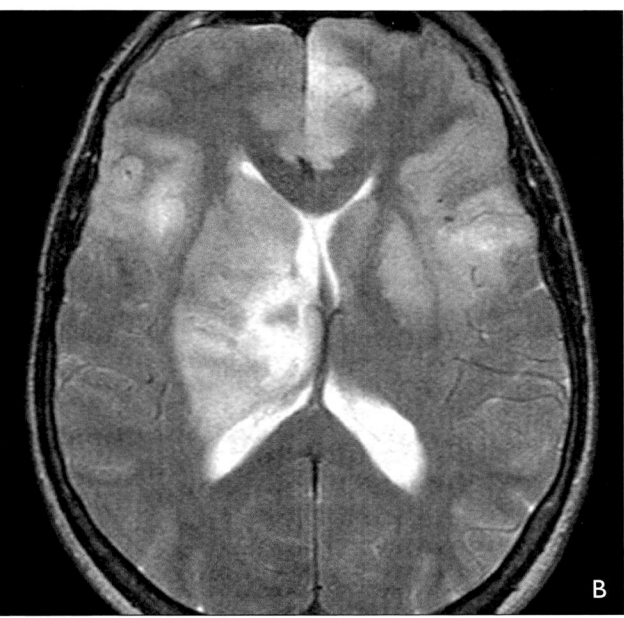

17-52B. Antemortem T2WI in the same case shows the involvement of white matter, deep gray matter, and cortex. GCs infiltrate and expand but maintain the underlying cerebral architecture. (Courtesy R. Hewlett, MD.)

tiology

GENERAL CONCEPTS. GC can arise de novo or from extension of a previously diagnosed diffusely infiltrating astrocytoma or (less commonly) oligodendroglioma.

GENETICS. There are very few reports defining the genetic alterations of GC. *IDH1* gene mutations similar to those of diffuse astrocytoma have been identified in some cases. In oligodendroglial GCs, codeletion of chromosomes 1p and 19q is common.

athology

LOCATION. GCs have been described in virtually all parts of the brain. Over 75% of cases involve the cerebral hemispheres, and an equal number are bilateral. The thalami and basal ganglia are commonly affected. Tumor extends into the midbrain in 50% of cases.

Posterior fossa GCs typically involve the pons, cerebellum, and/or medulla. Superior extension into the mesencephalon and diencephalon is common.

SIZE AND NUMBER. GCs are typically so extensive, widely infiltrating, and poorly marginated that it is difficult to identify their exact borders. Therefore, grossly visible tumor often underestimates lesion size.

GROSS PATHOLOGY. The pathologic diagnosis of GC depends not only on its histologic features but also its extent. Widespread neoplastic overgrowth with preservation of the underlying brain architecture is present. Existing normal structures are infiltrated and expanded but generally still recognizable. The gray-white matter junctions are blurred in some places while remaining intact in others (17-52). Bilateral involvement is common, but hemorrhage, necrosis, and cyst formation are rare (17-53).

MICROSCOPIC FEATURES. A wide range of predominantly astrocyte-like or oligodendroglial cells are present. Elongated glial cells with hyperchromatic nuclei and larger tumor cells with irregular pleomorphic nuclei are often interspersed along myelinated axons. Cellularity is generally low. Mitotic activity is variable but usually absent or minimal.

STAGING, GRADING, AND CLASSIFICATION. GC is a biologically aggressive neoplasm with tumor grades ranging from II-IV. The majority correspond to WHO grade III. Because GCs are so extensively infiltrating, grading and histologic subtyping can be based on nonrepresentative tissue sampling. Undergrading from small biopsy specimens is not uncommon.

Clinical Issues

EPIDEMIOLOGY. GC is a rare but probably underreported diffusely infiltrating tumor that represents approximately 1% of all astrocytomas. Prior to the advent of MR, most cases were diagnosed at autopsy.

DEMOGRAPHICS. GC can occur at any age, including in infants and children, but peak presentation is between 40-50 years.

PRESENTATION. Clinical signs and symptoms vary widely and are often nonspecific. Cognitive and behav-

17-53. *Autopsy case shows gliomatosis cerebri infiltrating the WM ⬌, cortex of both frontal lobes. Compare the effaced GM-WM interfaces ⬌ with the more normal-appearing parietal cortex. (Courtesy R. Hewlett, MD.)*
17-54A. *Axial T1WI in a patient with gliomatosis cerebri shows asymmetry between the normal-appearing right parietal cortex ⬌ and the thickened cortex in the rest of the hemispheres.*

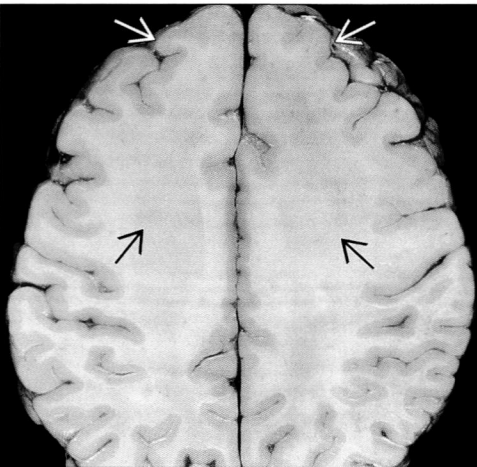
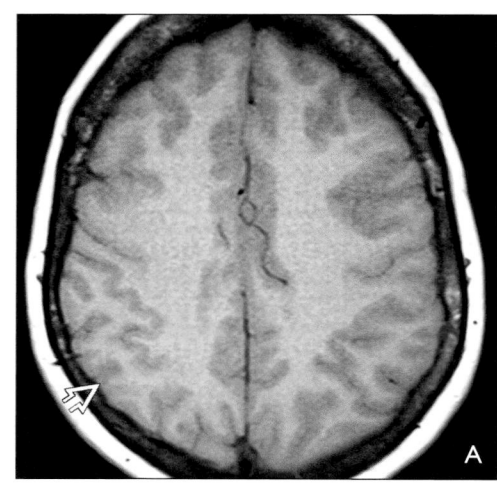

17-54B. *T2WI in the same patient shows hyperintensity in both temporal lobes, thalami, and cortex of both hemispheres ⬌. Only the right parietal cortex ⬌ appears spared.*
17-54C. *Scan through the upper corona radiata shows expanded hyperintense cortex, "hazy" hyperintensity in the underlying WM. Again, only the right parietal lobe ⬌ appears relatively spared. Although abnormal, the basic underlying cerebral architecture is preserved.*

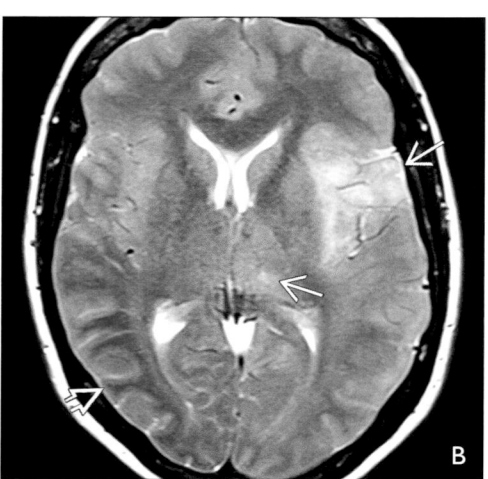
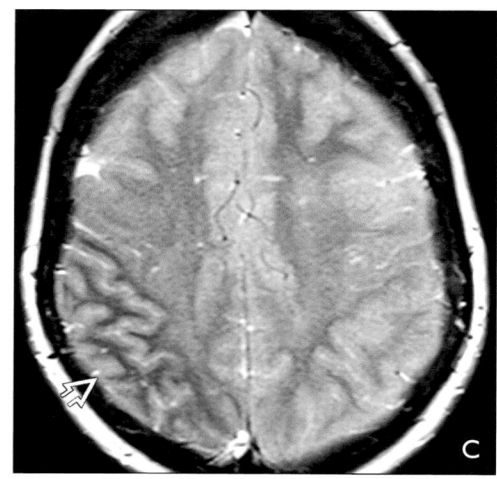

17-54D. *FLAIR scan demonstrates that the diffusely infiltrating mass extends throughout the cortex and corona radiata of both hemispheres. Only the right parietal lobe appears relatively uninvolved ⬌.* **17-54E.** *MRS shows almost normal appearance. Because GC infiltrates between and around normal tissue, spectra are often unrevealing. WHO grade II gliomatosis cerebri was found at biopsy.*

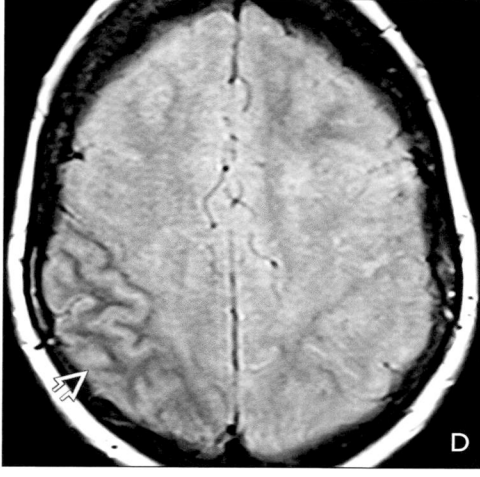
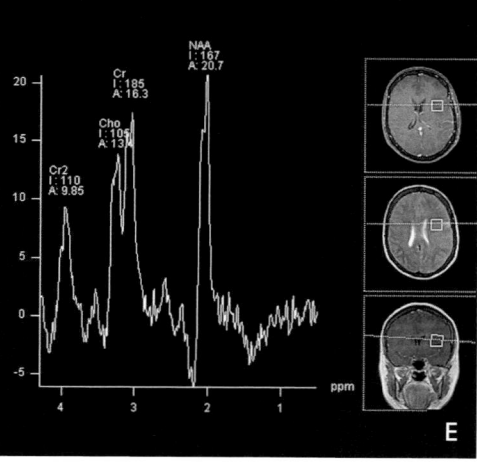

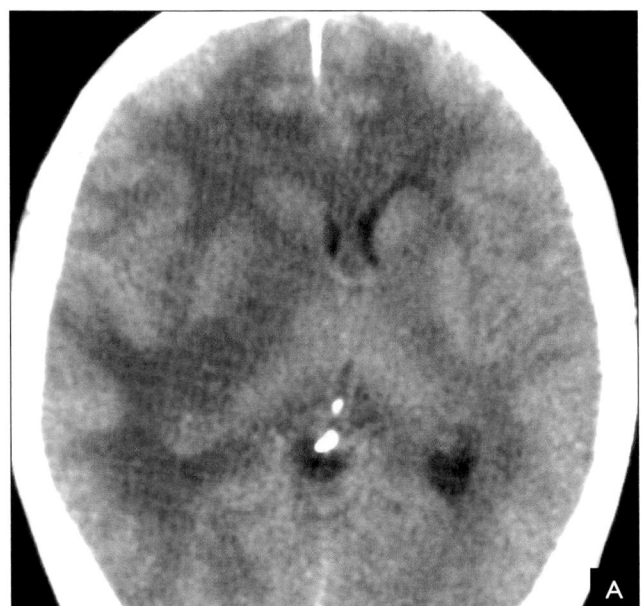

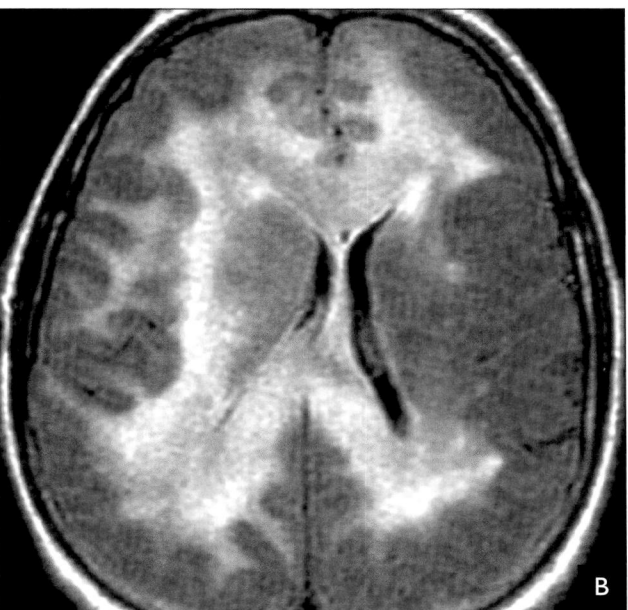

17-55A. CECT in a 45-year-old man with headaches, no focal neurological abnormality. Widespread hypodensity in the WM of both hemispheres with mild mass effect is present.

17-55B. FLAIR in the same patient shows diffuse confluent hyperintensity that thickens the corpus callosum, extends into the subcortical WM. Gliomatosis cerebri found at biopsy. (Courtesy C. Sutton, MD.)

ioral alterations are common. Seizure, focal neurologic deficits, lethargy, and headaches are frequent.

NATURAL HISTORY. GC is a relentlessly progressive neoplasm, and prognosis is poor. Median progression-free survival is 14 months. Overall mortality is 50% at one year and 75% by three years. Relatively favorable prognostic factors include *IDH1* gene mutation and unilateral, nonenhancing disease on MR imaging.

TREATMENT OPTIONS. Because GCs are widespread tumors, surgical resection is not a viable option. Whole brain radiation and standard chemotherapy generally have not changed patient survival. Procarbazine and lomustine therapy may be a promising option for primary therapy of GC.

Imaging

MR is the imaging modality of choice as CT can appear normal or only subtly abnormal.

CT FINDINGS. Little or no mass effect relative to the size of the lesion is typical. Mildly swollen hypodense brain with loss of differentiation between gray and white matter can be seen in some cases. Multifocal or confluent white matter hypodensities may mimic changes of small vessel vascular or acquired metabolic disease **(17-55)**. CECT scans usually show no enhancement.

MR FINDINGS. T1 scans can appear normal or minimally abnormal. The underlying brain architecture is distorted but relatively well preserved **(17-54)**. The hemispheric white matter and gyri may show mildly increased volume

with effaced sulci and poor gray-white matter discrimination. Posterior fossa GCs show diffuse expansion of the brainstem **(17-56), (17-57)**.

T2WI and FLAIR show diffuse hyperintense infiltrating mass effect with small ventricles and effaced sulci. T1 C+ scans usually show no enhancement. Patchy, poorly marginated, mildly enhancing foci typically represent areas of higher grade neoplasm.

DWI is usually normal. In rare cases, areas of high cellularity may show mildly to moderately restricted diffusion **(17-58)**.

MRS may appear almost normal, with mildly elevated choline and decreased NAA. Myoinositol (mI) may be elevated. Lipid-lactate peak is uncommon. As GC infiltrates yet preserves normal white matter architecture, DTI is usually normal.

Perfusion MR is helpful in selecting areas for stereotactic biopsy. Elevated rCBV suggests foci of malignant degeneration **(17-58F)**.

Differential Diagnosis

The difference between widely infiltrating **diffuse low-grade** and **anaplastic astrocytomas** and GC is largely one of disease extent. Once a diffuse astrocytoma spreads across the corpus callosum and involves three brain lobes or both thalami plus basal ganglia, the distinction becomes academic.

In middle-aged and older adults, the most important differential diagnosis is **arteriolosclerosis** (small vessel

17-56. Gliomatosis cerebri can sometimes begin in the posterior fossa and then extend upward through the midbrain into the thalami. In this autopsy specimen, the midbrain is expanded →, and both thalami are infiltrated by tumor. (Courtesy R. Hewlett, MD.) 17-57A. Sagittal T1WI in a 26-year-old neurologically normal woman with headaches. An extensive mass diffusely expands the midbrain, pons, medulla, and upper cervical spinal cord.

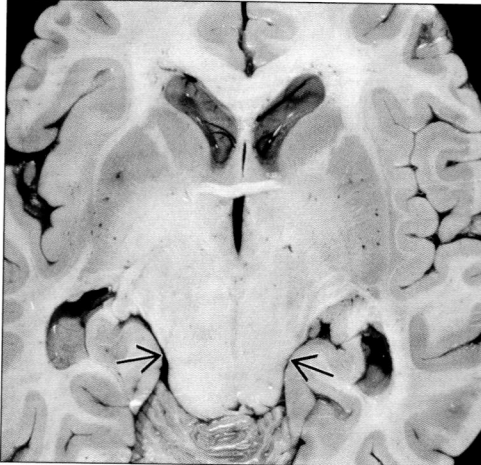
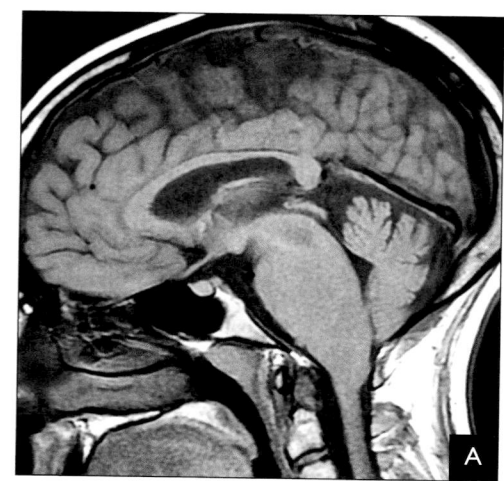

17-57B. Axial T2WI shows that the medulla is grossly enlarged but that its overall signal intensity is only slightly increased. 17-57C. T2WI through the middle of the pons shows striking enlargement without definite signal abnormality.

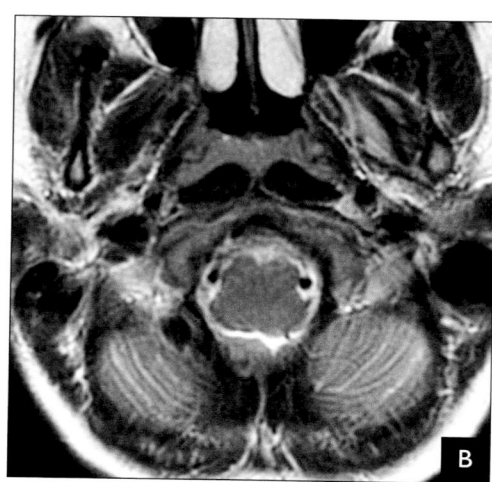
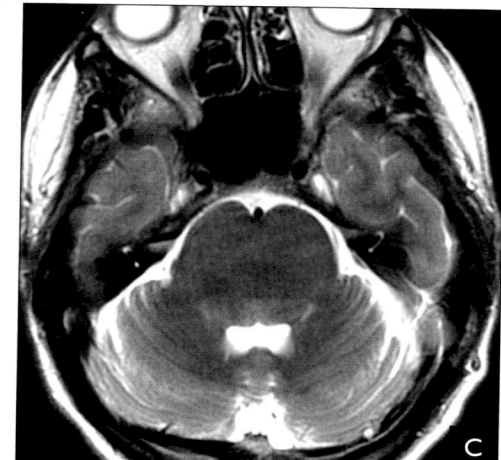

17-57D. More cephalad T2WI shows that the midbrain is almost twice its normal size, yet the aqueduct remains patent and there is no evidence of obstructive hydrocephalus. 17-57E. Coronal T1 C+ scan shows no evidence of enhancement, but slight hypointensity can be seen in the expanded medulla, pons, and midbrain →. Because the tumor involved the midbrain, hindbrain, and spinal cord, this was diagnosed as probable low-grade (WHO II) gliomatosis cerebri. No biopsy was performed.

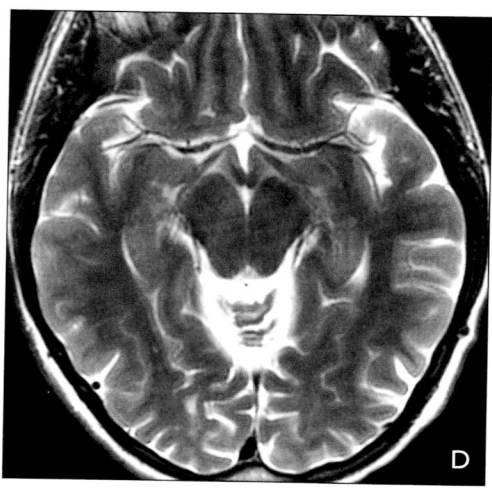
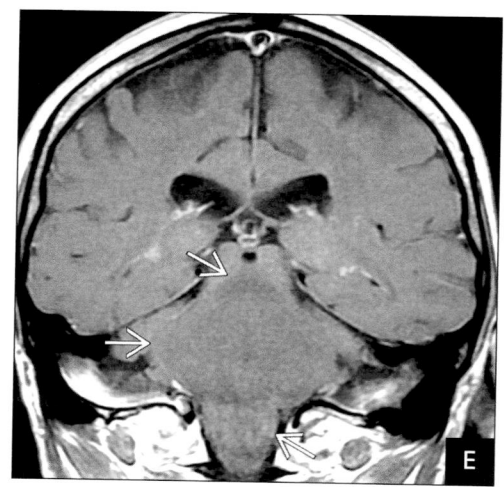

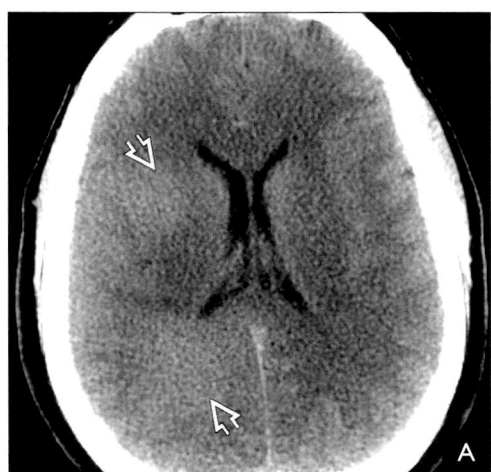

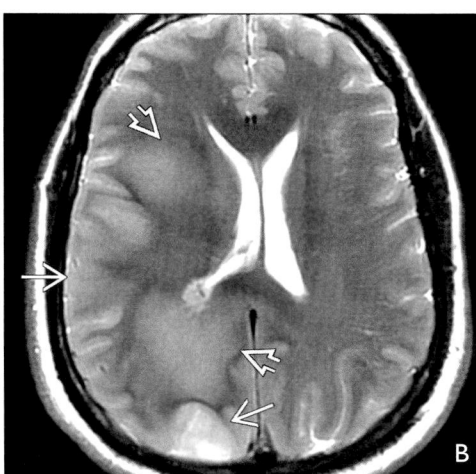

17-58A. *NECT scan in a 46-year-old man with left facial droop, altered mental status shows what appears to be a diffusely swollen brain. However, there are ill-defined hyperdensities* ⇨ *in the right hemisphere WM.* 17-58B. *T2WI shows that the hyperintensities in the right hemispheric WM* ⇨ *also involve the cortex in some areas* ➡, *effacing the gray-white matter interfaces.*

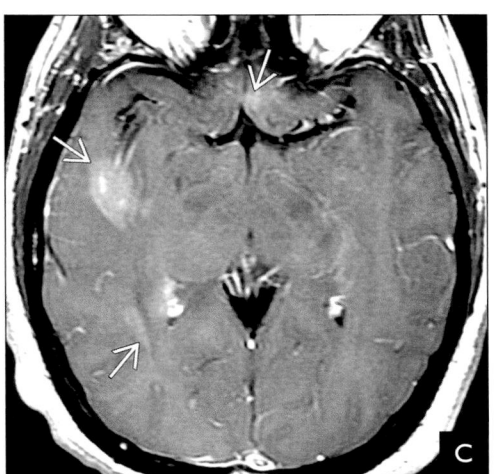

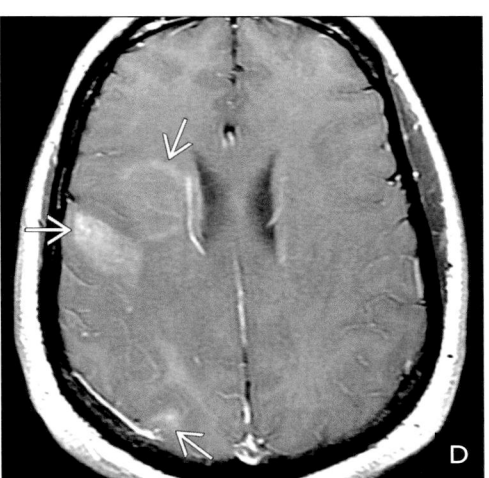

17-58C. *Axial T1 C+ scan shows scattered foci of mild to moderate enhancement* ➡. 17-58D. *More cephalad scan shows additional areas of faint, ill-defined enhancement in the right hemisphere* ➡.

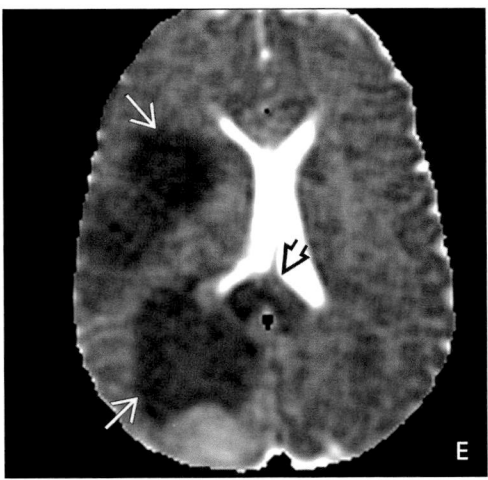

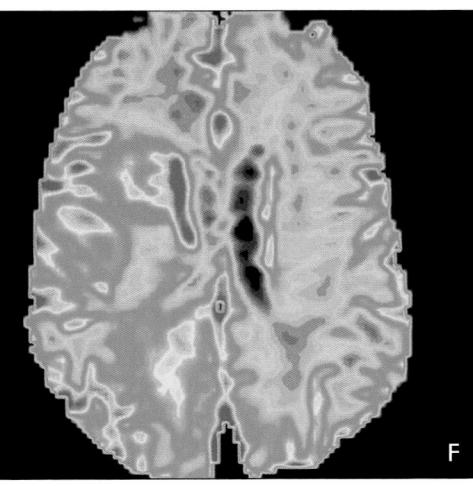

17-58E. *ADC map in the same patient demonstrates restricted diffusion* ➡ *in the hyperintense areas seen on T2WI. Moreover, an area of diffusion restriction* ⇨ *that was not apparent on T2WI is visible crossing the corpus callosum splenium.* 17-58F. *pMR shows elevated rCBV in most of the right hemisphere. Biopsy of the "hottest" areas disclosed foci of WHO grade IV neoplasm within the gliomatosis cerebri. (Courtesy P. Hildenbrand, MD.)*

or microvascular disease with white matter rarefaction). The confluent white matter changes in subcortical arteriosclerotic encephalopathy ("Binswanger disease") may closely resemble GC although infiltrating mass effect is absent.

Demyelinating disease (e.g., MS or ADEM) is typically patchy and asymmetric, showing little or no mass effect. **Progressive multifocal leukoencephalopathy** (PML) may demonstrate bilateral confluent but asymmetric white matter disease that can cross the corpus callosum and mimic GC. PML is generally seen in immunocompromised patients and rarely enhances.

Primary diffuse B-cell **lymphoma**, particularly intravascular (angiocentric) lymphoma, may appear diffusely infiltrating but typically is hypointense on T2WI and shows enhancement following contrast administration.

GC in children is rare and difficult to diagnose as it can resemble viral **encephalitis**. A flu-like prodrome, headache, fever, and mental status change may suggest an inflammatory etiology, but cognitive alterations occur in both diseases.

CT findings of mildly swollen brain with sulcal effacement and compressed ventricles may mimic **idiopathic intracranial hypertension ("pseudotumor cerebri")** in children as well as adults.

GLIOMATOSIS CEREBRI

Terminology
- Also known as diffuse cerebral gliomatosis

Pathology
- Gross pathology
  - Widespread infiltrating mass involving ≥ 3 lobes
  - Expands but doesn't destroy underlying cerebral architecture
  - Hemispheres (75%), bilateral (75%)
  - Often involves basal ganglia, thalami
  - Posterior fossa, spinal cord may be involved
- Microscopic pathology
  - Diffusely infiltrating
  - Generally low cellularity, few mitoses
  - Astrocytoma > oligodendroglioma
  - Majority are WHO grade III

Clinical Issues
- 1% of astrocytomas
- Any age, but peak = 40-50 years

Imaging
- Brain architecture expanded, distorted but preserved
- T2/FLAIR diffuse hyperintensity
- GM-WM interfaces may be effaced
- Any enhancement on T1 C+ suspicious for anaplasia
- DWI, MRS usually normal or near-normal

Differential Diagnosis
- Arteriolosclerosis with WM rarefaction
- Demyelinating disease
- Lymphoma
- Encephalitis

elected References

- Al-Hussaini M et al: Brain stem gliomas: a clinicopathological study from a single cancer center. Brain Tumor Pathol. Epub ahead of print, 2012
- Cage TA et al: High-grade gliomas in children. Neurosurg Clin N Am. 23(3):515-23, 2012
- Marsh JC et al: High-grade glioma relationship to the neural stem cell compartment: a retrospective review of 104 cases. Int J Radiat Oncol Biol Phys. 82(2):e159-65, 2012
- Poretti A et al: Neuroimaging of pediatric posterior fossa tumors including review of the literature. J Magn Reson Imaging. 35(1):32-47, 2012
- Kim TM et al: A developmental taxonomy of glioblastoma defined and maintained by MicroRNAs. Cancer Res. 71(9):3387-99, 2011
- Moser JJ et al: The microRNA and messengerRNA profile of the RNA-induced silencing complex in human primary astrocyte and astrocytoma cells. PLoS One. 5(10):e13445, 2010
- Kleihues P et al: WHO grading of tumours of the central nervous system. In Louis DN et al: WHO Classification of Tumours of the Central Nervous System. Lyon, France: IARC Press. 10-11, 2007

ocalized Astrocytic Tumors

Pilocytic Astrocytoma

- Hsieh MS et al: Cerebellar anaplastic pilocytic astrocytoma in a patient of neurofibromatosis type-1: Case report and review of the literature. Clin Neurol Neurosurg. 114(7):1027-9, 2012
- Kernagis D et al: 164 L1CAM as a marker of an aggressive tumor phenotype in children with juvenile pilocytic astrocytoma. Neurosurgery. 71(2):E565, 2012
- Ogiwara H et al: Long-term follow-up of pediatric benign cerebellar astrocytomas. Neurosurgery. 70(1):40-7; discussion 47-8, 2012
- Tabrizi RD et al: Radiologically typical pilocytic astrocytoma with histopathological signs of atypia. Childs Nerv Syst. 28(10):1791-4, 2012

Pilomyxoid Astrocytoma

- Horger M et al: T2 and DWI in pilocytic and pilomyxoid astrocytoma with pathologic correlation. Can J Neurol Sci. 39(4):491-8, 2012
- Forbes JA et al: Pediatric cerebellar pilomyxoid-spectrum astrocytomas. J Neurosurg Pediatr. 8(1):90-6, 2011
- Linscott LL et al: Pilomyxoid astrocytoma: expanding the imaging spectrum. AJNR Am J Neuroradiol. 29(10):1861-6, 2008

Subependymal Giant Cell Astrocytoma

- Komotar RJ et al: mTOR inhibitors in the treatment of subependymal giantcell astrocytomas associated with tuberous sclerosis. Neurosurgery. 68(4):N24-5, 2011
- Park KJ et al: Gamma knife surgery for subependymal giant cell astrocytomas. Clinical article. J Neurosurg. 114(3):808-13, 2011
- Adriaensen ME et al: Prevalence of subependymal giant cell tumors in patients with tuberous sclerosis and a review of the literature. Eur J Neurol. 16(6):691-6, 2009
- de Ribaupierre S et al: Subependymal giant-cell astrocytomas in pediatric tuberous sclerosis disease: when should we operate? Neurosurgery. 60(1):83-89; discussion 89-90, 2007

Pleomorphic Xanthoastrocytoma

- Bagriacik EU et al: Establishment of a primary pleomorphic xanthoastrocytoma cell line: in vitro responsiveness to some chemotherapeutics. Neurosurgery. 70(1):188-97, 2012
- Yu S et al: Pleomorphic xanthoastrocytoma: MR imaging findings in 19 patients. Acta Radiol. 52(2):223-8, 2011
- Crespo-Rodríguez AM et al: MR and CT imaging of 24 pleomorphic xanthoastrocytomas (PXA) and a review of the literature. Neuroradiology. 49(4):307-15, 2007

Diffusely Infiltrating Astrocytomas

Low-Grade Diffuse Astrocytoma

- Dahlback HS et al: Genomic aberrations in diffuse low-grade gliomas. Genes Chromosomes Cancer. 50(6):409-20, 2011
- Hartmann C et al: Molecular markers in low-grade gliomas: predictive or prognostic? Clin Cancer Res. 17(13):4588-99, 2011

Diffuse Intrinsic Pontine Gliomas

- Jansen MH et al: Diffuse intrinsic pontine gliomas: a systematic update on clinical trials and biology. Cancer Treat Rev. 38(1):27-35, 2012
- Reyes-Botero G et al: Adult brainstem gliomas. Oncologist. 17(3):388-97, 2012
- Khatua S et al: Diffuse intrinsic pontine glioma-current status and future strategies. Childs Nerv Syst. 27(9):1391-7, 2011

Anaplastic Astrocytoma

- Majós C et al: Proton MR spectroscopy provides relevant prognostic information in high-grade astrocytomas. AJNR Am J Neuroradiol. 32(1):74-80, 2011
- Chaichana KL et al: Prognostic significance of contrast-enhancing anaplastic astrocytomas in adults. J Neurosurg. 113(2):286-92, 2010

Glioblastoma Multiforme

- Hu LS et al: Reevaluating the imaging definition of tumor progression: perfusion MRI quantifies recurrent glioblastoma tumor fraction, pseudoprogression, and radiation necrosis to predict survival. Neuro Oncol. 14(7):919-30, 2012

- Jahangiri A et al: Pseudoprogression and treatment effect. Neurosurg Clin N Am. 23(2):277-87, viii-ix, 2012

- Sanghera P et al: The concepts, diagnosis and management of early imaging changes after therapy for glioblastomas. Clin Oncol (R Coll Radiol). 24(3):216-27, 2012

- Topkan E et al: Pseudoprogression in patients with glioblastoma multiforme after concurrent radiotherapy and temozolomide. Am J Clin Oncol. 35(3):284-9, 2012

- Ulmer S et al: Temporal changes in magnetic resonance imaging characteristics of Gliadel wafers and of the adjacent brain parenchyma. Neuro Oncol. 14(4):482-90, 2012

- Chamberlain MC: Radiographic patterns of relapse in glioblastoma. J Neurooncol. 101(2):319-23, 2011

- Kim TM et al: A developmental taxonomy of glioblastoma defined and maintained by MicroRNAs. Cancer Res. 71(9):3387-99, 2011

- Ohgaki H et al: Genetic profile of astrocytic and oligodendroglial gliomas. Brain Tumor Pathol. 28(3):177-83, 2011

Gliosarcoma

- Chikkannaiah P et al: De novo gliosarcoma occurring in the posterior fossa of a 11-year-old girl. Clin Neuropathol. 31(5):389-91, 2012

- Lee D et al: Clinicopathologic and genomic features of gliosarcomas. J Neurooncol. 107(3):643-50, 2012

- Zhang BY et al: Computed tomography and magnetic resonance features of gliosarcoma: a study of 54 cases. J Comput Assist Tomogr. 35(6):667-73, 2011

- Han SJ et al: Clinical characteristics and outcomes for a modern series of primary gliosarcoma patients. Cancer. 116(5):1358-66, 2010

- Han SJ et al: Secondary gliosarcoma after diagnosis of glioblastoma: clinical experience with 30 consecutive patients. J Neurosurg. 112(5):990-6, 2010

Gliomatosis Cerebri

- Rajz GG et al: Presentation patterns and outcome of gliomatosis cerebri. Oncol Lett. 3(1):209-213, 2012

- Zunz E et al: Gliomatosis cerebri presenting as idiopathic intracranial hypertension in a child. J Neuroophthalmol. 31(4):339-41, 2011

- Harrison JF et al: Gliomatosis cerebri: report of 3 cases. J Neurosurg Pediatr. 6(3):291-4, 2010

18

Nonastrocytic Glial Neoplasms

Nonastrocytic gliomas (NAGs) represent a broad spectrum of neoplasms derived from nonastrocytic glial cells or their progenitor neural stem cells. This group of neoplasms is significantly smaller than the astrocytomas but nevertheless comprises an important class of tumors that range from relatively well-circumscribed and biologically indolent neoplasms (e.g., choroid plexus papilloma) to highly malignant tumors such as anaplastic oligodendrogliomas and ependymomas.

As a group, NAGs occur in patients of all ages. Some—such as choroid plexus papilloma—are usually tumors of young children, often under the age of five. In contrast, oligodendrogliomas tend to be tumors of adults. Different ependymoma subtypes affect different ages. Cellular ependymoma is usually a childhood tumor whereas subependymoma is typically a tumor of older adults. Occasionally, a "pediatric" tumor such as ependymoma is found in adults and an "adult" tumor (such as anaplastic oligodendroglioma) is found in a child.

"Pure" gliomas consist of a single tumor type, but gliomas also can occur with mixed histologies of different cell lineages. Oligoastrocytoma is a classic example and the most common of the "mixed" gliomas.

The paramount importance of correct, specific glioma diagnosis relates to treatment decisions and prognosis. Gliomas within a single histological entity can be divided into subsets that show different clinical behaviors. For example, oligodendrogliomas that exhibit 1p,19q codeletions are particularly sensitive to chemotherapy. Even anaplastic oligodendrogliomas that harbor these deletions are often successfully treated without radiotherapy.

We first discuss oligodendroglial tumors and include "mixed" gliomas in this section, as they often contain oligodendroglial-like elements.

We follow with a discussion of ependymomas and their subtypes. Tumors of the choroid plexus, which itself is derived from modified ependymal cells, constitute the third group of neoplasms included in this chapter. Lastly, we briefly consider a miscellaneous group of uncommon nonastrocytic glial tumors, called "other neuroepithelial tumors" in the current WHO classification. To date, this group includes astroblastoma, chordoid glioma (of the third ventricle), and the recently described but still controversial angiocentric glioma.

Oligodendrogliomas and "Mixed" Gliomas

Oligodendrocytes are found predominantly in the white matter. Their primary function is the production and maintenance of myelin.

Tumors derived from oligodendrocytes—known as oligodendrogliomas—are the third most common type of glial neoplasm (after anaplastic astrocytoma and glioblastoma multiforme). Oligodendroglioma was originally defined in 1929 as a glioma subtype with cells that morphologically resembled normal oligodendro-

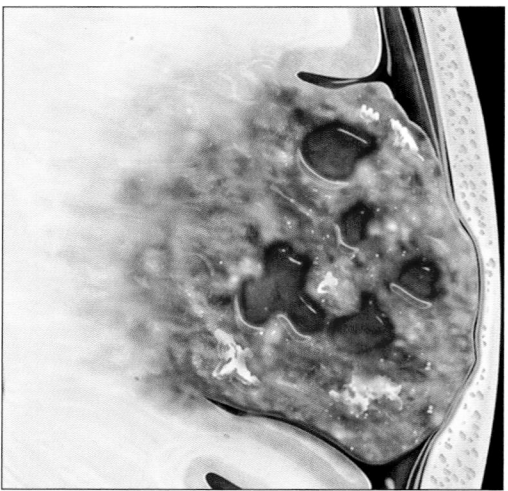

18-1. Oligodendrogliomas are poorly demarcated, "fleshy" masses that infiltrate cortex, subcortical WM. Remodeling of adjacent bone is common.

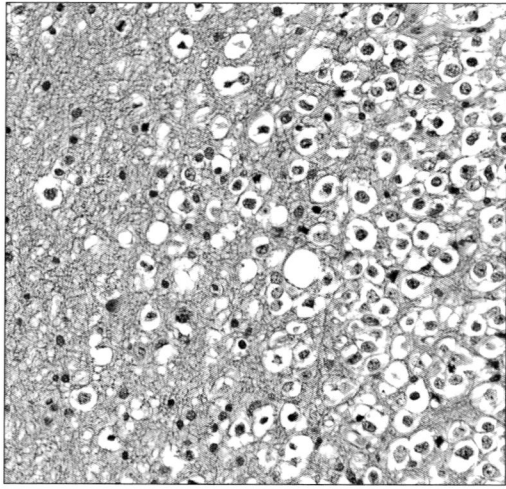

18-2. Oligodendroglioma cells have round uniform nuclei, perinuclear "halos" ("fried egg" appearance). (Courtesy P. Burger, MD.)

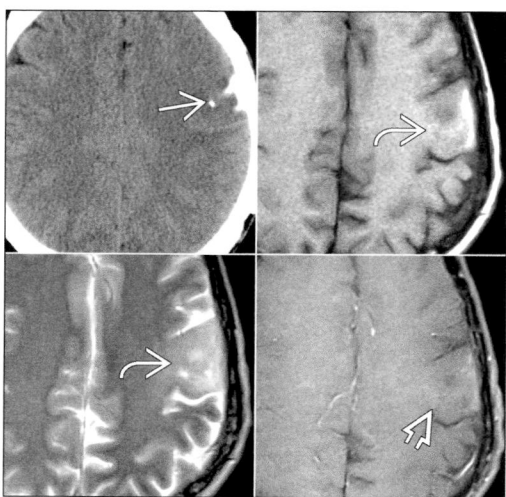

18-3. Hypodense cortical/subcortical mass with Ca++ ➡, heterogeneous signal ➡, and minimal enhancement ➡ on MR. Oligodendroglioma.

cytes. Oligodendrogliomas that are mixed with astrocytic-appearing elements are called oligoastrocytomas.

The common feature of both oligodendrogliomas and oligoastrocytomas is the predominance of cells that resemble normal oligodendrocytes. Histologically, oligodendroglial tumors range from well-differentiated to frankly malignant neoplasms. Oligodendrogliomas are currently classified into just two tiers: A well-differentiated tumor (oligodendroglioma) and a malignant variant (anaplastic oligodendroglioma). Both—along with oligoastrocytoma—are discussed in this section.

Oligodendroglioma

Terminology

Oligodendrogliomas (OGs) are well-differentiated, slow-growing but diffusely infiltrating hemispheric tumors that most likely arise from oligodendrocytes or immature glial stem cells.

Etiology

GENERAL CONCEPTS. Definitive proof that OGs actually arise from oligodendroglial cells is lacking. The putative origin of OGs is based on their morphologic similarities to normal oligodendrocytes.

GENETICS. In addition to their histologic features, OGs have specific genetic alterations that distinguish them from astrocytomas as well as from other gliomas. Allelic losses of chromosomes 1p and 19q are a distinct molecular "signature" of OGs and occur in 50-70% of both low-grade and anaplastic OGs.

IDH1 mutation is seen in 80% of cases. Concurrent cancer initiating cell mutations, *IDH* mutations, and 1p,19q loss are highly specific for OGs. *MGMT* gene promotor methylation is common in pediatric and young adult OGs whereas *IDH1* mutations are absent in most pediatric cases.

Pathology

LOCATION. Most OGs arise at the gray-white matter junction. The vast majority (85-90%) are supratentorial. The most common site is the frontal lobe (50-65%) followed by the parietal, temporal, and occipital lobes. Posterior fossa and spinal cord OGs are uncommon.

GROSS PATHOLOGY. Oligodendrogliomas are typically solid, soft, "fleshy," tan-to-pink masses. They tend to infiltrate the cortex and expand one or more gyri (18-1), (18-4). Extension through the glia limitans to the pial surface is common.

Most OGs are poorly circumscribed and blend gradually into adjacent structures. Cyst formation and necrosis are

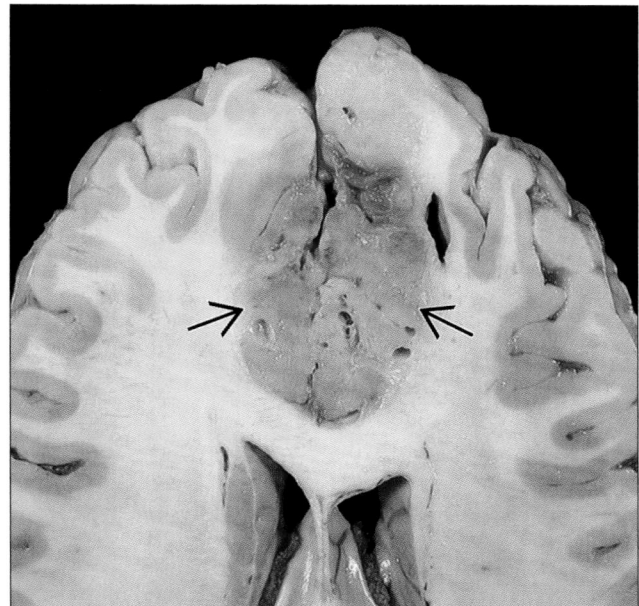

18-4. Autopsy specimen of oligodendroglioma shows typical cortical/subcortical "fleshy" mass ➡. (Courtesy R. Hewlett, MD.)

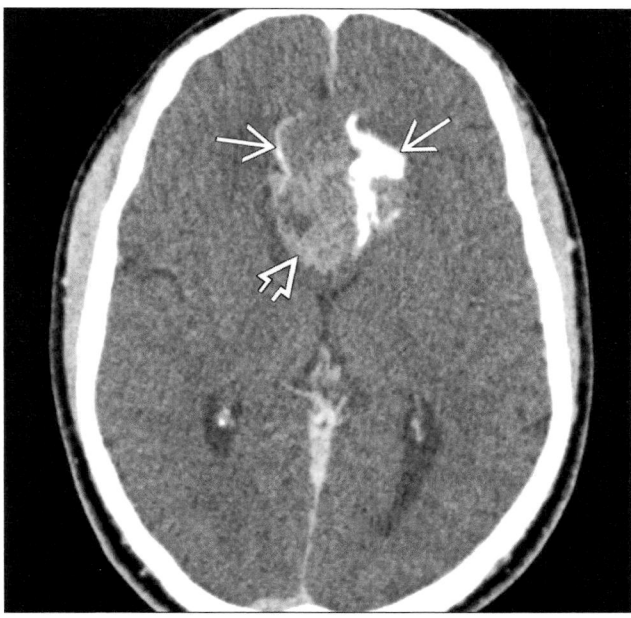

18-5. CECT scan shows calcification ➡, enhancement ➡ in this WHO grade II oligodendroglioma.

uncommon. Hemorrhage is rare in low-grade oligodendrogliomas.

MICROSCOPIC FEATURES. OGs vary in cellularity. Some are relatively paucicellular whereas others demonstrate "back to back" sheets of closely apposed cells. Uniform round or slightly oval hyperchromatic nuclei surrounded by a prominent perinuclear "halo" of clear watery cytoplasm give OGs a classic "fried egg" appearance **(18-2)**. Delicate angulated capillaries ("chicken wire" vascularity) are often present.

Immunohistochemistry is positive for Olig2 staining. GFAP is variable.

Cytogenetic and molecular data are key elements in OG evaluation. FISH analysis is essential to determine the presence or absence of 1p,19q codeletions, which in turn affects subsequent treatment planning.

STAGING, GRADING, AND CLASSIFICATION. Oligodendrogliomas are WHO grade II neoplasms.

linical Issues

EPIDEMIOLOGY. Oligodendrogliomas account for 2-5% of all primary CNS neoplasms and 5-20% of gliomas. Approximately half of oligodendroglial tumors are WHO grade II neoplasms. The remainder are anaplastic or histologically mixed tumors (see below).

OGs are primarily tumors of adults, with only 1-5% occurring in children. Most OGs arise between the ages of 35 and 55 with a peak between 40 and 45 years. There is a moderate male predominance.

PRESENTATION. Because OGs commonly involve the cortical gray matter, seizures are the most common presenting symptom. Headache is the second most common presentation.

NATURAL HISTORY. Oligodendrogliomas are slow-growing neoplasms. The five-year survival rate is 50-75%, and median survival time is 10 years. OGs are relatively indolent tumors but eventually fatal in most cases.

Local recurrence following resection is very common. Diffuse CSF dissemination is rare. Malignant degeneration to anaplastic oligodendroglioma or glioblastoma occurs in some patients.

TREATMENT OPTIONS. Gross total surgical resection is the primary treatment and independently improves outcome no matter the histological grade or genetic status. However, identifying the presence of 1p,19q deletion in the resected tumor is essential for treatment planning; OGs with these allelic deletions are chemosensitive and have a more favorable prognosis.

Imaging

GENERAL FEATURES. Oligodendrogliomas are seen as round or oval, relatively sharply delineated masses that involve the cortex and subcortical white matter.

CT FINDINGS. OGs are slow-growing tumors that are often peripheral and cortically based. Focal gyral expansion with thinning and remodeling of the overlying calvaria is common.

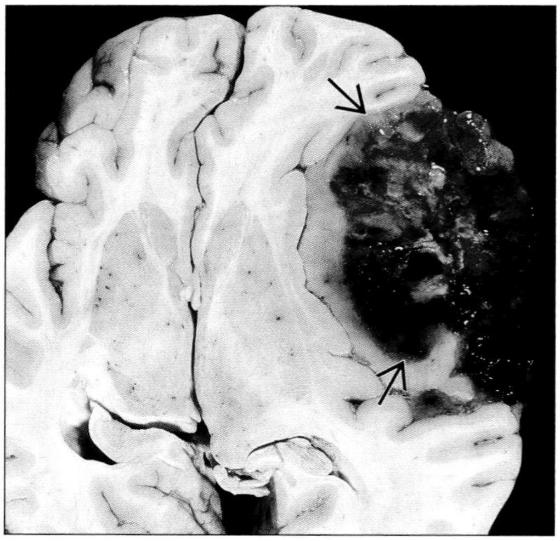

18-6. Occasionally, WHO grade II oligodendrogliomas exhibit hemorrhage, necrosis ➔. *(Courtesy R. Hewlett, MD.)*

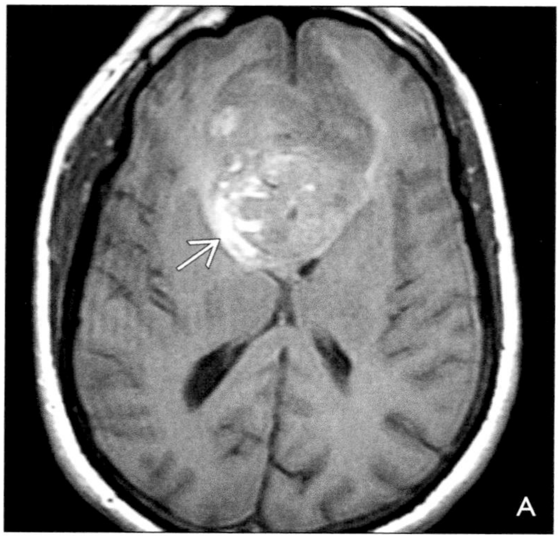

18-7A. T1WI shows an aggressive-appearing bifrontal neoplasm with heterogeneous signal intensity due to subacute hemorrhage ➔.

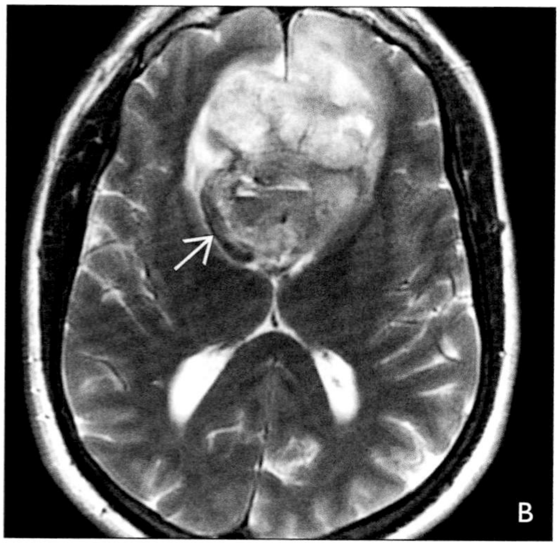

18-7B. T2WI shows subacute hemorrhage ➔, *heterogeneous signal. Preoperative diagnosis was GBM. Surgery disclosed oligodendroglioma.*

Almost two-thirds of OGs are hypodense on NECT scan. Mixed hypo- and isodense tumors are common. Coarse nodular or clumped calcification is seen in 70-90% of cases **(18-3)**. Cystic degeneration occurs in 20%. Gross hemorrhage and peritumoral edema are less common and, by themselves, do not indicate malignant degeneration **(18-6)**.

Enhancement varies from none to moderate; approximately 50% of OGs demonstrate some degree of enhancement **(18-5)**. A patchy multifocal pattern is typical.

MR Findings. OGs often appear relatively well-delineated and are usually hypointense relative to gray matter on T1WI. They are typically heterogeneously hyperintense on T2/FLAIR **(18-3)**, **(18-7)**. Vasogenic edema is uncommon. Calcification is seen as "blooming" foci on T2* sequences.

Moderate heterogeneous enhancement is seen in approximately half of all cases. There is no relationship between the presence or volume of enhancement and the presence or absence of 1p,19q deletion.

OGs do not restrict on DWI. Moderately elevated Cho and decreased NAA without a lactate peak is typical on MRS.

Perfusion MR imaging is often used to predict the WHO grade of brain neoplasms. Low-grade oligodendrogliomas are more highly vascular and metabolically active than astrocytomas of comparable grade. OGs may display high rCBV foci that reflect the prominent "chicken wire" vascularity so characteristic of low-grade 1p,19q-codeleted oligodendrogliomas. An elevated rCBV in an OG thus does not necessarily indicate high-grade histopathology.

Differential Diagnosis

The major differential diagnosis of OG is **low-grade diffuse astrocytoma**. Diffusely infiltrating fibrillary astrocytomas more commonly involve the white matter—not the cortex—and do not enhance. Differentiation of a WHO grade II OG from a mixed **oligoastrocytoma** or **anaplastic oligodendroglioma** (AO) may be difficult on the basis of imaging alone. Hemorrhage and necrosis are more common in AO than OG.

Other cortically based, slow-growing tumors that typically present with seizures include **ganglioglioma** and **dysembryoplastic neuroepithelial tumor (DNET)**. Both are more common in children and young adults. Gangliogliomas are more common in the temporal lobe with a "cyst + nodule" appearance. DNETs are typically "bubbly" and may have associated cortical dysplasia.

Central neurocytoma is indistinguishable from OG on light microscopy and requires immunohistochemical stains (e.g., synaptophysin) for diagnosis. Prior to the identification of central neurocytoma as a distinct entity, these neoplasms were usually called "intraventricular oligodendroglioma."

Extraventricular neurocytoma is a very rare, cortically based variant that does not necessarily exhibit the "bubbly" pattern so typical of its intraventricular counterpart; it may be indistinguishable from an OG on imaging.

OLIGODENDROGLIOMA

Pathology
- General features
  - Arise at gray-white matter junction
  - Hemispheric (85-90%)
  - Frontal lobe (50-65%)
  - Diffusely infiltrate cortex
  - Poorly circumscribed
- Microscopic features
  - "Fried egg" cells
  - WHO grade II

Clinical Issues
- Epidemiology
  - Third most common primary brain tumor (2-5%)
  - Most common in middle-aged adults
  - Rare in children
- Presentation
  - Seizures
- Treatment, prognosis
  - Chemosensitive if 1p,19q codeletion

Imaging
- Round/ovoid cortical mass
- Relatively well-delineated
- Ca++ (70-90%)
- Hemorrhage, peritumoral edema uncommon
- 50% enhance

Anaplastic Oligodendroglioma

Terminology

Anaplastic oligodendroglioma (AO) is the malignant counterpart of oligodendroglioma in the two-tiered WHO classification of oligodendroglial neoplasms.

Etiology

AOs can develop de novo or arise from progression of a preexisting WHO grade II oligodendroglioma. 1p,19q codeletions are present in 30-40% of cases. Between 20-25% exhibit *EGFR* gene amplification.

Pathology

LOCATION. AOs demonstrate the same preference for the frontal lobe as do OGs. The temporal lobe is the second most common site.

GROSS PATHOLOGY. Other than the presence of necrotic foci **(18-8)**, the macroscopic features of AO are similar to those of grade II oligodendrogliomas.

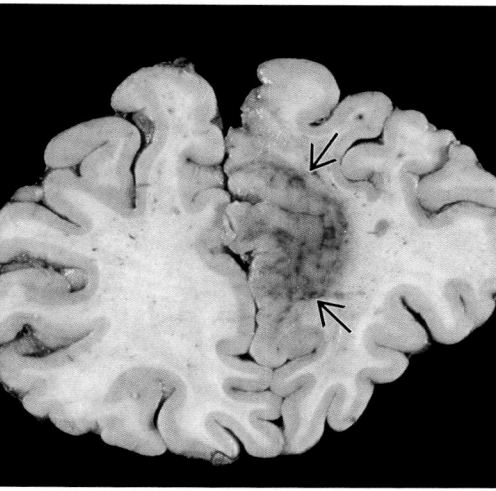

18-8. Autopsy of diffusely infiltrating anaplastic oligodendroglioma shows necrosis, hemorrhage ➡. (Courtesy R. Hewlett, MD.)

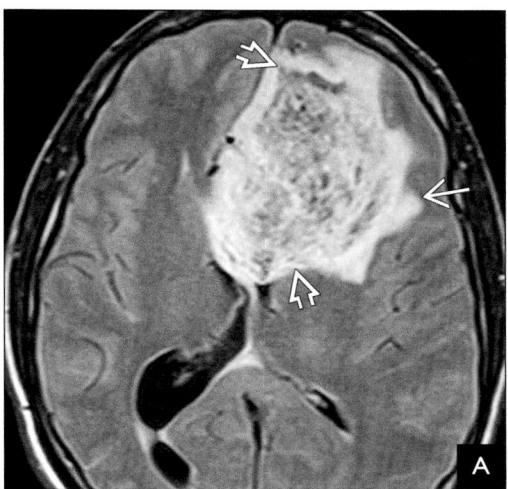

18-9A. FLAIR scan in a patient with anaplastic oligodendroglioma shows very heterogeneous signal intensity ➡, peritumoral edema ➡.

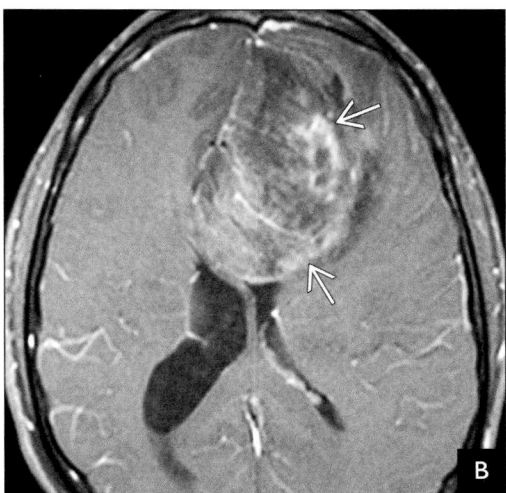

18-9B. T1 C+ FS shows linear and patchy enhancement ➡. Anaplastic oligodendroglioma (WHO grade III) was found at histopathology.

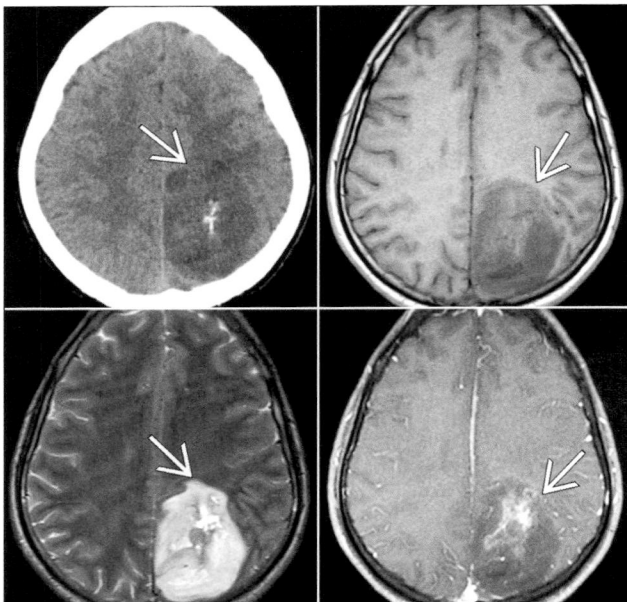

18-10. NECT, series of MR images in a 37-year-old man with new-onset seizures shows relatively well-demarcated left parietal mass ➡. Histologically proven WHO grade II oligodendroglioma.

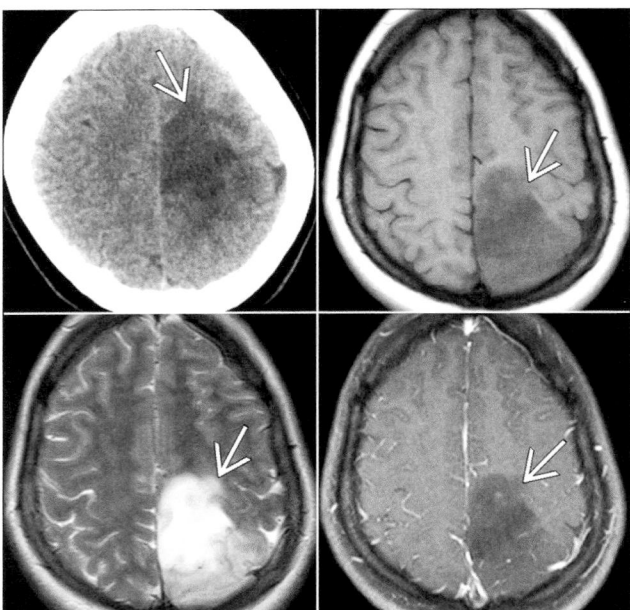

18-11. A 24-year-old woman presented to the emergency department with seizures. NECT, series of MR images show left parietal mass ➡, which looks like the oligodendroglioma in Figure 18-10. Anaplastic oligodendroglioma (WHO grade III).

MICROSCOPIC FEATURES. Focal or diffuse features of malignancy are present. AOs have higher cell density with more nuclear pleomorphism and hyperchromatism than OGs. Cystic degeneration and necrosis with or without pseudopalisading are common. Microvascular hypertrophy and proliferation are common.

Higher mitotic activity characterizes AOs. MIB-1 proliferation indices are elevated. Although there is no accepted cut-off value for distinguishing AO from OG, labeling indices in the 7-10% or higher range are typical.

STAGING, GRADING, AND CLASSIFICATION. AOs are WHO grade III tumors.

Clinical Issues

EPIDEMIOLOGY. Between 25-35% of all oligodendroglial tumors are anaplastic. AOs account for 1-2% of all primary brain tumors.

PRESENTATION. Patients with AOs are approximately seven or eight years older than patients with OGs. Mean age at presentation is 45-50 years. Clinical symptoms are indistinguishable from those of OG, with seizure and headache the most common presentations.

NATURAL HISTORY. Survival time varies from a few months to a few years. Mean survival is four years with an overall five-year survival rate of 20-40%. Patients with 1p,19q codeletions and chemosensitive tumors have a better prognosis.

TREATMENT OPTIONS. To date, there are no standard treatments for AOs. Maximal cytoreduction improves survival, so gross total resection remains the treatment mainstay. Chemotherapy with procarbazine, lomustine, and vincristine (PCV regimen) or temozolomide (TMZ) may be effective in AOs that show 1p,19q codeletion. Radiation therapy is an option for patients with residual or recurrent tumor.

Imaging

The general imaging features of AO are very similar to those of OG and do not reliably predict tumor grade (18-10), (18-11). Peritumoral edema, hemorrhage, and foci of cystic degeneration are more common. Enhancement is variable, ranging from none to striking (18-9).

As OGs are often quite vascular, rCBV may be misleading. MRS is more helpful, with a Cho:Cr ratio greater than 2.33 suggestive of anaplastic oligodendroglioma.

Differential Diagnosis

The major differential diagnosis of AO is **oligodendroglioma**. Tumor contrast enhancement is not helpful in distinguishing AO from low-grade oligodendroglioma. Histologic confirmation is necessary even in tumors without contrast enhancement.

Oligoastrocytoma and **anaplastic astrocytoma** or even **glioblastoma** may also be difficult to differentiate from AO on the basis of imaging findings alone.

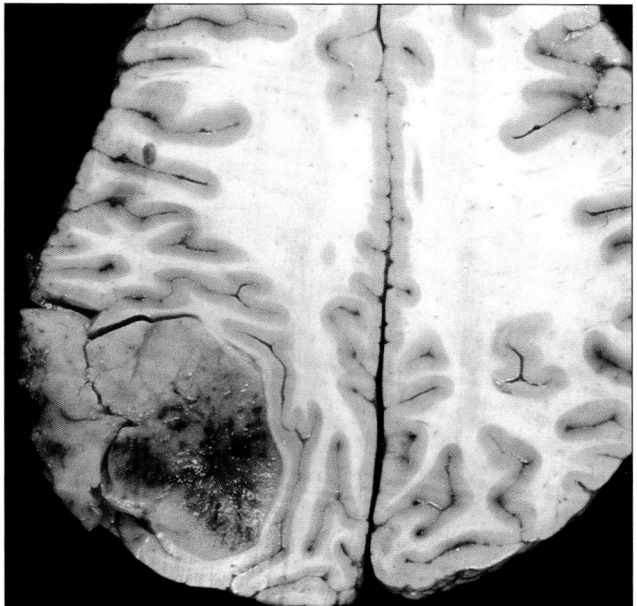

18-12. *Autopsy case of mixed oligoastrocytoma shows a seemingly well-demarcated parietal mass with hemorrhage, necrosis. (Courtesy R. Hewlett, MD.)*

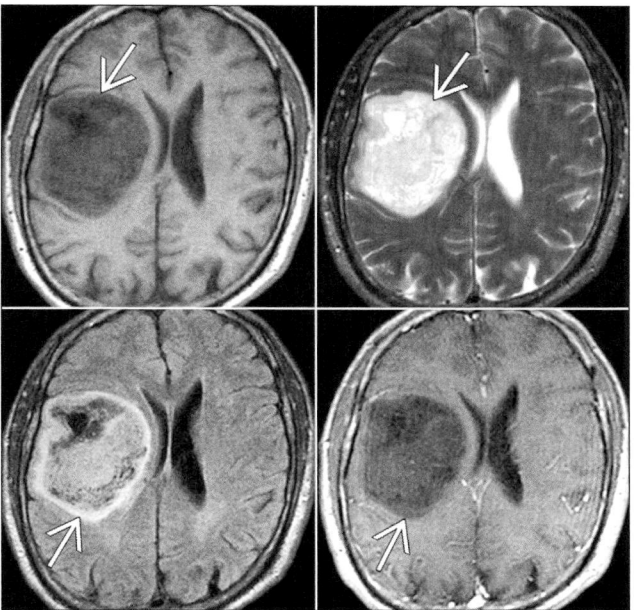

18-13. *Series of images in a patient with documented OA. The tumor* ➡ *looks relatively well-delineated, does not enhance, and is indistinguishable from oligodendroglioma or anaplastic oligodendroglioma on imaging.*

ligoastrocytomas

Oligoastrocytoma (OA) has a conspicuous admixture of two distinct neoplastic cell types. Tumor cells resembling those seen in oligodendroglioma and fibrillary astrocytoma are both present with varying degrees of anaplasia.

tiology

GENERAL CONCEPTS. Glial precursor cells, multipotential progenitor cells that are able to undergo both astrocytic and oligodendroglial differentiation, are the putative origin of OAs.

GENETICS. Between 30-50% of OAs demonstrate the 1p,19q codeletions that confer chemosensitivity and a relatively better prognosis.

athology

LOCATION. OA location is similar to that of oligodendroglioma. The frontal lobe is the most common site, accounting for 55-60% of all OAs. The temporal lobe is the second most common location.

GROSS PATHOLOGY. OAs have no gross features that distinguish them from other diffusely infiltrating glial neoplasms **(18-12)**.

MICROSCOPIC FEATURES. Neoplastic glial cells with both astrocytic and oligodendroglial phenotypes must be present for the histologic diagnosis of OA. Significant phenotypic heterogeneity is typical.

STAGING, GRADING, AND CLASSIFICATION. A two-tiered grading system is used, classifying OAs as either low-grade or anaplastic.

Low-grade OAs are moderately cellular neoplasms with no or low mitotic activity and are considered WHO grade II neoplasms; anaplastic oligodendrogliomas display classic features of malignancy and are designated WHO grade III.

If necrosis is present in a "mixed" tumor that contains both astrocytic and oligodendroglial elements, the current WHO classification suggests that the histologic diagnosis should be glioblastoma (with some oligodendroglial features), not OA.

Clinical Issues

EPIDEMIOLOGY. OA is the most common histologically mixed glioma, representing 5-10% of all gliomas.

DEMOGRAPHICS. OAs are typically tumors of young adults with mean age at diagnosis between 35-45 years.

PRESENTATION. Seizure is the most common presenting symptom, followed by focal neurologic deficit.

NATURAL HISTORY. The most malignant OA component—generally the astrocytoma—determines overall prognosis. The median survival time of 6.3 years for low-grade OA is in between that of pure low-grade and anaplastic oligodendrogliomas. Favorable prognostic factors include younger age, gross total tumor resection, and the presence of 1p,19q codeletions. The median survival time for anaplastic OA is 2.8 years.

TREATMENT OPTIONS. OAs respond less favorably to chemotherapy than pure oligodendroglial tumors, probably because the astrocytic component is generally chemoresistant. Nevertheless, the prognosis for patients with anaplastic OA is still better than for patients with glioblastoma multiforme.

Imaging

GENERAL FEATURES. Distinguishing pure oligodendroglial tumors from histologically mixed gliomas is not possible on imaging findings alone (18-13). In general, the imaging features of mixed oligoastrocytomas mirror the two grades of oligodendrogliomas. Low-grade OAs look very similar to WHO grade II oligodendrogliomas, and anaplastic OAs resemble WHO grade III AOs.

CT FINDINGS. OAs are heterogeneously hypodense on NECT and show variable enhancement on CECT.

MR FINDINGS. OAs are hypointense compared to cortical gray matter on T1WI. Heterogeneous hyperintensity is characteristic on T2WI and FLAIR.

Differential Diagnosis

The differential diagnosis of OA includes both **oligodendroglioma** and **diffusely infiltrating astrocytoma**.

Ependymal Tumors

Ependymal tumors arise from the ependymal lining of the cerebral ventricles or central canal of the spinal cord. Cancer progenitor/stem cells have also been posited as possible sources.

The WHO classifies tumors that exhibit ependymal differentiation as four distinct tumor types, in ascending order of malignancy: Subependymoma, myxopapil-

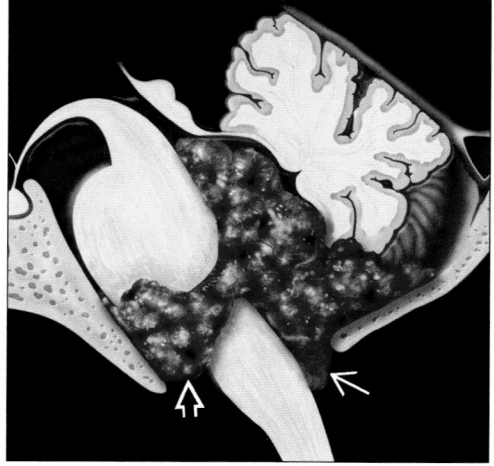
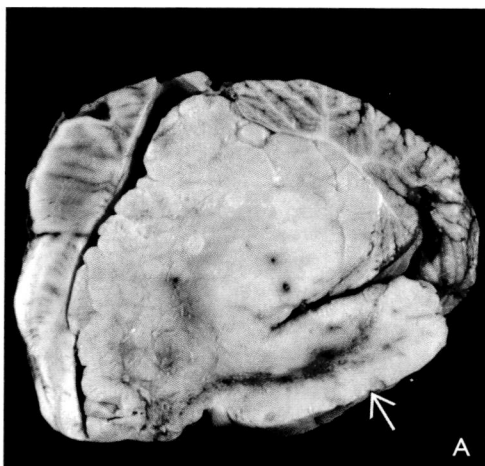

18-14. Graphic depicts "classic" cellular ependymoma of the fourth ventricle extending through the foramen of Magendie into the cisterna magna ➡, around the pons under the brachium pontis, and through the lateral recesses into the cerebellopontine angle cisterns ➡. 18-15A. Sagittal autopsy case shows ependymoma filling the fourth ventricle, elevating the vermis, extending posteroinferiorly to fill the cisterna magna ➡.

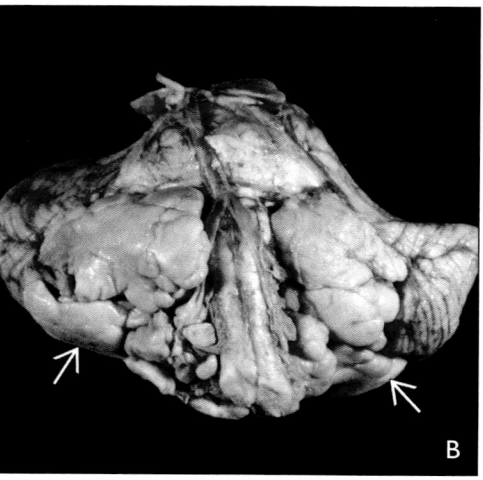
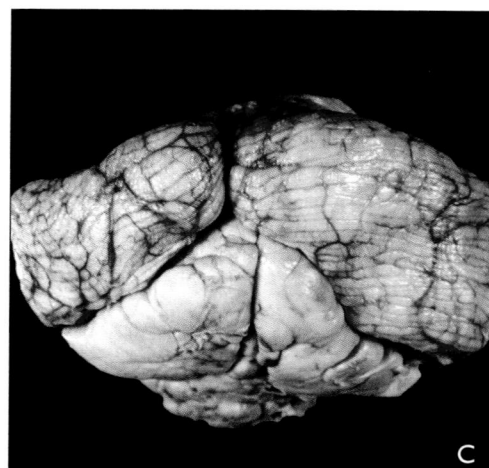

18-15B. Coronal view in the same case shows massive tumor extension through both foramina of Luschka into the cerebellopontine angle cisterns ➡. 18-15C. Posterior view shows tumor bulging through the foramen of Magendie, completely filling the cisterna magna. Posterior fossa ependymomas squeeze out the foramina of the fourth ventricle, oozing like toothpaste into the surrounding CSF spaces. (Courtesy E. Ross, MD.)

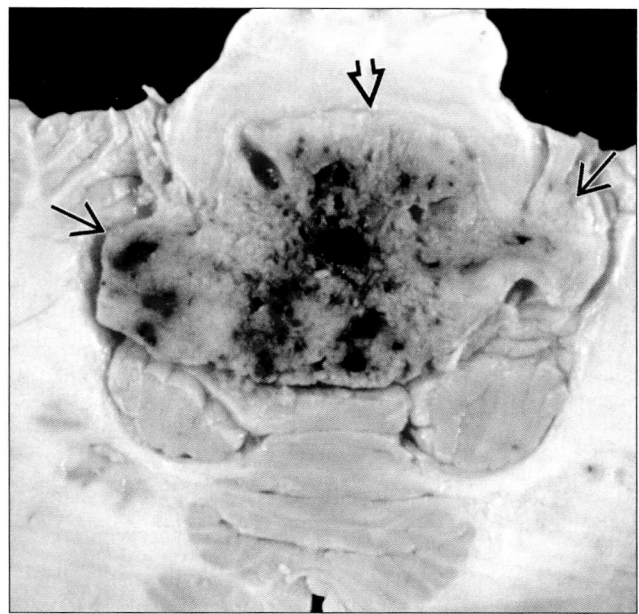

18-16. Axial section shows ependymoma filling the fourth ventricle ⊡, extending anterolaterally through the lateral recesses toward the foramina of Luschka ⊡.

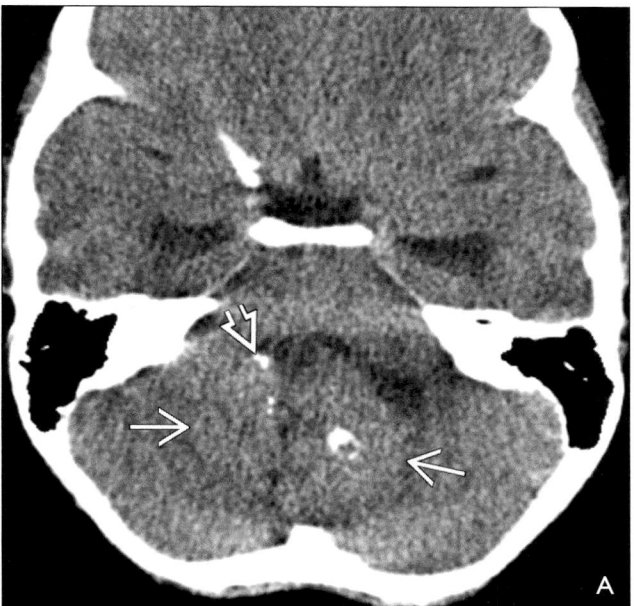

18-17A. NECT in a 3-year-old boy with ependymoma shows a mixed-density ➡, calcified ⊡ midline mass filling the fourth ventricle.

lary ependymoma, ependymoma, and anaplastic ependymoma.

Three WHO grades within the ependymoma tumor spectrum are recognized. Subependymoma and myxopapillary ependymoma are both WHO grade I neoplasms. Ependymoma is considered a grade II neoplasm, and anaplastic ependymoma is designated as a grade III tumor.

We discuss all these tumors in this section, starting with the most common subtype, **ependymoma**. We follow with a consideration of **anaplastic ependymoma** (AE). While AE is relatively uncommon, its imaging appearance is very similar to that of "classic" ependymoma. The last ependymoma subtype that occurs in the brain is **subependymoma**, which appears very different from ependymoma and anaplastic ependymoma.

Although it is almost exclusively an intraspinal tumor, we also briefly consider **myxopapillary ependymoma**. Ependymoblastoma, a WHO grade IV tumor, is classified as an embryonal neoplasm along with other primitive neuroectodermal tumors and is discussed in Chapter 21.

ʹpendymoma

ʹiology

GENETICS. The molecular alterations that lead to ependymoma oncogenesis have not been completely elucidated. Recent evidence suggests that ependymomas have localization as well as grade-specific expression

signatures, possibly related to different stem cell radial glia in all three craniospinal compartments. Mutant stem cells may not transform until they differentiate into more restricted progenitor cell types.

Each cell of origin is uniquely susceptible to some—but not other—genetic mutations. Various Notch and BMP receptor as well as hedgehog pathway alterations have been implicated in intracranial ependymoma tumorigenesis. Monosomy of chromosome 22 and homeobox-containing (*HOX*) mutations occur mostly with extracranial (spinal) ependymomas.

Pathology

LOCATION. Approximately 60-70% of ependymomas are *infratentorial*. Of these, 95% are found in the fourth ventricle. The remainder occur as cerebellopontine angle lesions.

Between 30-40% of ependymomas are *supratentorial*. The vast majority, between 80-85%, are hemispheric parenchymal neoplasms. Intraventricular location is rare.

SIZE AND NUMBER. Ependymomas are solitary neoplasms. Size varies, but most supratentorial ependymomas are large bulky neoplasms that exceed four centimeters in diameter at presentation.

GROSS PATHOLOGY. Posterior fossa ependymomas are reddish-tan or gray in color and form relatively well-demarcated, lobulated masses that extrude through the lateral recesses of the fourth ventricle **(18-14)**, **(18-15)**, **(18-16)**.

MICROSCOPIC FEATURES. Neuropathologists recognize four major histologic subtypes of ependymoma. From most to least common, they are cellular, clear cell, papillary, and tanycytic ependymoma. Rare variants include giant cell, lipidized, and melanotic ependymomas. In a few cases, malignant mesenchymal metaplasia occurs ("ependymosarcoma").

The most characteristic microarchitectural feature of ependymoma is the presence of perivascular pseudorosettes, in which tumor cells are arranged radially around blood vessels.

Typical ependymoma vasculature is relatively mature and shows little angiogenic activity compared to malignant gliomas or the anaplastic variant of ependymoma.

STAGING, GRADING, AND CLASSIFICATION. Ependymomas are WHO grade II neoplasms.

Clinical Issues

EPIDEMIOLOGY. Ependymomas represent 3-9% of all neuroepithelial tumors. Ependymoma accounts for approximately 10% of CNS neoplasms in children and 30% of all brain tumors in children under the age of three years. Ependymoma is the third most common posterior fossa tumor of childhood (after medulloblastoma and astrocytoma).

DEMOGRAPHICS. Ependymomas have a bimodal distribution. Although they are found in all age groups, most occur in children between one and five years of age. Mean age at presentation is between four and six years. A second, much smaller peak is seen in young adults between 20 and 30 years of age. Surveillance studies have shown a significant increase in the prevalence of adult ependymomas over the past three decades.

There is a moderate male predominance (57% of all ependymomas).

PRESENTATION. Symptoms are location-dependent. Fourth ventricle ependymomas commonly cause intraventricular obstructive hydrocephalus and present with headache, vomiting, and papilledema. Ataxia is common. Supratentorial parenchymal ependymomas present with seizures and focal neurologic deficits.

18-17B. FLAIR scan in the same patient shown on the previous page. The mixed signal intensity mass ➡ in the inferior fourth ventricle extends anterolaterally through both foramina of Luschka into the cerebellopontine angle cisterns ➡. 18-17C. Sagittal T1 C+ scan in the same patient shows the heterogeneously enhancing fourth ventricle mass ➡ extruding posteroinferiorly through the foramen of Magendie into the cisterna magna ➡.

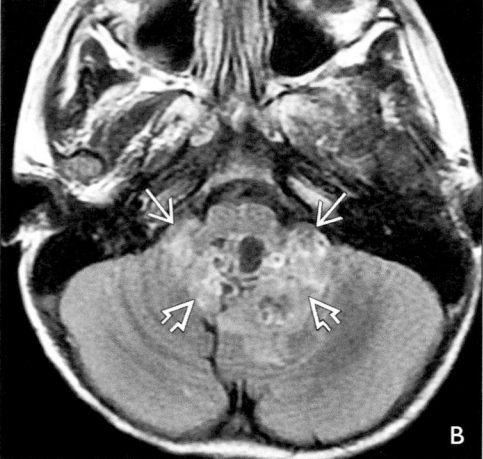

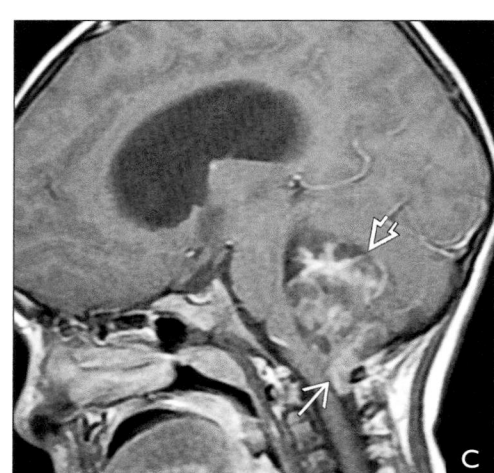

18-17D. Axial T1 C+ FS scan in the same patient shows mixed cystic, solid tumor with moderate rim ➡ and confluent ➡ and markedly enhancing portions. 18-17E. Coronal T1 C+ scan shows tumor extending inferiorly from the fourth ventricle into the cisterna magna ➡, laterally through the foramina of Luschka ➡. Note obstructive hydrocephalus ➡. Histopathology showed anaplastic ependymoma (WHO grade III).

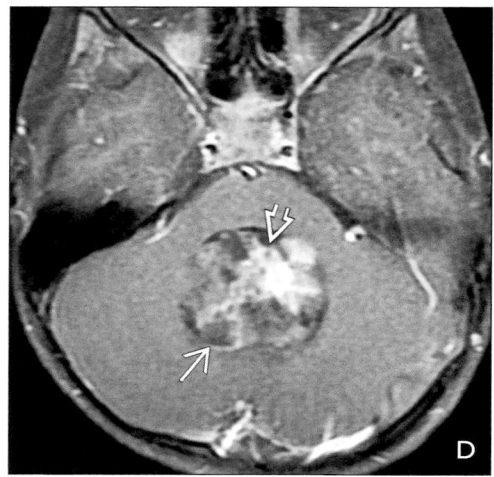

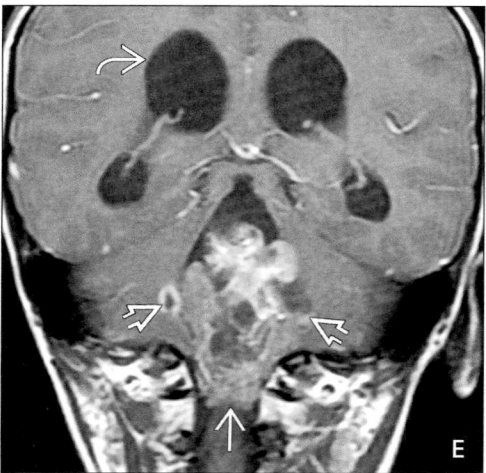

NATURAL HISTORY. Patients with ependymoma exhibit a wide range of clinical outcomes. Ependymoma is typically a slow-growing tumor. Nevertheless, overall prognosis is relatively poor with five-year survival rate of 50-60%. Extent of resection is the most important overall determining factor; the absence of demonstrable residual disease on postoperative imaging prolongs five-year survival to nearly 75%.

Correlation between tumor grade and outcome is controversial, but the overall survival rate of patients with WHO grade II ependymoma is better than that of patients with anaplastic ependymoma.

TREATMENT OPTIONS. Maximum cytoreduction surgery followed by conformal radiotherapy—not cranial spinal irradiation—is the standard treatment. Adjuvant therapy is generally reserved for recurrent tumor.

maging

GENERAL FEATURES. *Infratentorial* ependymomas are relatively well-delineated "plastic" tumors that typically arise from the floor of the fourth ventricle and extrude through the outlet foramina. They extend laterally through the foramina of Luschka toward the cerebellopontine angle (CPA) cistern and posteroinferiorly through the foramen of Magendie into the cisterna magna **(18-15)**.

Sagittal images disclose a mass that fills most of the fourth ventricle and extrudes inferiorly into the cisterna magna. Axial images show lateral extension toward or into the cerebellopontine angle cisterns **(18-17)**.

Obstructive hydrocephalus is a frequent accompanying feature of infratentorial ependymoma. Extracellular fluid often accumulates around the ventricles, giving the appearance of "blurred" margins.

CSF dissemination is a key factor in staging, prognosis, and treatment of ependymoma. The only statistically significant preoperative imaging predictor of patient outcome is evidence of tumor spread. Therefore, *preoperative imaging of the entire cranial-spinal axis should be performed in any child with a posterior fossa neoplasm,* especially if medulloblastoma or ependymoma is suspected.

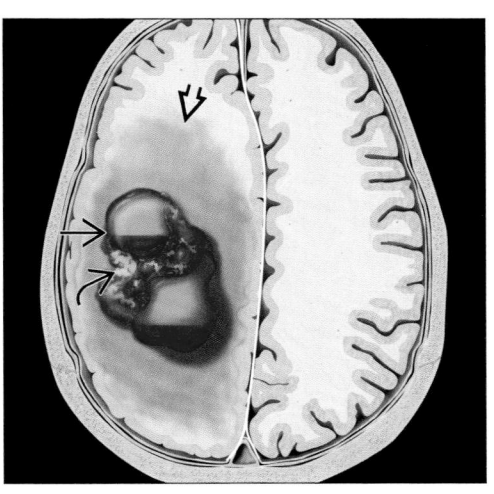

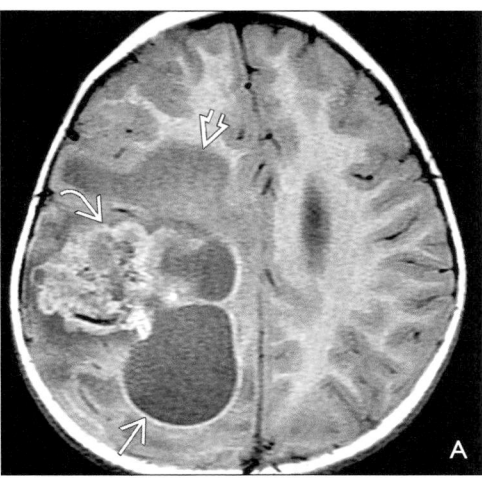

18-18. Graphic depicts supratentorial ependymoma as a large, hemorrhagic, hemispheric mass with multiple cysts, fluid-fluid levels ➡, calcification ➘, and significant peritumoral edema ➘. 18-19A. T1WI in a patient with a hemispheric ependymoma shows multiple cysts ➡ with mixed hyper-, hypointense solid components ➚, significant peritumoral edema ➡.

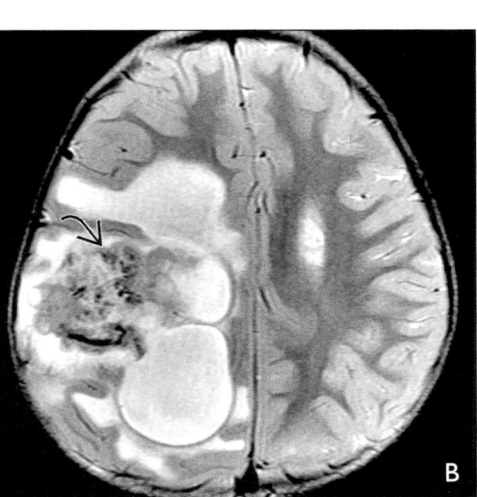

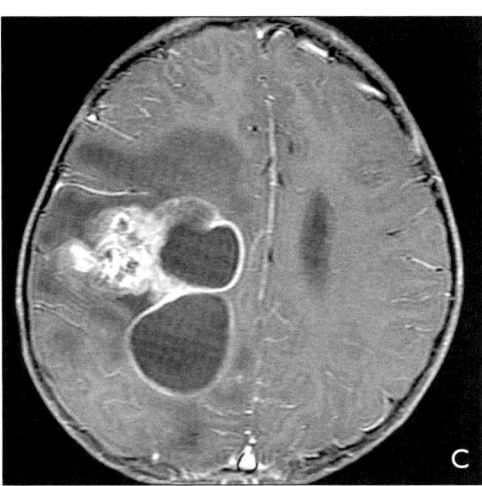

18-19B. T2WI shows the marked heterogeneous signal intensity of the solid part of the tumor mass ➚. 18-19C. T1 C+ FS scan shows heterogeneous, solid rim enhancement around the lesion. Most supratentorial ependymomas are in the brain parenchyma, not the ventricles.

Supratentorial ependymomas are generally large, bulky, aggressive-looking hemispheric tumors. Gross cyst formation, calcification, and hemorrhage are more common compared to their infratentorial counterparts **(18-18)**, **(18-19)**.

CT FINDINGS. Ependymomas are generally mixed density on NECT scans with hypodense intratumoral cysts intermixed with iso- and hyperdense soft tissue portions. Coarse calcification occurs in approximately half of all ependymomas **(18-17A)**. Macroscopic hemorrhage can be identified in approximately 10% of cases.

Most ependymomas show mild to moderate heterogeneous enhancement.

MR FINDINGS. Ependymomas are generally heterogeneously hypointense relative to brain parenchyma on T1WI and hyperintense on T2/FLAIR **(18-17)**. Following contrast administration, most ependymomas enhance. Areas of strong, relatively homogeneous enhancement are intermixed with foci of minimal or no enhancement.

T2* imaging (GRE, SWI) commonly demonstrates "blooming" foci that can be caused by calcification and/or old hemorrhage. An ependymoma may bleed, causing nonaneurysmal subarachnoid hemorrhage and siderosis around the tumor and along the pial surfaces of the cerebellum.

Most ependymomas do not restrict on DWI, although foci of restricted diffusion can be identified in some cases.

General MRS metabolite ratios are nonspecific. Elevated choline and reduced NAA are common in ependymoma, as in many other brain tumors. Perfusion MR generally demonstrates markedly elevated cerebral blood volume with poor return to baseline.

Differential Diagnosis

Differential diagnosis of ependymoma is location-dependent.

The major differential diagnosis of *infratentorial* ependymoma is **medulloblastoma (PNET-MB).** Medulloblastomas are more common and typically arise from the roof of the fourth ventricle (not from the floor, as is typical of ependymoma). PNET-MBs are hyperdense on NECT, often demonstrate diffusion restriction, and more frequently show evidence of CSF dissemination at the time of initial diagnosis. Cysts, hemorrhage, and calcification are less common in medulloblastoma compared with ependymoma.

The fourth ventricle is a relatively uncommon site for a **pilocytic astrocytoma**. A dorsally exophytic **brainstem glioma**, usually a diffusely infiltrating fibrillary astrocytoma, may project into the fourth ventricle, but

its intraaxial epicenter helps differentiate it from ependymoma.

The major differential diagnosis of *supratentorial* ependymoma is **anaplastic astrocytoma** or **glioblastoma multiforme**. **Astroblastoma** is typically a tumor of older children and young adults that has a mixed solid-cystic "bubbly" appearance. In very young children, **PNET** and **atypical teratoid/rhabdoid tumor** can cause hemispheric masses that closely resemble parenchymal ependymoma.

EPENDYMOMA

Location
- Infratentorial (60-70%)
  - Fourth ventricle (95%)
- Supratentorial (30-40%)
  - Hemispheres > > ventricles

Pathology
- Gross pathology
  - Extrudes from fourth ventricle into CPA, cisterna magna
- Histologic subtypes
  - Cellular (most common)
  - Clear cell
  - Papillary
  - Tanycytic (least common)
- Microscopic features
  - Perivascular pseudorosettes characteristic
  - WHO grade II

Clinical Issues
- 10% of childhood brain tumors
- Third most common posterior fossa tumor
  - After medulloblastoma, astrocytoma
- Bimodal age distribution
  - Most = 1-5 years old
  - Second small peak = 20-30 years old
- Presentation and natural history
  - Ataxia, symptoms of obstructive hydrocephalus
  - Relatively slow-growing
  - 5-year survival = 50-60%

Imaging
- Infratentorial ependymoma
  - Fills fourth ventricle
  - Extends into CPA, cisterna magna
  - Obstructive hydrocephalus
  - Cysts, Ca++ (50%), hemorrhage (10%) on NECT
  - Mixed signal intensity, strong enhancement on MR
  - "Blooming" foci on T2* common
  - Usually does not restrict on DWI
- Supratentorial ependymoma
  - Usually large, bulky, aggressive-looking
  - Gross cysts, Ca++, hemorrhage common

Differential Diagnosis
- Infratentorial ependymoma
  - Medulloblastoma (PNET-MB)
  - Pilocytic astrocytoma (relatively uncommon in fourth ventricle)
- Supratentorial ependymoma
  - Anaplastic astrocytoma, GBM
  - CNS-PNET
  - Atypical teratoid/rhabdoid tumor

naplastic Ependymoma

Anaplastic ependymoma (AE) is a malignant glioma that shows some ependymal differentiation but exhibits different genetic profiles. AEs have dysregulated Wnt/β pathways.

AE is characterized by more rapid growth, vascular proliferation, increased cellularity, higher mitotic activity, and less favorable outcome compared to the typical cellular ependymoma. AEs are designated WHO grade III neoplasms.

AE is a neuropathologic diagnosis as imaging findings are indistinguishable from those of cellular ependymoma.

ubependymoma

rminology

Subependymomas (SEs) are rare, benign, slow-growing, noninvasive tumors that are often found incidentally at imaging or autopsy.

iology

The origin of SEs is unclear. They may arise from pluripotential ependymal-glial precursor cells, astrocytes in the subependymal plate, or a preexisting hamartomatous lesion.

thology

Location. Subependymomas are usually located within or adjacent to an ependyma-lined space. They are most commonly found in the inferior fourth ventricle (50-60%) **(18-20)**, **(18-21)**, **(18-22)**, **(18-23)**, followed by the frontal horn of the lateral ventricle, often attached to the septi pellucidi (30-40%) **(18-25)**. Parenchymal SEs occur but are uncommon.

Size and Number. SEs are solitary tumors. Most are less than two centimeters, although some tumors may reach several centimeters in diameter. A few cases of very large biventricular SEs that fill both lateral ventricles have been reported. Because the posterior fossa is more anatomically constrained, infratentorial tumors are generally smaller than their supratentorial counterparts.

Gross Pathology. SEs are solid, round to somewhat lobulated, well-delineated, gray-tan masses. Calcification, cysts, and hemorrhage are common in larger lesions.

Microscopic Features. Bland nuclei in a dense fibrillary stroma with variable microcystic degeneration is typical. MIB-1 labeling is < 1%.

Staging, Grading, and Classification. Subependymomas are designated as WHO grade I neoplasms.

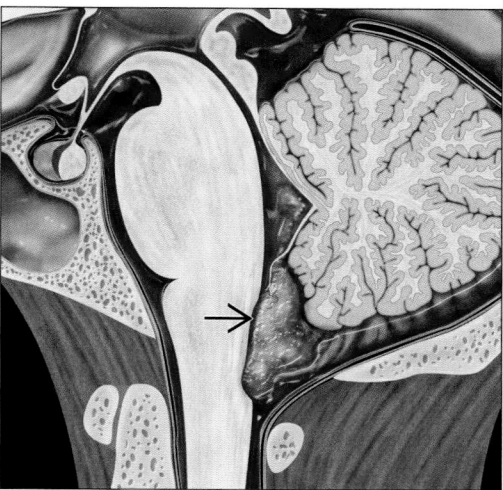

18-20. Graphic depicts subependymoma of the inferior fourth ventricle ⇥ at the level of the obex.

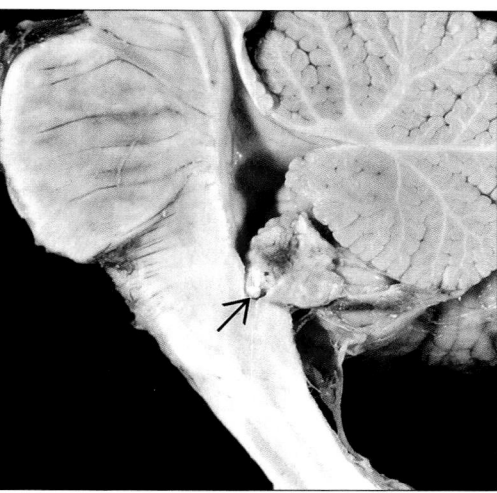

18-21. Sagittal autopsy section shows incidental finding of a small fourth ventricle subependymoma ⇥. (Courtesy P. Burger, MD.)

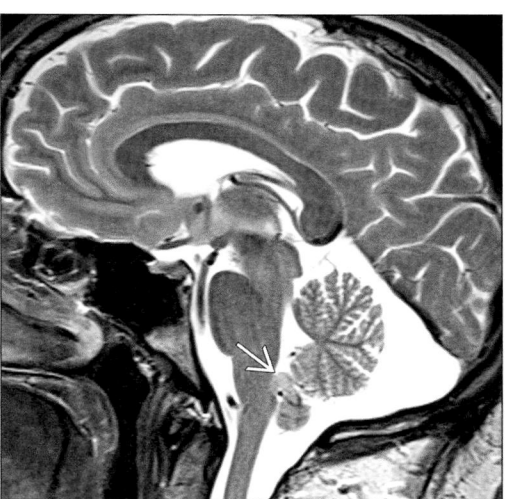

18-22. Sagittal T2WI shows incidental finding of fourth ventricle subependymoma in the obex ⇥.

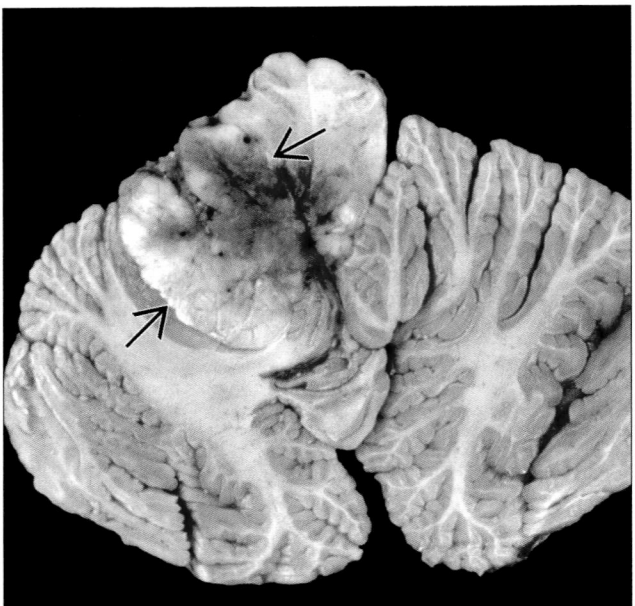

18-23. *Autopsy shows a large subependymoma of the fourth ventricle* ➡. *(Courtesy R. Hewlett, MD.)*

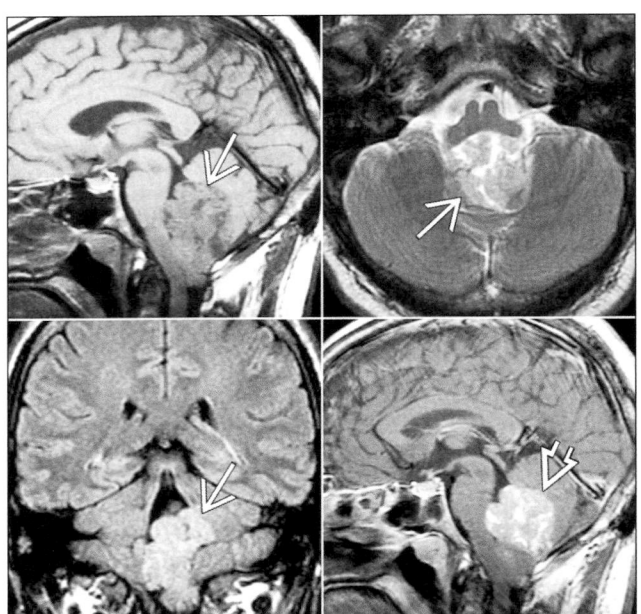

18-24. *Series of MR scans shows a large fourth ventricle subependymoma* ➡ *with mixed T1 iso-/hypointensity, T2/ FLAIR hyperintensity. The mass enhances strongly and relatively uniformly* ➡.

Clinical Issues

EPIDEMIOLOGY. SEs are found in 0.5-1% of autopsies and account for 8% of all ependymomas.

DEMOGRAPHICS. SEs are tumors of middle-aged and older adults. They are very rare in children. As with other ependymomas, there is a moderate male predominance.

PRESENTATION. The majority of subependymomas are asymptomatic and discovered incidentally. Approximately 40% cause symptoms, mostly related to CSF obstruction or mass effect.

NATURAL HISTORY. SEs exhibit an indolent growth pattern, expanding slowly into a ventricular space. Larger tumors may cause obstructive hydrocephalus, but they rarely invade adjacent brain. Recurrence is rare after gross total resection.

TREATMENT OPTIONS. "Watchful waiting" with serial imaging is appropriate in asymptomatic patients. Complete surgical resection of symptomatic SEs is the procedure of choice.

Imaging

GENERAL FEATURES. SEs are well-demarcated nodular masses that may expand the ventricle but usually cause little mass effect. Large lesions may cause obstructive hydrocephalus.

CT FINDINGS. SEs are iso- to slightly hypodense compared to brain on NECT scans. Calcification and intratumoral cysts may be present, especially in larger lesions.

Hemorrhage is rare. Little or no enhancement is seen on CECT.

MR FINDINGS. SEs are hypo- to isointense compared to brain on T1WI. Intratumoral cysts are common in larger lesions. SEs are heterogeneously hyperintense on T2/FLAIR (18-22), (18-24). Peritumoral edema is usually absent. T2* (GRE, SWI) may show "blooming" foci, probably secondary to calcification. Hemorrhage is seen in 10-12%. Enhancement varies from none or mild to moderate (18-26).

SEs do not restrict on DWI. MRS shows normal choline with mildly decreased NAA.

Differential Diagnosis

The differential diagnosis of SE varies with age and subependymoma location. In older patients, the major differential is intraventricular **metastasis**. Most intraventricular metastases arise in the choroid plexus. In young to middle-aged adults, **central neurocytoma** should be considered. Central neurocytoma is typically found in the body of the lateral ventricle, not the frontal horn or inferior fourth ventricle, and has a characteristic "bubbly" appearance. **Choroid plexus papilloma** usually occupies the body, not the inferior fourth ventricle.

In children, cellular **ependymoma** and (in patients with tuberous sclerosis) **subependymal giant cell astrocytoma** are considerations. **Choroid plexus papillomas** in children are usually in the atrium of the lateral ventricle. Choroid plexus papilloma also has a frond-like appearance and typically shows intense uniform enhancement.

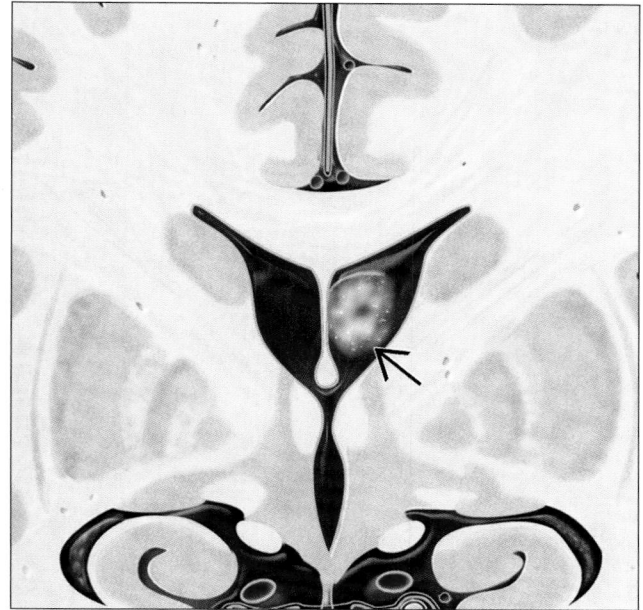

18-25. Coronal graphic depicts subependymoma in the frontal horn of the lateral ventricle ⮕, attached to the septi pellucidi.

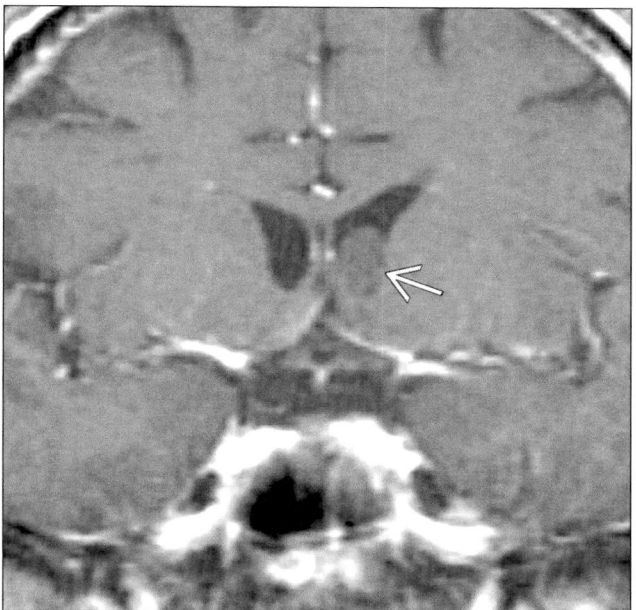

18-26. Coronal T1 C+ scan shows a nonenhancing mass in the left frontal horn ⮕. Presumed subependymoma, an incidental finding in this middle-aged male patient.

Myxopapillary Ependymoma

Myxopapillary ependymoma is a very slow-growing type of ependymoma that occurs mostly in young adults. It is almost exclusively a tumor of the conus medullaris, cauda equina, and filum terminale of the spinal cord.

Myxopapillary ependymomas correspond to WHO grade I. In the typical myxopapillary ependymoma, elongated GFAP-positive cells are in a papillary arrangement around a fibrovascular core that contains both hyalinized blood vessels and myxoid degeneration. MIB-1 labeling index is low, generally < 1%. No anaplastic variant of myxopapillary ependymoma is recognized.

Primary intracranial myxopapillary ependymomas are exceptionally rare but have been reported in the ventricles and brain parenchyma. Imaging findings are nonspecific but generally those of a cyst with enhancing nodule.

Choroid Plexus Tumors

Choroid plexus epithelium shares a common embryologic origin with ependymal cells. Hence choroid plexus tumors are considered tumors of neuroepithelial tissue and comprise an important subgroup of the nonastrocytic gliomas.

The most recent WHO classification recognizes three types of choroid plexus neoplasms: Choroid plexus papilloma, atypical choroid plexus papilloma, and choroid plexus carcinoma. In this section, we discuss each of these types with the major focus on choroid plexus papilloma—the most common primary choroid plexus tumor.

Choroid Plexus Papilloma

Terminology

Choroid plexus papilloma (CPP) is the most benign of the choroid plexus neoplasms.

Etiology

GENERAL CONCEPTS. Congenital CPPs are common and may develop when the differentiating fetal choroid plexus is transiently ciliated. Adult CPPs probably arise from differentiated choroid plexus epithelium.

GENETICS. Several genes that are differentially expressed in human choroid plexus papillomas have been identified. Among these, *TWIST1* is highly expressed and promotes proliferation and invasion.

Choroid plexus tumors—especially carcinomas—occur in patients with **Li-Fraumeni syndrome**, a cancer predisposition syndrome caused by *TP53* germline mutation. *SMARCB1* mutations with INI1 protein alterations and CPPs have been described in the **rhabdoid predis-**

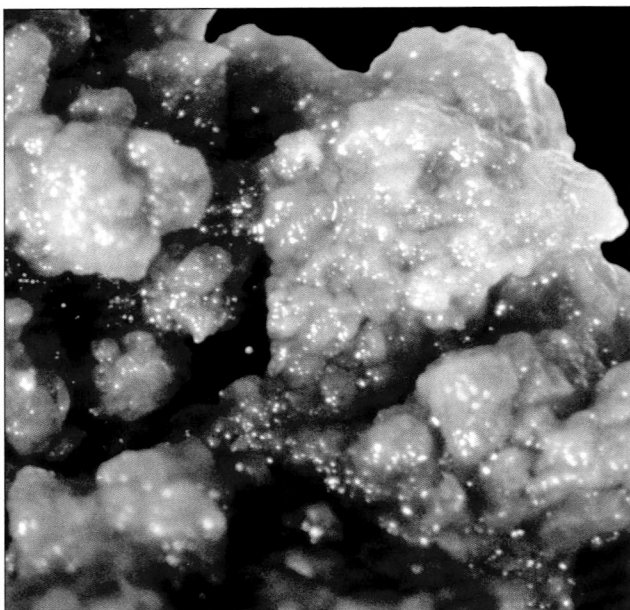

18-27. Close-up view of choroid plexus papilloma shows innumerable frond-like excrescences with CSF filling the crevices between the papillary projections. (Courtesy AFIP Archives.)

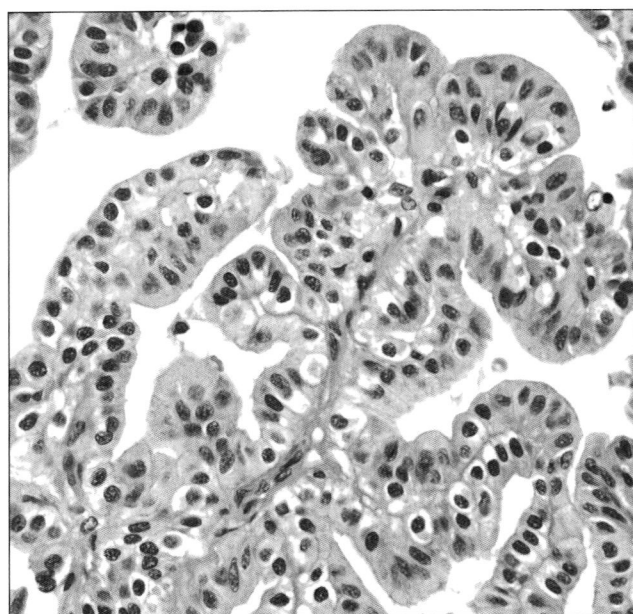

18-28. Typical microscopic appearance of choroid plexus papilloma is shown with redundant fronds, flattened papillae. No cellular atypia or mitotic figures are present. (Courtesy P. Burger, MD.)

position syndrome. Both mutations are very rarely identified in sporadic CPPs.

CPPs also occur as part of **Aicardi syndrome**, an X-linked dominant syndrome that occurs almost exclusively in females. Aicardi syndrome is defined by the triad of infantile spasms, corpus callosum agenesis, and pathognomonic chorioretinal abnormalities (lacunae). Since it was first described in 1965, new features such as cortical malformations, gray matter heterotopias, CPPs, and choroid plexus cysts have been identified and added to the Aicardi spectrum. The prevalence of CPPs in Aicardi syndrome is estimated at 3-5%. Bilateral and triventricular CPPs occur in 1% of cases.

Pathology

LOCATION. CPPs arise wherever choroid plexus is normally found, occurring in proportion to the amount of choroid plexus normally present in each location. Therefore, the vast majority arise in the lateral (50%) and fourth (40%) ventricles. The trigone is the most common overall site. A few large CPPs involve multiple locations. Triventricular CPP is seen in 5% of cases and originates in the third ventricle, extending cephalad through the foramen of Monro into both lateral ventricles.

Only 5-10% of all CPPs occur in locations other than the lateral and fourth ventricles. Just 5% are found in the third ventricle. CPPs are occasionally found as primary cerebellopontine angle (CPA) tumors, in which tufts of choroid plexus extrude through the foramina of Luschka into the adjacent CPA cisterns. Extraventricular CPPs are

extremely rare. They have been reported in the brainstem, cerebellum, pituitary fossa, and septi pellucidi.

There is a strong effect of age on CPP location. More than 80% of all CPPs in infants arise in the lateral ventricle. The fourth ventricle and CPA cisterns are more typical locations in adults with the lateral ventricle an exceptionally rare site of CPP in older patients.

SIZE AND NUMBER. CPPs are usually solitary tumors, varying in size from small to huge masses. Occasionally, multiple noncontiguous lesions are seen, but most represent CSF dissemination from the primary tumor site. Multiple CPPs arising independently as synchronous tumors are rarely seen.

GROSS PATHOLOGY. CPPs are well-circumscribed papillary or cauliflower-like masses that may adhere to—but usually do not invade through—the ventricular wall **(18-27)**. Cysts and hemorrhage are common.

MICROSCOPIC FEATURES. Histologically, the architecture of CPPs closely resembles that of normal nonneoplastic choroid plexus **(18-28)**. A core of fibrovascular connective tissue covered by a single layer of uniform benign-appearing epithelial cells is typical. Cytokeratins, vimentin, and podoplanin are expressed by virtually all CPPs.

Mitotic activity is very low, with MIB-1 < 1%. CPPs are generally confined to the ventricle of origin and rarely exhibit an infiltrative growth pattern.

Nonastrocytic Glial Neoplasms 509

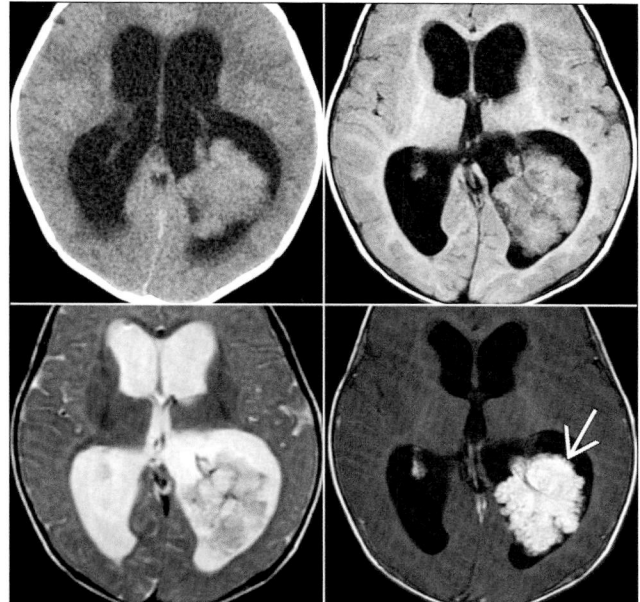

18-29. NECT scan and a series of MR images demonstrate the typical appearance of CPP. The lobulated intraventricular mass enhances strongly ➡. Note hydrocephalus caused by overproduction of CSF.

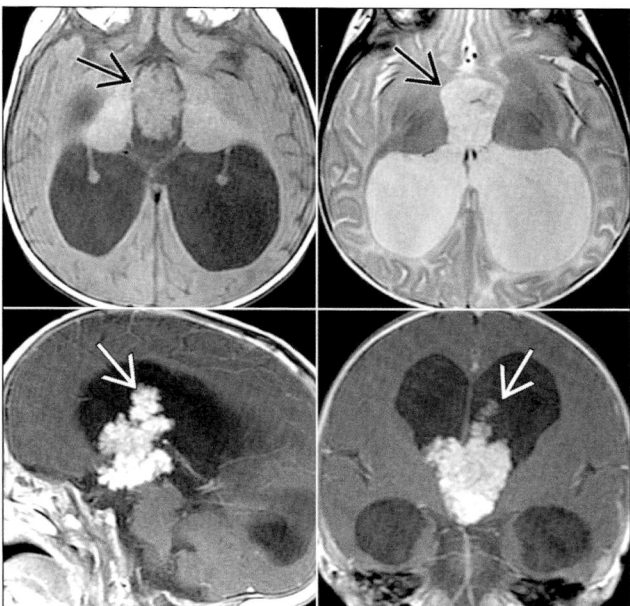

18-30. T1-, T2WIs show mass in the third ventricle ➡. Sagittal, coronal T1 C+ scans show the papillary nature of the mass ➡, which extends superiorly through the foramen of Monro into both lateral ventricles and causes obstructive hydrocephalus.

STAGING, GRADING, AND CLASSIFICATION. CPPs are WHO grade I neoplasms.

Clinical Issues

EPIDEMIOLOGY. CPPs are rare lesions, accounting for less than 1% of all primary intracranial neoplasms. However, CPPs represent 13% of brain tumors occurring in the first year of life.

DEMOGRAPHICS. Median age at presentation is 1.5 years for lateral and third ventricular CPPs, 22.5 years for fourth ventricle CPPs, and 35.5 years for CPA CPPs. There is a very slight male predominance.

PRESENTATION. CPPs tend to obstruct normal CSF pathways. Infants present with increased head size and raised intracranial pressure. Children and adults may experience headache, nausea, and vomiting.

CPP can also present as a fetal brain tumor and is the fifth most common congenital brain neoplasm (after teratoma, astrocytoma, craniopharyngioma, and primitive neuroectodermal tumor). Macrocephaly with a large intracranial mass and hydrocephalus is the most common presentation.

NATURAL HISTORY. Surgical resection is often curative. The recurrence rate following gross total resection is low, only about 5-6%. Malignant progression of CPP to choroid plexus carcinoma has been reported but is rare.

Imaging

GENERAL FEATURES. A well-delineated, lobulated intraventricular mass with frond-like papillary excrescences is typical. *Diffuse leptomeningeal dissemination is uncommon but does occur with histologically benign CPPs, so preoperative imaging of the entire neuraxis is recommended!*

CT FINDINGS. The majority of CPPs are iso- to hyperdense compared to brain on NECT scans **(18-29)**, **(18-31A)**. Calcification is seen in 25% of cases. Hydrocephalus—either obstructive or caused by CSF overproduction—is common. CECT scans show intense homogeneous enhancement **(18-31B)**.

MR FINDINGS. A sharply marginated lobular mass that is iso- to slightly hypointense relative to brain is seen on T1WI **(18-30)**. CPPs are iso- to hyperintense on T2WI and FLAIR **(18-31C)**. Linear and branching internal "flow voids" reflect the increased vascularity common in CPPs. T2* (GRE, SWI) may show hypointense foci secondary to calcification or intratumoral hemorrhage.

Intense homogeneous enhancement is seen following contrast administration **(18-30)**, **(18-31D)**. CPPs generally do not restrict on DWI. MRS may show elevated myoinositol (mI).

Rare CPP variants include purely cystic CPP and cystic extraaxial metastases from an intraventricular CPP. In purely cystic CPP a large, often mobile cyst with intensely enhancing mural nodules is attached to the choroid plexus. It can cause sudden obstructive hydrocephalus. Purely cystic extraaxial metastases from CPP are seen as nonenhancing cisternal CSF-like cysts that resemble multiple parasitic cysts, most commonly neurocysticercosis.

ULTRASOUND. CPPs appear as well-defined, lobular, hyperechoic intraventricular masses on transcranial US.

Differential Diagnosis

The major differential diagnoses of CPP are **atypical choroid plexus papilloma** and **choroid plexus carcinoma** (CPCa). Atypical CPP (WHO grade II neoplasm) and typical CPP (WHO grade I) share similar imaging features and must be differentiated histopathologically. CPCa is far more likely to invade brain parenchyma than CPP. CSF dissemination occurs with both CPP and CPCa and is therefore neither a distinguishing feature nor a reliable predictor of malignancy.

Choroid plexus hyperplasia, also called **villous hypertrophy of the choroid plexus**, is a very rare cause of CSF overproduction and shunt-resistant hydrocephalus. Diffuse villous hyperplasia may result in CSF production

exceeding three liters per day. Unlike CPP, most cases of choroid plexus hyperplasia are bilateral and diffusely enlarge the entire length of the choroid plexus.

Choroid plexus xanthogranulomas are benign incidental lesions that occur commonly in the lateral ventricular choroid plexus. They consist of desquamated epithelial cells with accumulated lipid together with macrophages and multinucleated foreign body giant cells. In contrast to most CPPs, they are found primarily in middle-aged and older patients. On imaging they appear as bilateral multiloculated cysts within the enhancing choroid plexus glomus.

Choroid plexus metastasis occurs in middle-aged and older adults and is not in the differential diagnosis of a pediatric CPP.

Atypical Choroid Plexus Papilloma

Atypical choroid plexus papilloma (aCPP) is a recently recognized neoplasm that is intermediate in malignancy between CPP (WHO grade I neoplasm) and choroid

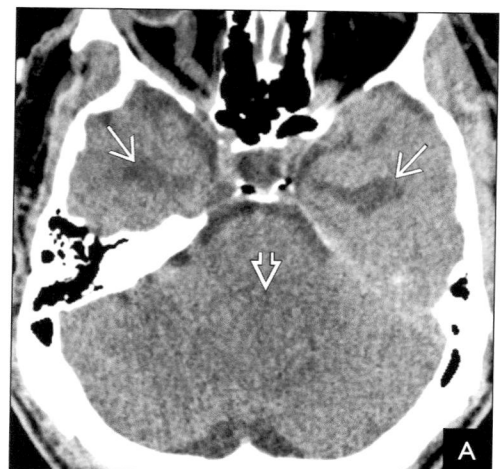

18-31A. *NECT scan in a 43-year-old man with severe headaches, nonfocal neurological examination shows moderately enlarged temporal horns of both lateral ventricles* ⇨. *The normal fourth ventricle is not visualized. Instead, a large nearly isodense mass* ⇨ *fills the barely visible fourth ventricle.* **18-31B.** *CECT scan shows that the mass enhances intensely and quite uniformly.*

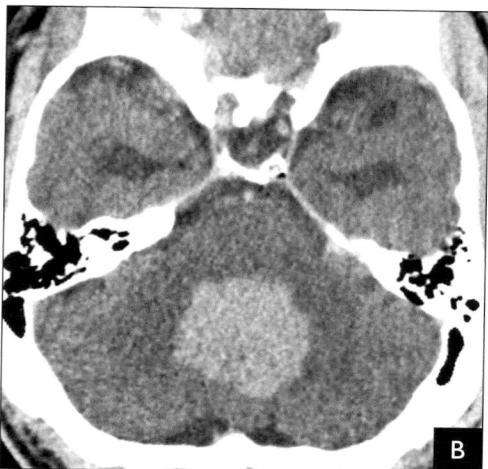

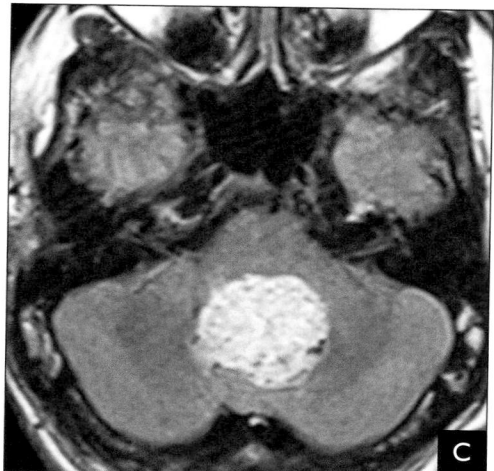

18-31C. *FLAIR scan in the same patient shows that the mass is hyperintense with some small internal hypointense foci.* **18-31D.** *T1 C+ FS scan shows the mass nicely. Note the frond-like enhancing excrescences with nonenhancing CSF in the interstices between the tumor fronds* ⇨. *WHO grade I choroid plexus papilloma was identified at histopathology.*

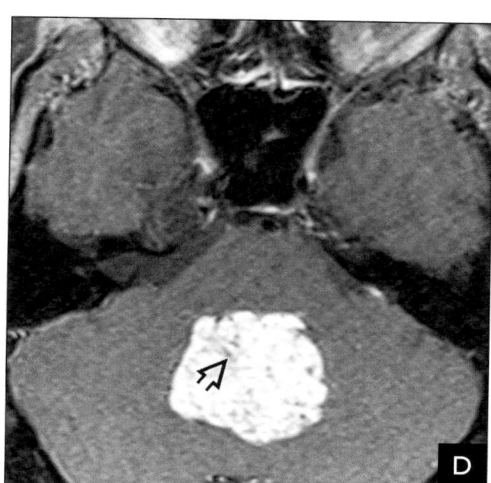

plexus carcinoma (WHO grade III neoplasm). aCPPs represent approximately 15% of all choroid plexus tumors.

The main distinguishing histopathologic feature of aCPP is increased mitotic activity with elevated MIB-1 labeling **(18-33)**. Increased cellularity and nuclear pleomorphism are common.

Only a few imaging cases of aCPP have been reported. All have the lobulated papillary appearance with strong uniform enhancement that also characterizes CPP **(18-32)**. Imaging findings to date do not discriminate between aCPP and CPP, so the definitive diagnosis depends on histopathology.

Choroid Plexus Carcinoma

Terminology

Choroid plexus carcinoma (CPCa) is a rare malignant tumor that occurs almost exclusively in young children.

Etiology

GENETICS. Nearly half of all CPCas harbor *TP53* mutations. The *TP53*-mutated tumor genome is associated with significant risk of progression and poor outcome. The reported five-year survival rate of TP53-immunopositive tumors is 0%.

Pathology

GROSS PATHOLOGY. CPCa almost always arises in the lateral ventricle. This heterogeneous, bulky intraventricular tumor often displays gross hemorrhage and necrotic foci. Invasion into adjacent brain parenchyma is common **(18-34)**.

MICROSCOPIC FEATURES. Frank cytologic features of malignancy are seen, including frequent mitoses (generally at least 5-10 per high-power field), increased cellular density, nuclear pleomorphism, loss of papillary architecture, and necrosis. MIB-1 is elevated, ranging from 15% to 20% **(18-35)**.

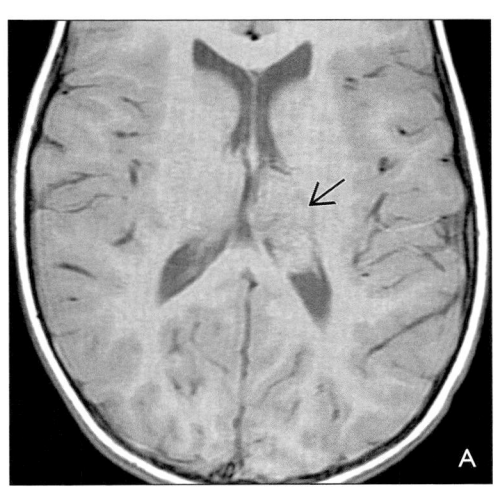
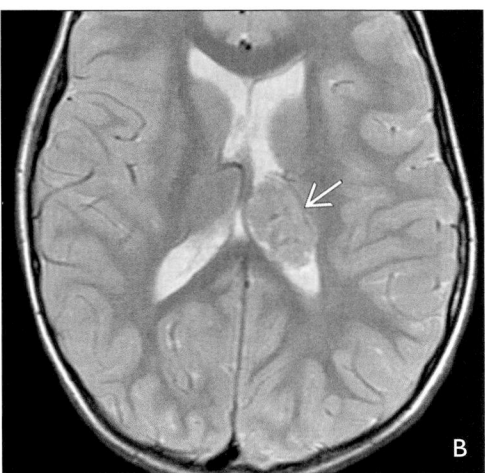

18-32A. T1WI shows a lobulated mass contained within the body of the left lateral ventricle →. 18-32B. T2WI shows that the mass → is isointense with gray matter.

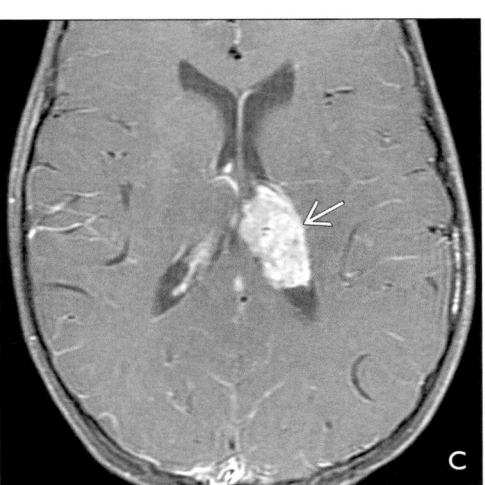
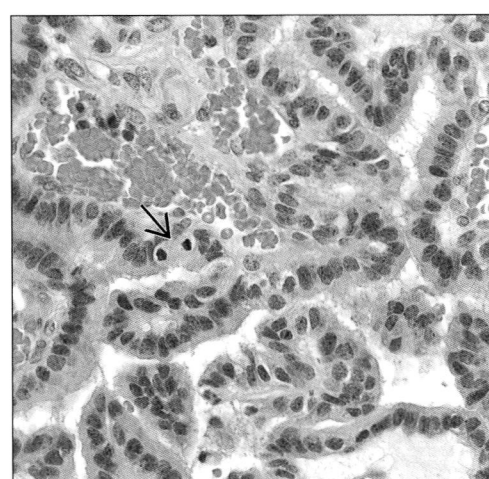

18-32C. The mass → enhances intensely on T1 C+ FS. Atypical CPP (WHO grade II) was histopathologically identified. 18-33. Papillary choroid plexus tumors are diagnosed as atypical on the basis of increased mitotic activity → (higher than that of WHO grade I CPPs). Two or more mitoses per 10 high-power fields is the suggested threshold, which this tumor meets. (Courtesy P. Burger, MD.)

Immunohistochemical and genetic features show some overlap between CPCa and atypical teratoid/rhabdoid tumor.

STAGING, GRADING, AND CLASSIFICATION. CPCa is a WHO grade III neoplasm.

Clinical Issues

EPIDEMIOLOGY. While CPCa is uncommon, representing less than 1% of all pediatric brain tumors, it accounts for 5% of supratentorial neoplasms. CPCa represents 20-40% of all primary choroid plexus neoplasms.

DEMOGRAPHICS. Between 70-80% of CPCas arise in children younger than three years. Median age at diagnosis is 18 months.

PRESENTATION. The most common symptoms—nausea, vomiting, headache, and obtundation—are caused by obstructive hydrocephalus.

NATURAL HISTORY. Prognosis in patients with these aggressive tumors is generally dismal, especially those with incomplete resection of a *TP53*-mutated genotype.

TREATMENT OPTIONS. Gross total resection is the primary treatment. Multimodality treatment with craniospinal radiation and neoadjuvant ICE (ifosfamide, carboplatin, etoposide) chemotherapy improves survival in some cases. Some TP53-immunonegative tumors have been successfully treated without radiation therapy.

Imaging

CPCa often invades through the ventricular ependyma into adjacent brain. Edema, necrosis, intratumoral cysts, and hemorrhage are common **(18-36)**. Enhancement is typically strong but heterogeneous **(18-37)**. CSF dissemination is common.

Differential Diagnosis

The major differential diagnoses are **choroid plexus papilloma** and **atypical choroid plexus papilloma**. Imaging features of all three primary choroid plexus tumors overlap. CSF spread occurs with both benign and malignant varieties. Choroid plexus papilloma rarely invades the brain, so the presence of frank parenchymal invasion and accompanying edema suggests CPCa.

18-34. Graphic depicts choroid plexus carcinoma. Hemorrhagic, highly vascular-appearing mass fills the atrium of the lateral ventricle, invades adjacent parenchyma. 18-35. Photomicrograph depicts choroid plexus carcinoma. Cellular atypia with multiple mitoses ➘ is indicative of CPCa. (Courtesy P. Burger, MD.)

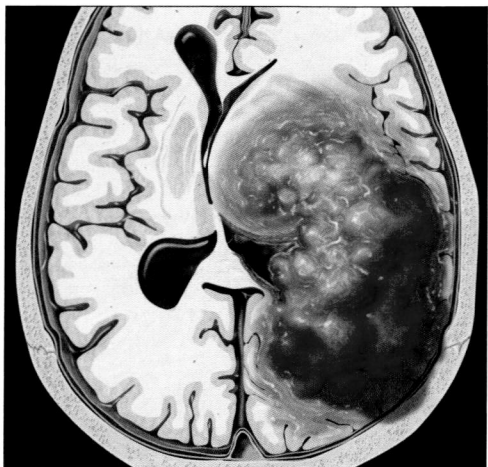

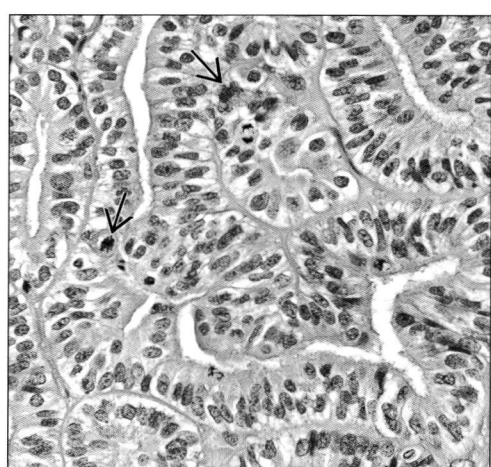

18-36A. Axial T2WI shows findings of typical choroid plexus carcinoma. The extremely heterogeneous signal intensity as well as lack of ependymal border between the tumor and adjacent brain are typical findings. 18-36B. Most choroid plexus carcinomas show significant intratumoral hemorrhage such as that seen on this T2* GRE scan as "blooming" hypointensity ➘. Note the siderosis from prior hemorrhage coating the surfaces of the cerebellum, medulla ➘.

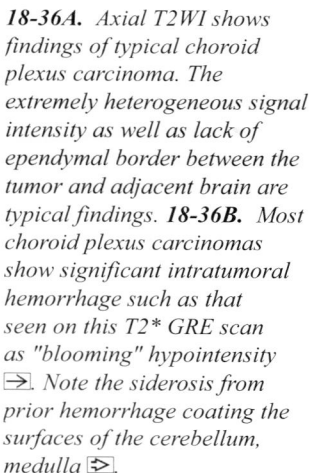

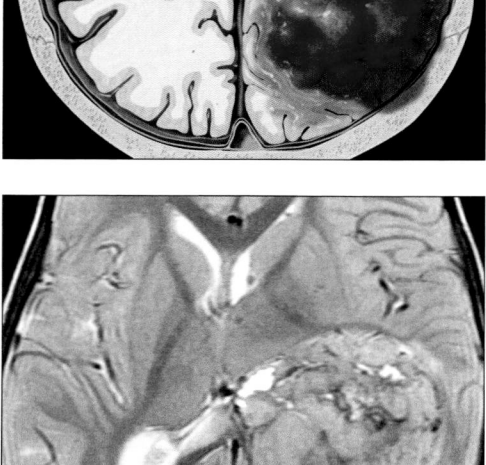

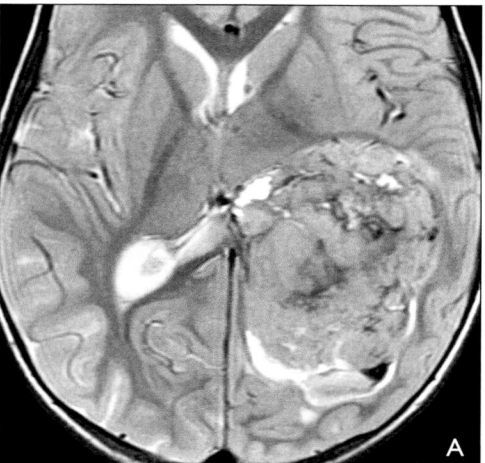

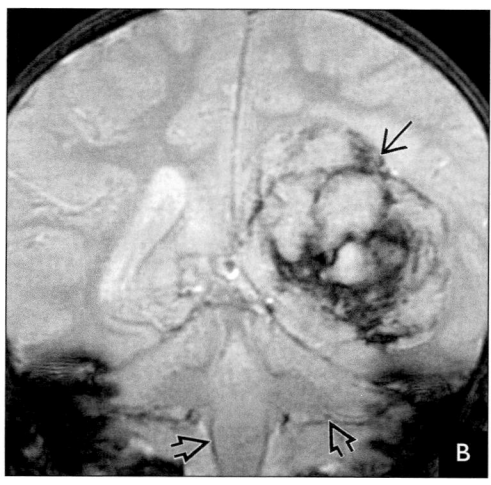

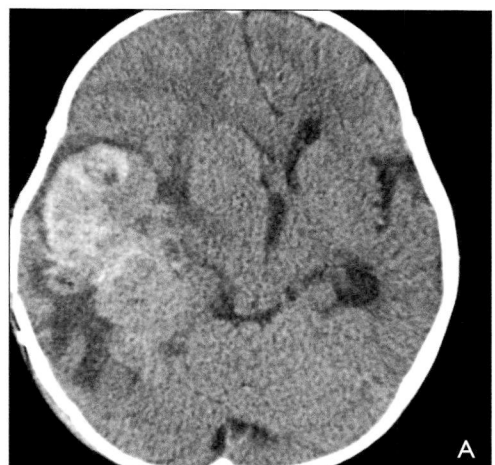

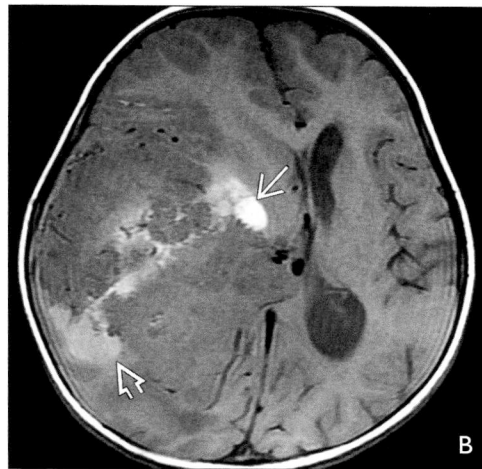

18-37A. *NECT scan in a 2-year-old girl with a large head, papilledema shows a predominantly hyperdense lobulated mass in the right lateral ventricle invading adjacent brain.* **18-37B.** *T1WI shows that the mass is mostly iso- and hypointense, but areas of variable hyperintensity suggest hemorrhage ⮕, proteinaceous fluid in cysts ⮕.*

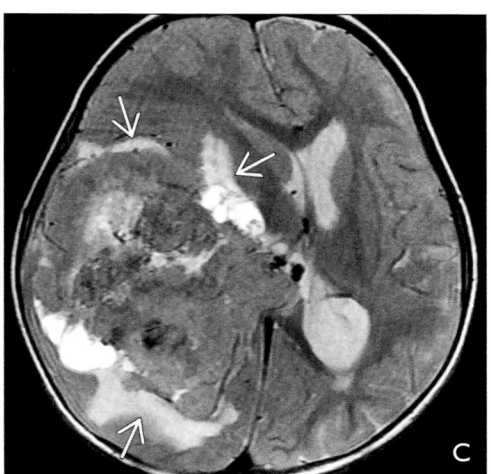

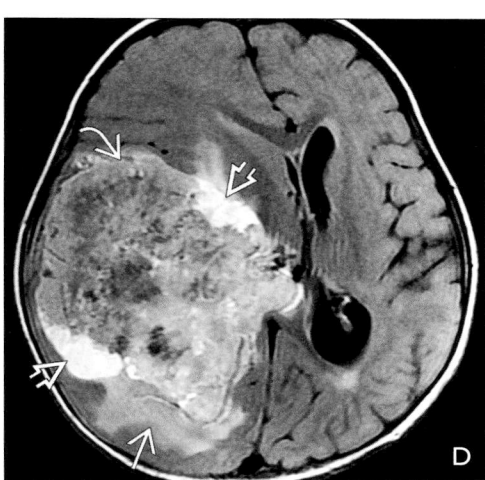

18-37C. *T2WI shows the extremely heterogeneous nature of the mass. Gross tumor invasion of the brain parenchyma with surrounding edema ⮕ is present.* **18-37D.** *FLAIR scan depicts the mass ⮕, surrounding edema ⮕, hemorrhage and/or cyst formation ⮕.*

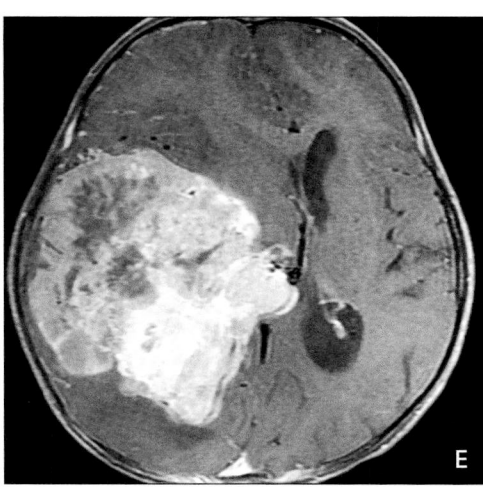

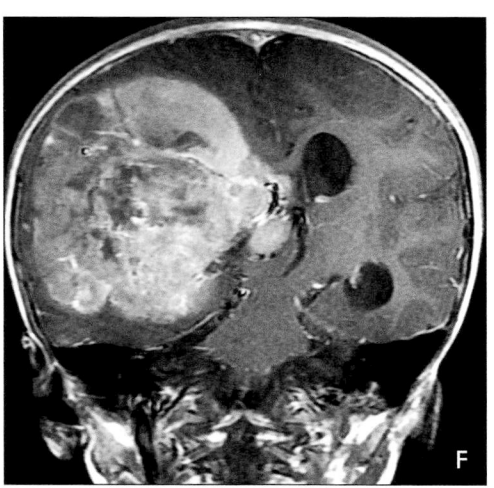

18-37E. *T1 C+ FS scan shows that the mass enhances intensely but heterogeneously.* **18-37F.** *Coronal T1 C+ scan shows the extent of tumor invasion into the adjacent parenchyma. Choroid plexus carcinoma.*

Most other supratentorial neoplasms in very young children are parenchymal rather than intraventricular. **Astrocytoma**, **ependymoma**, **primitive neuroectodermal tumor**, and **atypical teratoid/rhabdoid tumor** can all present as large, bulky, aggressive-appearing masses with hemorrhage and necrosis.

CHOROID PLEXUS TUMORS

Choroid Plexus Papilloma
- Pathology
  - Lateral ventricle (50%, usually children)
  - Fourth ventricle, CPA cistern (40%, usually adults)
  - Third ventricle (10%, children)
  - Lobulated, frond-like configuration
  - WHO grade I
- Clinical issues
  - 13% of brain tumors in first year of life
  - Mean age = 1.5 years for CPPs in lateral, third ventricle
  - Symptoms of obstructive hydrocephalus common
  - Occurs with Aicardi, Li-Fraumeni, rhabdoid predisposition syndromes
- CT
  - Iso-/hyperdense lobulated mass
  - Hydrocephalus common
  - Ca++ (25%)
  - CECT shows intense enhancement
- MR
  - Iso-/hypointense on T1
  - Iso-/hyperintense on T2/FLAIR
  - "Flow voids" common
  - May show "blooming" foci on T2*
  - Intense enhancement, no restriction
  - Occasionally demonstrates CSF dissemination (image entire neuraxis preoperatively!)

Atypical Choroid Plexus Papilloma
- WHO grade II
- Imaging findings similar to those of CPP

Choroid Plexus Carcinoma
- Rare
- Children < 3 years (70-80%)
- WHO grade III
- Imaging
  - Invades through ependyma
  - Edema, necrosis, cysts, hemorrhage common
  - Strong heterogeneous enhancement
  - CSF dissemination common

Other Neuroepithelial Tumors

"Other neuroepithelial tumors" is an eclectic group of uncommon neoplasms that currently includes astroblastoma, chordoid glioma of the third ventricle, and angiocentric glioma.

Astroblastoma

Terminology

Astroblastoma is a rare glial neoplasm that mainly affects younger patients. While its precise etiology and exact histogenesis are controversial, astroblastoma is now widely recognized as a distinct entity.

Pathology

Grossly, astroblastomas are firm, often cystic hemispheric parenchymal masses (18-38). Even though the name "astroblastoma" implies astrocytic lineage, it is histologically more similar to ependymoma with frequent perivascular pseudorosettes.

While some investigators recognize subsets of low-grade and high-grade astroblastomas, no WHO grade has been assigned to date.

Clinical Issues

Astroblastomas account for less than 1% of all primary brain tumors and 0.5-3% of gliomas. Although they can occur at any age, most astroblastomas are found in children and young adults. Peak onset is 10-30 years.

Despite its ominous-sounding name, the biological behavior of astroblastoma is quite variable. Patients with low-grade tumors and gross total resection often have good long-term survival rates.

Imaging

GENERAL FEATURES. Astroblastoma is almost exclusively a supratentorial hemispheric tumor that is typically well-demarcated. Surrounding edema is minimal or absent. Most astroblastomas exhibit both solid and cystic components, frequently giving them a characteristic "bubbly" appearance.

CT FINDINGS. Over 85% of astroblastomas demonstrate calcification on NECT. Punctate/psammomatous or dense globular calcification is typical.

MR FINDINGS. Astroblastoma is hypo- to isointense compared to white matter on T1WI and heterogeneously hyperintense on T2/FLAIR (18-39). A "bubbly" appearance, caused by intratumoral cysts, is common. Hemorrhage, including blood-fluid levels in the cystic components, can be present.

Heterogeneous enhancement following contrast administration is typical. The combination of peripheral rim and solid nodular enhancement gives some lesions a "signet ring" appearance. Some peripheral astroblastomas incite dural reaction, causing a "dural tail" sign.

ifferential Diagnosis

While the overall imaging findings of astroblastoma are somewhat nonspecific, the combination of age (10-30 years), anatomic location (cerebral hemisphere), and a "bubbly" appearance may suggest the diagnosis.

Other entities that resemble astroblastoma vary with age. In young children, **astrocytoma, hemispheric ependymoma**, and **atypical teratoid/rhabdoid tumor** should be considered. In older children and young adults, **oligodendroglioma** and **pleomorphic xanthoastrocytoma** are in the differential diagnosis.

hordoid Glioma of the Third entricle

Chordoid glioma (CG) is a rare adult tumor that is distinguished by its location (third ventricular region), stereotypical histology (both glial and chordoid elements), and characteristic imaging features.

Etiology

While the precise etiology of CGs is unclear, ultrastructural studies and the putative origin from the lamina terminalis of the third ventricle suggest an ependymal histogenesis of this unusual neoplasm. There are no known risk factors or syndromic associations.

Pathology

LOCATION. CGs arise in the anterior aspect of the third ventricle adjacent to the lamina terminalis. The smallest reported CG was 1.5 cm and the largest measured 7 cm in maximum diameter.

GROSS PATHOLOGY. CGs are solid, round or slightly lobulated, semitranslucent masses that are tan-gray and moderately vascular **(18-40)**. Many CGs are grossly encapsulated.

MICROSCOPIC FEATURES. The general appearance is that of a chordoid architecture with myxoid background. Cords and clusters of round or fusiform epithelioid neoplastic cells with abundant eosinophilic cytoplasm are

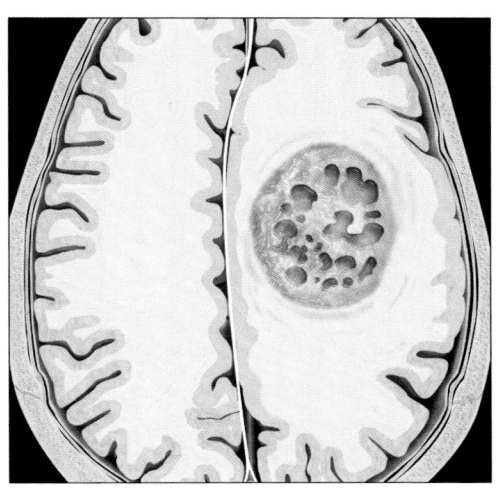

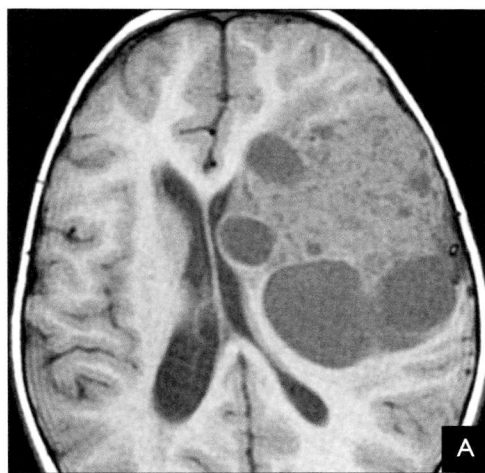

18-38. Graphic depicts astroblastoma as a relatively well-circumscribed hemispheric mass with multiple intratumoral cysts. 18-39A. Axial T1WI shows typical findings of astroblastoma with innumerable tiny and multiple large cysts.

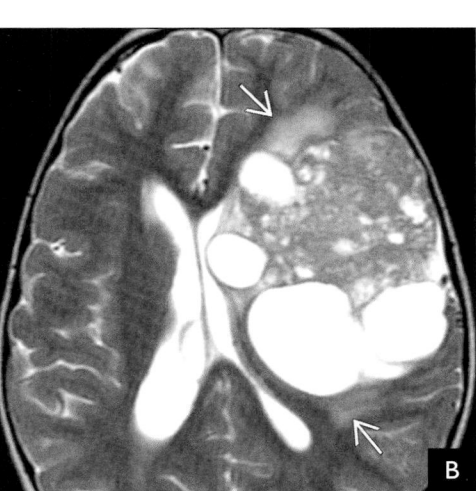

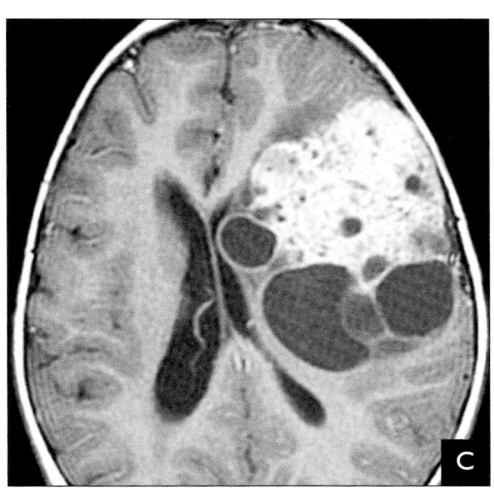

18-39B. T2WI shows that, relative to the size of the mass, there is little peritumoral edema ➡. 18-39C. T1 C+ shows that the solid portions of the mass enhance whereas the cysts do not.

suspended in a variably mucinous, often vacuolated, lymphoplasmacytic-rich matrix.

CGs resemble chordomas or chordoid meningiomas microscopically. However, unlike these similar-appearing tumors, CGs show strong diffuse immunoreactivity for the glial marker GFAP. Most are positive for an epithelial membrane antigen and CD34 but are usually negative for neurofilament protein.

Mitoses are rare, and MIB-1 labeling index is low.

STAGING, GRADING, AND CLASSIFICATION. CGs are WHO grade II neoplasms.

Clinical Issues

EPIDEMIOLOGY. CG is rare, representing less than 1% of all gliomas.

DEMOGRAPHICS. CG is a tumor of middle-aged adults (35-60 years old). There is a 2:1 F:M ratio.

PRESENTATION. Clinical presentation of CG varies. Headache, nausea, and memory impairment are common. On neurologic examination, visual field deficit is the most common abnormality. Endocrine disturbances are seen in 10-15% of patients.

NATURAL HISTORY AND TREATMENT. CGs are slow-growing tumors. Because they are frequently attached to the hypothalamus and floor of the third ventricle, resection is often subtotal. The most common postoperative complication is hypothalamic dysfunction with diabetes insipidus and obesity.

Imaging

GENERAL FEATURES. Radiological features of reported CGs are remarkably consistent. Most CGs are well-demarcated ovoid masses that are confined to the third ventricle and are clearly separate from the pituitary gland and infundibulum. While they often abut and may superficially adhere to the hypothalamus, gross brain invasion is rare. Enhancement is typically strong and relatively uniform.

CT FINDINGS. CGs are moderately hyperdense compared to brain on NECT. Strong, homogeneous enhancement is typical. Occasional cases with calcification have

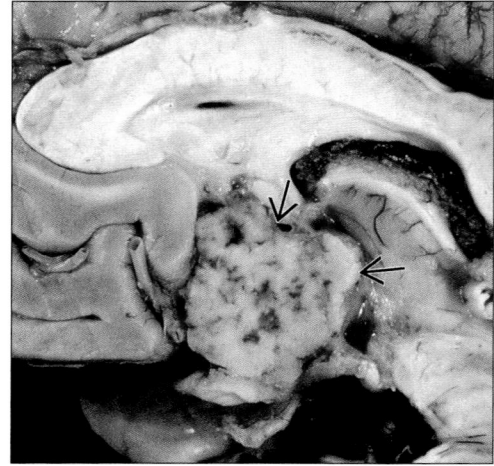

18-40. Midline sagittal autopsy specimen shows chordoid glioma as a lobulated mass ⇥ that fills the third ventricle. (Courtesy P. Burger, MD.) 18-41A. NECT scan shows a lobulated, hyperdense, partially calcified midline mass ⇥ in the inferior third ventricle.

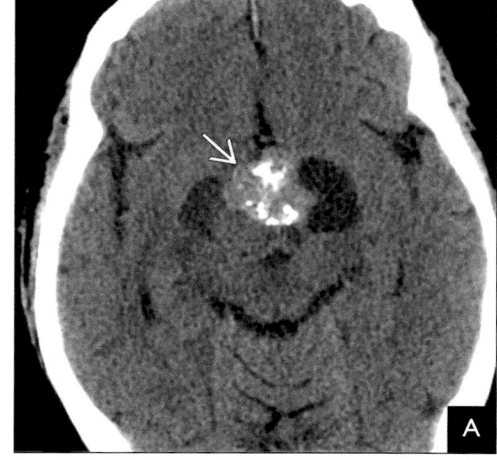

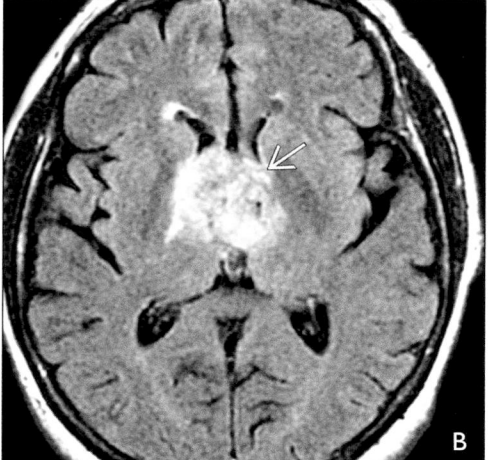

18-41B. FLAIR scan in the same patient shows that the mass ⇥ is heterogeneously hyperintense. 18-41C. Sagittal T1 C+ scan shows that the mass ⇥ is well-margined, enhances intensely but somewhat heterogeneously. The infundibular stalk, pituitary gland ⇥ appear entirely normal. Chordoid glioma of the third ventricle was the histopathologic diagnosis.

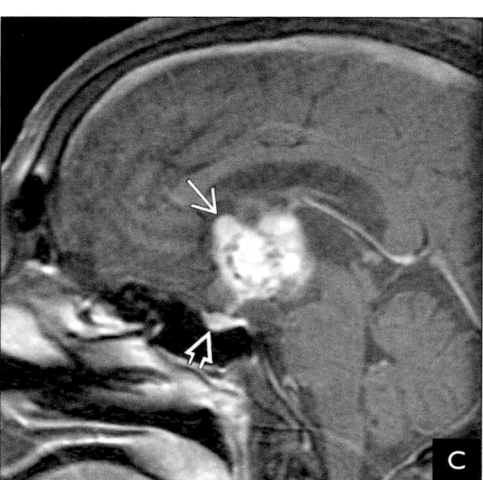

been reported. Hydrocephalus is present in 10-15% of cases.

MR FINDINGS. Sagittal MR demonstrates that the tumor is clearly separated from the pituitary gland and infundibular stalk **(18-41)**. CGs are typically isointense with brain on both T1- and T2WI. Strong uniform enhancement is typical. Intratumoral cysts are seen in 25% of cases, but hemorrhage is rare.

ifferential Diagnosis

Primary third ventricular tumors in adults are all uncommon, as are **metastases** in this location. As CGs are clearly separate from the pituitary gland, macroadenoma is usually not in the differential diagnosis although a few purely third ventricular **pituitary macroadenomas** and **craniopharyngiomas** have been reported. **Chordoid meningioma** can look just like a CG, but the third ventricle is a rarely reported site for a rare meningioma variant.

Tuber cinereum (TC) hamartomas are most common in preadolescent males with precocious puberty. While TC hamartomas are isointense with brain on T1- and T2WI, they do not enhance. As CGs are tumors of adults, childhood hypothalamic tumors such as adamantinomatous **craniopharyngioma** and **pilocytic astrocytoma** are not diagnostic considerations.

Angiocentric Glioma

Angiocentric glioma (AG) is a newly described epilepsy-associated tumor. Because of its uncertain histogenesis, the WHO groups AG together with astroblastoma and chordoid glioma in the category "other neuroepithelial tumors."

Terminology

Angiocentric glioma has also been called "angiocentric neuroepithelial tumor" (ANET).

Etiology

To date the etiology of AG is uncertain; both astrocytic and ependymal lineages have been suggested. Some investigators posit radial glia or neuronal precursors as possible origins.

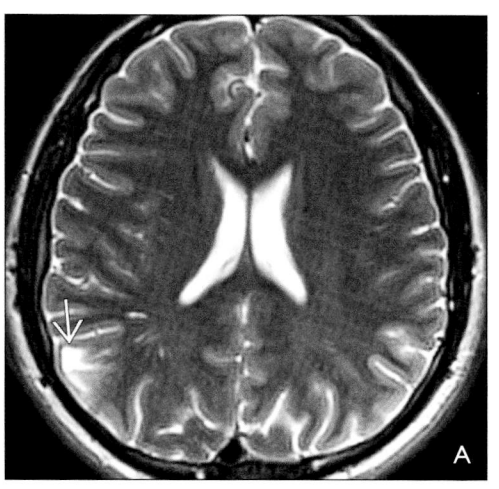

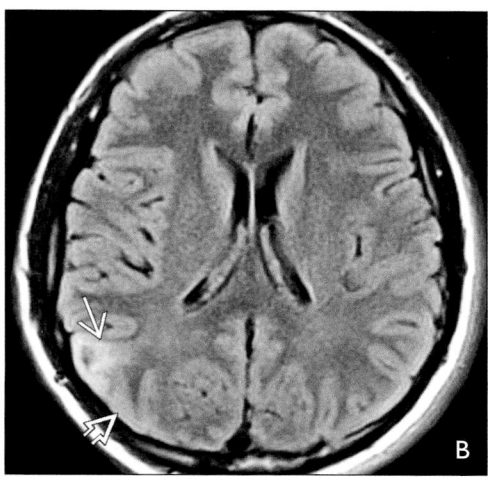

18-42A. Axial T2WI in a patient with seizures shows a wedge-shaped hyperintense cortical, subcortical mass in the right parietal lobe ➡. *18-42B. FLAIR scan shows the mass* ➡ *as well as thickening of the adjacent gyri* ➡.

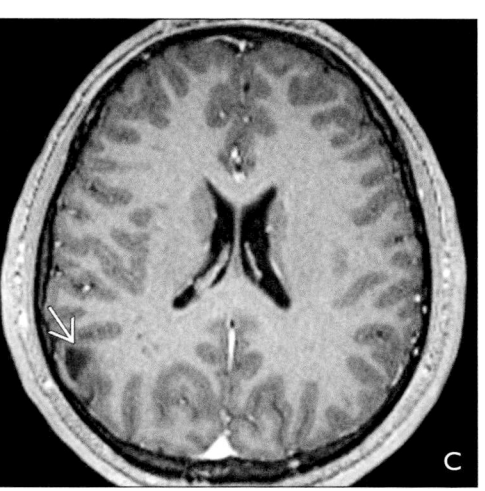

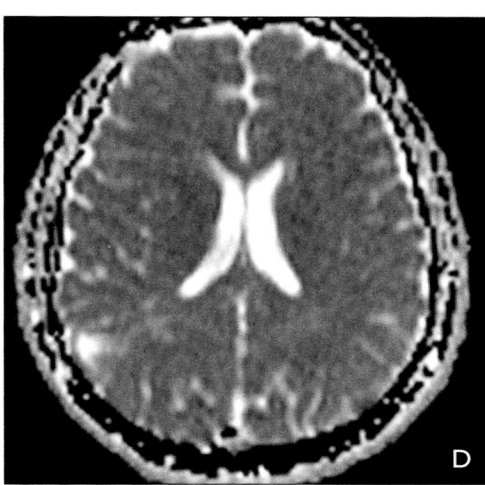

18-42C. T1 C+ shows that the mass ➡ *does not enhance. 18-42D. ADC map shows that the mass does not demonstrate diffusion restriction. Angiocentric glioma was the histologic diagnosis. The adjacent gyral thickening noted on the FLAIR scan probably represents associated focal cortical dysplasia, a finding commonly associated with angiocentric glioma. (Courtesy M. Castillo, MD.)*

Clinical Issues

While they can occur at any age, AGs are typically tumors of children and young adults. They are strongly epileptogenic with more than 95% of patients presenting with intractable focal epilepsy. AGs account for up to 8% of tumors discovered at epilepsy surgery.

Surgical excision is generally curative.

Pathology

AGs are superficial, cortically based tumors. The most common reported location is the frontal lobe, followed by the temporal lobe. AGs are characterized by elongated bipolar spindle cells with a striking radial or longitudinal angiocentric orientation. Adjacent focal cortical dysplasia is common.

The MIB-1 of AG is generally < 1%. AGs are designated as WHO grade I neoplasms.

Imaging

Imaging findings for only a few AG cases have been reported. The most common finding on CT is a solid, cortically based tumor. Necrosis, hemorrhage, intratumoral cysts, and calcification are absent.

MR shows a diffusely infiltrating expansile cortical mass without sharply demarcated borders. Most AGs are hyperintense on T2/FLAIR. A subtle rim of T1 shortening and stalk-like extension toward the ventricle has been described. Enhancement is typically absent. Focal cortical dysplasia can often be identified adjacent to the tumor **(18-42)**.

Differential Diagnosis

AG is very similar in appearance to other low-grade cortically based neoplasms in children/young adults who present with longstanding epilepsy. The major differential diagnoses include **dysembryoplastic neuroepithelial tumor (DNET)** as well as **ganglioglioma** and **oligodendroglioma**. All are more common than AG.

elected References

ligodendrogliomas and "Mixed" liomas

Oligodendroglioma

- Sankar T et al: Magnetic resonance imaging volumetric assessment of the extent of contrast enhancement and resection in oligodendroglial tumors. J Neurosurg. 116(6):1172-81, 2012
- Yip S et al: Concurrent CIC mutations, IDH mutations, and 1p/19q loss distinguish oligodendrogliomas from other cancers. J Pathol. 226(1):7-16, 2012
- Rodriguez FJ et al: Oligodendroglial tumors: diagnostic and molecular pathology. Semin Diagn Pathol. 27(2):136-45, 2010
- Larjavaara S et al: Incidence of gliomas by anatomic location. Neuro Oncol. 9(3):319-25, 2007
- Spampinato MV et al: Cerebral blood volume measurements and proton MR spectroscopy in grading of oligodendroglial tumors. AJR Am J Roentgenol. 188(1):204-12, 2007
- Jenkinson MD et al: Histological growth patterns and genotype in oligodendroglial tumours: correlation with MRI features. Brain. 129(Pt 7):1884-91, 2006
- Koeller KK et al: From the archives of the AFIP: Oligodendroglioma and its variants: radiologic-pathologic correlation. Radiographics. 25(6):1669-88, 2005
- Panageas KS et al: Initial treatment patterns over time for anaplastic oligodendroglial tumors. Neuro Oncol. 14(6):761-7, 2012

Anaplastic Oligodendroglioma

- Panageas KS et al: Initial treatment patterns over time for anaplastic oligodendroglial tumors. Neuro Oncol. 14(6):761-7, 2012
- Sankar T et al: Magnetic resonance imaging volumetric assessment of the extent of contrast enhancement and resection in oligodendroglial tumors. J Neurosurg. 116(6):1172-81, 2012
- Spampinato MV et al: Cerebral blood volume measurements and proton MR spectroscopy in grading of oligodendroglial tumors. AJR Am J Roentgenol. 188(1):204-12, 2007

Oligoastrocytomas

- Von Deimling A et al: Oligoastrocytoma and anaplastic oligoastrocytoma. In Louis DN et al: WHO Classification of Tumours of the Central Nervous System. Lyon, France: IARC Press. 60-5, 2007

Ependymal Tumors

Ependymoma

- Liu C et al: Developmental origins of brain tumors. Curr Opin Neurobiol. Epub ahead of print, 2012
- Pejavar S et al: Pediatric intracranial ependymoma: the roles of surgery, radiation and chemotherapy. J Neurooncol. 106(2):367-75, 2012
- McGuire CS et al: Incidence patterns for ependymoma: a surveillance, epidemiology, and end results study. J Neurosurg. 110(4):725-9, 2009
- Palm T et al: Expression profiling of ependymomas unravels localization and tumor grade-specific tumorigenesis. Cancer. 115(17):3955-68, 2009
- Yuh EL et al: Imaging of ependymomas: MRI and CT. Childs Nerv Syst. 25(10):1203-13, 2009

Anaplastic Ependymoma

- Phi JH et al: Pediatric infratentorial ependymoma: prognostic significance of anaplastic histology. J Neurooncol. 106(3):619-26, 2012

Subependymoma

- Ragel BT et al: Subependymomas: an analysis of clinical and imaging features. Neurosurgery. 58(5):881-90; discussion 881-90, 2006

Myxopapillary Ependymoma

- Chakraborti S et al: Primary myxopapillary ependymoma of the fourth ventricle with cartilaginous metaplasia: a case report and review of the literature. Brain Tumor Pathol. 29(1):25-30, 2012
- DiLuna ML et al: Primary myxopapillary ependymoma of the medulla: case report. Neurosurgery. 66(6):E1208-9; discussion E1209, 2010

Choroid Plexus Tumors

Choroid Plexus Papilloma

- Gozali AE et al: Choroid plexus tumors; management, outcome, and association with the Li-Fraumeni syndrome: the Children's Hospital Los Angeles (CHLA) experience, 1991-2010. Pediatr Blood Cancer. 58(6):905-9, 2012
- Ogiwara H et al: Choroid plexus tumors in pediatric patients. Br J Neurosurg. 26(1):32-7, 2012
- Lafay-Cousin L et al: Choroid plexus tumors in children less than 36 months: the Canadian Pediatric Brain Tumor Consortium (CPBTC) experience. Childs Nerv Syst. 27(2):259-64, 2011
- Severino M et al: Congenital tumors of the central nervous system. Neuroradiology. 52(6):531-48, 2010
- Hasselblatt M et al: TWIST-1 is overexpressed in neoplastic choroid plexus epithelial cells and promotes proliferation and invasion. Cancer Res. 69(6):2219-23, 2009
- Isaacs H: Fetal brain tumors: a review of 154 cases. Am J Perinatol. 26(6):453-66, 2009

- Frye RE et al: Choroid plexus papilloma expansion over 7 years in Aicardi syndrome. J Child Neurol. 22(4):484-7, 2007

Atypical Choroid Plexus Papilloma

- Ikota H et al: Clinicopathological and immunohistochemical study of 20 choroid plexus tumors: their histological diversity and the expression of markers useful for differentiation from metastatic cancer. Brain Tumor Pathol. 28(3):215-21, 2011
- Lee SH et al: Atypical choroid plexus papilloma in an adult. J Korean Neurosurg Soc. 46(1):74-6, 2009

Choroid Plexus Carcinoma

- Savage NM et al: The cytologic findings in choroid plexus carcinoma: report of a case with differential diagnosis. Diagn Cytopathol. 40(1):1-6, 2012
- Anselem O et al: Fetal tumors of the choroid plexus: is differential diagnosis between papilloma and carcinoma possible? Ultrasound Obstet Gynecol. 38(2):229-32, 2011
- Schittenhelm J et al: Atypical teratoid/rhabdoid tumors may show morphological and immunohistochemical features seen in choroid plexus tumors. Neuropathology. 31(5):461-7, 2011
- Tabori U et al: TP53 alterations determine clinical subgroups and survival of patients with choroid plexus tumors. J Clin Oncol. 28(12):1995-2001, 2010

Other Neuroepithelial Tumors

Astroblastoma

- Agarwal V et al: Cerebral astroblastoma: A case report and review of literature. Asian J Neurosurg. 7(2):98-100, 2012
- Bell JW et al: Neuroradiologic characteristics of astroblastoma. Neuroradiology. 49(3):203-9, 2007

Chordoid Glioma of the Third Ventricle

- Ni HC et al: Chordoid glioma of the third ventricle: Four cases including one case with papillary features. Neuropathology. Epub ahead of print, 2012
- Glastonbury CM et al: Masses and malformations of the third ventricle: normal anatomic relationships and differential diagnoses. Radiographics. 31(7):1889-905, 2011
- Wilson JL et al: Chordoid meningioma of the third ventricle: a case report and review of the literature. Clin Neuropathol. 30(2):70-4, 2011
- Desouza RM et al: Chordoid glioma: ten years of a low-grade tumor with high morbidity. Skull Base. 20(2):125-38, 2010

Angiocentric Glioma

- Koral K et al: Angiocentric glioma in a 4-year-old boy: imaging characteristics and review of the literature. Clin Imaging. 36(1):61-4, 2012
- Marburger T et al: Angiocentric glioma: a clinicopathologic review of 5 tumors with identification of associated cortical dysplasia. Arch Pathol Lab Med. 135(8):1037-41, 2011
- Mott RT et al: Angiocentric glioma: a case report and review of the literature. Diagn Cytopathol. 38(6):452-6, 2010
- Shakur SF et al: Angiocentric glioma: a case series. J Neurosurg Pediatr. 3(3):197-202, 2009
- Lellouch-Tubiana A et al: Angiocentric neuroepithelial tumor (ANET): a new epilepsy-related clinicopathological entity with distinctive MRI. Brain Pathol. 15(4):281-6, 2005

19

Neuronal and Glioneuronal Tumors

As previously discussed, neuroepithelial tumors are the largest group of CNS neoplasms. By definition, the term "neuroepithelial tumor" encompasses all neoplasms that are derived from glial cells, neurons, or their precursor stem cells.

Pure glial neoplasms—astrocytomas and the heterogeneous group of nonastrocytic gliomas—were considered in the preceding two chapters. We now turn our attention to the next major group of primary CNS neoplasms, i.e., neuroepithelial tumors with ganglion-like cells and/or differentiated neurocytes.

Pineal parenchymal tumors and embryonal tumors with poorly differentiated proliferating neuroblasts, the last two subgroups of neuroepithelial tumors, are discussed in chapters 20 and 21, respectively.

lioneuronal Tumors

The recognition of new low-grade gliomas that contain distinct neurocytic elements has broadened the spectrum of glioneuronal tumors. Glioneuronal tumors have varying morphologic patterns and biological behavior.

Glioneuronal tumors are less common than pure glial neoplasms, accounting for 0.5-2% of all primary brain tumors. As a group, glioneuronal neoplasms are often seizure-associated, less biologically aggressive than most glial tumors, and generally have a more favorable prognosis.

All tumors in the neuronal and mixed glioneuronal category are officially designated either WHO grade I or II. Some neuropathologists have identified a group of more aggressive glioneuronal tumors that morphologically resemble malignant gliomas but show immunohistochemical evidence of some neuronal differentiation; these have been provisionally assigned WHO grade III.

We begin this section by discussing histologically mixed tumors that display both neuronal and glial elements. One of these neoplasms (ganglioglioma) is among the most common tumors to cause epilepsy. We then briefly consider desmoplastic infantile tumors that have astrocytic and/or ganglion cell elements.

We next consider dysembryoplastic neuroepithelial tumor (DNET), a relatively new tumor that is now recognized as one of the more common causes of temporal lobe epilepsy. We conclude the section by discussing two tumors that were first included in the 2007 WHO classification: Rosette-forming glioneuronal tumor and papillary glioneuronal tumor.

Overview of Ganglion Cell Tumors

Ganglion cell tumors are well-differentiated neoplasms that contain mature but dysmorphic neurons. Most ganglion cell tumors are histologically mixed tumors that contain both ganglion cell and glial elements. These neoplasms are called **gangliogliomas**, which are WHO grade I or II neoplasms. More aggressive tumors (i.e., substantial mitotic activity, microvascular proliferation, occasional necrosis), called **anaplastic gangliomas**, have been provisionally assigned WHO grade III. WHO grade IV is not applied to ganglion cell tumors.

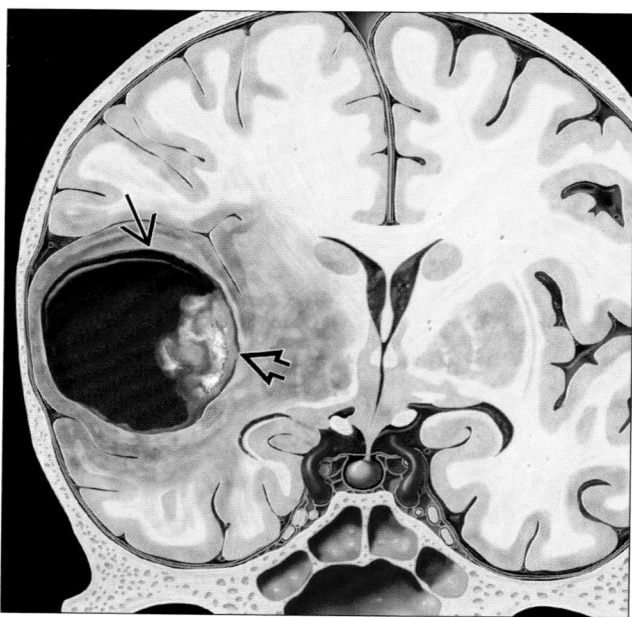

19-1. Coronal graphic depicts typical ganglioglioma of the temporal lobe with cyst ⇨, partially calcified mural nodule ⇨.

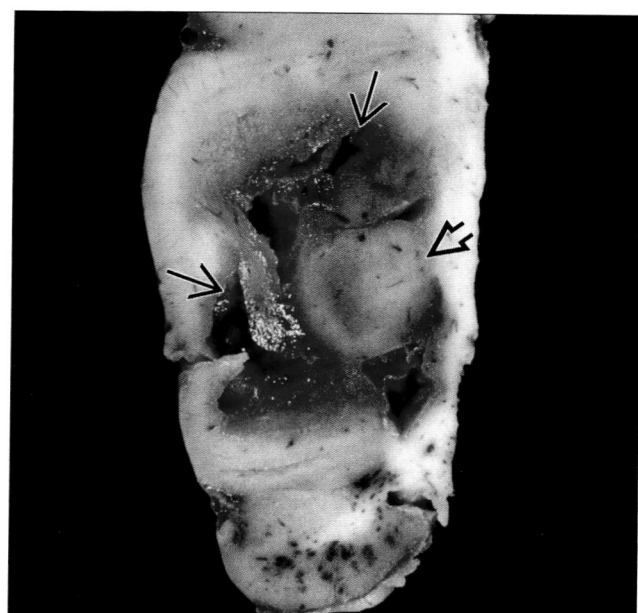

19-2. Partial temporal lobectomy specimen with ganglioglioma shows tumor nodule ⇨, partially collapsed cysts ⇨. Hemorrhage is primarily surgical. (Courtesy R. Hewlett, MD.)

Ganglion cell tumors that demonstrate *exclusive* ganglion cell composition are very rare. These neoplasms are designated as **gangliocytomas**. Gangliocytomas are all WHO grade I tumors.

We begin our discussion of ganglion cell tumors with ganglioglioma, which is the most common glioneuronal neoplasm in the CNS. They are also the most common cause of tumor-related temporal lobe epilepsy, accounting for 40% of all cases. As gangliocytomas are pure neuronal neoplasms, they are discussed in the following section.

Ganglioglioma

Terminology

Ganglioglioma (GG) is a well-differentiated, slow-growing tumor composed of dysplastic ganglion cells and neoplastic glial cells.

Etiology

GENERAL CONCEPTS. GGs probably arise from a malformative glioneuronal precursor lesion when the glial element undergoes neoplastic transformation. Some cases have been reported as arising from the dysplastic cortex.

GENETICS. Little is known about the molecular pathogenesis of GGs. Genomic imbalances with gains on chromosomes 7 and 12 and deletions of 22q in the neoplastic glial cells have been reported in up to two-thirds of all cases.

GG has been reported in Turcot syndrome as well as neurofibromatosis type 1 and neurofibromatosis type 2.

Pathology

LOCATION. GGs occur throughout the CNS, including the spinal cord. More than 75% arise in the temporal lobe **(19-1)**. The next most common site is the frontal lobe, the location for 10% of GGs.

Approximately 15% of GGs are found in the posterior fossa, usually either in the brainstem or cerebellum. A few GGs have been reported in the fourth ventricle and cerebellopontine angle. GGs also occur as intramedullary cord lesions.

SIZE AND NUMBER. GGs are solitary lesions that virtually never metastasize. They vary in size from one to six centimeters.

GROSS PATHOLOGY. GGs are superficially located, firm, grayish-tan neoplasms that often expand the cortex **(19-2)**. The most common appearance is that of a cyst with mural nodule or a solid tumor. Calcification is common, but gross hemorrhage and frank necrosis are rare. Extension into the adjacent subarachnoid space is common and does not indicate anaplasia.

MICROSCOPIC FEATURES. The histologic hallmark of GG is its combination of neuronal and glial elements, which can be mixed or geographically separated. Varying numbers of dysplastic neurons are intermixed with the glial component, which constitutes the proliferative and neoplastic element of the tumor. Astrocytic cells with

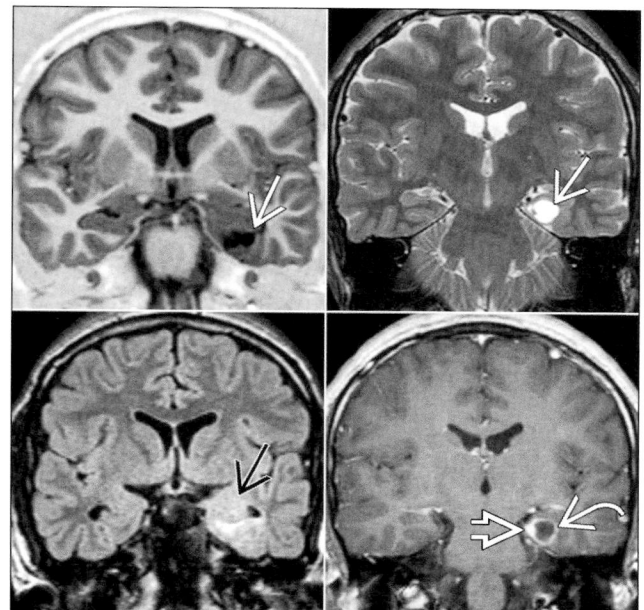

19-3. *Coronal MR scans in a 16-year-old boy with longstanding seizures shows a partially cystic, partially solid left temporal lobe mass* ➡ *with FLAIR hyperintensity* ➡, *nodule* ➡, *ring enhancement around cyst* ➡. *(Courtesy P. Rodriguez, MD.)*

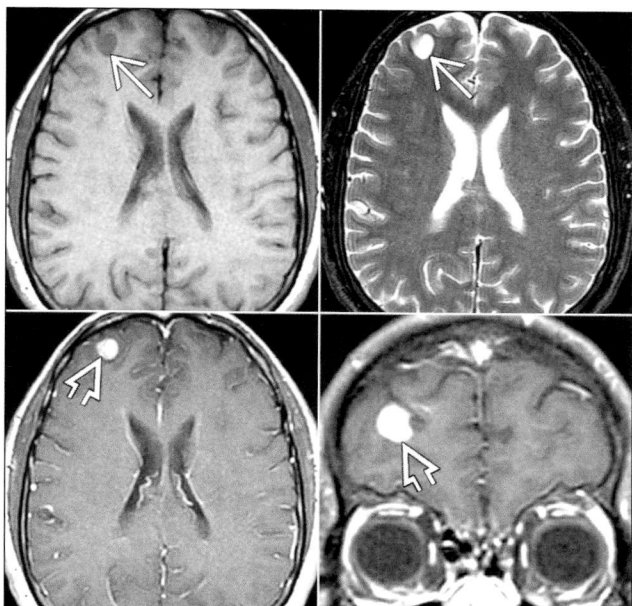

19-4. *Mostly solid T1 hypointense, T2 hyperintense frontal cortical/subcortical mass* ➡ *shows intense enhancement* ➡. *Ganglioglioma.*

pilocytic or fibrillary-like features are the most common glial element.

Mitotic figures are rare. MIB-1 reflects the proliferating glial component and varies from 1-3%.

Immunohistochemistry staining demonstrates both neuronal features (i.e., synaptophysin expression) and glial features (GFAP-positive cells). Approximately 75% of GGs exhibit immunoreactivity for the stem cell epitope CD34.

Malignant features in GGs are uncommon but—when present—almost invariably involve the glial component. Sarcomatous change occurs but is rare.

STAGING, GRADING, AND CLASSIFICATION. Gangliogliomas are generally benign, and most are designated as WHO grade I neoplasms. There are no established criteria to differentiate WHO grade I GGs from WHO grade II GGs.

Malignant transformation is rare. Very rarely, GGs with anaplastic features that correspond to WHO grade III have been reported.

inical Issues

EPIDEMIOLOGY. Ganglioglioma is the most common mixed glioneuronal tumor but causes just 1-1.5% of all primary brain tumors. GGs are more common in children and represent between 5-10% of pediatric CNS neoplasms.

DEMOGRAPHICS. GG is predominantly a tumor of children and young adults; 80% of patients are younger than 30 years. Peak presentation is 15-20 years. There is no gender predilection.

PRESENTATION. Chronic, pharmacologically resistant temporal lobe epilepsy (TLE) is present in 90% of cases. Seizures are generally the complex partial type.

NATURAL HISTORY. GGs are typically very slow-growing neoplasms. Malignant degeneration is uncommon, occurring in 1-5% of cases.

TREATMENT OPTIONS. Complete surgical resection is generally curative, with 80% of patients becoming seizure-free after tumor removal. The vast majority of patients experience a five-year recurrence-free survival.

Imaging

GENERAL FEATURES. GGs are cortically based superficial parenchymal lesions that have two general imaging patterns: (1) a partially cystic mass with mural nodule **(19-3)** or (2) a solid, relatively well-delineated tumor **(19-4)**. Diffusely infiltrating, poorly delineated GGs occur but are uncommon.

CT FINDINGS. GGs display varying attenuation on NECT. A cystic component is seen in nearly 60% of cases. Approximately 30% have a well-circumscribed hypodense cyst with isodense mural nodule while 40% are primarily hypodense. Between 30-50% of GGs calcify. Hemorrhage is rare.

Only 50% of GGs enhance following contrast administration. Patterns vary from solid, rim, or nodular to cystic with an enhancing nodule.

MR FINDINGS. Compared to cortex, GGs are hypo- to isointense on T1WI and hyperintense on T2/FLAIR. Surrounding edema is generally absent. Focal cortical dysplasia adjacent to the tumor occurs in some cases.

Enhancement varies from none or minimal to moderate but heterogeneous. The classic pattern is a cystic mass with an enhancing mural nodule. Homogeneous solid enhancement also occurs.

Differential Diagnosis

The major differential consideration is **low-grade fibrillary astrocytoma**. Note that low-grade diffusely infiltrating astrocytoma does not enhance. A supratentorial hemispheric **pilocytic astrocytoma** can present as a cyst with an enhancing nodule. Calcification in pilocytic astrocytoma is rare compared to GG.

Pleomorphic xanthoastrocytoma (PXA) often has a "cyst + mural nodule" and resembles GG. PXA often has a dural "tail," helping to distinguish it from other epilepsy-inducing cortical neoplasms.

Dysembryoplastic neuroepithelial tumor (DNET) is a superficial cortical neoplasm that typically has a multicystic "bubbly" appearance. A hyperintense rim surrounding the mass on FLAIR scan is common. In contrast to GG, enhancement is rare.

Oligodendroglioma is typically more diffuse and less well-delineated than GG. Oligodendrogliomas with a "cyst + mural nodule" configuration are uncommon. When they do occur, they are difficult to distinguish from GG on imaging studies alone.

CAUSES OF TEMPORAL LOBE EPILEPSY

Most common = mesial temporal sclerosis

Tumor-associated temporal lobe epilepsy
- Ganglioglioma (40%)
- DNET (20%)
- Diffuse low-grade astrocytoma (20%)
- Other (20%)
  - Pilocytic astrocytoma
  - Pleomorphic xanthoastrocytoma
  - Oligodendroglioma

Desmoplastic Infantile Astrocytoma/ Ganglioglioma

Terminology

Desmoplastic infantile tumors are rare, usually benign, mostly cystic lesions of young children that often have a radiologically aggressive appearance. Two histo-logic forms of desmoplastic infantile tumors have been described: Desmoplastic infantile astrocytoma (DIA) and desmoplastic infantile ganglioglioma (DIG). Because elements of both types are often present in a single lesion, the WHO considers DIA/DIG a single tumor entity.

Pathology

DIA/DIGs are large, bulky, supratentorial hemispheric masses with a median diameter approaching eight centimeters. They are sharply demarcated, mixed cystic-solid tumors that involve the superficial cortex and the adjacent leptomeninges, often appearing attached to the dura (19-5). The frontal and parietal lobes are the most common sites.

Microscopically, DIA/DIGs have three distinct components: Spindle cells in a "desmoplastic" stroma, plump astrocytes with glassy cytoplasm, and a variable neuronal component, usually clusters of undifferentiated neuronal or ganglion cells. Tumors without a ganglion cell component are termed "desmoplastic infantile astrocytoma."

Mitotic activity is rare. DIA/DIG is designated as a WHO grade I tumor.

Clinical Issues

DIA/DIGs occur in children under the age of five years, with a large majority presenting within the first year of life. Between 20-25% occur in children older than 24 months.

Increasing head circumference with tense bulging fontanelles in a lethargic infant with "sunset eyes" is the typical presentation.

Most intracranial neoplasms that present in infants and neonates are associated with poor outcome. In contrast, DIG/DIA has a benign prognosis and very rarely metastasizes. Gross total resection generally results in long-term survival. Some DIA/DIGs even regress spontaneously after partial debulking.

Approximately 15% of children with DIG/DIA develop leptomeningeal spread and die.

Imaging

Imaging discloses a massive, heterogeneous, mixed cystic-solid supratentorial mass. The cystic portion is usually located deep inside the hemispheric white matter whereas the solid portion is typically peripheral, often directly abutting the dura.

CT shows a cystic hypoattenuating portion with a mixed-density solid component. Calcification has been reported in a few cases but is uncommon. Hemorrhage, necrosis, and peritumoral edema are rare.

MR shows a large, often multilobulated or septated cystic mass with a solid plaque-like dura-based component. The solid mass enhances strongly but often heterogeneously (**19-6**). Adjacent dural thickening ("dural tail" sign) is common. Approximately 25% of cases show at least some cyst wall enhancement.

ifferential Diagnosis

The most common overall cause of a large, bulky, heterogeneous hemispheric mass in an infant is **teratoma**. Teratoma is much more heterogeneous appearing than DIA/DIG and often extends extracranially. **Primitive neuroectodermal tumor** (PNET) is another common congenital brain neoplasm. Teratomatous and PNET-related cysts are rarely as large as those of DIA/DIG, and their solid portions generally do not abut the dura.

Supratentorial ependymoma often calcifies, hemorrhages, and typically occurs in older children and adults.

NET

Ganglioglioma and dysembryoplastic neuroepithelial tumor (DNET or DNT) are the two most common long-term epilepsy-associated tumors. DNET was originally identified in the surgical specimens from young patients with medically refractory epilepsy. It was officially recognized as a distinct tumor entity in 1993 and included in the category of "neuronal and mixed neuronal-glial tumors."

erminology

DNET is a benign, usually cortically based lesion characterized by a multinodular architecture (**19-7**). Because DNET is often associated with cortical dysplasia, some neuropathologists believe it may be a congenital malformation rather than a true neoplastic lesion.

iology

The precise etiology of DNET is unknown. To date, no specific deletions or gene mutations have been detected. DNETs often express stem cell markers such as CD34, suggesting a possible developmental origin.

athology

LOCATION. Between 45-50% of DNETs are located in the temporal lobe; one-third occur in the frontal lobe. While most are found in the cortex, the white matter may be affected. Rare cases have been reported in other sites such as the lateral ventricle, and an unusual "diffuse" form of DNET has been described.

SIZE AND NUMBER. DNETs are generally solitary lesions although several cases with multiple tumor "microfoci" have been reported (**19-11**). DNETs vary in size from mil-

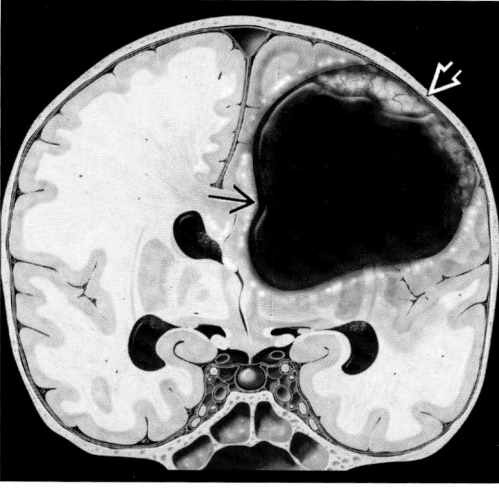

19-5. Graphic depicts desmoplastic infantile astrocytoma/ganglioma with large mixed cystic ➡, solid ➡ component abutting the dura.

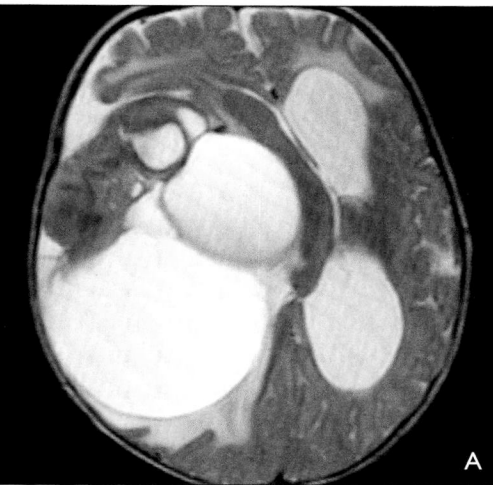

19-6A. T2WI in a 10-month-old infant shows obstructive hydrocephalus and a huge mixed cystic, solid mass in the right cerebral hemisphere.

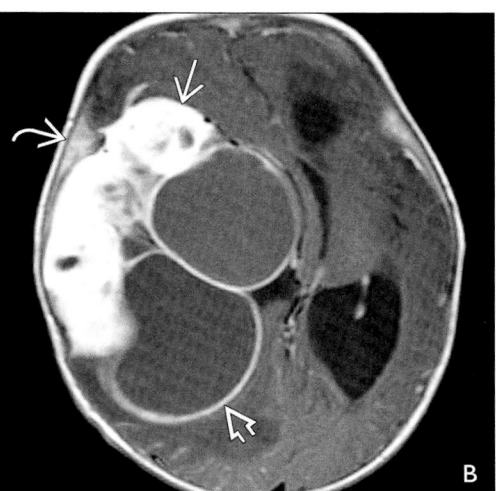

19-6B. T1 C+ shows the solid mass abuts, thickens the dura-arachnoid ➡ and enhances intensely ➡, as do the cyst walls ➡. DIA.

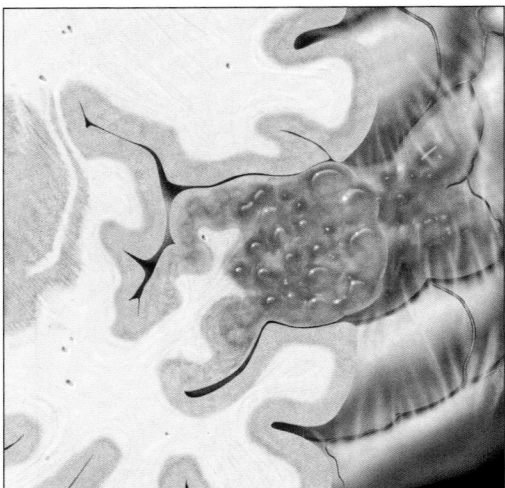

19-7. Graphic depicts DNET with multicystic, multinodular components.

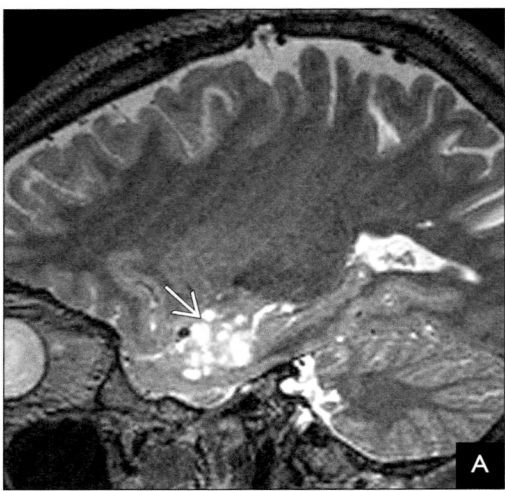

19-8A. Sagittal T2WI shows a "bubbly" temporal lobe mass ➡.

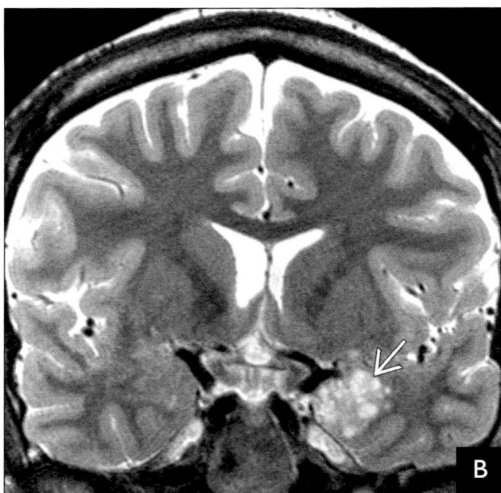

19-8B. Coronal T2WI in the same patient shows a cortically based, "bubbly" mass with the typical appearance of a DNET ➡.

limeters to several centimeters. A few tumors that involve a large portion of the affected lobe have been reported.

GROSS PATHOLOGY. DNETs are intracortical tumors that thicken and expand the gyri. The glioneuronal component often has a viscous consistency together with single or multiple firmer nodules **(19-9)**.

MICROSCOPIC FEATURES. The histologic hallmark of DNET is its "specific glioneuronal element" (SGNE). "Simple" DNETs consist of the SGNE and nodular areas. A multinodular architecture with columns or nodules of bundled axons oriented perpendicularly to the cortex and lined by oligodendrocyte-like cells is characteristic. Neurons appear to float in a pale, mucinous-appearing matrix adjacent to these columns. Cytologic atypia and mitoses are rare.

"Complex" DNETs have additional features, including cortical dysplasia. The adjacent cortex is dysplastic in nearly 80% of DNETs.

STAGING, GRADING, AND CLASSIFICATION. DNETs are WHO grade I neoplasms.

Clinical Issues

DNET is a tumor of children and young adults. The vast majority of patients present before age 20 years, typically with pharmacologically resistant partial complex seizures. While DNETs account for only 1% of all neuroepithelial tumors, they are second only to ganglioglioma as a cause of temporal lobe epilepsy.

DNETs show little or no growth over time. Malignant transformation is extremely rare.

Even simple lesionectomy is generally successful. Because cortical dysplasia is frequently associated with DNET, however, a more aggressive resection is advocated by many epilepsy surgeons. Removing epileptogenically active areas around the tumor increases seizure-free outcome.

Long-term clinical follow-up usually demonstrates no tumor recurrence, even in patients with subtotal resection.

Imaging

GENERAL FEATURES. DNET has a distinct appearance on neuroimaging studies. A well-demarcated, triangular, "pseudocystic" or "bubbly" cortical/subcortical mass in a young patient with longstanding complex partial epilepsy is highly suggestive of the diagnosis **(19-8)**.

CT FINDINGS. NECT scans disclose a hypodense cortical/subcortical mass. Calcification is seen in 20% of cases. Gross intratumoral hemorrhage is rare. Focal bony scalloping or calvarial remodeling is common with tumors adjacent to the inner table of the skull.

MR Findings. A multilobulated, hypointense, "bubbly" cortical mass that may involve the subcortical white matter is seen on T1WI. DNETs are strikingly hyperintense on T2WI with a multicystic or septated appearance **(19-10)**, **(19-11)**.

DNETs are hyperintense compared to normal cortex on FLAIR scans. A characteristic, even more hyperintense rim along the tumor periphery is present in 75% of cases. Peritumoral edema is absent.

"Blooming" on T2* (GRE, SWI) occurs in a few cases, more likely related to calcification than to hemorrhage.

DNETs generally show little or no enhancement on T1WI C+. When present, enhancement is generally limited to a mild nodular or punctate pattern.

MRS shows decreased NAA without elevated Cho or Cho:Cr ratio.

ifferential Diagnosis

The main imaging differential diagnoses are **focal cortical dysplasia** and **ganglioglioma**. The "bubbly" appear-

ance of DNET and FLAIR hyperintense rims are helpful distinguishing features. The rare **angiocentric glioma** closely resembles DNET on imaging, but a hyperintense rim is seen on T1WI rather than FLAIR.

DNET

Pathology
• Benign (WHO grade I)
• Rare (< 1% of all neuroepithelial tumors)
• Temporal lobe most common site
• Multinodular architecture
• Frequently associated with cortical dysplasia

Clinical Issues
• Patients < 20 years
  ∘ Complex partial epilepsy
  ∘ Second most common tumor-associated TLE
• Grows slowly, surgery usually curative

Imaging
• Wedge-shaped cortical/subcortical mass
• "Points" toward ventricle
• Multicystic/septated "bubbly" appearance
  ∘ Hyperintense on T2WI
  ∘ Rim of hyperintensity on FLAIR
  ∘ Edema absent
  ∘ Usually doesn't enhance

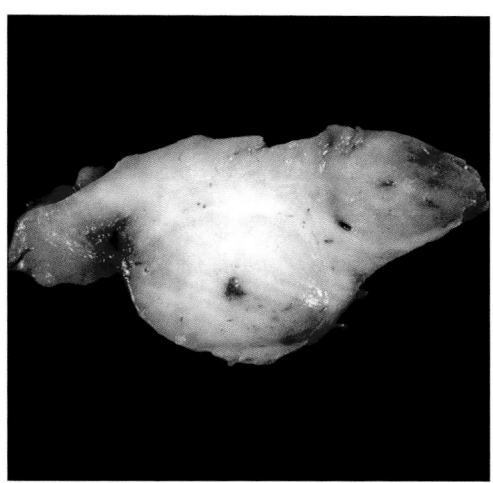

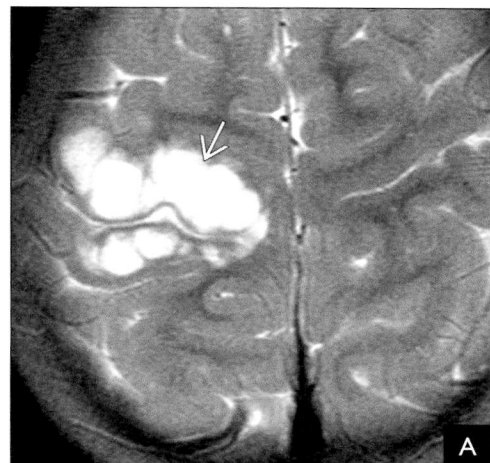

19-9. Resected surgical specimen shows the typical nodular, somewhat "mucinous" cysts of DNET. (Courtesy R. Hewlett, MD.) 19-10A. Axial T2WI shows expanded cortex with very hyperintense cysts ➡.

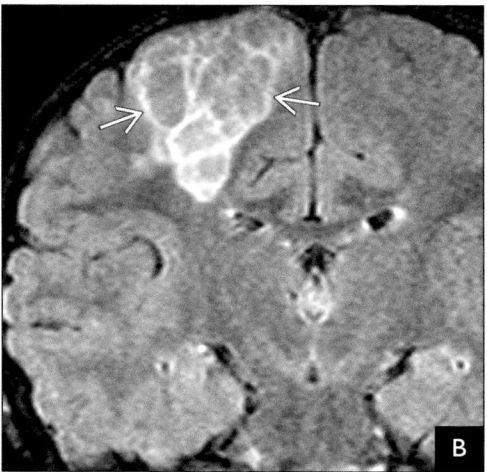

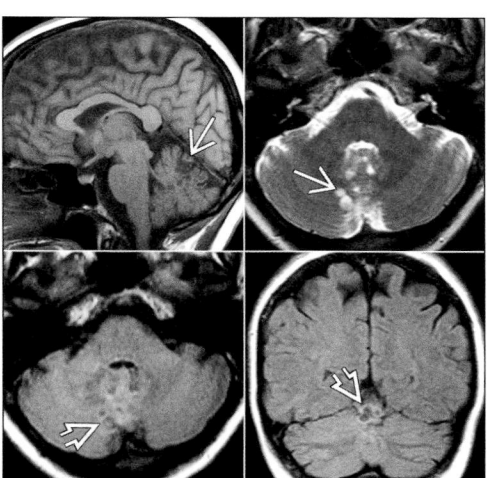

19-10B. FLAIR shows that the well-demarcated mass involves both cortex, subcortical white matter. Hyperintense rim ➡ is characteristic. (Courtesy L. Loevner, MD.) 19-11. Variant case of DNET shows diffuse vermian mass with multiple scattered cysts ➡. The FLAIR hyperintense rims around the cysts ➡ are highly suggestive of the diagnosis.

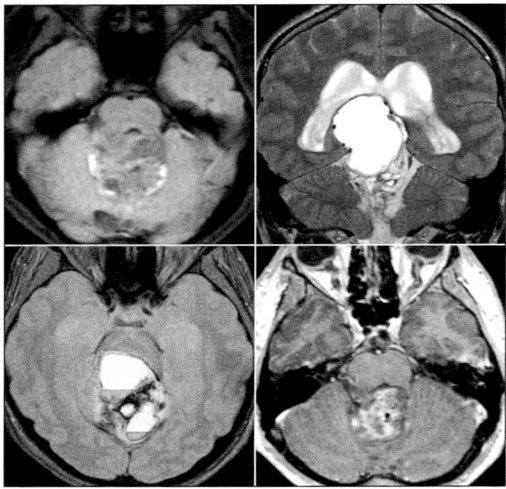

19-12. RGNT is a very heterogeneous tumor with cysts, hemorrhage, fluid-fluid levels, patchy enhancement. (Courtesy M. Thurnher, MD.)

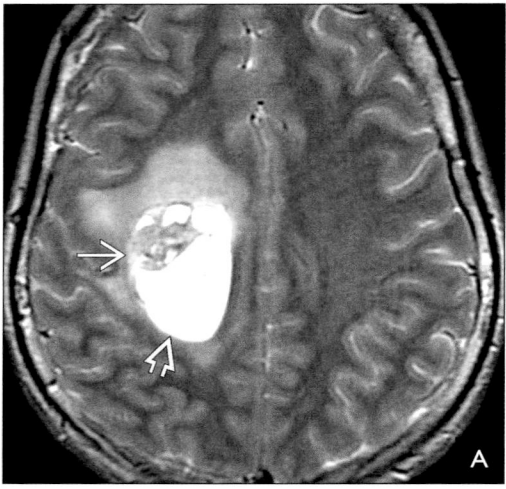

19-13A. T2WI of PGNT shows well-circumscribed cystic ➨ mass with mural nodule ➨ in the right hemisphere. (Courtesy F. J. Rodriguez, MD.)

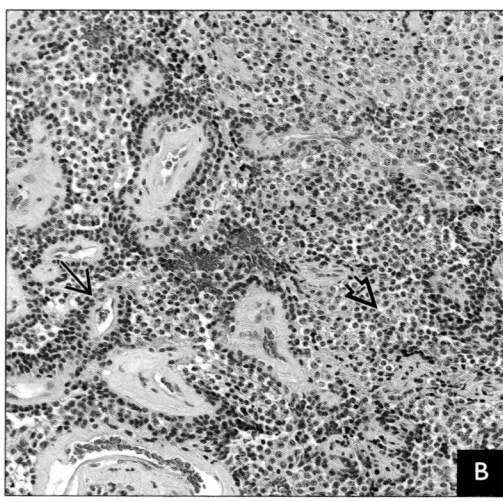

19-13B. Classic PGNT with dual population of glial perivascular layer ➨, round interpapillary neurocytes ➨. (Courtesy F. J. Rodriguez, MD.)

Rosette-Forming Glioneuronal Tumor

Rosette-forming glioneuronal tumor (RGNT) is a rare, slow-growing tumor of young and middle-aged adults that was first officially recognized in 2007. Mean age at diagnosis is 33 years. Typical presenting symptoms are headache and ataxia.

RGNTs are generally infratentorial lesions. The most common—but by no means the only—location is the fourth ventricle and/or cerebellar vermis. Size varies from one or two centimeters to large bulky tumors that occasionally exceed four centimeters in diameter.

The pathologic hallmark of RGNT is its biphasic histology with both neurocytic and astrocytic elements forming neurocytic perivascular pseudorosettes. MIB-1 labeling index is low. Local invasion and CSF dissemination are rare. RGNTs are WHO grade I neoplasms.

The imaging appearance of a classic RGNT is more ominous than its benign pathology and biological behavior would indicate. A heterogeneous-appearing mass centered within the fourth ventricle or vermis is the typical finding (19-12). A multicystic appearance with hemorrhage, blood-fluid levels, and calcification is common. Enhancement varies from none to inhomogeneous.

The differential diagnosis of RGNT is limited. **Metastasis** is always a consideration but rare in young adults. Primary infratentorial midline neoplasms in this age group are uncommon. **Ependymoma** with cysts and hemorrhage may resemble RGNT. **Pilocytic astrocytoma** is generally found in younger patients and rarely hemorrhages. **Choroid plexus papilloma** does occur in the fourth ventricle in adults but its intense contrast enhancement and distinctive frond-like papillary architecture help distinguish it from RGNT.

Papillary Glioneuronal Tumor

Initially considered a ganglioglioma variant, papillary glioneuronal tumor (PGNT) was recognized in 2007 as a distinct entity. It is a rare, relatively well-circumscribed, clinically indolent tumor of the cerebral hemispheres.

Similar to RGNTs, PGNTs are biphasic tumors with both astrocytic and neuronal elements. The distinguishing feature of PGNT is the presence of hyalinized vascular pseudopapillae. To date, PGNT has not been formally assigned a tumor grade, but its indolent behavior is characteristic of a grade I neoplasm.

Imaging findings in PGNT are nonspecific. A cyst with enhancing nodule is the most common reported appearance (19-13). The major differential diagnosis is ganglioglioma, which has a virtually identical imaging appearance to PGNT.

euronal Tumors

As a group, tumors that exhibit exclusive ganglion cell or neurocytic differentiation account for just 0.5-1% of all primary brain tumors. Two general categories of neuronal tumors are recognized: Gangliocytoma and neurocytoma.

angliocytoma Overview

Gangliocytomas are composed exclusively of ganglion cells. Gangliocytomas may appear more malformative (hamartomatous) than truly neoplastic and are often associated with adjacent cortical dysplasia. Supratentorial hemispheric gangliocytomas are very rare and are known simply as **gangliocytomas.**

Cerebellar gangliocytomas are more common. Also called "dysplastic cerebellar gangliocytoma," they are better known as **Lhermitte-Duclos disease** (LDD).

Gangliocytoma

Terminology

Gangliocytoma (GCyt) is a benign, well-circumscribed neoplasm that contains only differentiated ganglion cells. No glial component is present.

Etiology

The etiology of GCyt is unknown although it is considered a developmental tumor.

Pathology

LOCATION. Although they can occur anywhere, nearly three-quarters of supratentorial GCyts occur in the temporal lobe. Other reported sites include the brainstem, sellar region, and spinal cord.

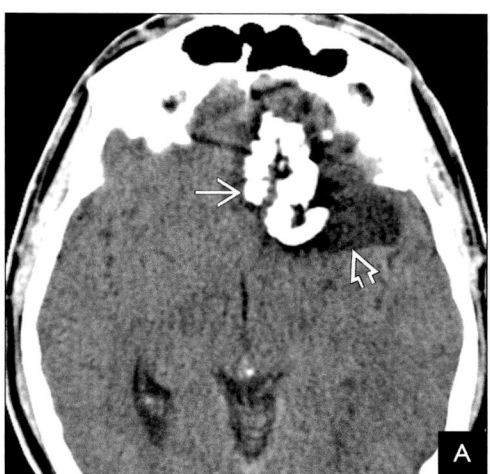
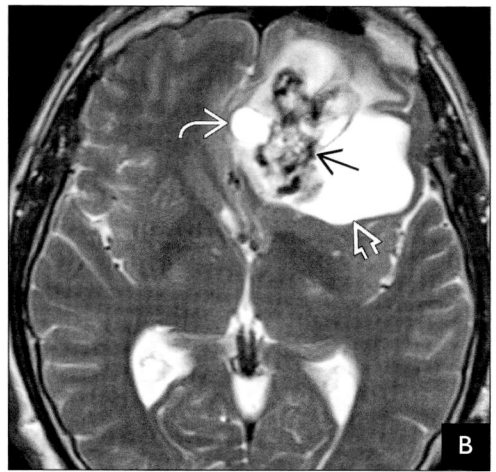

19-14A. NECT scan in a 29-year-old man with seizures shows a partially calcified ➡, partially cystic ➡ left frontal lobe mass. 19-14B. T2WI in the same patient shows that the partially calcified solid portion of the mass ➡ has very heterogeneous signal intensity. A large cyst ➡ and a smaller one ➡ are associated with the mass. Edema is minimal considering the large size of the tumor.

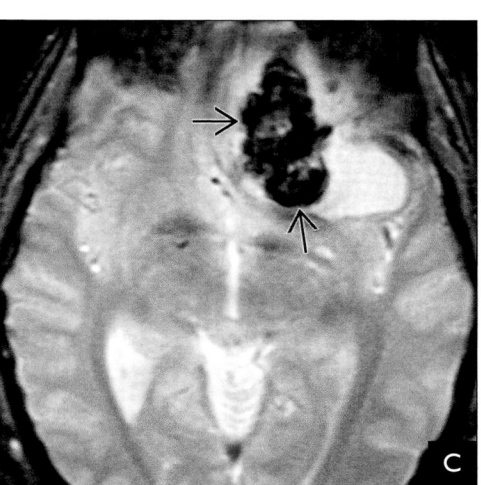
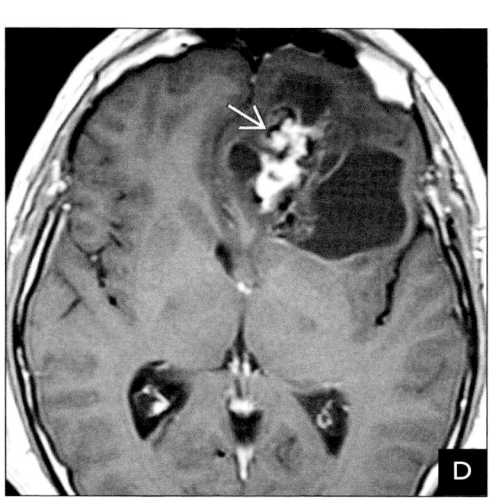

19-14C. T2* GRE shows that the densely calcified solid portion "blooms" ➡. 19-14D. The tumor nodule shows mild patchy enhancement ➡. Preoperative diagnosis was ganglioglioma. Pathologically proven gangliocytoma. (Courtesy N. Agarwal, MD.)

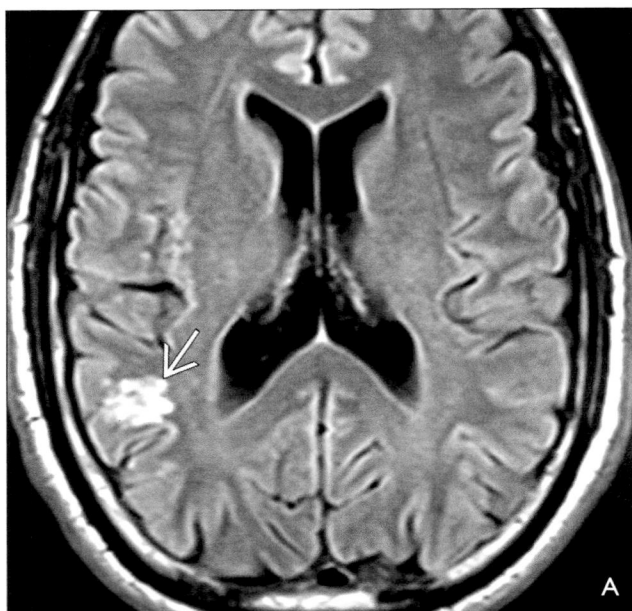

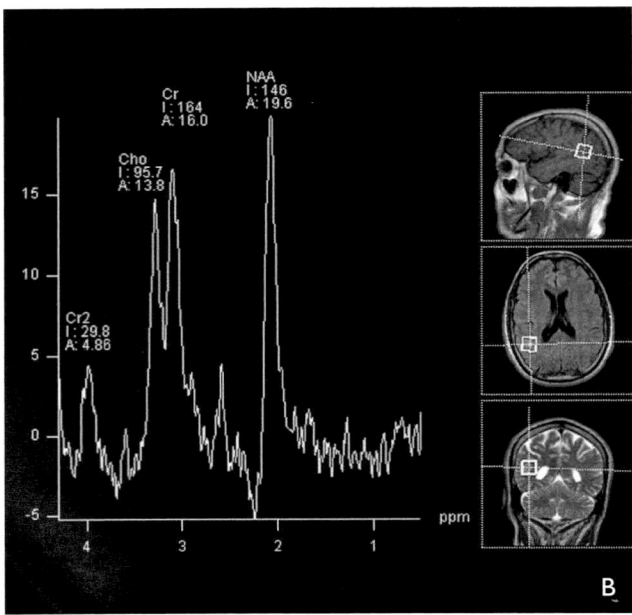

19-15A. FLAIR scan in a 55-year-old man with longstanding seizures shows a well-demarcated cortical/subcortical hyperintense lesion in the right parietal lobe ➔. The lesion did not enhance on T1 C+ (not shown).

19-15B. MRS shows normal-appearing metabolites. Gangliocytoma was diagnosed at histopathology.

GROSS AND MICROSCOPIC FEATURES. GCyts can be solid or mixed solid and cystic lesions. Microscopically, GCyts consist of bizarre-appearing mature ganglion cells. Mitoses are few or absent. Immunoreactivity to CD34, a stem cell marker, is positive in the majority of gangliocytomas.

GCyts are WHO grade I neoplasms.

Clinical Issues

GCyt occurs most frequently in children and young adults under the age of 30 years. Most patients present with pharmacoresistent epilepsy.

GCyts grow slowly, if at all. Surgical resection is generally curative and results in long-term progression-free survival.

Imaging

GCyts are mixed density on NECT, often containing both cystic and solid components **(19-14)**. Calcification is common, occurring in about one-third of cases. Hemorrhage and necrosis are absent.

GCyts are hypo- to isointense relative to cortex on T1WI and hyperintense on T2/FLAIR **(19-15)**. Enhancement varies from none to striking homogeneous enhancement in the solid portions of the tumor.

Differential Diagnosis

The major differential diagnosis of gangliocytoma is **ganglioglioma**. Gangliogliomas are often cortical,

epilepsy-inducing tumors with both a cystic and enhancing solid component. Ganglioglioma may be indistinguishable from GCyt on imaging studies. **Cortical dysplasia**, another common cause of refractory epilepsy in young patients, follows gray matter on all sequences and does not enhance.

Dysplastic Cerebellar Gangliocytoma

Terminology

Dysplastic cerebellar gangliocytoma is a rare benign cerebellar mass composed of dysplastic ganglion cells. Dysplastic cerebellar gangliocytoma is also known as **Lhermitte-Duclos disease** (LDD). Other terms for LDD include granular cell hypertrophy, granulomolecular hypertrophy of the cerebellum, cerebellar hamartoma, diffuse ganglioneuroma or gangliomatosis of the cerebellum.

LDD may occur as part of the multiple hamartoma syndrome called **Cowden syndrome** (CS). When LDD and CS occur together, they are sometimes called Cowden-Lhermitte-Duclos or **COLD syndrome**. CS is also known as **multiple hamartoma-neoplasia syndrome** or **PTEN hamartoma tumor syndrome**.

CS is an autosomal dominant phacomatosis. The vast majority of patients have hamartomatous neoplasms of the skin combined with neoplasms and hamartomas of multiple other organs. Breast, thyroid, endometrium, and gastrointestinal cancers are the most prevalent other neoplasms in CS.

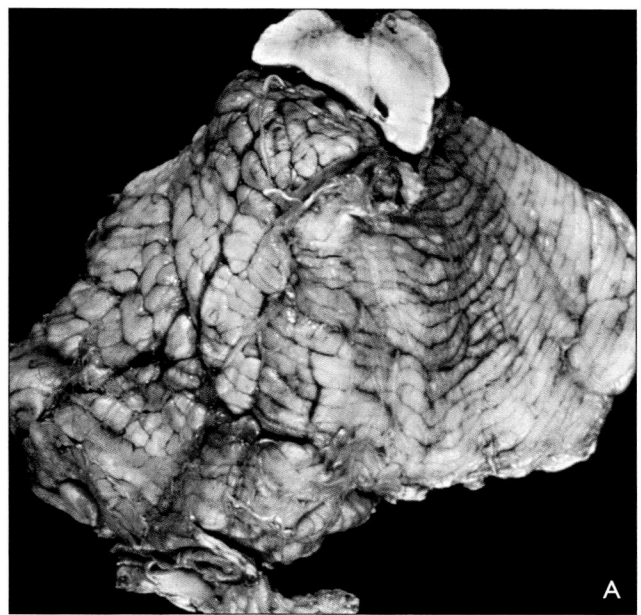

19-16A. *Autopsy specimen shows dysplastic cerebellar gangliocytoma expanding the cerebellar hemisphere.*

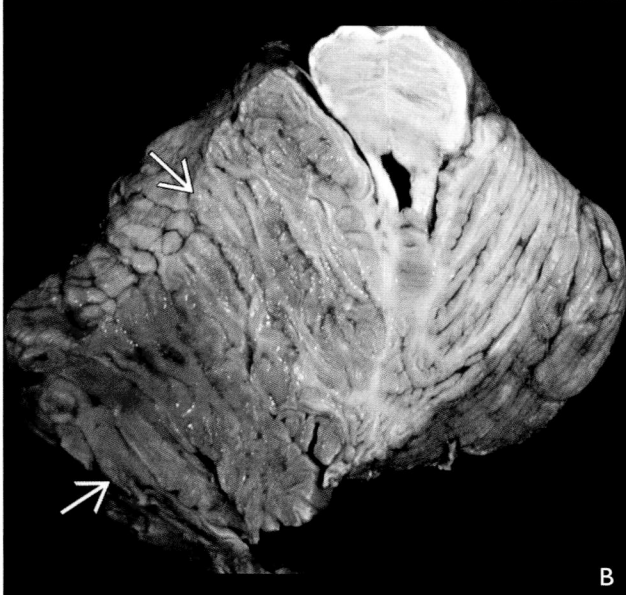

19-16B. *Cut section through the mass shows grossly thickened cerebellar folia* ➡. *(Courtesy AFIP Archives.)*

iology

GENERAL CONCEPTS. Whether LDD constitutes a neoplastic, malformative, or hamartomatous lesion is debated. The majority of LDD cases are sporadic, but the association of LDD with Cowden syndrome favors a hamartomatous origin.

Approximately 40% of dysplastic cerebellar gangliocytomas occur as part of CS.

GENETICS. Cowden syndrome is caused by a *PTEN* germline mutation that results in cellular proliferation of ectodermal, mesodermal, and endodermal tissues. CS is characterized by multiple hamartomas and malignant neoplasms.

thology

LOCATION. LDD is always infratentorial, usually involving the cerebellar hemisphere or the vermis. Large lesions involve both. The brainstem is a rare site for LDD.

SIZE AND NUMBER. Dysplastic cerebellar gangliocytomas often become very large, displacing the fourth ventricle and causing obstructive hydrocephalus. The vast majority are unilateral, although a few cases of LDD with bilateral lesions of the cerebellar hemispheres have been reported.

GROSS PATHOLOGY. The gross appearance of LDD is a tumor-like mass that expands and replaces the normal cerebellar architecture **(19-16)**. On cut section, the cere-

bellar folia are markedly widened and have a grossly "gyriform" appearance **(19-17)**.

MICROSCOPIC FEATURES. LDD is characterized by marked disruption of the normal cerebellar cortical layers. Diffuse hypertrophy of the granular cell layer with absence of the Purkinje layer of the cerebellum is typical **(19-18)**. Progressive hypertrophy of the granular cell neurons with increased myelination of their axons in an expanded molecular layer is also characteristic. Mitoses and necrosis are absent.

STAGING, GRADING, AND CLASSIFICATION. Although LDD is probably a hamartoma and not a true neoplasm, it is designated as WHO grade I.

Clinical Issues

EPIDEMIOLOGY. The prevalence of LDD is unknown. The incidence of Cowden syndrome with *PTEN* mutation is estimated at 1 in 250,000.

DEMOGRAPHICS. LDD occurs in all age groups, but most cases occur in adults between 20-40 years. The average age at diagnosis is 34 years. There is no gender predilection.

PRESENTATION. Patients may be asymptomatic or present with symptoms of increased intracranial pressure such as headache, nausea, and vomiting. Cranial nerve palsies, gait disturbance, and visual abnormalities are also common.

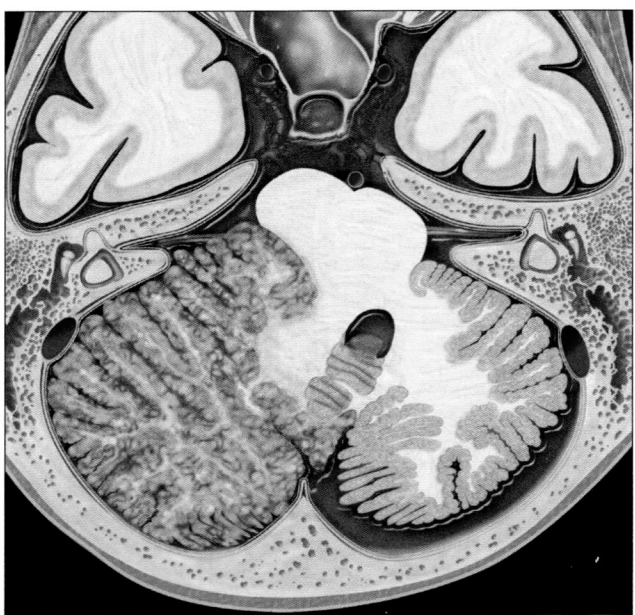

19-17. Graphic depicts dysplastic cerebellar gangliocytoma (Lhermitte-Duclos disease).

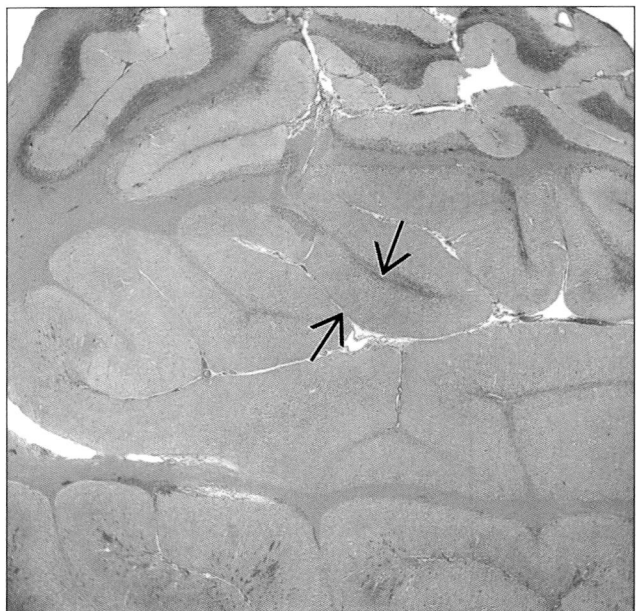

19-18. Folia expansion in LDD is best appreciated at low magnification, a view in which the thickness of the affected cerebellar cortex ➔, loss of dark-staining internal granule cells are readily apparent. (Courtesy F. J. Rodriguez, MD.)

NATURAL HISTORY. LDD enlarges very slowly over many years. No cases of metastatic spread or CSF dissemination have been reported.

TREATMENT OPTIONS. Shunting or surgical debulking are options for symptomatic patients with hydrocephalus. Because LDD is not encapsulated and blends gradually into normal cerebellar tissues, complete resection is difficult and the complication rate is high.

Imaging

GENERAL FEATURES. A nonenhancing unilateral cerebellar mass in a middle-aged patient that demonstrates a prominent "tiger stripe" pattern on MR is typical of LDD.

CT FINDINGS. Most cases of LDD are hypodense on NECT scans. Mass effect with compression of the fourth ventricle, effacement of the cerebellopontine angle cisterns, and obstructive hydrocephalus are common. Calcification is rare. Necrosis and hemorrhage are absent. CECT generally shows no appreciable enhancement.

LDD is moderately hypermetabolic on FDG PET/CT scans.

MR FINDINGS. An expansile cerebellar mass with linear hypointense bands on T1WI is typical. T2WI shows the pathognomonic "tiger stripe" pattern of alternating inner hyperintense and outer hypointense layers in enlarged cerebellar folia **(19-19)**.

T2* (GRE, SWI) demonstrates prominent venous channels surrounding the grossly thickened folia. T1 C+

shows striking linear enhancement of these abnormal veins.

DWI may show restricted diffusion, probably reflecting the hypercellularity and increased axonal density characteristic of LDD. PWI shows increased rCBV, reflecting the prominent enlarged interfolial veins, not malignancy.

MRS shows normal or slightly reduced NAA and normal Cho:Cr ratios. A lactate doublet may be present.

Differential Diagnosis

Imaging findings of LDD are so characteristic that the diagnosis can usually be established without biopsy confirmation. While the suggested differential diagnosis has sometimes included medulloblastoma and subacute cerebellar infarction, generally these should not be confused with LDD.

Medulloblastoma, especially the desmoplastic variant, may present as a lateral cerebellar mass but usually occurs in younger patients and rarely displays the "tiger stripes" so characteristic of LDD. **Cerebellar infarction** is confined to a specific vascular territory, and symptom onset is acute or subacute rather than chronic.

Occasionally **ganglioglioma** occurs in the posterior fossa and may mimic LDD. Gangliogliomas typically enhance and, although sometimes bizarre-appearing, rarely demonstrate prominent "tiger stripes."

A few rare **cerebellar cortical dysplasias** can mimic LDD. However, these malformations do not demonstrate

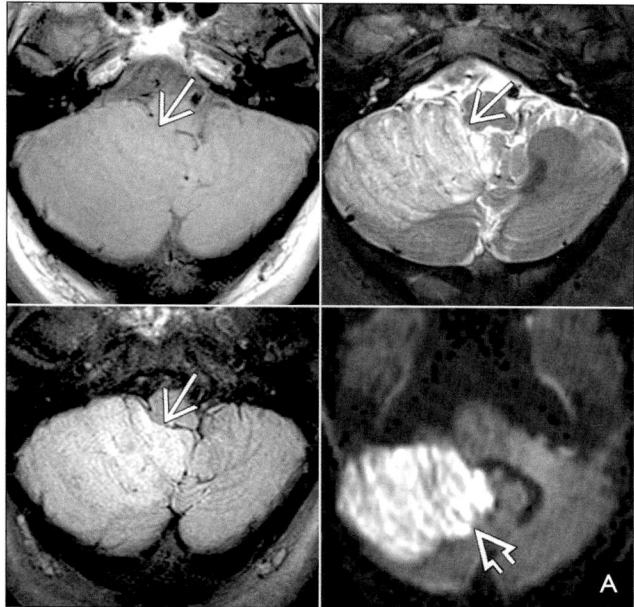

19-19A. *Series of MR images in a patient with LDD shows typical findings of thickened cerebellar folia, mass effect* ➡. *LDD is cellular, may show restricted diffusion* ➡.

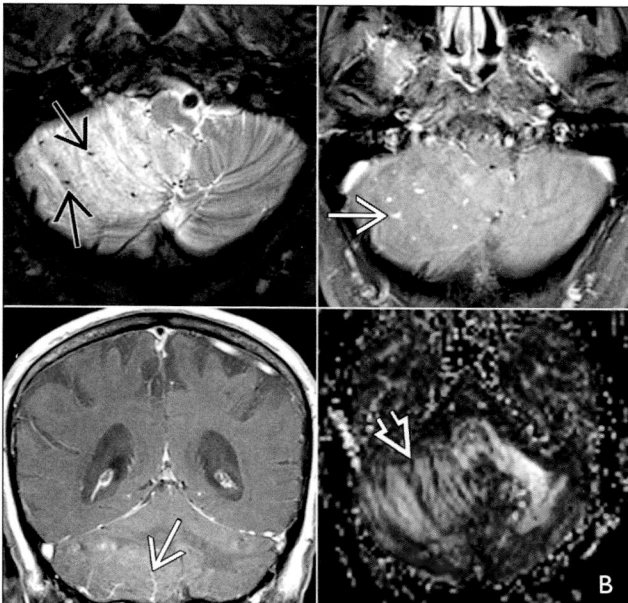

19-19B. *Additional images show numerous "flow voids"* ➡ *caused by enlarged veins that enhance on T1 C+* ➡. *DTI shows anterior-posterior orientation of the cerebellar folia* ➡.

progressive enlargement and rarely cause mass effect with hydrocephalus.

A few cases of posterior fossa **tuberous sclerosis complex** (TSC) that mimic LDD have been reported. However, these patients are generally younger and have other stigmata of TSC.

CEREBRAL GANGLIOCYTOMAS

Gangliocytoma
- Pathology
  - Rare tumor composed of differentiated ganglion cells
  - Temporal lobe (75%)
  - WHO grade I
- Clinical Issues
  - Most patients < 30 years
  - Epilepsy
- Imaging
  - "Cyst + nodule" or solid
  - No hemorrhage, necrosis
  - Ca++ frequent, enhancement variable

Dysplastic Cerebellar Gangliocytoma
- Terminology
  - Lhermitte-Duclos disease (LDD)
  - LDD + multiple hamartomas = Cowden disease (COLD)
- Pathology
  - Enlarged, thick "gyriform" cerebellar folia
  - Hypertrophied granular layer, absent Purkinje
  - WHO grade I
- Imaging
  - Mass with laminated, "tiger stripe" appearance
  - Linear enhancement of veins around thickened folia

Central Neurocytoma

An unusual benign-acting intraventricular neoplasm of young adults, originally thought to be an oligodendroglioma subtype, is now recognized as a tumor of neuronal lineage and has been given the name **central neurocytoma**. Similar-appearing neoplasms in the brain parenchyma are less common and are termed **extraventricular neurocytoma**. In this section we consider both these benign neurocytic neoplasms.

Terminology

Central neurocytoma (CNC) is a well-differentiated neuroepithelial tumor with mature neurocytic elements.

Etiology

The precise origin of CNCs is unknown. Bipotential precursor cells of the periventricular germinal matrix are capable of both neuronal and glial differentiation and may be the etiology of these unusual neoplasms. The 1p,19q codeletions characteristic of oligodendroglioma are absent.

Pathology

LOCATION. CNCs are tumors of the lateral ventricle body, usually attached to the septi pellucidi and arising near the foramen of Monro **(19-20)**.

SIZE AND NUMBER. CNCs vary in size from small to huge and extending through the foramen of Monro to involve the contralateral ventricle.

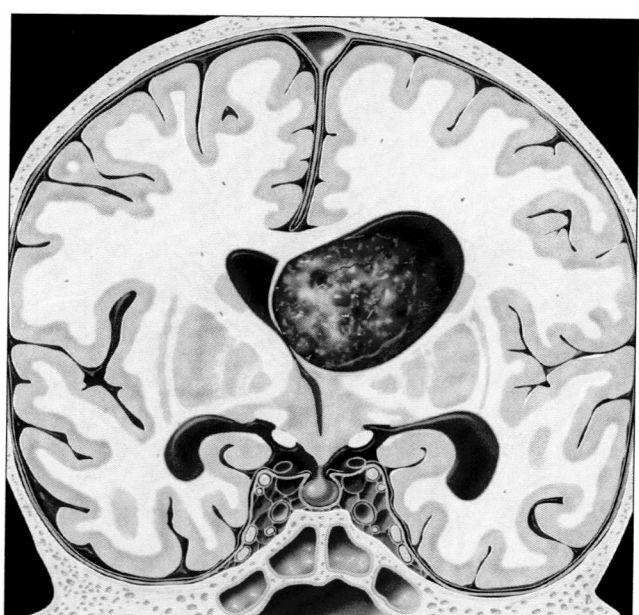

19-20. Coronal graphic depicts central neurocytoma as a multicystic, relatively vascular, occasionally hemorrhagic mass in the body of the lateral ventricle.

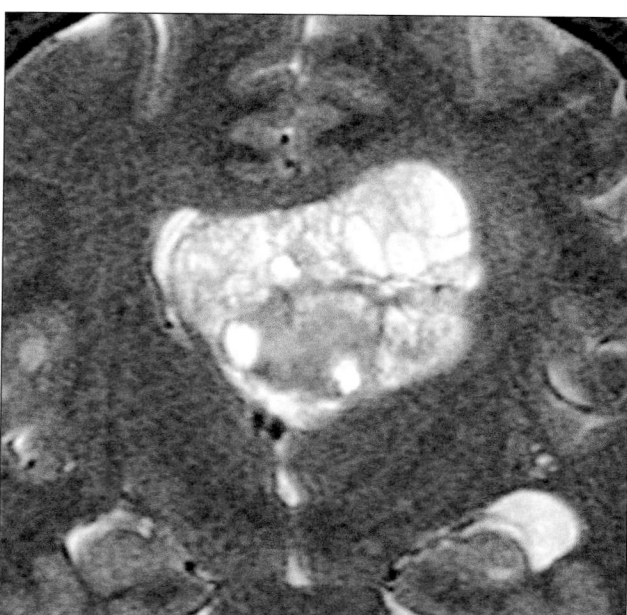

19-21. Coronal T2WI shows the classic appearance of a central neurocytoma with multiple hyperintense cysts causing a "soap bubble" appearance.

Gross Pathology. The gross appearance of CNC is similar to that of oligodendroglioma. A well-defined, lobulated, moderately vascular intraventricular mass is characteristic **(19-22)**.

Microscopic Features. The histologic hallmark of CNC is its remarkable nuclear uniformity with round uniform cells arranged in sheets or lobules. Prominent zones of fine delicate neuropil may be present in between the tumor lobules.

MIB-1 is generally less than 2%. A labeling index of more than 2% or increased mitoses with microvascular proliferation and necrosis have been associated with increased risk of tumor recurrence.

Immunohistochemistry is positive for synaptophysin. Olig2 is negative, which helps distinguish CNC from oligodendroglioma.

Staging, Grading, and Classification. Central neurocytoma is a WHO grade II neoplasm.

Clinical Issues

Epidemiology. CNC is the most common primary intraventricular neoplasm of young and middle-aged adults, accounting for nearly half of all cases. Overall, they are rare neoplasms that represent between 0.25-0.5% of intracranial neoplasms and 10% of all intraventricular tumors.

Demographics. CNCs are generally tumors of young adults and are rarely diagnosed in children or the elderly.

Nearly three-quarters of all patients present between the ages of 20 and 40 years. Mean age at presentation is 30 years. There is no gender predilection.

Presentation. Symptoms are usually those of increased intracranial pressure. Headache, mental status changes, and visual disturbances are common. Focal neurologic deficits are rare. Some CNCs are found incidentally at imaging.

Natural History. CNCs are slow-growing tumors that rarely invade adjacent brain parenchyma. Sudden ventricular obstruction or acute intratumoral hemorrhage may cause abrupt clinical deterioration and even death. CSF dissemination has been reported but is very rare.

Treatment Options. Complete surgical resection is the treatment of choice. The extent of resection is the most important prognostic factor. Recurrence is rare. Five-year survival rate is 90%.

Imaging

General Features. A "bubbly" mass in the body or frontal horn of the lateral ventricle is classic for CNC **(19-21)**.

CT Findings. NECT shows a mixed-density solid and cystic intraventricular neoplasm that is attached to the septi pellucidi. Obstructive hydrocephalus is common. Calcification is present in 50-70% of cases. Frank intratumoral hemorrhage occurs but is rare. CNCs show moderately strong but heterogeneous enhancement on CECT.

MR FINDINGS. CNCs are heterogeneous masses that are mostly isodense with gray matter on T1WI. Intratumoral cysts and prominent vascular "flow voids" are common. A "bubbly" appearance on T2WI is typical. CNCs are heterogeneously hyperintense on FLAIR and demonstrate moderate to strong but heterogeneous enhancement following contrast administration **(19-23)**.

Decreased NAA and modestly elevated Cho are present on MRS. The presence of some NAA and glycine along with an inverted alanine peak at 1.5 ppm with a TE of 135 msec is highly suggestive of neurocytoma.

Differential Diagnosis

The major differential diagnosis of CNC is **subependymoma**. Subependymoma is more common in the inferior fourth ventricle, but supratentorial subependymomas are typically located adjacent to the foramen of Monro and may appear very similar. CNCs are tumors of younger adults while subependymoma is more common in older adults.

Supratentorial cellular **ependymoma** occurs in children and is mostly a parenchymal, not intraventricular, lesion.

Subependymal giant cell astrocytoma also occurs in a similar location, adjacent to the foramen of Monro. Clinical and other imaging stigmata of tuberous sclerosis (i.e., subependymal nodules and cortical tubers) are usually present.

An intraventricular **metastasis** usually occurs in older patients. Choroid plexus is a more common site than the lateral ventricle body. **Meningioma** is also more common in the ventricular trigone (choroid plexus glomus) than the frontal horn or body.

True intraventricular **oligodendroglioma** is rare. As the imaging appearance is indistinguishable from CNC, the diagnosis of intraventricular oligodendroglioma is established on the basis of immunohistochemistry and genetic studies. Oligodendrogliomas are synaptophysin-negative and often show mutations of Olig2 and 1p,19q.

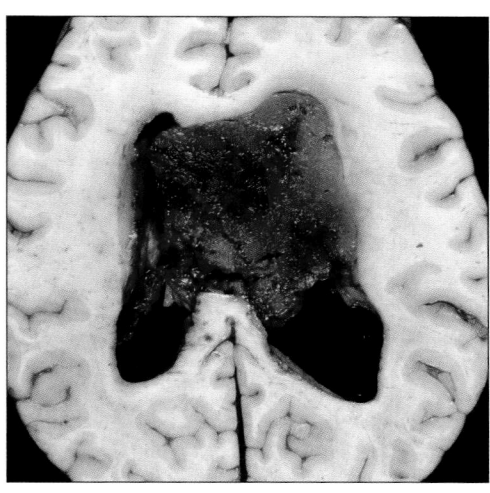

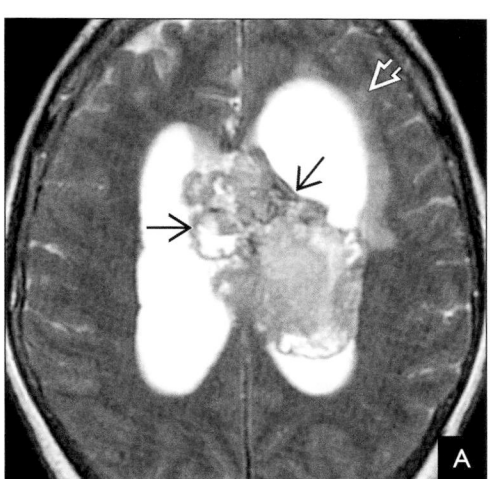

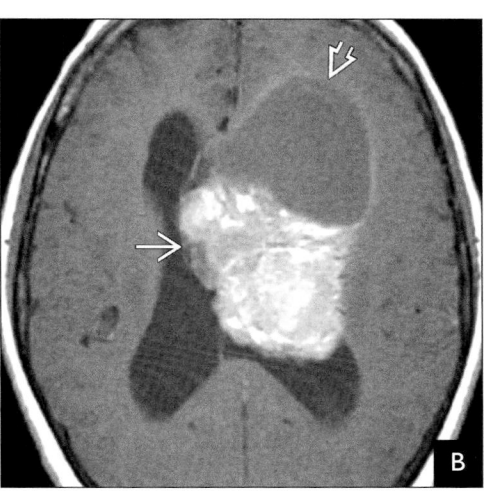

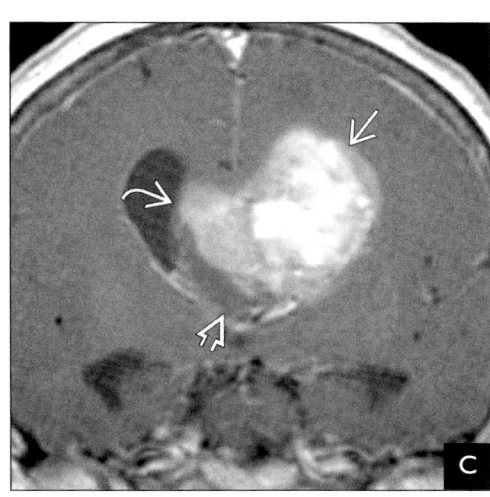

19-22. Autopsy case shows a large hemorrhagic neoplasm confined to the lateral ventricles. Central neurocytoma. (Courtesy R. Hewlett, MD.) 19-23A. Axial T2WI shows a biventricular mixed signal intensity mass ⇨ causing moderate obstructive hydrocephalus. Note subependymal fluid accumulation in the left frontal lobe ⧨. There is no periventricular "halo" around the remainder of the lateral ventricles.

19-23B. T1 C+ scan shows that the mass ⧨ enhances strongly but heterogeneously. The large "cyst" seen on the T2WI is an entrapped frontal horn of the left lateral ventricle that contains proteinaceous fluid ⧨. 19-23C. Coronal T1 C+ scan shows that the mass crosses from the body of the left lateral ventricle ⧨, passes through the foramen of Monro ⧨, and balloons into the right lateral ventricle ⧨. Central neurocytoma.

Extraventricular Neurocytoma

Terminology

Neoplasms that resemble central neurocytomas (CNCs) have been reported outside the ventricular system. In 2007, the WHO categorized these uncommon tumors as extraventricular neurocytoma (EVNCT).

Pathology

EVNCTs are histologically identical to CNCs. As the only definable distinguishing feature from CNC is location, both tumors are given the same pathologic code (WHO grade II).

Some authors have reported a wider variability in morphologic features, cellularity, proliferation rate, and outcome compared to CNCs. When atypical histologic features with necrosis, vascular proliferation, and mitoses (> 3 per 10 high-powered fields) are present, these variants are often called "atypical" EVNCT. A WHO grade has not been established for atypical EVNCT.

Clinical Issues

EVNCTs are generally tumors of young adults. The most common presenting symptom is epilepsy. Some studies have suggested that EVNCTs behave more aggressively than CNCs with poorer long-term outcome.

Imaging

EVNCTs vary widely in imaging appearance. They are usually located in the cerebral hemispheres or the parasellar region. Some tumors resemble CNCs or dysembryoplastic neuroepithelial tumors (DNETs) with a T2 hyperintense "bubbly" appearance (19-24). Others have a "cyst + nodule" configuration similar to ganglioglioma.

A few extraventricular neurocytomas appear as large, heterogeneous, enhancing parenchymal neoplasms that are difficult to distinguish from high-grade astrocytoma, primitive neuroectodermal tumor (PNET), or supratentorial ependymoma and probably represent "atypical" EVNCTs (19-25).

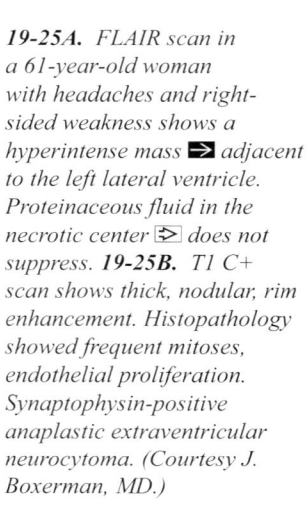

19-24A. Sagittal T2WI in a 7-year-old boy with seizures shows multiple hyperintense cysts in the inferior temporal gyrus ➡. 19-24B. Coronal T2WI in the same patient shows a relatively discrete cystic mass in the right medial temporal lobe ➡. Preoperative diagnosis was DNET. Extraventricular neurocytoma found by histopathology. (Courtesy A. Rossi, MD.)

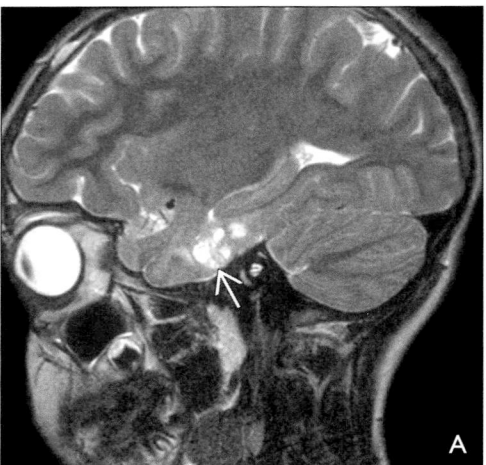

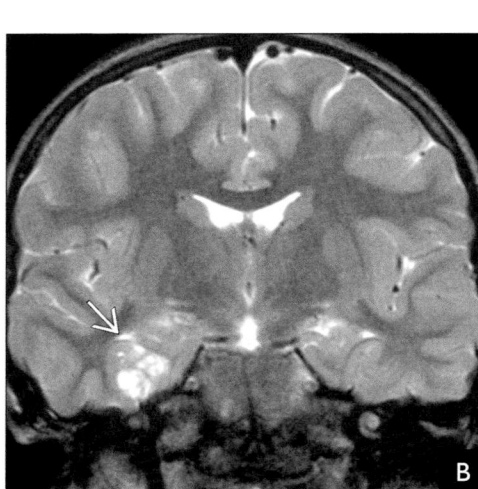

19-25A. FLAIR scan in a 61-year-old woman with headaches and right-sided weakness shows a hyperintense mass ➡ adjacent to the left lateral ventricle. Proteinaceous fluid in the necrotic center ⊳ does not suppress. 19-25B. T1 C+ scan shows thick, nodular, rim enhancement. Histopathology showed frequent mitoses, endothelial proliferation. Synaptophysin-positive anaplastic extraventricular neurocytoma. (Courtesy J. Boxerman, MD.)

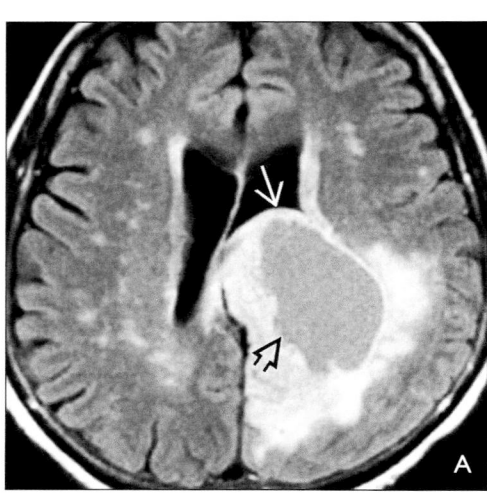

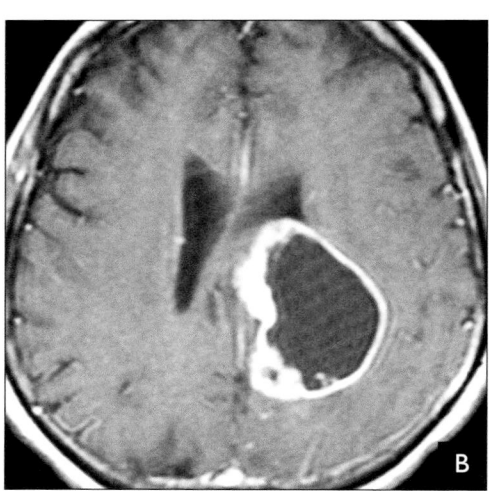

elected References

lioneuronal Tumors

- Chandrashekhar TN et al: Pathological spectrum of neuronal/ glioneuronal tumors from a tertiary referral neurological Institute. Neuropathology. 32(1):1-12, 2012
- Rodriguez FJ et al: Unusual malignant glioneuronal tumors of the cerebrum of adults: a clinicopathologic study of three cases. Acta Neuropathol. 112(6):727-37, 2006
- Varlet P et al: New variants of malignant glioneuronal tumors: a clinicopathological study of 40 cases. Neurosurgery. 55(6):1377-91: discussion 1391-2, 2004

Overview of Ganglion Cell Tumors

- Rodriguez FJ: Ganglion cell tumors. In Burger P et al: Diagnostic Pathology: Neuropathology. Salt Lake City: Amirsys Publishing. I.1.148-57, 2012

Ganglioglioma

- Lee CC et al: Malignant transformation of supratentorial ganglioglioma. Clin Neurol Neurosurg. Epub ahead of print, 2012
- Ortiz-González XR et al: Ganglioglioma arising from dysplastic cortex. Epilepsia. 52(9):e106-8, 2011
- Prayson RA: Brain tumors in adults with medically intractable epilepsy. Am J Clin Pathol. 136(4):557-63, 2011
- Ogiwara H et al: Pediatric epileptogenic gangliogliomas: seizure outcome and surgical results. J Neurosurg Pediatr. 5(3):271-6, 2010

Desmoplastic Infantile Astrocytoma/ Ganglioglioma

- Hummel TR et al: Clinical heterogeneity of desmoplastic infantile ganglioglioma: a case series and literature review. J Pediatr Hematol Oncol. 34(6):e232-6, 2012
- Gelabert-Gonzalez M et al: Desmoplastic infantile and non-infantile ganglioglioma. Review of the literature. Neurosurg Rev. 34(2):151-8, 2010
- Trehan G et al: MR imaging in the diagnosis of desmoplastic infantile tumor: retrospective study of six cases. AJNR Am J Neuroradiol. 25(6):1028-33, 2004

DNET

- Chandrashekhar TN et al: Pathological spectrum of neuronal/ glioneuronal tumors from a tertiary referral neurological institute. Neuropathology. 32(1):1-12, 2012
- Thom M et al: Long-term epilepsy-associated tumors. Brain Pathol. 22(3):350-79, 2012
- Thom M et al: One hundred and one dysembryoplastic neuroepithelial tumors: an adult epilepsy series with immunohistochemical, molecular genetic, and clinical correlations and a review of the literature. J Neuropathol Exp Neurol. 70(10):859-78, 2011
- Chang EF et al: Seizure control outcomes after resection of dysembryoplastic neuroepithelial tumor in 50 patients. J Neurosurg Pediatr. 5(1):123-30, 2010

Rosette-Forming Glioneuronal Tumor

- Hsu C et al: Rosette-forming glioneuronal tumour: Imaging features, histopathological correlation and a comprehensive review of literature. Br J Neurosurg. 26(5):668-73, 2012
- Shah MN et al: Rosette-forming glioneuronal tumors of the posterior fossa. J Neurosurg Pediatr. 5(1):98-103, 2010
- Louis DN et al: The 2007 WHO classification of tumours of the central nervous system. Acta Neuropathol. 114(2):97-109, 2007

Papillary Glioneuronal Tumor

- Xiao H et al: Papillary glioneuronal tumor: radiological evidence of a newly established tumor entity. J Neuroimaging. 21(3):297-302, 2011

Neuronal Tumors

- Chandrashekhar TN et al: Pathological spectrum of neuronal/ glioneuronal tumors from a tertiary referral neurological institute. Neuropathology. 32(1):1-12, 2012

Dysplastic Cerebellar Gangliocytoma

- Tutluer S et al: Cowden syndrome: a major indication for extensive cancer surveillance. Med Oncol. 29(2):1365-8, 2012
- Shinagare AB et al: Case 144: Dysplastic cerebellar gangliocytoma (Lhermitte-Duclos disease). Radiology. 251(1):298-303, 2009
- Cianfoni A et al: Morphological and functional MR imaging of Lhermitte-Duclos disease with pathology correlate. J Neuroradiol. 35(5):297-300, 2008
- Thomas B et al: Advanced MR imaging in Lhermitte-Duclos disease: moving closer to pathology and pathophysiology. Neuroradiology. 49(9):733-8, 2007

Central Neurocytoma

- Chen CL et al: Central neurocytoma: a clinical, radiological and pathological study of nine cases. Clin Neurol Neurosurg. 110(2):129-36, 2008

Extraventricular Neurocytoma

- Kane AJ et al: Atypia predicting prognosis for intracranial extraventricular neurocytomas. J Neurosurg. 116(2):349-54, 2012
- Myung JK et al: Clinicopathological and genetic characteristics of extraventricular neurocytomas. Neuropathology. Epub ahead of print, 2012
- Agarwal S et al: Extraventricular neurocytomas: a morphological and histogenetic consideration. A study of six cases. Pathology. 43(4):327-34, 2011
- Furtado A et al: Comprehensive review of extraventricular neurocytoma with report of two cases, and comparison with central neurocytoma. Clin Neuropathol. 29(3):134-40, 2010

Pineal and Germ Cell Tumors

The pineal region is located in the middle of the brain. Because there are so many critical structures that surround this small gland, operating on pineal region lesions poses a challenge to neurosurgeons. The posterior third ventricle, midbrain, thalamus, vein of Galen, internal cerebral vein, and quadrigeminal plate are all in the immediate "neighborhood."

The pineal gland itself consists of pineal parenchymal cells, astrocytes, and sympathetic neurons. Primitive germ cell rests are also often retained in midline structures (including the pineal gland), so the complete spectrum of germ cell tumor subtypes can also be found here.

A number of other cells can also be found adjacent to the pineal gland. These include ependymal cells (lining the third ventricle), choroid plexus cells, arachnoid cells that form the velum interpositum, and astrocytes in the brainstem, thalamus, and corpus callosum splenium.

Lesions of the pineal region include a broad spectrum of both neoplasms and nonneoplastic entities. This histologic diversity reflects the broad range of normal cell types that reside within the gland and its adjacent structures.

The pineal region may also be the site of neoplasms that are more commonly found elsewhere. Metastases, neuronal tumors, endothelial tumors, and lymphomas are all occasionally seen. Congenital lesions such as epidermoid and dermoid cysts as well as lipomas can also occur.

Overall, pineal region tumors are rare, accounting for 1-3% of all intracranial neoplasms. Despite their histological complexity, neoplasms in this region can be grouped into three simple overarching categories. The two most important groups arise from cells within the pineal gland itself: (1) tumors of pineal parenchymal cells and (2) germ cell tumors (GCTs).

The third group of pineal region lesions is composed of tumors of "other cell" origin. These are tumors and nonneoplastic masses that arise from adjacent structures, not from the pineal gland itself. They include entities such as tentorial apex meningioma, aneurysmal dilatation of the vein of Galen, and nonneoplastic cysts. These lesions are detailed elsewhere in the book but also included in a box at the end of this chapter that summarizes the differential diagnosis of a pineal region mass.

We begin our discussion with a brief review of normal gross and imaging anatomy of the pineal region. Understanding normal pineal region anatomy is critical for correct imaging diagnosis. The differential diagnoses are very different for a mass *inside* the pineal gland versus a mass that lies in the same region but is *outside* the gland.

We then turn our attention to the two major groups of neoplasms, pineal parenchymal and germ cell tumors. GCTs occupy a separate category in the WHO classification. However, because the pineal gland is by far the most common site for GCTs and because the differential diagnosis of an intrinsic pineal gland tumor includes both pineal parenchymal tumors and pineal germ cell tumors, we consider them together in this chapter.

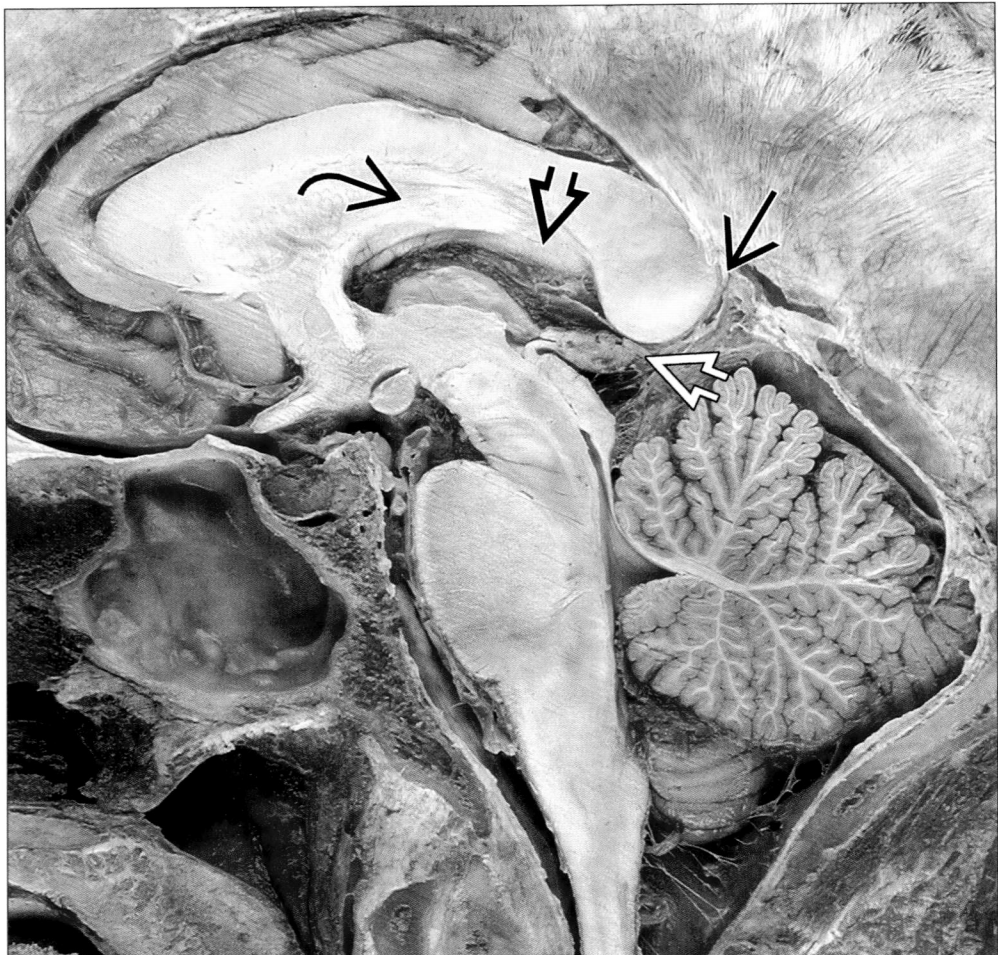

20-1. *Sagittal midline section demonstrates the anatomic complexity of the pineal region. The pineal gland* ⊵ *is adjacent to the tentorial apex and vein of Galen* ⊷*, lying behind the third ventricle below the velum interpositum (VI)* ⊵*. The VI lies below the fornix* ⊿*, contains the internal cerebral veins, and helps form the roof of the third ventricle. (Courtesy M. Nielsen, MS.)*

Pineal Region Anatomy

The pineal region is located under the falx cerebri, near its confluence with the tentorium cerebelli. This anatomically complex region encompasses the pineal gland itself, adjacent CSF spaces (the third ventricle and subarachnoid cisterns), brain parenchyma (corpus callosum splenium, quadrigeminal plate, upper vermis), arteries (medial and lateral posterior choroidal), veins (internal cerebral veins, vein of Galen), dural sinuses (inferior sagittal sinus, straight sinus), and meninges (dura and arachnoid) **(20-1)**.

Gross Anatomy

We begin our discussion of the pineal region with the pineal gland itself, then consider its relationship to the normal structures that surround it.

Pineal Gland

The pineal gland, also called the hypophysis cerebri, is a small round or triangular endocrine organ that nestles between the superior colliculi. It is attached to the diencephalon and posterior wall of the third ventricle by the pineal stalk. It has other connections to the habenular and posterior commissures. The pineal gland also connects with other important structures including the hypothalamus, hippocampi, amygdala, and brainstem.

The main vascular supply to the pineal gland is derived from branches of the medial posterior choroidal artery. The gland lacks a capillary blood-brain barrier.

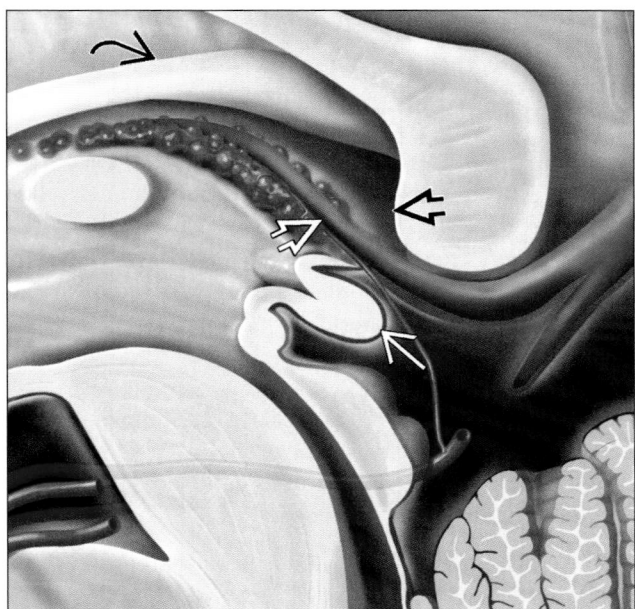

20-2. Sagittal graphic depicts the normal anatomy of the pineal region. The pineal gland ➡ *abuts the posterior third ventricle and lies below the fornix* ➡, *velum interpositum* ➡, *and internal cerebral vein* ➡.

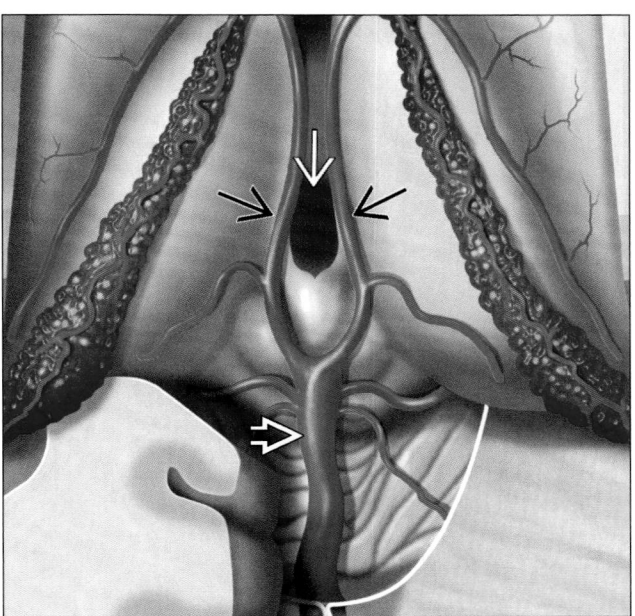

20-3. Axial graphic shows the velum interpositum ➡ *opened into the roof of the third ventricle, paired internal cerebral veins* ➡, *and vein of Galen* ➡.

Microscopically, 95% of the pineal gland consists of specialized neurons called **pinealocytes** that are arranged in cords or lobules separated by a fibrovascular stroma. Pinealocytes have both photosensory and neuroendocrine functions. The pinealocytes are interspersed with astrocytes and numerous blood vessels. Fine sand-like calcifications are commonly deposited within the pineal parenchyma.

The major hormone produced by the pineal gland is melatonin. **Melatonin** plays an important role in the synchronization of seasonal reproductive rhythms and entrainment of circadian cycles. Influenced by the dark/light cycle, the protein-coupled metabotropic melatonin receptors MT1 and MT2 are the primary mediators of its physiological actions.

Third Ventricle and Commissures

The pineal gland abuts the posterior third ventricle. The third ventricle has two small posterior CSF outpouchings that abut the pineal gland. The more prominent **suprapineal recess** lies above the pineal gland and below the corpus callosum splenium. The smaller **pineal recess** points posteriorly, directly into the gland.

Two commissural fiber tracts relate to the pineal gland. The **habenular commissure** lies just above the pineal gland, immediately below the suprapineal recess. The **posterior commissure** lies below the gland.

Fornix

The fornices are part of the limbic system. The two fornices, together with the fimbria, are the smallest and

innermost of three nested C-shaped arches that surround the diencephalon and basal ganglia. The fornices provide the primary efferent outputs from the hippocampus.

Each **fornix** has four parts. The **crura** arch under the corpus callosum splenium forms part of the medial wall of the lateral ventricles. The **commissure** connects the two crura, which then converge to form the body. The **body** is attached to the inferior surface of the corpus callosum. The bodies of the fornices curve inferiorly, forming the **columns** or "pillars" of the fornices. The fornices terminate in the mammillary bodies.

The commissure and bodies of the fornices lie above the velum interpositum, internal cerebral veins, and pineal gland **(20-2)**.

Velum Interpositum

The **tela choroidea** is a thin translucent bilaminar membrane that forms the **velum interpositum** (VI) **(20-1)**. The VI stretches (and thus is "interposed") between the bodies of the two fornices. The VI forms the roof of the third ventricle and is closed anteriorly at the foramen of Monro. If it is open posteriorly, it forms a CSF-filled space that communicates directly with the quadrigeminal cistern. This normal variant is called a **cavum of the velum interpositum** or **cistern of the velum interpositum.**

The VI extends laterally over the thalami where it becomes "tacked down" at the choroid fissures and continuous with the choroid plexus of the lateral ventricles.

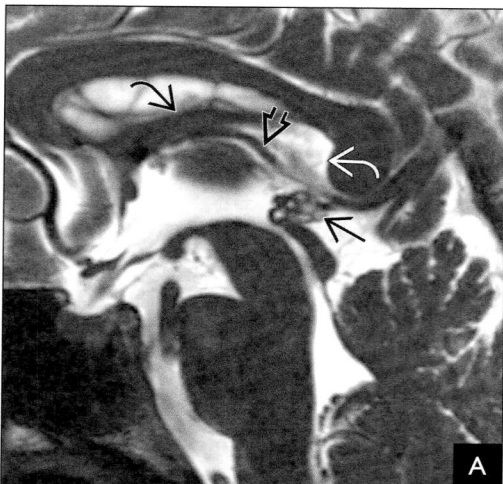

20-4A. Sagittal T2WI shows pineal gland ▢→ *behind third ventricle, below internal cerebral vein* ▢→ *, velum interpositum* ▢→ *, fornix* ▢→ *.*

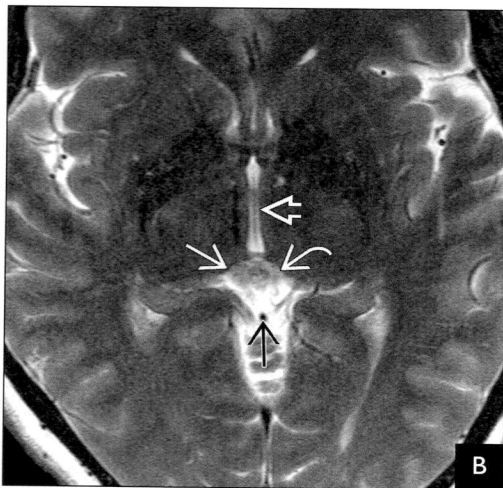

20-4B. Axial T2WI shows pineal gland ▢→ *behind the third ventricle* ▢→ *. The quadrigeminal cistern* ▢→ *, vein of Galen* ▢→ *are shown.*

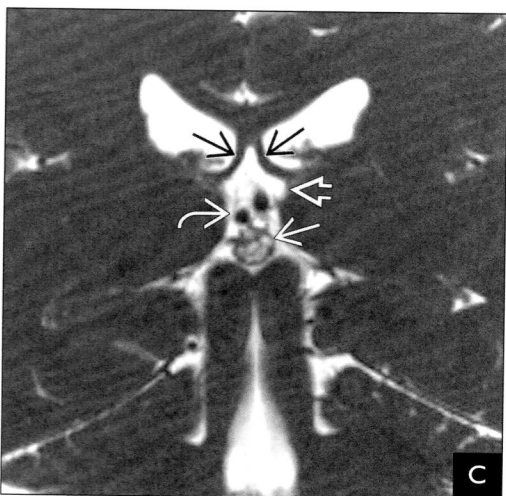

20-4C. Coronal T2WI shows pineal gland ▢→ *below internal cerebral veins* ▢→ *, velum interpositum* ▢→ *, fornices* ▢→ *.*

The VI covers the pineal gland and habenular commissure but is not directly attached to these structures.

Quadrigeminal Cistern

The **quadrigeminal cistern** is a rhomboid-shaped CSF space that lies dorsal to the tectal (quadrigeminal) plate and pineal gland. It is continuous inferiorly with the superior vermian cistern and laterally with the two ambient cisterns. Anteriorly it connects directly with the **cistern of the velum interpositum.**

Meninges

Infoldings of the inner (meningeal) layer of the dura form the **falx cerebri** and **tentorium cerebelli**. These two dural leaves unite just behind the corpus callosum splenium to form the **falcotentorial junction**.

A loosely adherent, thin, almost transparent layer of **arachnoid** closely follows the dura and forms the outer border of the subarachnoid spaces. The arachnoid does not invaginate into the sulci or CSF cisterns.

Veins and Venous Sinuses

The **internal cerebral veins** (ICVs) are paired, paramedian veins that course posteriorly between the dorsal and ventral membranous layers of the velum interpositum. The ICVs terminate in the quadrigeminal cisterns by uniting with each other and the basal veins of Rosenthal to form the great cerebral **vein of Galen (20-3)**. The ICVs lie above the pineal gland, which lies anteroinferior to the vein of Galen **(20-2)**.

The **inferior sagittal sinus** (ISS) courses posteriorly along the inferior (free) margin of the falx cerebri. The ISS and vein of Galen unite at the falcotentorial junction to form the **straight sinus**. The falcotentorial junction, together with the leaves of the tentorium cerebelli, forms the "roof" of the quadrigeminal cistern.

Arteries

The **medial posterior choroidal arteries** arise from the P2 segments of the posterior cerebral arteries. They curve laterally around the brainstem, enter the tela choroidea, and run anteromedially along the roof of the third ventricle. Branches of the medial posterior choroidal arteries provide the main arterial supply to the pineal gland.

Parenchyma

The **corpus callosum splenium** lies above and behind the pineal gland. The **tectal (quadrigeminal) plate** lies below it. The **thalami** lie inferolateral to the pineal gland.

ormal Imaging

ineal Calcification on NECT

Physiologic pineal gland calcification ("concretions") is common. Primary mineralization occurs in an organic matrix formed by pinealocytes. Pineal calcification increases with age. Reported prevalence is 1% in children under age six years, 8% in patients under age 10, and 40% in patients under 30. More than half of all adults have calcified pineal glands.

The diameter of normal pineal glands is usually ≤ 10 mm, but glands measuring 14-15 mm are not uncommon.

R of the Pineal Region

Thin-section, small field-of-view sagittal T2WI is the ideal sequence for imaging the pineal gland and adjacent structures. The contrast between CSF in the posterior third ventricle in front, the velum interpositum above, and the quadrigeminal cistern posteriorly allow maximum delineation of the gland (20-4).

An easy way to recall the relationship of the pineal gland to its adjacent structures can be identified using sagittal T2WI. From top down, the mnemonic "famous **V.I.P.**" identifies the **f**ornix, **v**elum interpositum, **i**nternal cerebral veins, and **p**ineal gland. Lesions in the fornix, VI, and ICVs will all displace the pineal gland inferiorly.

Lesions that arise from the tectal plate displace the pineal gland anterosuperiorly whereas third ventricle masses displace it posteriorly. Knowing the normal gross anatomy helps make it simple!

ineal Parenchymal Tumors

In North America and Europe, pineal *region* tumors represent less than 1% of all primary intracranial neoplasms but 3-8% of pediatric tumors. In Asia, they account for 3-3.5% of brain tumors.

Most tumors of the pineal *gland* are germ cell neoplasms, which account for 40% of all pineal tumors. Pineal parenchymal tumors (PPTs) account for less than 0.2% of all brain tumors but cause approximately 15-30% of pineal gland tumors.

PPTs are neuroepithelial neoplasms that arise from pinealocytes or their precursors. PPT grading is based on the presence or absence of mitoses and neurofilament staining. Three grades are recognized: (1) **pineocytoma**, the most common of all pineal parenchymal tumors; (2) **pineal parenchymal tumor of intermediate differenti-**

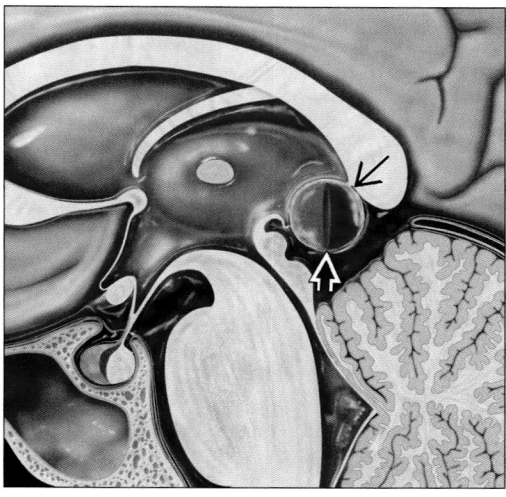

20-5. *Graphic depicts pineocytoma. The cystic center is lined by a rim of solid, partially calcified tumor ➡. Hemorrhage ⇒ is not uncommon.*

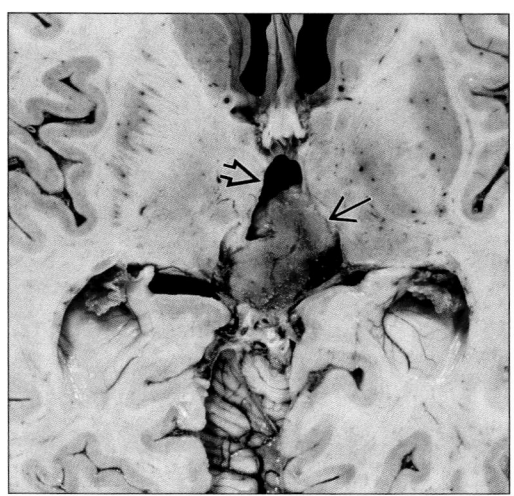

20-6. *Autopsy case shows pineocytoma as a well-demarcated lobulated mass ➡ behind the third ventricle ⟐. (Courtesy B. Horten, MD.)*

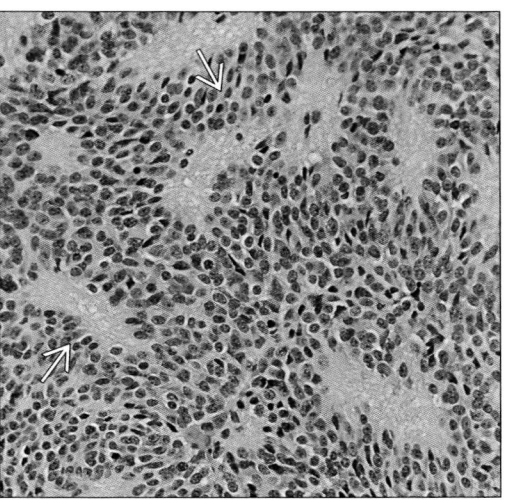

20-7. *Pineocytomatous rosettes are typical ➡. Unlike perivascular pseudorosettes, there is no central vessel. (Courtesy B. K. DeMasters, MD.)*

ation; and (3) **pineoblastoma**, the rarest but most malignant parenchymal cell tumor.

We conclude our discussion of PPTs with the newly recognized **papillary tumor of the pineal region** (PTPR). Macroscopically, PTPR resembles pineocytoma but actually arises from the subcommissural organ.

Pineocytoma

Terminology

Pineocytoma is a slow-growing and well-differentiated pineal parenchymal tumor composed of mature cells that resemble normal pinealocytes.

Etiology

Pineocytomas arise from pinealocytes or their precursors. No consistent genetic mutations have been described to date.

Pathology

LOCATION AND SIZE. Pineocytomas are located behind the third ventricle and rarely invade it or adjacent structures (20-5). Pineocytomas vary in size. Although "giant" tumors have been reported, most are smaller than three centimeters in diameter.

GROSS PATHOLOGY. Pineocytomas are well-circumscribed, round or lobular, gray-tan masses that may display intratumoral cysts or hemorrhagic foci on cut section (20-6).

MICROSCOPIC FEATURES. Pineocytomas are composed of small uniform cells that closely resemble pinealocytes. Large "pineocytomatous rosettes" are the most characteristic feature (20-7).

Immunopositivity for neuronal markers such as synaptophysin and neurofilament protein is common.

STAGING, GRADING, AND CLASSIFICATION. Pineocytoma is positive for both synaptophysin and neurofilament and shows no mitoses. Pineocytomas are WHO grade I neoplasms.

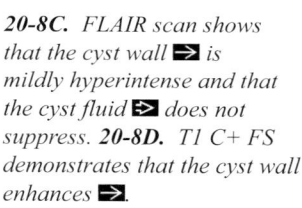

20-8A. NECT scan shows the typical findings of pineocytoma. The cystic-appearing pineal mass "explodes" calcifications toward the periphery of the lesion ➡. 20-8B. T2WI in the same patient shows a cyst ➡ surrounded by a thin rim of solid tissue ➡.

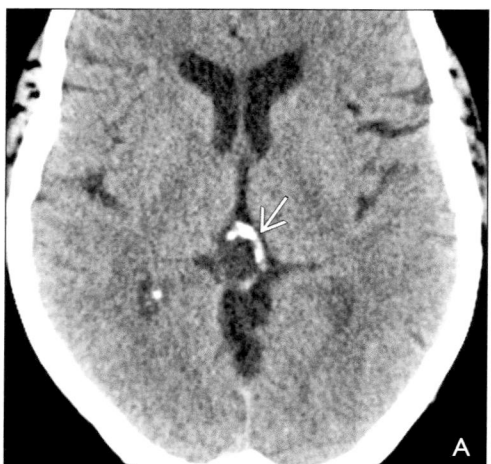

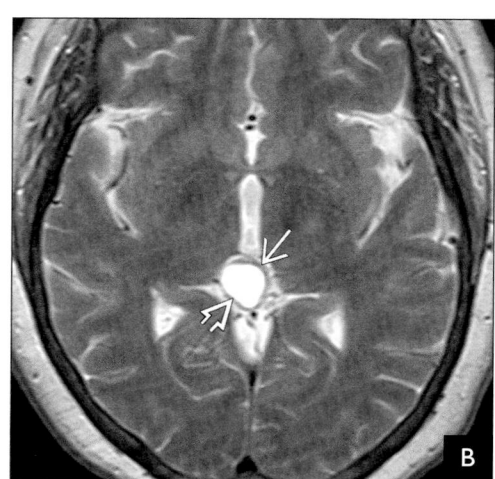

20-8C. FLAIR scan shows that the cyst wall ➡ is mildly hyperintense and that the cyst fluid ➡ does not suppress. 20-8D. T1 C+ FS demonstrates that the cyst wall enhances ➡.

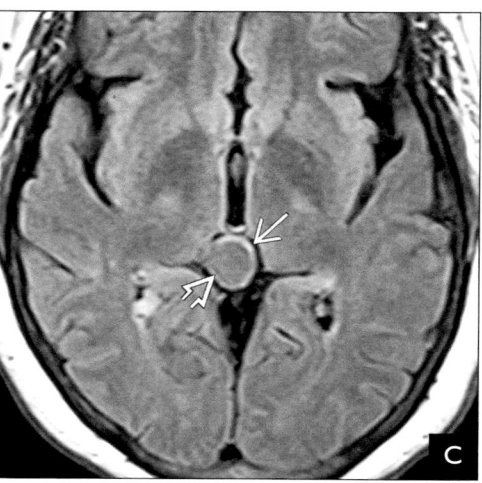

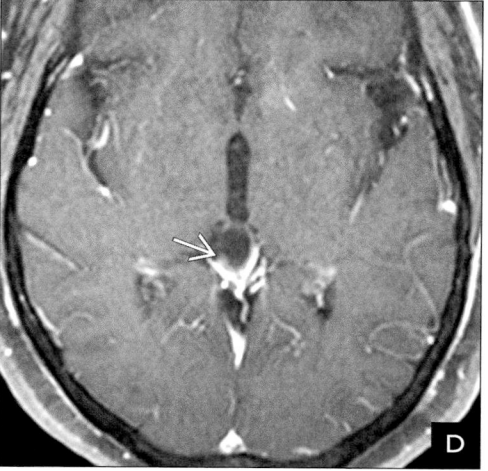

linical Issues

EPIDEMIOLOGY. Pineocytoma is the most common pineal parenchymal tumor (PPT), accounting for 15-60% of all primary PPTs.

DEMOGRAPHICS. Pineocytomas occur at all ages but are mostly tumors of adults. Mean age at diagnosis is approximately 40 years. There is no gender predilection.

PRESENTATION. Many small pineocytomas are discovered incidentally on imaging studies. Large lesions may compress adjacent structures or cause hydrocephalus. Headache and Parinaud syndrome (paralysis of upward gaze) are common in symptomatic patients.

NATURAL HISTORY. Pineocytomas grow very slowly and often remain stable in size over many years. The five-year survival rate is 85-100%.

TREATMENT OPTIONS. "Watchful waiting" is common with small lesions. Imaging is obtained only if the patient's symptoms change. Complete surgical resection is generally curative, without recurrence or CSF dissemination.

maging

CT FINDINGS. Pineocytomas are mixed iso- to hypodense lesions on NECT scans. Calcifications appear "exploded" toward the periphery of the pineal gland **(20-8A)**.

MR FINDINGS. Pineocytomas are well-demarcated round or lobular masses that are iso- to hypointense on T1WI and hyperintense on T2WI and FLAIR **(20-8B)**, **(20-8C)**. T2* GRE may show "blooming" foci secondary to calcification or hemorrhage. Pineocytomas typically enhance avidly with solid, rim, or even nodular patterns **(20-8D)**.

ifferential Diagnosis

The major differential diagnosis of pineocytoma is **pineal cyst**. Pineal cysts may be indistinguishable from pineocytomas on imaging studies. **Germinoma** typically "engulfs" rather than "explodes" the pineal calcifications, is most common in adolescent males, and enhances intensely and uniformly. **Pineal parenchymal tumor of intermediate differentiation** (PPTID) is a tumor of middle-aged and older patients. The imaging appearance of PPTIDs is more "aggressive" than that of pineocytoma (see below).

PINEOCYTOMA

Pathology
- Most 1-3 cm
- Well-demarcated, round/lobulated
- WHO grade I

Clinical Issues
- Most common pineal parenchymal tumor
- Adults (mean = 40 years)
- Grows very slowly, often stable for years

Imaging
- CT
  - Mixed iso-/hypodense
  - Pineal Ca++ "exploded"
- MR
  - Iso-/hypointense on T1, hyperintense on T2
  - Cysts common, may hemorrhage
  - Variable enhancement (solid, rim, nodular)
- Differential diagnosis
  - Benign pineal cyst (may be indistinguishable)
  - Germinoma ("engulfs" Ca++, adolescent males)
  - PPTID (more "aggressive looking")

Pineal Parenchymal Tumor of Intermediate Differentiation

Some pineal lesions both look worse and behave more aggressively than pineocytomas but are still less malignant than pineoblastomas. In 2007, the WHO formally recognized a new tumor, pineal parenchymal tumor of intermediate differentiation, which is intermediate in malignancy between pineocytoma and pineoblastoma.

Terminology

"Pineal parenchymal tumor of intermediate differentiation" (PPTID) supersedes the terms "atypical" or "aggressive" pineocytoma.

Pathology

Grossly, PPTID is a large, heterogeneous mass with peripheral calcification and variable cystic changes. Microscopically, PPTIDs are moderate to highly cellular tumors that exhibit dense lobular architecture. Areas of intermediate differentiation combined with pineocytomatous rosettes are common.

PPTIDs are either WHO grade II or III. Tumors with a Ki-67 between 3-7%, < 6 mitoses per 10 high-power fields (HPFs), and neurofilament protein positivity are grade II neoplasms. Tumors that are either NFP-negative with < 6 mitoses per HPF or NFP-positive with ≥ 6 mitoses are grade III lesions.

Clinical Issues

EPIDEMIOLOGY AND DEMOGRAPHICS. PPTIDs represent at least 20% of all pineal parenchymal tumors and are typically tumors of middle-aged adults.

NATURAL HISTORY. Relatively few documented cases of PPTID have been reported. Diplopia, Parinaud syndrome, and headache are the most common presenting symptoms.

Biological behavior is variable, and long-term survival—even with subtotal resection—is common. Tumors tend to enlarge slowly over many years and recur locally. CSF dissemination has been reported in a few cases.

TREATMENT OPTIONS. Treatment of PPTID is controversial. Stereotactic biopsy followed by surgical resection is the most common treatment. The role of adjuvant chemotherapy or radiotherapy is undetermined.

Imaging

GENERAL FEATURES. PPTIDs have a more "aggressive" imaging appearance than pineocytoma **(20-9)**. Extension into adjacent structures (e.g., the ventricles and thalami) is common. Size varies from less than one centimeter to large masses that are four to six centimeters in diameter. CSF dissemination is uncommon but does occur, so imaging evaluation of the entire neuraxis should be performed prior to surgical intervention.

CT FINDINGS. NECT scans show a hyperdense mass that "engulfs" pineal gland calcifications **(20-10)**. PPTIDs generally enhance strongly and uniformly.

MR FINDINGS. PPTIDs are mixed iso- and hypointense on T1WI, isointense with gray matter on T2WI, and hyperintense on FLAIR. T2* (GRE, SWI) scans may show hypointense "blooming" foci. Enhancement is generally strong but heterogeneous on T1 C+.

MRS shows elevated Cho and decreased NAA. A lactate peak may be present.

Differential Diagnosis

The major differential diagnosis of PPTID is **pineocytoma**. A more aggressive-appearing pineal mass in a middle-aged or older adult is most consistent with PPTID. Patients with a long history of "atypical pineocytoma" or a pineocytoma that grows over time may harbor a PPTID. **Pineoblastoma** is typically a tumor of younger patients.

20-9A. T1WI in a 57-year-old woman with headaches, intermittent visual problems shows a 2 cm, well-delineated, slightly hypointense mass → in the pineal gland. 20-9B. T2WI shows that the mass → is heterogeneously hyperintense with some areas of cystic degeneration →.

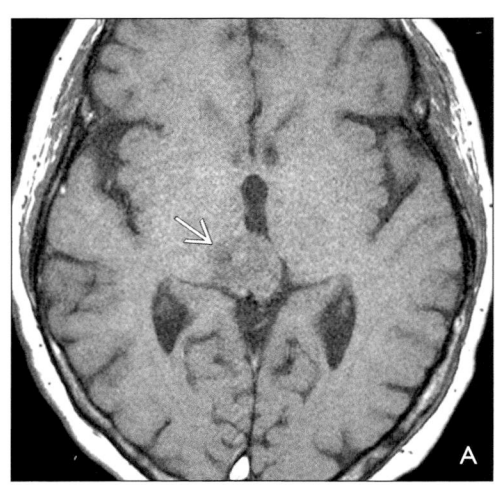
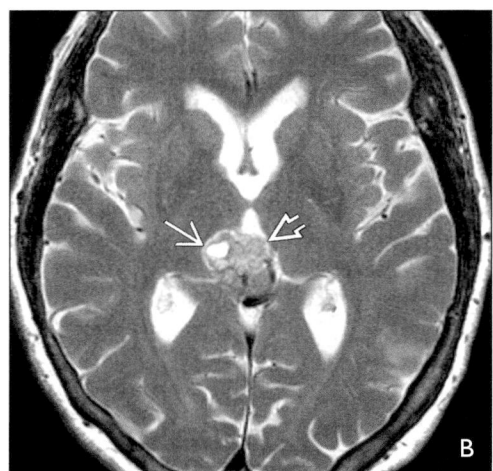

20-9C. Moderate heterogeneous enhancement → is seen on T1 C+. 20-9D. MRS shows elevated Cho →, decreased NAA →, lactate doublet →. Pineal parenchymal tumor of intermediate differentiation, WHO grade II, was diagnosed on imaging and confirmed at histopathology.

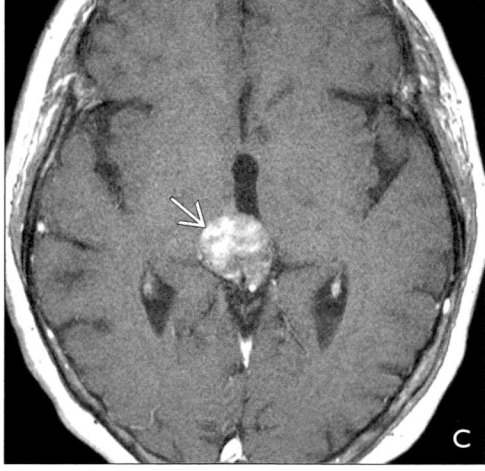
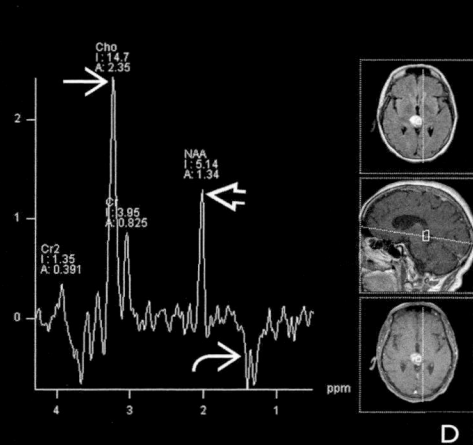

Germinoma is more common in adolescent males. **Papillary tumor of the pineal region** can appear identical but is very rare.

PINEAL PARENCHYMAL TUMOR OF INTERMEDIATE DIFFERENTIATION

Pathology
- PPTID: In between pineocytoma, pineoblastoma
- 20% of pineal parenchymal tumors
- WHO grade II or III
  - Varies with mitoses, neurofilament positivity

Clinical Issues
- Middle-aged adults
- Prognosis variable

Imaging
- Appears more "aggressive" than pineocytoma
- Usually larger, more heterogeneous
- May disseminate via CSF

Differential Diagnosis
- Pineocytoma > > pineoblastoma
- Germinoma
- Papillary tumor of the pineal region

Pineoblastoma

Terminology

Pineoblastoma (PB) is a highly malignant primitive neuroectodermal tumor (PNET) of the pineal gland.

Etiology

PBs are thought to arise from primitive embryonic precursor cells that express some features of pineal parenchymal cells ("pinealocytes").

Pathology

GROSS PATHOLOGY. A soft, friable, diffusely infiltrating tumor that invades adjacent brain and obstructs the cerebral aqueduct is typical **(20-11)**. Necrosis and intratumoral hemorrhage are common, as is CSF dissemination with sheet-like coating of the brain and spinal cord **(20-12)**.

MICROSCOPIC FEATURES. PBs are highly cellular embryonal neoplasms that resemble other PNETs. Small undifferentiated cells with hyperchromatic nuclei and scanty cytoplasm are the dominant histologic feature

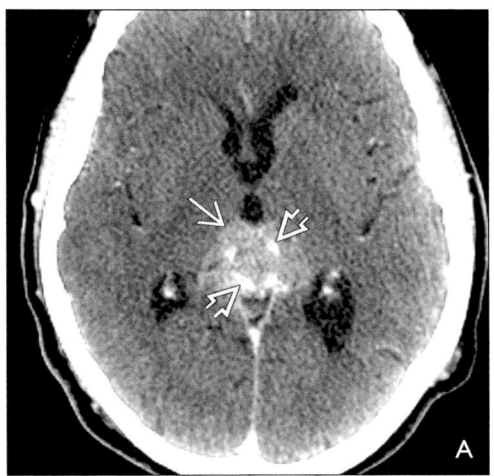
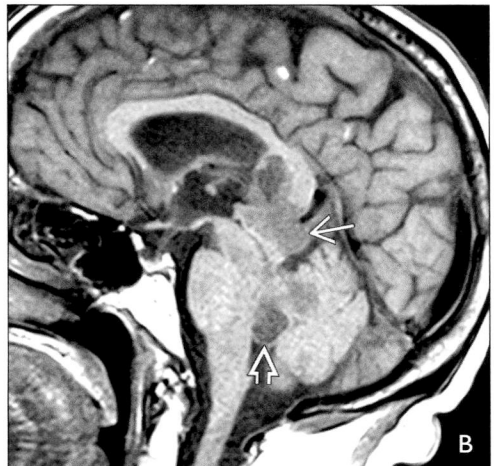

20-10A. CECT scan in a 75-year-old woman shows a lobulated enhancing pineal mass ⮕ with calcifications ⮕ "exploded" toward the periphery of the tumor.
20-10B. Sagittal T1WI shows that the lesion ⮕ is mixed iso-, hypointense. Another lesion is seen in the fourth ventricle ⮕.

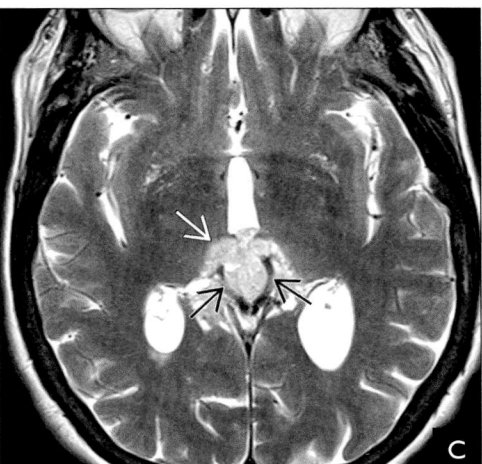
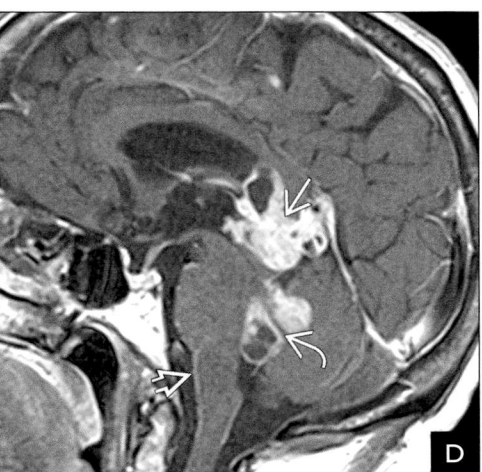

20-10C. T2WI shows that the lesion ⮕ is heterogeneously hyperintense and contains multiple cysts. The internal cerebral veins ⮕ appear encased by the mass.
20-10D. T1 C+ scan shows enhancement of the pineal mass ⮕ and the fourth ventricle lesion ⮕. Note subtle coating of the pons, medulla by enhancing tumor ⮕. Lumbosacral MR (not shown) demonstrated multiple "drop metastases." PPTID, grade III. (Courtesy P. Hildenbrand, MD.)

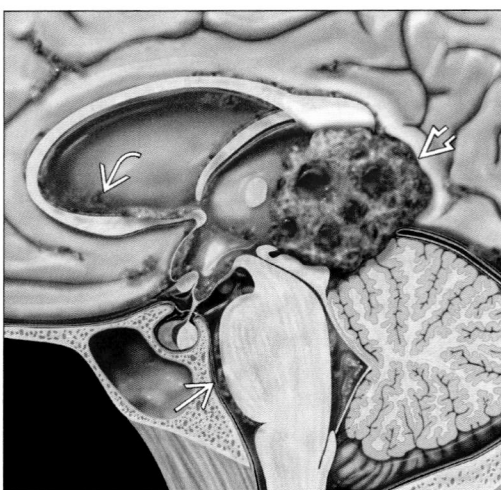

20-11. *Sagittal graphic depicts pineoblastoma* ⇨ *with CSF dissemination into ventricles* ⇒, *subarachnoid spaces* ⇒.

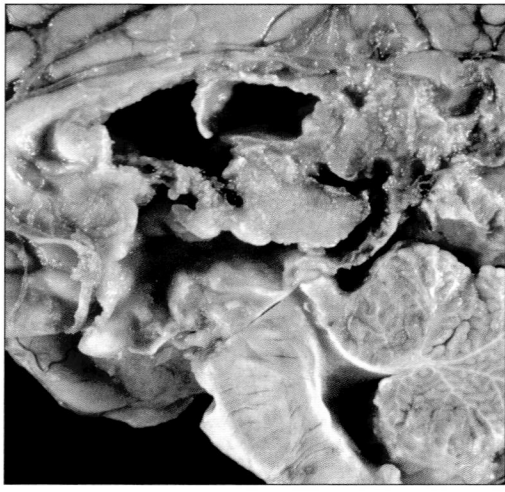

20-12. *Autopsy of pineoblastoma shows dissemination with nodular metastases coating the lateral, third ventricles. (Courtesy B. Horten, MD.)*

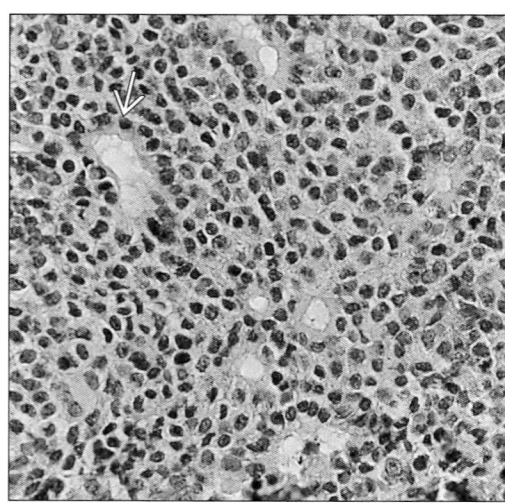

20-13. *Pineoblastoma is composed of sheets of small blue undifferentiated cells with occasional rosettes* ⇒. *(Courtesy B. K. DeMasters, MD.)*

of PB. Occasional Homer-Wright rosettes (neuroblastic differentiation) or Flexner-Wintersteiner rosettes (retinoblastic differentiation) can be identified **(20-13)**.

STAGING, GRADING, AND CLASSIFICATION. Pineoblastomas are WHO grade IV neoplasms.

Clinical Issues

EPIDEMIOLOGY. Pineoblastomas comprise 0.5-1% of primary brain tumors, 15% of pineal region neoplasms, and 30-45% of pineal parenchymal tumors.

DEMOGRAPHICS. Although they can occur at any age, PBs are decidedly more prevalent in children. Most present in the first two decades.

PRESENTATION. Symptoms of elevated intracranial pressure such as headache, nausea, and vomiting are typical. Parinaud syndrome is common.

NATURAL HISTORY. Pineoblastomas are the most primitive and biologically aggressive of all the pineal parenchymal tumors. Prognosis is poor with a median survival of 16-25 months. CSF dissemination is frequent at the time of initial diagnosis and the most common cause of death.

TREATMENT OPTIONS. Surgical debulking with adjuvant chemotherapy and craniospinal radiation is the typical regimen.

Imaging

GENERAL FEATURES. PBs are large, bulky, aggressive-looking pineal region masses that invade adjacent brain and usually cause obstructive hydrocephalus. CSF dissemination is common, so the entire neuraxis should be imaged prior to surgical intervention.

CT FINDINGS. A large, hyperdense, inhomogeneously enhancing mass with obstructive hydrocephalus is typical. If pineal calcifications are present, they appear "exploded" toward the periphery of the tumor **(20-14A)**.

MR FINDINGS. PBs are heterogeneous tumors that frequently demonstrate necrosis and intratumoral hemorrhage. They are usually mixed iso- to hypointense compared to brain on T1WI and mixed iso- to hyperintense on T2WI **(20-15)**. They enhance strongly but heterogeneously. Because they are densely cellular tumors, restriction on DWI is common **(20-14B)**.

Differential Diagnosis

The major differential diagnosis of pineoblastoma is **PPTID**. PBs tend to occur in children. CSF dissemination at diagnosis is more common. **Germinoma** may mimic PB on imaging studies as it also frequently demonstrates CSF spread. Germinomas are more common in adolescent and young adult males. They tend to "engulf" rather than "explode" pineal calcifications.

Nongerminomatous malignant germ cell tumors are a heterogeneous group of tumors that may be indistinguishable on imaging studies from PBs. Elevated tumor markers such as α-fetoprotein and β-human chorionic gonadotropin—all usually negative in germinoma and PB—are helpful in establishing the diagnosis.

PINEOBLASTOMA

Pathology
- Most primitive, malignant of all PPTs
- Embryonal PNET
- Diffusely infiltrates adjacent structures
- CSF dissemination common, early
- WHO grade IV

Clinical Issues
- 15% of pineal region tumors
- 30-45% of PPTs
- Affects children (< 20 years old)
- Prognosis generally poor

Imaging
- CT
  - Inhomogeneously hyperdense
  - Ca++ "exploded"
- MR
  - Large, bulky, aggressive-looking
  - Necrosis, intratumoral hemorrhage common
  - Enhances strongly, heterogeneously
  - Restricts on DWI (densely cellular)
  - Look for CSF spread (image entire neuraxis)

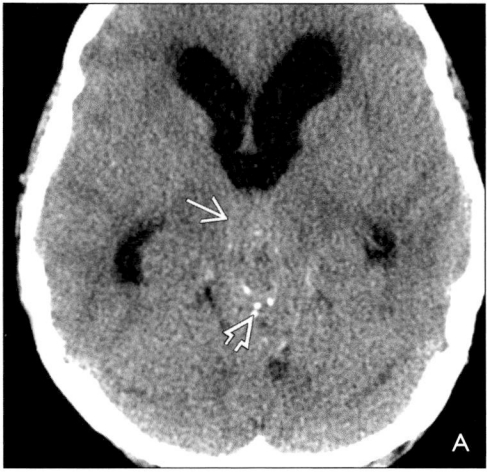
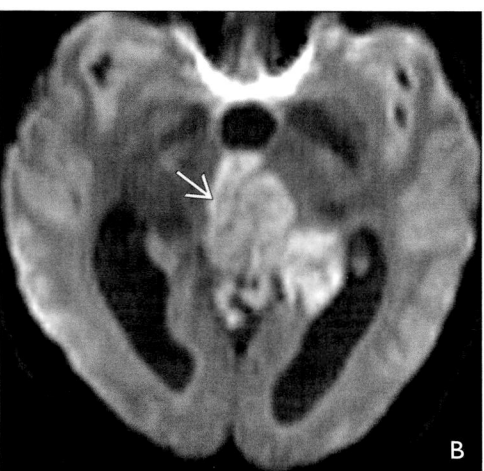

20-14A. *NECT of pineoblastoma shows an ill-defined, slightly hyperdense pineal region mass* ➡ *causing obstructive hydrocephalus. Some calcifications* ➡ *are seen toward the periphery of the mass.* *20-14B.* *DWI in the same patient shows moderate diffusion restriction* ➡*, consistent with high cellularity.*

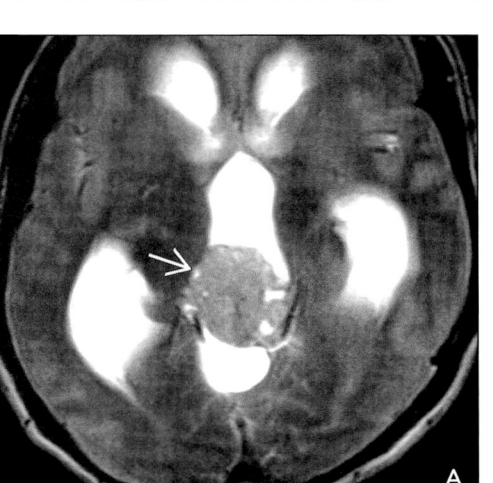
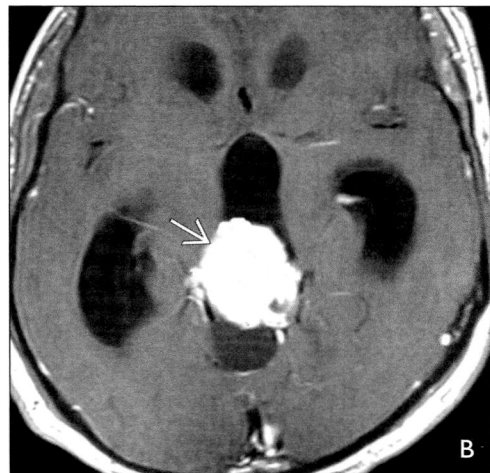

20-15A. *T2WI in another patient with pineoblastoma shows a large pineal mass* ➡ *that causes severe obstructive hydrocephalus.* *20-15B.* *T1 C+ scan in the same patient shows that the lesion* ➡ *enhances intensely, uniformly. (Courtesy R. Hewlett, MD.)*

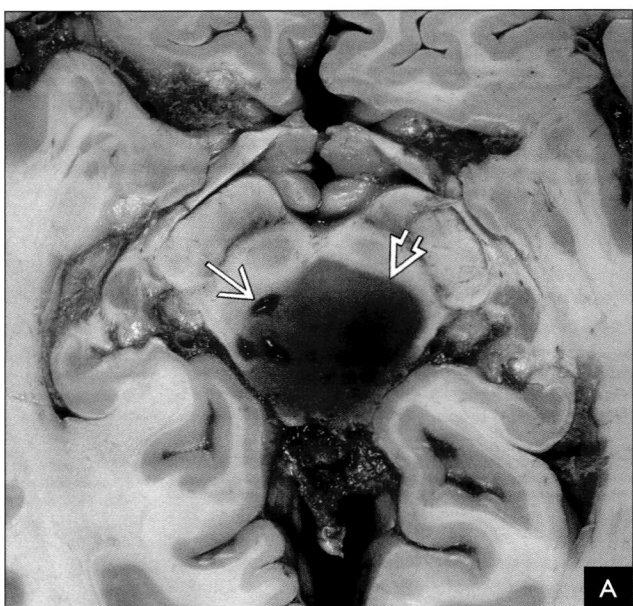

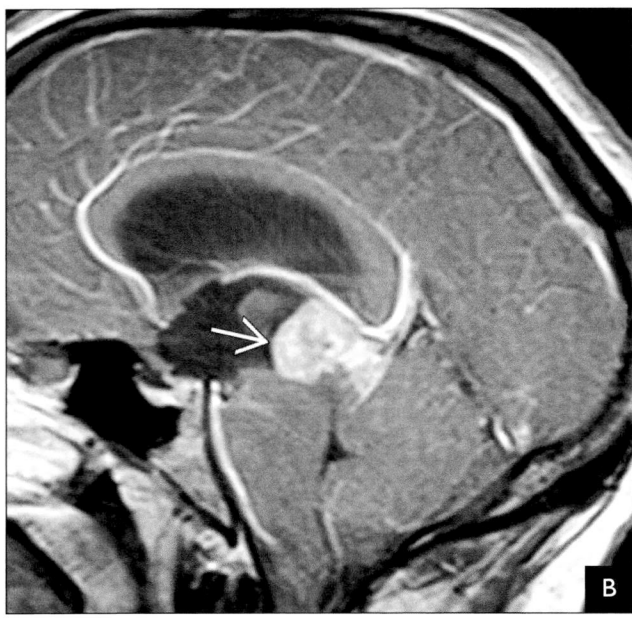

20-16A. Autopsy of a posterior third ventricular mass that invades midbrain tegmentum shows cysts ➡, hemorrhage ➡. Microscopy showed ependymal differentiation. Tumor would now likely be classified as PTPR. (Courtesy R. Hewlett, MD.)

20-16B. Sagittal T1 C+ scan of a PTPR shows an enhancing pineal mass ➡ causing obstructive hydrocephalus. Imaging findings are nonspecific. (Courtesy P. Burger, MD.)

Papillary Tumor of the Pineal Region

Papillary tumor of the pineal region (PTPR) is a rare, newly recognized neuroepithelial tumor that arises from specialized ependyma of the subcommissural organ in the posteroinferior wall of the third ventricle (20-16A). PTPRs are adult tumors; mean age at diagnosis is 32 years.

Macroscopically, PTPRs are indistinguishable from pineocytoma; microscopically, they are easily differentiated. PTPRs share morphologic features with both papillary ependymoma and choroid plexus tumors. PTPRs show distinct papillary architecture with pseudostratified columnar epithelium. Ultrastructural features suggest ependymal differentiation. Immunohistochemistry is positive for cytokeratins.

Grading of PTPRs has yet to be defined, but most neuropathologists consider these WHO grade II or III neoplasms. Thus the pathologic differentiation from pineocytoma, a WHO grade I neoplasm, is important for treatment purposes.

Only a few PTPRs with imaging findings have been reported. PTPRs tend to be large, relatively well-circumscribed, and often partially cystic. Strong but inhomogeneous enhancement is typical (20-16B). No features that would distinguish these tumors from pineal parenchymal tumors of intermediate differentiation, the major imaging differential diagnosis, have been described.

PAPILLARY TUMOR OF THE PINEAL REGION

Etiology and Pathology
- Newly recognized (2007 WHO)
- Probably arises from subcommissural organ
  - In wall of posterior third ventricle
  - Ependymal differentiation
- WHO grade II or III
  - Local recurrence, CSF dissemination

Imaging
- Nonspecific
- Large, lobulated, enhancing mass

Differential Diagnosis
- Pineal parenchymal tumor of intermediate differentiation

Germin Cell Tumors

Overview of Germ Cell Tumors

Intracranial germ cell tumors (GCTs) are rare neoplasms that vary in histological differentiation, prognosis, and clinical behavior.

GCTs are divided into two basic groups. Germinomas comprise the larger group. The smaller group consists of *non*germinomatous GCTs, which include both teratomas and a heterogeneous group of "other" nongerminomatous malignant germ cell neoplasms.

We begin with an overview of intracranial GCTs, then discuss germinomas, teratomas, and the "other" germ cell tumors in greater detail.

erminology

Intracranial GCTs are morphological and immunophenotypic homologues of similar neoplasms that arise in the gonads and extragonadal sites. They are given the same names as their extracranial counterparts, i.e., germinoma, teratoma, embryonal carcinoma, yolk sac tumor, choriocarcinoma, and mixed GCT.

tiology

GCTs arise from either totipotential stem cells or aberrant migration of cells from at least one of the three primordial germ layers (ectoderm, mesoderm, and endoderm). Recent studies evaluating mRNA profiles show that malignant GCTs most closely resemble embryonic stem cells.

Pathology

While GCTs can arise in many intracranial locations, they have a distinct affinity for the midline (i.e., the pineal region, around the third ventricle, and the pituitary infundibulum) or very near the midline (i.e., basal ganglia).

GCTs are classified and graded according to histological features and immunohistochemical profiles. They vary in malignancy from mature teratomas with fully differentiated tissue to poorly differentiated, highly aggressive neoplasms such as embryonal carcinoma, choriocarcinoma, and endodermal sinus (yolk sac) tumors.

Germ cell tumors often exhibit mixed histology (i.e., both germinomatous and nongerminomatous elements).

Clinical Issues

As a group, GCTs account for 0.5-3.5% of all brain tumors but cause 3-8% of primary CNS neoplasms in children. Prevalence varies with geographic location. In Asia, GCTs cause 9-15% of pediatric brain tumors.

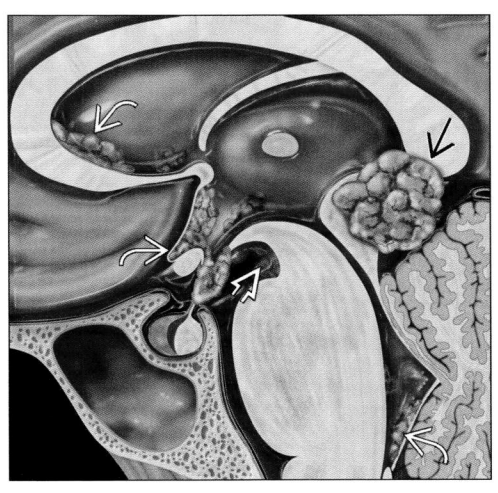

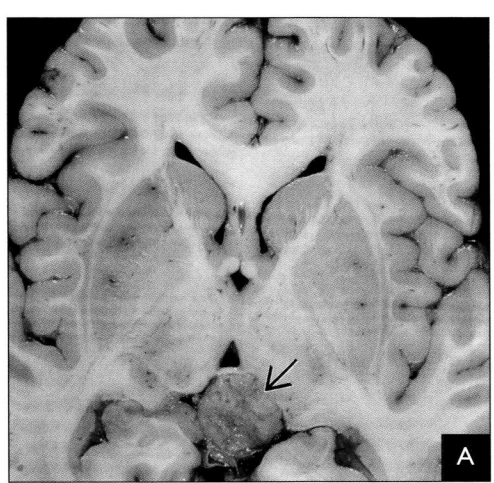

20-17. Sagittal graphic depicts typical pineal germinoma ➡. CSF dissemination to the third, lateral, and fourth ventricles ➡ is common, as is subarachnoid tumor spread ➡. 20-18A. Autopsy specimen shows a pineal germinoma ➡.

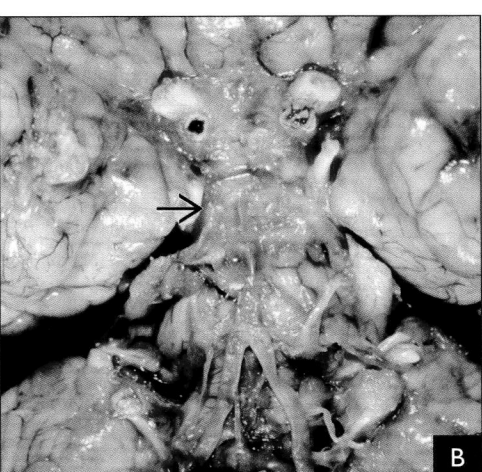

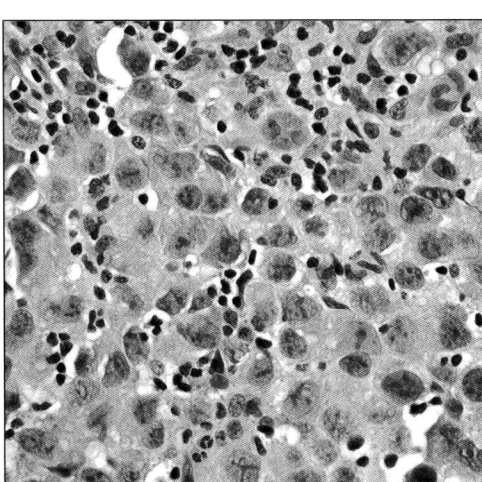

20-18B. Submentovertex view of the basal cisterns in the same case shows diffuse CSF tumor ("carcinomatous meningitis") filling the suprasellar cistern ➡ and coating the brain. (Courtesy R. Hewlett, MD.) 20-19. Classic germinoma consists of large round cells with prominent nucleoli, admixed with small lymphocytes. (Courtesy T. Tihan, MD.)

GCTs are generally tumors of children and young adults; 80-90% of patients are younger than 20 years of age. Many GCTs secrete oncoproteins such as α-fetoprotein or β-hCG, so laboratory as well as imaging evaluation is key to establishing the diagnosis.

Prognosis and treatment varies with tumor type. Localized germinomas are treated with radiation therapy and have a relatively good prognosis. Chemotherapy is reserved for disseminated germinomas. Mature teratomas are treated with surgery. The other GCTs are managed with various combinations of surgery, chemotherapy, and radiotherapy.

INTRACRANIAL GERM CELL TUMORS

Pathology
- Homologues of gonadal neoplasms
  - Germinoma, teratoma, choriocarcinoma, etc.
- Neoplastic correlates of primitive ectoderm, mesoderm, endoderm
- Propensity to arise in/near midline

Clinical Issues
- 3-8% of primary CNS tumors in children
  - More common in Asia (9-15% of pediatric brain tumors)
- Generally affect children, young adults
  - 80-90% < 20 years old
- Many secrete oncoproteins (α-fetoprotein, β-hCG)
- Treatment, prognosis varies with tumor type

Germinoma

Terminology

While germinomas are also called dysgerminoma or extragonadal seminoma, "germinoma" is the preferred term. The old name "atypical teratoma" is confusing and no longer used.

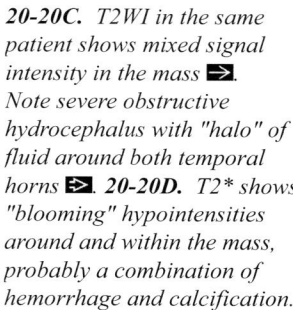

20-20A. Post-ventriculostomy NECT scan shows hyperdense pineal mass ➡ "engulfing" pineal gland calcifications ⧈. 20-20B. Sagittal T1WI in the same patient shows a well-defined pineal mass ➡ compressing the tectal plate inferiorly ⧈, causing severe obstructive hydrocephalus.

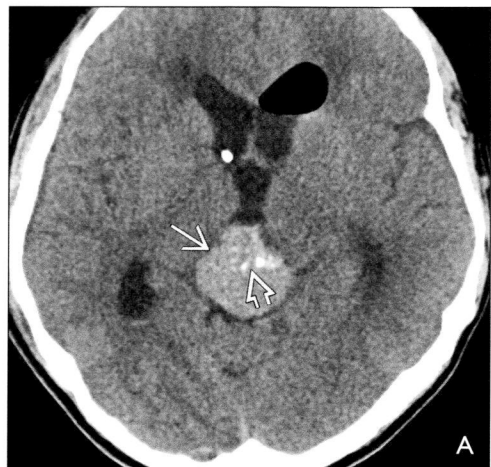

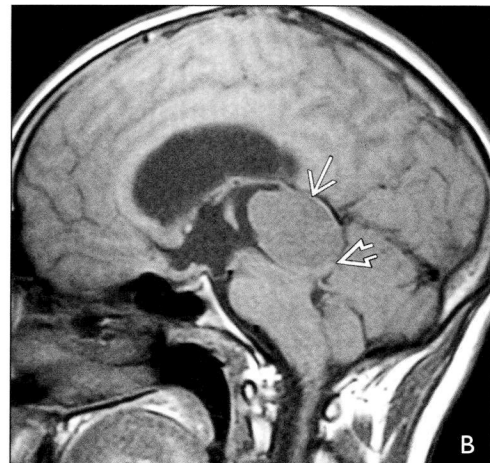

20-20C. T2WI in the same patient shows mixed signal intensity in the mass ➡. Note severe obstructive hydrocephalus with "halo" of fluid around both temporal horns ⧈. 20-20D. T2* shows "blooming" hypointensities around and within the mass, probably a combination of hemorrhage and calcification.

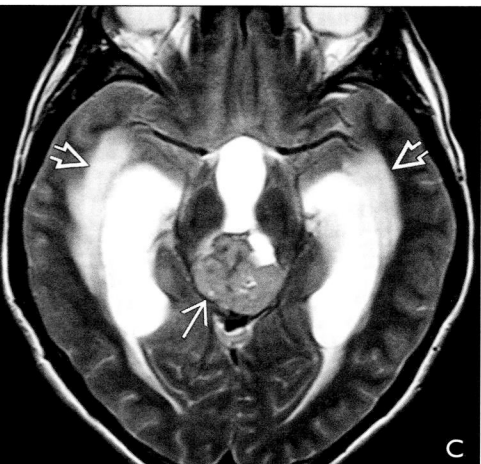

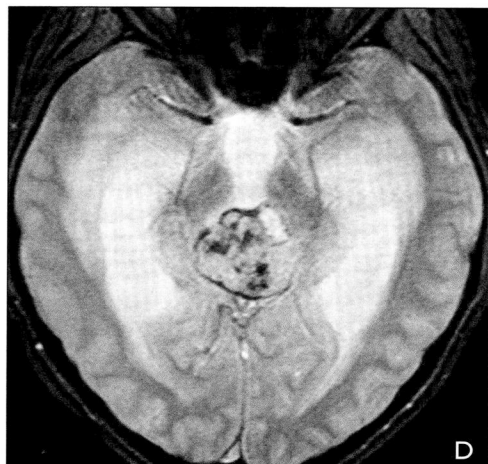

thology

LOCATION. Intracranial germinomas have a distinct predilection for midline structures. Between 80-90% "hug" the midline. One-half to two-thirds are found in the pineal region with the suprasellar region the second most frequent location, accounting for one-quarter to one-third of germinomas. Off-midline germinomas occur in 5-10% of cases. The basal ganglia are the most common off-midline site.

SIZE AND NUMBER. Size at diagnosis varies with location. Some infundibular stalk germinomas become symptomatic (usually causing central diabetes insipidus) before they can be detected on high-resolution contrast-enhanced MRs. Pineal germinomas that do not invade the tectum or cause hydrocephalus can be as large as several centimeters at the time of initial diagnosis.

Approximately 20% of intracranial germinomas are multiple. The most frequent combination is a pineal plus a suprasellar ("bifocal" or "double midline") germinoma **(20-17)**. Whether these are metastatic or synchronous lesions is debated.

GROSS PATHOLOGY. Germinomas are generally solid, friable, tan-white masses that often infiltrate adjacent structures. Intratumoral cysts, small hemorrhagic foci, and CSF dissemination are common **(20-18)**.

MICROSCOPIC FEATURES. Germinomas are histologically similar to ovarian dysgerminoma and testicular seminoma. A pure germinoma consists of large, relatively undifferentiated cells with prominent nucleoli arranged in monomorphous sheets or lobules separated by fine fibrovascular septa. Many germinomas have a biphasic pattern of abundant mature lymphocytes intermixed with larger germinoma cells. Mitoses are common, but necrosis is rare **(20-19)**.

STAGING, GRADING, AND CLASSIFICATION. Pure germinomas are WHO grade II neoplasms.

Clinical Issues

EPIDEMIOLOGY. Germinoma is the most common intracranial GCT and accounts for 1-2% of all primary brain tumors.

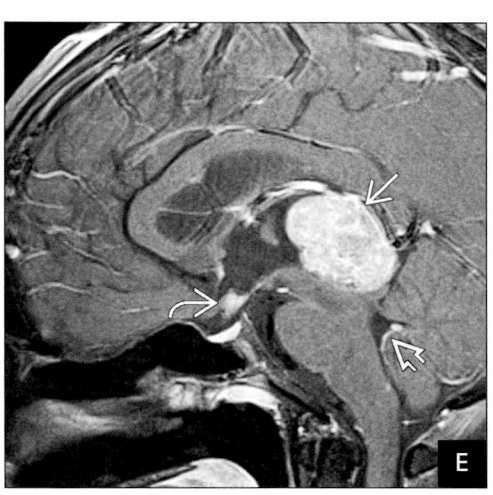
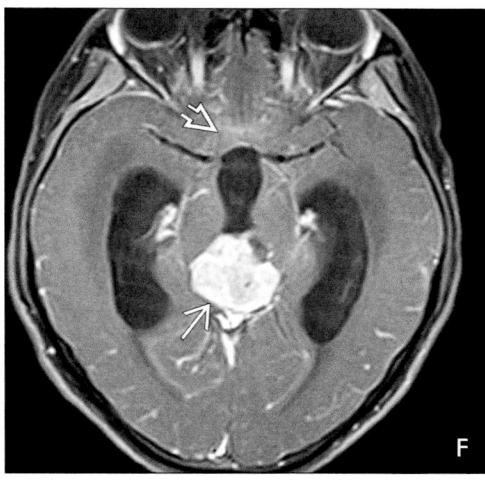
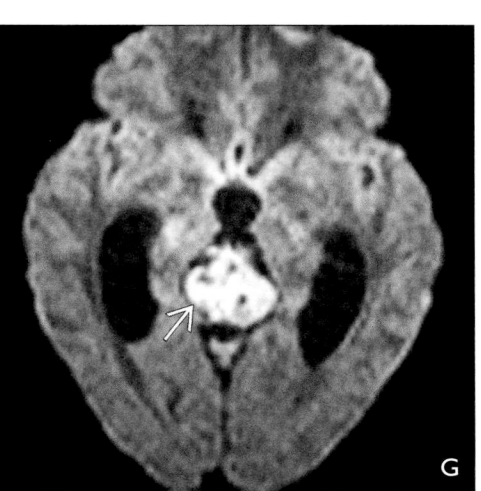
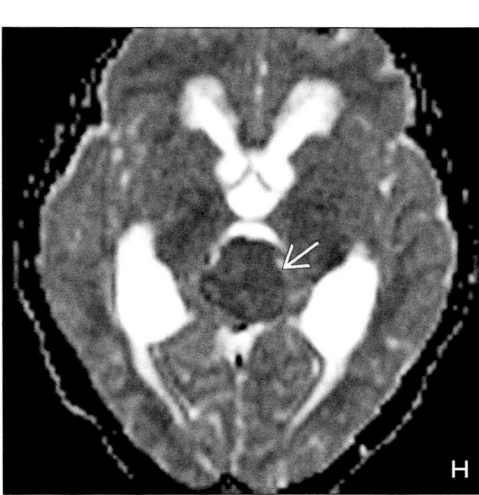

20-20E. Sagittal T1 C+ FS scan in the same patient shows that the mass ➡ enhances intensely. Note tumor in the anterior recesses of the third ventricle ➡ and along the floor of the fourth ventricle ➡. 20-20F. Axial T1 C+ FS shows the enhancing mass ➡, sulcal-cisternal enhancement ➡ suggesting CSF dissemination.

20-20G. DWI shows diffusion restriction ➡. 20-20H. ADC map shows moderate restriction ➡ consistent with a highly cellular mass. Germinoma.

DEMOGRAPHICS. More than 90% of patients are younger than 20 years of age at initial diagnosis. Peak presentation is 10-12 years. The M:F ratio for pineal germinoma is 10:1. Suprasellar germinomas have no gender predilection.

PRESENTATION. Presentation varies with location. Pineal germinomas typically present with headache and Parinaud syndrome. The most common presentation for suprasellar germinoma is central diabetes insipidus. Visual loss and precocious puberty are other presentations.

NATURAL HISTORY. CSF dissemination and invasion are common, but pure germinomas have a very favorable response to radiation therapy. The five-year survival for treated patients with pure germinoma is > 90%.

Germinomas that contain syncytiotrophoblastic giant cells have a higher recurrence rate and reduced long-term survival.

TREATMENT OPTIONS. Histologic documentation followed by radiation therapy is the standard treatment. Adjuvant chemotherapy is reserved for disseminated tumors.

GERMINOMA: PATHOLOGY AND CLINICAL ISSUES

Pathology
- Involve midline structures (80-90%)
- Pineal > > suprasellar > basal ganglia
- Multiple (20%, usually pineal + suprasellar)
- Germinoma cells + numerous lymphocytes

Clinical Issues
- 1-2% of all neoplasms (more common in Asia)
- Most common intracranial GCT
- > 90% of patients under age 20
- Pineal germinoma, M:F = 3-10:1; suprasellar, M = F
- May cause diabetes insipidus before infundibular lesion seen at imaging!

Imaging

GENERAL FEATURES. CSF dissemination is common, so the entire neuraxis should be imaged in patients with suspected germinoma. MR is the procedure of choice for complete delineation of germinoma extent. Caution: Some suprasellar germinomas may present with diabetes insipidus long before lesions are visible on MR. In such cases, serial imaging should be performed.

CT FINDINGS. Because many germinomas contain numerous lymphocytes, they are typically hyperdense compared to brain on NECT. They appear to be "draped" around the posterior third ventricle. Obstructive hydrocephalus is variable. Pineal calcifications are "engulfed" and surrounded by tumor **(20-20A)**. Strong uniform

enhancement is typical. Look for a second lesion in the suprasellar region!

MR FINDINGS. Germinomas are iso- to slightly hyperintense to cortex on T1- and T2WI. Variably sized intratumoral cysts are common, especially in larger lesions. Hemorrhage is generally uncommon except in basal ganglionic germinomas. T2* (GRE, SWI) may show "blooming" due to intratumoral calcification. Enhancement is strong and usually homogeneous **(20-20B)**, **(20-20C)**, **(20-20D)**, **(20-20E)**, **(20-20F)**.

Because of their high cellularity, germinomas may show restricted diffusion **(20-20G)**, **(20-20H)**.

Differential Diagnosis

The major differential diagnosis of pineal germinoma is **mixed germ cell tumor** as well as **nongerminomatous germ cell tumors**. Some **pineoblastomas** may appear similar to germinoma but "explode" rather than "engulf" pineal calcifications. **Pineal parenchymal tumor of intermediate differentiation** usually occurs in middle-aged and older adults.

The major differential diagnosis of suprasellar germinoma is **Langerhans cell histiocytosis** (LCH). Both are common in children, often cause diabetes insipidus, and may be indistinguishable on imaging studies alone. However, LCH does not produce oncoproteins. **Neurosarcoidosis** in an adult can cause a suprasellar mass that resembles germinoma.

GERMINOMA: IMAGING

CT
- NECT: Hyperdense, "engulfs" pineal Ca++
- CECT: Enhances strongly, uniformly

MR
- T1 iso-/hypo, T2 iso-/hyperintense
- GRE shows Ca++, hemorrhage
- Often restricts on DWI
- Enhances intensely, heterogeneously
- CSF spread common (look for other lesions)
- Image entire neuraxis before surgery!

Differential Diagnosis
- Nongerminomatous GCT
- PPTs (pineoblastoma, PPTID)
- Histiocytosis (stalk lesion in child)
- Neurosarcoidosis (stalk lesion in adult)

Teratoma

Teratomas are tridermic masses that originate from "misenfolded" or displaced embryonic stem cells. Teratomas recapitulate somatic development and differentiate along ectodermal, mesodermal, and endodermal cell types.

Although they may originate anywhere in the body, teratomas are most commonly found in sacrococcygeal, gonadal, mediastinal, retroperitoneal, cervicofacial, and intracranial locations. Teratomas preferentially involve the midline; intracranial lesions most often arise in the pineal or suprasellar region.

Teratomas account for 2-4% of primary brain tumors in children and almost half of all congenital (perinatal) brain tumors. They account for more than 60% of prenatally detected parenchymal brain tumors.

Teratomas are more common in Asians and males. They have two peaks in age distribution. Ten percent occur before age five; nearly half occur from 5-15 years of age. Age at diagnosis is an important prognostic feature, independent of tumor location. Peri- or antenatal presentation is associated with higher risk of adverse outcome. Clinical behavior also varies significantly with tumor size.

There are three recognized types of teratoma. These range from a benign well-differentiated "mature" teratoma to an immature teratoma to a teratoma with malignant differentiation. All three share some imaging features, viz., complex masses with striking heterogeneity in density and/or signal intensity. Cysts and hemorrhage are common.

ature Teratoma

Mature teratomas are well-demarcated lobulated tumors that contain well-differentiated mature elements from all three embryonic germ layers. Ectodermal elements such as skin, hair, and dermal appendages (e.g., sebaceous glands) are common (20-21). Mesodermal tissues such as cartilage, bone, fat, and muscle may be prominent features. Respiratory or enteric epithelium often lines intratumoral cysts (20-22).

Mitotic activity is low or absent. A mature teratoma is a WHO grade I lesion.

The size of a mature teratoma varies from relatively small pineal lesions to huge holocranial lesions with massive extracranial extension into the orbit, face, ears, and oral cavity. The intracranial component of these craniofacial teratomas may become so large that there is virtually complete loss of normal intracranial architecture. In such cases, normal brain structures are basically unrecognizable.

Imaging shows a complex-appearing multiloculated lesion with fat, calcification, numerous cysts, and other tissues (20-23). Hemorrhage is common. Enhancement is variable.

mature Teratoma

Immature teratomas contain a complex admixture of at least some fetal-type tissues from all three germ cell layers in combination with more mature tissue elements (20-24), (20-25). It is common to have cartilage, bone, intestinal mucous, and smooth muscle intermixed

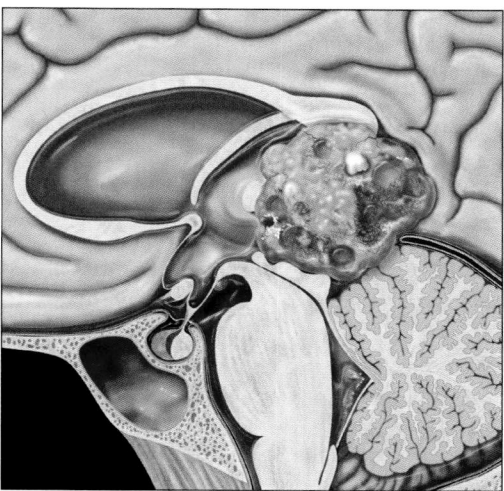

20-21. Graphic depicts pineal teratoma with the typical heterogeneous tissue components (cysts, solid tumor, calcifications, fat, etc.).

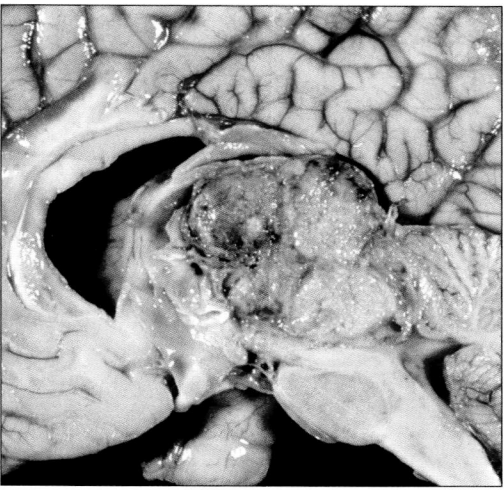

20-22. Autopsy case shows typical pineal teratoma with very heterogeneous-appearing components. (Courtesy B. Alvord, MD.)

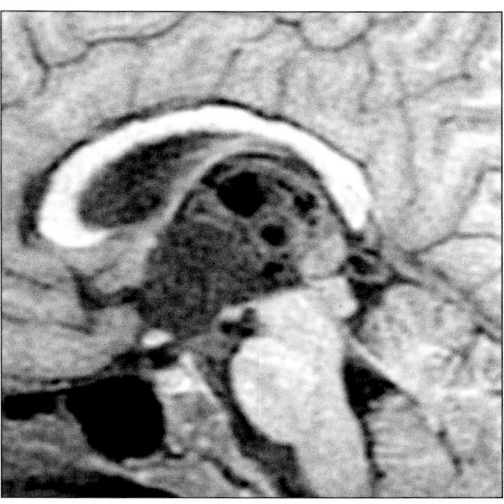

20-23. T1WI of mature pineal teratoma shows expected heterogeneous signal intensity. No frank lipomatous component with short T1 is seen.

with primitive neural ectodermal tissue. Hemorrhage and necrosis are common.

Giant immature teratomas are congenital lesions usually seen in a fetus or newborn. Most are associated with stillbirth, perinatal death, or significant morbidity after attempted surgical resection.

The fetal ultrasound diagnosis of intracranial teratoma can generally be established relatively early in pregnancy (15-16 weeks). Macrocephaly, progressive hydrocephalus, and polyhydramnios are common. A rapidly growing heterogeneous mass with mixed hyper- and hypoechogenic features is typical.

CT or MR demonstrate almost complete replacement of brain tissue by a complex mixed-density or signal intensity mass **(20-26)**, **(20-27)**.

Teratoma with Malignant Transformation

Teratomas with malignant transformation generally arise from immature teratomas and contain somatic-type cancers such as rhabdomyosarcoma or undifferentiated sarcoma.

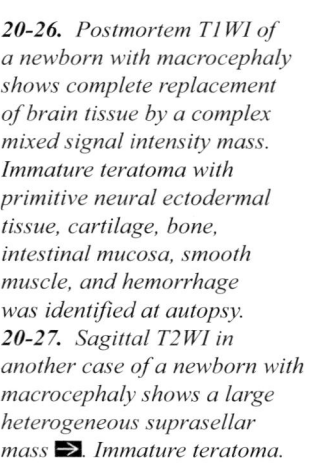
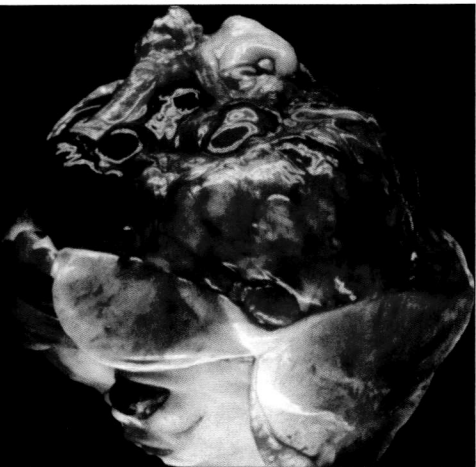
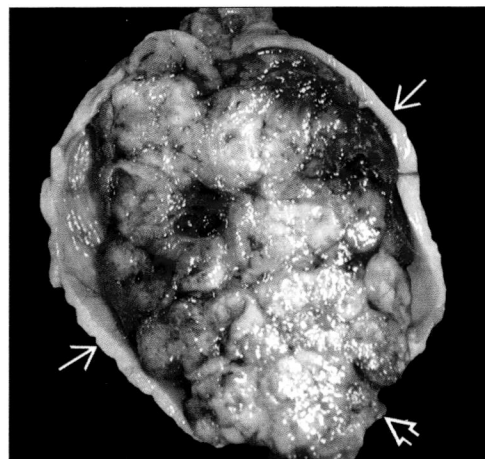

20-24. *Fetal autopsy case shows a large intra- and extracranial immature teratoma with multiple cysts and hemorrhage.* *20-25. Gross autopsy specimen of a congenital teratoma shows a heterogeneous mass occupying virtually all of the intracranial cavity* ⬧. *Only a thin rim of brain is present* ➡, *which has been displaced peripherally by the huge tumor. (Courtesy T. Tihan, MD.)*

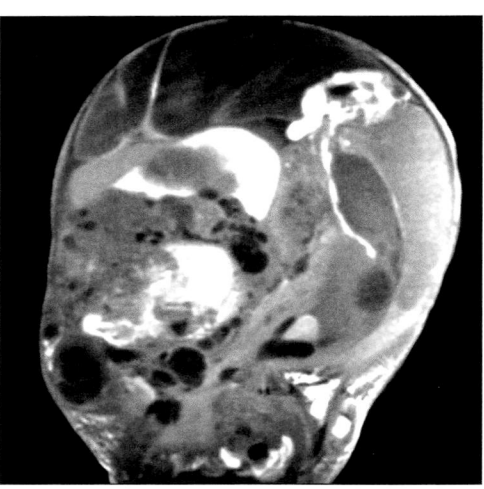
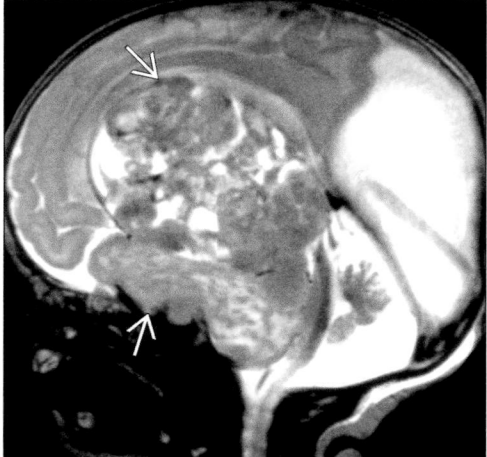

20-26. *Postmortem T1WI of a newborn with macrocephaly shows complete replacement of brain tissue by a complex mixed signal intensity mass. Immature teratoma with primitive neural ectodermal tissue, cartilage, bone, intestinal mucosa, smooth muscle, and hemorrhage was identified at autopsy.* *20-27. Sagittal T2WI in another case of a newborn with macrocephaly shows a large heterogeneous suprasellar mass* ➡. *Immature teratoma.*

ther Germ Cell Neoplasms

Germinomas are by far the most common of the germ cell neoplasms. Nongerminomatous malignant germ cell tumors (NGMGCTs) are rare neoplasms that contain undifferentiated epithelial cells and are often mixed with other germ cell elements (most often germinoma). These include **yolk sac (endodermal sinus) tumor**, **embryonal carcinoma**, **choriocarcinoma**, and **mixed germ cell tumor**.

NGMGCTs generally occur in adolescents with a peak incidence at 10-15 years of age. Prognosis is usually poor with overall survival less than two years.

Differentiating intracranial germ cell neoplasms on the basis of imaging studies alone is problematic. All intracranial GCTs—whether benign or malignant—tend to "hug" the midline. Many express different oncoproteins, so immunohistochemical profiling is an essential part of diagnosis.

olk Sac Tumor

Yolk sac (endodermal sinus) tumors represent just 2% of all intracranial GCTs. Yolk sac tumors are composed of primitive epithelial cells in a loose, variably cellular myxoid matrix. Peak occurrence is in the second decade. Imaging features are nonspecific.

nbryonal Carcinoma

Embryonal carcinoma is another tumor that contains large, anaplastic epithelioid cells that are arranged in sheets, cords, and nests.

Imaging findings are nonspecific. A large mixed-density/signal intensity, heterogeneously enhancing mass is the common appearance **(20-28)**.

horiocarcinoma

Most choriocarcinomas develop within or outside the uterus following a gestational event ("gestational" choriocarcinoma). Nongestational choriocarcinomas can arise from germ cells in gonadal or extragonadal midline locations.

CNS choriocarcinoma can be primary or metastatic, arising from an extracranial site such as the retroperitoneum or mediastinum. Primary intracranial choriocarcinoma (PICCC) is the rarest, most malignant of all the intracranial GCTs.

PICCCs are dimorphic tumors characterized by extraembryonic differentiation along cytrophoblastic and syncytiotrophoblastic lines. They are composed of mononucleated trophoblastic cells admixed with large multinucleated syncytiotrophoblastic cells. Hemorrhage, necrosis, fibrosis, and neovascularity are common.

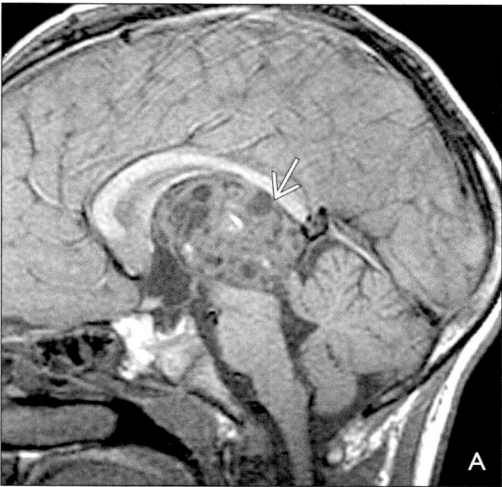

20-28A. Sagittal T1WI in an 8-year-old boy with headaches shows mixed signal intensity pineal mass ➡.

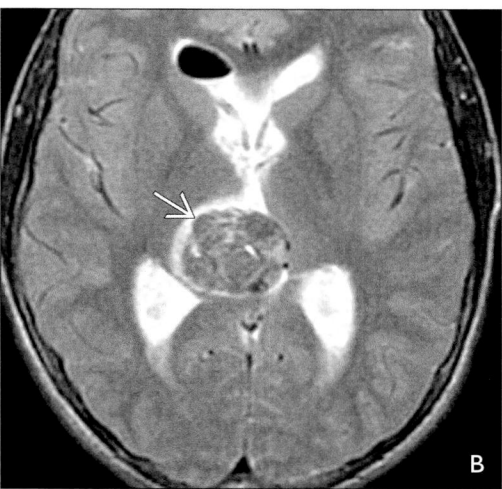

20-28B. Post-shunt T2WI shows that the mass ➡ retains its mixed signal characteristics.

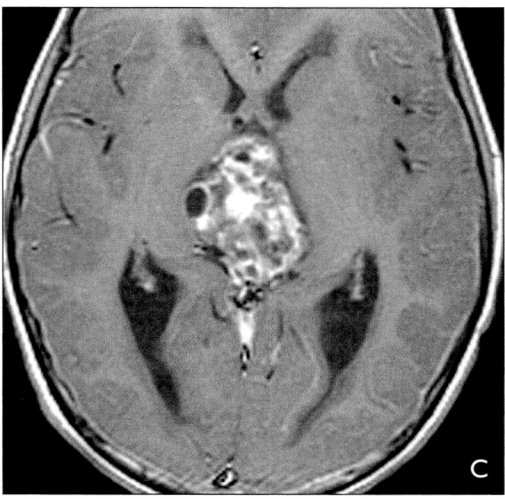

20-28C. T1 C+ shows areas of solid, ring, and nonenhancing foci. Preoperative diagnosis was teratoma. Pathology showed embryonal carcinoma.

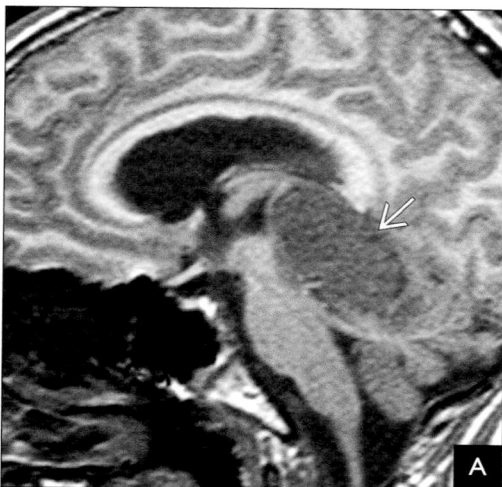

20-29A. *Sagittal T1WI in a 13-year-old boy with Parinaud syndrome shows a hypointense pineal mass* ➡.

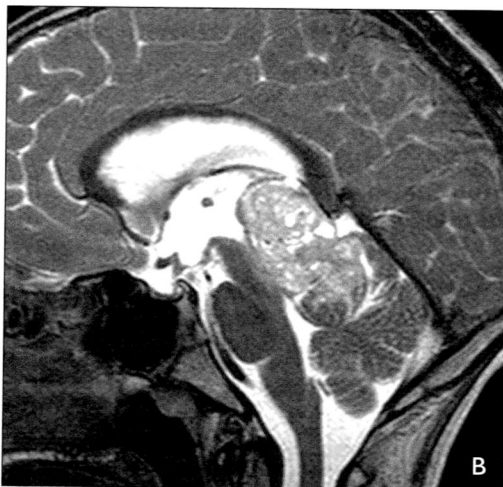

20-29B. *The mass is heterogeneously hyperintense on T2WI.*

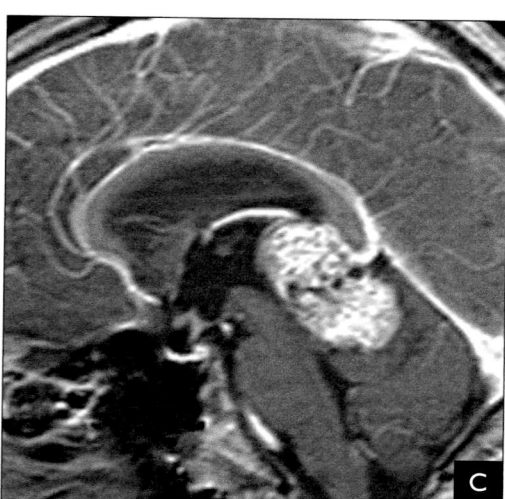

20-29C. *Strong but heterogeneous enhancement is seen on T1 C+ FS. Mixed germ cell tumor. (Courtesy M. Thurnher, MD.)*

PICCCs typically present in patients 3-20 years of age. There is a nearly 4:1 male predominance. Precocious puberty is the most common presentation in males. Markedly elevated serum hCG/β-hCG levels are strongly suggestive of PICCC.

The most common sites of PICCC are the pineal and suprasellar regions. MR imaging is helpful for tumor localization, characterization, and preoperative evaluation, but the findings are nonspecific. Intratumoral hemorrhage with stripe-like or patchy hypointensities on T2WI are common. Heterogeneous rim and nodular enhancement is seen in most cases. Extraneural/CSF metastases are common.

Mixed Germ Cell Tumor

Mixed GCTs are composed of any of the above histologic subtypes, often together with germinomatous elements. Mixed GCTs are more common than any pure germ cell lesion except for germinoma. Imaging findings are nonspecific **(20-29)**.

APPROACH TO PINEAL REGION MASSES
Three Key Questions to Consider
- Is the mass in the pineal gland itself?
- What is the patient's age, gender?
- Is there evidence of oncoproteins?

Pineal Gland Mass
- Common
  - Pineal cyst (nonneoplastic)
- Less common
  - Pineocytoma
  - Germinoma
- Rare but important
  - PPTID
  - Pineoblastoma
  - Nongerminomatous malignant GCT
  - Papillary tumor of the pineal region
  - Astrocytoma
  - Metastasis

Pineal Region Mass
- Common
  - Pineal gland masses
- Less common (masses *outside* pineal gland)
  - Other nonneoplastic cysts (arachnoid, dermoid, etc.)
  - Neoplasm (astrocytoma, meningioma, metastasis)
  - Lipoma
- Rare but important
  - Vascular lesions (vein of Galen malformation, aneurysm, dural arteriovenous fistula)

elected References

neal Region Anatomy
Gross Anatomy

- Zhang XA et al: The distribution of arachnoid membrane within the velum interpositum. Acta Neurochir (Wien). 154(9):1711-5, 2012
- Rios ER et al: Melatonin: pharmacological aspects and clinical trends. Int J Neurosci. 120(9):583-90, 2010
- Tubbs RS et al: The velum interpositum revisited and redefined. Surg Radiol Anat. 30(2):131-5, 2008

Normal Imaging

- Kennedy BC et al: Surgical approaches to the pineal region. Neurosurg Clin N Am. 22(3):367-80, viii, 2011
- Sun B et al: The pineal volume: a three-dimensional volumetric study in healthy young adults using 3.0 T MR data. Int J Dev Neurosci. 27(7):655-60, 2009
- Doyle AJ et al: Physiologic calcification of the pineal gland in children on computed tomography: prevalence, observer reliability and association with choroid plexus calcification. Acad Radiol. 13(7):822-6, 2006
- Hamilton BE: Pineal region. In Harnsberger HR et al: Diagnostic and Surgical Imaging Anatomy: Brain, Head and Neck, Spine. Salt Lake City: Amirsys Publishing. I.98.101, 2006

neal Parenchymal Tumors

- Parker JJ et al: Preoperative evaluation of pineal tumors. Neurosurg Clin N Am. 22(3):353-8, vii-viii, 2011
- Gaillard F et al: Masses of the pineal region: clinical presentation and radiographic features. Postgrad Med J. 86(1020):597-607, 2010
- Smith AB et al: From the archives of the AFIP: lesions of the pineal region: radiologic-pathologic correlation. Radiographics. 30(7):2001-20, 2010
- Sato K et al: Pathology of pineal parenchymal tumors. Prog Neurol Surg. 23:12-25, 2009

Pineal Parenchymal Tumor of Intermediate Differentiation

- Fukuoka K et al: Pineal parenchymal tumor of intermediate differentiation with marked elevation of MIB-1 labeling index. Brain Tumor Pathol. Epub ahead of print, 2012
- Han SJ et al: Pathology of pineal parenchymal tumors. Neurosurg Clin N Am. 22(3):335-40, vii, 2011
- Komakula S et al: Pineal parenchymal tumor of intermediate differentiation: imaging spectrum of an unusual tumor in 11 cases. Neuroradiology. 53(8):577-84, 2011

Pineoblastoma

- Smith AB et al: From the archives of the AFIP: lesions of the pineal region: radiologic-pathologic correlation. Radiographics. 30(7):2001-20, 2010

Papillary Tumor of the Pineal Region

- Wong YS et al: 45 year old man with a pineal region tumor for over 15 years. Brain Pathol. 22(2):255-8, 2012
- Murali R et al: Papillary tumour of the pineal region: cytological features and implications for intraoperative diagnosis. Pathology. 42(5):474-9, 2010

Germ Cell Tumors
Overview of Germ Cell Tumors

- Wang HW et al: Pediatric primary central nervous system germ cell tumors of different prognosis groups show characteristic miRNome traits and chromosome copy number variations. BMC Genomics. 11:132, 2010
- Kyritsis AP: Management of primary intracranial germ cell tumors. J Neurooncol. 96(2):143-9, 2010
- Kreutz J et al: Intracranial germ cell tumor. JBR-BTR. 93(4):196-7, 2010

Germinoma

- Wang Y et al: Intracranial germinoma: clinical and MRI findings in 56 patients. Childs Nerv Syst. 26(12):1773-7, 2010

Teratoma

- Isik N et al: Surgical treatment of huge congenital extracranial immature teratoma: a case report. Childs Nerv Syst. 27(5):833-9, 2011
- Barksdale EM Jr et al: Teratomas in infants and children. Curr Opin Pediatr. 21(3):344-9, 2009
- Isaacs H: Fetal brain tumors: a review of 154 cases. Am J Perinatol. 26(6):453-66, 2009
- Saada J et al: Early second-trimester diagnosis of intracranial teratoma. Ultrasound Obstet Gynecol. 33(1):109-11, 2009
- Woodward PJ et al: From the archives of the AFIP: a comprehensive review of fetal tumors with pathologic correlation. Radiographics. 25(1):215-42, 2005

Other Germ Cell Neoplasms

- Park SA et al: 18F-FDG PET/CT imaging for mixed germ cell tumor in the pineal region. Clin Nucl Med. 37(3):e61-3, 2012
- Verma R et al: Primary skull-based yolk-sac tumour: case report and review of central nervous system germ cell tumours. J Neurooncol. 101(1):129-34, 2011
- Lv XF et al: Primary intracranial choriocarcinoma: MR imaging findings. AJNR Am J Neuroradiol. 31(10):1994-8, 2010
- Davaus T et al: Pineal yolk sac tumor: correlation between neuroimaging and pathological findings. Arq Neuropsiquiatr. 65(2A):283-5, 2007

21

Embryonal and Neuroblastic Tumors

The growing use of molecular genetic profiling in neuropathology has had an enormous impact on the identification and treatment of CNS neoplasms. A classic example is the now-routine determination of 1p,19q status in oligodendrogliomas.

The rapidly evolving molecular classification of brain tumors has also greatly influenced our understanding of embryonal neoplasms, perhaps more so than any other group of neoplasms.

Embryonal brain tumors are a heterogeneous group of primitive neoplasms with protean histopathologic manifestations. Most consist of poorly differentiated stem-like cells whereas others show some degree of differentiation along neuronal, glial, or (less commonly) other lineages such as myogenic cell lines.

All embryonal tumors are designated as WHO grade IV neoplasms. Most occur preferentially in infants and young children and are generally characterized by aggressive clinical behavior. Most such tumors have an inherent tendency to metastasize early and widely via CSF pathways.

The WHO classification recognizes three categories of embryonal tumors: (1) medulloblastoma, (2) CNS primitive neuroectodermal tumors (PNETs), and (3) atypical teratoid/rhabdoid tumor. All three groups are discussed in this chapter, together with a newly recognized subtype of

CNS PNETs known as embryonal tumor with abundant neuropil and true rosettes (ETANTR).

Medulloblastoma

Medulloblastoma Overview

Significant variability in biological behavior exists among medulloblastomas (MBs), which are currently classified by histology alone, prompting an intense search for molecular markers that might facilitate recognition and treatment of this important childhood cancer.

We now understand clearly that medulloblastoma is not a single disease. Recent transcriptomic approaches demonstrated that the pathologically defined entity historically known as medulloblastoma is composed of multiple clinically and molecularly distinct subgroups. In addition, each subgroup contains at least one further level of hierarchy, and some have multiple levels and subtypes. Each distinct MB molecular subgroup differs in its demographics, transcriptomes, somatic genetic events, and clinical outcomes.

Understanding medulloblastoma in the context of a changing histologic classification and rapidly evolving molecular profiling is difficult. Attempting to correlate imaging manifestations with histology and molecular profiling compounds the challenge. This section provides a general overview of medulloblastoma, its pathology, and the current status of molecular diagnostics.

The following sections then discuss the specific MB subtypes and their imaging appearances. If you expect a 1:1 relationship between MB histologic variants, molecular subgroups, and specific imaging findings, you will be disappointed. It simply isn't possible. But if you want to improve your understanding of these fascinating tumors and their imaging appearances, read on.

Epidemiology

Medulloblastoma (MB) is the most common malignant CNS neoplasm of childhood and the second most common overall pediatric brain tumor (after astrocytoma).

Pathologic Classification of Medulloblastoma and MB Subtypes

Medulloblastomas are a pathologically diverse group of tumors. The 2007 WHO histologic classification recognized **classic medulloblastoma** (called simply "medulloblastoma") and four medulloblastoma variants: (1) **desmoplastic/nodular medulloblastoma**, (2) **medulloblastoma with extensive nodularity**, (3) **anaplastic medulloblastoma**, and (4) **large cell medulloblastoma**. The latter two are sometimes grouped together and referred to as "large cell/anaplastic medulloblastoma."

All medulloblastomas—regardless of subtype—are designated as WHO grade IV neoplasms.

Molecular Classification of MBs

A 2010 consensus conference identified four main molecular subgroups, each arising from different cytogenetic pathways. The two named pathways are the Shh and Wnt pathways. Two non-Wnt, non-Shh groups are called simply "group 3" and "group 4." All four subtypes have different origins, preferred anatomic locations, demographics, metastatic potential, and clinical outcomes.

SHH PATHWAY MBs. Between 25-30% of MBs arise from granule neuron precursor cells (GNPCs) after activation of the Shh pathway. GNPCs are found in the external granular layer of the cerebellum until early in the second year of life.

Shh MBs exhibit a bimodal age distribution, arising in infants (younger than four years) and adults (older than 16 years). There is no gender predilection.

Shh MBs are often located laterally within the cerebellar hemispheres. Although they can give rise to both classic and variant MB subtypes, they most often display large cell, anaplastic, or desmoplastic histology. Patients with Shh MBs have a relatively poor prognosis.

Individuals with germline mutations in the Shh receptor *PTCH* have basal cell nevus (Gorlin) syndrome and are predisposed to develop medulloblastoma.

WNT PATHWAY MBs. Wnt medulloblastomas are the smallest MB subgroup (10%) and are strikingly different from Shh MBs. Wnt MBs arise from and infiltrate the dorsal brainstem and fourth ventricle.

Wnt MBs are very rare in infants but more common in children and adults. They almost always exhibit classic MB histology and confer a significantly better long-term prognosis than MBs of other subgroups. They occur almost equally in males and females.

GROUP 3. Group 3 is the third largest MB subgroup (20-25%). Group 3 tumors usually exhibit classic MB histology, although this category also encompasses the majority of large cell/anaplastic tumors.

Group 3 MBs are most common in infants, rarely occur in adults, exhibit a nearly 2:1 M:F predominance, metastasize frequently, and have the worst outcome of all four molecular subtypes.

GROUP 4. Group 4 is the largest (about 35%) of the four molecular MB subgroups. Classic, anaplastic, and large cell variants occur while desmoplastic MBs are relatively uncommon. These MBs affect all ages but are more common in children. The M:F ratio is 2:1. Group 4 MBs frequently metastasize.

MEDULLOBLASTOMA CLASSIFICATION

Histopathologic Classification
- Medulloblastoma ("classic," CMB)
- Medulloblastoma variants
  - Desmoplastic/nodular medulloblastoma (DMB)
  - Medulloblastoma with extensive nodularity (MBEN)
  - Anaplastic medulloblastoma (AMB)
  - Large cell medulloblastoma (LCMB)

Molecular Classification
- Shh pathway medulloblastomas
  - Second largest subgroup (25-30%)
  - Arise from granule neuron precursor cells
  - Shh pathway activated
  - Most common in infants < 4 years, adults > 16 years
  - All histologic types but DMB, LCMB, AMB most common
- Wnt pathway medulloblastomas
  - Smallest subgroup (10%)
  - Arise from/infiltrate dorsal brainstem, fourth ventricle
  - Rare in infants; most common in children, adults
  - > 97% CMB
  - Best prognosis
- Group 3 medulloblastomas
  - Third largest subgroup (20-25%)
  - Infants; rare in adults
  - Mostly CMB, but most AMBs/LCAs are in group 3
  - Worst outcome
- Group 4 medulloblastomas
  - Largest subgroup (35%)
  - All histologic types; DMB rare
  - All ages but more common in children
  - Frequently metastasize

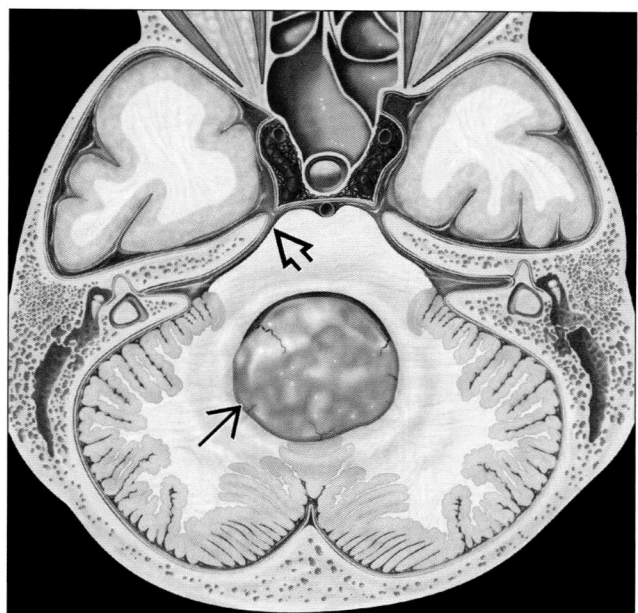

21-1. *Graphic illustrates classic MB as densely cellular "small round blue cell tumor" in the fourth ventricle ⊡. CSF dissemination ⊡ with diffuse "sugar icing" coating of brain surfaces is often present at initial diagnosis.*

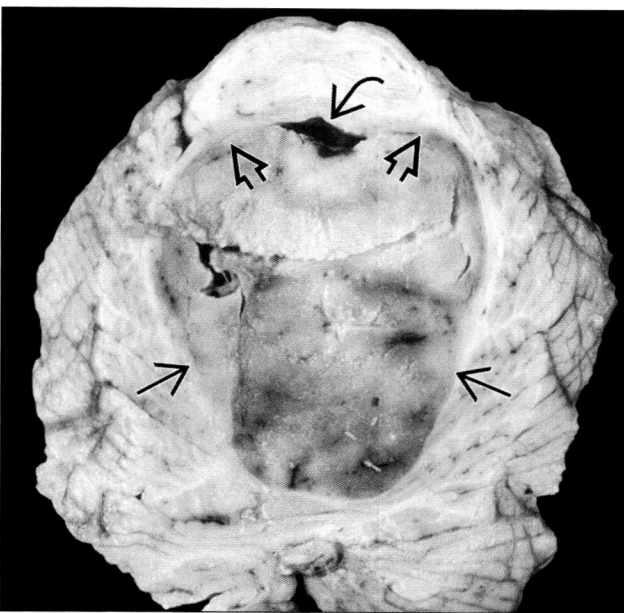

21-2. *Autopsy specimen demonstrates a large medulloblastoma ⊡ in the fourth ventricle with some sparing of the uppermost aspect of the ventricle ⊡. Pons is compressed anteriorly ⊡. (Courtesy R. Hewlett, MD.)*

Classic Medulloblastoma

Terminology

Classic medulloblastoma (CMB) is a primitive neuroectodermal tumor (PNET) that arises in the cerebellum. Classic posterior fossa MBs are also designated as PNET-MBs to distinguish them from PNETs that occur elsewhere in the CNS (see below).

Biology

CMBs occur in all four principal molecular subgroups.

Pathology

LOCATION. More than 85% of CMBs arise in the midline. They are located within the fourth ventricle and focally infiltrate the dorsal brainstem (21-1). Occasionally, CMB occurs as a diffusely infiltrating lesion without a focal dominant mass.

Posteroinferior extension into the cisterna magna is common. Unlike ependymoma, lateral extension into the cerebellopontine angle is rare.

SIZE AND NUMBER. CMBs vary in size. Most tumors are between two and four centimeters at the time of initial diagnosis.

GROSS PATHOLOGY. CMBs are relatively well-defined pink or grayish masses that typically fill the fourth ventricle, displacing and compressing the pons anteriorly (21-2). Small scattered foci of necrosis and hemorrhage may be present.

MICROSCOPIC FEATURES. CMBs are highly cellular tumors. Dense sheets of uniform cells with round or oval hyperchromatic pleomorphic nuclei surrounded by scanty cytoplasm is the typical appearance ("small round blue cell tumor"). Neuroblastic (Homer-Wright) rosettes—radial arrangements of tumor cells around fibrillary processes—are found in 40% of cases.

Clinical Issues

EPIDEMIOLOGY AND DEMOGRAPHICS. MBs cause 10% of all pediatric brain tumors and are the most common malignant posterior fossa childhood neoplasm. CMBs account for 70% of MBs. Most occur before age 10 years. There is a second, smaller peak in adults aged 20-40 years.

PRESENTATION. The most common clinical manifestations of MB are vomiting (90%) and headache (80%). Psychomotor regression, ataxia, strabismus, and spasticity are common. The median interval between symptom onset and diagnosis is two months.

Because of their location, MBs tend to compress the fourth ventricle and cause obstructive hydrocephalus. In one-third of children younger than three years, the diagnosis is made only after life-threatening signs of intracranial hypertension appear.

NATURAL HISTORY. Significant improvement in treatment has increased the five-year survival rate in patients

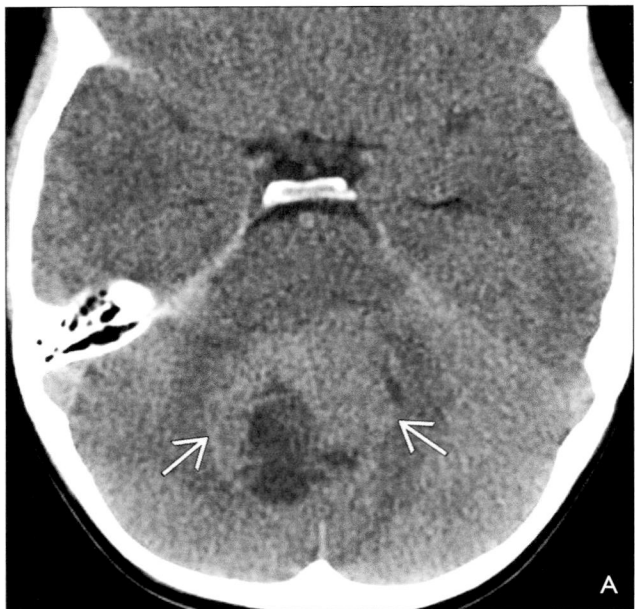

21-3A. NECT scan shows classic medulloblastoma. A mostly hyperdense midline posterior fossa mass ➡ is typical. Intratumoral cysts are present in 40% of cases.

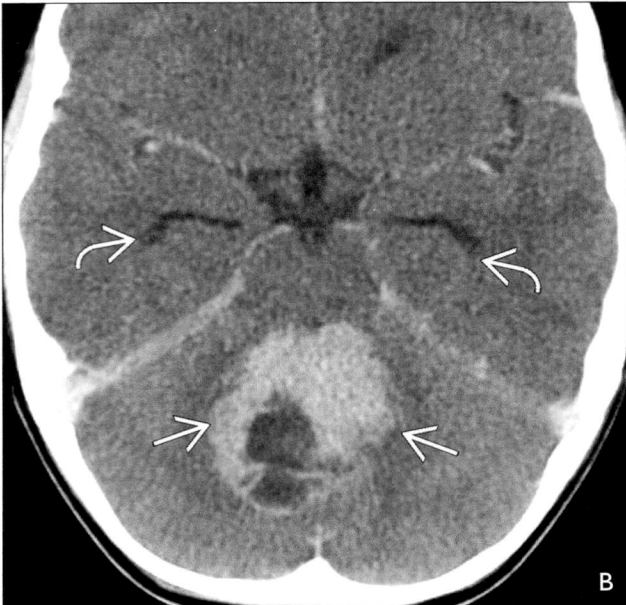

21-3B. CECT scan shows strong enhancement ➡. Note the mild enlargement of the temporal horns ➡. Obstructive hydrocephalus is a common finding with medulloblastoma.

with CMB to 60-70%. Classic MBs that show activation of the Wnt signaling pathway have a more favorable prognosis with a five-year survival of 95% in children and 100% in adults.

Treatment Options. Surgical resection is the primary treatment. Adjuvant chemotherapy increases survival rates in high-risk patients (i.e., children younger than three years, those with incomplete resection, and patients with CSF dissemination). Because of its significant adverse effects on the developing CNS, craniospinal radiation is generally avoided, especially in children under the age of two.

With recent advances in gene expression profiling, treatment decisions increasingly rely on identifying the specific molecular subtype in individuals with MB. For example, as most patients with documented Wnt-type MB survive, therapies that have significant associated morbidities may be unnecessary for these patients.

CLASSIC MEDULLOBLASTOMA

Terminology
- Classic medulloblastoma (CMB); PNET-MB

Etiology
- All 4 molecular subtypes represented
- CMBs from dorsal midbrain → fourth ventricle

Pathology
- Midline (> 85%, fourth ventricle)
- "Small round blue cell tumor"
- Neuroblastic (Homer-Wright) rosettes
- WHO grade IV

Epidemiology and Demographics
- MB: 10% of all pediatric brain tumors
- CMBs: 70% of all MBs
- Most common malignant posterior fossa childhood neoplasm
- Most CMBs in patients < 10 years; second peak in patients 20-40 years

---

Imaging

General Features. CMBs have relatively defined margins on imaging studies. Despite this appearance, 40-50% have CSF dissemination at the time of initial diagnosis. Preoperative contrast-enhanced MR imaging of the entire neuraxis is recommended.

CT Findings. NECT scans show a moderately hyperdense, relatively well-defined mass in the midline posterior fossa. Cyst formation (40%) and calcification (20-25%) are common. Gross hemorrhage is rare. Strong but heterogeneous enhancement is seen on CECT **(21-3)**.

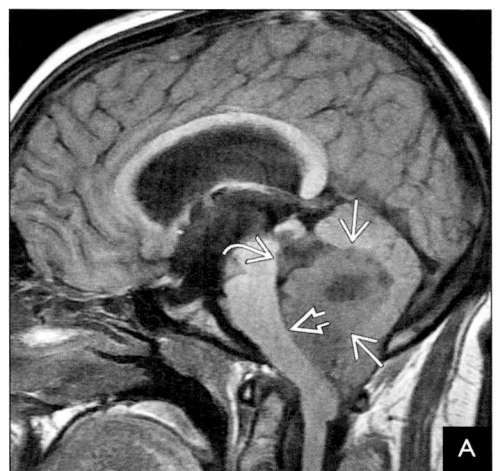

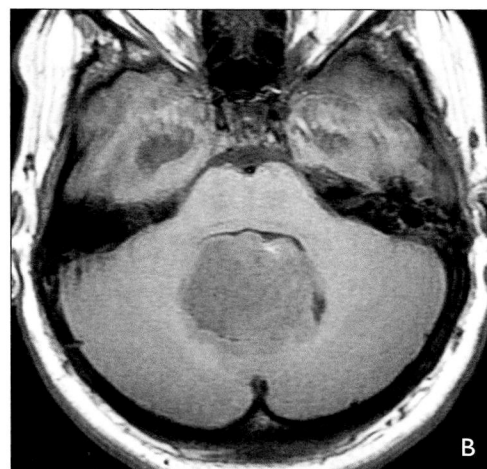

21-4A. Series of MR scans demonstrates typical findings of classic medulloblastoma. Sagittal T1WI shows a large hypointense mass ➡ expanding, filling most of the fourth ventricle but sparing its uppermost aspect ➡. The pons is compressed anteriorly ➡. Moderate obstructive hydrocephalus is present. 21-4B. Axial T1WI shows that the hypointense midline mass expands, fills the fourth ventricle.

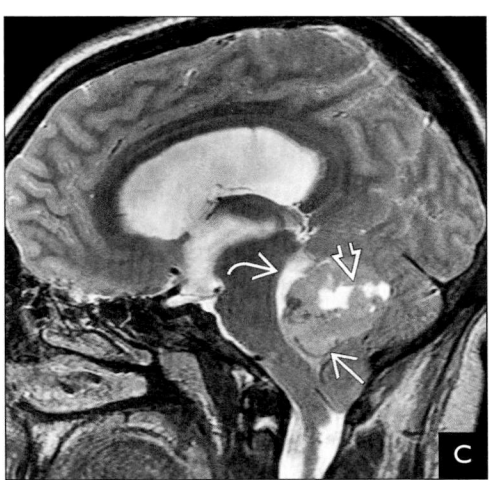

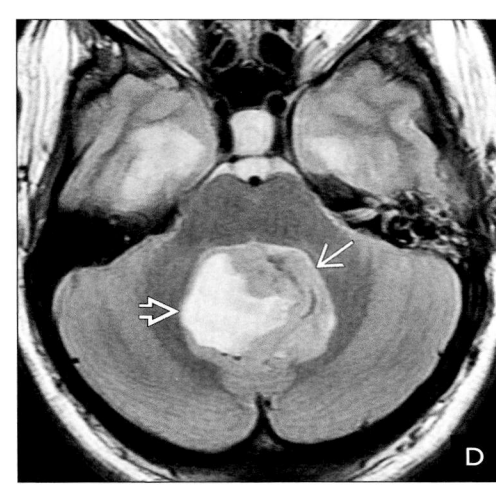

21-4C. Sagittal T2WI shows that the mass ➡ is mildly hyperintense on T2WI and contains several hyperintense cysts ➡. Note sparing of the upper fourth ventricle ➡. 21-4D. Axial T2WI shows the cyst ➡, heterogeneous hyperintensity of the mass ➡, dilated temporal horns from obstructive hydrocephalus.

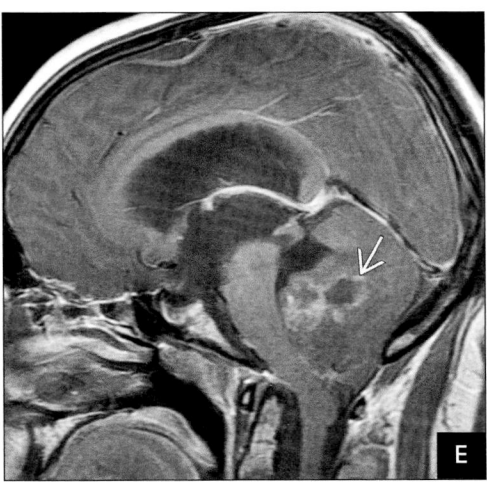

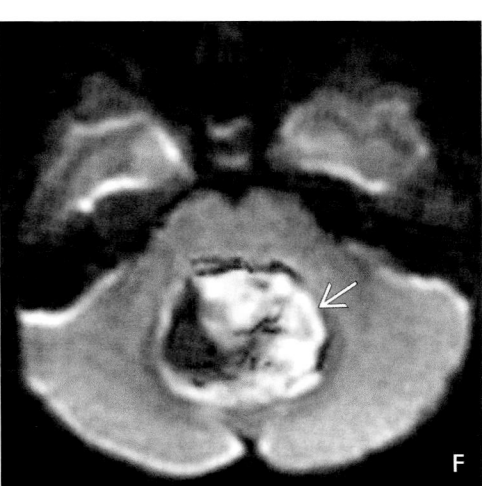

21-4E. Sagittal T1 C+ scan shows that the mass has partial patchy and ring enhancement ➡ but also that much of the tumor does not enhance. Enhancement of medulloblastoma is highly variable. 21-4F. DWI shows restricted diffusion in the densely cellular part of the mass ➡.

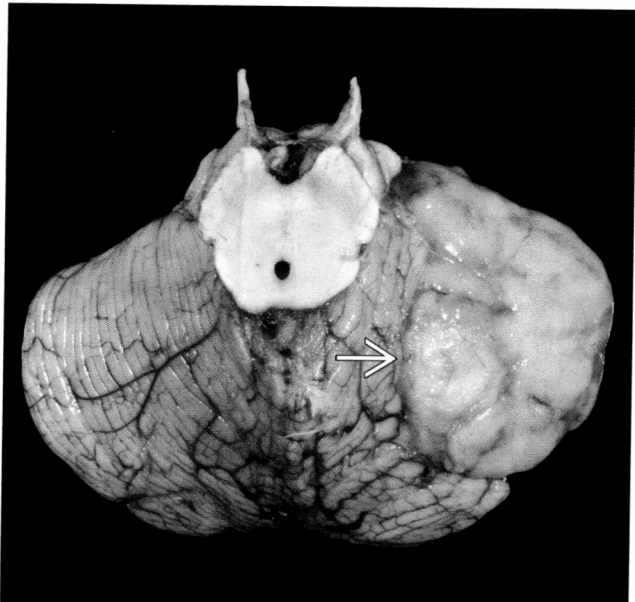

21-5. Autopsy specimen from an adult shows desmoplastic medulloblastoma as a fibrous-appearing, laterally located mass ➡ in the cerebellar hemisphere. (Courtesy R. Hewlett, MD.)

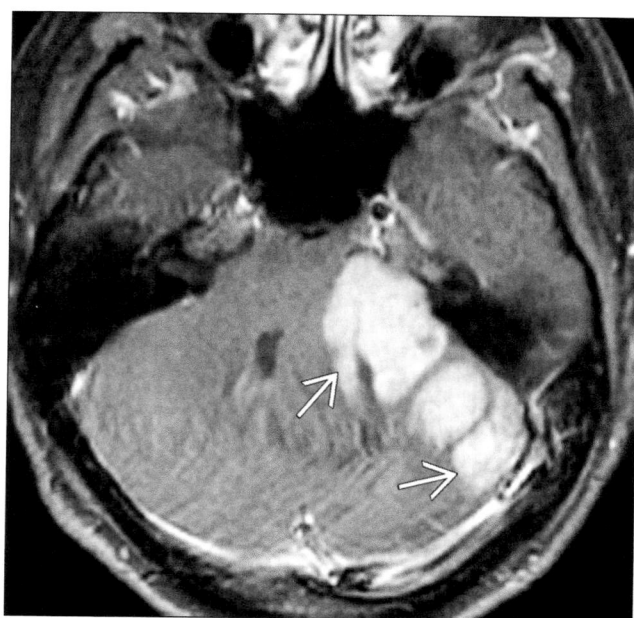

21-6. T1 C+ FS scan in an adult with a desmoplastic medulloblastoma shows strong enhancement, lateral cerebellar location of the mass ➡.

If dense tentorial or falcine calcifications are present, the patient should be evaluated for basal cell nevus (Gorlin) syndrome.

MR FINDINGS. Almost all CMBs are hypointense relative to gray matter on T1WI and hyperintense on T2WI. Peritumoral edema is present in one-third of cases. Obstructive hydrocephalus with transependymal CSF migration is common and best delineated on FLAIR.

Enhancement patterns show striking variation, ranging from minimal to patchy to marked. Two-thirds of CMBs show marked enhancement while one-third show only subtle, marginal, or linear enhancement.

Because of their dense cellularity, CMBs often show moderate restriction on DWI (21-4).

Differential Diagnosis

The major differential diagnosis of CMB in children is a **medulloblastoma variant**. A posterior fossa **atypical teratoid/rhabdoid tumor (AT/RT)** may be indistinguishable from CMB on imaging studies alone.

The differential diagnosis of MB in adults differs. The most common parenchymal posterior fossa mass in adults is metastasis.

Lhermitte-Duclos disease (LDD) can be seen in children but is more common in young adults. LDD and cerebellar medulloblastoma may resemble one another although the striated pattern of LDD is quite characteristic.

> **CLASSIC MEDULLOBLASTOMA: IMAGING**
> **CT**
> • Hyperdense on NECT
> • Cysts (40%)
> • Ca++ (20-25%)
> • Hemorrhage rare
> • Enhances strongly, heterogeneously
> **MR**
> • Hypo- on T1, hyperintense on T2
> • Often restricts on DWI
> • Enhancement: None to strong
> **Differential Diagnosis**
> • Medulloblastoma variant
> • Atypical teratoid/rhabdoid tumor
> • Lhermitte-Duclos disease (adults)

Medulloblastoma Variants

Desmoplastic Medulloblastoma

Desmoplastic medulloblastoma (DMB) is an MB variant characterized by nodules of neuronal maturation in a dense intercellular reticulin fiber network. There is a strong association between desmoplastic histology and Shh subtype; almost all adult and 90% of infant DMBs belong to the Shh subgroup.

DMBs account for 15-20% of medulloblastomas, but prevalence varies significantly with patient age. DMBs cause about 40% of MBs in infants but only 10% of adult MBs.

The vermis is the preferred location in children. Adult DMBs are often located laterally within the cerebellar

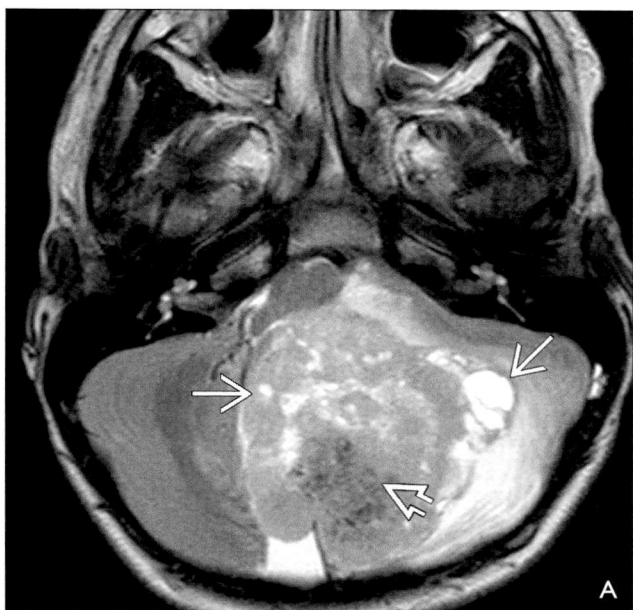

21-7A. *Axial T2WI in a 4 year old with desmoplastic medulloblastoma shows multiple small and peripheral cysts* ➡, *focal hypointense areas* ➡.

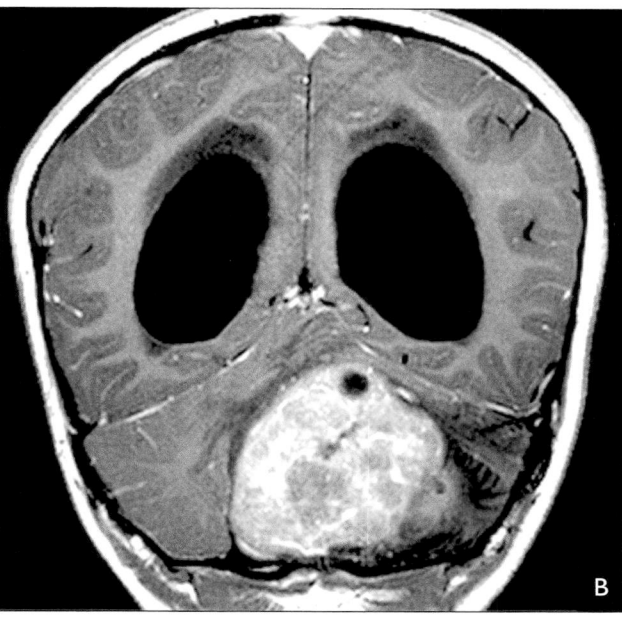

21-7B. *Coronal T1 C+ scan shows that the tumor enhances strongly but heterogeneously. The vermis is the preferred location for DMBs in children. (Courtesy S. Blaser, MD.)*

hemispheres **(21-5)**. DMBs have a somewhat better prognosis than classic, anaplastic, or large cell MBs.

Imaging findings that suggest DMB include off-midline location (adults) **(21-6)**, multiple peripheral small cysts **(21-7)**, and focal areas of T2/FLAIR iso- or hypointensity that enhance on T1 C+.

Medulloblastoma with Extensive Nodularity

Medulloblastomas with extensive nodularity (MBENs) occur almost exclusively in infants, and most are Shh pathway medulloblastomas. The expanded lobular ("nodular") architecture of MBENs is the major histologic feature that differentiates them from CMB and DMB.

Imaging studies demonstrate striking nodularity. Off- or paramidline location is more common. T1 C+ MR scans show multifocal grape-like tumor masses that enhance strongly and uniformly **(21-8)**.

Anaplastic Medulloblastoma

Anaplastic medulloblastoma (AMB) shows marked nuclear pleomorphism and high mitotic activity. Cysts, necrosis, and intratumoral hemorrhage are common. Marked but inhomogeneous enhancement is typical.

Large Cell Medulloblastoma

Large cell medulloblastoma (LCMB) is the rarest histologic variant, accounting for just 2-4% of cases. LCMBs have considerable cytologic overlap with AMBs and are often grouped together as "large cell/anaplastic medulloblastoma" (LCAMB). LCAMBs are generally Shh,

group 3, or group 4 molecular subtypes. Both LCMBs and AMBs have a dismal prognosis.

Monomorphic cells with large round nuclei, prominent nucleoli, and variable amounts of eosinophilic cytoplasm suggest the diagnosis of LCMB. There are no reported imaging features that distinguish LCMB from AMB **(21-9)**.

MEDULLOBLASTOMA VARIANTS

Desmoplastic Medulloblastoma
- Arises from granule neuron precursor cells
- Shh pathway activated
- Intranodular neuropil, dense reticulin fiber network
- Young children, second peak in young adults
- Off-midline location in adults, vermis in children
- Better prognosis

Medulloblastoma with Extensive Nodularity
- Infants
- Off-midline or paramidline > midline
- Multifocal grape-like tumor masses

Anaplastic Medulloblastoma
- Cysts, necrosis, hemorrhage common

Large Cell Medulloblastoma
- Rare
- Pathology and imaging overlap with anaplastic MB
- No imaging findings to distinguish from anaplastic MB

The bottom line when imaging medulloblastoma variants? There really are no pathognomonic imaging findings that reliably distinguish one variant from the others. Even the nodular pattern of MBENs can be mimicked by another subtype **(21-10)**.

21-8A. Axial T2WI in an infant with MBEN shows extensively nodular, almost gyriform pattern of the huge holocerebellar mass. 21-8B. Coronal T1 C+ shows nodular, grape-like enhancement of the tumor ➡. (Courtesy B. Jones, MD.)

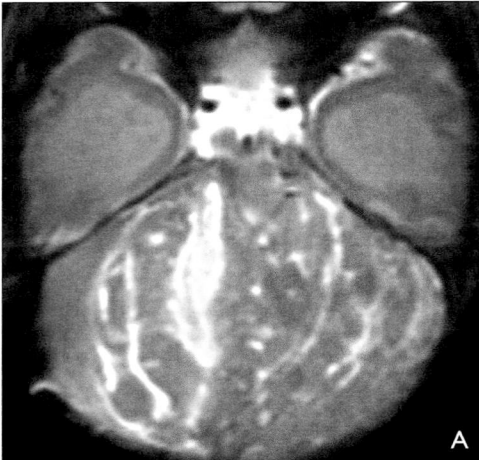
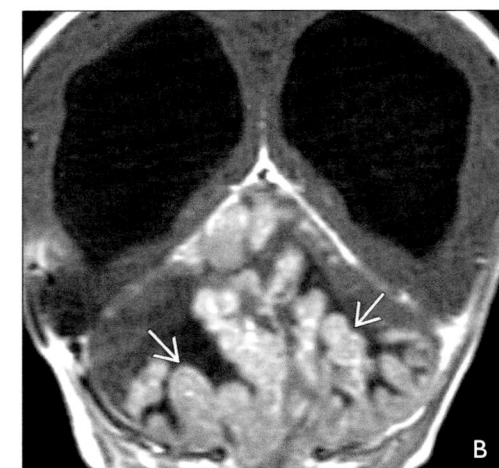

21-9A. Axial T2WI in a 5-year-old girl with unsteady gait shows a laterally located, mixed signal intensity mass ➡ with central hypointensity suggesting hemorrhage ⇨. 21-9B. T1 C+ shows that the mass enhances strongly but very heterogeneously. Histopathology disclosed large cell anaplastic medulloblastoma. (Courtesy S. Blaser, MD.)

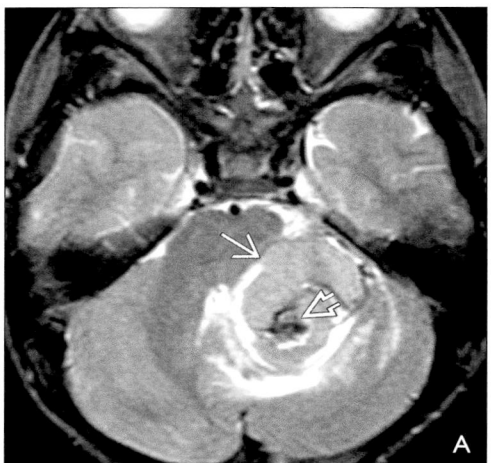
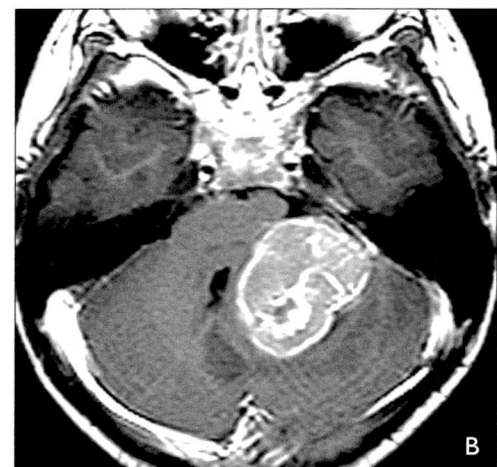

21-10A. Axial T2WI in a 2 year old shows a nodular-appearing, mixed intensity mass ➡ in vermis, extending laterally into both cerebellar hemispheres. 21-10B. The nodular components ➡ enhance strongly but somewhat heterogeneously. Except for the midline location, the imaging appearance suggests MBEN. Histopathology demonstrated desmoplastic medulloblastoma. This case illustrates the difficulty of predicting MB histology based on imaging findings alone.

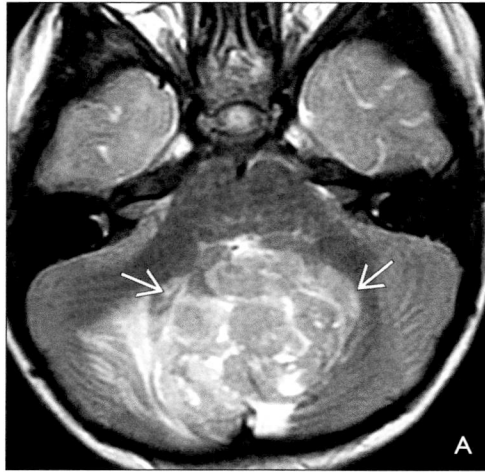
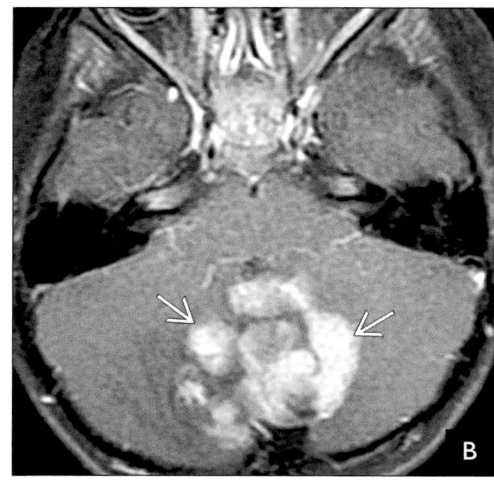

'NS Primitive Neuroectodermal umors (PNETs)

Primitive neuroectodermal tumors (PNETs) are the second major grouping of CNS embryonal neoplasms. They are a histologically heterogeneous group composed of poorly differentiated neuroepithelial cells. PNETs have the capacity to differentiate along embryonic neuronal, astrocytic, or ependymal lines. Some PNETs display multilineal differentiation.

All CNS PNETs are WHO grade IV neoplasms. Despite sharing some histopathologic features with medulloblastomas, CNS PNETs have different genetic characteristics and are comparatively more aggressive. Prognosis is generally poor.

CNS PNET has three major recognized subtypes: (1) **supratentorial PNET**, (2) **medulloepithelioma**, and

(3) **ependymoblastoma**. There is also a new tumor entity—embryonal tumor with abundant neuropil and true rosettes (ETANTR)—that is not yet officially recognized by the WHO as a PNET subtype. It is included here because of its general acceptance by neuropathologists, but its relationship to ependymoblastoma is debated.

Other primitive round cell tumors such as pineoblastoma are sufficiently unique that they retain their own separate diagnostic headings and are discussed in other chapters. We begin this section with supratentorial PNETs and then consider all the other less common CNS PNET subtypes together as "CNS PNET variants."

Supratentorial PNET

The terms "CNS PNET" or "supratentorial PNET" are applied to embryonal tumors that occur in *extracerebellar* CNS locations. *Cerebellar* PNETs are designated as medulloblastomas. Supratentorial PNET has predominantly glial features whereas medulloblastoma generally follows a pattern of neuronal differentiation.

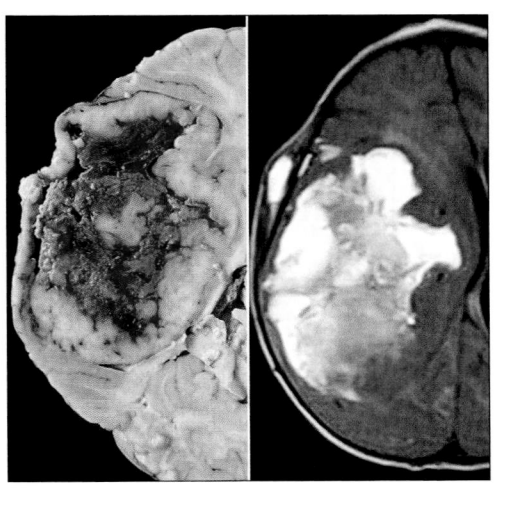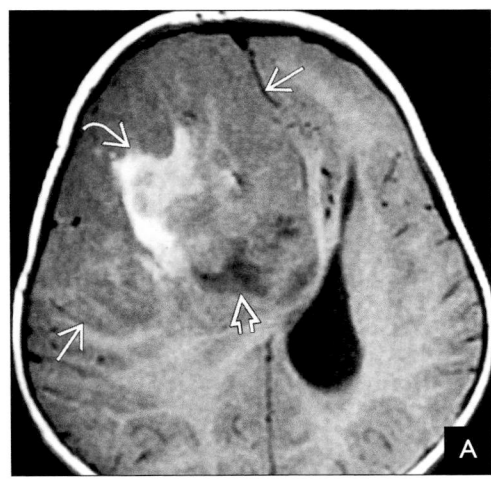

21-11. Autopsy (left) and antemortem FLAIR scan (right) in an 8-month-old infant with a supratentorial PNET shows a large, aggressive-looking hemispheric mass with confluent areas of necrosis and hemorrhage. There is relatively little peritumoral edema. (Courtesy R. Hewlett, MD.) 21-12A. Axial T1WI in another infant shows a very large right frontal mass ➡ with areas of necrosis ➡ and hemorrhage ➡.

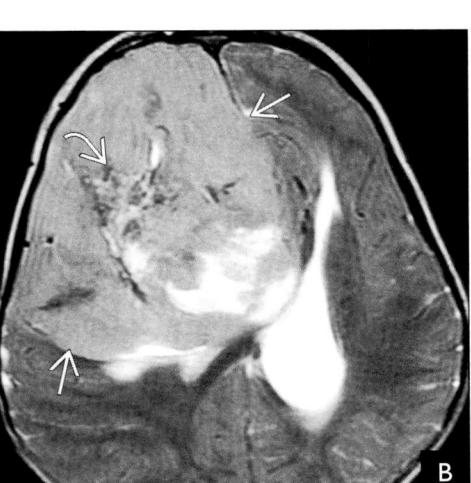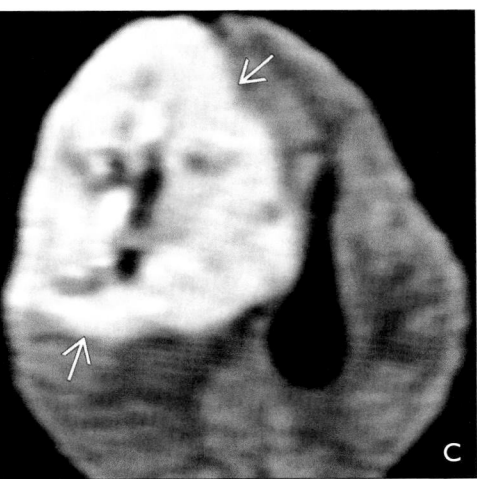

21-12B. T2WI in the same patient shows that the mass is relatively well-demarcated ➡ and mostly hyperintense with heterogeneously hypointense foci of hemorrhage ➡. 21-12C. The lesion restricts on DWI ➡. Supratentorial PNET. (Courtesy G. Hedlund, DO.)

Terminology

Supratentorial PNET is an embryonal tumor composed of undifferentiated or poorly differentiated neuroepithelial cells. Some differentiation along neuronal, astrocytic, muscular, or melanocytic cell lineages may occur. If a supratentorial PNET displays exclusively neuronal differentiation, it is called a **cerebral neuroblastoma**. If immature ganglion cells are present, the tumor is called a **ganglioneuroblastoma**.

Etiology

As with solid embryonal tumors at other sites, CNS PNETs are thought to arise from tumor-initiating stem-like cells. A few cases of "secondary" PNET have been reported in patients with a previously irradiated primary brain tumor.

A number of genetic alterations have been identified in CNS PNETs. Some of the more common cytogenetic abnormalities are 19q, 2p, and 1q gains. There are also genetic differences in the rare adult-onset CNS PNET. Adult sPNETs show a high incidence of *TP53* mutations.

c-myc and *n-myc* gene amplifications are common in children with sPNET but rare in adults. Amplification at chromosome 19q occurs in a subset of PNETs, including ETANTR.

Pathology

LOCATION. The cerebral hemispheres are the most common site for supratentorial PNETs. The suprasellar and pineal regions are less common locations. Rarely, PNETs arise as primary diffuse leptomeningeal neoplasms without an identifiable focal lesion.

GROSS PATHOLOGY. Supratentorial PNETs vary in size, but most are more than five centimeters in diameter. Some are massive lesions that occupy much of the cerebral hemisphere. Despite their size, PNETs often appear relatively well-demarcated and incite relatively little edema. On cut section, supratentorial PNETs are soft pink-red to purplish masses that often contain cysts and hemorrhages **(21-11)**.

MICROSCOPIC FEATURES. CNS PNETs are highly cellular tumors composed of poorly differentiated cells with

21-13A. NECT scan in a 13 month old with persistent vomiting and increasing lethargy shows a large, mixed hypo-, iso-, and hyperdense bifrontal mass ➡ with scattered calcifications.
21-13B. T1WI in the same patient shows a mixed signal intensity mass with predominantly iso- and hypointense areas.

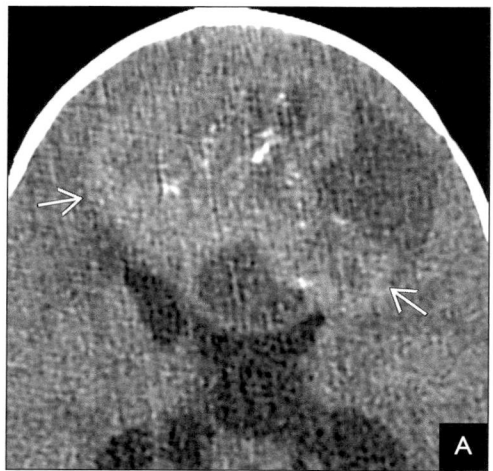
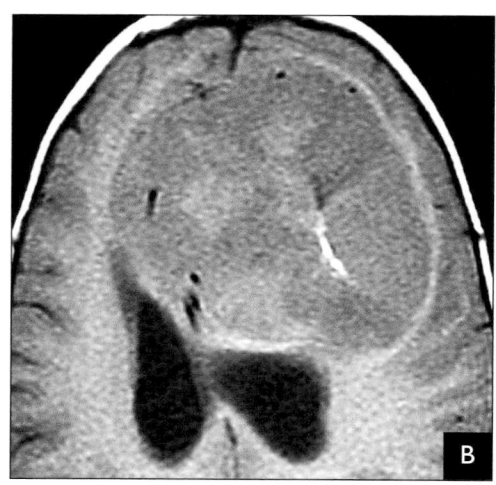

21-13C. T2WI shows that the mass is heterogeneously hyperintense. The lesion appears relatively well-demarcated from the surrounding brain, and there is no peritumoral edema.
21-13D. T1 C+ shows a heterogeneous pattern with rim enhancement around the nonenhancing cystic areas, linear streaks and patchy foci of enhancement. Supratentorial PNET was proven at pathology. (Courtesy G. Hedlund, DO.)

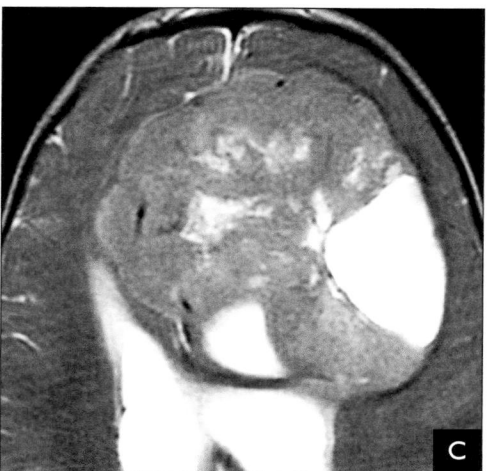
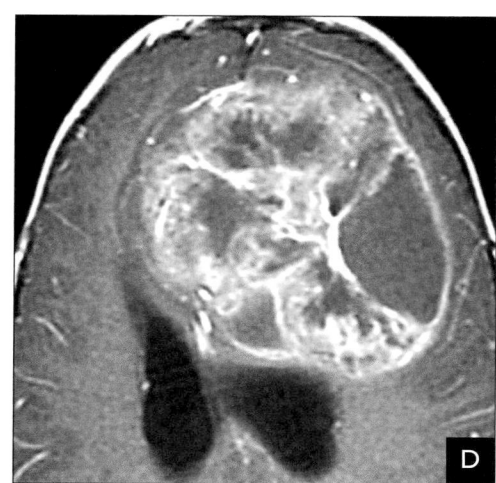

elevated nuclear to cytoplasmic ratios ("small round blue cells"). PNETs should express at least one immunohistochemical marker (e.g., synaptophysin) reflecting neuronal differentiation. Nuclear INI1 labeling is uniformly present. GFAP expression is variable. Mitotic activity is elevated.

STAGING, GRADING, AND CLASSIFICATION. All CNS PNETs are WHO grade IV neoplasms.

linical Issues

CNS PNETs occur mostly in children under the age of five years. They are the fourth most common fetal brain tumor (after teratoma, astrocytoma, and choroid plexus papilloma) but account for only 5% of all pediatric CNS neoplasms.

Infants with supratentorial PNET have increasing head circumference and signs of elevated intracranial pressure.

Prognosis is dismal with a worse five-year survival rate than medulloblastoma. Children younger than two years fare especially poorly. Early CSF dissemination occurs

in 25% of supratentorial PNETs and is an ominous prognostic factor.

Imaging

GENERAL FEATURES. Cerebral PNETs share a number of common imaging features. Tumors grow rapidly and are often very large, heterogeneous-appearing masses that cause gross distortion and effacement of the underlying brain architecture **(21-12)**.

CT FINDINGS. All CNS PNETs are complex, heterogeneously iso- to hyperdense lesions with mixed cystic and solid components **(21-13)**. Necrosis and intratumoral hemorrhages are common. At least 70% show dystrophic calcifications. Moderate but heterogeneous enhancement following contrast administration is typical.

MR FINDINGS. Heterogeneous signal intensity is present on all sequences. Supratentorial PNETs are predominantly hypointense to gray matter on T1WI, but areas of T1 shortening secondary to intratumoral hemorrhage are common.

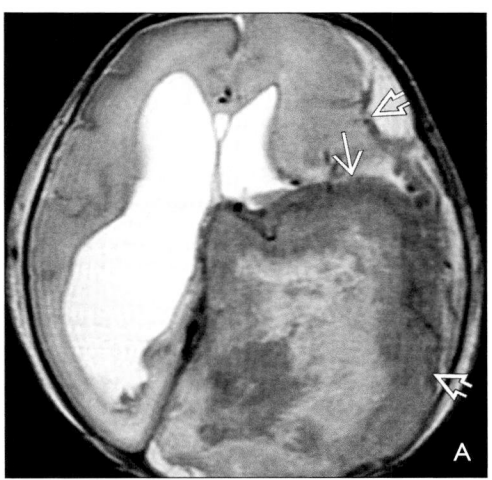
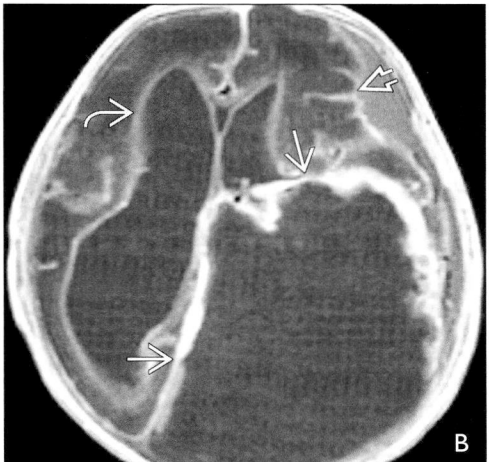

21-14A. T2WI in a newborn with macrocrania, nystagmus, periodic breathing, and bulging fontanelle shows a predominantly necrotic, partially hemorrhagic hemisphere mass ➡ with hemosiderin staining ➡ around the mass and over the cerebrum. 21-14B. This T1WI C+ shows that the rim of the tumor enhances ➡. Note the enhancement over the pia ➡ and around the ventricular ependyma ➡.

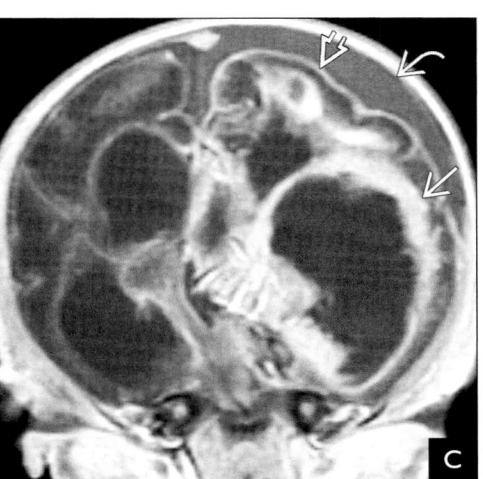
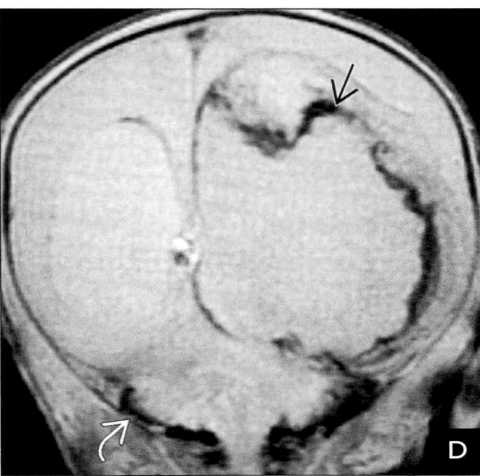

21-14C. Coronal T1 C+ scan shows the irregular enhancing "rind" of tumor ➡, pial enhancement indicating CSF dissemination ➡. There is a proteinaceous extraaxial fluid collection ➡ over the left hemisphere. 21-14D. Coronal T2 GRE shows "blooming" from hemosiderin deposition around the tumor ➡, cerebellum ➡. PNET was diagnosed at histopathology. (Courtesy G. Hedlund, DO.)*

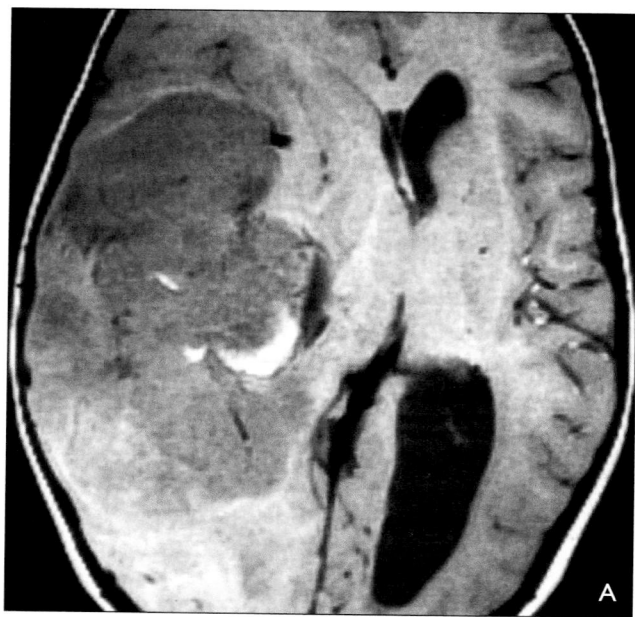

21-15A. Axial T1WI shows a nearly holohemispheric mass with mixed signal intensity occupying most of the right hemicranium.

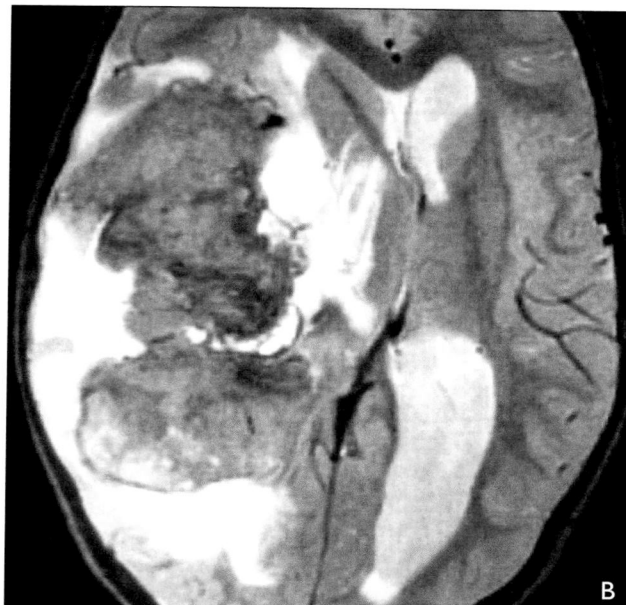

21-15B. T2WI shows the exceptionally heterogeneous nature of the mass with mixed hyper- and very hypointense foci. The histopathologic diagnosis was medulloepithelioma.

T2WI and FLAIR show areas of hyperintensity intermixed with hypointense hemorrhagic foci. Peritumoral edema is generally minimal or absent. Enhancement is variable and heterogeneous (21-14).

Because of their relatively dense cellularity, supratentorial PNETs generally show moderate diffusion restriction. Perfusion MR shows areas of increased cerebral blood volume (CBV) and vascular permeability.

Differential Diagnosis

The major differential diagnosis of supratentorial PNET is malignant **astrocytoma**. Astrocytomas in infants and young children are often highly aggressive, bulky tumors that may be difficult to distinguish from supratentorial PNET on the basis of imaging findings alone.

Other large hemispheric masses that occur in young children and can resemble supratentorial PNET are **supratentorial ependymoma** and **atypical teratoid/rhabdoid tumor**. **Teratoma** is the most common congenital brain tumor but usually arises in the midline, not in the cerebral hemispheres.

When intracranial neoplasms in newborns and infants become very large, their origin may be difficult to determine; the definitive diagnosis is based on histology, not imaging.

SUPRATENTORIAL PNETs

Terminology
- Embryonal tumor in an *extracerebellar* site
  - vs. *cerebellar* embryonal tumor (medulloblastoma a.k.a. PNET-MB)

Etiology
- Composed of poorly differentiated or undifferentiated neuroepithelial cells
  - Probably arises from tumor-initiating stem cells
  - Variable differentiation along divergent cell lineages
  - Can display neuronal, glial, other differentiation

Pathology
- Relatively well-demarcated hemispheric mass
- Pink-red with cysts, hemorrhages
- Primitive "small round blue cell tumor"

Clinical Issues
- Infants, children < 5 years
- Only 5% of all pediatric CNS neoplasms
  - *But* fourth most common fetal tumor

Imaging
- Bulky supratentorial mass with relatively little edema
  - Cysts, hemorrhage common
- Markedly heterogeneously hyperdense on NECT
- Mixed density/signal intensity on all MR sequences
- Patchy enhancement, DWI restriction

Differential Diagnosis
- Astrocytoma (AA, GBM)
- Supratentorial ependymoma
- Atypical teratoid/rhabdoid tumor
- Teratoma

'NS PNET Variants

Several CNS PNET variants are recognized and distinguished based on their distinctive patterns of differentiation. All are rare, highly malignant neoplasms that originate from primitive stem cells. All tend to affect infants and young children. They typically present as large, bulky supratentorial hemispheric masses that are characterized by similar imaging findings.

ledulloepithelioma

Medulloepithelioma (ME) is an embryonal tumor characterized by papillary tubular arrangements of neoplastic neuroepithelium that mimic the embryonic neural tube. Areas with MIB-1 exceeding 50% are common.

Almost all patients are younger than five years at the time of diagnosis. Half are under the age of two. Symptoms of elevated intracranial pressure are the typical presentation.

Like sPNETs, MEs are often massive tumors that replace much of the affected hemisphere and appear very heterogeneous on both CT and MR. Cysts, calcification, and sometimes hemorrhagic foci are common **(21-15)**. There

are no imaging features that distinguish MEs from other PNETs.

Ependymoblastoma

Ependymoblastoma is an ill-defined category, and its existence as a separate entity has been fiercely challenged (e.g., Judkins et al: Ependymoblastoma: dear, damned, distracting diagnosis, farewell! Brain Pathol. 20(1):133-9, 2010).

ETIOLOGY AND PATHOLOGY. At surgery and autopsy, ependymoblastoma usually appears as a large, soft, fleshy, rather friable hemispheric mass. Ependymoblastomas are highly vascular lesions, so macroscopic cystic and hemorrhagic changes are common.

The putative histologic hallmark is the presence of "ependymoblastomatous" rosettes, although these can also be seen in other PNETs. Many so-called ependymoblastomas have been reclassified as ETANTRs (see below).

CLINICAL ISSUES. Almost all reported patients are under five years of age. Ependymoblastomas generally grow

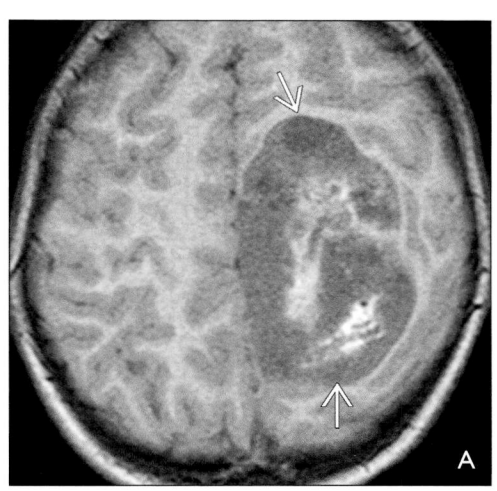
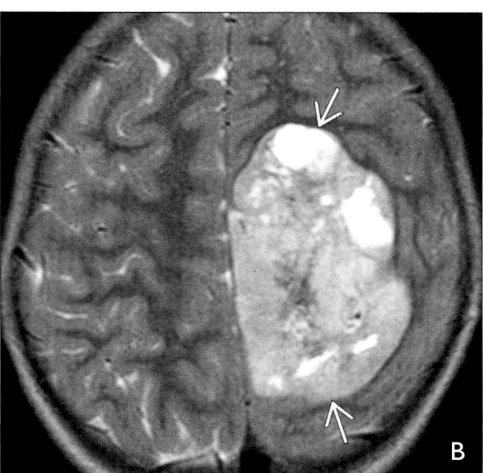

21-16A. Axial T1WI in a 4-year-old boy shows a well-marginated left parietal mass with mixed hyper-, hypo-, and isointense signal components ➡. 21-16B. T2WI confirms the well-delineated nature of the mass ➡. Note striking heterogeneous signal intensity yet complete lack of peritumoral edema.

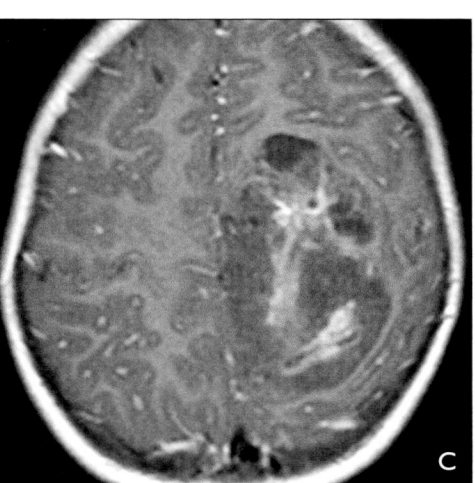
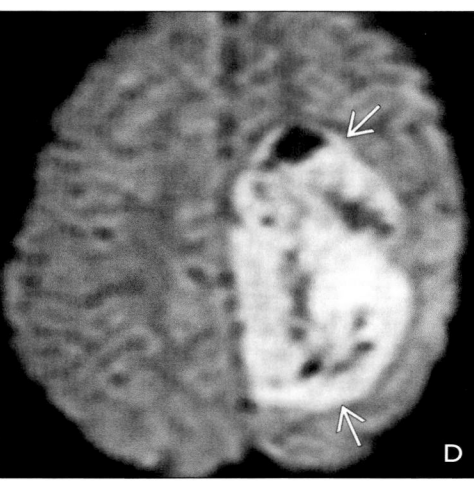

21-16C. T1 C+ FS shows that most of the mass does not enhance but that there are linear and solid enhancing foci scattered throughout the core of the tumor. 21-16D. The lesion restricts on DWI ➡. Histologic diagnosis was ependymoblastoma. (Courtesy M. Warmuth-Metz, MD.)

21-17A. *Series of images in a 3-year-old girl with proven ETANTR. T1WI shows a large, mixed signal intensity bifrontal mass.* **21-17B.** *Axial FLAIR shows that the mass is very heterogeneous and appears to contain foci of cystic degeneration* ➡ *and several vascular "flow voids"* ➡. *Note obstructive hydrocephalus with blocked drainage of interstitial fluid around the left lateral ventricle. Peritumoral edema is minimal.*

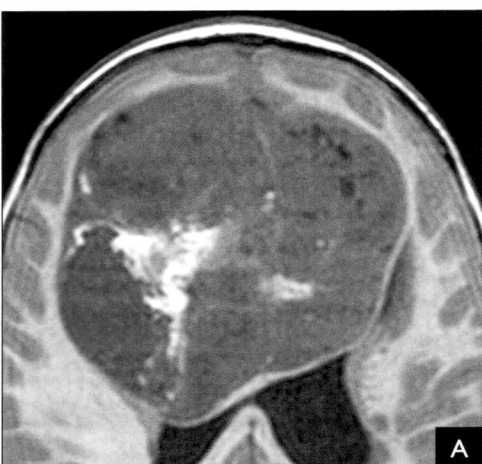

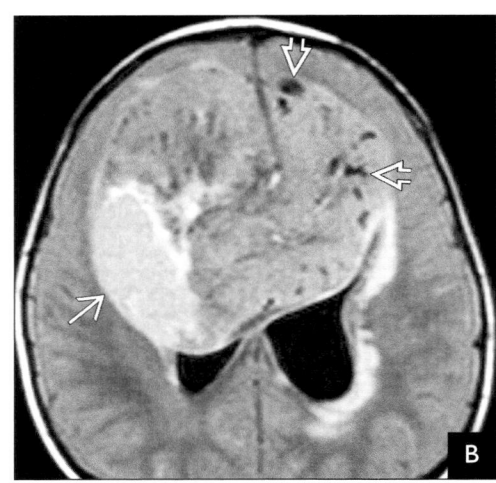

21-17C. *T2* GRE scan demonstrates "blooming" due to intratumoral hemorrhage* ➡. **21-17D.** *T1 C+ reveals that most of the lesion does not enhance. Slow flow in enlarged tumor vessels* ➡ *is present.*

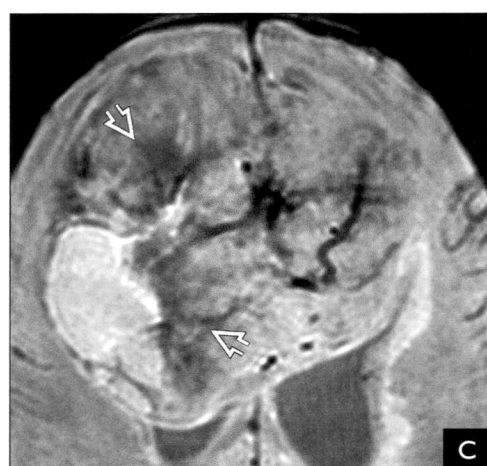

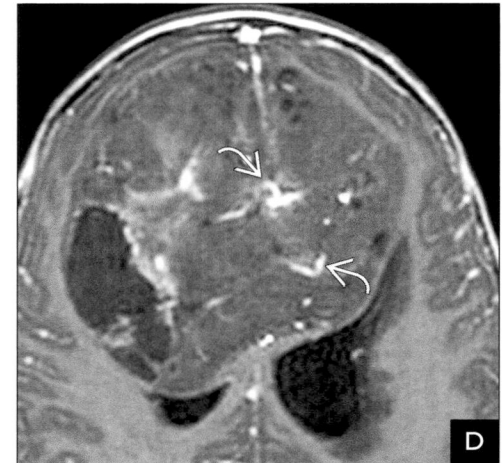

21-17E. *The solid portions of the tumor are highly cellular and restrict strongly on DWI* ➡. *Imaging findings of ETANTR are indistinguishable from those of other supratentorial PNETs. (Compare with figures 21-11 and 21-12.)* **21-17F.** *pMR shows only mildly elevated rCBV in the solid rim of the mass* ➡. *(Courtesy M. Thurnher, MD.)*

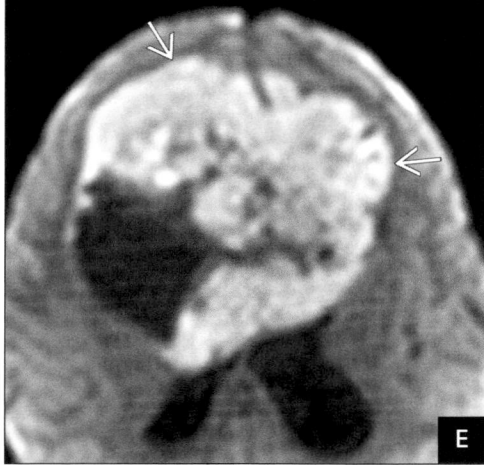

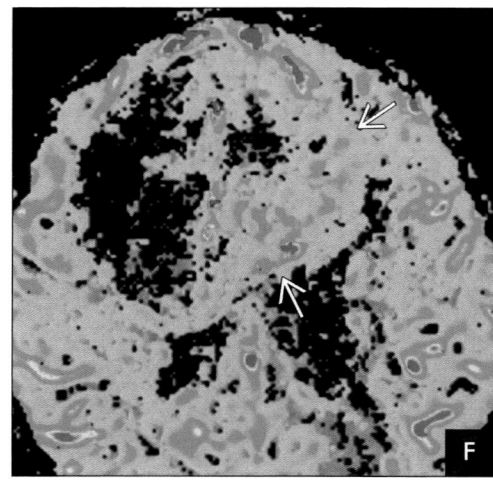

rapidly, so infants present with enlarging head circumference and older children with signs of increased intracranial pressure. CSF dissemination is common, and prognosis is generally poor even with aggressive treatment.

IMAGING AND DIFFERENTIAL DIAGNOSIS. Imaging findings are similar to those of other primitive embryonal tumors, i.e., a large, very heterogeneous hemispheric mass that appears relatively well-demarcated from adjacent brain. Peritumoral edema varies from none to extensive. Enhancement following contrast is also quite variable **(21-16)**.

The major differential diagnoses of ependymoblastoma are **CNS PNET** and other **PNET variants** such as medulloepithelioma and **ETANTR** (see below). All supratentorial PNETs and embryonal neoplasms appear similar on imaging studies, so definitive diagnosis depends on histopathology and immunohistochemical characterization.

Anaplastic ependymoma is a histologically distinct nonastrocytic glial neoplasm that should not be confused with ependymoblastoma.

Embryonal Tumor with Abundant Neuropil and True Rosettes

Embryonal tumor with abundant neuropil and true rosettes (ETANTR) is a rare subtype of CNS PNET that combines the microscopic features of neuroblastoma (see below) with those of ependymoblastoma. The presence of abundant fine fibrillary neuropil distinguishes ETANTR pathologically from other PNETs. ETANTRs are considered WHO grade IV neoplasms.

All reported ETANTRs have occurred in children younger than four years. In contrast to medulloblastoma, ETANTR occurs predominantly in females (F:M = 2:1). ETANTRs are highly malignant tumors with uniformly poor clinical outcome despite aggressive treatment.

Imaging findings are indistinguishable from those of other PNETs. A large, bulky, heterogeneous-appearing hemispheric mass that shows little edema and restricts on DWI is typical **(21-17)**.

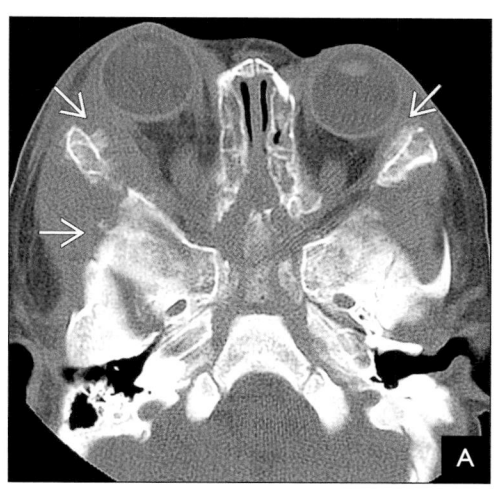
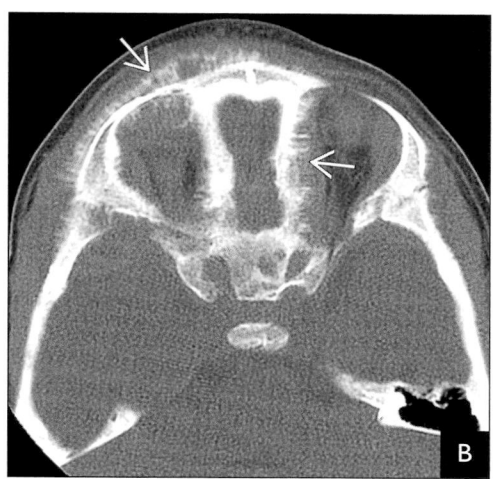

21-18A. Axial bone CT in a 9-month-old boy with proptosis, stage IV suprarenal neuroblastoma identified on abdominal CT (not shown). Note the striking orbital spiculated periostitis with adjacent soft tissue masses ➡. *21-18B. More cephalad scan in the same patient shows the classic "hair on end" appearance* ➡ *of metastatic neuroblastoma. (Courtesy S. Blaser, MD.)*

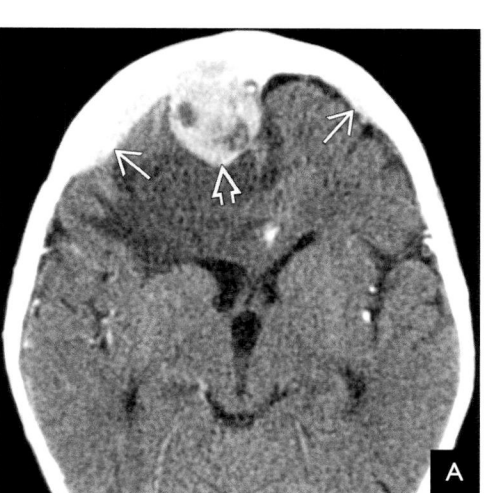
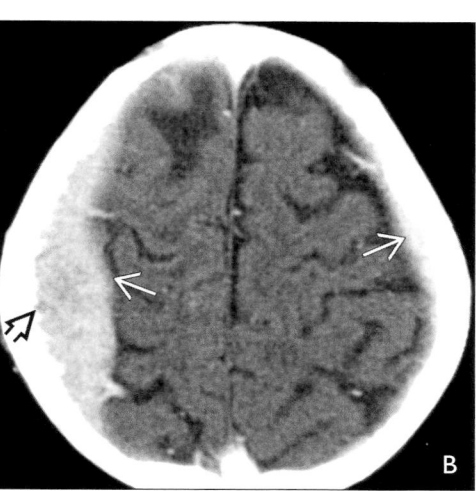

21-19A. Axial CECT in a 2-year-old boy with known neuroblastoma shows strongly enhancing dura-arachnoid metastases ➡ *with parenchymal extension* ➡. *21-19B. More cephalad scan in the same patient shows more extensive dura-arachnoid metastases* ➡. *Note the irregular "hair on end" pattern of calvarial involvement* ➡. *Bone CT (not shown) demonstrated multiple lytic and "hair on end" calvarial lesions.*

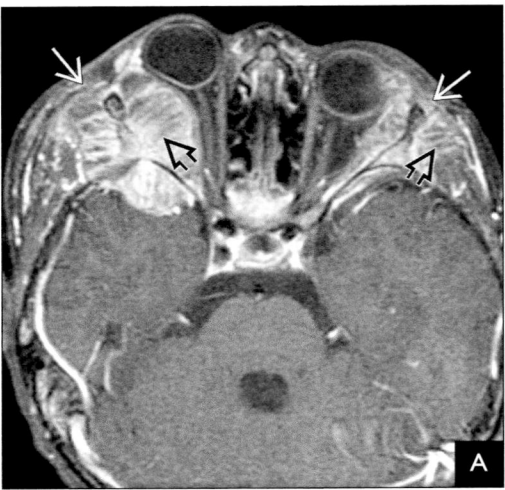

21-20A. *T1 C+ FS in metastatic neuroblastoma shows bilateral enhancing soft tissue masses* ➡️, *"hair on end" neoplastic periostitis* ▷.

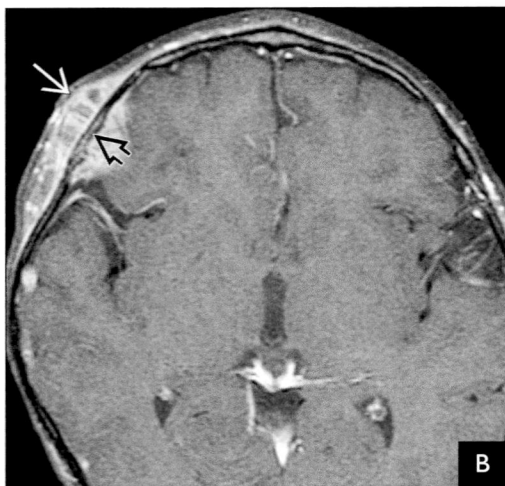

21-20B. *More cephalad T1 C+ FS scan shows the calvarial enhancement* ▷ *associated with both extracranial and intracranial tumor spread* ➡️.

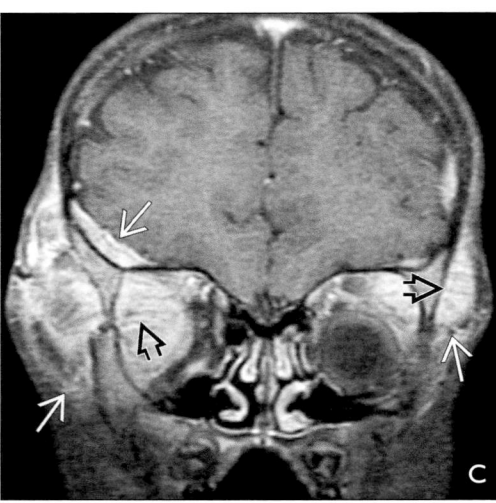

21-20C. *Coronal T1 C+ FS shows the extent of the metastases* ➡️, *striking "hair on end" neoplastic periosteitis* ▷. *(Courtesy C. Y. Ho, MD.)*

CNS Neuroblastoma

Craniocerebral neuroblastoma can be either secondary or primary. Secondary disease is far more common than primary CNS neuroblastoma and so is discussed first. Neuroblastoma is notorious for its diverse manifestations (one of the "great mimickers") and can masquerade as primary neurologic disease in a child with an unexplained neurologic disorder.

SECONDARY (METASTATIC) NEUROBLASTOMA. Neuroblastoma (NB) is a neuroendocrine tumor that arises from neural crest elements, usually within the adrenal gland or sympathetic nervous system. It is the most common extracranial solid cancer in childhood and the most common overall cancer of infants. NB accounts for 10-15% of all childhood malignancies, following leukemia and primary brain tumors in prevalence.

Clinical issues. Metastases are present in almost 70% of NB patients at the time of initial diagnosis. Skeletal metastases are the most common manifestation. Approximately 25% occur in the orbit, calvaria, and skull base. The classic clinical manifestation of orbital metastatic MB is a child with proptosis and "raccoon eyes."

CNS involvement by metastatic NB is uncommon and generally occurs as a late complication of stage IV disease (three-year risk = 8%). CNS NB metastases are usually detected at the time of disease recurrence rather than initial diagnosis.

Imaging. NECT shows one or more hyperdense soft-tissue masses with orbit, skull, scalp, and/or extradural components. Bone CT shows fine "hair on end" spicules of periosteal bone that project from the skull or greater sphenoid wings **(21-18)**. Multiple bilateral lesions involving both the inner and outer tables of the skull are typical **(21-19)**. Lytic defects and widened indistinct sutures are other common findings.

MR shows an extraaxial mass that is heterogeneously hypointense to brain on both T1- and T2WI. Strong enhancement following contrast administration is typical. Linear hypointensities that represent the "hair on end" bony spicules can sometimes be identified within the strongly enhancing masses **(21-20)**.

CNS lesions are uncommon, appearing as a parenchymal, an intraventricular, or even a spinal cord mass. Disseminated leptomeningeal disease is rare.

Nuclear medicine studies are helpful in the early evaluation of NB. Metaiodobenzylguanidine (MIBG) imaging is the most sensitive and specific imaging modality to determine primary and metastatic disease. F18 FDG PET is helpful in depicting stage I and II NB.

The major imaging differential diagnosis of neuroblastoma metastatic to the calvaria is **leukemia**. Both often have dura- or calvaria-based masses, but parenchymal lesions are much more common with leukemia than with NB.

Other lesions that can present with lytic bone lesions include **Langerhans cell histiocytosis** (LCH). Both can present with dura-based masses, but the spiculated periosteal reaction of metastatic NB is absent in LCH.

PRIMARY CNS NEUROBLASTOMA. Primary CNS neuroblastoma is much less common than secondary disease. If a supratentorial PNET displays *only* neuronal differentiation, then by definition it is a cerebral neuroblastoma. Imaging findings are indistinguishable from those of other sPNETs, i.e., a large hemispheric mass with necrosis, hemorrhage, and strong but heterogeneous enhancement following contrast administration.

sthesioneuroblastoma

TERMINOLOGY. Esthesioneuroblastoma (ENB) is a rare neuroectodermal tumor that arises in the superior nasal cavity **(21-21)**. It is also known as olfactory neuroblastoma.

ETIOLOGY. ENBs are tumors of neural crest origin that arise in the olfactory mucosa. There are no known risk factors.

PATHOLOGY. ENBs appear grossly as lobulated, moderately vascular masses. Microscopically, they feature a neurofibrillary intercellular matrix and rosette formation. Mild nuclear pleomorphism with infrequent mitoses is typical. Electron microscopy demonstrates neurosecretory granules.

As they are primarily extracranial neoplasms, ENBs are not graded according to WHO criteria. Histologic grading uses Hyams's system with grades 1-4 based on nuclear pleomorphism, mitoses, necrosis, etc. The Kadish classification is used for staging and recognizes three stages: Stage A, tumors that are localized to the nasal cavity; stage B, nasal cavity and paranasal sinuses; and stage C, extension beyond the sinonasal cavities, including intracranial involvement.

CLINICAL ISSUES. ENBs have a wide age range with a bimodal peak in the second and sixth decades of life. ENB is usually not a diagnostic consideration in children.

The most common symptoms are nasal obstruction and epistaxis. ENBs with intracranial extension may present with headache, proptosis, and cranial neuropathies.

Five-year survival rate is approximately 75% although local recurrence is common. Hematogenous or lymphatic metastases develop in 10-30% of patients.

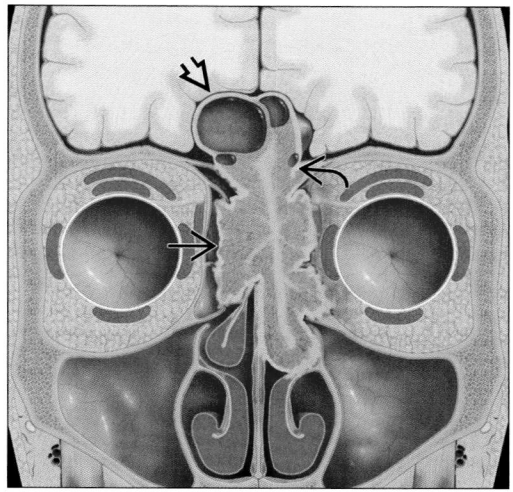

21-21. Coronal graphic depicts ENB as a large nasal mass ⇨ with cephalad intracranial extension ⇨ through the cribriform plate ⇨.

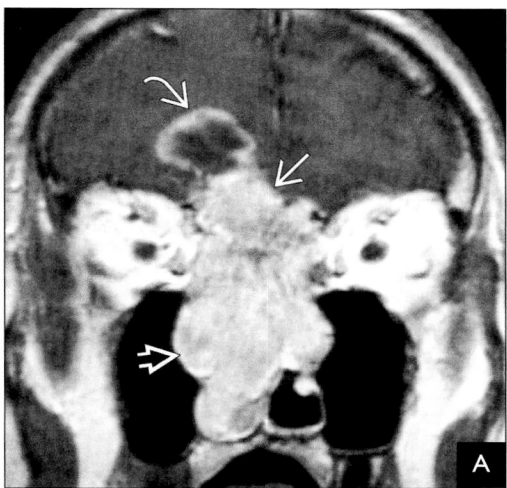

21-22A. Coronal T1 C+ shows a huge "dumbbell" ENB with large nasal mass ⇨, smaller intracranial mass ⇨, area of cystic degeneration ⇨.

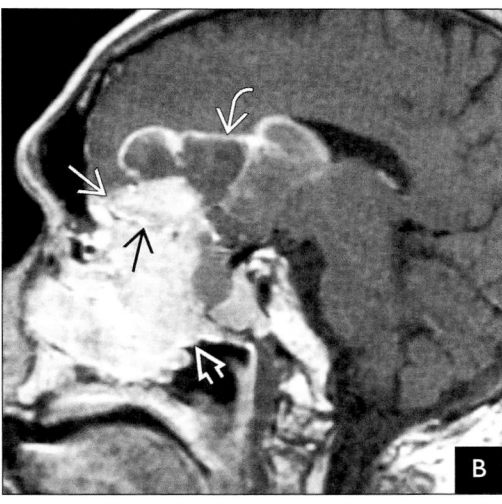

21-22B. Sagittal T1 C+ shows true extent of extra- ⇨, intracranial mass ⇨, cystic areas ⇨. Cribriform plate ⇨ is mostly destroyed.

IMAGING. The typical finding in ENB is a superior nasal cavity mass at the cribriform plate. A "dumbbell" shape—the upper portion in the anterior cranial fossa and the lower portion in the nose with the narrowest aspect at the cribriform plate—is seen with large masses **(21-22)**.

CT findings. Bone CT shows bone remodeling mixed with bone destruction, especially of the cribriform plate. Speckled intratumoral calcification is unusual. A homogeneously enhancing mass on CECT is typical.

MR findings. ENB is hypo- to isointense compared with brain on T1WI and iso- to hyperintense on T2WI. Areas of cystic degeneration and intratumoral hemorrhage are common. Some large ENBs that extend intracranially have benign nonneoplastic tumor-associated cysts around their superior and lateral margins at the tumor-brain interface. ENBs generally enhance strongly and relatively uniformly.

ENB spread to cervical lymph nodes is common, typically spreading first to level II nodes, with frequent involvement of level I, level III, and retropharyngeal nodal groups at later stages. Nodes harboring metasta-tic disease are predominantly solid and demonstrate avid contrast enhancement.

PET/CT. 18F FDG PET/CT is a useful adjunct to conventional imaging in the initial staging or subsequent restaging of ENB. Nodal and distant metastatic disease, as well as local recurrence obscured by treatment changes on standard imaging, can be depicted. PET/CT changes previously assigned disease stage and alters patient management in nearly 40% of cases with more than one-third of tumors upstaged.

DIFFERENTIAL DIAGNOSIS. The major differential diagnoses of ENB with intracranial extension are **sinonasal squamous cell carcinoma** (SCCa) and **adenocarcinoma**. Sinonasal SCCa is more common in the maxillary antrum than in the nose and does not enhance as intensely as ENB. Patients with sinonasal adenocarcinoma often have a history of occupational or wood dust exposure. **Undifferentiated sinonasal carcinoma** may be difficult to distinguish from ENB on imaging alone. **Sinonasal lymphoma** is typically hyperdense on NECT and rarely extends directly superiorly into the skull base and anterior fossa.

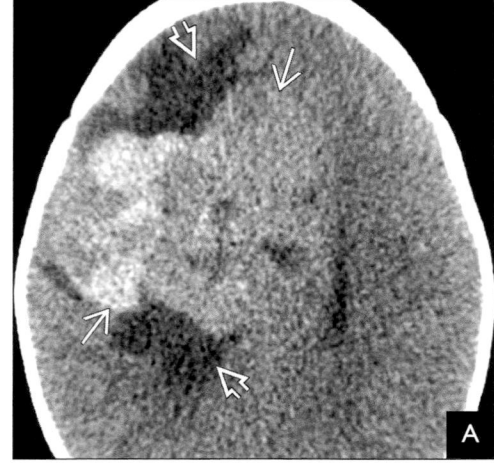 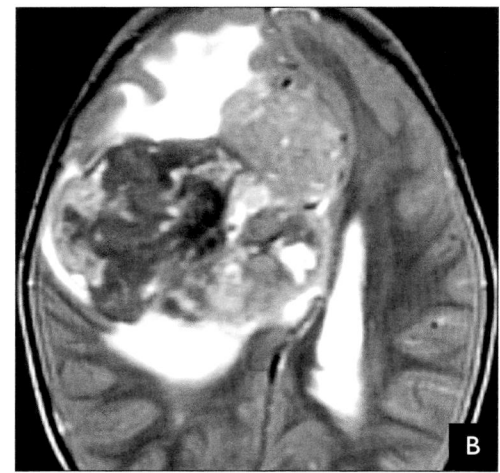

21-23A. NECT in an 18-month-old girl with vomiting for 1-2 weeks shows a mixed, mostly hyperdense right frontal mass ➡ with marked vasogenic edema ➡. 21-23B. T2WI shows that the mass has mixed, mostly hypo- and isointense signal intensity.

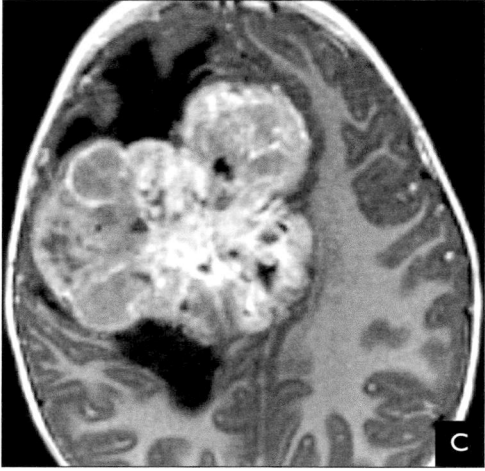 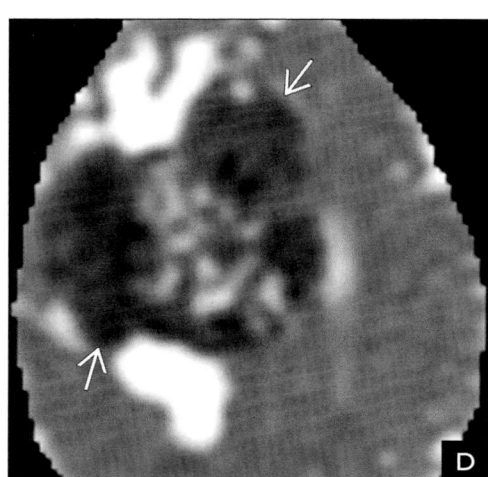

21-23C. T1 C+ shows diffuse but very heterogeneous enhancement. 21-23D. ADC map shows marked diffuse restriction ➡ due to the high cellularity of the tumor. MRS (not shown) demonstrated elevated Cho, lactate. Histologic diagnosis was AT/RT. (Courtesy B. Jones, MD.)

Malignant Rhabdoid Tumors

Malignant rhabdoid tumors (MRTs) are aggressive tumors that were first described in the kidneys and soft tissues of infants and young children. Cranial rhabdoid tumors were subsequently recognized as a distinct pathologic entity and termed atypical teratoid/rhabdoid tumor (AT/RT). AT/RTs are separated from PNETs and non-CNS MRTs by distinct immunohistochemical, histopathological, and molecular features.

Atypical Teratoid/Rhabdoid Tumor

Etiology

Atypical teratoid/rhabdoid tumor is one of the CNS tumors in which a pathognomonic alteration of a tumor-suppressor gene has been identified. Deletions in the *INI1/hSNF5/BAF47* gene occur in almost all cases and are considered diagnostic of AT/RT, differentiating this tumor from PNET and other CNS neoplasms with rhabdoid features.

Pathology

LOCATION. AT/RTs occur in both the supra- and infratentorial compartments. Approximately half of AT/RTs are supratentorial, usually occurring in the cerebral hemispheres. Posterior fossa AT/RTs preferentially occur in the cerebellar hemispheres.

GROSS PATHOLOGY. The gross appearance—a large, soft, fleshy, hemorrhagic, necrotic mass—is similar to that of other CNS PNETs.

MICROSCOPIC FEATURES. AT/RTs are composed of poorly differentiated neural, epithelial, and mesenchymal elements together with prominent rhabdoid cells.

Clinical Issues

EPIDEMIOLOGY. AT/RT accounts for 1-2% of all pediatric brain tumors. Most occur in children under five years of age. Peak incidence is between birth and two

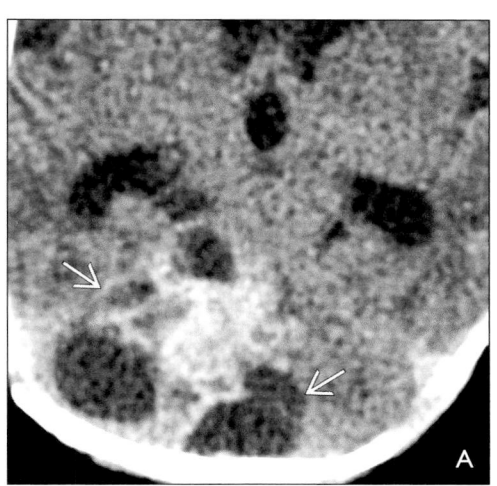
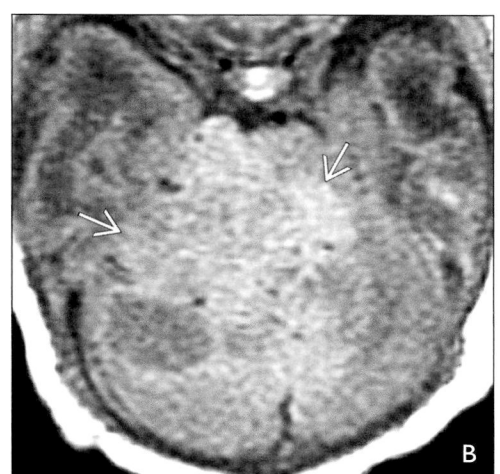

21-24A. NECT scan in a 5-year-old boy with morning nausea and vomiting shows a mixed hyperdense, cystic-appearing posterior fossa mass ➡ centered in the right cerebellar hemisphere. 21-24B. T1WI in the same patient shows that the mass is very large, exhibits mixed signal intensity ➡.

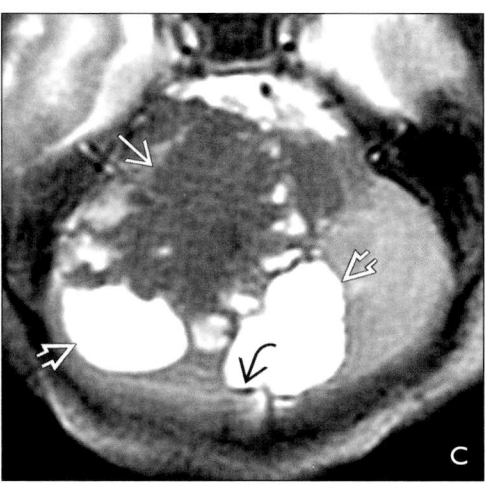
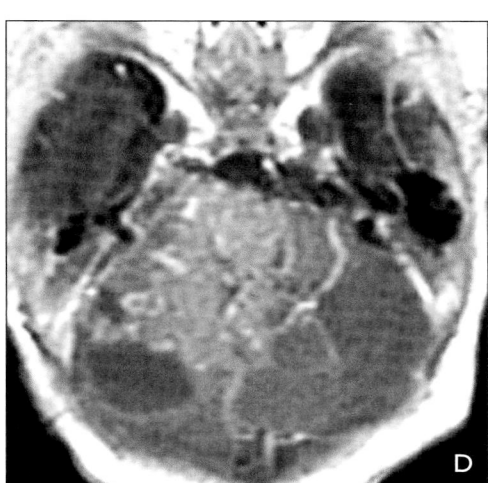

21-24C. T2WI shows that the solid portion ➡ is very hypointense whereas multiple cysts of varying sizes are hyperintense ➡. Note the blood-fluid levels ➡ in some of the cysts. 21-24D. T1WI C+ shows mild to moderate heterogeneous enhancement. MRS (not shown) demonstrated markedly elevated Cho. Histologic diagnosis was AT/RT. (Courtesy G. Hedlund, DO.)

years, a period during which AT/RT approaches PNET and medulloblastoma in frequency. AT/RT does occur in adults but is rare. There is a moderate male predominance.

Rhabdoid tumor predisposition syndrome (RTPS) is a familial cancer syndrome characterized by a markedly increased risk of developing MRTs—including AT/RT—caused by loss or inactivation of the *INI1* gene. Pedigree analysis supports an autosomal dominant inheritance pattern with incomplete penetrance.

Patients with RTPS may develop an AT/RT with a synchronous renal or extrarenal MRT. Children with RTPS and AT/RT are even younger, have more extensive disease, and experience more rapid progression. Other CNS tumors associated with RTPS include choroid plexus carcinoma and rhabdoid meningioma.

NATURAL HISTORY. AT/RT is a highly malignant tumor that is almost invariably fatal. Most children die within six to eight months despite aggressive therapy. Survival in adults is somewhat better, averaging two years.

Imaging

GENERAL FEATURES. AT/RT shares many imaging features with other embryonal tumors, i.e., they are densely cellular neoplasms that frequently contain hemorrhage, necrosis, cysts, and calcifications. A moderately large, bulky tumor with mixed solid and cystic components and heterogeneous density/signal intensity is typical.

CSF dissemination is common, so the entire neuraxis should be imaged prior to surgical intervention.

CT FINDINGS. NECT scan shows a mildly to moderately hyperdense mass with cysts and hemorrhagic foci (21-23). Calcification and obstructive hydrocephalus—especially with posterior fossa AT/RT—are common. Enhancement is typically strong but heterogeneous.

MR FINDINGS. AT/RTs are heterogeneously hypo- to isointense to brain on T1WI and iso- to hyperintense on T2WI (21-24). "Blooming" foci on T2* (GRE, SWI) are common. Mild to moderate diffusion restriction is present. MRS shows elevated Cho and decreased or absent NAA.

Enhancement on T1 C+ is strong but heterogeneous. Leptomeningeal spread is present in 15-20% of cases at the time of initial imaging.

Differential Diagnosis

The differential diagnosis of AT/RT varies with location.

The major differential diagnosis for supratentorial AT/RT includes **CNS PNET**, **supratentorial ependymoma**, **teratoma**, and **malignant astrocytoma**. As all of these

may be bulky—even massive—tumors with very heterogeneous imaging appearance, definitive diagnosis requires biopsy and INI1 staining.

The major differential diagnosis for posterior fossa AT/RT is **medulloblastoma**. Although these tumors can look virtually identical, medulloblastoma usually occur in the midline whereas AT/RTs are most often off-axis, near the cerebellopontine angle.

ATYPICAL TERATOID/RHABDOID TUMOR

Etiology
- Loss of tumor-suppressor gene *INI1/hSNF5/BAF47* on chromosome 22

Pathology
- Infratentorial (~ 50%), supratentorial (~ 50%)
  - Often off-midline (cerebral, cerebellar hemispheres)
- Poorly differentiated neuroepithelial elements + rhabdoid cells
- WHO grade IV

Clinical Issues
- 1-2% of pediatric brain tumors
- Children < 5 years, most < 2 years; rare in adults
- Rhabdoid tumor predisposition syndrome
  - Malignant rhabdoid tumors
  - Choroid plexus carcinoma

Imaging
- Heterogeneous, hyperdense on NECT
- Heterogeneous on both T1, T2
- Enhances strongly but heterogeneously
- CSF spread in 15-20% at diagnosis
- Restricts on DWI

Differential Diagnosis
- DDx of *supratentorial* AT/RT
  - CNS PNET
  - Ependymoma, teratoma, malignant astrocytoma
- DDx of *posterior fossa* AT/RT
  - Medulloblastoma (midline AT/RT may be indistinguishable)

Other CNS Neoplasms with Rhabdoid Features

Other than AT/RT, CNS tumors with rhabdoid or rhabdomyoblastic features are very rare. **Rhabdoid glioblastoma** is a recently described entity in which a glioblastoma (GBM) is associated with a definite rhabdoid component. Primary rhabdoid tumor with a low-grade glioma component has also been described. Immunohistochemistry in both tumors is positive for GFAP and INI1.

Rhabdoid meningioma is an uncommon WHO grade III meningioma subtype that contains sheets of rhabdoid cells. Most have high proliferative indices and exhibit other cytological features of malignancy. Rhabdoid meningiomas are very rare in infants and retain INI1 staining, which differentiates them histopathologically from AT/RT.

elected References

- Eberhart CG: Molecular diagnostics in embryonal brain tumors. Brain Pathol. 21(1):96-104, 2011
- Severino M et al: Congenital tumors of the central nervous system. Neuroradiology. 52(6):531-48, 2010

Medulloblastoma

Medulloblastoma Overview

- Kool M et al: Molecular subgroups of medulloblastoma: an international meta-analysis of transcriptome, genetic aberrations, and clinical data of WNT, SHH, Group 3, and Group 4 medulloblastomas. Acta Neuropathol. 123(4):473-84, 2012
- Northcott PA et al: The clinical implications of medulloblastoma subgroups. Nat Rev Neurol. 8(6):340-51, 2012
- Robinson G et al: Novel mutations target distinct subgroups of medulloblastoma. Nature. 488(7409):43-8, 2012
- Eberhart CG: Molecular diagnostics in embryonal brain tumors. Brain Pathol. 21(1):96-104, 2011
- Ellison DW et al: Medulloblastoma: clinicopathological correlates of SHH, WNT, and non- SHH/WNT molecular subgroups. Acta Neuropathol. 121(3):381-96, 2011
- Remke M et al: Adult medulloblastoma comprises three major molecular variants. J Clin Oncol. 29(19):2717-23, 2011
- Gibson P et al: Subtypes of medulloblastoma have distinct developmental origins. Nature. 468(7327):1095-9, 2010

Classic Medulloblastoma

- Taylor MD et al: Molecular subgroups of medulloblastoma: the current consensus. Acta Neuropathol. 123(4):465-72, 2012
- Fruehwald-Pallamar J et al: Magnetic resonance imaging spectrum of medulloblastoma. Neuroradiology. 53(6):387-96, 2011
- Northcott PA et al: Pediatric and adult sonic hedgehog medulloblastomas are clinically and molecularly distinct. Acta Neuropathol. 122(2):231-40, 2011
- Castillo M: Stem cells, radial glial cells, and a unified origin of brain tumors. AJNR Am J Neuroradiol. 31(3):389-90, 2010

Medulloblastoma Variants

- Liu HQ et al: MRI features in children with desmoplastic medulloblastoma. J Clin Neurosci. 19(2):281-5, 2012
- Fruehwald-Pallamar J et al: Magnetic resonance imaging spectrum of medulloblastoma. Neuroradiology. 53(6):387-96, 2011

CNS Primitive Neuroectodermal Tumors (PNETs)

- Behdad A et al: Central nervous system primitive neuroectodermal tumors: a clinicopathologic and genetic study of 33 cases. Brain Pathol. 20(2):441-50, 2010

Supratentorial PNET

- Rodriguez FJ: CNS primitive neuroectodermal tumors. In Burger P et al: Diagnostic Pathology: Neuropathology. Salt Lake City: Amirsys Publishing. I.1.234-9, 2012
- Dahlback HS et al: Genomic aberrations in pediatric gliomas and embryonal tumors. Genes Chromosomes Cancer. 50(10):788-99, 2011
- Gessi M et al: Supratentorial primitive neuroectodermal tumors of the central nervous system in adults: molecular and histopathologic analysis of 12 cases. Am J Surg Pathol. 35(4):573-82, 2011
- Phi JH et al: Upregulation of SOX2, NOTCH1, and ID1 in supratentorial primitive neuroectodermal tumors: a distinct differentiation pattern from that of medulloblastomas. J Neurosurg Pediatr. 5(6):608-14, 2010

CNS PNET Variants

- Broski SM et al: The Added Value of 18F-FDG PET/CT for Evaluation of Patients with Esthesioneuroblastoma. J Nucl Med. 53(8):1200-6, 2012
- Nobusawa S et al: Analysis of chromosome 19q13.42 amplification in embryonal brain tumors with ependymoblastic multilayered rosettes. Brain Pathol. 22(5):689-697, 2012
- Howell MC et al: Patterns of regional spread for esthesioneuroblastoma. AJNR Am J Neuroradiol. 32(5):929-33, 2011
- D'Ambrosio N et al: Imaging of metastatic CNS neuroblastoma. AJR Am J Roentgenol. 194(5):1223-9, 2010
- Judkins AR et al: Ependymoblastoma: dear, damned, distracting diagnosis, farewell!. Brain Pathol. 20(1):133-9, 2010

Malignant Rhabdoid Tumors

Atypical Teratoid/Rhabdoid Tumor

- Burger PC: Atypical teratoid/rhabdoid tumor. In Diagnostic Pathology: Neuropathology. Salt Lake City: Amirsys Publishing. I.1.248-55, 2012
- Harris TJ et al: Case 168: rhabdoid predisposition syndrome-- familial cancer syndromes in children. Radiology. 259(1):298-302, 2011

Other CNS Neoplasms with Rhabdoid Features

- Endo S et al: Primary rhabdoid tumor with low grade glioma component of the central nervous system in a young adult. Neuropathology. Epub ahead of print, 2012
- Bruggers CS et al: Clinicopathologic comparison of familial versus sporadic atypical teratoid/rhabdoid tumors (AT/

RT) of the central nervous system. Pediatr Blood Cancer. 56(7):1026-31, 2011

- He MX et al: Rhabdoid glioblastoma: case report and literature review. Neuropathology. 31(4):421-6, 2011
- Momota H et al: Rhabdoid glioblastoma in a child: case report and literature review. Brain Tumor Pathol. 28(1):65-70, 2011

22

Tumors of the Meninges

The cranial meninges give rise to a broad spectrum of neoplasms that usually occur as extraaxial masses (i.e., outside the brain parenchyma but inside the skull). Tumors of the cranial meninges are divided into four basic pathologic subgroups: (1) meningothelial neoplasms (i.e., meningiomas), (2) nonmeningothelial mesenchymal tumors, (3) primary melanocytic lesions, and (4) in the WHO terminology, "other neoplasms related to the meninges."

Meningioma is the most common type of intracranial neoplasm. Meningiomas (benign, atypical, and anaplastic) are by far the largest group of meningothelial neoplasms. While meningiomas are physically attached to the dura, they actually arise from arachnoid "cap" cells rather than from the dura itself.

Both benign and malignant mesenchymal tumors can originate within the CNS. These uncommon **nonmeningothelial mesenchymal tumors** correspond histologically to tumors of soft tissue or bone found elsewhere in the body. **Hemangioma** and **hemangiopericytoma** are included in this subgroup.

The third subgroup features the rare **primary melanocytic lesions** of the cranial meninges, including focal melanocytoma and diffuse leptomeningeal melanocytosis.

While the histogenesis of hemangioblastoma is uncertain, these highly vascular neoplasms contain both stromal and blood vessel elements. Because investigators have identified the stromal (not the vascular) cells as the neoplastic element, the WHO classification considers hemangioblastoma as part of the fourth and last category, **"other neoplasms related to the meninges."**

Anatomy of the Cranial Meninges

The cranial meninges consist of the dura mater, the arachnoid, and the pia.

Dura

The dura mater—also called the pachymeninx—is a continuous fibrous sheet that lines the calvaria and spine. As its name implies (Latin for "tough mother"), the dura is a comparatively tough covering that provides significant protection against injury and infection. It is also the most important site for CSF turnover.

Neurosurgeons traditionally view the cranial dura as a simple bilaminar structure with an **outer ("periosteal") layer** and an **inner ("meningeal") layer**. The periosteal layer is firmly attached to the cranial vault, especially at sutures. The inner (meningeal) layer folds inward to form the falx cerebri, tentorium cerebelli, and diaphragma sellae. The two layers separate to contain the dural venous sinuses (see Chapter 9).

Anatomists have identified *three* different layers of dura at light microscopy. The **outer dural border layer**,

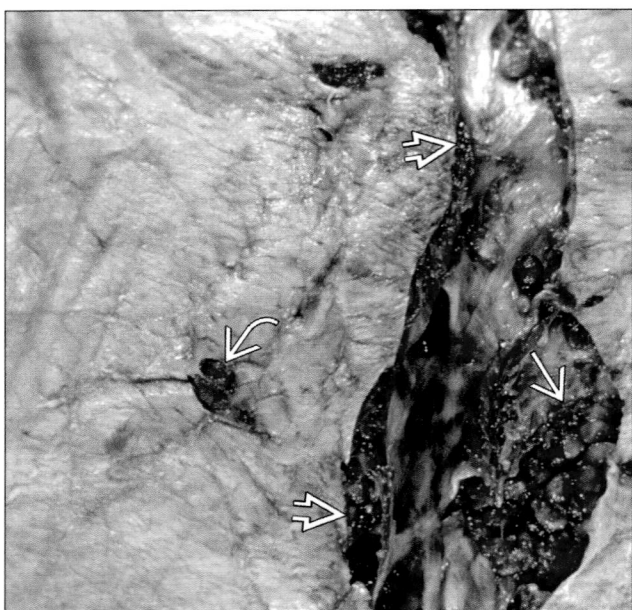

22-1. Close-up view of dura ➡, *opened to show the superior sagittal sinus with numerous arachnoid granulations protruding into the sinus* ➡. *Note the small parasagittal venous lake with arachnoid granulation* ➡. *(Courtesy E. Ross, MD.)*

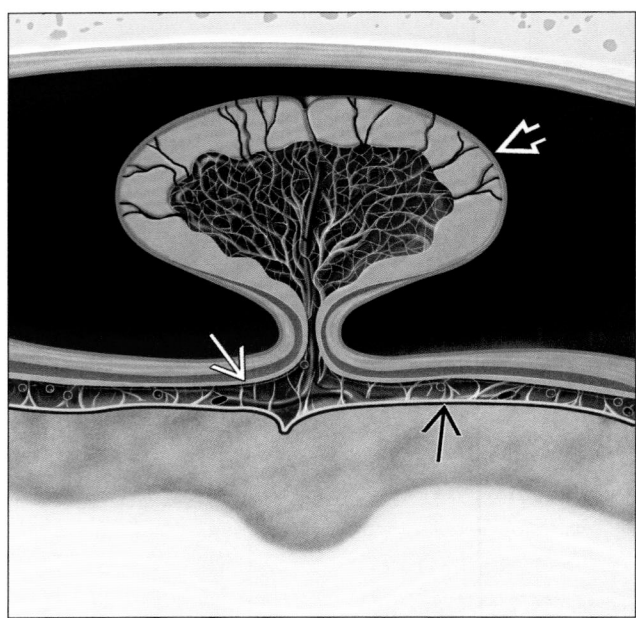

22-2. Graphic depicts pia ➡, *arachnoid* ➡, *arachnoid granulation projecting into venous sinus* ➡. *CSF from subarachnoid space is covered by a "cap" of arachnoid cells.*

which is just 2 μm thick, is the thinnest layer and consists of fibroblasts, collagen, and elastic fibers. The middle layer, called the **fibrous dura**, is well-vascularized. Its thickness varies according to location and patient age (more prominent in infants than in adults). The innermost layer is called the **dural border cell layer**. This inner layer is 8 μm thick and is composed of only cells that adhere to the arachnoid trabeculae.

Scanning electron microscopy reveals that the dura actually consists of *five* layers, each with different constituents and patterns of organization. The outermost (**bone surface layer**) abuts the inner table of the skull. The next three components (an **external median layer**, a **vascular layer**, and an **internal median layer**) comprise the middle layer recognized by anatomists as the fibrous dura. Highly ordered collagen fibers in the median layer are arranged in three directions to form the three different layers.

The innermost layer, which is called the **arachnoid layer**, faces the arachnoid membrane itself. The arachnoid layer consists of tortuous collagen bundles that are not oriented in any common direction.

Arachnoid and Arachnoid Granulations

The **arachnoid** is a thin translucent membrane that is loosely attached to the innermost dural layer and follows its contours all the way around the inside of the skull. The outermost layer of arachnoid cells intermingles with

cells of the inner dura but can be easily detached from the dura, forming a space (subdural or interdural space) between these two layers of the meninges.

Specialized villous outpouchings of the arachnoid protrude into dural venous sinuses **(22-1)**. These arachnoid granulations (AGs) are covered with a layer of specialized cells, arachnoid "cap" cells, that permits resorption of CSF into the venous system. **(22-2)**.

The largest AGs lie along the superior sagittal sinus but are present in other venous sinuses as well. AGs are also common in the temporal bone. Approximately 10-15% completely penetrate the dura to make direct contact with the inner cortical surface.

Pia Mater

The **pia** is the innermost layer of the cranial meninges. The pia covers the surface of the brain and adheres to the cortex relatively tightly, following gyral convolutions. The pia invaginates along penetrating vessels to form the perivascular (Virchow-Robin) spaces (PVSs).

Recent studies have shown that the PVSs form a complicated intraparenchymal network distributed over the whole brain, connecting the cerebral convexities, basal cisterns, and ventricular system. PVSs may play a significant role both in providing drainage routes for cerebral metabolites and in maintaining normal intracranial pressure.

Meningothelial Tumors

Meningiomas are one of the most common of all brain tumors, accounting for one-quarter to one-third of all primary intracranial neoplasms. The WHO divides meningiomas into three groups based on tumor grade and likelihood of recurrence. WHO grade I meningiomas have low risk of recurrence and aggressive growth. These histologically and biologically benign meningiomas are by far the most common type.

Certain meningioma subtypes are associated with more aggressive clinical behavior and less favorable outcomes. **Atypical meningioma** corresponds to WHO grade II. The most aggressive form of meningioma, corresponding to WHO grade III, is **anaplastic ("malignant") meningioma**. We consider all three grades of meningioma in this section.

Meningioma

Terminology

Benign meningiomas are also called common or typical meningiomas (TM).

Etiology

Meningiomas arise from arachnoid meningothelial ("cap") cells. Between 50-60% of meningiomas have inactivation of the *NF2* gene product Merlin due to 22q loss. Allelic losses on 1p and 3p are also common in sporadic meningiomas, particularly higher grade lesions.

Meningiomas can also be induced by radiation, with a dose-related time interval to tumor development that varies from 20 to 40 years. Many of these tumors have chromosome 7 monosomy.

Most meningiomas have progesterone or estrogen receptors. Meningioma is one of the few brain tumors that exhibits a female predominance.

Pathology

LOCATION. Meningiomas can occur at virtually any site within the CNS **(22-3)**. Over 90% of intracranial meningiomas are supratentorial. The most common location is parasagittal/convexity, accounting for almost half of all meningiomas.

Between 15-20% are located along the sphenoid ridge. Other common locations near the skull base include the olfactory groove and sellar/parasellar region (including the cavernous sinus). Less common supratentorial sites include the ventricles (usually in the choroid plexus glomus) and pineal region (tentorial apex).

Approximately 8-10% of intracranial meningiomas occur in the posterior fossa. The cerebellopontine angle is the most common infratentorial site followed by the jugular foramen and foramen magnum.

Between 1-2% of meningiomas are extradural. Sites include the orbit (optic nerve sheath), paranasal sinuses, and nose. A few TMs arise within the skull ("intradiploic" or "intraosseous" meningioma).

MENINGIOMA: LOCATION

General
- Supratentorial (90%), infratentorial (8-10%)
- Multiple (10%; NF2, meningiomatosis)

Sites
- Most common (60-70%)
  - Parasagittal (25%)
  - Convexity (20%)
  - Sphenoid ridge (15-20%)
- Less common (20-25%)
  - Posterior fossa (8-10%)
  - Olfactory groove (5-10%)
  - Parasellar (5-10%)
- Rare (2%)
  - Intraventricular
  - Pineal region/tentorial apex
  - Extradural (optic nerve sheath, sinuses, nose, intraosseous)

SIZE AND NUMBER. Meningiomas vary widely in size. Most are small (less than one centimeter) and found incidentally. Some—especially those arising in the anterior fossa from the olfactory groove—may attain large size before causing symptoms.

Meningiomas can be solitary or multiple. Multiple meningiomas occur in **NF2** as well as in **multiple meningiomatosis syndrome**.

GROSS PATHOLOGY. Meningiomas have two general configurations: A round ("globose") **(22-4)**, **(22-5)**, **(22-6)** and a flat, sheet- or carpet-like ("en plaque") appearance **(22-11)**. Most TMs are well-demarcated firm, rubbery, or gritty masses that have a broad base of dural attachment. As they grow, TMs typically invaginate toward adjacent brain. A CSF-vascular "cleft" is usually present between the tumor and underlying cortex **(22-5)**, **(22-6)**. While histologically benign meningiomas very occasionally invade the brain, this is uncommon.

Meningiomas often cause reactive nonneoplastic thickening of the adjacent dura ("dural tail" sign on imaging) **(22-7)**, **(22-8)**. They commonly invade dural venous sinuses and may extend through the dura to involve the skull, inducing calvarial hyperostosis.

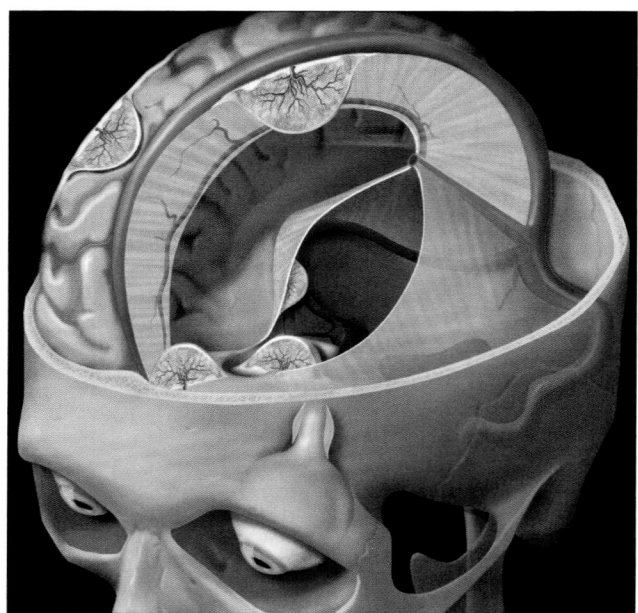

22-3. The most common meningioma sites are convexity, parafalcine, followed by sphenoid ridge, olfactory groove, sella/parasellar region. About 8-10% are infratentorial. Extracranial sites include optic nerve sheath, nose, paranasal sinuses.

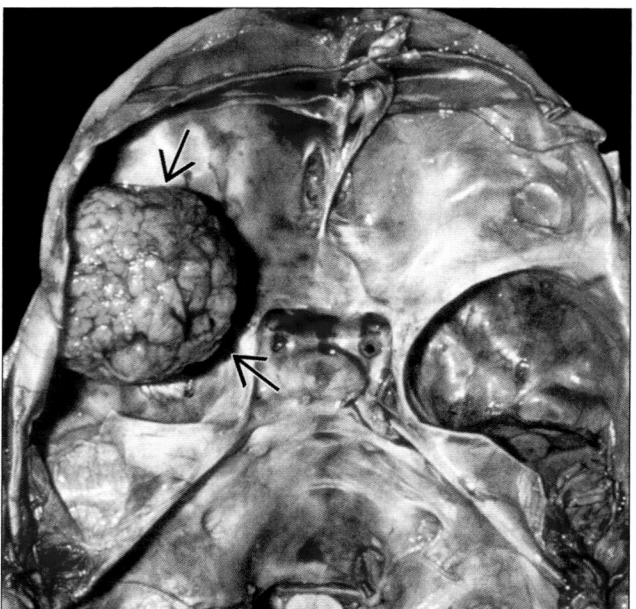

22-4. Autopsy specimen shows classic globose meningioma ⊡ as a round, "bosselated" mass with a flat surface toward the dura. (Courtesy R. Hewlett, MD.)

While small "microcysts" are not uncommon in TMs, gross cystic change is rare. Frank hemorrhage is uncommon, occurring in only 1-2% of cases.

Rarely, metastasis from an extracranial primary to a meningioma occurs. Such **"collision tumors"** are typically lung or breast metastases to a histologically typical meningioma.

MICROSCOPIC FEATURES. Meningiomas exhibit a wide spectrum of histologic appearances. Indeed, the WHO classification lists many subtypes of typical meningioma. The most common are the meningothelial, fibrous, and mixed or "transitional" variants.

All typical meningiomas are benign WHO grade I tumors and by definition carry a low risk of recurrence and aggressive growth. Their mitotic index is low, with MIB-1 usually < 1%.

Although there is no clinical difference among meningioma subtypes that share the same WHO grade, the most recent WHO classification suggests that histologically benign TMs that show gross or microscopic brain invasion should be designated as grade II neoplasms.

Clinical Issues

EPIDEMIOLOGY. Historically, meningioma was considered the second most common intracranial primary brain tumor (after astrocytoma). Recent epidemiologic data suggest that it is the most frequently diagnosed primary brain tumor, accounting for nearly one-third of all reported CNS tumors. Typical meningiomas account for 90-95% of these tumors.

Many TMs are small and discovered incidentally at imaging or autopsy. The prevalence of subclinical lesions is 1-3%.

Multiple meningiomas are common in patients with neurofibromatosis type 2 (NF2) and non-NF2 hereditary multiple meningioma syndromes. Sporadic multiple (i.e., not syndromic) meningiomas occur in about 10% of cases.

DEMOGRAPHICS. Meningiomas are classically tumors of middle-aged and older adults. Peak occurrence is in the sixth and seventh decades. Although meningioma accounts for less than 3% of primary brain tumors in children, meningioma still represents the most common dura-based neoplasm in this age group. Many (but by no means all) are related to NF2. NF2-related meningiomas occur at a significantly younger age compared to nonsyndromic meningiomas.

Women are almost twice as likely men to develop typical meningiomas. The F:M ratio varies with age, peaking at 3.5-4:1 in middle-aged patients.

PRESENTATION. Symptoms relate to size and tumor site. Less than 10% of meningiomas become symptomatic.

NATURAL HISTORY. Longitudinal studies have demonstrated that most meningiomas under 2.5 cm grow very slowly—if at all—over five years. The majority of small, asymptomatic, incidentally discovered menin-

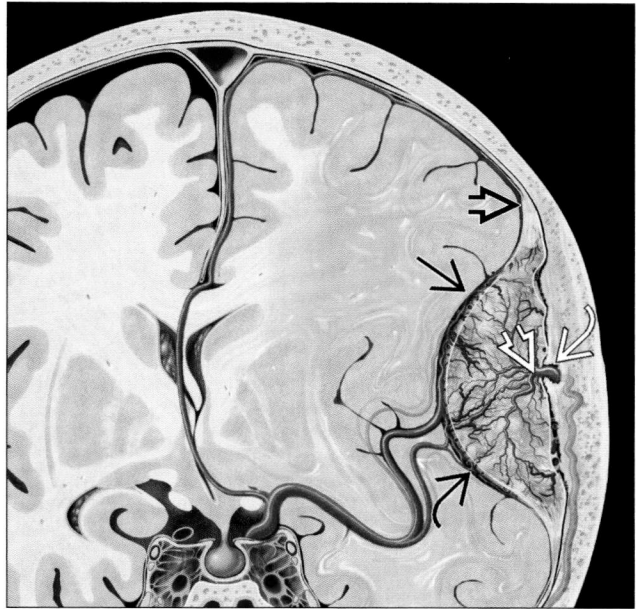

22-5. *Classic meningioma has a broad base toward dura, reactive dural thickening (dural "tail")* ⊳, *enostotic "spur"* ⊅, *CSF-vascular "cleft"* ⊳. *MMA supplies tumor core in "sunburst" pattern* ⊳; *pial vessels supply periphery* ⊳.

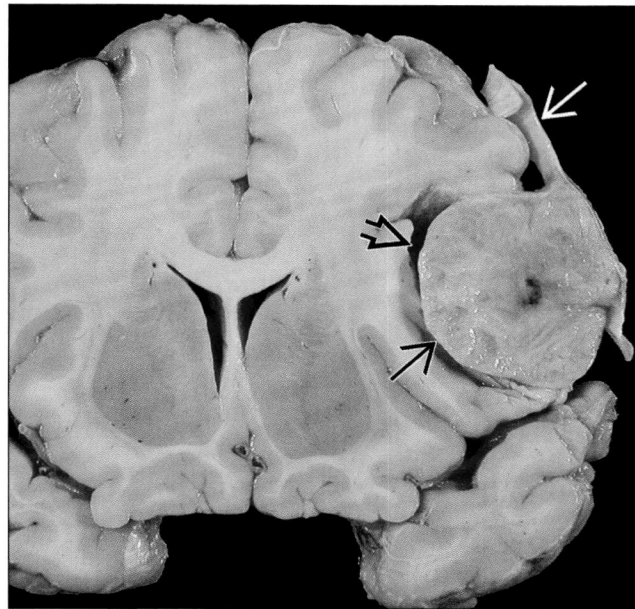

22-6. *Autopsy specimen shows classic globose meningioma* ⊳. *Note prominent CSF-vascular cleft* ⊳, *reactive dural thickening* ⊳ *("dural tail" sign).*

giomas show minimal growth and are usually followed with serial imaging.

Malignant degeneration of a TM into an atypical or anaplastic meningioma is rare. Extracranial metastases are exceptionally rare, occurring in 1 in 1,000 cases. When they do occur, metastases are generally to the lung or axial skeleton. Metastases from both benign and atypical/malignant meningiomas have been reported.

TREATMENT OPTIONS. A neurosurgeon once stated, "Like the impressions on a finger tip, each meningioma is different." Stratified treatment risk-benefit ratios vary not just with tumor type and grade, but also with size and location, vascular supply, and presence or absence of a brain/tumor cleavage plane.

Image-guided surgery with resection of symptomatic lesions is generally curative. Although the major factor associated with meningioma recurrence is subtotal resection, recent studies show that leaving small amounts of tumor adhering to crucial structures such as vessels and cranial nerves does not significantly affect outcome.

Stereotactic radiosurgery or chemotherapy with progesterone antagonists may be options in patients with TMs in critical locations such as the cavernous sinus.

MENINGIOMA: CLINICAL ISSUES

Epidemiology
- Most common intracranial primary neoplasm
- Most are asymptomatic
  - Found incidentally at imaging/autopsy (1-3%)
- Solitary (90%)
  - Multiple in NF2, meningiomatosis

Demographics
- F:M = 2:1
- Peak age = 40-60 years
- Rare in children unless NF2

Natural History
- Grows slowly
- Rarely metastasizes

Imaging

GENERAL FEATURES. The general appearance of a TM is a round or lobulated, sharply demarcated, extraaxial dura-based mass that buckles the cortex inward. A discernible CSF-vascular "cleft" is usually present, especially on MR. Parenchymal invasion is uncommon. Rarely, a meningioma is pedunculated and invaginates into the brain, which may make it difficult to distinguish from an intraaxial primary tumor.

Meningioma-associated cysts are found in 4-7% of cases. These can be intra- or extratumoral. Occasionally pools of CSF are trapped between the tumor and adjacent brain.

CT FINDINGS.

NECT. Almost three-quarters of meningiomas are mildly to moderately hyperdense compared to cortex

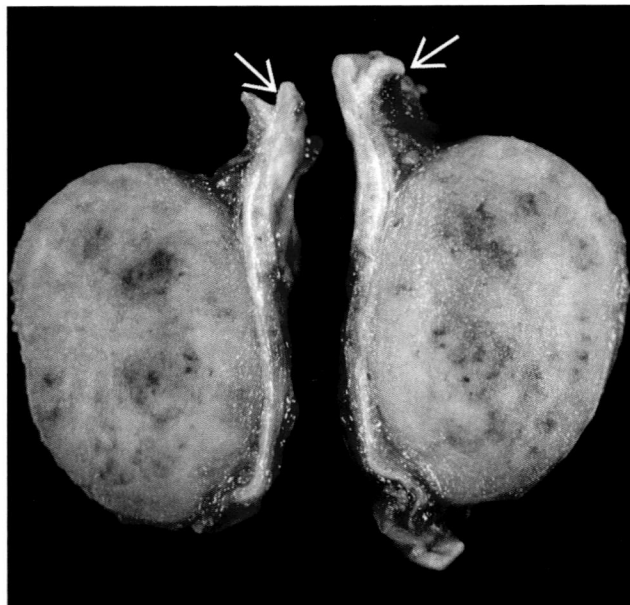

22-7. *Meningioma in cut section shows attachment to dura, reactive dural thickening* ➡ *("dural tail" sign.) (Courtesy R. Hewlett, MD.)*

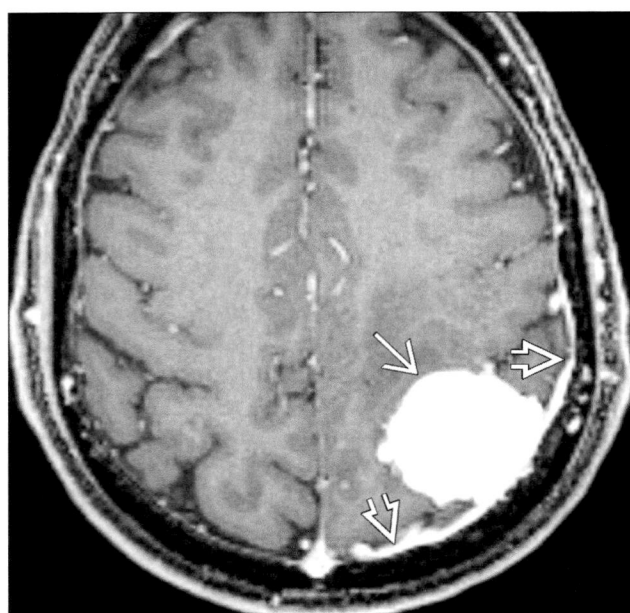

22-8. *T1 C+ scan shows that typical meningioma enhances strongly, quite uniformly* ➡. *Adjacent dural thickening* ➡ *("dural tail" sign) is common and usually reactive, not neoplastic.*

(22-9A). About one-quarter are isodense. Hypodense meningiomas are uncommon. Frank necrosis or hemorrhage is rare.

Peritumoral vasogenic edema, seen as confluent hypodensity in the adjacent brain, is present in about 60% of all cases.

Approximately 25% of TMs demonstrate calcification. Focal globular or more diffuse sand-like ("psammomatous") calcifications occur.

Bone CT may show hyperostosis that varies from minimal to striking. Hyperostosis is often but not invariably associated with tumor invasion **(22-12)**. Bone lysis or frank destruction can also occur. Bone involvement by meningioma occurs with both benign and malignant meningiomas and is not predictive of tumor grade.

CECT. The vast majority of meningiomas enhance strongly and uniformly **(22-9B)**.

MR FINDINGS.

General features. Most meningiomas are inhomogeneously isointense with cortex on all sequences. Between 10-25% of cases demonstrate changes suggestive of cyst formation or necrosis although frank hemorrhage is uncommon.

T1WI. Meningiomas are typically iso- to slightly hypointense compared to cortex **(22-10A)**, **(22-13A)**. Predominant hypointensity on T1WI suggests the microcystic variant of TM.

T2WI. Most TMs are iso- to moderately hyperintense compared to cortex **(22-10B)**, **(22-13B)**, **(22-15)**. These are associated with a "soft" consistency at surgery, whereas T2/FLAIR hypointense tumors tend to be "hard" and somewhat gritty. Densely fibrotic and calcified meningiomas can be very hypointense.

The CSF-vascular "cleft" is especially well-delineated on T2WI and is seen as a hyperintense rim interposed between the tumor and brain. A number of "flow voids" representing displaced vessels are often seen within the "cleft."

Sometimes a "sunburst" pattern that represents the dural vascular supply to the tumor can be identified radiating toward the periphery of the mass **(22-14)**.

FLAIR. Meningioma signal intensity varies from iso- to hyperintense **(22-10C)**, **(22-13C)**. FLAIR is very useful for depicting peritumoral edema, which is found with approximately half of all TMs. Peritumoral edema is related to the presence of pial blood supply and VEGF expression, not tumor size or grade. Some small meningiomas incite striking peritumoral edema while some very large masses exhibit virtually none.

Pools of CSF trapped in the cleft between tumor and brain ("peritumoral cysts") are usually proteinaceous and may not suppress completely on FLAIR.

T2* (GRE, SWI). T2* sequences are helpful to depict intratumoral calcification **(22-10D)**. "Blooming" secondary to intratumoral hemorrhage is rare.

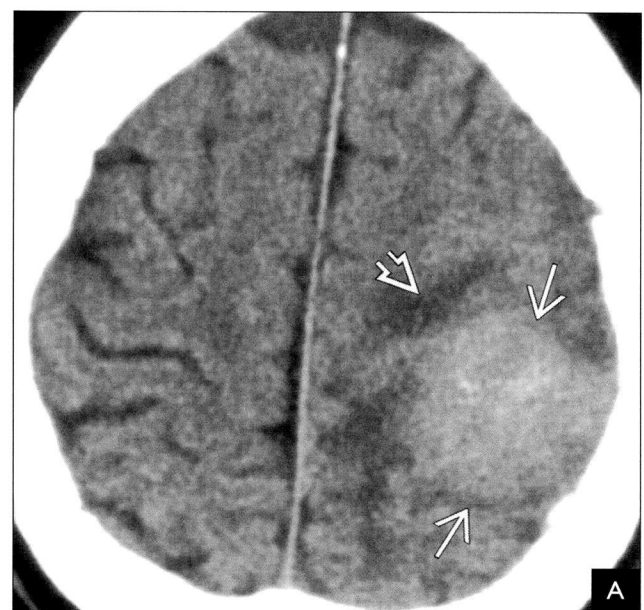

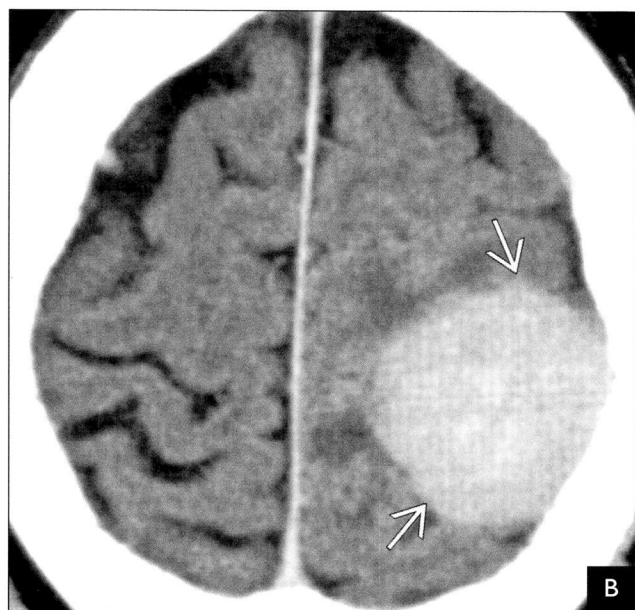

22-9A. *NECT scan shows the typical findings of meningioma. A mild to moderately hyperdense mass* ⮞ *is associated with hypodense peritumoral edge* ⮞.

22-9B. *CECT shows that the tumor* ⮞ *enhances strongly, uniformly.*

T1 C+. Virtually all meningiomas, including densely calcified "brain rocks" and intraosseous tumors, demonstrate at least some enhancement following contrast administration. Over 95% enhance strongly and homogeneously **(22-10E)**, **(22-10F)**, **(22-13D)**.

A dural "tail" is seen in the majority of meningiomas and varies from a relatively focal area adjacent to the tumor **(22-8)** to extensive dural thickening and enhancement extending far beyond the site of tumor attachment. The dural "tail" often enhances more intensely and more uniformly than the tumor itself. A "dural tail" sign is not pathognomonic of meningioma.

Most of the enhancing dural "tail" represents benign, reactive dural thickening. Tumor extending one centimeter beyond the base of the tumor is rare.

Nonenhancing *intratumoral* cysts are seen in 5% of cases. Nonneoplastic *peritumoral* cysts do not enhance. Enhancement around the rim of a peripherally located cyst suggests the presence of tumor in the cyst wall.

DWI. Most meningiomas do not restrict on DWI.

Perfusion MR. Perfusion MR may be helpful in distinguishing TM from atypical/malignant meningiomas. High rCBV in the lesion or in the surrounding edema suggests a more aggressive tumor grade.

MRS. Alanine (Ala, peak at 1.48 ppm) is often elevated in meningioma although glutamate-glutamine (Glx, peak at 2.1-2.6 ppm) and glutathione (GSH, peak at 2.95 ppm) may be more specific potential markers.

ANGIOGRAPHY.

CTA, MRA/MRV. CTA is very helpful in detecting dural venous sinus invasion or occlusion. While it may be helpful in depicting the general status of the vascular supply to a meningioma, DSA is best for detailed delineation of tumor vascularity prior to embolization or surgery. Tumor invasion of major dural venous sinuses is especially well-depicted on MRV.

DSA. The classic angiographic appearance of a meningioma is a radial "sunburst" of vessels extending from the base of the tumor toward its periphery. Dural vessels supply the core or center of the lesion, radiating outward from the vascular pedicle of the tumor **(22-16A)**. Pial vessels from internal carotid artery branches may become "parasitized" and supply the periphery of the mass **(22-16C)**.

A prolonged vascular "blush" that persists late into the venous phase is typical. In some cases, arteriovenous shunting with the appearance of "early draining" veins occurs **(22-16B)**. Careful examination of the venous phase should be conducted to detect dural sinus invasion or occlusion.

Preoperative embolization with tumor devascularization may substantially reduce operative time and blood loss. Careful delineation of tumor blood supply, including "dangerous" extra- to intracranial anastomoses, is essential to procedure success.

22-10A. *Large convexity meningioma with typical MR findings. The tumor has flat base toward the dural surface, "buckles" the cortex and GM-WM interface inward ➡. Meningiomas are most commonly isointense with cortex on T1WI. **22-10B.** T2 signal intensity varies. Here the tumor is iso-/slightly hyperintense relative to cortex. "Sunburst" of dural vessels ➡ is well seen. Note CSF-vascular "cleft," clearly seen here ➡, as is the displaced GM-WM interface ➡.*

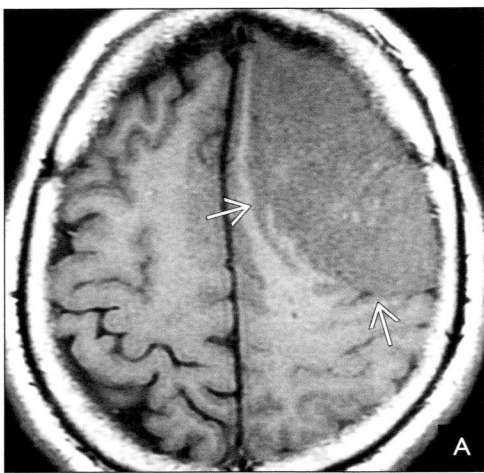

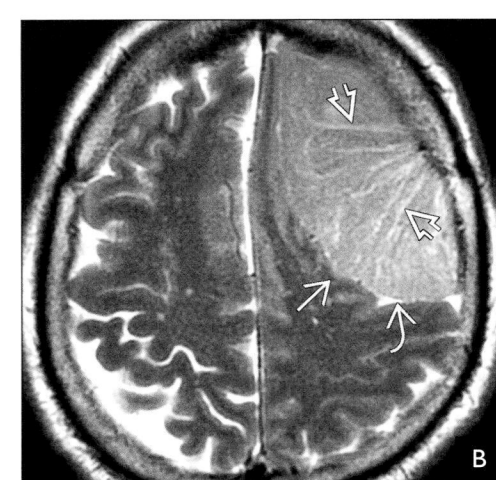

22-10C. *Signal intensity on FLAIR also varies. Here the tumor varies from iso- ➡ to slightly hyperintense ➡. **22-10D.** T2* GRE scans may show scattered "blooming" foci ➡, but these are usually related to calcification rather than hemorrhage. Gross hemorrhage in typical WHO grade I meningioma is rare.*

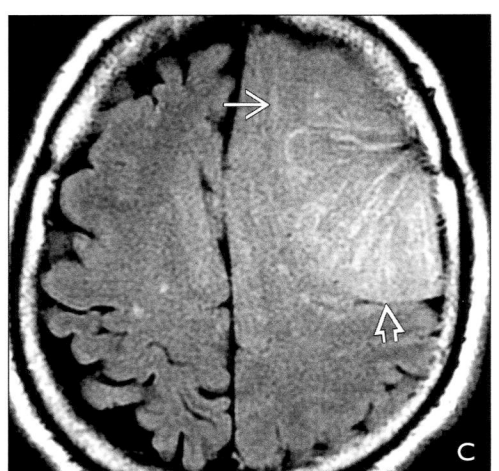

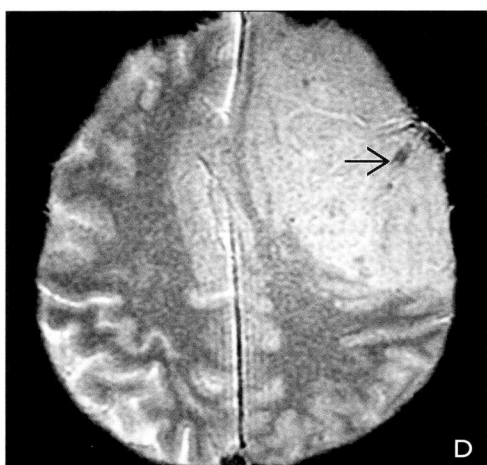

22-10E. *T1 C+ FS scan shows that the tumor enhances intensely. Especially well seen is the even more hyperintense "sunburst" of vessels ➡ that supplies the tumor, radiating outward from the enostotic "spur" ➡. **22-10F.** Coronal T1WI shows the "sunburst" of vessels especially well. Enlarged branches of the middle meningeal artery enter the tumor mass at the enostotic "spur" ➡.*

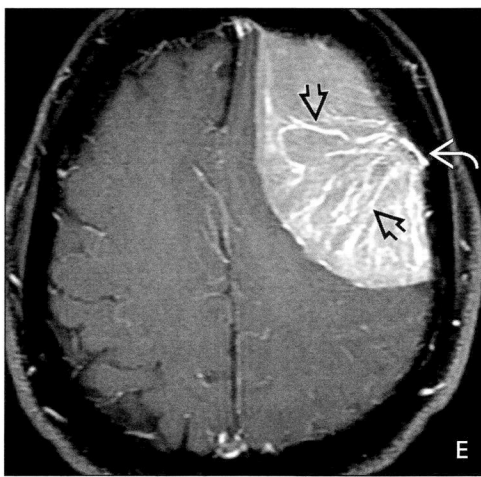

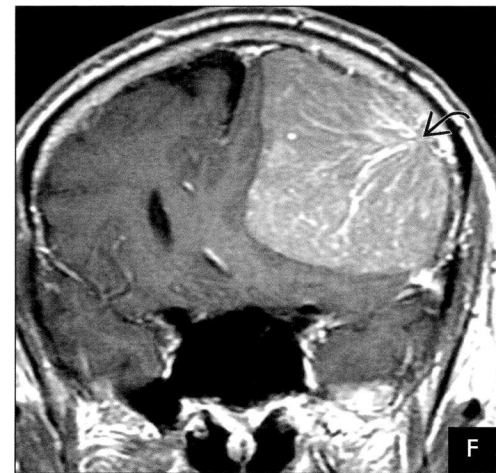

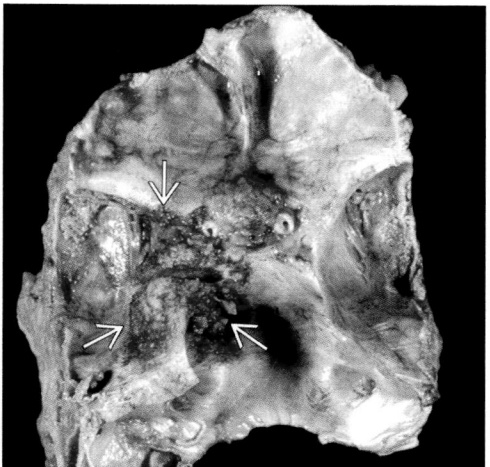

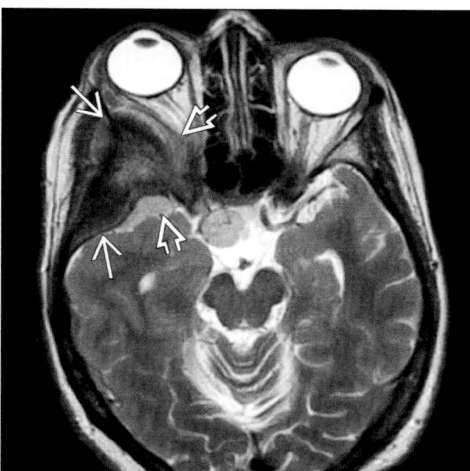

22-11. Autopsy specimen shows an extensive skull base "en plaque" meningioma ➡. Such tumors often affect more than one compartment, infiltrate and thicken bone. The sphenoid wing and orbit are favored sites. (Courtesy R. Hewlett, MD.) *22-12.* T2WI shows marked thickening of the greater sphenoid wing ➡ with "en plaque" meningioma ➡ in the orbit, middle cranial fossa, suprasellar cistern. (Courtesy S. Hetal, MD.)

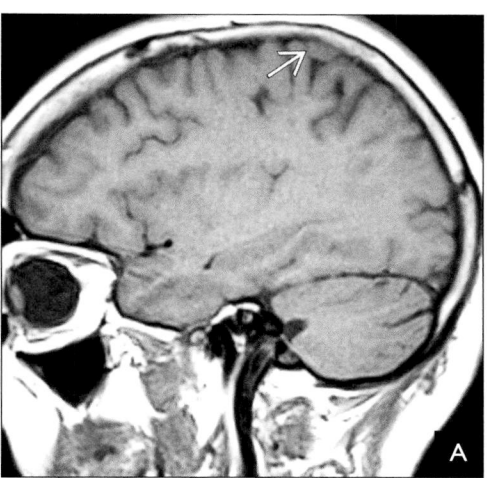

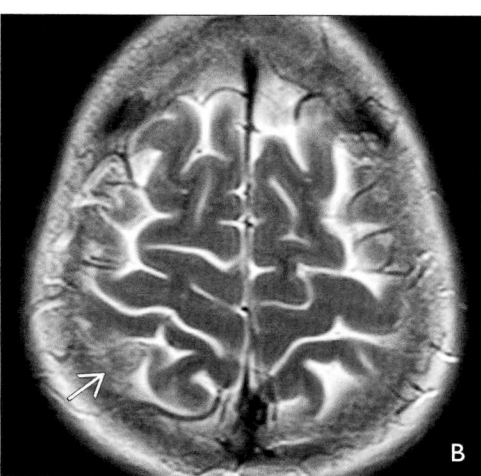

22-13A. Sagittal T1WI in a 54-year-old woman with headaches appears normal except for a tiny isointense convexity meningioma ➡, seen here "hiding" in a slightly widened sulcus. *22-13B.* Axial T2WI in the same patient shows that the meningioma ➡ is nearly isointense with underlying cortex, making it difficult to identify.

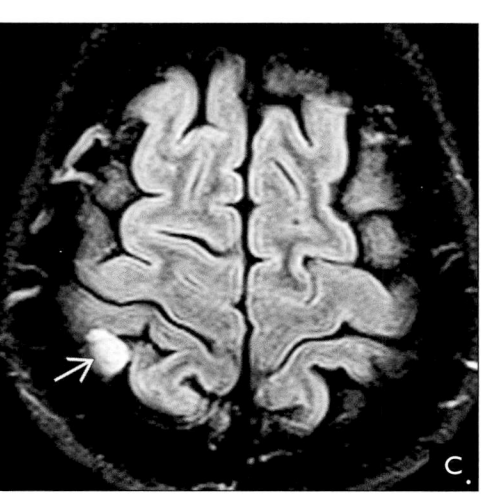

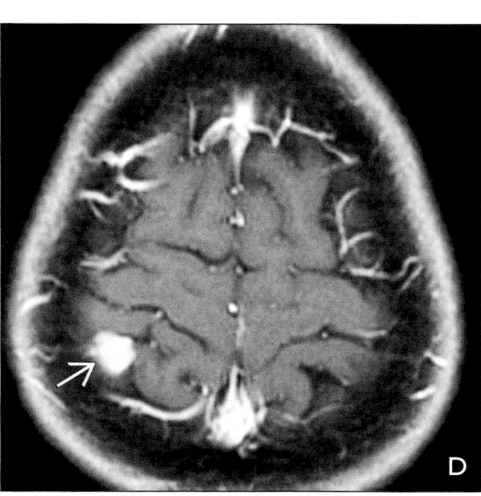

22-13C. The meningioma is hyperintense on FLAIR ➡, demonstrates no edema in the adjacent cortex. *22-13D.* T1 C+ FS scan shows that the small meningioma ➡ enhances strongly, uniformly. This lesion has been followed for 2 years with no change in size.

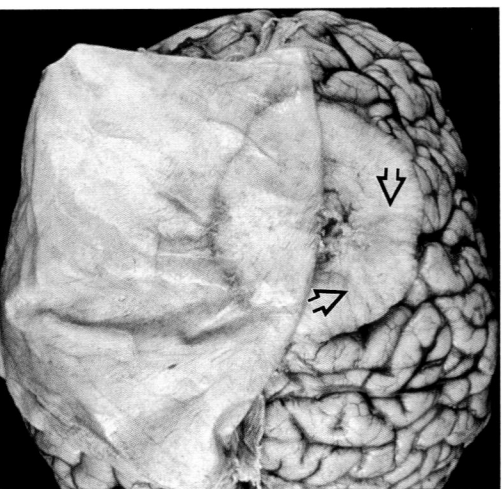

22-14. Autopsy case shows convexity meningioma with dural attachment, "sunburst" of vessels radiating outward ⊳. (Courtesy AFIP Archives).

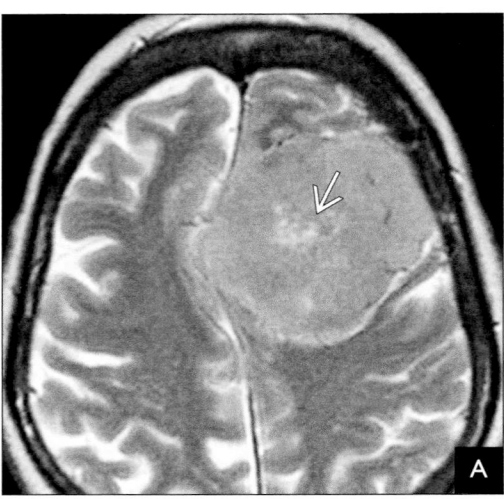

22-15A. T2WI shows an isointense convexity meningioma. Central hyperintensity ⟹ is where dural vessels enter the mass (compare 22-14).

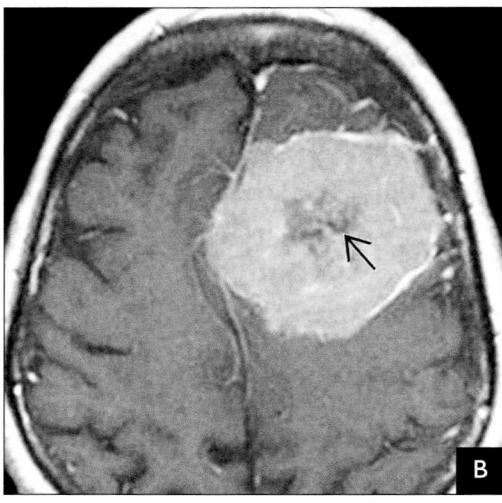

22-15B. T1 C+ shows that the mass enhances intensely. Note the "flow voids" in vascular center of the mass ⟹.

MENINGIOMA: IMAGING

General
- Round or flat ("en plaque"), dura-based
- Extraaxial mass with "cleft" between tumor, brain

CT
- Hyperdense (70-75%)
- Calcified (20-25%)
- Cysts (peri- or intratumoral) (10-15%)
- Hemorrhage rare
- > 90% enhance

MR
- Usually isointense with gray matter
- CSF-vascular "cleft"
- ± vascular "flow voids"
- Strong, often heterogeneous enhancement (> 98%)
- Dural "tail" (60%)

Angiography
- "Sunburst" vascularity
- Dural arteries to outside, pial to inside
- Prolonged, dense vascular "blush"

Differential Diagnosis

The major differential diagnosis of typical meningioma is **atypical** or **malignant meningioma**. While there are no pathognomonic imaging features that reliably distinguish TM from these more aggressive variants, TMs are statistically far more common. Malignant meningiomas typically invade brain and may exhibit a "mushrooming" configuration (see below).

Dural metastasis, usually from a breast or lung primary, may be virtually indistinguishable from meningioma on imaging studies.

Other meningioma mimics include **granuloma** (TB, sarcoid) and focal **idiopathic hypertrophic pachymeningitis**. Solitary dural granulomas are rare. Idiopathic hypertrophic pachymeningitis is uncommon. Most cases are found in or around the skull base, particularly the orbit, cavernous sinus, and posterior fossa (clivus/cerebellopontine angle). Idiopathic hypertrophic pachymeningitis can invade bone and may be virtually indistinguishable from "en plaque" meningioma.

Rare entities that can closely resemble meningioma include hemangioma and solitary fibrous tumors. A **hemangioma of the dura** or **venous sinuses** is a true vasoformative neoplasm that can resemble meningioma. Most hemangiomas are very hyperintense on T2WI whereas most meningiomas are iso- to mildly hyperintense. Delayed slow centripetal "filling in" of the mass on dynamic contrast-enhanced MR is suggestive of hemangioma.

Intracranial solitary fibrous tumor is very rare. Most are found adjacent to the dura, venous sinuses, or choroid plexus. Solitary fibrous tumor may be indistinguishable on imaging studies from typical meningioma.

Extramedullary hematopoiesis (EMH) can present as confluent or multifocal dura-based disease resembling "en plaque" solitary or multiple meningiomatosis. EMH occurs in the setting of chronic anemia or marrow depletion disorders.

MENINGIOMA MIMICS

Common
- Dural metastasis

Less Common
- Granuloma

Rare but Important
- Idiopathic hypertrophic pachymeningitis
- Dural/venous sinus hemangioma
- Solitary fibrous tumor
- Extramedullary hematopoiesis

---

typical Meningioma

rminology

Atypical meningioma (AM) is defined histopathologically (see below).

iology

There is a significant correlation between the number of inactivating *NF2* mutations and tumor grade. Almost 60% of AMs show gain of chromosome arm 1q.

thology

LOCATION. Most atypical and malignant meningiomas arise from the calvaria. The skull base is a relatively uncommon location for these more aggressive lesions.

GROSS PATHOLOGY. Although atypical meningiomas frequently invade adjacent brain, brain invasion alone is insufficient to establish the diagnosis of an AM. Irregular strands of histologically more atypical tumor cells infiltrate the brain parenchyma, without an intervening layer of leptomeninges.

MICROSCOPIC FEATURES. An atypical meningioma exhibits increased mitotic activity (≥ 4 mitoses per 10 high-power fields) or three or more of the following histologic features: Increased cellularity, small cells with high nuclear:cytoplasmic ratio, prominent nucleoli, patternless or sheet-like growth, and necrotic foci. A MIB-1 labeling index > 4 is typical.

Some meningioma subtypes are classified as WHO grade II tumors simply because of their greater likelihood of recurrence and/or more aggressive behavior. These include the chordoid and clear cell subtypes.

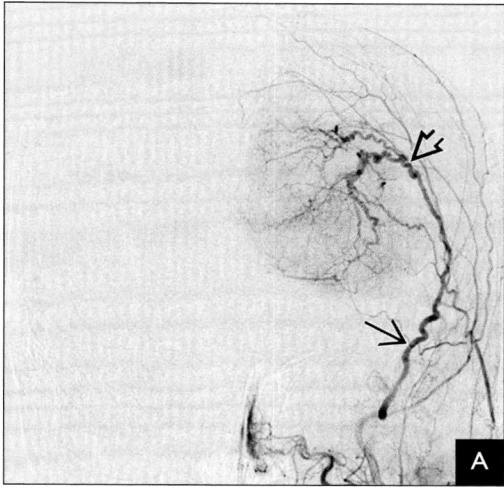

22-16A. AP DSA of ECA shows enlarged middle meningeal artery ➡ with "sunburst" of vessels ⇒ supplying meningioma.

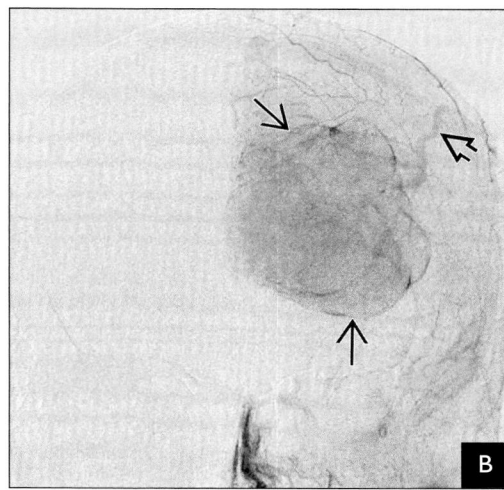

22-16B. Later phase of ECA DSA shows prolonged vascular "blush" ➡ characteristic of meningioma. "Early draining" vein is seen ⇒.

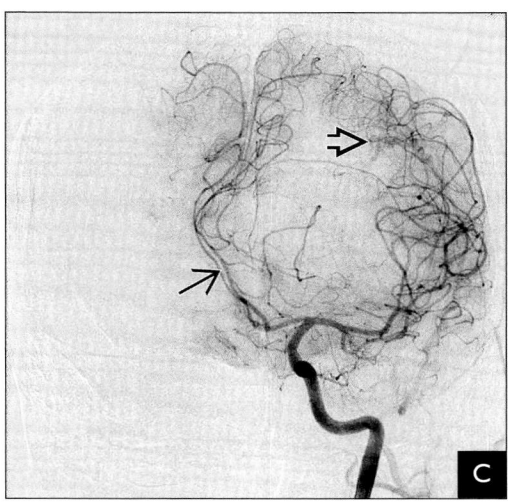

22-16C. ICA DSA shows mass effect with the ACA shifted ➡. Only minimal supply to periphery of tumor ⇒ is coming from pial MCA branches.

Clinical Issues

EPIDEMIOLOGY. AMs represent 4-8% of all meningiomas.

DEMOGRAPHICS. AMs tend to occur in slightly younger patients compared to TMs. Pediatric meningiomas tend to be more aggressive. In contrast with TMs, AMs display a slight male predominance.

NATURAL HISTORY. AMs are generally associated with a higher recurrence rate (25-30%) and shorter recurrence-free survival compared to TMs. The tendency of intrinsic cranial base meningiomas to recur depends more on surgical limitations than biological factors.

Imaging

GENERAL FEATURES. A good general rule is that it is difficult—if not impossible—to predict meningioma grade on the basis of imaging findings. However, because brain invasion is a frequent (but not invariable) feature of AMs, the CSF-vascular "cleft" typically seen in TMs is often absent.

CT FINDINGS. AMs are usually hyperdense with irregular margins. Minimal or no calcification is seen, and frank bone invasion with osteolysis is common. Tumor may invade through the skull into the scalp.

MR FINDINGS. Tumor margins are usually indistinct with no border between the tumor and the underlying cortex. A CSF-vascular "cleft" is often absent or partially effaced. Peritumoral edema is a common but nonspecific finding. Contrast enhancement is strong but often quite inhomogeneous.

ADC is significantly lower in atypical and malignant meningiomas compared to TMs. Perfusion MR may show elevated rCBV, especially in the peritumoral edema (22-17). MRS often shows elevated alanine.

Differential Diagnosis

Because it is difficult to determine meningioma tumor grade on the basis of imaging findings alone, the major differential diagnosis of AM is **typical meningioma**. **Dural metastasis** and **malignant meningioma** can also be indistinguishable from AM. **Sarcomas,** such as

22-17A. FLAIR scan in a 68-year-old woman with right-sided weakness shows a hyperintense, lobulated convexity mass ➡ with numerous "flow voids" ⟐, edema ➡. 22-17B. T1 C+ FS demonstrates that the mass ➡ enhances intensely and uniformly. Coronal T1 C+ (not shown) demonstrated that the mass was attached to the dura and exhibited a "dural tail" sign.

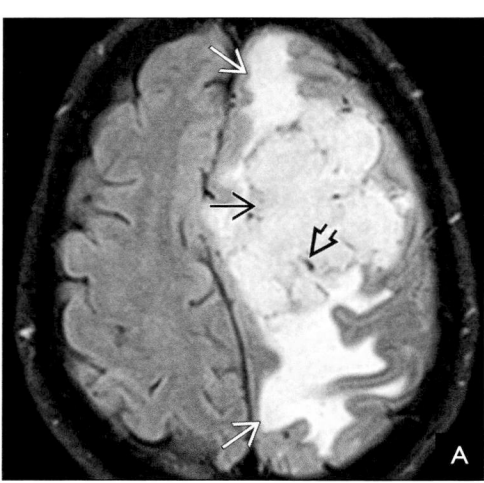
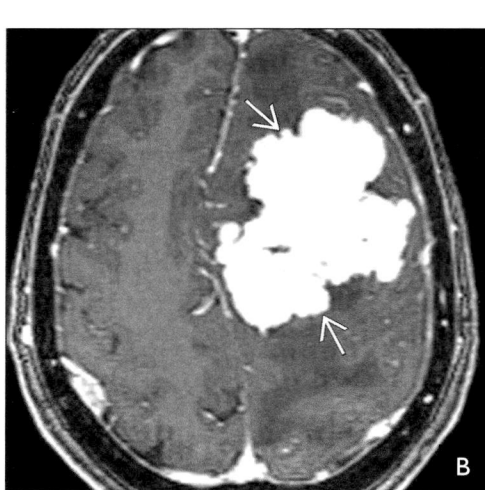

22-17C. The mass ➡ shows restricted diffusion, consistent with high cellularity. 22-17D. MRS showed markedly elevated Cho, decreased NAA. Choline map shows the elevated Cho ⟐ with the highest levels in the center of the lesion ➡. Atypical meningioma, clear cell type, WHO grade II. (Courtesy M. Thurnher, MD.)

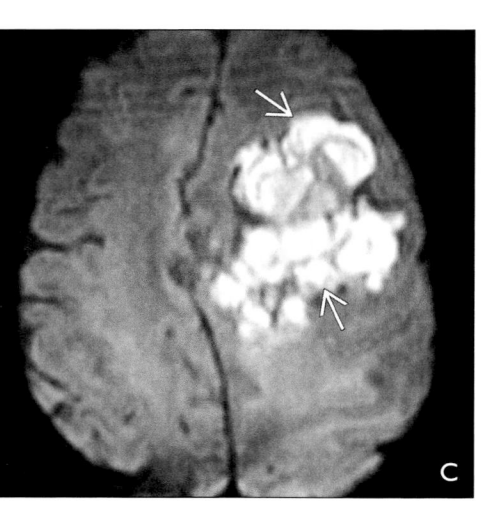
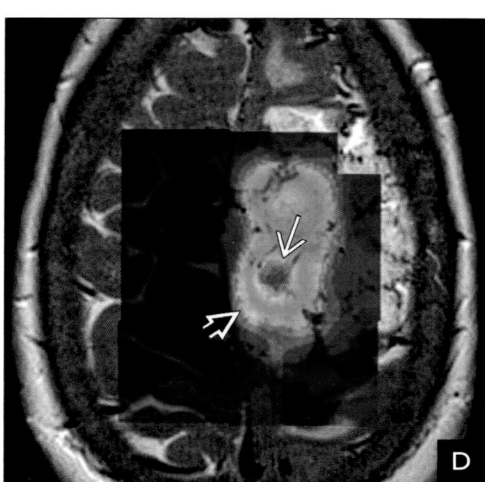

gliosarcoma in older patients and Ewing and osteogenic sarcoma in young patients, may also be difficult to distinguish from biologically aggressive meningiomas.

Malignant Meningioma

Terminology

Anaplastic or malignant meningioma (MMen) corresponds histologically to WHO grade III.

Biology

Chromosomal mutations are increased compared to AMs. HOXA methylation levels are significantly higher in WHO II/III meningiomas compared to grade I neoplasms.

Pathology

Most MMens invade the brain and exhibit histologic features of frank malignancy **(22-18)**. These include increased cellular atypia with bizarre nuclei and markedly elevated mitotic index (> 20). MMen subtypes include papillary and rhabdoid meningiomas.

Clinical Issues

EPIDEMIOLOGY. Frankly malignant meningiomas are rare, representing only 1-3% of all meningiomas. MMens have a striking male predominance.

NATURAL HISTORY. Prognosis is poor. Recurrence rates following MMen resection range from 50-95%. Survival times are short with median reported survival in some series under two years. A parasagittal-falcine location is also a significant predictor of decreased recurrence-free survival.

Imaging

GENERAL FEATURES. The imaging triad of extracranial mass, osteolysis, and "mushrooming" intracranial tumor is present in most—but not all—cases of MMen **(22-19)**, **(22-20)**.

Differential Diagnosis

The main differential diagnosis of MMen is **metastasis**. **Atypical meningioma** and **sarcomas** can be indistinguishable from MMen.

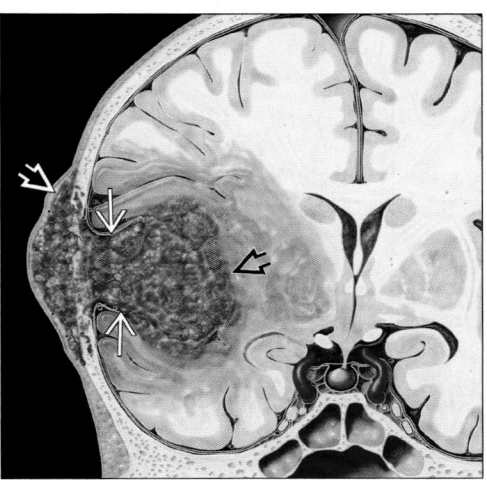

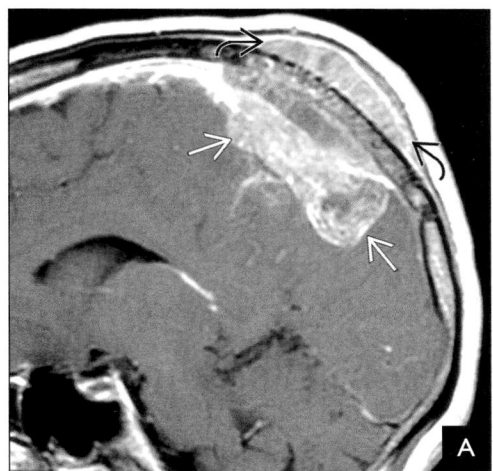

22-18. Graphic depicts malignant meningioma invading brain ⇨ with no clear-cut CSF-vascular "cleft." The tumor also penetrates the dura, invades the calvaria, and has a significant extracranial component ⇨. Note "mushroom" configuration ⇨, which may be more characteristic of aggressive versus benign meningiomas. 22-19A. Sagittal T1WI shows aggressive transcalvarial mass with both intra- ⇨ and extracranial ⇨ tumor.

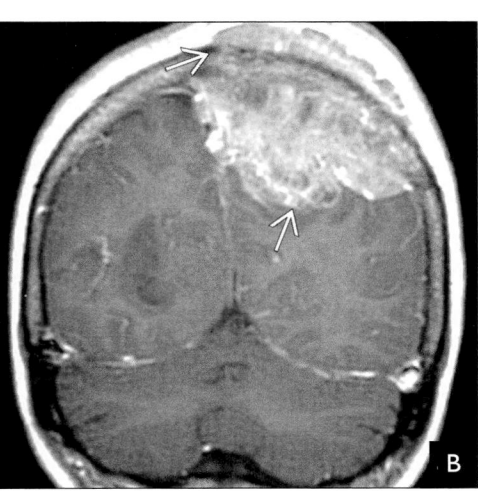

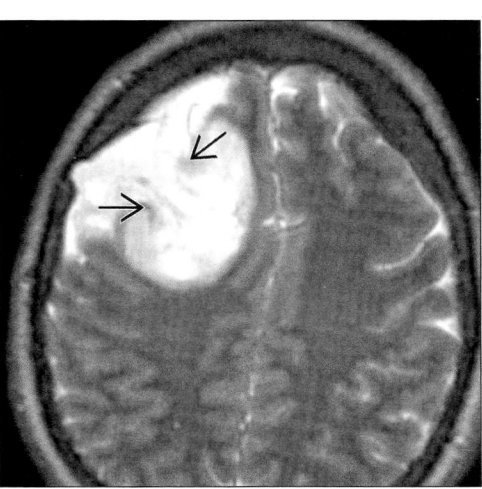

22-19B. Coronal T1 C+ scan in the same patient shows the transdural, transcranial invasive tumor ⇨. No border between neoplasm and brain is discernible. WHO grade III (malignant) meningioma was the histopathologic diagnosis. 22-20. T2WI in another patient with anaplastic (malignant) meningioma shows "mushroom" configuration ⇨.

Nonmeningothelial Mesenchymal Tumors

CNS nonmeningothelial mesenchymal neoplasms correspond to soft tissue or bone tumors found elsewhere in the body. They can be tumors of adipose, fibrous, histiocytic, cartilaginous, or vascular tissues and can also arise from muscle or bone. Both benign and malignant varieties of each type occur, ranging from benign (WHO grade I) to highly malignant (WHO grade IV) neoplasms.

Nonmeningothelial mesenchymal tumors rarely involve the CNS. When they do, they are usually extraaxial lesions. We discuss these tumors in two groups, benign and malignant neoplasms.

Benign Mesenchymal Tumors

Terminology

Benign mesenchymal tumors (BMTs) correspond in name and histology to their extracranial counterparts. Osteocartilaginous tumors such as chondroma, osteochondroma, and osteoma are the most common BMTs that occur within the CNS. Pure fibrous tumors such as fibromatosis and solitary fibrous tumor are rare, as are mixed fibrohistiocytic tumors such as benign fibrous histiocytoma (also termed fibrous xanthoma).

Etiology

Intracranial BMTs usually originate from the meninges (typically the dura), choroid plexus, or skull base. The cranial meninges contain primitive pluripotential mesenchymal cells that can give rise to a broad spectrum of nonmeningothelial mesenchymal tumors. Most are supratentorial; the falx is the most common site.

The skull base and clivus develop by enchondral ossification. **Chondromas** and **enchondromas** usually arise from cartilaginous synchondroses in the skull base (22-21). Therefore, the central skull base, especially the sella/parasellar region, is the most common site. Less commonly, chondromas can arise from the dura or falx. **Osteochondromas** also typically arise in or near the skull base.

In contrast to the skull base, the calvarial vault develops by membranous ossification. **Osteomas** are benign tumors that arise from membranous bone. In the head, the paranasal sinuses (22-22) and calvaria (22-23) are the most common sites.

Pathology

The macro- and microscopic appearance of BMTs depends on their cell type and is similar to their extracranial soft tissue counterparts. For example, **chondromas** are sharply demarcated "bosselated" tumors that gener-

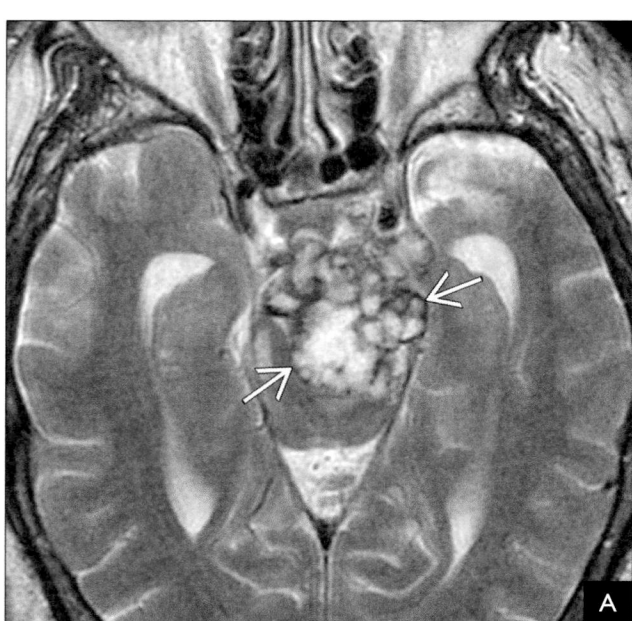

22-21A. T2WI shows a well-delineated suprasellar mass ➡ with hypointense arcs surrounding hyperintense lobulated areas.

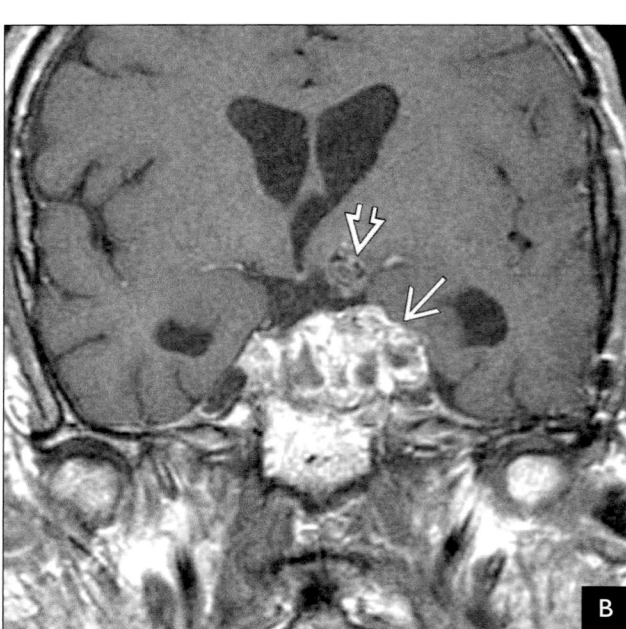

22-21B. Coronal T1 C+ shows that the mass involves the left cavernous sinus and enhances strongly but heterogeneously ➡. Small suprasellar component is seen ➡. Enchondroma was the histologic diagnosis. (Courtesy P. Sundgren, MD.)

ally have a broad flat base and grossly resemble carti-lage. **Osteochondromas** appear as a sessile or pedunculated cartilage-capped bony exostosis. **Osteomas** resemble dense lamellar bone.

Solitary fibrous tumors can arise anywhere but are generally dura-based. They present as solitary, firm, well-circumscribed masses that closely resemble meningioma.

BMTs are all WHO grade I neoplasms.

inical Issues

EPIDEMIOLOGY. With the exception of hemangiomas and lipomas, cranial mesenchymal non-meningothelial tumors are all rare. Together, these BMTs account for less than 1% of all intracranial neoplasms. Overall, **chondroma** is the most common benign osteocartilaginous tumor of the skull base. **Osteoma** is the most common benign osseous tumor of the calvaria.

Most BMTs occur as solitary nonsyndromic lesions. Multiple BMTs generally occur as part of inherited tumor syndromes. Multiple osteomas occur as part of **Gardner syndrome** (together with skin tumors and colon polyps). Multiple enchondromas or "enchondromatosis" is part of **Ollier disease**. Enchondromas associated with soft tissue hemangiomas are found in **Maffucci syndrome**.

DEMOGRAPHICS. BMTs can occur at any age. The peak age for chondroma is the second to fourth decades. Osteomas are more common in middle-aged patients. In general, there is no gender predilection.

PRESENTATION. Most BMTs are asymptomatic and discovered incidentally. Others such as osteomas may present as a longstanding skull "bump." Occasionally large BMTs, especially those arising within or near the skull base, cause cranial nerve palsies.

NATURAL HISTORY. Most BMTs can be completely resected and have a favorable prognosis. Malignant degeneration is generally rare. Multiple osteochondromas ("osteochondromatosis") have a higher propensity to undergo malignant transformation. The risk increases as the number and size of the lesions increase.

TREATMENT OPTIONS. Unless cosmetically deforming, small BMTs such as osteomas are generally of no clinical significance and are left alone. The treatment for symptomatic BMTs is complete surgical resection.

Imaging

GENERAL FEATURES. Imaging findings vary with tumor type. Most BMTs are benign-appearing nonaggressive masses of the scalp, skull, or dura that resemble their counterparts found elsewhere in the body.

CT FINDINGS. Chondromas are sessile, smoothly lobulated, expansile masses that contain curvilinear matrix calcifications. Slight enhancement on CECT may occur.

Osteochondromas are sessile or pedunculated bony masses that are contiguous with and project from their underlying bone of origin. Osteochondromas may

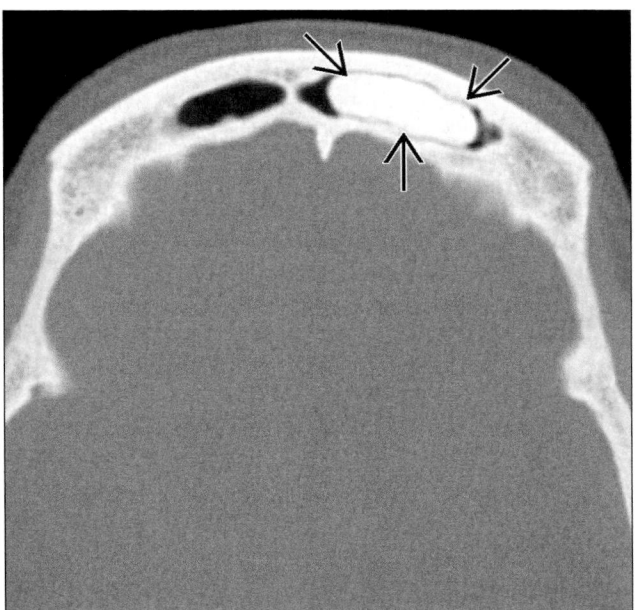

22-22. Bone CT shows a typical osteoma of the left frontal sinus ➡.

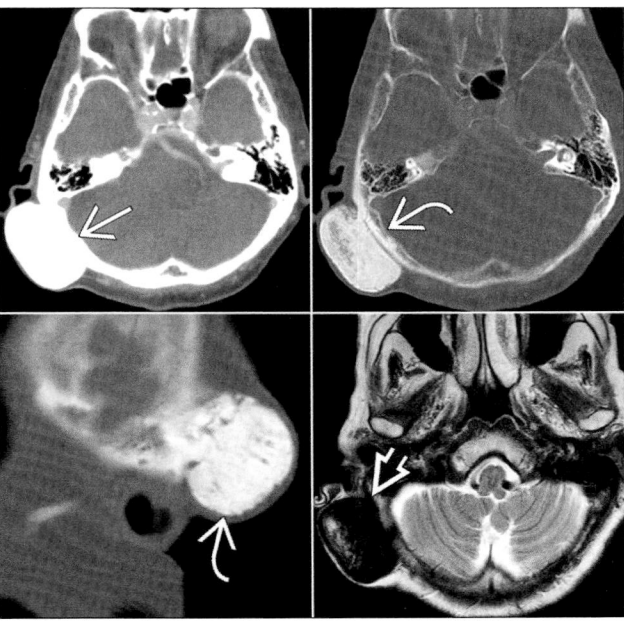

22-23. NECT shows a hyperdense mass arising from the right occipital bone ➡. *The mass is nicely seen on bone CT* ➡ *and looks like dense cortical bone. The mass is very hypointense on T2WI* ➡.

exhibit a "cap" of matrix with speckled calcification that enhances mildly following contrast administration.

Osteomas are seen as dense masses of well-demarcated mature lamellar bone. They occur in paranasal sinuses—the most common site—or the calvaria.

MR Findings. All BMTs are typically well-delineated, non-invasive-appearing masses with variable signal intensity on both T1- and T2WI. A "ring and arc" pattern of contrast enhancement can be seen with chondromas. BMTs generally do not incite dural reaction, so a "dural tail" sign is absent.

Hemangioma

Terminology

Hemangiomas are benign nonmeningothelial mesenchymal tumors. They are common vascular neoplasms that closely resemble normal vessels and are found in all organs of the body (22-24). Hemangiomas are completely different from—and should not be confused

with—cavernous angiomas, which are vascular malformations rather than neoplasms.

Etiology

Hemangiomas probably arise by endothelial hyperplasia and hamartomatous-like proliferation.

Pathology

Location. Intracranial hemangiomas can be located in different cranial compartments but are almost always extraaxial. They are found in the calvaria, dural venous sinuses, and dura.

Size and Number. Hemangiomas vary in size from microscopic to massive. Transspatial extension across different anatomic compartments (e.g., scalp and skull, soft tissues and orbit and cavernous sinus) is common. Multicentric lesions are uncommon in the CNS.

Gross Pathology. Hemangiomas are nonencapsulated, vascular-appearing, reddish-brown lesions. When they involve the calvaria, radiating spicules of lamellar bone are interspersed with vascular channels of varying

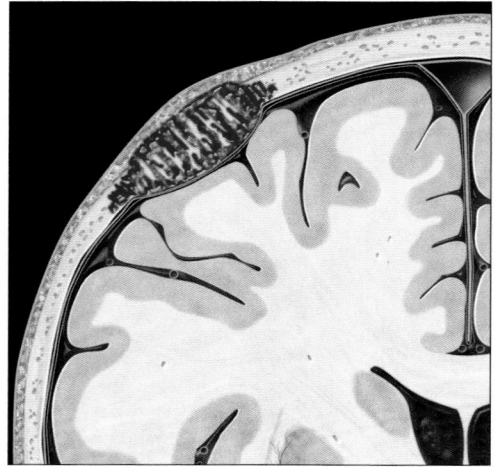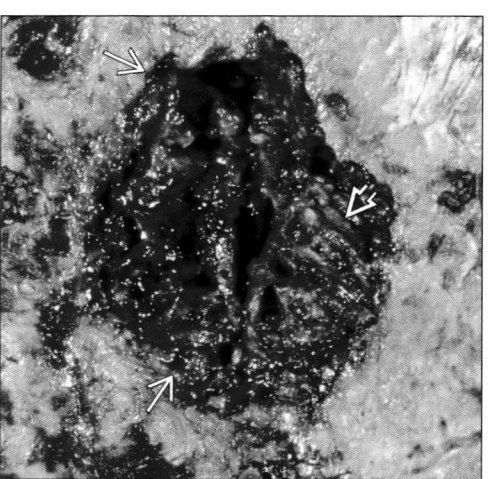

22-24. Coronal graphic depicts typical hemangioma of the calvaria as spicules of lamellar bone interspersed with vascular channels.
22-25. Photograph of resected calvarial hemangioma shows an unencapsulated, very vascular-appearing mass ➡ with radiating spicules of bone ➡.

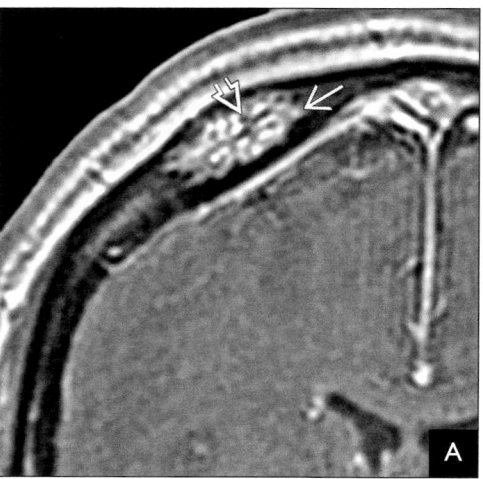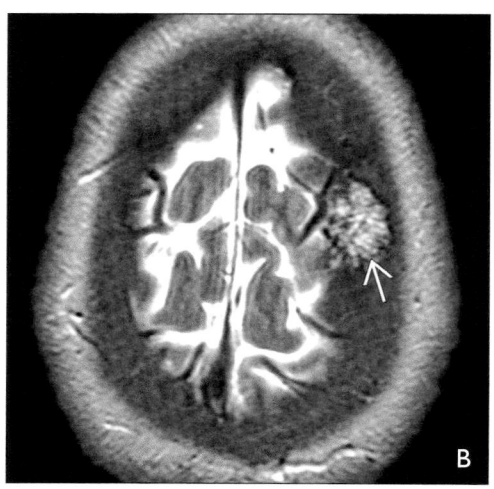

22-26A. Coronal T1 C+ FS scan shows a typical calvarial hemangioma ➡ that slightly expands the diploic space. The vascular channels enhance intensely, while the "dots" of bone spicules within the lesion ➡ do not. 22-26B. Axial T2WI of another calvarial hemangioma shows that the mass ➡ is mostly very hyperintense. The hypointense "dots" of radiating bone spicules give the lesion a striped appearance.

sizes **(22-25)**. Hemangiomas of the venous sinuses and dura do not contain bone but otherwise resemble calvarial hemangiomas, consisting of large vascular channels in a soft, compressible mass.

MICROSCOPIC FEATURES. Hemangiomas are classified on the basis of their dominant vessels and can be capillary, cavernous, or mixed lesions. Most intracranial hemangiomas are cavernous and contain large, endothelium-lined spaces separated by fibrous septa. True intracranial capillary hemangiomas are very rare and consist of smaller vessels without fibrous septa.

STAGING, GRADING, AND CLASSIFICATION. Hemangiomas are WHO grade I neoplasms.

linical Issues

DEMOGRAPHICS. Hemangiomas represent only about 1% of all bone tumors. Most are found in the spine; the diploic space of the calvaria is the most common intracranial site. Dural and venous sinus hemangiomas are rare.

Hemangiomas can occur at any age although the peak presentation is between the fourth and fifth decades. The M:F ratio is 1:2-4.

PRESENTATION. Most calvarial hemangiomas are asymptomatic, limited to the diploic space, and do not extend beyond the inner and outer tables **(22-26)**. Large lesions may present as painless firm masses. Scalp hemangiomas presenting with Kasabach-Merritt syndrome (consumptive coagulopathy due to sequestration and destruction of clotting factors within the lesion) have been reported.

Cavernous sinus hemangiomas can be asymptomatic but often present with headache, diplopia, or other cranial neuropathies such as anisocoria.

Intracranial hemangiomas occasionally occur as part of **POEMS** syndrome, a rare multisystem disease with typical features of **p**olyneuropathy, **o**rganomegaly, **e**ndocrinopathy, **m**onoclonal plasmaproliferative disorders, and **s**kin changes.

NATURAL HISTORY. Hemangiomas typically grow very slowly and do not undergo malignant degeneration. Pregnancy or hormone administration may trigger enlargement.

Capillary hemangiomas of infancy (usually in the skin, scalp, orbit, or oral mucosa) appear within a few months of birth, grow rapidly, plateau, and then involute **(22-27)**.

TREATMENT OPTIONS. Calvarial hemangiomas are typically left alone unless tumor growth is demonstrated. The treatment of venous sinus hemangiomas is much more problematic. These highly vascular lesions bleed easily, and surgical mortality is high. Radiation (gamma

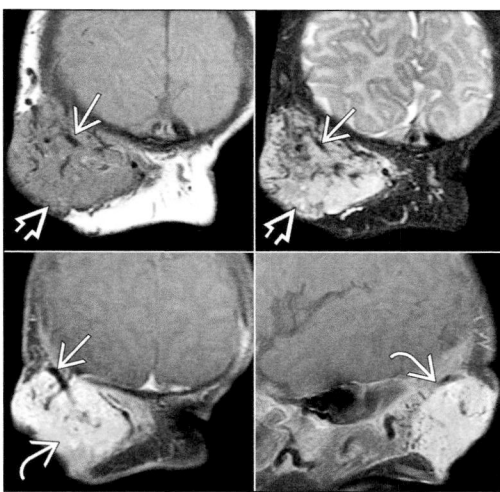

22-27. Large infantile soft tissue hemangioma ➡ is T1 iso-, T2 hyperintense and enhances intensely ➡. Note numerous "flow voids" ➡.

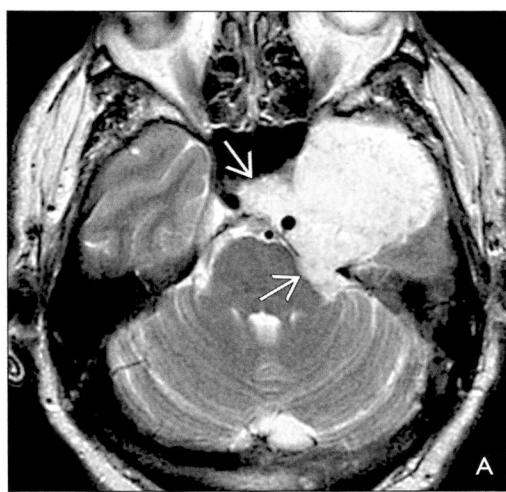

22-28A. Axial T2WI shows an exceptionally hyperintense mass ➡ in the left cavernous sinus extending into the sella, posterior fossa.

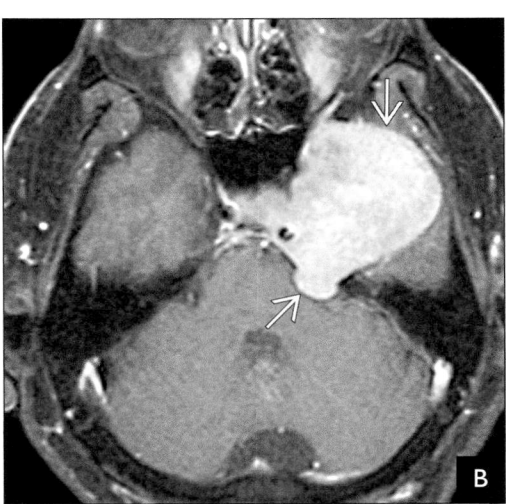

22-28B. T1 C+ FS shows that the mass enhances intensely and homogeneously ➡. Hemangioma was found at surgery. (Courtesy P. Chapman, MD.)

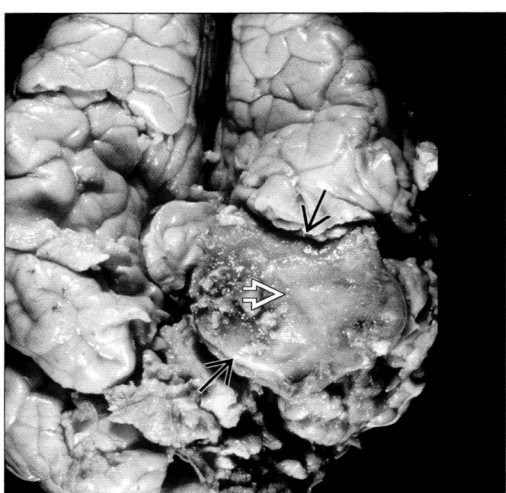

22-29. *Large skull base mass* ➪ *invading brain. Note cartilaginous-appearing components* ➥. *Chondrosarcoma. (AFIP Archives.)*

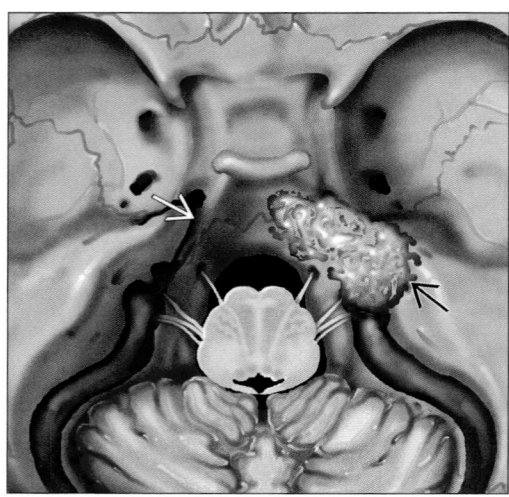

22-30. *Graphic depicts skull base chondrosarcoma* ➪ *centered in the left petrooccipital fissure (compare to the normal right side* ➥*).*

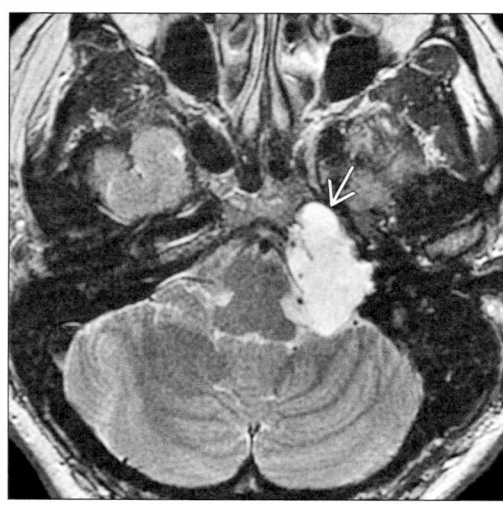

22-31. *T2WI shows typical skull base chondrosarcoma as hyperintense mass* ➥ *centered in the petrooccipital fissure, eroding petrous apex.*

knife surgery) has been used with some success in a few reported cases and may become the primary treatment choice for hemangiomas in critical locations such as the cavernous sinus.

Imaging

CT FINDINGS. A calvarial hemangiomas is seen as a sharply marginated, expansile diploic mass on NECT. Some lesions isolated to the scalp may have no underlying bony involvement.

Bone CT shows that the inner and outer tables are thinned but usually intact. A thin sclerotic margin may surround the lesion. "Spoke-wheel" or reticulated hyperdensities caused by fewer but thicker trabeculae are present within the hemangioma, giving it a "honeycomb" or "jail bars" appearance.

On CECT, foci of intense enhancement interspersed with focal hypodensities caused by the residual thickened trabeculae is typical.

MR FINDINGS. Mixed hypo- to isointensity is the dominant pattern on T1WI. Scattered hyperintensities usually are caused by fat—not hemorrhage—within the lesion. Most hemangiomas are markedly hyperintense on T2WI **(22-28A)**.

Contrast-enhanced scans show diffuse intense enhancement **(22-28B)**. Dynamic scans show slow centripetal "filling in" of the lesion.

ANGIOGRAPHY. Dural and venous sinus hemangiomas can closely resemble meningiomas, with slow, persistent contrast accumulation in the capillary and venous phases of the angiogram.

Differential Diagnosis

The differential diagnosis of calvarial hemangioma includes "holes in the skull" caused by venous lakes and arachnoid granulations, burr holes, dermoids, eosinophilic granuloma, and metastasis. The major differential diagnosis for dural/venous sinus hemangiomas is **meningioma**. Meningiomas do not display the marked hyperintensity on T2WI seen in most hemangiomas.

Malignant Mesenchymal Tumors

Malignant mesenchymal nonmeningothelial tumors are the malignant version of the soft tissue and bone tumors described above. Most are WHO grade IV neoplasms.

Terminology

Malignant mesenchymal tumors (MMTs) include mostly **sarcomas** (of many histologic types) and other neoplasms such as **malignant fibrous histiocytoma** (MFH).

iology

Most investigators posit pluripotential meningeal mesenchymal cells as the origin of MMTs. These cells are capable of giving rise to the spectrum of histologic types seen in nonmeningothelial neoplasms.

Prior radiation therapy is a known cause of MMTs, most commonly fibrosarcomas. The Epstein-Barr virus may play a role in developing smooth muscle tumors, which occasionally occur in immunocompromised patients.

thology

LOCATION. Most intracranial MMTs arise in the dura or skull base (22-29). Some arise in the scalp or calvaria. Chondrosarcomas classically arise from the petrooccipital fissure (22-30).

GROSS PATHOLOGY. Most intracranial sarcomas invade the brain. Necrosis and gross hemorrhage are common.

MICROSCOPIC FEATURES. Most MMTs are composed of small, undifferentiated mesenchymal cells that may be difficult to distinguish from one another by light microscopy. Electron microscopy and immunohistochemistry may be helpful.

linical Issues

EPIDEMIOLOGY. MMTs are rare tumors. In the aggregate, they represent 0.5-2% of intracranial neoplasms.

DEMOGRAPHICS. MMTs can occur at any age. Some (such as rhabdomyosarcoma and Ewing sarcoma) are much more common in children than adults. Chondrosarcomas are tumors of young adults with a mean age of 37 years at presentation. Fibrosarcomas are more common in middle-aged adults.

There is no gender predilection for most MMTs. Ewing sarcoma is more common in males.

PRESENTATION. Clinical symptoms vary with tumor location.

NATURAL HISTORY. Prognosis depends on tumor type and grade. Most MMTs grow rapidly, and prognosis is generally poor. Many recur locally, sometimes years after initial treatment, and metastases outside the CNS are not uncommon.

The exception to this general rule is skull base chondrosarcomas. Most are well- to moderately differentiated low-grade lesions and are slow-growing, locally invasive tumors that rarely metastasize (22-31). High-grade chondrosarcomas are more aggressive tumors that frequently metastasize and have a much poorer prognosis.

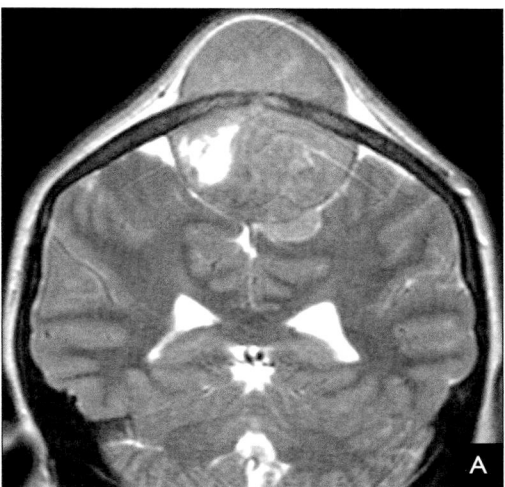

22-32A. Coronal T2WI in a child with a head "lump" shows an invasive transdural, transcalvarial, mixed signal intensity mass.

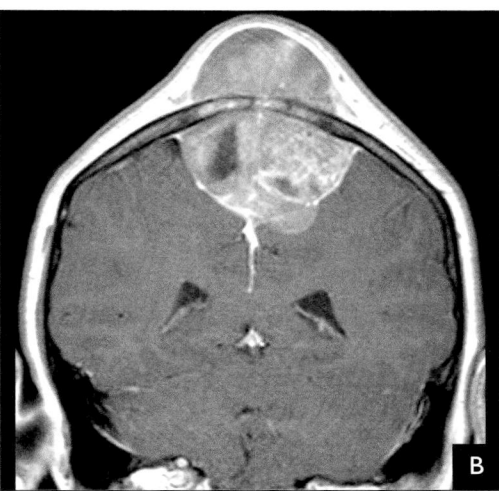

22-32B. The mass enhances strongly but very heterogeneously on T1 C+.

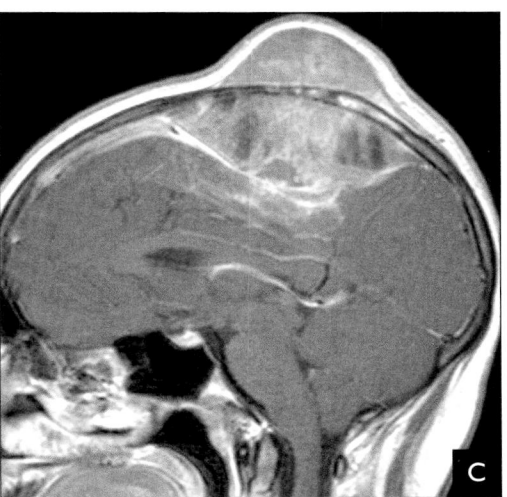

22-32C. Sagittal T1 C+ scan shows the heterogeneous, aggressive appearance of the mass. Ewing sarcoma.

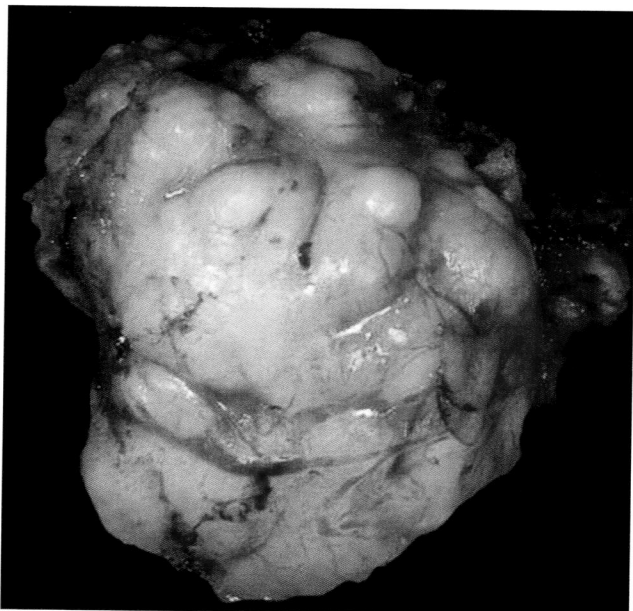

22-33. *Solitary fibrous tumors are firm, well-circumscribed masses that can appear identical to meningioma. (Courtesy E. Rushing, MD.)*

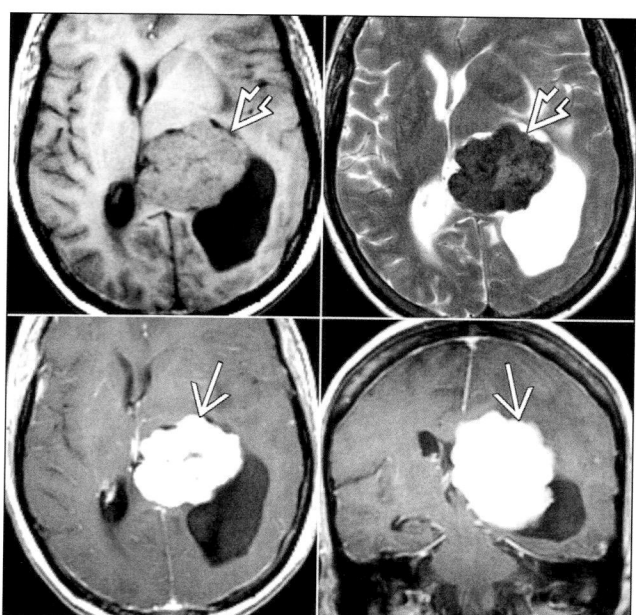

22-34. *A T1 iso-, T2 hypointense mass ▧ that enhances strongly, uniformly ▧ is seen in the atrium of the left lateral ventricle. Preoperative diagnosis was intraventricular meningioma. Postoperative diagnosis was solitary fibrous tumor.*

Imaging

GENERAL FEATURES. Imaging findings of MMTs are those of highly aggressive dural, skull base, calvarial, or scalp lesions that invade adjacent structures (22-32). Although intracranial sarcomas may appear grossly circumscribed, local parenchymal invasion is present at surgery.

CT FINDINGS. NECT scans show a mixed-density soft tissue mass that causes lysis of adjacent bone. Chondrosarcoma may have stippled calcifications or classic "rings and arcs." Sometimes "sunburst" calcifications can be seen in osteosarcomas. Periosteal reaction is generally absent, with the exception of Ewing sarcoma.

Most MMTs enhance strongly but quite heterogeneously.

MR FINDINGS. Other than suggesting a highly aggressive mass, there are no MR findings specific for MMTs. Fibrous, chondroid, and osteoid tissue are often very hypointense on both T1- and T2WI. FLAIR is very helpful in demonstrating brain invasion.

Most MMTs enhance strongly but heterogeneously. Foci of necrosis are common.

ANGIOGRAPHY. Some MMTs such as angiosarcomas are highly vascular. Others show little or no neovascularity and are seen primarily as a nonspecific avascular mass.

Differential Diagnosis

There are no characteristic radiologic findings that distinguish most MMTs from other aggressive neoplasms such as **malignant meningioma** or **metastases**. Sarcoma subtypes are difficult to identify on the basis of imaging findings alone. For example, a histologically definite liposarcoma may demonstrate virtually no imaging features that would suggest the presence of fat.

Solitary Fibrous Tumor and Hemangiopericytoma

Terminology

Solitary fibrous tumor (SFT) represents a continuum of mesenchymal tumors with increasing cellularity. The most malignant end of the SFT spectrum encompasses tumors previously termed **hemangiopericytoma** (HPC). Hemangiopericytoma is now called "solitary fibrous tumor, hemangiopericytoma type" or "cellular SFT."

Although relatively rare, HPC is the most common primary malignant mesenchymal nonmeningothelial neoplasm. These tumors are very cellular, highly vascular neoplasms known for their aggressive clinical behavior, high recurrence rates, and distant metastases even after gross total surgical resection.

Etiology

GENERAL CONCEPTS. Once thought to derive from blood vessel pericytes—contractile cells that abut capillaries—HPC is now considered a fibroblastic sarcoma.

athology

LOCATION. Most SFTs are dura-based, usually arising from the falx or tentorium. Intraparenchymal SFTs occur in the cerebrum and spinal cord, often without a discernible dural attachment. The cerebral ventricles are another common site.

The most common site for HPCs is the occipital region, where they often straddle the transverse sinus.

SIZE AND NUMBER. SFTs are almost always solitary lesions. They are relatively large tumors, reaching up to 10 cm in diameter. Lesions more than 4-5 cm are not uncommon.

GROSS PATHOLOGY. SFTs are solid, lobulated, relatively well-demarcated neoplasms **(22-33)**. HPCs contain abundant vascular spaces **(22-36)**. Intratumoral hemorrhage is common.

MICROSCOPIC FEATURES. SFTs demonstrate variable cellularity with a patternless fascicular architecture. Variable amounts of wire-like collagen and reticulin are present. Tumor vessels can be prominent. Mitoses are

rare, with Ki-67 mostly in the 1-4% range. Anaplasia is uncommon. Most SFTs are low-grade lesions.

Histologic features of HPC overlap those of SFT with no distinct cutoff between the two ends of the SFT spectrum. In general, HPCs are highly cellular tumors that contain dense masses of swirling cells, dilated slit-like "staghorn" blood vessels, and an abundant network of reticulin fibers. Necrosis is common. Nuclear atypia and mitotic activity vary, but > 5 mitoses per 10 high-power fields is common. Ki-67 is usually 10% or more. Both typical (WHO grade II) and anaplastic (WHO grade III) HPCs occur.

Clinical Issues

EPIDEMIOLOGY. HPCs are rare tumors, accounting for less than 1% of all primary intracranial neoplasms and 2-4% of all meningeal tumors.

DEMOGRAPHICS. Meningeal HPCs generally occur at a slightly younger age than meningiomas. Mean age at diagnosis is 43 years. There is a slight male predominance.

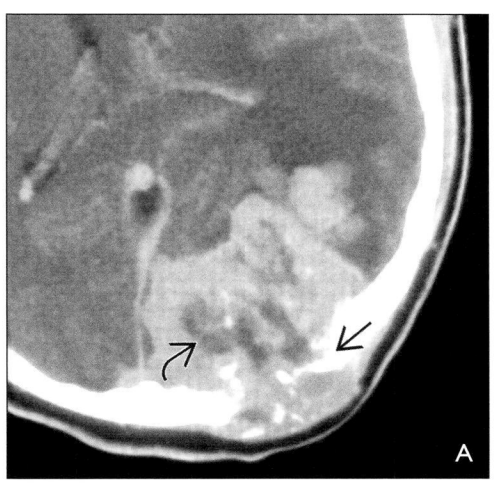

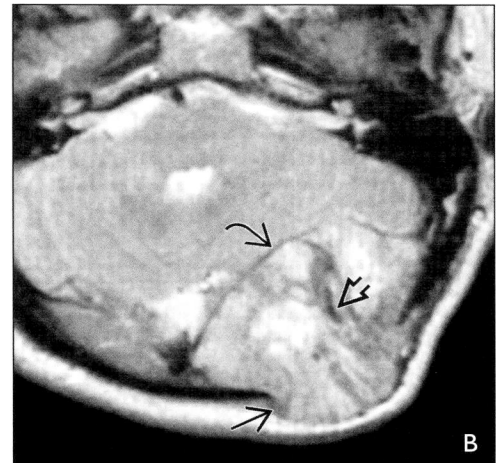

22-35A. CECT scan shows an aggressive enhancing transcalvarial mass that destroys bone ⇨, invades both brain and scalp. Nonenhancing areas ⇲ probably represent necrosis. 22-35B. T2WI shows that the mass displaces the dura inward ⇲, erodes through the skull into the subgaleal soft tissue ⇨. The lesion is heterogeneously hyperintense with hypointense foci ⇲, which may represent necrosis.

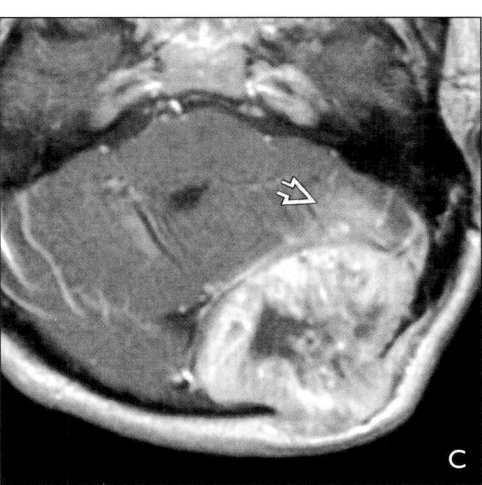

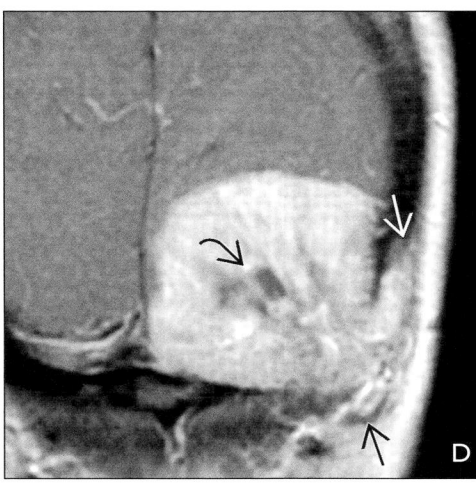

22-35C. T1 C+ scan shows that the mass enhances intensely but heterogeneously. Adjacent enhancement deep to the dura ⇨ suggests parenchymal invasion. 22-35D. Close-up view of coronal T1 C+ scan shows central hypointensity ⇲, "mushrooming" of tumor through the skull ⇨ into the subgaleal space ⇲. Hemangiopericytoma (cellular SFT).

NATURAL HISTORY. Even with complete resection, local recurrence is the rule. The majority of meningeal HPCs eventually metastasize extracranially to bone, lung, and liver. There is no significant difference in survival between grade II and grade III HPCs.

TREATMENT OPTIONS. Surgical resection with radiation therapy or radiosurgery is the treatment of choice.

Imaging

CT FINDINGS. HPCs are hyperdense extraaxial masses that invade and destroy bone. Extracalvarial extension under the scalp is common. Calcification and reactive hyperostosis are absent.

Strong but heterogeneous enhancement is typical.

MR FINDINGS. Low-grade intracranial SFTs are circumscribed masses that are usually dura-based and resemble meningioma. Lesions are isointense with GM on T1WI and show variable signal intensity on T2WI. A mixed hyper- and hypointense pattern is common. Collagen-rich areas can be very hypointense. Avid enhancement following contrast administration is typical **(22-34)**.

Most HPCs demonstrate mixed signal intensity on all sequences. They tend to be predominantly isointense to gray matter on T1 scans and iso- to hyperintense on T2 scans **(22-35)**. Prominent "flow voids" are almost always present.

Contrast enhancement is marked but heterogeneous. Nonenhancing necrotic foci are common.

ANGIOGRAPHY. HPCs may invade and occlude dural sinuses, so CTV or MRV are helpful noninvasive techniques for delineating patency.

DSA shows HPCs as hypervascular masses with prominent vascularity, "early draining" veins, and intense prolonged tumor "staining" **(22-35E), (22-35F)**. HPCs usually recruit blood supply from both dural and pial vessels.

Differential Diagnosis

The major differential diagnosis of low-grade SFT is typical (WHO grade I) meningioma. The major differential of HPC is a highly vascular aggressive meningioma, particularly an **atypical** or **malignant meningioma**. HPCs rarely calcify or cause hyperostosis.

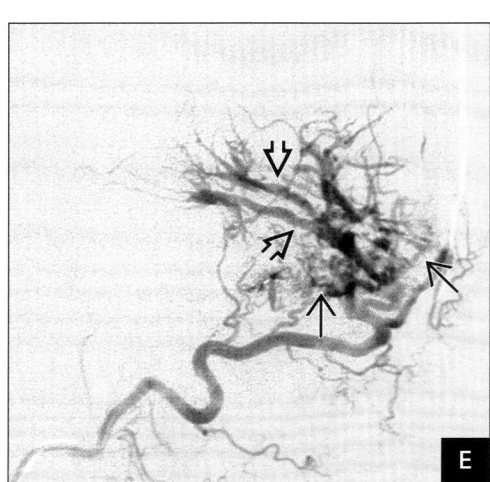
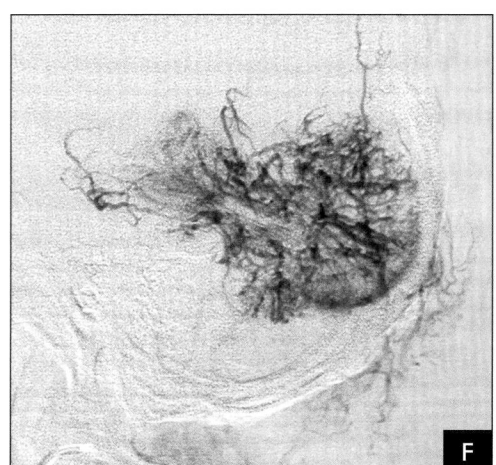

22-35E. Selective occipital artery angiogram in the same patient shown on the previous page demonstrates multiple enlarged transosseous branches ▷ supplying the tumor →. 22-35F. Later phase of the DSA shows intense, prolonged vascular "blush" in the tumor. Unlike benign SFTs, HPCs are very vascular neoplasms.

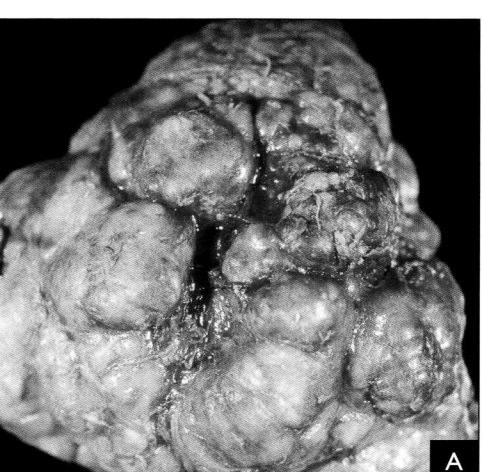
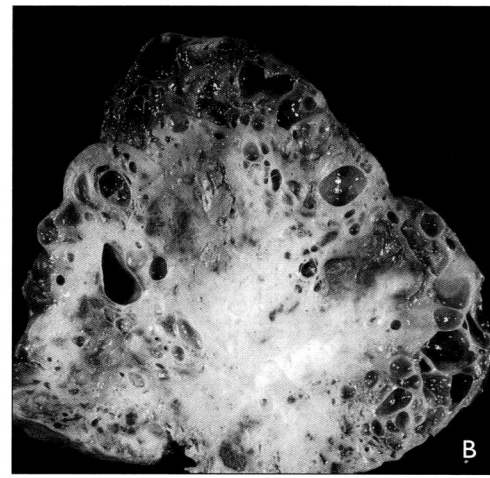

22-36A. Resected specimen shows "bosselated" nature of HPC. Note similarity to solitary fibrous tumor illustrated in Figure 22-33. 22-36B. Cut section through the specimen shows multiple cysts, enlarged vascular channels. (Courtesy R. Hewlett, MD.)

Dural metastases with skull invasion can be indistinguishable from HPC. Rare neoplasms that can resemble HPC include **gliosarcoma** and **malignant fibrous tumors**.

rimary Melanocytic Lesions

Primary melanocytic neoplasms of the CNS are rare neural crest neoplasms that are derived from leptomeningeal melanocytes. They can present as focal nodular masses or diffuse leptomeningeal infiltrates.

Focal masses span a morphologic spectrum from low-grade melanocytoma to malignant melanoma. Diffuse leptomeningeal melanotic infiltrates occur in meningeal melanocytosis/melanomatosis (neurocutaneous melanosis) **(22-37)**.

Most melanocytic CNS lesions are metastases from extracranial malignant melanomas. Primary melanocytic tumors of the CNS are very rare with an estimated incidence of 0.9 per 10 million. Primary melanocytic neoplasms vary from benign melanocytoma to melanocytic tumor of intermediate differentiation to malignant melanoma.

Melanocytoma

Melanocytomas account for less than 0.1% of all CNS neoplasms. Melanocytomas are solitary, darkly pigmented, low-grade tumors that do not invade adjacent brain. Preferred sites are the posterior fossa (skull base, cerebellopontine angle), Meckel cave (with nevus of Ota), and spinal cord/nerve roots.

Melanocytomas rarely undergo malignant transformation. Prognosis is variable for melanocytic tumors of intermediate differentiation and poor for melanoma.

Melanotic lesions are hyperdense on NECT and enhance strongly on CECT. The paramagnetic properties of melanin cause T1 shortening, so hyperintensity on T1WI and hypointensity on T2WI is characteristic.

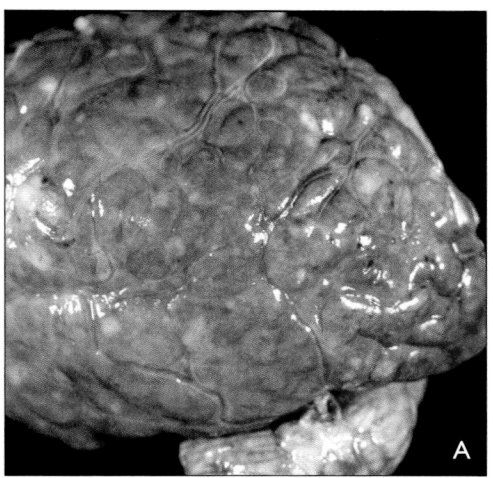
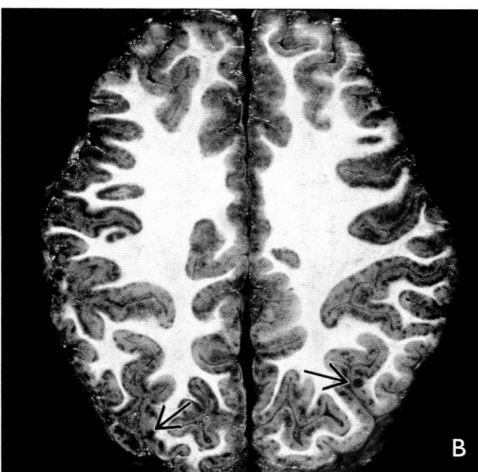

22-37A. Autopsy specimen shows diffuse leptomeningeal melanosis with gray-black discoloration of the entire brain surface. 22-37B. Axial section from the same specimen shows that the gyri are enlarged, studded with innumerable tiny black nodules ⇨ representing tumor extension via perivascular spaces. Diffuse primary leptomeningeal malignant melanocytosis. (Courtesy R. Hewlett, MD.)

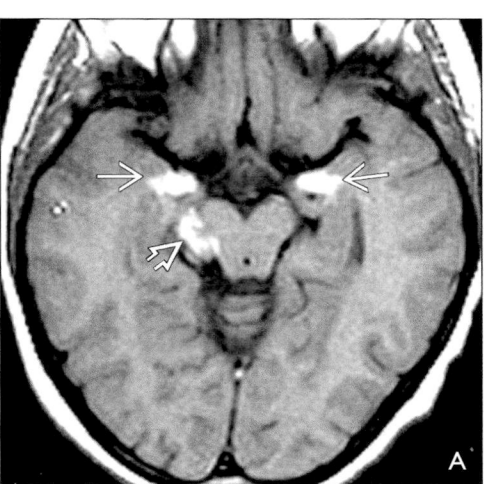
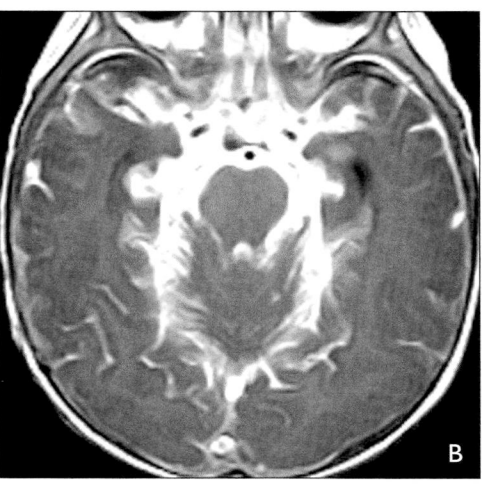

22-38A. T1WI in a patient with neurocutaneous melanosis shows characteristic ovoid hyperintensities in the amygdala of both temporal lobes ⇨. Another focus of melanotic deposition with T1 shortening ⇨ is seen along the midbrain. 22-38B. T1 C+ scan in the same patient shows diffuse, thick leptomeningeal enhancement. (Courtesy S. Blaser, MD.)

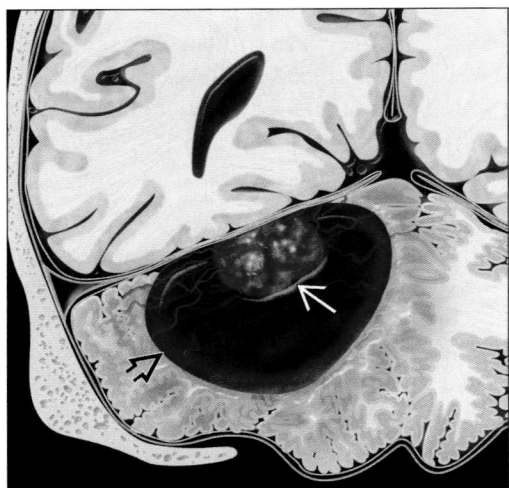

22-39. *Graphic depicts typical HGBL with cyst wall ⊵ composed of compressed cerebellum. Vascular tumor nodule ➡ abuts pial surface.*

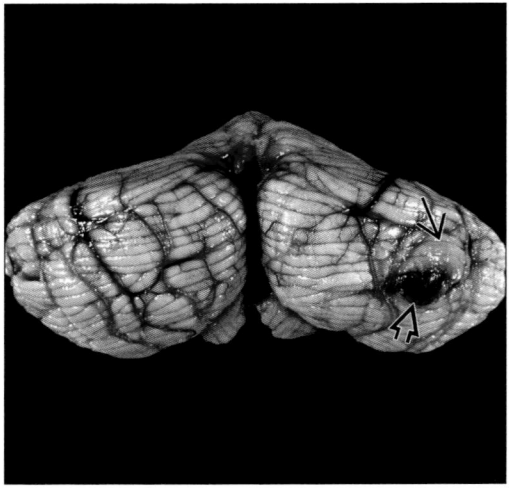

22-40. *Autopsy specimen shows nodule ➡, hemorrhagic cyst ⊵ of a typical HGBL. (Courtesy E. Ross, MD.)*

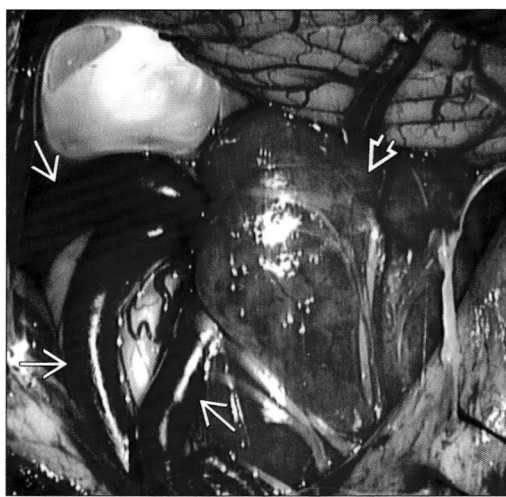

22-41. *Intraoperative photograph shows the enlarged vessels ➡ that supply a beefy-red solid HGBL ➡.*

The major differential diagnosis for primary melanocytic lesions of the brain is **metastatic malignant melanoma**.

Diffuse Meningeal Melanocytosis/ Melanomatosis

Diffuse leptomeningeal melanocytosis and melanomatosis are usually features of neurocutaneous melanosis (NCM), a rare neurocutaneous syndrome of childhood. Most patients present with numerous congenital melanotic nevi of the skin.

Diffuse melanocytic lesions appear as dense, thick, black confluent aggregates that fill the subarachnoid spaces and coat the pia.

Bilateral T1 hyperintense foci in the amygdala is an early sign of NCM **(22-38A)**. Diffuse leptomeningeal enhancement and extension into the brain parenchyma via the perivascular spaces can occur and usually indicates malignant transformation with poor prognosis **(22-38B)**.

Other Related Neoplasms

Hemangioblastoma

Terminology

Hemangioblastoma (HGBL) is also known as capillary hemangioma. Although the term "blastoma" suggests malignant, highly aggressive lesions, HGBLs are benign, slow-growing, relatively indolent vascular neoplasms. HGBL occurs in both sporadic and multiple forms.

Multiple HGBLs are almost always associated with the autosomal-dominant inherited cancer syndrome **von Hippel-Lindau disease** (VHL). A rare non-VHL form of multiple disseminated HGBLs is termed **leptomeningeal hemangioblastomatosis**.

Etiology

The precise etiology of HGBLs remains unknown. *VHL gene mutations (losses or inactivations) are present in 20-50% of sporadic HGBLs.*

Pathology

LOCATION. HGBLs can occur in any part of the CNS, although the vast majority (90-95%) of intracranial HGBLs are located in the posterior fossa. The cerebellum is by far the most common site (80%) followed by the vermis (15%). Approximately 5% occur in the brainstem, usually the medulla. The nodule of an HGBL is superficially located and typically abuts a pial surface **(22-39)**.

Supratentorial tumors are rare, accounting for 5-10% of all HGBLs. Most are clustered around the optic pathways and occur in the setting of VHL.

SIZE AND NUMBER. Hemangiomas vary in size from tiny to large, especially when associated with a cyst. Unless they are syndromic, HGBLs are solitary lesions.

GROSS PATHOLOGY. The common appearance is that of a beefy-red, vascular-appearing nodule that abuts a pial surface **(22-40)**. A variably sized cyst is present in 50-60% of cases. Cyst fluid is typically yellowish, and the cyst wall is usually smooth. Approximately 40% of HGBLs are solid tumors **(22-41)**.

MICROSCOPIC FEATURES. HGBLs contain two different cell types: Stromal and vascular cells. Generally it is the stromal (not the vascular) cells that are the neoplastic element of an HGBL.

The cyst wall of most HGBLs is nonneoplastic, composed of compressed brain with fibrillary neuroglia devoid of tumor cells. The intratumoral cyst fluid shares a proteomic fingerprint with normal serum and has no proteins in common with HGBL tumor tissue. Cyst formation in HGBLs is therefore a result of vascular leakage from tumor vessels, not tumor liquefaction or active secretion.

Mitoses in HGBLs are few or absent, so proliferation rates (usually MIB-1 < 1). HGBL is a WHO grade I neoplasm. There is no recognized atypical or anaplastic variant.

HEMANGIOBLASTOMA: PATHOLOGY AND CLINICAL ISSUES

Pathology
- Location
  - Posterior fossa (90-95%)
  - Cerebellum most common site
- Gross pathology
  - "Cyst + nodule" (60%), solid (40%)

Clinical Issues
- Epidemiology
  - Uncommon (1-2.5% of primary brain tumors)
  - 7% of all adult primary posterior fossa tumors
- Demographics
  - Peak age = 30-65 years (younger with VHL)
  - Rare under 15 years
- Natural history
  - Slow, "stuttering" growth
  - Metastasis rare

---

linical Issues

EPIDEMIOLOGY. HGBL accounts for 1-2.5% of primary CNS neoplasms and approximately 7% of all primary posterior fossa tumors in adults. It is the second most common infratentorial parenchymal mass in adults (after metastasis).

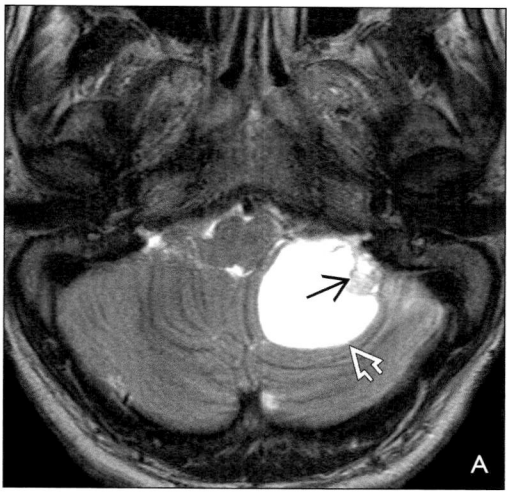

22-42A. *T2WI shows classic HGBL with a hyperintense cyst* ⬗*, tumor nodule* ⮕ *abutting pial surface.*

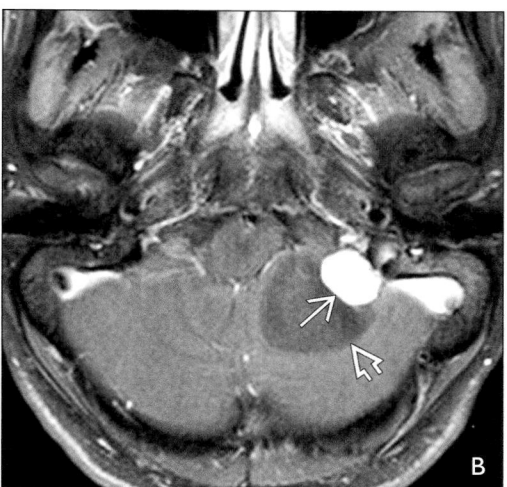

22-42B. *T1 C+ FS MR in the same patient shows that the tumor nodule* ⮕ *enhances intensely while the cyst wall* ⬗ *does not.*

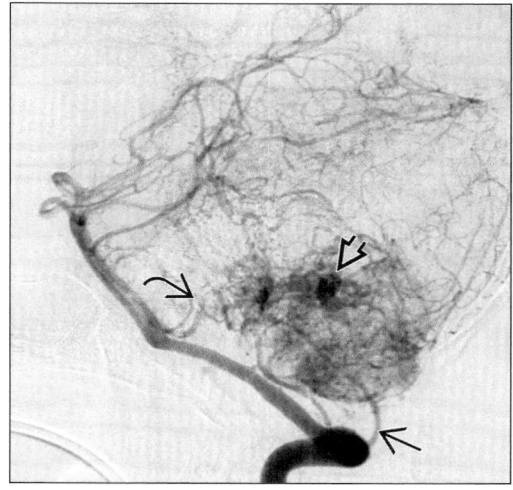

22-43. *DSA of typical HGBL shows the characteristic prolonged tumor "blush"* ⬗ *coming from branches of enlarged PICA* ⮕*, AICA* ⮕*.*

Between 25-40% of HGBLs are associated with VHL.

DEMOGRAPHICS. HGBL is generally a tumor of adults between the ages of 30 and 65 years. Pediatric HGBLs are rare. VHL-associated HGBLs tend to present at a significantly younger age but are still relatively rare in children under the age of 15. There is a slight male predominance.

PRESENTATION. Most symptoms in patients with the cystic form of HGBL are caused by the cyst, not the neoplastic nodule. Headache is the presenting symptom in 85% of cases.

NATURAL HISTORY AND TREATMENT OPTIONS. Because HGBLs exhibit a "stuttering" growth pattern, they frequently are stable lesions that can remain asymptomatic for long intervals. Imaging progression alone is not an indication for treatment although tumor/cyst growth rates can be used to predict symptom formation and future need for treatment.

While HGBLs show no intrinsic tendency to metastasize, there are sporadic reports of intraspinal dissemination. Complete en bloc resection is the procedure of choice.

Total resection eliminates tumor recurrence although new hemangioblastomas may develop in the setting of VHL.

Imaging

GENERAL FEATURES. HGBLs have four basic imaging patterns: (1) solid HGBLs without associated cysts, (2) HGBLs with intratumoral cysts, (3) HGBLs with peritumoral cysts (nonneoplastic cyst with solid tumor nodule), and (4) HGBLs associated with both peri- and intratumoral cysts (nonneoplastic cyst with cysts in the tumor nodule). A nonneoplastic peritumoral cyst with solid nodule is the most common pattern, seen in 50-65% of cases. The second most common pattern is the solid form, seen in about 40% of cases.

CT FINDINGS. The most common appearance is a well-delineated iso- to slightly hyperdense nodule associated with a hypodense cyst. Calcification and gross hemorrhage are absent. The nodule enhances strongly and uniformly following contrast administration.

MR FINDINGS. An isointense nodule with prominent "flow voids" is seen on T1WI. If an associated peri-

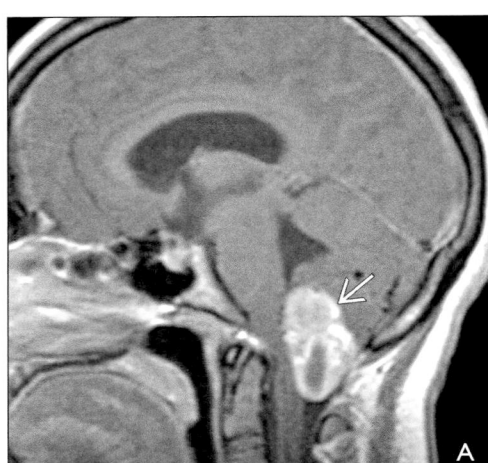
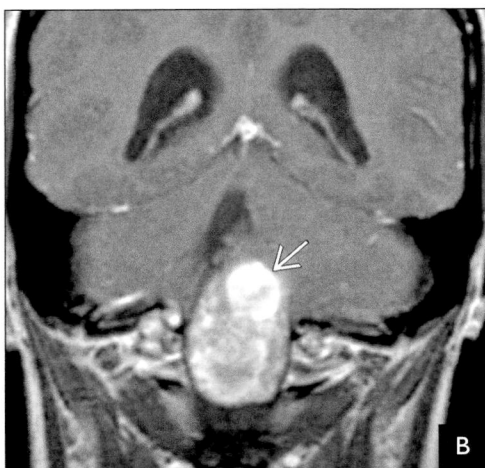

22-44A. Sagittal T1WI C+ shows the typical appearance of solid hemangioblastoma ➜. 22-44B. Coronal T1WI C+ shows the intensely but heterogeneously enhancing HGBL ➜. Compare with the intraoperative photograph shown as Figure 22-42. HGBLs in the medulla tend to be solid whereas those in the cerebellar hemispheres often have the "cyst + nodule" appearance.

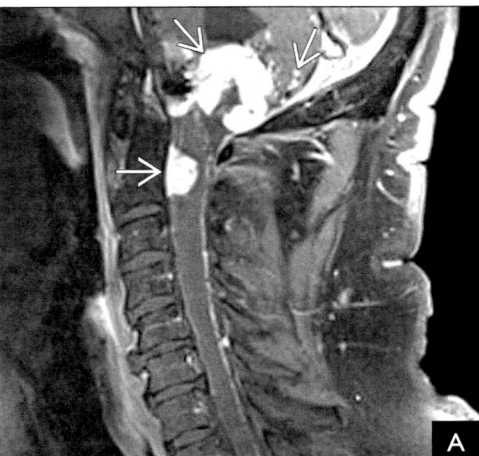
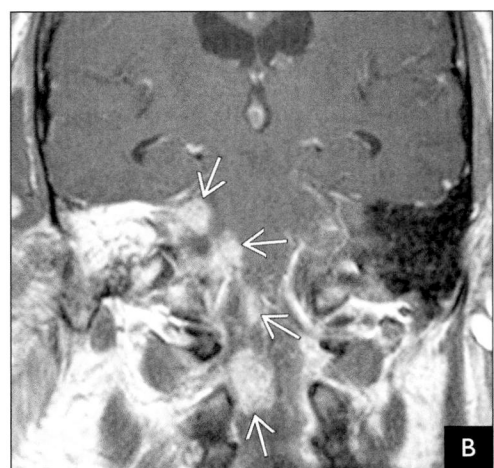

22-45A. Sagittal T1 C+ FS in a patient with VHL shows multiple hemangioblastomas in the cerebellum, spinal cord ➜. 22-45B. Coronal T1 C+ scan in the same patient shows at least 4 separate HGBLs ➜.

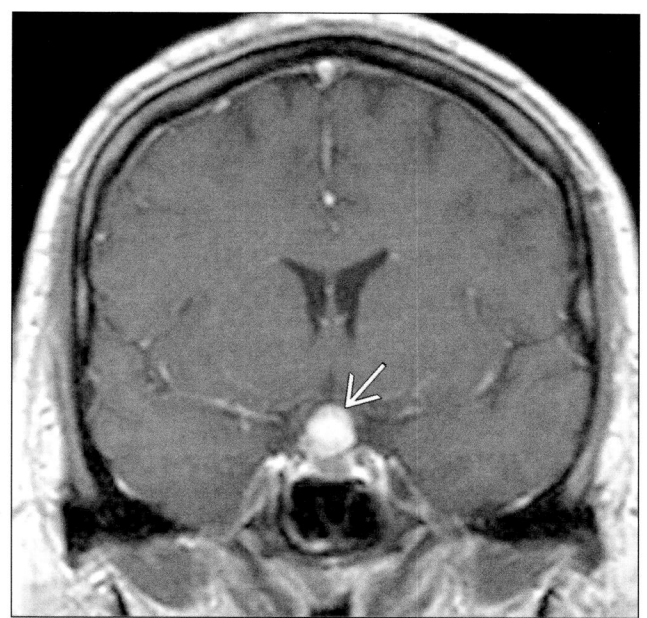

22-46. Coronal T1 C+ scan shows an enhancing suprasellar mass ➔. Biopsy-proven hemangioblastoma. (Courtesy R. Bert, MD.)

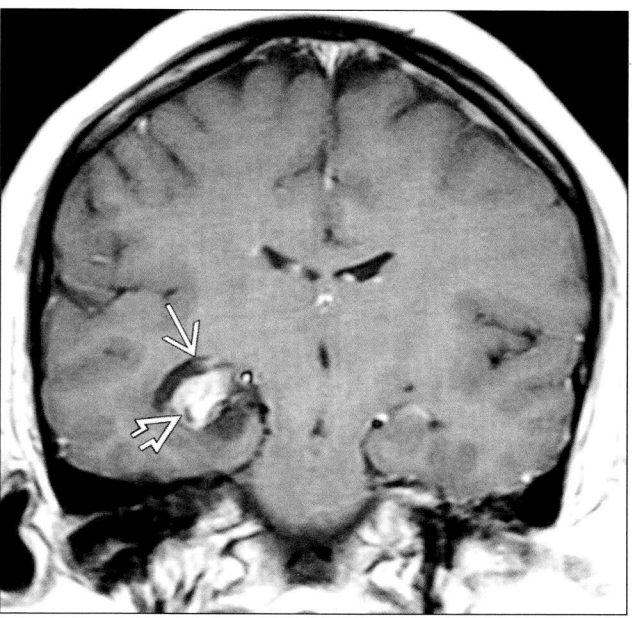

22-47. Coronal T1 C+ scan shows temporal lobe mass with enhancing cyst ➔, nodule ➔. Proven hemangioblastoma. (Courtesy C. Sutton, MD.)

tumoral cyst is present, it is typically hypointense to parenchyma on T1WI but hyperintense compared to CSF.

Compared to brain parenchyma, the tumor nodule of an HGBL is moderately hyperintense on T2WI and FLAIR. Intratumoral cysts and prominent "flow voids" are common. The cyst fluid is very hyperintense on both T2WI and FLAIR (22-42A).

Occasionally an HGBL hemorrhages. If present, blood products "bloom" on T2*.

Intense enhancement of the nodule—but not the cyst itself—is typical (22-42B). Cyst wall enhancement should raise the possibility of tumor involvement as compressed, nonneoplastic brain does not enhance.

Noncystic HGBLs enhance strongly but often heterogeneously (22-44). Multiple HGBLs are seen in VHL and vary from tiny punctate to large solid tumors (22-45).

Supratentorial HGBLs are rare. Most occur around the optic nerves or chiasm (22-46). HGBL occasionally occurs as a hemispheric mass with a "cyst + nodule" appearance (22-47).

ANGIOGRAPHY. The most common appearance is that of an intensely vascular tumor nodule that shows a prolonged vascular "blush" (22-43). "Early draining" veins are common. If a tumor-associated cyst is present, vessels appear displaced and "draped" around an avascular mass.

Differential Diagnosis

The differential diagnosis of HGBL varies with age. In a middle-aged or older adult, the statistically most common cause of an enhancing posterior fossa intraaxial (parenchymal) mass is **metastasis**, not HGBL!

A cerebellar mass with "cyst + nodule" in a child or young adult is most likely a **pilocytic astrocytoma**, not HGBL or metastasis. Occasionally a **cavernous malformation** can mimic an HGBL with hemorrhage.

If more than one HGBL is present, the patient by definition has VHL. A positive family history or presence of other VHL markers (such as visceral cysts, retinal angioma, renal cell carcinoma) should prompt genetic screening.

HEMANGIOBLASTOMA: IMAGING

General Features
- "Cyst + nodule" (60%)
  - Nodule abuts pial surface
- Solid (40%)

CT
- Low-density cyst
- Strongly enhancing nodule

MR
- Cyst
  - Fluid slightly hyperintense to CSF
  - Wall usually nonneoplastic
- Nodule
  - Isointense to brain
  - "Flow voids" common
  - Enhances intensely

Selected References

Anatomy of the Cranial Meninges

Dura

- Adeeb N et al: The cranial dura mater: a review of its history, embryology, and anatomy. Childs Nerv Syst. 28(6):827-37, 2012
- Protasoni M et al: The collagenic architecture of human dura mater. J Neurosurg. 114(6):1723-30, 2011

Arachnoid and Arachnoid Granulations

- Tubbs RS et al: Arachnoid granulations of the middle cranial fossa. Surg Radiol Anat. 33(3):289, 2011
- Yew M et al: Arachnoid granulations of the temporal bone: a histologic study of dural and osseous penetration. Otol Neurotol. 32(4):602-9, 2011

Pia Mater

- Tsutsumi S et al: The Virchow-Robin spaces: delineation by magnetic resonance imaging with considerations on anatomofunctional implications. Childs Nerv Syst. 27(12):2057-66, 2011

Meningothelial Tumors

- Perry A et al: Meningiomas. In Louis DN et al: WHO Classification of Tumours of the Central Nervous System. 4th ed. Lyon, France: IARC Press. 164-72, 2007

Meningioma

- Sitthinamsuwan B et al: Predictors of meningioma consistency: A study in 243 consecutive cases. Acta Neurochir (Wien). 154(8):1383-9, 2012
- Crisi G: 1H MR spectroscopy of meningiomas at 3.0T: the role of glutamate-glutamine complex and glutathione. The Neuroradiol Journal 24: 846-853, 2011
- Kotecha RS et al: Pediatric meningioma: current approaches and future direction. J Neurooncol. 104(1):1-10, 2011
- Lee Y et al: Genomic landscape of meningiomas. Brain Pathol. 20(4):751-62, 2010
- Sughrue ME et al: The relevance of Simpson Grade I and II resection in modern neurosurgical treatment of World Health Organization Grade I meningiomas. J Neurosurg. 113(5):1029-35, 2010
- Sughrue ME et al: Treatment decision making based on the published natural history and growth rate of small meningiomas. J Neurosurg. 113(5):1036-42, 2010
- Wiemels J et al: Epidemiology and etiology of meningioma. J Neurooncol. 99(3):307-14, 2010

Atypical Meningioma

- Jansen M et al: Gain of chromosome arm 1q in atypical meningioma correlates with shorter progression-free survival. Neuropathol Appl Neurobiol. 38(2):213-9, 2012
- Kane AJ et al: Anatomic location is a risk factor for atypical and malignant meningiomas. Cancer. 117(6):1272-8, 2011

Malignant Meningioma

- Di Vinci A et al: HOXA7, 9, and 10 are methylation targets associated with aggressive behavior in meningiomas. Transl Res. Epub ahead of print, 2012
- Herrmann A et al: Proteomic data in meningiomas: post-proteomic analysis can reveal novel pathophysiological pathways. J Neurooncol. 104(2):401-10, 2011
- Sughrue ME et al: Outcome and survival following primary and repeat surgery for World Health Organization Grade III meningiomas. J Neurosurg. 113(2):202-9, 2010
- Vranic A et al: Mitotic count, brain invasion, and location are independent predictors of recurrence-free survival in primary atypical and malignant meningiomas: a study of 86 patients. Neurosurgery. 67(4):1124-32, 2010
- Perry A et al: Meningiomas. In Louis DN et al: WHO Classification of Tumours of the Central Nervous System. 4th ed. Lyon, France: IARC Press. 164-72, 2007

Nonmeningothelial Mesenchymal Tumors

Hemangioma

- Jinhu Y et al: Dynamic enhancement features of cavernous sinus cavernous hemangiomas on conventional contrast-enhanced MR imaging. AJNR Am J Neuroradiol. 29(3):577-81, 2008

Malignant Mesenchymal Tumors

- Lin L et al: Diagnostic pitfall in the diagnosis of mesenchymal chondrosarcoma arising in the central nervous system. Neuropathology. 32(1):82-90, 2012

Solitary Fibrous Tumor and Hemangiopericytoma

- Demicco EG et al: Solitary fibrous tumor: a clinicopathological study of 110 cases and proposed risk assessment model. Mod Pathol. 25(9):1298-306, 2012
- Kumar N et al: Intracranial meningeal hemangiopericytoma: 10 years experience of a tertiary care institute. Acta Neurochir (Wien). 154(9):1647-51, 2012
- Zhou JL et al: Thirty-nine cases of intracranial hemangiopericytoma and anaplastic hemangiopericytoma: A retrospective review of MRI features and pathological findings. Eur J Radiol. Epub ahead of print, 2012
- Schiariti M et al: Hemangiopericytoma: long-term outcome revisited. Clinical article. J Neurosurg. 114(3):747-55, 2011
- Rutkowski MJ et al: Predictors of mortality following treatment of intracranial hemangiopericytoma. J Neurosurg. 113(2):333-9, 2010

Primary Melanocytic Lesions

- Smith AB et al: Pigmented lesions of the central nervous system: radiologic-pathologic correlation. Radiographics. 29(5):1503-24, 2009
- Bratt DJ et al: Melanocytic lesions. In Louis DN et al: WHO Classification of Tumours of the Central Nervous System. 4th ed. Lyon, France: IARC Press. 181-3, 2007

Other Related Neoplasms

Hemangioblastoma

- Micallef J et al: Proteomics: present and future implications in neuro-oncology. Neurosurgery. 62(3):539-55; discussion 539-55, 2008
- Ammerman JM et al: Long-term natural history of hemangioblastomas in patients with von Hippel-Lindau disease: implications for treatment. J Neurosurg. 105(2):248-55, 2006

23

Cranial Nerves and Nerve Sheath Tumors

The WHO classification of primary CNS tumors designates a separate category for nerve sheath tumors as "tumors of the cranial and paraspinal nerves." With the exception of vestibular schwannoma, all intracranial nerve sheath tumors are rare. They can occur ether sporadically or as part of two common tumor-associated neurocutaneous syndromes, neurofibromatosis types 1 and 2.

The vast majority of all nerve sheath neoplasms are benign. The two major tumor types that are found intracranially or near the skull base are schwannomas and neurofibromas. Both are discussed in detail here, along with the rare intracranial malignant peripheral nerve sheath tumor (MPNST).

A third type of benign tumor, perineurioma, is primarily a tumor of peripheral nerves and soft tissues, although rare cases involving cranial nerves have been reported. Perineurioma is briefly considered at the end of this chapter.

More than 99% of intracranial nerve sheath tumors are associated with a cranial nerve. Because characteristic imaging findings of these tumors are location-specific rather than generic, we begin this chapter with a review of normal cranial nerve anatomy.

Cranial Nerve Anatomy

In this section we briefly cover cranial nerve (CN) anatomy, beginning our discussion with the upper cranial nerves (CNs I-VI). We then turn to the lower cranial nerves (CNs VII-XII). The function, anatomy, and key clinical/imaging points are delineated for the individual cranial nerves.

The intracranial anatomy of each nerve is discussed segment by segment, from its intraaxial location and exit from the brain, passage through the adjacent CSF cisterns, entrance into or exit from the skull base, and extracranial course. Remember: Cranial nerves do *not* stop at the skull base! When imaging cranial neuropathies, it is critically important to image—and carefully evaluate—each segment, following the affected nerve all the way from its origin to its "functional endplate."

Upper Cranial Nerves

Olfactory Nerve (CN I)

FUNCTION. The olfactory nerve is a special visceral afferent involved with the sense of smell.

ANATOMY. Unmyelinated fibers from bipolar receptor cells high in the nasal vault gather into fascicles, pierce the cribriform plate of the ethmoid bone, and then synapse in the olfactory bulb. The olfactory bulb passes posteriorly to the olfactory trigone. Olfactory stria from the trigone pass into the brain with the largest tract, the lateral olfactory stria, terminating in the temporal lobe **(23-1)**.

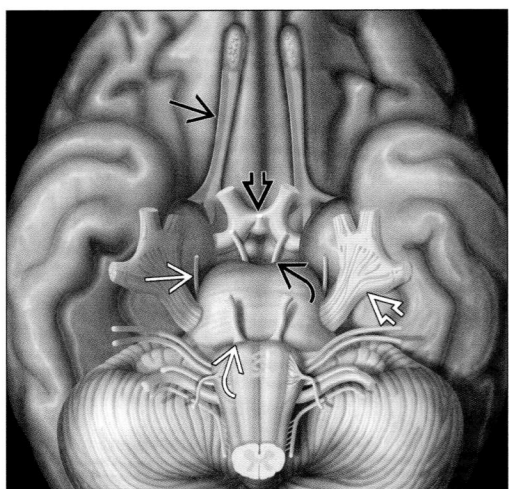

23-1. Olfactory tracts (CN I) ⮕*, optic chiasm* ⮕*, oculomotor (CN III)* ⮕*, trochlear (CN IV)* ⮕*, trigeminal* ⮕*, abducens (CN VI)* ⮕ *nerves.*

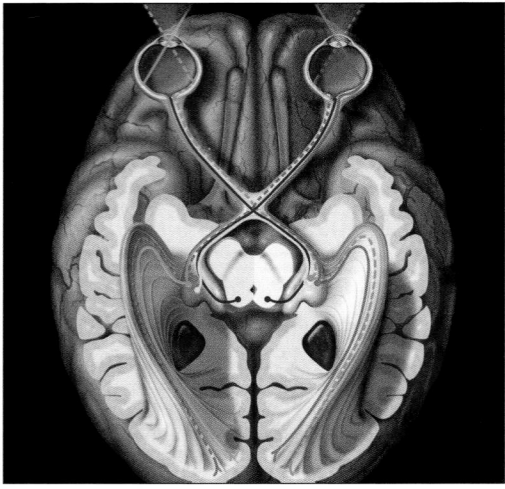

23-2. Graphic depicts the visual system with the fields from the globes to the calcarine cortex.

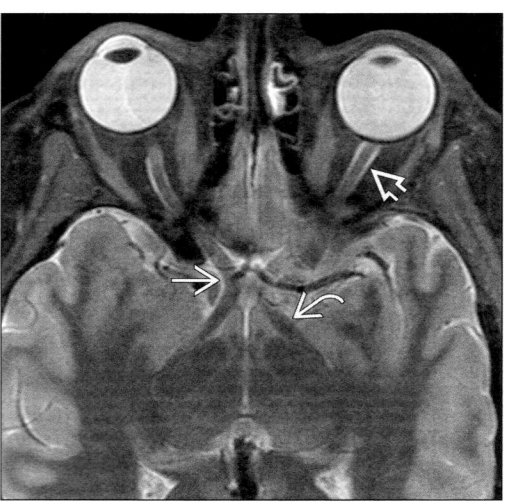

23-3. Axial T2WI shows optic nerves surrounded by CSF in optic nerve sheath ⮕*. Optic chiasm* ⮕*, tracts* ⮕ *are also visible.*

Olfactory nerves lack a layer of Schwann cells. Special cells called "olfactory ensheathing cells" (OECs) lie in the olfactory mucosa and olfactory bulb and surround the axons of the olfactory nerve. OECs resemble Schwann cells on light microscopy, but immunohistochemical staining distinguishes the two. OECs are special populations of astrocytic cells that can migrate and regenerate, enhancing axonal extension after injury.

KEY CONCEPTS. Coronal sinus CT that focuses on the nasal vault and cribriform plate is the best examination for isolated anosmia. MR of the nose, anterior cranial fossae, and medial temporal lobes is the best examination for clinically complicated anosmia.

Optic Nerve (CN II)

The optic nerve is technically a brain tract, not a true cranial nerve; it is ensheathed and myelinated by oligodendrocytes, not Schwann cells. Tumors of the optic nerve are astrocytomas, not schwannomas, and were discussed in Chapter 17.

FUNCTION. The optic nerve is the nerve of vision.

ANATOMY. The visual pathway consists of the globe/retina, optic nerve, optic chiasm, and retrochiasmal structures. The **intraocular segment** of CN II is surrounded by a sleeve of CSF that connects directly with the intracranial subarachnoid space (SAS). It is covered by the same three meningeal layers as the brain (dura, arachnoid, pia). The **intracanalicular segment** of the optic nerve passes through the optic canal (23-4), (23-6). The **intracranial (cisternal) segment** extends from the optic canal to the optic chiasm.

The **optic chiasm** is an X-shaped structure that lies in the upper suprasellar cistern. Nerve fibers from the medial half of both retinas cross here, running posterolaterally to the opposite side (23-2), (23-3).

The **optic tracts** are posterior extensions of the optic chiasm that curve around the cerebral peduncles. Their lateral bands synapse in the lateral geniculate body (LGB). Efferent axons from the LGB form the optic radiations (geniculocalcarine tracts). The **optic radiations** fan out as they pass posteriorly to terminate in the calcarine cortex (primary visual cortex) along the medial occipital lobes.

KEY CONCEPTS. Globe or optic nerve pathology results in **monocular visual loss**. Imaging focus should extend from the globe to the optic chiasm. Intrinsic or extrinsic lesions of the optic chiasm cause **bitemporal heteronymous hemianopsia**, i.e., loss of both temporal visual fields. Retrochiasmal pathology causes **homonymous hemianopsia**, i.e., vision loss that involves either the two right or the two left halves of both visual fields. A left-sided lesion causes *right* homonymous hemianopsia whereas a right-sided lesion causes *left* homonymous hemianopsia.

Papilledema is the ocular manifestation of increased intracranial pressure that is transmitted along the SAS of the optic nerve sheath complex. On imaging studies with moderate to severe papilledema, the posterior sclerae become flattened and the optic nerve head may appear elevated. Accentuated tortuosity and elongation with dilatation of the perioptic SAS are common.

culomotor Nerve (CN III)

FUNCTION. The oculomotor nerve has both motor and parasympathetic functions. It innervates all the extraocular muscles except the lateral rectus and superior oblique muscles. Its parasympathetic fibers control pupillary sphincter function and accommodation.

ANATOMY. The oculomotor nerve has four segments. Its **intraaxial segment** is in the midbrain. The oculomotor nucleus lies just in front of the periaqueductal gray matter. The fascicles of CN III course anteriorly through the red nucleus and substantia nigra, then exit the midbrain medial to the cerebral peduncles **(23-1)**.

The **cisternal segment** courses anteriorly toward the cavernous sinus, passing between the posterior cerebral and superior cerebellar arteries.

The **intracavernous segment** lies in the superolateral wall of the cavernous sinus and is surrounded by a thin sleeve of CSF (the **oculomotor cistern**) **(23-7)**, **(23-8)**, **(23-9)**. The oculomotor nerve exits the cavernous sinus through the superior orbital fissure **(23-4)**. Its **extracranial segment** passes through the tendinous annulus and then divides into superior and inferior branches **(23-10)**. Preganglionic parasympathetic fibers follow the inferior branch to the ciliary ganglion.

KEY CONCEPTS. The pupilloconstrictor fibers of CN III are located in the periphery of the nerve, predominantly along its superolateral aspect. The cisternal segment of the oculomotor nerve lies in close proximity to the posterior communicating artery (PCoA). PCoA aneurysms often compress the third nerve, causing **a pupil-involving third nerve palsy. Pupil-sparing third nerve palsy** is commonly caused by microvascular infarction of the core of the nerve with relative sparing of its peripheral fibers.

rochlear Nerve (CN IV)

FUNCTION. The trochlear nerve is a pure motor nerve that innervates the superior oblique muscle.

ANATOMY. Like the oculomotor nerve, CN IV has four segments. Its **intraaxial segment** is also in the midbrain, anterior to the periaqueductal gray matter lying just below the oculomotor nerve nuclei. Its fascicles then course pos-

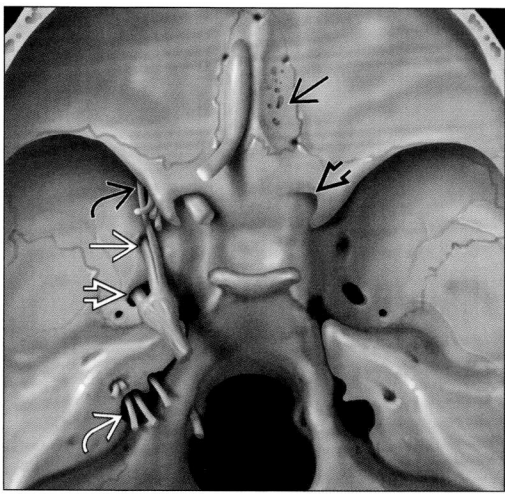

23-4. Cribriform plate (CN I) ➔, *optic canal (CN II)* ➔, *SOF (III, IV, V₁)* ➔, *rotundum (V₂)* ➔, *ovale (V₃)* ➔, *jugular foramen (IX-XI)* ➔.

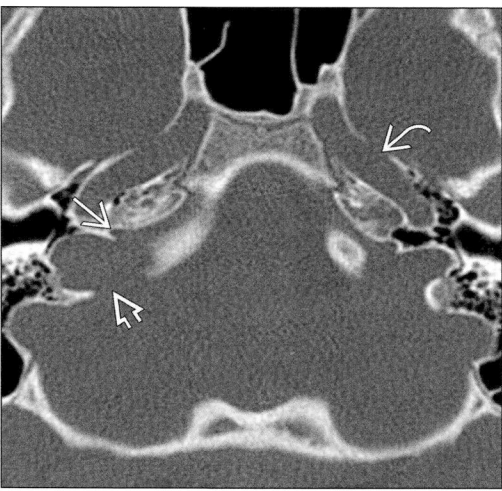

23-5. Bone CT shows the jugular foramen with pars nervosa ➔, *and pars vascularis* ➔. *The petrous carotid canal* ➔ *is also visible.*

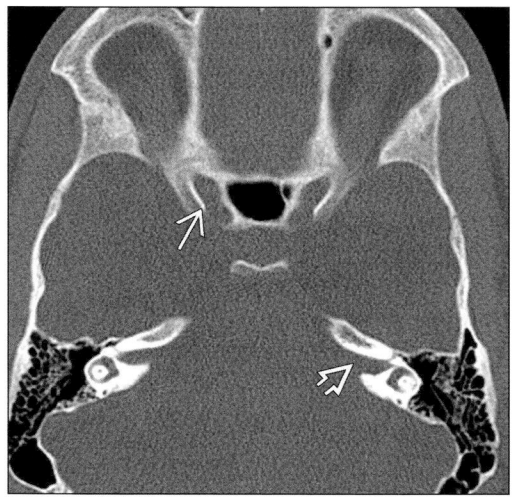

23-6. Bone CT shows the optic canals ➔ *and internal auditory canals* ➔.

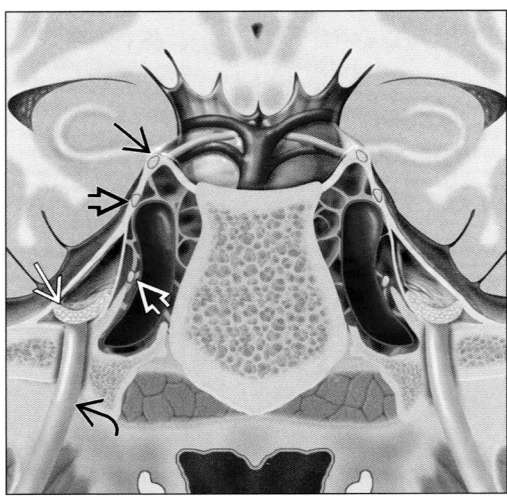

23-7. *CN III* ➡, *CN IV* ⇗, *gasserian (trigeminal) ganglion* ➡, *V₃* ⇗, *CN VI* ➡.

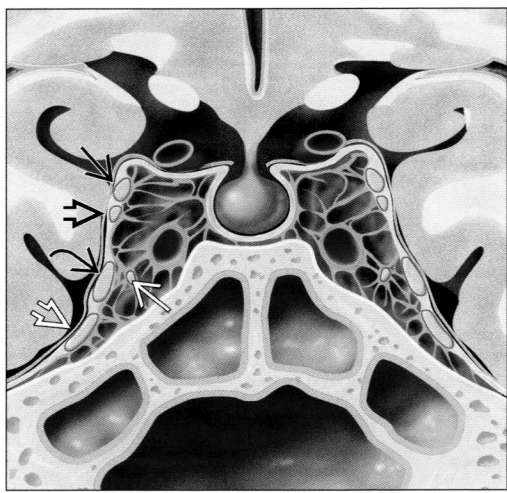

23-8. *With the exception of CN VI* ➡, *cavernous sinus CNs are in the lateral dural wall. CNs III* ➡, *IV* ⇗, *V₁* ⇗, *V₂* ➡.

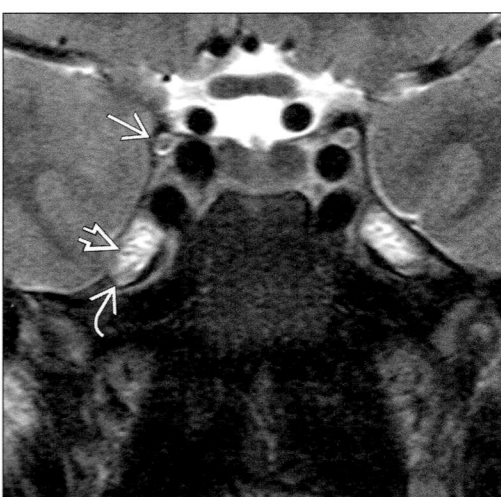

23-9. *Coronal T2 shows CN III in the oculomotor cistern* ➡, *the fascicles of trigeminal nerve in Meckel cave* ➡, *the gasserian ganglion* ➡.

teroinferiorly around the cerebral aqueduct and decussate within the superior medullary velum. The trochlear nerve exits the dorsal midbrain just below the inferior colliculi **(23-10)**.

The **cisternal segment** courses anteriorly in the ambient cistern, adjacent to the free edge of the tentorium. It then passes between the posterior cerebral and superior cerebellar arteries, just inferior to the oculomotor nerve, and enters the cavernous sinus (CS). The **cavernous segment** lies in the lateral dural wall, just below CN III **(23-8)**.

The trochlear nerve exits the CS through the superior orbital fissure together with CNs III and VI. The **extracranial segment** then passes above the tendinous annulus of Zinn (CNs III and VI pass through the ring).

KEY CONCEPTS. The long course of the cisternal segment and its proximity to the hard knife-like edge of the tentorium make the trochlear nerve especially vulnerable to injury during closed head trauma. Trochlear palsy causes superior oblique paralysis, resulting in outward rotation (extorsion) of the affected eye. The resulting diplopia and weakness of downward gaze causes most patients to compensate by tilting their heads away from the affected side. Look for trochlear neuropathy in patients with torticollis ("wry neck").

Trigeminal Nerve (CN V)

FUNCTION. The trigeminal nerve is a mixed sensory and motor nerve. It is the major sensory nerve of the head and face and innervates the muscles of mastication.

ANATOMY. The trigeminal nerve has four segments: A ganglion (the semilunar ganglion) and three postganglionic divisions **(23-11)**.

The **intraaxial segment** has four nuclei (three sensory and one motor) that are located in the brainstem and upper cervical spinal cord (between C2 and C4).

CN V emerges from the lateral pons at the root entry zone. The **cisternal segment** courses anteriorly through the prepontine cistern. It then passes through a dural ring, the porus trigeminus, to enter Meckel cave **(23-12)**.

The **interdural segment** lies entirely within **Meckel cave**, a CSF-filled, dura-arachnoid-lined outpouching from the prepontine subarachnoid space. Once inside Meckel cave, CN V separates into several discrete fascicles **(23-9)**. It then synapses in the **trigeminal (gasserian or semilunar) ganglion**, a small crescent of tissue that lies at the bottom of Meckel cave **(23-7)**.

The **postganglionic segment** of CN V consists of three divisions: CN V₁ (ophthalmic nerve), CN V₂ (maxillary nerve), and CN V₃ (mandibular nerve).

The **ophthalmic nerve** lies in the lateral cavernous sinus wall just below CN IV. It passes anteriorly toward the orbital apex and exits the CS through the **superior orbital fissure** (SOF). The ophthalmic nerve is a pure sensory nerve, innervating the scalp, forehead, nose, and globe.

The **maxillary nerve** courses anteriorly in the lateral dural wall of the CS, just below CN V_1. It exits through the **foramen rotundum**, traversing the upper aspect of the pterygopalatine fossa. It enters the orbit and courses anteriorly in the infraorbital groove, exiting through the infraorbital foramen. The maxillary nerve supplies sensation to the cheek and upper teeth.

The **mandibular nerve** exits Meckel cave directly from the semilunar ganglion, passing inferiorly through the foramen ovale. Unlike the other two postganglionic divisions, CN V_3 does *not* pass through the cavernous sinus. The mandibular nerve is both motor and sensory, supplying the muscles of mastication, the mylohyoid, and the anterior belly of the digastric. Its most important sensory innervations involves the teeth and tongue.

KEY CONCEPTS. Be alert for denervation atrophy (shrinkage, fatty infiltration) of the muscles of mastication. That may be the first imaging indication of CN V_3 neuropathy and should prompt further evaluation. (Meckel cave lesions are a common cause.)

bducens Nerve (CN VI)

FUNCTION. The abducens nerve is a pure motor nerve. It provides innervation to the lateral rectus muscle (abduction).

ANATOMY. The abducens nerve has five segments. The **intraaxial segment** begins in the CN VI nuclei, which are located in the pons, just anterior to the fourth ventricle. Axons of CN VII loop around the abducens nuclei, creating the "bump" in the floor of the fourth ventricle called the facial colliculus **(23-13)**.

Fibers from the abducens nuclei course directly anteriorly, emerging from the brainstem just lateral to the midline at the pontomesencephalic junction.

The **cisternal segment** of CN VI ascends anterosuperiorly through the prepontine cistern, then penetrates the clival dura. The **interdural segment** of CN VI courses superiorly between the two layers of dura in a shallow channel known as **Dorello canal**. The abducens nerve then crosses over the top of the petrous apex just below the petrosphenoidal ligament to enter the cavernous sinus.

The **cavernous segment** courses anteriorly within the CS itself, the only cranial nerve to do so (the others are embedded within the lateral dural wall). Inside the CS, the abducens nerve lies along the inferolateral aspect of the internal carotid artery **(23-7)**, **(23-8)**.

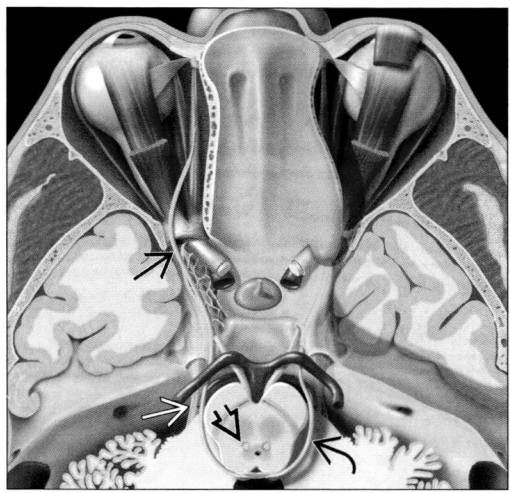

23-10. Oculomotor nerve (CN III) ⇥, trochlear nucleus ⇥, trochlear nerve ⇗, and trigeminal nerve (CN V) ⇥.

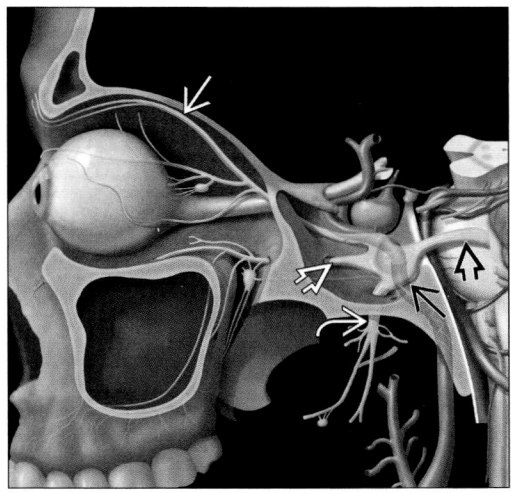

23-11. Graphic shows trigeminal nerve branches V_1 ⇥, V_2 ⇥, and V_3 ⇥, cisternal segment ⇥, gasserian ganglion in Meckel cave ⇥.

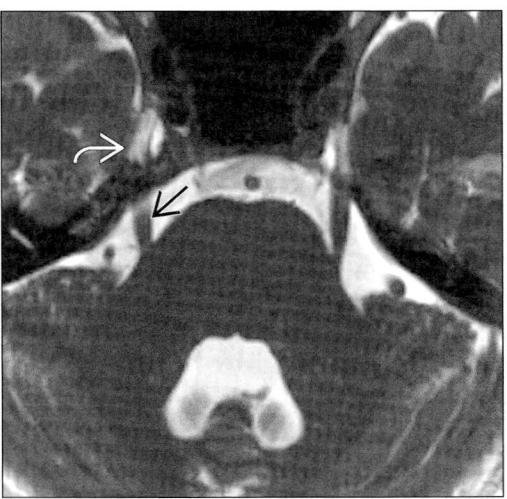

23-12. Axial T2WI shows the cisternal ⇥ and Meckel cave segments ⇥ of the trigeminal nerve.

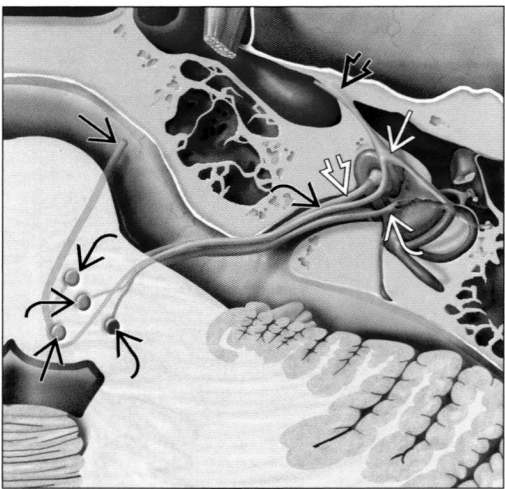

23-13. *CN VI nerve/nucleus ⮕. CN VII nuclei/IAC segment ⬀, geniculate ganglion ⮕, GSPN ⮔, and CN VIII cochlear ⮕, vestibular ⮕ nerves.*

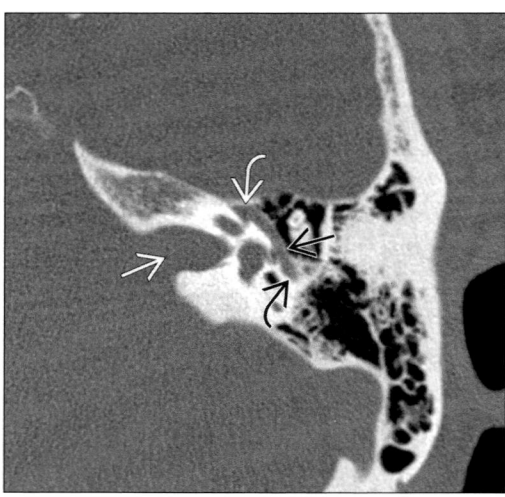

23-14. *Image shows IAC ⮕, bony facial nerve canal with anterior genu, geniculate ganglion ⮕, tympanic segment ⮔, posterior genu ⮔.*

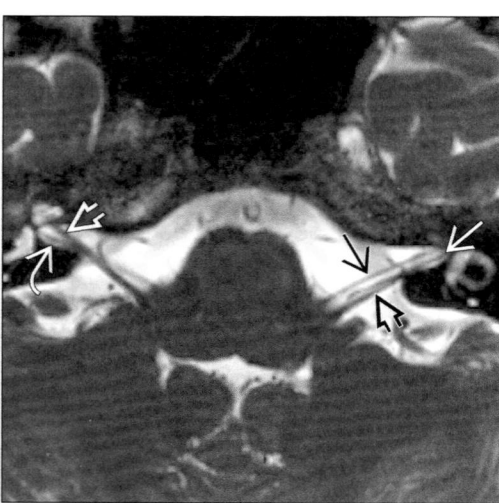

23-15. *T2WI shows left CN VII ⮕, vestibulo-cochlear ⮕, superior vestibular ⮕ nerves and right cochlear ⮕, inferior vestibular ⮕ nerves.*

CN VI exits the CS through the superior orbital fissure. The **intraorbital segment** passes anteriorly through the tendinous ring that attaches the extraocular muscles.

KEY CONCEPTS. Simple (i.e., isolated) abducens palsy is the most common ocular motor nerve palsy. A "pseudo" sixth nerve palsy (inability to abduct the eye) is usually caused by an infiltrative lesion in the lateral rectus muscle itself.

In its course over the petrous apex, the abducens nerve is vulnerable to increased intracranial pressure and inflammation in the adjacent temporal bone ("apical petrositis").

UPPER CRANIAL NERVES (CNs I-VI)

Olfactory Nerve (CN I)
- Function = visceral afferent for smell
- Skull entrance = cribriform plate
- Key concept
  - Image the coronal plane from upper nose to temporal lobes

Optic Nerve (CN II)
- Function = vision
- Skull entrance = optic canal
- Key concepts
  - Myelinated brain tract
  - Not ensheathed by Schwann cells
  - Tumors are astrocytomas, not schwannomas

Oculomotor Nerve (CN III)
- Function
  - Innervates all extraocular muscles, except lateral rectus, superior oblique
- Skull exit = superior orbital fissure
- Key concept
  - Is neuropathy pupil-involving or pupil-sparing?

Trochlear Nerve (CN IV)
- Function = innervates superior oblique muscle
- Skull exit = superior orbital fissure (SOF)
- Key concept
  - Head tilt/torticollis can be caused by CN IV injury

Trigeminal Nerve (CN V)
- Function (mixed motor, sensory)
  - Innervates muscles of mastication
  - Sensory from head, face
- Skull exits
  - Ophthalmic (CN V_1) = SOF
  - Maxillary (CN V_2) = foramen rotundum
  - Mandibular (CN V_3) = foramen ovale
- Key concepts
  - Look at face!
  - Denervation atrophy of masticator muscles

Abducens Nerve (CN VI)
- Function = innervates lateral rectus
- Skull exit = SOF
- Key concepts
  - Intrinsic lateral rectus disease can mimic CN VI palsy
  - ↑ intracranial pressure, apical petrositis can cause abducens palsy

ower Cranial Nerves

cial Nerve (CN VII)

FUNCTION. The facial nerve has multiple functions. It provides motor innervation to the muscles of facial expression. It provides parasympathetics innervation to the lacrimal, submandibular, and sublingual glands. It also provides a special sensory function, i.e., taste, to the anterior two-thirds of the tongue.

ANATOMY. The facial nerve has four segments. The **intraaxial segment** consists of the facial nerve nuclei that lie in the ventrolateral pons. Efferent fibers from the motor nucleus loop dorsally around the abducens nucleus, then pass anterolaterally to exit the brainstem at the pontomedullary junction **(23-13)**.

The **cisternal segment** of CN VII courses laterally through the cerebellopontine angle (CPA) together with the vestibulocochlear nerve (CN VIII) to the internal auditory canal (IAC) **(23-15)**.

The **intratemporal facial nerve** follows a complex course, first coursing laterally as the *IAC segment* and the most anterosuperior of the four nerves within the IAC. It then exits the bony IAC, bending anteriorly and becoming the *labyrinthine segment*. At its most anterior bend (which is called the "anterior genu"), the facial nerve synapses in the geniculate ganglion and then courses posteriorly under the lateral semicircular canal as the *tympanic segment* **(23-14)**. It curves inferiorly at the "posterior genu" and descends in the mastoid as the *mastoid segment* **(23-18)**.

The important intratemporal branches of the facial nerve from top to bottom are the **greater superficial petrosal nerve** (GSPN) (parasympathetic fibers that supply the lacrimal gland), the **stapedius nerve** (innervation of the stapedius muscle), and the **chorda tympani** (taste from the anterior two-thirds of the tongue) **(23-16)**, **(23-17)**.

The facial nerve exits the skull at the stylomastoid foramen, then enters the parotid gland. Once inside the gland the **extracranial facial nerve** ramifies into its terminal motor branches, which innervate the muscles of facial expression **(23-16)**.

KEY CONCEPTS. Facial nerve enhancement within the CPA cistern or internal auditory canal is always abnormal. With the exception of the labyrinthine segment, a robust vascular plexus surrounds most of the intratemporal facial nerve. Therefore, the facial nerve is the only cranial nerve with segments that may exhibit some enhancement following contrast administration.

If the bony intratemporal CN VII canal is normal, mild enhancement of the geniculate ganglion and tympanic and mastoid segments is considered normal. The genic-

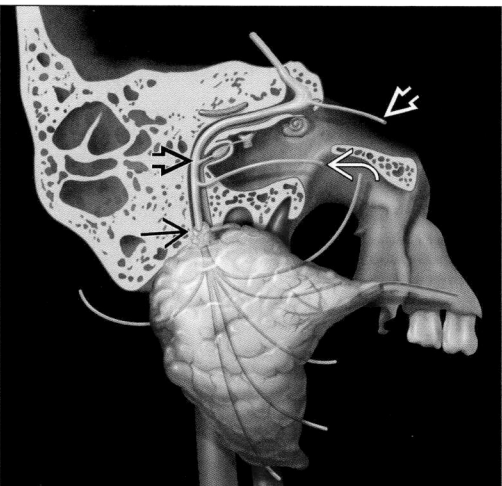

23-16. *CN VII GSPN* ⇒*, chorda tympani* ⇒*, stapedius nerve* ⇒*, stylomastoid foramen* ⇒*. Distal branches ramify within parotid gland.*

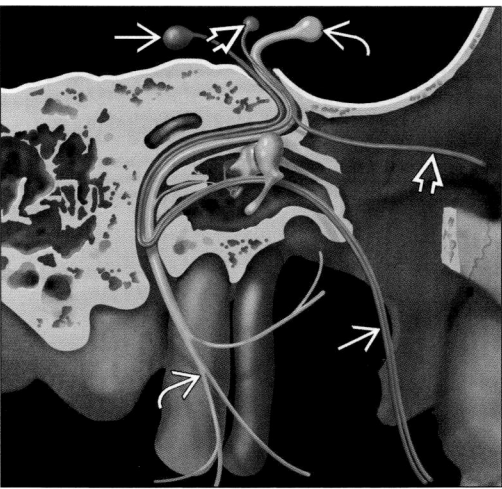

23-17. *Solitary nucleus to chorda tympani (taste)* ⇒*, superior salivatory nucleus to GSPN (lacrimation)* ⇒*, motor nucleus/nerve* ⇒*.*

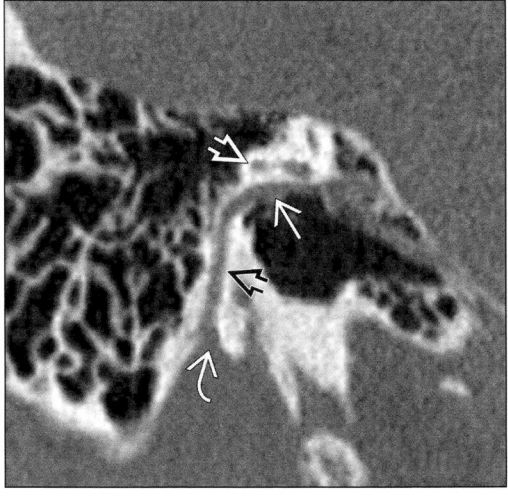

23-18. *Bone CT shows tympanic segment* ⇒ *under lateral semicircular canal* ⇒*, mastoid segment* ⇒ *descending to stylomastoid foramen* ⇒*.*

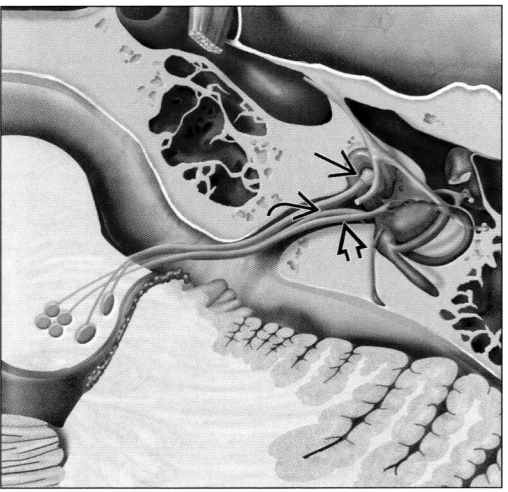

23-19. *CN VIII. Cochlear nerve/modiolus* ➡️, *inferior* ➡️/*superior* ➡️ *vestibular nerves. Nuclei in medulla, tracts in inferior cerebellar peduncle.*

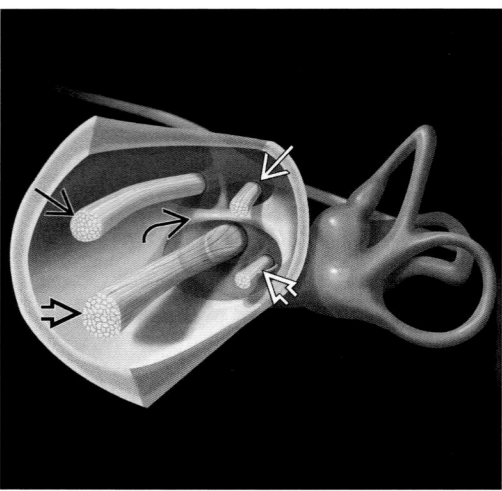

23-20. *Bony IAC with facial nerve (CN VII)* ➡️, *cochlear nerve (CN VIII)* ➡️, *superior* ➡️/*inferior* ➡️ *vestibular nerves, crista falciformis* ➡️.

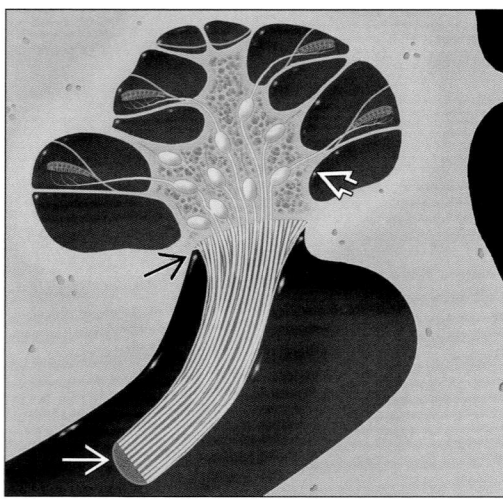

23-21. *Cochlea with modiolus* ➡️, *cochlear nerve* ➡️, *and aperture* ➡️. *Spiral ganglion cells are shown in yellow within the modiolus.*

ulate ganglion enhances in 75% of cases, and tympanic segment enhancement occurs in half of all cases. The mastoid segment nearly always enhances. Segmental facial nerve enhancement is more conspicuous at higher field strengths (3.0 T).

The first step in facial nerve imaging requires clinical input. When imaging is requested for "facial nerve palsy," detailed information is key. Typical Bell palsy (i.e., of short duration, uncomplicated by other CN neuropathy) does not need imaging.

It is essential to know whether a facial nerve deficit is central ("upper motor neuron") or peripheral ("lower motor neuron"). *Upper* (central or supranuclear) motor neuron injury, due to a parenchymal lesion above the brainstem, results in paralysis of the contralateral muscles of facial expression but spares the forehead. Stroke is a common cause of upper motor neuron facial palsy.

Lower motor neuron injury can involve CN VII at any point from its brainstem nucleus through its peripheral branches. Lower motor neuron facial palsy involves paralysis of all ipsilateral muscles of facial expression. In such cases, imaging should extend from the brainstem through the parotid gland.

If a lower motor neuron facial injury is present, further information regarding the so-called special functions of the facial nerve is essential. Are taste and lacrimation intact? Does the patient have hyperacusis? If these special functions are spared, the cause of a lower motor neuron facial palsy is extracranial.

If the special functions are affected, knowing exactly which ones are involved helps localize lesion extent. Malignant parotid tumors—especially adenoid cystic carcinoma—have a marked propensity to enter the stylomastoid foramen and invade up the intratemporal facial nerve.

The most distal of the intratemporal facial nerve branches is the chorda tympani, which is affected first. Loss of taste in the anterior tongue results. As tumor progresses more cephalad, the next affected branch is the stapedius nerve. Hyperacusis results. As tumor reaches the geniculate ganglion, the greater superficial petrosal nerve is compromised, resulting in problems with lacrimation.

A lesion proximal to the geniculate ganglion will cause facial paralysis and affect all three special functions.

If a complete lower neuron facial palsy is complicated by CN VI and/or CN VIII involvement, the lesion is most likely in the pons (CN VI) or CPA-IAC (CN VIII).

Vestibulocochlear Nerve (CN VIII)

FUNCTION. The vestibulocochlear nerve is purely sensory. It is the afferent sensory nerve responsible for hearing and the sense of balance.

ANATOMY. CN VIII has two major components, the **cochlear nerve** and the **vestibular nerve (23-19), (23-20)**. Unlike the other cranial nerves, CN VIII is best described from outside to inside (peripheral to central).

The **cochlear nerve** arises from the spiral ganglion in the modiolus of the cochlea. Its fibers pass through the cochlear aperture into the IAC **(23-21)**. The cochlear nerve is the most anteroinferior of the four nerves in the IAC **(23-24)**. Near the opening of the IAC, the porus acusticus, the cochlear nerve joins the superior and inferior vestibular nerves to form the vestibulocochlear nerve.

The **vestibular nerve** arises from bipolar neurons in the vestibular ganglion at the IAC fundus. Its fibers coalesce to form the **superior** and **inferior vestibular nerves**, which are separated by a bony bar called the falciform (transverse) crest. The superior and inferior vestibular nerves course medially in the posterior aspect of the IAC **(23-22), (23-23)**. At the porus acusticus, they join with the cochlear nerve to form CN VIII.

CN VIII passes medially through the CPA cistern and enters the lateral brainstem at the pontomedullary junction to become the **intraaxial segment**. The cochlear nuclei are found in the restiform body at the lateral surface of the inferior cerebellar peduncle. The vestibular nuclei lie along the inferior floor of the fourth ventricle.

KEY CONCEPTS. At least 90-95% of all lesions that cause unilateral sensorineural hearing loss (SNHL)—and are detected on imaging—are vestibulocochlear schwannomas. Isolated vestibular nerve dysfunction (dizziness, vertigo, balance problems) usually does not have positive findings on MR. "Conductive" (intracochlear) hearing loss is best evaluated by high-resolution multiformatted temporal bone CT.

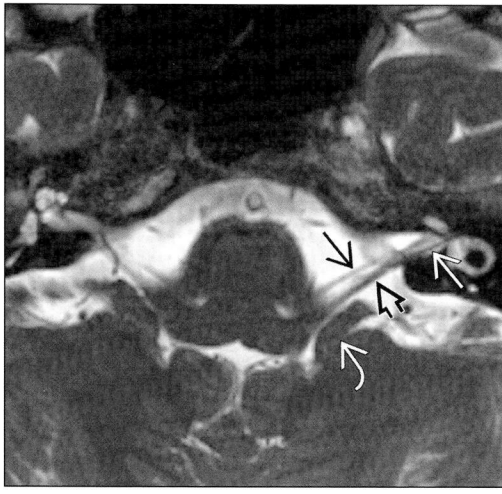

23-22. Axial T2WI shows CN VII ➡, vestibulocochlear nerve (CN VIII) ⬧➡, superior vestibular nerve ➡. Flocculus of cerebellum ➡.

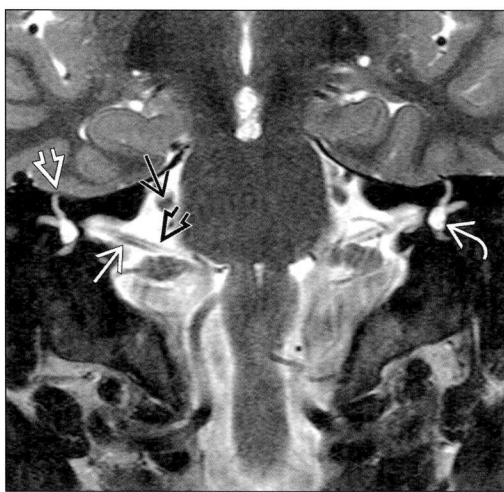

23-23. Coronal T2WI shows CN V ➡, CN VII ⬧➡, CN VIII ➡, vestibule ➡, superior semicircular canal ⬧➡.

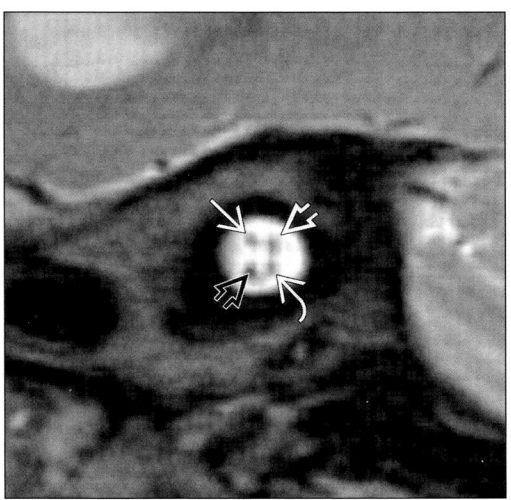

23-24. Sagittal T2WI of mid IAC shows 4 nerves as "dots" in CSF: CN VII ➡, superior ⬧➡ and inferior ➡ vestibular nerves, cochlear nerve ⬧➡.

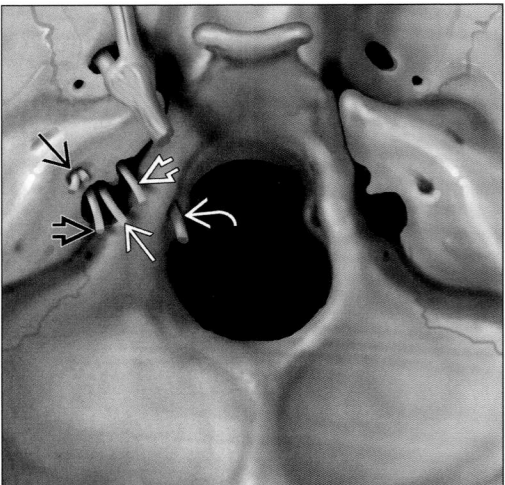

23-25. *Lower CNs, foramina: CNs VII and VIII in IAC ➔, CNs IX ⇒, X ➔, XI ⇒ in jugular foramen, CN XII ⇗ in hypoglossal canal.*

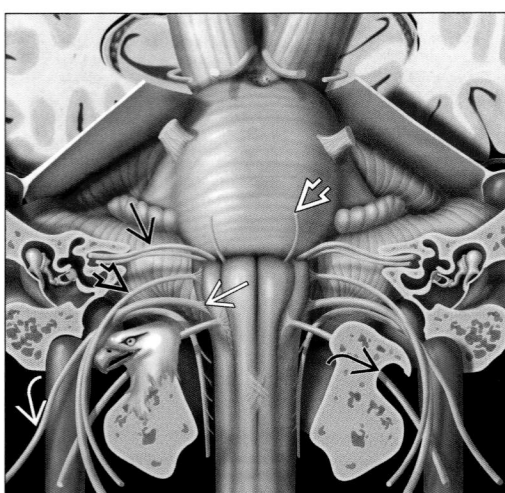

23-26. *CNs VI ⇒, VII and VIII ➔, IX ⇒, X ➔, XI ➔, XII ⇗. Jugular tubercle looks like the head of an eagle.*

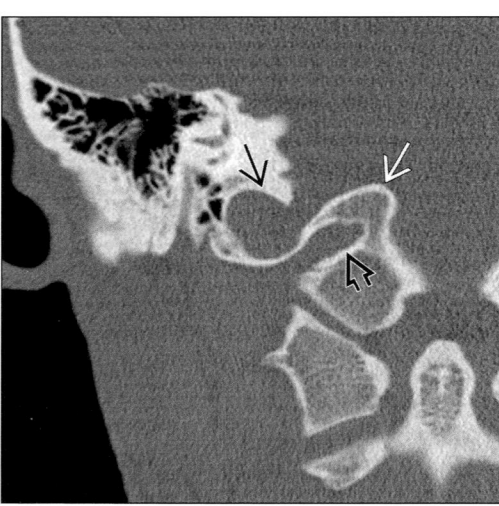

23-27. *CNs IX/X/XI exit jugular foramen ➔ on top of jugular tubercle ➔ (eagle's "head"). CN XII exits hypoglossal canal ⇒ under eagle's "beak."*

CRANIAL NERVES VII AND VIII

Facial Nerve (CN VII)
- Functions
  - Motor (muscles of facial expression)
  - Special sensory (taste, anterior 2/3 of tongue)
  - Parasympathetics (lacrimal, submandibular, sublingual glands)
- Skull exit
  - Exits through stylomastoid foramen into IAC along with CN VIII
- Key concepts
  - Typical Bell palsy does not require imaging
  - CN VII neuropathy? Ask if upper or lower motor neuron
  - Parotid malignancies "creep up" facial nerve
  - Special functions affected (taste, hyperacusis, lacrimation)?

Vestibulocochlear Nerve (CN VIII)
- Function = afferent sensory nerve
  - Hearing (cochlear nerve)
  - Balance (vestibular nerve)
- Skull entrance = IAC
  - Most anteroinferior = cochlear nerve
  - Posterior = superior, inferior vestibular nerves
- Key concepts
  - MR in vestibular nerve dysfunction usually negative
  - Unilateral SNHL with lesion on MR → 95% VS

Glossopharyngeal Nerve (CN IX)

FUNCTION. The glossopharyngeal nerve is small but has complex functions. It is a special sensory nerve (responsible for taste in the posterior third of the tongue) as well as a regular sensory nerve (innervating middle ear, pharynx). It carries parasympathetic fibers to the parotid gland and is the motor supply to the stylopharyngeus muscle. Last but by no means least, it is viscerosensory to the carotid body and sinus.

ANATOMY. Like most of the other cranial nerves, CN IX has four segments: Intraaxial, cisternal, skull base, and extracranial.

CN IX has four nuclei. All are in the upper and middle medulla, anterolateral to the inferior fourth ventricle. The **intraaxial segment** consists of these nuclei plus their tracts. The tracts course anterolaterally from the nuclei to exit or enter the medulla in the postolivary sulcus.

The **cisternal segment** travels toward the jugular foramen (JF), coursing just above the vagus nerve. The glossopharyngeal nerve exits the skull by passing into the anterior aspect (pars nervosa) of the jugular foramen **(23-5)**, **(23-25)**. In its **skull base segment**, the glossopharyngeal nerve lies adjacent to the inferior petrosal sinus. Its **extracranial segment** courses inferiorly through the carotid space.

KEY CONCEPTS. In the coronal plane, the jugular tubercles and basiocciput form a construct that resembles the head, beak, and body of an eagle. CN IX (together with

CNs X and XI) courses through the jugular foramen, which lies superolateral to the eagle's "head" and "beak." The hypoglossal canal lies under the eagle's "head," at the "neck" formed by the "beak" above and the "body" below **(23-26)**, **(23-27)**.

Vagus Nerve (CN X)

FUNCTION. The vagus nerve is also a mixed nerve with sensory (ear, larynx, viscera), special (taste from epiglottis), motor (most of soft palate, superior and recurrent laryngeal nerves), and parasympathetic (regions of head/neck, thorax, abdominal viscera) functions.

ANATOMY. The **intraaxial segment** of the vagus nerve lies in the inferior medulla. Its nuclei lie in front of the inferior fourth ventricle. Fibers to and from the nuclei exit the medulla in the postolivary sulcus. Its **cisternal segment** courses anterolaterally through the medullary cistern, lying between the glossopharyngeal nerve above and the bulbar portion of the spinal accessory nerve (CN XI) below.

Its **skull base segment** begins where CN X enters the posterior aspect (pars vascularis) of the jugular foramen. It lies anteromedial to the jugular bulb. CN X exits the jugular foramen into the carotid space. It descends, passing under the aortic arch on the left and the subclavian artery on the right. The recurrent laryngeal nerves on both sides then turn cephalad to course superiorly in the tracheoesophageal groove.

KEY CONCEPTS. Proximal vagal neuropathy requires imaging from the medulla to the level of the hyoid. If multiple cranial nerves (CNs IX-XII) are affected, the culprit lesion is usually in the medullary cistern or skull base (jugular foramen) where all four nerves are in close proximity.

Distal vagal neuropathy is usually isolated and manifests as laryngeal dysfunction (look for a paramedian vocal cord). It requires imaging from the level of the hyoid all the way to the carina/aortopulmonary window on the left and the subclavian artery on the right.

Spinal Accessory Nerve (CN XI)

FUNCTION. The spinal accessory nerve is a pure motor nerve that innervates the sternomastoid and trapezius muscles.

ANATOMY. CN XI has **two intraaxial segments** that arise from two different sets of nuclei, one in the medulla and the other in the proximal cervical cord. Bulbar fibers arise from the nucleus ambiguus in the medulla **(23-28)**. Spinal fibers originate from the spinal nucleus, a column of cells along the anterior horn extending from C1-C5 **(23-29)**.

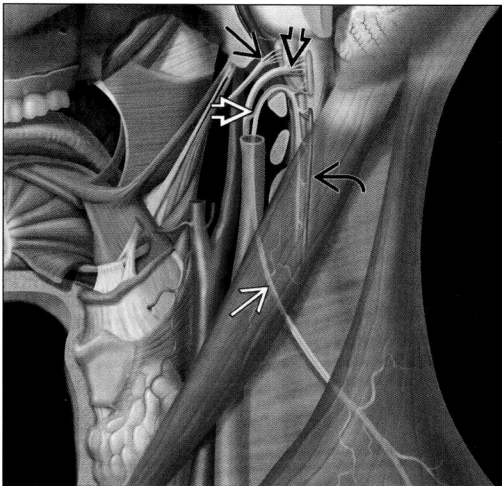

23-28. CNs IX ⇨, X ⇨, XI ⇨. Bulbar CN XI ⇨ crosses to CN X, joins spinal root from spinal accessory nucleus of CN XI ⇨ in jugular foramen.

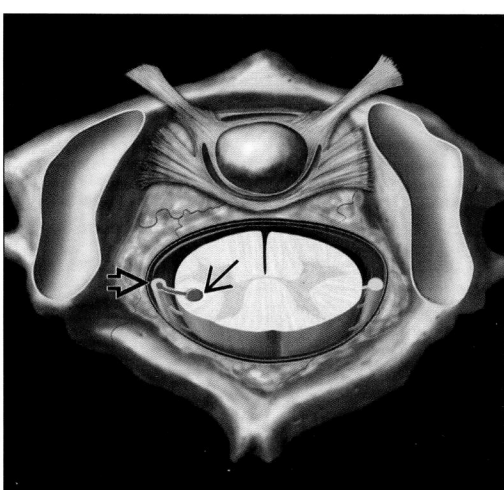

23-29. The spinal nucleus of CN XI ⇨ sends rootlets to form the spinal root of the accessory nerve ⇨.

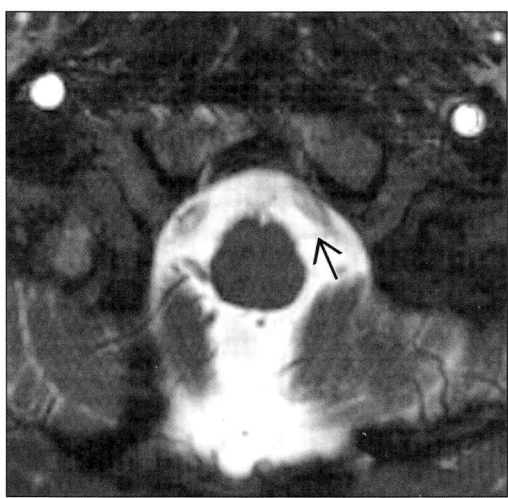

23-30. Axial T2WI shows the left bulbar CN XI segment ⇨ exiting the postolivary sulcus.

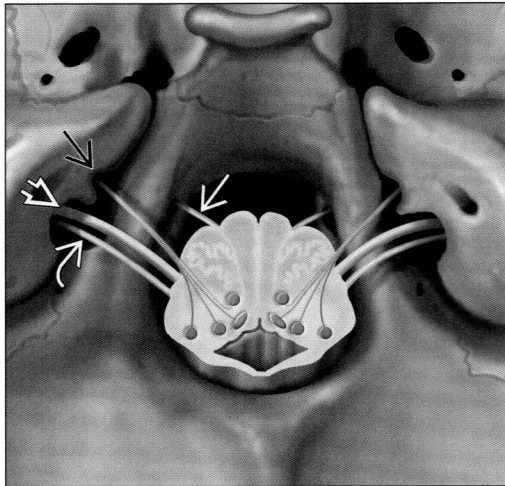

23-31. *CN XII* ➡ *exits the medulla at the preolivary sulcus. CN IX is in the pars nervosa of JF* ➡. *CNs X* ➡, *XI* ➡ *are in the pars vascularis.*

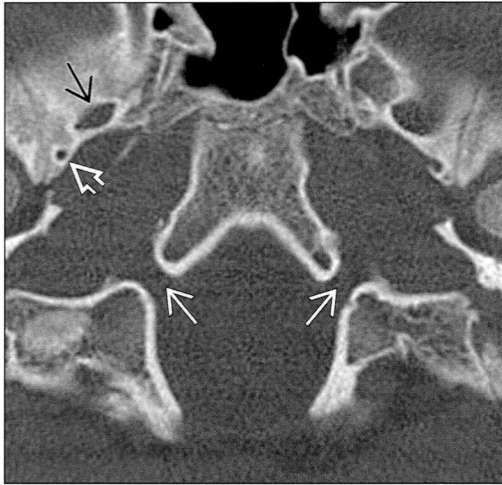

23-32. *Axial bone CT shows hypoglossal canals* ➡. *Foramen ovale* ➡ *(CN V₃), foramen spinosum* ➡ *(middle meningeal artery) are also seen.*

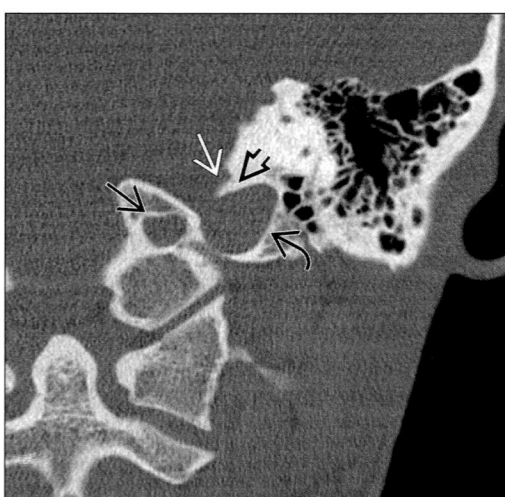

23-33. *Hypoglossal canal* ➡ *(CN XII exit), jugular foramen + jugular spine* ➡. *CN IX exits pars nervosa* ➡, *CNs X and XI exit pars vascularis* ➡.

The **two cisternal segments** of CN XI initially follow different courses. The bulbar fibers exit the medulla at the postolivary sulcus **(23-30)** and course anterolaterally through the basal cistern together with CNs IX and X. The spinal fibers emerge from the lateral aspect of the cervical spinal cord and course superiorly **(23-31)**. Both fiber bundles then unite in the basal cistern. The **skull base segment** of CN XI passes through the posterior part (pars vascularis) of the jugular foramen, together with the vagus nerve and jugular bulb **(23-34)**.

The **extracranial segment** begins as the glossopharyngeal nerve exits the jugular foramen into the carotid space.

KEY CONCEPTS. CN XI is often injured during radical neck dissection. Look for trapezius atrophy and compensatory hypertrophy of the ipsilateral levator scapulae.

CRANIAL NERVES IX, X, AND XI

Glossopharyngeal Nerve (CN IX)
- Functions
  - Taste/sensation to posterior 1/3 of tongue
  - Sensory to middle ear/pharynx
  - Parasympathetic to parotid gland
  - Motor to stylopharyngeus
  - Viscerosensory to carotid body/sinus
- Skull exit
  - Jugular foramen (pars nervosa)
- Key concepts
  - Isolated CN IX neuropathy very rare
  - Usually occurs with CNs X, XI neuropathy
  - Look for medullary cistern, skull base lesion

Vagus Nerve (CN X)
- Functions
  - Sensory (ear, larynx, viscera)
  - Taste (epiglottis)
  - Motor (innervates soft palate, pharyngeal constrictors, larynx)
  - Parasympathetic (head/neck, thorax, abdomen)
- Skull exit
  - Jugular foramen (pars vascularis)
- Key concepts
  - Proximal neuropathy: Image medulla to hyoid
  - Distal neuropathy: Image through subclavian artery (right), aortopulmonary window (left)

Spinal Accessory Nerve (CN XI)
- Function
  - Motor to sternomastoid, trapezius
- Skull exit/entrance
  - Spinal component enters through foramen magnum
  - Unites with bulbar portion
  - Both exit through jugular foramen (pars vascularis)
- Key concepts
  - May be injured during radical neck dissection
  - Look for ipsilateral trapezius atrophy

Hypoglossal Nerve (CN XII)

FUNCTION. The hypoglossal nerve is a pure motor nerve that innervates both the intrinsic and most of the extrinsic (styloglossus, hyoglossus, genioglossus) tongue muscles.

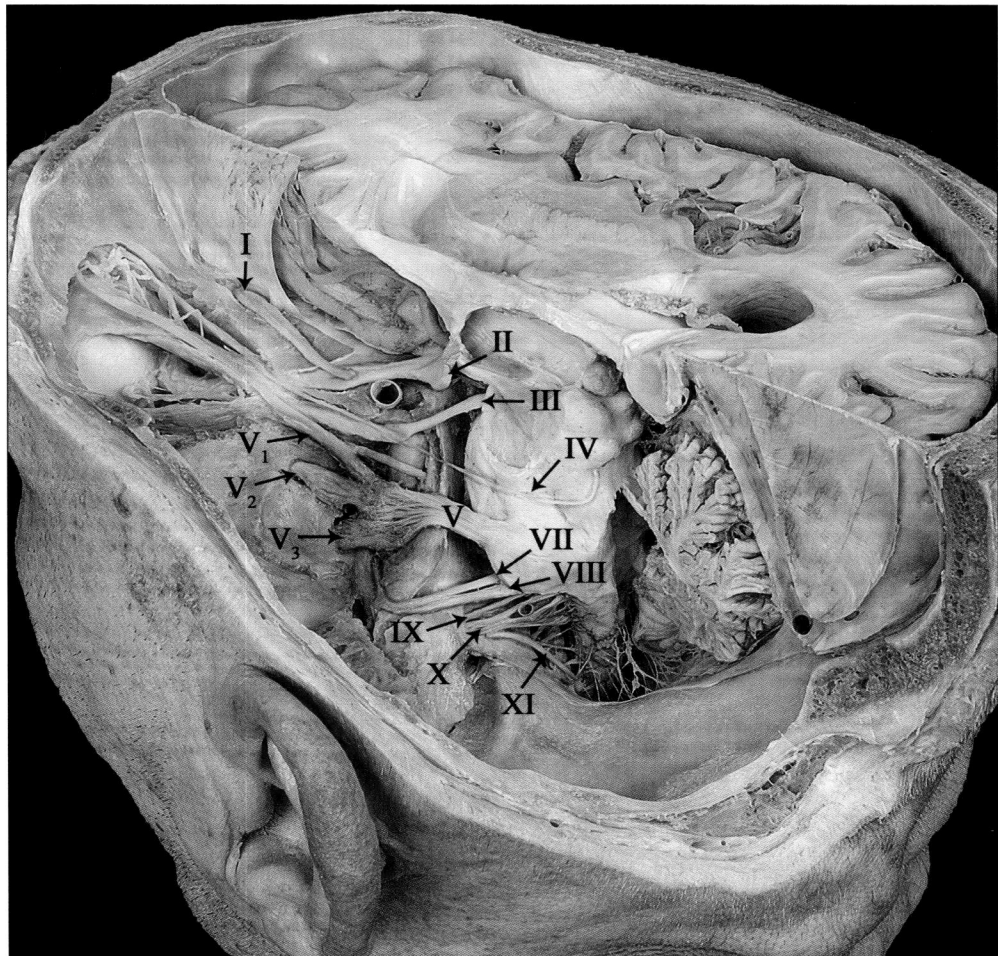

23-34. *Olfactory nerve (I), optic chiasm (II), oculomotor nerve (III), trochlear nerve (IV) coursing anteriorly in the ambient cistern, trigeminal nerve (V) with its ophthalmic (V₁), maxillary (V₂), and mandibular (V₃) branches. Abducens (VI), hypoglossal (XII) nerves are not visualized. CPA segments of the facial (VII) and vestibulocochlear (VIII) nerves are shown. Glossopharyngeal (IX), vagus (X), and spinal accessory (XI) nerves course toward the jugular foramen. (Courtesy M. Nielsen, MS.)*

The only exception is the geniohyoid muscle, which is innervated by the C1 spinal nerve.

ANATOMY. The hypoglossal nerve has four distinct segments. The intraaxial, cisternal, and skull base segments are relatively short. The extracranial segment is by far the longest and most complex portion of CN XII.

The **intraaxial segment** of CN XII begins at the hypoglossal nucleus. The hypoglossal nucleus lies just under the hypoglossal eminence of the inferior fourth ventricle. Fibers course anteriorly across the medulla and exit at the preolivary (ventrolateral) sulcus to enter the medullary (basal) cistern.

The **cisternal segment** extends from its exit at the medulla through the basal cistern to the entrance of the hypoglossal canal (**23-31**). Accompanied by a prominent venous plexus, the **skull base segment** of CN XII passes through the **hypoglossal canal**, which is located in the occipital bone beneath the jugular tubercle and jugular foramen.

The **extracranial segment** of the hypoglossal nerve descends in the posterior aspect of the carotid space. It exits the carotid space between the carotid artery and the internal jugular vein, then runs anteroinferiorly toward the hyoid bone to provide motor innervation to the tongue muscles.

KEY CLINICAL/IMAGING CONCEPTS. CN XII is most readily identified on axial images. The clival cortex takes an abrupt right-angle turn anterolaterally and forms the medial wall of the short, obliquely oriented hypoglossal canal (**23-32**).

In the coronal plane, the jugular tubercle and occipital condyle form a visual construct that resembles the head, beak, and body of an eagle. The hypoglossal canal and nerve are located between its "head" and "beak" (**23-27**), (**23-33**).

A hypoglossal lesion causes atrophy of the ipsilateral tongue muscles. Look for fatty infiltration and volume loss.

HYPOGLOSSAL NERVE (CN XII)
- Function
  - Motor to tongue muscles
- Skull exit = hypoglossal canal
  - At base of occipital bone
  - Below jugular tubercle, jugular foramen
- Key concepts
  - Look for ipsilateral denervation tongue atrophy
  - Shrunken, fatty infiltration

Schwannomas

Neuropathologists recognize four histologic subtypes of schwannoma: Conventional, cellular, plexiform, and melanocytic. The vast majority of schwannomas that involve cranial nerves are the conventional type. With the exception of melanotic schwannoma, imaging findings do not distinguish between histologic subtypes. Rather, conventional intracranial schwannomas are distinguished—and discussed here—according to their cranial nerve of origin.

Because the pathology of intracranial schwannomas is similar, we discuss it and other shared features before delving into specific schwannomas.

Schwannoma Overview

Terminology

Schwannomas are benign slow-growing encapsulated tumors that are composed entirely of well-differentiated Schwann cells. Less common terms are neurinoma and neurilemmoma.

Etiology

GENERAL CONCEPTS. Schwannomas originate from Schwann cells, which are derived from the neural crest. Because the olfactory and optic nerves do not contain Schwann cells, schwannomas do not arise from CNs I and II. The rare reported cases of "olfactory groove schwannomas" are probably tumors that arise from olfactory ensheathing cells.

Schwann cells are also not a component of normal parenchyma. The exceptionally rare intraparenchymal schwannoma is thought to arise from neural crest remnants that later express aberrant Schwann cell differentiation. Intramedullary (spinal cord) schwannomas are more common than intraparenchymal brain schwannomas.

GENETICS. The NF2 tumor suppressor Merlin is a protein whose loss results in defective morphogenesis and

tumorigenesis in multiple tissues. Genetic studies have linked both sporadic and NF2-associated schwannomas (especially vestibular schwannomas [VSs]) to the *NF2* tumor suppressor gene located on chromosome 22. Approximately half of NF2 cases represent new mutations, suggesting a high mutation rate in this gene.

Biallelic inactivation (the classic "two-hit mechanism") of the *NF2* gene is also detected in nearly all sporadic vestibular schwannomas and 50-70% of meningiomas.

INHERITED TUMOR SYNDROMES. The most common tumor predisposition syndrome that causes multiple schwannomas is **neurofibromatosis type 2 (NF2)**. The presence of bilateral vestibular schwannomas is pathognomonic of NF2. One VS and a first-degree relative with NF2 or a VS in combination with another cranial nerve schwannoma, meningioma, or glioma is also indicative of NF2.

Schwannomatosis is a condition with multiple peripheral, often painful schwannomas without other features of NF2. These patients have no evidence of VS, no first-degree relative with NF2, and no known constitutional *NF2* mutation.

Schwannomatosis occurs in 2-4% of patients with schwannomas. Both sporadic and familial forms of schwannomatosis occur and can be associated with both nonvestibular intracranial and spinal schwannomas.

Patients with schwannomatosis tend to be younger than those who present with solitary schwannomas. The average age at onset is 28.5 years.

Plexiform schwannoma, also known as **multinodular schwannoma**, is a Schwann cell tumor in which multiple (2-50) circumscribed lesions occur along an affected nerve fascicle. Most are dermal-subcutaneous tumors of the extremities, trunk, head, and neck. Brain lesions have not been reported.

Approximately 90% of plexiform schwannomas are sporadic with 5% associated with NF2 and 5% with schwannomatosis. Unlike patients with neurofibromatosis type 1 and plexiform neurofibromas, there is no known predilection for malignant degeneration of plexiform schwannomas.

Pathology

LOCATION. Schwannomas arise at the glial-Schwann cell junction of CNs III-XII. The distance from the brain to the interface where the glial covering terminates and Schwann cell ensheathing begins varies with each cranial nerve. In some—such as the oculomotor nerve (CN III)—the junction is in close proximity to the brain. Here schwannomas arise close to the exit of the parent nerve from the brain. In others—such as the vestibulocochlear

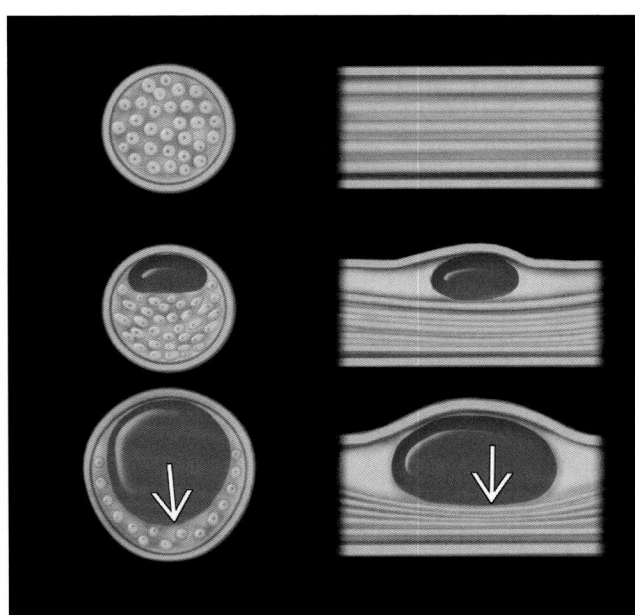

23-35. Axial (left) and sagittal (right) graphics show a schwannoma arising within a unifascicular nerve. The tumor displaces other nerve fibers peripherally ➡.

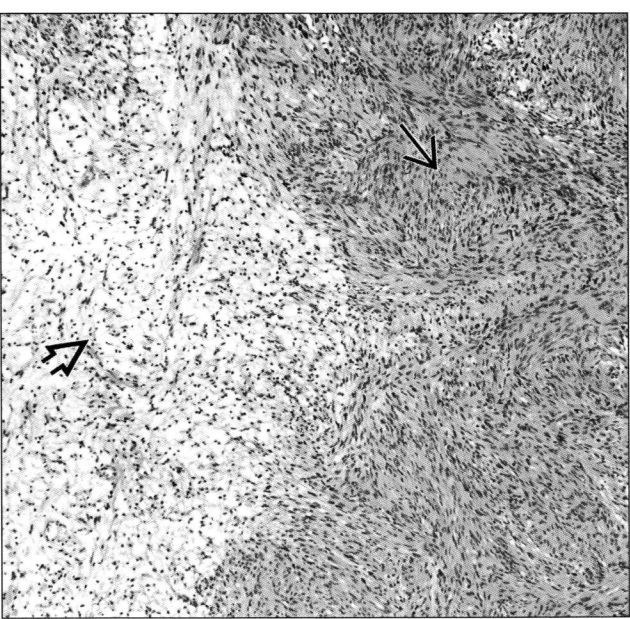

23-36. The juxtaposition of the cellular "Antoni A" ➡ and loose "Antoni B" ➤ patterns is classic for conventional schwannoma. (Courtesy A. Ersen, MD, B. Scheithauer, MD.)

nerve (CN VIII)—the junction lies at some distance from the nerve exit or entrance into the brainstem.

Sensory nerves are much more commonly affected by schwannomas compared to pure motor cranial nerves. The vestibulocochlear nerve is by far the most common intracranial site (95%). The second most common site is the trigeminal nerve (CN V) (2-4%).

Schwannomas of cranial nerves other than CN VIII and CN V are very rare, accounting for just 1-2%. As a group, jugular foramen schwannomas (i.e., schwannomas arising from the glossopharyngeal, vagal, and spinal accessory nerves) are the third most common, followed by facial (CN VII) and hypoglossal (CN XII) schwannomas. In the absence of NF2, schwannomas of CNs III, IV, and VI are all very rare. Intraparenchymal schwannomas occur but are extremely uncommon.

SIZE AND NUMBER. Most intracranial schwannomas are small, especially those that arise from motor nerves. Some, especially trigeminal schwannomas, can attain huge size and involve both intra- and extracranial compartments.

Most schwannomas occur singly in otherwise healthy individuals and are termed "sporadic" or "solitary" schwannomas. The presence of multiple schwannomas in the same individual suggests an underlying tumor predisposition syndrome.

GROSS PATHOLOGY. Schwannomas arise eccentrically from their parent nerves and are smooth or nodular well-encapsulated lesions **(23-35)**, **(23-37)**. Cystic change

is common, as is yellow discoloration due to lipidization **(23-38)**. Hemorrhage occurs, but gross macroscopic bleeds are rare.

MICROSCOPIC FEATURES. A biphasic pattern is typical of **conventional schwannoma**. The "Antoni A" pattern consists of compact fascicles of elongated spindle cells that demonstrate occasional nuclear palisading (Verocay bodies). A less cellular, loosely textured, more haphazard arrangement with clusters of lipid-laden cells is called the "Antoni B" pattern **(23-36)**. Mitotic figures are rare. Immunohistochemistry is characterized by strong diffuse positivity for S100 protein.

Cellular schwannoma consists mostly of "Antoni A" tissue but lacks Verocay bodies. Such tumors may demonstrate hypercellularity and minor nuclear atypia. Frequent mitotic figures and increased proliferative indices can be seen in young children. Cellular schwannomas do not undergo malignant transformation.

Plexiform schwannoma can be either conventional or cellular type. **Melanotic schwannoma** can be benign or malignant (10%) with frequent mitoses, macronucleoli, and distant metastases.

STAGING, GRADING, AND CLASSIFICATION. Conventional schwannomas correspond to WHO grade I.

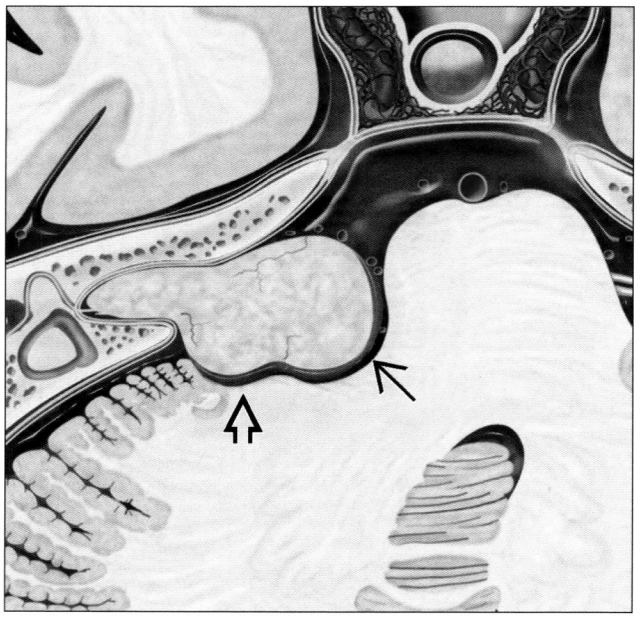

23-37. Graphic of a large vestibular schwannoma shows the typical "ice cream on cone" morphology. Note the prominent CSF-vascular "cleft" between the middle cerebellar peduncle ⊟, the cerebellar hemisphere ⊟.

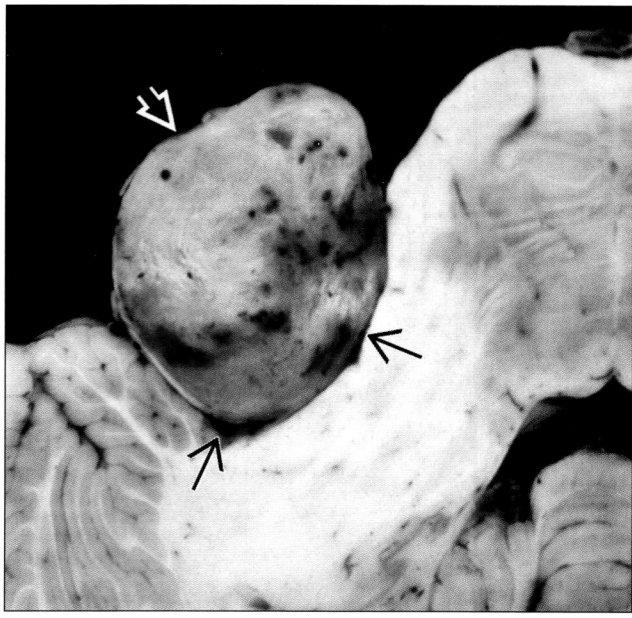

23-38. Autopsy specimen shows vestibulocochlear schwannoma ⊟. Yellow discoloration and petechial hemorrhages are common. Note the CSF-vascular "cleft" ⊟ between tumor, brain. (Courtesy B. Horten, MD.)

INTRACRANIAL SCHWANNOMAS

Synonyms
- Neurilemoma, neurinoma

Epidemiology
- Vestibular (CN VIII) most common (95%)
  - All other sites combined (1-5%)
- Trigeminal (CN V) second most common
- Jugular foramen (CNs IX, X, XI) third
- Hypoglossal (CN XII) fourth
- All others rare except in NF2
- Intraparenchymal schwannomas very rare

Pathology
- Arise at glial-Schwann cell junction
  - Distance from brain varies according to CN
- Benign encapsulated nerve sheath tumor
- Well-differentiated neoplastic Schwann cells
- Biphasic histology with 2 components
  - Compact, highly ordered cellularity ("Antoni A")
  - Less cellular, myxoid matrix ("Antoni B")

Clinical Issues

EPIDEMIOLOGY. The vast majority of schwannomas occur outside the CNS, most often in the skin and subcutaneous tissues. Intracranial schwannomas are relatively uncommon, constituting about 7% of all primary neoplasms.

DEMOGRAPHICS. All ages are affected, but the peak incidence is in the fourth to sixth decades. Schwannomas occur in children but are uncommon unless associated with NF2. There is no gender predilection.

PRESENTATION. Many schwannomas are asymptomatic, and any symptoms are location-specific. As schwannomas favor sensory nerves, motor symptoms are rare. Vestibulocochlear schwannoma, the most common intracranial schwannoma, presents with sensorineural hearing loss (see below).

NATURAL HISTORY. Schwannomas are benign tumors that tend to grow very slowly. The exception is VSs in young patients with NF2. These tumors have higher MIB-1 indices.

Recurrence after surgical removal of a conventional schwannoma is generally uncommon. Roughly 30-40% of cellular schwannomas recur after subtotal resection but do not undergo malignant transformation.

Schwannomas rarely—if ever—undergo malignant degeneration. Most "malignant intracerebral schwannomas" are probably malignant peripheral nerve sheath tumors (see below).

Approximately 10% of melanotic schwannomas are malignant. In approximately half of these cases, the patients have **Carney complex**, an autosomal dominant disorder characterized by lentiginous facial pigmentation, cardiac myxoma, and endocrine overactivity (e.g., precocious puberty, pituitary adenoma with acromegaly, Cushing syndrome with multinodular adrenal hyperplasia).

TREATMENT OPTIONS. Depending on size, location, and symptoms, treatment options range from watchful waiting to surgery and stereotactic radiosurgery.

Imaging

GENERAL FEATURES. Neuroimaging demonstrates a well-circumscribed extraaxial mass that originates within or near a cranial nerve.

CT FINDINGS. Most schwannomas are heterogeneous on NECT scans. Cystic change is common. Hemorrhage is uncommon. Calcification is rare. Strong moderately heterogeneous enhancement after contrast administration is typical.

MR FINDINGS. Schwannomas are generally isointense with brain on T1WI and heterogeneously hyperintense on T2WI and FLAIR **(23-39)**, **(23-41)**. Although macroscopic intratumoral hemorrhage is rare, T2* (GRE, SWI) scans often reveal "blooming" foci of microbleeds.

Virtually all schwannomas enhance intensely. Approximately 15% have nonenhancing intratumoral cysts. Nonneoplastic peritumoral cysts occur in 5-10% of cases, especially with larger lesions.

Differential Diagnosis

The differential diagnosis of a **solitary enlarged enhancing cranial nerve** includes schwannoma, multiple sclerosis, viral and post-viral neuritis, Lyme disease, sarcoid, ischemia, and malignant neoplasm (metastases, lymphoma, leukemia).

The most common cause of **multiple enhancing cranial nerves** is metastasis. NF2, neuritis (especially Lyme disease), lymphoma, and leukemia are significantly less common than metastasis. Rare but important causes include multiple sclerosis and chronic inflammatory demyelinating polyneuropathy, a disorder that usually affects spinal nerves but may involve cranial nerves.

Vestibular Schwannoma

Terminology

Vestibular schwannoma (VS) is the preferred term for a CN VIII schwannoma. VSs are also known as **acoustic schwannomas** and **acoustic neuromas**.

Focal **intralabyrinthine schwannomas**, also known as **inner ear schwannomas**, form a special subgroup of CN VIII schwannomas **(23-40)**. Intralabyrinthine schwannomas are named according to sublocation. Schwannomas within the cochlea are termed **intracochlear**. Lesions within the vestibule are called **intravestibular** schwannomas **(23-42)**. If a schwannoma involves *both* the vestibule and the cochlea, it is termed **vestibulocochlear**. A schwannoma that crosses the modiolus from the cochlea into the internal auditory canal (IAC) fundus is a **transmodiolar** schwannoma. If a lesion crosses from the vestibule into the IAC fundus, it is termed **transmac-**

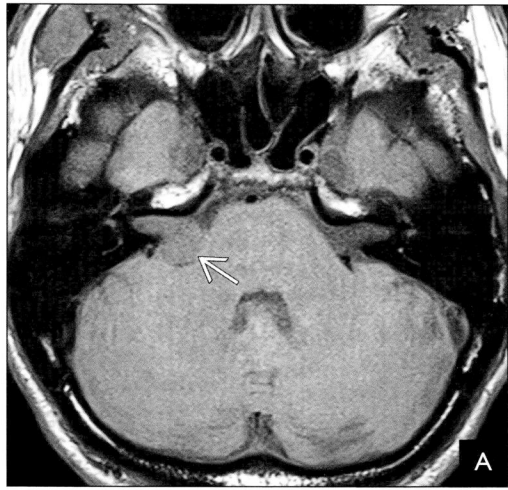

23-39A. *Series of images depicts a classic VS. T1WI shows that the lesion* ➡ *is isointense with GM, looks like "ice cream on a cone."*

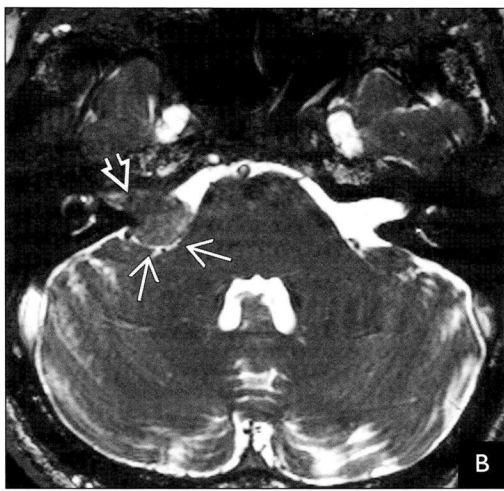

23-39B. *Thin-section CISS demonstrates the lesion* ➡, *CSF-vascular "cleft"* ➡.

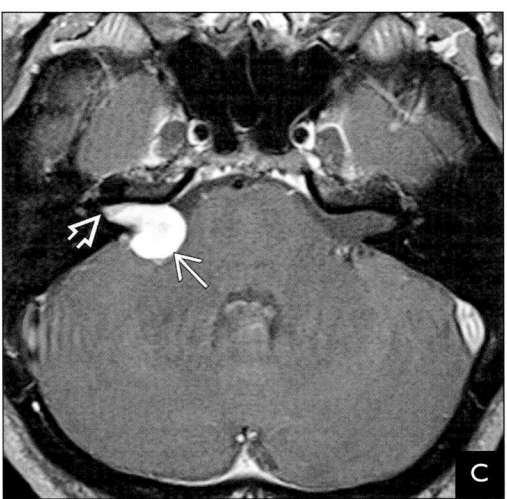

23-39C. *Strong, relatively uniform enhancement* ➡ *is seen on T1 C+ FS scan. The tumor extends to the IAC fundus* ➡.

ular. Finally, an extensive schwannoma that crosses the entire inner ear from the IAC fundus to the middle ear is called **transotic (23-43).**

Etiology

GENERAL CONCEPTS. VSs arise from the vestibular portion of CN VIII at the glial-Schwann cell junction, inside the internal auditory canal near the porus acusticus. Schwannomas rarely arise from the cochlear portion of CN VIII.

GENETICS. The pathogenesis underlying both familial and most sporadic VSs has been linked to mutation in a single gene, the neurofibromin 2 *(NF2)* gene located on chromosome 22. Nearly 60% of sporadic VSs have inactivating mutations of *NF2*.

Pathology

LOCATION. VSs may occur at any location along the course of the nerve. Small VSs are often completely intracanalicular. Larger lesions frequently protrude medi-

ally through the porus acusticus into the cerebellopontine angle (CPA) cistern.

SIZE AND NUMBER. Small VSs are round or ovoid lesions that generally measure 2-10 mm in length. VSs that extend into the CPA cistern can become very large, up to five centimeters in diameter. Bilateral VSs are pathognomonic of NF2.

Clinical Issues

EPIDEMIOLOGY. VS is by far the most common intracranial schwannoma. VS is also the most common cerebellopontine cistern mass, accounting for 85-90% of lesions in this location.

DEMOGRAPHICS. Peak presentation is 40-60 years of age. There is no gender predilection.

PRESENTATION. The most common presentation is in an adult with slowly progressive unilateral sensorineural hearing loss (SNHL). Small VSs may present initially with tinnitus. Large lesions often present with trigeminal and/or facial neuropathy.

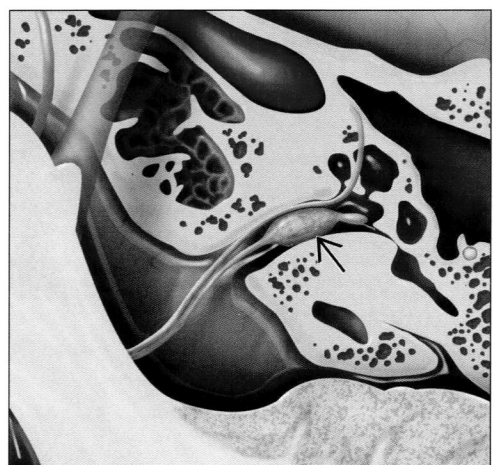

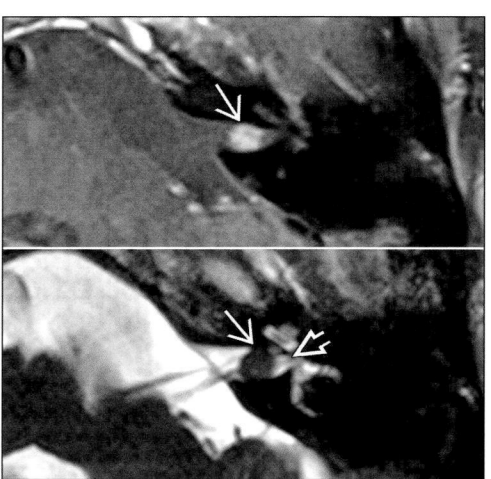

23-40. Graphic depicts an intracanalicular VS as round or fusiform enlargement of the nerve ➡. 23-41. (Top) Small intracanalicular VS ➡ is shown on axial T1 C+ scan. (Bottom) High-resolution axial T2WI in the same patient nicely shows the VS as a round isointense mass in the IAC ➡. Note the fundal "cap" of CSF ➡.

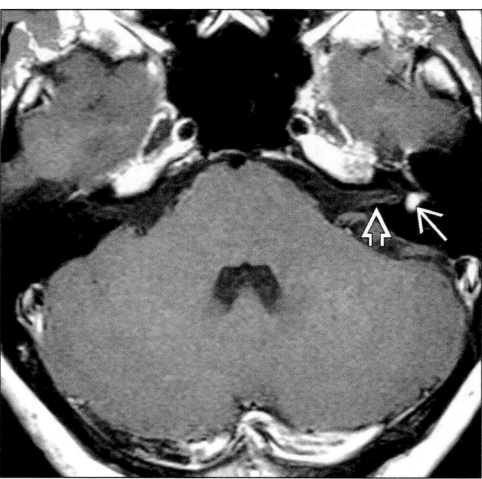

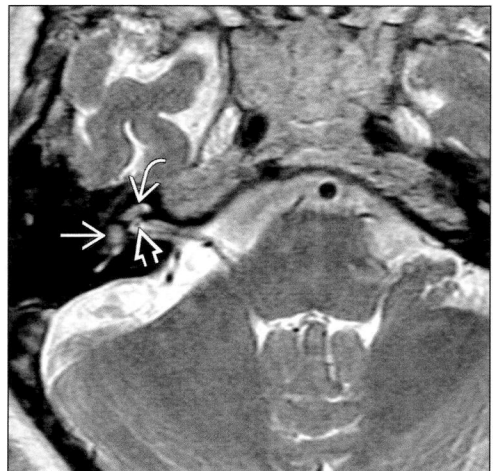

23-42. Axial T1 C+ shows a tiny enhancing intralabyrinthine schwannoma ➡. Because the tumor involves only the vestibule, it is called an intravestibular schwannoma. The IAC ➡ is normal. 23-43. Axial T2WI shows a schwannoma that involves both the vestibule ➡ and the cochlea ➡. A tiny nodule of tumor ➡ can be seen at the IAC fundus, so this is a transotic schwannoma.

NATURAL HISTORY. The growth rate of VSs varies. On average, they tend to enlarge between one or two millimeters per year. Approximately 60% grow very slowly (under one millimeter per year) whereas 10% of patients experience rapid enlargement of their lesions (more than three millimeters per year).

The growth rate of NF2-associated VSs is generally considered more aggressive compared to that of sporadic VSs.

TREATMENT OPTIONS. Treatment options vary. Watchful observation of small lesions with interval follow-up imaging is common, especially in older patients. Surgical removal or stereotactic radiotherapy are other possibilities. The surgical approach of choice varies with tumor size and location, as well as whether hearing preservation is possible.

Imaging

GENERAL FEATURES. The classic imaging appearance of VS is an avidly enhancing mass that looks like "ice cream on a cone" **(23-37)**. Many VSs extend medially from their origin within the IAC. The intracanalicular part of the tumor represents the "cone." If a VS passes through the porus acusticus, it typically expands when it enters the CPA, forming the "ice cream" on the cone.

Precisely defining the size and extent of a VS is one of the most important goals of imaging. Some VSs remain as small slow-growing lesions that are entirely intracanalicular. Many intracanalicular VSs have a distinctive fundal "cap" of CSF interposed between the lesion and the modiolus. Others grow laterally, extending deep into the IAC fundus, and may eventually pass through the cochlear aperture into the modiolus.

CT FINDINGS. CT is generally negative unless lesions are large enough to expand the IAC or protrude into the CPA cistern. VSs are generally noncalcified, appear mildly hyperdense on NECT, and enhance strongly and relatively uniformly on CECT. Bone CT may show IAC enlargement on the symptomatic side.

MR FINDINGS. Full brain FLAIR with axial and coronal fat-saturated T1 C+ imaging of the CPA and ICA is the standard. A "screening" study for adults with uncomplicated unilateral SNHL is a common option and is generally limited to high-resolution T2WI, CISS, or FIESTA sequences. Detailed evaluation of the CPA/ICA can be performed with these sequences, reserving contrast-enhanced studies for patients with equivocal screening studies.

VSs are generally isointense with brain on T1WI **(23-39A)**. An intracanalicular VSs appears as a hypointense filling defect within the bright CSF on CISS **(23-39B)**. Larger VSs are iso- to heterogeneously hyperintense on T2WI. Microhemorrhage on T2* is common although macroscopic hemorrhage is rare.

Virtually all VSs enhance strongly following contrast administration **(23-39C)**. A schwannoma-associated "dural tail" sign occurs but is rare compared to CPA meningiomas.

Special imaging sequences may be helpful in the preoperative planning for VS surgery. MR tractography with three-dimensional tumor modeling can depict the precise location of the CNs that surround large VSs.

Differential Diagnosis

The major differential diagnosis of VS is **CPA meningioma**. Most meningiomas "cap" the IAC and do not extend deep to the porus. However, a reactive dural "tail" in the IAC may make distinction between VS and meningioma difficult unless other dural "tails" along the petrous ridge are also present.

A **facial nerve schwannoma** confined to the IAC may be difficult to distinguish from a VS. Facial nerve schwannomas are much less common and usually have a labyrinthine segment "tail." Beware: Extension along the labyrinthine segment of the facial nerve means the schwannoma arises from CN VII and is not a VS.

Metastases can coat the facial and vestibulocochlear nerves within the IAC. Metastases are usually bilateral with other lesions present.

Other CPA masses such as **epidermoid cysts**, **arachnoid cysts**, and **aneurysms** can usually be distinguished easily from VS. VSs occasionally have prominent intramural cysts, but a completely cystic schwannoma without an enhancing tumor rim is very rare.

Trigeminal Schwannoma

Although trigeminal schwannomas are the second most common intracranial schwannoma, they are rare tumors. They may involve any part of the CN V complex, including extracranial peripheral divisions of the nerve. Nearly two-thirds of all Meckel cave tumors are schwannomas.

The principal presenting symptoms involve sensory impairment in one or more of the three divisions. Trigeminal neuralgia can occur but is uncommon.

Imaging

Trigeminal schwannomas arise from the junction of the gasserian ganglion and the trigeminal nerve root **(23-44)**. Small lesions may be confined to Meckel cave. They have a very characteristic appearance on coronal T2WI, the "winking Meckel cave" sign. Because at least 90% of each Meckel cave is normally filled with CSF, any lesion that fills the cave with soft tissue contrasts sharply with the bright signal on the opposite normal side **(23-45)**.

Bicompartmental tumors are common. Schwannomas that originate in Meckel cave can extend into the posterior fossa (through the porus trigeminus). These tumors have a characteristic "dumbbell" configuration **(23-46)**. Less commonly, bicompartmental tumors extend from the middle fossa anteroinferiorly through the foramen ovale into the masticator space. Tumors that involve all three locations are uncommon and are termed "three-compartment" trigeminal schwannomas **(23-47)**.

Schwannomas that involve the mandibular division (CN V₃) may cause denervation atrophy of the muscles of mastication.

Differential Diagnosis

The appearance of a bi- or tricompartmental CN V schwannoma is distinctive. The major differential diagnoses of a Meckel cave schwannoma are **meningioma** and **metastasis**.

Jugular Foramen Schwannoma

Although schwannomas account for approximately 40% of all jugular foramen (JF) neoplasms, JF schwannomas constitute only 2-4% of all intracranial schwannomas.

Glossopharyngeal schwannomas are the most common JF schwannoma but are still rare, with just 42 cases reported between 1908 and 2008. The vast majority (85%) presented with vestibulocochlear symptoms secondary to compression and displacement, not CN IX symptoms. Glossopharyngeal schwannomas can occur anywhere along the course of CN IX, but the majority of symptomatic cases are intracranial/intraosseous.

Compared to their extracranial counterpart, intracranial **vagal schwannomas** are rare. Purely intracisternal ones are even more unusual. Most vagal schwannomas are "dumbbell" lesions that extend from the basal cistern through the jugular foramen into the high deep carotid space **(23-48)**, **(23-49)**. When large, they may compress the ventrolateral medulla and cause refractory neurogenic hypertension.

23-44. "Dumbbell" trigeminal schwannoma. The cisternal tumor segment ⧴ is constricted as it passes through the porus trigeminus ➡. The schwannoma then expands again ⧨ when it enters Meckel cave. 23-45. (Top) Coronal T2WI of left CN V schwannoma illustrates "winking Meckel cave" sign. CSF-filled right side ⧴ contrasts with tumor-filled left Meckel cave ➡. (Bottom) Schwannoma enhances ➡ while the right side ⧴ is normal.

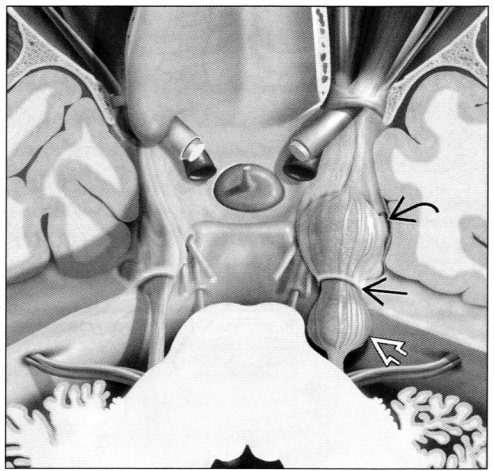

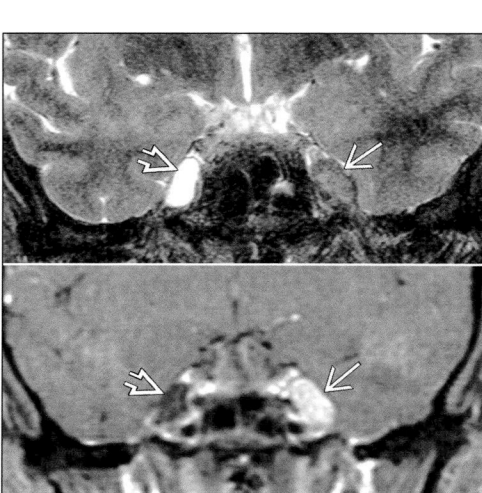

23-46. Large "dumbbell" trigeminal schwannoma. The tumor is hyperintense on T2WI, and FLAIR ➡ enhances strongly on T1 C+ ⧴. Note prominent constriction by the dural ring of the porus trigeminus ⧨. 23-47. Giant "tricompartmental" schwannoma of CNs V₂ and V₃ with cystic and hemorrhagic changes enlarges the pterygopalatine fossa ⧴, extends from posterior fossa ➡ into middle fossa ⧨, through foramen ovale into the masticator space ⧴.

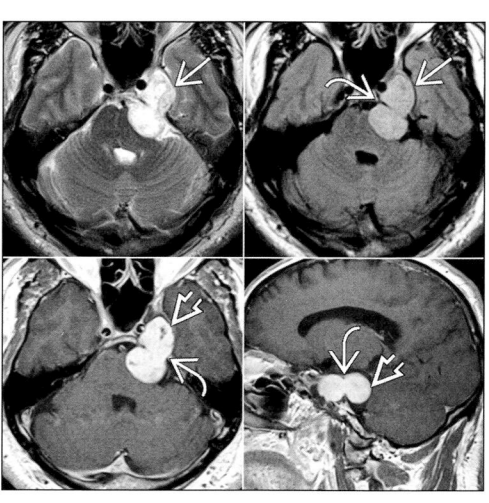

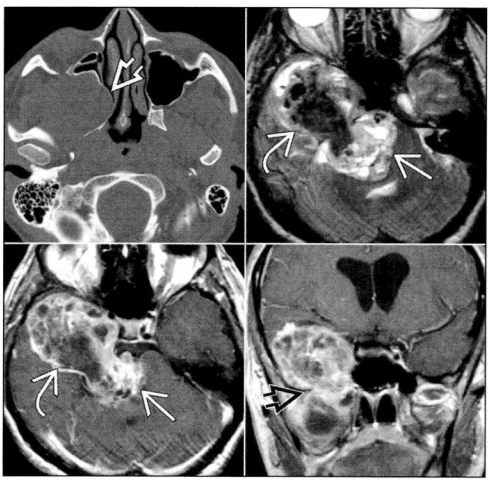

Spinal accessory nerve schwannomas not associated with neurofibromatosis are very rare. They can be either intrajugular or intracisternal.

The major differential diagnoses of JF schwannoma include **meningioma**, **glomus jugulare tumor**, and **metastasis**. Only a JF schwannoma smoothly enlarges and remodels the jugular fossa.

Facial Nerve Schwannoma

Facial nerve schwannomas (FNSs) are rare lesions that can arise anywhere along the course of the facial nerve, from its origin in the cerebellopontine angle to its extracranial ramifications in the parotid space **(23-50)**, **(23-51)**. Depending on their location along CN VII, FNSs display several imaging patterns. The most common presentation is facial neuropathy.

CPA-IAC FNSs are radiologically indistinguishable from vestibular schwannomas if they do not demonstrate extension into the labyrinthine segment of the facial nerve canal. Lesions that traverse the labyrinthine segment often have a "dumbbell" appearance.

Almost 90% of FN schwannomas involve more than one facial nerve segment **(23-52)**. The **geniculate fossa** is the most common site, involved in more than 80% of all FN schwannomas. The **labyrinthine** and **tympanic segments** are each involved in slightly over half of FN schwannomas.

Geniculate fossa FNSs typically appear as a round or tubular enhancing mass in a smoothly enlarged facial nerve canal.

FNSs that tract along the **greater superficial petrosal nerve** are seen as a round middle cranial fossa extraaxial mass **(23-53)**.

Tympanic segment FNSs often pedunculates into the middle ear cavity, losing its tubular configuration.

When the **mastoid segment** is involved, tumor may break into adjacent mastoid air cells and assume a more aggressive appearance, mimicking a malignant invasive tumor.

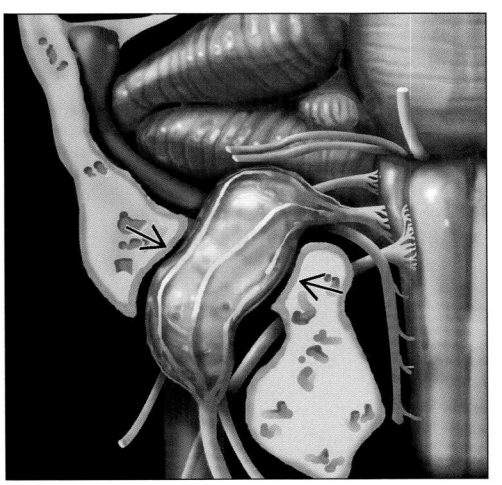

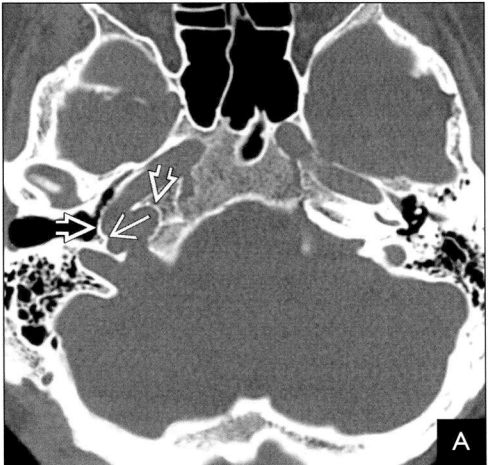

23-48. Coronal graphic of a vagal schwannoma shows the tumor enlarging and remodeling the bony margins of the jugular foramen ➡. The "beak" of the "eagle" is eroded. 23-49A. NECT scan shows osseous remodeling of the right jugular foramen. The jugular spine ➡ is eroded, but the surrounding cortex ➡ appears intact (compare with Figure 23-6).

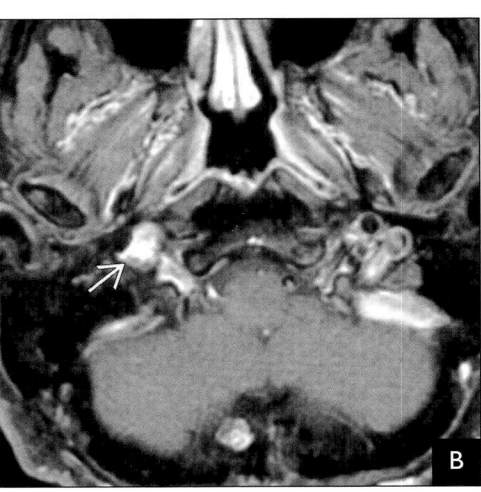

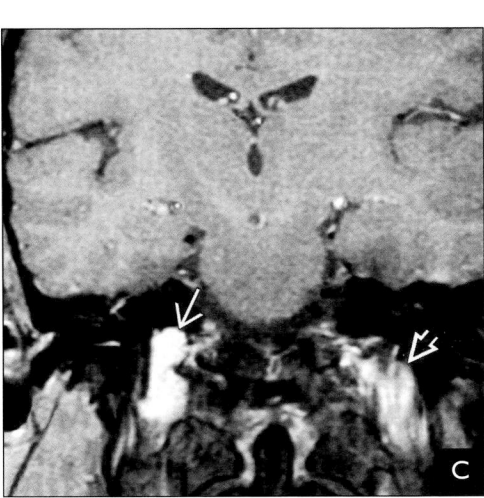

23-49B. Axial T1 C+ FS scan shows an enhancing mass in the jugular foramen ➡. 23-49C. Coronal T1 C+ FS shows the intensely enhancing mass ➡. Contrast this with the normally enhancing left jugular bulb and vein ➡. At surgery, this jugular foramen schwannoma proved to be arising from the vagal nerve (CN X).

Schwannomas of Other Intracranial Nerves

Motor nerve schwannomas are much less common than those arising from sensory or mixed sensory-motor nerves. Less than 1% of intracranial schwannomas arise from CNs III, IV, VI, and XII.

"Other" cranial schwannomas resemble their more common counterparts on imaging studies. Most motor nerve schwannomas are small, round or ovoid, well-delineated, strongly enhancing lesions.

Olfactory (CN I) "Schwannoma"

The cells that ensheathe the intracranial olfactory nerve are actually modified glial cells, not Schwann cells (see above). Primary tumors of the CN I nerve sheath are very rare. Once termed "olfactory groove schwannoma" or "subfrontal schwannoma," these neoplasms are more accurately called "olfactory ensheathing cell (OEC) tumors." The distinction between OEC and a true schwannoma can only be made using immunohistochemical staining.

Tumors of CN I typically present with anosmia. Many reach large size, causing frontal lobe signs such as emotional lability and complex partial seizures (23-54).

Esthesioneuroblastoma, also known as olfactory neuroblastoma, is a rare malignant tumor that arises in the superior nasal cavity from olfactory mucosa. Esthesioneuroblastoma is discussed with embryonal and neuroblastic tumors (see Chapter 21).

Optic Nerve (CN II) "Schwannoma"

Neoplasms of the optic nerve (a brain tract) are astrocytomas, not schwannomas. Intraorbital schwannomas arise from peripheral branches of CNs IV, V_1, or VI or from sympathetic or parasympathetic fibers (not the optic nerve).

Oculomotor (CN III) Schwannoma

Oculomotor schwannomas are rare but are the most common of all the pure motor nerve schwannomas (23-55). They can be asymptomatic or present with diplopia.

The most frequent location of a CN III schwannoma is in the interpeduncular cistern near the nerve exit from

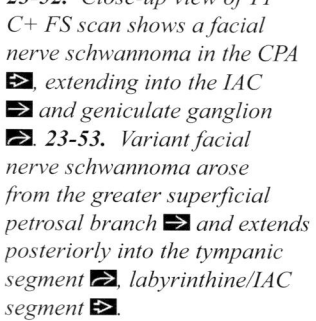

23-50. Axial graphic depicts a small tubular facial nerve schwannoma involving the labyrinthine segment ➡, geniculate ganglion ➡, and anterior tympanic segment ➡ on CN VII. 23-51. Graphic depicts a larger facial nerve schwannoma with CPA ➡, IAC ➡ segments. This can mimic a vestibular schwannoma ("ice cream on cone" appearance) except for the "tail" of tumor ➡ extending into the labyrinthine segment.

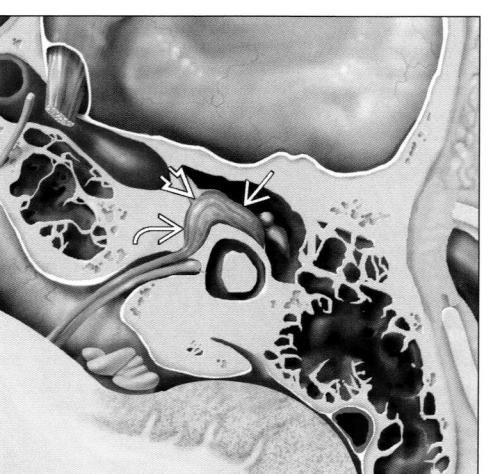

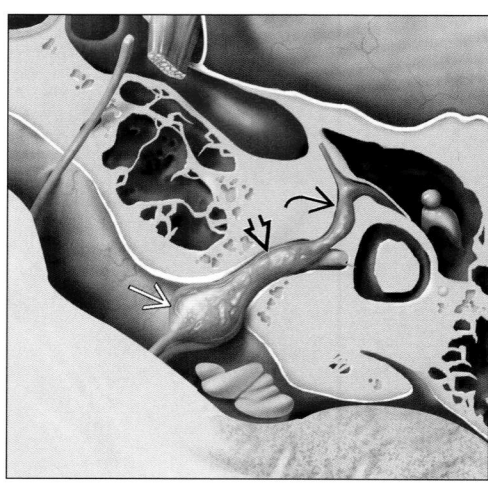

23-52. Close-up view of T1 C+ FS scan shows a facial nerve schwannoma in the CPA ➡, extending into the IAC ➡ and geniculate ganglion ➡. 23-53. Variant facial nerve schwannoma arose from the greater superficial petrosal branch ➡ and extends posteriorly into the tympanic segment ➡, labyrinthine/IAC segment ➡.

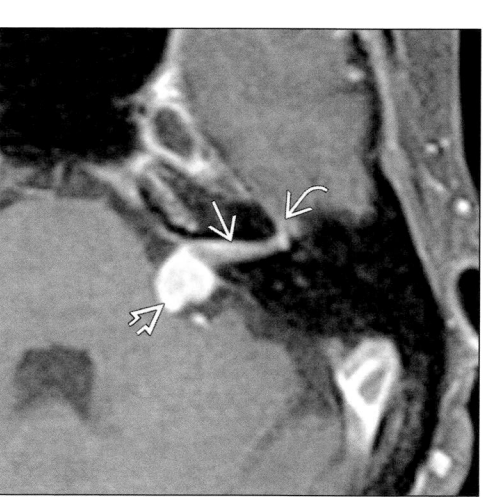

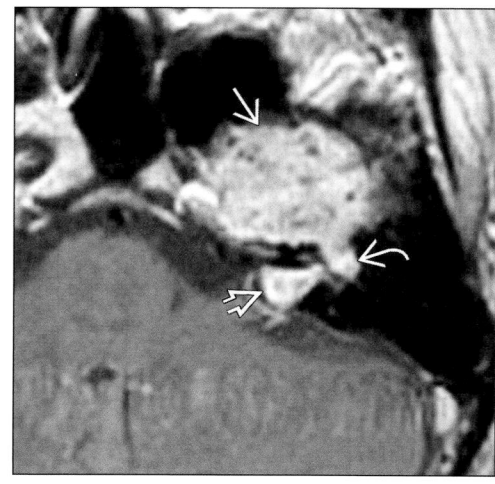

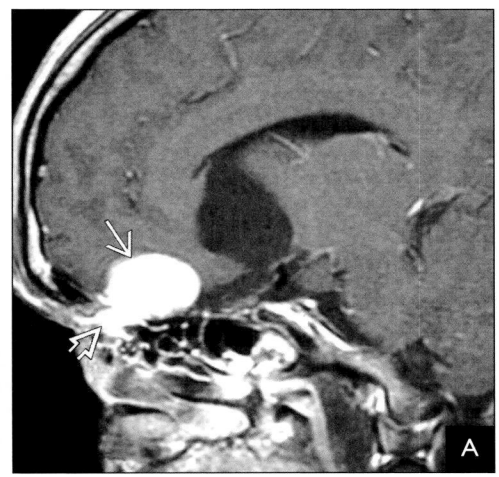

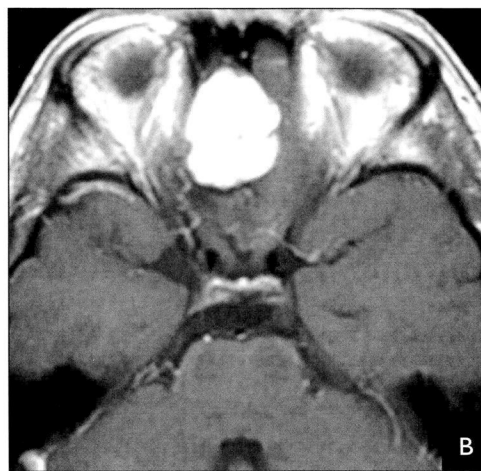

23-54A. Sagittal T1 C+ FS shows an intensely enhancing, subfrontal, "dumbbell" mass ➡ that extends through an eroded cribriform plate into the nasal cavity ➡. 23-54B. Axial T1 C+ in the same patient shows that the well-circumscribed, intensely enhancing mass is centered on the cribriform plate. Histologic diagnosis was olfactory nerve schwannoma. Most similar-appearing cases are probably olfactory ensheathing cell tumors, not true schwannomas. (Courtesy G. Parker, MD.)

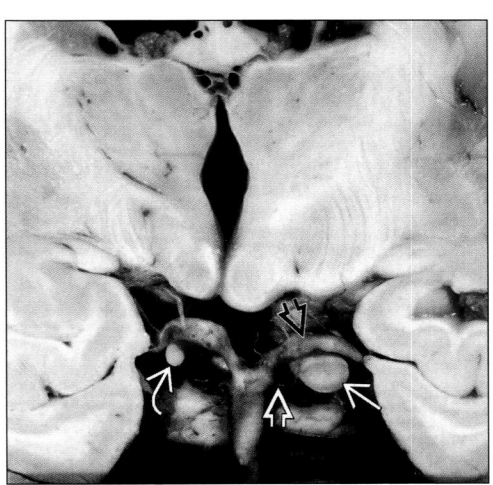

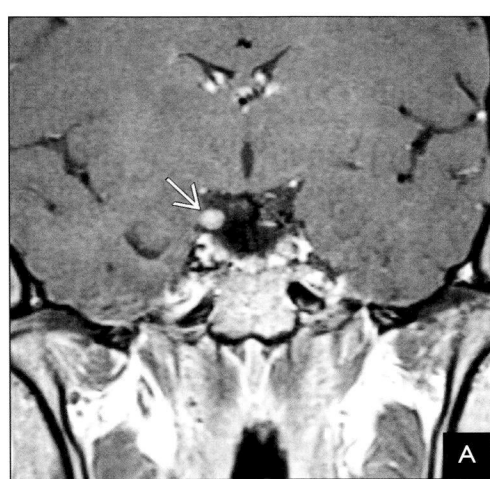

23-55. Coronal autopsy case of incidental left oculomotor schwannoma ➡ seen between posterior cerebral artery above ➡, superior cerebellar artery below ➡. Contrast with the normal right CN III ➡. (Courtesy E. T. Hedley-Whyte, MD.) 23-56A. Coronal T1WI C+ demonstrates the enlarged, enhancing right oculomotor nerve ➡.

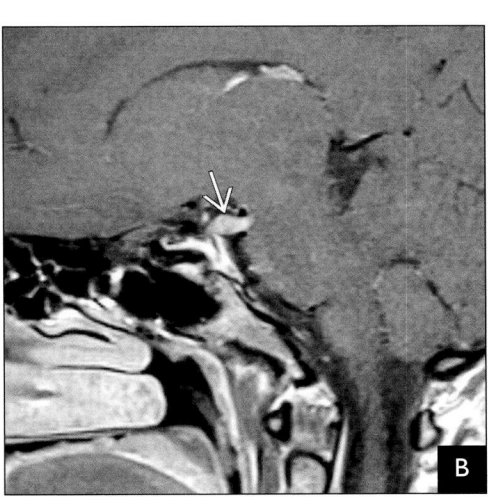

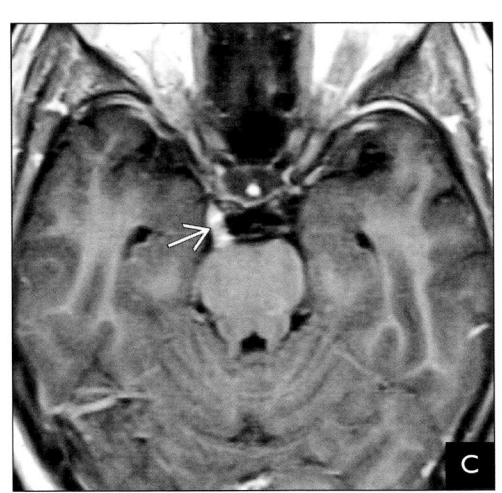

23-56B. Sagittal T1 C+ scan in the same patient shows tubular enlargement of the oculomotor nerve ➡ extending from its midbrain exit to the cavernous sinus. 23-56C. Axial T1 C+ scan in the same patient shows the enlarged, intensely enhancing right oculomotor nerve ➡. The lesion was unchanged after 3 years. Presumed schwannoma.

23-57A. *Axial T1 C+ FS scan shows a small enhancing tumor in the left ambient cistern* ➡. ***23-57B.*** *Coronal T1 C+ FS scan in the same patient shows that the tumor* ➡ *lies along the expected course of CN IV. Probable trochlear schwannoma.*

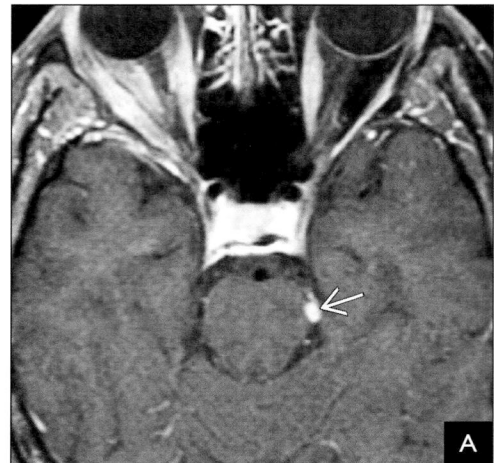

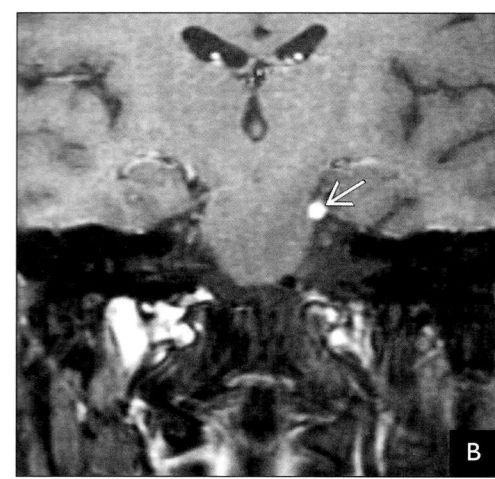

23-58. *Graphic depicts hypoglossal schwannoma. CN XII schwannomas have a "dumbbell" shape with a cisternal segment* ➡, *relative constriction in the bony hypoglossal canal* ➡, *larger extracranial component* ➡. ***23-59.*** *Close-up view of coronal bone CT with hypoglossal schwannoma shows enlarged hypoglossal canal* ➡ *with thinning, remodeling of the jugular tubercle* ➡ *("head" and "beak" of the "eagle," as seen in Figure 23-27).*

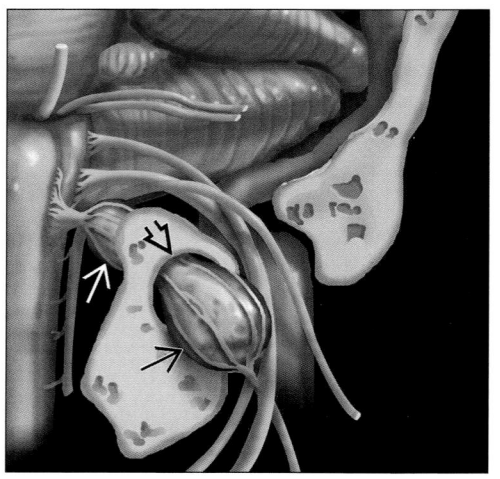

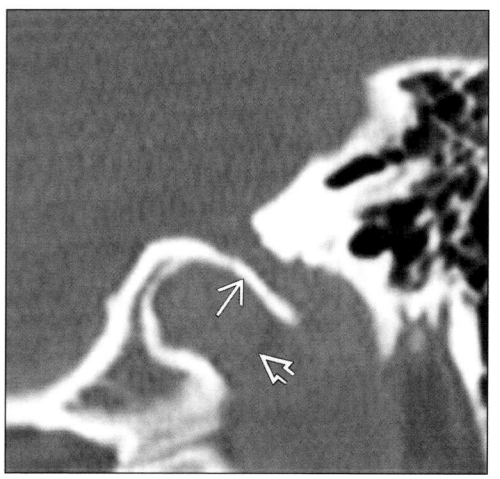

23-60A. *Axial T1WI shows tongue atrophy with hyperintense fatty infiltration of the left side of the tongue* ➡. ***23-60B.*** *Axial T1 C+ FS scan in the same patient shows hypoglossal schwannoma with a small cisternal segment* ➡, *an enlarged bony hypoglossal canal* ➡, *a large extracranial tumor mass* ➡. *Contrast with the normal right hypoglossal canal* ➡.

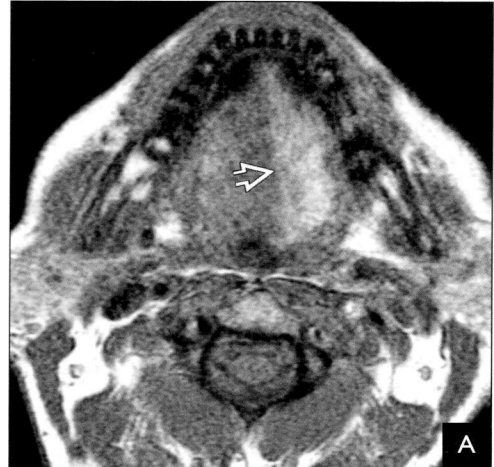

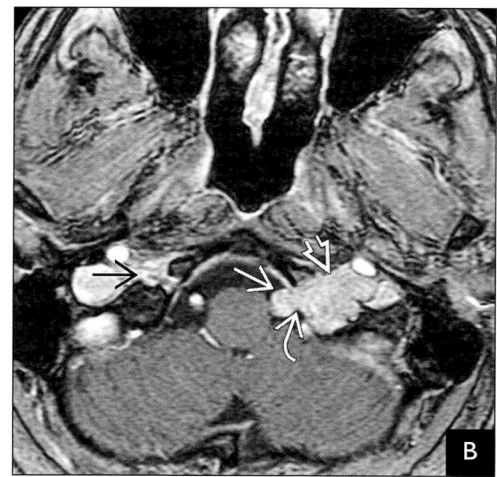

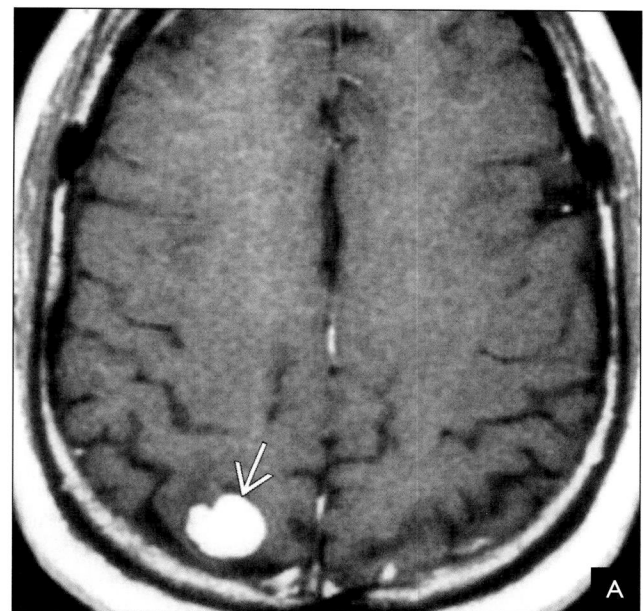

23-61A. Axial T1 C+ scan shows a well-demarcated, enhancing parenchymal mass ➡ without edema.

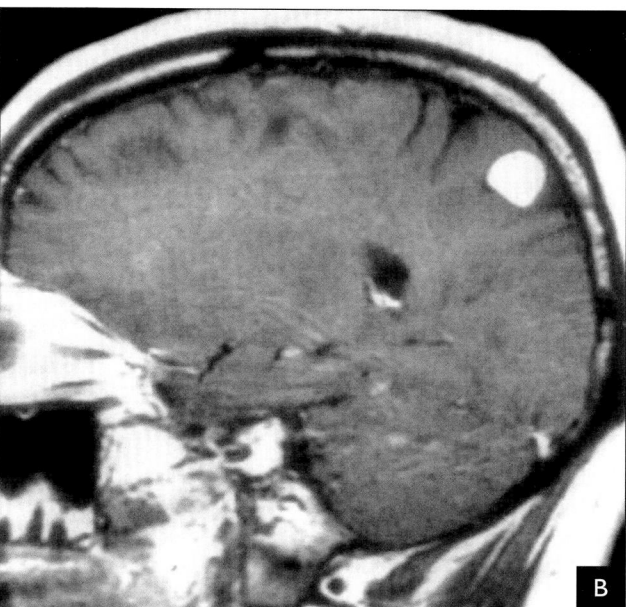

23-61B. Sagittal T1 C+ scan in the same patient shows that the lesion is clearly intraaxial. Parenchymal schwannoma was diagnosed at histopathology.

the midbrain **(23-56)**. The second most common site is the cavernous sinus. Most intracranial oculomotor schwannomas are small, generally measuring less than 0.5 cm in diameter. Combined orbitocavernous sinus schwannomas are somewhat larger, extending from the orbit through the superior orbital fissure into the cavernous sinus.

Intraorbital schwannomas are rare. As a group, they account for just 1% of all orbital tumors. They typically present with slowly progressive proptosis and seldom develop diplopia.

rochlear (CN IV) Schwannoma

Trochlear nerve schwannomas are uncommon **(23-57)**. They cause diplopia (isolated unilateral superior oblique palsy) and compensatory head tilt that may be misdiagnosed clinically as "wry neck." Most CN IV schwannomas are small and are either simply watched or treated with prism spectacles.

bducens (CN VI) Schwannoma

Schwannomas of the abducens nerve are extremely rare. Most patients present with a history of diplopia.

Schwannomas can occur anywhere along the entire length of the nerve, including its intracavernous and orbital segments. Most are found in the cerebellopontine angle cistern, adjacent to the pontomesencephalic junction. They typically displace the facial/vestibulocochlear nerve complex posterosuperiorly and may be difficult to distinguish on imaging studies from schwannomas that arise from the cisternal segments of these nerves.

Hypoglossal (CN XII) Schwannoma

Hypoglossal tumors are the rarest of the "other" schwannomas, accounting for only 5% of all nonvestibular intracranial schwannomas **(23-58)**. Over 90% present with denervation hemiatrophy of the tongue **(23-60)**.

Most CN XII schwannomas originate intracranially but can also extend extracranially as a "dumbbell" tumor that expands and remodels the hypoglossal canal **(23-59)**. Most are solid enhancing masses **(23-60)**, although cystic and even hemorrhagic CN XII schwannomas have been reported.

Parenchymal Schwannomas

Because the brain parenchyma does not contain Schwann cells, schwannomas not associated with cranial nerves are very rare. Most reported cases of intraparenchymal schwannoma are found in the frontal and temporal lobes. Parenchymal schwannomas have also been described in the cerebellar hemispheres, vermis, brainstem, and cerebral ventricles.

Parenchymal schwannomas may arise from ectopic neural crest cells that become displaced during embryogenesis. Other possible etiologies include origin in the sympathetic nerve plexus that surrounds cerebral blood vessels.

Pathologically, two-thirds of cases are either cystic or contain areas of cystic degeneration. The histology of parenchymal schwannoma is indistinguishable from that of other schwannomas.

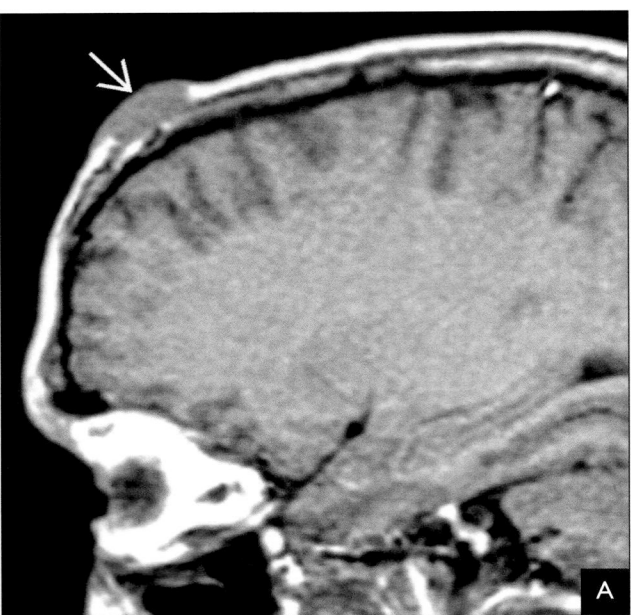

23-62A. *Sagittal T1WI in a 17-year-old male with a longstanding painless scalp mass shows a well-demarcated isointense soft tissue mass* ➡.

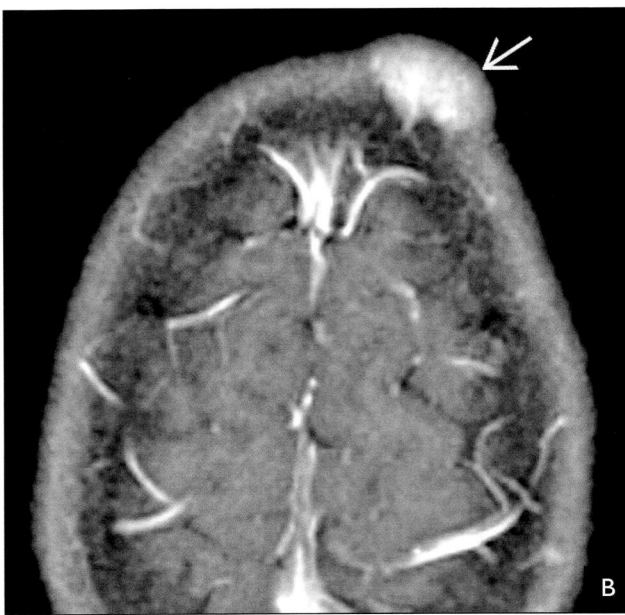

23-62B. *Axial T1 C+ FS scan in the same patient shows that the lesion enhances intensely* ➡. *Solitary neurofibroma was found at surgery.*

On imaging studies, most intracranial parenchymal schwannomas appear well-demarcated. The most common imaging pattern is that of a cyst with a mural nodule and peripheral enhancement. One-third are solid tumors with strong homogeneous or heterogeneous enhancement **(23-61)**. Peritumoral edema varies from none to moderate.

Neurofibromas

Intracranial neurofibromas (NFs) are much less common than schwannomas. NFs can affect the scalp, skull, some cranial nerves (especially CN V$_1$), or—rarely—the brain. They are found at all ages. Both sexes are affected equally.

NFs can be solitary or multiple. Multiple NFs and plexiform NFs occur only in connection with neurofibromatosis type 1 (NF1).

The gross appearance of NFs is different from that of schwannomas. Schwannomas are well-delineated encapsulated lesions that arise eccentrically from their parent nerve. Schwannomas typically displace elements of the normal parent nerve to one side. In contrast, neurofibromas generally present as more diffuse nerve expansions. They display single or multiple fascicles that enter and leave the affected nerve. Axons of the parent nerve pass through neurofibromas and are intermixed with tumor cells, distinguishing them from schwannoma.

The microscopic appearance of NFs also differs from that of schwannomas. Schwannomas are pure Schwann cell tumors. Neurofibromas consist of both Schwann cells and fibroblasts. NFs also contain other cell types, including perineural cells, mast cells, pericytes, endothelial cells, and smooth muscle cells. NFs also typically have a large amount of extracellular matrix with collagen.

In this section, we discuss both solitary and plexiform neurofibromas. Both neurofibromatosis types 1 and 2 are discussed in Chapter 39.

Solitary Neurofibroma

A solitary neurofibroma in the head and neck rarely—if ever—involves cranial nerves. Solitary neurofibromas affect patients of all ages and are usually sporadic (nonsyndromic). Most occur in the absence of NF1 and present as a painless scalp or skin mass.

Solitary neurofibromas are round or ovoid unencapsulated masses composed of Schwann cells and fibroblasts in a myxoid or collagenous matrix. Solitary neurofibromas are WHO grade I neoplasms.

Scalp solitary neurofibromas are seen on imaging studies as well-delineated, focal, enhancing masses that abut but do not invade the calvaria **(23-62)**.

Plexiform Neurofibroma

Terminology and Etiology

Plexiform neurofibromas (PNFs) are infiltrative intra- and extraneural neoplasms that occur almost exclusively in patients with NF1 **(23-63)**. Rarely, these tumors occur without other signs of NF1. Biallelic inactivation of the NF1 gene has been identified in sporadic PNFs.

Pathology

LOCATION. Approximately one-third of PNFs are found in the head and neck. Cranial PNFs usually involve CNs V, IX, or X. The most typical locations are the scalp, orbit, pterygopalatine fossa, and parotid gland. Scalp and orbital PNFs most commonly involve the ophthalmic branches of the trigeminal nerve. Parotid PNFs involve peripheral branches of the facial nerve.

Extracranial PNFs are often multicompartmental and do not respect fascial boundaries. Orbital PNFs may enlarge the superior orbital fissure and extend into the cavernous sinus as far as Meckel cave **(23-64)**.

SIZE AND NUMBER. PNFs are typically extensive, diffusely infiltrating lesions. Multiple variably sized lesions are typical.

GROSS AND MICROSCOPIC FEATURES. Grossly, PNFs have a distinctive "bag of worms" appearance **(23-65)**. PNFs demonstrate a predominant intrafascicular growth pattern, with redundant loops of expanded nerve fascicles intermixed with collagen fibers and mucoid material **(23-66)**.

STAGING, GRADING, AND CLASSIFICATION. PNFs are WHO grade I neoplasms.

Clinical Issues

PNFs are a major cause of morbidity in patients with NF1. Approximately 5% of PNFs eventually degenerate into malignant peripheral nerve sheath tumors.

Imaging

GENERAL FEATURES. PNFs are poorly delineated worm-like soft tissue masses that diffusely infiltrate the scalp, orbit, or parotid gland.

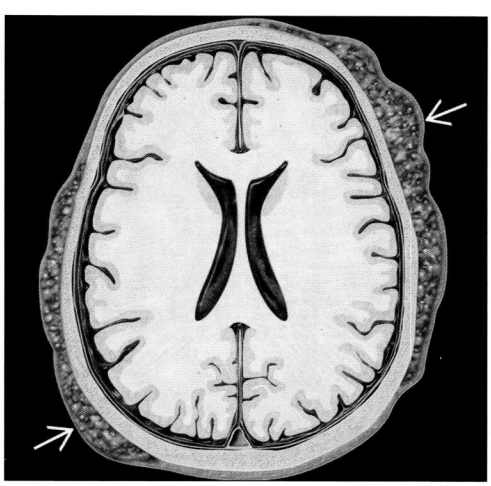

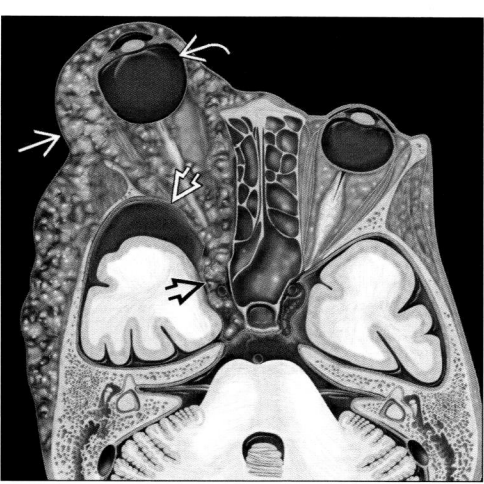

23-63. Graphic depicts plexiform neurofibromas (PNFs) diffusely infiltrating, deforming the scalp ➡. 23-64. Axial graphic depicts extensive PNF ➡ of the right face and orbit, infiltrating the cavernous sinus ▷ in a patient with NF1. Buphthalmos ("cow eye") ➘, sphenoid wing hypoplasia ▷ are other features of NF1 that are illustrated here.

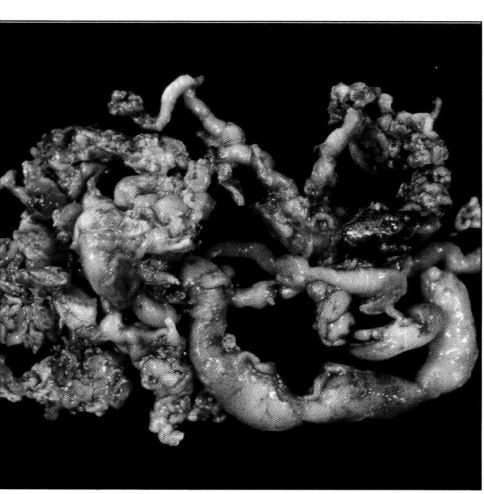

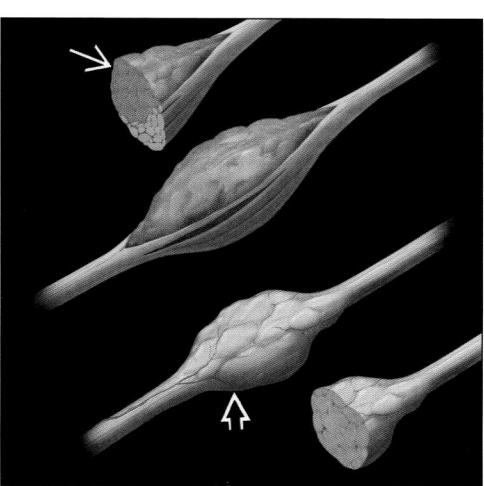

23-65. Gross pathology shows plexiform neurofibroma with multiple enlarged, worm-like tumor fascicles. (Courtesy R. Hewlett, MD.) 23-66. Graphic depicts the difference between schwannoma (above) and neurofibroma (below). Schwannomas ➡ displace nerve fascicles whereas neurofibromas ➡ infiltrate between fascicles.

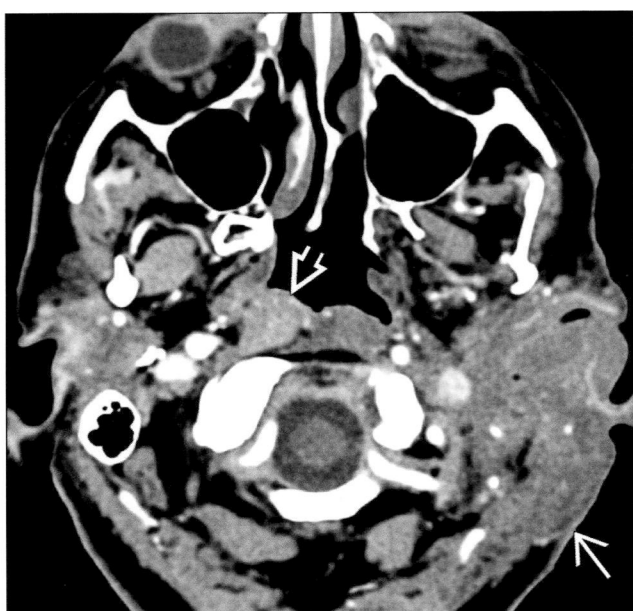

23-67. *CECT shows PNF as a minimally enhancing infiltrating mass ▷ that involves the subcutaneous soft tissues, parotid gland. Another PNF is seen in the right prevertebral muscle ▷. (Courtesy C. Glastonbury, MBBS.)*

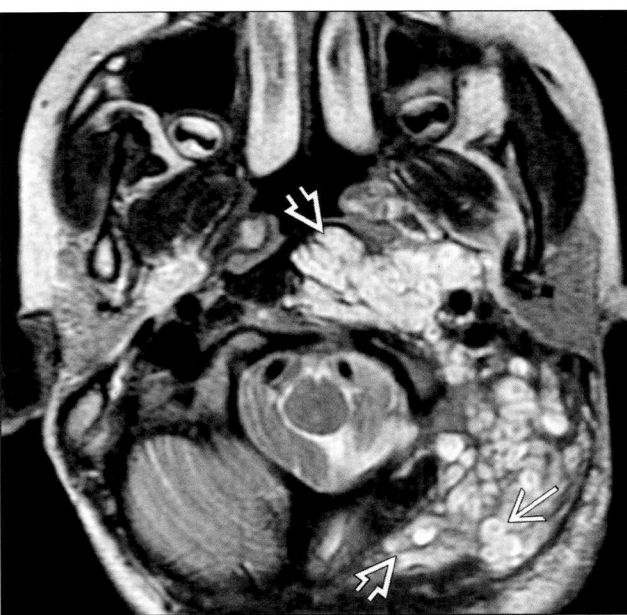

23-68. *T2WI in a patient with NF1 shows the characteristic findings of PNF. Multilobulated hyperintense masses ▷ with central hypointense ▷ "dots" are typical. (Courtesy C. Glastonbury, MBBS.)*

CT FINDINGS. PNFs infiltrate and enlarge soft tissues, typically the scalp and periorbita. They are generally isodense with muscle. Calcification and hemorrhage are rare.

CECT shows heterogeneous enhancement **(23-67)**. Bone CT may show expansion of the superior orbital fissure and pterygopalatine fossa.

MR FINDINGS. PNFs are isointense on T1WI and hyperintense on T2WI. Strong, sometimes heterogeneous enhancement is typical. A "target" sign of hypointensity within an enhancing tumor fascicle is seen in some PNFs but is not considered pathognomonic **(23-68)**.

Differential Diagnosis

The major differential diagnosis of PNF is **malignant peripheral nerve sheath tumor (MPNST)**. As many MPNSTs arise from PNFs, early differentiation may be difficult. If a previously quiescent PNF enlarges rapidly or becomes painful, malignant degeneration into MPNST should be suspected. Most MPNSTs are invasive as well as infiltrating lesions.

Schwannomas are well-circumscribed solitary lesions that involve cranial nerves, especially CN VIII. In contrast to PNF, scalp and orbital schwannomas are uncommon. **Basal cell carcinoma** and infiltrating skin/scalp **metastases** without concomitant involvement of the underlying skull are rare. Scalp **sarcomas** and **lymphomas** are likewise rare. When present, they are more diffusely infiltrating, homogeneous lesions without normal-appearing tissue interspersed within the mass.

NEUROFIBROMA

Solitary Neurofibroma
- Most are sporadic (nonsyndromic)
- All ages (children to adults)
- Nodular to polypoid
- Scalp, skin
- Rarely (if ever) involves cranial nerves

Plexiform Neurofibroma
- Pathology
  - Composed of Schwann cells + fibroblasts, mucoid material
  - Fusiform, infiltrates nerve
  - Often multicompartmental
  - Does not respect fascial boundaries
- Clinical issues
  - Usually diagnostic of NF1
  - "Sporadic" PNFs can occur without other signs of NF1, but most have NF1 gene alterations
  - Risk of malignant degeneration in PNF = 5%
  - Rapid/painful enlargement, invasion? Suspect MPNST!
- Imaging
  - Multifocal scalp, orbit lesions most common
  - "Bag of worms" appearance
  - May enlarge SOF, extend into cavernous sinus
  - Intracranial involvement rare unless malignant degeneration
- Differential diagnosis
  - MPNST (invasive)
  - Schwannoma (usually solitary; skin/scalp lesions, plexiform schwannoma rare)
  - Metastases

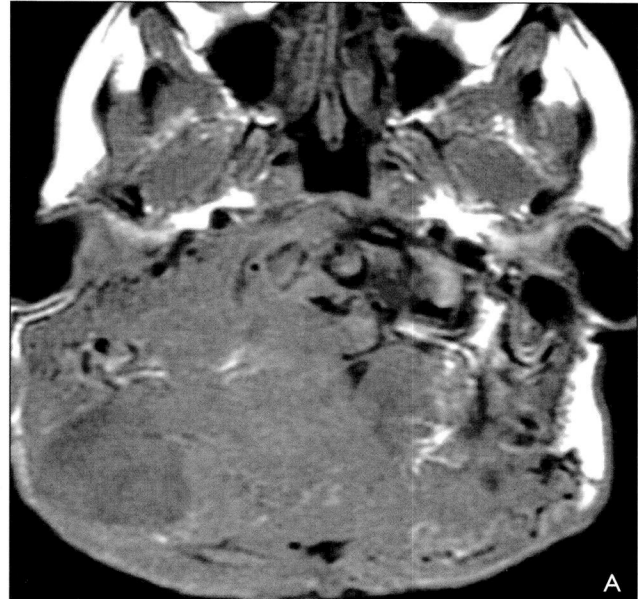

23-69A. *An NF1 patient with a longstanding PNF experienced rapid enlargement of the mass, which became painful. T1WI shows a massive soft tissue mass invading the skull base and upper cervical spine.*

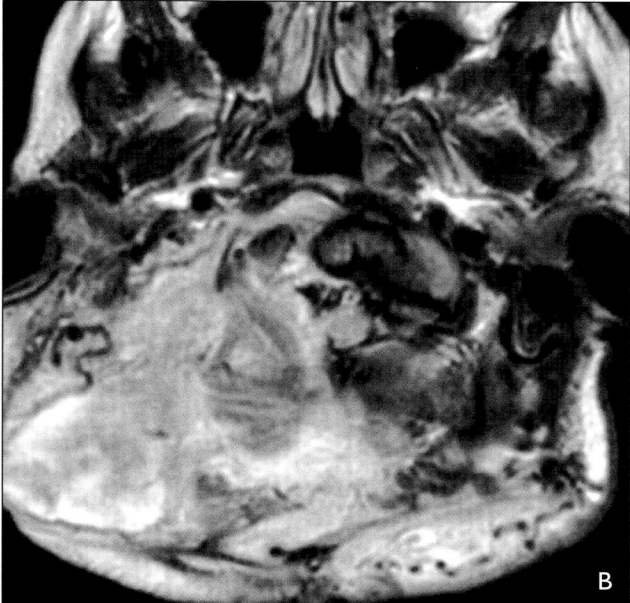

23-69B. *T1 C+ shows that the mass enhances intensely but very heterogeneously. The size, extent, and invasive nature of the mass were significantly different from prior baseline studies. MPNST was found at biopsy.*

Malignant Nerve Sheath Neoplasms

Malignant Peripheral Nerve Sheath Tumor

Terminology

A malignant peripheral nerve sheath tumor (MPNST) is any malignant tumor that arises from a peripheral nerve or shows nerve sheath differentiation. This term replaces designations such as malignant schwannoma, malignant neurofibroma, neurosarcoma, and neurofibrosarcoma.

When it occurs intracranially, an MPNST is sometimes called a malignant intracerebral nerve sheath tumor or a primary malignant intracranial nerve sheath tumor.

Etiology

Approximately half of all cranial MPNSTs occur sporadically, most likely from pluripotent neural crest cells. The other half arise from a preexisting benign nerve sheath tumor. Identifiable precursor lesions reported with MPNSTs include both plexiform and solitary intraneural neurofibroma. Malignant transformation of conventional or cellular schwannomas is exceptionally rare.

Approximately two-thirds of *peripheral* MPNSTs are associated with malignant degeneration of tumors associated with NF1. The overall lifetime risk of developing an MPNST at any location in patients with NF1 is estimated at 8-13%.

In a recent series of *intracranial* MPNSTs, 5 of 17 patients had NF1. Four had post-irradiation MPNSTs.

Pathology

LOCATION. MPNST is much more common in the peripheral or spinal nerves than in the cranial nerves. The most commonly affected cranial nerves are the vestibular, facial, and trigeminal nerves. Intracranial MPNSTs not associated with cranial nerves are extremely rare.

SIZE AND NUMBER. The majority of MPNSTs are over five centimeters, although intracranial lesions may be smaller at initial diagnosis.

MICROSCOPIC FEATURES. MPNST is a widely infiltrating, hypercellular lesion that shows proliferating malignant spindle cells with numerous mitoses. Immunohistochemistry differentiates tumors of nerve sheath derivation from soft tissue sarcomas. The majority of cases show diffuse, strong immunoreactivity for p53 protein along with S100 and collagen IV-laminin staining.

Triton tumor is an MPNST subtype that demonstrates rhabdomyosarcomatous differentiation.

STAGING, GRADING, AND CLASSIFICATION. Peripheral MPNSTs are often graded according to the Enneking classification of bone and soft tissue extremity sarcomas. In contrast, intracranial MPNSTs are graded (as are all brain tumors) on the WHO scale. Virtually all intracranial MPNSTs are histologically high grade and are designated as WHO grade III and IV neoplasms.

Clinical Issues

EPIDEMIOLOGY. MPNSTs are rare, accounting for only 0.001% of malignant neoplasms. MPNSTs that arise from cranial nerves are even rarer. Intracranial MPNSTs not associated with cranial nerves are exceptionally rare.

DEMOGRAPHICS. Although they can occur at almost any age, sporadic MPNSTs are primarily tumors of middle-aged and older adults. Peak occurrence is in the fifth and sixth decades. NF1-associated MPNSTs occur earlier, with mean age 20-35 years. MPNSTs show a slight female predominance.

NATURAL HISTORY. Intracranial MPNSTs are fast-growing, aggressive, highly invasive tumors that generally have the same poor prognosis as those of spinal and peripheral nerves. MPNSTs are fatal in two-thirds of all patients. Most die as a result of disseminated metastases despite surgery, radiation, and chemotherapy.

TREATMENT OPTIONS. Total tumor resection with adjuvant radiotherapy is the treatment mainstay. Even with tumor-free margins, recurrence is common (40-70%). Survival of patients with subtotal tumor removal is generally less than one year.

Imaging

There are no obvious characteristics that would differentiate MPNST from benign nerve sheath tumor on a single baseline imaging study. Gross necrosis or hemorrhage is rare. A few tumors may initially show frank brain or skull invasion, poor margination, and edema. MRS findings are nonspecific. Elevated choline is common.

It is the behavior on *serial* imaging studies that helps distinguish MPNST from benign nerve sheath tumors. Aggressive growth with brain and bone invasion is typical **(23-69)**. CSF dissemination often rapidly ensues after the initial diagnosis is established. Distant extracranial metastases, most often to the lung, are common.

Differential Diagnosis

Small MPNSTs may be indistinguishable from benign nerve sheath tumors. The major differential diagnosis of a scalp or skull base MPNST is **plexiform neurofibroma** (PNF). Both are diffusely infiltrating, poorly marginated lesions. When PNFs extend intracranially, they expand natural foramina and fissures but do not directly invade bone or brain. Rapid enlargement and bone destruction are more consistent with MPNST.

The rare brain parenchymal MPNST that is not associated with a cranial nerve is indistinguishable from other highly aggressive, invasive malignant neoplasms. The major differential diagnoses include **glioblastoma multiforme**, **gliosarcoma**, **fibrosarcoma**, and **malignant fibrous histiocytoma**.

MALIGNANT PERIPHERAL NERVE SHEATH TUMOR

Terminology
- MPNST is the accepted term (replaces malignant schwannoma, neurofibrosarcoma)

Pathology
- Location
  ○ Peripheral/spinal > > cranial nerves
  ○ Vestibular, facial, trigeminal most common intracranial locations
- Features
  ○ Widely infiltrating
  ○ Malignant spindle cells, numerous mitoses
  ○ IHC distinguishes MPNST from other sarcomas
  ○ WHO grade III or IV

Clinical Issues
- Rare; usually middle-aged, older adults
- Younger if NF1-associated
- Many arise de novo or from malignant degeneration of neurofibroma
- 8-13% risk of MPNST in plexiform neurofibroma

Imaging
- No distinctive imaging features
- Behavior on serial imaging best indicator
- Rapid aggressive growth
- Invasion, CSF dissemination

Other Nerve Sheath Tumors

A number of other neoplasms occasionally involve cranial nerves, though most are much more common in peripheral nerves and soft tissues. Examples include perineurioma, solitary fibrous tumor, and neurofibrosarcoma. WHO grades vary from benign (grade I) to malignant (WHO grades II and III).

Intraneural **perineuriomas** account for just 1% of nerve sheath tumors. Perineuriomas involving cranial nerves are very rare. Reported cases primarily involved extracranial branches of the trigeminal or facial nerves.

A subpopulation of **solitary fibrous tumors** (SFTs) arise directly from nerves rather than the meninges, where they mimic dura-based lesions such as meningioma. SFTs that arise from intracranial CNs are indistinguishable from schwannomas on imaging studies, so the definitive diagnosis is histopathological.

Neurofibrosarcomas are more properly considered malignant nerve sheath tumors (whether peripheral or intracranial). Intracranial extension from malignant degeneration of a scalp plexiform neurofibroma is a common source of these lesions.

elected References

Cranial Nerve Anatomy

Upper Cranial Nerves

- Honoré A et al: Isolation, characterization, and genetic profiling of subpopulations of olfactory ensheathing cells from the olfactory bulb. Glia. 60(3):404-13, 2012
- Kralik SF et al: Evaluation of orbital disorders and cranial nerve innervation of the extraocular muscles. Magn Reson Imaging Clin N Am. 20(3):413-34, 2012

Lower Cranial Nerves

- Hong HS et al: Enhancement pattern of the normal facial nerve at 3.0 T temporal MRI. Br J Radiol. 83(986):118-21, 2010
- Sheth S et al: Appearance of normal cranial nerves on steady-state free precession MR images. Radiographics. 29(4):1045-55, 2009. Erratum in: Radiographics. 29(5):1544, 2009
- Harnsberger HR: Cranial nerves. In Diagnostic and Surgical Imaging Anatomy: Brain, Head and Neck, Spine. Salt Lake City: Amirsys Publishing. I.174-254, 2006

Schwannomas

- Ersen A et al: Conventional schwannoma. In Burger P et al: Diagnostic Pathology: Neuropathology. Salt Lake City: Amirsys Publishing. I.4.2-11, 2012
- Scheithauer BW et al: Schwannoma. In Louis DN et al: WHO Classification of Tumours of the Central Nervous System. Lyon, France: IARC Press. 152-5, 2007

Schwannoma Overview

- Gonzalvo A et al: Schwannomatosis, sporadic schwannomatosis, and familial schwannomatosis: a surgical series with long-term follow-up. J Neurosurg. 114(3):756-62, 2011

Vestibular Schwannoma

- Kohno M et al: Is an acoustic neuroma an epiarachnoid or subarachnoid tumor? Neurosurgery. 68(4):1006-16; discussion 1016-7, 2011
- Sughrue ME et al: Molecular biology of familial and sporadic vestibular schwannomas: implications for novel therapeutics. J Neurosurg. 114(2):359-66, 2011

Trigeminal Schwannoma

- Muto J et al: Meckel's cave tumors: relation to the meninges and minimally invasive approaches for surgery: anatomic and clinical studies. Neurosurgery. 67(3 Suppl Operative):291-8; discussion 298-9, 2010
- Sharma BS et al: Trigeminal schwannomas: experience with 68 cases. J Clin Neurosci. 15(7):738-43, 2008
- Moffat D et al: Surgical management of trigeminal neuromas: a report of eight cases. J Laryngol Otol. 120(8):631-7, 2006

Jugular Foramen Schwannoma

- Vorasubin N et al: Glossopharyngeal schwannomas: a 100 year review. Laryngoscope. 119(1):26-35, 2009
- Bulsara KR et al: Microsurgical management of 53 jugular foramen schwannomas: lessons learned incorporated into a modified grading system. J Neurosurg. 109(5):794-803, 2008

Facial Nerve Schwannoma

- Wiggins RH 3rd et al: The many faces of facial nerve schwannoma. AJNR Am J Neuroradiol. 27(3):694-9, 2006

Schwannomas of Other Intracranial Nerves

- Nonaka Y et al: Microsurgical management of hypoglossal schwannomas over 3 decades: a modified grading scale to guide surgical approach. Neurosurgery. 69(2 Suppl Operative):ons121-40; discussion ons140, 2011
- Darie I et al: Olfactory ensheathing cell tumour: case report and literature review. J Neurooncol. 100(2):285-9, 2010
- Elmalem VI et al: Clinical course and prognosis of trochlear nerve schwannomas. Ophthalmology. 116(10):2011-6, 2009
- Park JH et al: Abducens nerve schwannoma: case report and review of the literature. Neurosurg Rev. 32(3):375-8; discussion 378, 2009
- Fisher LM et al: Distribution of nonvestibular cranial nerve schwannomas in neurofibromatosis 2. Otol Neurotol. 28(8):1083-90, 2007

Parenchymal Schwannomas

- Muzzafar S et al: Imaging and clinical features of an intra-axial brain stem schwannoma. AJNR Am J Neuroradiol. 31(3):567-9, 2010
- Casadei GP et al: Intracranial parenchymal schwannoma. A clinicopathological and neuroimaging study of nine cases. J Neurosurg. 79(2):217-22, 1993

Neurofibromas

- Gottfried ON et al: Molecular, genetic, and cellular pathogenesis of neurofibromas and surgical implications. Neurosurgery. 58(1):1-16; discussion 1-16, 2006

Plexiform Neurofibroma

- Bechtold D et al: Plexiform neurofibroma of the eye region occurring in patients without neurofibromatosis type 1. Ophthal Plast Reconstr Surg. Epub ahead of print, 2012
- Beert E et al: Biallelic inactivation of NF1 in a sporadic plexiform neurofibroma. Genes Chromosomes Cancer. 51(9):852-7, 2012
- Yoon SH et al: A study of 77 cases of surgically excised scalp and skull masses in pediatric patients. Childs Nerv Syst. 24(4):459-65, 2008

- Park WC et al: The role of highresolution computed tomography and magnetic resonance imaging in the evaluation of isolated orbital neurofibromas. Am J Ophthalmol. 142(3):456-63, 2006

Malignant Nerve Sheath Neoplasms

Malignant Peripheral Nerve Sheath Tumor

- Guo A et al: Malignant peripheral nerve sheath tumors: differentiation patterns and immunohistochemical features - a mini-review and our new findings. J Cancer. 3:303-309, 2012
- Ziadi A et al: Malignant peripheral nerve sheath tumor of intracranial nerve: a case series review. Auris Nasus Larynx. 37(5):539-45, 2010
- Scheithauer BW et al: Malignant peripheral nerve sheath tumors of cranial nerves and intracranial contents: a clinicopathologic study of 17 cases. Am J Surg Pathol. 33(3):325-38, 2009
- Kozic D et al: Malignant peripheral nerve sheath tumor of the oculomotor nerve. Acta Radiol. 47(6):595-8, 2006

Other Nerve Sheath Tumors

- Rodriguez FJ et al: Pathology of peripheral nerve sheath tumors: diagnostic overview and update on selected diagnostic problems. Acta Neuropathol. 123(3):295-319, 2012
- Abreu E et al: Peripheral tumor and tumor-like neurogenic lesions. Eur J Radiol. Epub ahead of print, 2011
- Waldron JS et al: Solitary fibrous tumor arising from Cranial Nerve VI in the prepontine cistern: case report and review of a tumor subpopulation mimicking schwannoma. Neurosurgery. 59(4):E939-40; discussion E940, 2006

24

Lymphomas, Hematopoietic and Histiocytic Tumors

The spectrum of hematopoietic neoplasms and tumor-like disorders ranges from nonneoplastic lesions such as extramedullary hemapoiesis and the histiocytoses to frankly malignant neoplasms like lymphoma.

We begin our discussion with the most common of these lesions, CNS lymphoma. We first focus on **primary CNS lymphoma**. We then consider other primary CNS lymphoma subtypes, including **intravascular (angiocentric) lymphoma**, a very special CNS lymphoma that spreads through blood vessels and along perivascular spaces.

Nonmalignant and premalignant lymphomatoid conditions, including **lymphomatoid granulomatosis** and **post-transplant lymphoproliferative disorder**, can occasionally affect the CNS. Both are discussed in the lymphoma section.

Histiocytic tumors can involve the CNS. These neoplasms and nonneoplastic tumor-like masses are composed of histiocytes that are microscopically identical to their extracranial counterparts. Both **Langerhans cell histiocytosis** and **non-Langerhans histiocytoses** are considered.

We then turn our attention to **leukemia**. While the most recent WHO classification of CNS neoplasms includes only malignant lymphomas and histiocytic tumors in the group of hematopoietic neoplasms, we include leukemia in this chapter even though CNS involvement is almost always secondary to systemic disease. **Plasmacytoma** and **multiple myeloma** affecting the skull and brain are also usually secondary to extracranial disease, but they too are included here rather than in Chapter 27 on metastases.

We conclude this chapter with a discussion of **extramedullary hematopoiesis**—benign, nonneoplastic proliferations of blood-forming elements—which can appear virtually identical to malignant hematopoietic neoplasms and is discussed with nonneoplastic tumor-like conditions

Lymphomas

The CNS can be involved by a variety of lymphoid lesions that occur either as primary tumors or metastatic deposits from extracranial disease. Together, lymphoid neoplasms comprise the sixth most common group of CNS malignancies.

All lymphoid neoplasms, including lymphoma, myeloma, and lymphoid leukemia, arise from malignant transformation of normal lymphoid cells. As the CNS lacks lymphatics and lymphoid tissue, how and why lymphomas can arise as primary CNS neoplasms is unknown. What is clearly evident is that lymphoma cells—regardless of whether they originate within or outside the brain—exhibit a distinct, highly selective neurotropism for the CNS microenvironment and its vasculature.

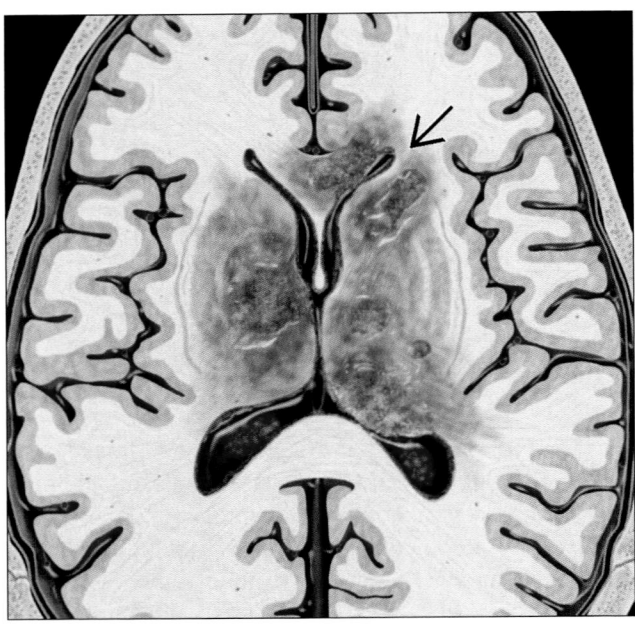

24-1. Multiple periventricular lesions with involvement of the basal ganglia, thalamus, and corpus callosum, typical of primary PCNSL. Note the extensive subependymal spread of disease ⇨; PCNSL typically extends along ependymal surfaces.

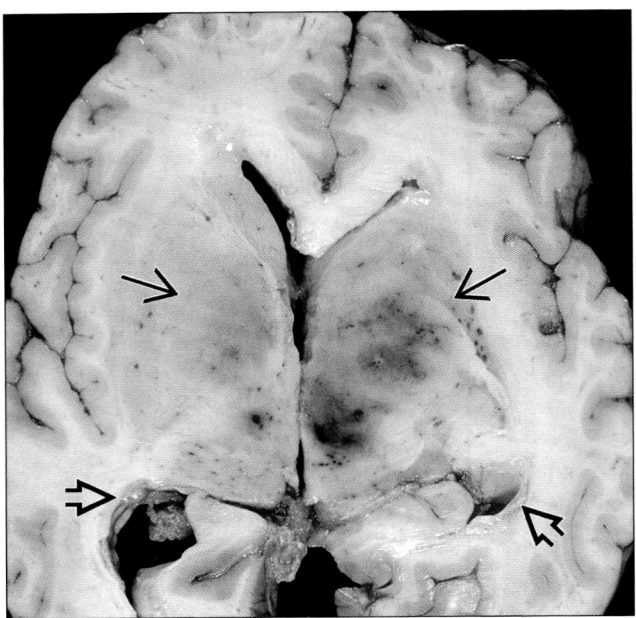

24-2. Autopsy specimen shows PCNSL with bilateral deep basal ganglionic, thalamic masses ⇨, tumor spread around the ependyma of the lateral ventricles ⇨. (Courtesy R. Hewlett, MD.)

More than 95% of primary CNS lymphomas (PCNSLs) are diffuse large B-cell lymphomas (DLBCLs). Other PCNSL subtypes accounting for less than 5% of cases. CNS Hodgkin-type lymphomas (HLs) are uncommon. Most are seen in the setting of advanced systemic disease, but rare primary CNS lesions have been described. Extranodal natural killer (NK) T-cell lymphomas typically involve the nasal cavity and affect the CNS only when they extend into the anterior cranial fossa through the cribriform plate.

We begin our discussion of primary CNS lymphoma by focusing on DLBCL. We then consider a few of the non-DLBCL lymphomas, including intravascular lymphoma, lymphomatosis cerebri, MALT lymphoma, and post-transplant lymphoproliferative disorder (PTLD). We close the section with a brief review of CNS metastatic lymphoma. (Metastatic lymphoma is included here instead of in Chapter 27 with other metastatic disease as its imaging appearance differs from that of other systemic cancers that spread to the brain.)

Primary CNS Lymphoma

Terminology

Primary CNS lymphoma (PCNSL) is a rare variant of extranodal non-Hodgkin lymphoma restricted to the brain, spinal cord, eye, and meninges. By definition, disease outside the nervous system is absent at the time of initial diagnosis.

Etiology

GENERAL CONCEPTS. Although the precise etiology of PCNSL is unknown, many investigators believe it probably arises from germinal center lymphoid precursor cells.

PCNSL develops in both immunocompetent and immunodeficient patients. **Autoimmune diseases** linked to PCNSL include rheumatoid arthritis, Sjögren syndrome, and systemic lupus erythematosus.

Some lymphomas are linked to viral infections. PCNSLs associated with **Epstein-Barr virus** (EBV) account for 10-15% of all cases.

Congenital immunodeficiency syndromes increase the risk of lymphoma, as does severe acquired immunosuppression. Congenital immunodeficiency syndromes include **Wiskott-Aldrich syndrome** and **severe combined immunodeficiency**.

CNS involvement occurs in 20-25% of **immunosuppressed** patients who develop post-transplant lymphomas (see below). Between 2-12% of **HIV/AIDS** patients on highly active antiretroviral therapy (HAART) eventually develop CNS lymphoma, generally during the later stages of their disease. These patients can exhibit elevated levels of B-cell-stimulatory cytokines and other markers of immune activation several years prior to the diagnosis of systemic AIDS-associated non-Hodgkin B-cell lymphomas.

GENETICS. PCNSL is associated with three distinct genetic "signatures" that parallel those of systemic

DLBCL: Germinal center B-cell, activated B-cell, and type 3 large B-cell lymphoma. Several genes associated with interleukin-4, a B-cell growth factor, are highly expressed in PCNSL.

athology

LOCATION. PCNSL can affect any part of the neuraxis. Over 95% of PCNSLs contact a CSF surface, either the ventricular ependyma or pia **(24-1)**. The cerebral hemispheres are the preferred site (85%). Lesions are often deep-seated with a predilection for the periventricular white matter, especially the corpus callosum. The basal ganglia and thalami are the next most common locations. Tumor spread along the ventricular ependyma and into the choroid plexus is seen in some cases **(24-2)**.

The hypothalamus, infundibulum, and pituitary gland are less common sites for PCNSL. Posterior fossa lesions are relatively rare (15% of cases).

PCNSL may develop in the dura, leptomeninges, calvarial vault, and central skull base although these areas are more commonly involved by metastatic spread from extracranial primary tumors.

Primary dura-based lymphomas are very rare. Most consist of T-cell lymphomas and low-grade B-cell lymphomas, often the lymphoplasmacytic or MALT types.

Ocular lymphomas are almost always high-grade B-cell lymphomas. In contrast, lymphomas of the orbital adnexa are most often MALT type tumors (see below).

SIZE AND NUMBER. PCNSL lesions vary in size from microscopic implants to large bulky masses.

An estimated 40-60% of PCNSLs are solitary lesions. Of the PCNSLs with multiple lesions, half are bilateral. Widely disseminated lesions—a condition termed "lymphomatosis cerebri"—are uncommon, occurring in 5% of cases (see below).

GROSS PATHOLOGY. Single or multiple hemispheric masses are typical. In contrast to astrocytomas, lymphomas tend to be relatively well-demarcated rather than diffusely infiltrating lesions. Most are solid, pale lesions with occasional small hemorrhagic foci. Frank necrosis

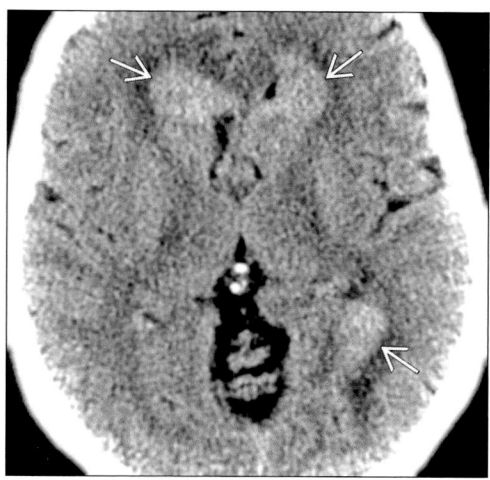
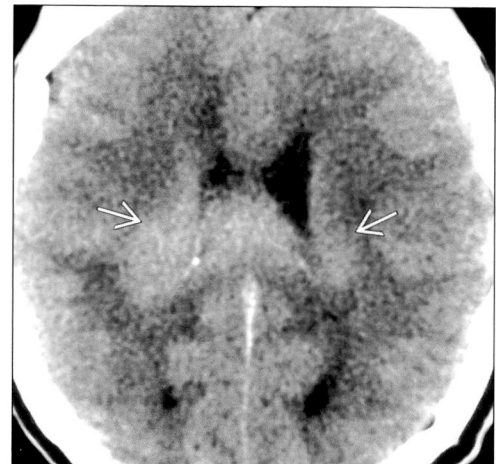

24-3. NECT scan shows multiple hyperdense masses bordering the lateral ventricles ➡, a characteristic finding in PCNSL. 24-4. NECT scan in another patient with PCNSL shows a "butterfly" hyperdense mass ➡ crossing the corpus callosum.

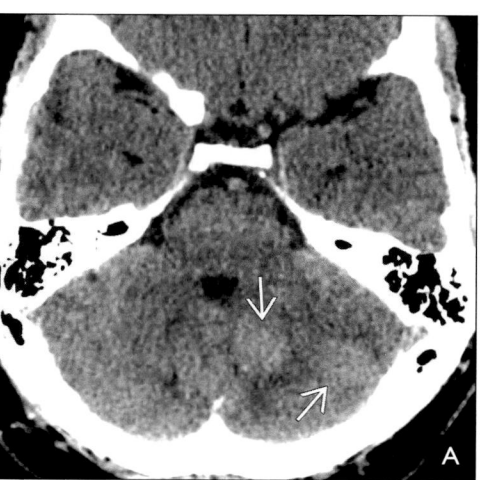
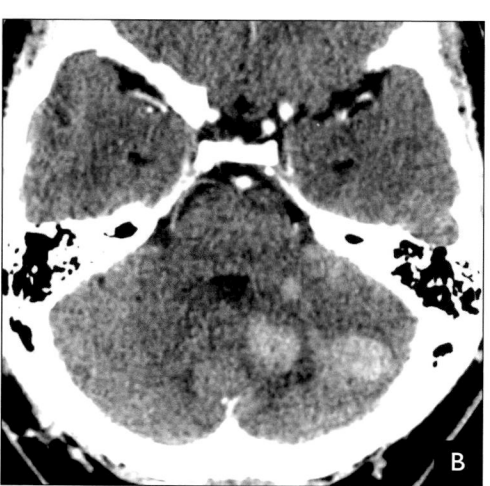

24-5A. NECT scan in a patient with PCNSL shows hyperdense masses in the left cerebellum ➡. 24-5B. CECT shows multiple moderately enhancing masses in the cerebellum. (Courtesy P. Hildenbrand, MD.)

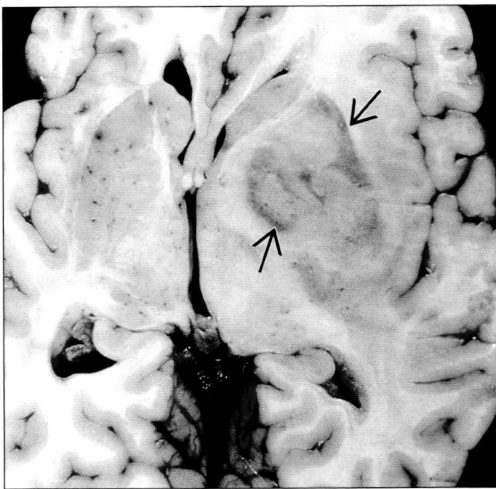

24-6. Autopsy specimen from an HIV/AIDS patient with PCNSL shows hemorrhagic, necrotic left basal ganglia mass ⤳. (Courtesy R. Hewlett, MD.)

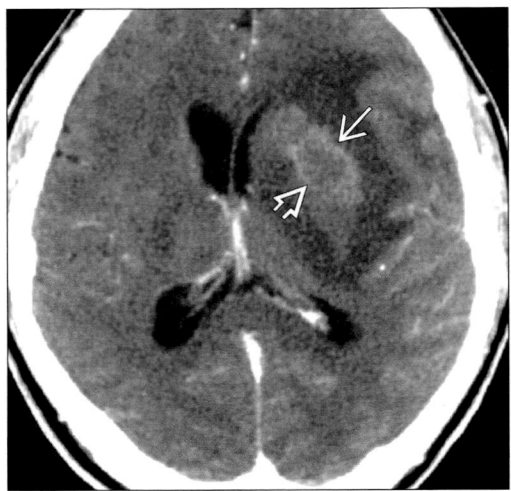

24-7. CECT scan shows necrosis ⇥, only faint rim enhancement ⇥ in this HIV-positive patient with PCNSL.

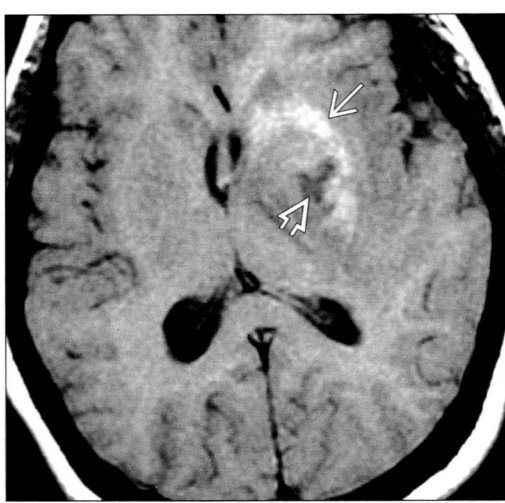

24-8. T1WI shows T1 shortening due to subacute hemorrhage ⇥ with more acute hemorrhage in the necrotic core of the lesion ⇥.

and gross intratumoral hemorrhage are more common in AIDS-related PCNSL (24-6).

MICROSCOPIC FEATURES. PCNSLs exhibit a predilection for blood vessels, resulting in a characteristic lymphoid clustering around small cerebral vessels. Tumor cells extend from these perivascular cuffs into the adjacent parenchyma.

Most PCNSLs are high-grade B-cell lymphomas that demonstrate predominance of immature blastic cells with large pleomorphic nuclei. MIB-1 is high, often exceeding 50 (significantly higher than with glioblastoma multiforme). Low-grade PCNSLs are uncommon and correspond histologically to their systemic counterparts.

PCNSL: ETIOLOGY AND PATHOLOGY

Etiology
- Precise origin unknown
- CNS lacks lymphatics, lymphocytes
- Increased risk with
  - Viruses (EBV, HIV/AIDS)
  - Congenital immunodeficiency syndromes
  - Severe immunosuppression (chemotherapy, long-term steroids)

Pathology
- 6% of all primary CNS neoplasms but increasing
- Predilection for deep brain
  - Periventricular WM, basal ganglia
  - Perivascular lymphoid clusters common
- Solitary (2/3), multiple (1/3)
  - Multiple compartments may be involved
- Focal > diffusely infiltrating lesions
- Hemorrhage, necrosis rare in immunocompetent
- Vast majority are non-Hodgkin lymphomas
- Diffuse large B-cell lymphomas (90-95%)
  - Immature blastic cells
  - MIB-1 > 50
- Low-grade, Burkitt, T-cell lymphomas (5-10%)
- Primary CNS Hodgkin lymphoma rare

Clinical Issues

EPIDEMIOLOGY. While PCNSL accounts for only 6% of all malignant CNS neoplasms, prevalence is increasing as a result of the HIV/AIDS epidemic and the use of immunosuppressive therapies.

DEMOGRAPHICS. Although PCNSLs can occur at all ages, they are generally tumors of middle-aged and older adults. Peak age in immunocompetent patients is 60 years. By comparison, mean age at onset in patients with HIV/AIDS is 40 years. Lymphomas in transplant recipients generally occur between the ages of 35 and 40. Mean age of onset in children with inherited immunodeficiencies is 10 years. There is an overall 3:2 male predominance in PCNSL.

PRESENTATION. Most patients with PCNSL present with focal neurologic deficits, altered mental status, and neuropsychiatric disturbances. Seizures are less common than in patients with other primary brain tumors.

NATURAL HISTORY. Regardless of immune status, prognosis is generally poor. PCNSL is an aggressive tumor with a median survival of only a few months. Even with conventional chemo- and radiation therapy, the five-year survival rate is less than 10%. Immunocompetent patients younger than 60 years fare better than older patients with PCNSL. Overall survival in HIV/AIDS and other immunocompromised patients with PCNSL is substantially diminished, no matter the age at presentation.

TREATMENT OPTIONS. Early diagnosis is crucial for proper management of PCNSL. As gross surgical resection does not improve prognosis, stereotactic biopsy for diagnostic confirmation and histologic tumor typing is recommended.

As with systemic NHLs, treatment options for PCNSL include corticosteroids, chemotherapy, and radiation. Approximately 70% of PCNSLs initially respond to treatment, but relapse is very common. Only 20-40% of patients experience prolonged progression-free survival.

Antineoplastic agents designed specifically to treat B-cell malignancies and B-cell-driven diseases such as rheumatoid arthritis have been used with some success in selected cases. Rituximab is a chimeric murine/human monoclonal immunoglobulin G1 antibody that targets CD20, a cell-surface marker specifically found on B lymphocytes.

Autologous stem cell transplants have yielded mixed results but may be effective, especially in younger patients with newly diagnosed PCNSL.

aging

GENERAL FEATURES. Imaging findings of PCNSL vary with immune status.

Contrast-enhanced cranial MR is the modality of choice in evaluating patients with suspected PCNSL. As isolated spinal cord involvement is rare (3-4% of cases), spinal imaging is indicated only in patients with myelopathy or suspected diffuse meningeal dissemination.

CT FINDINGS. PCNSLs are highly cellular tumors. White matter or basal ganglia lesions in contact with a CSF surface are typical. Most lesions appear hyperdense compared to normal brain on NECT scans **(24-3)**, **(24-4)**. Marked peritumoral edema is common, but necrosis, hemorrhage, and calcification are rare (2-5%) unless the patient is immunocompromised **(24-7)**.

CNS lymphomas in immunocompetent patients show mild to moderate, relatively homogeneous enhancement **(24-5)**. Irregular ring enhancement is rare unless the patient is immunocompromised.

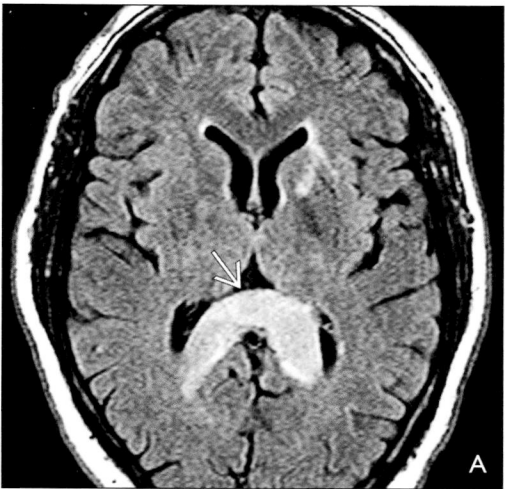

24-9A. FLAIR scan in a patient with primary large B-cell lymphoma shows a hyperintense mass in the corpus callosum splenium ⇥.

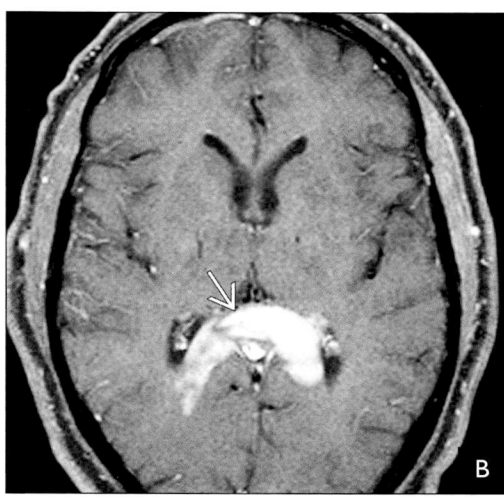

24-9B. T1 C+ FS in the same patient shows that the mass ⇥ enhances strongly, mostly uniformly.

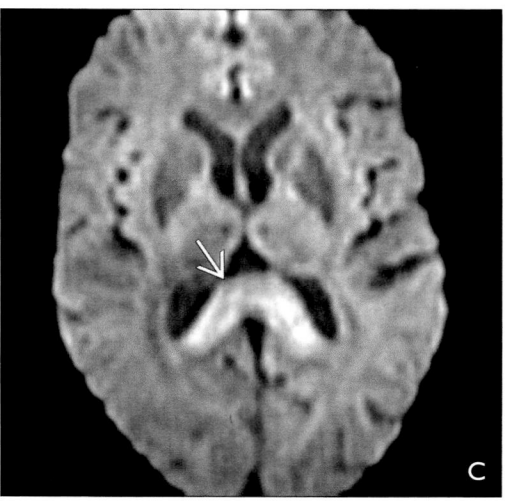

24-9C. DWI shows diffusion restriction ⇥ characteristic of a densely cellular mass.

24-10A. *Multicompartmental (dura, parenchymal) primary DLBCL in an 81-year-old immunocompetent man is illustrated in this series of images. Axial T1WI shows an isointense dura-based right frontal mass* ➡ *with significant peritumoral edema* ⬎. *24-10B.* *T2WI shows that the mass* ⬎ *is iso- to slightly hyperintense relative to gray matter.*

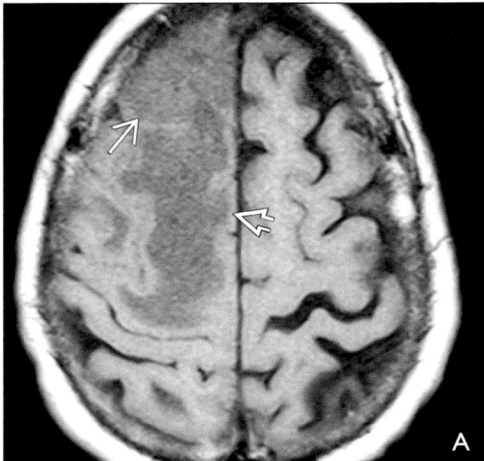
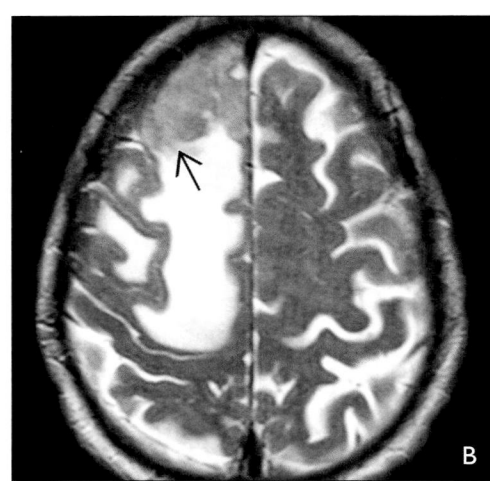

24-10C. *The lesion* ➡ *restricts strongly on DWI. 24-10D. Axial T1 C+ FS shows that the lesion* ➡ *enhances intensely, uniformly.*

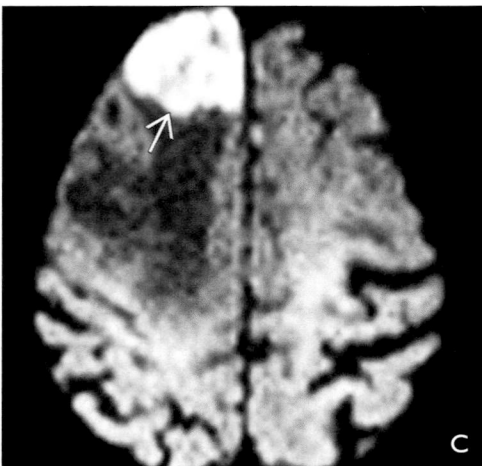
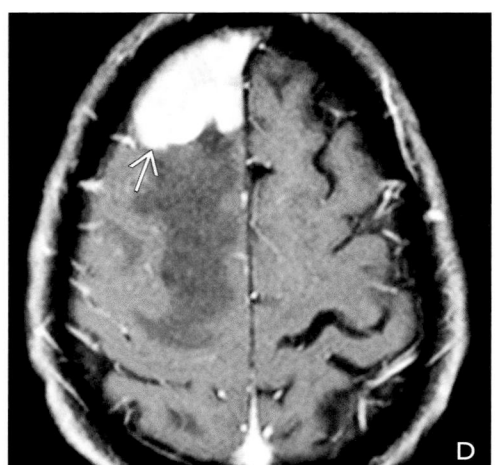

24-10E. *Axial T1 C+ FS through the lateral ventricles shows an ill-defined but strongly enhancing parenchymal mass* ➡ *and a smaller left frontal lesion* ⬎. *24-10F.* *Coronal T1 C+ in the same patient shows patchy multifocal enhancement.*

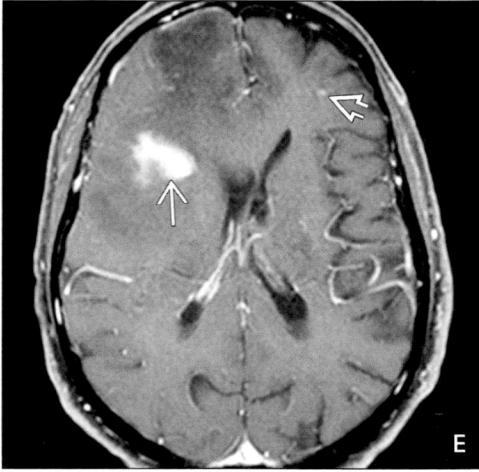
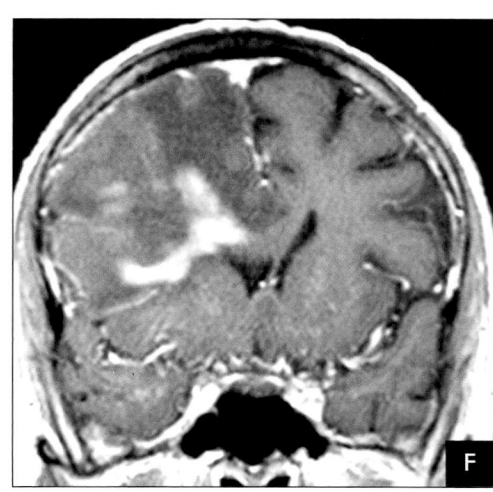

MR FINDINGS. Over three-quarters of DLBCLs in **immunocompetent** patients are iso- or slightly hypointense compared to gray matter on T1WI and isointense on T2WI **(24-10)**. T-cell lymphomas are mildly to moderately hyperintense on T2WI **(24-11)**.

FLAIR signal is variable but usually iso- or hyperintense. Microhemorrhages with intratumoral "blooming" on T2* are present in 5-8% of cases. Because of their high cellularity, over 95% of PCNSLs show mild to moderate diffusion restriction **(24-9)**.

Nearly all PCNSLs in immunocompetent patients enhance. Solid homogeneous or heterogeneous enhancement is common; ring enhancement is rare. On perfusion MR, rCBV is relatively low compared with glioblastoma.

In **immunocompromised** patients, intratumor hemorrhage with T1 shortening and "blooming" on T2* scans is common **(24-8)**. Enhancement is variable but often mild. Ring enhancement surrounding a nonenhancing core of necrotic tissue is typical.

FDG PET FINDINGS. Occult systemic lymphomas are found in 5-8% of patients with putative PCNSL. FDG PET and PET/CT fusion imaging are helpful in looking for extracranial lymphoma.

ifferential Diagnosis

The major differential diagnosis of PCNSL is **glioblastoma multiforme** (GBM). Although both tumors often cross the corpus callosum, hemorrhage and necrosis are rare in PCNSL. Enhancement in immunocompetent patients with PCNSL is strong and relatively homogeneous whereas a peripheral ring pattern is more typical of GBM.

The second most common differential diagnosis of PCNSL is **metastasis**. Dura-based PCNSLs may resemble **meningioma** or—due to their hyperdensity—even look like an acute epi- or subdural hematoma.

If the patient is immunocompromised, the major differential diagnosis of PCNSL is **toxoplasmosis**. *A solitary ring-enhancing lesion in an HIV/AIDS patient is most often lymphoma* whereas multiple lesions are more characteristic of toxoplasmosis. An "eccentric target" sign is suggestive of toxoplasmosis although necrotic lymphomas occasionally show an enhancing "ring with a nodule" pattern. Toxoplasmosis is hypometabolic on PET and pMR.

Progressive multifocal leukoencephalopathy (PML) usually does not enhance. However, **acute PML** lesions and JC virus-associated **immune reconstitution inflammatory syndrome** (IRIS) may show ring enhancement. Enhancement often looks quite bizarre with multifocal

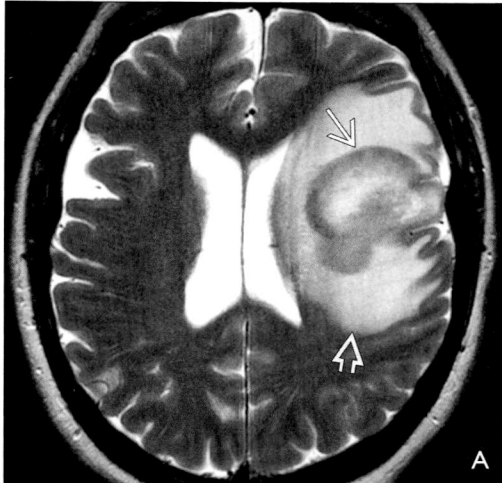

24-11A. *T2WI in a 52 yo woman with PCNSL, diffuse large T-cell type, shows hyper-, hypointense mass* ➡ *with striking peritumoral edema* ⇥.

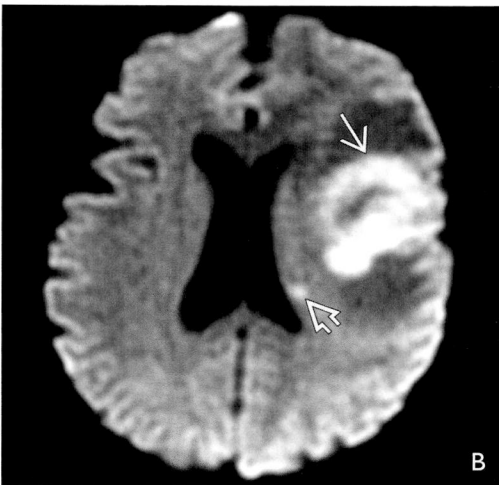

24-11B. *The hypercellular mass* ➡ *shows diffusion restriction on DWI. Note the second small periventricular tumor nodule* ⇥.

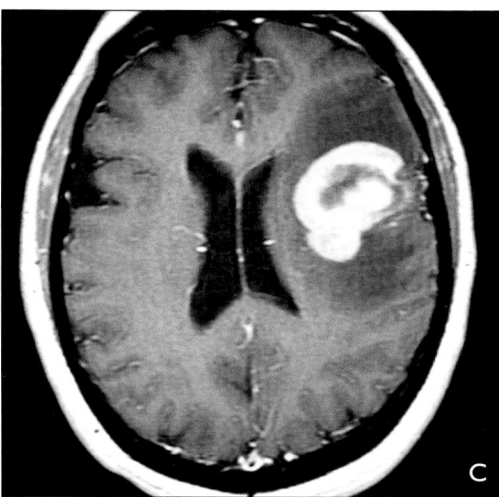

24-11C. *T1 C+ scan shows that the mass enhances strongly and uniformly.*

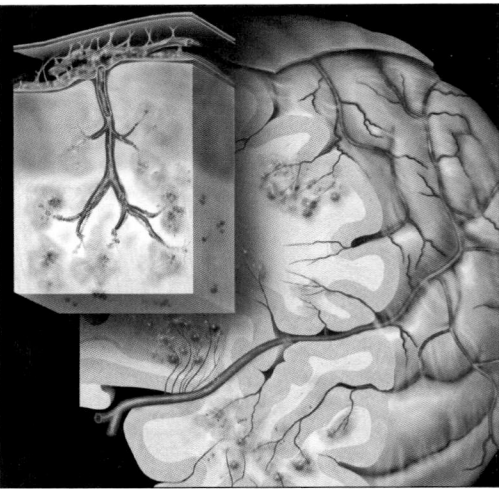

24-12. Graphic depicts IVL. Malignant cells plug vessels, causing perivascular infiltrates and petechial hemorrhages.

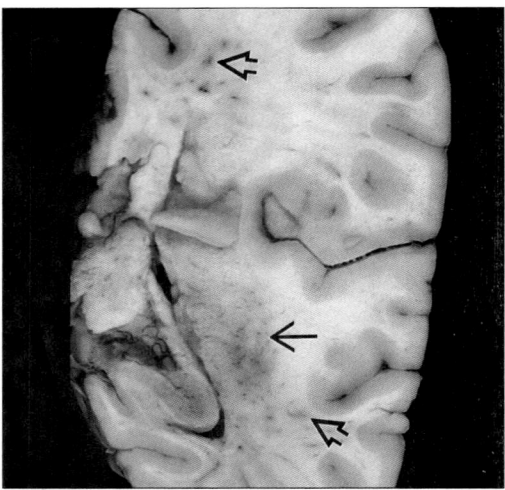

24-13. Autopsy of IVL shows punctate, linear grayish infiltrates ⊵ with petechial and perivascular hemorrhages ➔.

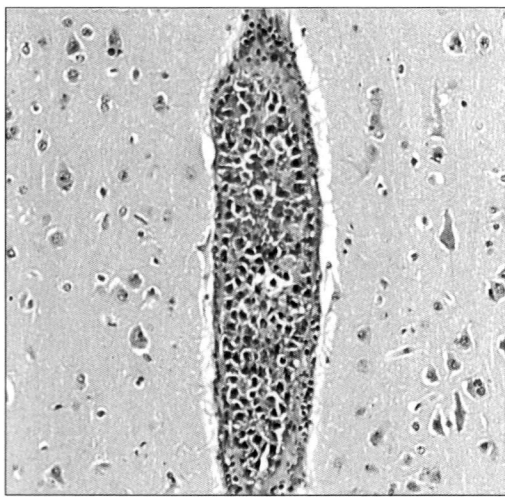

24-14. Intravascular lymphoma completely fills brain arteriole with "small round blue cells." (Courtesy T. Tihan, MD.)

poorly delineated partial rings of enhancement surrounding the demyelinating foci.

In the setting of solid organ or hematopoietic stem cell transplants, **lymphomatoid granulomatosis** and **post-transplant lymphoproliferative disorder** (PTLD) may closely resemble PCNSL. Biopsy is necessary for confirmation and patient management.

PCNSL: IMAGING

General Features
- Findings vary with immune status
- Steroids may mask/↓ imaging findings
- Periventricular WM, basal ganglia common sites

CT
- Hyperdense on NECT (immunocompetent)
- Hemorrhage, necrosis rare unless immunocompromised

MR
- Generally isointense with GM on T1-, T2WI
- Petechial hemorrhage in immunocompetent
- Gross hemorrhage, necrosis in immunocompromised
- Strong uniform enhancement (ring in immunocompromised)
- Often restricts on DWI

Differential Diagnosis
- Glioblastoma multiforme, metastasis in immunocompetent
- Toxoplasmosis in immunocompromised
- Lymphomatoid granulomatosis, PTLD in transplant patients

Intravascular (Angiocentric) Lymphoma

Intravascular lymphoma (IVL) is a rare type of lymphoma characterized by proliferating malignant cells within small and medium-sized vessels. Although it can involve any organ, IVL typically affects the skin and the CNS.

Terminology

IVL is also called angiocentric or angioendotheliotropic lymphoma, angiotropic large cell lymphoma, endovascular lymphoma, and malignant angioendotheliomatosis.

Etiology

IVL is an aggressive malignant lymphoma that usually arises from B cells. T cells or NK cells may occasionally be the cell of origin. A possible association of IVL (especially the NK type) with EBV has been reported.

Pathology

The gross macroscopic appearance varies from normal to small multifocal infarcts of varying ages scattered throughout the cortex and subcortical white matter **(24-12)**.

Focal cerebral masses are rare. Petechial microhemorrhages may be present and are more common than confluent macroscopic bleeds **(24-13)**.

At histologic examination, markedly atypical cells with large round nuclei and prominent nuclei are found in small and medium-sized vessels **(24-14)**. Extension into the adjacent perivascular spaces is minimal or absent. CD20 staining is helpful in identifying tumor cells, especially when they are sparse and widely scattered.

inical Issues

EPIDEMIOLOGY. IVL is rare. CNS involvement occurs in 75-85% of patients.

DEMOGRAPHICS. IVL is typically a tumor of middle-aged and elderly patients. Mean age at presentation is 60-65 years.

PRESENTATION. Sensory and motor deficits, neuropathies, and multiple stroke-like episodes are common symptoms. Some patients present with progressive neurological deterioration and cognitive decline characterized by confusion and memory loss. Skin changes with elevated plaques or nodules are present in half of all cases.

NATURAL HISTORY. Outcome is generally poor. By the time of initial presentation, most patients have advanced disseminated disease. IVL is a relentless, rapidly progressive disease with high mortality rate. Mean survival is 7-12 months.

TREATMENT OPTIONS. Because IVL is a widely disseminated disease, systemic chemotherapy is the recommended treatment. High-dose chemotherapy with autologous stem cell transplantation is often used in younger patients.

aging

There are no pathognomonic neuroimaging findings for IVL. Ischemic foci are the most common imaging finding. CT may be normal or nonspecific, demonstrating only scattered white matter hypodensities. MR shows multiple T2/FLAIR hyperintensities **(24-15)**. Microhemorrhages are common, so "blooming" foci on T2* (GRE, SWI) are often present **(24-16)**. Linear/punctate enhancement oriented along perivascular spaces is suggestive of IVL. Multifocal areas of diffusion restriction may be present **(24-16D)**.

fferential Diagnosis

IVL is a "great imitator," both clinically and on imaging studies. Stereotactic biopsy is thus necessary to establish the definitive diagnosis. **Vasculitis** with punctate and linear enhancing foci may be virtually indistinguishable from IVL on imaging studies alone.

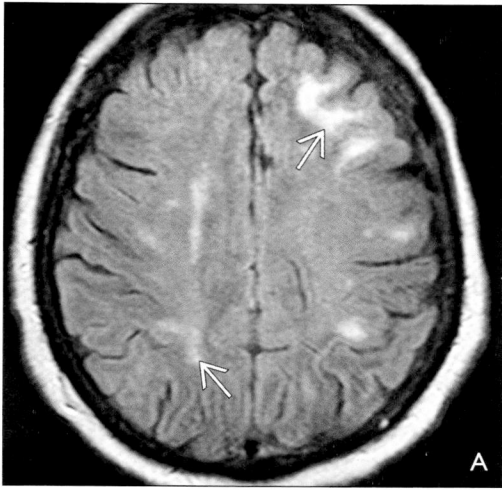

24-15A. FLAIR scan in 78 yo woman with confusion, declining mental status shows multiple bilateral subcortical, deep WM hyperintensities ➡.

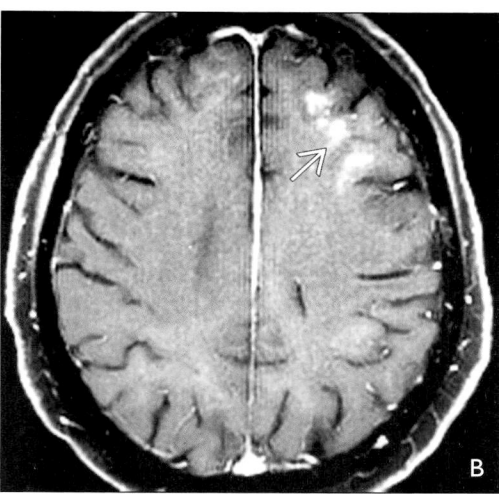

24-15B. T1 C+ FS shows patchy enhancement of the lesions ➡.

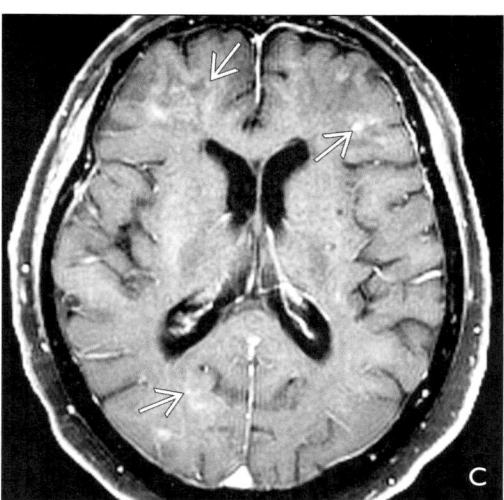

24-15C. T1 C+ FS through the lateral ventricles shows numerous additional enhancing lesions ➡. *Biopsy disclosed intravascular lymphoma.*

PCNSL, especially in the setting of immunodeficiency syndromes, may mimic IVL. IVL is most often multifocal whereas two-thirds of PCNSLs are solitary lesions. Diffuse multifocal PCNSL, especially when it occurs in the form of **lymphomatosis cerebri**, may be difficult to distinguish from IVL. Lymphomatosis cerebri often shows little or no enhancement.

Rapidly progressive leukoencephalopathy with confluent nonenhancing white matter lesions is a rare presentation of diffusely infiltrating CNS IVL and may mimic a cerebral **demyelinating disorder**.

Diffuse **subacute viral encephalitis** can likewise mimic IVL, especially on biopsy. Parenchymal **neurosarcoid** with perivascular nodular spread may also resemble IVL on imaging studies.

INTRAVASCULAR (ANGIOCENTRIC) LYMPHOMA

Pathology
- Small/medium-sized vessels filled with tumor
- Little/no parenchymal tumor
- Multifocal infarcts, microhemorrhages common

Clinical Issues
- Older patients with dementia, cognitive decline, TIAs
- Skin lesions (50%)

Imaging
- Multifocal T2/FLAIR hyperintensities
- Hemorrhages, foci of restricted diffusion
- Linear/punctate enhancement

Common Differential Diagnoses
- PCNSL
- Vasculitis

Lymphomatosis Cerebri

Lymphomatosis cerebri is an uncommon form of PCNSL. Diffuse infiltration of lymphoma cells in both gray and white matter without a focal mass lesion is characteristic.

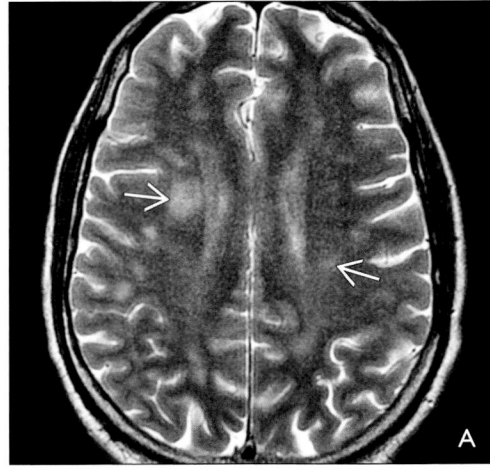
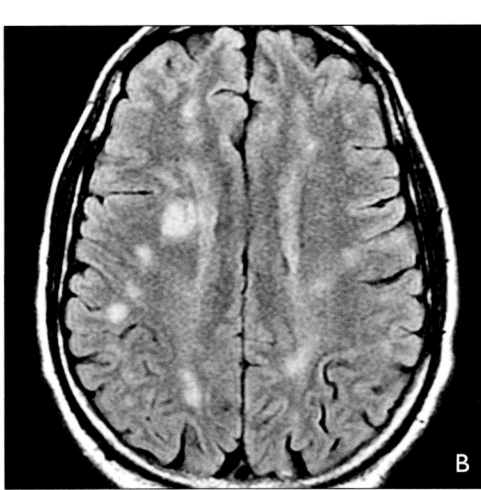

24-16A. *T2WI in a 60-year-old man with several-month history of increasing confusion, decreasing mental status shows multifocal ill-defined hyperintensities in the hemispheric WM➡. 24-16B. FLAIR scan in the same patient shows several additional lesions. There was no evidence of cortical or basal ganglia hyperintensities.*

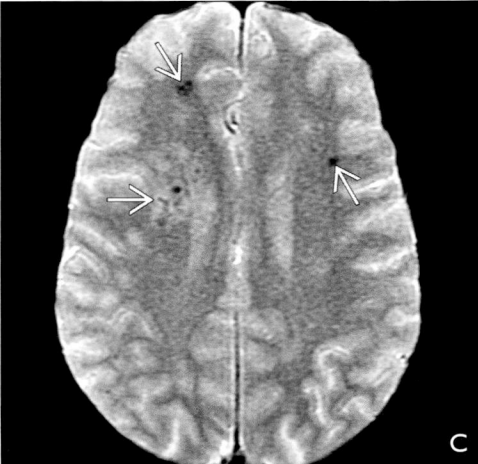
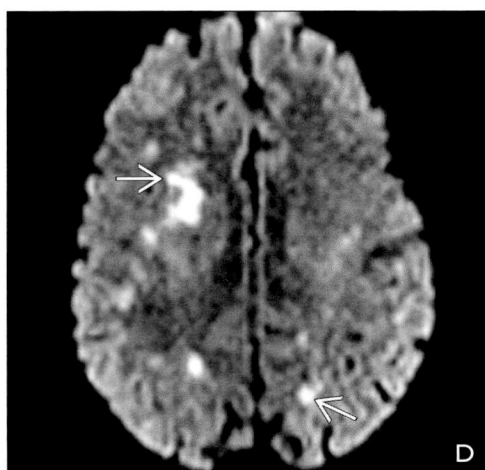

24-16C. *T2* GRE shows multiple tiny hemorrhagic foci ➡. 24-16D. DWI shows multiple foci of restricted diffusion in both hemispheres ➡. The patient died shortly after the scan was obtained. Autopsy demonstrated intravascular lymphoma.*

Most patients are middle-aged or elderly and present with subacute encephalopathy or rapidly progressive dementia. Personality changes and ataxia are common.

Imaging findings are nonspecific with patchy and confluent T2/FLAIR hyperintensities. Little or no enhancement is typical (24-17). The major differential diagnosis is **gliomatosis cerebri**.

MALT Lymphoma

Mucosa-associated lymphoid tissue (MALT) lymphomas in the head and neck are most often ocular adnexal tumors, occurring in the conjunctiva, lacrimal glands, orbit, and eyelids (24-18). The cranial meninges, especially the dura, are occasional sites. Parenchymal lesions are rare.

Lymphomatoid Granulomatosis

Terminology

Lymphomatoid granulomatosis (LYG) is a rare multisystem angiocentric and angioinvasive lymphoproliferative disorder characterized by atypical B-cell proliferations of uncertain malignant potential.

Etiology

EBV infection is a feature of most reported cases. LYG also occurs in the setting of HIV/AIDS and in patients on maintenance immunosuppression following solid organ transplantation. Inherited disorders such as Wiskott-Aldrich disease and congenital immunodeficiency syndrome are rare but reported causes of LYG.

Pathology

The lung is the most commonly involved site, followed by the skin. The CNS is involved in about 25% of cases.

Lesions range in size from a few millimeters up to one or two centimeters in diameter. Large focal masses are rare.

LYG shares several histologic similarities with post-transplantation lymphoproliferative disorders (see below). Angiocentric and angiodestructive polymorphous infiltrates consisting predominantly of lympho-

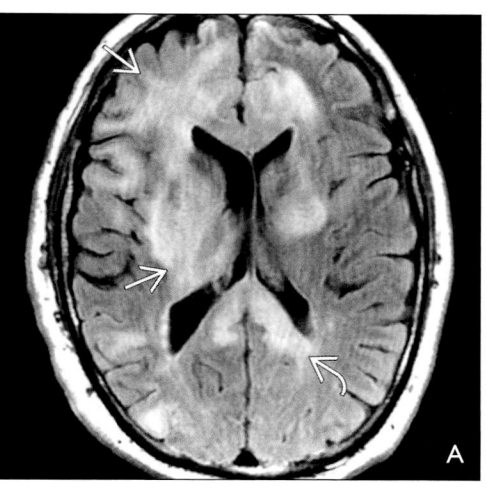
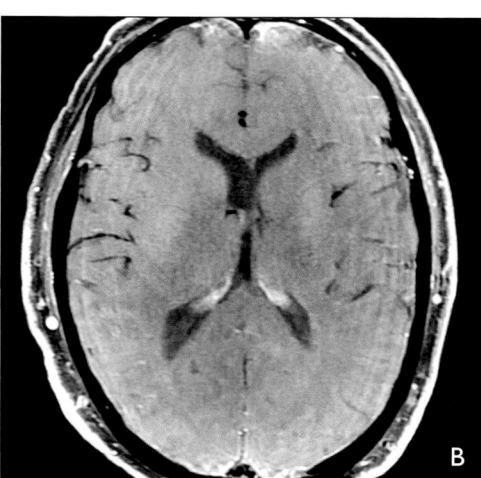

24-17A. FLAIR scan in an elderly patient with confusion, mental status changes shows extensive, confluent WM and basal ganglia hyperintensities in both hemispheres →. Note the involvement of the corpus callosum splenium →. 24-17B. T1 C+ FS scan shows no enhancement. Histopathologic diagnosis was lymphomatosis cerebri. (Courtesy T. Tihan, MD.)

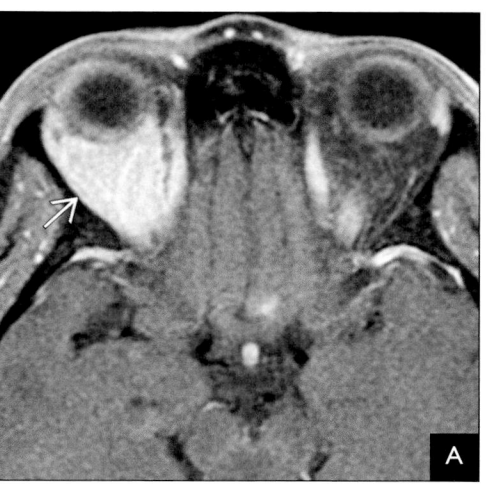
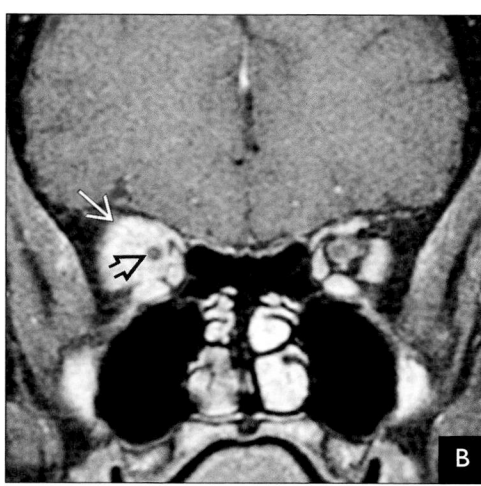

24-18A. Axial T1 C+ FS in a 63-year-old woman with right-sided proptosis shows an intensely enhancing multicompartmental mass → that involves the intraconal retrobulbar space, extraocular muscles, and lacrimal gland. 24-18B. Coronal T1 C+ FS shows that the lesion fills the orbit →, surrounds the optic nerve →. Biopsy demonstrated MALT lymphoma. (Courtesy L. Ginsberg, MD.)

cytes mixed with plasma cells, immunoblasts, and histiocytes are present.

LYG is graded on a scale of 1 to 3 based on the numbers of atypical EBV-positive B cells and the amount of necrosis present.

Clinical Issues

Patients of all ages are affected, but peak occurrence is between the fourth and sixth decades. Clinical manifestations, laboratory data, and imaging are all nonspecific, so biopsy is required for definitive diagnosis.

Prognosis is generally poor. Between 10-60% of patients with LYG eventually develop large B-cell lymphomas. Mean survival time after malignant transformation is 20 months. Radiation, chemotherapy, and anti-CD20 monoclonal antibodies have been used with limited success.

Imaging

Nearly half of patients with LYG have demonstrable brain lesions on MR imaging. Imaging findings are non-specific, and there is no direct correlation with LYG grade.

The most common abnormalities are multifocal T2/FLAIR nodular hyperintensities in the cerebral hemispheres, cerebellum, or spinal cord. The second most common imaging finding in LYG is involvement of the leptomeninges and cranial nerves. Dura-based masses and choroid plexus lesions also occur.

LYG typically enhances strongly. Both solid and ring-like patterns as well as multifocal punctate and linear enhancing foci have been described (24-19).

Post-Transplant Lymphoproliferative Disorder

Post-transplant lymphoproliferative disorder (PTLD) is one of the life-threatening complications of immunosuppressive therapy in patients with solid organ or hematopoietic cell transplantation.

The PTLD disease spectrum ranges from an infectious mononucleosis-like illness with reactive lymph node

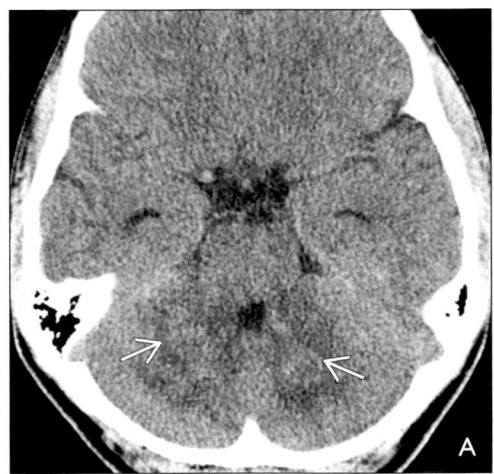
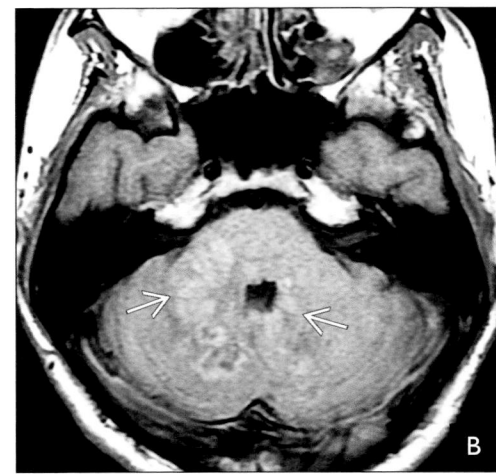

24-19A. NECT scan in a 16-year-old male with fever, cough, and ataxia shows heterogeneous hypo-, isodense infiltrate ➡ in the WM of both cerebellar hemispheres. 24-19B. Axial T1WI in the same patient shows that the multifocal cerebellar lesions are slightly hyperintense ➡.

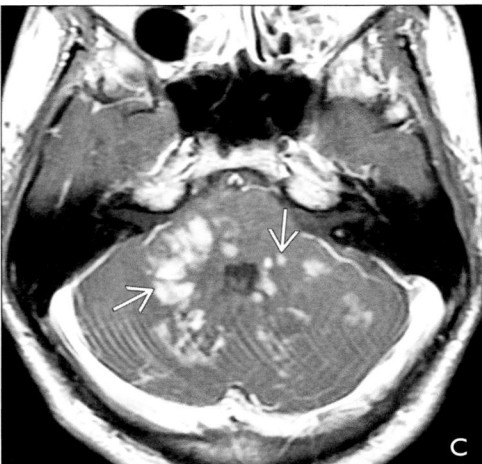
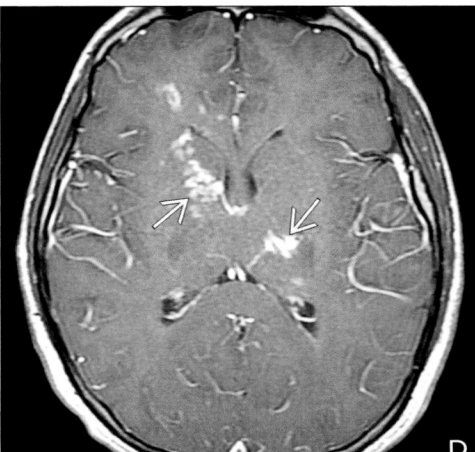

24-19C. T1 C+ shows strong enhancement of the lesions ➡. 24-19D. More cephalad T1 C+ scan shows additional enhancing foci ➡ in the basal ganglia, hemispheric WM. Imaging diagnosis was hemophagocytic lymphohistiocytosis. Biopsy disclosed lymphomatoid granulomatosis.

hyperplasia to malignant lymphoma. Most PTLDs are EBV-related.

Pathology

PTLDs can be polymorphic or monomorphic. Polymorphic PTLD consists of a heterogeneous cell population that may reflect the full range of B-cell maturation from prominent plasmacytic infiltrates to proliferating immunoblasts with necrosis. Polymorphic PTLD does not fulfill the histologic criteria for lymphoma.

Monomorphic PTLDs consist of large blastic cells with prominent nucleoli. Most are classified as large B-cell lymphomas.

Clinical Issues

EPIDEMIOLOGY. The overall prevalence of PTLD following solid organ transplantation is 0.5-2.5%. CNS involvement is rare, occurring in less than 0.5% of transplant cases. However, up to 15-20% of patients who do develop PTLD have CNS involvement.

DEMOGRAPHICS. Pediatric transplant recipients develop PTLD more frequently than adult patients because children are less likely to have EBV-specific immunity at transplantation. The frequency varies with the type of transplant, with the highest prevalence reported with multiorgan or intestinal (20%), lung or heart (8-20%), liver (4-15%), and kidney (1-8%) transplants. PTLD after hematopoietic cell transplantation accounts for less than 2% of cases.

PRESENTATION. PTLD typically presents several years following transplantation. Symptoms relate to tumor location.

TREATMENT OPTIONS. Because treatment regimens vary significantly, distinguishing polymorphic from monomorphic PTLD and malignant lymphoma is essential, often requiring biopsy for definitive diagnosis.

Reduction or cessation of immunosuppression is generally the first step in treating PTLD. Polymorphic PTLD usually responds well within two to four weeks. PTLD that fails to respond to reduced immunosuppression has a very high mortality rate (50-90%).

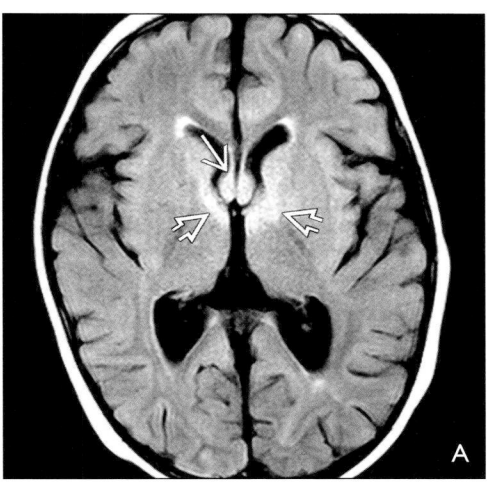

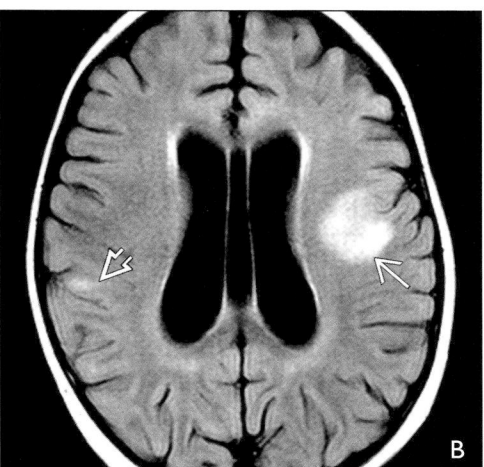

24-20A. FLAIR scan in a 4-year-old boy who underwent multiorgan transplant and then developed seizure and tremors. Note thickening, hyperintensity of the fornices ➡, medial basal ganglia, and genu of both internal capsules ➡. 24-20B. More cephalad scan shows a large lesion at the GM-WM junction in the left hemisphere ➡ and a smaller lesion in the right hemisphere ➡.

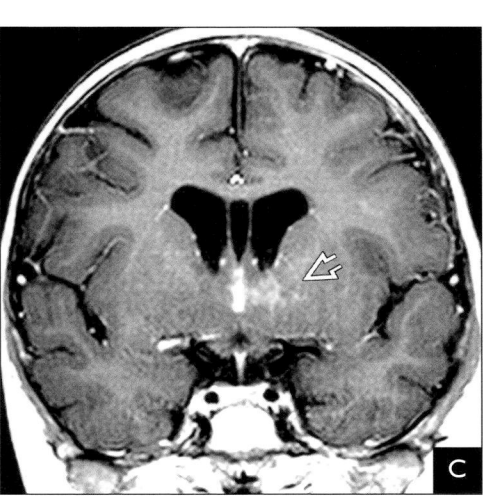

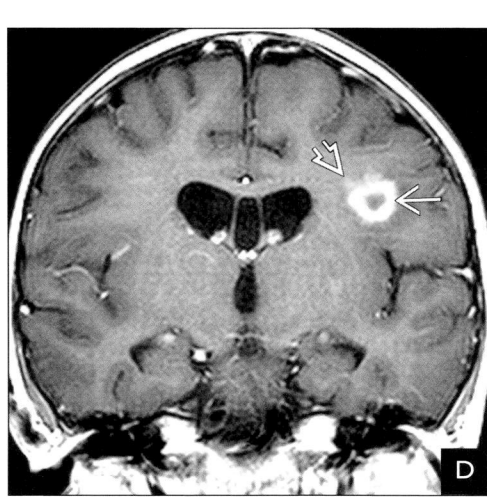

24-20C. Coronal T1 C+ shows heterogeneous enhancement ➡ in the basal ganglia, hypothalamus. 24-20D. The left hemisphere lesion shows strong ring enhancement ➡ with faint tendrils of tumor extending into the adjacent WM ➡. ADC map (not shown) demonstrated moderate diffusion restriction. Biopsy disclosed PTLD with large B-cell lymphoma. (Courtesy S. Blaser, MD.)

Most cases of monomorphic PTLD are unresponsive to immunosuppression withdrawal and require additional therapeutic modalities. Surgical resection, chemotherapy, and radiation therapy are possibilities.

Because CNS PTLD lesions are often resistant to CHOP, radiotherapy is generally used in combination with agents such as high dose methotrexate. High-dose rituximab, an anti-CD20 monoclonal antibody, may be effective in some patients.

Imaging

Imaging features of CNS PTLD resemble those of AIDS-related lymphoma. Most lesions are solitary masses that are hypointense to cortex on T1WI and heterogeneously hypo-/hyperintense on T2WI. Peripheral, ring-like enhancement is common following contrast administration (24-20). Lymphoma-related PTLDs usually show moderate restriction on DWI.

Extracranial head and neck PTLD results in a spectrum of findings. Bilateral cervical lymphadenopathy occurs in 75% of cases. Nodes often appear necrotic. Other manifestations include orbital involvement and sinonasal lesions that resemble polyposis or sinusitis.

Differential Diagnosis

The major differential diagnosis of PTLD is **primary CNS lymphoma**—especially AIDS-related lymphoma. The imaging differential diagnosis of CNS lesions in transplant recipients also includes **opportunistic infections** such as toxoplasmosis.

POST-TRANSPLANT LYMPHOPROLIFERATIVE DISORDER

Terminology and Etiology
- Complication of organ or stem cell transplants
  ○ Long-term maintenance immunosuppression
- Ranges from benign mono-like illness to malignant lymphoma

Pathology
- Monomorphic or polymorphic lymphoid proliferations
- Polymorphic PTLD has plasmacytic B-cell elements of varying maturity
- Monomorphic PTLD has blastic cells → large B-cell lymphoma

Clinical Issues
- 0.5-2.5% of patients with solid organ transplants
- 15-20% with PTLD have CNS involvement
- Presents several years after transplantation
- Children > adults

Imaging
- Brain findings resemble those of AIDS-related lymphoma
- Extracranial PTLD
  ○ Bilateral cervical adenopathy common
  ○ Orbital, sinonasal lesions

Metastatic Intracranial Lymphoma

Terminology

Metastatic intracranial lymphoma is also called secondary CNS lymphoma (SCNSL). Here the skull, meningeal, and brain lesions are all secondary to systemic lymphoma (24-21), (24-22), (24-23), (24-24), (24-25), (24-26).

Clinical Issues

Aggressive high-grade tumors increase the risk of CNS spread. Between 3-5% of patients with diffuse large B-cell systemic lymphomas eventually develop CNS involvement. Approximately 80% of SCNSLs are caused by DLBCL.

Peak prevalence of metastatic CNS lymphoma is in the sixth and seventh decades. Prognosis is poor, especially in elderly patients. Systemic methotrexate has been recommended as the optimal treatment for isolated CNS relapse involving the brain parenchyma. Rituximab treatment may be effective in some cases.

Imaging

SCNSL is typically identified with neuroimaging. Skull and dural involvement is much more frequent than with PCNSL (24-27). Both calvarial vault and skull base metastases are common (24-28). Skull base metastases may extend inferiorly into the nose and paranasal sinuses or spread superolaterally into the cavernous sinus, Meckel cave, and pituitary gland/stalk.

Calvarial lesions often involve the adjacent scalp and epidural space. Dural "tails" are common. Involvement of the leptomeninges and underlying brain parenchyma may occur as late complications. Parenchymal lesions in the absence of skull and dural disease are uncommon.

Diffuse leptomeningeal tumor spread and disseminated CSF lesions are relatively uncommon (24-29). Tumor spread along the optic nerve sheath is rare. Cranial neuropathies with multifocal enhancing cranial nerves occur as a late complication. Intradural lesions in the spine ("drop metastases") occur in 3-5% of cases.

SECONDARY (METASTATIC) INTRACRANIAL LYMPHOMA

80% from high-grade systemic B-cell lymphomas
Skull, dural lesions > > brain parenchyma
- Multicompartmental disease common
- Calvaria + epidural, scalp lesions
- Skull base + nose, cavernous sinus/pituitary

Leptomeningeal, CSF spread uncommon
Spine "drop mets" (3-5%)

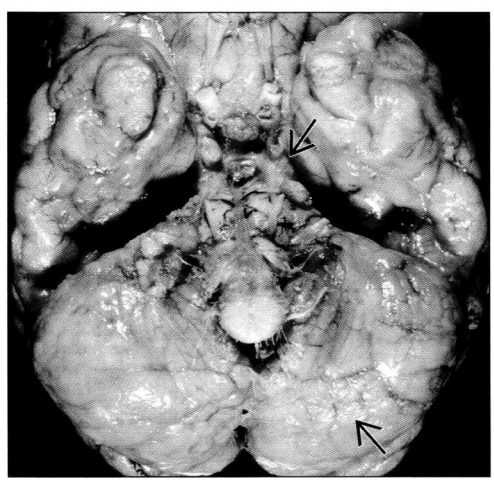

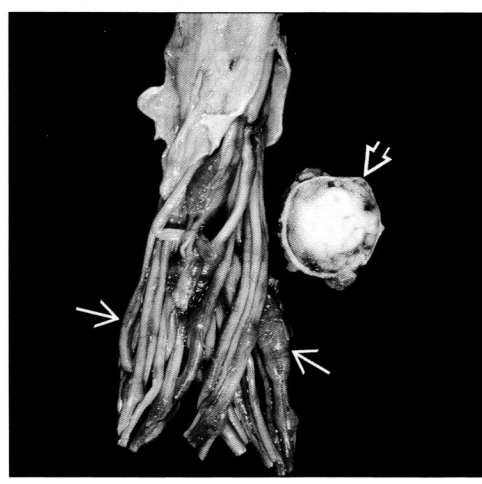

24-21. *Gallery of autopsy cases demonstrates the broad spectrum of metastatic lymphoma appearances in the CNS. Here the leptomeninges are diffusely coated with tumor, giving them a glistening "sugar icing" appearance* ➡. **24-22.** *Multiple nodular, linear metastases from systemic lymphoma diffusely thicken the nerve roots of the cauda equina* ➡. *Axial section through the thoracic cord shows that the intradural, extramedullary space is filled with tumor* ➡.

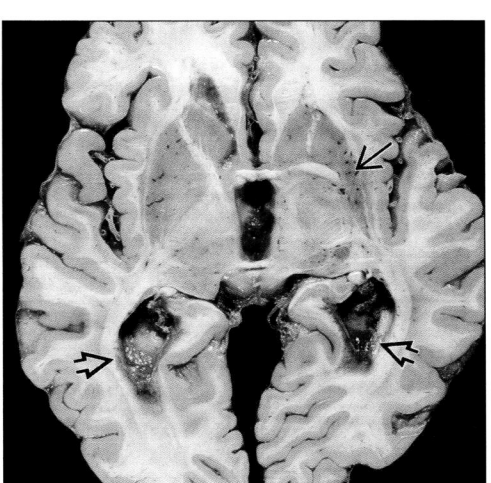

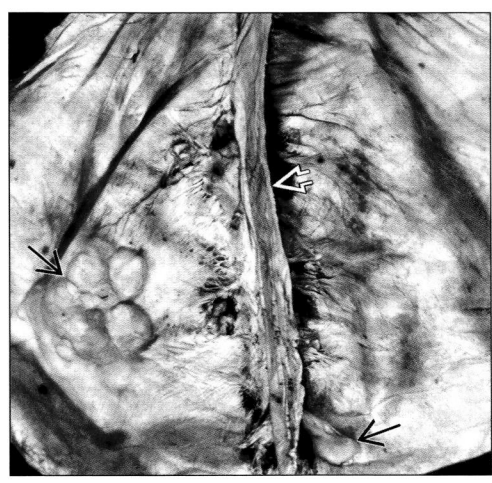

24-23. *Cut section through the ventricles shows that the ependymal surfaces of the lateral ventricles are coated with glistening tumor* ➡. *The perivascular spaces in the basal ganglia are enlarged by cords of intravascular malignant lymphoma* ➡. **24-24.** *Diffuse dural thickening* ➡ *with multiple focal deposits of lymphoma* ➡ *resembles meningiomatosis.*

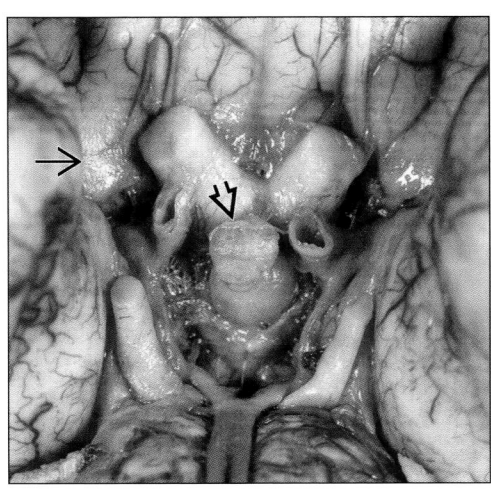

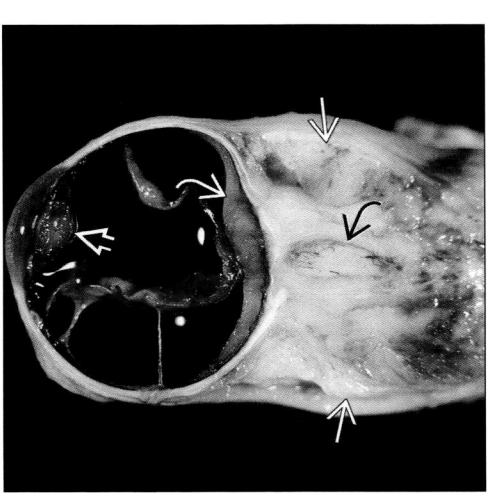

24-25. *Close-up view shows leptomeningeal metastases* ➡. *Metastatic lymphoma also thickens the infundibular stalk* ➡. *The pituitary gland (not shown) was also involved by tumor.* **24-26.** *Metastatic lymphoma fills, expands optic nerve sheath* ➡ *and surrounds the optic nerve* ➡. *The retina is detached, and the choroid is thickened by tumor* ➡. *There is a focal nodule of lymphoma just behind the lens* ➡. *(Cases courtesy R. Hewlett, MD.)*

24-27A. *Axial T1 C+ FS shows diffuse dural thickening ➡, scalp mass ➡. 24-27B. Coronal T1 C+ scan in the same patient shows that the diffuse dural thickening is most striking just under the scalp mass. The calvaria shows diffuse tumor involvement, seen as patchy enhancement ➡. Systemic large B-cell lymphoma.*

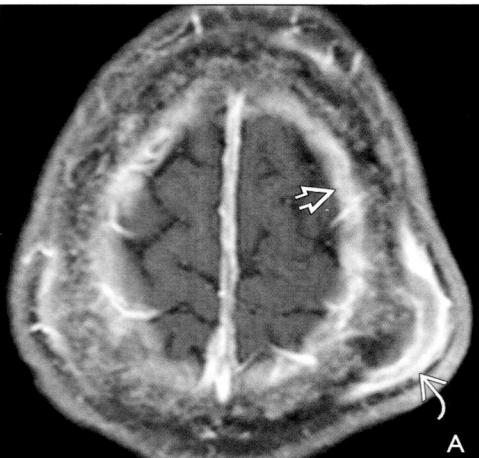
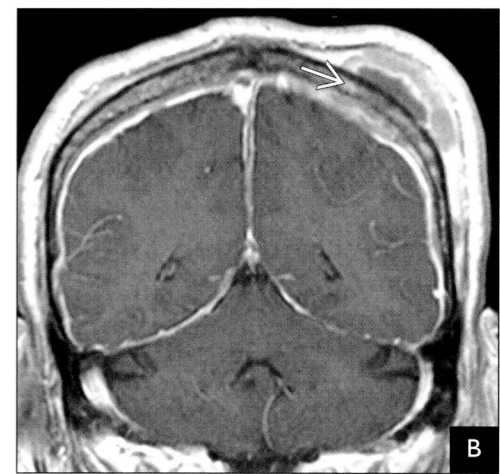

24-28A. *Axial bone CT shows diffuse lytic lesions throughout ➡ the central skull base, clivus ➡. 24-28B. T1 C+ shows diffuse enhancement with an extradural tumor extending into both middle cranial fossae ➡. Tumor has eroded through the clivus into the prepontine cistern ➡. Both internal auditory canals are filled with enhancing tumor as well ➡. Multiple metastases from systemic diffuse B-cell lymphoma.*

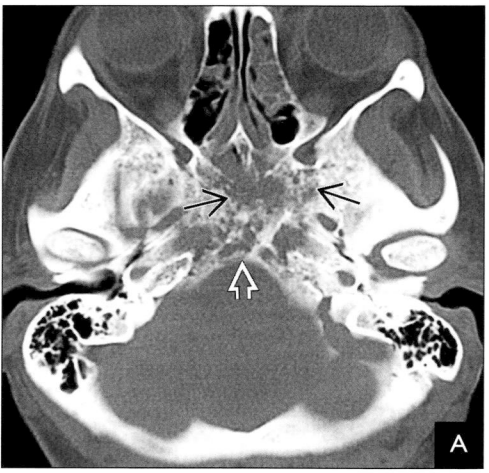
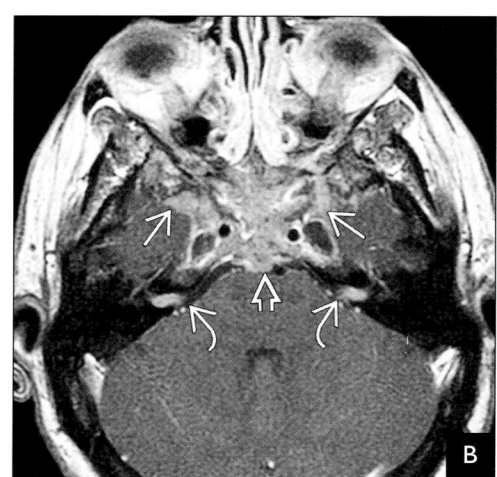

24-29A. *Axial T1 C+ scan in another patient with metastatic B-cell lymphoma shows extensive linear and nodular enhancing tumor ➡ in the ependyma of both lateral ventricles. Note the left frontal dural thickening and enhancement ➡. 24-29B. Coronal T1 C+ scan shows extensive ependymal and subependymal enhancement along the walls of both lateral ventricles ➡. Diffuse dural thickening ➡, a focal mass in the fourth ventricular choroid plexus ➡ are also seen.*

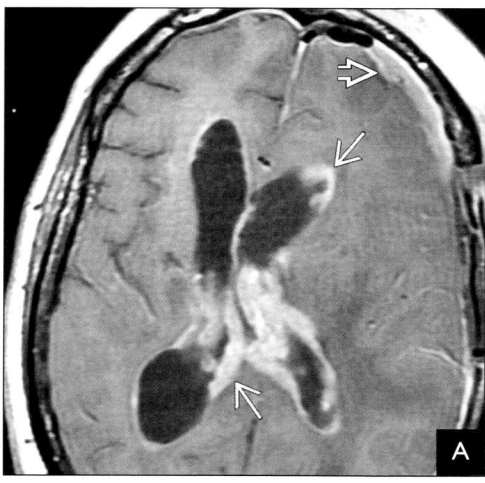
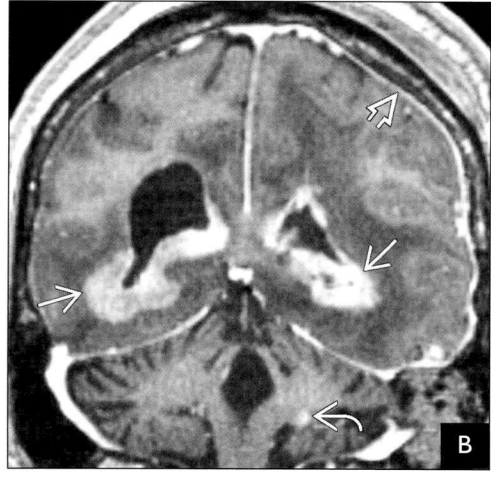

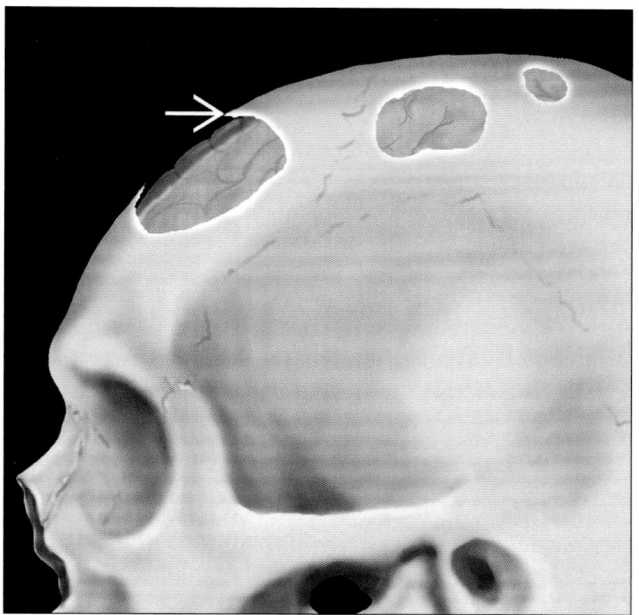

24-30. Graphic depicts the well-defined lytic skull lesions that are characteristic of LCH. The lesions lack marginal sclerosis and show "beveled" edges ➡.

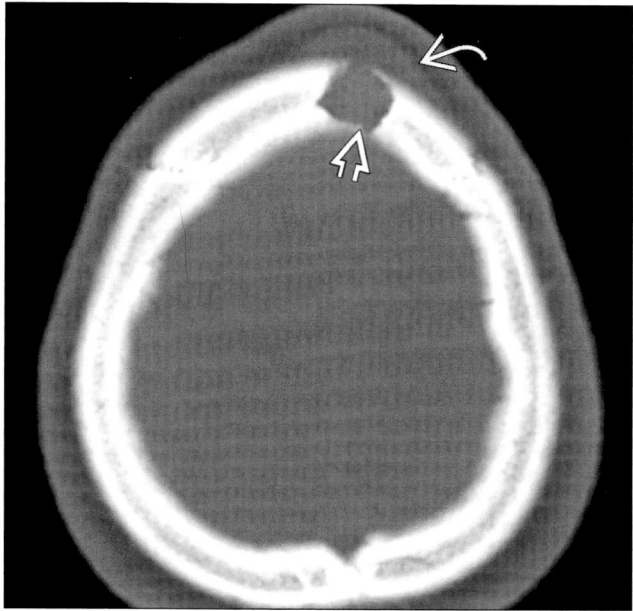

24-31. Bone CT shows the classic appearance of LCH as a sharply marginated lytic calvarial lesion ➡. Note the associated soft tissue mass ➡.

istiocytic Tumors

Histiocytic tumors are a heterogeneous group of tumors and tumor-like masses composed of histiocytes and commonly associated with histologically identical extracranial lesions.

Histiocytic proliferations are identified by their component cells and are classified into three groups. The first consists of dendritic cell-related disorders, of which Langerhans cell histiocytosis is the most common type. The second is a diverse group of macrophage-related non-Langerhans cell histiocytic disorders. The third group comprises malignant histiocytic disorders such as monocytic leukemia and histiocytic sarcoma. These are usually found in the skin, lymph nodes, and intestinal tract. They rarely occur as primary CNS tumors and so are not discussed further.

We begin this section by discussing Langerhans cell histiocytosis. We follow with four non-Langerhans cell histiocytoses that affect the CNS, namely Rosai-Dorfman disease, Erdheim-Chester disease, hemophagocytic lymphohistiocytosis, and juvenile xanthogranuloma. We close with a brief consideration of the malignant histiocytoses.

Langerhans Cell Histiocytosis

Terminology

Langerhans cell histiocytosis (LCH) was previously referred to as histiocytosis X and included eosinophilic granuloma, Hashimoto-Pritzker disease, Hand-Schüller-Christian disease, and Abt-Letterer-Siwe disease.

Etiology

The etiology of the histiocytic lesions remains unknown although an abnormal immune response between T-cells and macrophages is posited.

LCH cells represent immature, partially activated dendritic Langerhans cells. Microglial cells are the intrinsic histiocytes of the brain and may participate in causing secondary neuronal damage such as LCH-associated neurodegeneration of the cerebellum and basal ganglia.

Pathology

LOCATION. Bone lesions are the most frequent manifestation of LCH, occurring in 80-95% of cases **(24-30)**. Half of these cases are monostotic.

The craniofacial bones and skull base are the most commonly affected sites (55%), followed by the hypothalamic-pituitary region (50%), cranial meninges (30%), and choroid plexus (5%). Approximately one-third of patients exhibit parenchymal lesions. Associated neurodegenerative changes in the cerebellum and brainstem are seen in 5-10% of cases.

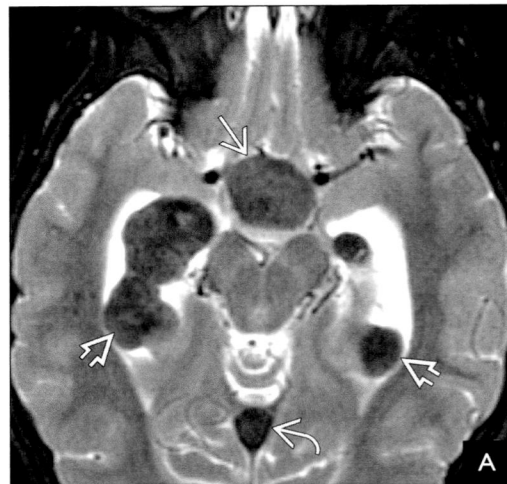

24-32A. T2WI in a patient with LCH shows hypointense suprasellar ➡, choroid plexus ➡, and dural masses ➡.

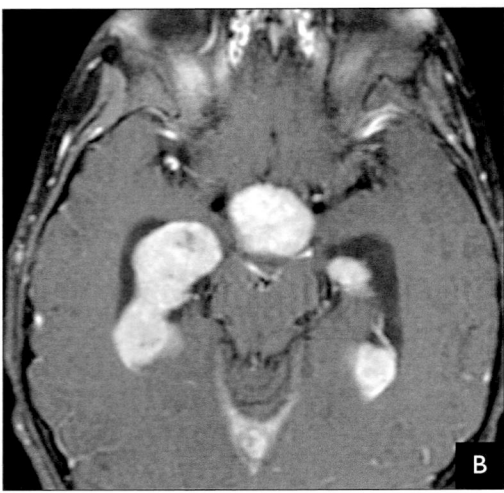

24-32B. T1 C+ FS scan in the same patient shows that the lesions enhance intensely, slightly heterogeneously.

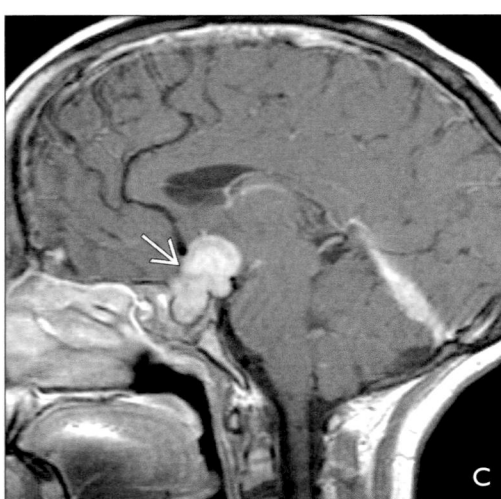

24-32C. Sagittal T1 C+ scan shows the suprasellar mass involving the hypothalamus, infundibular stalk and infiltrating the pituitary gland ➡.

SIZE AND NUMBER. Size ranges from small calvarial lesions to extensive infiltrating masses that involve most of the skull base. Multiple lesions are found in 50% of cases.

GROSS PATHOLOGY. Lesions are yellowish-white and vary from discrete dura-based nodules to granular, poorly defined parenchymal infiltrates.

MICROSCOPIC FEATURES. LCH lesions contain a mixture of Langerhans cells, macrophages, lymphocytes, plasma cells, and occasionally eosinophils. Nuclear grooves and clefts help distinguish Langerhans cells from generic histiocytes. Langerhans cells express S100 and vimentin as well as several histocyte markers.

STAGING, GRADING, AND CLASSIFICATION. LCH is now classified on the basis of disease extent as unifocal, multifocal (usually polyostotic), and disseminated disease.

Clinical Issues

EPIDEMIOLOGY. LCH is rare. The prevalence in children is estimated at 0.5 per 100,000 per year.

DEMOGRAPHICS. Most cases with isolated lesions present in young children under two years of age with a M:F predominance of 2:1. Multifocal disease onset is generally between two and five years of age.

PRESENTATION. The most common neurologic sign of LCH is diabetes insipidus, which is present in 12% of patients with multifocal LCH. Other CNS-related findings include symptoms of increased intracranial pressure, cranial nerve palsies, seizures, visual disturbances, and ataxia.

NATURAL HISTORY. Natural history and prognosis vary according to age at onset and whether the disease is isolated, multifocal, or disseminated. In general, there is an inverse relationship between severity of involvement and age of onset. Overall survival rates are good although mortality in young children with multisystem disease approaches 15-20%. Solitary osseous lesions have the best prognosis as spontaneous remission is relatively common.

TREATMENT OPTIONS. Therapeutic options depend on symptoms, location, and disease extent, ranging from simple surgical excision to radiation and chemotherapy.

Imaging

CT FINDINGS. One or more sharply marginated lytic skull or facial bone defects are the most common manifestations on NECT **(24-31)**. A "beveled" appearance with the inner table more affected than the outer is typical. Geographic skull base destruction, often centered on the temporal bone, may be extensive **(24-33)**. Associated soft tissue lesions may be small and relatively discrete, or they may be large, extensively infiltrating masses.

MR FINDINGS. Soft tissue masses adjacent to calvarial vault or skull base lesions may show mild T1 shortening secondary to the presence of lipid-laden histiocytes.

Abnormalities of the hypothalamus and pituitary stalk are common. The posterior pituitary "bright spot" is often absent, and the infundibular stalk may appear thickened and nontapering. Lesions are slightly hyperintense on T2WI. Secondary cerebellar degeneration occurs in 25% of cases and is seen as confluent T2/FLAIR hyperintensities.

LCH enhances strongly and uniformly on T1 C+ scans. Look for a thickened enhancing infundibulum, dura-based masses, and choroid plexus involvement **(24-32)**.

fferential Diagnosis

The differential diagnosis varies with lesion site. Lytic calvarial lesions that may mimic LCH include **burr holes** and other **surgical defects**, **dermoid** and **epidermoids**, **leptomeningeal cysts**, and **infection**. With the exception of neuroblastoma, osseous **metastases** are relatively rare in children.

A thickened infundibular stalk can be seen with **germinoma**, the most important differential consideration. Less common lesions with a thick nontapering stalk include **neurosarcoid** (uncommon in children), **astrocytoma**, and **hypophysitis**.

Skull base destruction centered on the temporal bone occurs with severe **otomastoiditis** and **rhabdomyosarcoma**.

Non-Langerhans Cell Histiocytoses

Tumors and tumor-like lesions in this group lack dendritic Langerhans cells. Most non-LCH disorders arise from bone marrow-derived mononuclear macrophages at various stages of development and activation.

Rosai-Dorfman Disease

TERMINOLOGY AND ETIOLOGY. Rosai-Dorfman disease (RDD), also called sinus histiocytosis with massive lymphadenopathy, is a rare benign pseudolymphomatous

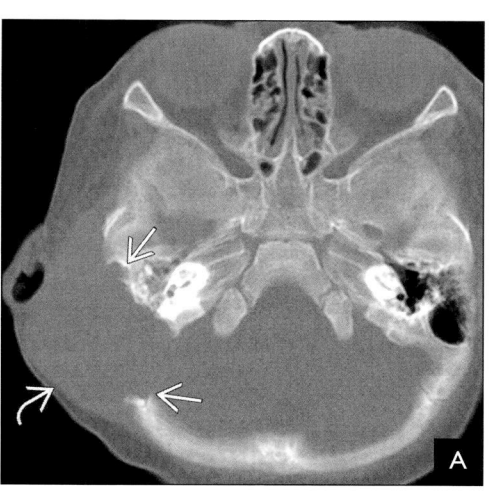

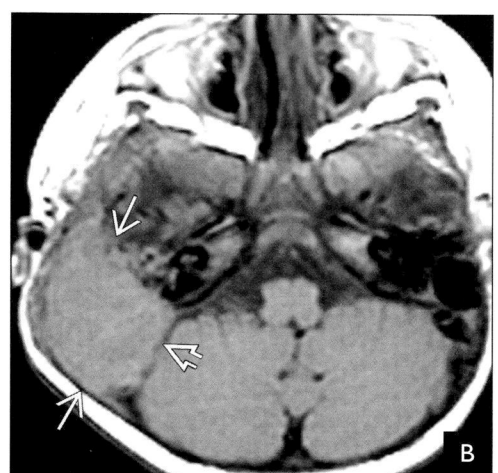

24-33A. *Bone CT in a child with LCH shows lytic skull base destruction centered in the right temporal bone* ➡️. *Note the large associated soft tissue mass* ➡️. **24-33B.** *T1WI in the same patient shows that the destructive mass* ➡️ *is isointense with brain. Note the medially displaced thin black line of dura* ➡️.

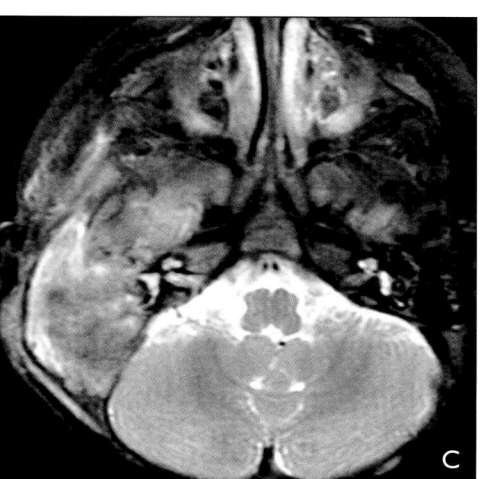

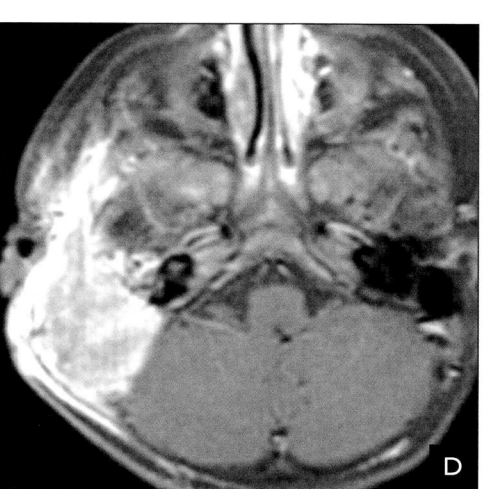

24-33C. *T2WI shows that the mass is heterogeneously hyper-, isointense relative to white matter.* **24-33D.** *The lesion enhances strongly, somewhat heterogeneously.*

entity of unknown etiology. Benign proliferating histiocytes cause striking lymphatic sinus enlargement.

CLINICAL ISSUES. Almost 80% of patients with RDD are younger than 20 years at the time of initial diagnosis. Prognosis is generally favorable after surgical resection and/or corticosteroid treatment.

IMAGING. RDD has a protean imaging appearance but most frequently presents as bilateral cervical lymphadenopathy. Extranodal involvement is seen in 50% of cases. The skin, nose, sinuses, and orbit (especially the eyelids and lacrimal glands) are often affected.

Intracranial RDD occurs in 5% of cases. Solitary or multiple dura-based masses that are moderately hyperdense on NECT and enhance strongly on CECT are typical findings. Sellar/suprasellar and intraspinal lesions are even less common. They can be isolated or occur in concert with more typical dura-based and/or orbital lesions.

RDD is typically isointense with gray matter on T1WI and iso- to slightly hypointense on T2WI **(24-34)**. Lesions demonstrate high fractional anisotropy, low ADC, and mild "blooming" on SWI. Intense homogeneous enhancement occurs following contrast administration. pMR is decreased.

FDG PET shows variable uptake. Nodal and lacrimal disease shows avid uptake, but other sites are often "cold" on FDG PET.

DIFFERENTIAL DIAGNOSIS. *Extra*cranial RDD closely resembles **non-Hodgkin lymphoma**. Reactive lymphadenopathy and TB adenopathy are common in children and may mimic RDD. Biopsy with histopathology is necessary for definitive diagnosis.

The major imaging differential diagnosis of *intra*cranial RDD is **meningioma**. pMR is helpful in distinguishing RDD, which is generally hypometabolic. **Neurosarcoid** with dura-based and sellar/suprasellar involvement can mimic RDD.

Erdheim-Chester Disease

TERMINOLOGY AND ETIOLOGY. Erdheim-Chester disease (ECD) is a rare non-LCH histiocytosis characterized by xanthomatous infiltrates of foamy histiocytes. Its etiology is unknown.

24-34A. T1WI shows effaced sulci, GM-WM interfaces in both frontal lobes ➔ and along the interhemispheric fissure ⤴. 24-34B. T2WI shows lobulated parafalcine masses ➔ that are iso- to slightly hyperintense relative to cortex.

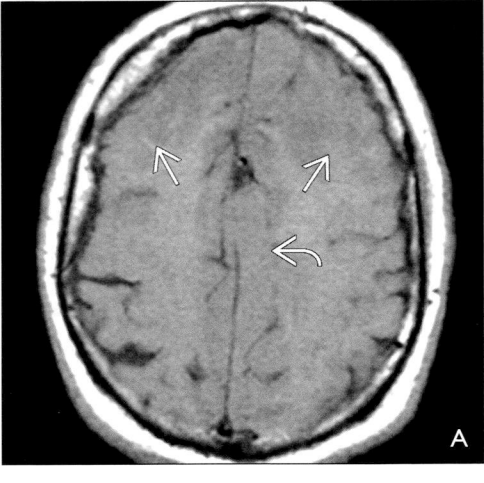

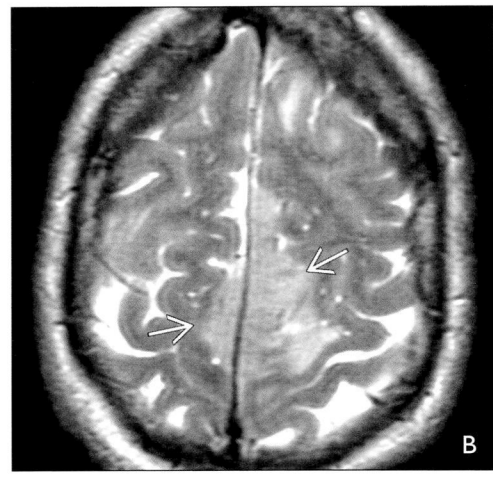

24-34C. Axial T1 C+ shows extensive, lobulated, intensely enhancing frontal and parafalcine masses ➔. 24-34D. Coronal T1 C+ scan shows additional lesions over the convexity ➔ and along the leaves of the tentorium cerebelli ⇥. The patient had Rosai-Dorfman disease diagnosed by cervical lymph node biopsy.

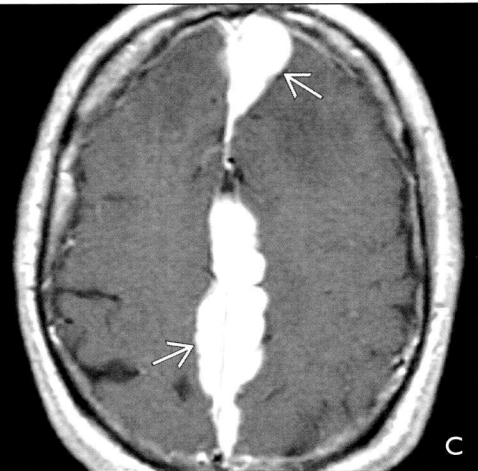

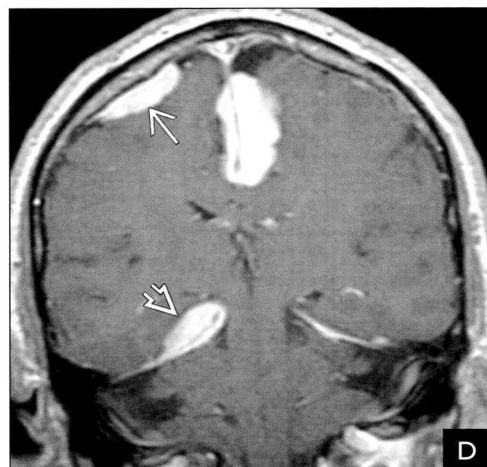

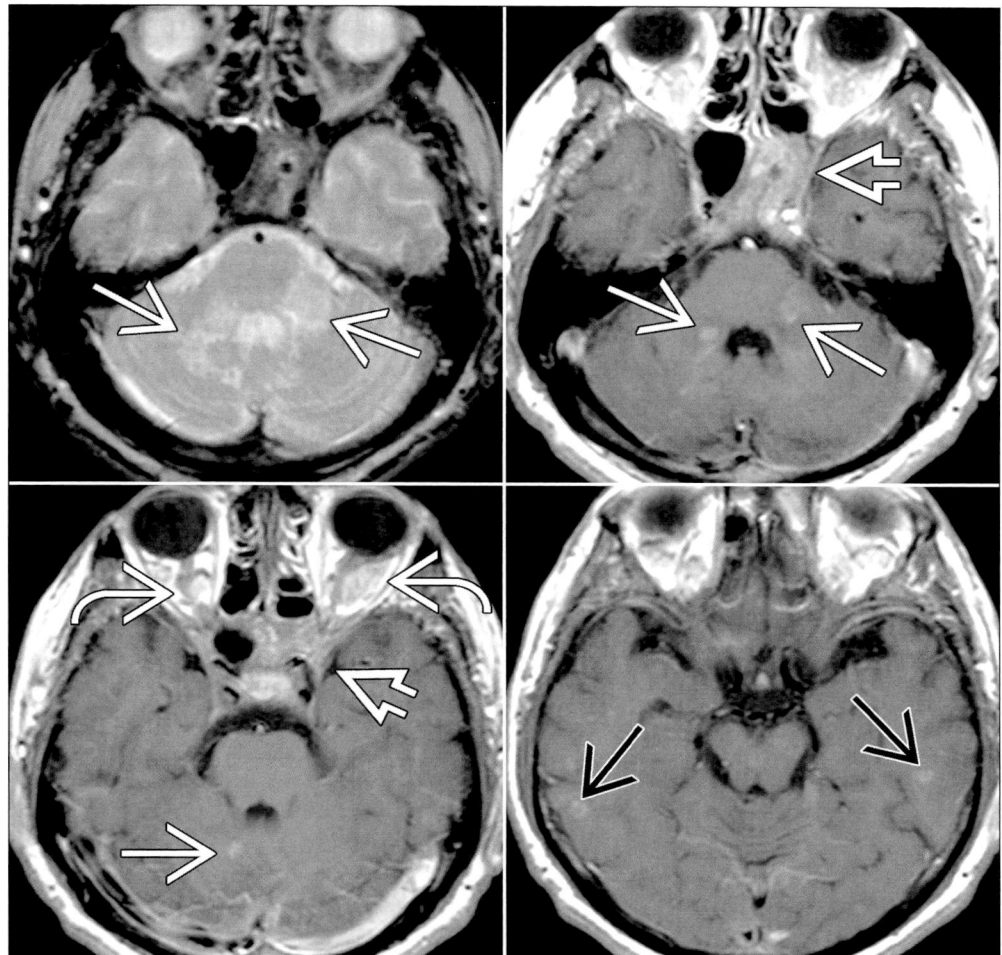

24-35. *(Upper left) T2WI shows patchy hyperintensities in the dentate nuclei, brachium pontis of both cerebellar hemispheres* ➡. *(Upper right) Patchy enhancement* ➡ *is seen on T1 C+. (Bottom) Additional lesions are present in the cavernous sinus* ➡, *superior cerebellum* ➡, *both temporal lobes* ➡, *and orbits* ➡. *Biopsy-proven Erdheim-Chester disease. (Courtesy M. Warmuth-Metz, MD.)*

CLINICAL ISSUES. ECD usually occurs in adults over 55 years of age. Prognosis in ECD is generally poor although treatment with interferon-α has improved survival in some patients.

PATHOLOGY. ECD is characterized by infiltrates of lipid-laden macrophages, giant cells, and histiocytes.

Although it may affect multiple organs, ECD is most typically a disease of long bones. Extraskeletal manifestations occur in 50% of cases. Intracranial lesions are present in 10% of patients. The brain, meninges, orbits, and sellar/juxtasellar region are all reported sites of ECD. Almost all patients with intracranial ECD have facial and/or calvarial thickening.

IMAGING. The hypothalamic-pituitary axis is involved in 50-55% of intracranial ECD. The pons and cerebellum—especially the dentate nuclei—are the second most common intraaxial location. Solitary or multiple dura-based masses with or without diffuse pachy-

meningeal thickening occurs in almost 25% of cases. Osteosclerosis of the facial bones, calvaria, or vertebral column may be a specific feature suggesting the diagnosis.

Imaging in patients with hypothalamic-pituitary involvement shows absent posterior pituitary "bright spot" on T1WI. A focal suprasellar mass or nodular thickening of the infundibular stalk is common.

Meningioma-like dural masses are isointense on T1WI and iso- to hypointense on T2WI. Strong homogeneous enhancement is typical.

Between 15-20% of ECD cases demonstrate parenchymal lesions. Multifocal areas of T2/FLAIR hyperintensity that show mild nodular enhancement on T1 C+ are typical findings **(24-35)**. Ependymal enhancement with deep linear extension into the lentiform nuclei has been described as a finding suggestive of ECD.

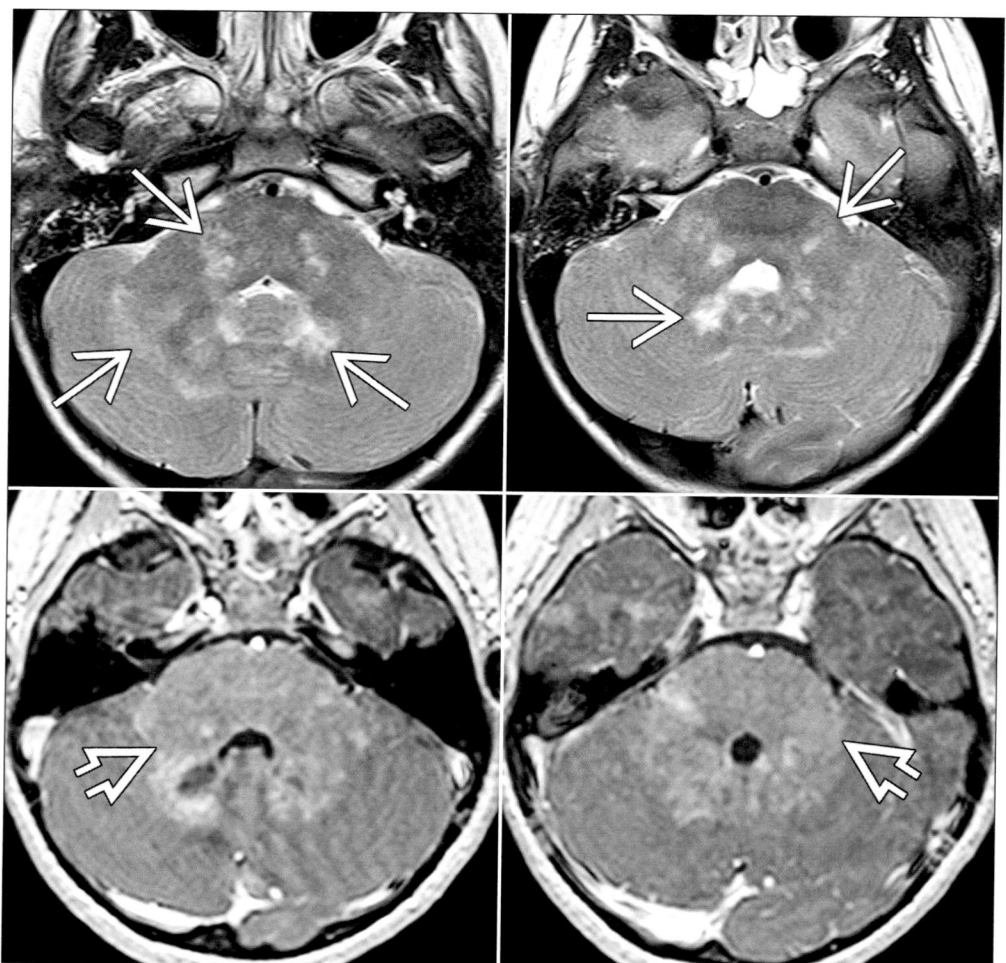

24-36. *(Top) T2 scans in a 2 year old with high fever and seizures show multiple patchy hyperintensities ⇥ expanding the pons and both middle cerebellar peduncles, extending into the dentate nuclei and cerebellar hemispheres. (Bottom) T1 C+ SPGR scans for stereotactic localization prior to biopsy show diffuse confluent and patchy enhancement ⇥. Histopathologic diagnosis was hemophagocytic lymphohistiocytosis.*

A unique finding with ECD is perivascular disease. Periaortic fibrosis and perivascular infiltration along the carotid arteries extending into the cavernous sinus may occur. These lesions are very hypointense on T2WI and enhance strongly and intensely.

DIFFERENTIAL DIAGNOSIS. The differential diagnosis of ECD includes **meningioma** and **LCH**. LCH is generally a disease of children whereas ECD primarily affects middle-aged and older adults. Osteosclerosis of the facial bones and/or calvaria may be a unique feature of ECD although histologic analysis plays the definitive role in differentiating ECD from other histiocytoses. **Wegener granulomatosis** (WG) may mimic ECD with sinus, orbital, and meningeal lesions, but WG usually causes osteolysis, not osteosclerosis.

Hemophagocytic Lymphohistiocytosis

TERMINOLOGY AND ETIOLOGY. Hemophagocytic lymphohistiocytosis (HLH) is a rare systemic disease characterized by aggressive proliferation of activated macrophages and histiocytes that show hemophagocytosis. It consists of two distinct forms: (1) primary or familial HLH, which usually occurs in infancy as an autosomal recessive disorder, and (2) secondary HLH, which is a reactive infection-associated process caused by viruses such as EBV, H1N1, and Bunyavirus.

CLINICAL ISSUES. HLH is primarily a disease of infants and young children. Fever, hepatosplenomegaly, and cytopenias characterize the disease. The typical clinical presentation includes irritability, bulging fontanelle, seizures, cranial nerve palsies, ataxia, and hemiplegia.

Primary HLH is lethal without allogenic stem cell transplantation. Secondary HLH is usually self-limited.

IMAGING. CNS involvement is present in at least 75% of all HLH patients at the time of initial diagnosis. Imaging shows extensive confluent T2/FLAIR hyperintense infiltrates in the cerebellum and cerebral white matter **(24-36)**.

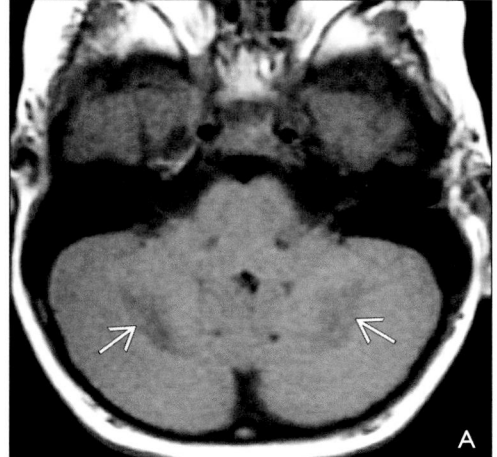

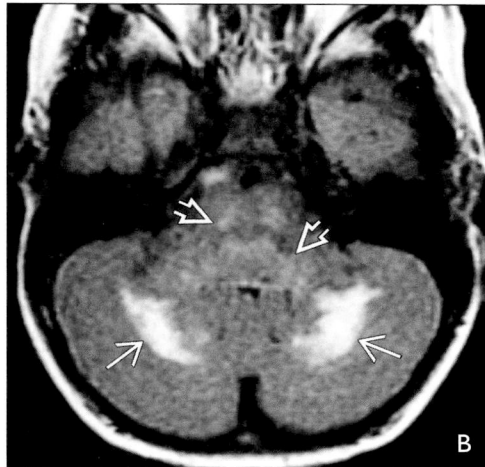

24-37A. Series of images demonstrates typical findings in a patient with juvenile xanthogranuloma. Axial T1WI shows bilateral symmetric hypointensities ➡ in the white matter of both cerebellar hemispheres. *24-37B.* The lesions ➡ are hyperintense on FLAIR. Additional lesions are seen in the lower pons, medulla ⇥.

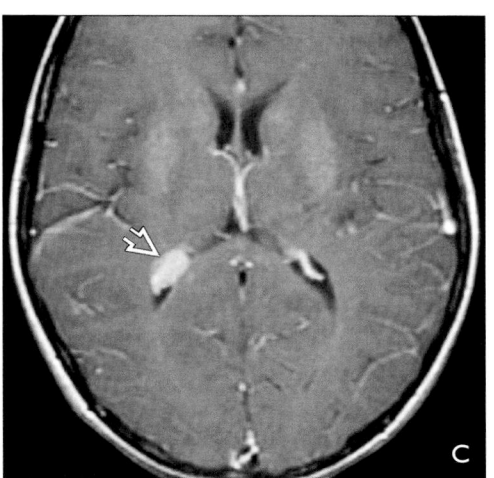

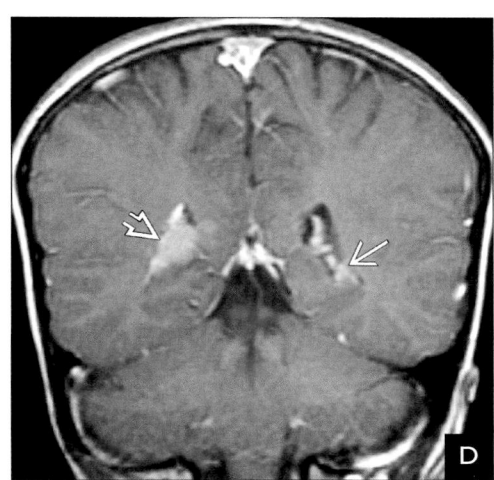

24-37C. T1 C+ shows enlarged, enhancing choroid plexus ⇥. *24-37D.* Coronal T1 C+ shows the large right choroid plexus lesion ⇥ and a smaller one in the left choroid plexus ➡.

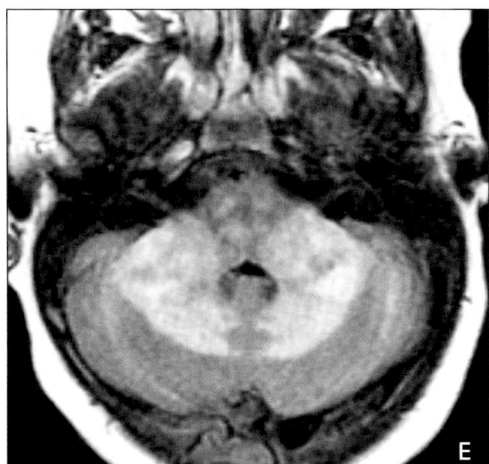

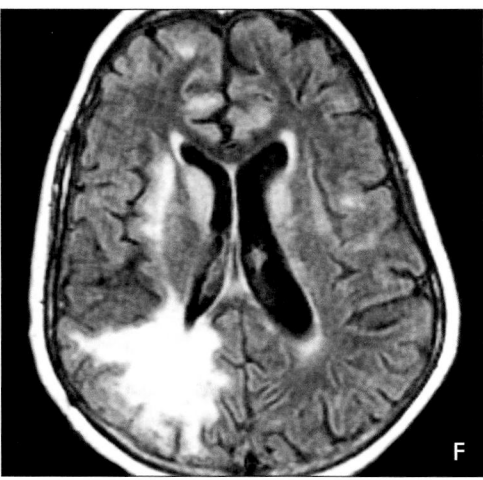

24-37E. The patient's condition worsened. Repeat FLAIR scan several months later shows that the cerebellar, brainstem lesions are now confluent. *24-37F.* More cephalad scan shows interval development of extensive supratentorial WM lesions. Biopsy-proven juvenile xanthogranuloma.

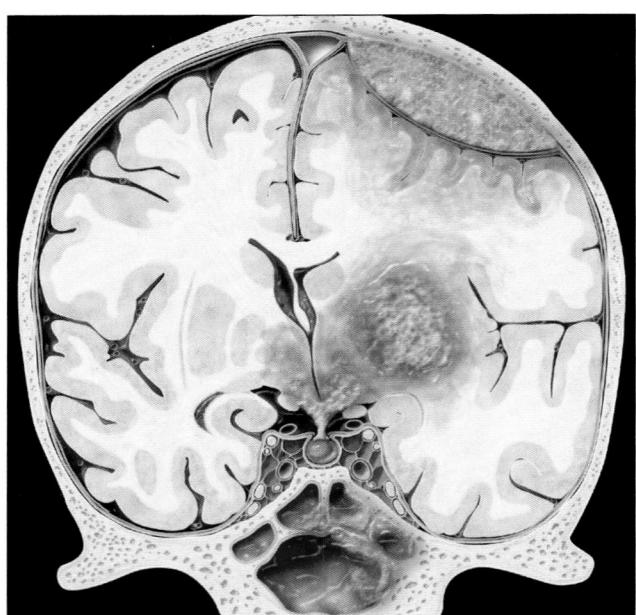

24-38. Coronal graphic depicts the typical greenish discoloration of granulocytic sarcoma. Extradural and sinus disease is common. Parenchymal lesions in the basal ganglia, hypothalamus, infundibular stalk are also illustrated.

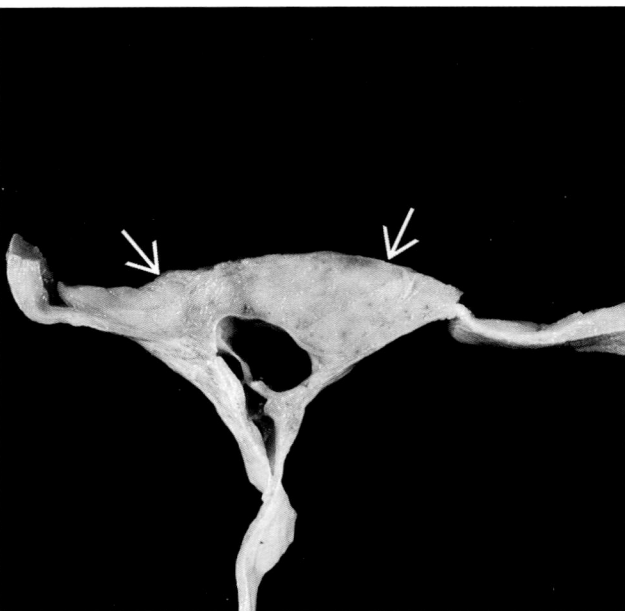

24-39. Autopsy specimen shows dural thickening, infiltration, focal masses ➤ in a patient who died from AML. (Courtesy R. Hewlett, MD.)

Symmetric periventricular lesions without thalamic and brainstem involvement are common in primary HLH.

Linear and nodular enhancement of parenchymal lesions and the pial surfaces of the brain is typical.

DIFFERENTIAL DIAGNOSIS. The major differential diagnoses of HLH are **Langerhans cell histiocytosis** and **juvenile xanthogranuloma**, an uncommon non-LCH histiocytosis. Biopsy is required for definitive diagnosis and appropriate treatment planning.

Acute disseminated encephalomyelitis (ADEM) can mimic secondary HLH clinically but often involves the thalami and brainstem and lacks symmetric periventricular lesions.

Juvenile Xanthogranuloma

Juvenile xanthogranuloma (JXG) is an uncommon benign histiocytic disease that generally affects young children and is usually limited to the skin. JXG may arise in the brain or cranial meninges, either with or without cutaneous manifestations. Cerebral lesions have been associated with multifocal or systemic forms of the disease, with an occasionally fulminant or relentless progressive clinical course.

Imaging findings with JXG vary. Disseminated white matter lesions resemble those of HLH (24-37). Lesions may also affect the sellar region, choroid plexus, orbits, and paranasal sinuses.

A rare disseminated form of xanthoma, called xanthoma disseminatum, preferentially affects young adults. The pituitary-hypothalamic axis and dura are most commonly affected by this variant.

Malignant Histiocytoses

Malignant histiocytosis is a rare neoplasm of the reticuloendothelial system characterized by neoplastic proliferation of tissue histiocytes. Malignant fibrous histiocytoma is now considered a high-grade undifferentiated pleomorphic sarcoma and is no longer regarded as a true histiocytic lesion. Only isolated cases have been reported to involve the brain. Sarcomas and malignant mesenchymal tumors are discussed in Chapter 22.

Hematopoietic Tumors and Tumor-like Lesions

Leukemia

Leukemia is the most common form of childhood cancer, representing approximately one-third of all cases. Acute lymphoblastic leukemia (ALL) accounts for 80% and acute myeloid leukemia (AML) for most of the remaining 15-20%. Chronic myelocytic leukemia (CML) and lymphocytic leukemia are much more common in adults. Regardless of specific type, the general clinical features of leukemias are similar.

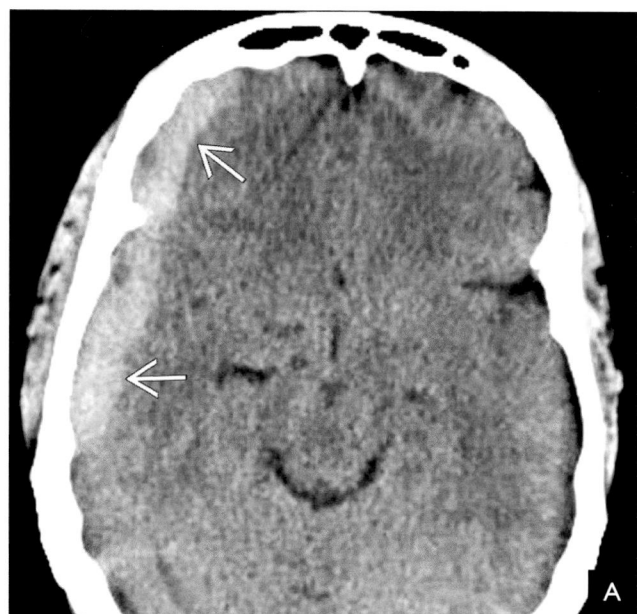

24-40A. *NECT scan in a patient with granulocytic sarcoma shows a hyperdense extraaxial mass* ➔ *that resembles a subdural hematoma.*

24-40B. *More cephalad scan in the same patient shows multiple additional hyperdense extraaxial masses* ➔.

Once relatively uncommon, the prevalence of CNS involvement has risen with treatment advances that result in prolonged overall survival. Neurological symptoms in leukemia patients may be due to CNS involvement (direct or primary effects) or occur as treatment complications (secondary effects).

Treatment-related complications include white matter lesions, mineralizing microangiopathy, posterior reversible encephalopathy syndrome (PRES), secondary tumors, infections, and brain volume loss. These are considered separately in Chapter 30, "Toxic Encephalopathy." Here we consider the direct effects of leukemia on the CNS.

Terminology

Leukemic masses containing primitive myeloblasts, promyelocytes, or myelocytes were initially called **chloromas** (for the greenish discoloration caused by high levels of myeloperoxidase in these immature cells). As 30% of the cells are other colors (white, gray, or brown), these tumors have been renamed **granulocytic (myeloid) sarcomas**.

Etiology

Granulocytic sarcoma is often diagnosed simultaneously with or immediately after the onset of acute leukemia. In patients without overt leukemia, granulocytic sarcoma usually presages the development of AML by several months. Other conditions that predispose to the development of granulocytic sarcoma are myelodysplastic syndromes and nonneoplastic myeloproliferative disorders such as polycythemia vera, hypereosinophilia, and myeloid metaplasia.

Intracranial granulocytic sarcomas probably develop when neoplastic cells in the calvaria migrate via haversian canals through the periosteum and into the dura to form focal leukemic masses. If the pial-glial barrier is breached, tumor can spread directly or via the perivascular spaces into the underlying brain.

Extramedullary leukemia (EML) is common in children with leukemia. CNS involvement is rare and occurs either as leukemia cells within the CSF or as focal aggregates of immature myeloid cells that infiltrate bone and soft tissues.

Pathology

LOCATION. EML can affect virtually any part of the body, including the skin, lymph nodes, stomach, and colon. Multiple lesions are common. Lesions of the vertebrae, orbits, and calvaria are more common than intracranial deposits, which are relatively rare.

Between 5-7% of patients with AML have asymptomatic CNS involvement as evidenced by positive CSF cytological analysis. Overt CNS leukemia presents in three forms: (1) meningeal disease ("carcinomatous meningitis"), (2) intravascular tumor aggregates with diffuse brain disease ("carcinomatous encephalitis"), and (3) focal tumor masses (granulocytic sarcoma).

Most intracranial lesions are located adjacent to malignant deposits in the orbits, paranasal sinuses, skull base, or calvaria. Intraaxial granulocytic sarcomas occur but are less common (24-38).

SIZE AND NUMBER. Multifocal involvement is typical. Extraaxial lesions are generally large and seen as extensive bony infiltrates and dura-based masses (24-39). Parenchymal lesions are usually smaller, ranging from a few millimeters to one or two centimeters.

MICROSCOPIC FEATURES. Granulocytic sarcomas are highly cellular tumors that consist of leukemic myeloblasts and myeloid precursors embedded in a rich reticulin-fiber network. Monotonous tumor cells with large nuclei, prominent nucleoli, and scanty eosinophilic cytoplasm are typical. Nuclei are often pleomorphic. Multiple mitoses are typical, with MIB-1 labeling exceeding 50%.

Clinical Issues

EPIDEMIOLOGY AND DEMOGRAPHICS. Granulocytic sarcoma occurs in 3-10% of patients with AML and 1-2% of patients with CML. Intracranial and intraspinal lesions in the absence of systemic disease are very rare. Although granulocytic sarcoma can affect patients of virtually any age, 60% are younger than 15 years at the time of initial diagnosis.

PRESENTATION. The typical clinical setting is that of a child with AML who develops headache or focal neurologic deficits. Meningeal disease may occur in adults with either acute or chronic myelogenous leukemia. Cranial nerve palsies are typical symptoms.

NATURAL HISTORY. Although the overall survival in treated AML is 40-50%, development of granulocytic sarcoma implies blastic transformation and poor prognosis. Transformation of chronic lymphocytic leukemia (CLL) into diffuse large non-Hodgkin lymphoma ("Richter syndrome") is a rare but serious complication. Median survival in transformed CLL is five or six months despite multiagent therapy.

TREATMENT OPTIONS. Patients with AML presenting with granulocytic sarcoma may benefit from individually tailored regimens with risk-adapted chemotherapy,

24-41A. NECT scan in a child with acute myeloid leukemia, scalp mass shows a hyperdense midline frontal mass ➡ with peritumoral edema, bone destruction ⊒. *24-41B.* T2WI in the same patient shows the scalp mass ➡, permeative destructive bone lesion ➡, parenchymal mass ⊒ that is isointense with cortex.

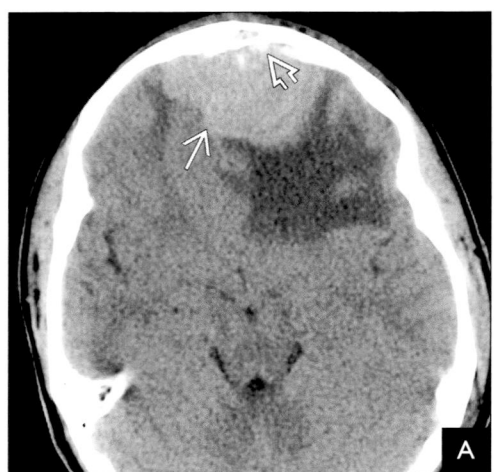
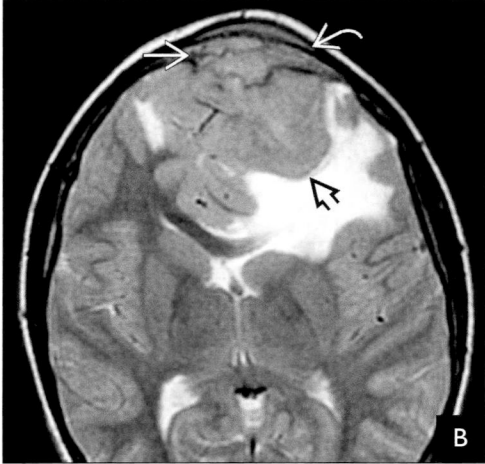

24-41C. The lesion is highly cellular, showing moderate diffusion restriction ➡ on DWI. *24-41D.* The lesion enhances strongly, mostly uniformly on T1 C+. Granulocytic sarcoma.

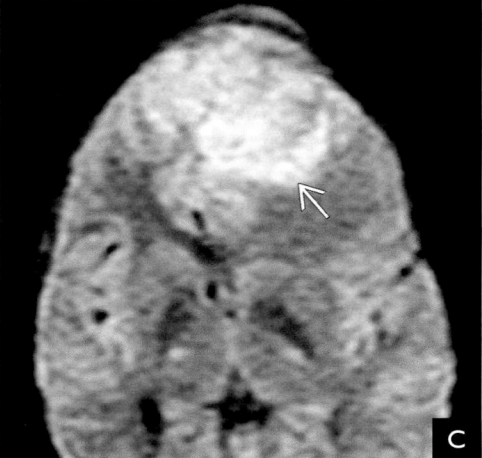
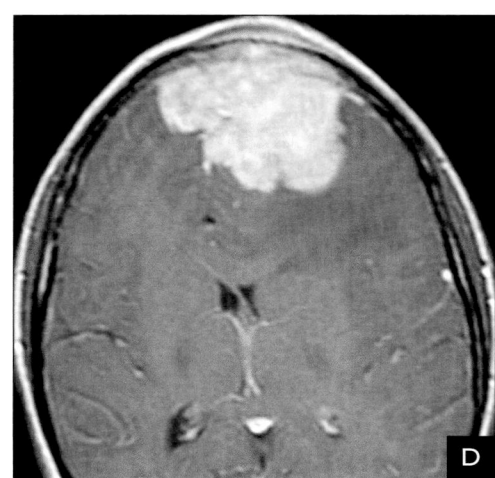

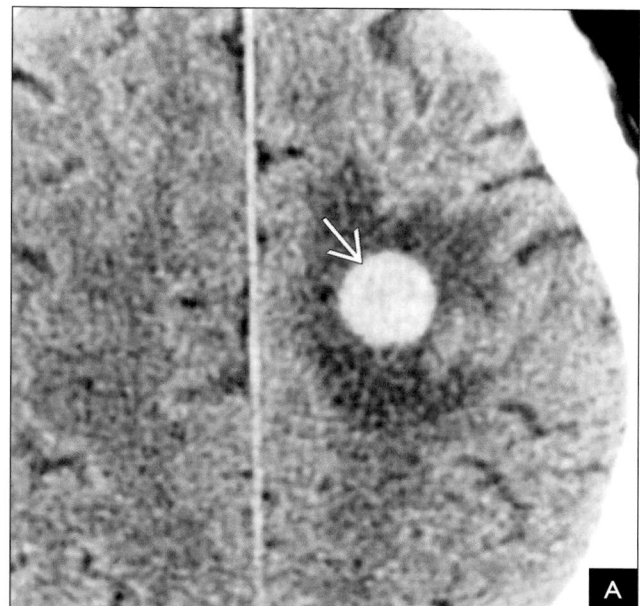

24-42A. NECT scan in a child with AML shows a round, very hyperdense mass ➡ in the left corona radiata.

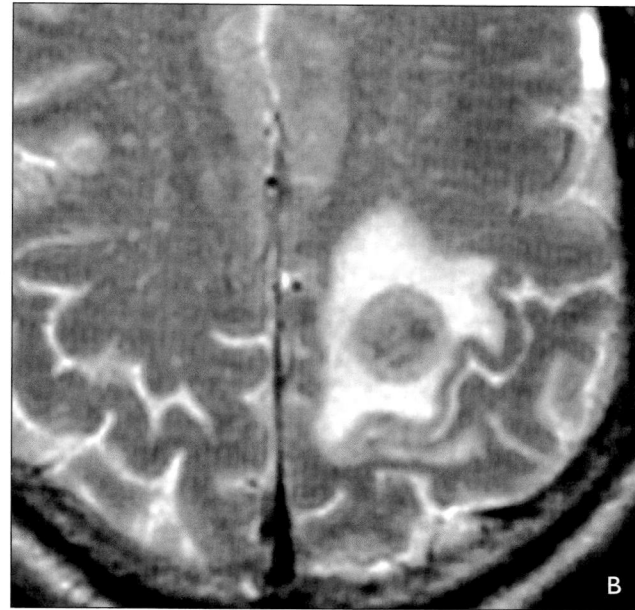

24-42B. The lesion is hypointense on T2WI. "Chloroma" (granulocytic sarcoma) was found at biopsy.

post-induction intensification of therapy, hematopoietic stem cell transplantation, and prolonged treatment maintenance.

Imaging

Imaging is key to the diagnosis of CNS involvement, as CSF studies may be negative.

CT Findings. Granulocytic sarcomas typically present as one or more iso- or hyperdense dura-based masses on NECT **(24-40)**. Strong uniform enhancement is typical. Bone CT often shows infiltrating, permeative, destructive lucent lesions. An adjacent soft tissue mass may be present.

MR Findings. Lesions are hypo- to isointense on T1WI and heterogeneously iso- to hypointense on T2/FLAIR **(24-41)**, **(24-42)**. FLAIR is helpful in detecting pial, perivascular, and CSF spread. Hemorrhage is common and easily detected on T2* (GRE, SWI) imaging.

Enhancement is typically strong and relatively homogeneous. Fat-saturated post-contrast T1 scans are especially helpful in detecting osseous involvement and delineating its extent. Because of its cellularity, granulocytic sarcoma often demonstrates diffusion restriction.

Nuclear Medicine Findings. Tc-99m MDP is commonly used to detect bone disease. Whole-body FDG PET or fused PET/CT shows avid uptake and is useful for initial staging as well as assessing treatment response.

Differential Diagnosis

Differential diagnosis depends on location. Dura-based granulocytic sarcomas may resemble **extraaxial hematoma**, **lymphoma**, or **meningioma**.

In younger children, **metastatic neuroblastoma** and **Langerhans cell histiocytosis** can mimic granulocytic sarcoma. **Extramedullary hematopoiesis** is a diagnostic consideration but is typically more hypointense than granulocytic sarcoma on T2WI.

Parenchymal granulocytic sarcomas or "chloromas" are much less common than dura-based lesions. The major differential diagnosis of granulocytic sarcoma is **lymphoma** or (in older patients) **metastasis**.

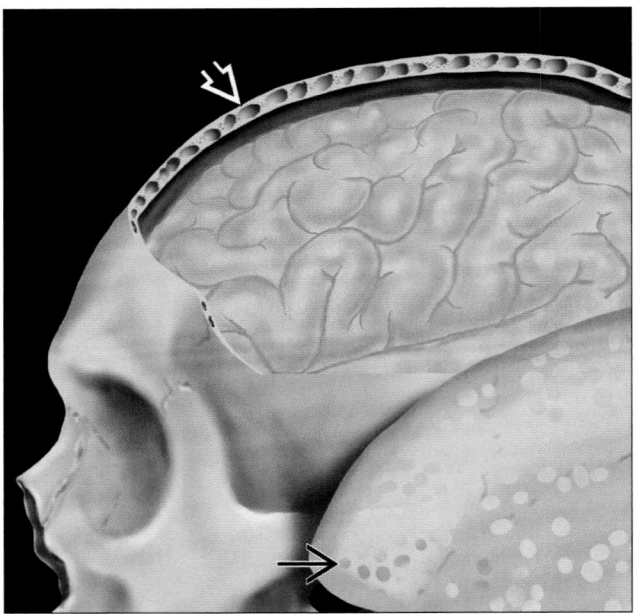

24-43. Graphic shows calvaria with multiple lytic foci ➡️ *characteristic of multiple myeloma. Sagittal section shows the "punched-out" lesions in the diploic space* ⏩.

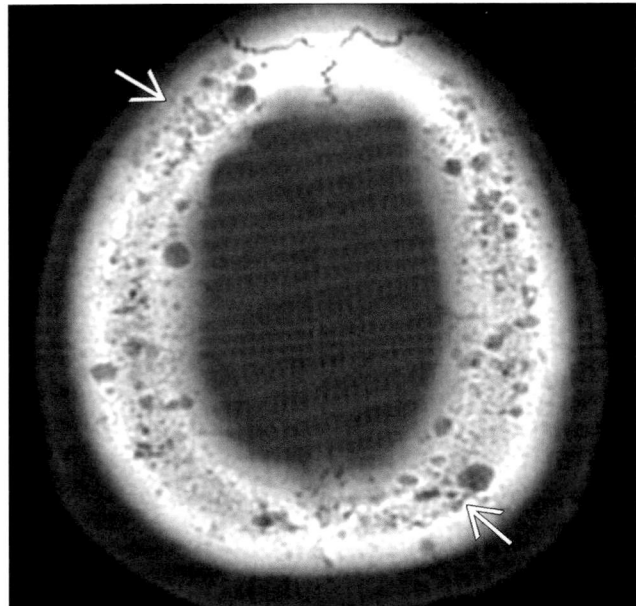

24-44. Bone CT shows typical findings in MM. Innumerable lytic "punched-out" lesions ➡️ *give the calvaria the characteristic "salt and pepper" appearance of MM.*

CNS LEUKEMIA

Terminology and Etiology
- Leukemia = most common childhood cancer
  - Acute lymphoblastic leukemia (ALL) (80%)
  - Acute myeloid leukemia (AML) (20%)
  - Chronic leukemias generally in adults
- CNS leukemias are extramedullary leukemias

Pathology and Clinical Issues
- CNS leukemia disease spectrum
  - Meningeal disease
  - Diffuse parenchymal disease (rare)
  - Granulocytic sarcoma (focal leukemic mass)
- Location
  - Extraaxial, dura-based > parenchymal
  - Typically by malignant deposits in skull, orbit, sinuses
  - Multiple lesions, multiple compartments typical
- Presentation varies; asymptomatic, positive CSF (5-7%)
  - CNS involvement in 3-10% of patients with AML

Imaging
- NECT
  - Permeative destructive bone lesions
  - Hyperdense dural masses (parenchymal disease rare)
- MR
  - Hypo-/isointense to brain on T1
  - Heterogeneously iso-/hyperintense on T2
  - ± hemorrhage on T2* (GRE, SWI)
  - Enhances strongly
  - DWI often positive
- Whole-body FDG PET, PET/CT
  - Useful for staging, assessing treatment response

Plasma Cell Tumors

Plasma cell myeloma and related immunosecretory disorders are a group of B-cell clonal proliferations characterized by production of monoclonal immunoglobulin from immortalized plasma cells.

Three major forms of neoplastic plasma cell proliferations are recognized: (1) solitary bone plasmacytoma, (2) solitary extramedullary plasmacytoma, and (3) multiple myeloma.

Solitary bone plasmacytomas (SBPs) are sometimes simply called plasmacytoma or solitary plasmacytoma (SP). SPs are characterized by a mass of neoplastic monoclonal plasma cells in either bone or soft tissue without evidence of systemic disease. SPs are rare (5-10% of all plasma cell neoplasms) and are most commonly found in the vertebrae and skull.

Solitary extramedullary plasmacytoma (EMP) is usually seen in the head and neck, typically in the nasal cavity or nasopharynx.

Multifocal disease is termed **multiple myeloma** (MM) **(24-43)**. **Plasmablastic lymphoma** is an uncommon, aggressive lymphoma that most frequently arises in the oral cavity of HIV-infected patients. Rarely, **atypical monoclonal plasma cell hyperplasia** occurs as an intracranial inflammatory pseudotumor (discussed in Chapter 28, "Nonneoplastic Cysts").

tiology

While the etiology of plasma cell tumors remains unknown, there is good evidence for a multistep transformation process that corresponds to clinically discernible disease stages.

Monoclonal gammopathy is a common asymptomatic precursor lesion that carries a 1% annual risk for progression to frank plasma cell neoplasms. Terminal stages in plasma cell neoplasms are characterized by increasing genetic complexity and independence from bone marrow stromal cells.

athology

LOCATION. SBPs almost always occur in red marrow, most frequently in the spine. The skull is the next most common location in the head and neck. Extramedullary plasmacytomas and EMPs in the presence of MM are uncommon (4-5% of cases) and rarely involve the CNS.

GROSS AND MICROSCOPIC FEATURES. Gelatinous red-brown tissue replaces normal-appearing yellow marrow. Trabecular bone loss is usually apparent. Microscopic examination discloses monotonous sheets of uniform well-differentiated neoplastic plasma cells with eccentric nuclei and basophilic cytoplasm. In general, at least 10% of the cells in a bone marrow biopsy specimen must be plasma cells for definitive diagnosis of MM.

Plasma cell tumors that express immunoglobulin light and heavy chains. Approximately 60% of MMs produce IgG, 20-25% produce IgA, and 15-20% produce free immunoglobulin light chains.

STAGING, GRADING, AND CLASSIFICATION. The two most commonly used myeloma staging systems are the Durie-Salmon PLUS classification and the International Staging System (ISS). Durie-Salmon PLUS integrates clinical, laboratory, and histopathologic parameters with imaging features (see box below).

Clinical Issues

EPIDEMIOLOGY. MM is the most common primary bone malignancy, accounting for approximately 10% of all hematologic malignancies. Almost half of all solitary bone plasmacytomas eventually progress to MM.

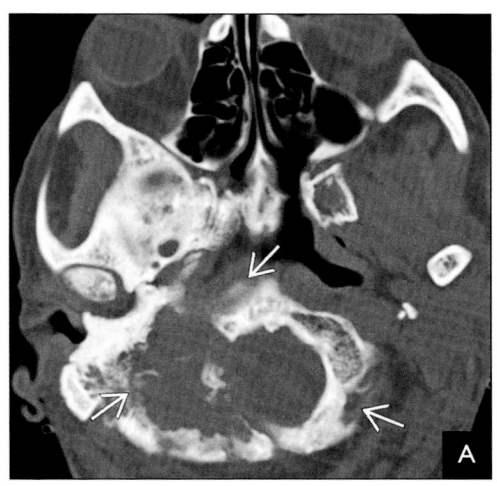
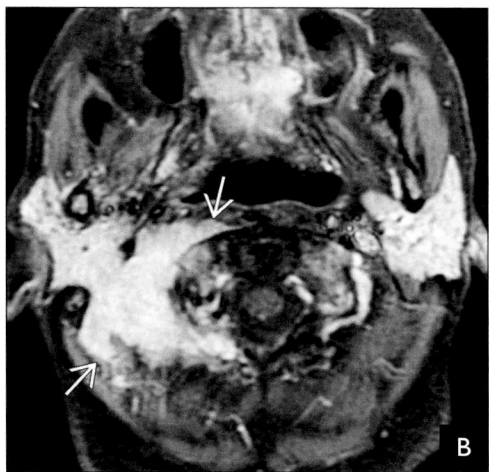

24-45A. Bone CT shows extensive permeative destructive lesions in the skull base ➡ characteristic of multiple myeloma. 24-45B. T1 C+ FS MR in the same patient shows that the lesions ➡ enhance strongly, uniformly.

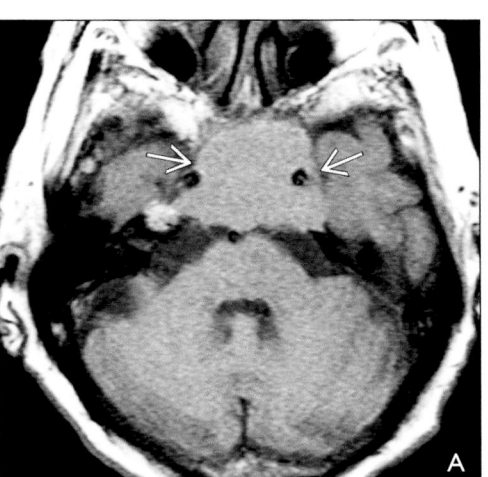
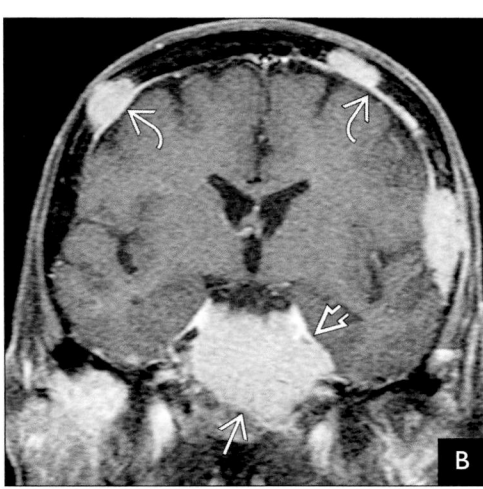

24-46A. Axial T1WI in a patient with MM, multiple cranial nerve palsies shows an isointense mass ➡ infiltrating, destroying the central skull base and extending laterally into both cavernous sinuses. 24-46B. Coronal T1 C+ FS shows that the skull base lesion enhances strongly, extends into the upper nasopharynx ➡ and into the left Meckel cave ➡. Additional lesions are present in the calvarial vault and demonstrate dural "tails" ➡.

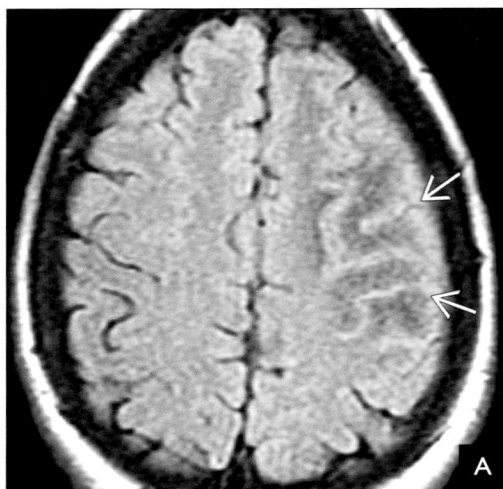

24-47A. *FLAIR scan in a patient with Waldenström macroglobulinemia shows hyperintense sulci, edema in the left hemisphere* ➡.

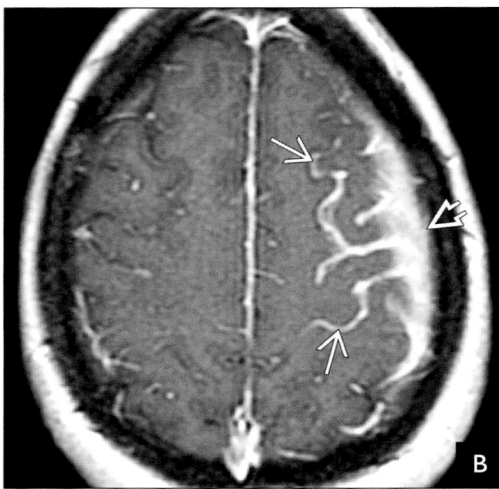

24-47B. *T1 C+ scan shows an enhancing dura-arachnoid mass* ➡ *with enhancement of the underlying sulci* ➡.

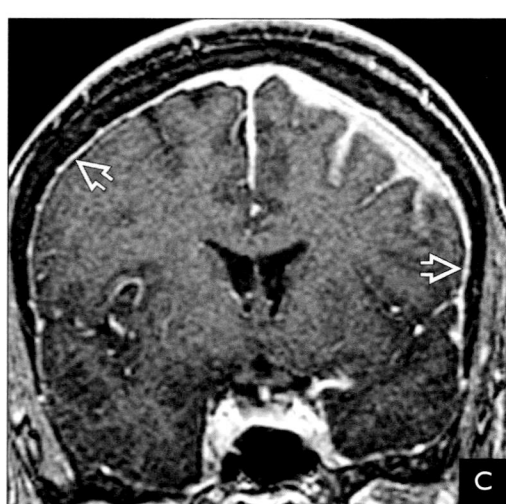

24-47C. *Coronal T1 C+ FS shows diffuse dura-arachnoid thickening* ➡. *Lymphoplasmacytic infiltrate in meninges. (P. Hildenbrand, MD.)*

Intracranial MM is uncommon and is usually secondary, occurring mostly as extension into the dura and leptomeninges from osseous lesions in the calvaria, skull base, nose, or paranasal sinuses.

Primary CNS plasmacytoma is very rare. Waldenström macroglobulinemia (a.k.a. Bing-Neel syndrome) may form dural lesions that then invade the brain parenchyma.

DEMOGRAPHICS. Prevalence varies with the type of plasma cell proliferation but generally rises with advancing age. Median age of patients with SBP or EMP is 55 years. The vast majority of patients with MM are older than 40 years with peak age at presentation in the seventh decade. There is a slight female predominance for SBP and a moderate male predominance in EMP and MM.

PRESENTATION. The most common presentation is bone pain. Constitutional symptoms such as fever of unknown origin are common with MM. Cranial nerve involvement is rare but may develop secondary to skull base plasmacytoma.

Immunoelectrophoresis detects M protein in the serum and/or urine from 99% of patients.

NATURAL HISTORY. Many plasma cell tumors eventually transform into MM. The five-year survival rate of MM is 20%. With newer treatment regimens, median survival has increased from two or three years to four years. Death is usually secondary to renal insufficiency, infection, and thromboembolic events.

TREATMENT OPTIONS. Diagnosis is made on biopsy, and treatment depends on disease stage. Careful evaluation of clinical, morphological, immunophenotypical, and cytogenetic features is necessary for individual risk assessment and appropriate therapy.

Common options for solitary plasmacytic lesions are radiotherapy followed by thalidomide plus dexamethasone. Autologous stem cell transplantation has prolonged survival in some patients with MM.

Treatment complications include osteonecrosis and bisphosphonate complications (mandibular osteonecrosis and subtrochanteric insufficiency fractures).

Imaging

Although radiography can only detect trabecular bone loss of more than 30-50%, skeletal surveys are still widely used for staging and surveillance of plasma cell tumors. CT is the best procedure for delineating lytic lesions in the skull base or calvaria.

MR is best used to evaluate the presence of diffuse marrow infiltration and define the extent of soft tissue disease. Whole-body MR is helpful in detecting systemic disease that would indicate the diagnosis of multiple myeloma instead of solitary plasmacytoma.

CT Findings. Solitary bone plasmacytomas are intramedullary soft tissue masses that produce lytic lesions centered in bone marrow. NECT shows a "punched-out" lesion without sclerotic margins or identifiable internal matrix. Cortical breakthrough with formation of a soft tissue mass adjacent to the lytic lesion may be present.

Multiple myeloma shows numerous lytic lesions, usually centered in the spine, skull base, calvarial vault, or facial bones. A variegated "salt and pepper" pattern is typical **(24-44)**.

Diffuse osteopenia without focal lesions is seen in 10% of MM cases.

MR Findings. In staging multiple myeloma, extent of bone marrow involvement is assessed on T1WI. Wholebody MR has emerged as the most sensitive imaging modality for detecting diffuse and focal bony lesions.

Osseous lesions replace normal hyperintense fatty marrow and are typically hypointense on T1WI **(24-46)**. Fatsaturated sequences such as T2-weighted STIR imaging also highlight the extent of marrow infiltration. Focal and diffuse lesions appear hyperintense. Both SBPs and MM enhance strongly following contrast administration **(24-45)**. Leptomeningeal and parenchymal disease occurs but is uncommon **(24-47)**.

Nuclear Medicine. Bone scintigraphy is not useful in evaluating MM, as lesions are often "cold" on Tc-99m scans. PET/CT is especially helpful for identifying and localizing extramedullary lesions. Sensitivity is 96% with a specificity of almost 80%.

Differential Diagnosis

Multiple "punched-out" destructive myeloma lesions can appear virtually identical to lytic **metastases**.

Spine and skull base MM can resemble **leukemia** or non-Hodgkin **lymphoma.** Both leukemia and lymphoma generally show increased activity on bone scan.

Sphenoclival **chordoma** can mimic MM but is typically very hyperintense on T2WI and contains intratumoral calcified bony sequestra.

Invasive pituitary macroadenoma may be difficult to distinguish from MM as both are isointense with gray matter. An elevated prolactin is often present. The pituitary gland cannot be separated from the mass.

PLASMA CELL TUMORS

Terminology
- Solitary bone plasmacytoma (SBP)
- Multifocal disease = multiple myeloma (MM)

Pathology
- Preferential involvement of red marrow sites
- Spine > skull

Durie-Salmon PLUS Staging (Multiple Myeloma)
- Monoclonal gammopathy
  ○ < 10% plasma cells in bone marrow
  ○ Normal marrow on MR, PET/CT
- Smoldering multiple myeloma
  ○ ≥ 10% plasma cells in bone marrow
  ○ Limited marrow disease on MR, PET/CT
- Multiple myeloma
  ○ ≥ 10% plasma cells and/or plasmacytoma + endorgan damage
  ○ Focal or diffuse lesions on MR
  ○ ↑ FDG marrow uptake (multifocal or diffuse)

Clinical Issues
- Monoclonal gammopathy is common precursor lesion
- 1% annual risk of developing plasma cell neoplasm
- Generally older adults
- Approximately 50% of SBPs progress to MM
- MM 5-year survival = 20%

Imaging
- NECT
  ○ Solitary or multiple "punched-out" lytic lesion(s)
  ○ ± soft tissue mass
- MR
  ○ Lesions replace normal fatty marrow
  ○ Hypointense on T1-, T2WI
  ○ Enhance on T1 C+ FS

Differential Diagnosis
- Lytic metastases (extracranial primary)
- Leukemia, lymphoma
- Invasive pituitary macroadenoma (central skull base)

Extramedullary Hematopoiesis

Extramedullary hematopoiesis (EMH) is the compensatory formation of blood elements due to decreased medullary hematopoiesis. Various anemias (thalassemia, sickle cell disease, hereditary spherocytosis, etc.) are the most common etiologies, accounting for 45% of cases. Myelofibrosis/myelodysplastic syndromes (35%) are the next most common underlying causes associated with EMH.

Multiple smooth, juxtaosseous, circumscribed, hypercellular masses are typical **(24-48)**, **(24-49)**. The most common site is along the axial skeleton **(24-51)**. The face and skull are the most common head and neck sites. The subdural space is the most common intracranial location.

EMH is hyperdense on NECT, enhances strongly and homogeneously on CECT **(24-50)**, and may show findings of underlying disease on bone CT (e.g., "hair on end" pattern in thalassemia, dense bone obliterating the diploic space in osteopetrosis).

Round or lobulated subdural masses that are iso- to slightly hyperintense relative to GM on T1WI and hypointense on T2WI are typical **(24-52A)**, **(24-52B)**. EMH enhances strongly and uniformly on post-contrast T1WI **(24-52C)**.

The major differential diagnoses of intracranial EMH are **dural metastases** and **meningioma**. **Neurosarcoid** and **lymphoma** are other considerations.

EXTRAMEDULLARY HEMATOPOIESIS

Etiology
- Decreased medullary hematopoiesis
- Compensatory formation of blood elements
- Anemias (45%), myelofibrosis/myelodysplasia (35%)

Pathology
- Multiple smooth juxtaosseous masses
- Spine, face, skull, dura

Imaging
- Hyperdense on NECT
- T1 iso-/hypo-, T2 hypointense
- Enhances strongly

Differential Diagnosis
- Dural metastases
- Meningioma
- Neurosarcoid
- Lymphoma

24-48. Graphic depicts extramedullary hematopoiesis. The diploic space converts from fatty to hematopoietic ("red") marrow ➡. Multiple lobulated extraaxial masses ▷, usually subdural, can occur in severe cases. *24-49.* Resected nodule of EMH shows hematopoietic tissue as red marrow, scattered between fatty foci. (Courtesy R. Hewlett, MD.)

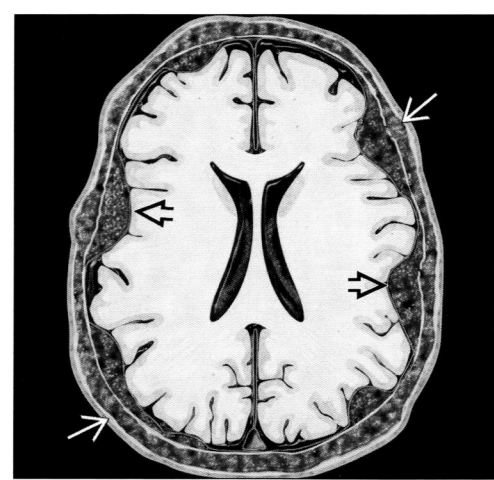

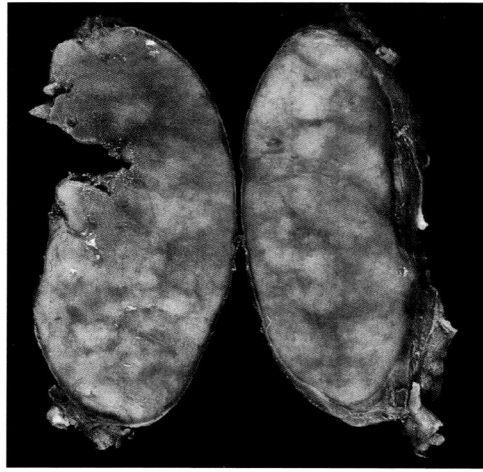

24-50. CECT scan shows enhancing dura-based masses ➡ in a teenage male with thalassemia, extramedullary hematopoiesis. *24-51.* Coronal T1 C+ FS scan in a teenage female with thalassemia, extramedullary hematopoiesis shows multiple lobulated enhancing paraspinal masses ➡. (Courtesy S. Blaser, MD.)

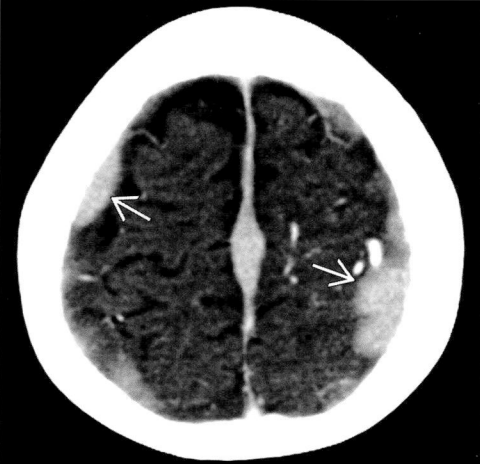

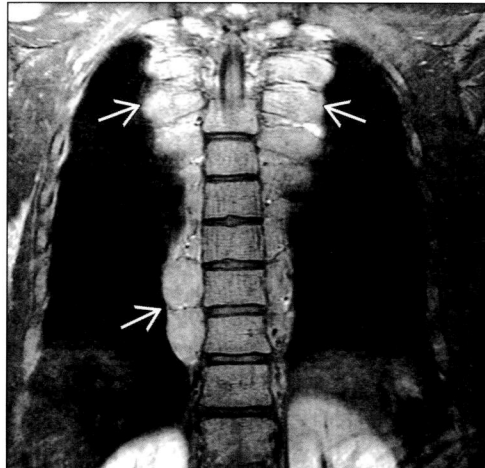

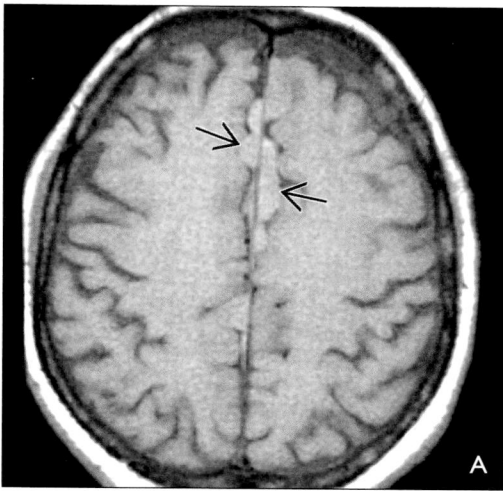

24-52A. *MR findings in intracranial EMH. On T1WI, well-defined dura-based masses ⇒ are iso- to slightly hyperintense compared to GM on T1WI.*

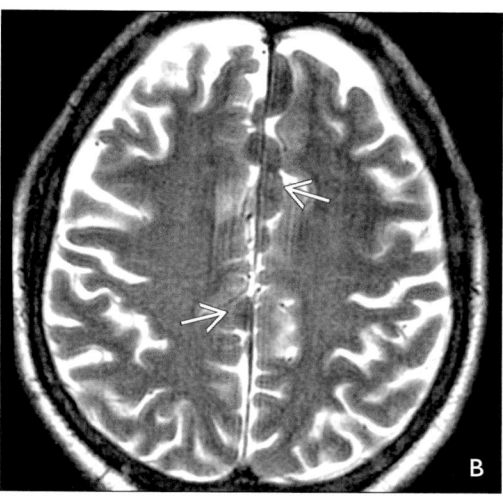

24-52B. *The lobulated lesions are very hypointense on T2WI ➡.*

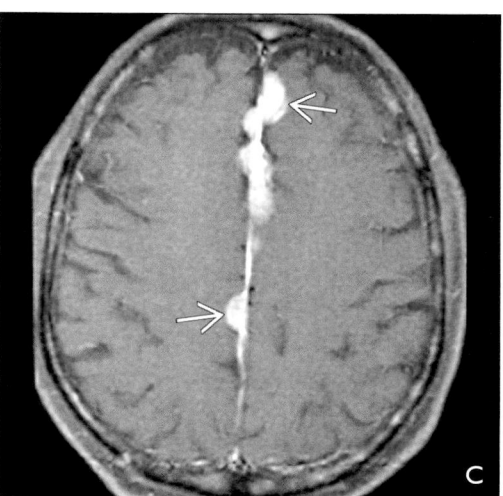

24-52C. *EMH enhances strongly, uniformly ➡ as shown on this T1 C+ FS scan in the same patient.*

elected References

ymphomas

Primary CNS Lymphoma

- Papanicolau-Sengos A et al: Rare case of a primary non-dural central nervous system low grade Bcell lymphoma and literature review. Int J Clin Exp Pathol. 5(1):89-95, 2012
- Ricard D et al: Primary brain tumours in adults. Lancet. 379(9830):1984-96, 2012
- Yap KK et al: Magnetic resonance features of primary central nervous system lymphoma in the immunocompetent patient: a pictorial essay. J Med Imaging Radiat Oncol. 56(2):179-86, 2012
- Breen EC et al: B-cell stimulatory cytokines and markers of immune activation are elevated several years prior to the diagnosis of systemic AIDS-associated non-Hodgkin B-cell lymphoma. Cancer Epidemiol Biomarkers Prev. 20(7):1303-14, 2011
- Lim T et al: Primary CNS lymphoma other than DLBCL: a descriptive analysis of clinical features and treatment outcomes. Ann Hematol. 90(12):1391-8, 2011
- Gerstner ER et al: Primary central nervous system lymphoma. Arch Neurol. 67(3):291-7, 2010
- Jiang L et al: Selective central nervous system tropism of primary central nervous system lymphoma. Int J Clin Exp Pathol. 3(8):763-7, 2010

Intravascular (Angiocentric) Lymphoma

- Orwat DE et al: Intravascular large B-cell lymphoma. Arch Pathol Lab Med. 136(3):333-8, 2012
- Mihaljevic B et al: Intravascular large B-cell lymphoma of central nervous system: a report of two cases and literature review. Clin Neuropathol. 29(4):233-8, 2010

Lymphomatosis Cerebri

- Keswani A et al: Lymphomatosis cerebri presenting with orthostatic hypotension, anorexia, and paraparesis. J Neurooncol. 109(3):581-6, 2012
- Kitai R et al: Lymphomatosis cerebri: clinical characteristics, neuroimaging, and pathological findings. Brain Tumor Pathol. 29(1):47-53, 2012

MALT Lymphoma

- Papanicolau-Sengos A et al: Rare case of a primary non-dural central nervous system low grade B-cell lymphoma and literature review. Int J Clin Exp Pathol. 5(1):89-95, 2012
- Bayraktar S et al: Primary ocular adnexal mucosa-associated lymphoid tissue lymphoma (MALT): single institution experience in a large cohort of patients. Br J Haematol. 152(1):72-80, 2011

Lymphomatoid Granulomatosis

- Dunleavy K et al: Lymphomatoid granulomatosis and other Epstein-Barr virus associated lymphoproliferative processes. Curr Hematol Malig Rep. 7(3):208-15, 2012
- Kobayashi Z et al: Differential diagnosis of CNS lymphomatoid granulomatosis. Neuropathology. 30(3):302; author reply 302-3, 2010
- Lucantoni C et al: Primary cerebral lymphomatoid granulomatosis: report of four cases and literature review. J Neurooncol. 94(2):235-42, 2009
- Patsalides AD et al: Lymphomatoid granulomatosis: abnormalities of the brain at MR imaging. Radiology. 237(1):265-73, 2005

Post-Transplant Lymphoproliferative Disorder

- Ghigna MR et al: Epstein-Barr virus infection and altered control of apoptotic pathways in posttransplant lymphoproliferative disorders. Pathobiology. 80(2):53-59, 2012
- Patrick A et al: High-dose intravenous rituximab for multifocal, monomorphic primary central nervous system post-transplant lymphoproliferative disorder. J Neurooncol. 103(3):739-43, 2011
- Arita H et al: Post-transplant lymphoproliferative disorders of the central nervous system after kidney transplantation: single center experience over 40 years: two case reports. Neurol Med Chir (Tokyo). 50(12):1079-83, 2010

Metastatic Intracranial Lymphoma

- Baraniskin A et al: Current strategies in the diagnosis of diffuse large B-cell lymphoma of the central nervous system. Br J Haematol. 156(4):421-32, 2012
- Pui CH et al: Central nervous system disease in hematologic malignancies: historical perspective and practical applications. Semin Oncol. 36(4 Suppl 2):S2-S16, 2009

Histiocytic Tumors

- Gill-Samra S et al: Histiocytic sarcoma of the brain. J Clin Neurosci. 19(10):1456-8, 2012

Langerhans Cell Histiocytosis

- Spagnolo F et al: Neurodegeneration in the course of Langerhans cell histiocytosis. Neurol Sci. 33(3):605-7, 2012
- Laurencikas E et al: Incidence and pattern of radiological central nervous system Langerhans cell histiocytosis in children: a population based study. Pediatr Blood Cancer. 56(2):250-7, 2011
- Shioda Y et al: Analysis of 43 cases of Langerhans cell histiocytosis (LCH)-induced central diabetes insipidus registered in the JLSG-96 and JLSG-02 studies in Japan. Int J Hematol. 94(6):545-51, 2011
- Paulus W et al: Histiocytic tumours. In Louis DN et al: WHO Classification of Tumours of the Central Nervous System. Lyon, France: IARC Press. 193-6, 2007

Non-Langerhans Cell Histiocytoses

- Camp SJ et al: Intracerebral multifocal Rosai-Dorfman disease. J Clin Neurosci. 19(9):1308-10, 2012
- Lou X et al: MR findings of Rosai-Dorfman disease in sellar and suprasellar region. Eur J Radiol. 81(6):1231-7, 2012
- Arnaud L et al: CNS involvement and treatment with interferon-α are independent prognostic factors in Erdheim-Chester disease: a multicenter survival analysis of 53 patients. Blood. 117(10):2778-82, 2011
- Lalitha P et al: Extensive intracranial juvenile xanthogranulomas. AJNR Am J Neuroradiol. 32(7):E132-3, 2011
- Raslan OA et al: Rosai-Dorfman disease in neuroradiology: imaging findings in a series of 10 patients. AJR Am J Roentgenol. 196(2):W187-93, 2011
- Sedrak P et al: Erdheim-Chester disease of the central nervous system: new manifestations of a rare disease. AJNR Am J Neuroradiol. 32(11):2126-31, 2011
- Drier A et al: Cerebral, facial, and orbital involvement in Erdheim-Chester disease: CT and MR imaging findings. Radiology. 255(2):586-94, 2010
- Hingwala D et al: Advanced MRI in Rosai-Dorfman disease: correlation with histopathology. J Neuroradiol. Epub ahead of print, 2010

Malignant Histiocytoses

- Black J et al: Fibrohistiocytic tumors and related neoplasms in children and adolescents. Pediatr Dev Pathol. 15(1 Suppl):181-210, 2012

Hematopoietic Tumors and Tumor-like Lesions

Leukemia

- Pauls S et al: Use of magnetic resonance imaging to detect neoplastic meningitis: limited use in leukemia and lymphoma but convincing results in solid tumors. Eur J Radiol. 81(5):974-8, 2012
- Akhaddar A et al: Acute myeloid leukemia with brain involvement (chloroma). Intern Med. 50(5):535-6, 2011
- Vanderhoek M et al: Early assessment of treatment response in patients with AML using [(18)F]FLT PET imaging. Leuk Res. 35(3):310-6, 2011
- Porto L et al: Granulocytic sarcoma in children. Neuroradiology. 46(5):374-7, 2004
- Guermazi A et al: Granulocytic sarcoma (chloroma): imaging findings in adults and children. AJR Am J Roentgenol. 178(2):319-25, 2002

Plasma Cell Tumors

- Kilciksiz S et al: A review for solitary plasmacytoma of bone and extramedullary plasmacytoma. ScientificWorldJournal. 2012:895765, 2012
- Lu YY et al: FDG PET or PET/CT for detecting intramedullary and extramedullary lesions in multiple

- myeloma: a systematic review and meta-analysis. Clin Nucl Med. 37(9):833-7, 2012
- Walker RC et al: Imaging of multiple myeloma and related plasma cell dyscrasias. J Nucl Med. 53(7):1091-101, 2012
- Healy CF et al: Multiple myeloma: a review of imaging features and radiological techniques. Bone Marrow Res. 2011:583439, 2011
- Fend F: Molecular pathology of plasma cell neoplasms. Pathologe. 31 Suppl 2:188-92, 2010
- Hanrahan CJ et al: Current concepts in the evaluation of multiple myeloma with MR imaging and FDG PET/CT. Radiographics. 30(1):127-42, 2010

Extramedullary Hematopoiesis

- Ginzel AW et al: Mass-like extramedullary hematopoiesis: imaging features. Skeletal Radiol. 41(8):911-6, 2012

25

Sellar Neoplasms and Tumor-like Lesions

Overview

The sellar region is one of the most anatomically complex areas in the brain. It encompasses the bony sella turcica and pituitary gland plus all the normal structures that surround it. Virtually any of these can give rise to pathology that ranges from unimportant and innocuous to serious, potentially life-threatening disease.

At least 30 different lesions occur in or around the pituitary gland, arising from either the pituitary gland itself or the structures that surround it. These include the cavernous sinus and its contents, arteries (the circle of Willis), cranial nerves, meninges, CSF spaces (the suprasellar cistern and third ventricle), and brain parenchyma (the hypothalamus).

Despite the overwhelming variety of lesions that can occur in this region, at least 75-80% of all sellar/juxtasellar masses are due to one of the "Big Five": Macroadenoma, meningioma, aneurysm, craniopharyngioma, and astrocytoma. All other lesions combined account for less than one-quarter of sellar region masses. Entities such as germinoma, Rathke cleft cyst, and hypophysitis each cause 1-2% or less.

Some authors recommend using a mnemonic (such as SATCHMO for **s**arcoid, **a**neurysm or **a**denoma, **t**eratoma or **t**uberculosis, **c**raniopharyngioma or **c**yst, **h**ypophysitis or **h**amartoma or **h**istiocytosis, **m**eningioma or **m**etastasis, and **o**ptic glioma) to remember the spectrum of lesions that can occur in/around the sella. However, this list mixes rare with common lesions and is unhelpful in establishing a clinically tailored, radiologically appropriate differential diagnosis.

The previous chapters in this part focus on specific neoplasms as defined histopathologically. This chapter is different. It's defined by geography and location. The goal of this discussion is to present the anatomy of the sellar region and then discuss the various lesions that make their home in this anatomically varied "neighborhood."

We begin the chapter with a general overview that includes keys to diagnosis, clinical considerations, and helpful findings on imaging studies. We then consider the normal gross and imaging anatomy of the sellar region.

Next we discuss normal variants such as physiologic hypertrophy that can mimic pituitary pathology. Congenital lesions (such as tuber cinereum hamartoma) that can be mistaken for more ominous pathology are also delineated. Pituitary gland and infundibular stalk neoplasms are then discussed. A brief consideration of miscellaneous lesions such as lymphocytic hypophysitis, pituitary apoplexy, and the postoperative sella follows.

The goal of imaging is to determine precisely the location and characteristics of a sellar mass, delineate its relation-

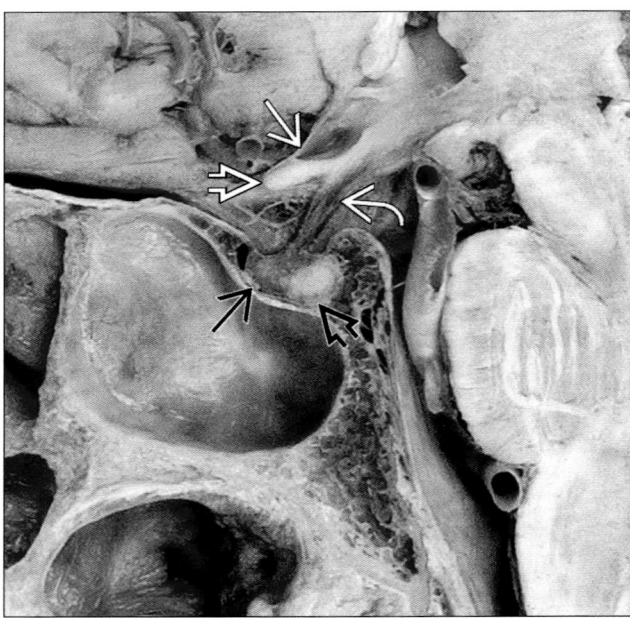

25-1. Midline anatomic section depicts sella, surrounding structures. Adenohypophysis ➡, neurohypophysis ⇉ are shown, along with the optic chiasm ⇶, optic ➡ and infundibular ➹ recesses of the third ventricle. (Courtesy M. Nielsen, MS.)

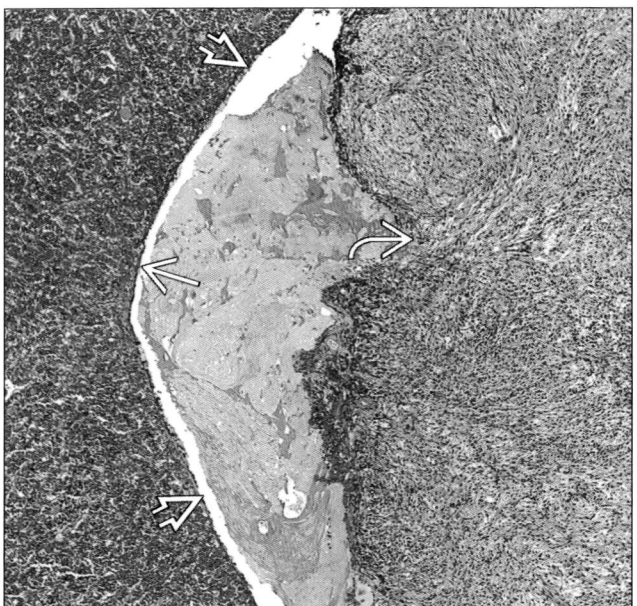

25-2. Photomicrograph of a sectioned normal pituitary gland shows Rathke pouch remnant as a "cleft" ⇉ between the anterior (left ➡), posterior (right ➡) lobes of the pituitary gland. (Courtesy A. Ersen, MD, B. Scheithauer, MD.)

ship to—and involvement with—surrounding structures, and construct a reasonable, limited differential diagnosis to help direct patient management. So we conclude the chapter with a summary of—and approach to—a differential diagnosis of sellar masses.

When you finish this discussion, you should be able to look at an unknown sellar mass and offer a focused differential diagnosis, not simply a recital of all the possible lesions that can be found in this anatomically complex region!

Diagnostic Considerations

Anatomic sublocation is the single most important key to establishing an appropriate differential diagnosis of a sellar region mass. The first step is assigning a lesion to one of three anatomic compartments, identifying it as a (1) intrasellar, (2) suprasellar, or (3) infundibular stalk lesion.

The key to determining anatomic sublocation accurately is the question, "Can I find the pituitary gland separate from the mass?" If you can't, and the gland *is* the mass, the most likely diagnosis is macroadenoma.

If the mass is clearly *separate* from the pituitary gland, it is extrapituitary and therefore not a macroadenoma. Other pathologies such as meningioma or craniopharyngioma should be considered in such cases.

Clinical Considerations

The single most important clinical feature in establishing an appropriate differential diagnosis for a sellar

region mass is patient age. Lesions that are common in adults (macroadenoma, meningioma, and aneurysm) are generally rare in children. A lesion in a prepubescent child—especially a boy—that looks like a macroadenoma almost never is a neoplasm. Nonneoplastic pituitary gland enlargement in children is much more common than tumors. Therefore, a "fat" pituitary gland in a child is almost always either normal physiologic hypertrophy or nonphysiologic nonneoplastic hyperplasia secondary to end-organ failure (most commonly hypothyroidism).

Some lesions that are common in children (e.g., optic-ochiasmatic/hypothalamic pilocytic astrocytoma and craniopharyngioma) are relatively uncommon in adults.

Gender is also important. Imaging studies of young menstruating females and postpartum women often demonstrate plump-appearing pituitary glands due to temporary physiologic hyperplasia.

Imaging Considerations

Imaging appearance is very helpful in evaluating a lesion of the sellar region. After establishing the anatomic sublocation of a lesion, look for imaging clues. Are other lesions present? Is the lesion calcified? Does it appear cystic? Does it contain blood products? Is it focal or infiltrating? Does it enhance?

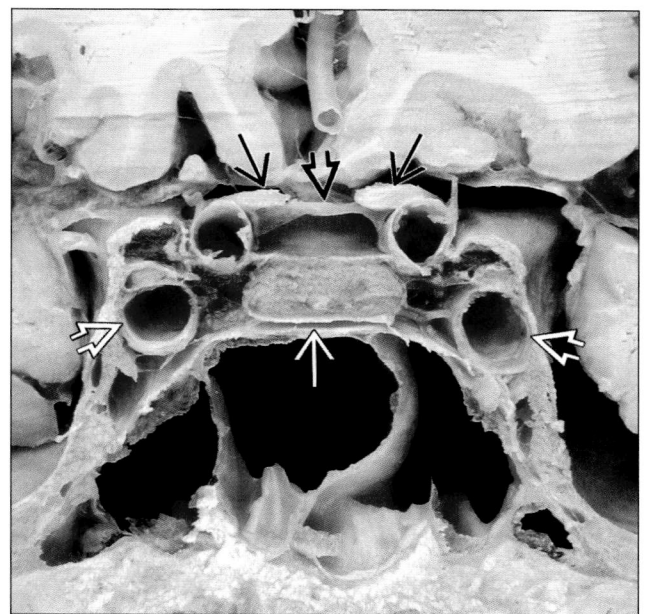

25-3. *Coronal gross section shows important structures adjacent to the pituitary gland ➡. Cavernous ⧉, supraclinoid ICAs are shown, as are the diaphragma sellae ⧈, optic nerves ➡. (Courtesy M. Nielsen, MS.)*

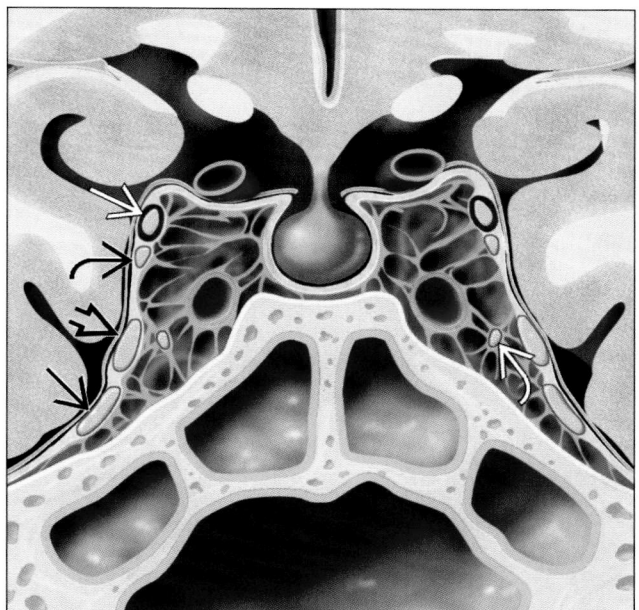

25-4. *Cranial nerves in the lateral dural wall of cavernous sinus include CNs III ➡, IV ➡, V₁ ⧈, V₂ ➡. Only CN VI ➡ is inside the cavernous sinus itself.*

ellar Region Anatomy

We briefly review the normal gross and imaging anatomy of the sellar region. Understanding normal anatomy forms the foundation for our subsequent consideration of sellar neoplasms and tumor-like lesions, the major topics of this chapter.

ross Anatomy

ony Anatomy

The **sella turcica** ("Turkish saddle") is a midline concavity in the basisphenoid that contains the pituitary gland. The anterior borders of the sella are formed by the anterior clinoid processes of the lesser sphenoid wing while the posterior border is formed by the dorsum sellae. The top of the dorsum sellae expands slightly to form the posterior clinoid processes, which in turn form the upper margin of the clivus **(25-1)**.

The sellar floor is part of the sphenoid sinus roof, which is partially or completely aerated. The cavernous segments of the internal carotid arteries lie in shallow bony grooves (the **carotid sulci**) located inferolateral to the pituitary fossa **(25-3)**.

Meninges

The meninges in and around the sella form important anatomic landmarks. **Dura** covers the bony floor of the sella, separating it from the pituitary gland. A thin dural reflection borders the pituitary fossa laterally and forms the medial cavernous sinus wall.

A small circular dural shelf, the **diaphragma sellae (25-3)**, forms a roof over the sella that almost covers the pituitary gland. The diaphragma sellae has a variably sized central opening, the **diaphragmatic hiatus**, that transmits the pituitary stalk **(25-5)**. The mean diameter of the diaphragmatic hiatus is seven millimeters.

A prominent basal **arachnoid** membrane, called the Liliequist membrane, forms trabeculae that cross the suprasellar cistern and cover the hypothalamus and diaphragma sellae. A sleeve of arachnoid reflects over the pituitary stalk, forming a thin hypophyseal cistern that can provide a surgical dissection plane in approaching suprasellar masses.

Pituitary Gland

The pituitary gland, also called the hypophysis, is a reddish-gray, bean-shaped gland with two distinct parts (sometimes called "lobes"): The anterior pituitary, also called the **adenohypophysis** (AH), and the posterior pituitary or **neurohypophysis** (NH) **(25-37)**.

The anterior and posterior pituitaries differ in embryologic origin, structure, and function but are joined together into a single gland, the hypophysis.

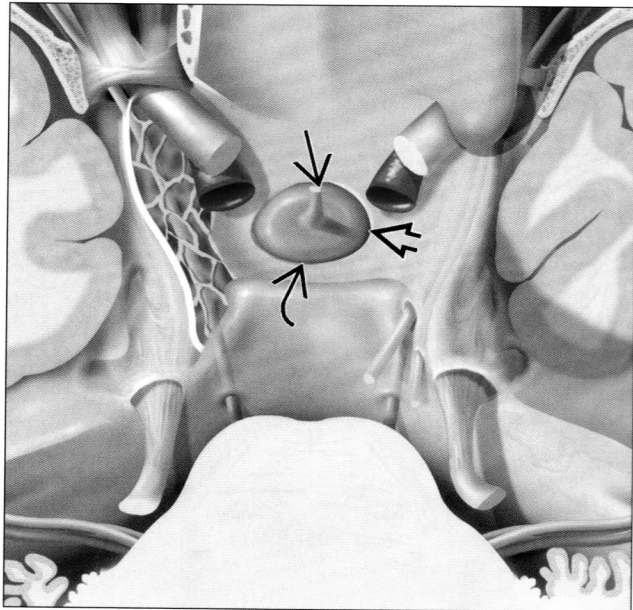

25-5. Axial graphic depicts the pituitary gland ⇗, stalk ⇒ seen through the opening of the diaphragma sellae ⇲.

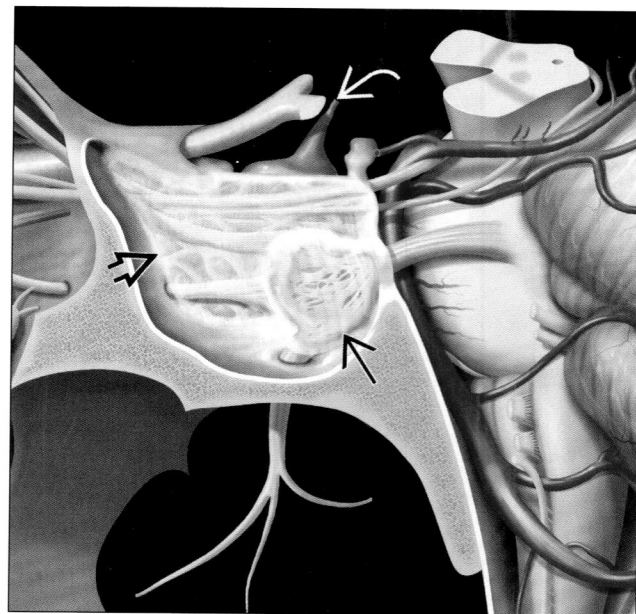

25-6. Sagittal graphic depicts cranial nerves of the cavernous sinus ⇒ lateral to the pituitary gland, stalk ⇒. Meckel cave is filled with CSF, contains fascicles of CN V and the gasserian (semilunar) ganglion ⇒.

ANTERIOR PITUITARY (ADENOHYPOPHYSIS). The AH, formerly called the anterior lobe, accounts for 75-80% of the total pituitary gland volume. The AH wraps antero-laterally around the NH in a U-shaped configuration. The AH is subdivided into three parts: The pars distalis (pars anterior), pars intermedia (PI), and pars tuberalis.

The AH develops as an outgrowth—called **Rathke pouch**—of embryonic ectoderm that lines the roof of the buccal cavity (25-2). This outgrowth subsequently detaches from the buccal cavity, and its anterior wall thickens to become the largest part of the AH called the **pars distalis**. The posterior wall differentiates into the **pars intermedia**, while the dorsolateral portions extend around the infundibulum as the **pars tuberalis**.

All three parts of the AH produce hormones. Most are tropins that regulate the function of other endocrine cells such as secretary cells in the gonads, thyroid, and adrenal cortex. All of the anterior pituitary hormones are regulated by hypothalamic-releasing hormones except prolactin, which is under control of a dopaminergic circuit.

Cells in the pars distalis of the AH produce five different hormones: Somatotropin (also known as growth hormone or GH), prolactin, thyroid-stimulating hormone (TSH), follicle-stimulating hormone/luteinizing hormone (FSH/LH), and adrenocorticotrophic hormone (ACTH). In addition, the AH also has a substantial proportion of cells that do not express hormonal markers. These non-hormone-secreting cells are called chromophobes.

The pituitary gland of newborns already presents a full set of terminally differentiated hormone-producing cells. However, the postnatal gland undergoes extensive remodeling. Soon after birth, the AH enters a dramatic growth phase that significantly increases the size of the gland.

The adult pituitary gland can adapt its cellular composition in response to changing physiological conditions.

POSTERIOR PITUITARY (NEUROHYPOPHYSIS). The posterior pituitary or neurohypophysis develops from the embryonic diencephalon (forebrain) as a downward extension of the hypothalamus. The posterior pituitary is subdivided into a large **pars nervosa** and smaller **infundibulum** (pituitary stalk).

The NH comprises 20-25% of the overall pituitary gland volume. The NH remains attached to the brain via the infundibulum, which inserts into the **median eminence of the hypothalamus**.

Most of the pars nervosa parenchyma consists of axonal terminations of neurons whose cell bodies are located in the hypothalamus. Neurons constitute approximately 75% of the posterior lobe. The remaining 25% of the posterior lobe consists of glial cells called **pituicytes**.

There are no intrinsic hormone-producing cells in the pars nervosa or pituitary stalk. Instead, the pars nervosa secretes two hormones that are formed in the hypothalamus: **Antidiuretic hormone** (ADH, also called **vasopressin**) and **oxytocin**. Both are synthesized as a larger precursor prohormone that also contains a carrier protein, **neurophysin**. The prohormone is transported down the axons of the hypothalamo-hypophyseal tract in the infundibulum, cleaved to its active form in the NH, and stored as secretory granules in the axon terminals.

Blood Supply

VEINS. The **hypophyseal portal system** consists of a primary capillary plexus in the median eminence and infundibulum and a secondary capillary plexus in the pars distalis of the AH. These are connected by long hypophyseal portal veins. Venous blood from both the anterior and posterior pituitary drains into the cavernous sinus.

The portal system forms an essential link between the hypothalamus and endocrine system: It is the route by which hypothalamic releasing and inhibitory hormones reach their target cells in the pars distalis of the AH to control pituitary function. The portal system also carries hypophyseal hormones from the gland to their endocrine targets and facilitates feedback control of secretion.

ARTERIES. Two sets of branches arise from the **internal carotid arteries** (ICAs) to supply the neurohypophysis. Single **inferior hypophyseal arteries** arise from the cavernous ICAs and supply most of the neurohypophysis. Several **superior hypophyseal arteries** arise from the supraclinoid ICAs with smaller contributions from the anterior and posterior cerebral arteries. The superior hypophyseal arteries mostly supply the median eminence of the hypothalamus and infundibular stalk.

There is no direct arterial supply to the adenohypophysis.

Hypothalamus and Third Ventricle

The **hypothalamus** lies directly above the pituitary gland, extending posteriorly from the lamina terminalis (anterior wall of the third ventricle) to the mammillary bodies. The **tuber cinereum** is part of the hypothalamus. It is the thin convex mass of gray matter that lies between the mammillary bodies and the optic chiasm. The infundibular stalk extends inferiorly from the tuber cinereum, gradually tapering as it descends to become continuous with the posterior pituitary lobe.

The **third ventricle** lies in the midline just above the hypothalamus. Two CSF-filled recesses of the third ventricle, the **optic** and **infundibular recesses**, project inferiorly toward the hypothalamus. The optic recess is more rounded and lies just in front of the **optic chiasm**. The infundibular recess is more conical and pointed, extending into the upper part of the pituitary stalk.

Cavernous Sinus, Cranial Nerves

CAVERNOUS SINUS. The **cavernous sinuses** (CSs) are irregularly shaped, trabeculated venous compartments that lie along the sides of the sella turcica. The CSs are contained within a prominent lateral and a thin (often inapparent) medial dural wall. Important CS contents include the **cavernous ICA** segments and several cranial nerves.

CRANIAL NERVES. Here we briefly review the cranial nerves that course through the cavernous sinus. (Anatomy of all the cranial nerves is discussed in detail in Chapter 23.)

The **abducens cranial nerve** (CN VI) is the only cranial nerve that actually lies within the CS, inferolateral to the cavernous ICA. Cranial nerves III, IV, V_1, and V_2 all lie within the lateral dural wall (25-4). The **oculomotor nerve** (CN III) is the most cephalad of the cavernous CNs and is contained within a thin sleeve of CSF-filled arachnoid called the **oculomotor cistern**. The **trochlear nerve** (CN IV) lies just below CN III.

Two divisions of the **trigeminal nerve** (CN V), the ophthalmic (V_1) and maxillary (V_2) divisions, lie below the trochlear nerve. The mandibular nerve (CN V_3) does not enter the CS. The trigeminal ganglion lies within another arachnoid-lined CSF space, **Meckel cave**. CN V_3 exits inferiorly from the trigeminal (gasserian or semilunar) ganglion and passes through the foramen ovale into the masticator space (25-6).

Imaging Technique and Anatomy

Technical Considerations

Appropriate imaging of the hypothalamic-pituitary axis is based on specific endocrine testing as suggested by clinical signs and symptoms. Thin-section multiplanar MR with small field of view obtained before and after contrast administration (dynamic as well as static sequences) is the best procedure, especially for hypothalamic abnormalities (25-7). CTA, MRA, DSA, and petrosal sinus sampling are supplemental techniques in selected cases.

Contrast-enhanced CT occasionally facilitates diagnosis of neuroendocrine abnormalities but is less sensitive than MR. Bone CT may be helpful in depicting the extent of bony involvement with invasive adenomas.

Pituitary Size and Configuration

Overall height of the pituitary gland on coronal T1-weighted MR scans varies with both age and gender. In prepubescent children, six millimeters or less is normal. The upper limit of normal in adult males and postmenopausal females is eight millimeters.

Physiologic hypertrophy in pubertal and young menstruating females is common, with normal gland height reaching 10 mm. Pregnant and postpartum lactating females have even larger, superiorly convex pituitary glands that may measure up to 14-15 mm in height.

25-7A. *3.0 T sagittal T2WI depicts pituitary gland, surrounding structures: Optic chiasm ⇉, optic ➔ and infundibular ➔ recesses.*
25-7B. *T1 C+ scan shows intensely enhancing venous blood, dura of the cavernous sinus ➔, slightly less intensely enhancing pituitary gland ⇉. Right CN III is seen as a nonenhancing linear structure ➔ coursing anteriorly in the lateral dural wall. "Flow voids" of cavernous ICA normally lie in the carotid sulci lateral to the pituitary gland.*

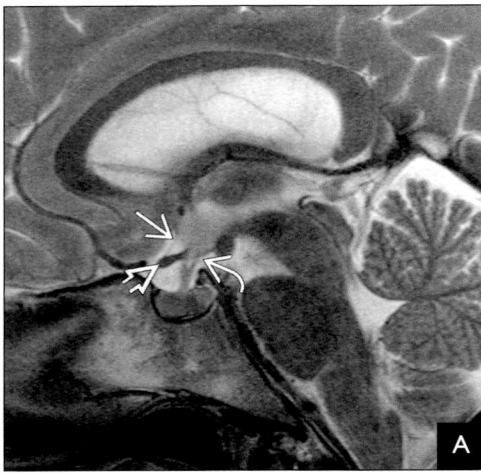
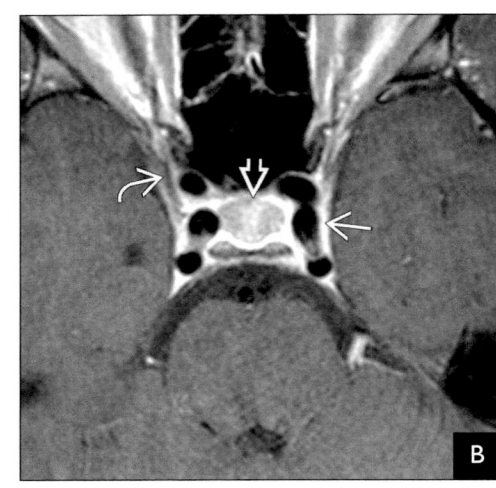

25-7C. *Coronal T2WI shows hyperintensity of CSF in the oculomotor cisterns ➔, Meckel caves ⇉. The "dots" inside Meckel caves are fascicles of the trigeminal nerve. Diaphragma sellae ➔ covers the sella.* **25-7D.** *Coronal T1 C+ FS shows CN III as nonenhancing rounded filling defects ➔ at the upper outer corners of the cavernous sinus. The infundibular stalk ➔, pituitary gland ⇉ enhance but less intensely than venous blood in the cavernous sinus.*

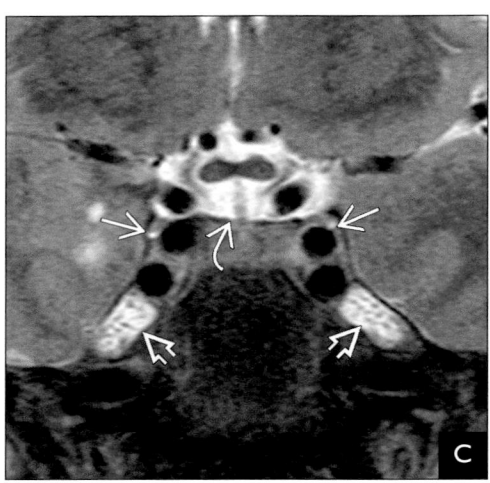
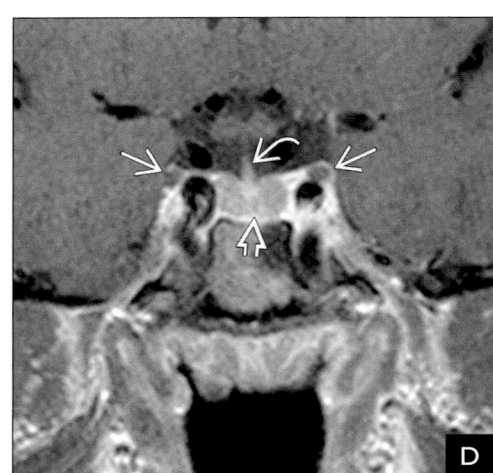

25-7E. *Sagittal T1WI with fat saturation shows that the neurohypophysis ➔ remains bright, indicating that its hyperintensity is not fat but neurosecretory granules.* **25-7F.** *Sagittal T1 C+ FS shows that the infundibular stalk ➔, tuber cinereum of the hypothalamus ⇉ lack blood-brain barrier, enhance. Note normal tapering of the infundibulum as it courses inferiorly from the hypothalamus to the pituitary gland.*

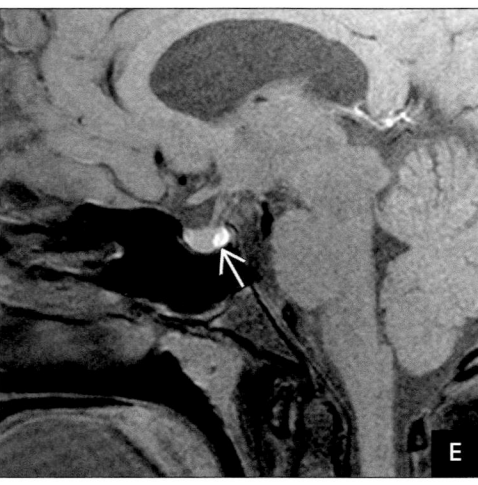
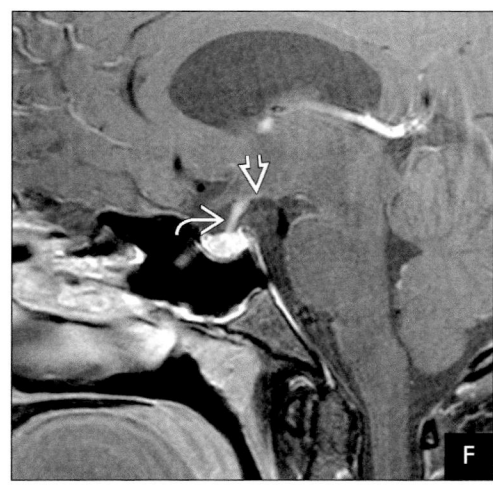

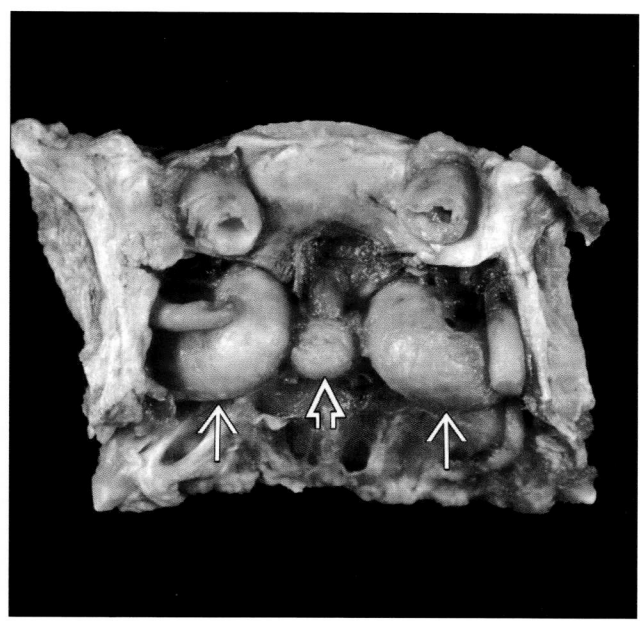

25-8. *Autopsy dissection of the central skull base shows medially positioned cavernous carotid arteries ➡ abutting, slightly compressing the pituitary gland ⇨. (Courtesy A. Ersen, MD, B. Scheithauer, MD.)*

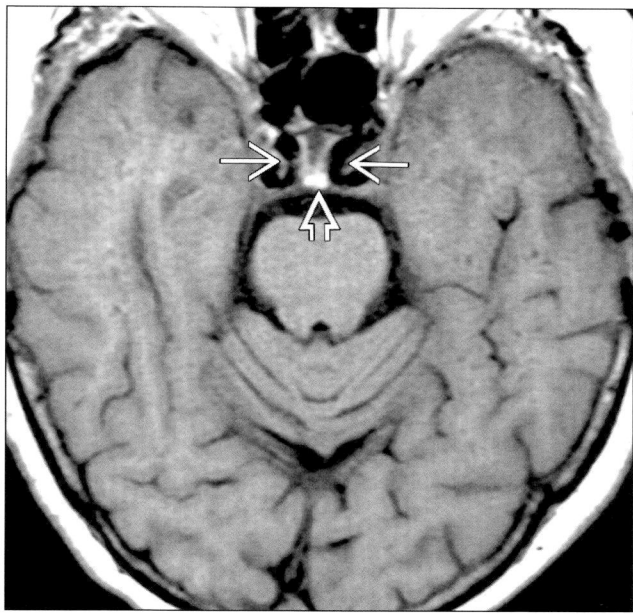

25-9. *Axial T1WI shows "kissing" carotids ➡ with compressed pituitary gland between them. The posterior pituitary "bright spot" ⇨ is seen squeezed upward between the carotid arteries.*

The infundibular stalk measures approximately 3.3 mm in diameter at the level of the optic chiasm and gradually tapers to about 2 mm as it descends to its insertion into the pituitary gland **(25-7F)**.

gnal Intensity of the Pituitary Gland

Pituitary gland signal intensity varies. With the exception of neonates (in whom the AH can be large and *very* hyperintense), the AH is typically isointense compared to cortex on both T1- and T2WI. The NH usually has a short T1 (the so-called posterior pituitary "bright spot" or PPBS) caused by the presence of neurosecretory granules. The PPBS does not contain lipid and does not suppress on fat-suppression techniques **(25-7E)**. Up to 20% of endocrinologically normal patients lack a PPBS.

The infundibular stalk is isointense with the pituitary except for a central hyperintensity on T2WI. The infundibular recess of the third ventricle extends inferiorly into the stalk for a variable distance.

hancement Patterns

The pituitary gland does not have a blood-brain barrier, so it enhances rapidly and intensely following contrast administration. Pituitary gland enhancement is slightly less intense than that of venous blood in the adjacent cavernous sinuses **(25-7D)**.

The infundibular stalk and tuber cinereum also lack a blood-brain barrier and enhance on T1 C+ **(25-7F)**.

Pituitary "Incidentalomas"

Focal areas of hypointensity or nonenhancement are common on contrast-enhanced scans of the pituitary gland. They are seen in 15-20% of asymptomatic patients and have been dubbed pituitary "incidentalomas." Most are less than one centimeter in diameter ("microincidentalomas"). They can be caused by intrapituitary cysts as well as nonfunctioning microadenomas. Both are common at autopsy.

While most pituitary "incidentalomas" are unsuspected imaging findings and generally of no clinical significance, recent endocrinologic guidelines recommend that patients with microincidentalomas undergo a thorough history, physical examination, and limited laboratory evaluation (i.e., prolactin and IGF-1 levels). Patients with "macroincidentalomas" (more than one centimeter) should be evaluated for hypopituitarism and have formal visual field evaluation if the lesion abuts the optic nerves or chiasm.

If patients do not meet specified surgical criteria for removal, follow-up MR is recommended at six months for a "macroincidentaloma," one year for a "microincidentaloma," and progressively less frequently thereafter if the "incidentaloma" remains unchanged in size.

Normal Imaging Variants

A number of variants occur in the pituitary gland and around the sella turcica; these should not be mistaken for disease on imaging studies. Not all enlarged pituitary glands are abnormal! Pseudoenlargement of the pituitary gland can be caused by "kissing" carotids or an unusually shallow bony sella. Pituitary hyperplasia can be abnormal, but it can also be physiologic and normal. An empty sella is a common normal variant but can also be a manifestation of idiopathic intracranial hypertension (pseudotumor cerebri).

"Kissing" Carotid Arteries

The cavernous internal carotid arteries normally lie lateral to the pituitary gland in the parasellar carotid sulci. Occasionally, the ICAs are positioned medially and actually course *inside* the bony sella (25-8). These "kiss-

ing" carotid arteries may compress the pituitary gland, squeezing it upward and making it appear modestly enlarged. The presence of medially positioned ICAs is highly important in presurgical planning for transsphenoidal hypophysectomy as normally positioned ICAs are not encountered in this approach (25-9).

Pituitary Hyperplasia

Terminology

Pituitary hyperplasia is a nonneoplastic increase in adenohypophysial cell number. It can be normal (physiologic) or pathologic.

Etiology

PHYSIOLOGIC HYPERPLASIA. Physiologic increase in pituitary volume is common and normal in many circumstances. Physiological hypertrophy of puberty and enlarged pituitary glands in young menstruating females are very common (25-10), (25-11), (25-12), (25-13). Pituitary gland enlargement secondary to prolactin cell hyperpla-

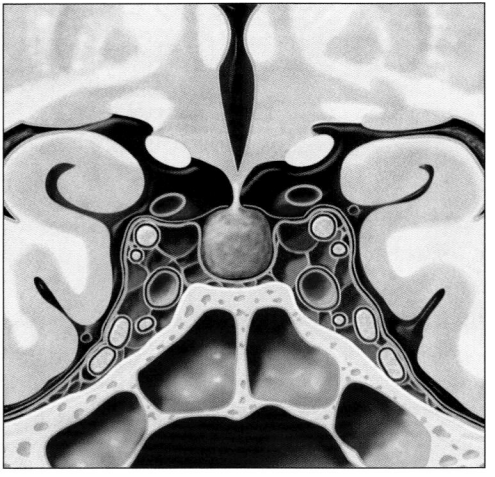

25-10. Coronal graphic shows physiologic pituitary hyperplasia. The gland is uniformly enlarged and has a mildly convex superior margin. 25-11. Low-power photomicrograph shows an axial section of a pituitary gland with hyperplasia. The diffusely enlarged anterior lobe ➡ dwarfs the neurohypophysis ⧗. (Courtesy A. Ersen, MD, B. Scheithauer, MD.)

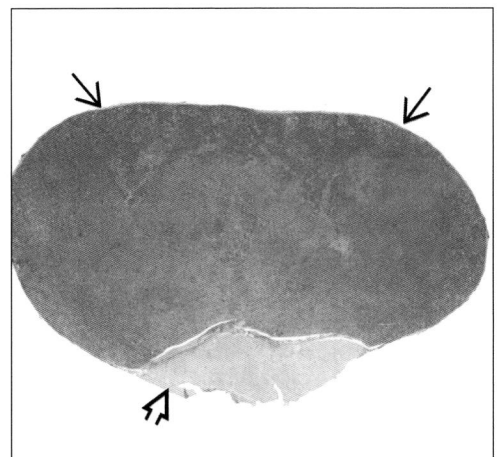

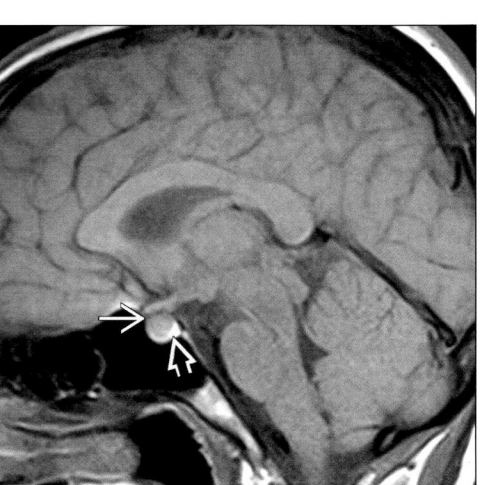

25-12. Sagittal T1WI in a 16-year-old female shows normal upward bulging of the pituitary gland ➡. The sellar floor is intact. Note the normal hyperintensity of the neurohypophysis ⧗. 25-13. Coronal T1 C+ in the same patient shows the upwardly convex gland ➡ almost touching the optic chiasm. The overall volume of the pituitary gland is almost twice the size of one in a postmenopausal woman.

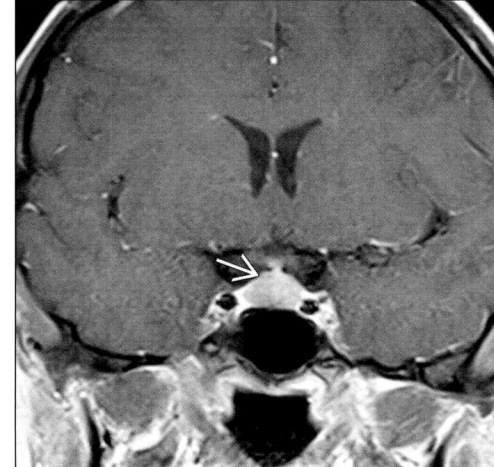

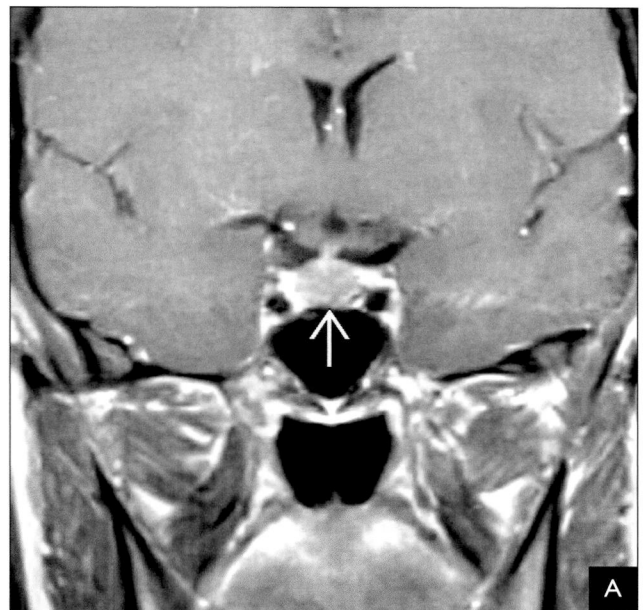

25-14A. *Coronal T1 C+ scan in a prepubescent male shows pituitary hyperplasia* ➔ *with an upwardly bulging gland that mimics macroadenoma.*

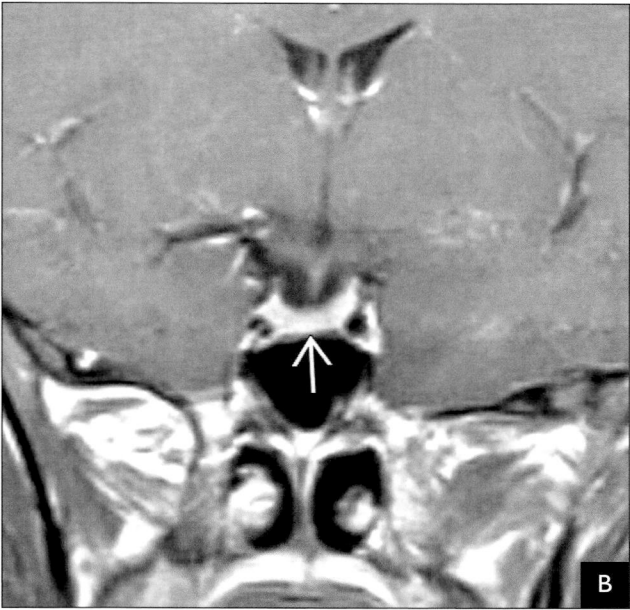

25-14B. *Endocrine evaluation revealed hypothyroidism. Repeat scan obtained a few weeks following initiation of hormone replacement now appears normal* ➔.

sia also occurs during pregnancy and lactation or in response to exogenous estrogen treatment.

PATHOLOGIC HYPERPLASIA. Pathologic hyperplasia most commonly occurs in response to **end-organ failure.** TSH cell hyperplasia can be induced by longstanding primary hypothyroidism **(25-14)**. ACTH cell hyperplasia occurs with hypocortisolism in Addison disease. Gonadotroph hyperplasia occurs as a response to primary hypogonadism (Klinefelter or Turner syndromes).

Pathologic hyperplasia can also be induced by ectopic excess of releasing hormones. GH cell hyperplasia occurs with increased GHRH secreted by pancreatic islet cell tumor, pheochromocytoma, bronchial carcinoma, and thymic carcinoid tumor.

ACTH cell hyperplasia may be secondary to CRH secretion from a hypothalamic hamartoma (see below), neuroendocrine tumor, or ACTH-dependent Cushing disease. Mammosomatotroph hyperplasia occurs in McCune-Albright syndrome and gigantism.

athology

GROSS PATHOLOGY. The most common physiologic form of pituitary hyperplasia is diffuse prolactin (PRL) cell hyperplasia during pregnancy and lactation. The adenohypophysis is symmetrically enlarged, sometimes nearly twice or three times normal size, but otherwise appears grossly normal.

Clinical Issues

EPIDEMIOLOGY. With the exception of PRL cell hyperplasia in pregnancy, pituitary hyperplasia is rare.

DEMOGRAPHICS. Most patients are children or young adults. PRL cell hyperplasia is the most common etiology.

PRESENTATION. Symptoms vary with the specific hormone. PRL cell hyperplasia causes hyperprolactinemia whereas GH cell hyperplasia causes gigantism or acromegaly. ACTH cell hyperplasia causes Cushing disease.

NATURAL HISTORY. Normal physiologic hypertrophy does not require treatment. Pathologic hyperplasia is treated medically, and prognosis is excellent. There is no increase in prevalence of adenoma.

Imaging

Symmetric increase in pituitary gland size and overall volume without focal mass effect or bony erosion is the classic finding.

NECT scans show that the superior margin of the gland is convex upward, measuring 10-15 mm in height. There is no evidence of erosion of the bony sella turcica. Enhancement is strong and generally uniform on CECT.

MR demonstrates an enlarged gland that bulges upward and may even contact the optic chiasm. The enlarged pituitary is isointense with cortex on both T1- and T2WI. Dynamic contrast-enhanced MR scans with three millimeters slice thickness and small field of view show that the gland enhances homogeneously. Occasionally focal nodular enhancement is present, especially with ACTH-cell hyperplasia.

Differential Diagnosis

Pituitary hyperplasia may be difficult to distinguish from **macroadenoma**. Age, gender, and endocrine status are helpful. Primary neoplasms of the pituitary gland are rare in children whereas physiological enlargement is common. Remember: *An enlarged pituitary gland in a prepubescent male is almost always hyperplasia, not adenoma!*

Lymphocytic hypophysitis can cause an enlarged pituitary gland. Lymphocytic hypophysitis is most common in pregnant and postpartum females and may be difficult to distinguish from physiologic PRL cell hyperplasia on imaging studies alone. If stalk enlargement is present, hypophysitis is more likely than hyperplasia.

Empty Sella

Terminology

An **empty sella** (ES) is an arachnoid-lined, CSF-filled protrusion that extends from the suprasellar cistern through the diaphragma sellae into the sella turcica (25-15). An ES is rarely completely "empty"; a small remnant of flattened pituitary gland is almost always present at the bottom of the bony sella, even if it is inapparent on imaging studies. Therefore, the term "partially empty sella" is anatomically more accurate.

Etiology

An ES can be primary or secondary. A **primary empty sella** occurs when an unusually wide (sometimes called "incompetent") opening in the diaphragma sellae allows intrasellar herniation of arachnoid and CSF from the suprasellar cistern above into the sella turcica below (25-16). Pulsatile CSF may gradually enlarge and deepen the sella, but the bony lamina dura separating the sella from the sphenoid sinus remains intact (25-17).

25-15. Graphic depicts primary empty sella ➡ with CSF-filled arachnoid cistern protruding inferiorly into the enlarged sella, flattening the pituitary gland posteroinferiorly against the sellar floor ➡. 25-16. Autopsy specimen seen from above shows a wide opening of the diaphragma sellae ➡ with CSF-filled sella below ➡. (Courtesy M. Sage, MD.)

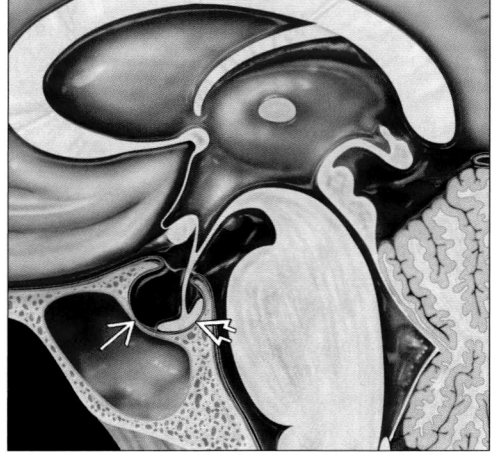
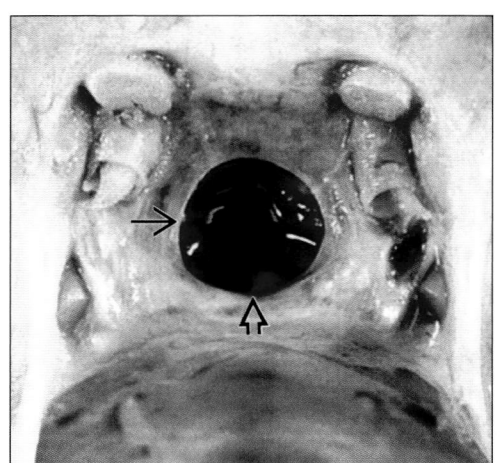

25-17. Sagittal low-power photomicrograph shows a partially empty sella as an enlarged, mostly CSF-filled sella ➡ with the pituitary gland ➡ flattened against the sellar floor. (Courtesy W. Kucharczyk, MD.) 25-18. Sagittal T1WI in an asymptomatic patient shows the classic empty sella as a CSF-filled space ➡. The pituitary gland is thinned and flattened against the sellar floor ➡. The patient was endocrinologically normal.

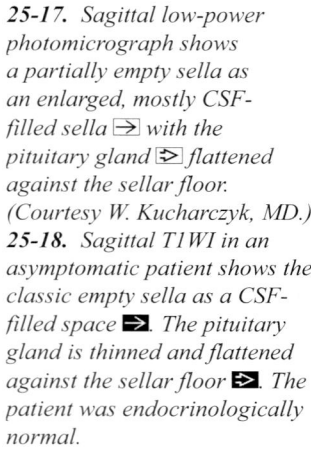
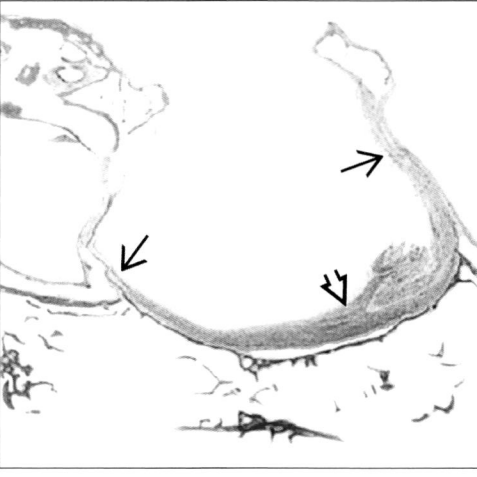
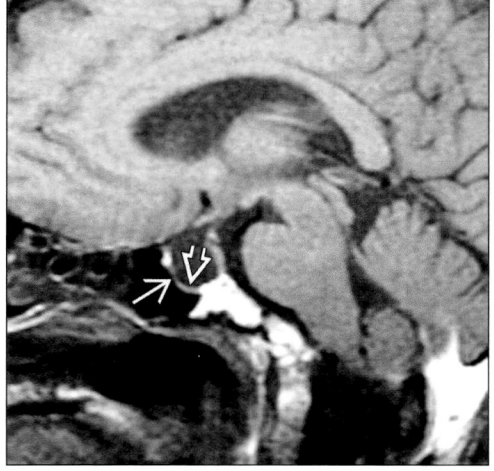

A **secondary empty sella** occurs when pituitary volume is reduced with surgery, bromocriptine therapy, or radiation treatment. Less often, pituitary apoplexy (usually with pituitary macroadenoma) may leave the expanded bony sella largely empty with only a small remnant of infarcted hemorrhagic gland at the posteroinferior aspect of the sella.

Rarely, a child with perinatal insult resulting in diffuse neuronal necrosis in the hypothalamus may have a very thin hypophyseal stalk and a partially empty sella.

A rare but important cause of secondary ES is **Sheehan syndrome**. Sheehan syndrome is one of the most common causes of hypopituitarism in underdeveloped countries. It results from ischemic pituitary necrosis due to severe postpartum hemorrhage. The great majority of patients with Sheehan syndrome have an empty sella on CT or MR scan.

Clinical Issues

EPIDEMIOLOGY. The exact prevalence of ES is unknown. An ES is identified in 5-10% of cranial MR scans.

DEMOGRAPHICS. While ES can occur at any age, peak presentation is in the fifth decade. There is a 4:1 female predominance. The mean body mass index of patients with an empty or partially empty sella is significantly higher than of those without an ES.

PRESENTATION. Most patients with ES are asymptomatic or have nonspecific symptoms such as headache **(25-18)**, **(25-19)**. However, primary ES may be associated with various clinical conditions ranging from mild endocrine disturbances to rhinorrhea or otorrhea. Between 18-20% of patients with primary ES have hyperprolactinemia, 5% have global anterior hypopituitarism, and 4% have isolated GH deficiency. Almost 80% of middle-aged obese females with spontaneous CSF otorrhea or rhinorrhea have an associated ES demonstrated on preoperative MR **(25-20)**.

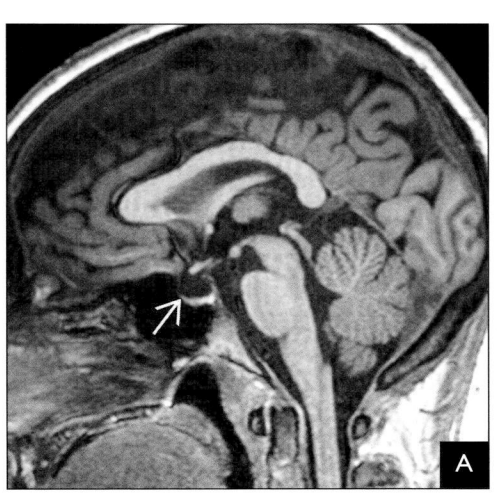

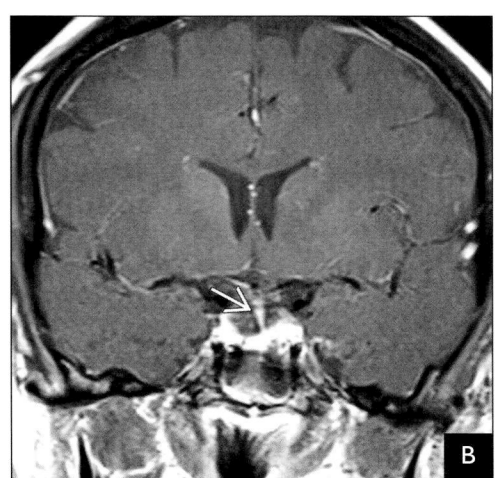

25-19A. Sagittal T1WI in a 28-year-old woman with complex partial seizures shows an empty sella ➡. 25-19B. Coronal T1 C+ in the same patient shows that the stalk ➡ inserts off-midline, a normal variant. The patient's endocrine profile was normal.

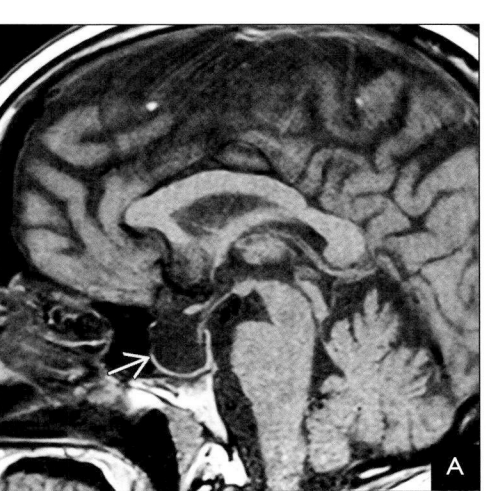

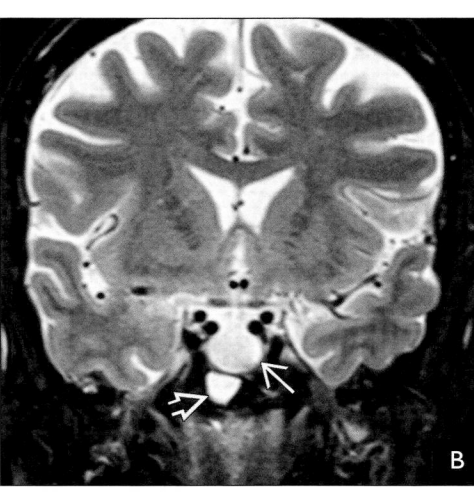

25-20A. An empty sella is not always benign, as illustrated by this case of a 56-year-old woman with a CSF leak. The enormous CSF-filled empty sella ➡ is much larger than the usual normal variant. 25-20B. Coronal T2WI in the same patient shows the CSF-filled sella ➡ with a fluid collection ➡ below the thinned floor. Surgery confirmed a bony dehiscence, which was repaired.

Occasionally, patients present with visual disturbances caused by inferior displacement of the optic chiasm into the empty sella. Most such cases are secondary ES following transsphenoidal hypophysectomy for pituitary adenoma resection.

TREATMENT OPTIONS. Primary and secondary ES generally do not require definitive treatment. Hormone replacement may be needed in some cases. CSF rhinorrhea/otorrhea or optic chiasm displacement with severe visual compromise may necessitate surgical intervention.

Imaging

GENERAL FEATURES. Imaging studies show intrasellar CSF with a thinned pituitary gland flattened against the sellar floor.

CT FINDINGS. CSF-density fluid fills a sella that may be of normal size or moderately enlarged. The bony floor of the sella is intact in primary ES, but in secondary ES, it often shows a surgical defect caused by transsphenoidal hypophysectomy. The infundibular stalk and pituitary remnant enhance normally on CECT scans. The

stalk may be displaced off midline, appearing somewhat "tilted."

MR FINDINGS. The intrasellar fluid behaves exactly like CSF on T1- and T2WI and suppresses completely on FLAIR. DWI shows no diffusion restriction. In severe cases, the optic chiasm and/or anterior third ventricle may appear herniated into—or retracted toward—the sella. If the ES is secondary to surgery, fat packing and scarring with adhesions may distort the imaging findings.

Differential Diagnosis

The major differential diagnosis of ES is **idiopathic intracranial hypertension** (IIH), also sometimes called "pseudotumor cerebri." Both have an increased prevalence in obese females. Imaging findings also show some overlap, as both conditions often demonstrate an empty sella. In IIH, the optic nerve sheaths are often dilated and the ventricles and CSF cisterns often appear smaller than normal.

Increased intracranial pressure (↑ ICP) caused by obstructive hydrocephalus usually results in dis-

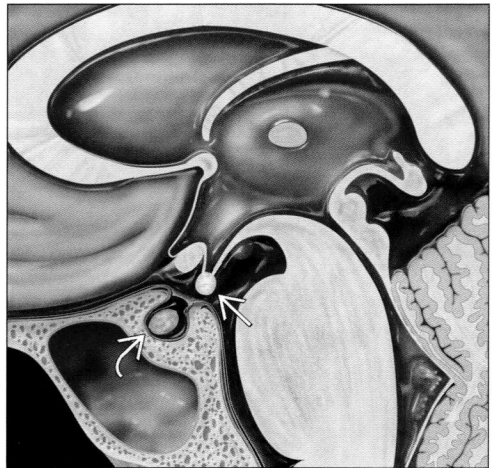
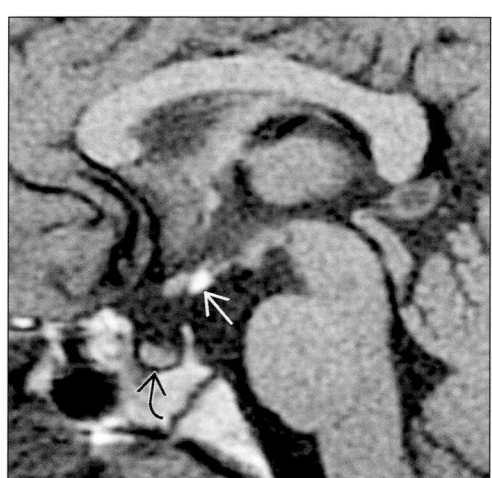

25-21. Sagittal graphic demonstrates ectopia of the posterior pituitary gland ➡, located at the distal end of a truncated pituitary stalk. The sella turcica and adenohypophysis ➡ are both small!. 25-22. Sagittal T1WI shows an ectopic posterior pituitary gland at the median eminence ➡. The infundibulum is absent, and the anterior pituitary gland ➡ is small. The normal posterior pituitary "bright spot" is absent.

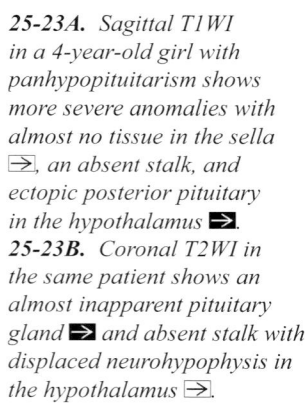
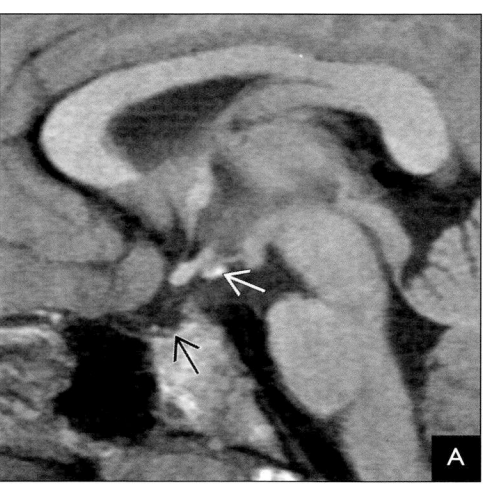
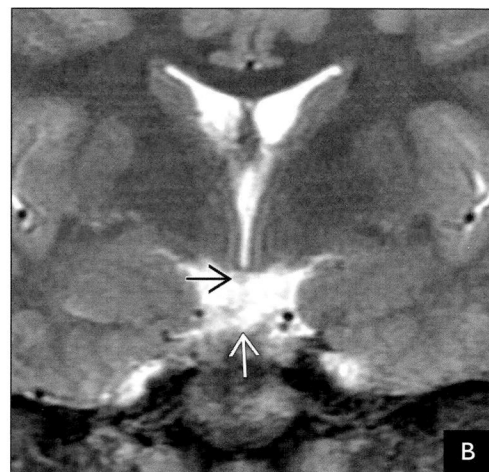

25-23A. Sagittal T1WI in a 4-year-old girl with panhypopituitarism shows more severe anomalies with almost no tissue in the sella ➡, an absent stalk, and ectopic posterior pituitary in the hypothalamus ➡. 25-23B. Coronal T2WI in the same patient shows an almost inapparent pituitary gland ➡ and absent stalk with displaced neurohypophysis in the hypothalamus ➡.

placement of the enlarged anterior third ventricle recesses—not the suprasellar cistern—toward or into the bony sella. Transependymal CSF migration is common in ↑ ICP but absent in ES.

A **suprasellar arachnoid cyst** (SSAC) may herniate into the sella turcica. The bony sella is often not simply enlarged but eroded and flattened. Sagittal T2WI shows an elevated, compressed third ventricle draped over the SSAC.

ongenital Lesions

ituitary Anomalies

Complete absence of the pituitary gland and stalk is rare and nearly always fatal at or soon after birth. Pituitary hypoplasia is much more common **(25-21)**. Many affected children have growth hormone deficiency and short stature, i.e., they are "pituitary dwarfs." These patients can be treated with hormone replacement therapy, so accurate diagnosis and early recognition of this disorder is essential.

tuitary Hypoplasia

A **hypoplastic pituitary gland** is the most frequent abnormality in children with *isolated* growth hormone deficiency (IGHD) whereas **stalk abnormalities** are more common in children with *multiple* hormone deficiencies. Nearly 75% of children with hypopituitarism are male.

Imaging abnormalities include a small sella and anterior pituitary lobe, hypoplasia or absence of the stalk, and an "ectopic" posterior pituitary "bright spot" seen as displacement of the T1 hyperintense posterior lobe into the infundibulum or median eminence of the hypothalamus **(25-22), (25-23)**.

In general, the extent of MR abnormalities correlates with the severity of hormone deficiency. Patients with isolated GH deficiency are more likely to have a normal-sized adenohypophysis and infundibulum than those with multiple endocrine deficiencies.

Kallmann syndrome, also known as hypogonadotropic hypogonadism, is a neuronal migration disorder that results in hypoplastic or absent olfactory nerves and sulci. Various visual and septal anomalies as well as pituitary gland hypoplasia are common.

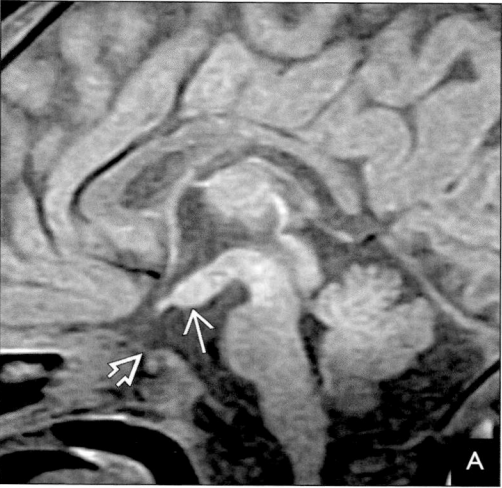

25-24A. *Sagittal T1WI MR shows the thickened floor of the third ventricle* ➡ *and a very shallow, almost inapparent sella turcica* ➡.

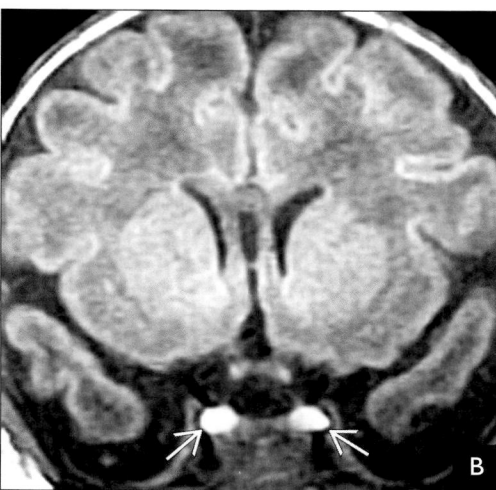

25-24B. *Coronal T1WI in the same patient shows 2 hyperintense pituitary glands* ➡.

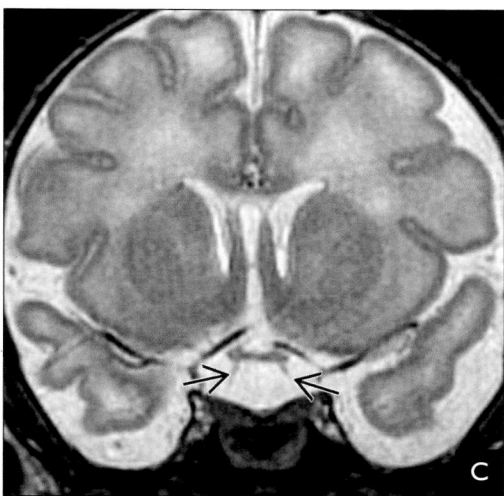

25-24C. *Coronal T2WI in the same patient shows duplicated stalks* ➡. *The presence of duplicated pituitary gland, stalks is a rare congenital anomaly.*

Pituitary Duplication

Pituitary duplication is a rare anomaly in which two pituitary stalks can be identified on the coronal view **(25-24B)**, **(25-24C)**. The tuber cinereum and mammillary bodies are fused into a single thick mass that is best visualized on midline sagittal views **(25-24A)**. Associated craniofacial and craniocervical anomalies are common in these cases.

Unlike pituitary hypoplasia, pituitary duplication rarely causes hormone deficiencies. Instead, a spectrum of midline craniofacial and craniocervical segmentation and fusion anomalies are often seen. Females are more commonly affected.

Hypothalamic Hamartoma

Terminology

Hypothalamic hamartoma (HH), also known as diencephalic or **tuber cinereum hamartoma**, is a nonneoplastic congenital malformation associated with precocious puberty, behavioral disturbances, and gelastic seizures.

Etiology

HHs are an anomaly of neuronal migration that probably occurs between gestational days 33 and 41. A syndromic abnormality that occurs with HH, **Pallister-Hall syndrome** (PHS), is caused by *GLI3* frameshift mutations on chromosome 7p13.

Pathology

LOCATION. The majority of HHs are located in the tuber cinereum, i.e., between the infundibular stalk in front and the mammillary bodies behind **(25-25)**, **(25-26)**. They can be pedunculated **(25-27)** or sessile **(25-28)**. Pedunculated lesions extend inferiorly from the hypothalamus into the suprasellar cistern whereas sessile HHs project from the floor of the third ventricle into its lumen.

SIZE AND NUMBER. HHs are solitary lesions that vary in size from a few millimeters **(25-29)** to huge mixed solid-cystic lesions measuring several centimeters in diameter **(25-30)**, **(25-31)**.

GROSS AND MICROSCOPIC FEATURES. HHs are well-defined round or ovoid soft tissue masses that resemble

25-25. Sagittal graphic shows a pedunculated hypothalamic hamartoma ⇗ interposed between the infundibulum anteriorly, the mammillary bodies posteriorly. The mass resembles gray matter. *25-26.* Submentovertex view shows a classic "collar button" pedunculated HH ⇢ positioned between the infundibular stalk ➡ in front, mammillary bodies (not visible) and pons ➡ behind. (Courtesy R. Hewlett, MD.)

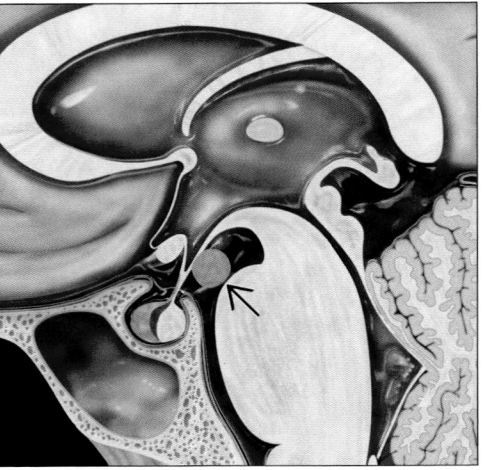

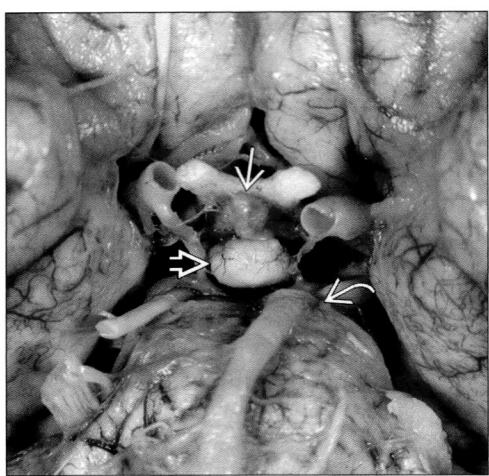

25-27A. Sagittal T2WI in a 12-month-old child with central precocious puberty shows a classic "collar button" hypothalamic hamartoma ➡ between the infundibular stalk ⇗ and the mammillary bodies ⇲. The mass is isointense with gray matter. *25-27B.* Sagittal T1 C+ in the same patient shows that the hypothalamic hamartoma ➡ does not enhance.

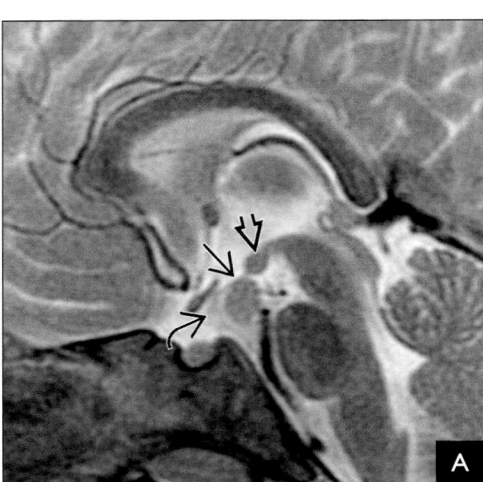

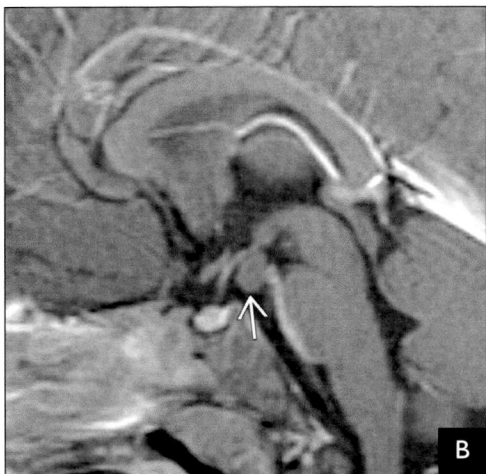

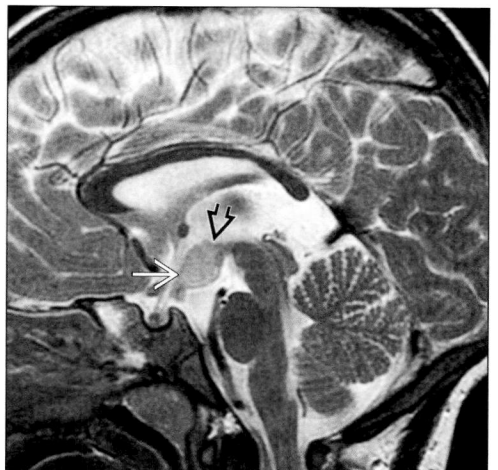

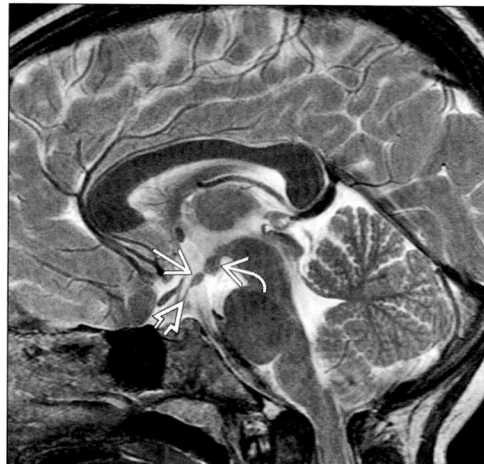

25-28. Sagittal T2WI shows a classic sessile HH ➡ bulging into the floor of the third ventricle ⤵. 25-29. Sagittal T2WI shows a tiny sessile HH ➡ just behind the infundibulum ⤵ and in front of the mammillary bodies ➡.

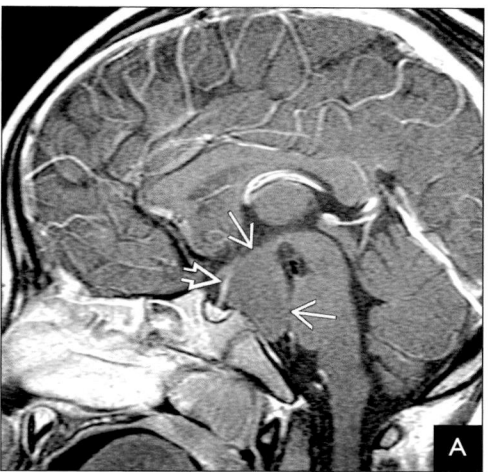

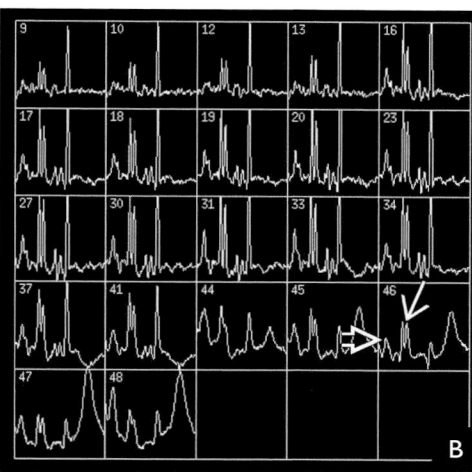

25-30A. T1WI C+ scan in a teenage male with hypogonadotropic hypogonadism shows a huge, lobulated, nonenhancing lesion ➡ in the suprasellar and prepontine cistern. The infundibular stalk ⤵ is displaced anteriorly. 25-30B. Multivoxel MRS of the lesion shows decreased NAA ➡ with elevated myoinositol ⤵ in the voxel directly over the lesion. Findings and clinical history are consistent with a large hypothalamic hamartoma.

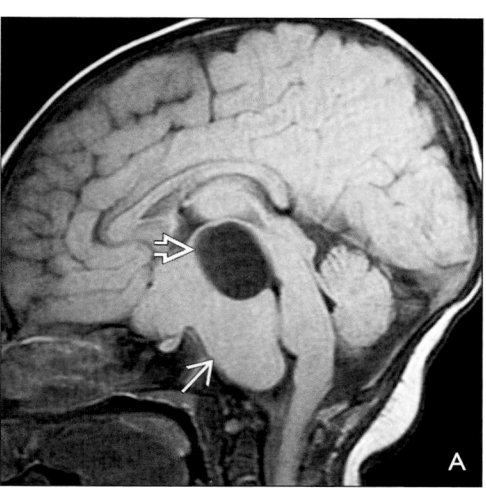

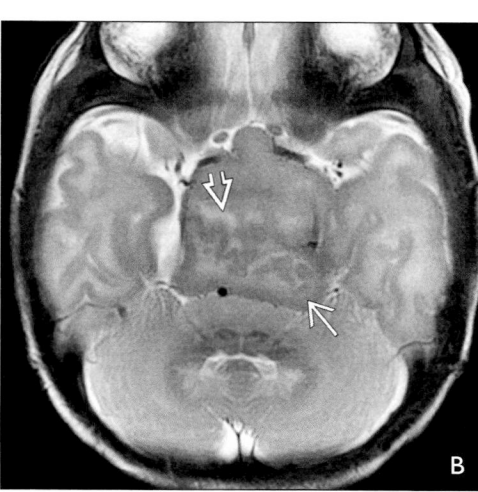

25-31A. Sagittal T1WI shows an enormous hypothalamic hamartoma extending posteriorly behind the clivus ➡. A CSF-like cyst ⤵ is associated with the mass. 25-31B. T2WI in the same patient shows that the hamartoma is composed of dysplastic, disorganized gray matter ➡ with some unmyelinated white matter ➡ inside the lesion. (Courtesy R. Nguyen, MD.)

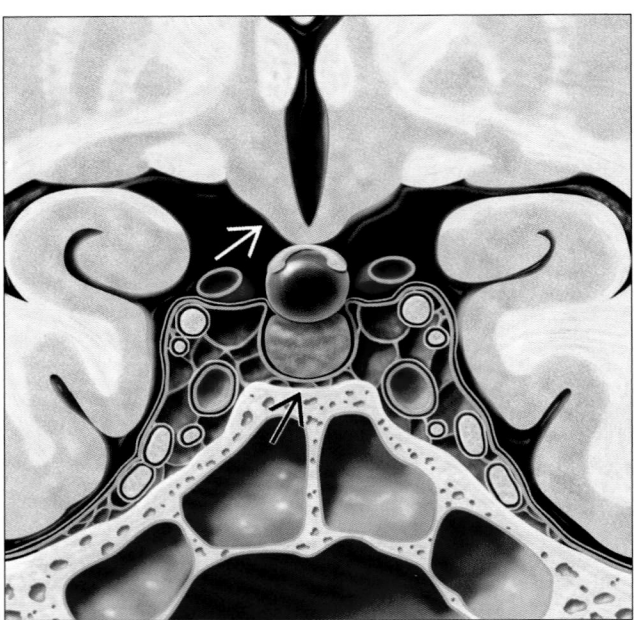

25-32. Coronal graphic shows a typical suprasellar Rathke cleft cyst interposed between the pituitary gland ⇒ and the optic chiasm ➡.

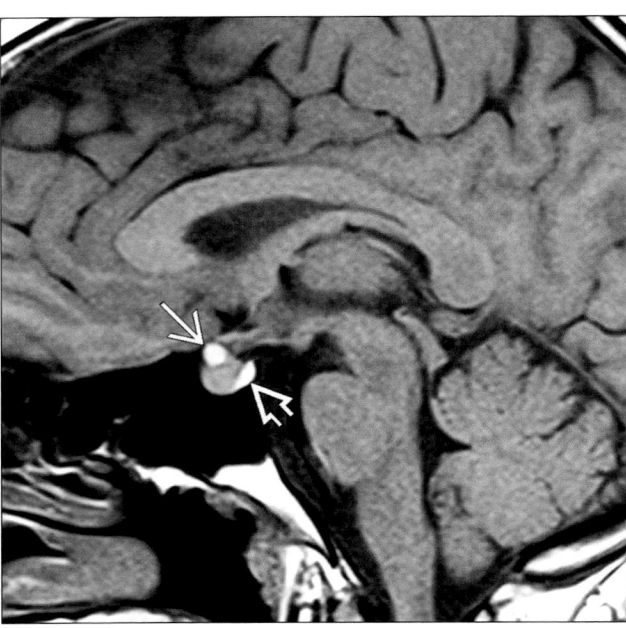

25-33. Sagittal T1WI in an asymptomatic patient shows a tiny hyperintense suprasellar mass ➡ that appears separate from the pituitary gland, "bright spot" of the neurohypophysis ➡. Presumed Rathke cleft cyst.

normal brain parenchyma. Histologically, HHs consist of well-differentiated small and large neurons interspersed with variable amounts of glial cells. Calcification, hemorrhage, and necrosis are rare although very large lesions often contain well-delineated cysts.

STAGING, GRADING, AND CLASSIFICATION. The most common classification of HHs is morphologic. HHs can be pedunculated or sessile. **Pedunculated** HHs are attached to the tuber cinereum and project into the suprasellar cistern. **Sessile** HHs are attached to the floor of the third ventricle and often incorporate the mammillary bodies. Projection into the suprasellar cistern is variable.

Clinical Issues

DEMOGRAPHICS. HHs are rare lesions although up to one-third of patients with central precocious puberty have an HH. There is a moderate male predominance.

PRESENTATION. Most HHs present between one and three years of age. Three-quarters of patients with histologically verified HHs have precocious puberty and 50% have seizures.

HH-associated seizures are highly variable, age dependent, and often refractory to treatment. Gelastic seizures (ictal laughing fits) are the most common type and vary from facial grinning to intense contractions of the diaphragm accompanied by body shaking.

Anomalies associated with HH include holoprosencephaly. Patients with PHS have digital malformations

and other midline (epiglottis/larynx) and cardiac, renal, or anal anomalies in addition to the hypothalamic hamartoma.

NATURAL HISTORY. HHs generally remain stable in size. Hormonal suppressive therapy, i.e., LHRH-agonists, is helpful in some cases. Failure of medical therapy or rapid lesion growth may necessitate surgery.

Imaging

GENERAL FEATURES. A nonenhancing hypothalamic mass between the infundibular stalk and mammillary bodies is the classic imaging appearance of HH (25-27).

CT FINDINGS. NECT scan shows a homogeneous suprasellar mass that is iso- to slightly hypodense compared to brain. Intralesional cysts may be present in larger HHs. HHs do not enhance on CECT.

MR FINDINGS. Pedunculated HHs are shaped like a collar button on sagittal T1WI, extending inferiorly into the suprasellar cistern. Signal intensity is usually isointense to normal gray matter on T1WI and iso- to slightly hyperintense on T2/FLAIR. The degree of T2 hyperintensity is directly related to the proportion of glial versus neuronal tissue in the lesion.

HHs do not enhance following contrast administration.

MRS shows mildly decreased NAA and slightly increased choline, consistent with reduced neuronal density and relative gliosis. Myoinositol is elevated, which is consistent with increased glial component compared to normal brain.

Differential Diagnosis

The differential diagnoses of HH are craniopharyngioma and chiasmatic/hypothalamic astrocytoma. Clinical features are very helpful in distinguishing HH from these lesions.

Craniopharyngioma is the most common suprasellar mass in children. Over 90% of craniopharyngiomas are cystic, 90% calcify, and 90% show nodular and rim enhancement.

Optic pathway/hypothalamic pilocytic astrocytoma is the second most common pediatric suprasellar mass. Astrocytomas are hyperintense on T2/FLAIR and often enhance on T1 C+.

Rathke Cleft Cyst

Terminology

Rathke cleft cyst (RCC) is a benign endodermal cyst of the sellar region.

Etiology

RCCs are thought to arise from remnants of the fetal Rathke pouch. When the embryonic stomodeum (the primitive oral cavity) invaginates and extends dorsally, it forms the endoderm-lined craniopharyngeal duct. It meets an outgrowth from the third ventricle, giving rise to the hypophysis. The anterior wall of the pouch forms the anterior lobe and pars tuberalis while the posterior wall forms the pars intermedia. The interposed lumen forms a narrow "cleft"—Rathke cleft—that normally regresses by the twelfth gestational week. If it persists and expands, it forms an RCC.

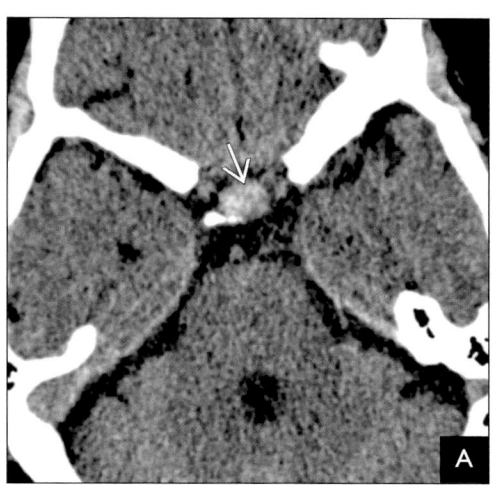
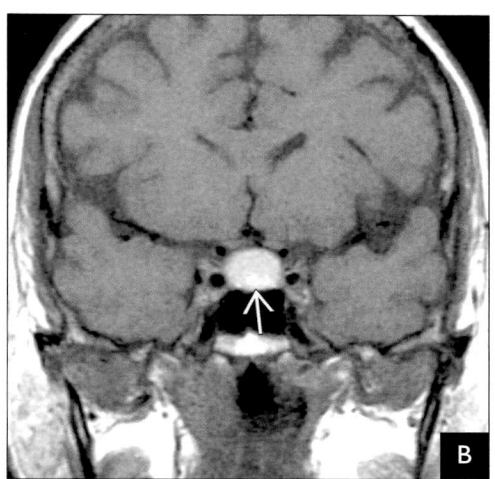

25-34A. *NECT scan shows a hyperdense mass projecting superiorly into the suprasellar cistern* ➡. **25-34B.** *Coronal T1WI scan in the same patient shows that the mass* ➡ *is hyperintense.*

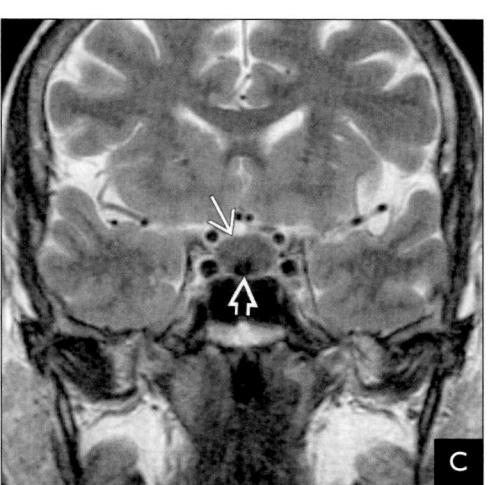
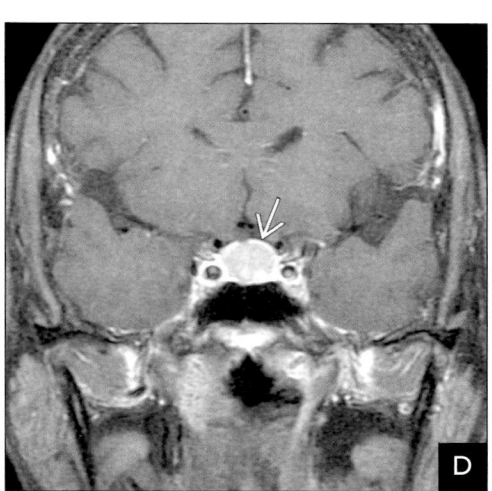

25-34C. *T2WI in the same patient shows that the cyst* ➡ *is hypointense and contains an even more hypointense intracystic nodule* ➡. **25-34D.** *A rim ("claw") of enhancing pituitary gland* ➡ *is seen around the cyst. Rathke cleft cyst with intracystic nodule was found at surgery.*

Pathology

LOCATION. RCCs are limited to the sellar region. Approximately 40% are completely intrasellar, generally positioned between the anterior lobe and pars intermedia whereas 60% are suprasellar **(25-32), (25-33)**.

SIZE AND NUMBER. Most symptomatic RCCs are 5-15 mm in diameter. Occasionally, an RCC becomes very large and can compress the adjacent brain and erode into the skull base.

GROSS PATHOLOGY. RCCs are smoothly lobulated, sharply marginated cysts. Cyst contents vary from clear and CSF-like to thick yellow inspissated mucoid material.

MICROSCOPIC FEATURES. RCCs are endodermal (not ectodermal) cysts. They are lined by a single layer of ciliated cuboidal or columnar epithelium together with various amounts of goblet cells. On immunohistochemical studies, RCCs express cytokeratins 8 and 20.

Clinical Issues

DEMOGRAPHICS. Although RCCs occur at all ages, mean age at presentation is 45 years.

PRESENTATION. Most RCCs are asymptomatic and discovered incidentally at imaging or autopsy. Symptomatic RCCs cause pituitary dysfunction, visual disturbances, and headache.

Occasionally RCCs present with "cyst apoplexy," usually—but not invariably—caused by sudden intracystic hemorrhage. Symptoms are generally indistinguishable from those of pituitary apoplexy.

NATURAL HISTORY. Most RCCs are stable and do not change in size or intensity characteristics. RCCs do not undergo malignant degeneration.

Imaging

CT FINDINGS. NECT scans show a well-delineated round or ovoid mass within or just above the sella turcica. Three-quarters of RCCs are hypodense on NECT whereas 20% are mixed hypo- and isodense. Between

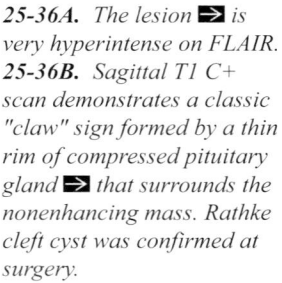

25-35A. Sagittal T1WI in a patient with visual problems shows that the optic chiasm ➨ is elevated by an intra- and suprasellar mass ➨, which is isointense with gray matter. 25-35B. The mass ➨ is very hyperintense on T2WI. Note elevation, draping of the optic chiasm ➨ over the lesion.

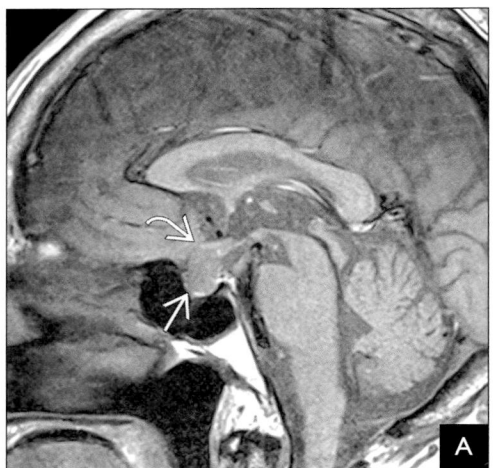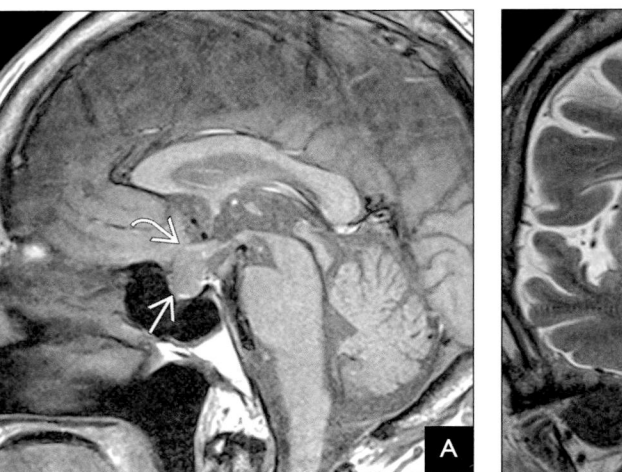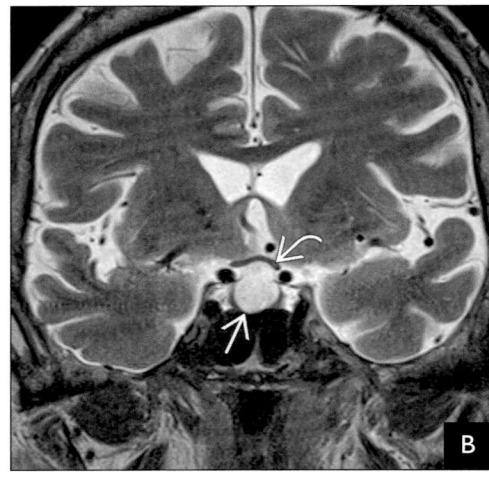

25-36A. The lesion ➨ is very hyperintense on FLAIR. 25-36B. Sagittal T1 C+ scan demonstrates a classic "claw" sign formed by a thin rim of compressed pituitary gland ➨ that surrounds the nonenhancing mass. Rathke cleft cyst was confirmed at surgery.

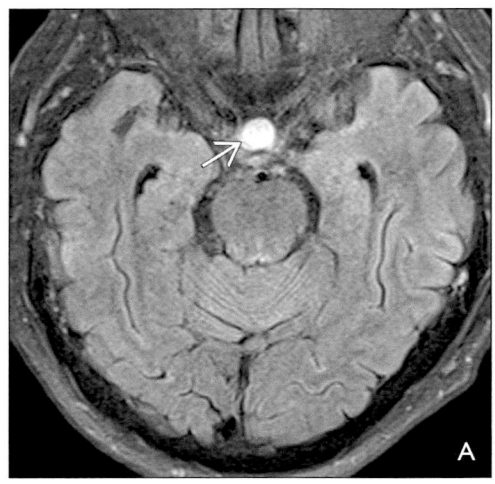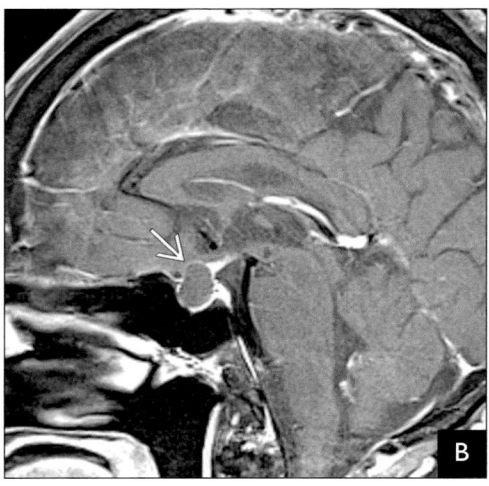

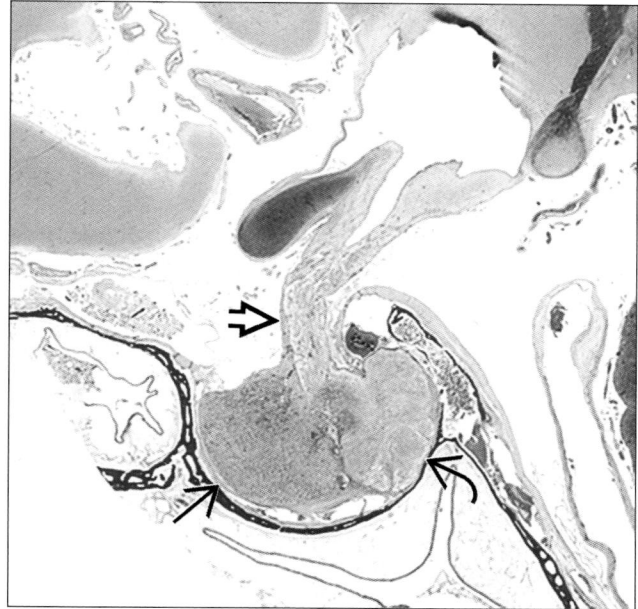

25-37. Sagittal section through the pituitary gland demonstrates the anterior ⊒, posterior ⊘ pituitary lobes, as well as the infundibular stalk ⊛ connecting the hypothalamus to the neurohypophysis. (Courtesy A. Ersen, MD, B. Scheithauer, MD.)

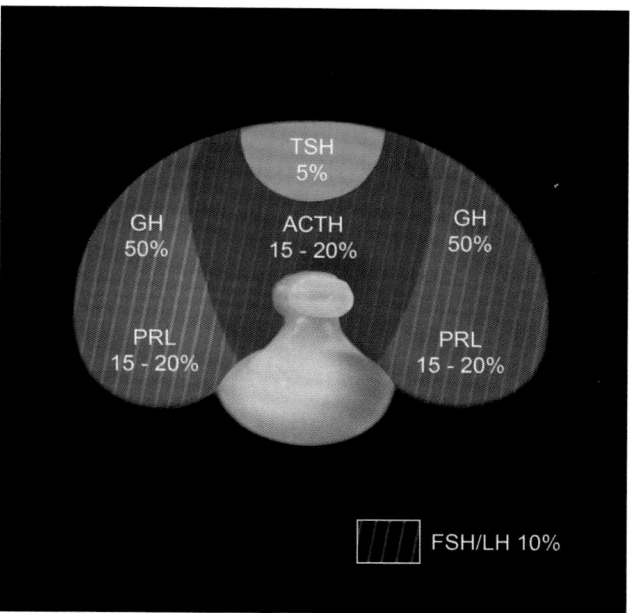

25-38. Graphic depicts localization of anterior pituitary lobe cells. Lateral wings contain mainly GH and PRL cells. Corticotrophs, thyrotrophs are in the median mucoid wedge (green). FSH/LH cells are distributed diffusely.

5-10% are hyperdense **(25-34A)**. Calcification is uncommon compared to craniopharyngioma.

MR FINDINGS. Signal intensity varies with cyst contents. Half of all RCCs are hypointense on T1WI, and half are hyperintense **(25-34)**. The majority of RCCs are hyperintense on T2WI **(25-35)** whereas 25-30% are iso- to hypointense. Careful inspection reveals an intracystic nodule in 40-75% of cases **(25-34C)**, **(25-34D)**.

RCCs are almost always hyperintense on FLAIR **(25-36A)**. An enhancing rim ("claw" sign) of compressed pituitary gland can often be seen surrounding the nonenhancing cyst **(25-36B)**.

ifferential Diagnosis

The major differential diagnosis of RCC is **craniopharyngioma**. Floccular, rim, or nodular calcifications are common in craniopharyngioma whereas RCCs rarely calcify. The rim or nodular enhancement in craniopharyngioma is generally thicker and more irregular than the "claw" of enhancing pituitary gland that surrounds the nonenhancing RCC.

A cystic pituitary adenoma—especially a **nonfunctioning cystic microadenoma**—can be difficult to distinguish from a small intrasellar RCC. Both rarely calcify; both are common etiologies for pituitary "incidentalomas" on MR scans. Neither requires treatment, so the distinction is largely academic.

Other nonneoplastic cysts that can occur in the sellar region are dermoid (fat, calcification common) and epi-

dermoid cysts (rarely midline, usually CSF-like), arachnoid cysts (larger, CSF-like, lacking an intracystic nodule), and inflammatory cysts (e.g., neurocysticercosis; multiple far more prevalent than solitary cysts).

RATHKE CLEFT CYST
Etiology and Pathology
- Remnant of embryonic Rathke cleft
- Intrasellar (40%), suprasellar (60%)
- Contents vary (CSF-like to thick mucoid)
- Endodermal lining + goblet cells

Imaging
- Hypointense (50%), hyperintense (50%) on T1WI
- Hyperintense on T2/FLAIR
- Look for
  ○ Intracystic nodule (40-75%)
  ○ "Claw" of enhancement

Neoplasms

Pituitary Adenomas

Terminology

Pituitary adenomas (PAs) are adenohypophysial tumors composed of secretory cells that produce pituitary hormones **(25-37)**, **(25-38)**. **Microadenomas** are defined as tumors ≤ 10 mm in diameter, while larger adenomas are designated **macroadenomas (25-39), (25-40), (25-41), (25-42)**.

Etiology

GENERAL CONCEPTS. Cells with multipotent progenitor/stem-cell-like properties have been identified in the adult pituitary gland and may play a key role in tumorigenesis. Alterations in the normal microenvironment of pituitary stem cells may trigger uncoordinated proliferation and subsequent formation of pituitary adenomas.

GENETICS. Adenomagenesis is a multistep, multicausal process that includes both initiation and progression phases. A number of activated oncogenes and loss of tumor suppressor gene functions are involved. In addition, several endocrine factors at either the hypothalamic or systemic level may induce adenohypophysial cell proliferation.

Mutations in the aryl hydrocarbon receptor-interacting protein gene (*AIP*) have been identified in patients with familial isolated pituitary adenoma syndrome (see below) but are rare in patients with sporadic PAs.

FAMILIAL PITUITARY TUMOR SYNDROMES. Most PAs are sporadic tumors and occur in adults. Approximately 5% of all PAs are familial.

Four recognized inherited familial tumor syndromes with specific identified genetic defects are associated with pituitary adenomas: Multiple endocrine neoplasia type 1, Carney complex, McCune-Albright syndrome, and familial isolated PA syndrome.

Multiple endocrine neoplasia type 1 (MEN1) is an autosomal dominant disease with highly penetrant germline mutations that predisposes patients to develop tumors in hormone-secreting cells. MEN1 is characterized by combinations of more than 20 different endocrine and nonendocrine tumors. Pituitary tumors occur in 15-40% of MEN1 patients. MEN1-associated adenomas are often plurihormonal (most commonly secreting prolactin and growth hormone), larger, and more invasive neoplasms.

Carney complex is associated with spotty skin pigmentation, myxomas, endocrine tumors, and schwannomas. Adrenal involvement causing ACTH-independent Cush-

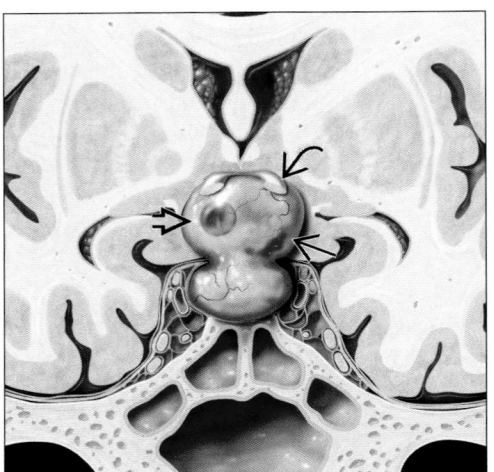

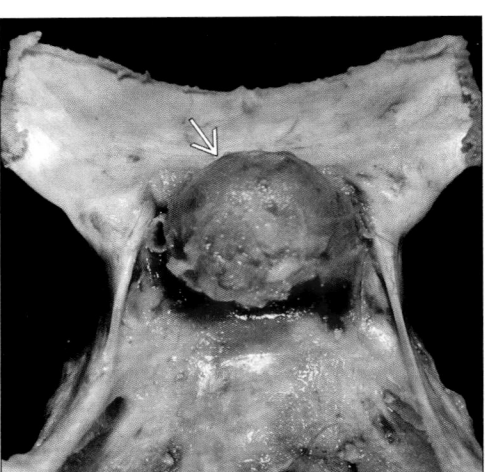

25-39. Coronal graphic shows a snowman-shaped or "figure eight" sellar/suprasellar mass. Small foci of hemorrhage and cystic change are present within the lesion. The pituitary gland cannot be identified separate from the mass; indeed, the gland is the mass. 25-40. Autopsy specimen shows a macroadenoma protruding superiorly through the diaphragma sellae into the suprasellar cistern.

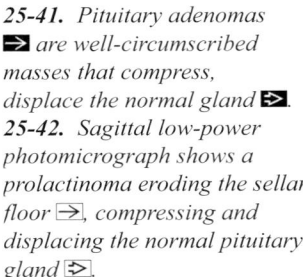

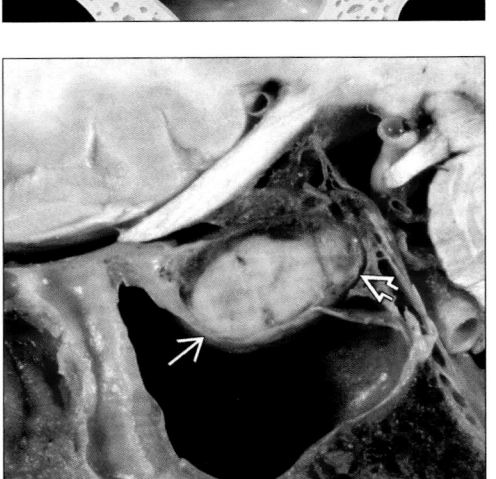

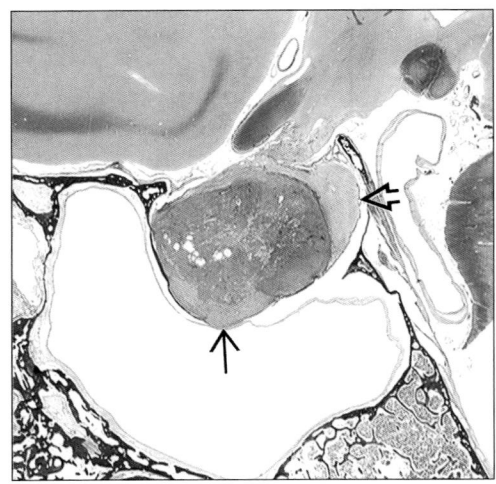

25-41. Pituitary adenomas are well-circumscribed masses that compress, displace the normal gland. 25-42. Sagittal low-power photomicrograph shows a prolactinoma eroding the sellar floor, compressing and displacing the normal pituitary gland.

Functional Classification of Pituitary Adenomas

Adenoma Type	%	M:F	IHC Profile	Clinical Presentation
Sparsely granulated PRL cell adenoma	27.0	1:2.5	PRL	Females: Amenorrhea-galactorrhea syndrome; males: Sellar mass, hypogonadism
Densely granulated PRL cell adenoma	0.04	N/A	PRL	
Densely granulated GH cell adenoma	7.1	1:0.7	GH, α-subunit (PRL, TSH, LH, FSH)	Acromegaly (adult) or gigantism (child)
Sparsely granulated GH cell adenoma	6.2	1:1.1	GH (PRL, α-subunit)	Acromegaly (adult) or gigantism (child)
Mixed GH-PRL cell adenoma	3.5	1:1.1	GH, PRL (α-subunit, TSH)	Acromegaly + hyperprolactinemia
Mammosomatotroph adenoma	1.2	1:1.1	GH, PRL (α-subunit, TSH)	Acromegaly + hyperprolactinemia
Acidophil stem cell adenoma	1.6	1:1.5	PRL, GH	Hyperprolactinemia; acromegaly is uncommon
Densely granulated corticotroph adenoma	9.6	1:5.4	ACTH (LH, α-subunit)	Cushing disease, Nelson syndrome
Sparsely granulated corticotroph adenoma	Rare	N/A	ACTH	Cushing disease, Nelson syndrome
Thyrotroph adenoma	1.1	1:1.3	TSH (GH, PRL, α-subunit)	Hyperthyroidism
Gonadotroph adenoma	9.8	1:0.8	FSH, LH, α-subunit (ACTH)	Nonfunctioning sellar mass
Silent "corticotroph" adenoma subtype 1	1.5	1:1.7	ACTH	Nonfunctioning sellar mass, pituitary
Silent "corticotroph" adenoma subtype 2	2.0	1:0.2	β-endorphin, ACTH	Nonfunctioning sellar mass
Silent adenoma subtype 3	1.4	1:1.1	Any combination of anterior pituitary hormones	Females: Mimics PRL-secreting adenoma; males: Nonfunctioning sellar mass
Null cell adenoma	12.4	1:0.7	Immunoreactive (FSH, LH, TSH, α-subunit)	Nonfunctioning sellar mass
Oncocytoma	13.4	1:0.5	Immunonegative (FSH, LH, TSH, α-subunit)	Nonfunctioning sellar mass
Unclassified adenomas	1.8	N/A	N/A	Variable

Table 25-1. *N/A = not available.*

ing syndrome is seen in one-third to one-half of patients with Carney complex. GH-producing pituitary tumors are seen in 10%.

McCune-Albright syndrome (MAS) is defined by the triad of gonadotropin-independent sexual precocity, café au lait skin lesions, and fibrous dysplasia. Tumors or nodular hyperplasia of a number of endocrine glands lead to hypersecretory syndromes such as acromegaly, hyperprolactinemia, and Cushing syndrome. MAS is caused by a postzygotic mutation in the *GNAS* gene.

Familial isolated pituitary adenoma syndrome (FIPA) is a recently described condition in which affected family members develop only pituitary tumors. It includes familial pituitary tumors that are *not* associated with MEN1 and Carney complex.

Prolactinomas are found in 40% of all FIPA patients, somatotropinomas in 30%, and nonsecreting adenomas in 13%. In general, pituitary tumors in FIPA present earlier than sporadic PAs, are significantly larger, and more often demonstrate cavernous sinus invasion.

Two FIPA subgroups have been identified based on genetic and phenotypic features. In 15-25% of cases, affected families have *AIP* gene mutations and autosomal dominant inheritance. They typically develop growth hormone-secreting adenomas and prolactinomas, often in childhood. The second, much larger group has adult-

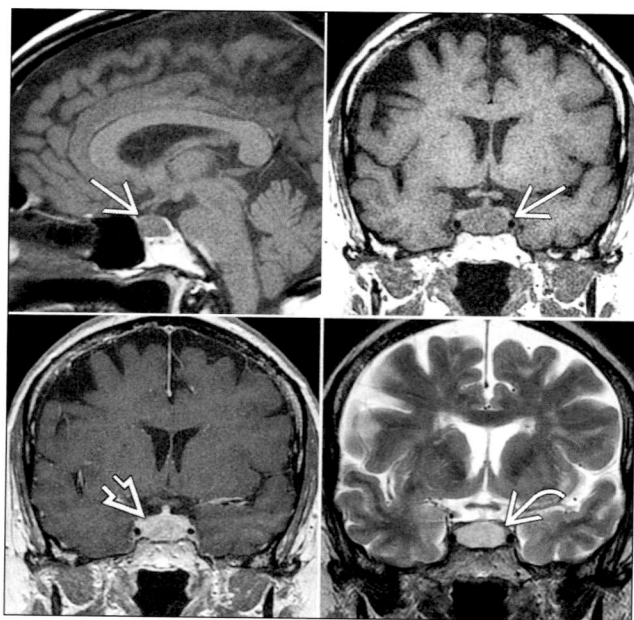

25-43. *Series of scans shows a small macroadenoma that measured 12 mm in height. The mass is isointense with GM* ➤ *on T1-, T2WI* ➤ *and enhances strongly, uniformly* ➤.

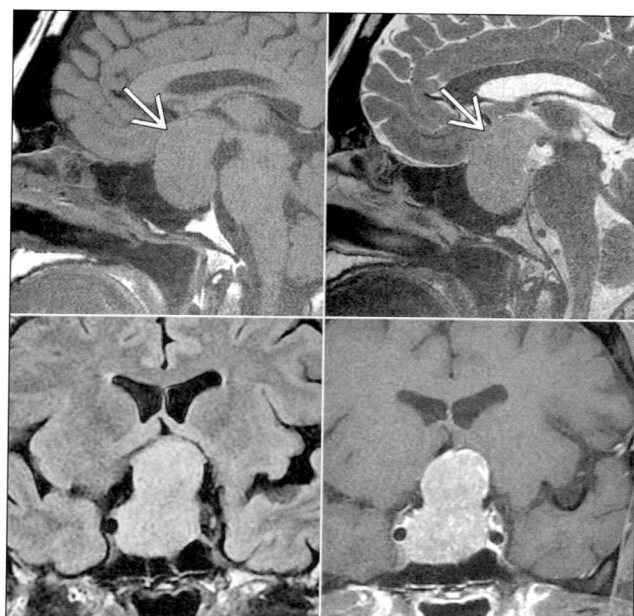

25-44. *Sagittal T1WI (top left), T2WI (top right), FLAIR (bottom left), T1 C+ (bottom right) show a very large "snowman" or "figure eight" intra-/suprasellar mass* ➤. *The pituitary gland cannot be identified as separate from the mass (macroadenoma).*

onset disease and more varied types of adenoma. To date, no causative gene has been identified.

Pathology

LOCATION. With rare exceptions, adenomas arise within the sella turcica. Reported sites include the sphenoid sinus (the most common site), nasopharynx, third ventricle, and suprasellar cistern. Such cases are designated **ectopic pituitary adenoma**.

Adenomas arise from the adenohypophysis. Specific sublocation follows the normal distribution of peptide-containing cells. Prolactinomas and growth-hormone secreting tumors—the two most common PAs—tend to arise laterally within the AH whereas TSH- and ACTH-secreting tumors are more often midline.

SIZE AND NUMBER. Adenomas vary in size from microscopic lesions **(25-47)**, **(25-48)** to giant tumors more than five centimeters that invade the skull base and extend into multiple cranial fossae. PAs are usually solitary lesions. Multiple synchronous pituitary adenomas are unusual. "Double" or even "triple" adenomas are found in 1% of autopsies but rarely diagnosed on preoperative MR scans.

GROSS PATHOLOGY. Macroadenomas are red-brown, lobulated masses that often bulge upward through the opening of diaphragma sella **(25-40)**, or less commonly, extend laterally toward the cavernous sinus. Approximately half of macroadenomas contain cysts and/or hemorrhagic foci.

MICROSCOPIC FEATURES. Histologic examination shows a uniform population of round, polygonal, or elongated cells with moderately abundant cytoplasm and inconspicuous nucleoli. Cellular atypia is uncommon, and mitoses are rare.

STAGING, GRADING, AND CLASSIFICATION. Adenoma classification is now based on immunohistochemical profile and clinical presentation. The "tinctorial" characteristics of cells as seen on H&E preparations ("acidophilic," "basophilic," "chromophobic") are not precisely correlated with specific hormone production and are no longer used as diagnostic terms.

Pituitary adenomas are all WHO grade I tumors. MIB-1 and p53 immunoreactivity correlate with tumor invasion but do not indicate malignant transformation. Most adenomas are "typical" lesions with both MIB-1 and p53 under 3%. Elevated indices correlate with early recurrence and more rapid regrowth.

Clinical Issues

EPIDEMIOLOGY. Pituitary adenomas are among the most common of all CNS neoplasms, accounting for 10-15% of primary intracranial neoplasms. Approximately 60% of patients undergoing surgery have macroadenomas, and 40% have microadenomas. However, microadenomas are much more common than macroadenomas at autopsy. Clinically silent incidental microadenomas are identified in 15-25% of autopsies.

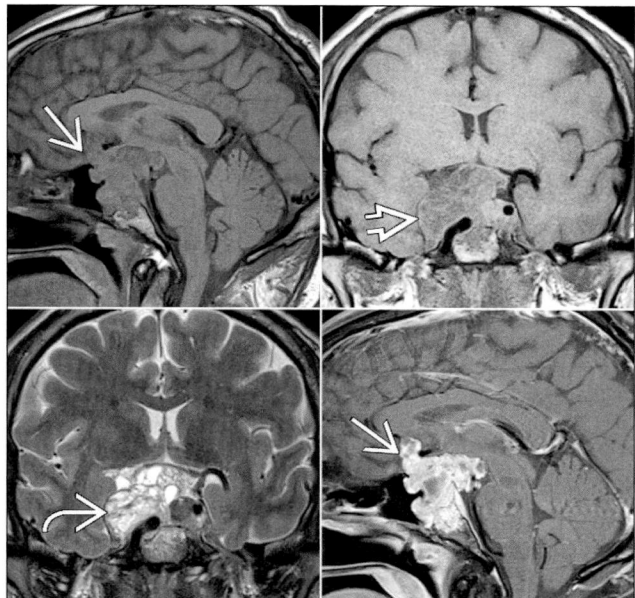

25-45. Lobulated, invasive sellar/suprasellar mass ➡ shows multiple medium/small-sized hyperintense cysts ➡. Macroadenoma also invades the right cavernous sinus ➡.

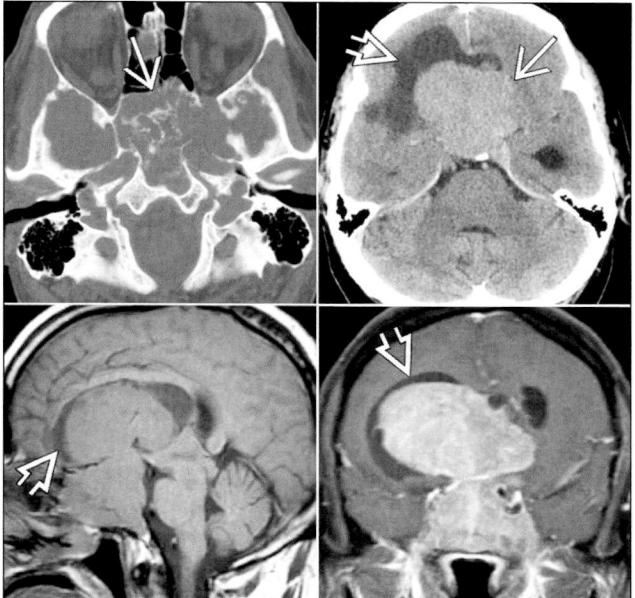

25-46. Bone CT (top left), CECT (top right) show a huge invasive pituitary macroadenoma ➡. The CECT, sagittal T1WI, coronal T1 C+ FS show trapped pools of CSF adjacent to the tumor ➡. These are nonneoplastic peritumoral cysts.

DEMOGRAPHICS. Peak age of presentation is between the fourth and seventh decades. Only 2% of PAs are found in children. Most of these occur in adolescent females. PAs in prepubescent males are very rare.

PRESENTATION. Almost two-thirds of pituitary adenomas secrete a hormone (48% prolactin, 10% growth hormone, 6% corticotropin, 1% thyrotropin) and cause typical hypersecretory syndromes. The remaining one-third do not produce a hormone and are referred to as nonfunctioning (or nonsecreting) adenomas **(Table 25-1)**.

Females with prolactinomas present with amenorrhea-galactorrhea syndrome whereas males present with hypogonadism and impotence. GH-secreting tumors cause acromegaly in adults and gigantism in children. Patients with corticotroph tumors present with Cushing disease or Nelson syndrome (rapid enlargement of an adenoma following bilateral adrenalectomy). TSH-secreting adenomas cause hyperthyroidism.

Macroadenomas generally present with mass effect. Headache and visual disturbances are common. Diabetes insipidus is rarely associated with PA, so its presence should prompt consideration of an alternative diagnosis.

NATURAL HISTORY AND TREATMENT. Although PA growth rates are quite variable, most enlarge slowly over a period of years. Malignant transformation is exceptionally rare.

Treatment options are numerous and include surgical resection, medical management, stereotactic radio-

surgery, and conventional radiation therapy. Management strategy should be individualized for each patient.

Imaging

GENERAL FEATURES. A sellar or combined intra- and suprasellar mass that cannot be identified separately from the pituitary gland—the mass *is* the gland—is the most characteristic imaging finding.

CT FINDINGS. Bone CT may show an enlarged, remodeled sella turcica. The lamina dura of the sellar floor is generally intact. Note, however, that "giant" PAs may erode and extensively invade the skull base, mimicking metastasis or aggressive infection.

PAs demonstrate variable attenuation on NECT scans. Macroadenomas are usually isodense with gray matter, but cysts (15-20%) and hemorrhage (10%) are common. Calcification is rare (less than 2%). Moderate but heterogeneous enhancement of macroadenomas is typical on CECT, but small microadenomas may be invisible.

MR FINDINGS.

Macroadenomas. Macroadenomas are usually isointense with cortex **(25-43)**, **(25-44)**. The posterior pituitary "bright spot" is absent (20%) or displaced into the supradiaphragmatic cistern (80%) on T1-weighted sagittal scans. Small cysts and hemorrhagic foci are common. Fluid-fluid levels can be present but are more common in patients with pituitary apoplexy.

PAs are generally isointense with gray matter on T2WI but can also demonstrate heterogeneous signal intensity (25-45). Hyperintensity along the optic pathways on T2/FLAIR occurs in 15-20% of cases in which macroadenomas compress the optic chiasm. Hemorrhagic adenomas "bloom" on T2*.

Most macroadenomas enhance strongly but heterogeneously on T1 C+ (25-46). Subtle dural thickening (a dural "tail") is present in 5-10% of cases.

Microadenomas. Unless they hemorrhage, small microadenomas may be inapparent on standard nonenhanced sequences. Many microadenomas appear slightly hypointense on T1 C+. Others enhance more strongly and become isointense with the enhancing pituitary gland, rendering them virtually invisible.

Microadenomas enhance more slowly than the normal pituitary tissue. This discrepancy in enhancement timing can be exploited by using thin-section coronal dynamic contrast-enhanced scans. Fast image acquisition during contrast administration can often discriminate between the slowly enhancing microadenoma and rapidly enhancing normal gland. Between 10-30% of microadenomas are seen only on dynamic T1 C+ imaging (25-49).

ANGIOGRAPHY. CTA in patients with suprasellar extension of macroadenoma may show the supraclinoid internal carotid and anterior choroidal arteries displaced laterally. DSA may demonstrate an enlarged meningohypophyseal trunk with prolonged vascular "stain" or "blush" in the tumor.

Cavernous/inferior petrosal venous sampling may be helpful in evaluating patients with ACTH-dependent Cushing syndrome.

Differential Diagnosis

The differential diagnosis of PA varies with size and patient demographics.

PITUITARY MACROADENOMA. The major differential diagnosis of pituitary macroadenoma is **pituitary hyperplasia**. Between 25-50% of endocrinologically normal females who are 18-35 years old have an upwardly convex pituitary gland on MR or CT examination. The height of the gland is usually ≤ 10 mm unless the patient is pregnant or lactating. Less commonly, end-organ failure (such as hypothyroidism) results in compensatory pituitary enlargement. *As adenomas are very rare in children, if a prepubescent female or young male has an "adenoma-looking" pituitary gland, endocrine work-up is mandatory!*

Tumors that can resemble PA include meningioma, metastasis, and craniopharyngioma. Meningioma and metastasis are very rare in children. **Meningioma** of the diaphragma sellae can usually be identified as clearly separate from the pituitary gland below. True isolated intrasellar meningiomas are very rare.

Metastasis to the stalk and/or pituitary gland from an extracranial primary neoplasm is uncommon. Lung and breast are the most common sources. Most pituitary metastases are secondary to spread from adjacent bone or the cavernous sinus, generally occurring as a late manifestation of known systemic tumor. Hematogenous metastases to the pituitary gland do occur but are rare. CNS metastases elsewhere in the brain are common but not invariably present.

Craniopharyngioma is the most common suprasellar tumor of childhood whereas PAs are rare. Craniopharyngiomas in middle-aged adults are typically solid papillary tumors that do not calcify as the adamantinomatous ones do. Regardless, the pituitary gland can generally be identified as anatomically separate from the mass.

Pituitary carcinoma is exceedingly rare (see below). Because of this rarity, even the most aggressive-looking pituitary tumors are statistically far more likely to be macroadenomas than carcinomas.

Nonneoplastic entities that can mimic macroadenoma include aneurysm and hypophysitis. An **aneurysm** arises eccentrically from the circle of Willis and is usually not in the midline directly above the sella. Paramedian saccular aneurysms are hyperdense on NECT and may demonstrate rim calcification whereas PAs rarely calcify. A "flow void" with or without laminated clot along the aneurysm wall is common on MR.

Hypophysitis is much less common than macroadenoma but can appear virtually identical to PA on imaging studies. Lymphocytic hypophysitis—the most common type—typically occurs in peripartum or postpartum females or as an autoimmune hypophysitis in patients treated with immunomodulating therapies (e.g., ipilimumab for metastatic malignant melanoma).

PITUITARY MICROADENOMA. Pituitary microadenoma may be difficult to distinguish from incidental nonneoplastic intrapituitary cysts such as **Rathke cleft cyst** or **pars intermedia cyst**. Microadenomas enhance; cysts are seen as nonenhancing foci within the intensely enhancing pituitary gland. A small hemorrhagic microadenoma may appear identical to an RCC that contains proteinaceous fluid as both are hyperintense on T1WI.

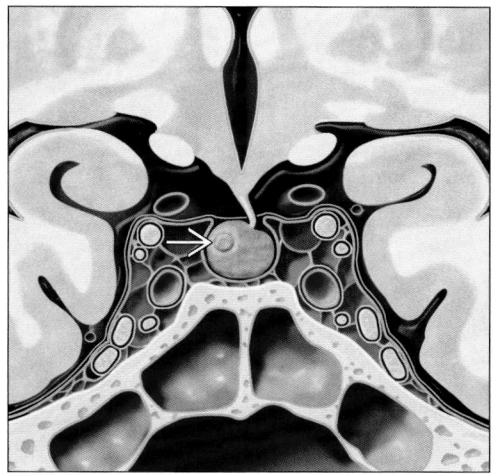

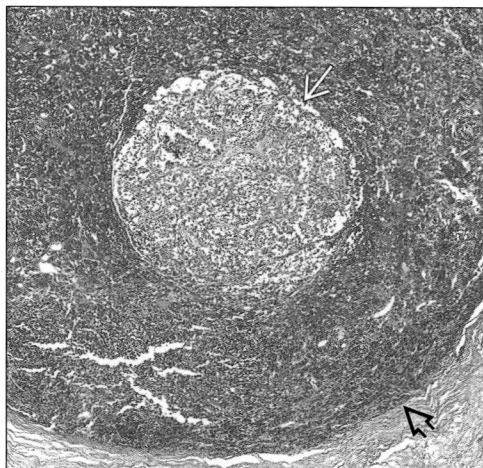

25-47. Coronal graphic depicts a pituitary microadenoma ➡. 25-48. Low-power photomicrograph of a pituitary gland at autopsy shows a small nonsecreting microadenoma ➡ surrounded by the normal adenohypophysis ⬈. Incidental asymptomatic microadenomas are common on imaging studies and at autopsy. (Courtesy J. Townsend, MD.)

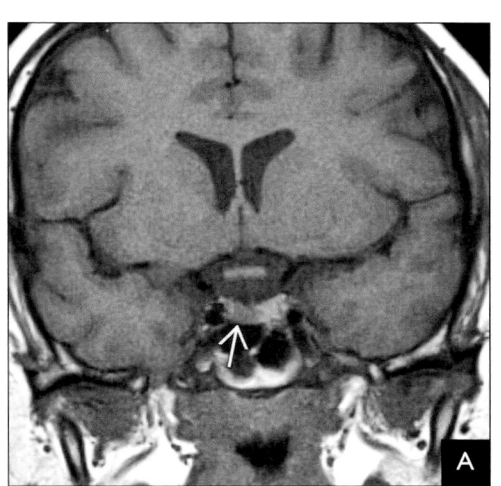

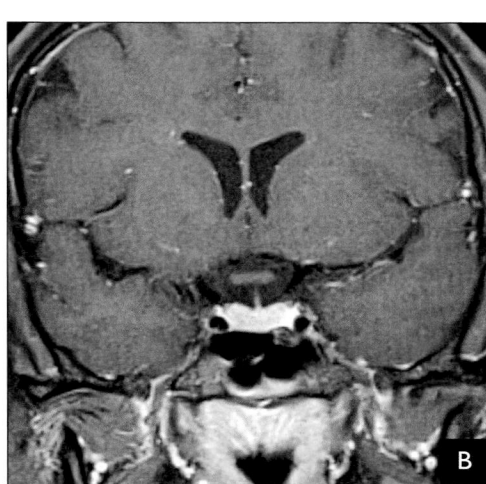

25-49A. Coronal T1WI in a patient with headache, amenorrhea, elevated prolactin demonstrates a hypointense mass ➡ in the right lateral pituitary gland. 25-49B. Standard T1 C+ FS shows no abnormality.

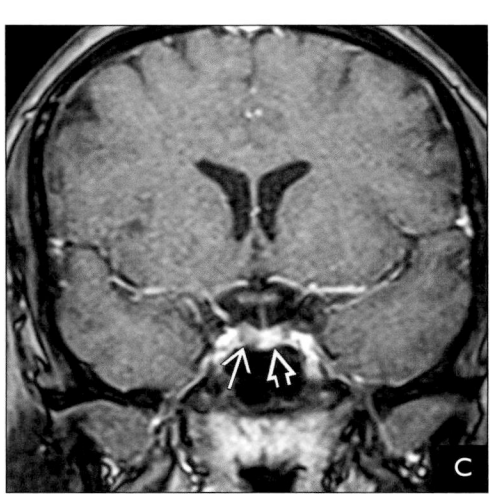

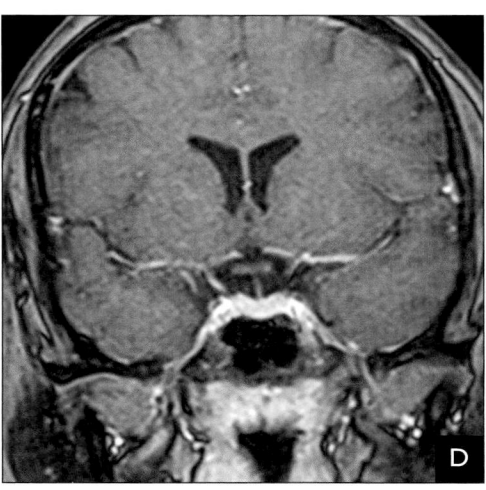

25-49C. Early coronal image from a dynamic contrast-enhanced sequence shows the intensely, rapidly enhancing normal gland ➡. The mass enhances more slowly and so appears relatively hypointense ➡. 25-49D. Late scan in the dynamic sequence shows that the mass has enhanced to isointensity with the remainder of the gland and is invisible. Pituitary microadenoma was found at surgery.

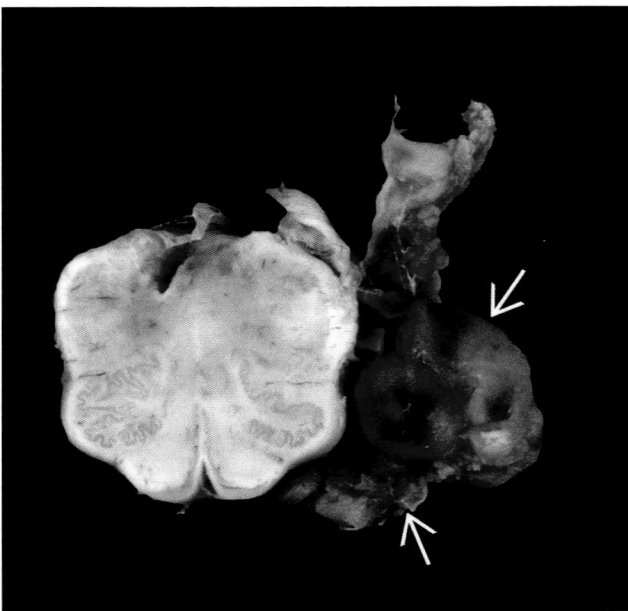

25-50. Autopsy specimen of pituitary carcinoma with CSF spread shows "drop metastasis" ➡ adjacent to the medulla. CSF or systemic dissemination is required for the diagnosis. (Courtesy A. Ersen, MD, B. Scheithauer, MD.)

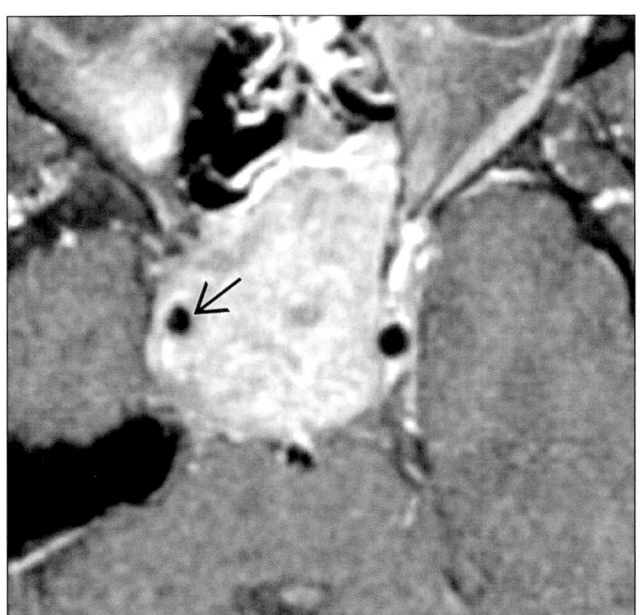

25-51. T1 C+ shows pituitary carcinoma as a heterogeneously enhancing mass invading clivus, encasing cavernous carotid artery ➡. Imaging findings are indistinguishable from invasive macroadenoma. (Courtesy A. Ersen, MD, B. Scheithauer, MD.)

PITUITARY ADENOMA: IMAGING

CT
- Sella usually enlarged, remodeled, cortex intact
- Invasive PAs erode, destroy bone
- Majority are isodense with brain
  - Cysts (15-20%)
  - Hemorrhage (10%)
  - Ca++ rare (1-2%)

MR
- Usually isointense with cortex
- Heterogeneous SI common (cysts, hemorrhage)
- Strong but heterogeneous enhancement
- 10-30% of microadenomas seen only with dynamic T1 C+

Differential Diagnosis
- Pituitary hyperplasia (know patient age, gender!)
  - Physiologic (young/pregnant/lactating females)
  - Nonphysiologic (end-organ failure)
- Other tumors
  - Meningioma, craniopharyngioma, metastasis
  - Pituitary carcinoma *exceptionally* rare
  - Aggressive-looking PA is almost never malignant!
- Nonneoplastic lesions
  - Aneurysm
  - Hypophysitis

Pituitary Carcinoma

Pituitary carcinoma (PCa) is very rare, representing less than 0.2% of all operated adenohypophysial neoplasms. Its estimated prevalence is four per one million person-years. Most PCas arise as metastases from multiple recurring invasive adenomas; de novo malignancy is unusual. Survival is inversely proportionate with increasing age.

Conventional histologic criteria for malignancy (necrosis, nuclear atypia, pleomorphism, mitotic activity) are insufficient for diagnosis. A true PCa must exhibit either frank brain invasion or CSF/systemic metastases **(25-50)**.

PCa has no unique imaging features and may be indistinguishable from an invasive but histologically typical adenoma **(25-51)**. Only documentation of craniospinal metastases or systemic tumor spread can confirm the diagnosis.

Pituitary Blastoma

Pituitary blastoma is a recently described pituitary tumor in neonates and infants characterized by large glandular structures that resemble Rathke epithelium and adenohypophysial cells. Arrested pituitary development and unchecked proliferation is the likely etiology of this unusual tumor.

Histology shows small undifferentiated blastema-like cells interspersed with large pituitary secretory cells. Mitotic activity is variable. Imaging findings are nonspecific and resemble those of macroadenoma. The few described cases show a heterogeneously enhancing sellar/suprasellar mass, often invading the cavernous sinus.

Craniopharyngioma

Terminology and Etiology

Craniopharyngioma (CP) is a benign, often partly cystic sellar/suprasellar mass that probably arises from epithelial remnants of Rathke pouch. The molecular pathogenesis of CP is unknown. Reactivation of the Wnt signal-

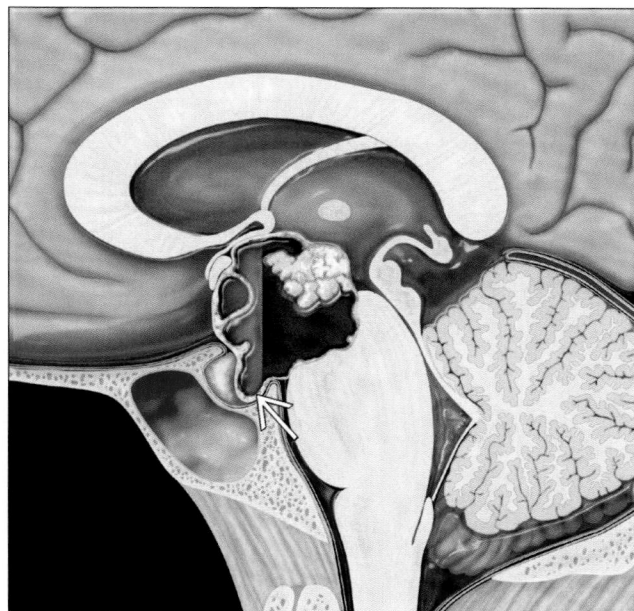

25-52. *Sagittal graphic shows a predominantly cystic, partially solid suprasellar mass with focal rim calcifications. Note the small intrasellar component* ➡ *and fluid-fluid level. The fluid, rich in cholesterol, is dark and viscous.*

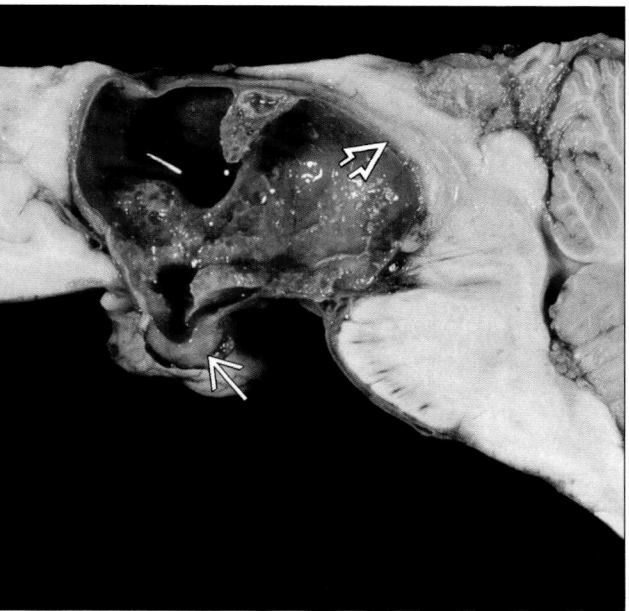

25-53. *Sagittal autopsy specimen of adamantinomatous craniopharyngioma shows a small solid intrasellar component* ➡, *a large suprasellar cystic component that adheres to adjacent brain* ⧨. *(Courtesy R. Hewlett, MD.)*

ing pathway may be one factor in the pathogenesis of adamantinomatous CPs.

athology

LOCATION. Completely intrasellar CPs are rare. CPs are primarily suprasellar tumors (75%). A small intrasellar component is present in 20-25% of cases **(25-52)**. Occasionally, CPs (especially the papillary type) arise mostly or entirely within the third ventricle **(25-58)**, **(25-61)**.

SIZE AND NUMBER. CPs are solitary lesions that range in size from a few millimeters to several centimeters. Lesions larger than five centimeters are common. Giant craniopharyngiomas may extend into both anterior and middle cranial fossae **(25-57)**. Posteroinferior extension between the clivus and pons down to the foramen magnum can be seen in exceptionally large lesions.

GROSS PATHOLOGY. Two types of craniopharyngiomas are recognized: Adamantinomatous and papillary. About 90% of all CPs are adamantinomatous; 10% are papillary.

The typical gross appearance of an **adamantinomatous craniopharyngioma** is that of a multilobulated, partially solid but mostly cystic suprasellar mass **(25-53)**, **(25-54)**. Multiple loculated cysts are common. The cysts often contain dark, viscous, "machinery oil" fluid rich in cholesterol crystals **(25-52)**. The surfaces of adamantinomatous CPs are often irregular and infiltrative, adhering to adjacent structures such as the hypothalamus.

Papillary craniopharyngioma is usually a discrete encapsulated mass with a smooth surface that does not adhere to adjacent brain. Papillary CPs are often solid, with a cauliflower-like configuration. When they contain cysts, the fluid is clear (unlike the "machinery oil" cholesterol-rich contents of adamantinomatous CPs).

MICROSCOPIC FEATURES. Adamantinomatous CPs have a peripheral layer of palisading stratified squamous epithelium surrounding nodules of "wet" keratin. Cholesterol "clefts" and squamous debris are typical. Calcification is common.

Papillary CPs have solid sheets of well-differentiated squamous epithelium. Crude epithelial pseudopapillae form around fibrovascular stromal cores. Occasional goblet cells are present.

STAGING, GRADING, AND CLASSIFICATION. Both adamantinomatous and papillary craniopharyngiomas are WHO grade I neoplasms. MIB-1 is low.

Clinical Issues

EPIDEMIOLOGY. CP is the most common nonglial neoplasm in children, accounting for 6-10% of all pediatric brain tumors and slightly more than half of suprasellar neoplasms.

DEMOGRAPHICS. CPs occur nearly equally in children and adults. Adamantinomatous CPs have a bimodal age distribution with a large peak between 5-10 years and a second, smaller peak at 50-60 years. CPs are rare in newborns and infants; only 5% arise in patients between birth and five years of age.

25-54. Axial autopsy specimen shows a mostly cystic craniopharyngioma ⇗ in the suprasellar cistern. A small tumor nodule is present ⇒. (Courtesy R. Hewlett, MD.) **25-55A.** Axial NECT scan in a 7-year-old boy with a 2-month history of visual problems presents with acute near-total vision loss shows a typical cystic suprasellar mass with rim calcification ⇒ suggesting craniopharyngioma.

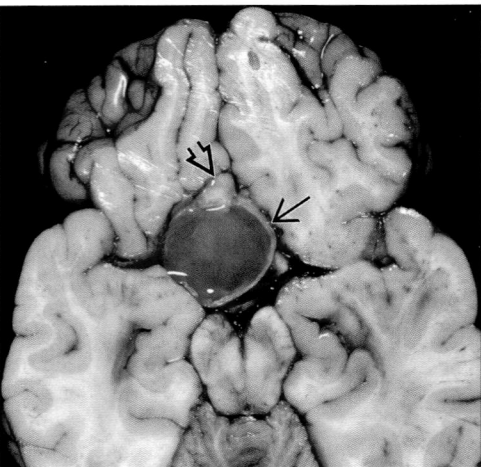
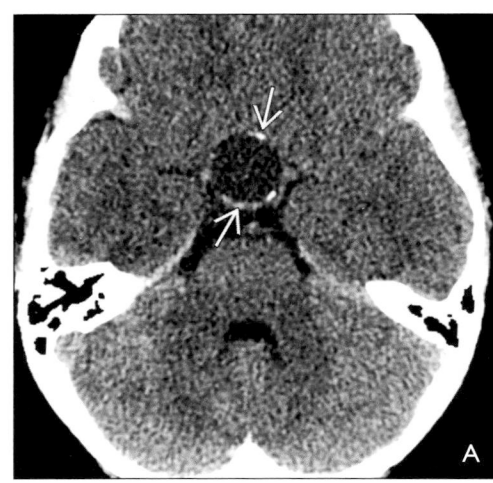

25-55B. Sagittal T1WI shows a lobulated intra-, suprasellar mass ⇒ that is nearly isointense with white matter in the corpus callosum. **25-55C.** The mass ⇒ is very hyperintense on sagittal T2WI. Some hypointense debris ⇒ is present at the bottom of the mostly cystic mass.

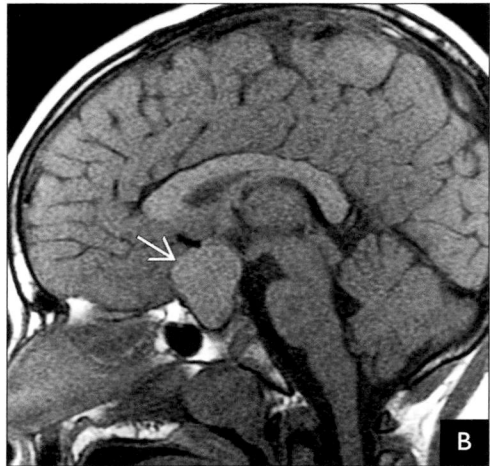
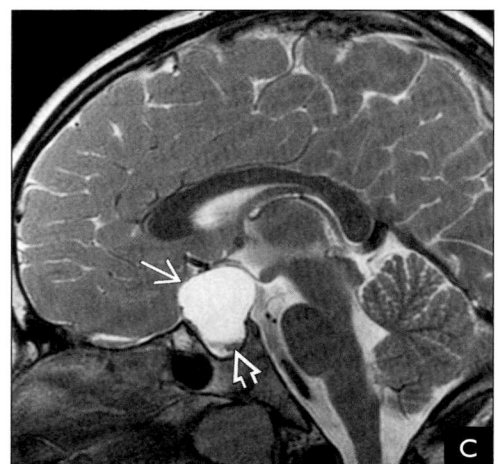

25-55D. Sagittal T1 C+ shows thin rim enhancement around the mass ⇒. **25-55E.** Coronal T1 C+ shows the thin enhancing tumor rim ⇒ with a small tumor nodule ⇒. Adamantinomatous craniopharyngioma was found at surgery.

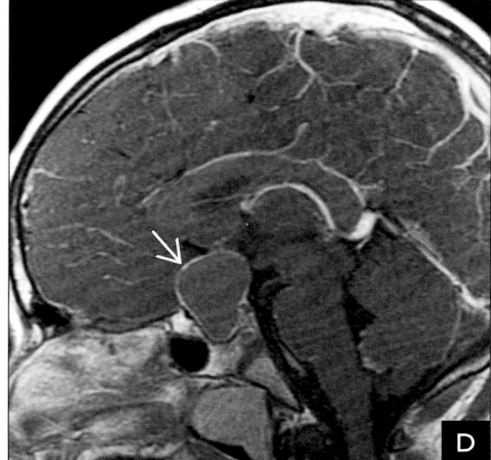
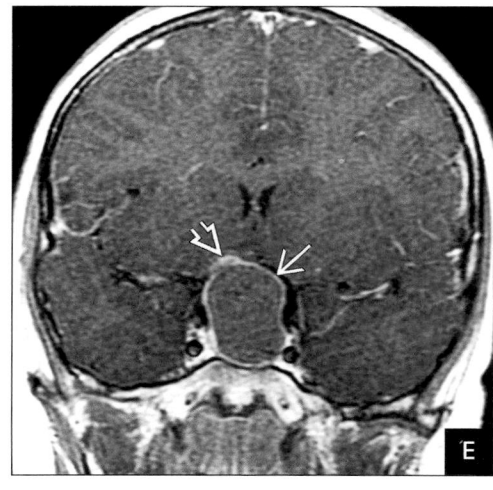

Papillary CPs almost always occur in adults with a peak incidence between 40 and 44 years.

PRESENTATION. Symptoms vary with tumor size and patient age. Patients most commonly present with visual disturbances, either with or without accompanying headache. Large tumors compress the infundibular stalk ("stalk effect"). Endocrine deficiencies including growth failure, delayed puberty, and diabetes insipidus are common.

NATURAL HISTORY. CPs are slow-growing neoplasms with a propensity to recur following surgery. More than 85% of patients survive at least three years following diagnosis. However, the recurrence rate at 10 years approaches 20% even in patients with gross total resection. Recurrence is significantly more common with larger and incompletely excised lesions.

Approximately half of long-term survivors experience reduced quality of life, mostly due to morbid hypothalamic obesity. Spontaneous malignant transformation is rare. Most cases of CP malignant degeneration occur in patients with multiple recurrences and prior radiotherapy.

TREATMENT OPTIONS. Gross total resection is the best treatment option. Hypothalamic injury is the major risk, especially with large adamantinomatous CPs.

Imaging

GENERAL FEATURES. A partially calcified, mixed solid and cystic extraaxial suprasellar mass in a child is the classic appearance. A compressed, displaced pituitary gland can sometimes be identified as separate from the mass.

CT FINDINGS. Adamantinomatous CPs follow a "rule of ninety," i.e., 90% are mixed cystic/solid, 90% are calcified, and 90% enhance (25-55).

Papillary CPs rarely calcify. They are often solid or mostly solid. When they contain intratumoral cysts, the cysts are usually smaller and less complex-appearing than those seen with adamantinomatous CPs.

MR FINDINGS. Signal intensity varies with cyst contents (25-56). Multiple cysts are common, and intracystic fluid within each cyst varies from hypo- to hyperintense compared to brain on T1WI (25-55).

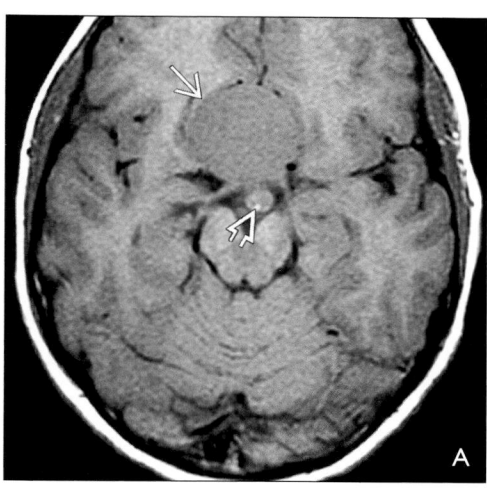
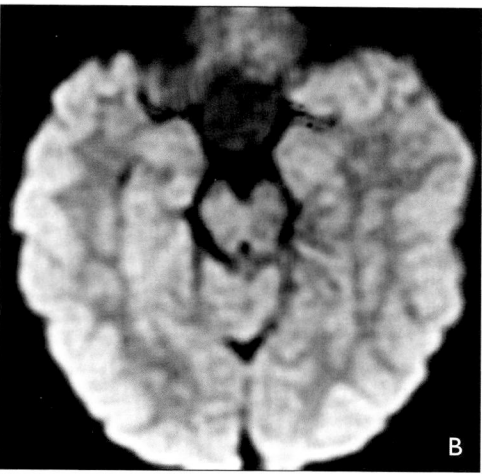

25-56A. Axial T1WI in a 14-year-old male shows a large suprasellar mass ➡ that is mostly isointense with cortex except for a small nodular posterior excrescence that has a tiny hyperintense focus ➡. 25-56B. DWI shows no restriction.

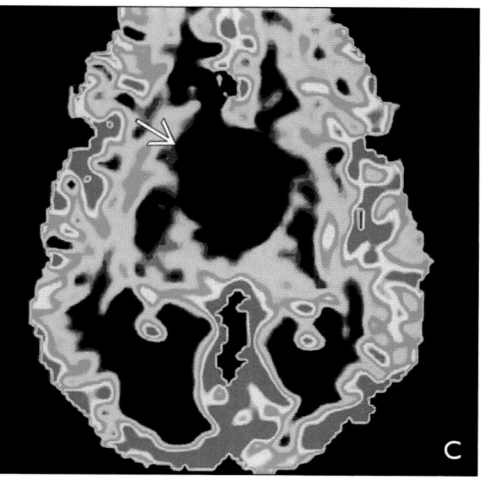
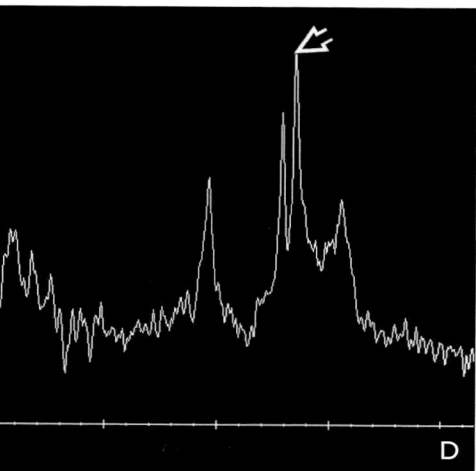

25-56C. pMR shows no evidence of elevated rCBV. The mass ➡ is essentially as avascular as the CSF-containing occipital horns of the lateral ventricles. 25-56D. MRS shows a very large lipid-lactate peak ➡ characteristic of the cholesterol and lipid contents of craniopharyngioma. Adamantinomatous craniopharyngioma was found at surgery.

25-57A. Axial NECT scan in a 9-year-old boy shows an extensive hypodense mass involving the anterior, middle, and posterior cranial fossae ⭢. A small focus of calcification ⮑ is present inside the mass. **25-57B.** Axial T2WI shows that the cysts are mostly hyperintense ⭢.

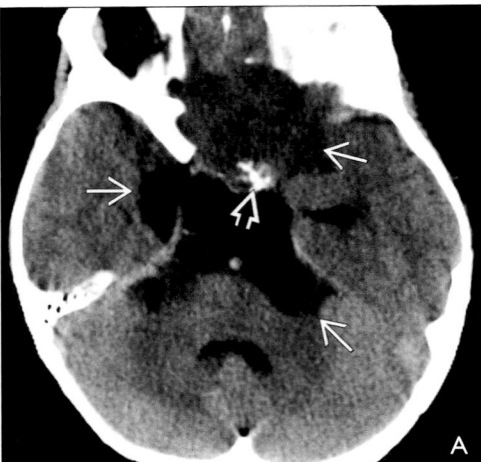
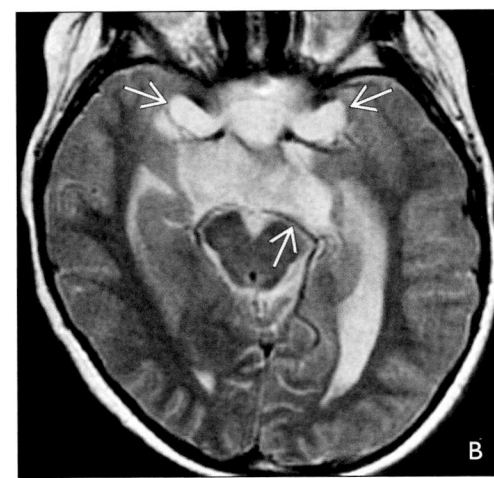

25-57C. Sagittal T1 C+ demonstrates some thin rim enhancement ⭢ around parts of the mass. **25-57D.** Axial T1 C+ confirms that thin rims of enhancement are present ⭢. When a multicystic, bizarre-appearing mass in a child extends into several fossae, craniopharyngioma should be a consideration.

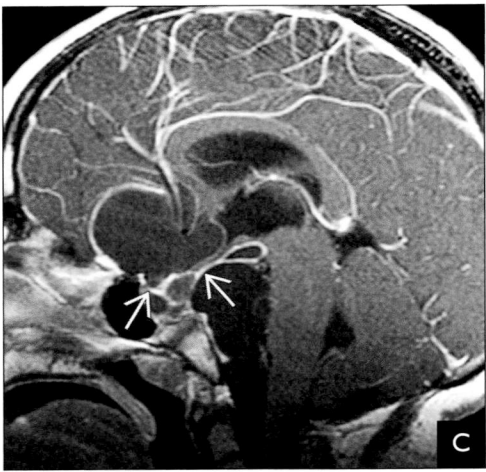
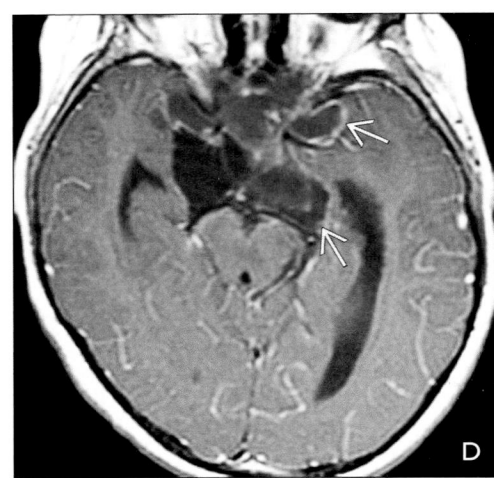

25-58. Midline sagittal section shows a solid mass filling the third ventricle. Papillary craniopharyngioma. (Courtesy B. Scheithauer, MD.) **25-59.** Sagittal T1 C+ scan in a 37-year-old man shows a solidly enhancing mass in the third ventricle ⭢. Papillary craniopharyngioma. (Courtesy C. Sutton, MD.)

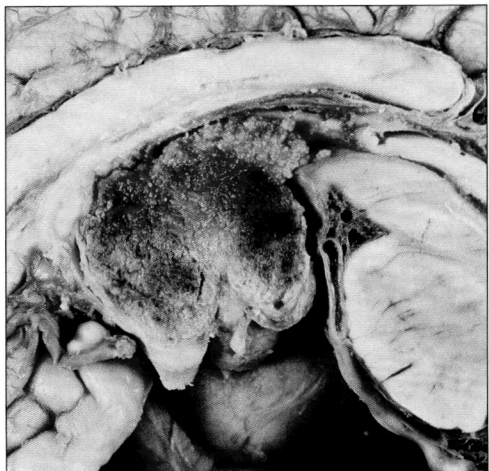
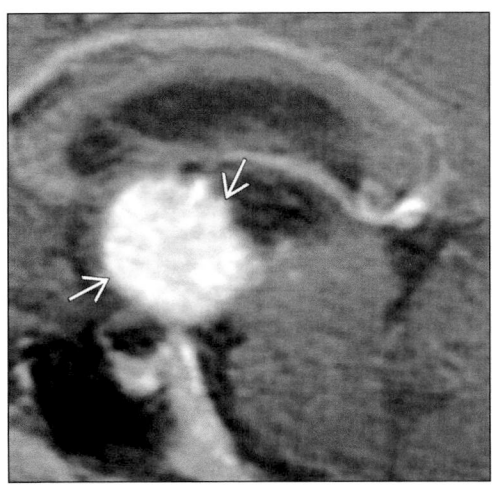

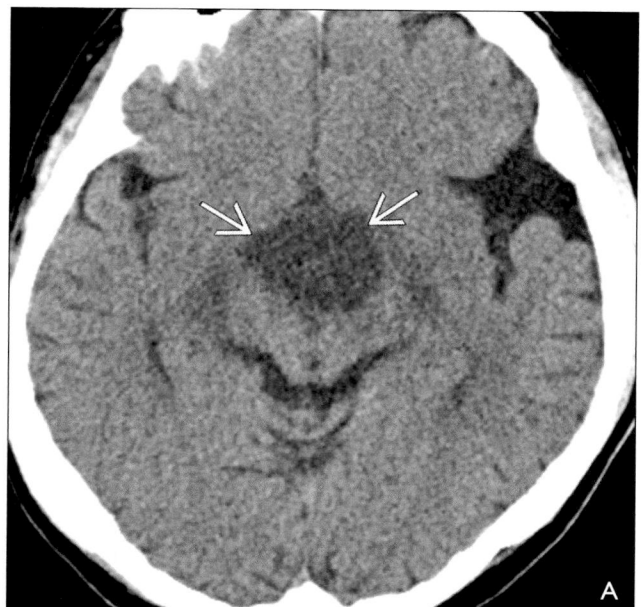

25-60A. A 44-year-old man with headaches, psychiatric symptoms. NECT shows a well-defined, hypodense, noncalcified mass ⇒ in the suprasellar cistern.

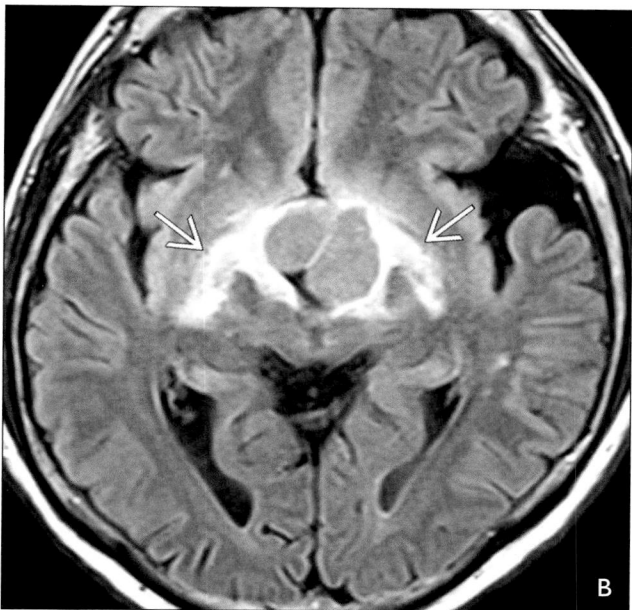

25-60B. FLAIR scan demonstrates that the mass does not suppress. Note the hyperintensity in the hypothalamus, optic tracts ⇒. Papillary craniopharyngioma was found at surgery. No parenchymal tumor invasion was present.

CP cysts are variably hyperintense on T2WI and FLAIR. The solid nodule is often calcified and moderately hypointense. Hyperintensity extending along the optic tracts is common and usually represents edema, not tumor invasion **(25-60)**.

The cyst walls and solid nodules typically enhance following contrast administration **(25-55)**, **(25-59)**.

MRS shows a large lipid-lactate peak, characteristic of the cholesterol and lipid constituents of a CP. pMR shows low rCBV **(25-56)**.

ifferential Diagnosis

The major differential diagnosis of CP is **Rathke cleft cyst** (RCC). RCCs do not calcify, appear to be much less heterogeneous, and do not show nodular enhancement. The ADC of RCC is significantly increased compared to that of cystic CPs. Immunohistochemistry is helpful, as RCCs express specific cytokeratins that CPs do not.

Hypothalamic/chiasmatic astrocytoma is usually a solid suprasellar mass that is clearly intraparenchymal. Calcifications and cysts are uncommon.

Pituitary adenoma is rare in prepubescent children (peak age period for CP). A **dermoid cyst** can be hyperintense on T1WI and may demonstrate calcification. An **epidermoid cyst** (EC) is usually off-midline; suprasellar ECs are uncommon. Neither dermoid nor epidermoid cysts enhance.

CRANIOPHARYNGIOMA

Etiology
- Epithelial remnants of Rathke pouch

Pathology
- 2 types
  - Adamantinomatous (90%)
  - Papillary (10%)
  - Both are WHO grade I
- Adamantinomatous
  - Multiple cysts
  - Squamous epithelium, "wet" keratin
  - Cholesterol-rich "machinery oil" fluid
- Papillary
  - Solid > > cystic (clear fluid)
  - Almost always adults

Clinical Issues
- > 50% of pediatric suprasellar neoplasms
- Occurs equally in children, adults
  - Peak in children = 5-10 years
  - Peak in adults = 40-44 years
- Slow growth
  - Recurrence common
  - Malignant transformation rare

Imaging
- CT
  - Can be giant (> 5 cm), involve multiple fossae
  - Adenomatous: 90% cystic, 90% calcify, 90% enhance
  - Papillary: Solid > cystic
- MR
  - Variable signal on T1WI
  - Usually hyperintense on T2/FLAIR
  - MRS: Large lipid-lactate peak

Differential Diagnosis
- Rathke cleft cyst

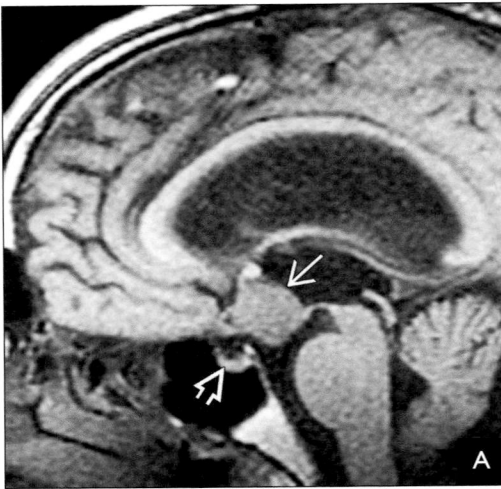

25-61A. Sagittal T1WI in a 64-year-old man with dizziness shows a mass ➡ *in the anterior third ventricle clearly separate from normal pituitary* ➡.

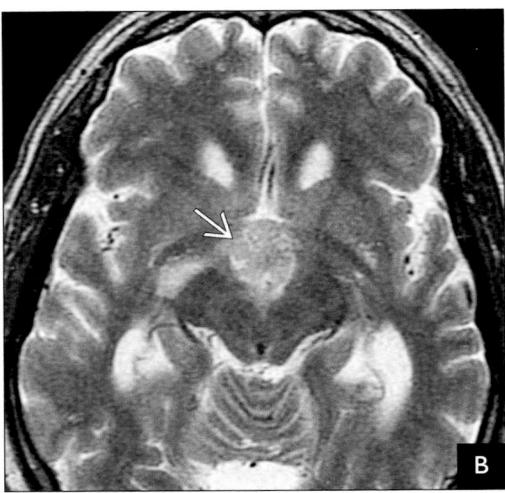

25-61B. T2WI shows that the third ventricle mass ➡ *is solid, isointense with cortex.*

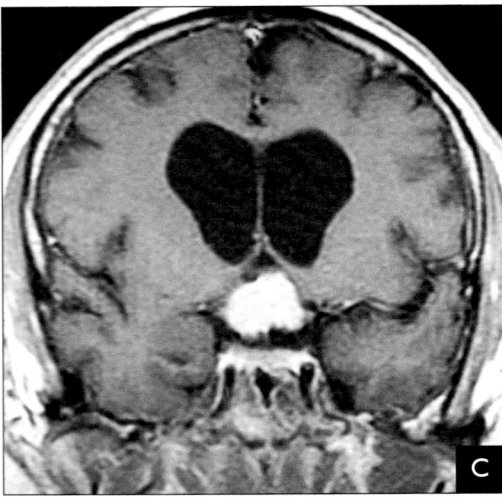

25-61C. Coronal T1 C+ shows the mass enhancing intensely, homogeneously. Adamantinomatous craniopharyngioma was found at surgery.

Nonadenomatous Pituitary Tumors

Primary nonadenomatous pituitary gland tumors are rare, poorly understood entities with confusing nomenclature. The 2007 WHO Classification of Tumors of the Central Nervous System clarified matters, formally recognizing three histologically distinct neoplasms: Pituicytoma, spindle cell oncocytoma (SCO), and granular cell tumor. All are WHO grade I tumors.

Pituicytoma

Previously also known as "choristoma" and "infundibuloma," pituicytoma arises from modified glial cells ("pituicytes") that reside in the infundibular stalk and neurohypophysis (25-62).

Visual disturbance with or without headache is the most common presenting symptom. Patients with pituicytoma almost never present with diabetes insipidus, galactorrhea, or prolactinemia.

Pituicytoma can appear as either an intra- or a suprasellar mass. The majority of pituicytomas are isointense with brain on T1WI and hyperintense on T2WI. They enhance homogeneously following contrast enhancement (25-63).

Pituicytoma is the only one of the nonadenomatous tumors that can present as a purely intrasellar mass. An intrasellar mass that is clearly separate from the anterior pituitary gland and enhances homogeneously is most likely a pituicytoma.

Spindle Cell Oncocytoma

SCO, also known as folliculostellate cell tumor, arises from the adenohypophysis. SCOs consist of "spindled" oncocytes containing granular, mitochondria-rich cytoplasm.

Visual disturbance, panhypopituitarism, and headache are the most common presenting symptoms. SCOs do not appear to cause diabetes insipidus.

To date, all pathologically proven cases have presented as mixed intra- and suprasellar infiltrating pituitary lesions. Imaging findings are similar to—and cannot be distinguished from—those of pituitary adenoma or lymphocytic hypophysis (25-64).

Granular Cell Tumor

Like pituicytoma, granular cell tumor is a tumor of the neurohypophysis. Many Granular cell tumors are asymptomatic and discovered incidentally at autopsy. Some enlarge with time, becoming symptomatic in middle-aged or older adults. Visual disturbance, headache, and amenorrhea are common. Similar to pituicytoma and SCO, granular cell tumors rarely present with diabetes insipidus, prolactinemia, or galactorrhea.

Granular cell tumors are typically suprasellar masses. They are hyperdense on NECT and isointense with brain on both T1- and T2WI. Granular cell tumors enhance strongly and homogeneously following contrast administration.

Miscellaneous Lesions

Hypophysitis

Hypophysitis is an inflammation of the pituitary gland that comprises an increasingly complex group of disorders. There are two main histologic forms of hypophysitis: Lymphocytic hypophysitis and nonlymphocytic hypophysitis. Recent reports of other variants broaden the hypophysitis spectrum even further. In this section, we focus on lymphocytic hypophysitis, the most common form. We then briefly discuss nonlymphocytic hypophysitis, including granulomatous hypophysitis and

some of the newly described entities that are often characterized by plasma cell infiltrates.

Lymphocytic Hypophysitis

TERMINOLOGY. Lymphocytic hypophysitis (LH) is also called lymphocytic adenohypophysitis, primary hypophysitis, and stalkitis. A variant form of LH is called lymphocytic infundibuloneurohypophysitis (LINH).

ETIOLOGY. LH is an uncommon autoimmune inflammatory disorder of the pituitary gland that most often occurs in women of child bearing age, usually late in pregnancy or shortly after childbirth. Immune competence is reestablished in the late pregnancy/peripartum period. Antipituitary antibodies co-react with both the pituitary gland and the placenta.

LH is also associated with other autoimmune disorders. Approximately 25% of patients have coexistent systemic inflammatory/autoimmune disease. Thyroiditis, polymyositis, type 1 diabetes, and psoriasis have all been associated with LH.

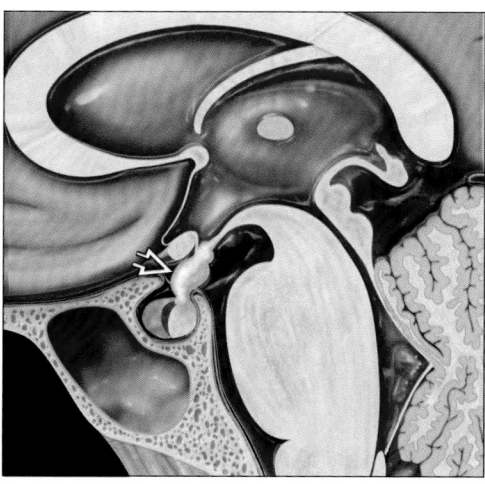

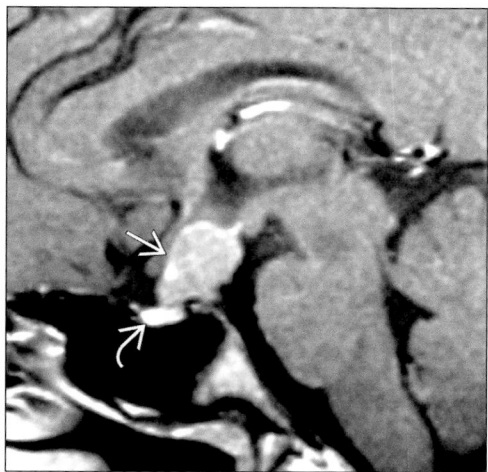

25-62. Sagittal graphic shows a pituicytoma ⇨ involving the infundibular stalk and neurohypophysis. 25-63. Sagittal T1 C+ scan in a 22-year-old woman with delayed growth and hypopituitarism shows an enhancing infundibular mass ⇨ that is clearly separate from the pituitary gland ⇗. Imaging findings have remained stable over many years. Presumed pituicytoma.

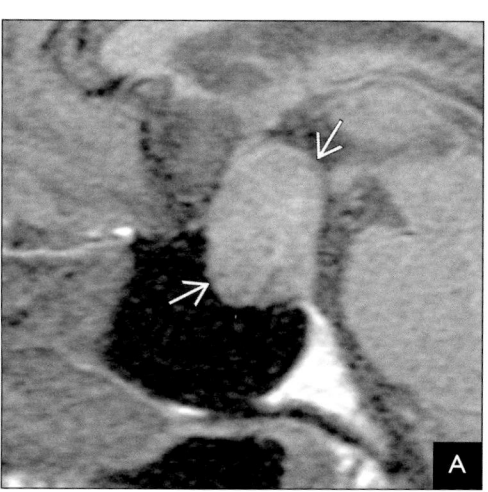

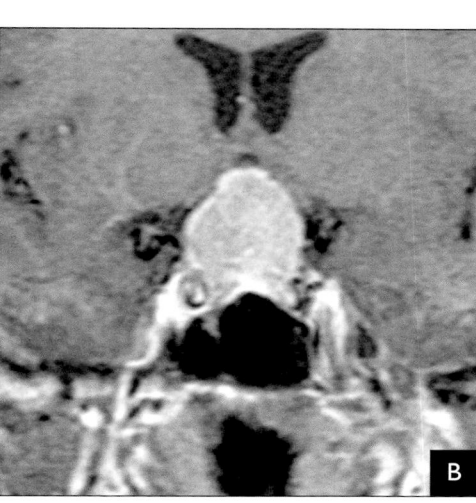

25-64A. Sagittal T1WI in a 69-year-old woman with headaches, bitemporal hemianopsia shows a sellar-suprasellar mass ⇨ that is well-delineated and isointense with brain. The pituitary gland cannot be distinguished as separate from the mass. 25-64B. Coronal T1 C+ scan shows that the lesion enhances strongly and uniformly. Preoperative diagnosis was pituitary macroadenoma. Spindle cell oncocytoma was diagnosed at histologic examination.

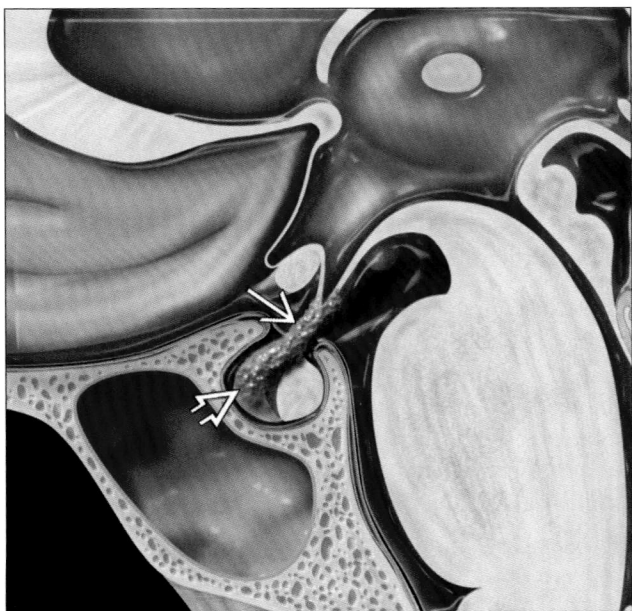

25-65. Sagittal graphic shows lymphocytic hypophysitis. Note thickening of the infundibulum ➡, infiltration into the anterior lobe of the pituitary gland ➡.

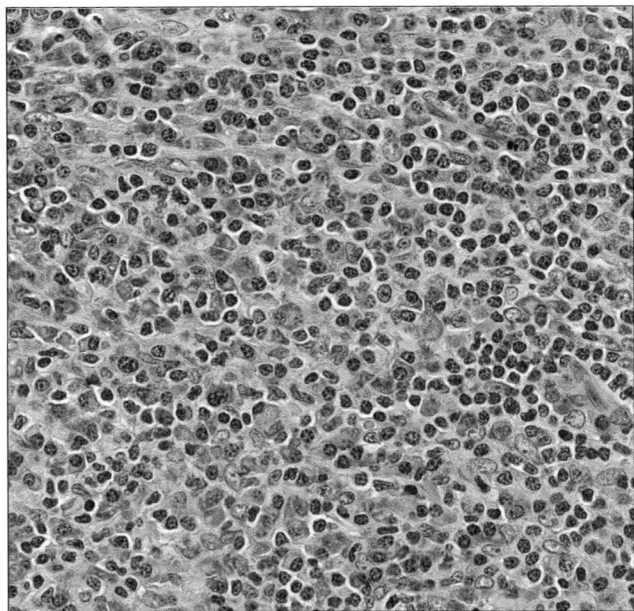

25-66. Lymphocytic adenohypophysitis is typified by numerous infiltrating cytologically benign lymphocytes overrunning the gland. (Courtesy B. K. DeMasters, MD.)

PATHOLOGY. The pituitary gland and stalk in LH appear diffusely enlarged and firm although inflammatory changes are predominantly or exclusively in the anterior lobe **(25-65)**. Microscopic features include a dense infiltrate mostly composed of T-cell lymphocytes **(25-66)**. Varying degrees of gland destruction and fibrosis may be present. Granulomas and giant cells are absent.

LINH typically involves *both* the neuro- and the adenohypophysis.

CLINICAL ISSUES. Between 80-90% of patients with LH are female; 30-60% of cases occur in the peripartum period. There is no adverse effect on the fetus.

The most common presenting symptoms are headache and multiple endocrine deficiencies with partial or total hypopituitarism. Diabetes insipidus is common. ACTH deficits often appear first. Hyperprolactinemia occurs in one-third of all patients, probably secondary to stalk compression.

Men, women past child bearing age, and children are affected in 10-20% of cases. Middle-aged men typically present with diabetes insipidus.

Treatment is hormone replacement with or without corticosteroids.

IMAGING. LH is typically both intra- and suprasellar. Adjacent dural or sphenoid sinus mucosal thickening is common.

Imaging shows a thickened, nontapering infundibular stalk. A rounded, symmetrically enlarged pituitary gland

is common **(25-67)**. The sellar floor is intact, not expanded or eroded. The posterior pituitary "bright spot" is absent in 75% of cases. LH enhances intensely and uniformly.

DIFFERENTIAL DIAGNOSIS. The major differential diagnosis for LH is nonsecreting **pituitary macroadenoma**. The distinction is important as treatment differs significantly. LH is treated medically whereas surgical resection is the primary treatment for pituitary macroadenoma. Macroadenomas can be giant, but LH only occasionally exceeds three centimeters in diameter. Clinical findings are also helpful as LH commonly presents with diabetes insipidus **(25-69)**.

The stalk is usually normal in **pituitary hyperplasia**, although patient age and gender are similar. **Metastasis** usually occurs in older patients with known systemic primary tumor.

Granulomatous hypophysitis may occur secondary to infection, sarcoidosis, or Langerhans cell histiocytosis. GH is less common than LH, has a different epidemiological profile, and tends to enhance more heterogeneously. **IgG4-** and **drug-related hypophysitis** are very rare.

Granulomatous Hypophysitis

Granulomatous hypophysitis (GH) has different epidemiological characteristics than LH does. GH is equally common in both genders, and there is no association with pregnancy.

GH can be primary (idiopathic) or secondary **(25-68)**. **Secondary GH** (sGH) is far more common than primary GH and typically results from necrotizing granulomatous inflammation. Infectious/inflammatory sGH can be caused by TB, sarcoid, fungal infection, syphilis, Langerhans cell histiocytosis, Wegener granulomatosis, Erdheim-Chester disease, granulomatous autoimmune hypophysitis, ruptured Rathke cleft cyst, or craniopharyngioma. sGH may also occur as a reaction to systemic inflammatory disorders such as Crohn disease. Imaging findings are nonspecific, resembling those of LH or pituitary adenoma.

Primary GH (pGH) is a rare inflammatory disease without identifiable infectious organisms. The precise etiology of pGH is unknown. Nonnecrotizing granulomas with multinucleated giant cells, histiocytes, and various

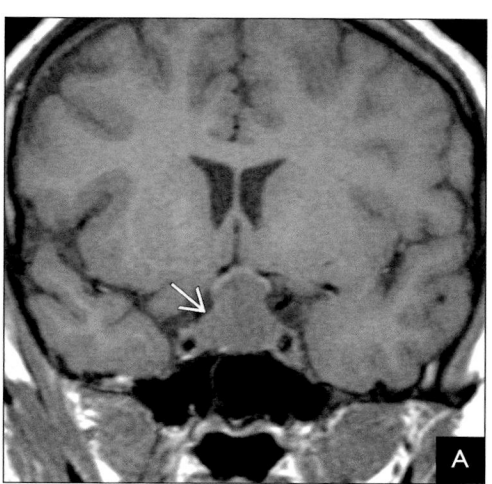

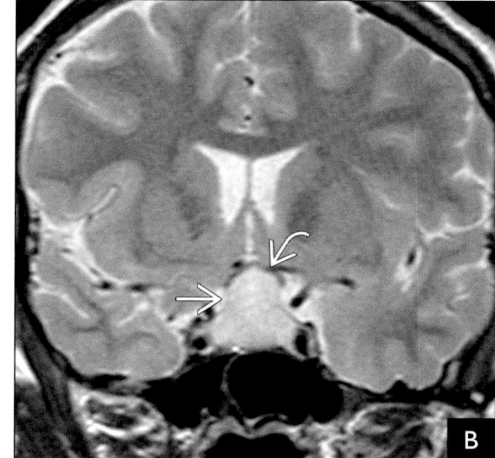

25-67A. *A 19-year-old pregnant woman developed acute vision problems in the late third trimester. Coronal T1WI shows a "figure eight" or snowman-shaped intra- and suprasellar mass* ➡. *25-67B. Coronal T2WI shows that the lesion* ➡ *is mildly hyperintense. Note elevation and draping of the optic chiasm* ➡ *over the mass.*

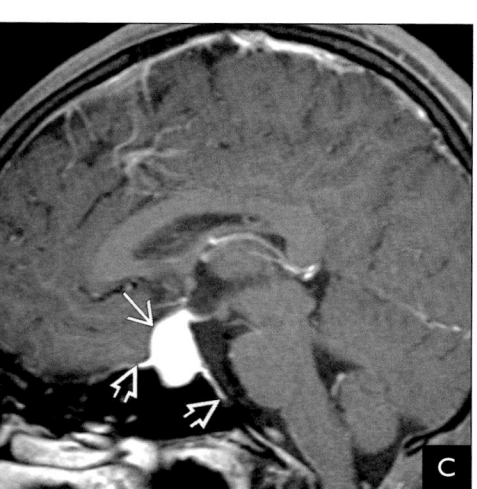

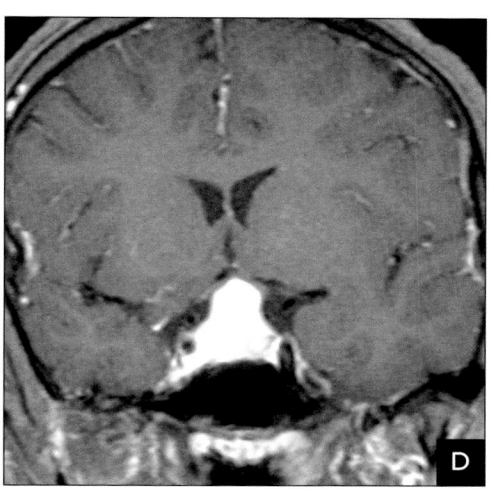

25-67C. Sagittal T1 C+ FS shows that the mass ➡ *enhances intensely, uniformly. Note the dural "tails"* ➡ *adjacent to the mass. 25-67D. Coronal T1 C+ shows that the mass has a "figure eight" appearance virtually identical to that seen with pituitary macroadenoma. However, the dural "tails" seen on the sagittal scan are unusual findings in macroadenomas. Lymphocytic hypophysitis.*

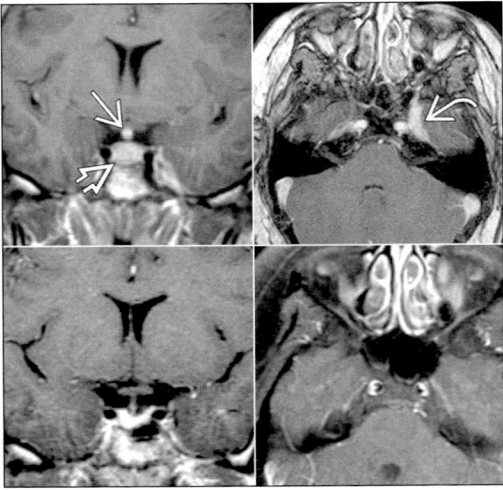

25-68. *Granulomatous hypophysitis. (Top) "Fat" pituitary gland* ➡, *stalk* ➡, *pseudotumor* ➡. *(Bottom) Resolution after steroids.*

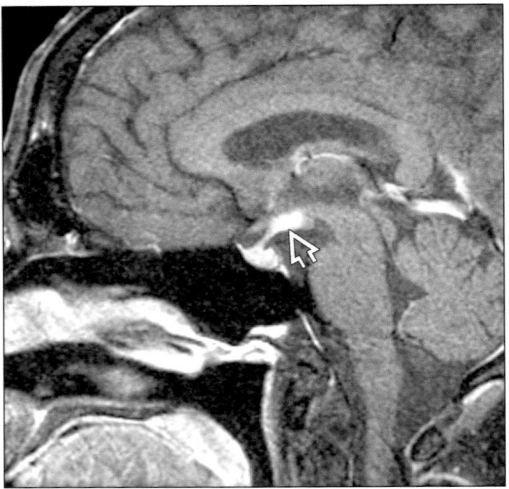

25-69. *LINH in a middle-aged man with diabetes insipidus is seen here as an enhancing mass* ➡ *in the hypothalamus.*

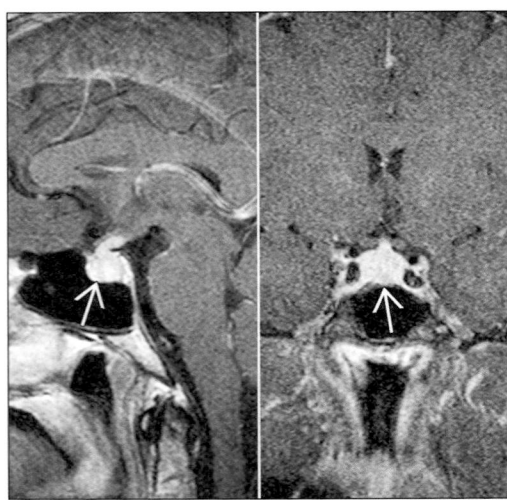

25-70. *Patient on ipilimumab for metastatic melanoma developed drug-induced hypophysitis with infiltration of the stalk, pituitary gland* ➡.

numbers of plasma cells and lymphocytes are typical. pGH usually presents with diabetes insipidus. A symmetric sellar mass that enhances strongly but heterogeneously is seen on imaging studies.

Other Hypophysitis Variants

A number of new hypophysitis variants have been recently described. **IgG4-related hypophysitis** has a marked mononuclear infiltrate mainly characterized by increased numbers of IgG4-positive plasma cells. Imaging findings resemble those of lymphocytic infundibuloneurohypophysitis. The pituitary stalk and posterior pituitary lobe are enlarged and enhance intensely following contrast administration.

Drug-related hypophysitis has been reported in cases of cancer immunotherapy with antibodies that stimulate T-cell responses (e.g., ipilimumab) (25-70). Clinicians and radiologists should be aware of autoimmune-induced hypophysitis as a complication of new treatments.

Pituitary Apoplexy

Pituitary apoplexy (PAP) is a well-described acute clinical syndrome with headache, visual defects, and variable endocrine deficiencies. In some cases, profound pituitary insufficiency develops and may become life-threatening.

Etiology

PAP is caused by hemorrhage into—or ischemic necrosis of—the pituitary gland. A preexisting macroadenoma is present in 65-90% of cases, but PAP can also occur in microadenomas or histologically normal pituitary glands. What precipitates the hemorrhage or necrosis is unknown.

In rare cases, patients undergoing treatment with bromocriptine or cabergoline for pituitary adenoma have developed life-threatening PAP.

Pathology

The most common gross appearance of PAP is that of a large intra- or combined intra- and suprasellar mass (25-71). Between 85-90% of cases demonstrate gross hemorrhagic infarction (25-72). Nonhemorrhagic ("bland") pituitary infarction causes an enlarged, edematous-appearing pituitary gland.

Absent findings of an underlying neoplasm (60% are nonfunctioning null-cell adenomas), microscopic features are nonspecific and generally unremarkable.

Clinical Issues

EPIDEMIOLOGY AND DEMOGRAPHICS. PAP is rare, occurring in approximately 1% of all patients with pituitary macroadenomas. Peak age is 55-60 years. PAP is rare in patients under the age of 15. The M:F ratio is 2:1.

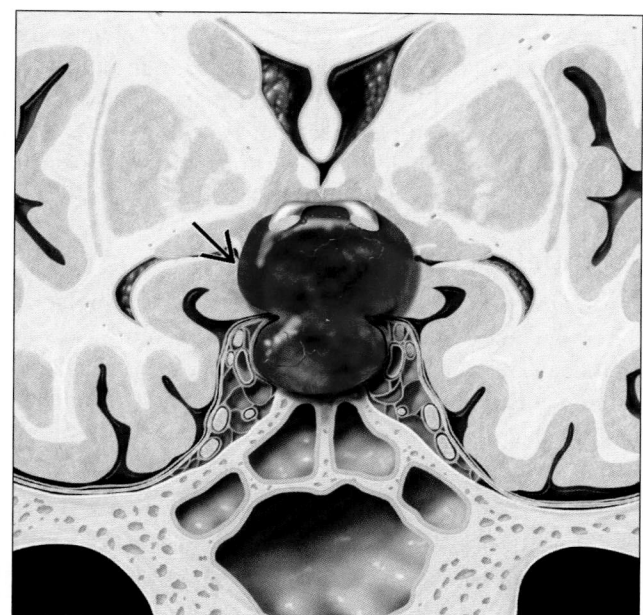

25-71. Coronal graphic shows a macroadenoma with acute hemorrhage ⇨ causing pituitary apoplexy.

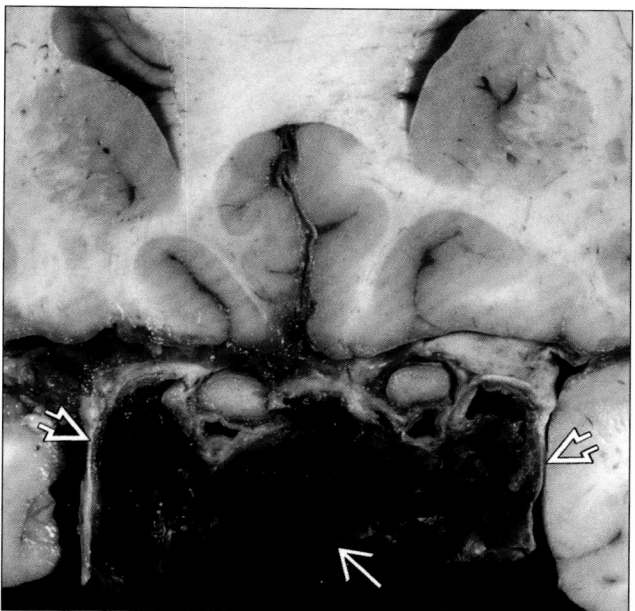

25-72. Autopsy specimen of pituitary apoplexy shows hemorrhagic macroadenoma ⇨ extending into both cavernous sinuses ⇨. (Courtesy R. Hewlett, MD.)

PRESENTATION. Headache is almost universal in patients with PAP and is the most common presenting symptom, followed by nausea (80%) and visual field disturbance (70%). Hemorrhagic tumors that extend into the cavernous sinus may compress cranial nerves III, IV, V, and VI.

Almost 80% of patients with PAP have panhypopituitarism. Acute adrenal crisis with hypovolemia, shock, and disseminated intravascular coagulation may occur.

Rarely, pituitary apoplexy with panhypopituitarism and diabetes insipidus develops in patients with **h**emolysis, **e**levated **l**iver enzymes, and **l**ow **p**latelet count (HELLP) syndrome.

NATURAL HISTORY. PAP varies from a clinically benign event to catastrophic presentation with permanent neurologic deficits. Coma or even death may ensue in severe cases.

Long-term survivors often have permanent pituitary insufficiency requiring hormone replacement (most commonly steroids or thyroid hormone). Almost half of all males with PAP require testosterone replacement.

Patients with pituitary adenomas and PAP may show recurrent pituitary tumor growth and therefore merit continued postoperative surveillance.

A rare variant of PAP is **Sheehan syndrome** (SS). Sheehan syndrome is acute postpartum ischemic necrosis of the anterior pituitary gland, typically caused by blood loss and hypovolemic shock during or after childbirth.

SS may result in long-term loss of hormone function. Remote SS is a rare cause of partially empty sella on imaging studies.

TREATMENT OPTIONS. Surgical decompression is generally necessary in patients with compromised visual acuity. Supportive therapy with steroids and fluid/electrolyte/hormone replacement is often required.

Imaging

GENERAL FEATURES. An enlarged pituitary gland with peripheral rim enhancement is typical **(25-73)**. Gross intraglandular hemorrhage is common but not invariably present.

CT FINDINGS. NECT scans are often normal. Hemorrhage into the pituitary gland with a hyperdense sellar/suprasellar mass can be identified in 20-25% of cases. Occasionally, subarachnoid hemorrhage into the basilar cisterns can be identified.

MR FINDINGS. MR is the procedure of choice to evaluate suspected PAP. Signal intensity depends on whether the PAP is hemorrhagic or nonhemorrhagic. Hemorrhage can be identified in 85-90% of cases **(25-74)**.

Signal intensity depends on clot age. Acute PAP is heterogeneously iso- to hypointense to brain on T1WI. Initially iso- to mildly hyperintense on T2WI, PAP rapidly becomes hypointense on T2WI. Acute compression of the hypothalamus and optic chiasm may cause visible edema along the optic tracts on T2/FLAIR scans.

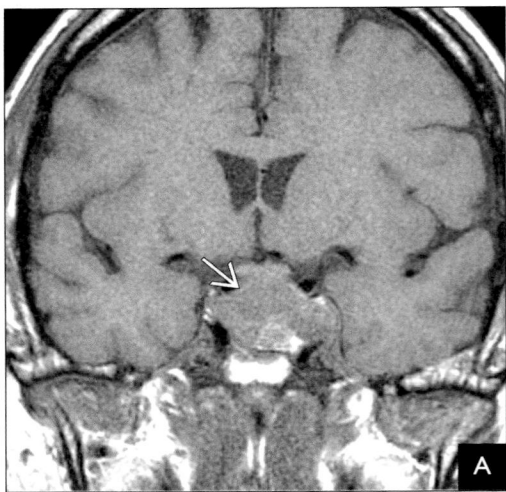

25-73A. T1WI in a 68-year-old man with "thunderclap" headache, visual changes shows mostly isointense intra- and suprasellar mass ➡.

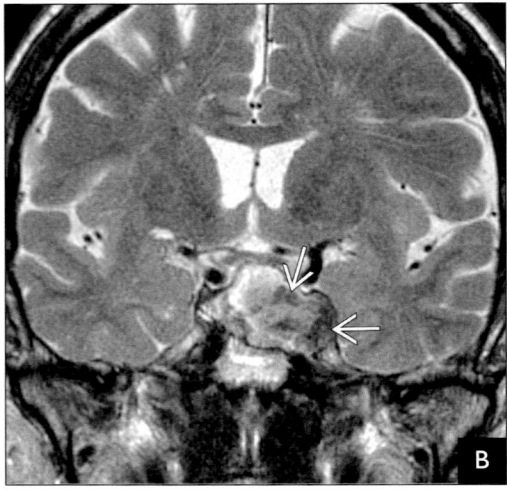

25-73B. Coronal T2WI shows that the mass is very heterogeneous in signal intensity with multiple hemorrhagic foci ➡.

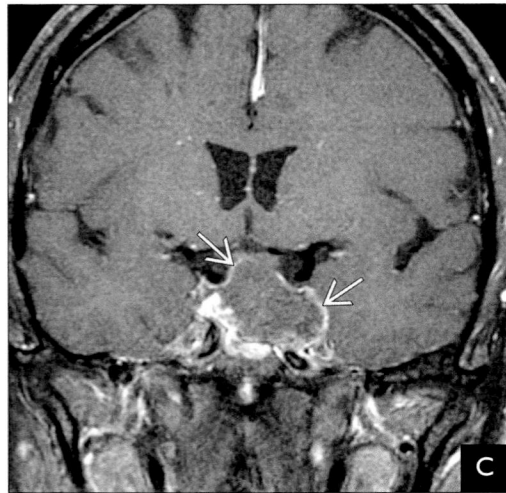

25-73C. Coronal T1 C+ FS shows a thin peripheral rim of enhancement ➡. Pituitary apoplexy. Mostly necrotic, hemorrhagic adenoma found at surgery.

"Blooming" on T2* is common if blood products are present but may be obscured by artifact from the adjacent paranasal sinuses. T1 C+ shows rim enhancement (25-75). Dural thickening and enhancement is seen in 50%, and mucosal thickening in the adjacent sphenoid sinus occurs in 80% of all patients. PAP usually restricts on DWI.

Differential Diagnosis

The major differential diagnosis of pituitary apoplexy is **hemorrhagic macroadenoma**. Focal hemorrhages in adenomas are common, but in contrast to PAP, the clinical course is typically subacute or chronic. Most adenomas enhance strongly but heterogeneously whereas PAP demonstrates rim enhancement around a predominantly nonenhancing, expanded pituitary gland.

Lymphocytic **hypophysitis** can cause relatively sudden onset of symptoms and thus mimic PAP. LH usually causes only modest gland enlargement. The pituitary enhances intensely and uniformly.

Rathke cleft cyst (RCC) can contain thick proteinaceous fluid that appears hyperintense on T1WI and mimic intrapituitary hemorrhage. Most RCCs are asymptomatic and found incidentally. With some exceptions, RCCs that become symptomatic typically follow a subacute/chronic course. Apoplexy is a rare but distinct presentation caused by sudden hemorrhage into the cyst. RCC with apoplexy can mimic the symptoms of PAP, but the cyst can usually be identified as separate from the pituitary gland.

Pituitary abscess is a rare entity that may be difficult to distinguish from PAP with "bland" (ischemic) infarction. Clinical signs of infection may be minimal or absent. T1 shortening around the rim rather than the center of the mass is characteristic of abscess. Rim enhancement with restriction on DWI is typical for both pituitary abscess and PAP.

Acute thrombosis of a large intra- or parasellar **aneurysm** can present with panhypopituitarism and subarachnoid hemorrhage. "Mixed age" laminated clot is common, and a small residual "flow void" from the residual patent lumen can often be identified.

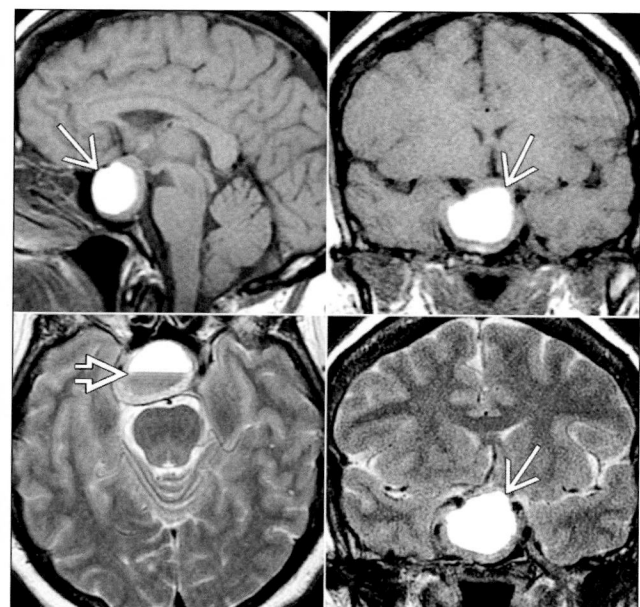

25-74. *Pituitary apoplexy in a 50-year-old woman with 4 days of visual changes shows subacute hemorrhage in the pituitary gland* ➡ *with a blood-fluid level* ⬂.

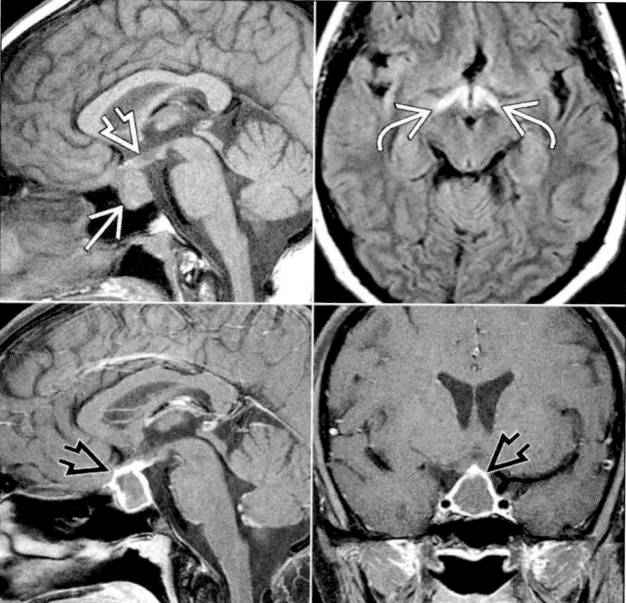

25-75. *(Top left) T1WI shows an enlarged pituitary gland* ➡, *thick hypothalamus* ➡. *(Top right) FLAIR hyperintensity along both optic tracts* ➡. *(Bottom) Rim enhancement* ⬂. *Nonhemorrhagic pituitary apoplexy.*

PITUITARY APOPLEXY

Etiology
- Hemorrhagic or nonhemorrhagic pituitary necrosis
- Preexisting macroadenoma (65-90%)

Clinical Issues
- Sudden onset
- Headache, visual defects
- Hypopituitarism (80%)
- Can be life-threatening
- Can result in permanent pituitary insufficiency
- Sheehan syndrome = postpartum pituitary necrosis

Imaging
- Enlarged pituitary
  - ± hemorrhage
- Rim enhancement around nonenhancing gland
- May cause hypothalamic, optic tract edema

Differential Diagnosis
- Hemorrhagic macroadenoma without apoplexy
- Hypophysitis
- Rathke cleft cyst apoplexy
- Pituitary abscess
- Acute thrombosed aneurysm

---

e- and Postoperative Sella

Two approaches are almost universally used in sellar surgery: Traditional sublabial transsphenoidal surgery and minimally invasive completely endoscopic surgery. Image-guided surgery with robotics and stereotactic intraoperative MR is increasingly used with microsurgical and endoscopic techniques. Subfrontal craniotomy is now relatively uncommon and is generally used only for lesions with uncommonly large supradiaphragmatic tumors.

Each of these techniques requires careful preoperative imaging evaluation. In this section, we focus on the preoperative evaluation for—and postoperative imaging of—transsphenoidal and endoscopic surgery. Both involve safely navigating the sphenoid sinus and avoiding the many critical structures in and around the sella.

Preoperative Evaluation

Most surgical approaches (transethmoid, transnasal, or transseptal) pass through the sphenoid sinus to reach the sella. Regardless of which operative technique—microscopic or endoscopic—is used, delineating sphenoid sinus anatomy and identifying anatomic variants that might impact surgery is important to successful patient outcome.

CT and MR each has a unique contribution to the full preoperative evaluation of sellar lesions. Multiplanar MR is the procedure of choice to characterize the lesion and define its extent. In concert with MR, preoperative CT helps define relevant bony anatomy.

Four key features of sphenoid sinus anatomy should be identified: The location and extent of pneumatization, the sellar configuration, any septation, and the intercarotid distance.

PNEUMATIZATION. Location and extent of sphenoid sinus pneumatization is the major concern. Pneumatization is classified as sellar (57%), postsellar (22%), presel-

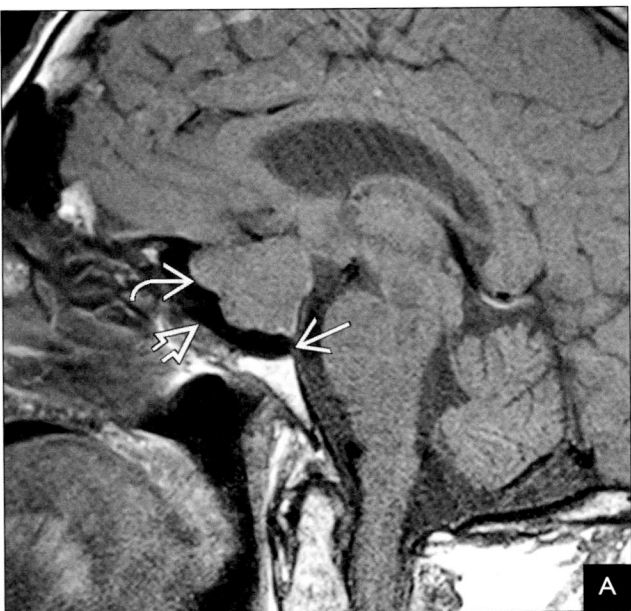

25-76A. Sagittal T1WI in a patient with longstanding acromegaly shows well-aerated sphenoid sinus ⇥ extending posteriorly to clivus ⇥. Pneumatization is classified as postsellar. Note well-defined sellar bulge ⇥ into sphenoid sinus.

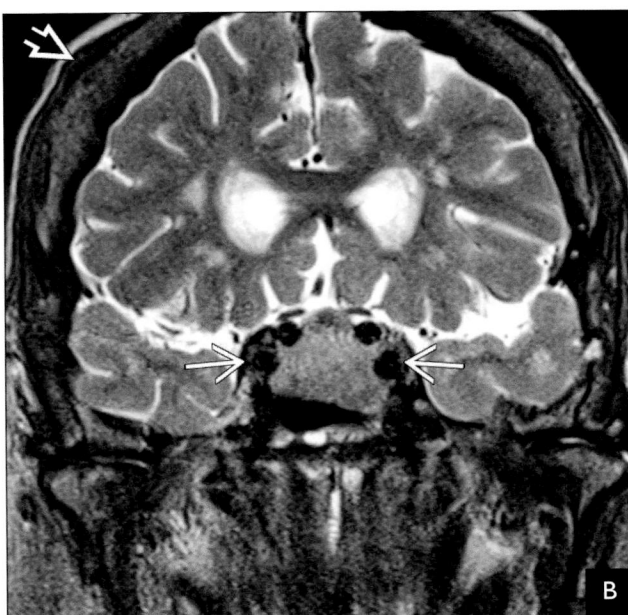

25-76B. Coronal T2WI shows the exceptionally thick skull ⇥ of this patient. The intercarotid distance ⇥ measured 24 mm. Transsphenoidal surgery was successful because of the favorable anatomy.

lar (21%), or conchal (2%). The specific type of pneumatization is generally determined from sagittal MR images **(25-76)**.

The rare conchal nonpneumatized sphenoid is important to recognize preoperatively as it makes transsphenoidal surgery more difficult. At the opposite end of the spectrum, a highly pneumatized sphenoid sinus may make the surgery technically easier but also distorts the anatomic configuration, attenuating the bone and potentially uncovering the carotid arteries and optic nerves.

A pneumatized dorsum sellae can be penetrated during surgery, resulting in CSF leak.

SELLAR CONFIGURATION. The presence (well-defined) or absence (ill-defined) of sellar bulging in relationship to the sellar floor and the degree of sphenoid pneumatization should be reported. Pneumatization of the planum sphenoidale and dorsum sellae should also be noted. These are determined from sagittal MR imaging.

A prominent sellar bulge into a pneumatized sphenoid sinus is seen in 75% of patients **(25-76A)**. The other 25% have an absent or ill-defined sellar bulge. A well-pneumatized sphenoid sinus with a prominent sellar bulge facilitates surgery, which is further eased if the sellar floor is thinned or disrupted by tumor. Dorsum sellae pneumatization is present in the majority.

SEPTATION. The presence or absence of an intersphenoid septum should be determined. If present, note whether there is a single intersinus septum or more than one septa. The position of the septal insertion (in the sellar floor, at

the carotid canal, or at the optic canal) should be identified. This is best evaluated on both axial and coronal bone CT.

Axial scans show no septum in 10-11% of patients and a single intersphenoid septum in 70%. An accessory septum is seen in 10% of patients, and 7-9% have multiple septa.

The intersphenoid septum must be removed to expose the sellar floor, so determining its location is crucial. The septum is rarely located in the midline. It typically deviates to one side or the other, dividing the sphenoid sinus into two unequal cavities. This results in an asymmetric appearance of the sellar floor. In 30-40% of patients, the septum deviates quite laterally and terminates adjacent to the internal carotid artery.

INTERCAROTID DISTANCE. The intercarotid distance is measured between the medial aspects of the two signal "voids" of the cavernous ICA segments as seen on midsellar coronal MR. Intercarotid distance varies widely, ranging from 10-12 mm to 30 mm (mean of 23 mm). Narrow distances (< 12 mm) increase the chance of vascular injury during transsphenoidal surgery.

Postoperative Evaluation

To evaluate the postoperative sella, thin-section, small FOV imaging in both the sagittal and coronal planes is mandatory. Pre-contrast T1- and T2WI images plus postcontrast fat-saturated sequences are standard.

The appearance on postoperative MR scans is complicated by hemorrhage, use of hemostatic agents, packing materials (muscle, fat, fascia lata), and residual tumor. Typical findings include a bony defect in the anterior sphenoid sinus wall, fluid and mucosal thickening in the sinus, fat packing within the sella turcica, hemorrhage, and varying amounts of residual mass effect (25-77).

The first postoperative scan provides the baseline against which subsequent imaging is compared. With time, hemorrhage evolves and resorbs, fat packing fibroses and retracts, and mass effect decreases. A partially empty sella with or without traction on the infundibular stalk and optic chiasm is typical in the months and years following the initial surgery.

Complications such as diabetes insipidus, stalk transection, and electrolyte disturbances are usually temporary. Long-term complications include CSF leaks and cranial neuropathy.

Differential Diagnosis of a Sellar Region Mass

We close this chapter by recapping the approach to constructing a helpful and targeted differential diagnosis for a sellar region mass.

Determining anatomic sublocation is the first, most important step. Is the lesion (1) intrasellar, (2) suprasellar, or (3) in the infundibular stalk? Or is it a combination of these locations?

Whether a sellar/suprasellar mass *is* the pituitary gland itself or is separate from the mass is the most important imaging task and the most helpful finding (25-78), (25-79), (25-80), (25-81). Masses that can be clearly distinguished as separate from the pituitary gland are rarely—if ever—macroadenomas.

The most helpful clinical feature is patient age. Some lesions are common in adults but rarely occur in children. Gender and endocrine status are helpful ancillary clues. For example, pituitary macroadenomas rarely cause diabetes insipidus, but it is one of the most common presenting symptoms of hypophysitis.

Lastly, consider some specific imaging findings. Is the mass cystic? Is it calcified? What is its signal intensity?

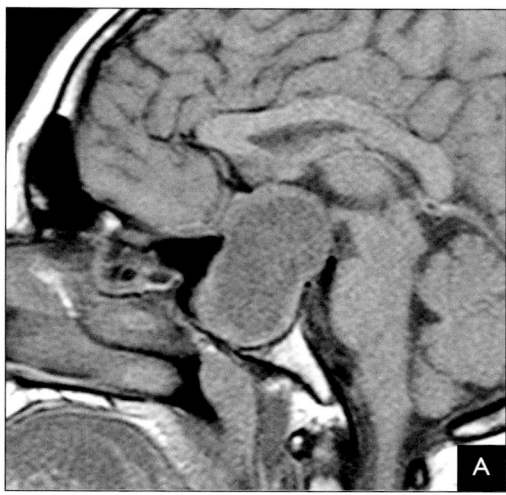

25-77A. Preoperative sagittal T1WI shows a large intra- and suprasellar mixed solid and cystic mass that expands, erodes, deepens the sella turcica.

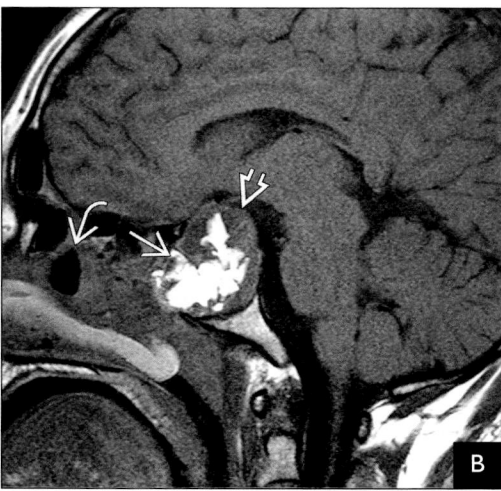

25-77B. Postoperative T1 C+ scan after tumor debulking shows fat packing ➡, residual tumor ➡, and sphenoid air-fluid level ➡.

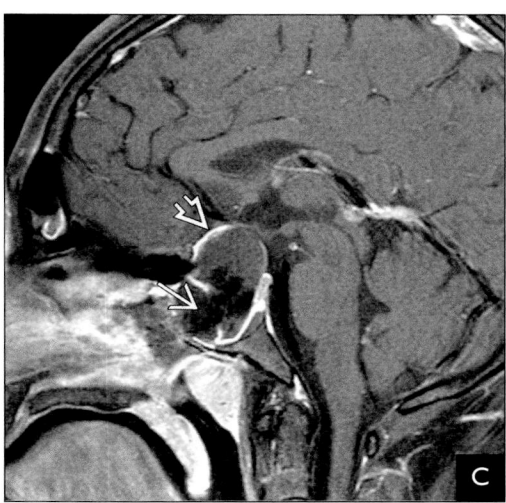

25-77C. T1 C+ FS scan shows suppressed fat ➡ and a thin rim of enhancing tumor ➡.

WHEN THE MASS *CANNOT* BE SEPARATED FROM THE PITUITARY GLAND

Common
- Pituitary hyperplasia
- Pituitary macroadenoma

Less Common
- Neurosarcoid
- Langerhans cell histiocytosis
- Hypophysitis

Rare but Important
- Metastasis
- Lymphoma
- Germinoma

INTRASELLAR LESION

Common
- Pituitary hyperplasia (physiologic, nonphysiologic)
- Pituitary microadenoma
- Empty sella

Less Common
- Pituitary macroadenoma
- Rathke cleft (or other) cyst
- Craniopharyngioma
- Neurosarcoid

Rare but Important
- Lymphocytic hypophysitis
- Intracranial hypotension (venous congestion)
- Vascular ("kissing" carotids, aneurysm)
- Meningioma
- Metastasis
- Lymphoma

Intrasellar Lesions

Intrasellar lesions can be mass-like or non-mass-like. Keep two concepts in mind: (1) Not all "enlarged pituitary glands" are abnormal. Pituitary size and height vary with gender and age. A "fat" pituitary can also occur with intracranial hypotension. (2) Pituitary "incidentalomas" are common (identified in 15-20% of normal MR scans).

Common Suprasellar Masses

The five most common overall suprasellar masses, i.e., the "Big Five," are pituitary macroadenoma, meningioma, aneurysm, craniopharyngioma, and astrocytoma. Together they account for 75-80% of all sel-

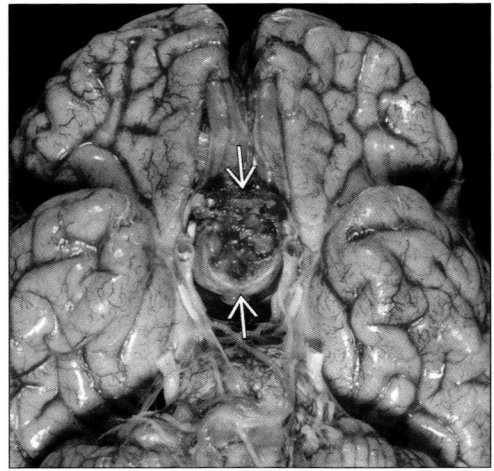

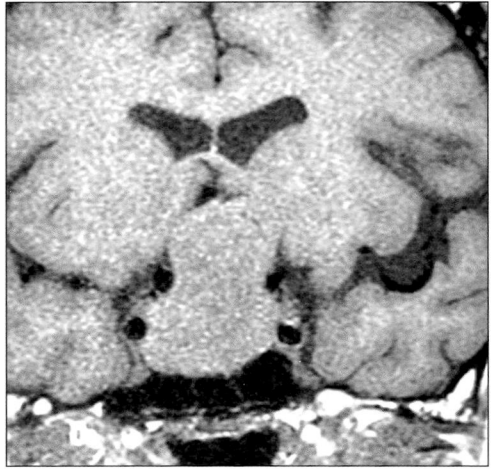

25-78. Submentovertex view of autopsied brain with large intra- and suprasellar mass ➡. The pituitary gland cannot be separated from the mass and indeed is the mass. (Courtesy R. Hewlett, MD.) 25-79. Coronal T1WI shows the classic "snowman" shape of macroadenoma. The mass and gland are indistinguishable from each other.

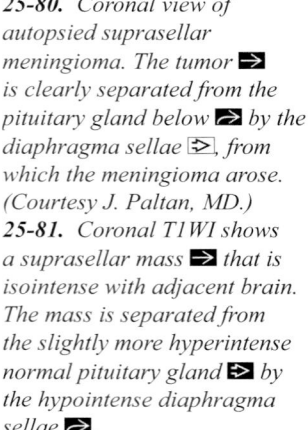

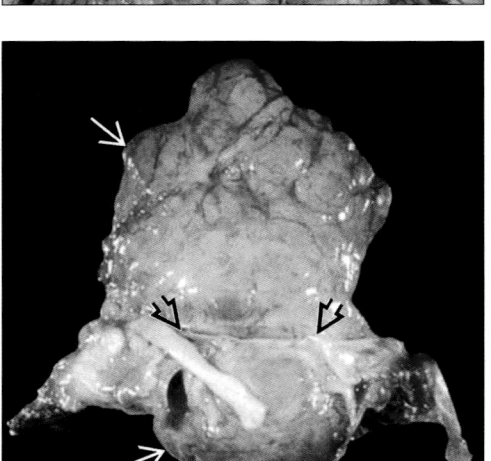

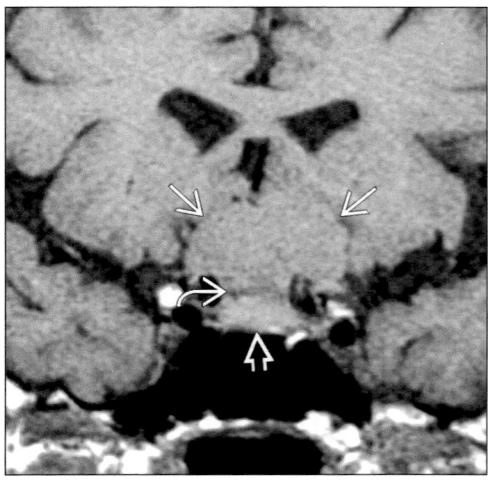

25-80. Coronal view of autopsied suprasellar meningioma. The tumor ➡ is clearly separated from the pituitary gland below ➡ by the diaphragma sellae ➡, from which the meningioma arose. (Courtesy J. Paltan, MD.) 25-81. Coronal T1WI shows a suprasellar mass ➡ that is isointense with adjacent brain. The mass is separated from the slightly more hyperintense normal pituitary gland ➡ by the hypointense diaphragma sellae ➡.

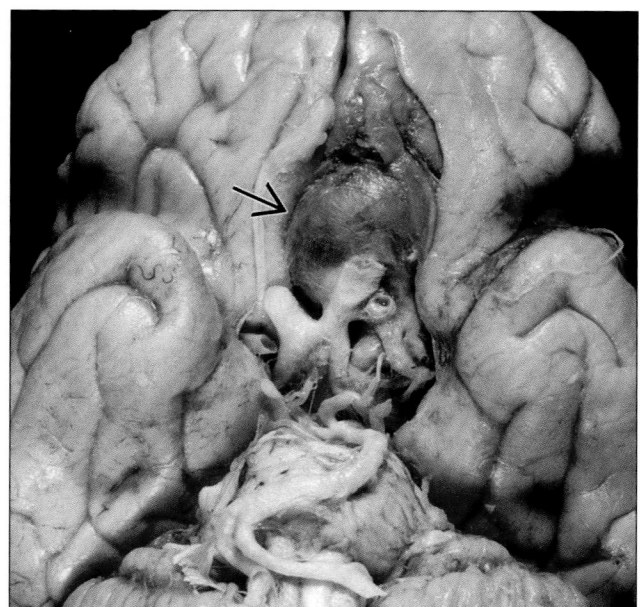

25-82. Autopsy specimen demonstrates an unruptured suprasellar aneurysm ⇨.

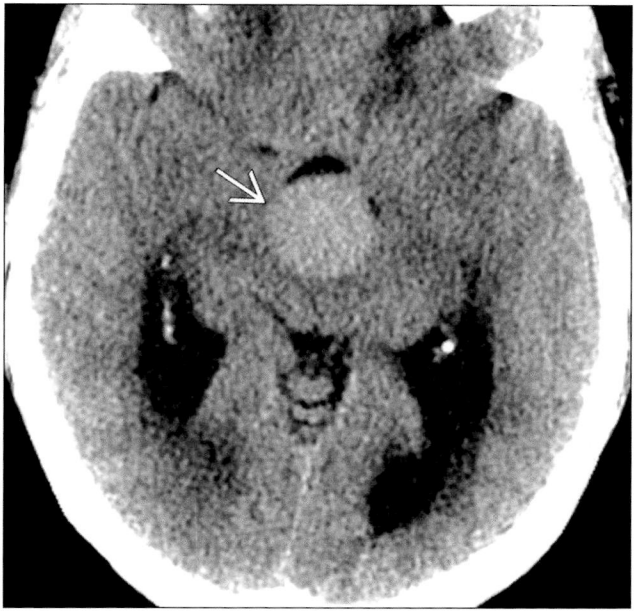

25-83. NECT in 55-year-old man with headaches shows hyperdense noncalcified mass ⇨ in the suprasellar cistern. Considerations in an adult include macroadenoma, meningioma, aneurysm. Large basilar tip aneurysm.

lar region masses. Three of the "Big Five" (the "Big Three")—adenoma, meningioma, aneurysm—are common in adults but rare in children **(25-82)**, **(25-83)**. Craniopharyngioma and hypothalamic/optic chiasm pilocytic astrocytoma are the "Big Two" in children.

COMMON SUPRASELLAR MASSES

Adults
- Pituitary adenoma (mass = gland)
- Meningioma (mass separate from gland)
- Aneurysm ("flow void," pulsation artifact)

Children
- Craniopharyngioma (90% cystic, 90% calcify, 90% enhance)
- Hypothalamic/optic chiasm pilocytic astrocytoma (solid, no calcification)

---

ess Common Suprasellar Masses

The presence of some less common lesions can often be inferred from imaging studies.

LESS COMMON SUPRASELLAR MASSES

Rathke cleft cyst (well-delineated, separate from pituitary)

Arachnoid cyst (behaves just like CSF)

Dermoid cyst (looks like fat)

Neurocysticercosis (usually multiple)

Rare but Important Suprasellar Masses

Keep these lesions in mind—they can mimic more common lesions or the appropriate treatment differs sharply.

RARE BUT IMPORTANT SUPRASELLAR MASSES

Hypophysitis (may look like adenoma)

Hypothalamic hamartoma ("collar button" between stalk, mammillary bodies)

Metastasis (systemic cancer; look for other lesions)

Lymphoma (often infiltrates adjacent structures)

Infundibular Stalk Masses

These include entities whose primary manifestation is infundibular stalk thickening. Age is again pertinent.

INFUNDIBULAR STALK MASSES

Adults
- Neurosarcoid (isolated stalk lesion rare)
- Hypophysitis ("stalkitis")
- Metastasis
- Lymphoma
- Pituicytoma
- Stalk transection (can make stalk look "stubby")

Children
- Germinoma (diabetes insipidus may occur before lesion is visible on MR!)
- Histiocytosis (look for other lesions)
- Ectopic neurohypophysis (displaced PPBS)
- Leukemia

Cystic Intra-/Suprasellar Mass

If an intra- or suprasellar mass is primarily or exclusively cystic, the differential diagnosis considerations change. The key issue is to distinguish a cystic mass that originates *within* the sella versus intrasellar extension *from* a suprasellar lesion. Other than Rathke cleft cyst, completely intrasellar nonneoplastic cysts are rare, as is a totally intrasellar craniopharyngioma without suprasellar extension.

CYSTIC *INTRASELLAR* MASS

Common
- Empty sella
- Idiopathic intracranial hypertension

Less Common
- Rathke cleft cyst
- Neurocysticercosis cyst

Rare but Important
- Craniopharyngioma
- Epidermoid cyst
- Arachnoid cyst
- Pituitary apoplexy
- Thrombosed aneurysm

CYSTIC *SUPRASELLAR* MASS

Common
- Enlarged third ventricle
  - Obstructive hydrocephalus (generic)
  - Aqueductal stenosis
- Arachnoid cyst
- Craniopharyngioma
- Neurocysticercosis cyst

Less Common
- Rathke cleft cyst
- Dermoid cyst
- Epidermoid cyst
- Enlarged perivascular spaces (basal ganglia)

Rare but Important
- Pituitary macroadenoma
- Pituitary apoplexy
- Astrocytoma (usually solid)
- Ependymal cyst
- Thrombosed saccular aneurysm

---

elected References

ellar Region Anatomy

Gross Anatomy

- Buchfelder M et al: Modern imaging of pituitary adenomas. Front Horm Res. 38:109-20, 2010
- Song-tao Q et al: The arachnoid sleeve enveloping the pituitary stalk: anatomical and histologic study. Neurosurgery. 66(3):585-9, 2010

Imaging Technique and Anatomy

- Orija IB et al: Pituitary incidentaloma. Best Pract Res Clin Endocrinol Metab. 26(1):47-68, 2012
- Freda PU et al: Pituitary incidentaloma: an endocrine society clinical practice guideline. J Clin Endocrinol Metab. 96(4):894-904, 2011
- Seidenwurm DJ: Expert Panel on Neurologic Imaging: neuroendocrine imaging. AJNR Am J Neuroradiol. 29(3):613-5, 2008

ormal Imaging Variants

Pituitary Hyperplasia

- Han L et al: Pituitary tumorous hyperplasia due to primary hypothyroidism. Acta Neurochir (Wien). 154(8):1489-92, 2012
- Aquilina K et al: Nonneoplastic enlargement of the pituitary gland in children. J Neurosurg Pediatr. 7(5):510-5, 2011
- Karaca Z et al: Pregnancy and pituitary disorders. Eur J Endocrinol. 162(3):453-75, 2010

Empty Sella

- Goddard JC et al: New considerations in the cause of spontaneous cerebrospinal fluid otorrhea. Otol Neurotol. 31(6):940-5, 2010
- De Marinis L et al: Primary empty sella. J Clin Endocrinol Metab. 90(9):5471-7, 2005

ongenital Lesions

Pituitary Anomalies

- Dutta P et al: Clinico-radiological correlation in childhood hypopituitarism. Indian Pediatr. 47(7):615-8, 2010

Hypothalamic Hamartoma

- Oehl B et al: Semiologic aspects of epileptic seizures in 31 patients with hypothalamic hamartoma. Epilepsia. 51(10):2116-23, 2010
- Amstutz DR et al: Hypothalamic hamartomas: correlation of MR imaging and spectroscopic findings with tumor glial content. AJNR Am J Neuroradiol. 27(4):794-8, 2006

Rathke Cleft Cyst

- Trifanescu R et al: Rathke's cleft cysts. Clin Endocrinol (Oxf). 76(2):151-60, 2012

Neoplasms

Pituitary Adenomas

- Cazabat L et al: Germline AIP mutations in apparently sporadic pituitary adenomas: prevalence in a prospective single-center cohort of 443 patients. J Clin Endocrinol Metab. 97(4):E663-70, 2012
- Mete O et al: Clinicopathological correlations in pituitary adenomas. Brain Pathol. 22(4):443-53, 2012
- Rostad S: Pituitary adenoma pathogenesis: an update. Curr Opin Endocrinol Diabetes Obes. 19(4):322-7, 2012
- Scheithauer BW: Pituitary adenomas. In Burger P: Diagnostic Pathology: Neuropathology. Salt Lake City: Amirsys Publishing. I.2.2-11, 2012
- Thompson LD et al: Ectopic sphenoid sinus pituitary adenoma (ESSPA) with normal anterior pituitary gland: a clinicopathologic and immunophenotypic study of 32 cases with a comprehensive review of the english literature. Head Neck Pathol. 6(1):75-100, 2012
- Vasilev V et al: Familial pituitary tumor syndromes. Endocr Pract. 17 Suppl 3:41-6, 2011
- de Almeida JP et al: Pituitary stem cells: review of the literature and current understanding. Neurosurgery. 67(3):770-80, 2010
- Xekouki P et al: Anterior pituitary adenomas: inherited syndromes, novel genes and molecular pathways. Expert Rev Endocrinol Metab. 5(5):697-709, 2010

Pituitary Carcinoma

- Ersen A et al: Pituitary carcinoma. In Burger P: Diagnostic Pathology: Neuropathology. Salt Lake City: Amirsys Publishing. I.2.46-9, 2012
- van der Zwan JM et al: Carcinoma of endocrine organs: Results of the RARECARE project. Eur J Cancer. 48(13):1923-1931, 2012
- Dudziak K et al: Pituitary carcinoma with malignant growth from first presentation and fulminant clinical course: case report and review of the literature. J Clin Endocrinol Metab. 96(9):2665-9, 2011

Pituitary Blastoma

- Scheithauer BW et al: Pituitary blastoma: a unique embryonal tumor. Pituitary. 15(3):365-73, 2012

Craniopharyngioma

- Müller HL: Childhood craniopharyngioma. Pituitary. Epub ahead of print, 2012
- Zacharia BE et al: Incidence, treatment and survival of patients with craniopharyngioma in the surveillance,

epidemiology and end results program. Neuro Oncol. 14(8):1070-8, 2012

- Elliott RE et al: Efficacy and safety of radical resection of primary and recurrent craniopharyngiomas in 86 children. J Neurosurg Pediatr. 5(1):30-48, 2010

Nonadenomatous Pituitary Tumors

- Secci F et al: Pituicytomas: radiological findings, clinical behavior and surgical management. Acta Neurochir (Wien). 154(4):649-57; discussion 657, 2012
- Covington MF et al: Pituicytoma, spindle cell oncocytoma, and granular cell tumor: clarification and meta-analysis of the world literature since 1893. AJNR Am J Neuroradiol. 32(11):2067-72, 2011

Miscellaneous Lesions

Hypophysitis

- Juszczak A et al: Mechanisms in endocrinology: Ipilimumab: a novel immunomodulating therapy causing autoimmune hypophysitis: a case report and review. Eur J Endocrinol. 167(1):1-5, 2012
- Leporati P et al: IgG4-related hypophysitis: a new addition to the hypophysitis spectrum. J Clin Endocrinol Metab. 96(7):1971-80, 2011
- Su SB et al: Primary granulomatous hypophysitis: a case report and literature review. Endocr J. 58(6):467-73, 2011
- Gutenberg A et al: A radiologic score to distinguish autoimmune hypophysitis from nonsecreting pituitary adenoma preoperatively. AJNR Am J Neuroradiol. 30(9):1766-72, 2009

Pituitary Apoplexy

- Kerr JM et al: Pituitary apoplexy. BMJ. 342:d1270, 2011

Pre- and Postoperative Sella

- Hamid O et al: Anatomic variations of the sphenoid sinus and their impact on trans-sphenoid pituitary surgery. Skull Base. 18(1):9-15, 2008
- Har-El G: Endoscopic transnasal trans-sphenoidal pituitary surgery: comparison with the traditional sublabial trans-septal approach. Otolaryngol Clin North Am. 38(4):723-35, 2005

26

Miscellaneous Tumors and Tumor-like Conditions

Some important neoplasms that affect the calvaria, skull base, and cranial meninges are not included in the most recent standardized WHO classification of CNS tumors. This chapter covers several of these intriguing tumors as well as tumor-like lesions that do not easily fit into other sections of this text. Although infections, granulomatous disease, demyelinating disorders, and vascular diseases (among others) may sometimes mimic CNS neoplasms, they are treated separately in their own respective chapters.

We begin with *extra*cranial tumors and tumor-like conditions. These lesions mostly arise within the calvaria or skull base. We then turn our attention to an interesting group of *intra*cranial lesions that all mimic neoplasms, i.e., they are pseudotumors. These tumor-like lesions may arise within the meninges, CSF cisterns, or brain parenchyma. Some lesions—especially idiopathic inflammatory pseudotumor—may involve multiple compartments and can be intracranial, extracranial, or a combination of both.

Extracranial Tumors and Tumor-like Conditions

Fibrous Dysplasia

Benign fibroosseous lesions of the craniofacial complex are represented by a variety of intraosseous disease processes. These include bone dysplasias, the most common of which is fibrous dysplasia.

Terminology

Fibrous dysplasia (FD) is a benign dysplastic fibroosseous lesion that is also known as fibrocartilaginous dysplasia, osteitis fibrosa, and generalized fibrocystic disease of bone.

Etiology

GENERAL CONCEPTS. FD is a developmental dysplasia with local arrest of normal structural/architectural development. Abnormal differentiation of osteoblasts results in replacement of normal marrow and cancellous bone by immature "woven" bone and fibrous stroma.

GENETICS. FD results from somatic mutations of the *GNAS1* gene, which is involved in skeleton-forming mesenchymal tissue.

Pathology

LOCATION. Virtually any bone in the head and neck can be affected by FD. The skull and facial bones are the location of 10-25% of all monostotic FD lesions. The frontal bone is the most common calvarial site, followed by the temporal bone, sphenoid, and parietal bones. Involvement of the clivus is rare. The orbit, zygoma, maxilla, and mandible are the most frequent sites in the face **(26-1)**.

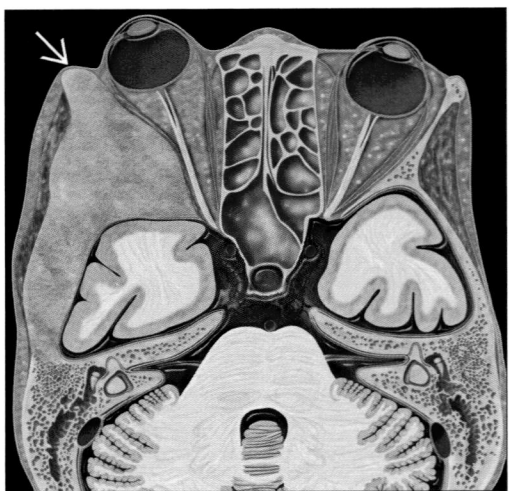

26-1. *FD with expansion of the lateral orbital rim* ➡, *sphenoid wing, and temporal squamosa. Note exophthalmos, stretching of the optic nerve.*

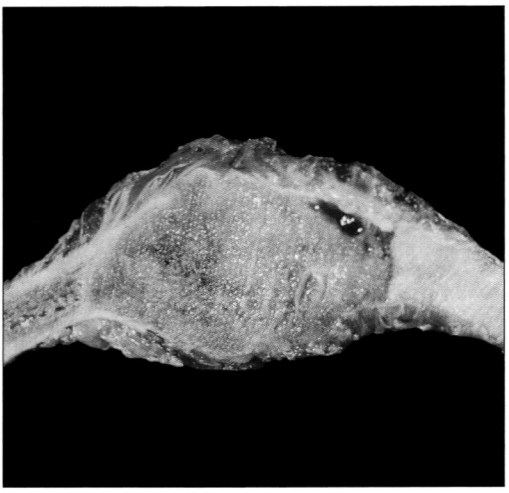

26-2. *FD in a rib is a solid tan tumor that expands bone, has "ground-glass" appearance. (Courtesy A. Rosenberg, MD, G. P. Nielsen, MD.)*

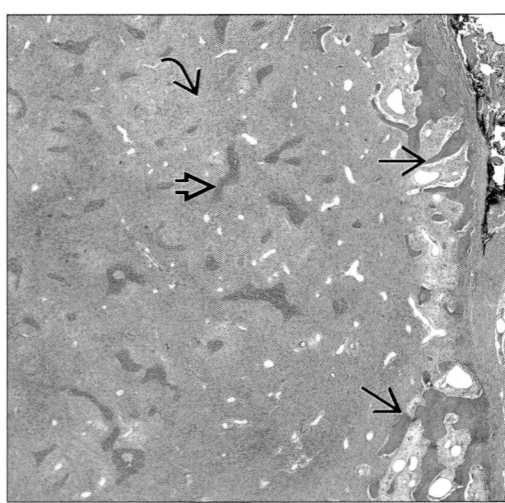

26-3. *FD shows "woven" bony trabeculae* ➤, *fibrous stroma* ➘, *reactive subperiosteal new bone* ➘. *(A. Rosenberg, MD, G. P. Nielsen, MD.)*

SIZE AND NUMBER. FD lesions range in size from relatively small—less than one centimeter—to massive lesions that involve virtually an entire bone. Altered osteogenesis may occur within a single bone ("monostotic FD") or multiple bones ("polyostotic FD"). Solitary FD accounts for 80-85% of all lesions; polyostotic FD occurs in 15-20% of cases.

Polyostotic FD with endocrinopathy is known as **McCune-Albright syndrome** (MAS) and occurs in 3-5% of cases. The classic MAS triad consists of multiple FD lesions, endocrine dysfunction (typically precocious puberty), and cutaneous hyperpigmentation ("café au lait spots").

GROSS PATHOLOGY. FD is tan to whitish gray **(26-2)**. Depending on the relative amount of fibrous versus osseous content, texture varies from firm and rubbery to "gritty."

MICROSCOPIC FEATURES. Fibrous and osseous tissues are admixed in varying proportions **(26-3)**. In the early stages, pronounced osteogenesis with thin osteoid anastomosing trabeculae rimmed with osteoblasts is seen. A stromal fibroblastic element with variable vascularity is interspersed between trabeculae of immature "woven" bone that resembles "Chinese letters."

Almost 60% of cases demonstrate different stromal patterns admixed with the usual fibroblastic elements. These include focal fatty metamorphosis (20-25%), myxoid stroma (15%), and calcifications (12%). Cystic degeneration occurs but is uncommon.

Clinical Issues

EPIDEMIOLOGY. FD is rare, representing approximately 1% of all biopsied primary bone tumors. It is the second most common pediatric primary skull lesion (after dermoid cysts).

DEMOGRAPHICS. Although FD can present at virtually any age, most patients are younger than 30 years at the time of initial diagnosis. Polyostotic FD presents earlier; the mean age is eight years. With the exception of FD as part of MAS, which affects females more than males, there is no gender predilection.

PRESENTATION. Symptoms of craniofacial FD depend on lesion location. Painless osseous expansion with calvarial or facial asymmetry is common. Proptosis and optic neuropathy are common in patients with orbital disease. Conductive hearing loss and facial weakness are typical in patients with temporal bone FD. Mandibular FD typically presents with "cherubism."

Polyostotic FD may cause "leontiasis ossea" (lion-like physiognomy) or complex cranial neuropathies (secondary to severe narrowing of the neural foramina).

NATURAL HISTORY. Disease course varies. Monostotic lesions do not regress or disappear, but they usually stabilize at puberty. In contrast, polyostotic FD generally becomes less active after puberty, although long bone deformities may progress and microfractures may develop. Whether monostotic or polyostotic, FD rarely undergoes malignant transformation.

TREATMENT OPTIONS. Treatment options for FD are limited. Recurrence is very high following curettage and bone grafting. Radiation therapy is generally avoided as it may induce malignant transformation. Intravenous bisphosphonate therapy has been used to ameliorate the disease course with some reported success.

FIBROUS DYSPLASIA: PATHOLOGY AND CLINICAL ISSUES

Pathology
- Location, number
  - Any bone
  - Craniofacial (10-25%)
  - Solitary (80-85%) or polyostotic
- Gross pathology: "Woven" bone
- Microscopic pathology
  - Variable admixture of fibrous, osseous components
  - Less common: Fat, myxoid tissue, Ca++, cysts

Clinical Issues
- Rare (< 1% of biopsied bone tumors)
  - One of most common fibroosseous lesions
- Monostotic patients < 30 years
- Polyostotic FD
  - Younger (mean age = 8 years)
  - McCune-Albright (3-5%)
  - Craniofacial involvement common

Imaging

GENERAL FEATURES. Most craniofacial lesions are monostotic. However, skeletal survey or whole-body MR is recommended to detect asymptomatic lesions in other bones that would indicate polyostotic disease or McCune-Albright syndrome.

Imaging findings depend on disease stage. In general, very early lesions are radiolucent and then undergo progressive calcification, resulting in a "ground-glass" appearance. Mixed patterns are common.

CT FINDINGS. Nonaggressive osseous remodeling and thickening of the affected bone are typical. NECT shows a geographic expansile lesion centered in the medullary cavity. Abrupt transition between the lesion and adjacent normal bone is typical.

Bone CT appearance varies with the relative content of fibrous versus osseous tissue. FD can be sclerotic, cystic,

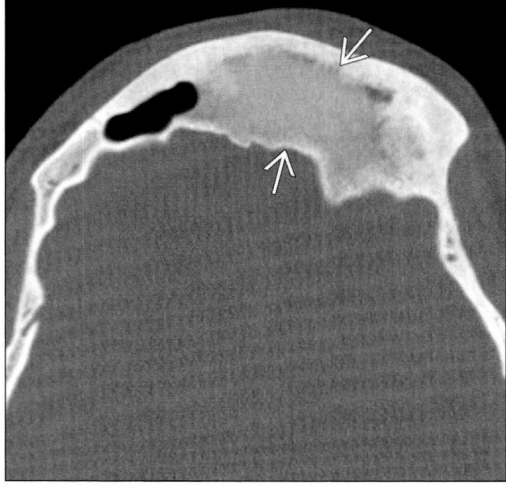

26-4. Bone CT shows FD as expansile lesion with "ground-glass" appearance ➡. *The frontal bone is the most common site of FD in the calvaria.*

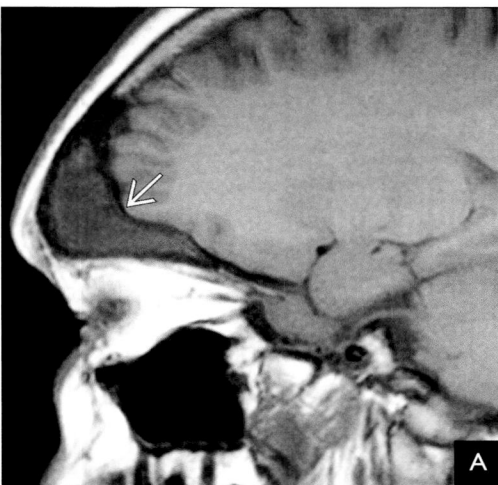

26-5A. Sagittal T1WI in the same patient shows that the expanded frontal bone is filled with homogeneously hypointense tissue ➡.

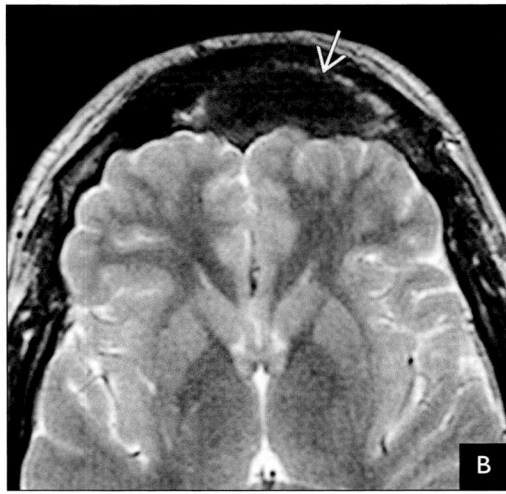

26-5B. Moderate hypointensity on T2WI ➡ *is characteristic of FD with extensive ossified/fibrous portions.*

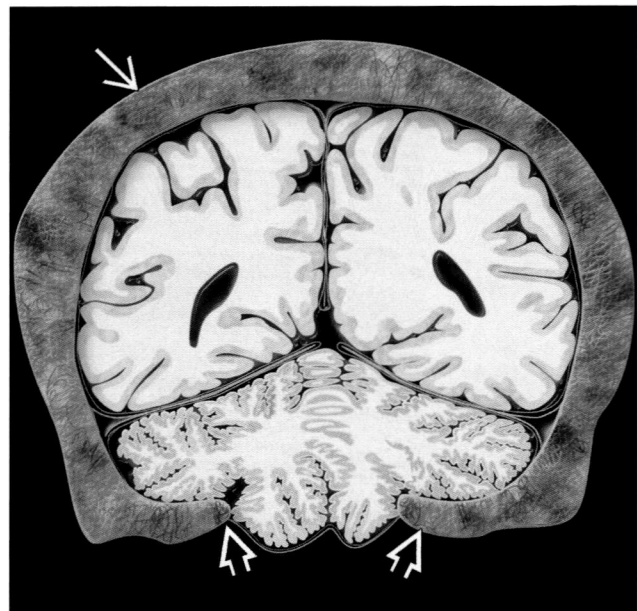

26-6. Coronal graphic illustrates diffuse Paget disease of the skull with severe diploic widening ⟶, basilar invagination ⟹ crowding the contents of the posterior fossa.

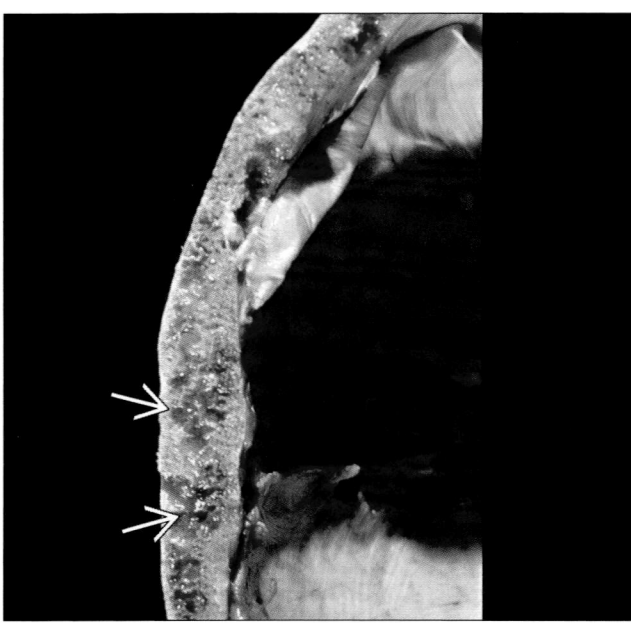

26-7. Autopsy specimen shows pagetoid changes in the calvaria with diffuse thickening, replacement of fatty marrow with fibrovascular tissue ⟶. (Courtesy E. T. Hedley-Whyte, MD.)

or mixed (sometimes called "pagetoid"). A pattern with mixed areas of radiopacity and radiolucency is found in almost half of all cases. The classic relatively homogeneous "ground-glass" appearance occurs in 25% **(26-4)**. Densely sclerotic lesions are common in the skull base. Almost one-quarter of all FD cases have some cystic changes, seen as central lucent areas with thinned but sclerotic borders.

MR FINDINGS. FD is usually homogeneously hypointense on T1WI **(26-5A)**. Signal intensity on T2WI is variable. Moderate hypointensity is characteristic of ossified and/or fibrous portions of the lesion **(26-5B)**. Active lesions may be heterogeneous and may have hyperintense areas on FLAIR. Cysts appear as rounded high signal foci.

Signal intensity following contrast administration varies depending on the lesion stage and ranges from no enhancement to diffuse, avid enhancement in active lesions.

NUCLEAR MEDICINE. FDG PET shows increased metabolic activity in one or more sites.

Differential Diagnosis

The major differential diagnoses for craniofacial FD are Paget disease and ossifying fibroma.

Paget disease typically occurs in elderly patients and usually involves the calvaria and temporal bone. A "cotton wool" appearance is typical on digital skull radiographs and bone CT.

Ossifying fibroma (OF) may mimic the cystic monostotic form of FD. OF has a thick, bony rim with a lower density center on bone CT and generally appears more mass-like and localized. Diffuse **sclerosing osteomyelitis** of the mandible may also resemble FD.

Intraosseous meningioma is another differential consideration. Intraosseous meningiomas are more common in the calvaria than in the skull base and facial bones. A strongly enhancing "en plaque" soft tissue mass is often associated with the bony lesion. A mixed sclerotic-destructive skull base **metastasis** may mimic FD. In most cases, an extracranial primary site is known.

The differential diagnosis of FD includes rare fibroosseous disorders that can affect the craniofacial bones. These include **osteitis deformans**, **florid osseous dysplasia**, **focal cementoosseous dysplasia**, and **periapical cemental dysplasia**.

Facial bone changes associated with hyperparathyroidism and **renal osteodystrophy** may present with a classic "ground-glass" appearance on both conventional radiography and CT. However, in contrast to FD, these changes are generalized and diffuse.

<table>
<tr><td colspan="1">

FIBROUS DYSPLASIA: IMAGING

Imaging
- CT
  - Bone remodeled, expanded
  - "Ground-glass" appearance classic
  - Sclerotic, cystic, mixed ("pagetoid") changes
- MR
  - T1 hypointense, T2 variable (usually hypointense)
  - Enhancement varies from none to intense

Differential Diagnosis
- Paget disease (older patients)
- Ossifying fibroma, other benign fibroosseous lesions
- Intraosseous meningioma
- Renal osteodystrophy

</td></tr>
</table>

Paget Disease

Terminology

Paget disease (PaD) of bone, also called osteitis deformans, is the most exaggerated example of abnormal osseous remodeling. PaD is characterized by rapid bone turnover within one or more discrete skeletal lesions.

Etiology

Genetic alterations occur in both classic Paget disease of the elderly and the uncommon familial Paget-like bone dysplasias that arise during childhood. All involve defective function of the molecular pathway that regulates osteoclastogenesis (the osteoprotegerin/TNFRSF11A or B/RANKL/RANK pathway).

Mutations in the gene encoding sequestosome 1 (*SQSTM1*) have been identified in one-third of patients with the familial form of FD and in a smaller proportion of patients with sporadic PaD. *SQSTM1* mutations affect functioning of the p62 phenotype, which increases the sensitivity of osteoclast precursors to osteoclastogenic cytokines, thus causing a predisposition to PaD. *SQSTM1* mutations are also strongly associated with PaD disease severity and complications.

Mutations in the valosin-containing protein gene (*VCP*) cause a unique disorder characterized by classic PaD, inclusion body myopathy, and frontotemporal dementia.

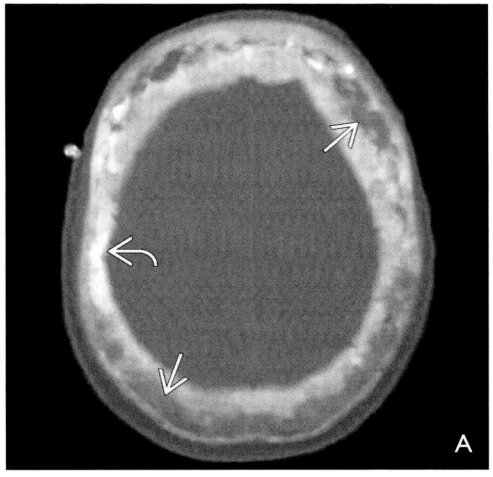
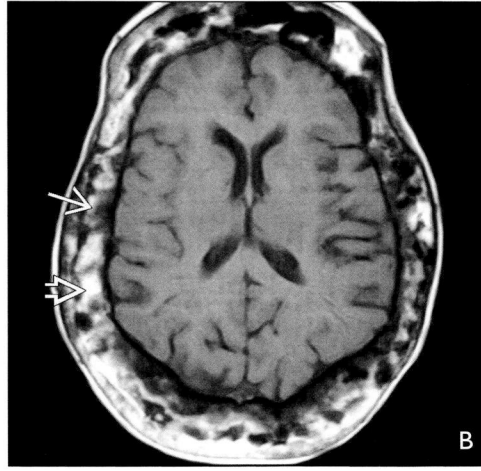

26-8A. *Bone CT shows a thick calvaria with mixed lytic ➡, sclerotic ➡ components ("cotton wool" appearance) characteristic of the mixed active, sclerotic stage of Paget disease.* **26-8B.** *T1WI shows mixed hyper- ➡, hypointense ➡ diploic lesions in a massively expanded calvaria in this elderly patient with Paget disease.*

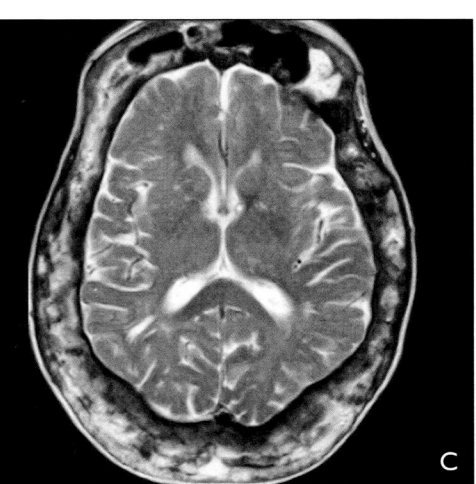
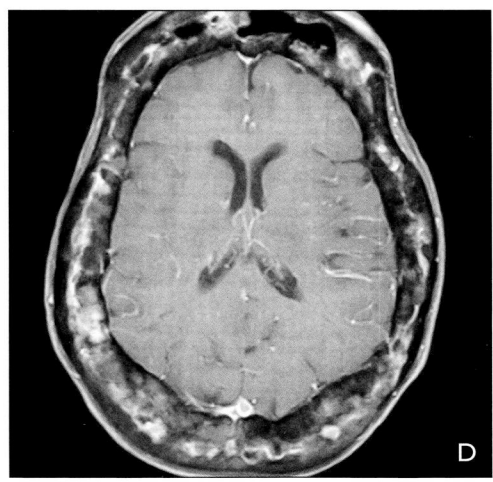

26-8C. *T2WI shows the extremely "mottled" heterogeneous appearance of calvarial Paget disease.* **26-8D.** *Patchy enhancement is seen on T1 C+ FS, indicating that some active disease is present in this longstanding case.*

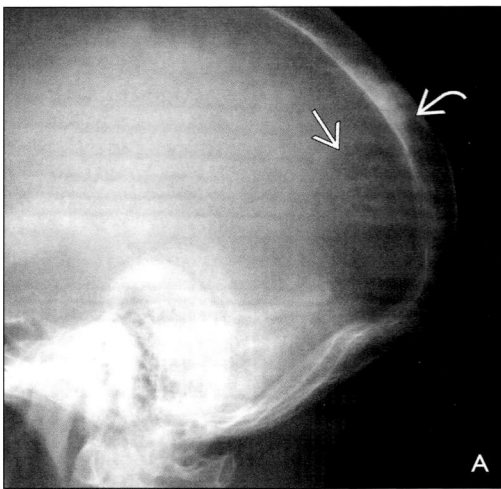

26-9A. Lateral skull film shows the lytic phase of PaD ➔, "osteoporosis circumscripta," together with an area of skull thickening ➔.

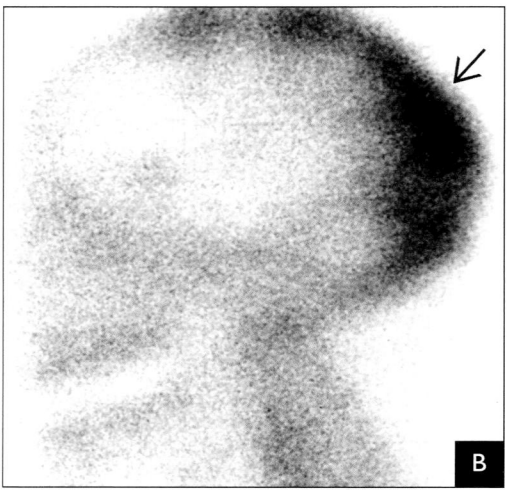

26-9B. Bone scan in the same patient shows an area of abnormal uptake in the occiput ➔, a typical PaD location in the calvaria.

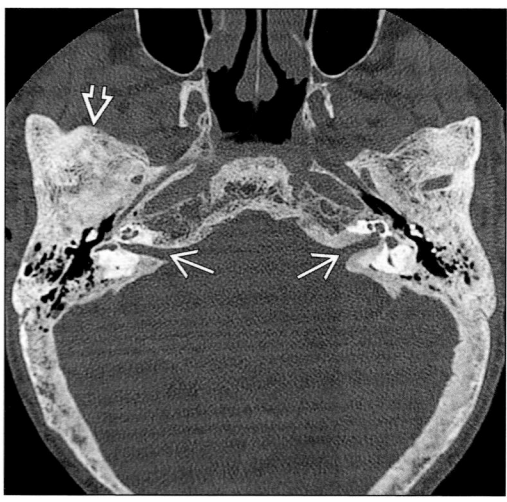

26-10. Temporal bone CT shows quiescent skull base sclerosis ➔ with bony expansion, cortical thickening, narrowing of both IACs ➔.

Pathology

LOCATION, SIZE, AND NUMBER. The skull (both calvaria and skull base) is affected in 25-65% of patients (26-6). In contrast to FD, PaD is more commonly polyostotic (65-90% of cases).

GROSS PATHOLOGY. The pagetoid skull shows diffuse thickening. Patches of fibrovascular tissue initially replace fatty marrow (26-7).

MICROSCOPIC FEATURES. In the early lytic stage, active PaD is characterized by cellular fibroosseous lesions with minimally calcified osteoid trabeculae. Increased vascularity is common. Osteoblastic rimming is present together with osteoclastic resorptive lacunae. Osteoclasts are numerous and larger than normal; they also have increased numbers of nuclei.

In the inactive stage, bone turnover and excessive vascularity decrease and the trabeculae coarsen.

Clinical Issues

EPIDEMIOLOGY. PaD is common, affecting up to 10% of individuals over the age of 80. It is especially prevalent in the United States and the British Isles, Canada, Australia, and some parts of Western Europe. PaD is rare in Asia and Africa.

DEMOGRAPHICS. Classic PaD is a disease of the elderly. Most patients are 55-85 years of age with less than 5% of cases occurring in patients under the age of 40. There is a moderate male predominance.

Juvenile Paget disease, also known as idiopathic hyperphosphatasia, is an autosomal recessive bone dysplasia. It begins in infancy or early childhood and is characterized by long bone widening, acetabular protrusion, pathologic fractures, and skull thickening.

PRESENTATION. Presentation varies with location, and all bones of the craniofacial complex can be affected. Patients with calvarial PaD may experience increasing hat size. Cranial neuropathy is common with skull base lesions, most commonly affecting CN VIII. Patients may present with either conductive (ossicular involvement) or sensorineural hearing loss (cochlear involvement or bony compression).

Markedly elevated serum alkaline phosphatase is a constant feature, while calcium and phosphate levels remain within normal range.

NATURAL HISTORY. In the extracranial skeleton, osseous expansion with progressive skeletal deformity is typical. Osseous weakening leads to long bone deformities and fractures. In comparison, craniofacial PaD generally has a more benign course and may remain asymptomatic for many years.

Two neoplastic processes are associated with PaD: Giant cell tumor (benign) and sarcoma (malignant). **Giant cell tumor** is an expansile intraosseous mass that usually occurs in the epiphyses and metaphyses of long bones in patients with longstanding polyostotic PaD. Giant cell tumors that arise secondarily in pagetoid bone are rare. Just 2% occur in the skull, where the most common site is the sphenoid bone. Involvement of the calvarial vault is rare.

Malignant transformation to **osteosarcoma** occurs in 0.5-1% of cases and is generally seen in patients with widespread disease. Most osteosarcomas are high grade and have already metastasized at the time of diagnosis. Only 15% of patients survive beyond two or three years.

TREATMENT OPTIONS. Bisphosphonates reduce bone turnover and have been effective in many cases of PaD.

maging

GENERAL FEATURES. Imaging findings in PaD vary with disease stage. In the early active stage, radiolucent lesions develop in the calvaria, a condition termed **"osteoporosis circumscripta"** (26-9A). Enlarged bone with mixed lytic and sclerotic foci and confluent nodular calcifications follows (the **"cotton wool"** appearance) in the mixed active stage (26-11). The final inactive or quiescent stage is seen as **dense bony sclerosis (26-10)**.

CT FINDINGS. In early PaD, bone CT shows well-defined lytic foci (osteoporosis circumscripta). Mixed areas of bony lysis and sclerosis then develop, producing the "cotton wool" appearance (26-8A), (26-12). Varying degrees of dense bony sclerosis can develop.

In severe cases, the softened expanded skull base can produce basilar invagination.

MR FINDINGS. Multifocal T1 hypointense lesions replace fatty marrow (26-8B). Signal intensity on T2WI is often heterogeneous (26-8C). Patchy enhancement on T1 C+ can occur in the advancing hypervascular zone of active PaD (26-8D).

NUCLEAR MEDICINE. The active stage of PaD shows markedly increased uptake on Tc-99m bone scan (26-9B), (26-13).

ifferential Diagnosis

Fibrous dysplasia may appear very similar to craniofacial PaD. However, PaD occurs mostly in the elderly and does not have the typical "ground-glass" appearance that often characterizes FD.

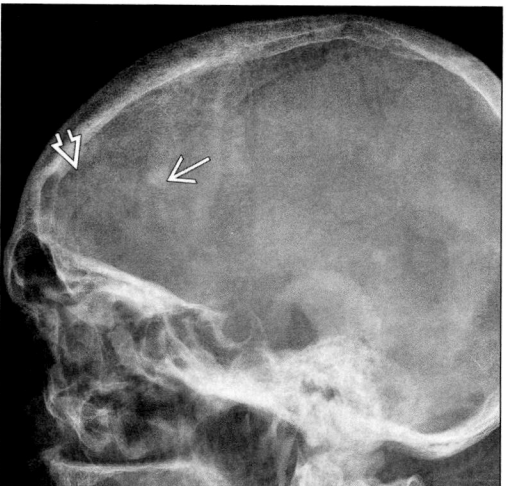

26-11. *Lateral skull radiograph shows mixed lytic ➡, sclerotic ➡ bone, the "cotton wool" appearance of PaD in the mixed active phase.*

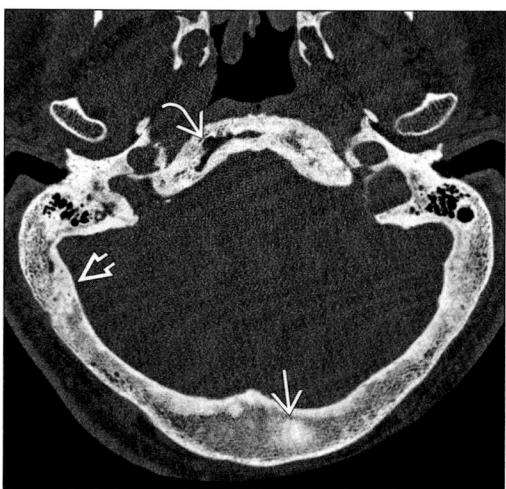

26-12. *Bone CT shows lytic foci ➡ mixed with bone thickening ➡, ill-defined sclerosis ➡ ("cotton wool" stage of PaD).*

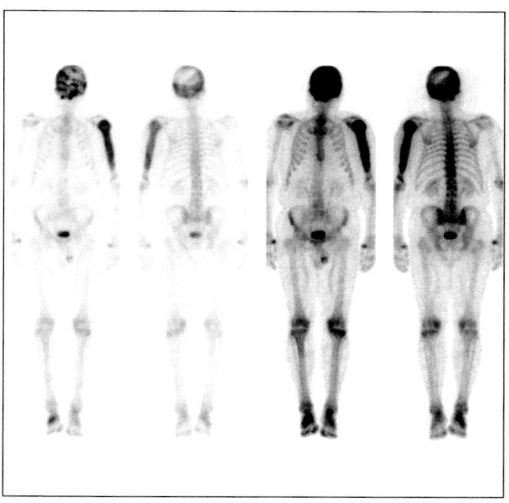

26-13. *Bone scan shows multiple areas of increased uptake in a patient with polyostotic PaD.*

Sclerotic metastases may resemble PaD, but no trabecular coarsening or bony enlargement is present. The early lytic phase of PaD may resemble lytic metastases or multiple myeloma; neither enlarges the affected bone.

PAGET DISEASE

Pathology
- Monostotic (65-90%)
- Calvaria, skull base affected (25-60%)
- Fibroosseous tissue replaces fatty marrow

Clinical Issues
- Affects up to 10% of patients > 80 years
- Enlarging skull, CN VIII neuropathy common
- Malignant transformation (0.5-1%)
  - Sarcoma > giant cell tumor

Imaging
- Early: Lytic ("osteoporosis circumscripta")
- Mid: Mixed lytic, sclerotic ("cotton wool")
- Late: Dense bony sclerosis

Differential Diagnosis
- Fibrous dysplasia (younger patients)
- Metastases, myeloma

Aneurysmal Bone Cyst

Terminology

Aneurysmal bone cysts (ABCs) are benign expansile multicystic lesions that typically develop in childhood or early adulthood. At least 70% of ABCs are primary lesions; the rest arise secondarily within a preexisting benign tumor such as giant cell tumor or osteoblastoma.

Pathology

The most common overall ABC location is the metaphysis of long bones (70-80% of cases) with the vertebrae (generally the posterior elements) the site of 15% of lesions.

The craniofacial bones are a relatively uncommon location. Lesions can occur in the jaws (maxilla, mandible), petrous temporal bone, basisphenoid, and paranasal sinuses. ABCs of the skull and orbit are rare, accounting for less than 1% of all cases.

ABCs consist of blood-filled cavernous spaces with intracystic hemorrhages of variable ages. Multiple vari-

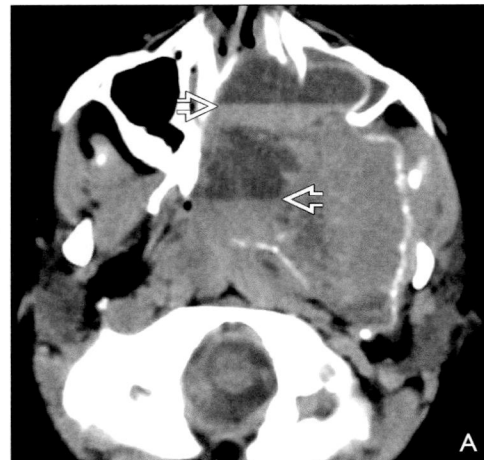
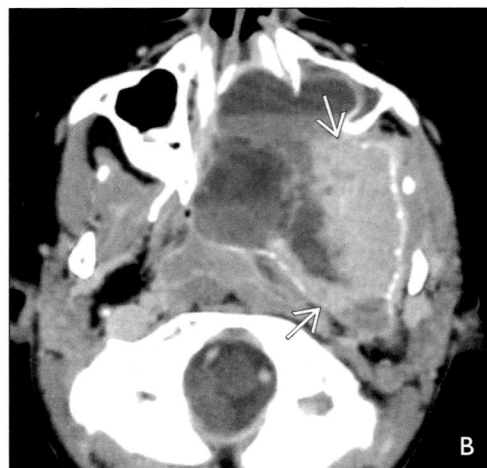

26-14A. NECT in a 7-year-old girl with left proptosis, mouth breathing shows a huge expansile mass in the deep face involving the left skull base. Note the fluid-fluid levels ⧨. 26-14B. CECT shows that the lateral aspect of the lesion demonstrates solid, relatively uniform enhancement ➔.

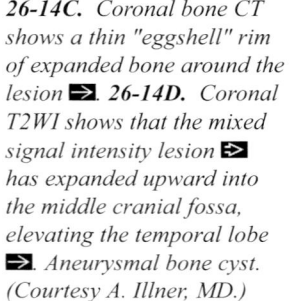
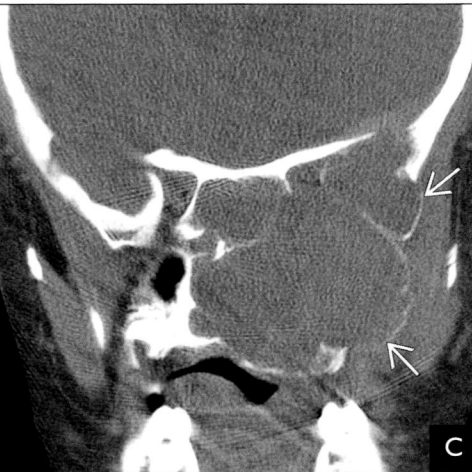
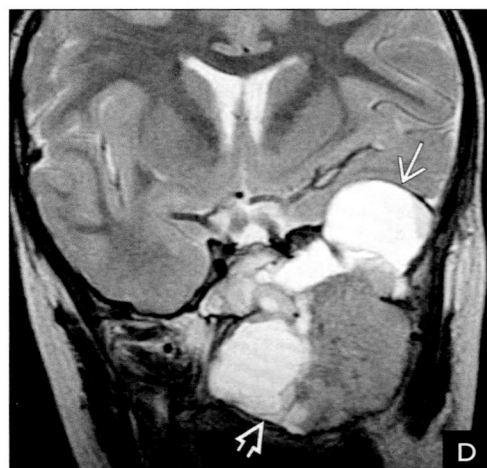

26-14C. Coronal bone CT shows a thin "eggshell" rim of expanded bone around the lesion ➔. 26-14D. Coronal T2WI shows that the mixed signal intensity lesion ➔ has expanded upward into the middle cranial fossa, elevating the temporal lobe ➔. Aneurysmal bone cyst. (Courtesy A. Illner, MD.)

ably sized cysts are separated by septa lined by endothelium, spindle-shaped fibroblasts, and scattered multinucleated giant cells.

Clinical Issues

ABCs represent 5% of all primary bone tumors and are the second most common pathologically proven bone tumor of childhood. About 70% occur in the first two decades, with a slight male predominance. Symptoms vary with location. Many lesions are asymptomatic or present with slowly progressive swelling.

Treatments for symptomatic ABC are curettage, cryosurgery, and bone graft. Recurrence rates are high, varying from 20-50%. Preoperative embolization may be helpful in selected cases.

Imaging

NECT scans show an eccentric lesion with expanded, remodeled, ballooned ("aneurysmally dilated") bone surrounded by a thin sclerotic rim **(26-14)**. Multiple cystic spaces with fluid-fluid levels are present.

MR shows a multicystic lesion with a hypointense rim surrounding multiple fluid-filled spaces. Hemorrhages of varying ages with fluid-fluid levels are a prominent imaging feature, as are smaller cysts ("diverticula") that project from larger lesions. The surrounding rim and fibrous septa enhance following contrast administration **(26-15)**.

Differential Diagnosis

Some ABCs may have a phase of relatively rapid growth and can be mistaken clinically for a more aggressive lesion. The most important imaging differential diagnosis of ABC is **telangiectatic osteosarcoma** (OS), which may have fluid-fluid levels that resemble those of ABC. Incomplete margination, soft tissue mass, cortical destruction, and significant solid portions should suggest telangiectatic OS instead.

Giant cell tumor and **osteoblastoma** are associated with secondary ABC and both show significant solid components.

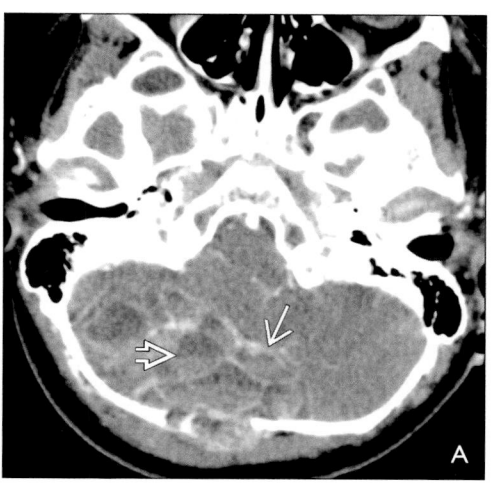

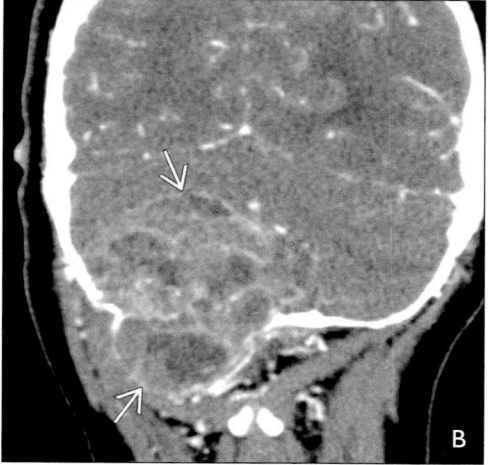

26-15A. Axial CECT of an aneurysmal bone cyst demonstrates multiple cysts with fluid-fluid levels ➡, enhancing rims ➡. 26-15B. Coronal CECT shows that the mass ➡ is both intra- and extracranial. The dependent blood-fluid levels in the cysts are better appreciated on the axial scan.

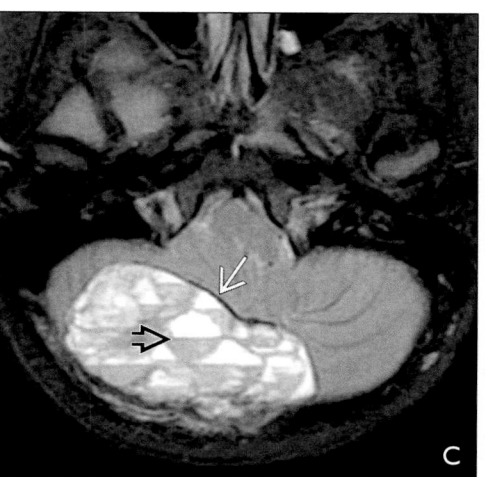

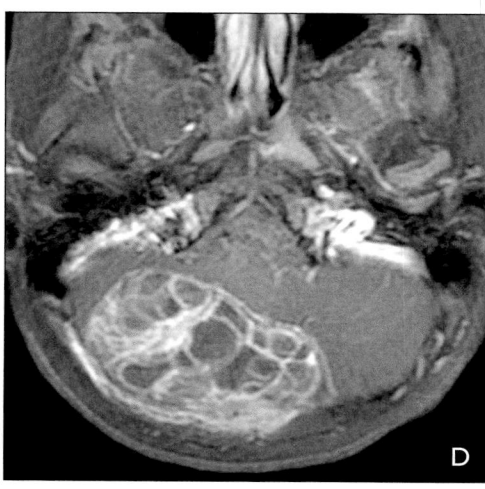

26-15C. T2WI shows multiple cysts with blood-fluid levels ➡. The thin black line draped over the mass ➡ is the displaced dura. 26-15D. T1 C+ FS shows the characteristic enhancement of the cyst walls, septations within the tumor.

Chordoma

Terminology and Etiology

Chordomas are rare, locally aggressive primary malignant neoplasms with a phenotype that recapitulates the notochord. Skull base (clival) chordomas (CCh) probably arise from the cranial end of primitive notochordal remnants. Subpopulations of cancer stem-like cells have been identified in some chordomas.

Pathology

Chordomas are midline tumors that may arise anywhere along the primitive notochord. The sacrum is the most common site (50% of all chordomas) followed by the sphenooccipital (clival) region (35%) and spine (15%).

Most sphenooccipital chordomas are midline lesions (26-16). Occasionally, a chordoma is predominantly extraosseous and arises off-midline, usually in the nasopharynx or cavernous sinus.

Two major histologic forms of chordoma are recognized: Typical ("classic") and chondroid. Typical or classic chordoma consists of physaliphorous cells that contain mucin and glycogen vacuoles, giving a characteristic "bubbly" appearance to its cytoplasm. Chondroid chordomas have stromal elements that resemble hyaline cartilage with neoplastic cells nestled within lacunae. A third type, dedifferentiated chordoma, represents less than 5% of chordomas and typically occurs in the sacrococcygeal region.

Both typical and chondroid chordomas are strongly immunopositive for the epithelial markers cytokeratin and epithelial membrane antigen (EMA).

Clinical Issues

Chordomas account for 2-5% of all primary bone tumors but cause almost 40% of sacral tumors. While chordomas may occur at any age, peak prevalence is between the fourth and sixth decades. There is a moderate male predominance.

Clival chordomas typically present with headaches and diplopia secondary to CN VI compression. Large chor-

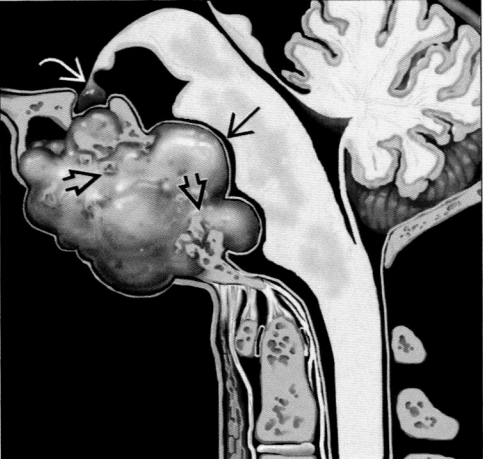
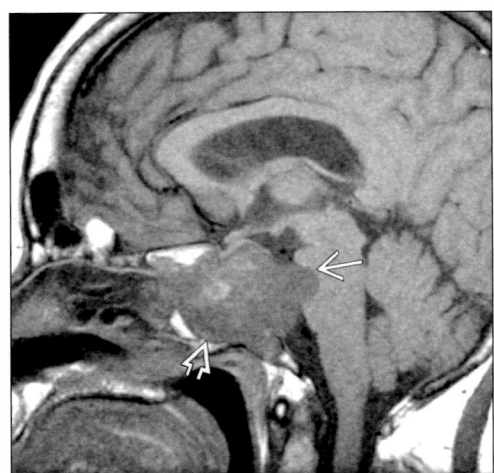

26-16. Sagittal graphic shows an expansile, destructive, lobulated clival mass with a "thumb" of tumor ➡ indenting the pons. The pituitary gland ➡ is elevated by the tumor. Note the bone fragments ▷ "floating" in the chordoma.
26-17. Sagittal T1WI shows the clivus almost completely replaced by an expansile chordoma ➡ with a classic "thumb" of tissue indenting the pons ➡.

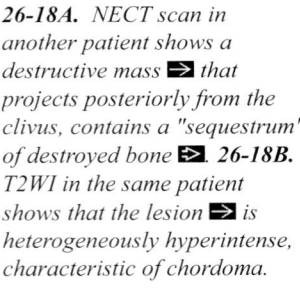

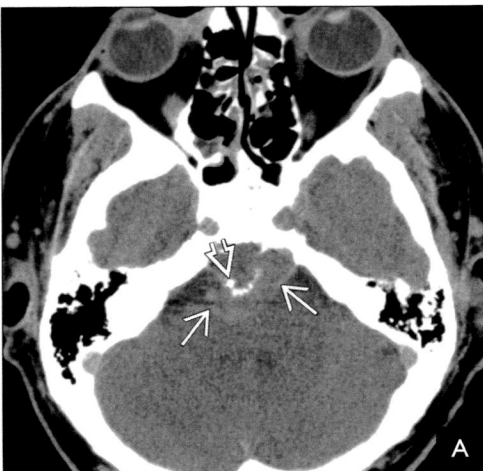
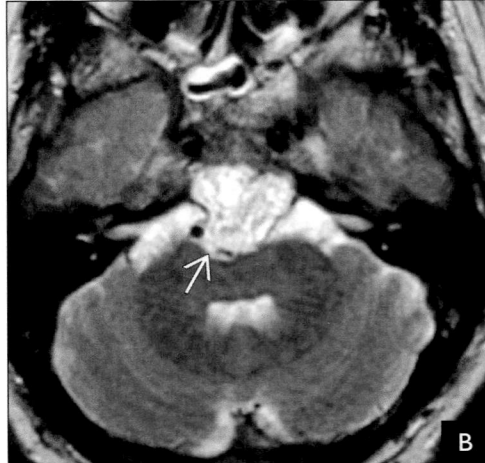

26-18A. NECT scan in another patient shows a destructive mass ➡ that projects posteriorly from the clivus, contains a "sequestrum" of destroyed bone ▷. 26-18B. T2WI in the same patient shows that the lesion ➡ is heterogeneously hyperintense, characteristic of chordoma.

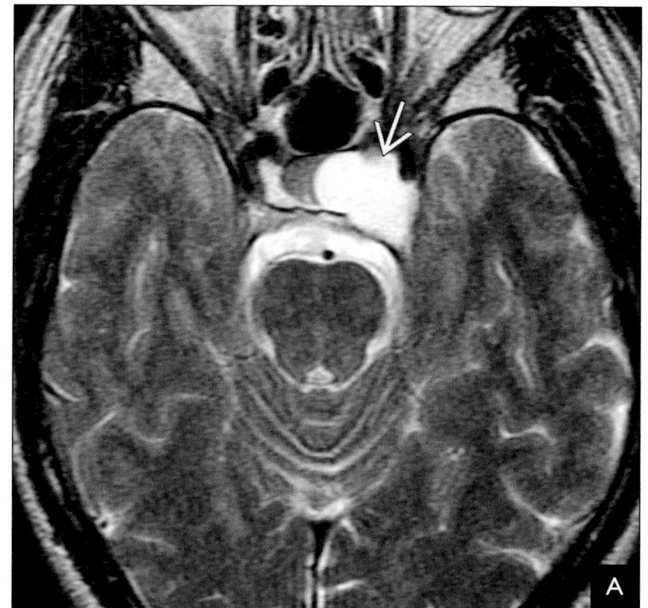

26-19A. *Axial T2WI shows a hyperintense mass* ➡ *in the left cavernous sinus invading the sphenoid bone.*

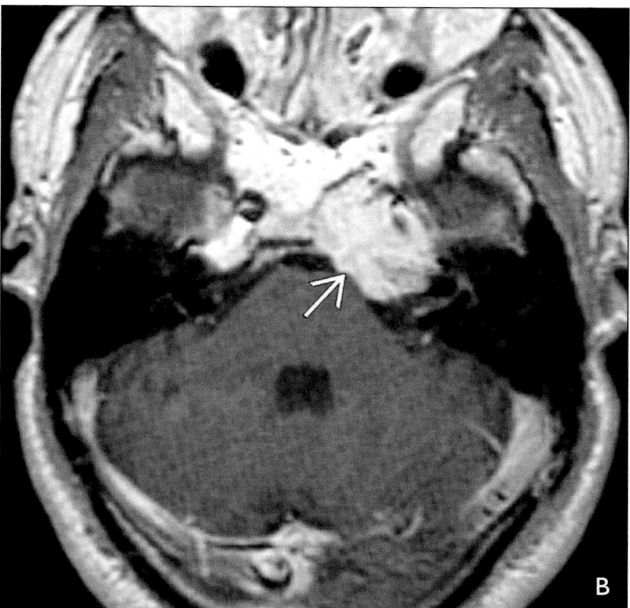

26-19B. *The mass* ➡ *enhances strongly on T1 C+. Lateral clival chordomas are less common than midline lesions. (Courtesy J. Curé, MD.)*

domas may cause multiple cranial neuropathies, including visual loss and facial pain.

Although they grow slowly, chordomas are eventually lethal unless treated with aggressive resection and proton beam irradiation. The overall five-year survival rate of patients following radical resection is 75%.

Imaging

NECT shows a relatively well-circumscribed, moderately hyperdense midline clival mass with permeative lytic bony changes. Intratumoral calcifications generally represent sequestrations from destroyed bone **(26-18)**.

Chordomas are typically intermediate to low signal intensity on T1WI. On sagittal images, a "thumb" of tumor tissue is often seen extending posteriorly through the cortex of the clivus and indenting the pons **(26-17)**.

Typical chordomas are very hyperintense on T2WI **(26-19)**, reflecting high fluid content within the physaliphorous cells. Intratumoral calcifications and hemorrhage may cause foci of decreased signal within the overall hyperintense mass. Moderate to marked but heterogeneous enhancement is typical after contrast administration.

Differential Diagnosis

The major differential diagnosis of clival chordoma is **invasive pituitary macroadenoma**. CChs typically displace but do not invade the pituitary gland whereas macroadenomas cannot be identified separate from the gland.

Signal intensity of a **skull base chondrosarcoma** is very similar to that of CCh. Chondrosarcomas typically arise off-midline, along the petrooccipital fissure. **Ecchordosis physaliphora** is a rare nonneoplastic notochordal remnant that may arise anywhere from the skull base to the sacrum. Most are small and found incidentally at autopsy or imaging. They usually lie just in front of the pons and have a thin stalk-like connection to a smaller intraclival component.

Skull base **metastases** and **plasmacytoma** are destructive lesions that are usually isointense with brain on all sequences. Predominantly intraosseous **meningioma** is rare in the skull base. It usually causes sclerosis and hyperostosis rather than a permeative destructive pattern.

Intracranial Pseudotumors

Ecchordosis Physaliphora

Ecchordosis physaliphora (EP) is a small gelatinous soft tissue mass that represents an ectopic notochordal remnant **(26-20)**. Ectopic notochordal rests can occur anywhere along the midline craniospinal axis from the dorsum sellae to the sacrococcygeal region. EPs are more

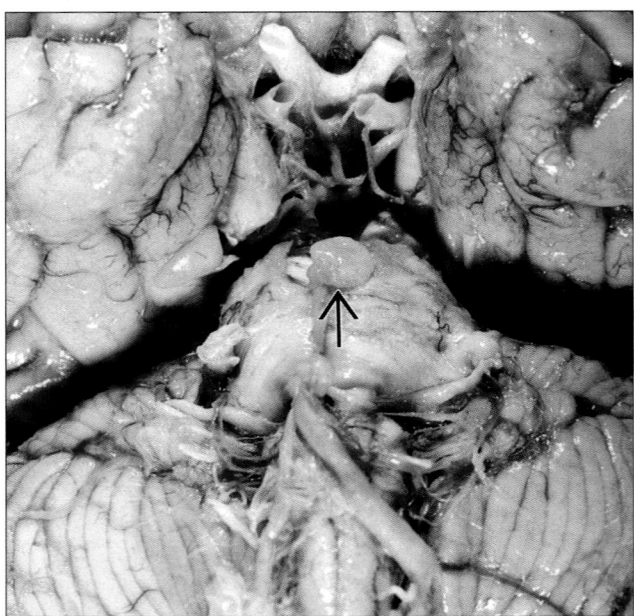

26-20. Autopsy specimen shows a glistening, gelatinous-appearing nodule ⤳ in front of the pons. Incidental finding of physaliphorous ecchordosis. (Courtesy R. Hewlett, MD.)

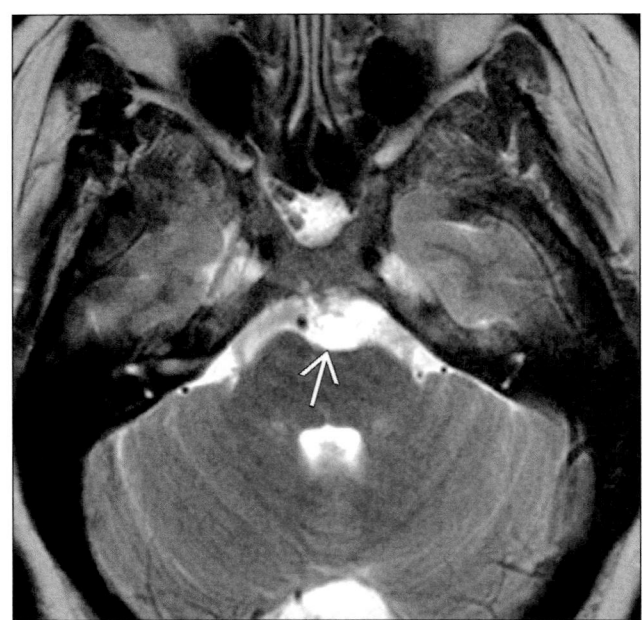

26-21. Axial T2WI shows a lobulated, well-delineated, hyperintense midline mass ⤳ that indents the pons. Physaliphorous ecchordosis.

common in the spine than the skull and are generally incidental findings at imaging or autopsy.

CT demonstrates a well-delineated nonenhancing midline intraclival mass with scalloped sclerotic margins.

The key imaging feature of EP that distinguishes it from other similar-appearing lesions is the presence of a small pedicle or stalk that connects the clival lesion to an intradural component in the prepontine cistern. Best demonstrated on MR, EPs are iso- to slightly hyperintense to CSF on T1WI and hyperintense on T2WI **(26-21)**.

The major differential diagnosis of EP in the basisphenoid bone is **clival chordoma.** Chordomas are permeative destructive lesions. Other prepontine cistern lesions that can mimic EP include arachnoid, neurenteric, epidermoid, and dermoid cysts. **Arachnoid cysts** are much more common in the cerebellopontine angle cisterns and behave exactly like CSF on all sequences.

Neurenteric cysts are often slightly off-midline and somewhat lower, adjacent to the pontomedullary junction. **Epidermoid cysts** (ECs) are irregular, somewhat frond-like lesions that restrict on DWI. ECs are more common in the cerebellopontine angle cisterns. **Dermoid cysts** usually follow fat signal, not CSF.

Textiloma

Hemostatic elements that are introduced into the central nervous system occasionally induce an excessive inflammatory reaction that may be difficult to distinguish from recurrent or residual tumor on neuroimaging studies.

Terminology

Textiloma refers to a mass created by a retained surgical element and its associated foreign body inflammatory reaction. The terms "gossypiboma," "gauzoma," and "muslinoma" refer specifically to retained nonresorbable cotton or woven materials.

Etiology

Hemostatic agents can be resorbable or nonresorbable. Resorbable agents include gelatin sponge, oxidized cellulose, and microfibrillar collagen. Nonresorbable agents include various forms of cotton pledgets, cloth (i.e., muslin), and synthetic rayon. While bioabsorbable hemostats are often left in place, nonresorbable agents are typically removed prior to surgical closure. Any of these materials may induce an inflammatory reaction, creating a textiloma.

Pathology

Most textilomas occur within surgical resection sites or around muslin-reinforced aneurysms. Histologic examination typically shows a core of degenerating inert hemostatic agent surrounded by inflammatory reaction. Foreign body giant cells and histiocytes are often present. Each agent exhibits distinctive histologic features, often permitting specific identification **(26-22C)**.

Clinical Issues

Textilomas are uncommon. The highest reported prevalence is following abdominal and orthopedic surgery.

Intracranial textilomas are rare with fewer than 75 reported cases.

Textilomas may be asymptomatic or cause symptoms that suggest tumor recurrence.

Imaging

Intracranial textilomas are almost always iso- or hypointense on T1WI. Approximately 45% are iso- and 40% are hypointense on T2/FLAIR **(26-22A)**. Some "blooming" on T2* may be present. All reported cases of textiloma enhance on post-contrast scans. Ring and heterogeneous solid enhancement patterns occur almost equally **(26-22B)**.

Differential Diagnosis

The major differential diagnosis is **recurrent neoplasm** or **radiation necrosis**. Residual or recurrent tumor can coexist with textiloma. If present, T2 hypointensity helps distinguish textiloma from neoplasm or **abscess**. Definitive diagnosis typically requires biopsy and histologic examination with both routine stains and polarized light.

Calcifying Pseudoneoplasm of the Neuraxis

Calcifying pseudoneoplasm of the neuraxis (CAPNON) is a rare but distinctive nonneoplastic lesion of the CNS. Calcifying pseudoneoplasms are also known as fibroosseous lesions, cerebral calculi, "brain stones," and "brain rocks."

CAPNONs are nonneoplastic, noninflammatory lesions. They are discrete masses that contain various combinations of chondromyxoid and fibrovascular stroma, metaplastic calcification, and ossification.

CAPNONs are usually asymptomatic and discovered incidentally on imaging studies. The most common symptom is seizure. A few cases have been reported in association with meningioangiomatosis and neurofibromatosis type 2.

NECT scans demonstrate a densely calcified leptomeningeal, deep intrasulcal, or brain parenchymal "rock." The temporal lobe is the most common site **(26-23A)**.

On MR, CAPNONs demonstrate little mass effect, are isointense on T1WI, and are uniformly hypointense on T2WI and FLAIR **(26-23B)**. Mild "blooming" is seen on T2* GRE. Perilesional edema varies from none to extensive. Enhancement varies from none to moderate. Solid, linear, serpiginous, and peripheral rim-like enhancement patterns have all been reported **(26-23C)**.

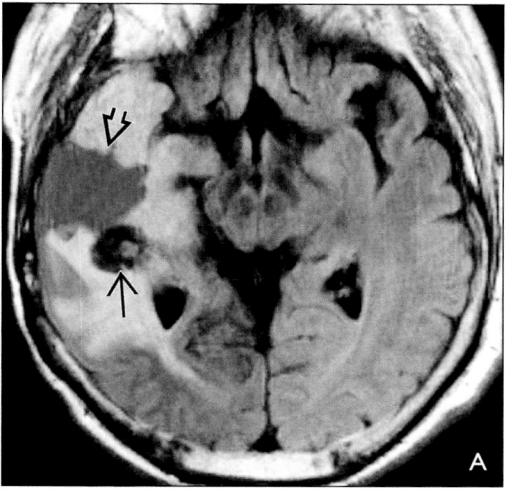

26-22A. *Axial FLAIR scan shows a hypointense mass ⇨ adjacent to the tumor resection cavity ⇨.*

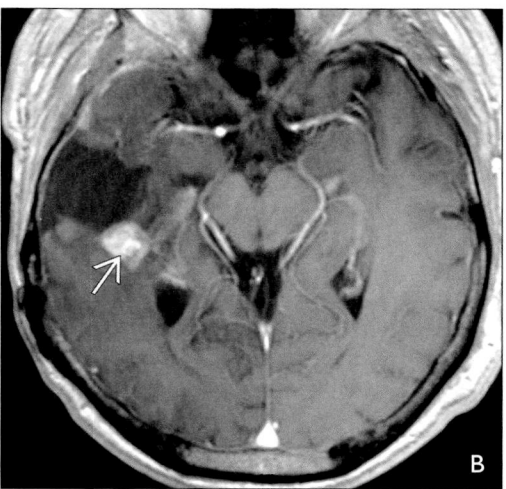

26-22B. *The lesion ➡ demonstrates solid but heterogeneous enhancement on T1 C+ FS.*

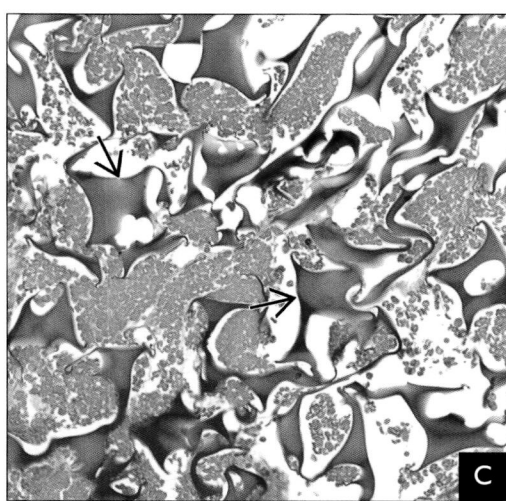

26-22C. *Histology (same case) shows amorphous spicules ⇨ surrounded by blood. Gelfoam textiloma. (Courtesy B. K. DeMasters, MD.)*

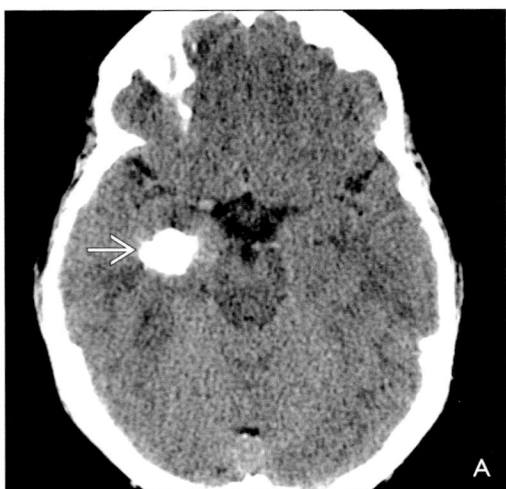

26-23A. *NECT scan shows a densely calcified mass in the right temporal lobe* ➡.

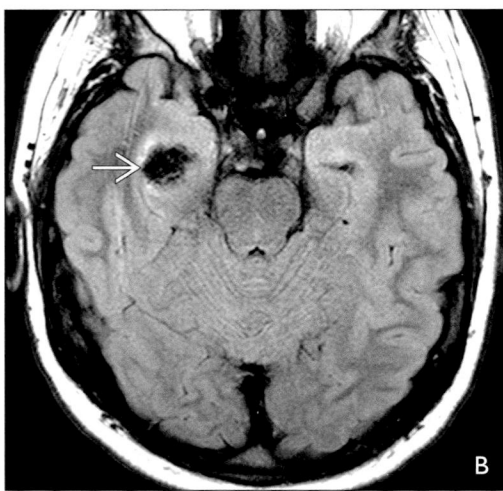

26-23B. *FLAIR scan shows absent signal in the mass* ➡.

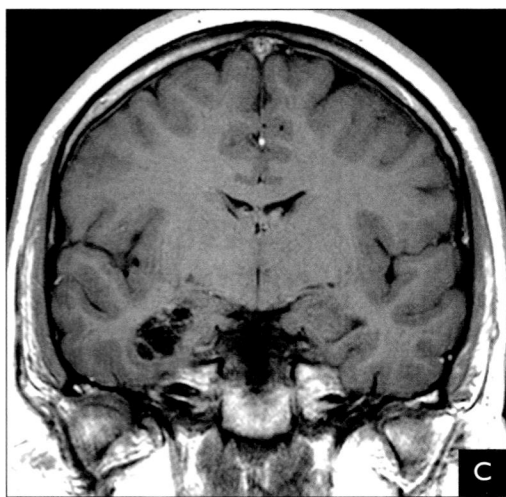

26-23C. *Coronal T1 C+ scan shows faint enhancement in the septations within the lesion. CAPNON. (Courtesy S. Blaser, MD.)*

The differential diagnosis of CAPNON includes an ossified vascular lesion—most often a **cavernous malformation**—and densely calcified neoplasm such as **oligodendroglioma**, **meningioma**, and **choroid plexus papilloma** with osseous metaplasia. Although cavernous malformations can often be distinguished by their "popcorn" mixed hyperintensity on T2WI, biopsy is usually necessary for definitive diagnosis.

Idiopathic Inflammatory Pseudotumor

Inflammatory pseudotumors are uncommon lesions that may be virtually indistinguishable from true neoplasms. Although they are most common in the lung, inflammatory pseudotumors have been described in virtually all body parts. Head and neck pseudotumors typically involve the orbit, where they represent 5-8% of orbital masses.

Extraorbital (skull base and intracranial) pseudotumors are rare. They often behave aggressively, simulating more ominous lesions such as invasive fungal infection or malignant neoplasm.

Terminology

Intracranial idiopathic inflammatory pseudotumor (IIP) is a benign nonneoplastic inflammatory process that is also known as inflammatory myofibroblastic tumor, plasma cell granuloma, xanthogranuloma, idiopathic hypertrophic cranial pachymeningitis, and Tolosa-Hunt syndrome.

Etiology

IIPs typically occur without identifiable local or systemic causes, and their true origin remains unknown. Many investigators have posited an exaggerated immunological process mediated by both B and T lymphocytes as a possible etiology for these unusual lesions. Others have suggested that viral infection (e.g., Epstein-Barr) may play a significant role in the pathogenesis of inflammatory pseudotumors.

Pathology

LOCATION. Intracranial pseudotumors are divided into five types by location: Parenchymal, meningeal, mixed meningeal/parenchymal, intraventricular, and cavernous sinus (often but not invariably extension from orbital disease). Nearly 60% of IIPs arise from the meninges. Invasion of underlying brain parenchyma occurs in approximately 10% of cases.

SIZE AND NUMBER. Intracranial lesions vary from small focal infiltrations to large multifocal dura-based masses with extensive parenchymal involvement (**26-24C**), (**26-24D**).

GROSS PATHOLOGY. The classic IIP is a firm, yellowish, somewhat lobulated mass that thickens the dura-arachnoid (**26-24D**). Some cases show local infiltration of the underlying brain (**26-24C**).

MICROSCOPIC FEATURES. The usual appearance of IIP on standard hematoxylin-and-eosin-stained slides is that of proliferating but benign-appearing myofibroblastic cells admixed with inflammatory infiltrates (**26-25C**). Variable amounts of polyclonal lymphocytes, macrophages, polymorphonuclear cells, plasma cells, eosinophils, and occasional histiocytes are present within the fibrous stroma.

The amount of fibrosis within an IIP generally increases with chronicity. No neoplastic cells are present, and stains for infectious agents are negative. MIB-1 is low, generally under 1%.

Immunohistochemistry shows expression of smooth muscle actin, but stains for anaplastic lymphoma kinase (ALK) are generally negative.

Clinical Issues

Orbital pseudotumors can occur at any age and cause painful proptosis. Skull base and intracranial inflammatory pseudotumors typically present in adults. Headache, visual symptoms, and cranial neuropathy are common symptoms.

With some exceptions, most IIPs—especially those with dense fibrous sclerosis—often respond poorly to steroids alone. The treatment of choice is thus surgical resection. Radiation and chemotherapy have been used with modest success.

Imaging

GENERAL FEATURES. IIPs usually cause mass-like dural thickening. Skull base IIPs often extend into or through the orbit, cavernous sinus, Meckel cave, and adjacent dura. Posterior fossa lesions may invade the clivus and temporal bone. Thickening and enhancement of one or more cranial nerves have been reported.

CT FINDINGS. NECT scans typically show one or more slightly hyperdense extraaxial masses (**26-24A**). Focal

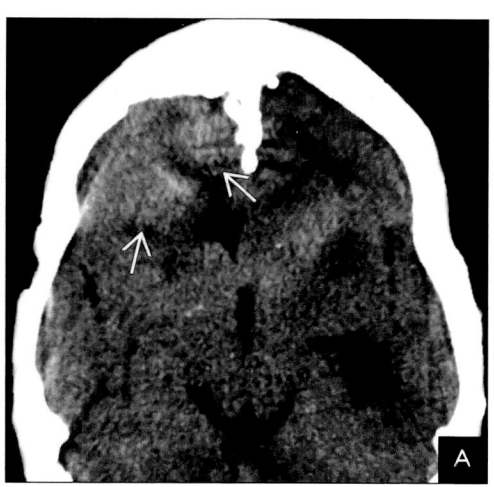
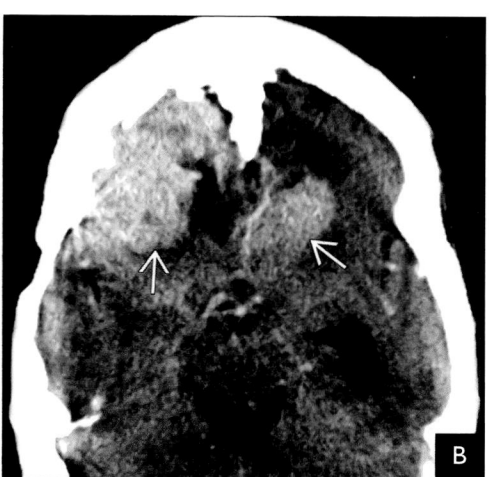

26-24A. NECT scan shows a hyperdense right frontal mass ➡ with associated thickening of the adjacent calvaria. 26-24B. CECT scan shows that the extensive mass involves both frontal lobes, enhances moderately and relatively uniformly ➡.

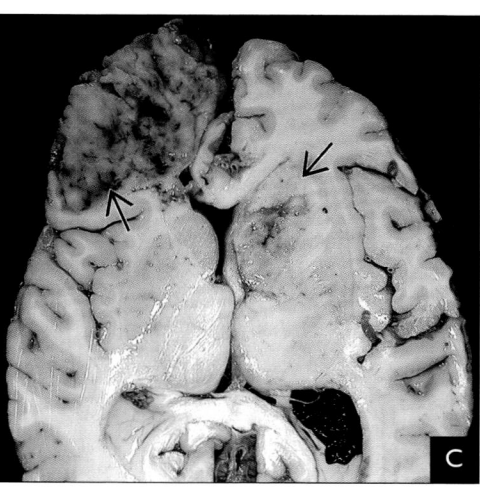
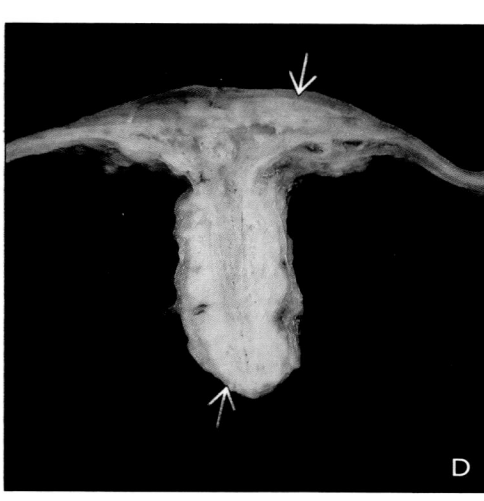

26-24C. Autopsy specimen from the same patient shows a heterogeneous, extensively infiltrating mass in the right frontal lobe, left caudate nucleus ➡. 26-24D. The dura is markedly infiltrated and thickened ➡. Histology showed idiopathic invasive inflammatory pseudotumor without evidence of neoplasm or infection. (Courtesy R. Hewlett, MD.)

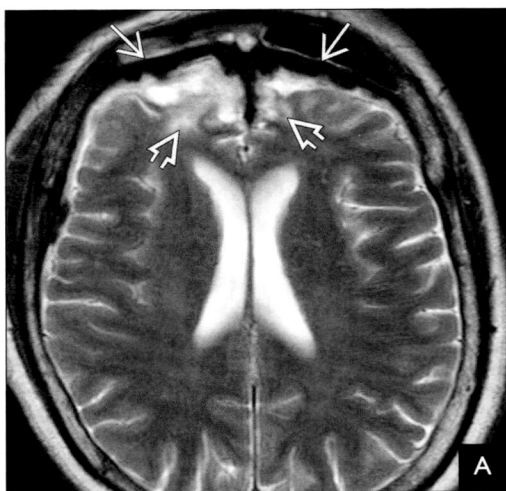

26-25A. T2WI shows a very hypointense, lobulated, bifrontal dural mass ➡️ with underlying hyperintensity in both frontal lobes ➡️.

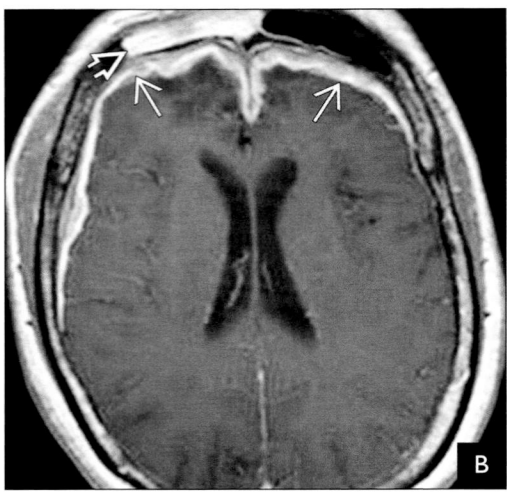

26-25B. T1 C+ in the same patient shows extensive dural thickening ➡️ with invasion of the right frontal sinus ➡️.

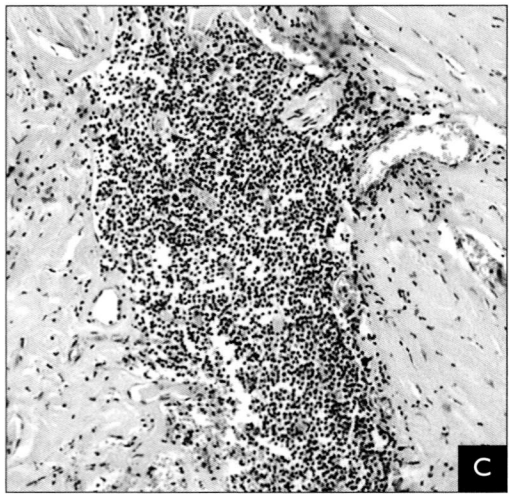

26-25C. Biopsy shows monotonous inflammatory infiltrate, no evidence of neoplasia. Inflammatory pseudotumor. (Courtesy P. J. van Rensburg, MD.)

bone remodeling, erosion, and even frank destruction may occur but are unusual. Strong uniform enhancement following contrast administration is typical **(26-24B)**.

MR FINDINGS. IIPs are usually isointense to cortex on T1WI and moderately to strikingly hypointense on T2WI **(26-25A)**. T2 hypointensity correlates with the amount of fibrosis present in the lesion.

Strong uniform enhancement is characteristic of IIPs and is best demonstrated on T1 C+ FS sequences **(26-25B)**. The appearance of a smooth or lobulated enhancing dura-based mass is typical **(26-26)**.

Cortical vein and/or dural sinus thrombosis is a frequent secondary finding in patients with more extensive IIPs. Focal parenchymal edema, seen as increased signal intensity on T2WI and FLAIR, is common and may reflect venous congestion or frank pseudotumor invasion into the underlying brain.

Differential Diagnosis

Definitive diagnosis of IIP requires biopsy and histologic confirmation; there are no pathognomonic imaging characteristics of IIP. Findings may be very similar to "en plaque" **meningioma** and meningeal non-Hodgkin **lymphoma**. Signal intensity and enhancement in all three lesions may be virtually identical although profound hypointensity on T2WI is more typical of IIP.

Other intracranial lesions that may mimic IIP are **neurosarcoid, atypical mycobacterial spindle cell pseudotumor**, skull and meningeal **metastases**, and cephalad invasion by **nasopharyngeal carcinoma**. **Meningitis**, especially secondary to tuberculosis or fungal infection, may cause focal meningeal thickening that closely resembles IIP with or without adjacent bone erosion.

elected References

xtracranial Tumors and Tumor-like onditions

Fibrous Dysplasia

- Cai M et al: Clinical and radiological observation in a surgical series of 36 cases of fibrous dysplasia of the skull. Clin Neurol Neurosurg. 114(3):254-9, 2012
- Hayden Gephart MG et al: Primary pediatric skull tumors. Pediatr Neurosurg. 47(3):198-203, 2011
- Lui YW et al: Sphenoid masses in children: radiologic differential diagnosis with pathologic correlation. AJNR Am J Neuroradiol. 32(4):617-26, 2011
- Eversole R et al: Benign fibro-osseous lesions of the craniofacial complex: a review. Head Neck Pathol. 2(3):177-202, 2008

Paget Disease

- Farpour F et al: Radiological features of Paget disease of bone associated with VCP myopathy. Skeletal Radiol. 41(3):329-37, 2012
- Goode A et al: Recent advances in understanding the molecular basis of Paget disease of bone. J Clin Pathol. 63(3):199-203, 2010

Aneurysmal Bone Cyst

- Senol U et al: Aneurysmal bone cyst of the orbit. AJNR Am J Neuroradiol. 23(2):319-21, 2002

Chordoma

- Aydemir E et al: Characterization of cancer stem-like cells in chordoma. J Neurosurg. 116(4):810-20, 2012
- Sen C et al: Clival chordomas: clinical management, results, and complications in 71 patients. J Neurosurg. 113(5):1059-71, 2010

tracranial Pseudotumors

Ecchordosis Physaliphora

- Ciarpaglini R et al: Intradural clival chordoma and ecchordosis physaliphora: a challenging differential diagnosis: case report. Neurosurgery. 64(2):E387-8; discussion E388, 2009
- Srinivasan A et al: Case 133: Ecchordosis physaliphora. Radiology. 247(2):585-8, 2008
- Mehnert F et al: Retroclival ecchordosis physaliphora: MR imaging and review of the literature. AJNR Am J Neuroradiol. 25(10):1851-5, 2004

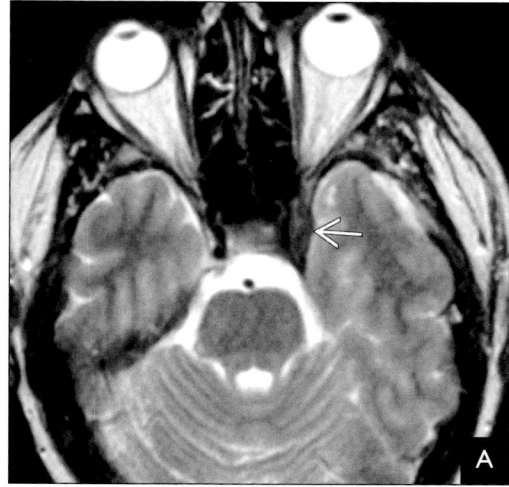

26-26A. T2WI in a patient with left-sided proptosis, ophthalmoplegia shows a hypointense mass infiltrating the left cavernous sinus.

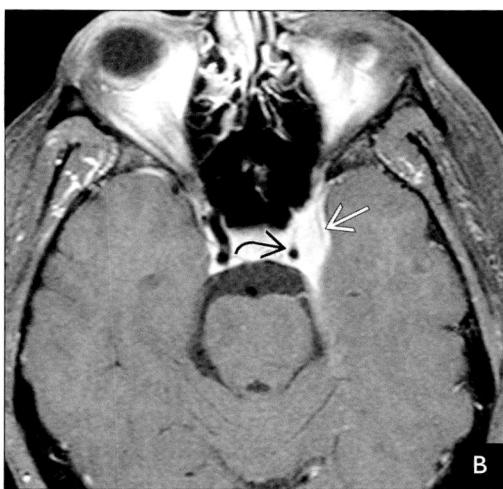

26-26B. The lesion enhances intensely, encases the left cavernous carotid artery.

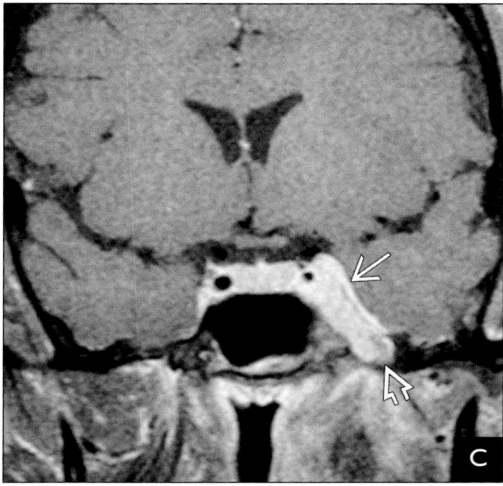

26-26C. Coronal T1 C+ shows that lesion infiltrates cavernous sinus, extends inferiorly into foramen ovale. Inflammatory pseudotumor.

Textiloma

- Warren A et al: Intracranial textiloma: Meta-analysis of the world literature and four new cases. Presented at the 50th Annual Scientific Meeting, American Society of Neuroradiology, New York, April 2012

- Ribalta T et al: Textiloma (gossypiboma) mimicking recurrent intracranial tumor. Arch Pathol Lab Med. 128(7):749-58, 2004

Calcifying Pseudoneoplasm of the Neuraxis

- Fletcher AM et al: Endoscopic resection of calcifying pseudoneoplasm of the neuraxis (CAPNON) of the anterior skull base with sinonasal extension. J Clin Neurosci. 19(7):1048-9, 2012

- Mohapatra I et al: Calcifying pseudoneoplasm (fibroosseous lesion) of neuraxis (CAPNON) - a case report. Clin Neuropathol. 29(4):223-6, 2010

- Aiken AH et al: Calcifying pseudoneoplasms of the neuraxis: CT, MR imaging, and histologic features. AJNR Am J Neuroradiol. 30(6):1256-60, 2009

Idiopathic Inflammatory Pseudotumor

- Carswell C et al: The successful long-term management of an intracranial inflammatory myofibroblastic tumor with corticosteroids. Clin Neurol Neurosurg. 114(1):77-9, 2012

- Ginat DT et al: Inflammatory pseudotumors of the head and neck in pathology-proven cases. J Neuroradiol. 39(2):110-5, 2012

- Lui PC et al: Inflammatory pseudotumors of the central nervous system. Hum Pathol. 40(11):1611-7, 2009

- Park SB et al: Imaging findings of head and neck inflammatory pseudotumor. AJR Am J Roentgenol. 193(4):1180-6, 2009

Metastases and Paraneoplastic Syndromes

CNS metastatic disease arises from numerous sources and has many different imaging "faces." We begin with an overview that focuses on general features, including how and from where cranial metastases arise, the effect of age on primary tumor type and CNS location, symptomatology, treatment options, and prognosis.

We follow with a discussion of cranial metastases by anatomic location, beginning with the parenchyma, the most common location overall. We conclude with a consideration of the remote effects of cancer on the CNS and the increasingly important group of so-called paraneoplastic syndromes.

Metastatic Lesions

Brain metastases are not only a leading cause of cancer mortality but as a group have become the most common CNS neoplasm in adults. Since 1960, there has been nearly a five-fold increase in the overall prevalence of brain metastases; the ratio between metastatic to primary brain tumors is now almost 50:50. Worldwide population aging, improved diagnosis, and new treatment regimens that allow patients with primary systemic cancers to sur-

vive longer all contribute to this striking increase. In the United States, more than 40% of cancer patients eventually develop brain metastases.

Overview

Terminology

Metastases are secondary tumors that arise from primary neoplasms at another site.

Etiology

ROUTES OF SPREAD. CNS metastases can arise from both extra- and intracranial primary tumors. Metastases from **extracranial primary neoplasms** ("body-to-brain metastases") most commonly spread via **hematogenous dissemination**.

A rare variant of body-to-brain hematogenous metastasis is **tumor-to-tumor metastasis** (TTM). TTM typically occurs when an aggressive "donor" extracranial epithelial neoplasm (most often breast or lung carcinoma) metastasizes to an existing "recipient" benign or low-grade intracranial tumor (usually a meningioma). TTM is sometimes called a **collision tumor**, i.e., two different tumor types are juxtaposed within a single mass, but this term more correctly refers to two neighboring neoplasms that invade each other.

Direct geographic extension from a lesion in an adjacent structure (such as squamous cell carcinoma in the nasopharynx) also occurs but is much less common than hematogenous spread. Invasion usually proceeds along paths of least resistance, i.e., through natural foramina and fissures where bone is thin or absent. **Perineural** and **perivascular spread** are less common but important direct geographic routes by which head and neck tumors gain access to the CNS.

Primary intracranial neoplasms sometimes spread from one CNS site to another, causing brain-to-brain or brain-to-spine metastases. One typical example is spread of a malignant astrocytoma (e.g., glioblastoma multi-

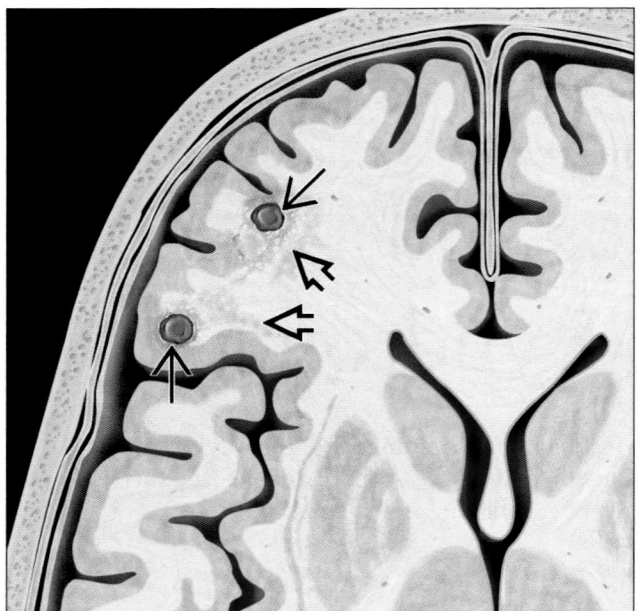

27-1. Graphic shows parenchymal metastases ➡ with surrounding edema ⊟. The gray-white matter junction is the most common location. Most metastases are round, not infiltrating.

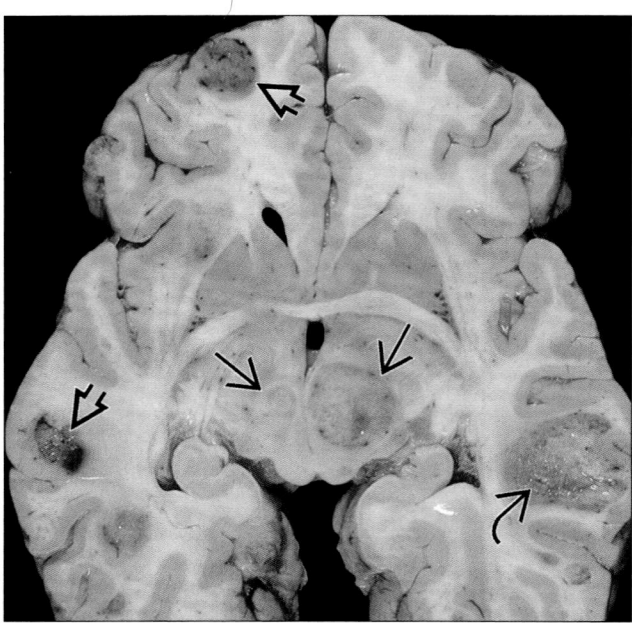

27-2. Metastases from bronchogenic carcinoma show varied locations, appearances. GM-WM lesions show hemorrhage ⊟, midbrain lesions are gray-tan ➡, and another parenchymal metastasis shows necrosis ➢. (Courtesy R. Hewlett, MD.)

forme) to other CNS sites. Spread occurs preferentially along compact white matter tracts such as the corpus callosum and internal capsule but can also involve the ventricular ependyma, pia, and perivascular spaces.

CSF dissemination with "carcinomatous meningitis" and "drop metastases" to the brain and spine occurs with both extra- and intracranial primary neoplasms.

METASTASIS FORMATION. While vascular dissemination of systemic tumor cells occurs readily, the development of brain metastases is far more complex than simply delivering a tumor embolism to an end organ. The brain is a biologically "relatively protected site" because of the blood-brain barrier. Most disseminated tumor cells do not immediately produce brain metastases.

The establishment, growth, and survival of metastases all depend on the interaction of tumor cells with multiple different host factors in the target organ microenvironment. Metastasis formation is a biologically complicated, genetically mediated process. A veritable cascade of events is required before brain metastases develop. Specific receptors mediate attachment and subsequent infiltration of circulating tumor cells into the CNS. Once tumor cells enter the brain, they are surrounded and infiltrated by activated astrocytes. These astrocytes upregulate "survival genes" in tumor cells, rendering them highly resistant to chemotherapy.

If metastatic cells manage to colonize the inhospitable brain habitat, matrix proteins, cytokines, and various growth factors may create a microenvironment that actu-

ally promotes tumor growth. Inactivation of tumor suppressor genes with simultaneous activation of protooncogenes is typical. Upregulation and amplification of some genes such as *EGFR* is also common.

ORIGIN OF CNS METASTASES. Both the source and the intracranial location of metastases vary significantly with patient age. Approximately 10% of all brain metastases originate from an unknown primary neoplasm at the time of initial diagnosis. In 10% of patients, the brain is the only site involved.

Children. The most common sources of cranial metastases in children are hematologic malignancies. In descending order of frequency, they are leukemia, lymphoma, and sarcoma (osteogenic sarcoma, rhabdomyosarcoma, and Ewing sarcoma).

The preferential location is the skull and dura. Parenchymal metastases are much less common in children compared to adults.

Adults. The overall most common extracranial primary tumor that metastasizes to the brain parenchyma is lung cancer (especially small cell and adenocarcinoma). Breast cancer is the second most common primary source, followed by melanoma, renal carcinoma, and colon cancer.

Skull, dura, and spine metastases are typically caused by prostate, breast, or lung cancer, followed by non-Hodgkin lymphoma, multiple myeloma, and renal cancers.

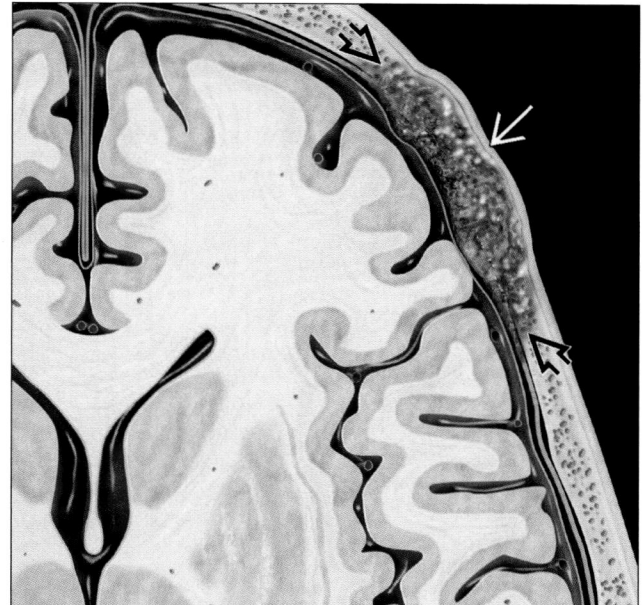

27-3. *Axial graphic illustrates a destructive skull metastasis ⇒ expanding the diploic space and invading/thickening the underlying dura (light blue linear structure) ⊵.*

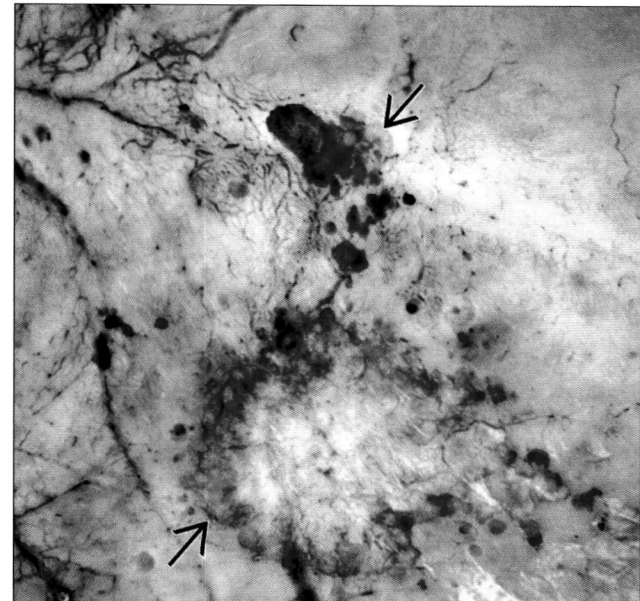

27-4. *Skull metastases are seen here as permeative, lytic, destructive lesions ⇥.*

CNS METASTASES: EPIDEMIOLOGY AND ETIOLOGY

Epidemiology
- Adults > > children
  - Mets = most common CNS neoplasm in adults
  - 5x increase in past 50 years
  - Brain mets in > 40% of cancer patients

Routes of Spread
- Most common = extracranial primary to CNS via
  - Hematogenous dissemination
  - Direct geographic extension (nasopharynx, sinuses)
  - Perineural, perivascular spread
- Less common
  - Brain-to-brain from CNS primary
  - Brain-to-CSF from CNS primary
- Least common
  - Tumor-to-tumor metastasis
  - Juxtaposition of 2 unique tumor types within single mass
  - Sometimes called "collision tumor"
  - Most common "donor" tumor = breast, lung
  - Most common "recipient" tumor = meningioma

Origin
- 10% unknown primary at initial diagnosis
  - Children: Leukemia, lymphoma, sarcoma
  - Adults: Lung, breast cancer; melanoma, renal carcinoma, colon cancer

athology

LOCATION. The brain parenchyma is the most common site (80%), followed by the skull and dura (15%). Diffuse leptomeningeal (pial) and subarachnoid space infiltration is relatively uncommon, accounting for just 5% of all cases.

The vast majority of parenchymal metastases are located in the cerebral hemispheres. Hematogenous metastases have a special predilection for arterial border zones and the junction between the cortex and subcortical white matter (27-1). Between 3-5% are found in the basal ganglia. Rarely, tumor cells diffusely infiltrate the brain perivascular spaces, a process termed "carcinomatous encephalitis."

Only 15% of metastases are found in the cerebellum. The midbrain, pons, and medulla are uncommon sites (especially for solitary lesions) and account for less than 1% of metastases.

Other rare sites include the choroid plexus, ventricular ependyma, pituitary gland/stalk, and retinal choroid.

SIZE AND NUMBER. While parenchymal metastases vary in size from microscopic implants to a few centimeters in diameter, most are between a few millimeters and 1.5 centimeters. Large hemispheric metastases are rare. In contrast, skull and dural metastases can become very large.

Approximately half of all metastases are solitary lesions, and half are multiple. About 20% of patients have two lesions, 30% have three or more, and only 5% have more than five lesions.

GROSS PATHOLOGY. The gross pathologic appearance of metastases varies according to tumor site.

Parenchymal metastases. Parenchymal metastases are generally round, relatively discrete lesions (27-2).

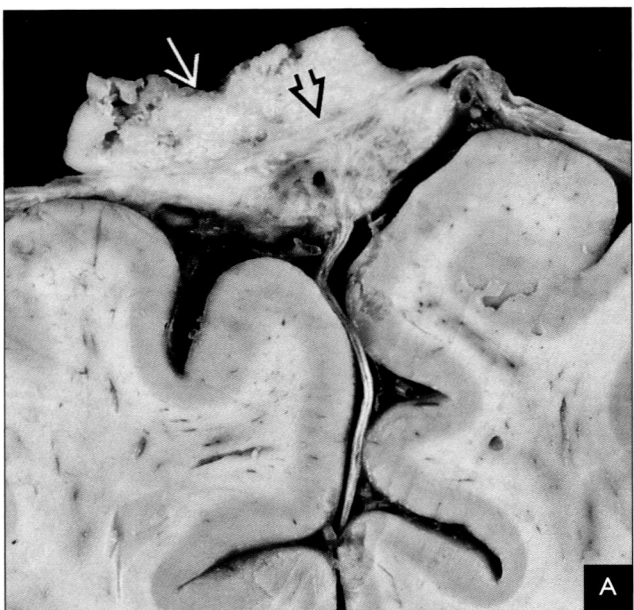

27-5A. Metastatic tumor ➡ *penetrates the dura* ⇨, *invades the superior sagittal sinus. The overlying skull (not shown) was involved.*

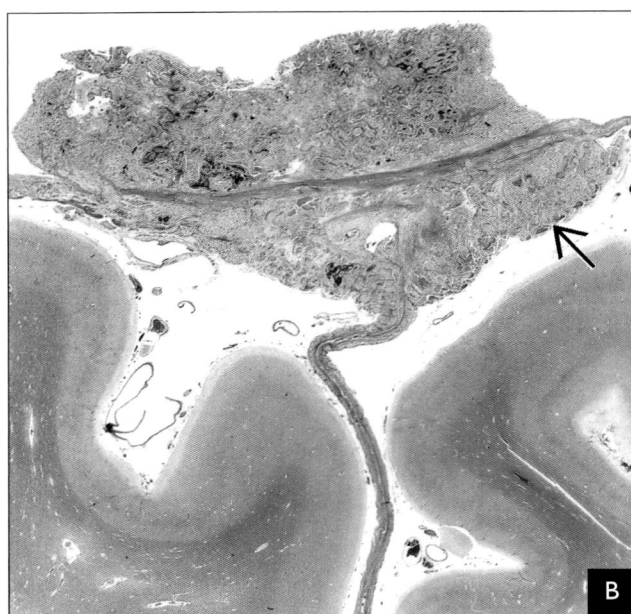

27-5B. Low-power photomicrograph shows that the endocranial aspect of the tumor involves both the dura and underlying arachnoid ⇨. *(Courtesy P. Burger, MD.)*

Peritumoral edema, necrosis, and mass effect range from none to striking. With the exception of melanotic melanoma, which is black, most are tan or grayish white. Some mucin-producing adenocarcinomas have a gelatinous appearance.

The spatial distribution of parenchymal metastases is nonuniform, suggesting that vulnerability to metastases may differ among brain regions. For example, the parietooccipital lobes are the most common site for non-small cell lung cancers. Hemorrhage also varies with primary tumor type. Melanoma, renal cell carcinoma, and choriocarcinoma are especially prone to develop intratumoral hemorrhages. For example, compared to lung cancer, metastatic melanoma is five times more likely to hemorrhage.

Diffusely infiltrating parenchymal metastases are rare. When they occur, they may be grossly indistinguishable from anaplastic astrocytoma or glioblastoma multiforme. Small cell lung carcinoma is the most common tumor that causes pseudogliomatous infiltration.

Skull/dural metastases. Calvarial and skull base metastases can be relatively well-circumscribed or diffusely destructive, poorly marginated lesions (27-3), (27-4). Head and neck tumors that extend intracranially by direct geographic invasion generally cause significant local bony destruction.

Dural metastases usually occur in combination with adjacent skull lesions, appearing as focal nodules or more diffuse, plaque-like sheets of tumor (27-5), (27-6), (27-7),

(27-8). Dural metastasis without skull involvement is much less common.

Leptomeningeal metastases. The term "leptomeningeal metastases" actually describes metastases to the subarachnoid spaces and pia. Diffuse opacification of the leptomeninges with sugar-like coating of the pia is typical (27-9). Infiltration of the perivascular (Virchow-Robin) spaces with extension into the adjacent cortex is common (27-10).

MICROSCOPIC FEATURES. Although metastases may display more marked mitoses and elevated labeling indices compared to their primary systemic source, they generally preserve the same cellular features.

Some metastases are more difficult than others to characterize on standard histopathological studies. Immunohistochemical characterization and new microRNA-based tests can identify the tumor tissue of origin in the majority of such cases.

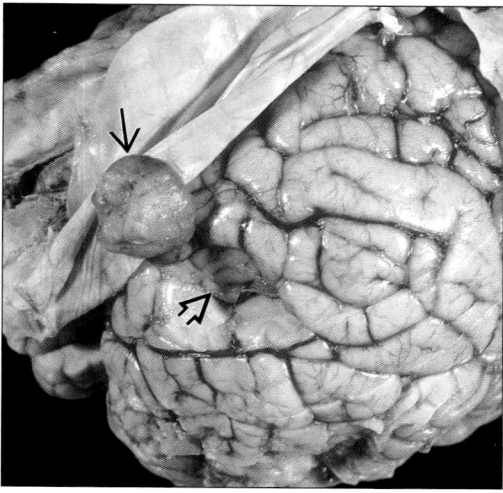

27-6. *Solitary dural metastasis* ➔ *indents the brain* ➔, *appears identical to a meningioma. (Courtesy R. Hewlett, MD.)*

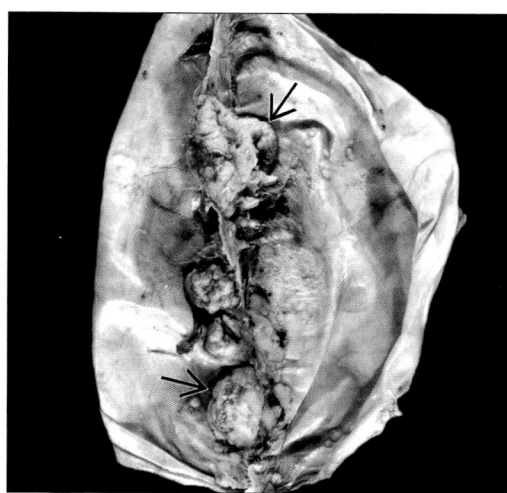

27-7. *Multiple dural metastases from breast carcinoma* ➔. *(Courtesy B. Horten, MD.)*

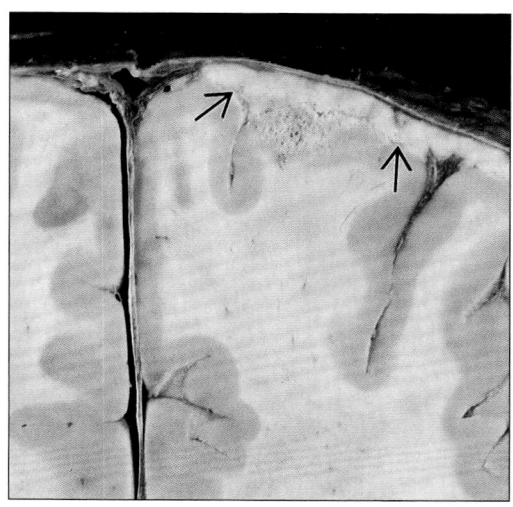

27-8. *Dura-arachnoid metastasis from prostate primary obliterates subarachnoid space, extends to pial surface of brain* ➔. *(Courtesy P. Burger, MD.)*

CNS METASTASES: PATHOLOGY

Location
- Adults
  - Brain (80%, cerebral hemispheres > > cerebellum)
  - Skull/dura (15%)
  - Pia ("leptomeningeal"), CSF (5%)
  - Other (1%)
- Children
  - Skull/dura > > brain parenchyma

Size
- Parenchymal metastases
  - Microscopic to a few centimeters (most 0.5-1.5 cm)
- Skull/dura metastases
  - Variable; can become very large

Number
- Solitary (50%)
- 2 lesions (20%)
- ≥ 3 lesions (30%)
  - Only 5% have > 5 lesions

Gross Pathology
- Round, well-circumscribed > > > infiltrating
- Variable edema, necrosis, hemorrhage

Microscopic Features
- Preserves general features of primary tumor
- May have more mitoses, elevated labeling indices

Clinical Issues

DEMOGRAPHICS. As treatments for primary systemic cancers improve, patients live longer and the incidence of brain metastasis continues to increase.

Currently, up to 40% of patients with treated systemic cancers eventually develop brain metastases. The incidence is strongly age-related, ranging from less than 1:100,000 in patients younger than 25 years to more than 30:100,000 at age 60 years.

Peak prevalence is in patients over 65 years of age. Only 6-10% of children with extracranial malignancies develop brain metastases.

Skull/dura metastases have a bimodal distribution. There is a smaller peak in children and a much larger peak in middle-aged and older adults. Overall average age is 50 years, skewed by pediatric cases and young women with aggressive breast cancers.

PRESENTATION. Symptoms vary with tumor site. Seizure and focal neurologic deficit are the most common presenting symptoms of parenchymal metastases. Half of all patients with skull/durae metastases present with headache. Seizure, sensory or motor deficit, cranial neuropathy, or a palpable mass under the scalp are other common symptoms.

NATURAL HISTORY. The natural history of parenchymal metastases is grim. Relentless progressive increase in both number and size of metastases is typical.

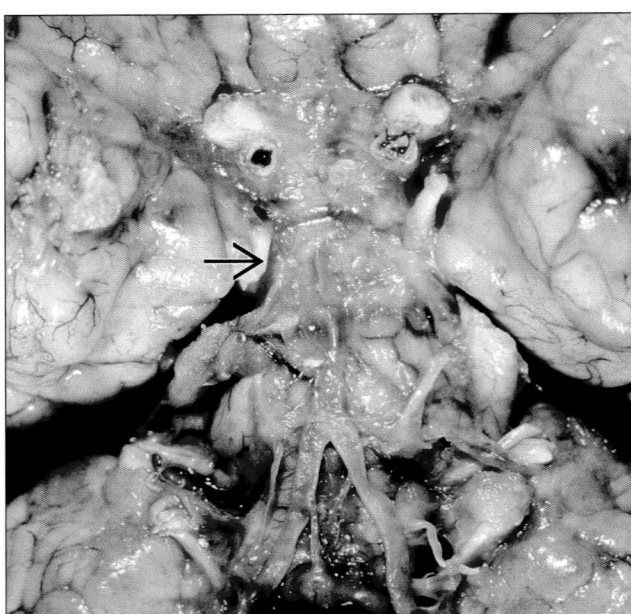

27-9. Pia-subarachnoid ("leptomeningeal") metastases coat the brain, fill the basilar subarachnoid cisterns ➡. (Courtesy R. Hewlett, MD.)

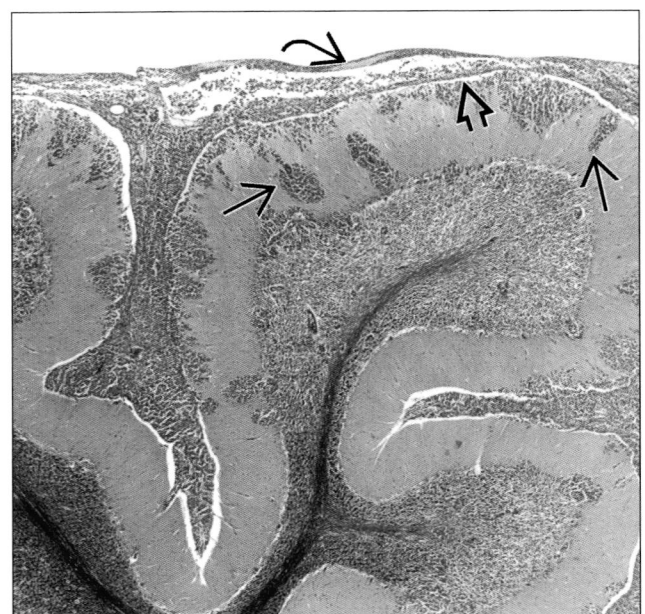

27-10. Metastases fill the subarachnoid space between the arachnoid ➢ and pial surface of the brain ➡, extend along the perivascular spaces into the cortex ➡. (Courtesy P. Burger, MD.)

Median survival after diagnosis is short, generally averaging between three and six months. For example, median survival in patients with untreated metastases from lung cancer is around one month.

TREATMENT OPTIONS. Treatment aims are symptom prevention/palliation, improvement in quality of life, and prolonged survival. Surgical resection, fractionated stereotactic radiosurgery, whole-brain radiation, and chemotherapy are the common options.

Treatment choice varies with the number and location of metastases. Patients with a solitary metastasis may experience improved quality of life and modestly prolonged survival from surgical resection and/or stereotactic radiosurgery.

Imaging

Imaging findings and differential diagnosis vary with metastasis location. Each anatomic site has special features; each is discussed separately below.

Parenchymal Metastases

Terminology

Parenchymal metastases are secondary tumor implants that involve the brain parenchyma. Tumor in the perivascular (Virchow-Robin) spaces is included in our discussion of parenchymal metastases; intraventricular (ependymal and choroid plexus) metastases are discussed as miscellaneous metastases (see below).

Imaging

Conventional CT and MR are the most commonly used techniques for detecting brain metastases and monitoring treatment response.

CT FINDINGS. Both soft tissue and bone algorithm reconstructions should be performed as subtle calvarial lesions can easily be overlooked. Soft tissue reconstructions should be viewed with both narrow and intermediate ("subdural") window widths (27-11).

NECT. Most metastases are iso- to slightly hypodense relative to gray matter (27-12A). In the absence of edema or intratumoral hemorrhage, even moderately large metastases may be virtually invisible on NECT scans. With the exception of treated metastases, calcification is rare.

Occasionally, the first manifestation of an intracranial metastasis is catastrophic brain bleeding. An underlying metastasis is a not uncommon cause of spontaneous intracranial hemorrhage in older adults (27-13).

CECT. The vast majority of parenchymal metastases enhance strongly following contrast administration (27-12B). Double dose delayed scans may increase lesion conspicuity. Solid, punctate, nodular, or ring patterns can be seen.

MR FINDINGS.

T1WI. Most metastases are iso- to mildly hypointense on T1WI (27-14A). The exception is melanoma metastasis, which has intrinsic T1 shortening

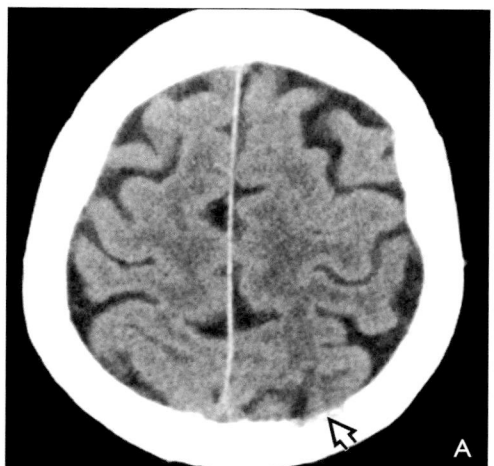
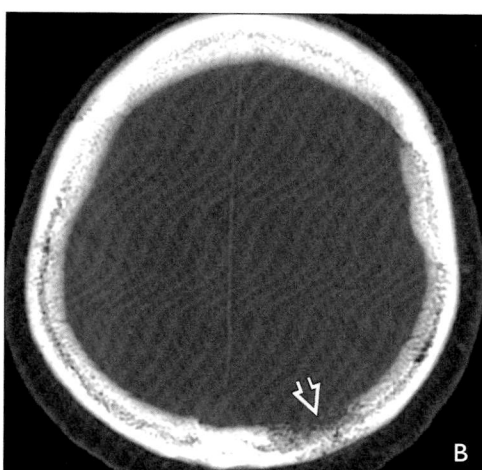

27-11A. *NECT scan in a 64-year-old man with headache, no focal neurologic signs shows no abnormality of the brain parenchyma. A subtle irregularity of the left posterior parietal bone* ⇨ *can be seen on soft tissue reconstruction (80 HU).* **27-11B.** *Bone algorithm reconstruction shows a solitary permeative destructive lesion that extends through the inner, outer tables of the skull* ⇨. *Metastasis from lung carcinoma.*

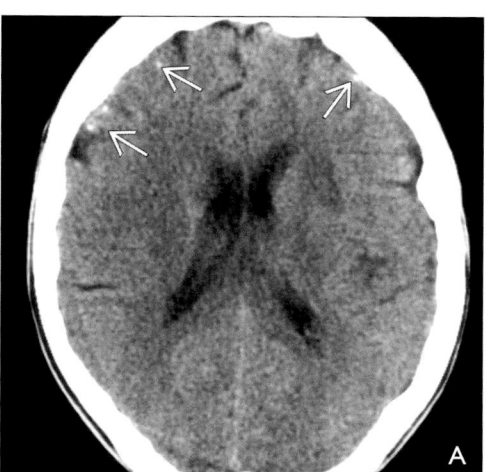
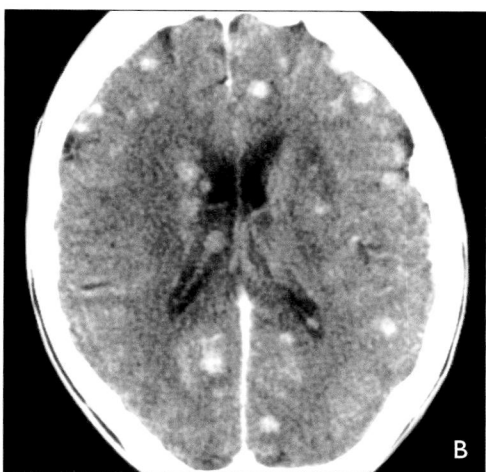

27-12A. *Axial NECT in a 63-year-old woman with known breast carcinoma shows a few scattered bifrontal hyperdensities* ⇨. **27-12B.** *CECT scan shows "too numerous to count" enhancing metastases, most of which were isodense and completely invisible on the pre-contrast study.*

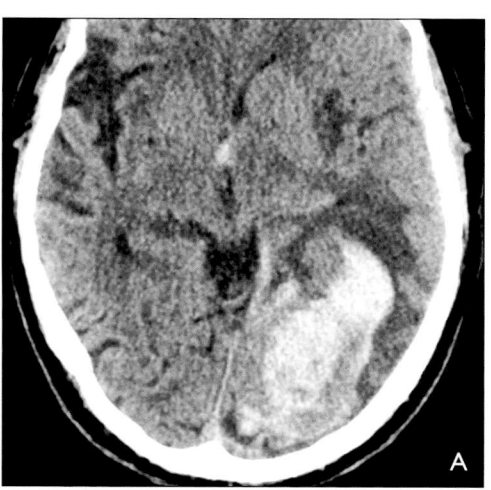
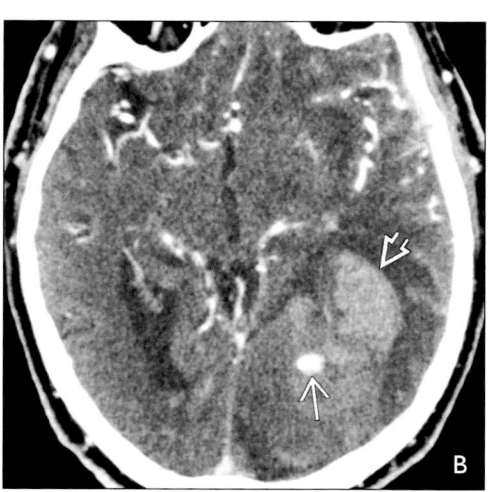

27-13A. *An 80-year-old man in the emergency department for "brain attack." NECT shows a large heterogeneously hyperdense left parietooccipital hematoma.* **27-13B.** *CT perfusion study (not shown) and CTA were performed. CTA shows a "spot" sign of contrast accumulation* ⇨ *within the expanding hematoma* ⇨. *Preoperative diagnosis was hypertensive hemorrhage with bleeding pseudoaneurysm. Actively bleeding metastatic adenocarcinoma, unknown primary, was found at surgery.*

and thus appears moderately hyperintense **(27-15)**. Subacute hemorrhagic metastases show disordered, heterogeneous signal intensity, often with bizarre-appearing intermixed foci of T1 hyper- and hypointensities **(27-16)**.

T2/FLAIR. Signal intensity on T2WI varies widely depending on tumor type, lesion cellularity, presence of hemorrhagic residua, and amount of peritumoral edema. Many metastases are very cellular neoplasms with high nuclear to cytoplasmic ratios and thus appear hypointense on T2WI and FLAIR **(27-14B)**, **(27-14C)**. Exceptions are mucinous tumors, cystic metastases, and tumors with large amounts of central necrosis, all of which can appear moderately hyperintense.

Some hyperintense metastases show little or no surrounding edema. Multiple small hyperintense metastases ("miliary metastases") can be mistaken for small vessel vascular disease unless contrast is administered.

T2*. Blood products and melanin contain metal ions including iron, copper, manganese, and zinc. Both subacute hemorrhage and melanin cause prominent signal intensity loss ("blooming") on T2* (GRE, SWI) images **(27-16)**, **(27-19)**. Nearly 75% of melanoma metastases have either T1 hyperintensity or demonstrate susceptibility effect; 25% demonstrate both. Nonhemorrhagic nonmelanotic metastases do not become hypointense on T2* **(27-15)**.

T1 C+. Virtually all nonhemorrhagic metastases enhance following contrast administration **(27-14D)**. Patterns vary from solid, uniform enhancement to nodular, "cyst + nodule," and ring-like lesions **(27-17)**, **(27-18)**. Multiple metastases in the same patient may exhibit different patterns **(27-16)**.

Longitudinal studies have demonstrated that, in older patients, multifocal hyperintensities identified on T2-weighted or FLAIR scans that do not enhance following contrast administration virtually never turn out to be metastases.

The conspicuity of metastases can be increased on T1 C+ scans with fat suppression and magnetization transfer sequences. The use of double- and even triple-dose contrast-enhanced scans has been reported to increase sensitivity but is not in standard use. Contrast-enhanced T2 FLAIR is a new technique that improves sensitivity compared to contrast-enhanced inversion recovery (IR) and IR-prepared fast spoiled gradient echo (FSPGR) sequences.

DWI. With the exception of highly cellular neoplasms such as medulloblastoma and lymphoma, most *primary* brain tumors do not show restriction on DWI. Metastasis behavior on diffusion-weighted imaging is much more unpredictable. Well-differentiated adeno-

carcinoma metastases tend to be hypointense (nonrestricting) whereas more aggressive small and large cell neuroendocrine carcinomas are hyperintense on DWI **(27-17A)**. ADC values inversely reflect tumor cellularity, i.e., low ADC indicates high cellularity.

DTI with a combination of fractional anisotropy (FA) and ADC calculations may be helpful in distinguishing metastases from glioblastoma.

PWI. The differentiation of primary from solitary metastatic brain tumors using pMR is controversial. Some studies suggest the diagnostic accuracy of MR—including rCBV measurement—is better at grading glial neoplasms than differentiating high-grade gliomas from solitary parenchymal metastases.

MRS. Prominent lipid signal is the dominating peak on MRS in the majority of brain metastases. However, lipid signal is also common in many cellular processes including inflammation and necrosis. Choline is generally elevated, and Cr is depressed or absent in most metastases.

Molecular MR. Some MR contrast agents specifically target markers such as endothelial vascular cell adhesion molecule-1 (VICAM-1) that are upregulated in vessels associated with brain metastases. Their use may permit early detection of micrometastases before lesions become apparent on standard gadolinium-enhanced sequences.

NUCLEAR MEDICINE FINDINGS. Although it is effective for delineating systemic disease, standard PET/CT understages patients with brain metastases and fails to demonstrate a number of lesions easily detected on standard MR. Early results using new agents such as F18-DOPA show promise in detecting disease relapse after surgical treatment and/or radiotherapy.

Differential Diagnosis

The differential diagnosis of parenchymal metastases varies with imaging findings. The major differential diagnosis for punctate and ring-enhancing metastases is abscess. **Abscesses** and **septic emboli** typically restrict on DWI and show elevated amino acids and lactate on MRS.

Occasionally, **glioblastoma multiforme** (GBM) can mimic parenchymal metastases, especially a multifocal GBM with metachronous lesions or brain-to-brain tumor spread. Solitary GBM tends to be infiltrating, whereas metastases are almost always round and relatively well-demarcated. GBMs are generally solitary and preferentially located in the deep cerebral white matter whereas 50% of metastases are multiple, typically occurring at gray-white matter interfaces.

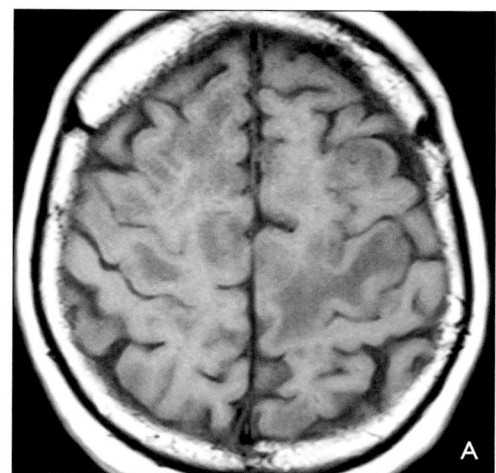

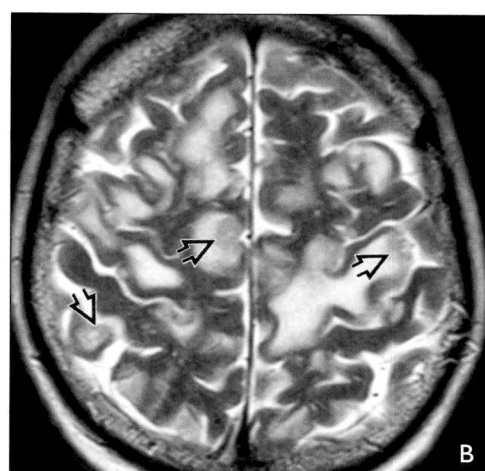

27-14A. T1WI in a 63-year-old man with a urogenital primary carcinoma and a normal scan 6 months prior to presenting with seizure. Multiple hypointensities are visible in the subcortical WM of both hemispheres. 27-14B. Iso-to slightly hyperintense nodules at the GM-WM interfaces ⊟ are surrounded by edema on this T2WI.

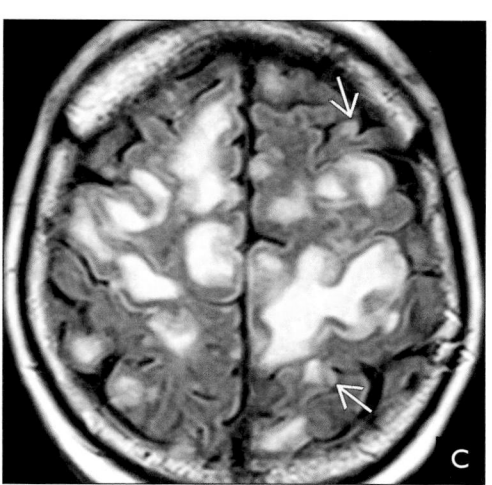

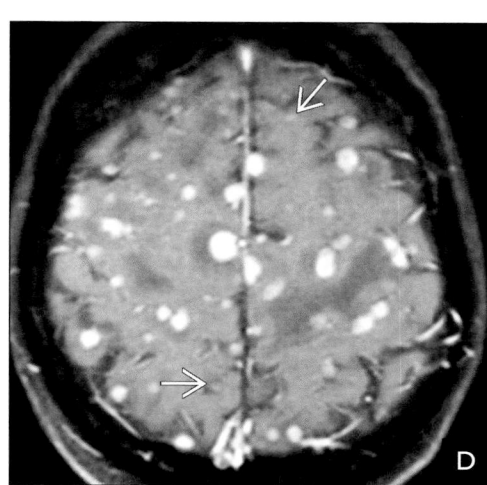

27-14C. The nodules appear hyperintense on FLAIR. Additional small lesions in the cortex-subcortical WM are seen ➡. 27-14D. The lesions enhance intensely on T1 C+ FS. A number of tiny enhancing foci ➡ that were not seen on T2 or FLAIR are identified.

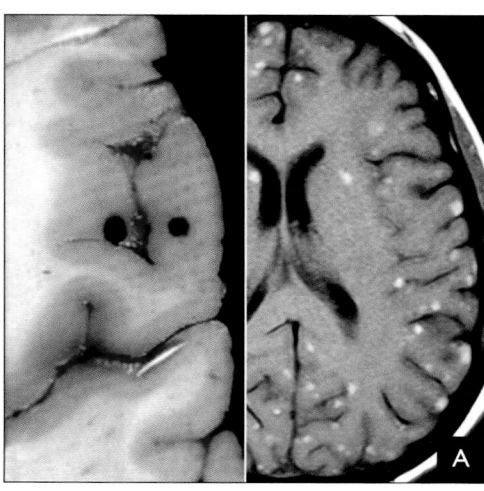

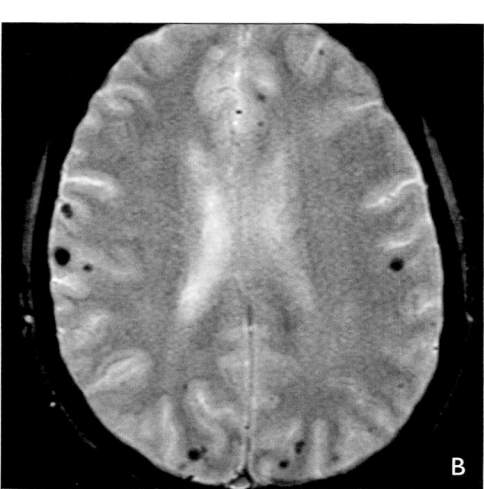

27-15A. (Left) Autopsy specimen shows typical round, black nodules in the cortex, GM-WM interface characteristic of melanoma metastases. (Right) T1WI in a patient with metastatic melanoma shows innumerable hyperintense metastases. 27-15B. T2* GRE scan in the same patient shows that only a few of the metastases visible on the T1WI "bloom," indicating that most of the T1 shortening was secondary to melanin, not subacute hemorrhage.

27-16A. *T1WI in another patient with metastatic melanoma demonstrates 3 metastases, each with a different appearance. One* ⇗ *has hemorrhages of different ages, resembles cavernous malformation. The second has central necrosis* ⇒*, and the infundibular metastasis* ⇒ *is isointense with white matter.* **27-16B.** *Slightly more cephalad T2WI in the same patient shows hemorrhage with fluid-fluid level* ⇒ *in the necrotic metastasis.*

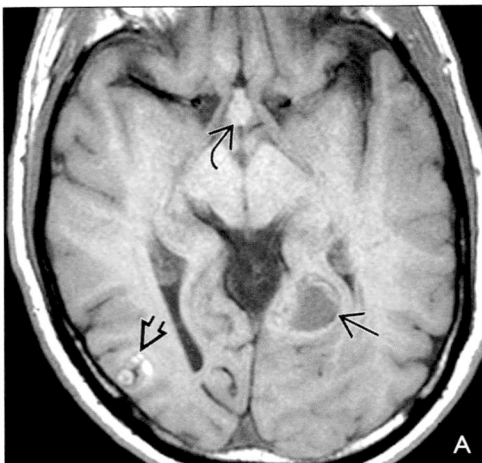
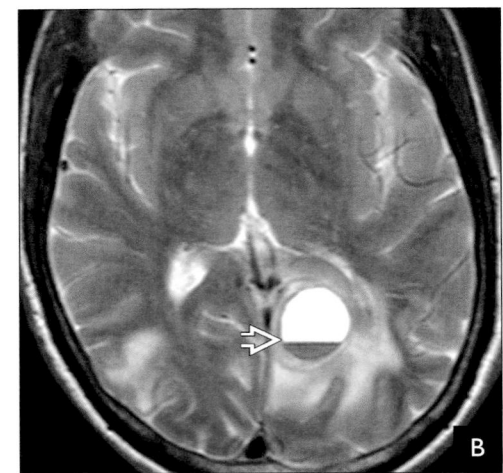

27-16C. *T2* GRE shows "blooming" around the rim of the necrotic metastasis* ⇗*, while the other hemorrhagic lesion* ⇒ *shows nearly homogeneous signal loss.* **27-16D.** *T1 C+ FS shows that the infundibular metastasis* ⇒ *enhances strongly, uniformly. The necrotic metastasis shows a "cyst + nodule" configuration* ⇒*, while the smaller hemorrhagic metastasis shows a tiny ring of enhancement* ⇒*.*

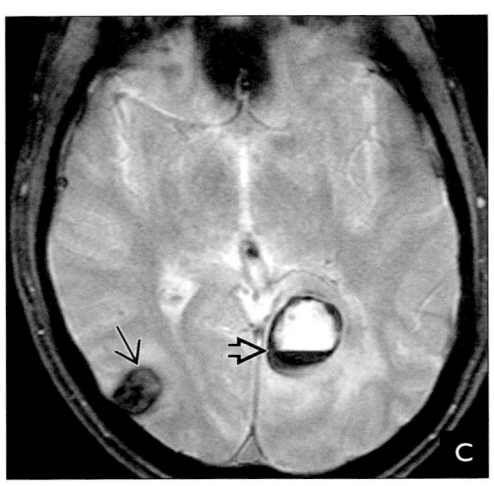
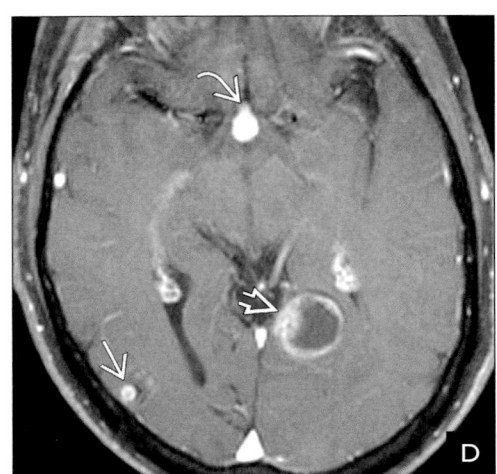

27-17A. *Two unusual cases show variant appearances of metastases. Metastases from lung carcinoma in an elderly patient appear as nonspecific T2 hyperintensities* ⇒ *but show punctate, ring enhancement on T1 C+ FS* ⇒*. Some show restriction on DWI* ⇒*.* **27-17B.** *(Left) T2WI shows infiltrating, cystic, hemorrhagic lesion* ⇒*. (Right) T1 C+ FS shows bizarre multiloculated ring enhancement* ⇒*. Preoperative diagnosis was GBM. Breast metastasis found at surgery.*

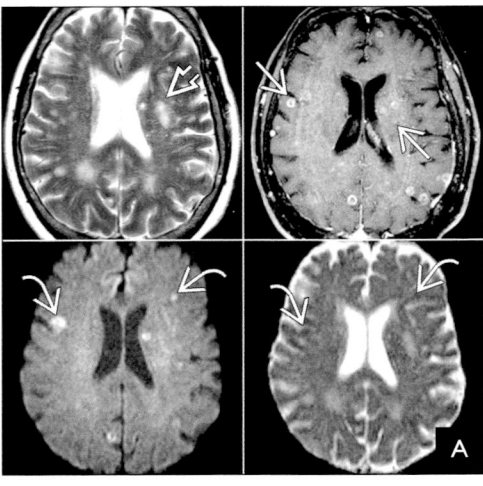
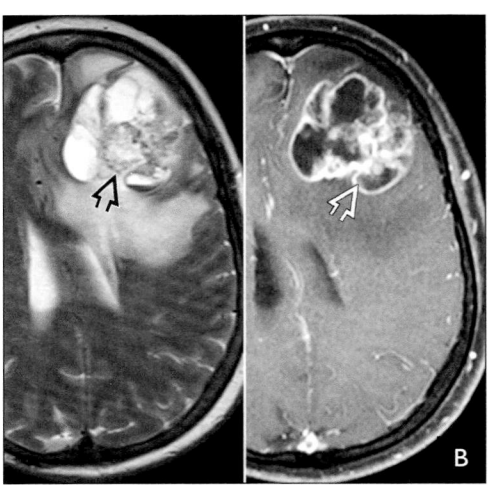

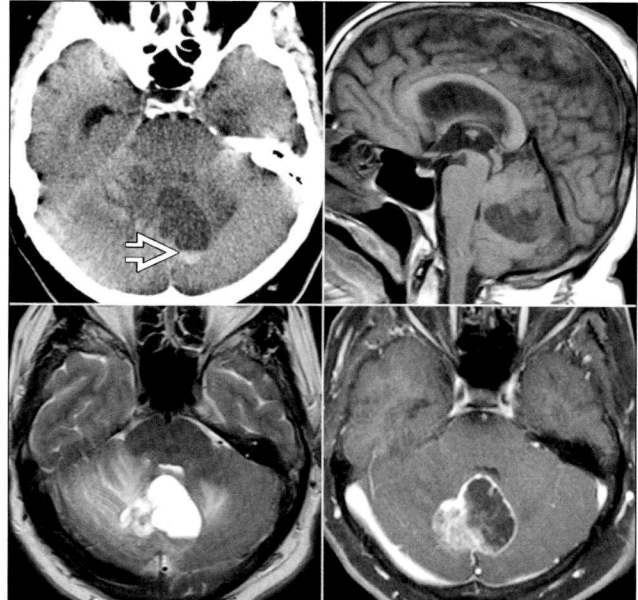

27-18. *A 63-year-old man presented with severe headaches, papilledema. NECT scan shows a solitary posterior fossa mass with hemorrhage* ➡. *MR scans show a "cyst + nodule" pattern. Adenocarcinoma, unknown primary.*

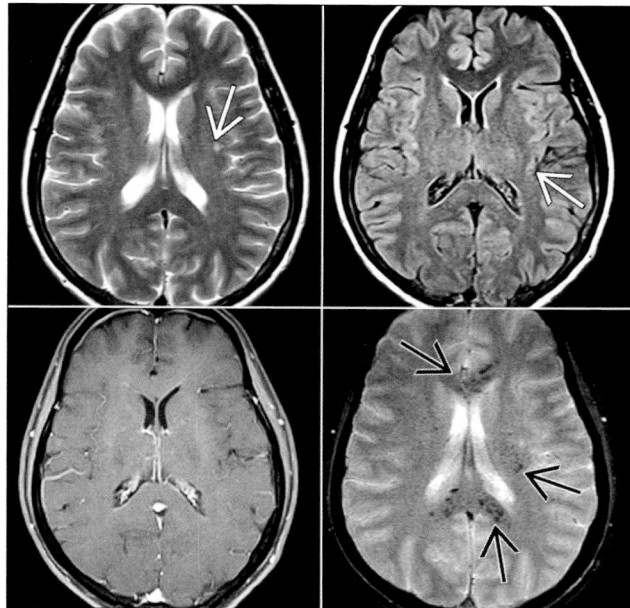

27-19. *Occasionally, metastases present with nonspecific encephalopathy. T2/FLAIR scans show a few scattered WM hyperintensities* ➡. *No definite enhancement on T1 C+, multiple "blooming" foci on T2** ➡. *Metastases from breast primary.*

Primary infratentorial parenchymal brain tumors in adults are rare. No matter what the imaging findings are, *a solitary cerebellar mass in a middle-aged or older adult should be considered a metastasis until proved otherwise!* Even with a "cyst + nodule" appearance, which is classic for **hemangioblastoma**, metastasis should still be at the top of the differential diagnosis list.

Both metastases and **multiple embolic infarcts** share a predilection for arterial "border zones" and the gray-white matter interfaces. Most acute infarcts restrict strongly on DWI and rarely demonstrate a ring-enhancing pattern on T1 C+ scans. Chronic infarcts and age-related **small vessel microvascular disease** are hyperintense on T2WI and do not enhance following contrast administration.

Multiple sclerosis (MS) occurs in younger patients and is preferentially located in the deep periventricular white matter. An incomplete ring or "horseshoe" pattern of enhancement is more characteristic of MS and other demyelinating disorders than of metastasis.

Multiple **cavernous angiomas** can mimic hemorrhagic metastases. Hemorrhagic metastases generally show disordered evolution of blood products and an incomplete hemosiderin rim.

PARENCHYMAL METASTASES: IMAGING

CT
- Variable density (most iso-, hypodense)
- Most enhance on CECT
- Perform bone CT for calvarial, skull base metastases

T1WI
- Most metastases: Iso- to slightly hypointense
- Melanoma metastases: Hyperintense
- Hemorrhagic metastases: Heterogeneously hyperintense

T2/FLAIR
- Varies with tumor type, cellularity, hemorrhage
- Most common: Iso- to mildly hyperintense
- Can resemble small vessel vascular disease

T2*
- Subacute blood, melanin "bloom"

T1 C+
- Almost all nonhemorrhagic metastases enhance strongly
- Solid, punctate, ring, "cyst + nodule"

DWI
- Variable; most common: No restriction
- Highly cellular metastases may restrict

MRS
- Most prominent feature: Lipid peak
- Elevated Cho, depressed/absent Cr

Differential Diagnosis
- Most common: Abscess, septic emboli
- Less common
  - Glioblastoma multiforme
  - Multiple embolic infarcts
  - Small vessel (microvascular) disease
  - Demyelinating disease
  - Multiple cavernous malformations

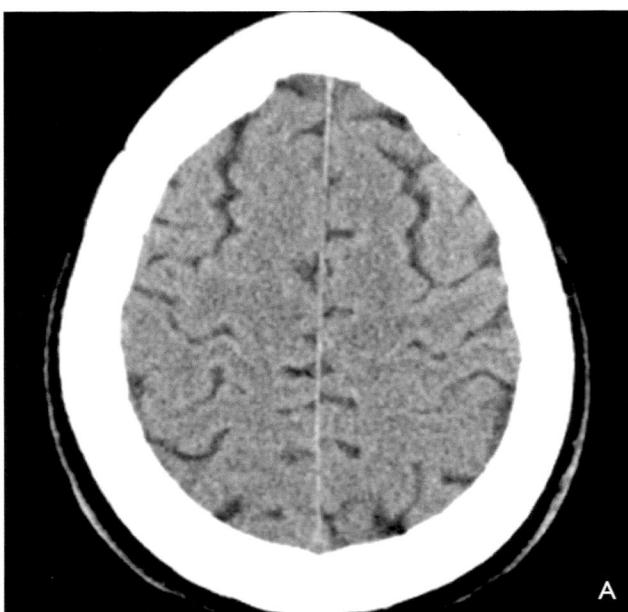

27-20A. NECT scan with a soft tissue algorithm reconstruction, soft tissue windows (80 HU) shows no abnormalities in this 53-year-old man with headaches.

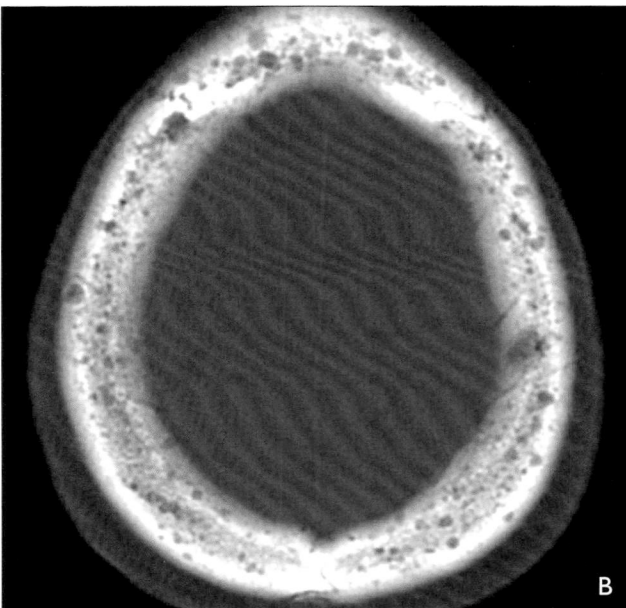

27-20B. Bone algorithm reconstruction shows innumerable well-defined lytic lesions in the skull. Multiple myeloma.

Skull and Dural Metastases

Terminology

The term "skull" refers both to the calvaria and to the skull base. As one cannot distinguish neoplastic involvement of the periosteal versus meningeal dural layers, we refer to these layers collectively as the "dura." The arachnoid—the outermost layer of the leptomeninges—adheres to the dura, so it too is almost always involved any time tumor invades the dura. For purposes of discussion, these structures are collectively referred to as the dura-arachnoid.

Overview

The skull and dura are the second most common sites of CNS metastases from extracranial primary tumors. Calvarial and skull base metastases and can occur either with or without dural involvement.

In contrast, dural metastases (DMs) without coexisting calvarial lesions are less common. Between 8-10% of patients with advanced systemic cancer have DMs. Breast (35%) and prostate (15-20%) cancers are the most frequent sources. Single lesions are slightly more common than multiple DMs.

Imaging

GENERAL FEATURES. Solitary or multiple focal lesions involve the skull, dura-arachnoid, or both. A less common pattern is diffuse neoplastic dura-arachnoid thicken-

ing, seen as a curvilinear layer of tumor that follows the inner table of the calvaria.

CT FINDINGS. Complete evaluation requires *both* soft tissue and bone algorithm reconstructions of the imaging data **(27-20)**. Scans with soft tissue reconstruction obscure skull lesions, which may be invisible unless bone algorithms are utilized. Soft tissue scans viewed with bone windows do not provide sufficient detail for adequate assessment.

NECT. Large dural metastases displace the brain inward, buckling the gray-white matter interface medially. Hypodensities in the underlying brain suggest parenchymal invasion or venous ischemia.

Bone CT usually demonstrates one or more relatively circumscribed intraosseous lesions. Permeative, diffusely destructive lesions are the second most common pattern. A few osseous metastases—mostly those from prostate and treated breast cancer—can be blastic and sclerotic.

CECT. The most common finding is a focal soft tissue mass centered on the diploic space. A biconvex shape with both subgaleal and dural extension is typical **(27-21)**. Most dural metastases enhance strongly.

MR FINDINGS.

T1WI. Hyperintense fat in the diploic space provides excellent, naturally occurring demarcation from skull metastases. Metastases replace hyperintense yellow marrow and appear as hypointense infiltrating foci **(27-22)**. Dural metastases thicken the dura-arachnoid and are typ-

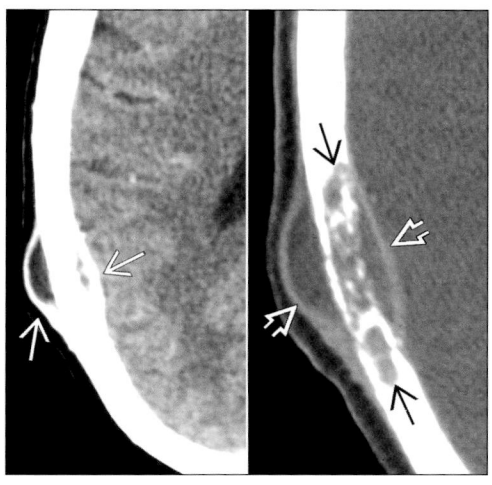

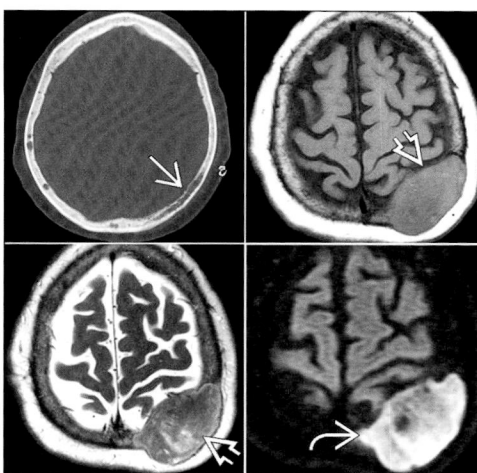

27-21. (Left) CECT scan with soft tissue windows shows a lesion ➡ centered on the diploic space of the calvaria. (Right) Intermediate windows show the extent of the lytic, destructive metastasis ⇥, better delineate the subgaleal and extradural components ⇒. *27-22.* Metastatic breast carcinoma to the skull, dura is seen as a permeative destructive lesion in the left parietal diploe ⇥. The lesion is mostly isointense to brain on T1-, T2WI ⇥ and restricts on DWI ➡.

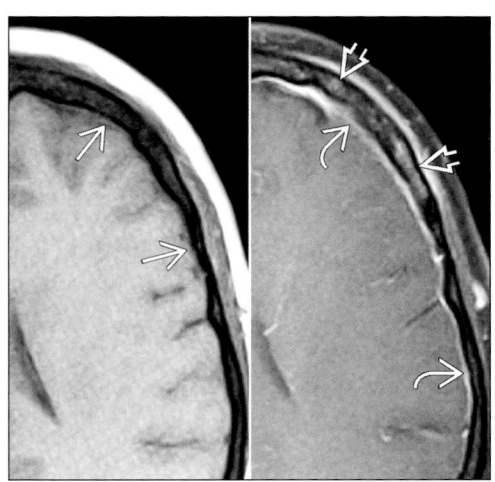

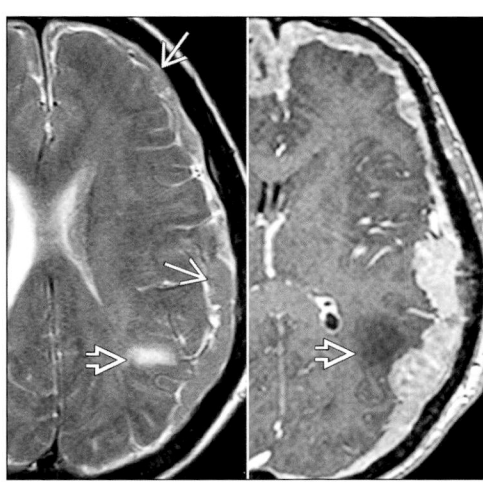

27-23. (Left) Subtle dura-arachnoid metastasis is seen here as mild thickening ⇥. (Right) Thickened dura ⇒ enhances on T1 C+ FS. Enhancing lesions in the diploic space can now be identified ⇥. *27-24.* Metastases from prostate cancer thicken the dura, fill the subarachnoid space ⇥. Edema ⇒ indicates infiltration along the perivascular spaces into the brain parenchyma. (Courtesy N. Agarwal, MD.)

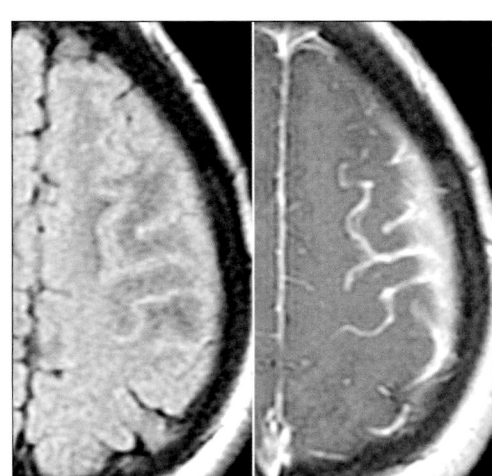

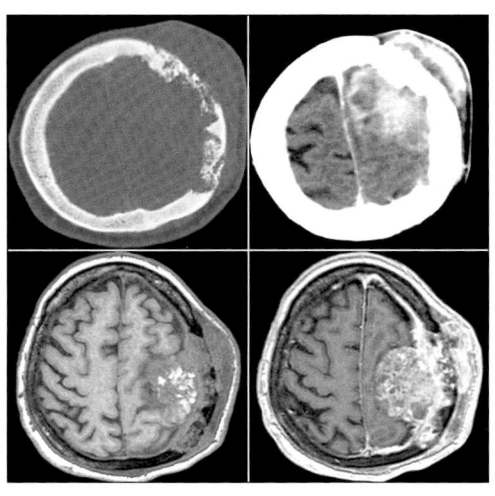

27-25. Dura-arachnoid metastasis from Waldenström macroglobulinemia extends into the subarachnoid space, effaces the sulci. (Courtesy P. Hildenbrand, MD.) *27-26.* Extensive calvarial, scalp, dural metastasis from lung carcinoma is illustrated.

ically iso- or hypointense to underlying cortex (27-23), (27-24).

T2/FLAIR. Most skull metastases are hyperintense to marrow on T2WI, but the signal intensity of dural metastases varies. FLAIR hyperintensity in the underlying sulci suggests pia-subarachnoid tumor spread (27-25). Hyperintensity in the underlying brain is present in half of all cases and suggests either tumor invasion along the perivascular spaces or compromise of venous drainage.

T1 C+. Nearly 70% of dural metastases are accompanied by metastases in the overlying skull (27-26). Involvement of the adjacent scalp is also common. Contrast-enhanced T1WI should be performed with fat saturation (T1 C+ FS) for optimal delineation as some calvarial lesions may enhance just enough to become isointense with fat.

Most DMs enhance strongly, appearing as biconvex masses centered along the adjacent diploic space. Dural "tails" are present in about half of all cases. Frank tumor invasion into the underlying brain is seen in one-third. Dural thickening can be smooth and diffuse or nodular and mass-like.

DWI. Hypercellular metastases with enlarged nuclei and reduced extracellular matrix may show diffusion restriction (hyperintense) and decreased ADC values (hypointense).

NUCLEAR MEDICINE FINDINGS. Skull metastases are intensely positive on Tc-99m scan. Integrated FDG PET/CT scans have a very high positive predictive value for bone metastases, including calvarial lesions. Dural lesions are less well-visualized.

Differential Diagnosis

The differential diagnosis of skull and dura-arachnoid metastases depends on which compartment is involved and whether solitary or multiple lesions are present.

The major differential diagnoses for skull metastases are surgical defects and normal structures. A **surgical defect** such as a burr hole or craniotomy can be distinguished from a metastasis by clinical history and the presence of defects in the overlying scalp. **Venous lakes**, **vascular grooves**, **arachnoid granulations**, and sometimes even **sutures** can mimic calvarial metastases. Normal structures are typically well-corticated, and the underlying dura is normal.

Myeloma can be indistinguishable from multiple lytic skull metastases. Skull base **osteomyelitis** is a rare but life-threatening infection that can resemble diffuse skull base metastases. ADC values are generally higher in infection than in malignant neoplasms.

The major differential diagnosis for solitary or multifocal dura-arachnoid metastases is **meningioma**. Metastases, especially from breast cancer, can be virtually indistinguishable from solitary or multiple meningiomas on the basis of imaging studies alone.

The differential diagnosis of diffuse dura-arachnoid thickening is much broader. Nonneoplastic pachymeningopathies such as meningitis, chronic subdural hematoma, and intracranial hypotension can all cause diffuse dura-arachnoid thickening. Metastatic dural thickening is generally—although not invariably—more "lumpy-bumpy" (27-23), (27-24).

SKULL/DURA-ARACHNOID METASTASES

General Features
- Second most common site of CNS metastases
- Skull alone or skull + dura > > isolated dural metastases
- "Dural" metastases usually dura *plus* arachnoid

CT
- Use both soft tissue, bone reconstructions
- Skull: Permeative lytic lesion(s)
- Scalp, dura: Biconvex mass centered on skull

MR
- T1WI: Metastases replace hyperintense fat
- T2WI: Most skull metastases hyperintense
- FLAIR: Look for
  - Underlying sulcal hyperintensity (suggests pia-subarachnoid space tumor)
  - Parenchymal hyperintensity (suggests brain invasion along perivascular spaces)
- T1 C+
  - Use fat-saturation sequence
  - Skull/scalp/dural lesion(s) can be focal or diffuse, enhance strongly
  - "Dural tail" sign (50%)
  - Less common: Diffuse dura-arachnoid thickening ("lumpy-bumpy" or smooth)
- DWI: Hypercellular metastases may restrict

Differential Diagnosis
- Skull metastases
  - Surgical defect, venous lakes/arachnoid granulations
  - Myeloma
  - Osteomyelitis
- Dural metastases
  - Meningioma (solitary or multiple)

Leptomeningeal Metastases

Leptomeningeal cancer dissemination is a metastatic complication with growing impact in clinical oncology. Recent advances in therapeutic management have been achieved, so early diagnosis is critical for optimal treatment. In addition to CSF examination, contrast-enhanced MR of the entire neuraxis is recommended for complete pre-treatment evaluation.

Terminology

The anatomic term "leptomeninges" refers to both the arachnoid *and* the pia. The widely used term "leptomeningeal metastases" is technically incorrect, as it is employed to designate the imaging pattern seen when tumor involves the pia and subarachnoid spaces (27-27). Arachnoid metastases are almost always secondary to dura involvement and look quite different (27-28).

For purposes of this discussion, pia-subarachnoid space metastases are referred to as leptomeningeal metastases (LMs). Other synonyms include meningeal carcinomatosis, neoplastic meningitis, and carcinomatous meningitis.

Epidemiology and Etiology

Leptomeningeal metastases are uncommon, seen in only 5% of patients with **systemic cancers** (27-9). The most common extracranial primary tumor causing LM is breast cancer. The second most common source is small cell lung carcinoma.

Intracranial primary tumors more commonly cause LM. In adults, the two most common are glioblastoma and lymphoma (27-29). The most common sources of childhood LM are primitive neuroectodermal tumor (PNET), medulloblastoma, ependymoma, and germinoma.

Imaging

GENERAL FEATURES. In contrast to dura-arachnoid metastases that "hug" the inner table of the calvaria, leptomeningeal metastases follow the brain surfaces, curving along gyri and dipping into the sulci. The general appearance on contrast-enhanced scans is as though the CSF "turns white" (27-29).

CT FINDINGS. NECT scans may be normal or show only mild hydrocephalus. Subtle sulcal-cisternal effacement with nearly isodense infiltrates can be seen replacing the hypodense CSF in some cases.

CECT scans may also be normal. Sulcal-cisternal enhancement, especially at the base of the brain, can be seen in some cases.

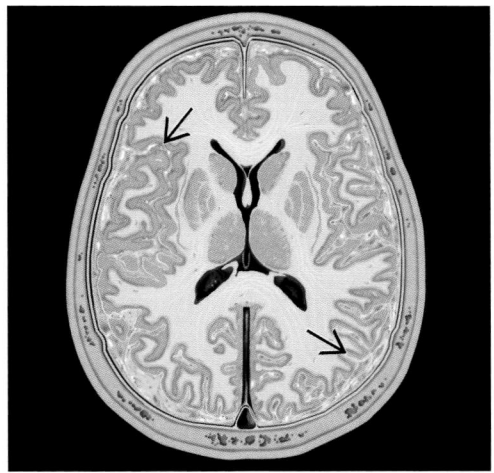
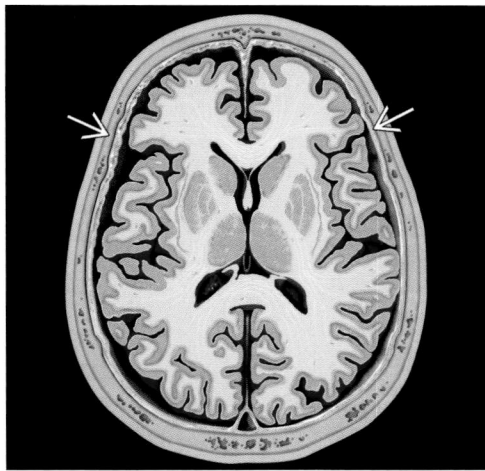

27-27. Series of 2 drawings displays the difference in imaging patterns between pia-arachnoid ("leptomeningeal") and dura-arachnoid metastases on contrast-enhanced scans. This graphic depicts pia-subarachnoid space metastases in white, covering the brain surface, sulci and filling the subarachnoid spaces ➡. 27-28. This graphic depicts dura-arachnoid metastases as curvilinear thickening that follows the inner table of the skull ➡.

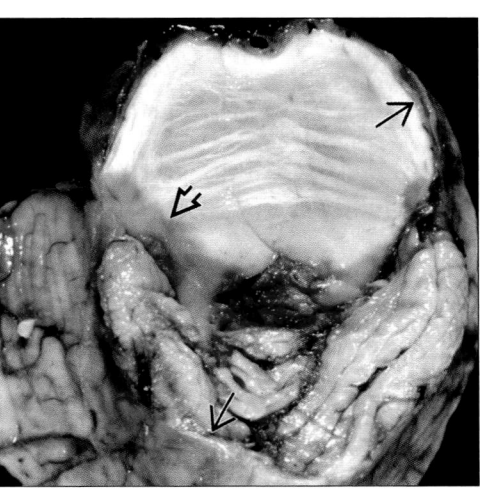
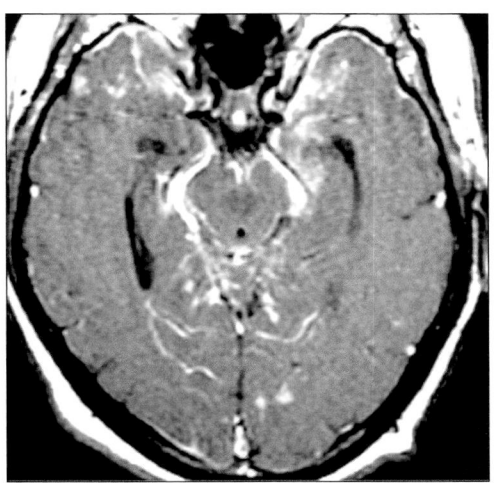

27-29. Autopsy specimen shows diffuse leptomeningeal metastases that look like "sugar icing" coating the brain surfaces ➡, filling the subarachnoid spaces ➡. Glioblastoma in adults and medulloblastoma in children are common causes of this pattern. 27-30. T1 C+ scan shows diffuse linear and nodular metastases from breast carcinoma coating the brain surfaces, filling the subarachnoid spaces.

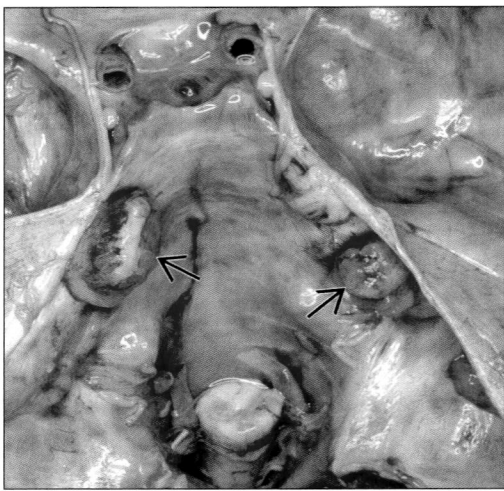

27-31. Autopsy specimen shows bilateral IAC/CPA metastases to CNs VII, VIII ▷. Colon carcinoma. (Courtesy R. Hewlett, MD.)

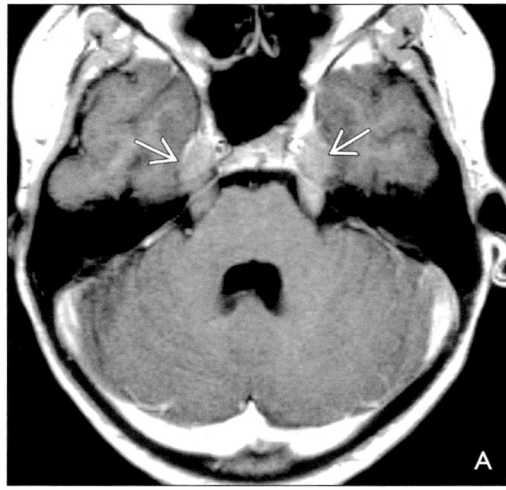

27-32A. Axial T1 C+ scan shows that the cisternal, Meckel cave segments of both trigeminal nerves are thickened, enhance ▷.

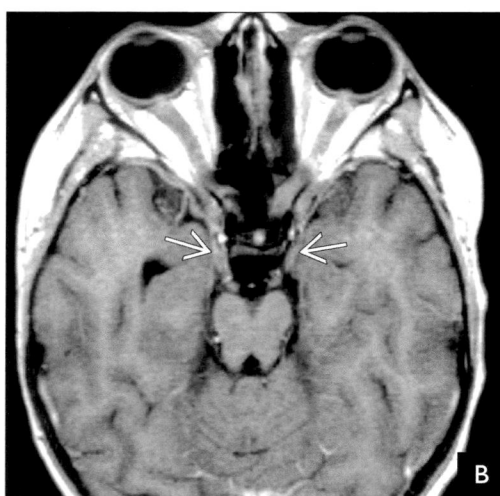

27-32B. Axial T1 C+ scan in the same patient shows that both oculomotor nerves are also thickened ▷. Acute lymphoblastic leukemia.

MR FINDINGS. T1 scans may be normal or show only smudged "dirty" CSF. Most LMs are hyperintense on T2WI and may be indistinguishable from normal CSF.

FLAIR imaging shows loss of CSF suppression, resulting in nonspecific sulcal-cisternal hyperintensity. If tumor has extended from the pia into the perivascular spaces, underlying brain parenchyma may show hyperintense vasogenic edema.

Post-contrast T1 scans show meningitis-like findings. Smooth or nodular enhancement seems to coat the brain surface and sometimes almost entirely fills the subarachnoid spaces (27-30). Cranial nerve thickening with linear, nodular, or focal mass-like enhancement may occur with or without disseminated disease (27-31), (27-32).

Tiny enhancing miliary nodules or linear enhancing foci in the cortex and subcortical white matter indicate extension along the penetrating perivascular spaces.

Differential Diagnosis

The major differential diagnosis of leptomeningeal metastases is **infectious meningitis**. It may be difficult or impossible to distinguish between carcinomatous and infectious meningitis on the basis of imaging findings alone. Other diagnostic considerations include **neurosarcoid**. Clinical history and laboratory features are essential elements in establishing the correct diagnosis.

LEPTOMENINGEAL METASTASES

General Features
- Pia + subarachnoid space metastases
- Uncommon
  - 5% of systemic cancers
  - More common with primary brain tumors (e.g., GBM, PNET, germinoma)

CT
- NECT: May be normal ± mild hydrocephalus
- CECT: Sulcal-cisternal enhancement (looks like pyogenic meningitis)

MR
- T1WI: Normal or "dirty" CSF
- T2WI: Usually normal
- FLAIR: Sulcal-cisternal hyperintensity (nonspecific)
- T1 C+: Sulcal-cisternal enhancement (nonspecific)

Differential Diagnosis
- Meningitis
- Neurosarcoid

Miscellaneous Metastases

The three areas covered above (brain parenchyma, skull/dura-arachnoid, and pia-subarachnoid spaces) are—by far—the most common sites for CNS metastatic deposits. Nevertheless, there are several "secret" sites that may also harbor metastases. The CSF, ventricles and choroid plexus, pituitary gland/infundibular stalk, pineal gland,

and eye are less obvious places where intracranial metastases occur and may escape detection **(27-33)**. In this section, we briefly consider the location and imaging appearances of these metastases.

CSF Metastases

Circulating tumors cells in the CSF can be difficult to detect using routine cytological examination and are typically identified on imaging studies in the later stages of disease dissemination.

Both extra- and intracranial metastases can seed the CSF. Intracranial CSF metastases are usually seen as "dirty" CSF on T1WI and FLAIR, often occurring together with diffuse pial spread. "Drop metastases" into the spinal subarachnoid space are a manifestation of generalized CSF spread.

Ependymal spread around the ventricular walls occurs with primary CNS tumors much more often than with extracranial sources.

Ventricles/Choroid Plexus Metastases

LOCATION. The lateral ventricle choroid plexus (CP) is the most common site for ventricular metastases, followed by the third ventricle. Only 0.5% of ventricular metastases occur in the fourth ventricle. Solitary CP metastases are more common than multiple lesions. CP metastases usually occur in the presence of multiple metastases elsewhere in the brain. Occasionally, a metastatic deposit can lodge in the choroid plexus before parenchymal lesions become apparent.

CLINICAL ISSUES. Intraventricular metastases from extracranial malignancies are rare, accounting for just 1-5% of cerebral metastases and 6% of all intraventricular tumors. Most involve the choroid plexus **(27-35)**; the ventricular ependyma is affected less frequently **(27-36)**.

The most common primary sources in adults are renal cell carcinoma and lung cancer. Melanoma, stomach and colon cancers, and lymphoma are less common causes of CP metastases. Neuroblastoma, Wilms tumor, and retinoblastoma are the most common primary tumors in children. Prognosis is generally poor with most patients

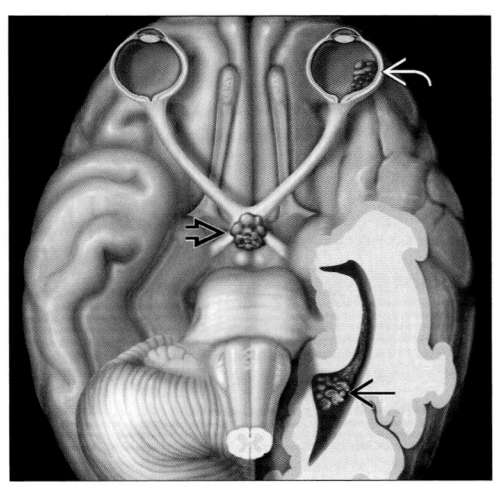
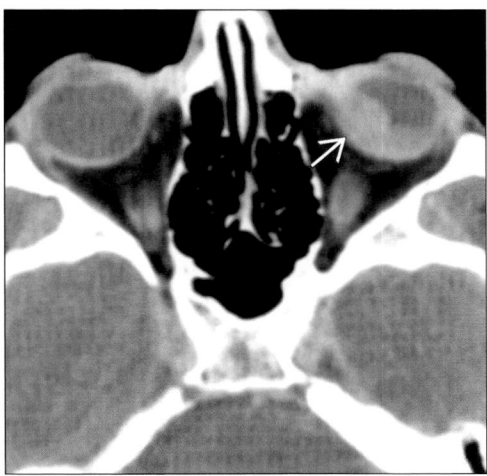

27-33. Submentovertex graphic shows the typical sites for miscellaneous nonparenchymal CNS metastases. These include the choroid plexus and ventricles ⇥, pituitary gland, infundibular stalk ⇛, and eye (choroid of the retina) ⇗. 27-34. CECT scan shows a lobulated enhancing mass in the posterior segment of the left globe ⇥. Metastatic breast carcinoma.

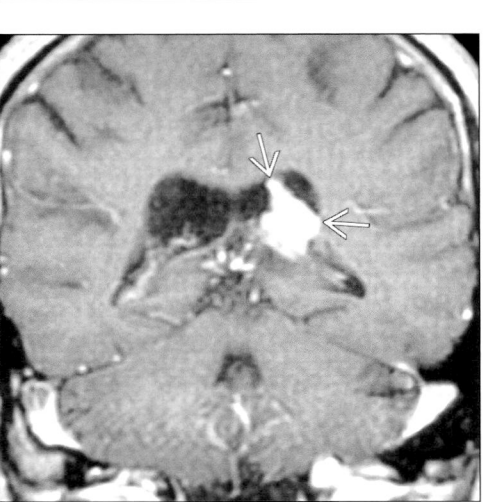
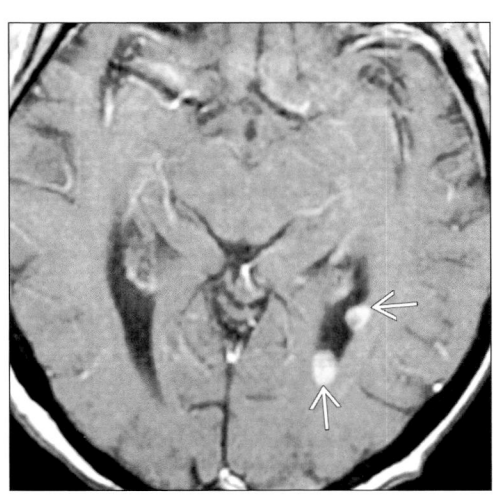

27-35. Coronal T1 C+ scan shows an enlarged, intensely enhancing glomus of the left choroid plexus ⇥. Metastatic breast carcinoma. 27-36. Axial T1 C+ scan in another patient shows 2 enhancing ependymal nodules ⇥. Metastatic breast carcinoma.

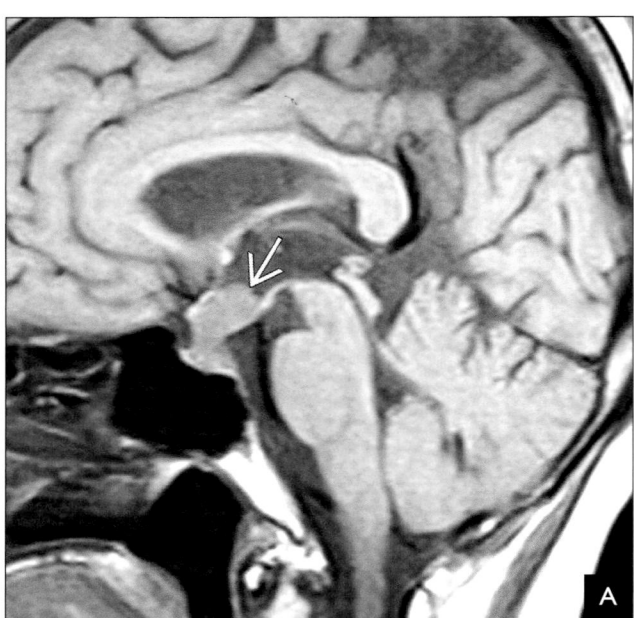

27-37A. Sagittal T1WI shows an infiltrating mass in the hypothalamus and infundibular stalk ➔.

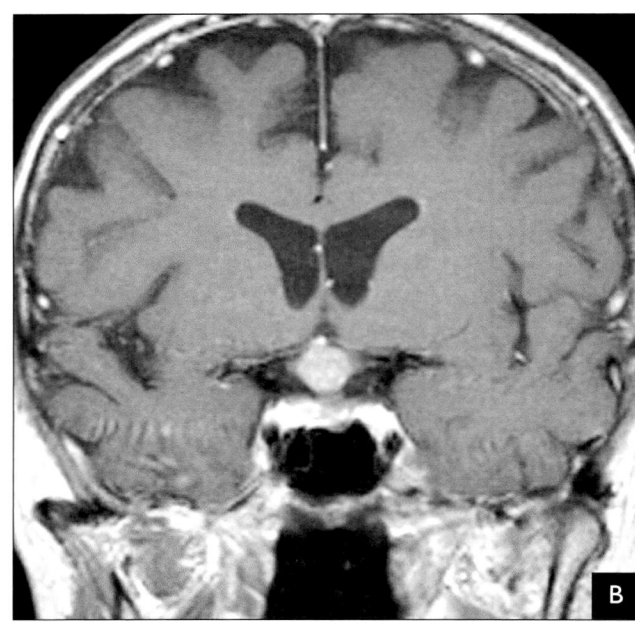

27-37B. T1 C+ shows that the mass enhances intensely, uniformly. Metastatic breast cancer.

succumbing to systemic disease progression or to multi-focal CNS disease.

IMAGING. CP metastases enlarge the choroid plexus and are iso- to hyperdense compared to normal choroid plexus on NECT scans. They enhance strongly but heterogeneously.

Choroid plexus metastases are often hypervascular, so hemorrhage is quite common. Most nonhemorrhagic CP metastases are hypointense to brain on T1WI and hyperintense on T2/FLAIR. Intense enhancement following contrast administration is typical. CP metastases display a prolonged vascular "blush" on DSA.

DIFFERENTIAL DIAGNOSIS. In an older patient (especially one with known systemic cancer such as renal cell carcinoma), the differential diagnosis of a choroid plexus mass should always include metastasis. Other common choroid plexus lesions in older patients are **meningioma** and **choroid plexus xanthogranuloma**. Choroid plexus meningiomas enhance strongly and generally uniformly. Choroid plexus cysts (xanthogranulomas) are usually bilateral, multicystic-appearing lesions.

While solitary metastasis to the third ventricle is rare, metastatic deposit to the choroid plexus in the foramen of Monro may mimic **colloid cyst**. Although the wall of a colloid cyst occasionally demonstrates rim enhancement, solid enhancement almost never occurs.

Pituitary Gland/Infundibular Stalk Metastases

CLINICAL ISSUES. Metastasis causes approximately 1% of all resected pituitary tumors and is found in 1-2% of autopsies. Breast and lung primaries account for two-thirds of cases, followed by GI tract adenocarcinomas. Most pituitary metastases involve the posterior lobe, probably because of its direct systemic arterial supply via the hypophyseal arteries (the anterior pituitary is mostly supplied by the hypophyseal portal venous system). Coexisting brain metastases are common, but solitary lesions do occur.

Signs and symptoms such as headache and visual disturbances can mimic those of pituitary macroadenoma, although they often progress much more rapidly in patients with metastases. Clinical diabetes insipidus is common.

IMAGING. A sellar mass with or without bone erosion, stalk thickening, loss of posterior pituitary "bright spot," and cavernous sinus invasion is typical but nonspecific. So too is an infiltrating pituitary and/or stalk mass with cysts, hemorrhage, and heterogeneous enhancement **(27-37)**. MR findings are nonspecific and closely resemble those of pituitary macroadenoma.

DIFFERENTIAL DIAGNOSIS. The major differential diagnosis of pituitary metastasis is **macroadenoma**. Macroadenomas rarely present with diabetes insipidus. In the setting of a known systemic cancer, rapid growth of a pituitary mass with onset of clinical diabetes insipidus

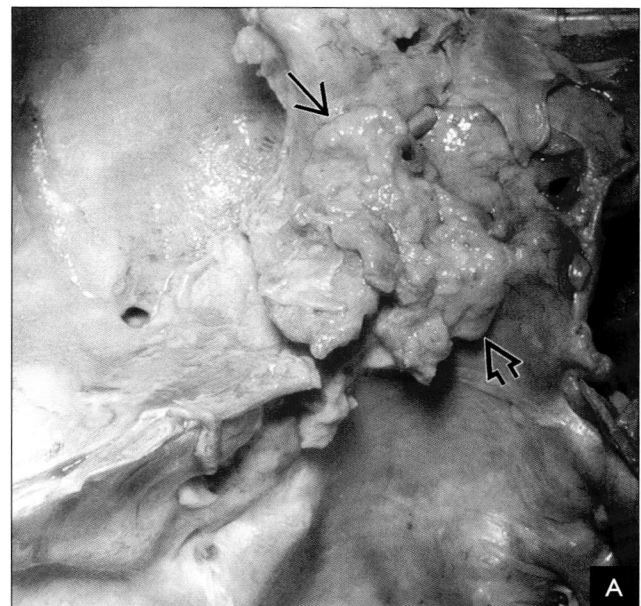

27-38A. Autopsy specimen shows nasopharyngeal squamous cell carcinoma extending cephalad, eroding through the central skull base into the cavernous sinus ⇒ and sellar floor ⧕.

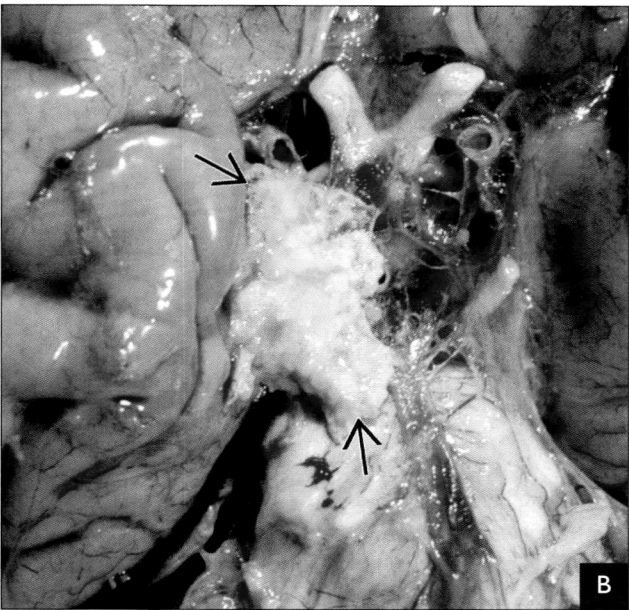

27-38B. Tumor extends from the cavernous sinus along CN III into the suprasellar, prepontine cistern ⇒. (Courtesy R. Hewlett, MD.)

is highly suggestive but certainly not diagnostic of metastasis. **Lymphocytic hypophysitis** can also resemble pituitary metastasis on imaging studies.

Pineal Gland Metastases

While the pineal gland is a relatively common source of primary CNS tumors that seed the CSF, it is one of the rarest sites to harbor a metastasis. Only 0.3% of intracranial metastases involve the pineal gland. Lung, breast, skin (melanoma), and kidney are the most frequent sources. When pineal metastases do occur, they are usually solitary lesions without evidence of metastatic deposits elsewhere and are indistinguishable on imaging studies from primary pineal neoplasms.

Ocular Metastases

CLINICAL ISSUES. Metastases to the eye are rare. The highly vascular uveal tract is the most common location if metastases are present. Within the uvea, the choroid is by far the most commonly affected site, accounting for nearly 90% of all ocular metastases. The iris (8-9%) and the ciliary body (2%) are other possible locations.

Breast cancer is the most common cause of ocular metastases, followed by lung cancer. The diagnosis of ocular metastases is based on clinical findings supplemented by imaging studies.

IMAGING. CT and MR findings are nonspecific, demonstrating a posterior segment mass that often enhances strongly after contrast administration **(27-34)**. Whole-brain imaging is recommended as 20-25% of patients with choroidal metastases have concurrent CNS lesions.

DIFFERENTIAL DIAGNOSIS. The differential diagnosis of choroidal metastasis includes other hyperdense posterior segment masses. Primary **choroidal melanoma** and **hemangioma** may appear similar on both CT and MR. Both metastasis and melanoma can penetrate the Bruch membrane. Ocular ultrasound may be helpful in diagnosing hemangioma. Melanoma and metastases may incite **hemorrhagic choroidal** or **retinal detachment**.

Direct Geographic Spread from Head and Neck Neoplasms

Cephalad spread from head and neck neoplasms such as **sinonasal squamous cell carcinoma, adenoid cystic carcinoma, non-Hodgkin lymphoma,** and **esthesioneuroblastoma** may extend intracranially. This direct extension is also called geographic or regional spread.

Sinonasal tumors gain access to the cranial cavity in three ways: (1) erosion superiorly through the relatively weak bone of the cribriform plate into the anterior cranial fossa, (2) direct extension into the pterygopalatine fossa (PTPF) with posterior spread into the cavernous sinus **(27-38)**, and (3) perineural tumor spread into the PTPF, cavernous sinus, and Meckel cave. We now briefly discuss sinonasal squamous cell carcinoma as the prototypical head and neck neoplasm with geographic intracranial spread. Perineural tumor spread is considered separately below.

Sinonasal Squamous Cell Carcinoma

Squamous cell carcinoma (SCCa) is an aggressive malignant epithelial tumor with squamous cell or epidermoid differentiation. SCCa is the most common sinonasal malignancy, accounting for 3% of all head and neck neoplasms. Almost all sinonasal SCCas occur in patients older than 40, with peak prevalence at 50-70 years. There is a moderate male predominance. Most patients present with symptoms of sinusitis refractory to medical therapy.

Risk factors for developing sinonasal SCCa include inhaled wood dust, metallic particles, and some chemicals. There is *no* direct link to smoking.

PATHOLOGY. Nearly three-quarters of sinonasal squamous cell carcinomas arise in the sinuses whereas 25-30% arise primarily in the nose. The maxillary antrum is the most common site for sinonasal SCCa overall. Approximately 10% of sinus SCCas arise in the ethmoid sinuses.

Sinonasal SCCa that involves the brain is classified according to American Joint Committee on Cancer (AJCC) criteria rather than given a WHO grade. Nasal-

ethmoidal SCCa that invades the cribriform plate is considered a T3 tumor. If the anterior cranial fossa is involved, the tumor is a T4a lesion. T4b tumors involve the dura, brain, middle cranial fossa, clivus, or cranial nerves other than the mandibular nerve (CN V_3).

IMAGING. CT scans show a solid mass with irregular margins and bone destruction. Sinonasal SCCa is isointense with mucosa on T1WI and mildly to moderately hypointense on T2WI.

SCCa shows mild to moderate enhancement following contrast administration but enhances to a lesser extent than adenocarcinoma, esthesioneuroblastoma, and melanoma. Axial and sagittal T1 C+ fat-saturated images are recommended to detect perineural tumor spread (see below). Coronal T1 C+ FS images are recommended to delineate extension through the cribriform plate into the anterior cranial fossae **(27-39)**.

DIFFERENTIAL DIAGNOSIS. The differential diagnosis of sinonasal SCCa with intracranial extension includes **other malignancies** such as sinonasal adenocarcinoma, undifferentiated carcinoma, and non-Hodgkin

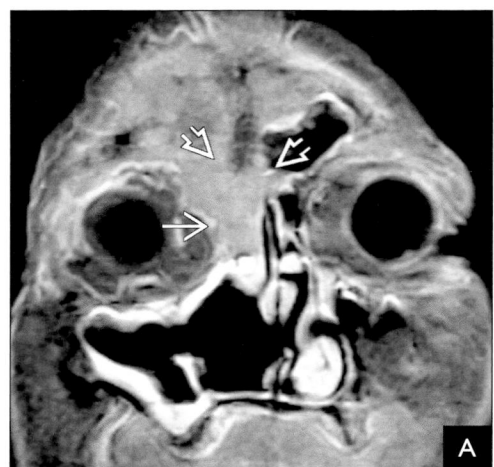
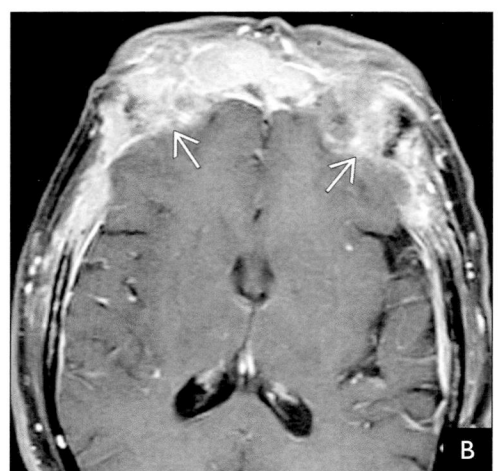

27-39A. Recurrent nasopharyngeal SCCa shows cephalad extension into the right ethmoid sinus ⇨, both anterior cranial fossae ⇨. 27-39B. Axial T1 C+ FS scan shows the massive extension of tumor into the frontal sinuses. The frontal bones are completely eroded. The dura is thickened and disrupted ⇨ with tumor extending into and obliterating the underlying subarachnoid space.

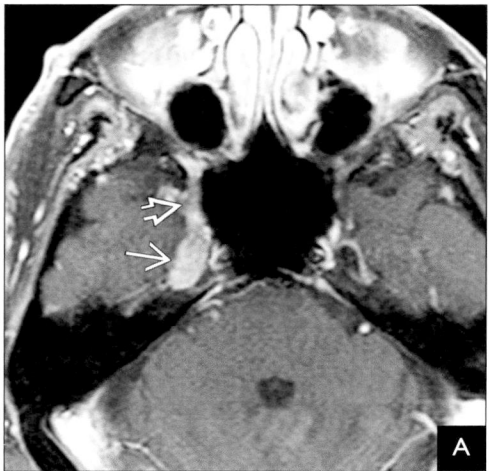
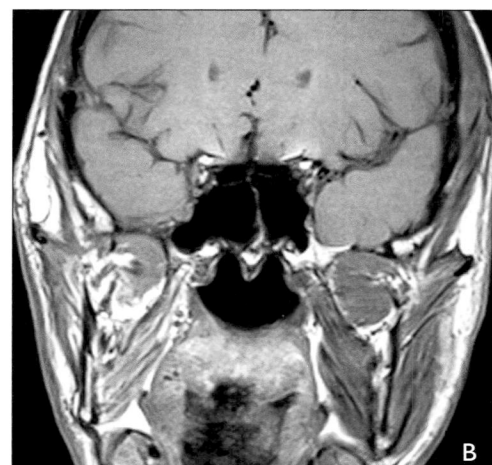

27-40A. Enhancing lesion fills the right Meckel cave ⇨, infiltrates and thickens CN V_2 ⇨. CN V_3 (not shown) also demonstrated tumor involvement. 27-40B. Coronal T1 C+ shows that the ipsilateral muscles of mastication including the temporalis muscle are atrophic, fatty infiltrated compared to the normal-appearing left side. Denervation atrophy.

lymphoma. Nonmalignant mimics of sinonasal SCCa that may extend intracranially include **invasive fungal sinusitis** and **Wegener granulomatosis**.

Perineural Metastases

Terminology

Perineural tumor (PNT) spread is defined as extension of malignant tumor along neural sheaths.

Etiology

Many head and neck cancers have a propensity to spread along nerve sheaths. Mucosal or cutaneous tumors such as SCCa and major/minor salivary gland malignancies such as adenoid cystic carcinoma all are prone to PNT spread. Other tumors such as melanoma and non-Hodgkin lymphoma also frequently spread along major nerve sheaths. Perineural invasion occurs in 2-6% of cutaneous head and neck basal and squamous cell carcinomas.

PNT spread may be anterograde, retrograde, or both. "Skip" lesions and lesions that cross from one nerve to another are common.

Pathology

Location. The most common nerves to be affected by PNT are the maxillary division of the trigeminal nerve (CN V$_2$) **(27-41)** and the facial nerve (CN VII) **(27-42)**. SCCa or melanoma of the cheek can infiltrate the infraorbital division of CN V$_2$. Posterior spread into the PTPF allows access to the cavernous sinus and Meckel cave via the foramen rotundum.

The mandibular nerve (CN V$_3$) can be invaded by any masticator space malignancy. Retrograde spread up the nerve from an oral cavity mucosal SCCa is a classic example **(27-43)**.

Parotid gland malignancies such as adenoid cystic carcinoma can "creep" up the facial nerve all the way into the internal auditory canal.

Microscopic Features. Tumor extends along a nerve via the epineurium, expressing neural cell adhesion molecules (N-CAMs) and eventually invading the nerve itself.

Clinical Issues

Early PNT spread is often asymptomatic. Trigeminal pain and paresthesia, including denervation atrophy of the muscles of mastication, are common with CN V lesions. CN VII lesions present with facial weakness or paralysis. CN VII special functions are lost as tumor gradually spreads upward along the facial nerve canal.

Imaging

General Features. Tubular enlargement of the affected nerve together with widening of its bony canal or foramen is typical. If the nerve passes through a structure such as the PTPF that is normally filled with fat, the fat becomes "dirty" or effaced. *Look for denervation atrophy*—common with CN V$_3$ lesions—seen as small, shrunken muscles of mastication with fatty infiltration **(27-40)**.

CT Findings. Bone CT shows smooth—not permeative destructive—enlargement of the affected foramen or canal. NECT may show abnormal soft tissue density replacing normal fat. CECT may show subtle soft tissue enhancement.

If tumor extends into the cavernous sinus, the walls may bulge outward and Meckel cave may be filled with soft tissue instead of CSF.

MR Findings. The natural contrast provided by fat on T1WI is extremely helpful in detecting possible PNT. Obliterated fat—especially in the PTPF—is a key finding. PNT is often isointense with nerve and difficult to see on T2WI. Tumor spread into Meckel cave replaces the normal hyperintense CSF with isointense soft tissue.

Post-contrast T1 scans should be performed with fat saturation to increase conspicuity of the enlarged, strongly and uniformly enhancing nerve.

Differential Diagnosis

The major differential diagnosis of a solitary enlarged, enhancing cranial nerve in a middle-aged or older adult is perineural metastasis versus **schwannoma**. Schwannomas are tubular or fusiform enlargements that enhance strongly but heterogeneously. The vast majority of schwannomas are vestibulocochlear while the trigeminal and facial nerves are the most common sites for perineural metastases. **Lymphoma** can involve a single cranial nerve but is more often multifocal.

Plexiform neurofibroma can infiltrate the orbital division of CN V but almost always occur with neurofibromatosis type 1.

Neurosarcoid and **invasive fungal sinusitis** can infiltrate one or more cranial nerves. **Chronic inflammatory demyelinating polyneuropathy** (CIDP) usually involves spinal nerves but occasionally affects cranial nerves. Multiple enhancing CNs are more common than solitary involvement in CIDP. Other causes of multifocal cranial nerve enhancement include **multiple sclerosis**, **viral/postviral neuritis**, and **Lyme disease**.

27-41A. *Sagittal graphic shows perineural tumor spread from a cheek malignancy "creeping" along the infraorbital nerve* ➡ *into the pterygopalatine fossa* ➡ *, through the foramen rotundum into the Meckel cave and gasserian ganglion* ➡ *. 27-41B. Sagittal T1 C+ FS shows tumor in the cheek spreading retrograde along the infraorbital nerve* ➡ *, filling the pterygopalatine fossa* ➡ *, extending into the foramen rotundum* ➡ *.*

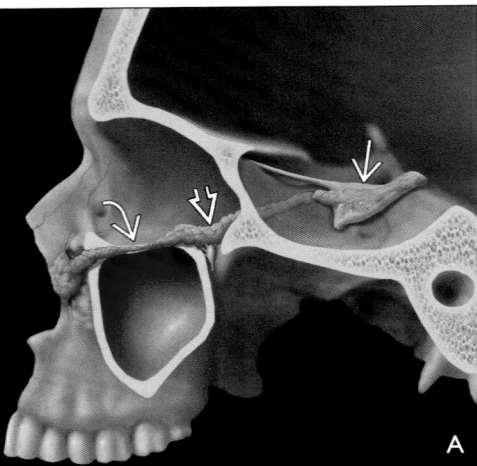
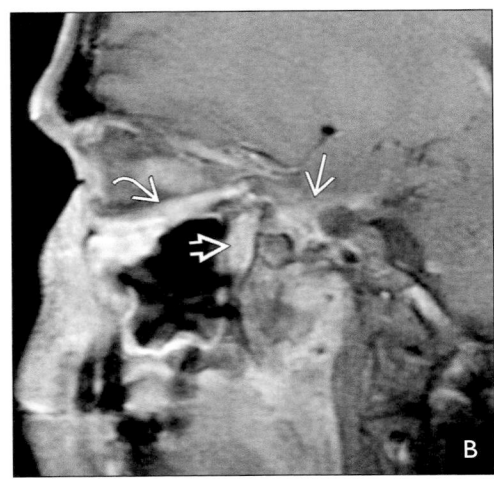

27-42A. *Oblique sagittal graphic depicts a parotid gland tumor* ➡ *spreading intracranially along the descending CN VII* ➡ *up to the posterior genu* ➡ *. 27-42B. Sagittal T1 C+ FS scan shows an enhancing parotid tumor* ➡ *extending along the descending portion of the facial nerve* ➡ *.*

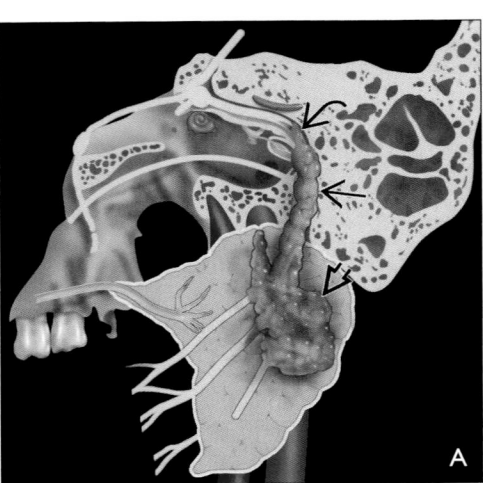
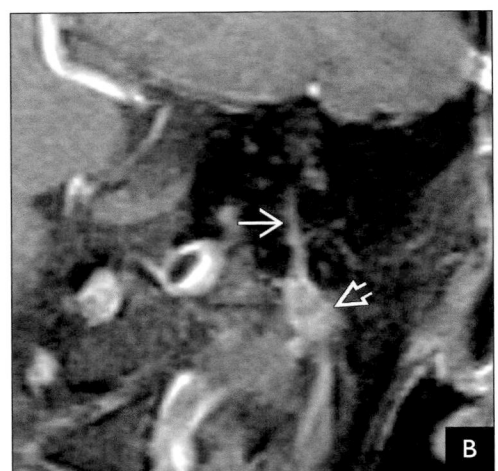

27-43A. *Coronal graphic depicts a perineural tumor extending from the masticator space into the mandible along the inferior alveolar nerve* ➡ *, then spreading along the mandibular nerve (V₃)* ➡ *through the foramen ovale* ➡ *into the Meckel cave and gasserian ganglion. 27-43B. Coronal T1 C+ FS scan shows a markedly thickened, enhancing mandibular nerve* ➡ *that extends proximally into the foramen ovale* ➡ *. Compare to the normal, nonenhancing left CN V* ➡ *.*

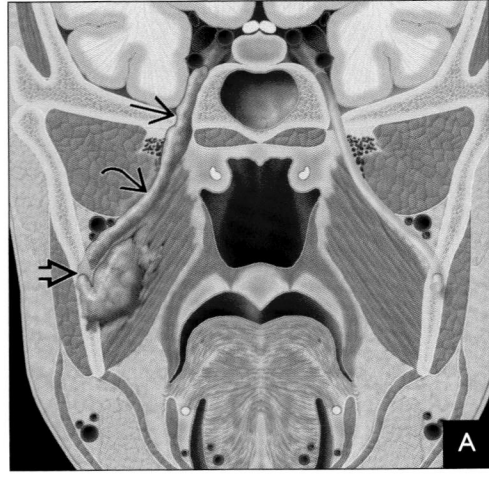
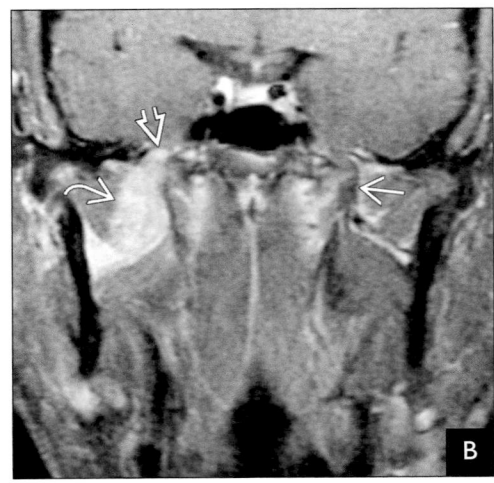

araneoplastic Syndromes

We close this chapter with a brief discussion of cancer-induced remote neurological effects, collectively called **paraneoplastic syndromes** or **paraneoplastic neurologic disorders** (PNDs). By definition, PNDs are not related to direct (local or metastatic) tumor invasion, adverse effects of chemotherapy, malnutrition, or infection. In a paraneoplastic syndrome, extra-CNS tumors exert their adverse influence on the brain not via metastasis but indirectly, largely through immune- or T-cell-mediated mechanisms. PNDs may involve the CNS (brain, spinal cord) or peripheral nervous system.

Paraneoplastic syndromes are rare, affecting less than 1% of all patients with systemic cancer. In such cases, a paraneoplastic syndrome is usually diagnosed only after other etiologies—primarily metastatic disease—have been excluded. In 70% of patients with PND, neurologic symptoms are the *first* manifestation of a tumor. At least 60% of PND patients have antineuronal antibodies that can be detected in the serum or CSF, but imaging may offer the first clues to the presence of a possible PND.

Several types of PND have been recognized. These include paraneoplastic limbic encephalitis, paraneoplastic encephalomyelitis, paraneoplastic cerebellar degeneration, paraneoplastic opsoclonus-myoclonus-ataxia, paraneoplastic sensory neuropathy, and Lambert-Eaton myasthenic syndrome.

We consider the most common paraneoplastic syndrome—paraneoplastic limbic encephalitis—and then discuss a few miscellaneous PNDs. We conclude with a brief mention of extralimbic paraneoplastic disorders and seronegative autoimmune syndromes that can mimic paraneoplastic limbic encephalitis.

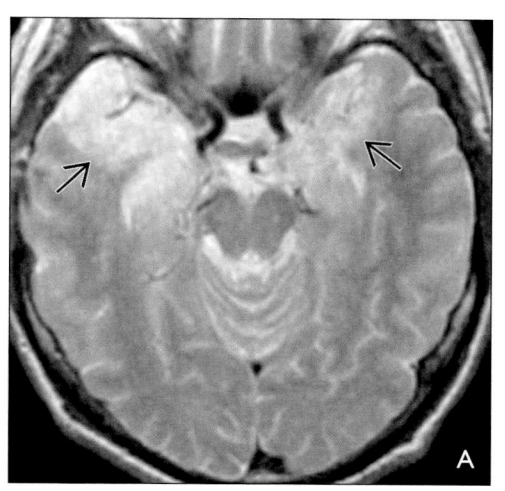
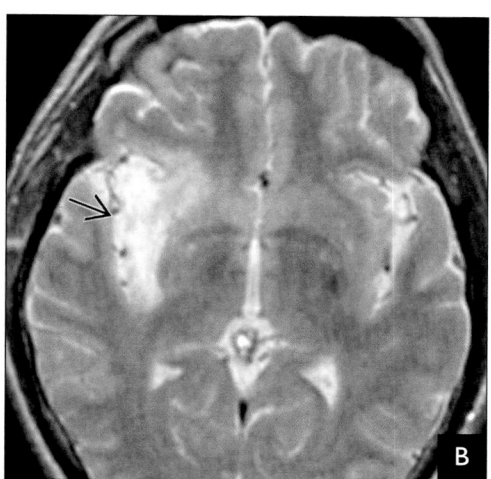

27-44A. *Axial T2WI in a 75-year-old man with small cell lung cancer and paraneoplastic limbic encephalitis shows bilateral confluent hyperintensity in both anteromedial temporal lobes* ⇒. **27-44B.** *More cephalad scan in the same patient shows that the right insular cortex, the extreme and external capsules are affected* ⇒.

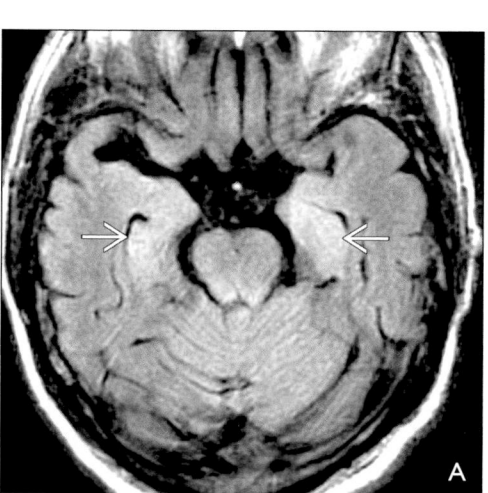
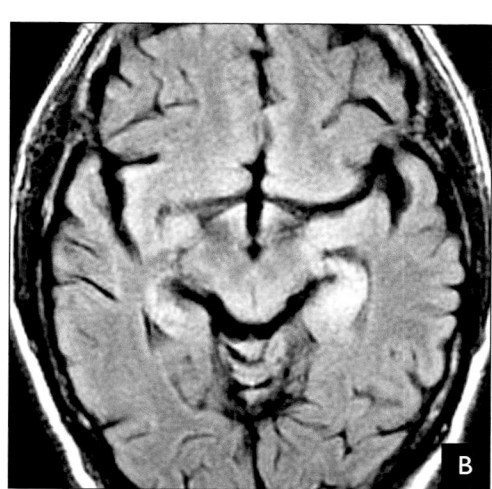

27-45A. *Axial FLAIR scan in a 67-year-old man with documented voltage-gated potassium channel complex (VGKC) antibodies shows hyperintensity in both medial temporal lobes* ➡. **27-45B.** *More cephalad scan shows the extent of the hyperintensity, including involvement of the right insula.*

Paraneoplastic Limbic Encephalitis

Terminology

By definition, paraneoplastic limbic encephalitis (PLE) is a limbic system disorder. The medial temporal lobes are preferentially involved, but the inferior frontal region, insular cortex, and cingulate gyrus can also be affected.

Etiology

The most frequent neoplasm associated with PLE is small cell lung cancer, identified in about half of all cases. Other associated tumors include testicular neoplasms (20%), breast carcinoma (8%), thymoma, and lymphoma.

Antineuronal antibodies are frequently but not invariably found in the CSF or serum of patients with PLE. The most common is the anti-Hu antibody, which is present in about half the patients with small cell lung cancer-associated PLE. Anti-Ta antibody has been associated with testicular cancer.

Clinical Issues

PRESENTATION. Neurological symptoms often precede identification of the inciting tumor by weeks or months. The nonspecific nature and diversity of symptoms add to the difficulty of diagnosing PLE. Symptoms gradually develop and evolve over a period of days to weeks. Confusion and short-term memory loss with relative preservation of other cognitive functions—with or without mood and behavioral changes—is typical. Complex partial seizures are common.

Pathology

The histologic features of PLE are similar to those of viral encephalitis and myelitis. A lymphoplasmacytic inflammatory infiltrate with variable degrees of neuronal loss is typical.

Imaging

MR is the procedure of choice in diagnosing PLE. T2/FLAIR shows hyperintensity in one or both medial temporal lobes (27-44).

Differential Diagnosis

The major differential diagnosis of PLE is **herpes encephalitis**. Other causes of limbic encephalitis that can mimic PLE include **post-transplant acute limbic encephalitis** (PALE) syndrome and **human herpesvirus 6 (HHV-6) encephalitis**. HHV-6 encephalitis is associated with hematological malignancies such as Hodgkin and angioimmunoblastic T-cell lymphoma and leukemia.

Gliomatosis cerebri occasionally crosses the anterior commissure and infiltrates both temporal lobes, mimicking PLE.

Miscellaneous Paraneoplastic Syndromes

Paraneoplastic Cerebellar Degeneration

Paraneoplastic cerebellar degeneration (PCD) selectively involves the cerebellum and typically presents with ataxia and gait instability, vertigo, dizziness, and oscillopsia. Anti-Yo antibodies or antibodies against P/Q voltage-gated calcium channels may be detected in the serum of affected patients.

No macroscopic abnormalities are generally visible. The microscopic hallmark of PCD is widespread severe loss of Purkinje cells with variable loss of granule cells. Inflammatory infiltrates are usually sparse or absent.

MR imaging is normal ("remarkably unremarkable") in most patients. Some cases demonstrate transient cerebellar enlargement with focal or diffuse hyperintensity on FLAIR. Mild cortical-meningeal enhancement may be present. Subacute or chronic PCD shows mild to moderate generalized cerebellar atrophy and hypometabolism on PET.

Voltage-Gated Potassium Channel Complex Antibody Disorders

Voltage-gated potassium channel complex (VGKC) antibodies are associated with both typical PLE and a less focal encephalitis that is primarily associated with psychiatric disturbances and symptoms of autonomic dysfunction (e.g., gastrointestinal motility disorders).

In childhood, CNS presentations associated with VGKC antibodies include limbic encephalitis, status epilepticus, epileptic encephalopathy, and autistic regression.

VGKC antibodies are also found in many nonparaneoplastic patients with limbic encephalitis. Only 30% of patients with antibodies against VGKC have systemic tumors, primarily small cell lung cancer and thymoma. Imaging findings are nonspecific and include T2/FLAIR hyperintensity in the limbic system and/or basal ganglia (27-45).

Lobar Extralimbic and Seronegative Autoimmune Paraneoplastic Encephalopathies

Lobar extralimbic paraneoplastic encephalopathies (LELPEs) and seronegative autoimmune limbic encephalitis (SNALE) have received less attention than the more classic PLE and PCD syndromes. In these syndromes, exhaustive searches for infectious pathogens and autoantibodies are negative.

Imaging findings are similar to those of herpes encephalitis and paraneoplastic limbic encephalitis with uncal-hippocampal T2/FLAIR hyperintensity **(27-46)**. Some cases can resemble glioma with a focal mass-like enhancing lesion.

Oncogenic Osteomalacia

Oncogenic osteomalacia, also called tumor-induced osteomalacia (TIO), is an uncommon acquired paraneoplastic syndrome. It usually affects the limbs or axial skeleton but occasionally involves the skull base. TIO is difficult to diagnose because of the insidious onset of symptoms—mostly systemic bone pain and muscle weakness.

Tumors that cause TIO are **phosphaturic mesenchymal tumors** with mixed connective tissue that secrete fibroblast growth factor 23 (FGF-23). FGF-23 inactivates sodium phosphate cotransporters in the proximal renal tubules. **Hemangiopericytoma** causes approximately 70-80% of TIO cases.

Hypophosphatemia results in severe osteopenia with multiple poorly healing fractures of the spine and extremities. The skull base, oral, and maxillofacial regions are occasionally affected.

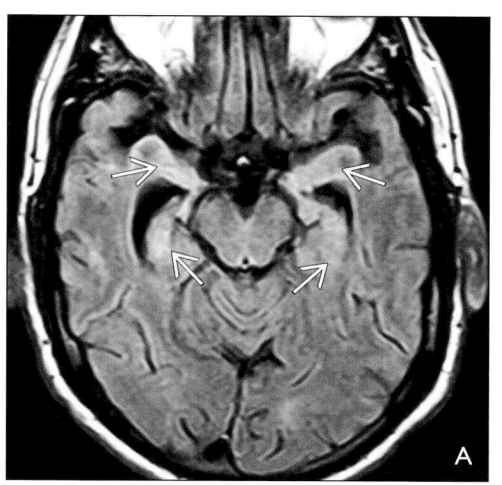

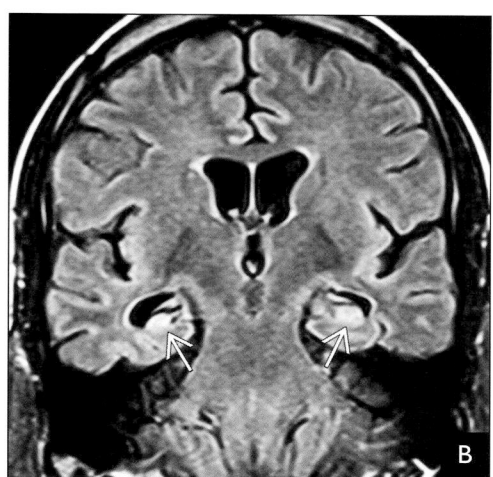

27-46A. Axial FLAIR scan in a 32-year-old man with a 6-month history of progressive dementia shows enlarged sylvian fissures, prominent temporal horns, and striking volume loss in both hippocampi. Bilaterally symmetric uncal-hippocampal hyperintensity is present ➡. *27-46B. Coronal FLAIR scan shows generalized supratentorial volume loss with symmetric hippocampal hyperintensity* ➡.

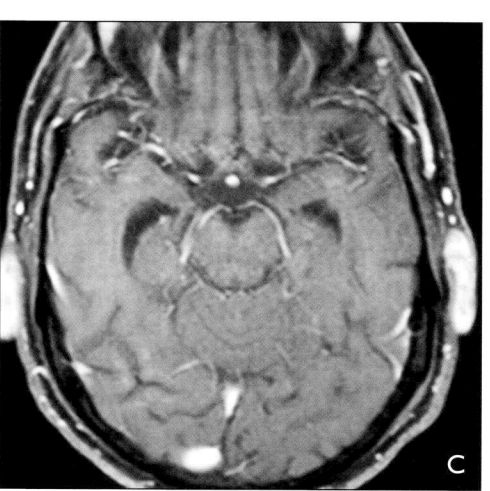

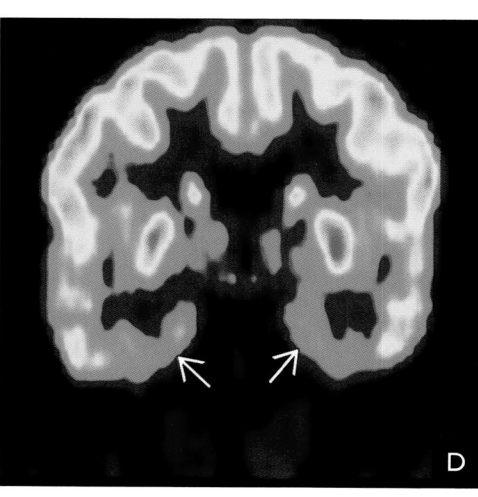

27-46C. T1 C+ FS scan shows no evidence of enhancement. 27-46D. Coronal FDG PET scan shows strikingly reduced uptake in both medial temporal lobes ➡. *Imaging diagnosis was paraneoplastic limbic encephalitis. Extensive evaluation for systemic neoplasm and infectious pathogens was negative. Final diagnosis was seronegative autoimmune limbic encephalitis (SNALE).*

Selected References

Metastatic Lesions

- Barajas RF Jr et al: Imaging diagnosis of brain metastasis. Prog Neurol Surg. 25:55-73, 2012
- Nayak L et al: Epidemiology of brain metastases. Curr Oncol Rep. 14(1):48-54, 2012

Overview

- Moody P et al: Tumor-to-tumor metastasis: pathology and neuroimaging considerations. Int J Clin Exp Pathol. 5(4):367-73, 2012
- Quattrocchi CC et al: Spatial brain distribution of intra-axial metastatic lesions in breast and lung cancer patients. J Neurooncol. 110(1):79-87, 2012
- Kim SJ et al: Astrocytes upregulate survival genes in tumor cells and induce protection from chemotherapy. Neoplasia. 13(3):286-98, 2011
- Mueller WC et al: Accurate classification of metastatic brain tumors using a novel microRNA-based test. Oncologist. 16(2):165-74, 2011

Parenchymal Metastases

- Chen W et al: Multicontrast single-slab 3D MRI to detect cerebral metastasis. AJR Am J Roentgenol. 198(1):27-32, 2012
- Chen XZ et al: Differentiation between brain glioblastoma multiforme and solitary metastasis: qualitative and quantitative analysis based on routine MR imaging. AJNR Am J Neuroradiol. Epub ahead of print, 2012
- Gaudino S et al: Magnetic resonance imaging of solitary brain metastases: main findings of nonmorphological sequences. Radiol Med. Epub ahead of print, 2012
- Serres S et al: Molecular MRI enables early and sensitive detection of brain metastases. Proc Natl Acad Sci U S A. 109(17):6674-9, 2012
- Hanssens P et al: Detection of brain micrometastases by high-resolution stereotactic magnetic resonance imaging and its impact on the timing of and risk for distant recurrences. J Neurosurg. 115(3):499-504, 2011
- Lee HY et al: Diagnostic efficacy of PET/CT plus brain MR imaging for detection of extrathoracic metastases in patients with lung adenocarcinoma. J Korean Med Sci. 24(6):1132-8, 2009

Skull and Dural Metastases

- Mitsuya K et al: Metastatic skull tumors: MRI features and a new conventional classification. J Neurooncol. 104(1):239-45, 2011
- Nayak L et al: Intracranial dural metastases. Cancer. 115(9):1947-53, 2009

Leptomeningeal Metastases

- Bruna J et al: Leptomeningeal metastases. Curr Treat Options Neurol. 14(4):402-15, 2012

Miscellaneous Metastases

- Post KD: Pituitary metastases: role of surgery. World Neurosurg. Epub ahead of print, 2012
- Faltas B: Circulating tumor cells in the cerebrospinal fluid: "tapping" into diagnostic and predictive potential. Oncotarget. 2(11):822, 2011
- Ikota H et al: Clinicopathological and immunohistochemical study of 20 choroid plexus tumors: their histological diversity and the expression of markers useful for differentiation from metastatic cancer. Brain Tumor Pathol. 28(3):215-21, 2011
- Siomin V et al: Stereotactic radiosurgical treatment of brain metastases to the choroid plexus. Int J Radiat Oncol Biol Phys. 80(4):1134-42, 2011
- Vianello F et al: Follicular thyroid carcinoma with metastases to the pituitary causing pituitary insufficiency. Thyroid. 21(8):921-5, 2011
- Asteriou C et al: Blurred vision due to choroidal metastasis as the first manifestation of lung cancer: a case report. World J Surg Oncol. 8:2, 2010
- Hassaneen W et al: Surgical management of lateral-ventricle metastases: report of 29 cases in a single-institution experience. J Neurosurg. 112(5):1046-55, 2010
- Cole B et al: 70-year-old man with enlarged pineal gland. Brain Pathol. 18(4):602-4, 2008
- Koeller KK et al: Cerebral intraventricular neoplasms: radiologic-pathologic correlation. Radiographics. 22(6):1473-505, 2002

Perineural Metastases

- Balamucki CJ et al: Skin carcinoma of the head and neck with perineural invasion. Am J Otolaryngol. 33(4):447-54, 2012
- Lee DH et al: Distant metastases and survival prediction in head and neck squamous cell carcinoma. Otolaryngol Head Neck Surg. Epub ahead of print, 2012
- Mendenhall WM et al: Cutaneous head and neck basal and squamous cell carcinomas with perineural invasion. Oral Oncol. 48(10):918-22, 2012

Paraneoplastic Syndromes

- Dalmau J et al: Paraneoplastic syndromes of the CNS. Lancet Neurol. 7(4):327-40, 2008

Paraneoplastic Limbic Encephalitis

- Fahim A et al: A case of limbic encephalitis presenting as a paraneoplastic manifestation of limited stage small cell lung cancer: a case report. J Med Case Reports. 4:408, 2010

Miscellaneous Paraneoplastic Syndromes

- Chokyu I et al: Oncogenic osteomalacia associated with mesenchymal tumor in the middle cranial fossa: a case report. J Med Case Rep. 6(1):181, 2012

- Hacohen Y et al: A clinico-radiological phenotype of voltage-gated potassium channel complex antibodymediated disorder presenting with seizures and basal ganglia changes. Dev Med Child Neurol. Epub ahead of print, 2012

- Sureka J et al: Clinico-radiological spectrum of bilateral temporal lobe hyperintensity: a retrospective review. Br J Radiol. 85(1017):e782-92, 2012

- Hendry DS et al: Case 165: oncogenic osteomalacia. Radiology. 258(1):320-2, 2011

- Najjar S et al: Spontaneously resolving seronegative autoimmune limbic encephalitis. Cogn Behav Neurol. 24(2):99-105, 2011

- Uno T et al: Osteomalacia caused by skull base tumors: report of 2 cases. Neurosurgery. 69(1):E239-44; discussion E244, 2011

- McKeon A et al: Reversible extralimbic paraneoplastic encephalopathies with large abnormalities on magnetic resonance images. Arch Neurol. 66(2):268-71, 2009

28

Nonneoplastic Cysts

There are many types of intracranial cysts. Some are incidental and of no significance. Others may cause serious—even life-threatening—symptoms.

In this chapter we consider a number of different intracranial cysts: Cystic-appearing anatomic variants that can be mistaken for disease, congenital/developmental cysts, and a variety of miscellaneous cysts. We exclude parasitic cysts, cystic brain malformations, and cystic neoplasms as they are discussed in their respective chapters.

The etiology, pathology, and clinical significance of nonneoplastic intracranial cysts is so varied that classifying them presents a significant challenge.

In a schema based on *etiology*, cysts are classified as normal anatomic variants (e.g., enlarged perivascular spaces), congenital lesions derived from embryonic ecto- or endoderm (colloid and neurenteric cysts), developmental inclusion cysts (e.g., dermoid and epidermoid cysts), and miscellaneous cysts that don't easily fit into any particular category (such as choroid plexus and tumor-associated cysts). Etiology is interesting but unhelpful in establishing an imaging-based diagnosis.

Categorizing cysts by the *histologic* characteristics of their walls—as is traditional in neuropathology texts—is again of little help when faced with the challenge of providing an appropriate differential diagnosis based on imaging findings alone.

An *imaging-based* approach to the classification of intracranial cysts is much more practical as most intracranial cysts are discovered on CT or MR examination. This approach takes into account three easily defined features: (1) anatomic location, (2) imaging characteristics (i.e., density/signal intensity of the contents, presence/absence of calcification and/or enhancement), and (3) patient age. Of these three, anatomic location is the most helpful.

While many types of intracranial cysts occur in more than one anatomic location, some sites are "preferred" by certain cysts. In this chapter, we discuss cysts from the outside in, beginning with scalp and intracranial extraaxial cysts before turning our attention to parenchymal and intraventricular cysts.

There are four key anatomy-based questions to consider about a cystic-appearing intracranial lesion (see below). A summary chart based on these simple questions, together with the cysts discussed throughout the text, is included on the next page (**Table 28-1**).

FOUR KEY ANATOMY-BASED QUESTIONS

Is the cyst extra- or intraaxial?

Is the cyst supra- or infratentorial?

Is the cyst midline or off-midline?

If the cyst is intraaxial, is it in the brain parenchyma or inside the ventricles?

Intracranial Cystic-appearing Lesions

EXTRAAXIAL	INTRAAXIAL
Supratentorial	**Supratentorial**
Midline	Parenchymal
Pineal cyst	Enlarged PVSs
Dermoid cyst	Neuroglial cyst
Rathke cleft cyst	Porencephalic cyst
Arachnoid cyst (suprasellar)	Hippocampal sulcus remnants
Off-midline	Intraventricular
Arachnoid cyst (middle cranial fossa, convexity)	Choroid plexus cysts
Epidermoid cyst	Colloid cyst
Tumor-associated cysts	Choroid fissure cysts
Trichilemmal ("sebaceous") cyst (scalp)	Ependymal cyst
Leptomeningeal cyst ("growing fracture")	
Infratentorial	**Infratentorial**
Midline	Parenchymal
Neurenteric cyst	Enlarged PVSs (dentate nuclei)
Arachnoid cyst (retrocerebellar)	
Off-midline	Intraventricular
Epidermoid (CPA)	Epidermoid (fourth ventricle, cisterna magna)
Arachnoid cyst (CPA)	Cystic ("trapped") fourth ventricle
Tumor-associated cysts	

Table 28-1. *CPA = cerebellopontine angle; PVS = perivascular space. Leptomeningeal cyst, Rathke cleft cyst, and cystic/trapped fourth ventricle are discussed in chapters 2, 25, and 34, respectively. All the other entities in the table are considered here.*

Scalp Cysts

Overview

A number of benign cutaneous cysts can present as scalp lesions. Most are not deliberately imaged, as the scalp is easily accessible to both visual and manual inspection. Nevertheless, scalp masses are not uncommonly identified on imaging studies intended to visualize intracranial structures. Imaging also becomes important when a scalp lesion is clinically felt to be potentially malignant, has a vascular component, or might be in anatomic continuity with intracranial contents.

Age is helpful in the differential diagnosis of nontraumatic scalp masses. In adults, the differential diagnosis includes skin carcinomas (basal and squamous cell), dermoid and epidermoid cysts, hemangiomas, and metastases. Trichilemmal ("sebaceous") cysts are common scalp masses in middle-aged and older patients.

The most common scalp mass in children is Langerhans cell histiocytosis, followed by epidermoid and dermoid cysts, scalp hemangiomas, and neurofibromas. Less common but important scalp lesions in children include cephalocele and sinus pericranii.

The three statistically most common scalp cysts are epidermoid cyst (50%), trichilemmal cysts (25-30%), and dermoid cysts (20-25%). Epidermoid and dermoid cysts are discussed later in the chapter. We discuss trichilemmal (pilar or "sebaceous") cysts of the scalp here.

Trichilemmal ("Sebaceous") Cyst

Terminology

While the term "sebaceous cyst" is commonly used by radiologists, this type of cyst does not actually contain sebaceous material. Such cysts are more accurately called trichilemmal cysts (TCs). Rarely, TCs enlarge and proliferate. Proliferating trichilemmal cysts are known as pilar ("turban") tumors. Malignant TCs are referred to as "proliferating trichilemmal cystic carcinoma."

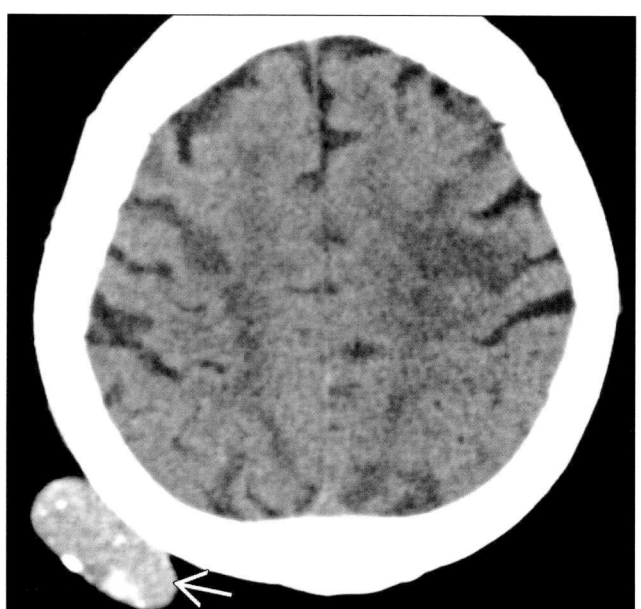

28-1. Axial NECT in a 79-year-old woman with a nontender scalp mass that had been present for years. The mass ➡ is hyperdense, partially calcified. Trichilemmal cyst.

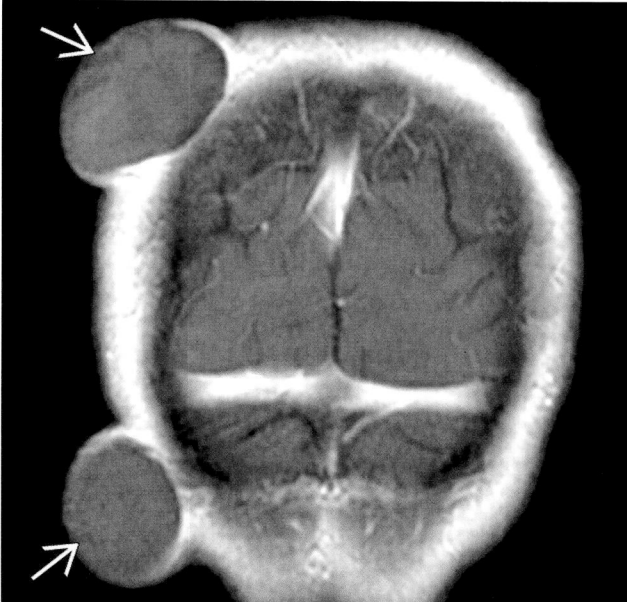

28-2. Two trichilemmal cysts ➡ are seen on this coronal T1WI C+ scan. The cysts are heterogeneous, isointense with brain, and incompletely surrounded by fat. They do not enhance.

athology

LOCATION, SIZE, AND NUMBER. Most TCs are found within the dermis or subcutaneous tissue. They can be single or multiple and vary from a few millimeters to several centimeters.

GROSS AND MICROSCOPIC FEATURES. TCs are characterized by a fibrous capsule lined by stratified squamous epithelium. The cyst contents consist primarily of waxy desquamated keratin. Microscopically, a TC resembles the root sheath of a hair follicle, not a sebaceous gland.

linical Issues

EPIDEMIOLOGY AND DEMOGRAPHICS. TCs affect 5-10% of the population. While they can occur at any age, most occur in elderly women.

PRESENTATION AND NATURAL HISTORY. TCs generally appear as hairless, mobile, slightly compressible, subcutaneous scalp masses.

TCs grow slowly and have often been present for years. Rarely, they become locally aggressive and may even invade bone. Malignant degeneration with distant metastasis is rare.

TREATMENT OPTIONS. Surgical excision is the major treatment. Incomplete excision may result in recurrence.

Imaging

GENERAL FEATURES. These scalp masses are generally large, well-delineated, round or ovoid, but somewhat complex-appearing lesions.

CT FINDINGS. TCs are sharply delineated solid, cystic, or mixed solid-cystic masses that are hyperdense compared to subcutaneous fat. Calcification is common and may be seen in punctate, curvilinear, or coarse forms (28-1). Sometimes calcifications layer in the dependent portion of larger cysts. Typical TCs do not enhance, nor do they remodel or invade the underlying calvaria.

MR FINDINGS. TCs are well-circumscribed scalp masses that appear incompletely surrounded by fat (28-2). They are generally isointense with brain and muscle on T1WI and inhomogeneously hypointense on T2WI.

TCs do not suppress on FLAIR. "Blooming" foci on T2* (GRE, SWI) are caused by calcifications, not hemorrhage.

Simple uncomplicated TCs do not enhance, although the proliferating variant may show significant enhancement with solid lobules interspersed with nonenhancing cystic foci.

Differential Diagnosis

In adults, the imaging differential diagnoses are benign and malignant scalp tumors. **Basal cell carcinomas** and **scalp metastases** are ill-defined, poorly delineated scalp masses that invade the subcutaneous soft tissues and may erode bone. Superficial ulceration is common. **Dermoid and epidermoid cysts** as well as **hemangiomas** are all much more common in the skull than in the scalp.

TCs are rare in children. In this age group, the most important lesions to differentiate from benign scalp cysts (usually dermoids/epidermoids, not TCs) are congenital brain malformations that protrude through skull defects and present as subcutaneous masses. **Cephaloceles** contain variable combinations of brain/meninges/vessels. They vary in size from very large to small lesions ("atretic cephalocele"). **Sinus pericranii** is a compressible, bluish-tinged scalp mass that communicates with the intracranial venous system through a skull defect.

Extraaxial Cysts

Extraaxial cysts are between the skull and brain. With few exceptions, most lie within the arachnoid membrane or in the subarachnoid space.

Determining sublocation of an extraaxial cyst (supra- vs. infratentorial, midline vs. off-midline) is helpful in establishing a meaningful differential diagnosis **(Table 28-1)**. For example, an arachnoid cyst is the only type that commonly occurs in the posterior fossa. Some extraaxial cysts are usually (although not invariably) off-midline. Others—pineal and Rathke cleft cysts—occur only in the midline.

We begin our discussion of extraaxial cysts with the most common type, arachnoid cyst.

28-3. Graphic depicts a middle cranial fossa AC. The arachnoid ⇥ splits and encloses CSF, the middle fossa is expanded, and the overlying bone is thinned. Note that the temporal lobe ⇥ is displaced posteriorly. 28-4. Autopsy specimen shows a classic middle fossa arachnoid cyst between layers of "duplicated" arachnoid ⇥. The temporal lobe ⇥ is displaced, hypoplastic. (Courtesy J. Townsend, MD.)

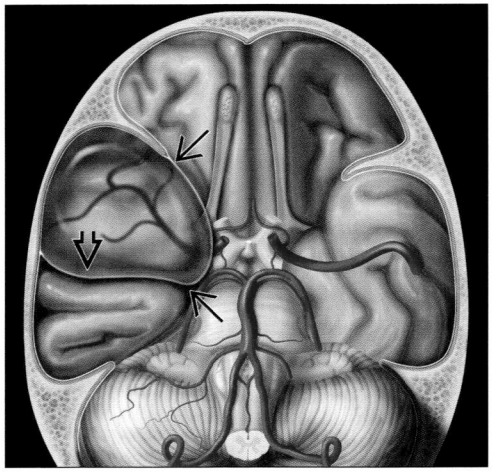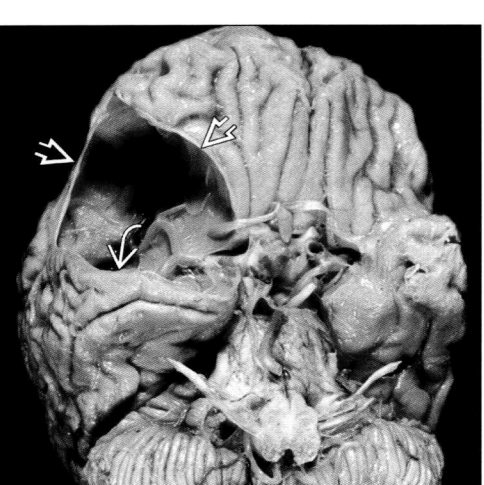

28-5. An arachnoid cyst is lined by a single layer of mature arachnoid cells ⇥ under a delicate fibrous membrane. (Courtesy P. Burger, MD.) 28-6. Arachnoid cysts often have scalloped margins and are CSF-like on T2WI ⇥. They suppress on FLAIR ⇥, remodel the skull ⇥, and do not enhance.

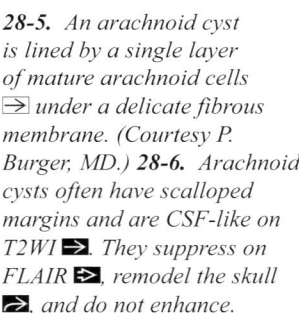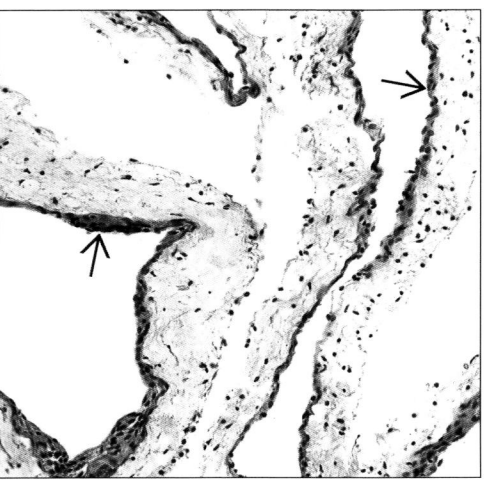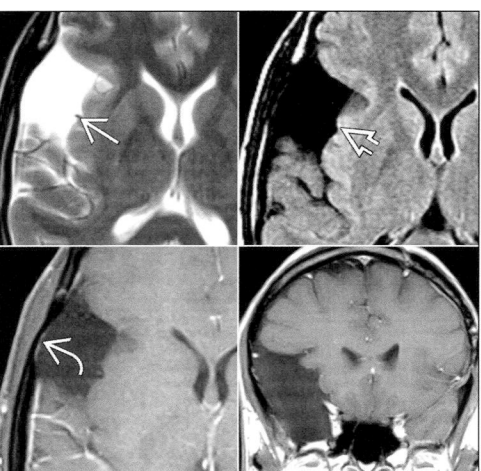

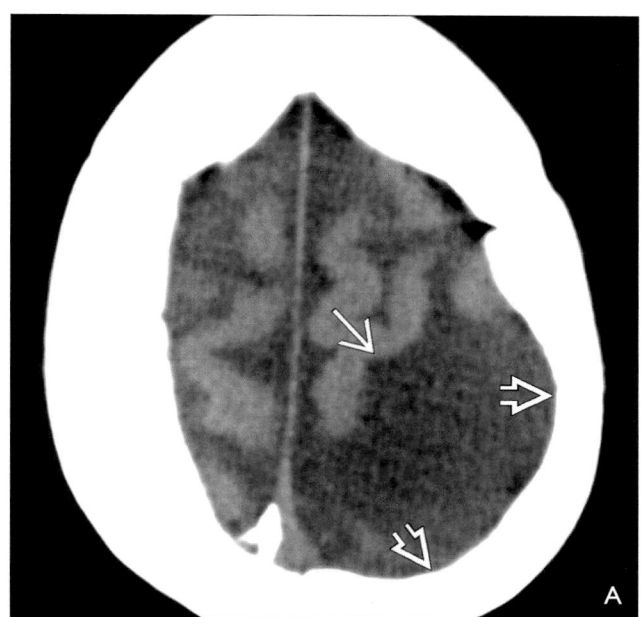

28-7A. NECT scan shows a convexity arachnoid cyst ➡ that expands, remodels the skull ▷.

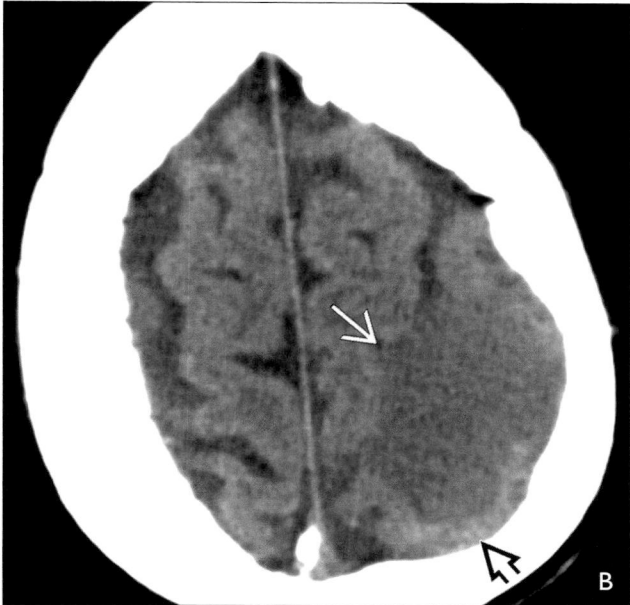

28-7B. Six months later, the patient had sudden onset of severe headache. The cyst ➡ is now hyperdense compared to CSF, shows a blood-fluid level ▷. Cyst apoplexy with sudden hemorrhage.

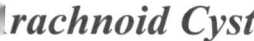

rachnoid Cyst

While arachnoid cysts occur throughout the neuraxis, the vast majority are intracranial.

erminology

An arachnoid cyst (AC), also known as a meningeal cyst, is a CSF-containing cyst lined by a layer of flattened arachnoid cells.

tiology

GENERAL CONCEPTS. The vast majority of ACs arise as anomalies of meningeal development. The embryonic endomeninges fail to merge and remain separated, forming a "duplicated" arachnoid. CSF is secreted by cells in the cyst wall and accumulates between the layers.

Less commonly, arachnoid loculations are acquired as a result of hemorrhage, infection, or surgery. Arachnoid-like cysts also sometimes arise adjacent to extraaxial tumors such as meningiomas, schwannomas, and pituitary macroadenomas. These benign fluid-containing tumor-associated cysts are discussed separately.

GENETICS. Most ACs are sporadic and nonsyndromic. Syndromic ACs have been reported in association with acrocallosal, Aicardi, and Pallister-Hall syndromes.

athology

LOCATION. Most ACs are supratentorial. They are usually off-midline and are the most common off-midline extraaxial supratentorial cyst **(28-3)**.

Nearly two-thirds are found in the middle cranial fossa, anteromedial to the temporal lobe **(28-4)**. Fifteen percent of ACs are found over the cerebral convexities, predominantly over the frontal lobes.

Midline ACs are relatively rare in the supratentorial compartment. The most frequent supratentorial midline location for ACs is the suprasellar cistern, followed by the quadrigeminal cistern and velum interpositum.

Between 10-15% of ACs are found in the posterior fossa. The most common location is the cerebellopontine angle cistern, where ACs are the second most common cystic-appearing extraaxial mass (after epidermoid). The next most frequent site is retrocerebellar.

SIZE AND NUMBER. ACs vary in size, ranging from small incidental cysts to large space-occupying lesions. ACs are almost always solitary. Multiple meningeal cysts have been reported but are probably acquired, resulting from undetected meningitis.

GROSS PATHOLOGY. ACs are well-marginated cysts filled with clear colorless fluid that resembles CSF. They are devoid of internal septations and are completely encased by a delicate translucent membrane.

MICROSCOPIC FEATURES. ACs consist of a delicate fibrous membrane lined by a single layer of mature, histologically normal arachnoid cells **(28-5)**. Small inflammatory infiltrates occur but are rare.

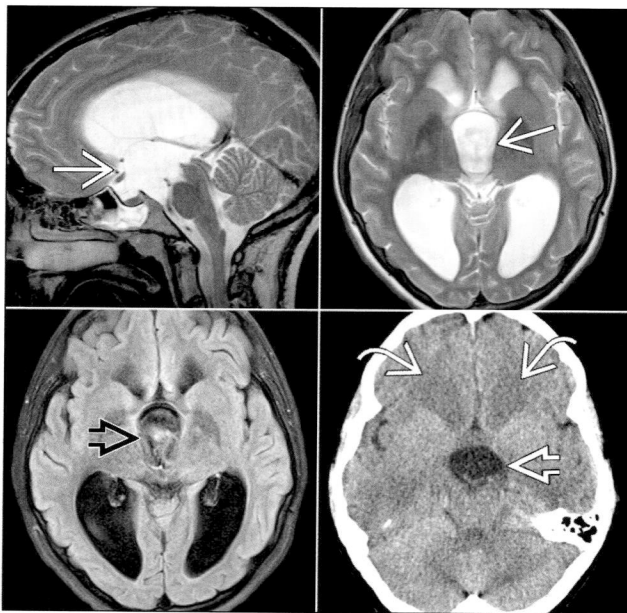

28-8. Suprasellar AC is isointense with CSF on T2WI ➡. CSF pulsations in the cyst do not suppress completely on FLAIR ➡. CT cisternogram shows dilute contrast in the lateral ventricles ➡, while the noncommunicating cyst ➡ does not opacify.

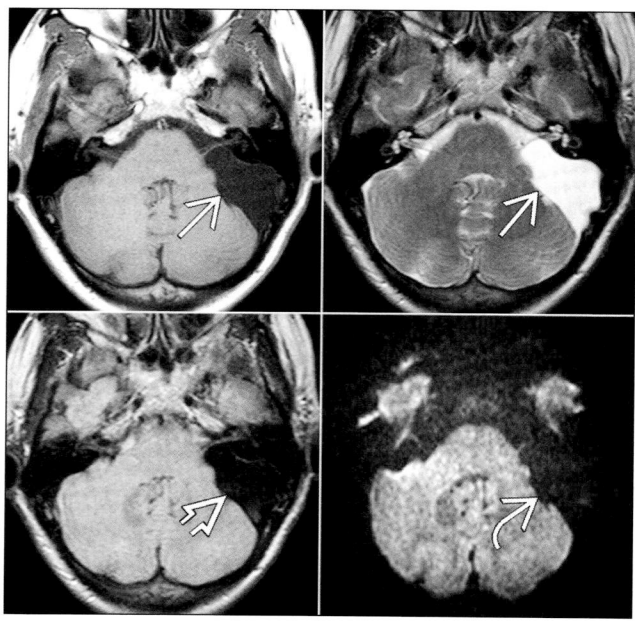

28-9. Left cerebellopontine angle AC is isointense with CSF on T1- and T2WI ➡ and suppresses completely on FLAIR ➡. No diffusion restriction is seen on DWI ➡.

ARACHNOID CYST: PATHOLOGY

Location
- Supratentorial (90%)
  - Middle fossa (67%)
  - Convexities (15%)
  - Other (5-10%): Suprasellar, quadrigeminal cisterns
- Infratentorial (10-12%)
  - Mostly CPA cistern (second most common cystic CPA mass)
  - Less common = cisterna magna

Gross Pathology
- Thin translucent cyst wall bulging with clear fluid
- Lined by mature arachnoid cells

Clinical Issues

EPIDEMIOLOGY. ACs are the most common of all congenital intracranial cysts. They account for approximately 1% of all space-occupying intracranial lesions and are identified on imaging studies in approximately 2% of patients.

DEMOGRAPHICS. ACs can be seen at any age. Most (nearly 75%) are found in children and young adults. There is a slight male predominance.

PRESENTATION. Most ACs are asymptomatic and found incidentally. Symptoms vary with size and location. Headaches are common in symptomatic ACs.

Some suprasellar arachnoid cysts become very large and cause obstructive hydrocephalus.

NATURAL HISTORY. Most ACs remain stable over many years. Enlargement—if any—is very gradual. Enlargement is strongly associated with younger age and rarely occurs in children older than four years at the time of initial diagnosis.

Hemorrhage into an AC is rare but may cause sudden enlargement.

TREATMENT OPTIONS. Asymptomatic ACs are usually "leave me alone" lesions. Surgical options for symptomatic ACs include endoscopic resection or fenestration, open fenestration/marsupialization, or cystoperitoneal shunting with a programmable valve. Following shunting, 60% of ACs disappear completely; in half of these patients, it is possible to remove the shunt without shunt dependence.

Imaging

GENERAL FEATURES. Uncomplicated ACs behave *exactly* like CSF on CT and MR **(28-6)**. FLAIR and DWI are the best sequences to distinguish cystic-appearing intracranial masses from one another.

CT FINDINGS. Uncomplicated ACs are CSF density **(28-7A)**. If intracystic hemorrhage has occurred, the cyst fluid may be moderately hyperdense compared to CSF **(28-7B)**. Large middle cranial fossa ACs expand the fossa and cause temporal lobe hypoplasia or displacement.

With moderately large ACs, bone CT may show pressure remodeling of the adjacent calvaria. ACs do not cause frank bone invasion.

ACs do not enhance. Installation of intrathecal contrast ("CT cisternography") may be helpful in demonstrating communication with the subarachnoid space (SAS) **(28-8)**. Most symptomatic ACs do not demonstrate direct, free communication with the SAS and may require microsurgical decompression. Patients with completely communicating ACs may not need surgical intervention.

MR FINDINGS. ACs are sharply marginated, somewhat scalloped-appearing lesions that parallel CSF signal intensity on all sequences **(28-6)**. They are therefore isointense with CSF on T1- and T2-weighted images **(28-9)**. ACs cause moderate focal mass effect, displacing but not engulfing adjacent brain, vessels, and cranial nerves.

The internal appearance of an AC is intrinsically featureless, containing neither septations nor vessels.

ACs suppress completely with FLAIR **(28-10)**. Occasionally, CSF pulsations within large lesions may cause spin dephasing, producing heterogeneous signal intensity and significant propagation of phase artifact across the scan.

ACs do not restrict on DWI and do not enhance. CSF flow imaging such as 2D cine PC may demonstrate communication between cyst and adjacent subarachnoid space.

Differential Diagnosis

The major differential diagnosis of AC is **epidermoid cyst** (EC). Epidermoid cysts are often almost—but not quite—exactly like CSF. They have a cauliflower-like, lobulated configuration instead of the sharply marginated borders of an AC. ECs engulf vessels and nerves, insinuating themselves along CSF cisterns. ECs do not suppress completely on FLAIR and typically show moderate to marked hyperintensity on DWI.

Enlarged subarachnoid spaces caused by brain volume loss are usually more diffuse CSF collections and do not cause mass effect on adjacent structures.

A **subdural hygroma** or **chronic subdural hematoma** (cSDH) is not precisely like CSF and is usually crescentic, not round or scalloped. cSDHs usually show evidence of prior hemorrhage, especially on T2* sequences, and may have enhancing encasing membranes.

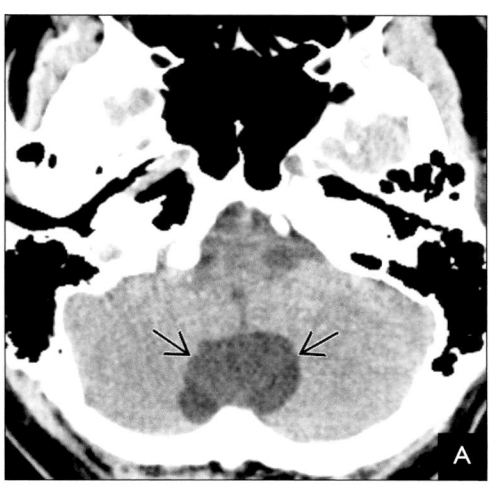

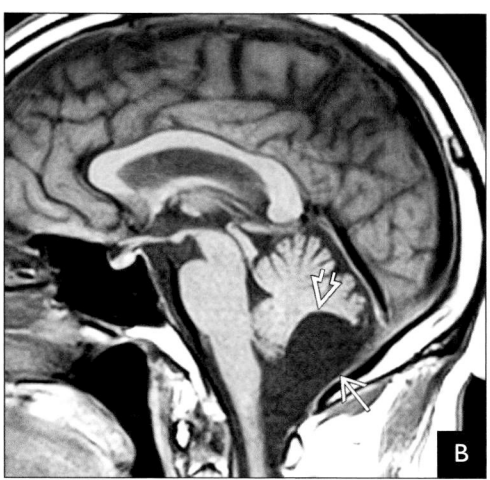

28-10A. Midline retrocerebellar AC ➡ is well-marginated, CSF density on NECT. 28-10B. Sagittal T1WI shows that the rounded cyst ➡ is isointense with CSF, elevates and deforms the cerebellar vermis ➡.

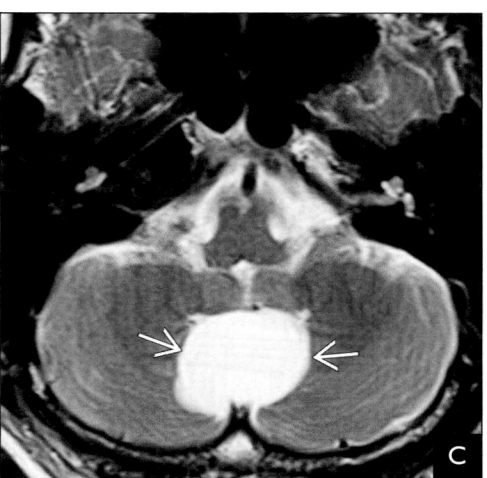

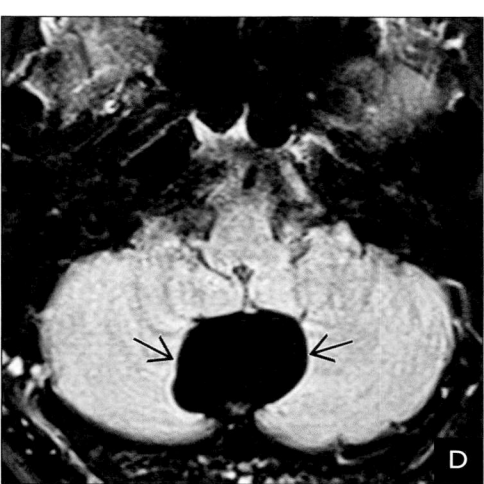

28-10C. The cyst ➡ is isointense with CSF on T2WI. 28-10D. The cyst ➡ suppresses completely on FLAIR. The second most common posterior fossa location for arachnoid cysts is the retrocerebellar aspect of the cisterna magna.

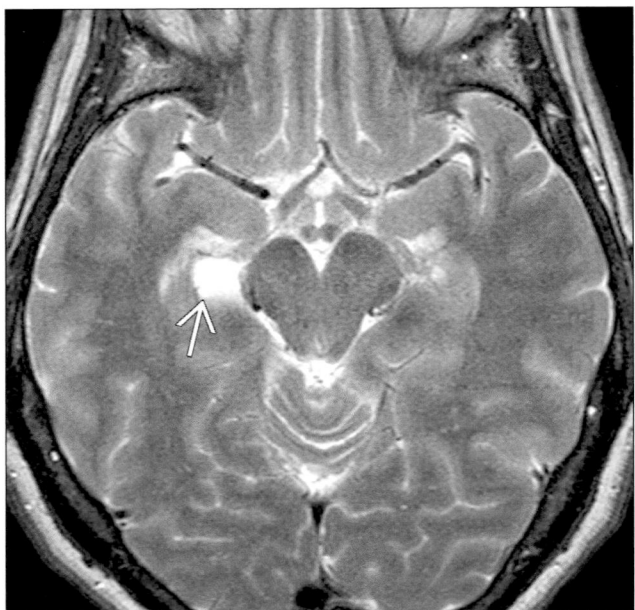

28-11. Axial T2WI shows a classic choroid fissure cyst ➡ as a well-delineated, CSF-like cyst medial to the temporal horn of the lateral ventricle.

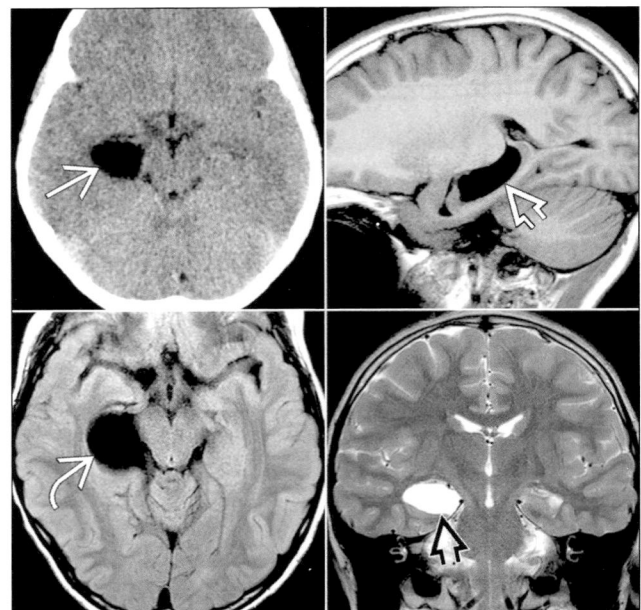

28-12. Choroid fissure cyst is isodense with CSF on NECT ➡. Sagittal T1WI shows classic elongated "spindle" shape of cyst ➡. The lesion suppresses completely on FLAIR ➡ and is isointense with CSF on T2WI ➡.

A **porencephalic cyst** looks just like CSF, but it is intraaxial and lined by gliotic white matter that is often hyperintense on FLAIR. Rarely, **neurenteric cysts** can resemble ACs although they are usually hyperintense compared to CSF. Supratentorial neurenteric cysts are rare.

ARACHNOID CYST: CLINICAL ISSUES AND IMAGING

Clinical Issues
- Most common nonneoplastic intracranial cyst
  - 1% of all intracranial masses
  - All ages; children + young adults (75%)
  - Prevalence = 2% on imaging studies
- Most do not communicate freely with SAS

Imaging
- Behaves *exactly* like CSF
- FLAIR/DWI best to distinguish from other cysts

Differential Diagnosis
- Most common = epidermoid cyst
- Less common
  - Enlarged subarachnoid spaces
  - Loculated subdural hygroma/hematoma
  - Porencephalic cyst
  - Neoplasm-associated cyst
- Rare = neurenteric cyst

Choroid Fissure Cyst

The choroid fissure is an infolding of CSF between the fornix and thalamus. It is normally a shallow, inconspicuous, C-shaped cleft that curves posterosuperiorly from the anterior temporal lobe all the way to the atrium of the lateral ventricle. The choroidal arteries and choroid plexus lie just medial to the choroid fissure.

A CSF-containing cyst can form anywhere along the choroid fissure. These "choroid fissure cysts" are probably caused by maldevelopment of the embryonic tela choroidea, a double layer of pia that invaginates through the choroid fissure to reach the lateral ventricles.

Choroid fissure cysts can therefore be regarded as a subtype of arachnoid cyst. We consider them separately because of their unique location and imaging appearance.

Imaging

Choroid fissure cysts lie just medial to the temporal horn of the lateral ventricle and follow CSF density/signal intensity on all sequences (28-11). On axial and coronal images they are round to oval but on sagittal images have a distinctive, somewhat elongated "spindle" shape (28-12).

Epidermoid Cyst

Both congenital and acquired epidermoid cysts are found in the CNS. While spinal epidermoid cysts are often acquired lesions, intracranial epidermoid cysts are always congenital in origin.

Terminology

An intracranial epidermoid cyst (EC) is an inclusion cyst that is derived from embryonic ectodermal elements. Epidermoid cysts have incorrectly been called "tumors," but

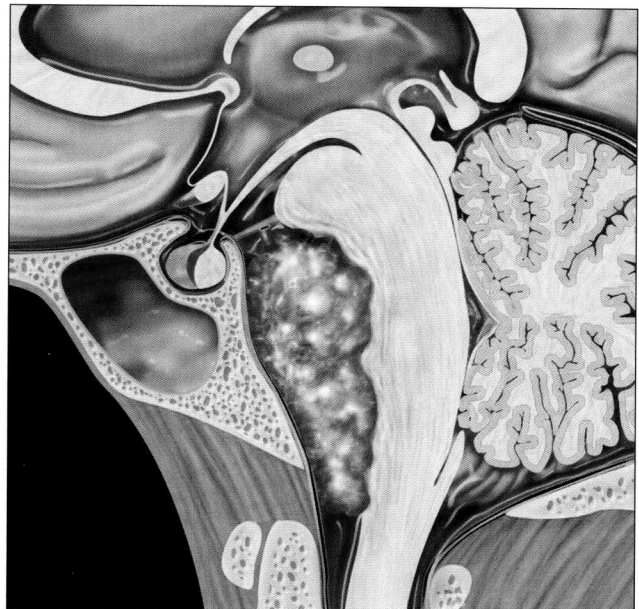

28-13. Sagittal graphic illustrates a multilobulated epidermoid cyst, primarily within the prepontine cistern. Significant mass effect displaces the pons, cervicomedullary junction, upper cervical spine.

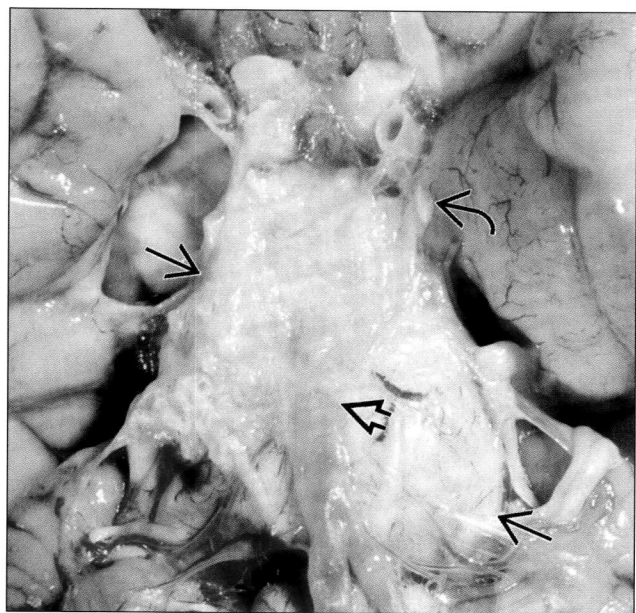

28-14. Autopsy specimen shows a posterior fossa epidermoid cyst as a white, "pearly" tumor in the cerebellopontine, prepontine cisterns ⇨. Note the encased basilar artery ⇘, oculomotor nerves ⇗.

they are not neoplastic. The term "cholesteatoma" should be reserved for an acquired lesion arising as a complication of chronic otitis media.

tiology

GENERAL CONCEPTS. ECs arise during the third to fifth gestational weeks. Ectodermal cellular remnants caused by incomplete cleavage of neural from cutaneous ectoderm result in the inclusion of epiblasts in the neural tube. Congenital CPA epidermoids are derived from cells of the first branchial groove.

athology

LOCATION. Extracranial ECs commonly involve the scalp, face, and neck. Over 90% of intracranial ECs are intradural and are almost always extraaxial **(28-13)**. ECs are more often off- or paramidline and have a predilection for the basal cisterns, where they insinuate themselves around cranial nerves and vessels.

The CPA cistern is the single most common site, accounting for nearly half of all intracranial ECs. The middle cranial fossa (sylvian fissure) and parasellar region together account for 10-15% of ECs. Less common locations are the cerebral ventricles, usually the fourth ventricle. Purely extradural intradiploic ECs account for 5-10% of cases. Parenchymal ECs do occur but are rare.

GROSS PATHOLOGY. The outer surface of an EC is often shiny, resembling mother of pearl **(28-14)**. Multiple "cauliflower" excrescences are typical **(28-15)**. The cyst is filled with soft, waxy, creamy, or flaky material.

MICROSCOPIC FEATURES. The cyst wall consists of an outer fibrous capsule lined by stratified squamous epithelium. The cyst contains concentric lamellae of keratinaceous debris and solid crystalline cholesterol. Dermal appendages (a characteristic of dermoid cysts) are absent.

Clinical Issues

EPIDEMIOLOGY. ECs represent 0.2-1.8% of primary intracranial tumors and tumor-like lesions. They are the most common intracranial developmental cyst and are four to nine times more common than dermoid cysts. Overall, EC is the third most common CPA mass (after vestibular schwannoma and meningioma) and the most common cystic mass in this location.

DEMOGRAPHICS. Peak age of presentation is 20-60 years. Symptomatic ECs are rare in children. There is no gender predominance.

PRESENTATION. ECs may remain clinically silent for many years. Symptoms are location-dependent. Headache and cranial neuropathy (especially involving CNs V, VII, and VIII) are common features.

NATURAL HISTORY. ECs grow very slowly via progressive accumulation of normally dividing epidermal cells and accretion of desquamated keratin. ECs often reach considerable size before becoming symptomatic. In contrast to dermoid cysts, rupture of an EC is rare. Malignant transformation is extremely rare.

TREATMENT OPTIONS. The insinuating characteristics of ECs make them difficult to resect. Although total

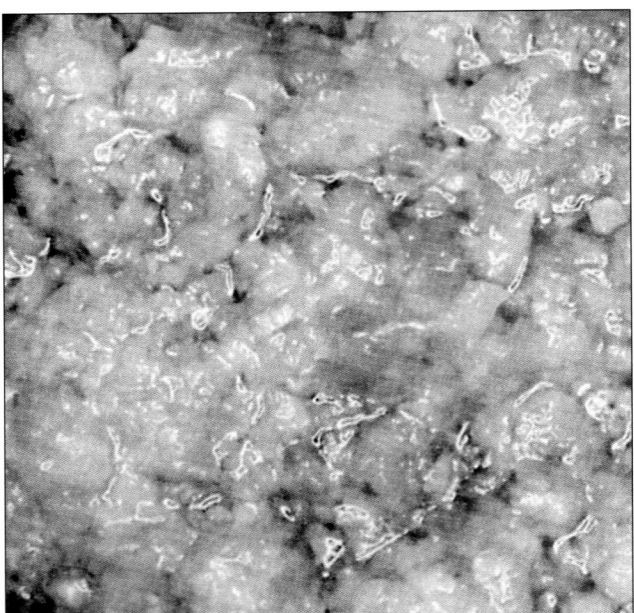

28-15. *Close-up view of a surgical specimen shows classic "cauliflower" appearance of the external surface of an epidermoid cyst.*

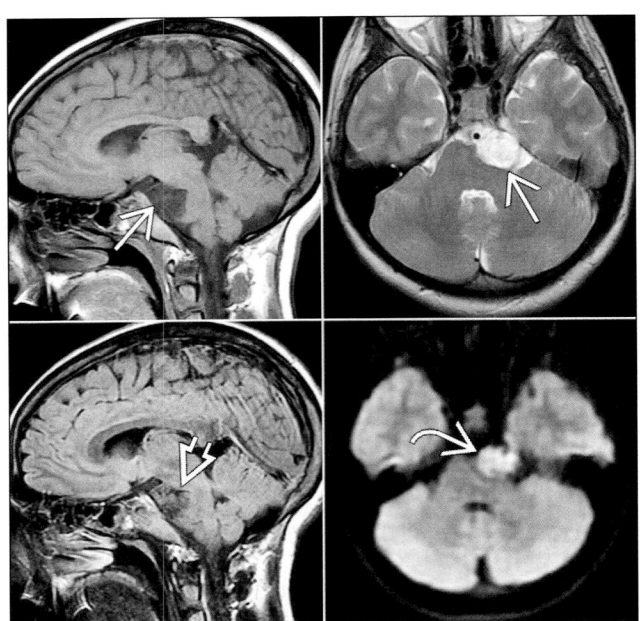

28-16. *Epidermoid cyst resembles CSF on T1- and T2WI ➡ but does not suppress on FLAIR ➡, demonstrates moderate restricted diffusion ➡.*

resection minimizes the risk of postoperative aseptic meningitis, hydrocephalus, and tumor recurrence, aggressive surgery may be associated with cranial nerve or ischemic deficits.

EPIDERMOID CYST: ETIOLOGY, PATHOLOGY, AND EPIDEMIOLOGY

Etiology
- Congenital inclusion cyst
- Epithelial remnants in neural tube

Pathology
- Gross pathology
  - Insinuating, wraps around vessels/cranial nerves
  - Surface lobulated with "pearly" excrescences
  - Waxy, creamy contents
- Microscopic pathology
  - Squamous epithelium + keratin debris, solid cholesterol
  - *NO* dermal appendages!

Epidemiology
- 0.2-1.8% of primary intracranial tumors

Imaging

GENERAL FEATURES. Epidermoid cysts resemble CSF on imaging (**28-16**). Irregular frond-like excrescences and an insinuating growth pattern in CSF cisterns are characteristic.

CT FINDINGS. Over 95% of ECs are hypodense and appear almost identical to CSF on NECT scans. Calcification is present in 10-25%. Hemorrhage is very rare. Hyperdense "white" epidermoids are uncommon, representing 3% of reported lesions. Enhancement is rare.

MR FINDINGS. ECs are iso- or slightly hyperintense compared to CSF on both T1- and T2-weighted sequences. Slight heterogeneity in signal intensity is often present (**28-17**).

"Atypical" epidermoids account for only 5-6% of cases. A "white" epidermoid is a rare type of epidermoid cyst that has a high protein content and may be hyperintense on T1WI and hypointense on T2WI. Enhancement is generally absent although mild peripheral enhancement can be seen in 25% of cases.

ECs either do not suppress at all or suppress incompletely on FLAIR. They restrict on DWI and are therefore moderately to strikingly hyperintense (**28-18**).

Differential Diagnosis

The major differential diagnosis is **arachnoid cyst**. ACs are smoothly marginated, behave *exactly* like CSF on all sequences, suppress completely on FLAIR, and do not restrict on DWI. The rare "white" epidermoid can mimic **neurenteric cyst**.

Parasitic cysts such as neurocysticercosis (NCC) are usually multiple and small and often contain a discernible scolex. Most NCC cysts are located within the depths of cerebral sulci or in the brain parenchyma. **Cystic neoplasms** are rarely mistaken for ECs as the cyst wall and/or nodule enhances.

Dermoid cysts should not be confused with ECs. Dermoid cysts contain fat and dermal appendages and do not resemble CSF on imaging studies.

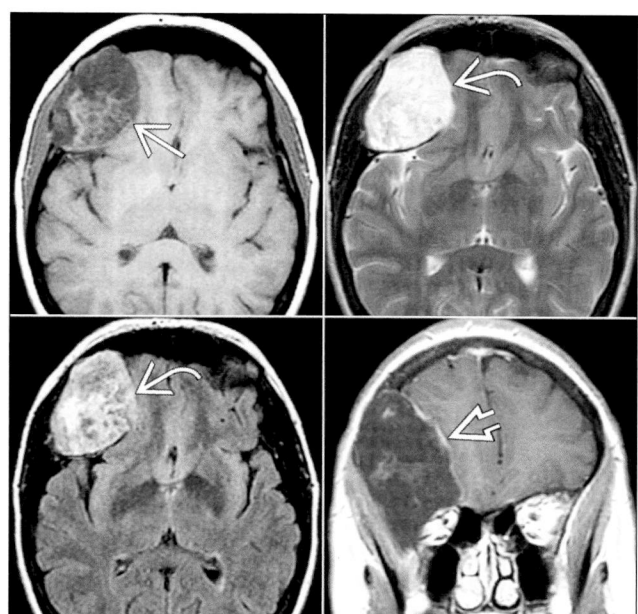

28-17. *Epidermoid cyst of the skull expands the diploic space, shows mottled iso-/hypointensity on T1WI ➡, heterogeneous hyperintensity on T2/FLAIR ➡, mild peripheral enhancement ➡.*

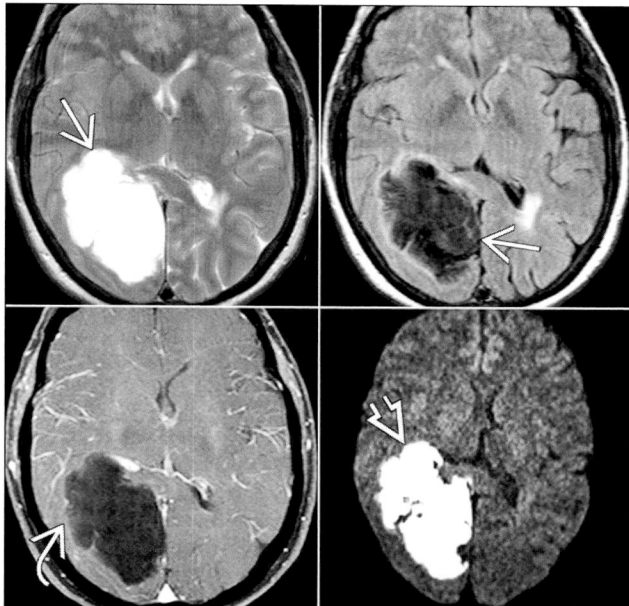

28-18. *Variant case shows a rare epidermoid cyst of the brain parenchyma. Cyst signal intensity is very similar to that of CSF on T2/FLAIR ➡, but the cyst shows faint rim enhancement ➡ and strongly restricted diffusion ➡.*

EPIDERMOID CYST: IMAGING

General Features
- Resembles CSF (vs. fat like dermoid)
- Insinuates around/along CSF cisterns

Location
- Intradural (90%), intradiploic (10%)
- CPA cistern most common site (~ 50%)

CT
- Hypodense (> 95%)

MR
- Slightly hyperintense to CSF on T1WI
- Does not suppress on FLAIR
- Restricts ("bright") on DWI

Differential Diagnosis
- Most common = arachnoid cyst
- Less common = inflammatory cyst

---

ermoid Cyst

rminology

A dermoid cyst (DC) is a histologically benign cystic mass with mature squamous epithelium, keratinous material, and adnexal structures (hair follicles, sebaceous and sweat glands).

iology

GENERAL CONCEPTS. Like epidermoid cysts, DCs are thought to arise from the inclusion of ectodermally committed cells at the time of neural tube closure (third to fifth week of embryogenesis). DCs grow slowly sec-

ondary to the production of hair and oils from the internal dermal elements.

GENETICS. Most DCs are sporadic although there is a reported association with Goldenhar and Klippel-Feil syndromes.

Pathology

LOCATION. DCs are usually extraaxial lesions that are most often found in the midline (28-19). The suprasellar cistern is the most common site, followed by the posterior fossa and frontonasal region.

GROSS PATHOLOGY. A dermoid cyst is a thick-walled unilocular cyst lined by stratified squamous epithelium. Sectioned DCs typically contain thick, greasy sebaceous material, keratin debris, and skin adnexa such as hair follicles (28-20). Lipid and cholesterol elements floating on proteinaceous material may be present.

MICROSCOPIC FEATURES. The outer wall of a DC consists of squamous epithelium. The inner lining contains multiple sebaceous and apocrine glands, fat, and hair follicles.

Clinical Issues

EPIDEMIOLOGY. DCs are much less common than epidermoid cysts, representing less than 0.5% of intracranial masses.

DEMOGRAPHICS. Presentation occurs at significantly younger ages compared to epidermoids, peaking in the second to third decades.

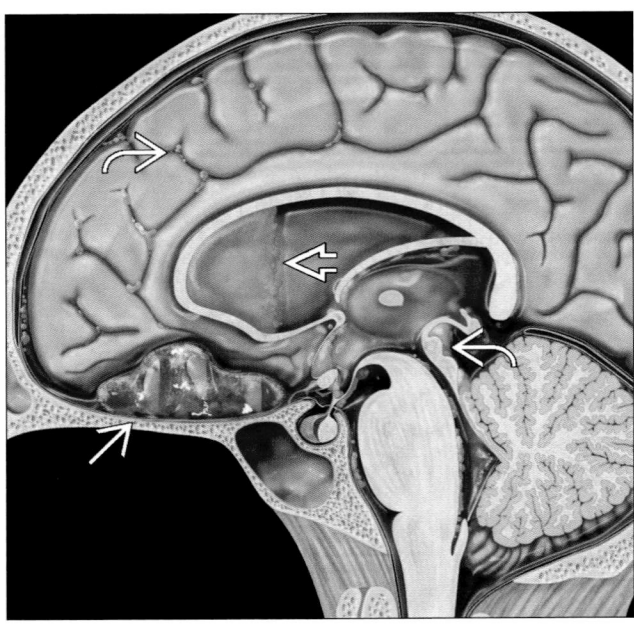

28-19. Inferior frontal dermoid cyst ➡ *is seen as a discrete, heterogeneous, fat-containing mass with squamous epithelium and dermal appendages. Note the ventricular fat-fluid level* ⇥ *and fat in the subarachnoid spaces* ⇥ *from cyst rupture.*

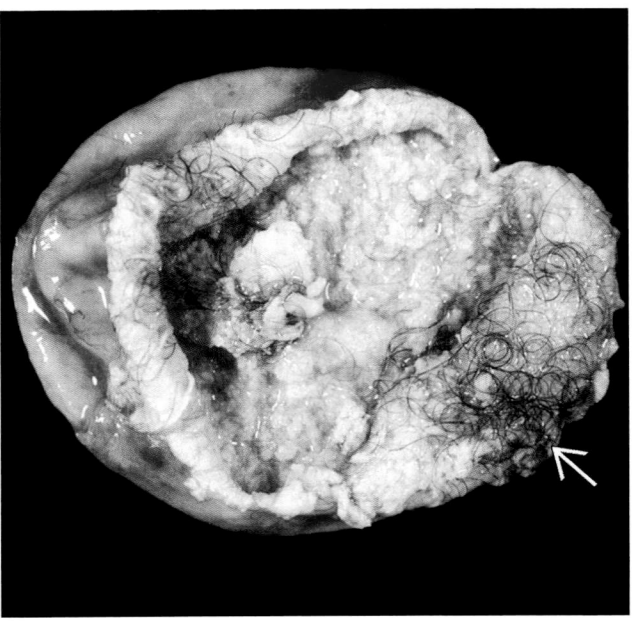

28-20. Dermoid cyst contains thick, greasy sebaceous material, keratin debris, hair ➡. *(Courtesy R. Hewlett, MD.)*

PRESENTATION. DCs often remain asymptomatic until they rupture. Although cyst rupture is usually not fatal, chemical meningitis with seizure, coma, vasospasm, infarction, and even death may ensue as a consequence.

NATURAL HISTORY. DCs typically grow very slowly, although rapid enlargement with rupture has been reported. Cyst rupture is usually spontaneous but has also been associated with head trauma. Fat from a ruptured DC may persist for years. DCs occasionally degenerate into squamous cell carcinomas.

TREATMENT OPTIONS. Complete surgical resection is the goal, but residual tumor adherent to neurovascular structures is often left behind to minimize postoperative complications. Unlike ECs, the recurrence rate after DC resection is very low.

Imaging

GENERAL FEATURES. DCs resemble fat. A round, well-circumscribed lipid-containing mass is the usual appearance.

CT FINDINGS. DCs are quite hypointense on NECT scans **(28-21)**. Calcification of the capsule is seen in 20% of cases. With rupture, hypodense fatty "droplets" disseminate in the CSF cisterns and may cause discernible fat-fluid levels in the ventricles.

In infants with frontal DC, bone CT usually discloses a bifid crista galli with a large foramen cecum and sinus tract.

MR FINDINGS. Signal intensity varies with fat content in the cyst. Most DCs are heterogeneously hyperintense on T1WI. T1WI is also the most sensitive sequence to detect disseminated fat "droplets" in the subarachnoid space, diagnostic of ruptured dermoid **(28-22)**. Fat suppression is helpful to confirm the presence of lipid elements.

Standard PD and T2 scans show increasingly more pronounced "chemical shift" artifact in the frequency-encoding direction as the TR is lengthened. Fat is very hypointense on standard T2WI but is "bright" (hyperintense) on fast spin echo T2-weighted sequences. DCs demonstrate heterogeneous hyperintensity with linear or striated laminations if hair is present within the cyst.

Uncomplicated DCs are heterogeneously hyperintense on FLAIR. Ruptured DCs demonstrate subtle FLAIR sulcal hyperintensity and "bloom" on T2* GRE.

Most DCs do not enhance, although ruptured DCs may cause significant chemical meningitis with extensive leptomeningeal reaction and enhancement.

Spectroscopy may show an elevated lipid peak at 0.9-1.3 ppm.

Differential Diagnosis

The major differential diagnosis of DC is **epidermoid cyst**. ECs behave like CSF whereas DCs resemble fat. **Lipoma** may resemble a DC but is generally much more homogeneous on imaging and is often associated with other congenital malformations such as callosal dysgenesis. **Craniopharyngioma** is often multicystic, extends

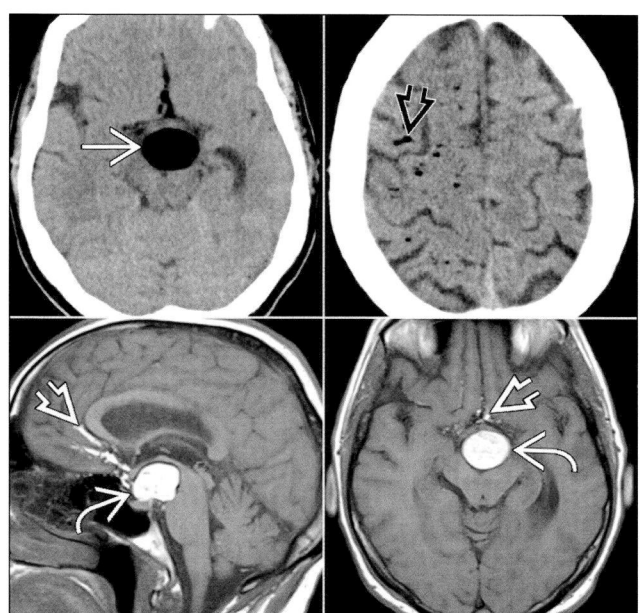

28-21. NECT scans of a ruptured dermoid show a hypodense suprasellar mass ➡️ and fat droplets in the sulci ▷. The cyst contents ➡️ and subarachnoid fat ➡️ are hyperintense on T1WI.

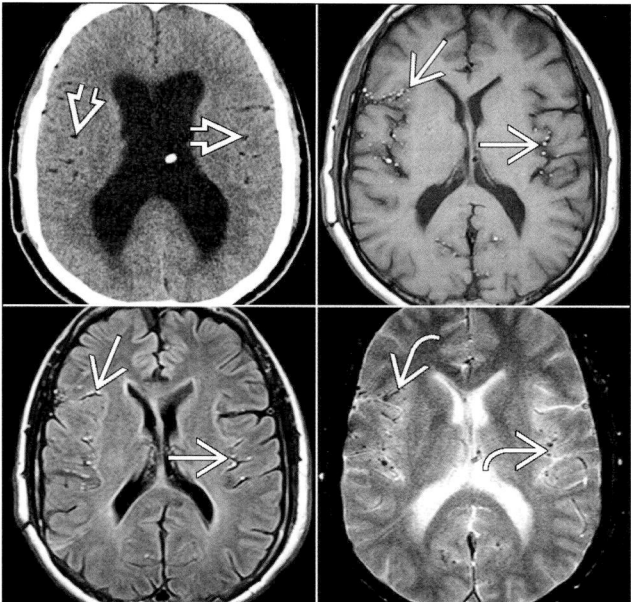

28-22. Ruptured dermoid in a 44-year-old man with sudden onset severe headache. NECT shows obstructive hydrocephalus, hypodense fat "droplets" in subarachnoid spaces ➡️. Fat is hyperintense on T1WI, FLAIR ➡️, "blooms" on T2* GRE ➡️.

into the sella, calcifies, and enhances. **Teratoma** may resemble a DC but most commonly occurs in the pineal gland and is much more heterogeneous on imaging than the typical DC.

DERMOID vs. EPIDERMOID CYST

Pathology
- Squamous epithelium + keratin debris (both dermoid, epidermoid)
- Plus fat, dermal appendages (only dermoid)

Clinical Issues
- At least 4x *less* common than epidermoid cyst
- More common in children, young adults
- Commonly ruptures

Imaging
- DC behaves like fat, EC like CSF

Neurenteric Cyst

Neurenteric cysts are rare endodermal-derived developmental CNS lesions. They are significantly more common in the spine than in the brain.

Terminology

Neurenteric (NE) cyst is also called enterogenous cyst, enteric cyst, and endodermal cyst. Other less common terms, primarily applied to intraspinal NE cysts, are gastrogenic and archenteric cysts.

Etiology

Neurenteric cysts, along with Rathke cleft and colloid cysts, are endodermally derived developmental lesions of the CNS. They probably arise from persistence of the embryonic neurenteric canal, a temporary connection between the amniotic and yolk sacs during the third week of embryogenesis. Primitive endodermal cells may then become incorporated into the notochord. These displaced nests of alimentary tissue may ultimately form an NE cyst.

The most cephalad aspect of the notochord forms the clivus, which is why most intracranial NE cysts are found in the midline posterior fossa. There are no reasonable theories to explain the development of the even rarer supratentorial NE cysts.

Pathology

LOCATION. The most common CNS site is the spine. Intracranial NE cysts are rare, accounting for less than 25% of all cases. Almost 75% of these occur in the posterior fossa, and almost all are extraaxial. The typical location is midline or slightly off-midline, just anterior to the pontomedullary junction **(28-23)**. The lower CPA cistern is also a common site.

Between 25-30% of intracranial NE cysts are supratentorial. Almost all reported cases are off-midline, located adjacent to the frontal lobes.

SIZE AND NUMBER. NE cysts vary in size. Most are relatively small (one to three centimeters in diameter). Occasionally, NE cysts can become very large (up to nine centimeters), especially when they occur in the supratentorial compartment.

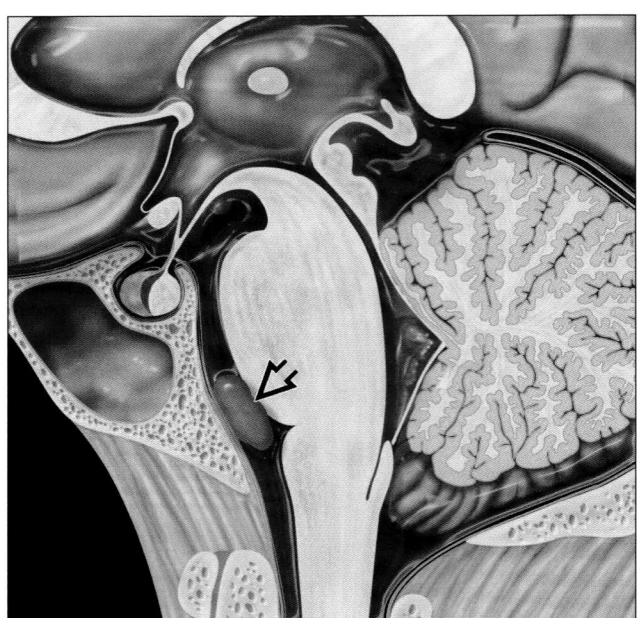

28-23. Sagittal graphic shows a classic neurenteric cyst ⬦. Intracranial neurenteric cysts are most often found near the midline, anterior to the brainstem.

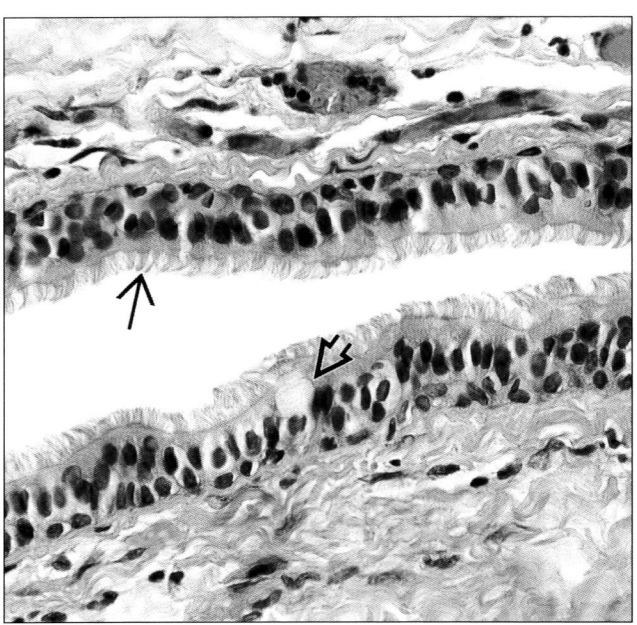

28-24. Neurenteric (endodermal) cysts are mostly lined with pseudostratified ciliated epithelium ⬦ and contain variable numbers of goblet cells ⬦. (Courtesy P. Burger, MD.)

NE cysts are almost always solitary. "Seeding" or wide dissemination with multiple cysts spreading throughout the spinal canal is reported but rare.

GROSS PATHOLOGY. NE cysts are typically well-delineated, smoothly marginated cysts. The wall is thin and translucent. Cyst contents range from clear colorless fluid that resembles CSF to thick viscous mucoid secretions.

MICROSCOPIC FEATURES. NE cysts are lined by pseudostratified columnar epithelium wtum heavily ciliated cells and variable amounts of mucin-secreting goblet cells **(28-24)**. A few cases of squamous metaplasia and even mucinous adenocarcinomas arising in an NE cyst have been reported.

Clinical Issues

DEMOGRAPHICS. NE cysts occur in patients of all ages. Age distribution is bimodal, with a large peak in the third and fourth decades and a smaller peak in the first decade. Average age at presentation is 34 years. There is a slight male predominance.

PRESENTATION. Posterior fossa NE cysts typically present with waxing and waning neck pain or occipital headaches. Headaches, behavior changes, and seizures have been reported with supratentorial lesions.

NATURAL HISTORY. NE cysts grow very slowly and are often stable for years.

TREATMENT OPTIONS. Small NE cysts are sometimes monitored with periodic imaging. Symptomatic cysts are

excised. Total surgical removal is the treatment goal but may be difficult due to adhesion of the cyst membrane to critical neurovascular structures.

NEURENTERIC CYST: PATHOLOGY AND CLINICAL ISSUES

Location
- Posterior fossa (75%)
  - Extraaxial, midline/slightly off-midline
  - Anterior to pontomedullary junction
- Supratentorial (25%)
  - Extraaxial, adjacent to frontal lobes

Pathology
- Endodermal-derived congenital inclusion cyst
- Size varies from 1-9 cm
- Round/ovoid shape, smoothly marginated
- Wall contains mucin-secreting goblet cells

Clinical Issues
- Spinal NE cyst 3-4x more common than intracranial
- Asymptomatic or headache, neck pain

Imaging

GENERAL FEATURES. NE cysts are all well-delineated and round to ovoid. Density and signal intensity vary according to protein content of the cyst fluid. Most NE cysts are moderately proteinaceous and therefore often do not precisely parallel CSF.

CT FINDINGS. Most NE cysts are iso- to slightly hyperdense compared to CSF. Hyperdense ("white") NE cysts are seen in about 25% of cases. Calcification and intracystic hemorrhage are absent. In contrast to spinal NE cysts, bony anomalies are rare. NE cysts do not enhance following contrast administration.

MR FINDINGS. NE cysts are sharply demarcated lesions that displace but do not engulf adjacent neurovascular structures. The cyst wall itself is often inapparent. Signal intensity of cyst contents varies widely, depending on imaging sequence and protein content.

Cyst fluid is almost always iso- to hyperintense compared to CSF on T1WI **(28-25)**. Over 90% are hyperintense to CSF on PD and T2WI. Between 5-10%—typically NE cysts with inspissated, significantly dehydrated contents—are hypointense.

NE cysts do not suppress on FLAIR and are almost always hyperintense relative to CSF. As NE cysts almost never calcify or hemorrhage, T2* (GRE, SWI) sequences do not demonstrate "blooming."

Only a few reports of NE cysts have included DWI findings. In those cases, diffusion restriction was mild or absent.

Most NE cysts do not enhance following contrast administration. A few cases of mild posterior rim enhancement at the cyst-brain interface have been reported.

Differential Diagnosis

Other endodermal-derived cysts such as Rathke cleft (sella) and colloid cyst (foramen of Monro) are easily differentiated from NE. They are very location-specific, and their anatomic sites do not overlap with those of NE.

The major differential diagnosis of NE cyst is **epidermoid cyst**. Epidermoid cysts are insinuating lesions that have lobulated frond-like surfaces. Most ECs restrict strongly on DWI. Posterior fossa ECs are usually more lateral than NE cysts, occurring more commonly in the CPA cistern than at the pontomedullary junction. Some reported cases of "white" epidermoids may actually have been NE cysts.

Arachnoid cyst follows CSF signal intensity on all sequences (e.g., suppresses completely on FLAIR) and does not restrict on DWI.

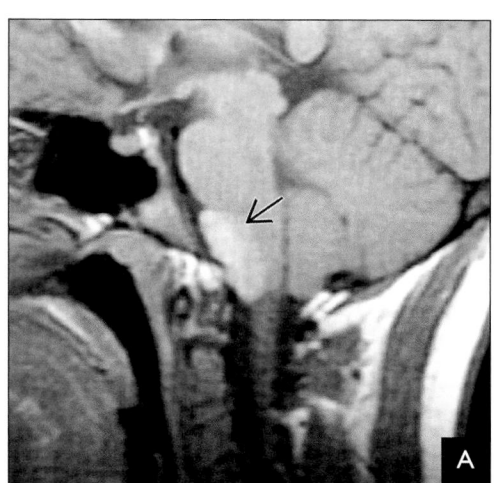

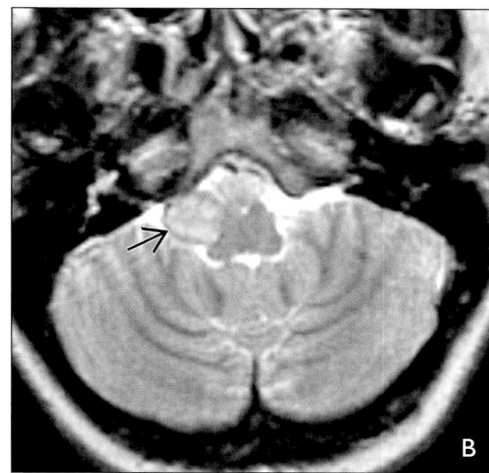

28-25A. Sagittal T1WI of a NE cyst shows a hyperintense ovoid midline mass ⇨ in front of the medulla. 28-25B. Axial T2WI shows that the mass ⇨ is well-delineated. It is heterogeneously hypointense to CSF, suggesting inspissated contents. More typically NE cysts are hyperintense to CSF.

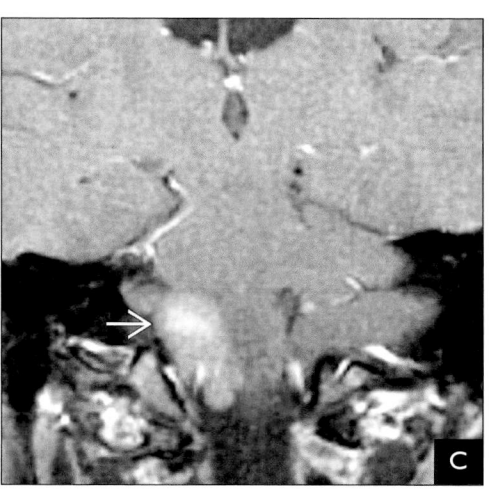

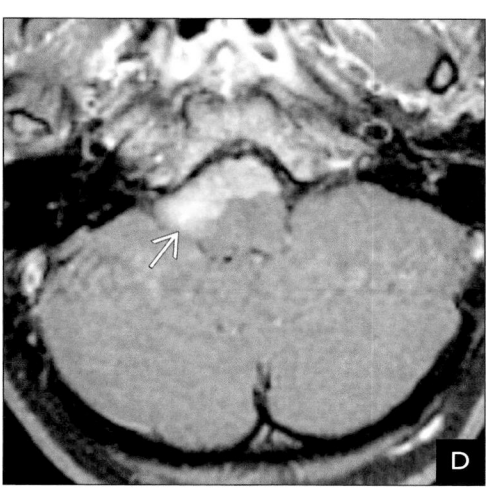

28-25C. Coronal T1 C+ scan shows that the ovoid mass ⇨ is well-demarcated, hyperintense. 28-25D. Axial T1 C+ FS shows that the mass ⇨ extends inferiorly to the lower medulla. The center of the mass is just slightly off-midline, a typical solution for a posterior fossa NE cyst.

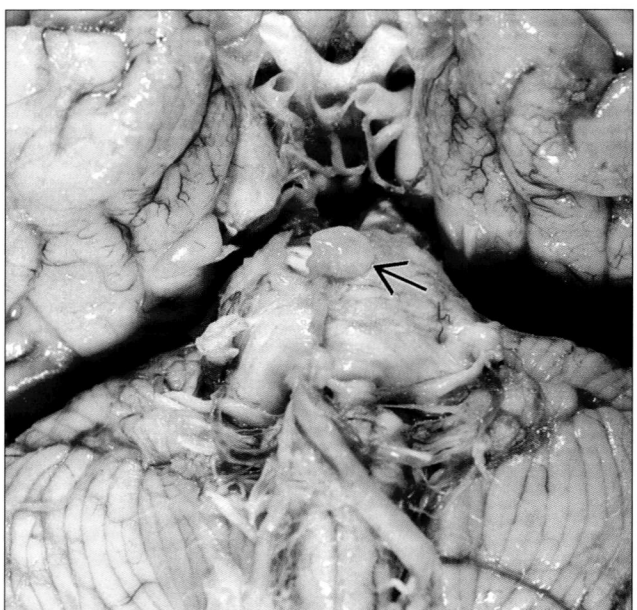

28-26. Autopsy specimen shows a round gelatinous-appearing mass in front of the pons ⮞. *Incidental finding of ecchordosis physaliphorous. (Courtesy R. Hewlett, MD.)*

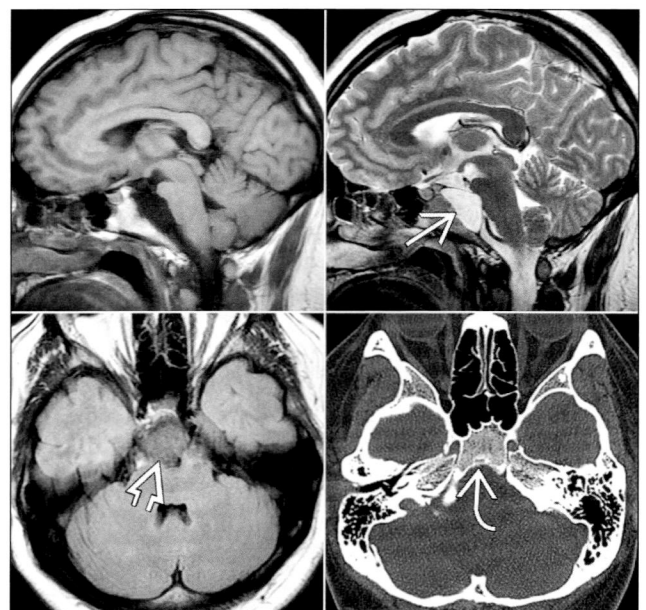

28-27. Physaliphorous ecchordosis is seen here as a lobulated prepontine mass that is slightly hyperintense to CSF on T2WI ⮞, *does not suppress on FLAIR* ⮞, *connects in the midline to the clivus* ⮞.

Schwannoma is the most common extraaxial posterior fossa mass in adults. It typically enhances strongly and rarely occurs in the midline.

A rare anatomic variant that can be confused with a posterior fossa NE cyst is **ecchordosis physaliphora**. An ecchordosis physaliphora (EP) is a gelatinous-appearing notochordal remnant that can appear anywhere from the dorsum sellae to the sacrococcygeal region. EPs are found in approximately 2% of autopsies. Intracranial EPs are well-demarcated midline lesions that typically occur in the prepontine cistern (28-26). They are attached to a visible defect in the dorsal clivus by a thin stalk-like pedicle (28-27). Chordoma is the malignant counterpart of ecchordosis.

NEURENTERIC CYST: IMAGING

CT
- NECT: Iso-/slightly hyperintense to CSF
- CECT: No enhancement

MR
- T1WI: Almost always iso-/slightly hyperintense to CSF
- PD, T2WI: Hyperintense to CSF (> 90%)
- FLAIR: Does not suppress
- DWI: Mild/no restriction

Differential Diagnosis
- Most common = epidermoid, arachnoid cysts
- Less common = schwannoma (cystic)
- Rare = ecchordosis physaliphora

Pineal Cyst

Modern imaging has resulted in a plethora of pineal "things" found on CT and especially MR. These lesions, often seen in patients with vague complaints and no symptoms referable to the pineal region, can be troublesome to both radiologists and referring clinicians.

Terminology

A pineal cyst (PC) is a benign glia-lined, fluid-containing cyst within the pineal gland parenchyma.

Etiology

The precise etiology of PCs is unknown. Theories include persistent coalescing embryonic pineal cavities and glial degeneration with cavitation.

Pathology

LOCATION. An easy way to remember the normal midline anatomic structures in the pineal region—from top to bottom—is "famous **V.I.P.**" for **f**ornix, **v**elum interpositum, **i**nternal cerebral veins, and **p**ineal gland (see Chapter 20). As expected, any pineal gland mass—including PCs—therefore lies below the fornix, velum interpositum, and internal cerebral veins, displacing them superiorly. While PCs may compress the posterior third ventricle, most PCs exert little or no mass effect on the tectum and aqueduct, so hydrocephalus is rare except with very large cysts.

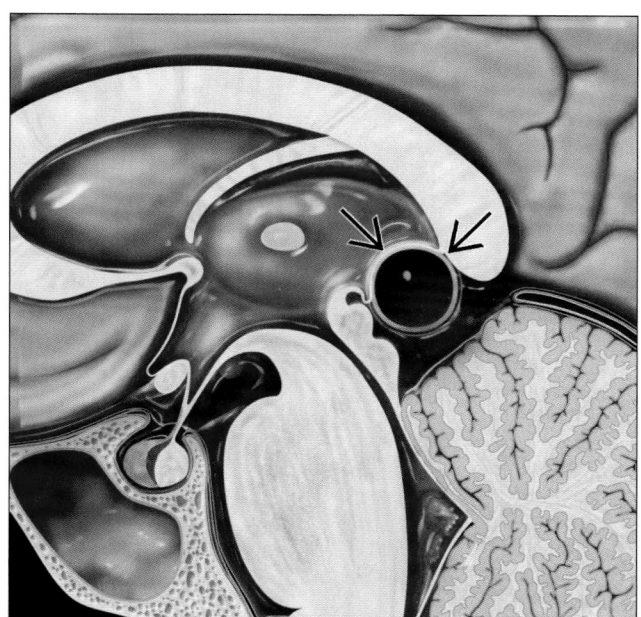

28-28. Sagittal graphic shows a small cystic lesion within the pineal gland ⇥. Small benign pineal cysts are often found incidentally at autopsy or imaging.

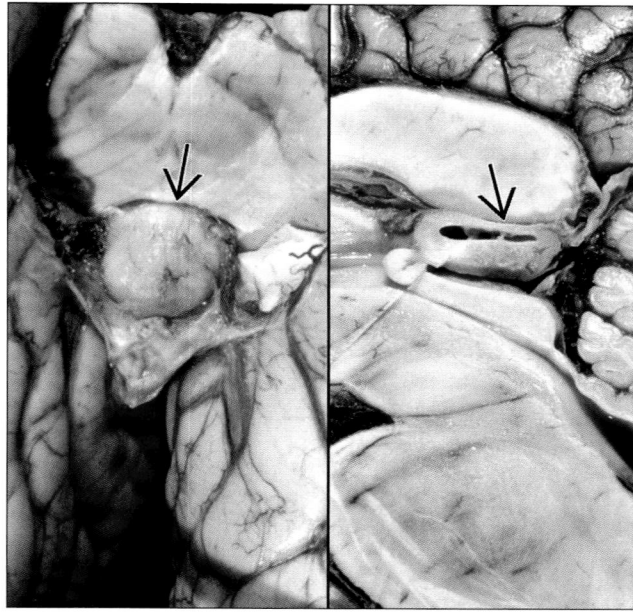

28-29. Axial (left), sagittal (right) autopsy views of pineal cyst ⇥ show the typical location behind the tectal plate. (Courtesy E. T. Hedley-Whyte, MD.)

SIZE AND NUMBER. PCs are well-demarcated round or ovoid expansions within an otherwise normal-appearing pineal gland **(28-28)**. Most PCs are less than 10 mm in diameter. The largest reported PC is 4.5 cm. Pineal cysts are usually unilocular, but lesions containing multiple smaller cysts do occur.

GROSS PATHOLOGY. The general appearance is that of a smooth, soft, tan-yellow pineal gland that contains a uni- or multilocular cyst **(28-29)**. Cyst fluid is clear to yellowish.

MICROSCOPIC FEATURES. Pineal cysts are cavities of various sizes surrounded by an outer layer of attenuated pineal parenchyma. The inner layer is a sharply defined zone of finely fibrillar glial tissue with Rosenthal fibers. PCs have no ependymal or epithelial lining. The inner surface of the cyst cavity is often hemosiderin-stained as the result of intralesional hemorrhage. There is no histologic difference between asymptomatic and symptomatic PCs.

Clinical Issues

EPIDEMIOLOGY. Cystic-appearing lesions in the pineal gland are common, seen in 23% of healthy adults on MR scans. Between 25-40% of autopsied pineal glands contain microscopic cysts.

DEMOGRAPHICS. PCs can occur at *any* age although they are more often discovered in middle-aged and older adults.

The overall F:M ratio is 3:1. The incidence among women ages 21-30 years is significantly higher than in any other group.

PRESENTATION. Most PCs are clinically benign and asymptomatic, discovered incidentally at imaging or autopsy. Large pineal cysts may obstruct the cerebral aqueduct, resulting in hydrocephalus and headache. Parinaud syndrome (tectal compression) is less common.

Pineal "apoplexy" occurs with sudden intracystic hemorrhage. Acute worsening of headaches combined with visual symptoms can occur. A "thunderclap" headache may mimic symptoms of aneurysmal subarachnoid hemorrhage. Pineal "apoplexy" can result in acute intraventricular obstructive hydrocephalus. Rare cases result in sudden death.

NATURAL HISTORY. Serial follow-up of indeterminate cystic lesions of the pineal region shows, in most lesions, no significant change in size or character over time intervals from months to years. Most investigators recommend that incidentally identified pineal cysts be followed clinically and do not require serial imaging.

TREATMENT OPTIONS. Most pineal cysts are "leave me alone" lesions. Symptomatic cysts may require stereotactic aspiration or biopsy/resection.

Imaging

CT FINDINGS. At least 25% of PCs show calcification within the cyst wall **(28-30)**. The cyst fluid is iso- to slightly hyperdense compared to CSF **(28-31)**. A very

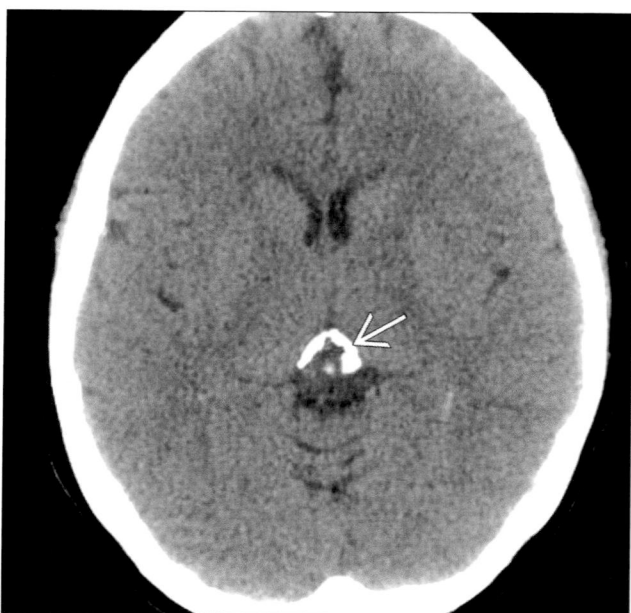

28-30. NECT scan shows rim calcification in the wall of an enlarged pineal gland ➡, characteristic for both pineal cyst and pineocytoma. Surgically proven nonneoplastic pineal cyst.

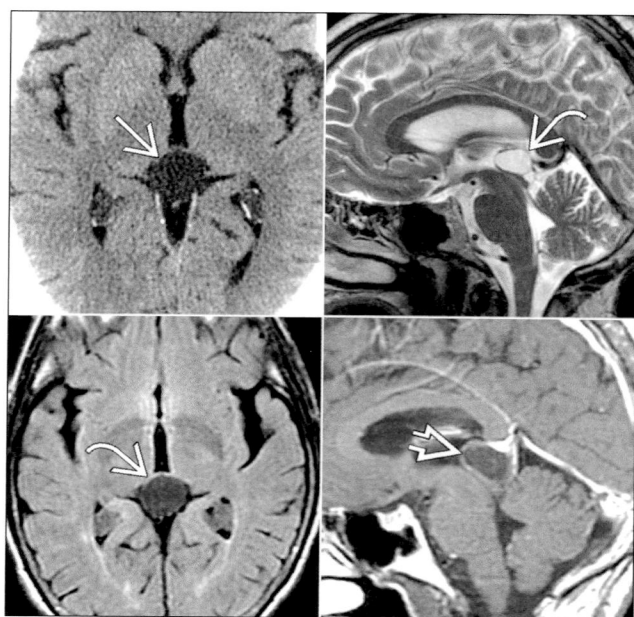

28-31. Large pineal cyst is slightly hyperdense to CSF on NECT ➡ and hyperintense on T2WI and FLAIR ➡, shows a thin enhancing rim ➡ on T1 C+.

hyperdense PC in a patient with severe headache should raise suspicion of hemorrhage with cyst "apoplexy."

The ventricles are usually normal. Large ventricles with "blurred" margins indicate acute obstructive hydrocephalus.

Enhancement is typical. Rim, crescentic, or nodular patterns have all been described with PCs.

MR FINDINGS. Thin-section high-resolution sagittal and axial T2 scans are especially helpful for detecting and characterizing lesions in the anatomically complex pineal region.

As with other cysts, PC signal intensity varies with imaging sequence and cyst contents.

Most pineal cysts are small and cause minimal or no mass effect. Large cysts—or PCs with acute intracystic hemorrhage—may cause obstructive hydrocephalus. In such cases, PD and T2/FLAIR scans show "fingers" of hyperintensity extending into the periventricular white matter due to subependymal accumulation of brain interstitial fluid. These are especially well-demonstrated on sagittal scans.

Between 50-60% of PCs are slightly hyperintense compared to CSF on T1WI. Approximately 40% are isointense with CSF. Approximately 1-2% are very hyperintense, which may indicate intracystic hemorrhage. A blood-fluid level may be present **(28-32)**.

The vast majority of PCs are hyperintense to CSF on intermediate (PD) sequences and iso- to slightly hyperin-

tense on T2WI. Internal septations are visible in 20-25% of cases. If acute hemorrhage has occurred, intracystic blood may appear very hypointense.

PCs do not suppress completely on FLAIR and are moderately hyperintense relative to brain parenchyma. If intracystic hemorrhage has occurred, cyst fluid "blooms" on T2* (GRE, SWI) **(28-33)**. Rim calcifications may show mild "blooming."

Over 90% of PCs enhance. The most common pattern is a thin circumferential rim of enhancement **(28-31)**. Less common patterns include nodular, crescentic, or irregular enhancement.

PCs typically do not restrict on DWI. Neuronal markers are absent on MRS.

Differential Diagnosis

The most common differential diagnosis is **normal pineal gland**. Normal pineal glands often contain one or more small cysts and can have nodular, crescentic, or ring-like enhancement.

The most important pathologic entity to be differentiated from a PC is **pineocytoma**. Pineocytoma is a WHO grade I pineal parenchymal tumor that is usually solid or at least partially solid/cystic. Purely cystic pineocytomas are much less common and can be indistinguishable from PC on imaging. As these are extremely slow-growing neoplasms, pineocytomas can remain stable for many years without significant change on serial imaging.

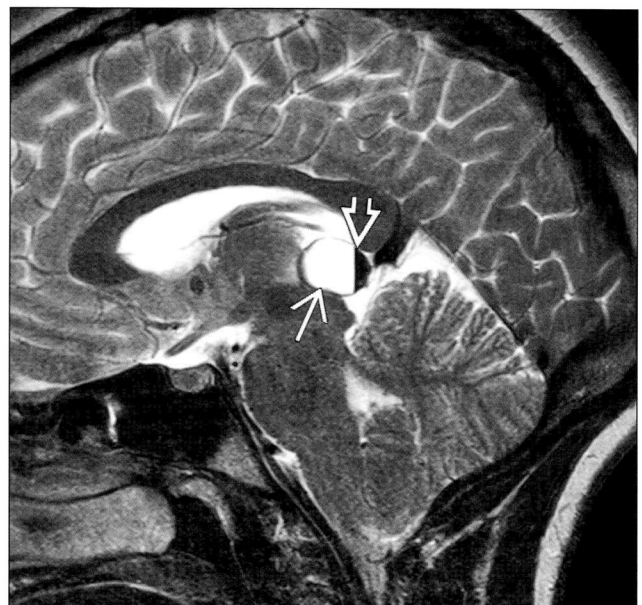

28-32. Sagittal T2WI in a 17-year-old female with sudden onset severe headache, visual difficulties shows a large pineal cyst ➡ with blood-fluid level ⇉ indicating hemorrhage (cyst "apoplexy").

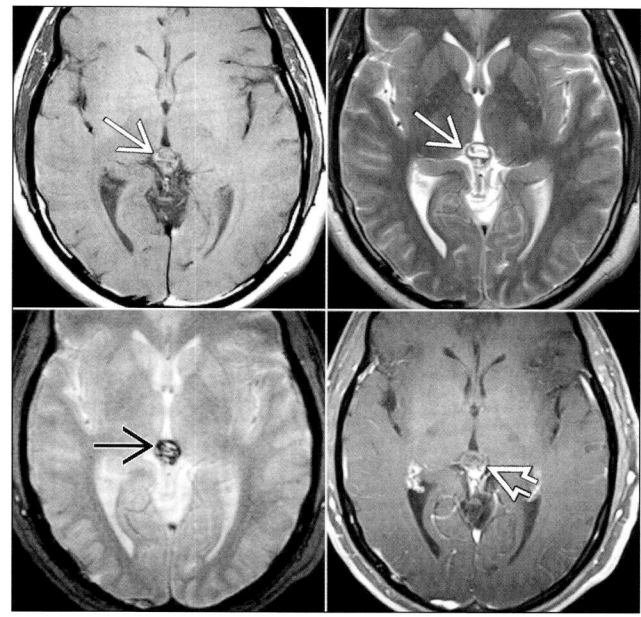

28-33. Small pineal cyst with hemorrhage ➡, "blooming" on T2* ⇒, rim and nodular enhancement on T1 C+ FS ⇉.

Atypical imaging findings, focal invasion, or significant interval change in a presumed pineal cyst or pineocytoma should raise suspicion for the more aggressive **pineal parenchymal tumor of intermediate differentiation** (PPTID).

Nonneoplastic cysts that occasionally occur in the vicinity of the pineal gland include **epidermoid cyst** and **arachnoid cyst** (of the quadrigeminal plate or velum interpositum). These extrapineal lesions should not be confused with PC.

PINEAL CYST

Pathology
- Below fornix, internal cerebral veins
- Usually < I cm, typically unilocular
- Wall contains attenuated pineal parenchyma
- Fluid clear to yellowish

Clinical Issues
- Common
  ○ 23% of normal MRs, 25-40% of autopsies
- Occur at any age; more common in adults
- Usually asymptomatic, found incidentally

Imaging
- Ca++ (25%)
- Rim, nodular, or crescentic enhancement

Differential Diagnosis
- Normal pineal gland
- Pineocytoma

Nonneoplastic Tumor-associated Cysts

Terminology

Tumor-associated cysts (TACs) are benign cysts that are adjacent to, but not contained within, a neoplasm.

TACs are also referred to as peritumoral cysts. Surgeons sometimes call them "herald" cysts, as they are immediately adjacent to (and thus "herald" the presence of) a tumor mass.

Etiology

Whether TACs are true arachnoid cysts or fluid collections mostly lined by compressed gliotic brain is debatable. Cyst formation may also relate to blood-brain-barrier deficiency with peritumoral extravasation of water, electrolytes, and plasma proteins from altered microvessels.

TACs are usually associated with benign extraaxial tumors such as meningioma, schwannoma, pituitary macroadenoma, and craniopharyngioma. TACs are found in both supra- and infratentorial compartments.

Pathology

Most TACs represent trapped, encysted "pools" of CSF adjacent to a large extraaxial neoplasm **(28-34)**. The contents of these peritumoral collections vary from clear CSF-like liquid to turbid proteinaceous fluid. The cyst wall generally consists of gliotic brain with reactive astrocytes and lymphocytes. No tumor cells are present.

LOCATION. TACs are usually positioned at the tumor-brain interface between the mass and adjacent cortex.

SIZE AND NUMBER. TACs vary from small insignificant collections to very large cysts. Most are solitary, but occasionally multiple loculated fluid collections are trapped at the tumor-brain interface.

Clinical Issues

Unless a TAC becomes unusually large, symptoms are generally related to the neoplasm itself, not the TAC.

Imaging

GENERAL FEATURES. The common appearance is one or more "pools" of trapped fluid surrounding an extraaxial tumor mass **(28-35)**.

CT FINDINGS. TACs are hypodense to brain and usually iso- to slightly hyperdense compared to CSF. No calcification, hemorrhage, or enhancement is present.

MR FINDINGS. As with other cysts, signal intensity varies with protein content. Most TACs are hypointense to brain on T1WI and very hyperintense on PD and T2WI **(28-36)**, **(28-37)**. Suppression on FLAIR is variable. Enhancement is minimal or absent and generally related to reactive inflammatory changes in the cyst wall, not tumor.

Differential Diagnosis

Tumor-associated cysts must be distinguished from **cystic neoplasms**. Other considerations include **arachnoid cyst** (not tumor-associated) and **enlarged perivascular (Virchow-Robin) spaces**. The latter are intraparenchymal clusters of variably sized cysts that contain interstitial fluid but behave like CSF on imaging studies.

28-34. Autopsy specimen shows a frontal meningioma ➡ with CSF-vascular "cleft" ➡, large tumor-associated cyst ⊳. 28-35. Coronal T2WI shows a typical sphenoid wing meningioma ➡ with hyperintense pools of trapped fluid ⊳ between the tumor, brain. (Courtesy M. Thurnher, MD.)

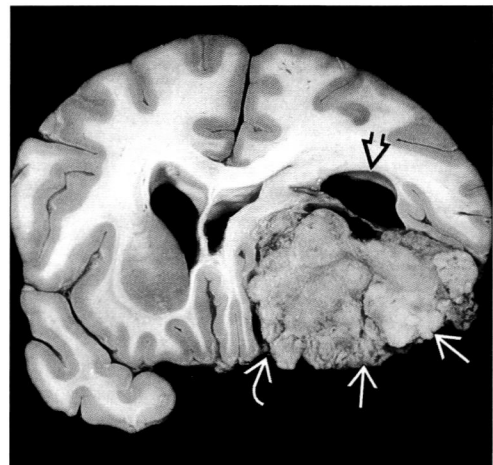
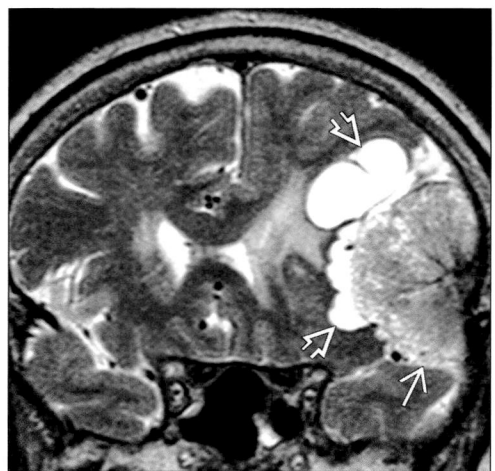

28-36. Axial T2WI shows a large vestibular schwannoma ➡ with a prominent cyst ⊳ interposed between the tumor, cerebellum. 28-37. Axial T2WI shows a pituitary macroadenoma with suprasellar extension ➡, a prominent tumor-associated cyst ➡ with a blood-fluid level ⊳.

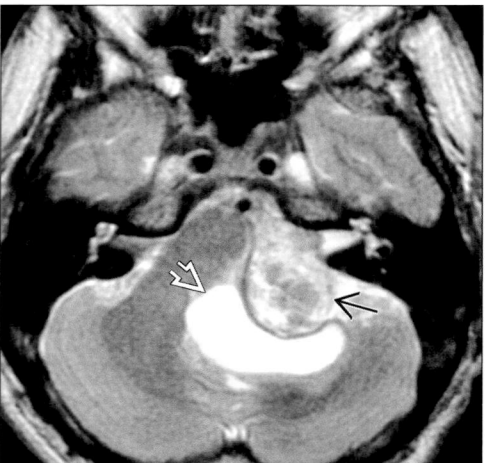
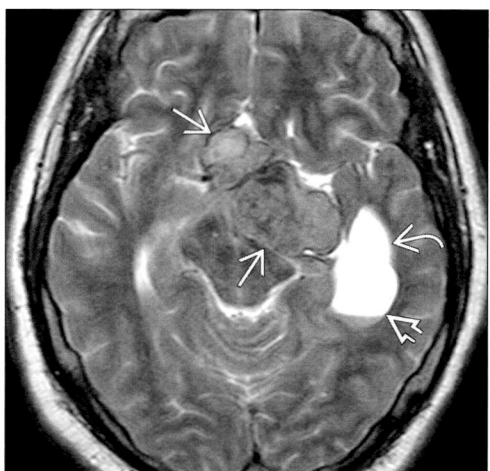

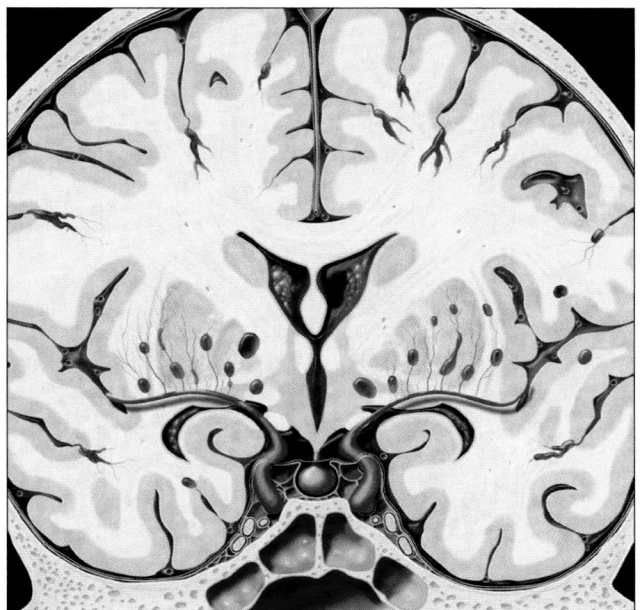

28-38. *Coronal graphic shows normal PVSs as they accompany penetrating arteries into the basal ganglia and subcortical white matter. Normal PVSs cluster around the anterior commissure but also occur in all areas.*

28-39. *Axial T2WI shows typical perivascular spaces* ➡️ *clustered around the anterior commissure* ➡️.

Parenchymal Cysts

Parenchymal (intraaxial) cysts are much more common than either their extraaxial or intraventricular counterparts. Once a cyst has been identified as lying within the brain itself, the differential diagnosis is limited. The most common parenchymal cysts—prominent perivascular spaces and hippocampal sulcus remnants—are anatomic variants. Neuroglial cysts and porencephalic cysts are relatively uncommon. All other nonneoplastic, noninfectious brain cysts are rare.

Enlarged Perivascular Spaces

By far the most common parenchymal brain "cysts" are enlarged perivascular spaces. They vary from solitary, small, inconspicuous, and unremarkable to multiple, large, bizarre, alarming-looking collections of CSF-like fluid. They are often asymmetric, may cause mass effect, and have frequently been mistaken for multicystic brain tumors.

Terminology

Perivascular spaces (PVSs) are also known as Virchow-Robin spaces. PVSs are pia-lined spaces that accompany penetrating arteries and arterioles into the brain parenchyma. The PVSs do not communicate directly with the subarachnoid space.

Etiology

GENERAL CONCEPTS. The brain PVSs form a complicated intraparenchymal network that is distributed throughout the cerebral hemispheres, midbrain, and cerebellum. They are filled with interstitial fluid (ISF), not CSF, and are thought to be a major pathway for ISF and cerebral metabolites to exit the brain. Recent evidence suggests the PVSs also perform an essential role in maintaining intracranial pressure homeostasis.

Precisely why some PVSs become enlarged is unknown. Most investigators believe ISF egress is blocked, causing cystic enlargement of the PVSs.

GENETICS. Sporadic PVS enlargement has no known genetic predilection. Patients with Hurler, Hunter, or Sanfilippo disease accumulate undegraded mucopolysaccharides within enlarged PVSs. A few congenital muscular dystrophies have also been associated with cystic PVSs.

Pathology

LOCATION. While PVSs can be found virtually anywhere in the brain, they have a striking predilection for the inferior third of the basal ganglia, especially near the anterior commissure **(28-38)**, **(28-39)**. They are also common in the subcortical and deep white matter as well as the midbrain and dentate nuclei of the cerebellum.

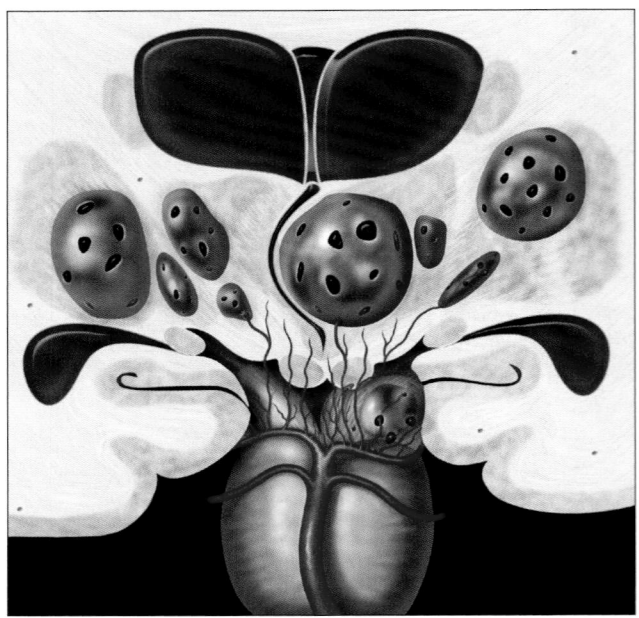

28-40. Coronal graphic shows enlarged perivascular spaces in the midbrain and thalami that cause mass effect on the third ventricle and aqueduct with resulting hydrocephalus.

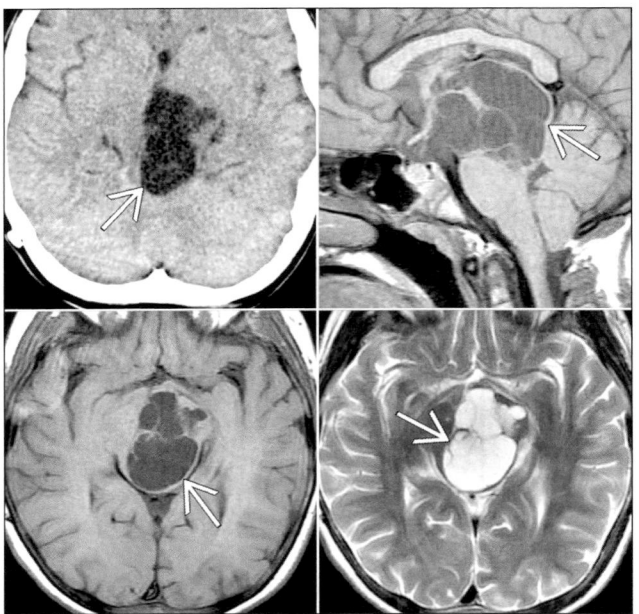

28-41. NECT, MR scans show a cluster of variably sized CSF-like cysts ➡ grossly expanding the midbrain. Giant "tumefactive" perivascular spaces.

SIZE AND NUMBER. Enlarged PVSs tend to occur in clusters. Collections of multiple variably sized PVSs are much more common than solitary unilocular lesions.

Most PVSs are smaller than two millimeters. PVSs increase in size and prevalence with age. Giant so-called tumefactive PVSs measuring up to nine centimeters in diameter have been reported.

GROSS PATHOLOGY. Enlarged PVSs appear as collections of smoothly demarcated cysts filled with clear colorless fluid **(28-40)**.

MICROSCOPIC FEATURES. PVSs are bounded by a single or double layer of invaginated pia. Cortical PVSs are lined by a single layer of pia, whereas two layers accompany lenticulostriate and midbrain arteries.

As a PVS penetrates into the subcortical white matter, it becomes fenestrated and discontinuous. The pial layer disappears completely at the capillary level.

The brain parenchyma surrounding enlarged PVSs is typically normal without gliosis, inflammation, hemorrhage, or discernible amyloid deposition.

Clinical Issues

EPIDEMIOLOGY. PVSs are the most common nonneoplastic parenchymal brain "cysts." With high-resolution 3.0 T MR, small PVSs are seen in nearly all patients, in virtually every location, and at all ages.

DEMOGRAPHICS. Enlarged PVSs are more common in middle-aged and older patients. Between 25-30% of chil-

dren demonstrate prominent PVSs on high-resolution MR scans.

PRESENTATION. Most enlarged PVSs do not cause symptoms and are discovered incidentally on imaging studies or at autopsy. Neuropsychological evaluation is typically normal. Nonspecific symptoms such as headache, dizziness, memory impairment, and Parkinson-like symptoms have been reported in some cases, but their relationship to enlarged PVSs is unclear. Large PVSs in the midbrain may cause obstructive hydrocephalus and present with headache.

NATURAL HISTORY. Enlarged PVSs tend to be stable in size and remain unchanged over many years. Only a few cases of progressively enlarging PVSs have been reported.

TREATMENT OPTIONS. Enlarged PVSs are "leave me alone" lesions that should not be mistaken for serious disease. If midbrain PVSs cause obstructive hydrocephalus, the generally accepted treatment is to shunt the ventricles, not the cysts.

Imaging

GENERAL FEATURES. The common pattern of enlarged PVSs is one or more clusters of variably sized CSF-like cysts. They commonly cause focal mass effect. For example, if they occur in the subcortical white matter, the overlying gyri are enlarged with concomitant compression of adjacent sulci.

CT FINDINGS. Enlarged PVSs are groups of round/ovoid/linear/punctate CSF-like lesions that do not demonstrate calcification or hemorrhage (28-41). PVSs do not enhance following contrast administration.

MR FINDINGS. Even though they are filled with interstitial fluid, PVSs closely parallel CSF signal intensity on all imaging sequences (28-41). Focal mass effect is common. Enlarged PVSs in the subcortical white matter expand overlying gyri (28-42), (28-43). Enlarged PVSs in the midbrain may compress the aqueduct and third ventricle, resulting in intraventricular obstructive hydrocephalus (28-41).

PVSs are isointense with CSF on T1-, PD, and T2WI. They suppress completely on FLAIR. Edema in the adjacent brain is absent although 25% of "tumefactive" PVSs have minimal increased signal intensity around the cysts.

PVSs do not hemorrhage, enhance, or demonstrate restricted diffusion.

ENLARGED PERIVASCULAR SPACES

Terminology
- Also known as Virchow-Robin spaces
- Found around penetrating blood vessels
- Lined by pia, filled with interstitial fluid
- Do not communicate directly with SAS

Pathology
- Normal PVSs common, < 2 cm
- Giant "tumefactive" PVSs up to 9 cm reported
- Basal ganglia, subcortical WM most common

Imaging
- Often bizarre-looking
- Occur in clusters
- Variably sized cysts
- Follow CSF

Differential Diagnosis

The major differential diagnosis is chronic **lacunar infarction**. While they often affect the basal ganglia and suppress on FLAIR, lacunar infarcts do not cluster around the anterior commissure, are often irregular in shape, and frequently exhibit hyperintensity in the adjacent brain.

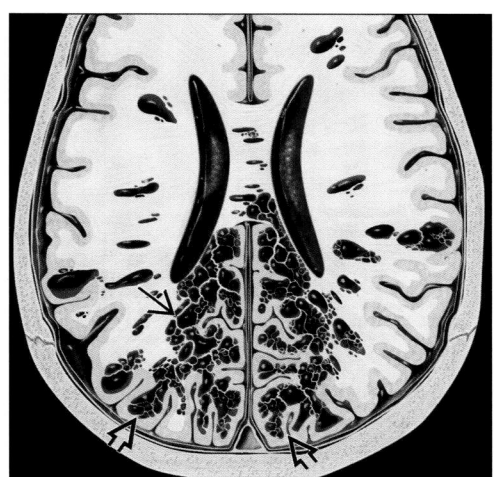

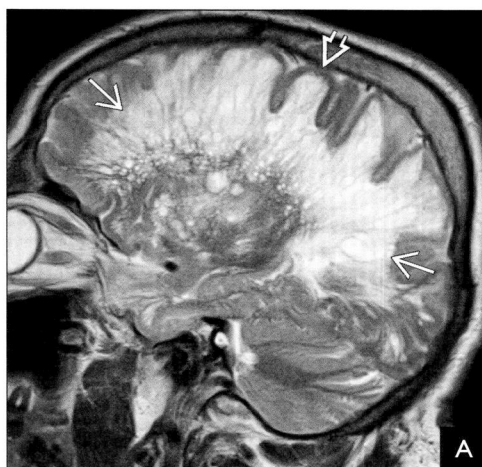

28-42. Graphic depicts innumerable hemispheric enlarged PVSs ⇥ in subcortical, deep WM. Note that the overlying gyri ⇥ are expanded but otherwise normal. 28-43A. Sagittal T2WI shows markedly enlarged PVSs involving most of the subcortical and deep hemispheric white matter ⇥. Overlying gyri are expanded ⇥, but the cortex is intact.

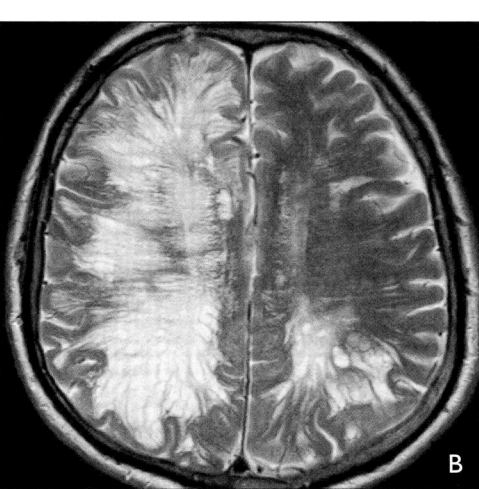

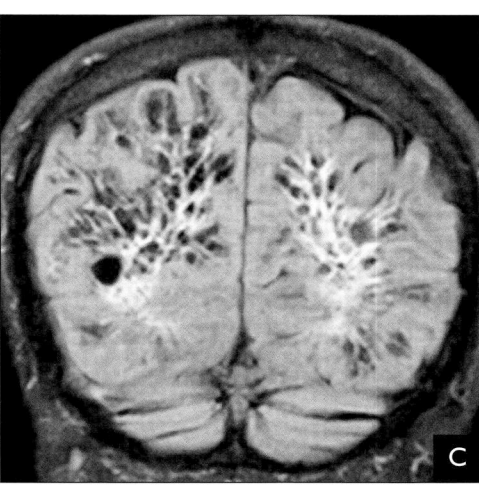

28-43B. Axial T2WI shows that both hemispheres are affected but that the distribution of enlarged PVSs is quite asymmetric. 28-43C. Coronal FLAIR scan in the same patient shows that fluid in the PVSs suppresses, but there is some hyperintensity around the cysts consistent with mild gliosis. (Courtesy M. Warmuth-Metz, MD.)

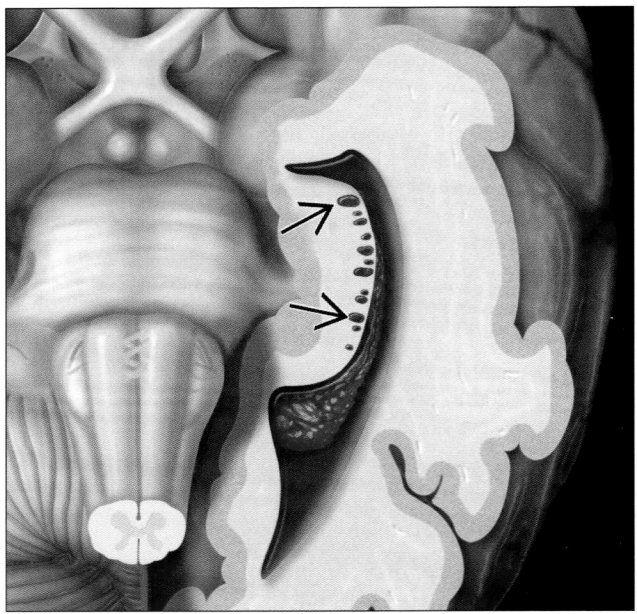

28-44. Graphic of normal temporal lobe shows a string of cysts within the lateral hippocampus, along the residual cavity of the primitive hippocampal sulcus ⇒. Hippocampal sulcus remnant cysts are incidental, a normal finding.

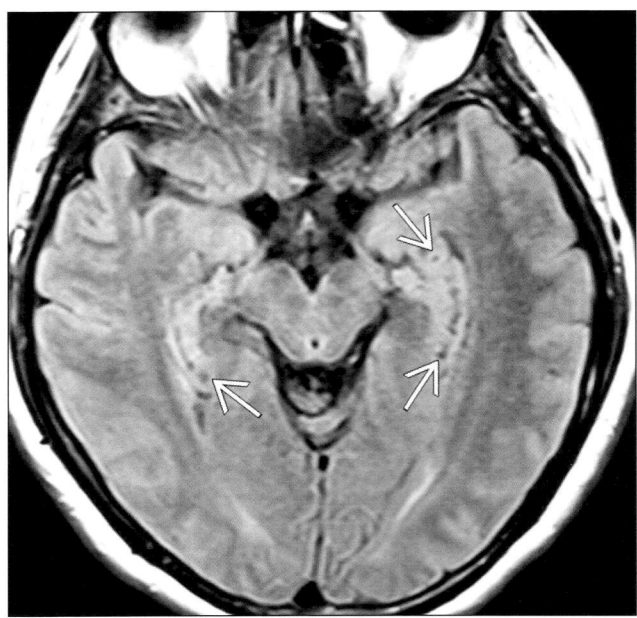

28-45. Axial FLAIR scan shows hippocampal sulcus remnants as lines of tiny cysts ➡ medial to both temporal lobes. These contain CSF and so suppress completely on FLAIR.

In some older patients, very prominent PVSs in the basal ganglia are present. This condition, called **"état criblé,"** should not be mistaken for multiple lacunar infarcts. PVSs are round/ovoid and regular in configuration, and the adjacent brain parenchymal is usually normal without gliosis or edema.

Infectious cysts (especially parenchymal neurocysticercosis cysts) are usually small. Although often multiple or multilocular, they typically do not occur in clusters of variably sized cysts as is typical for enlarged PVSs.

Hippocampal Sulcus Remnants

Terminology

Hippocampal sulcus remnants (HCSR) are also called hippocampal remnant cysts and hippocampal sulcal cavities.

Etiology

At 15 fetal weeks, the hippocampus normally unfolds and surrounds an "open" shallow fissure—the hippocampal sulcus—along the medial surface of the temporal lobe. The walls of the hippocampal sulcus gradually fuse, and the sulcus is eventually obliterated.

At times, some segments of the closing hippocampal sulcus fail to fuse. One or more residual cystic cavities remain and persist into adult life. These remnant cavities—hippocampal remnant cysts—are normal anatomic variants **(28-44)**.

Pathology

HCSRs are pia-lined cavities filled with CSF. Small blood vessels are often also included as the hippocampal sulcus forms, folds, and fuses.

Clinical Issues

HCSRs are incidental findings of no clinical significance. They do not cause seizures and are not related to trauma.

Imaging

HCSRs are seen in 10-15% of normal high-resolution MR scans. They appear as a "string of beads" with multiple small round or ovoid cysts curving along the hippocampus between the dentate gyrus and subiculum, just medial to the temporal horn of the lateral ventricle. HCSRs follow CSF in signal intensity on all sequences. They suppress completely on FLAIR **(28-45)**, do not enhance, and do not restrict on DWI.

Differential Diagnosis

The major differential diagnosis HCSRs is **enlarged perivascular spaces**. When they occur in the temporal lobe, enlarged PVSs are found in the subcortical white matter of the insula and anterior tip of the temporal lobe, not medial to the temporal horn of the lateral ventricle.

Neuroglial Cyst

Terminology

Neuroglial cysts (NGCs) are sometimes called **glioependymal cysts** or **neuroepithelial cysts**. They are benign fluid-containing cavities buried within the cerebral white matter.

Pathology

LOCATION. While NGCs occur throughout the neuraxis, they are usually supratentorial. The frontal lobe is the most common site. They often lie adjacent to—but do not communicate directly with—the cerebral ventricles.

SIZE AND NUMBER. Most NGCs are solitary unilocular cysts. They vary in size from a few millimeters up to several centimeters in diameter.

GROSS PATHOLOGY. NGCs are rounded, smooth, unilocular cysts that contain clear CSF-like fluid.

MICROSCOPIC FEATURES. Most NGCs are lined with a simple, nonstratified, low columnar/cuboidal epithelium (28-46). The epithelium usually sits directly on deep cerebral WM without an intervening capsule or basement membrane.

Clinical Issues

EPIDEMIOLOGY. Parenchymal neuroglial cysts are uncommon, representing less than 1% of all intracranial cysts.

DEMOGRAPHICS. NGCs occur in all age groups but are generally more common in adults. There is no gender predilection.

PRESENTATION. NGCs are often asymptomatic and found incidentally at imaging or autopsy. The most common presenting symptom, if any, is headache.

NATURAL HISTORY. Many—if not most—NGCs remain stable over many years.

TREATMENT OPTIONS. Serial observation with imaging studies is the usual course. Large NGCs have been fenestrated or drained.

Imaging

GENERAL FEATURES. NGCs are smooth, round or ovoid, fluid-containing cysts.

CT FINDINGS. NGCs are fluid density, typically resemble CSF, do not contain calcifications, and do not hemorrhage.

MR FINDINGS. Signal intensity varies with cyst content. Most NGCs are iso- or slightly hyperintense to CSF

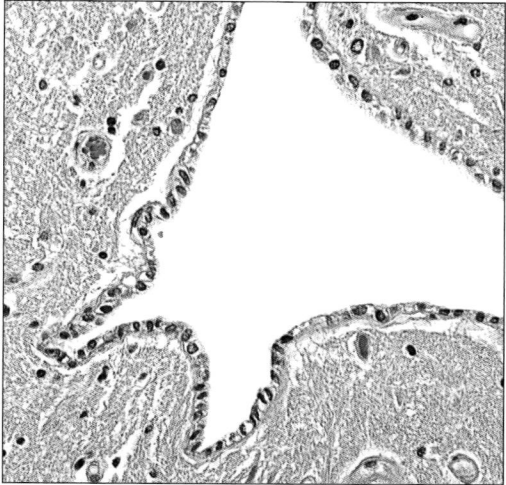

28-46. Neuroglial cysts are lined by a single layer of cuboidal/low columnar epithelium. Cilia are rare. (Courtesy P. Burger, MD.)

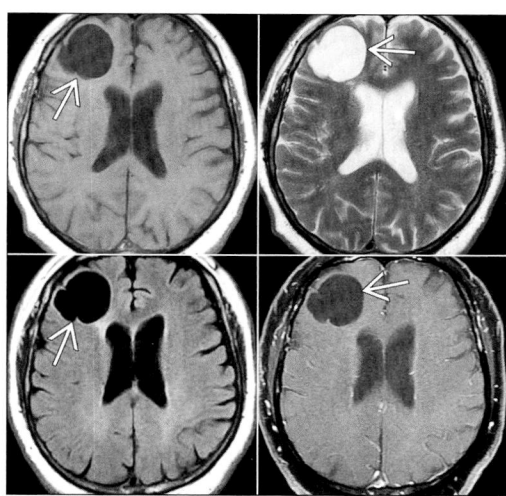

28-47. Right frontal neuroglial cyst ➡ in a 69-year-old man follows CSF signal intensity on all sequences, does not enhance.

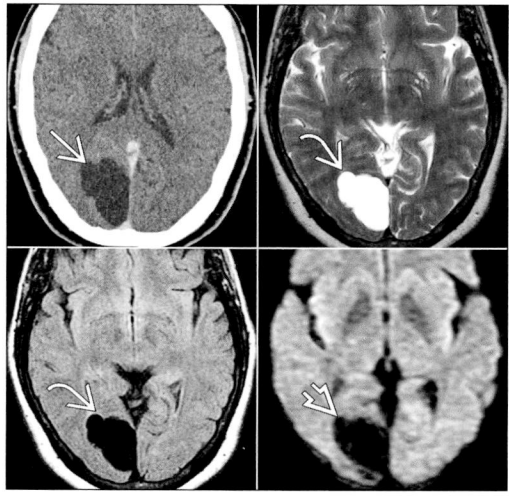

28-48. Proven neuroglial cyst in the right occipital lobe does not enhance on CECT ➡, follows CSF on T2/FLAIR ➡, does not restrict ➡.

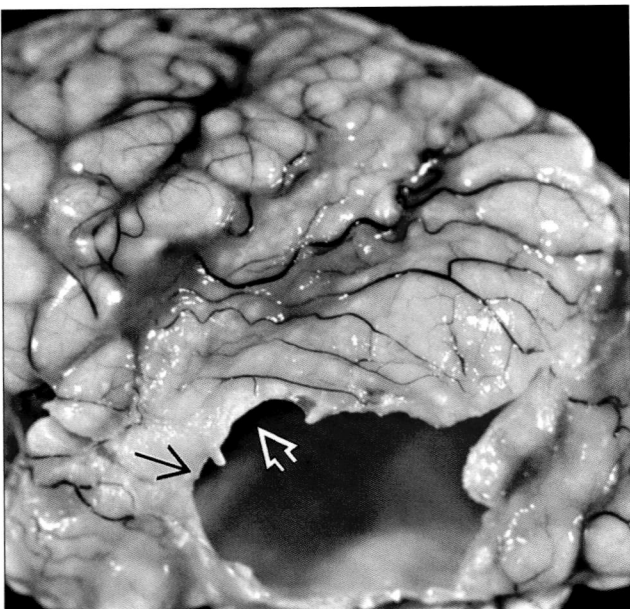

28-49. *Autopsy specimen shows a typical porencephalic cyst as a CSF-filled cavity that extends from the brain surface ⇨ to the ventricular ependyma ⇰. (Courtesy J. Townsend, MD.)*

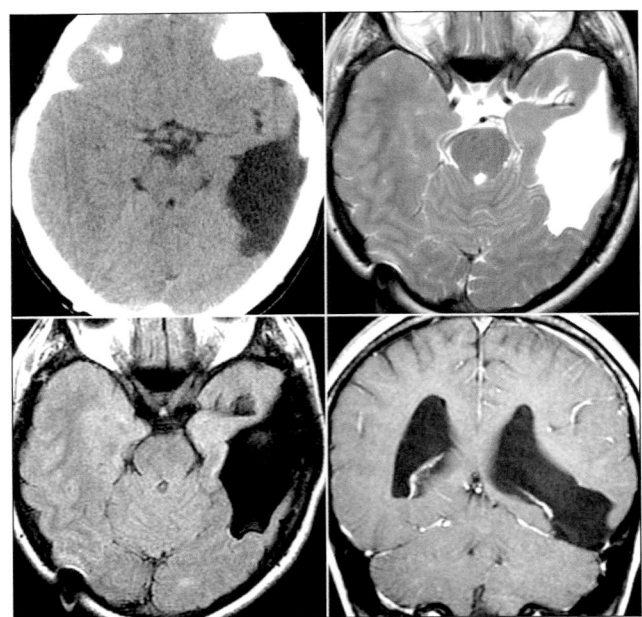

28-50. *NECT, MR scans show a post-traumatic porencephalic cyst extending from the surface of the temporal lobe to the temporal horn of the lateral ventricle. The cyst contains CSF.*

(28-47). They usually suppress on FLAIR, do not restrict, and do not enhance **(28-48)**. The parenchyma surrounding an NGC is usually normal or may show minimal gliosis.

Differential Diagnosis

The diagnosis of NGC is mostly a process of elimination, excluding other, sometimes more ominous possibilities.

The major differential diagnosis of NGC is an **enlarged perivascular space**. Most enlarged PVSs are multiple (not solitary) and occur as clusters of variably sized cysts. A **porencephalic cyst** is a result of an insult to the brain parenchyma. Porencephalic cysts communicate with the ventricle and are lined by gliotic or spongiotic white matter.

Arachnoid cysts are extraaxial, not intraaxial, and are lined with flattened arachnoid cells. **Epidermoid cysts** are almost always extraaxial, do not suppress on FLAIR, and restrict on DWI. **Ependymal cysts** are intraventricular.

Neoplastic and **inflammatory cysts** generally do not follow CSF, often demonstrate wall enhancement or calcification, and are frequently surrounded by edema.

A variety of miscellaneous periventricular cysts occur in newborns or children. Some may persist into adulthood. These include connatal cysts, germinolytic cysts, and cystic periventricular leukomalacia (PVL). **Connatal cysts** are cystic ependyma-lined areas adjacent to the superolateral margins of the body and frontal horns of the lateral ventricles. They are relatively common and gener-

ally innocuous lesions caused by coarctation or coaption of the walls of the frontal horns.

Germinolytic cysts are glia-lined cysts that lie along the caudothalamic groove. They are associated with inherited metabolic disorders (e.g., Zellweger) and congenital infections (e.g., CMV), often contain septations or hemosiderin, and do not enhance. **Cystic PVL** most frequently occurs in premature infants and is located dorsolaterally to the bodies of the lateral ventricles.

Porencephalic Cyst

Terminology

"Porencephaly" literally means a hole in the brain. Porencephalic cysts are congenital or acquired CSF-filled parenchymal cavities that usually—but not invariably—communicate with the ventricular system. These cysts or cavities also often communicate via a "pore" with the subarachnoid space.

Etiology

Porencephalic cysts are encephaloclastic lesions, the end result of a destructive process (e.g., trauma, infection, vascular insult, surgery) that compromises brain parenchyma.

Most porencephalic cysts are sporadic. A few inherited syndromes (e.g., autosomal dominant familial porencephaly) have been reported.

Pathology

Porencephalic cysts range in size from a few centimeters to cysts that involve virtually an entire cerebral hemisphere.

Porencephalic cysts are deep, uni- or bilateral, smooth-walled cavities or excavations within the brain parenchyma. They are often "full thickness" lesions, extending from the ventricle to the glia limitans of the cortex **(28-49)**. Occasionally, a thin rim of ependyma or subependymal white matter may separate the cyst from the ventricle.

Clinical Issues

EPIDEMIOLOGY. Porencephalic cysts are relatively common, especially in children, in whom they represent 2.5% of congenital brain lesions.

PRESENTATION. Spastic hemiplegia, medically refractory epilepsy, and psychomotor retardation are the most common symptoms.

NATURAL HISTORY. Most porencephalic cysts remain stable for many years. Occasionally a porencephalic cyst will continue to sequester fluid and expand, causing mass effect.

Imaging

CT FINDINGS. Porencephalic cysts are sharply marginated, smooth-walled, CSF-filled cavities that usually communicate directly with an adjacent ventricle **(28-50)**. The ipsilateral ventricle is often enlarged secondary to volume loss in the adjacent parenchyma.

Calcification is rare. Bone CT may show skull thinning and remodeling caused by chronic CSF pulsations.

A porencephalic cyst does not enhance.

MR FINDINGS. Porencephalic cysts follow CSF signal intensity on all sequences **(28-50)**. Large cysts may show internal inhomogeneities secondary to spin dephasing. These cysts suppress completely on FLAIR, although there is often a rim of hyperintense gliotic or spongiotic white matter around the cyst. No restriction on DWI is present.

Differential Diagnosis

The major differential diagnosis is **cystic encephalomalacia**. An encephalomalacic cavity is often more irregular and does not communicate with the adjacent ventricle.

Porencephalic cysts are lined by reactive gliosis (glial "scar"), which occurs when histologically benign astrocytes proliferate in and around damaged brain parenchyma. A porencephalic cyst with surrounding **reactive gliosis** must be distinguished from **spongiosis,** a process that represents tissue loss (not astrocytic proliferation) with formation of empty (spongiform) areas ("holes") in the brain. Gliosis is a low to medium cellularity lesion that is hyperintense on T2WI and does not suppress on FLAIR. Spongiosis is T2 hyperintense but suppresses on FLAIR.

An **arachnoid cyst** is extraaxial and does not communicate with the ventricle. **Schizencephaly** (literally "split brain") is a congenital lesion that can be either "open" or "closed lip." An "open lip" schizencephalic cleft can look very much like a porencephalic cyst but is lined with dysplastic gray matter, not gliotic white matter.

Hydranencephaly ("water on the brain") is a congenital lesion in which most of the supratentorial developing brain has been destroyed by arterial occlusion. Here the brain looks like a bag of water with little or no remnant cortex. Hydranencephaly is bilateral and symmetric whereas most porencephalic cysts are unilateral or bilateral but asymmetric.

Intraventricular Cysts

Intraventricular cysts include choroid plexus cysts, colloid cysts, and ependymal cysts.

Choroid Plexus Cysts

Choroid plexus cysts are one of the most common types of intracranial cyst. Most are small and unremarkable. Occasionally, large cysts may appear somewhat atypical and cause diagnostic concern.

Terminology

A choroid plexus cyst (CPC) is also often called a choroid plexus xanthogranuloma (CPX). CPCs are nonneoplastic noninflammatory cysts of the choroid plexus.

Etiology

GENERAL CONCEPTS. CPCs can be either congenital or acquired. Acquired lesions are much more common; lipid that accumulates from desquamating, degenerating choroid plexus epithelium coalesces into macrocysts and provokes a xanthomatous response.

GENETICS. Large (> 10 mm), congenital CPCs can be associated with aneuploidy, particularly trisomy 18. CPCs, together with choroid plexus papillomas, also occur as part of Aicardi syndrome.

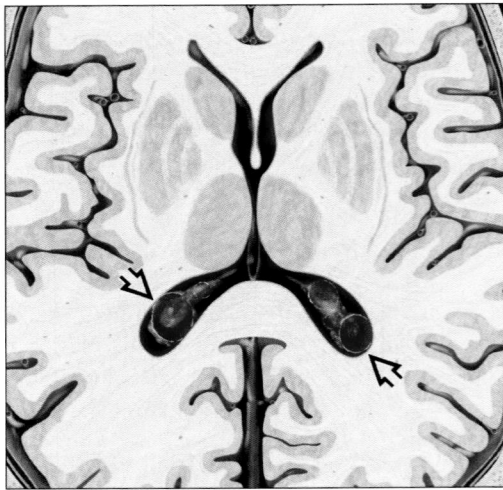

28-51. *Multiple cystic masses in the choroid plexus glomi* ⧨. *In adults, their prevalence increases with age. Most are degenerative xanthogranulomas.*

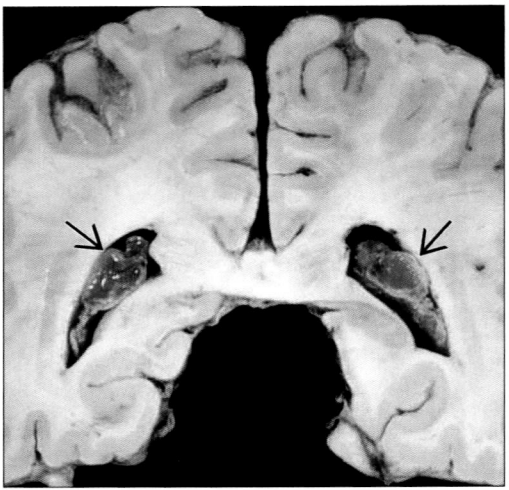

28-52. *Autopsy specimen shows multiple cysts in the choroid plexus glomi of both lateral ventricles* ⧨. *(Courtesy N. Nakase, MD.)*

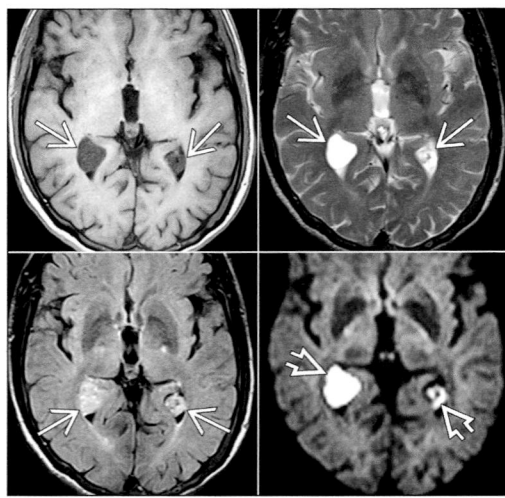

28-53. *Choroid plexus cysts are usually bilateral, hyperintense compared to CSF* ⧨ *and are often very bright on DWI* ⧨.

Pathology

LOCATION. Most CPCs are found in the atrium of the lateral ventricle, within the choroid plexus glomus **(28-51)**.

SIZE AND NUMBER. CPCs are mostly small, ranging from a few millimeters up to one centimeter, although occasionally larger cysts exceed two centimeters in diameter. Multiple bilateral lesions are significantly more common than solitary unilateral CPCs.

GROSS PATHOLOGY. CPCs are nodular, partly cystic, yellowish-gray masses that are most often found in the choroid plexus glomus **(28-52)**. They are highly proteinaceous and often gelatinous. Gross hemorrhage is rare.

Clinical Issues

DEMOGRAPHICS. CPCs are the most common of all intracranial cysts, occurring in up to 50% of autopsies. CPCs are found at both ends of the age spectrum. In adults, their prevalence increases with age whereas fetal CPCs decrease with gestational age. There is no gender predilection.

PRESENTATION AND NATURAL HISTORY. Most adult CPCs are found incidentally and are asymptomatic, remaining stable for many years. Congenital CPCs are detected on prenatal ultrasound in 1% of fetuses during the second trimester and generally resolve during the third trimester. When detected postnatally, CPCs are of no clinical significance in otherwise normal neonates.

Imaging

CT FINDINGS. CPCs are iso- to slightly hyperdense compared to intraventricular CSF. Irregular clumps of calcification around the margins are common findings. Enhancement varies from none to a complete rim surrounding each cyst.

MR FINDINGS. CPCs do not precisely follow CSF signal intensity. They are iso- to slightly hyperintense compared to CSF on T1WI and are hyperintense on PD and T2WI. FLAIR signal is variable **(28-53)**.

Enhancement following contrast administration varies from none to striking. Solid, ring, and nodular patterns occur.

Between 60-80% of CPCs appear quite bright on DWI but often remain isointense with parenchyma on ADC. This may therefore represent pseudorestriction rather than true restricted diffusion.

ULTRASOUND. Fetal ultrasound may show multiple cysts of variable sizes.

Differential Diagnosis

The major differential diagnosis of a CPC is an **ependymal cyst**. Ependymal cysts generally displace and compress the choroid plexus rather than arise from it. Ependymal cysts usually behave much more like CSF than CPCs do. Intraventricular parasitic cysts, specifically those of **neurocysticercosis**, are relatively uncommon. They are not associated with the choroid plexus. A scolex is often present.

Epidermoid cysts occasionally occur in the ventricles but are much more common in the fourth ventricle, a rare site for CPCs.

Choroid plexus papilloma of the lateral ventricle is a tumor of children younger than five years old and enhances intensely. An enhancing, enlarged choroid plexus without frank cyst formation can also be seen with **Sturge-Weber malformation**, **collateral venous drainage**, and **diffuse villous hyperplasia**. Sturge-Weber and collateral venous drainage usually cause unilateral choroid plexus enlargement. The entire choroid plexus is enlarged in diffuse villous hyperplasia.

CHOROID PLEXUS CYST

Etiology
- Congenital
  - Aicardi syndrome
  - Trisomy 18
- Acquired
  - Desquamated, degenerated epithelium
  - Xanthomatous response

Pathology
- Bilateral, usually multiloculated
- Most common in glomi of choroid plexus
- Proteinaceous, gelatinous contents

Clinical Issues
- Most common intracranial cyst
- Most found incidentally
- Most common in fetus/infants, older adults

Imaging
- CT
  - Iso-/mildly hyperdense
  - Ca++ common
  - Variable enhancement (rim enhancement most common)
- MR
  - Iso-/mildly hyperintense to CSF on T1WI
  - Hyperintense on PD/T2WI, FLAIR variable
  - Variable enhancement
  - Bright on DWI but isointense on ADC

Differential Diagnosis
- Most common
  - Ependymal cyst (unilateral)
- Uncommon/rare
  - Epidermoid cyst (rarely intraventricular)
  - Cystic metastasis

Colloid Cyst

Terminology

Colloid cysts (CCs) are also called paraphyseal cysts. They are unilocular, mucin-containing cysts that are almost always found wedged into the top of the third ventricle at the foramen of Monro **(28-54)**.

Etiology

GENERAL CONCEPTS. CCs are endodermal—rather than neuroectodermal—cysts. They are similar to the other intracranial foregut-derived cysts, i.e., Rathke cleft and neurenteric cysts. While their precise etiology is unknown, they are presumed to arise from ectopic endodermal elements that migrate into the embryonic diencephalic roof.

GENETICS. No specific gene mutations have been identified. A few rare familial colloid cysts have been described that appear to have an autosomal recessive pattern of inheritance with variable penetrance.

Pathology

LOCATION. More than 99% of CCs are wedged into the foramen of Monro, attached to the anterosuperior roof of the third ventricle. The posterior aspects of the frontal horns of the lateral ventricle are splayed laterally around the cyst, and the pillars of the fornix "straddle" the CC.

SIZE AND NUMBER. CCs are virtually always solitary lesions. Size varies from tiny (a few millimeters) up to three centimeters. Mean diameter is 1.5 cm.

GROSS PATHOLOGY. CCs are smooth-walled, well-demarcated, spherical or ovoid cysts that have a gelatinous center of variable viscosity **(28-55)**. Gross hemorrhage is very rare.

MICROSCOPIC FEATURES. The wall of a CC consists of a thin fibrous capsule that is lined with simple or pseudostratified columnar epithelium. Some ciliated and mucin-secreting goblet cells are interspersed throughout the cyst lining. Like other endodermal cysts, CCs are cytokeratin and EMA positive on immunohistochemistry.

Clinical Issues

EPIDEMIOLOGY. Colloid cysts account for about 1% of all intracranial tumors but cause 15-20% of all intraventricular tumors.

DEMOGRAPHICS. Most symptomatic CCs present between the third and fifth decades. The peak age is 40 years. Pediatric CCs are rare; less than 8% of all patients are younger than 15 years at the time of initial diagnosis. There is no gender predilection.

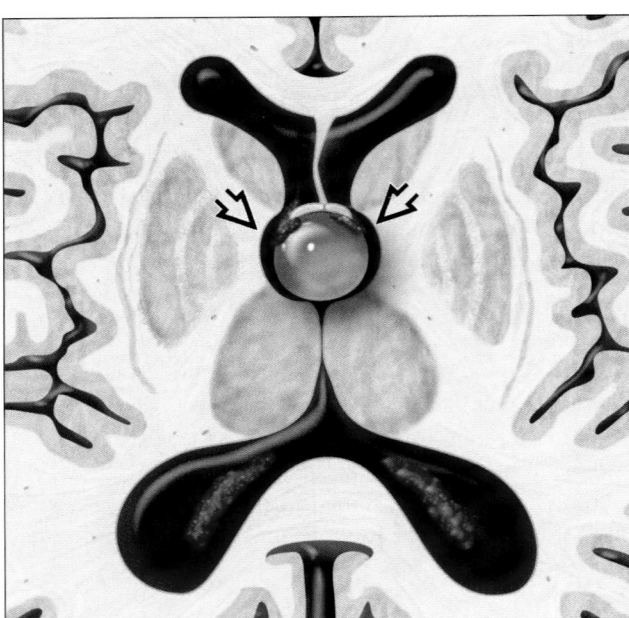

28-54. Axial graphic shows a classic colloid cyst at the foramen of Monro causing mild/moderate obstructive hydrocephalus. Note that the fornices and choroid plexus are elevated and stretched over the cyst ⧨.

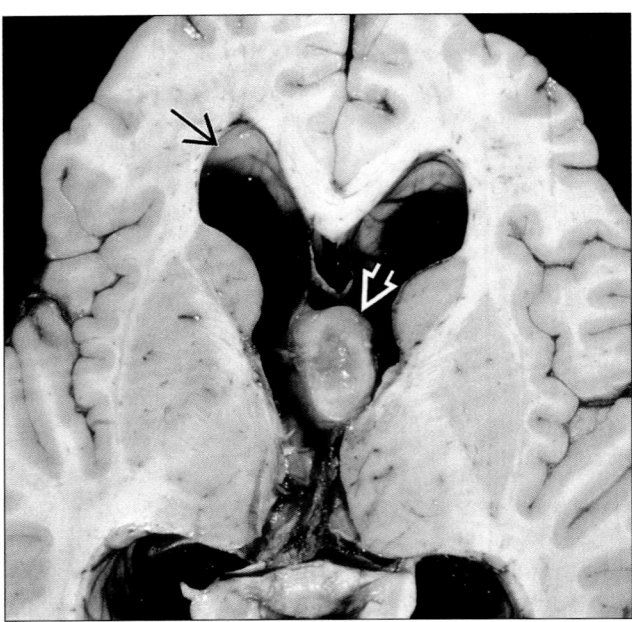

28-55. Autopsy specimen shows obstructive hydrocephalus ⧨, *a large gelatinous-appearing colloid cyst* ⧨ *in the foramen of Monro. (Courtesy R. Hewlett, MD.)*

PRESENTATION. The clinical presentation of CCs is diverse, ranging from asymptomatic, incidentally discovered cysts (nearly half of all patients) to acute deterioration, coma, and death. CCs cause symptoms when they obstruct CSF flow at the foramina of Monro. Headache is the presenting symptom in 50-60% of symptomatic patients.

NATURAL HISTORY. Over 90% of CCs—especially small cysts found in older patients—are stable and do not enlarge. The roughly 10% that *do* enlarge tend to be larger lesions, often causing hydrocephalus, and found in younger patients.

Cyst "apoplexy" with intracystic hemorrhage and sudden enlargement occurs but is rare.

TREATMENT OPTIONS. Small asymptomatic colloid cysts that are discovered incidentally and followed with serial imaging rarely grow or cause obstructive hydrocephalus. Yet their treatment is debated. Neuroendoscopic management has emerged as a safe, effective alternative to microsurgery with either a transcortical-transventricular or a transcallosal approach.

COLLOID CYST: PATHOETIOLOGY AND CLINICAL ISSUES

Etiology
- Endodermal cyst
- Probably derived from ectopic elements in diencephalic roof

Pathology
- Foramen of Monro (> 99%)
- Size varies from a few mm up to 3 cm
- Fibrous capsule
- Cyst lining
  - Columnar epithelium
  - Mucin-secreting goblet cells
- Gelatinous center (variable viscosity)

Clinical Issues
- Epidemiology
  - 1% of all intracranial tumors
  - 15-20% of intraventricular masses
- Peak age = 40 years (rare in children)
- Asymptomatic, found incidentally (50%)
- Headache most common symptom
- Sudden obstruction can cause coma, death
- Stable, do not enlarge (90%)

Imaging

GENERAL FEATURES. CCs are well-delineated round or ovoid masses. Imaging appearance depends on their viscosity and/or cholesterol content. The relative amounts of mucous material, cholesterol, protein, and water content all affect density/signal intensity. Desiccated, inspissated cysts appear very different from water-rich lesions.

CT FINDINGS. Density on NECT correlates directly with the hydration state of the cyst contents. Nearly two-thirds

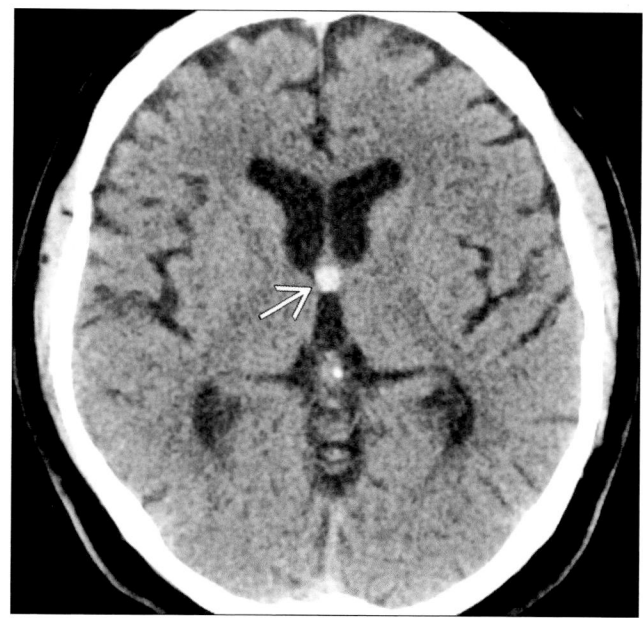

28-56. NECT scan shows a classic colloid cyst as a well-circumscribed hyperdense mass ➡ *in the foramen of Monro.*

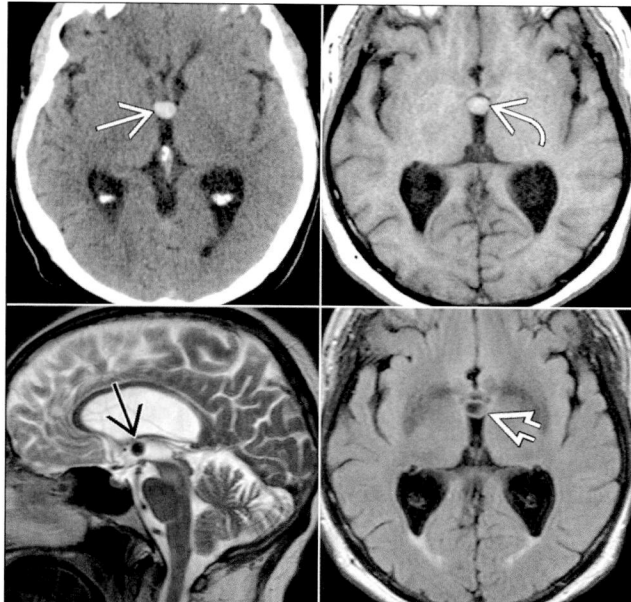

28-57. NECT scan shows hyperdense colloid cyst ➡ *that is hyperintense on T1WI* ➡, *hypointense on T2WI* ➡, *mixed signal intensity on FLAIR* ➡.

of all CCs are hyperdense compared to brain **(28-56)** while one-third are iso- to hypodense **(28-58)**. Hydrocephalus is variable. Hemorrhage and calcification are very rare.

Most CCs show no enhancement. Occasionally, a thin enhancing rim surrounds the cyst. Solid or nodular enhancement almost never occurs.

CTA/CTV demonstrates that the internal cerebral veins are displaced posterolaterally around the CC.

MR FINDINGS. Signal intensity varies with cyst content.

Signal intensity on T1WI reflects cholesterol concentration. Most CCs are hyperintense compared to brain **(28-57)**, but one-third are isointense. Small isointense CCs may be very difficult to identify on T1WI.

Signal on PD and T2WI is more variable, as it is more reflective of water content. Most CCs are minimally hyperintense to brain on PD and usually isointense on T2WI. A few CCs with inspissated contents are hypointense. Approximately 25% demonstrate mixed hypo- and hyperintensity (the "black hole" effect). Fluid-fluid levels are rare.

CCs do not suppress on FLAIR **(28-58)**, nor do they restrict on DWI.

CCs generally do not enhance. A thin peripheral rim of enhancement can be seen in some cases **(28-58)**.

ifferential Diagnosis

A well-delineated focal hyperdense lesion at the foramen of Monro on NECT scan is virtually pathogno-

monic of a CC. Occasionally, extreme **ectasia of an artery**—usually the basilar artery—can mimic a CC although serial sections easily demonstrate the tubular nature of the ectatic vessel.

On MR, the most common "lesion" that mimics a CC is artifact caused by **pulsatile CSF flow (28-59), (28-60)**. Phase artifact propagated across the image is helpful in establishing the etiology. Multiplanar imaging and other pulse sequences are also helpful.

Neoplasms such as **metastasis** and **subependymoma** (usually in the frontal horn or foramen of Monro, not anterosuperior third ventricle) can be hyperdense on NECT scans. Large **craniopharyngiomas** and pituitary **macroadenomas** occasionally extend superiorly almost to the foramen of Monro. Multiplanar MR shows that the origin of these tumors is inferior to the third ventricle.

Rarely, an **astrocytoma** or **lymphoma** can infiltrate and thicken the fornices and thus mimic a colloid cyst. Most all of these neoplasms are diffusely infiltrating, nonfocal lesions that often show moderate to marked enhancement following contrast administration.

Other third ventricle/foramen of Monro **choroid plexus masses** such as papilloma, xanthogranuloma, and choroid plexus cysts are rare.

28-58A. Patient had sudden onset severe headache before he became comatose. Emergency NECT scan shows an isodense mass at the foramen of Monro ➡️ with enlarged ventricles. Note the "blurred" ventricular margins ⬅️. *28-58B.* FLAIR shows that the cyst is hyperintense ➡️. The "halo" of fluid ⬅️ around the lateral ventricles is secondary to obstructed drainage of interstitial fluid in the deep cerebral WM.

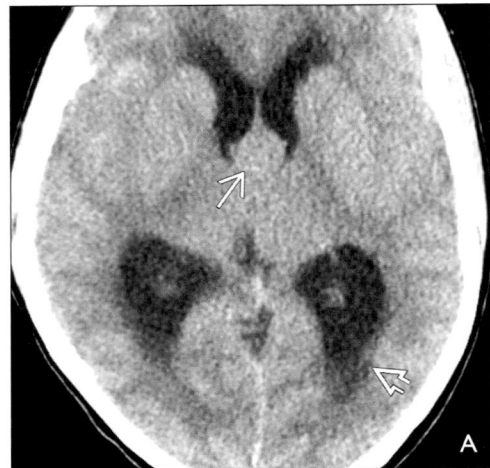

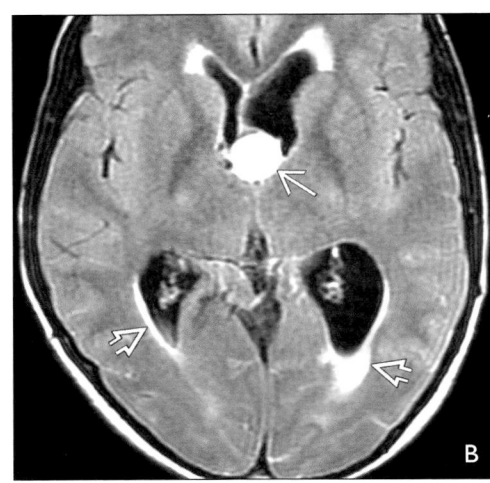

28-58C. T1 C+ FS demonstrates a rim of enhancement around the cyst ➡️. *28-58D.* Coronal T1 C+ also shows the enhancing rim ➡️. This is a variant colloid cyst.

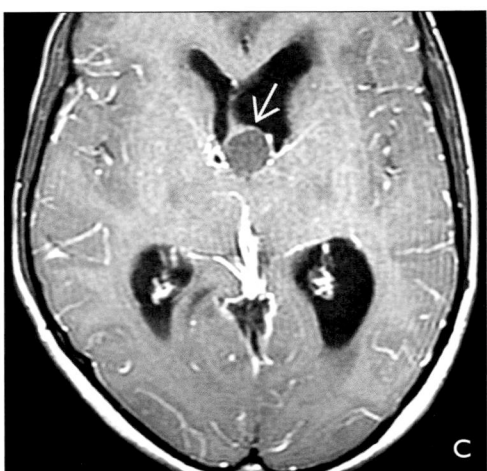

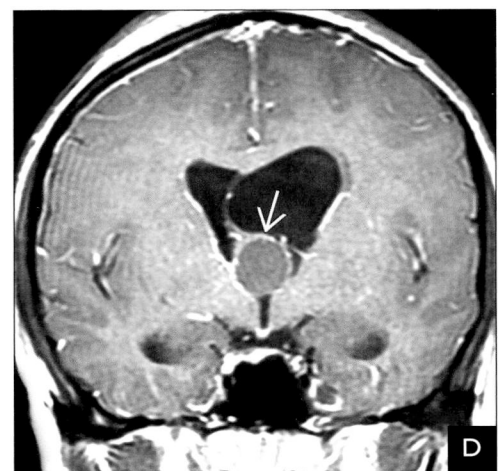

28-59. Axial FLAIR scan shows pulsatile CSF in the third ventricle ➡️, foramen of Monro ⬅️. *28-60.* Coronal T1 C+ shows CSF flow at the foramen of Monro ➡️ mimicking a colloid cyst. Note the normal position of the fornices ➡️, internal cerebral veins ➡️.

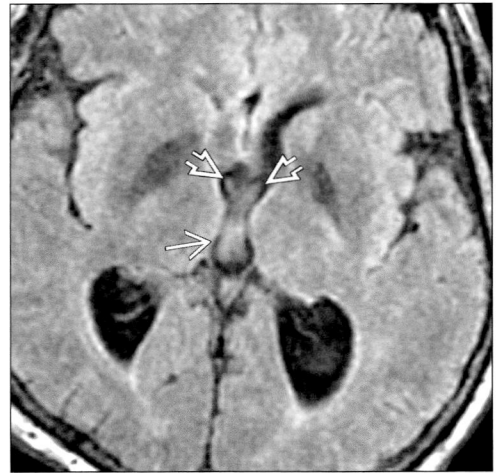

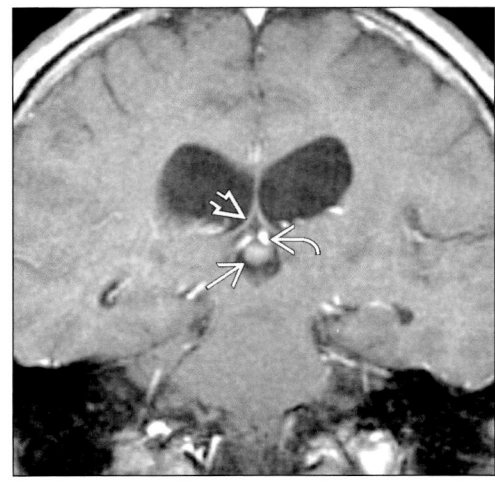

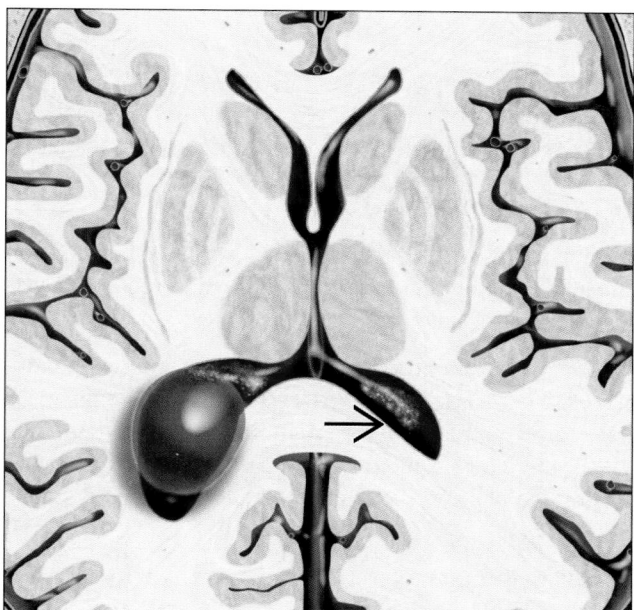

28-61. Axial graphic depicts a typical ependymal cyst of the lateral ventricle ⇥, seen here as a CSF-containing simple cyst that displaces the choroid plexus around it. Ependymal cysts typically follow CSF signal on all sequences.

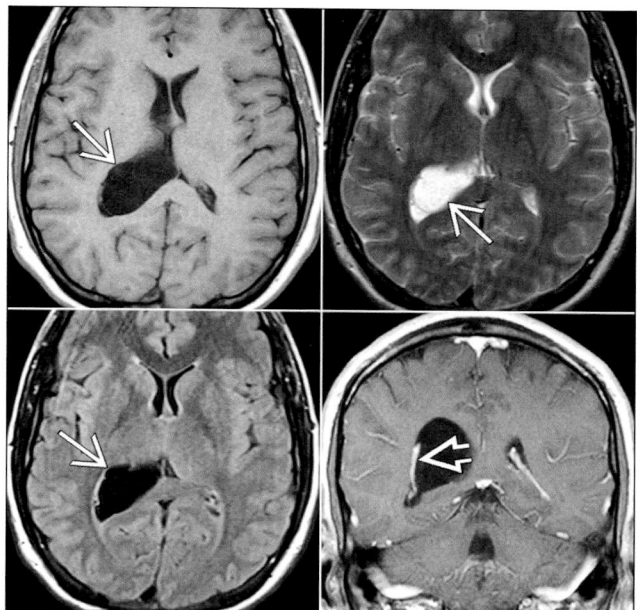

28-62. MR scans demonstrate the typical appearance of an ependymal cyst in the atrium of the right lateral ventricle. The cyst ⇥ behaves exactly like CSF on all sequences. Note choroid plexus ⇥ displaced around the mass.

COLLOID CYST: IMAGING

Imaging
- CT
  - 2/3 hyperdense
  - 1/3 iso- to hypodense
  - Usually do not enhance
- MR
  - Signal intensity varies with sequence, cyst contents
  - Typical: T1 hyper-, T2 hypointense
  - Inspissated: T2 hypointense
  - "Black hole" effect (25%)
  - Do not suppress on FLAIR
  - Generally do not enhance
  - Thin peripheral rim enhancement may occur
  - No restriction on DWI

Differential Diagnosis
- Most common
  - Ectatic basilar artery (NECT)
  - CSF flow artifact (MR)
- Less common
  - Metastasis
  - Subependymoma
  - Pituitary macroadenoma
  - Craniopharyngioma
- Rare but important
  - Low-grade astrocytoma
  - Lymphoma
  - Choroid plexus papilloma
  - Choroid plexus cyst
  - Xanthogranuloma

Ependymal Cyst

Terminology

Ependymal cysts are also called glioependymal cysts. Some authors consider ependymal cysts a subtype of neuroepithelial cyst.

Pathology

Ependymal cysts are solitary lesions that are most often found in the atrium of the lateral ventricles, where they may cause significant ventricular asymmetry (28-61). Less commonly they occur in the brain parenchyma.

Ependymal cysts are rare lesions, accounting for less than 1% of all nonneoplastic intracranial cysts. Their precise pathogenesis is unknown.

Ependymal cysts are usually unilocular, thin walled, and filled with clear CSF-like liquid. They are lined by a layer of simple columnar or cuboidal cells that are similar to the normal endoventricular lining.

Clinical Issues

Ependymal cysts are typically asymptomatic and discovered incidentally at imaging or autopsy. Most patients present as young adults (under 40 years of age). Nonspecific symptoms such as headache and cognitive dysfunction are common. Large ependymal cysts occasionally cause obstructive hydrocephalus and increased intracranial pressure.

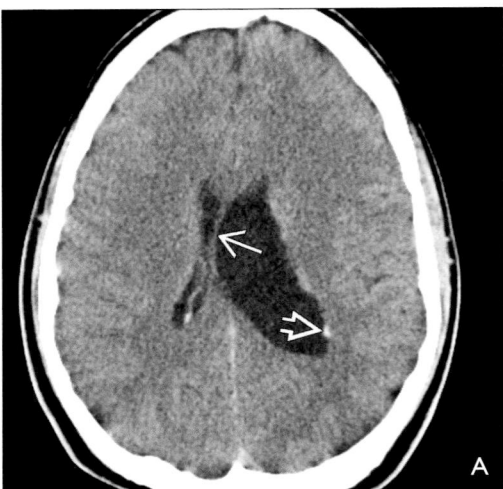

28-63A. NECT in a 22 yo with headaches shows a CSF-like intraventricular mass that displaces the cavum septi pellucidi ➔ and choroid plexus ➤.

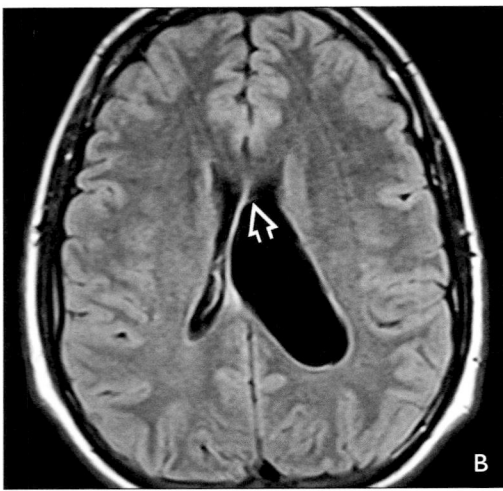

28-63B. FLAIR scan in the same patient shows that the fluid suppresses completely. The thin rim of the cyst ➤ is faintly visible.

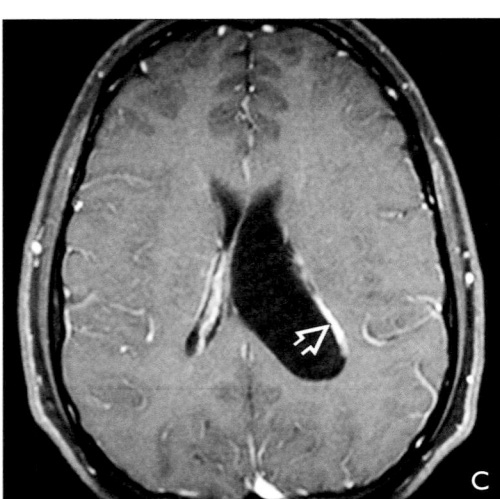

28-63C. T1 C+ FS shows that the cyst does not enhance and displaces the choroid plexus ➤ laterally. Ependymal cyst.

Imaging

Ependymal cysts parallel CSF in density/signal intensity. They suppress completely on FLAIR, do not enhance, and do not demonstrate diffusion restriction **(28-62), (28-63)**.

Differential Diagnosis

Except for location, ependymal cysts may be indistinguishable on imaging from other benign intracranial cysts such as neuroglial cysts.

The major intraventricular mass that can mimic ependymal cyst is a **choroid plexus cyst**. Choroid plexus cysts are typically bilateral, often multilocular, and located within the choroid plexus glomi. Ependymal cysts arise *outside* the choroid plexus and usually displace it superolaterally.

Epidermoid cysts are rare in the lateral ventricle. They do not suppress completely on FLAIR and demonstrate diffusion restriction on DWI. **Arachnoid cysts** are identical to ependymal cysts in density and signal intensity but are rarely intraventricular. **Cystic metastases** to the choroid plexus are rare; nodular or irregular rim enhancement is typical.

EPENDYMAL CYST

Terminology
- Also called glioependymal or neuroepithelial cyst

Pathology
- 1% of intracranial cysts
- Solitary, usually unilocular
- Lined by columnar epithelium
- Contain CSF

Clinical Issues
- Most asymptomatic, discovered incidentally
- All ages, but usually < 40 years

Imaging
- Density, signal intensity = CSF
- No enhancement, no restriction

Differential Diagnosis
- Most common
  ○ Choroid plexus cyst
- Uncommon/rare
  ○ Epidermoid cyst
  ○ Arachnoid cyst
  ○ Cystic metastasis

Selected References

- Osborn AG et al: Intracranial cysts: radiologic-pathologic correlation and imaging approach. Radiology. 239(3):650-64, 2006
- Lev S et al: Imaging of cystic lesions. Radiol Clin North Am. 38(5):1013-27, 2000

Scalp Cysts

Overview

- Al-Khateeb TH et al: Cutaneous cysts of the head and neck. J Oral Maxillofac Surg. 67(1):52-7, 2009
- Yoon SH et al: A study of 77 cases of surgically excised scalp and skull masses in pediatric patients. Childs Nerv Syst. 24(4):459-65, 2008

Trichilemmal ("Sebaceous") Cyst

- Garcia-Zuazaga J et al: Epidermoid cyst mimicry: report of seven cases and review of the literature. J Clin Aesthet Dermatol. 2(10):28-33, 2009
- Chang SJ et al: Proliferating trichilemmal cysts of the scalp on CT. AJNR Am J Neuroradiol. 27(3):712-4, 2006

Extraaxial Cysts

Arachnoid Cyst

- Wang X et al: CT cisternography in intracranial symptomatic arachnoid cysts: classification and treatment. J Neurol Sci. 318(1-2):125-30, 2012
- Al-Holou WN et al: Prevalence and natural history of arachnoid cysts in children. J Neurosurg Pediatr. 5(6):578-85, 2010
- Helland CA et al: Location, sidedness, and sex distribution of intracranial arachnoid cysts in a population-based sample. J Neurosurg. 113(5):934-9, 2010
- Liang C et al: MR imaging of the cisternal segment of the posterior group of cranial nerves: neurovascular relationships and abnormal changes. Eur J Radiol. 75(1):57-63, 2010
- Mottolese C et al: The parallel use of endoscopic fenestration and a cystoperitoneal shunt with programmable valve to treat arachnoid cysts: experience and hypothesis. J Neurosurg Pediatr. 5(4):408-14, 2010

Choroid Fissure Cyst

- Zemmoura I et al: The choroidal fissure: anatomy and surgical implications. Adv Tech Stand Neurosurg. 38:97-113, 2012
- Sherman JL et al: MR imaging of CSF-like choroidal fissure and parenchymal cysts of the brain. AJNR Am J Neuroradiol. 11(5):939-45, 1990

Epidermoid Cyst

- Lian K et al: Rare frontal lobe intraparenchymal epidermoid cyst with atypical imaging. J Clin Neurosci. 19(8):1185-7, 2012
- Ren X et al: Clinical, radiological, and pathological features of 24 atypical intracranial epidermoid cysts. J Neurosurg. 116(3):611-21, 2012
- Ahmed I et al: Neurosurgical management of intracranial epidermoid tumors in children: clinical article. J Neurosurg Pediatr. 4(2):91-6, 2009

Dermoid Cyst

- Ray MJ et al: Ruptured intracranial dermoid cyst. Proc (Bayl Univ Med Cent). 25(1):23-5, 2012
- Liu JK et al: Ruptured intracranial dermoid cysts: clinical, radiographic, and surgical features. Neurosurgery. 62(2):377-84; discussion 384, 2008

Neurenteric Cyst

- Gauden AJ et al: Intracranial neuroenteric cysts: a concise review including an illustrative patient. J Clin Neurosci. 19(3):352-9, 2012
- Wang L et al: Diagnosis and management of adult intracranial neurenteric cysts. Neurosurgery. 68(1):44-52; discussion 52, 2011
- Mittal S et al: Supratentorial neurenteric cysts- A fascinating entity of uncertain embryopathogenesis. Clin Neurol Neurosurg. 112(2):89-97, 2010
- Ciarpaglini R et al: Intradural clival chordoma and ecchordosis physaliphora: a challenging differential diagnosis: case report. Neurosurgery. 64(2):E387-8; discussion E388, 2009
- Preece MT et al: Intracranial neurenteric cysts: imaging and pathology spectrum. AJNR Am J Neuroradiol. 27(6):1211-6, 2006
- Mehnert F et al: Retroclival ecchordosis physaliphora: MR imaging and review of the literature. AJNR Am J Neuroradiol. 25(10):1851-5, 2004

Pineal Cyst

- Al-Holou WN et al: Prevalence and natural history of pineal cysts in adults. J Neurosurg. 115(6):1106-14, 2011
- Choy W et al: Pineal cyst: a review of clinical and radiological features. Neurosurg Clin N Am. 22(3):341-51, vii, 2011
- Smith AB et al: From the archives of the AFIP: lesions of the pineal region: radiologic-pathologic correlation. Radiographics. 30(7):2001-20, 2010
- Taraszewska A et al: Asymptomatic and symptomatic glial cysts of the pineal gland. Folia Neuropathol. 46(3):186-95, 2008
- Pu Y et al: High prevalence of pineal cysts in healthy adults demonstrated by high-resolution, noncontrast brain MR imaging. AJNR Am J Neuroradiol. 28(9):1706-9, 2007

Nonneoplastic Tumor-associated Cysts

- Osborn AG et al: Intracranial cysts: radiologic-pathologic correlation and imaging approach. Radiology. 239(3):650-64, 2006

Parenchymal Cysts

Enlarged Perivascular Spaces

- Mavridis I et al: Differential diagnosis of frontal lobe dilated perivascular spaces. Surg Radiol Anat. 34(3):289-90, 2012
- Tsutsumi S et al: The Virchow-Robin spaces: delineation by magnetic resonance imaging with considerations on anatomofunctional implications. Childs Nerv Syst. 27(12):2057-66, 2011
- Zhu YC et al: Frequency and location of dilated Virchow-Robin spaces in elderly people: a populationbased 3D MR imaging study. AJNR Am J Neuroradiol. 32(4):709-13, 2011
- Kwee RM et al: Virchow-Robin spaces at MR imaging. Radiographics. 27(4):1071-86, 2007
- Mathias J et al: Giant cystic widening of Virchow-Robin spaces: an anatomofunctional study. AJNR Am J Neuroradiol. 28(8):1523-5, 2007

Hippocampal Sulcus Remnants

- Kier EL et al: Limbic lobe embryology and anatomy: dissection and MR of the medial surface of the fetal cerebral hemisphere. AJNR Am J Neuroradiol. 16(9):1847-53, 1995
- Sasaki M et al: Hippocampal sulcus remnant: potential cause of change in signal intensity in the hippocampus. Radiology. 188(3):743-6, 1993

Neuroglial Cyst

- Savas Erdeve S et al: The endocrine spectrum of intracranial cysts in childhood and review of the literature. J Pediatr Endocrinol Metab. 24(11-12):867-75, 2011
- Epelman M et al: Differential diagnosis of intracranial cystic lesions at head US: correlation with CT and MR imaging. Radiographics. 26(1):173-96, 2006

Porencephalic Cyst

- Ryzenman JM et al: Porencephalic cyst: a review of the literature and management of a rare cause of cerebrospinal fluid otorrhea. Otol Neurotol. 28(3):381-6, 2007

Intraventricular Cysts

Choroid Plexus Cysts

- Naeini RM et al: Spectrum of choroid plexus lesions in children. AJR Am J Roentgenol. 192(1):32-40, 2009

Colloid Cyst

- Algin O et al: Radiologic manifestations of colloid cysts: a pictorial essay. Can Assoc Radiol J. Epub ahead of print, 2012
- Carrasco R et al: Acute hemorrhage in a colloid cyst of the third ventricle: A rare cause of sudden deterioration. Surg Neurol Int. 3:24, 2012
- Kumar V et al: Pediatric colloid cysts of the third ventricle: management considerations. Acta Neurochir (Wien). 152(3):451-61, 2010
- Pollock BE et al: Natural history of asymptomatic colloid cysts of the third ventricle. J Neurosurg. 91(3):364-9, 1999

Ependymal Cyst

- Talamonti G et al: Intracranial cysts containing cerebrospinal fluid-like fluid: results of endoscopic neurosurgery in a series of 64 consecutive cases. Neurosurgery. 68(3):788-803; discussion 803, 2011
- Xi-An Z et al: Endoscopic treatment of intraventricular cerebrospinal fluid cysts: 10 consecutive cases. Minim Invasive Neurosurg. 52(4):158-62, 2009

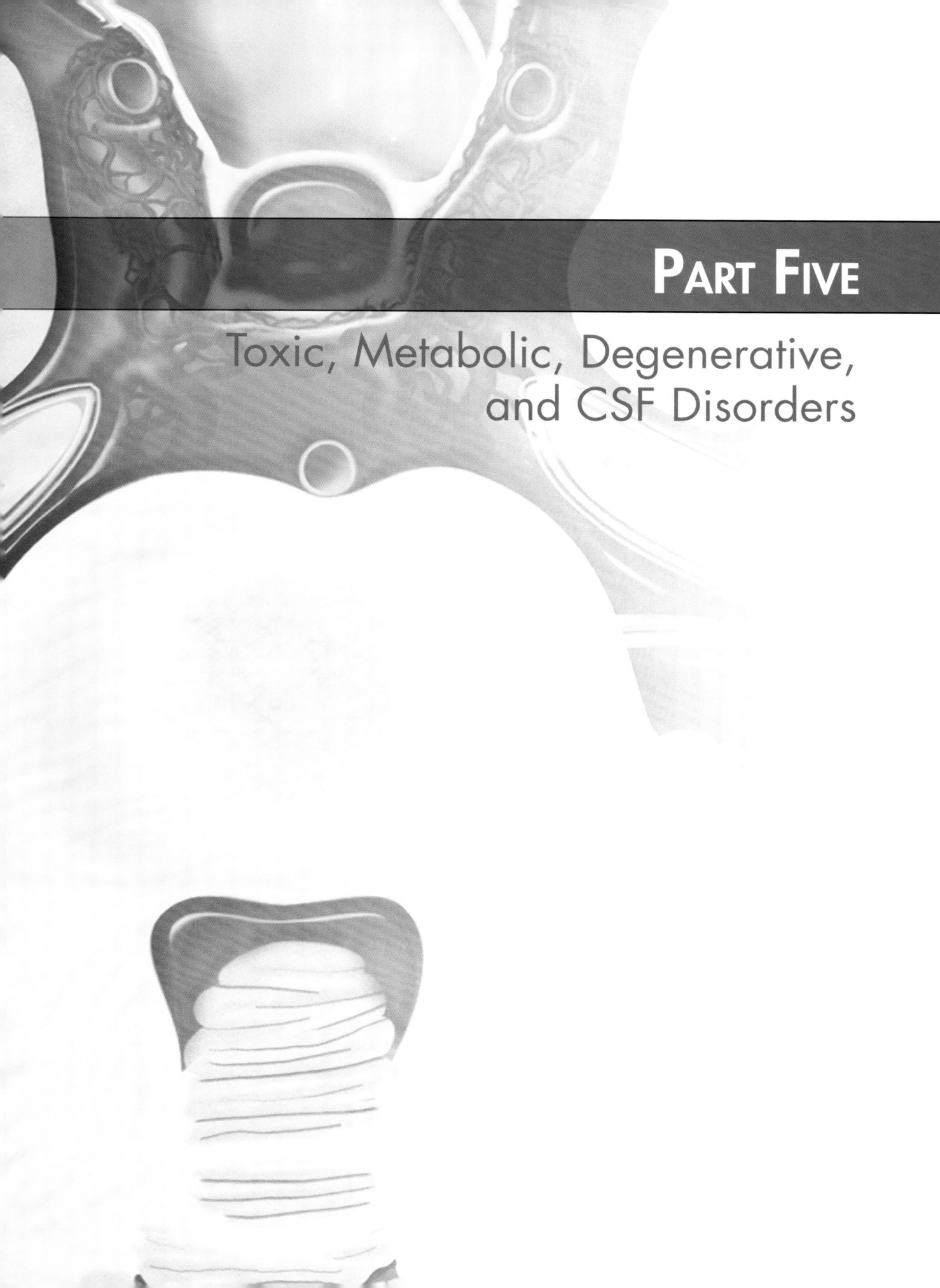

PART FIVE

Toxic, Metabolic, Degenerative, and CSF Disorders

29

Approach to Toxic, Metabolic, Degenerative, and CSF Disorders

This part, devoted to toxic, metabolic, degenerative, and CSF disorders, addresses some of the most difficult and challenging issues in neuroimaging. In contrast to many other brain diseases, here the CNS effects are often secondary to systemic disorders. Patients who present acutely with encephalopathy may have unknown or undiagnosed metabolic derangements.

Metabolic disorders are relatively uncommon but important diseases in which imaging can play a key role in early diagnosis and appropriate patient management. Drug and alcohol abuse are increasing around the world, and the list of environmental toxins that can affect the CNS continues to increase. Recognizing toxic and metabolic-induced encephalopathies has become a clinical and imaging imperative. The two etiologies are often linked, as many toxins induce metabolic derangements and some systemic metabolic diseases have a direct toxic effect on the brain.

With rapidly increasing numbers of aging people, the prevalence of dementia and brain degeneration is also becoming a global concern. Brain scans in elderly patients with mental status changes are now some of the most frequently requested imaging examinations. We also include hydrocephalus and related disorders in this part of the text.

Because inherited and acquired toxic, metabolic, and degenerative brain disorders often affect the deep gray nuclei in a bilaterally symmetric pattern, we begin this chapter by considering the normal physiology, gross anatomy, and imaging of the basal ganglia and dopaminergic striatonigral system.

We then present an anatomy-based approach to the differential diagnosis of toxic, metabolic, and degenerative disorders. Shaded text boxes and representative cases illustrate this approach to—and some supplemental considerations for—imaging diagnosis.

Lastly, we briefly discuss normal age-related changes in the CNS, which lays the foundation for an imaging approach to dementia, brain degeneration, and CSF disorders.

Anatomy and Physiology of the Basal Ganglia and Thalami

Physiologic Considerations

Basal Ganglia Metabolism

By weight and volume, the brain is a small structure. However, relative to its size, the brain is one of the most metabolically active of all organs. It normally receives about 15% of total cardiac output, consumes about 20% of blood oxygen, and metabolizes up to 20% of blood glucose.

Because of its high intrinsic metabolic demands, the brain is exquisitely sensitive to processes that decrease delivery or utilization of blood, oxygen, and glucose. A variety of toxic substances do exactly that.

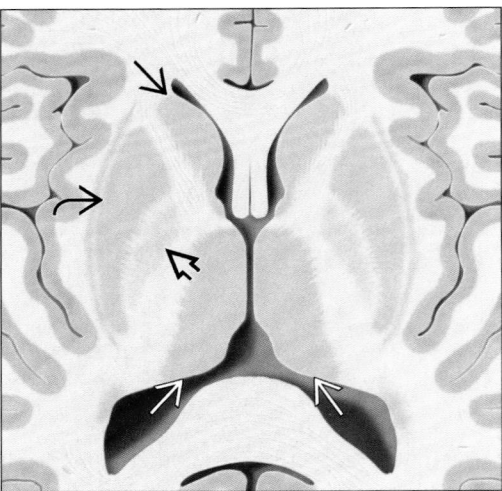

29-1. Graphic depicts basal ganglia. Caudate nucleus ➡, putamen ➚, globus pallidus ➤. Thalami ➡ form borders of the third ventricle.

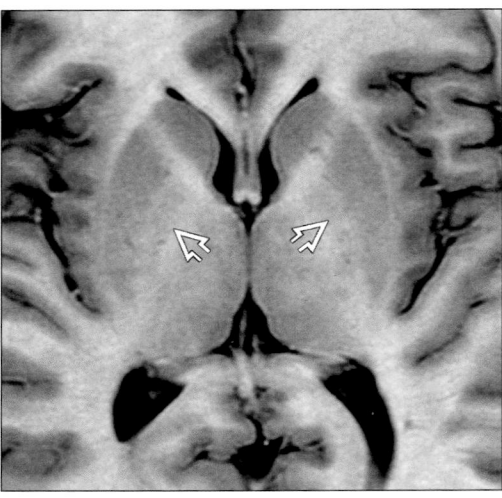

29-2. Axial T1WI shows basal ganglia, thalami as isointense with gray matter. Globi pallidi ➤ are slightly hyperintense to the caudate, putamen.

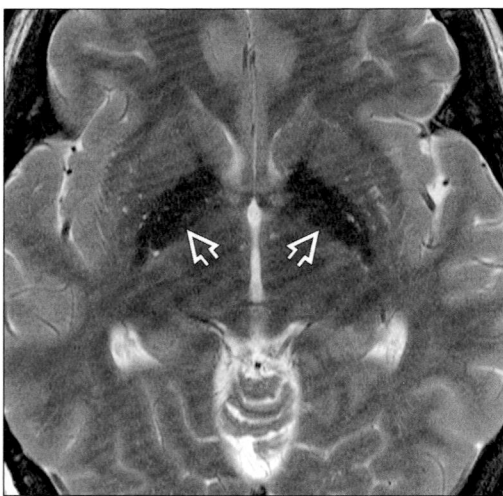

29-3. On T2WI, the globi pallidi ➤ are more hypointense than the putamen, caudate. Putamen reaches same hypointensity in 7th or 8th decade.

Two areas of the brain are especially susceptible to toxic and metabolic damage: The deep gray nuclei and the cerebral white matter. The basal ganglia (BG) are highly vascular, rich in mitochondria, and loaded with neurotransmitters. The BG—especially the putamen and globus pallidus—are particularly susceptible to hypoxia or anoxia and are also commonly affected by toxins and metabolic derangements. The cerebral white matter (WM) is particularly vulnerable to lipophilic toxic substances.

The Dopaminergic Striatonigral System

The substantia nigra pars compacta (SNPc) contains most of the dopaminergic neuron population of the midbrain. Mesencephalic dopaminergic neurons help regulate voluntary movement. Degeneration of dopaminergic neurons in the SNPc reduces dopaminergic input to the striatum and results in movement disorders such as Parkinson disease. The dopaminergic striatonigral system is discussed in greater detail in the chapter on dementias and brain degeneration.

Normal Gross Anatomy

The **basal ganglia** (BG) are symmetric paired subcortical (deep gray matter) nuclei that form the core of the extrapyramidal system and control motor activity. The BG consist of (1) the caudate nucleus (CNuc), (2) the putamen, and (3) the globus pallidus (GP).

The caudate nucleus and putamen form the **corpus striatum**. Two other structures—the substantia nigra and subthalamic nuclei—are functionally related to the striatum. Together these structures form the striatonigral system.

Because of their triangular or lens shape, the putamen and GP together are also called the **lentiform nuclei (29-1)**.

The lentiform nuclei lie just deep to the insular cortex and are separated from it (from medial to lateral) by the white matter (WM) of the external capsule, the gray matter of the claustrum, and the thin WM layer of the extreme capsule. Medially, the lentiform nuclei are separated from the caudate nucleus and thalamus by the anterior and posterior limbs of the internal capsule **(29-4)**.

The substantia nigra and subthalamic nuclei are considered next as they are an integral part of the striatonigral system.

The thalami are the largest and most prominent of the deep gray matter nuclei but are generally not included in the term "basal ganglia." The thalami are also considered separately below.

Caudate Nucleus

The CNuc is a C-shaped structure with a large head, tapered body, and down-curving tail. The CNuc parallels the lateral ventricle body, forming part of its floor and lateral wall. The tail follows the curve of the temporal horn, lying along its roof. Anteriorly, the tail expands and becomes continuous with the posteroinferior aspect of the putamen. The most anterior aspect of the tail abuts—but remains separate from—the amygdala.

A deep groove called the sulcus terminalis separates the CNuc from the thalamus and covers a band of fibers called the stria terminalis. The ST runs all the way around the lateral ventricle from the amygdala to the hypothalamus.

The CNuc together with the putamen receives input from the cerebral cortex and is connected to the substantia nigra and GP.

Putamen

The putamen is the outermost part of the BG. Medially, the putamen is separated from the GP by a thin layer of WM fibers, the lateral (external) medullary lamina.

Globus Pallidus

The GP consists of two segments. The lateral (external) segment is separated from the medial segment by a thin layer of myelinated axons, the internal medullary lamina.

Thalamus

The thalami are symmetric, obliquely oriented ovoid masses of gray matter that lie posteromedial to the lentiform nuclei. The two thalami form the lateral walls of the third ventricle (29-7). The anterior aspect of each thalamus abuts the foramen of Monro. The posterior thalamus bulges into the lateral ventricle atrium while the dorsal surface forms part of the lateral ventricle floor. The stria terminalis demarcates the border between the thalamus and the body of the CNuc. The fornix curves above the thalamus and is separated from it by the choroid fissure.

Laterally, the thalami are separated from the GP by the posterior limb of the internal capsule. The thalami act as sensory and motor relay stations to the cortex.

Each thalamus is subdivided into several groups of nuclei (anterior, medial, and lateral thalamic). The lateral geniculate nuclei (part of the visual system) and medial geniculate nuclei (part of the auditory system) are also considered part of the thalamus. The pulvinar is the most posterior aspect of the thalamus and is nestled within the curve of the lateral ventricle, just in front of the atrium.

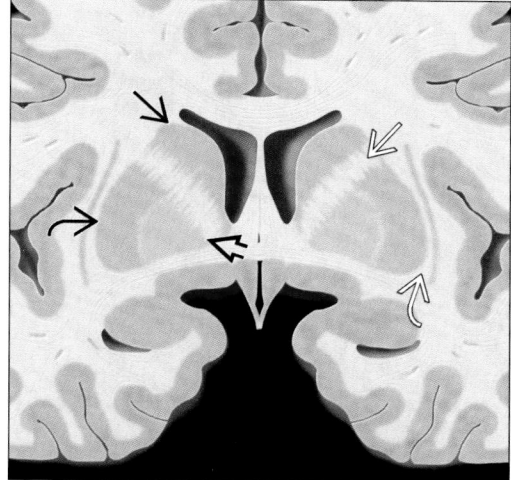

29-4. Coronal through frontal horns shows caudate nucleus ➘, putamen ➚, globus pallidus ➘, external capsule ➘, internal capsule ➜.

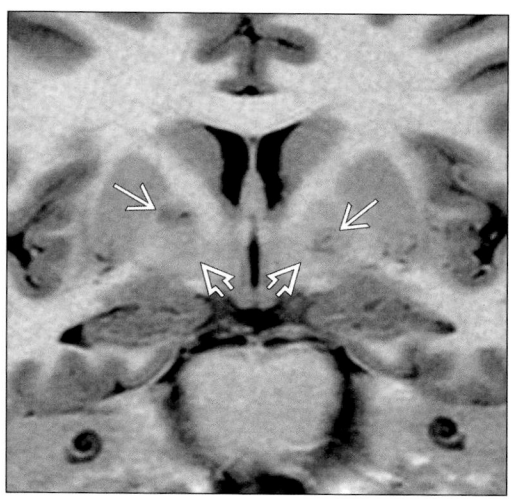

29-5. On coronal T1WI, the globi pallidi ➘ are slightly hyperintense to the putamina except for punctate hypointensities caused by Ca++ ➜.

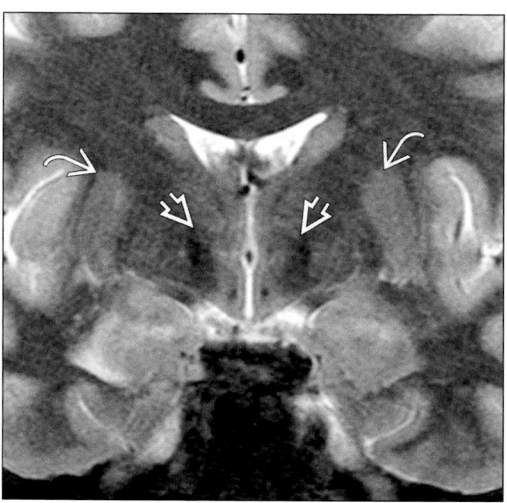

29-6. Coronal T2WI shows medial GP ➘ are the most hypointense of the basal ganglia. Putamina ➚ are isointense with cortex.

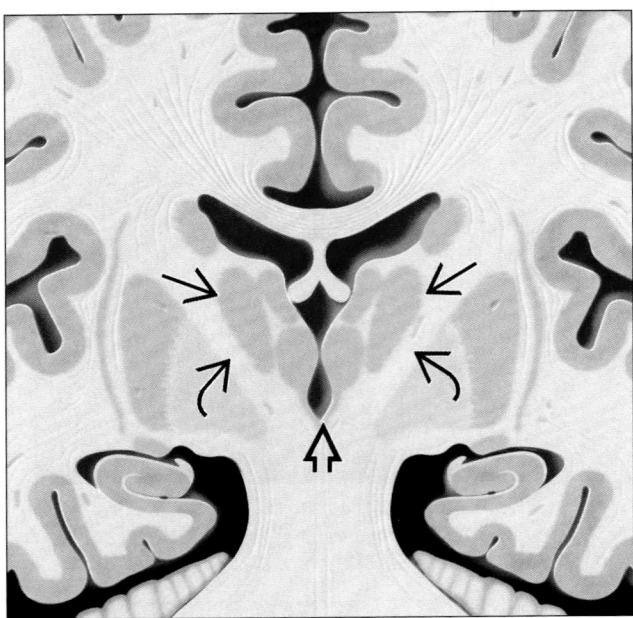

29-7. Coronal graphic depicts the major thalamic subnuclei ⇒ and their relationship to the third ventricle ⇒ and internal capsules ⇒.

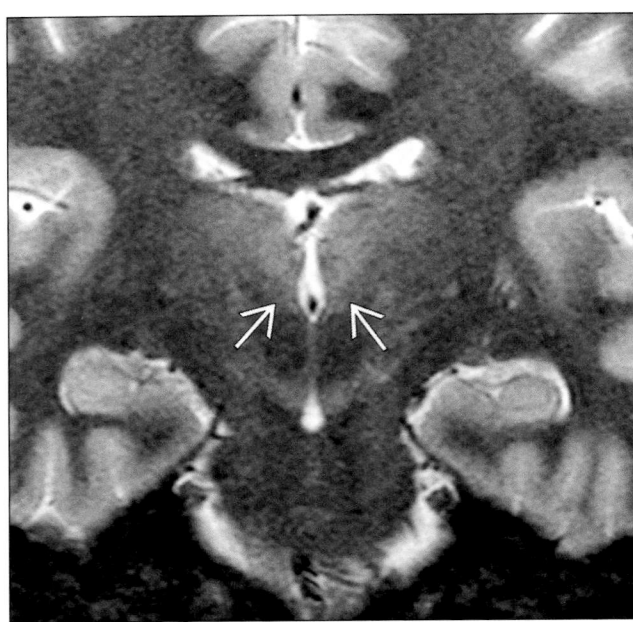

29-8. Coronal T2WI through the posterior third ventricle shows that thalami ➡ are mostly isointense with the cortex.

Substantia Nigra

The substantia nigra (SN) is located in the midbrain (mesencephalon). The SN appears black on gross anatomical sections because of high melanin levels in dopaminergic neurons. The SN is composed of two parts, a deep cell-rich pars compacta (SNPc) and a larger but less cellular segment, the pars reticulata.

Subthalamic Nucleus

The subthalamic nucleus (STN) is a small lens-shaped nucleus that lies in the upper midbrain, inferomedial to the thalamus and internal capsule and superolateral to the red nucleus. The STN is wrapped by fibers of the substantia nigra but receives its main input from the GP.

Normal Imaging Anatomy

While the lentiform nuclei, CNuc, thalami, and internal/external capsules can be identified on CT scans, their anatomy is best detailed on MR.

T1WI

The CNuc, putamina, and thalami are isointense with cortex on T1 scans. The globi pallidi are less cell-rich than either the putamen or caudate (29-2). As the site of both physiologic calcification and age-related iron deposition, the GP segments vary in signal intensity (29-5). Calcification may cause T1 shortening and mild hyperintensity in the medial segment. The fully myelinated, compact WM in the internal and external capsules appears hyperintense relative to the basal ganglia.

T2WI

The CNuc, putamina, and thalami are isointense with cortical gray matter on T2 scans (29-8). The myelin content in the GP is higher relative to the putamen (29-3), (29-6), so it appears relatively more hypointense on T2WI. Increasing iron deposition occurs with aging, and the putamen becomes progressively more hypointense. A "dark" putamen is normal by the seventh or eighth decade of life.

T2*

The GP is hypointense relative to cortex on GRE or SWI imaging. By the seventh or eighth decade of life, iron deposition in the putamen "blooms," and the lateral putamen appears hypointense relative to the thalami but not as intensely hypointense as the GP. The age-associated changes of brain iron deposition are discussed in greater detail in the chapter on dementias and brain degeneration.

Toxic and Metabolic Disorders

Many toxic, metabolic, systemic, and degenerative diseases affect the basal ganglia and thalami in a strikingly symmetric fashion.

When imaging discloses bilateral lesions that involve all the deep gray nuclei, the lesions are most often secondary to diffuse systemic or metabolic derangements. Patchy, discrete, focal, and asymmetric lesions are more commonly infectious, postinfectious, traumatic, or neoplastic in origin.

Bilateral basal ganglia lesions have many potential causes. Diseases that specifically affect the putamen or globi pallidi in a bilaterally symmetric pattern have a somewhat different pathoetiologic spectrum. Both patient age and imaging characteristics can also help establish a reasonable differential diagnosis.

In the subsequent chapters in this part, we consider toxic and metabolic disorders by diagnosis (e.g., chronic hepatic disease, acute hepatic encephalopathy, and hypoxic-ischemic encephalopathy).

Here we address the differential diagnosis of BG lesions first by general location (i.e., bilateral BG lesions) and then by sublocation. Entities within each differential diagnosis are categorized as common, less common, and rare but important.

Differential Diagnosis of Bilateral Basal Ganglia Lesions

The most common bilateral basal ganglia lesions are normal variants, such as physiologic calcification and prominent perivascular spaces. Vascular disease, hypoxic-ischemic insults, and common metabolic disorders, such as chronic liver failure, are the most frequent causes of abnormality.

Infection, toxins and drug abuse, or metabolic disorders, such as osmotic demyelination and Wernicke encephalopathy, are less common causes of bilateral basal ganglia lesions.

Careful evaluation of imaging findings outside the BG such as cortical or WM involvement—together with clinical correlation and laboratory data—is essential to differentiate among the many disorders that cause bilateral BG abnormalities **(29-9)**, **(29-10)**, **(29-11)**, **(29-12)**, **(29-13)**, **(29-14)**, **(29-15)**, **(29-16)**, **(29-17)**, **(29-18)**.

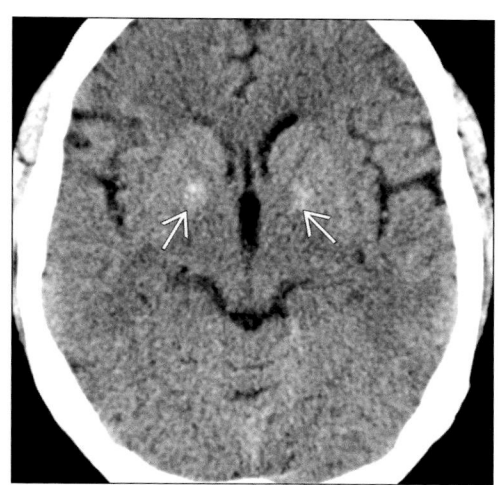
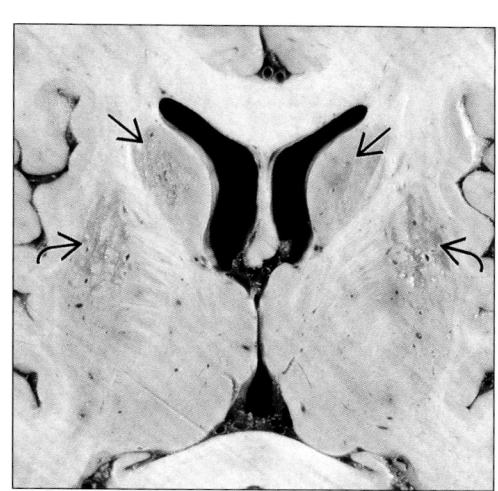

29-9. Axial NECT scan in a 34-year-old woman with headaches and normal neurologic examination shows normal bilateral symmetric physiologic calcifications in the medial globi pallidi ➡. 29-10. Autopsy case of hypoxia with acute striatal necrosis shows bilateral caudate nuclei ➡, putamina ⤳ lesions. The globi pallidi and thalami are spared. (Courtesy R. Hewlett, MD.)

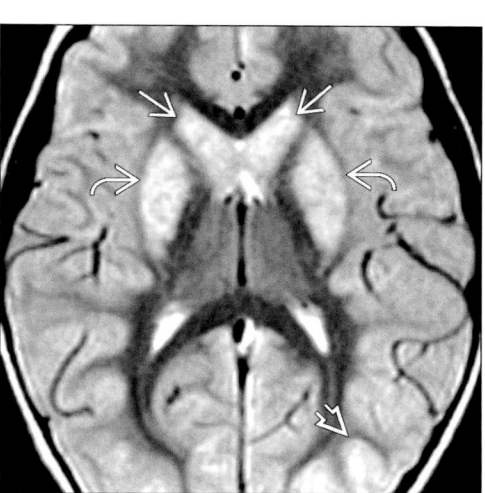
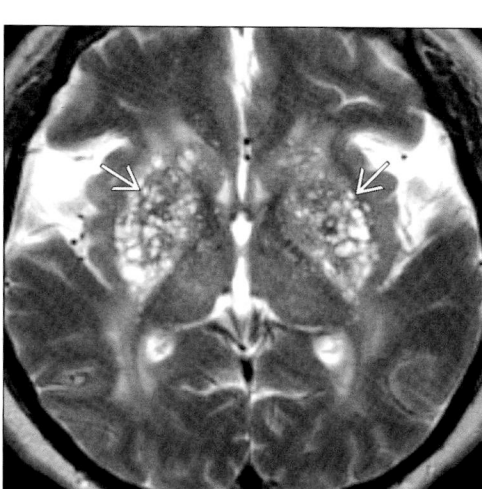

29-11. Axial T2WI in a patient with anoxia, basal ganglia necrosis shows bilateral hyperintensity in the caudate nuclei ➡, putamina and globi pallidi ⤳, and cortex ⇥. The thalamus is relatively spared. 29-12. Axial T2WI shows innumerable variably sized CSF-like cysts in the caudate nuclei, putamina, and globi pallidi ➡ with relative sparing of the thalamus. These are unusually prominent enlarged perivascular spaces (sometimes called "état criblé" or "cribriform state").

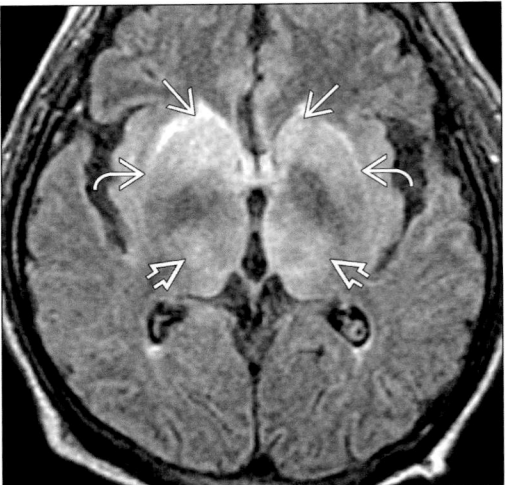

29-13. FLAIR scan shows bilateral CNuc ➡, putamina ➡, thalamic hyperintensity ➡. West Nile encephalitis. (Courtesy M. Colombo, MD.)

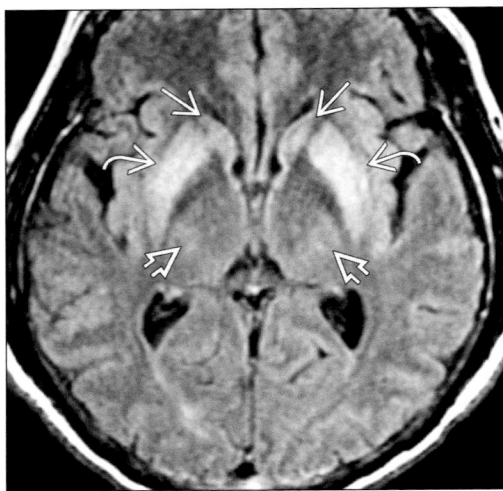

29-14. Axial FLAIR shows CNuc ➡, putamina ➡, thalamic ➡ symmetric hyperintensity. Extrapontine osmotic myelinolysis.

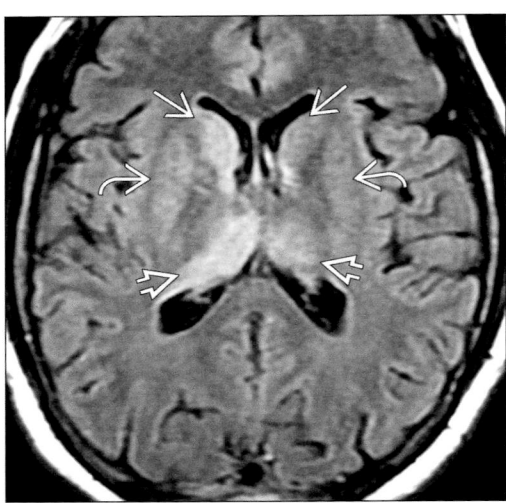

29-15. Axial FLAIR shows bilateral but asymmetric CNuc ➡, putamen ➡, thalamic ➡ hyperintensity. Deep vein occlusion.

COMMON BILATERAL BASAL GANGLIA LESIONS

Normal Variants
- Physiologic mineralization
  - Medial GP > > caudate, putamen
- Prominent perivascular spaces
  - Follow CSF, suppress on FLAIR

Vascular Disease
- Lacunar infarcts
  - Multiple bilateral, scattered, asymmetric
- Diffuse axonal/vascular injury
  - Hemorrhage, other lesions

Hypoxic-Ischemic Injury
- Hypoxic-ischemic encephalopathy (HIE)
  - BG ± cortex/watershed, hippocampi, thalami

Metabolic Disorders
- Chronic liver disease
  - GP, SN hyperintensity

LESS COMMON BILATERAL BASAL GANGLIA LESIONS

Infection/Post-Infection
- Viral
  - Especially flaviviral encephalitides (West Nile virus, Japanese encephalitis, etc.)
- Post-virus, post-vaccination
  - Acute disseminated encephalomyelitis (ADEM): Patchy > confluent; WM, thalami, cord often involved
  - Acute striatal necrosis

Toxic Poisoning and Drug Abuse
- Carbon monoxide
  - GP (WM may show delayed involvement)
- Heroin
  - BG, WM ("chasing the dragon")
- Methanol
  - Putamen, WM
- Cyanide
  - Putamen (often hemorrhagic)
- Nitroimidazole
  - Dentate nuclei, inferior colliculi, splenium, BG

Metabolic Disorders
- Osmotic ("extrapontine") demyelination
  - BG, ± pons, WM
- Wernicke encephalopathy
  - Medial thalami, midbrain (periaqueductal), mammillary bodies

Vascular Disease
- Internal cerebral vein/vein of Galen/straight sinus thrombosis
  - BG, deep WM
- Artery of Percheron infarct
  - Bilateral thalami, midbrain ("V" sign)

Neoplasm
- Primary CNS lymphoma
  - Periventricular (WM, BG)
- Astrocytoma
  - Bithalamic "glioma"

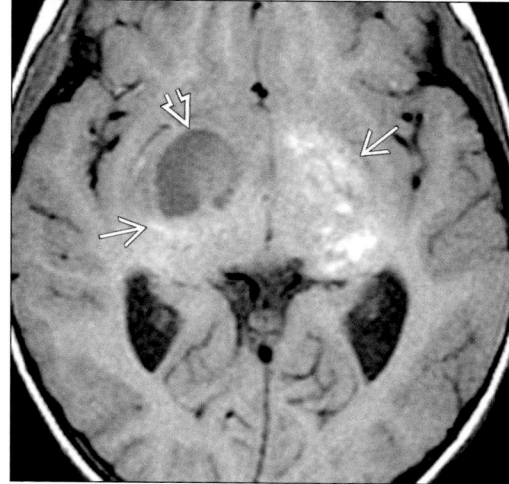

29-16. *Axial T1WI in a patient with NF1 shows multifocal BG hyperintensities* ➡, *large hyperintensity* ➡ *from myelin vacuolization.*

RARE BUT IMPORTANT BILATERAL BASAL GANGLIA LESIONS

Metabolic Disorders
- Acute hyperammonemia
  - Acute liver failure
  - Ornithine transcarbamylase deficiency, etc.
- Acute hyperglycemia
  - GP, caudate
- Severe hypoglycemia
  - Occipital cortex, hippocampi, ± WM

Infection and Inflammation
- Toxoplasmosis
  - Often HIV-positive, other ring-enhancing lesions
- Behçet disease
  - Midbrain often involved
  - Orogenital aphthous ulcers
- Chronic longstanding multiple sclerosis (MS)
  - BG become very hypointense
  - Putamina, thalami > GP, CNuc
  - Extensive WM disease, volume loss
- Creutzfeldt-Jakob disease (CJD)
  - Anterior BG (caudate, putamen)
  - Posteromedial thalami (T2/FLAIR hyperintense "hockey stick" sign)
  - Variable cortical (occipital = Heidenhain variant)

Inherited Disorders
- Neurofibromatosis type 1 (NF1)
  - GP T1 hyperintensity, T2 hyperintense foci
- Mitochondrial encephalopathies
  - Mitochondrial encephalopathy with lactic acidosis and stroke-like episodes (MELAS), myoclonic epilepsy with ragged red fibers (MERRF)
  - Leigh disease (putamen, periaqueductal region, cerebral peduncles)
- Wilson disease
  - Putamina, CNuc, ventrolateral thalami
- Pantothenate kinase-associated neurodegeneration (PKAN)
  - GP ("eye of the tiger")
- Huntington disease
  - Atrophic CNuc, putamina
- Fahr disease
  - Dense symmetric BG, thalami, dentate nuclei, subcortical WM Ca++
- Iron storage disorders
  - Symmetric BG "blooming" hypointensity

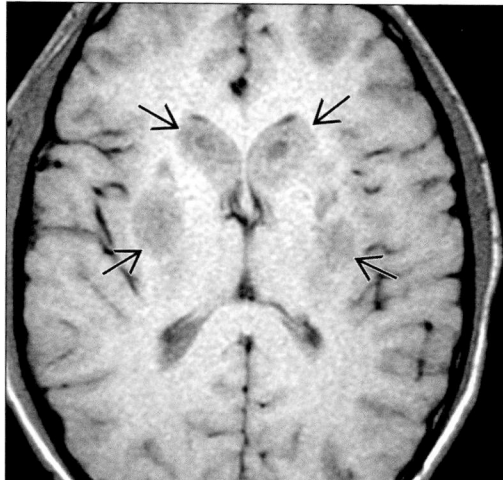

29-17. *Axial T1WI in patient with mitochondrial encephalopathy (MERRF) shows multifocal hypointensities in the BG* ➡.

Putamen Lesions

In general, the putamina are less commonly affected than either the globi pallidi or thalami. The most common lesion to affect the putamen is hypertensive hemorrhage. Acute hypertensive bleeds are usually unilateral although T2* scans often disclose evidence of prior hemorrhages.

Bilateral symmetric putamen lesions usually occur with more generalized BG involvement. However, there are some lesions that predominantly or almost exclusively involve the putamina.

Toxic, metabolic, hypoxic-ischemic events, and degenerative disorders account for the vast majority of symmetric putamen lesions (29-19), (29-20), (29-21).

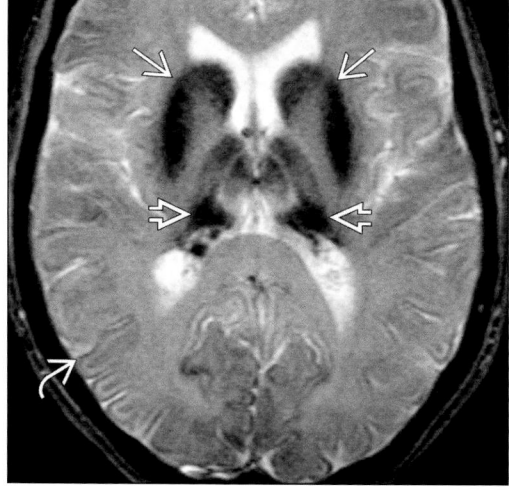

29-18. *T2* GRE in a patient with aceruloplasminemia shows symmetric "blooming" hypointensities in BG* ➡, *thalami* ➡, *cortex* ➡.

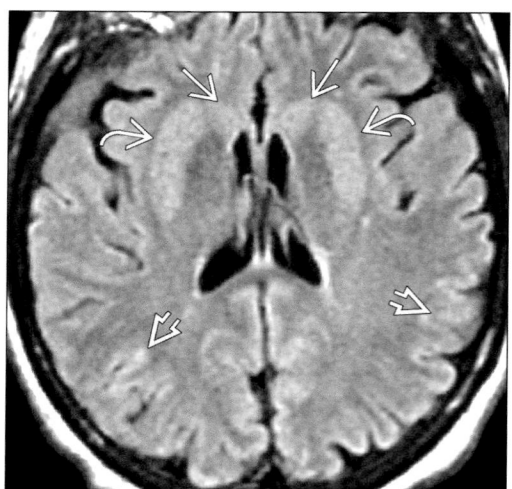

29-19. FLAIR scan in a patient with anoxia shows bilateral putamina ➨, caudate nuclei ➨, cortical ➨ hyperintensity.

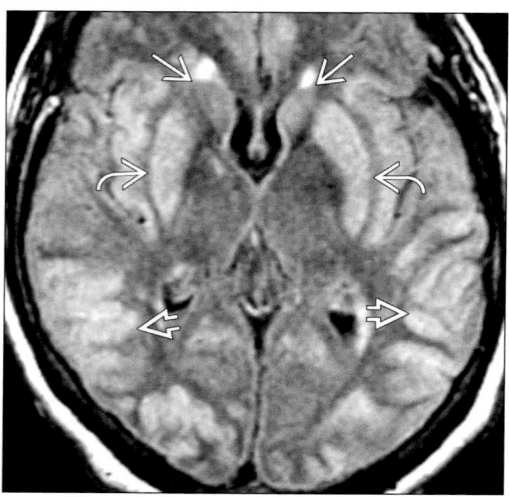

29-20. FLAIR shows symmetric hyperintensity in the CNuc ➨, putamina ➨, cortex ➨. Severe hypoglycemia. (Courtesy M. Castillo, MD.)

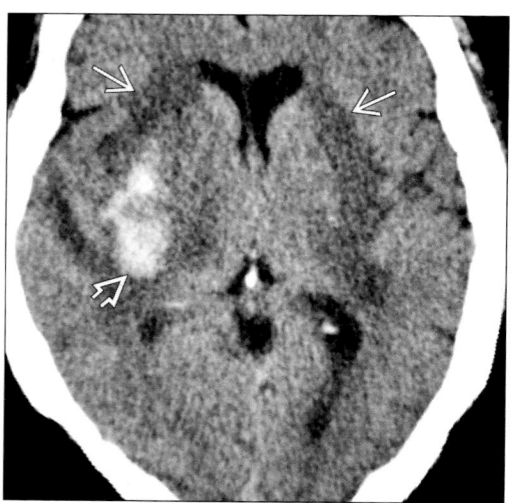

29-21. NECT shows bilaterally symmetric hypointense putaminal lesions ➨, hemorrhage ➨. Acute methanol toxicity. (Courtesy B. Hart, MD.)

COMMON PUTAMEN LESIONS

Metabolic Disorders
- Hypertensive hemorrhage
  - Lateral putamen/external capsule

Hypoxic-Ischemic Encephalopathy
- HIE in term infants
- Hypotensive infarction

LESS COMMON PUTAMEN LESIONS

Toxic Disorders
- Methanol toxicity*
  - Often hemorrhagic
  - ± subcortical WM
- Osmotic demyelination
  - Extrapontine myelinolysis

Inherited Disorders
- Leigh disease
- Neuroferritinopathy
  - Putamina, GP, dentate

* Predominantly or almost exclusively involves the putamina.

RARE BUT IMPORTANT PUTAMEN LESIONS

Degenerative Diseases
- Huntington disease
  - CNuc, putamina
- Parkinson disease
  - Putamen hypointensity
- Multiple system atrophy
  - Parkinsonian type* (hyperintense putaminal rim)

Miscellaneous
- Creutzfeldt-Jakob disease*
  - Anterior putamina, CNuc
  - Posteromedial thalami
  - Variable cortex (± predominant or exclusive involvement)

* Predominantly or almost exclusively involves the putamina.

Globus Pallidus Lesions

The globus pallidus (GP) is the part of the BG that is most sensitive to hypoxia. The vast majority of symmetric GP lesions are secondary to hypoxic, toxic, or metabolic processes. Most cause bilateral symmetric abnormalities on imaging studies **(29-22)**, **(29-23)**, **(29-24)**.

The differential diagnosis of GP lesions can be approached by prevalence (common, less common, rare but important), etiology, age, imaging appearance, or a combination of these factors.

COMMON GLOBUS PALLIDUS LESIONS
Normal Variant
- Physiologic calcification
  - Medial GP

Hypoxic-Ischemic Encephalopathy
- Anoxia, hypoxia (near-drowning, cerebral hypoperfusion)
- Neonatal HIE (profound acute)

Toxic/Metabolic Disorders
- Chronic liver disease
  - T1 hyper-, T2* hypointensity
- Carbon monoxide
  - T2 hyperintense medial GP

LESS COMMON GLOBUS PALLIDUS LESIONS
Toxic/Metabolic Disorders
- Post-opioid toxic encephalopathy
  - Often combined with HIE
- Hyperalimentation
  - Manganese deposition, short T1
- Chronic hypothyroidism
  - Punctate calcification
  - T1 hyper-, T2 hypointensity

Inherited Disorders
- NF1
- Leigh disease

RARE BUT IMPORTANT GLOBUS PALLIDUS LESIONS
Toxic/Metabolic Disorders
- Kernicterus
  - T1 shortening
- Cyanide poisoning
  - Hemorrhagic GP, laminar cortical necrosis

Inherited Disorders
- Fahr disease
  - Dense symmetric confluent calcification
- Wilson disease
  - T2 hyperintensity in GP, putamen
  - "Face of giant panda" sign in midbrain
- PKAN
  - "Eye of the tiger" (central T2 hyper-, peripheral hypointensity)
  - Not always present!
- Neurodegeneration with brain iron accumulation (NBIA)
  - GP, SN hypointensity ± putamen
- Maple syrup urine disease (MSUD)
  - Edema (GP, brainstem, thalami, cerebellar WM)
- Methylmalonic acidemia (MMA)
  - Symmetric GP T2 hyperintensity ± WM

Degenerative Diseases
- Hepatocerebral degeneration
  - 1% of patients with cirrhosis, portosystemic shunts
  - T1 shortening
- Progressive supranuclear palsy
  - Also affects STN, SN

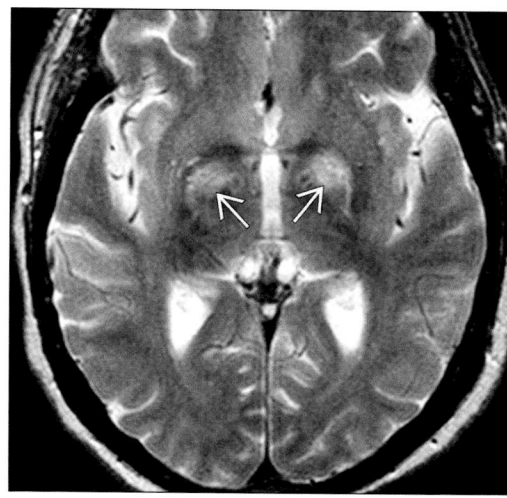

29-22. *T2WI in a patient with hypotensive infarct following narcotic overdose shows bilateral globus pallidus hyperintensities* ➔.

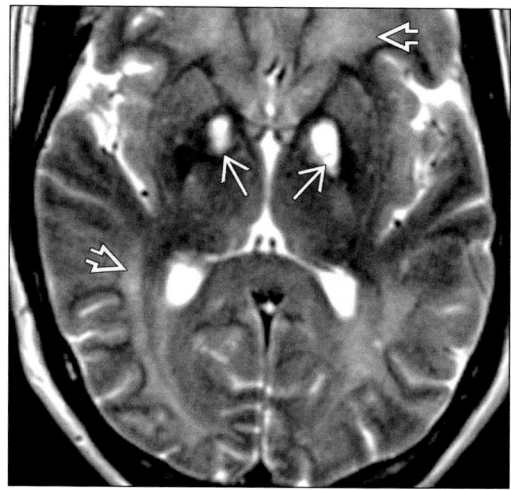

29-23. *T2WI shows bilateral medial GP hyperintensities* ➔ *as well as diffuse confluent WM hyperintensity* ➔. *Carbon monoxide poisoning.*

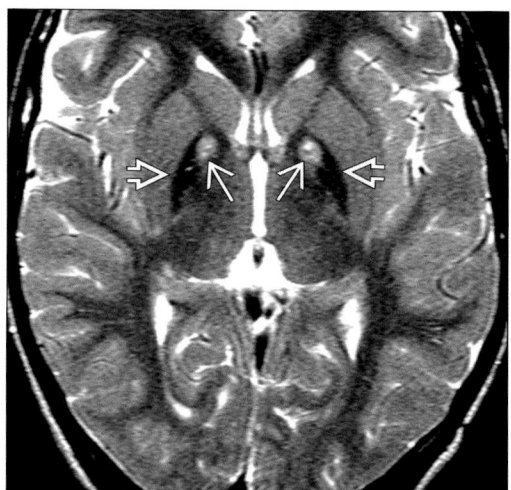

29-24. *T2WI shows classic "eye of the tiger" with medial GP hyperintensities* ➔ *surrounded by well-defined hypointensity* ➔. *PKAN.*

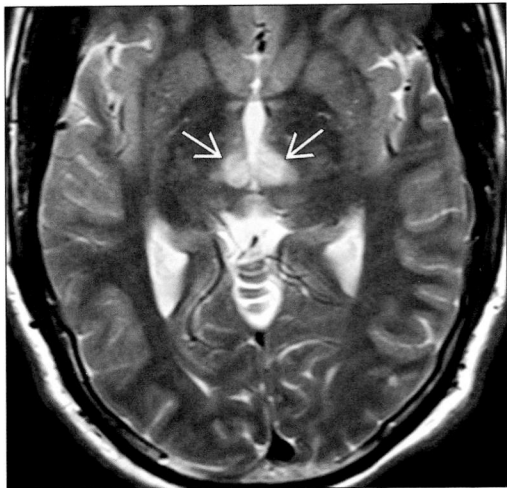

29-25. Axial T2WI shows bilateral medial thalamic infarcts ➡ caused by artery of Percheron occlusion.

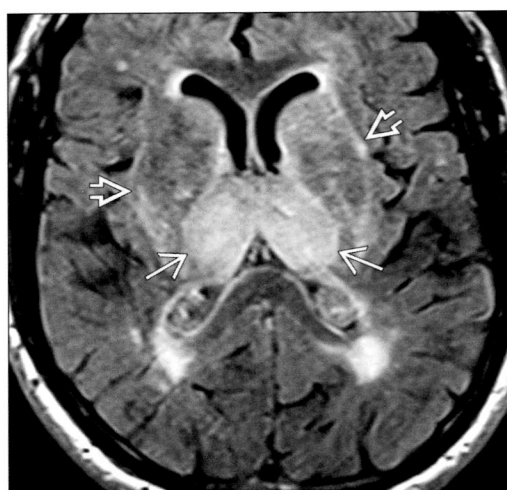

29-26. Axial FLAIR shows bithalamic lesions ➡ with less extensive involvement of putamina ⇉, GP. Internal cerebral vein occlusion.

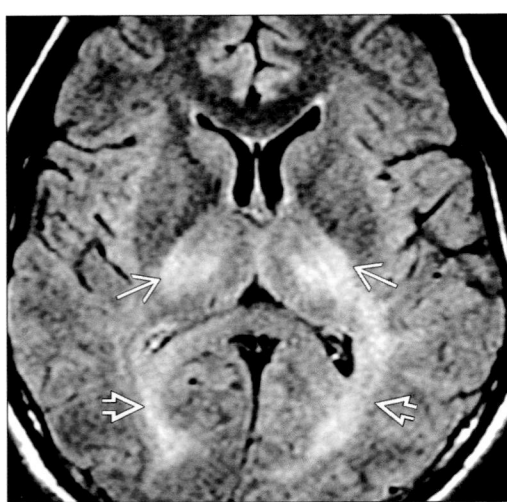

29-27. FLAIR scan in a patient with EBV encephalitis shows bithalamic ➡, occipital WM involvement ⇉.

Globus Pallidus Lesions by Age

Some GP lesions are common in adults but rare in children; others are seen primarily in the pediatric age group.

GLOBUS PALLIDUS LESIONS BY AGE
GP Lesions of Adulthood
• Hypoxia/anoxia
• Drug abuse
• Carbon monoxide poisoning
• Hepatic encephalopathy
• Hyperalimentation
• Hypothyroidism
• Wilson disease
• NBIA
GP Lesions of Childhood
• HIE
• NF1
• Leigh disease
• Wilson disease
• Kernicterus
• NBIA, PKAN
• MSUD
• MMA

Globus Pallidus Lesions by Appearance

Some GP lesions can be distinguished by their typical attenuation on CT or signal intensity on MR.

GLOBUS PALLIDUS LESIONS BY CHARACTERISTIC APPEARANCE
NECT Hypodensity
• HIE
• Carbon monoxide poisoning
NECT Hyperdensity
• Physiologic Ca++
• Hypothyroidism
• Fahr disease
T1 Hyperintensity
• Chronic hepatic encephalopathy
• Hyperalimentation (manganese deposition)
• NF1
• Hypothyroidism
• Kernicterus (acute)
• Wilson disease
T2 Hyperintensity
• HIE
• Drug abuse
• Carbon monoxide poisoning
• NF1
• Leigh disease
• Kernicterus (chronic)
• Wilson disease
• PKAN, MSUD, MMA

Thalamic Lesions

Because lacunar infarcts and hypertensive bleeds are so common, *unilateral* thalamic lesions are much more common than bilateral symmetric abnormalities.

In contrast, *bilateral* symmetric thalamic lesions are relatively uncommon and have a somewhat limited differential diagnosis. As with the symmetric basal ganglia lesions discussed previously, bilateral thalamic lesions tend to be toxic, metabolic, vascular, infectious, or hypoxic-ischemic **(29-25)**, **(29-26)**, **(29-27)**, **(29-28)**, **(29-29)**, **(29-30)**.

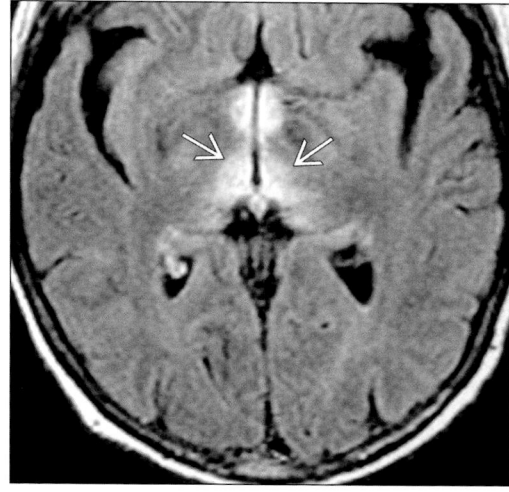

29-28. *FLAIR in a patient with Wernicke encephalopathy shows symmetric lesions in both medial thalami* ➡.

UNILATERAL THALAMIC LESIONS

Common
- Lacunar infarction
- Hypertensive intracranial hemorrhage

Less Common
- NF1
- Diffuse astrocytoma (low-grade fibrillary)
- Glioblastoma multiforme
- Anaplastic astrocytoma
- ADEM

Rare but Important
- MS
- Unilateral internal cerebral vein thrombosis
- Germinoma

COMMON BITHALAMIC LESIONS

Vascular Lesions
- Deep venous occlusion
  - Thalami > GP, putamina, CNuc ± deep WM
- Arterial ischemia
  - Artery of Percheron infarct
  - "Top of the basilar" thrombosis
- Vasculitis

Hypoxic-Ischemic Encephalopathy
- Profound hypoperfusion
  - BG, hippocampi, cortex
- Usually occurs in full-term neonates

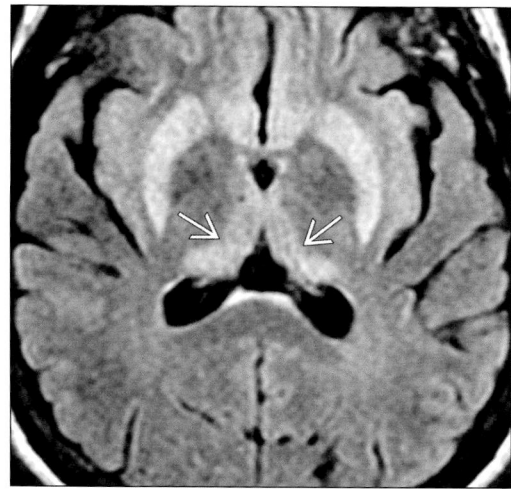

29-29. *FLAIR scan in a patient with CJD shows classic "hockey stick" sign* ➡ *as well as anterior caudate, putamen hyperintensity.*

LESS COMMON BITHALAMIC LESIONS

Infection/Post-Infection/Inflammatory Disorders
- ADEM
  - Usually with WM lesions
- Viral encephalitis
  - *Many* agents affect thalami (Epstein-Barr virus, West Nile virus, Japanese encephalitis, etc.)
- CJD
  - "Hockey stick" sign (pulvinar, medial thalami)

Toxic/Metabolic Disorders
- Osmotic myelinolysis (extrapontine)
  - Thalami, external capsules, putamina, CNuc
- Wernicke encephalopathy
  - Medial thalami, midbrain, mammillary bodies
- Solvent inhalation (toluene, etc.)
- Acute hypertensive encephalopathy (PRES)
  - Occipital lobes, watershed zones > BG
- Status epilepticus
  - Pulvinar, splenium
  - Often hippocampi ± cortex

Neoplasms
- Bithalamic low-grade astrocytoma
- Gliomatosis cerebri

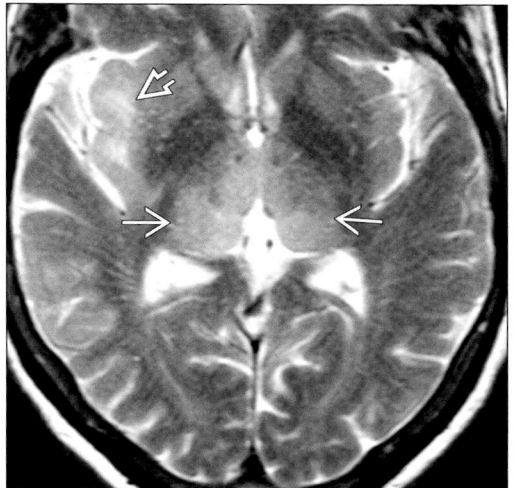

29-30. *T2WI shows bithalamic* ➡, *right insular* ➡ *hyperintensity in a patient with gliomatosis cerebri, WHO grade II astrocytoma.*

RARE BUT IMPORTANT BITHALAMIC LESIONS

Infection/Post-Infection/Inflammatory Disorders
- MS (severe, chronic)
  - Hypointense BG on T2*
- Acute necrotizing encephalopathy of childhood

Inherited Disorders
- Mitochondrial disorders
- Krabbe disease
  - Hyperdense on CT, hypointense on T2
- Wilson disease
  - Putamina, CNuc > thalami
- Fahr disease
  - GP > thalami
- Fabry disease
  - T1 hyperintense posterior thalamus ("pulvinar")
  - M >> F
  - Strokes (territorial, lacunar)
  - Renal, cardiac disease

Neoplasm
- Glioblastoma multiforme
- Anaplastic astrocytoma

Paraneoplastic Syndromes
- Can mimic prion disease

Bithalamic Lesions by Age

As with GP lesions, some symmetric bithalamic lesions—such as those caused by inherited metabolic disorders—are more common in infants and children. Others are seen primarily in adults. Some (e.g., acquired metabolic disorders, deep venous occlusion, ADEM) occur in all ages.

The most common and rare but important causes of bithalamic lesions in children and adults are shown in the box below.

BITHALAMIC LESIONS BY AGE

Childhood Bithalamic Lesions
- Hypoxic-ischemic encephalopathy
- ADEM
- Bithalamic astrocytoma
- Inherited metabolic disorder
- Acquired metabolic disorders
- Toxic encephalopathy
- Deep venous occlusion
- Acute necrotizing encephalitis

Adult Bithalamic Lesions
- Deep venous occlusion
- Artery of Percheron, "top of the basilar" occlusion
- Profound hypoperfusion
- ADEM
- Wernicke encephalopathy
- Osmotic demyelination
- Vasculitis
- CJD

Degenerative and CSF Disorders

Age-related Changes

Normal age-related changes in the brain occur throughout life. Understanding the different stages of brain formation and normal progression of myelination is essential to diagnosing inherited metabolic disorders.

At the opposite end of the age spectrum, volume is normally lost in some parts of the brain while others remain relatively intact. Abnormal mineral deposition in the basal ganglia can be a clue to degenerative and metabolic disorders. Understanding what is normal heavy metal deposition in different decades is a prerequisite to diagnosing these abnormalities on imaging studies.

Dementia and Brain Degeneration

Once an understanding of the normal aging brain is established, we discuss the pathology and imaging manifestations of dementia. While identifying a "lobar predominant" pattern of volume loss on CT and standard MR can be accomplished in many cases, these are usually late-stage manifestations. The early diagnosis of dementing disorders increasingly relies on functional MR and PET studies.

CNS degenerations from Parkinson disease to wallerian and hypertrophic olivary degeneration are considered. The anatomy and physiology of the brain dopaminergic system are briefly reviewed, as is the anatomy essential to evaluating pre- and postoperative deep brain stimulation.

Hydrocephalus and CSF Disorders

Because abnormalities of the brain CSF spaces are a common manifestation of brain degeneration in the elderly as well as a potentially treatable cause of encephalopathy, we devote the last chapter in this part to hydrocephalus and CSF disorders.

We first address the normal anatomy of the ventricles and CSF spaces as well as imaging variants that can be mistaken for disease.

Hydrocephalus, disorders of CSF production/circulation/absorption, and the newly described syndrome of inappropriately low-pressure acute hydrocephalus are then discussed. Lastly, we consider CSF leaks and sequelae including intracranial hypotension—conditions in which imaging plays an essential role in both diagnosis and patient management.

Selected References

Anatomy and Physiology of the Basal Ganglia and Thalami

Physiologic Considerations

- Rothwell JC: The motor functions of the basal ganglia. J Integr Neurosci. 10(3):303-15, 2011

Normal Gross Anatomy

- Rothwell JC: The motor functions of the basal ganglia. J Integr Neurosci. 10(3):303-15, 2011
- Salzman KL: Basal ganglia and thalamus. In Harnsberger HR et al: Diagnostic and Surgical Imaging Anatomy: Brain, Head and Neck, Spine. Salt Lake City: Amirsys Publishing. I.64-75, 2006

Normal Imaging Anatomy

- Salzman KL: Basal ganglia and thalamus. In Harnsberger HR et al: Diagnostic and Surgical Imaging Anatomy: Brain, Head and Neck, Spine. Salt Lake City: Amirsys Publishing. I.64-75, 2006

Toxic and Metabolic Disorders

- Johnstone D et al: Molecular genetic approaches to understanding the roles and regulation of iron in brain health and disease. J Neurochem. 113(6):1387-402, 2010

Differential Diagnosis of Bilateral Basal Ganglia Lesions

- Hegde AN et al: Differential diagnosis for bilateral abnormalities of the basal ganglia and thalamus. Radiographics. 31(1):5-30, 2011
- Fischbein NJ: Bilateral basal ganglia lesions. In Osborn AG et al: EXPERTddx: Brain and Spine. Salt Lake City: Amirsys Publishing. I.6.80-3, 2009
- Hantson P et al: The value of morphological neuroimaging after acute exposure to toxic substances. Toxicol Rev. 25(2):87-98, 2006
- Mas A: Hepatic encephalopathy: from pathophysiology to treatment. Digestion. 73 Suppl 1:86-93, 2006

Putamen Lesions

- Salzman KL: Putamen lesion(s). In Osborn AG et al: EXPERTddx: Brain and Spine. Salt Lake City: Amirsys Publishing. I.6.84-5, 2009

Globus Pallidus Lesions

- Salzman KL: Globus pallidus lesion(s). In Osborn AG et al: EXPERTddx: Brain and Spine. Salt Lake City: Amirsys Publishing. I.6.86-9, 2009

- Prockop LD et al: Carbon monoxide intoxication: an updated review. J Neurol Sci. 262(1-2):122-30, 2007

Thalamic Lesions

- Khalil M et al: Iron and neurodegeneration in multiple sclerosis. Mult Scler Int. 2011:606807, 2011
- Khanna PC et al: Imaging bithalamic pathology in the pediatric brain: demystifying a diagnostic conundrum. AJR Am J Roentgenol. 197(6):1449-59, 2011
- Tschampa HJ et al: Thalamus lesions in chronic and acute seizure disorders. Neuroradiology. 53(4):245-54, 2011
- Smith AB et al: Bilateral thalamic lesions. AJR Am J Roentgenol. 192(2):W53-62, 2009

Degenerative and CSF Disorders

Age-related Changes

- Maillard P et al: Coevolution of white matter hyperintensities and cognition in the elderly. Neurology. 79(5):442-8, 2012

Dementia and Brain Degeneration

- Doecke JD et al: Blood-based protein biomarkers for diagnosis of Alzheimer disease. Arch Neurol. Epub ahead of print, 2012
- Whitwell JL et al: Comparison of imaging biomarkers in the Alzheimer disease neuroimaging initiative and the Mayo Clinic study of aging. Arch Neurol. 69(5):614-22, 2012

Hydrocephalus and CSF Disorders

- Stadlbauer A et al: Magnetic resonance velocity mapping of 3D cerebrospinal fluid flow dynamics in hydrocephalus: preliminary results. Eur Radiol. 22(1):232-42, 2012

30

Toxic Encephalopathy

The list of toxins and poisons that affect the CNS is long and continues to grow. Some agents are deliberately injected, inhaled, or ingested whereas others are accidentally encountered or administered in a controlled medical setting. Some toxins accumulate slowly, so their clinical manifestations are subtle and onset insidious. Others cause profound, virtually immediate CNS toxicity with rapid onset of coma and death. Still others—such as ethanol—have both acute and chronic effects.

Many illicit "street" drugs have serious adverse impacts on the CNS. An accurate history is often difficult to obtain in affected patients, and clinical symptoms are frequently nonspecific. Presentation may be confounded by "polydrug" abuse and secondary effects such as hypoxia that mask the underlying pathology. Acute on chronic underlying disease in abusers also contributes to the difficulty in sorting out which clinical and imaging findings can be attributed to specific drugs.

The vast majority of toxins cause bilateral symmetric lesions that involve the deep gray nuclei (basal ganglia, thalamus) with varying white matter involvement.

We first focus on the most common types of toxic encephalopathies, beginning with the acute and long-term effects of alcohol on the brain followed by a discussion of drug abuse. Inhaled toxins (such as carbon monoxide and cyanide) and heavy metal poisoning are then considered. We conclude with treatment-related disorders.

Alcohol and Related Disorders

Alcohol (ethanol [EtOH]) is one of the most commonly abused substances in the world. EtOH causes different effects on different organs. While the gastrointestinal system is exposed to higher concentrations of alcohol than any other tissue, ethanol easily crosses the blood-brain barrier and is a potent neurotoxin. Both its short- and long-term effects on the central nervous system are profound.

Excessive alcohol consumption can result in chronic brain changes as well as acute, life-threatening neurologic disorders. Comorbid diseases such as malnutrition with vitamin deficiencies may lead to Wernicke encephalopathy. Altered serum osmolarity associated with alcohol abuse can cause acute demyelinating disorders.

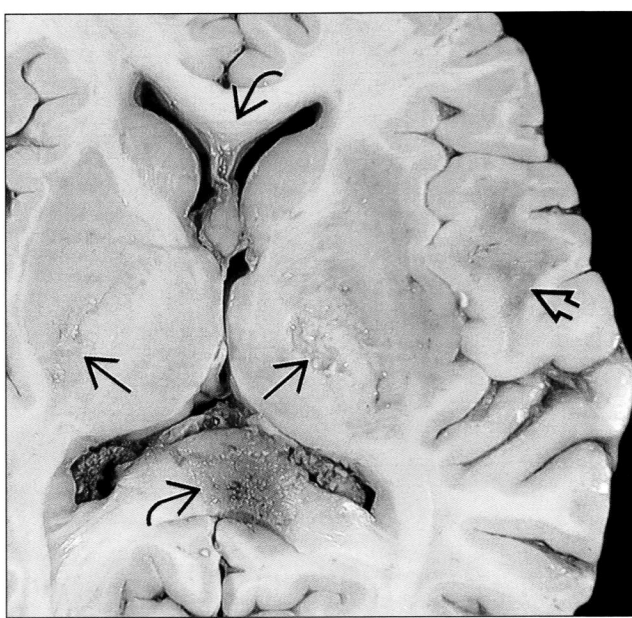

30-1. Autopsy of acute EtOH poisoning shows brain swelling with necrosis in subcortical/deep WM ⊵, especially marked in the corpus callosum ⊿. Basal ganglia/thalami are swollen, pale, infarcted ⊵. (Courtesy R. Hewlett, MD.)

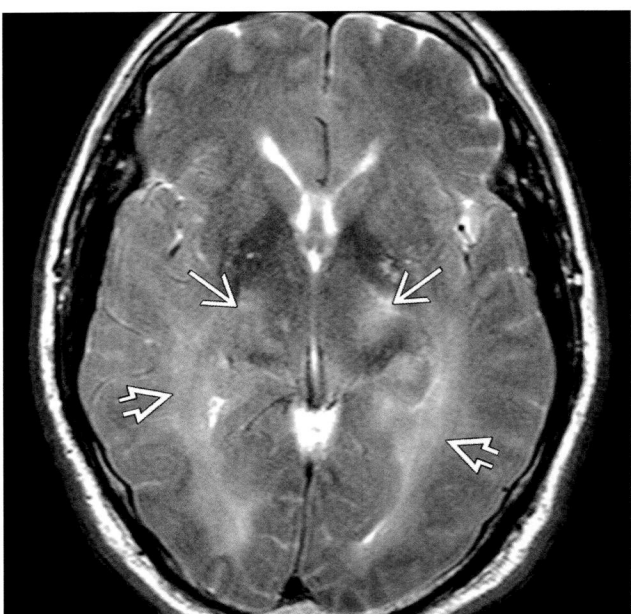

30-2. T2WI in a comatose patient who drank a 1 gallon of vodka or whisky daily for a full week shows diffuse brain swelling, hyperintense WM ➤, bithalamic lesions ➤. Acute alcohol poisoning.

We begin our discussion of alcohol and the brain by briefly considering the acute effects of alcohol poisoning. We then consider chronic alcoholic encephalopathy before turning to other complications of alcohol abuse, including alcohol-induced demyelination syndromes and Wernicke encephalopathy. We close the section with two less common forms of related abuse, i.e., methanol intoxication and ethylene glycol (antifreeze) ingestion.

Acute Alcohol Poisoning

Etiology

Acute alcohol poisoning is a complication of binge drinking and is most common in adolescents, who are especially vulnerable to alcohol neurotoxicity. The adolescent brain is undergoing structural maturation and has a unique sensitivity to alcohol. Adolescent binge drinking reduces adult neurotransmitter gene expression, reduces basal forebrain function, and decreases the density of cholinergic neurons.

The acute effects of binge drinking are striking. EtOH inhibits Na+/K+ activity. Cellular swelling, life-threatening cytotoxic cerebral edema, and nonconvulsive status epilepticus may ensue **(30-1)**. A blood alcohol concentration of 0.40% typically results in unconsciousness, and a level exceeding 0.50% is usually lethal.

Imaging

Imaging findings in patients with acute alcohol poisoning include diffuse brain swelling and confluent hyper-

intensity in the supratentorial subcortical and deep white matter on T2/FLAIR **(30-2)**. Seizure-induced changes in the cortex, with gyral hyperintensity and diffusion restriction, may also be associated. DTI can detect brain changes after acute alcohol consumption that are not visible on conventional MR imaging.

Chronic Alcoholic Encephalopathy

The long-term adverse effects of ethanol on the brain are much more common than those of acute alcohol poisoning.

Chronic alcohol-related brain damage can be divided into primary and secondary effects. We begin our discussion with the effects of EtOH itself on the brain and then consider secondary effects, which are mostly related to the sequelae of liver disease, malnutrition, malabsorption, and electrolyte disturbances.

Etiology

Alcohol is readily absorbed through the gastric and small intestinal mucosae. A normally functioning liver breaks down nearly 90% of alcohol.

EtOH readily crosses the blood-brain barrier, causing both direct and indirect neurotoxicity. Direct brain toxicity is caused by upregulation of NMDA receptors resulting in increased susceptibility to glutamate-mediated excitotoxicity. Other direct effects include the toxicity of acetaldehyde and related lipid peroxidation products, which can bind to brain tissue and initiate upregulation and expression of inflammatory factors. The resultant

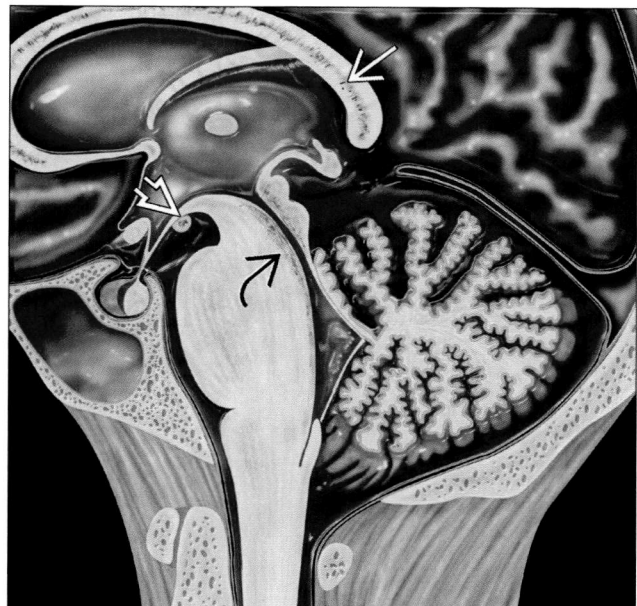

30-3. Sagittal graphic shows generalized and superior vermian atrophy, corpus callosum necrosis ➡ related to alcoholic toxicity. Mammillary body ➡, periaqueductal gray necrosis ⤳ is seen with Wernicke encephalopathy.

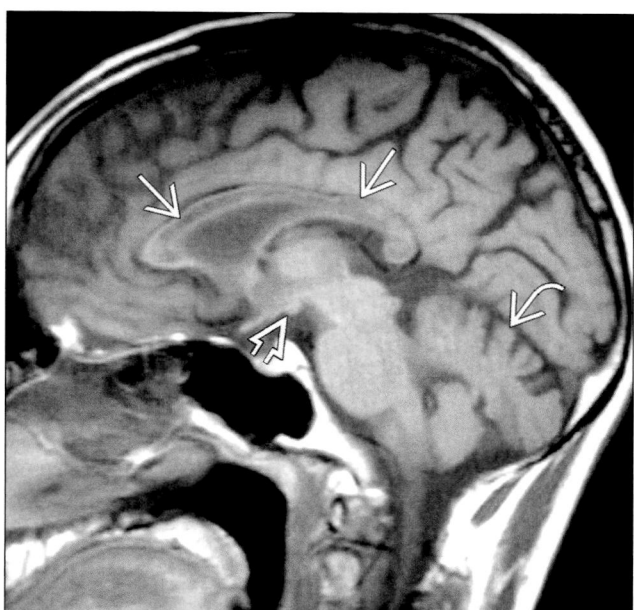

30-4. Sagittal T1WI in chronic alcoholic encephalopathy and Marchiafava-Bignami disease shows hypointensity in the entire middle corpus callosum ➡. Mammillary bodies ➡, superior vermis ➡ are atrophic. (Courtesy A. Datir, MD.)

membrane injury, neuronal loss, and reduction of white matter volume reflect the indirect effects of alcohol neurotoxicity.

Chronic EtOH abuse dysregulates synaptic connectivity, causes increased apoptosis, and decreases expression of myelin protein-encoding genes in the frontal cortex, hippocampus, and cerebellum.

Pathology

GROSS PATHOLOGY. The brain reflects the gross long-term effects of cumulative EtOH consumption (30-3). Cerebral atrophy is evidenced by enlarged ventricles and sulci, particularly in the frontal lobes, and is due predominantly to reduced white matter volume.

Alcohol-induced cerebellar degeneration is also common. The folia of the rostral vermis and anterosuperior aspects of the cerebellar hemispheres are atrophic, separated by widened interfolial sulci.

MICROSCOPIC FEATURES. Histologic changes in the cerebral hemispheres are nonspecific. Purkinje cell loss in the cerebellum, together with patchy loss of granular cells and molecular layer atrophy, reflects the alcohol-induced cerebellar degeneration.

Imaging

GENERAL FEATURES. A characteristic pattern of progressive brain volume loss is seen with chronic alcoholic encephalopathy. Initially, the superior vermis atrophies and the cerebellar fissures become prominent (30-4),

(30-5). In later stages, the frontal white matter becomes involved, reflected by widened sulci and enlarged lateral ventricles. In the final stages, global volume loss is present (30-6).

CT FINDINGS. NECT scans show generalized ventricular and sulcal enlargement. The cerebral white matter is often abnormally hypodense and reduced in volume. The great horizontal fissure of the cerebellum and the superior vermian folia are unusually prominent relative to the patient's age.

MR FINDINGS. Chronic liver failure secondary to cirrhosis may cause BG hyperintensity on T1WI, probably secondary to manganese accumulation. Focal and confluent cerebral white matter hyperintensities on T2/FLAIR sequences are common.

Alcohol-induced neurochemical changes can be detected before visible brain atrophy becomes apparent. MRS may demonstrate decreased concentration of NAA (a marker of neuronal viability) and choline-containing metabolites (membrane turnover markers), together with increased myoinositol (a putative marker of astrocyte proliferation).

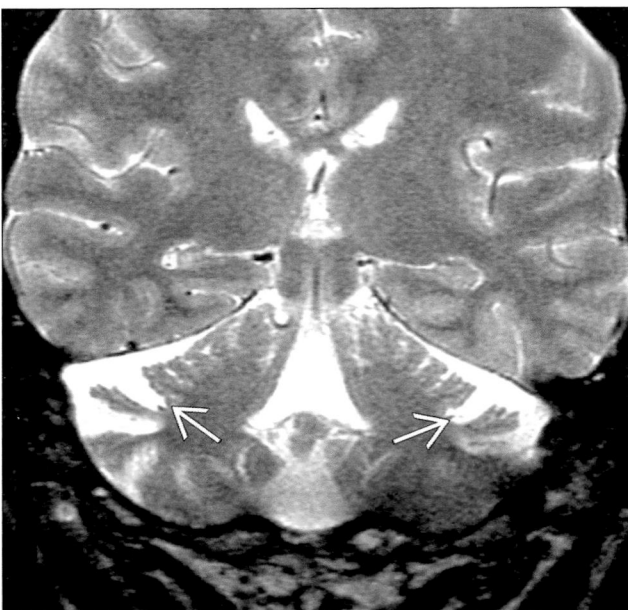

30-5. Coronal T2WI in a 41-year-old male chronic alcoholic shows marked atrophy of the superior cerebellum with striking widening of the horizontal fissures ➡. The supratentorial brain is relatively spared.

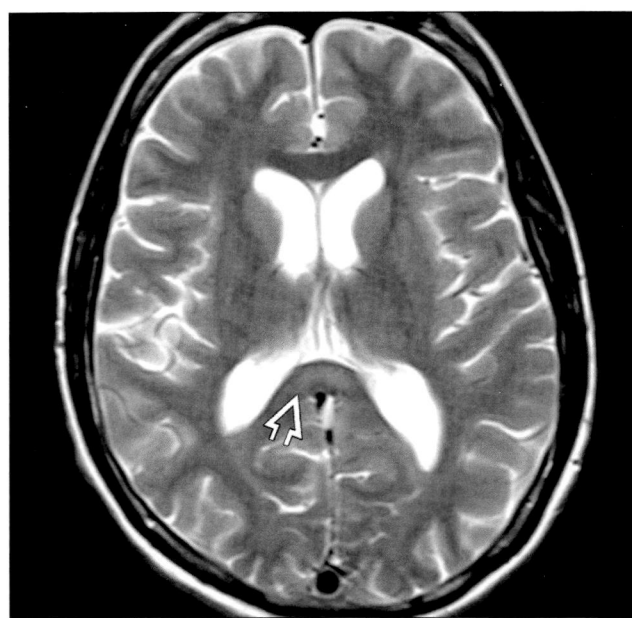

30-6. T2WI in a 30-year-old chronic alcoholic with acute deterioration shows generalized volume loss. Note corpus callosum splenium lesion ⇨; it restricted on DWI (not shown). Alcohol-induced atrophy with acute toxic demyelination.

ACUTE/CHRONIC ALCOHOLIC ENCEPHALOPATHY

Acute Alcohol Poisoning
- Rare
- Caused by binge drinking
- Imaging
  - Diffuse cerebral edema
  - Acute demyelination

Chronic Alcoholic Encephalopathy
- Common
- Primary toxic effect on neurons
  - Neurotransmitters, receptors
- Secondary effects related to liver, GI disease
  - Hepatic encephalopathy
  - Malnutrition, malabsorption
  - Electrolyte homeostasis
- Imaging
  - Volume loss (superior vermis, cerebellum, frontal lobes then generalized)
  - White matter myelinolysis

Wernicke Encephalopathy

Terminology

Wernicke encephalopathy (WE) is also known as Wernicke-Korsakoff syndrome. Both alcohol- and non-alcohol-related Wernicke encephalopathy can occur.

Etiology

GENERAL CONCEPTS. Thiamine (vitamin B1) is required to maintain membrane integrity and osmotic gradients across cell membranes. Inadequate thiamine results in lactic acidosis with intra- and extracellular edema.

Wernicke encephalopathy is caused by thiamine deficiency. Malnutrition with inadequate thiamine intake, decreased gastrointestinal absorption, and poor intracellular thiamine utilization may all contribute to the onset of alcoholic WE.

The underlying pathophysiology of *non*alcoholic WE is identical to that of alcoholic WE, but the etiology is different. Malnutrition secondary to eating disorders or gastric bypass surgery with drastically reduced thiamine intake is typical. Hyperemesis (e.g., pregnancy, chemotherapy) and prolonged hyperalimentation are other common causes of nonalcoholic WE.

Pathology

LOCATION. The mammillary bodies, hypothalamus, medial thalamic nuclei (adjacent to the third ventricle), tectal plate, and periaqueductal gray matter are most commonly affected **(30-7)**. Less commonly involved areas include the cerebellum (especially the dentate nuclei), red nuclei, corpus callosum splenium, and cerebral cortex.

GROSS PATHOLOGY. If WE occurs in the setting of chronic alcoholism, generalized brain atrophy (especially of the cerebellar vermis and frontal lobes) is present. Demyelination and petechial hemorrhages are common in the acute stage of WE. Callosal necrosis, white matter rarefaction, and mammillary body atrophy can be seen in chronic WE.

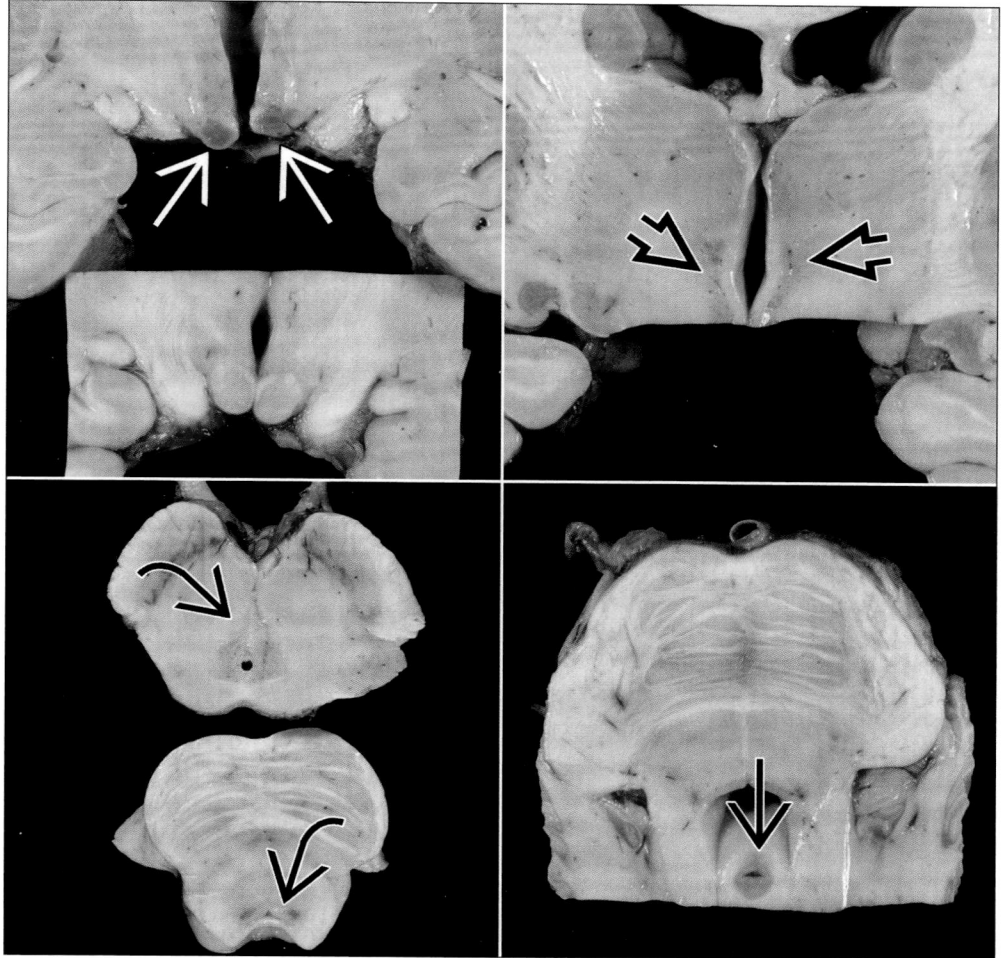

30-7. *Autopsy specimens from a patient with Wernicke encephalopathy shows hemorrhagic mammillary body necrosis* ➡ *(inset shows normal for comparison), bithalamic necrosis around walls of the third ventricle* ➡, *necrosis in periaqueductal gray matter* ➡ *and bottom of tectum* ➡. *(Courtesy R. Hewlett, MD.)*

Clinical Issues

DEMOGRAPHICS. Alcohol dependence occurs in all countries and all socioeconomic groups. Alcohol-related WE is dose-dependent and occurs without gender or ethnicity predilection. *Almost half of all WE cases occur in nonalcoholics.* Although WE is generally more common in adults, it *can and does occur in children!*

PRESENTATION. Only 30% of patients demonstrate the classic WE clinical triad of (1) ocular dysfunction (e.g., nystagmus, conjugate gaze palsies, ophthalmoplegia), (2) ataxia, and (3) altered mental status. The majority of patients have polyneuropathy.

NATURAL HISTORY. Mortality of untreated WE is high. Rapid intravenous thiamine replacement is imperative to prevent the most severe sequelae of Wernicke encephalopathy. Some survivors develop Korsakoff psychosis with severe amnesia, memory loss, and confabulation.

Imaging

Imaging—especially MR—is playing an increasingly important role in the early diagnosis of WE.

CT FINDINGS. CT has a low sensitivity for the detection of WE. NECT scans in acute WE are often normal. Subtle findings include bilateral hypodensities around the third ventricle and midbrain. CECT may show subtle enhancement in the affected areas.

MR FINDINGS. MR is much more sensitive than CT and is the procedure of choice in evaluating patients with possible WE. T1WI may show hypointensity around the third ventricle and cerebral aqueduct. In severe cases, petechial hemorrhages are present and may cause T1 hyperintensities in the medial thalami and mammillary bodies.

During the acute phase, T2/FLAIR hyperintensity can be seen in the affected areas **(30-8)**. Bilateral symmetric lesions in the mammillary bodies and around the third

30-8A. *FLAIR scan in a patient with acute Wernicke encephalopathy shows hyperintensity in the periaqueductal gray matter ➡, tectum ➡. **30-8B.** More cephalad FLAIR scan again shows the periaqueductal gray matter hyperintensity ➡. Both mammillary bodies are also hyperintense ➡.*

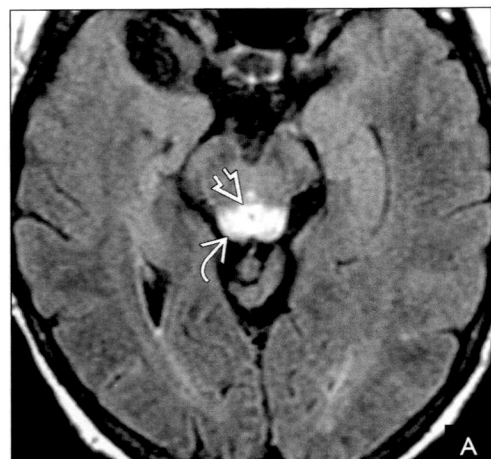

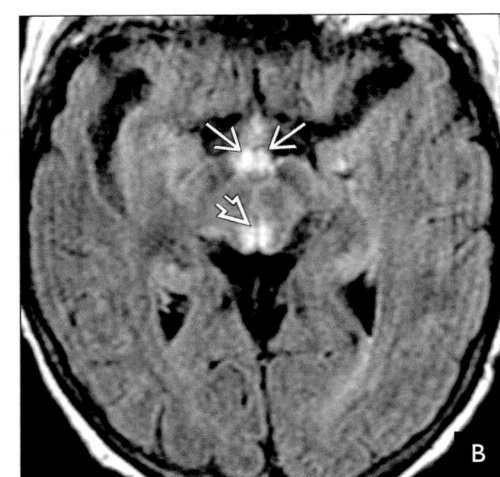

30-8C. *FLAIR scan shows hyperintensity in the medial thalami around the walls of the third ventricle ➡. The hypothalamus ➡ is also involved. **30-8D.** FLAIR scan through the cerebral convexities shows bilateral, relatively symmetric cortical hyperintensities ➡.*

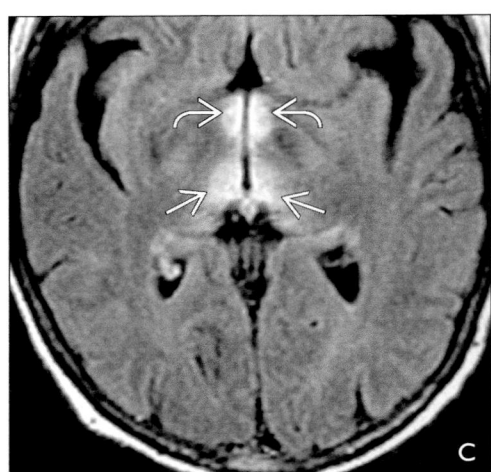

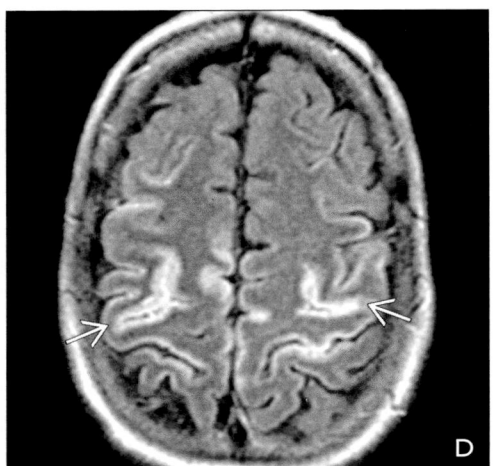

30-8E. *DWI in the same patient shows restricted diffusion in the mammillary bodies ➡. The periaqueductal GM does not restrict, suggesting that the midbrain lesions seen on FLAIR may be somewhat less acute. **30-8F.** Coronal T1 C+ demonstrates enhancement in the inferior colliculi ➡.*

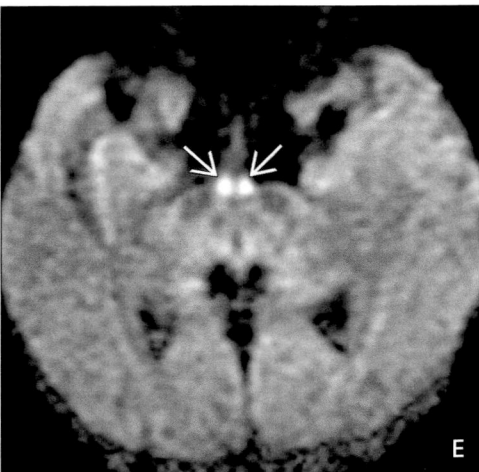

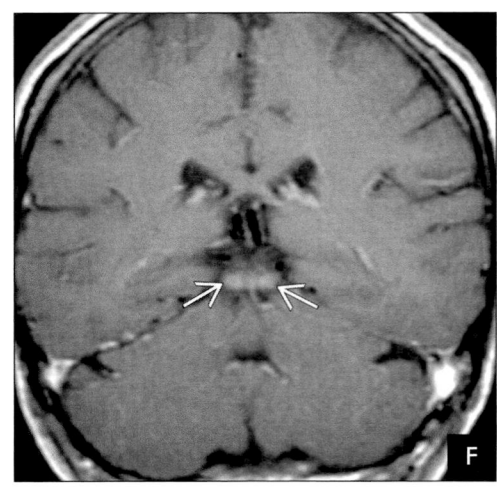

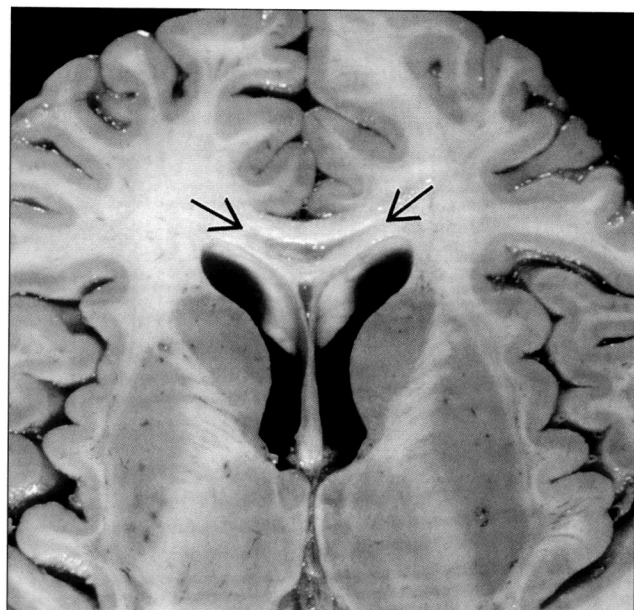

30-9. Autopsy specimen from a patient with Marchiafava-Bignami disease shows necrosis in the middle layers of the corpus callosum ⇥, the classic pathology in this disorder. (Courtesy R. Hewlett, MD.)

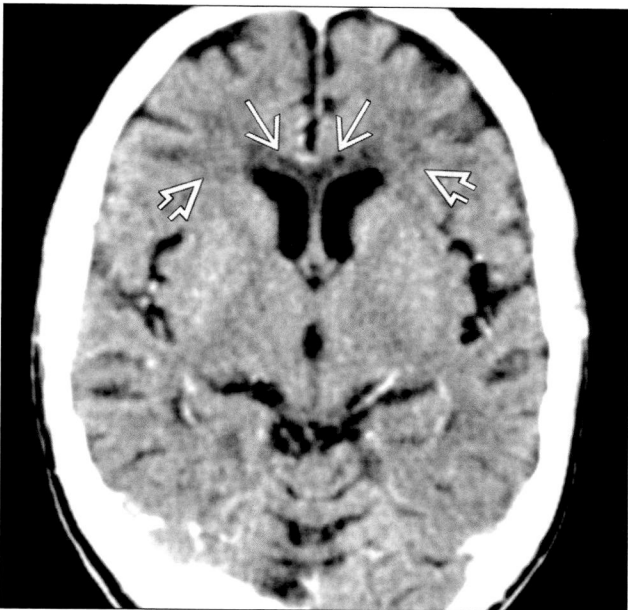

30-10. CECT scan in an alcoholic patient with Marchiafava-Bignami disease shows generalized cerebral atrophy, striking hypodensity in the corpus callosum genu ➡ and the adjacent white matter ⧫. (Courtesy A. Datir, MD.)

ventricle are typical. The tectal plate and periaqueductal gray matter are often involved. Less commonly, bilateral but asymmetric cortical hyperintensities are present, and DWI shows corresponding areas of restricted diffusion. Some cases show an isolated focus of diffusion restriction in the corpus callosum splenium.

In about half of all alcoholic WE cases, post-contrast scans demonstrate enhancement of the periventricular and periaqueductal lesions. Strong uniform enhancement of the mammillary bodies is seen in up to 80% of acute cases and is considered pathognomonic of WE. Nevertheless, some investigators report that enhancement is much less common in nonalcoholic WE.

With chronic WE, mammillary body atrophy ensues.

Differential Diagnosis

The differential diagnosis of classic WE is limited. The medial thalami and midbrain can be symmetrically involved in **artery of Percheron (AOP) infarct**. However, AOP infarcts do not affect the mammillary bodies and usually spare the tectal plate.

WERNICKE ENCEPHALOPATHY

Etiology
- Thiamine (vitamin B1) deficiency
- Alcohol-related (50%), nonalcoholic (50%)

Pathology
- Location
  - Common = mammillary bodies, medial thalami, tectum, periaqueductal GM
  - Less common = cortex, cerebellum, corpus callosum splenium

Clinical Issues
- Classic triad of ocular dysfunction, ataxia, altered mental status in < 30%
- Can occur in children!
- Intravenous thiamine imperative

Imaging
- T2/FLAIR hyperintensity, DWI restriction
- Enhancement varies; more common in alcoholic WE
  - Mammillary body enhancement pathognomonic

Marchiafava-Bignami Disease

Marchiafava-Bignami disease is a rare disorder that causes progressive demyelination and corpus callosum necrosis.

Terminology

Marchiafava-Bignami disease (MBD) is also (incorrectly) known as "red wine drinkers' encephalopathy."

Etiology

MBD is primarily associated with chronic EtOH abuse. There is an anecdotal (but unproven) association with red wine. Rare cases of MBD in nonalcoholic patients have been reported. Most investigators attribute MBD to vitamin B complex deficiency (i.e., all eight vitamins, in contrast to the more specific B1 deficiency of WE).

Pathology

LOCATION. The imaging diagnosis of MBD is based on the presence of callosal lesions. Selective involvement of the middle layers along the entire length of the corpus callosum is highly suggestive of MBD **(30-9)**.

Extracallosal lesions do occur with MBD. Hemispheric white matter, internal capsule, and middle cerebellar peduncle lesions have been reported. In addition, a specific type of cerebral cortical lesion, known as Morel laminar sclerosis, can be seen in the frontolateral cortex.

GROSS PATHOLOGY. Corpus callosum degeneration is the hallmark of MBD and varies from demyelination to frank cystic necrosis of the middle layers.

Clinical Issues

EPIDEMIOLOGY. MBD is rare. Most cases are found in middle-aged males.

PRESENTATION. The clinical diagnosis of MBD is difficult and often confused with WE. Some investigators report that both diseases often occur together.

MBD presents in two major clinical forms. In acute MBD, rapid decline with impaired consciousness, seizures, muscular rigidity, and death within several days is typical. In the chronic form, interhemispheric disconnection syndrome (e.g., apraxia, hemialexia, dementia) can be seen and lasts from months to several years.

NATURAL HISTORY. Most patients who survive MBD have severe neurologic sequelae, although a few cases with favorable outcome have been reported.

TREATMENT OPTIONS. If instituted quickly, intravenous vitamin B complex and methylprednisolone therapy may reverse the course of acute MBD.

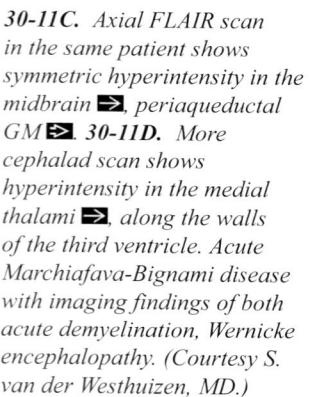

30-11A. Coronal T1 C+ in a patient who "drinks like a fish" shows enhancement in the corpus callosum ➡. 30-11B. Sagittal T1 C+ FS scan shows enhancing lesions in the corpus callosum ➡.

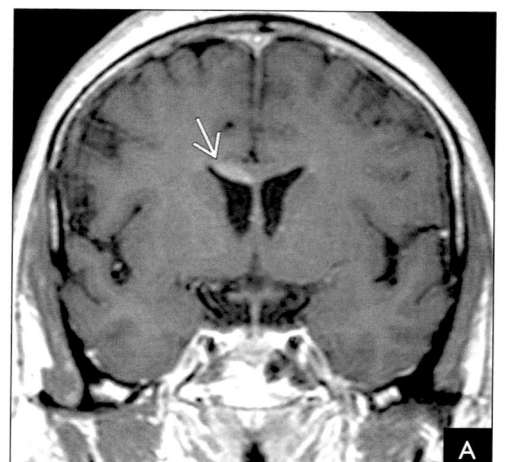
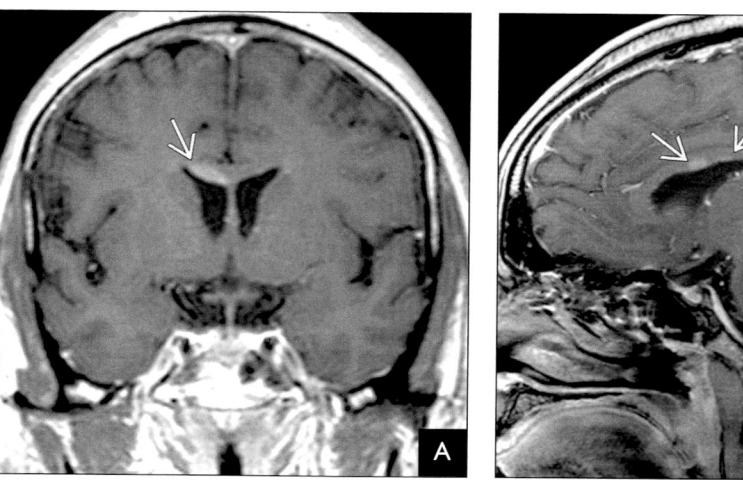

30-11C. Axial FLAIR scan in the same patient shows symmetric hyperintensity in the midbrain ➡, periaqueductal GM ➡. 30-11D. More cephalad scan shows hyperintensity in the medial thalami ➡, along the walls of the third ventricle. Acute Marchiafava-Bignami disease with imaging findings of both acute demyelination, Wernicke encephalopathy. (Courtesy S. van der Westhuizen, MD.)

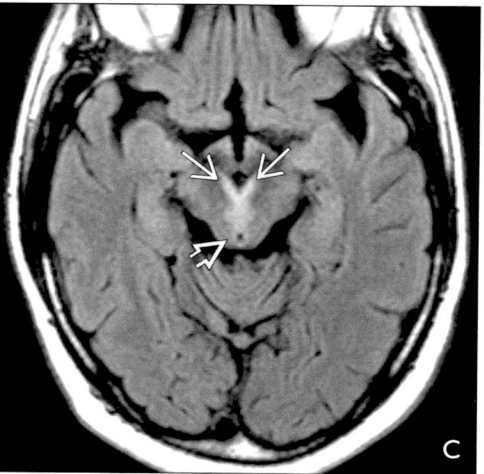
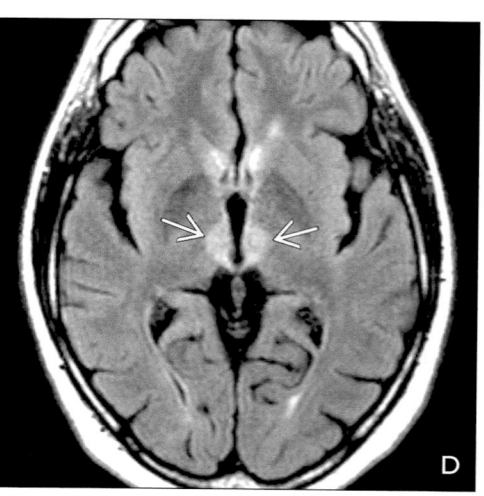

maging

GENERAL FEATURES. Selective involvement of the middle layers of the corpus callosum is typical. As with other alcohol-related disorders, MBD can also be accompanied by other alcohol-related pathologies. Chronic alcoholic encephalopathy with generalized brain volume loss is common. Electrolyte disturbances may cause osmotic demyelination.

CT FINDINGS. CT may be normal in the acute stage of MBD. Chronic MBD shows linear hypodensity in the corpus callosum genu that, in the setting of chronic alcohol abuse, is highly suggestive of the diagnosis **(30-10).**

MR FINDINGS. The initial changes of *acute* MBD are best seen on FLAIR. Hyperintensity in the corpus callosum genu and frontoparietal cortex appears first, followed by splenial lesions. DWI is initially negative, suggesting that the FLAIR changes probably reflect intramyelinic vasogenic (not cytotoxic) edema. Restriction subsequently develops in the corpus callosum splenium.

During the acute phase, the white matter lesions may enhance **(30-11).** Peripheral (rim) or solid confluent patterns have both been reported.

Chronic MBD with frank callosal necrosis is seen as thinning of the corpus callosum on sagittal T1WI with linear hypointensities in the middle layers **(30-4).** In patients with chronic MBD, T2* susceptibility-weighted imaging may demonstrate multiple hypointense areas in the cortical-subcortical regions and corpus callosum. Other changes associated with chronic alcohol abuse, such as cortical, cerebellar, and mammillary body atrophy, are common.

Differential Diagnosis

In the setting of EtOH abuse, callosal lesions are highly suggestive of MBD. Other diseases that may affect the corpus callosum include **multiple sclerosis, axonal stretch injuries**, and **lacunar infarction**. All have patchy discontinuous lesions that rarely involve the entire length of the corpus callosum.

Methanol Intoxication

Methanol is a strong CNS depressant. Patients are often comatose, and an accurate history may be impossible to obtain. Moreover, few hospitals include methanol in their standard toxicology screens. Therefore, delayed diagnosis is common, and morbidity and mortality remain high. Imaging may provide important clues to the diagnosis of possible methanol toxicity.

Terminology

Methanol (MtOH) intoxication or poisoning is also known as methanol encephalopathy.

Etiology

MtOH is a common component of solvents, varnishes, perfumes, paint removers, antifreeze, and gasoline mix-

30-12. Autopsy specimen from a patient with fatal methanol toxicity shows hemorrhagic necrosis in both putamina ➡, subinsular white matter ➡. (Courtesy R. Hewlett, MD.)

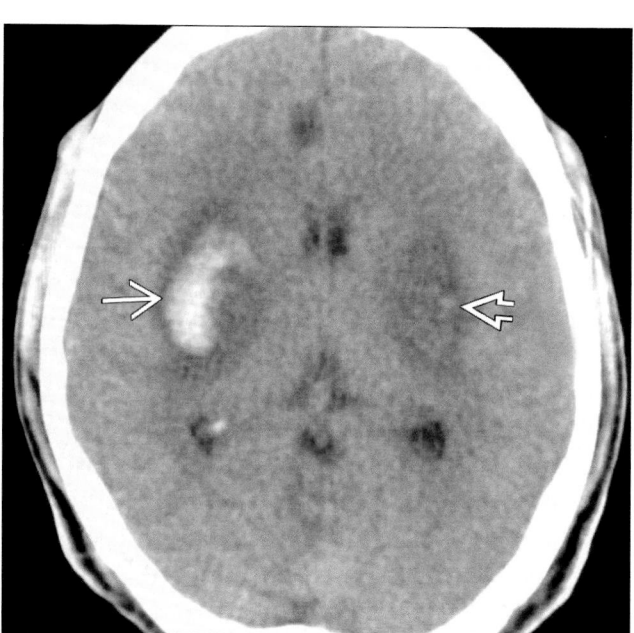

30-13. NECT scan in a patient with acute methanol poisoning shows confluent ➡ and patchy ➡ hemorrhagic putaminal necrosis. (Courtesy R. Ramakantan, MD.)

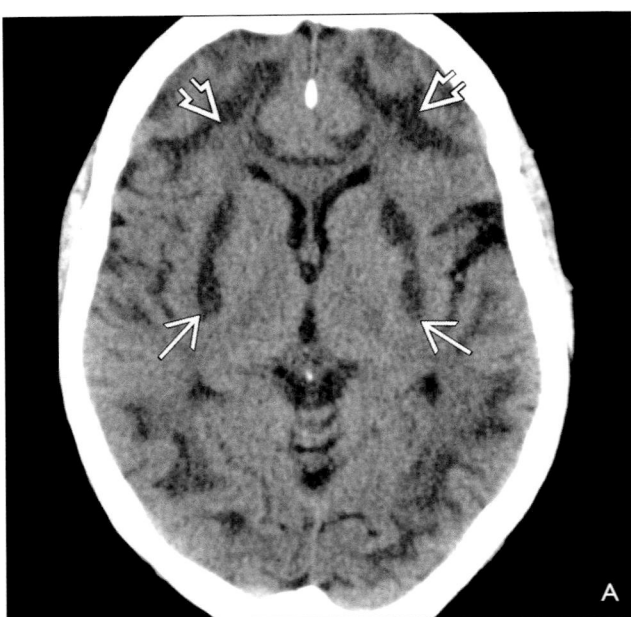

30-14A. *NECT scan in a patient who survived acute methanol poisoning shows shrunken, hypodense putamina* ➡ *and bilateral symmetric hypodensities in the subcortical WM* ➡.

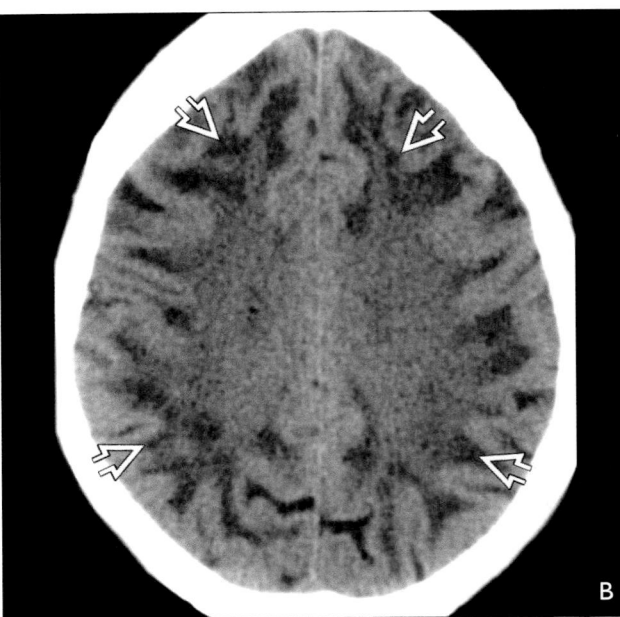

30-14B. *More cephalad NECT scan through the corona radiata shows striking hypodensity throughout the WM of both hemispheres* ➡.

tures. It can be accidentally or intentionally ingested, inhaled, or absorbed transdermally. Some cases of MtOH poisoning result from the intake of illicit spirits ("moonshine").

MtOH is metabolized to formic and lactic acid, causing severe metabolic acidosis with arterial pHs ranging from 6.8 to 7.1. Increased anion and osmolar gaps are important laboratory clues to the presence of MtOH toxicity.

Pathology

LOCATION. Bilateral basal ganglia necrosis is the most characteristic imaging feature of MtOH poisoning. Selective putamina involvement with relative sparing of the globi pallidi is common. Diffuse necrosis of the subinsular and subcortical white matter occurs in severe cases **(30-12).**

There is no consistent relationship between clinical outcome and the extent of imaging abnormalities.

Clinical Issues

EPIDEMIOLOGY. Compared to ethanol-induced encephalopathy, MtOH poisoning is rare.

DEMOGRAPHICS. Patients are overwhelmingly male. Peak age is between the third and fourth decades.

PRESENTATION. A peculiarity of MtOH poisoning is the latent period between ingestion and the appearance of clinical symptoms. Symptom onset is variable and often delayed, especially if ethanol is ingested simultaneously, as this slows MtOH metabolism. Between 85-90% of

patients present with visual disturbances. Three-quarters of all patients have nonspecific gastrointestinal symptoms such as nausea and vomiting. Approximately 25% are comatose on admission.

NATURAL HISTORY. Ingestion of 30 mL of pure MtOH usually results in death. As little as four mL can result in blindness. Blood MtOH levels above 200 mg/L are considered toxic, and levels above 1,500 mg/L are potentially fatal.

Although the latency in symptom onset is variable, symptom progression may be rapid. Respiratory arrest and death can occur within a few hours.

Putaminal hemorrhage and insular subcortical white matter necrosis are associated with poor clinical outcome.

TREATMENT OPTIONS. MtOH is effectively treated with alkali to combat acidosis, antidotes (ethanol or fomepizole) to block production of formic acid, and hemodialysis to remove MtOH and formate.

Imaging

CT FINDINGS. Initial NECT scan is normal in many patients with MtOH poisoning. Most patients who survive for more than 24 hours demonstrate bilateral symmetric hypodense lesions in the putamina and sometimes the deep cerebral white matter. Hemorrhagic putaminal necrosis is seen in 15-25% of cases **(30-13).** Enhancement is variable, ranging from none to peripheral enhancement of the putaminal lesions.

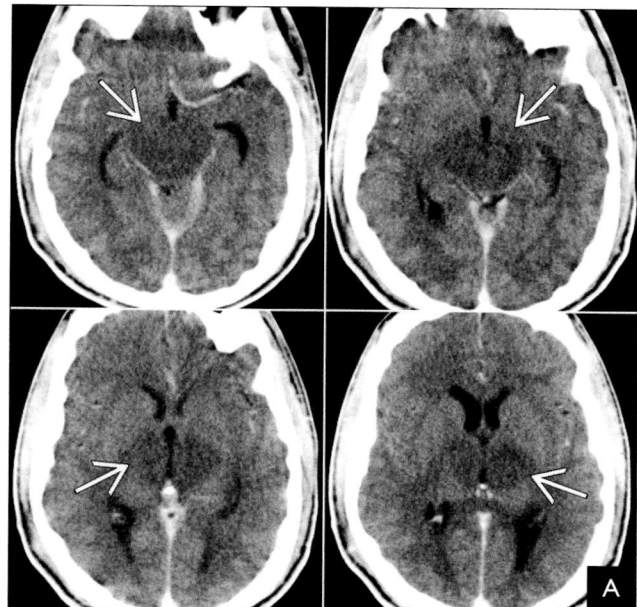

30-15A. *CECT scans in a patient who drank ethylene glycol shows symmetric hypodensity in the midbrain extending cephalad into both thalami* ➡.

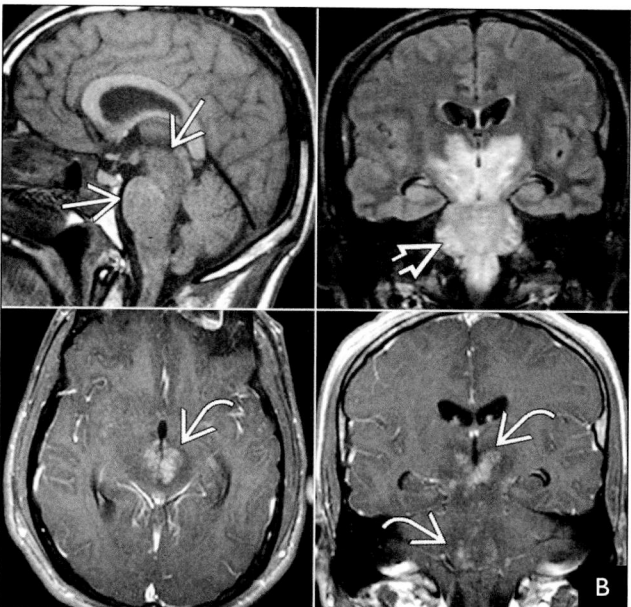

30-15B. *Sagittal T1WI shows pons, midbrain hypointensity* ➡, *which is better seen as hyperintensity on coronal FLAIR* ➡. *Patchy enhancement is seen on T1 C+* ➡.

If the patient survives, cystic cavities form within the putamina, representing the chronic sequelae of MtOH poisoning **(30-14)**.

MR FINDINGS. Bilateral putaminal necrosis with variable white matter involvement is present. T1 hyperintensity and patchy T2 hypointensity are present in the late acute/early subacute phase of hemorrhagic necrosis. "Blooming" on T2* is present. DWI shows restricted diffusion in the affected areas.

Surviving patients have symmetric T2/FLAIR hyperintense lesions in the putamina with variable involvement of the subcortical white matter.

ifferential Diagnosis

Bilateral symmetric putaminal lesions are not specific for MtOH and can be seen in **Wilson disease** and **mitochondrial encephalopathies** (e.g., Kearns-Sayre, Leigh). **Hypoxic-ischemic encephalopathy** involves the caudate and other deep gray nuclei in addition to the putamina. Acute **cyanide poisoning** is rare but can resemble MtOH encephalopathy. **Carbon monoxide poisoning** generally affects the globi pallidi rather than the putamina.

thylene Glycol Poisoning

Ethylene glycol is a colorless, odorless, sweet-tasting, but poisonous form of alcohol that is a common component in antifreeze and deicing fluids. It may be ingested by alcoholics or, because of its sweet taste and the ease of access, it is often accidentally ingested by children and animals.

When ingested, ethylene glycol causes metabolic acidosis and can damage the brain, liver, kidneys, and lungs. Ethylene glycol is metabolized to glycolate, which is the metabolite mainly responsible for the metabolic acidosis. Glycolate is then metabolized to oxalate, which precipitates with calcium as calcium oxalate and is deposited in various tissues. The high anion gap metabolic acidosis and osmolar gap resolve within 24 to 72 hours.

Early treatment with the alcohol dehydrogenase inhibitor 4-methylpyrazole (4MP, fomepizole) is very effective. Other treatment regimens include alkali to combat acidosis, ethanol as an antimetabolite, and dialysis.

Imaging findings of acute ethylene glycol toxicity include edema in the basal ganglia, thalami, midbrain, and upper pons **(30-15)**. Putaminal necrosis, similar to that observed in methanol intoxication, can be seen in subacute and chronic cases.

Amphetamines and Derivatives

The "hedonic" and addictive properties of drugs of abuse—particularly amphetamines and cocaine—are related to increased dopamine levels in the synapses of monoaminergic neurons. Most addictive drugs are excitotoxic and cause two major types of pathologies: Vascular events (e.g., ischemia, hemorrhage) and leukoencephalopathy.

Functional neuroimaging studies have also demonstrated that drugs of abuse are associated with dysfunctions in a range of overlapping brain regions. Working memory, inhibitory control, attention, and decision-making are all negatively impacted , the degree of which correlates with the severity and chronicity of abuse. In addition, CNS mitosis, migration, and cell survival in the fetus of a pregnant, substance-abusing woman are adversely affected.

Methamphetamine

Methamphetamine (MA or "meth") is a highly addictive psychostimulant drug. "Crystal" methamphetamine abuse has been steadily increasing over the past decade. Even a single acute exposure to MA can result in profound changes in cerebral blood flow. Both hemorrhagic and ischemic strokes occur (30-16).

MR imaging in chronic adult MA users demonstrates lower gray matter volumes on T1WI, especially in the frontal lobes, and more white matter hyperintensities on T2/FLAIR scans than are appropriate for the patient's age. MRS shows increased choline and myoinositol levels in the frontal lobes. DTI shows lower FA in the frontal lobes and higher ADC values in the basal ganglia.

MDMA ("Ecstasy")

3-, 4-methylenedioxymethamphetamine is also known as **MDMA** or **ecstasy**. Popular as a party drug, MDMA induces euphoria and sensory disturbances secondary to rapid release of potent vasoconstrictors from serotonergic synapses. MDMA can cause arterial constriction, vasculitis, or prolonged vasospasm with acute ischemic infarcts. MDMA-induced ischemia is most pronounced in serotonin-rich brain areas such as the globus pallidus and occipital cortex, which are especially vulnerable (30-17).

Acute hippocampal necrosis with subsequent atrophy has been reported in chronic ecstasy users.

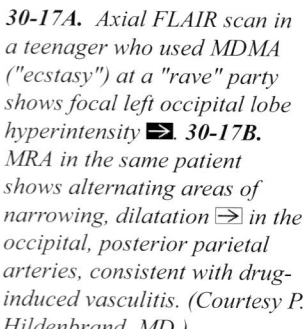

30-16A. A 32-year-old female methamphetamine abuser had sudden onset severe headache, followed by collapse and coma. NECT shows diffuse subarachnoid, intraventricular hemorrhage ➡. A focal interhemispheric hematoma ➡ surrounds a round hypodense focus caused by an anterior communicating artery aneurysm ➡. 30-16B. Sagittal reconstruction in the same case shows the ventricular system filled with clot. Subarachnoid hemorrhage, focal hemorrhage surrounds the aneurysm ➡.

30-17A. Axial FLAIR scan in a teenager who used MDMA ("ecstasy") at a "rave" party shows focal left occipital lobe hyperintensity ➡. 30-17B. MRA in the same patient shows alternating areas of narrowing, dilatation ➡ in the occipital, posterior parietal arteries, consistent with drug-induced vasculitis. (Courtesy P. Hildenbrand, MD.)

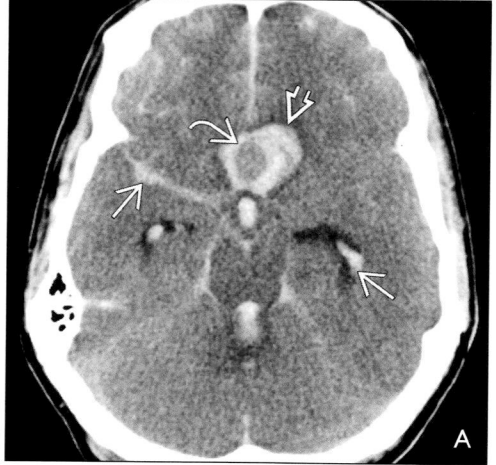

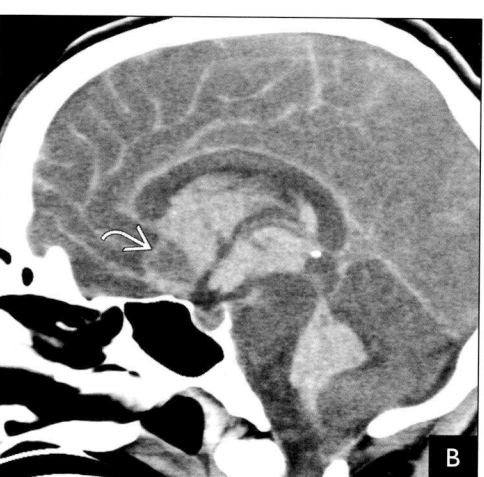

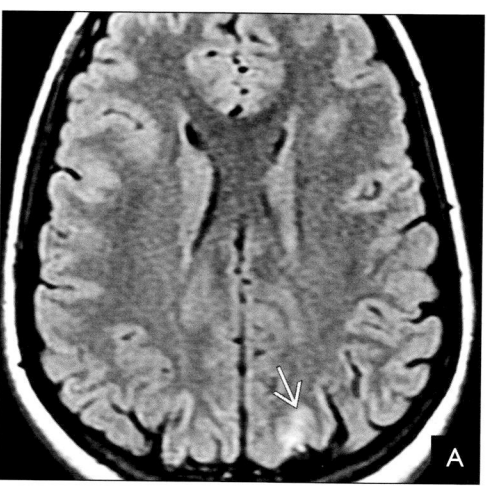

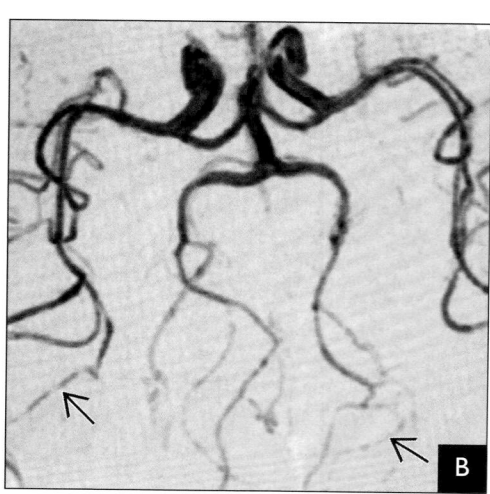

Benzodiazepines

Benzodiazepines, sometimes called **"benzo,"** are psychoactive drugs used to treat anxiety, insomnia, seizures, muscle spasms, and alcohol withdrawal. Benzodiazepine overdose has been associated with hypoxic-ischemic encephalopathy **(30-18)**, hemorrhagic ischemic strokes **(30-19)**, and delayed toxic leukoencephalopathy.

Cocaine

Cocaine can be sniffed/snorted, smoked, or injected. In its most common form (cocaine hydrochloride), it is ingested via the nasal mucosa. "Crack," the alkaloidal freebase form of cocaine hydrochloride, can also be smoked.

Etiology

Regardless of the route of administration, the adverse impact of cocaine on the brain is largely related to its vascular effects. Systemic hypertension can be extreme, causing spontaneous hemorrhagic strokes.

Rupture of a preexisting aneurysm or underlying vascular malformation accounts for nearly half of all cocaine-related hemorrhagic strokes. Cocaine also facilitates platelet aggregation and may lead to thrombotic vascular occlusion.

Acute cerebral vasoconstriction and/or cocaine-induced vasculopathy may lead to ischemic strokes. Snorted cocaine causes severe vasoconstriction in the vascular plexus of the nasal septal mucosa (Kiesselbach plexus). Chronic abuse may lead to septal necrosis and perforation.

Pathology

Macroscopic hemorrhages, particularly in the putamen and external capsule, are the most common gross pathologic findings and are twice as common as ischemic strokes.

Microscopically, cocaine arteriopathy is characterized by inflammatory changes and necrosis.

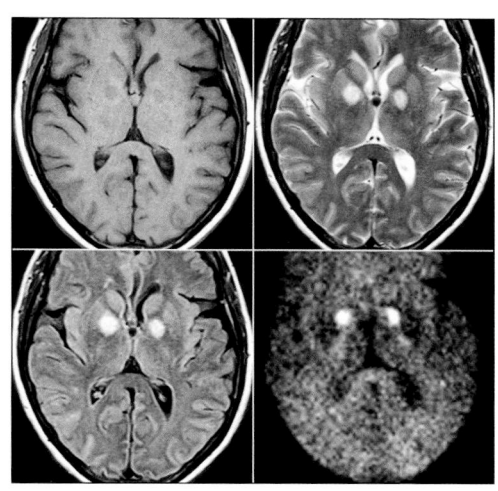
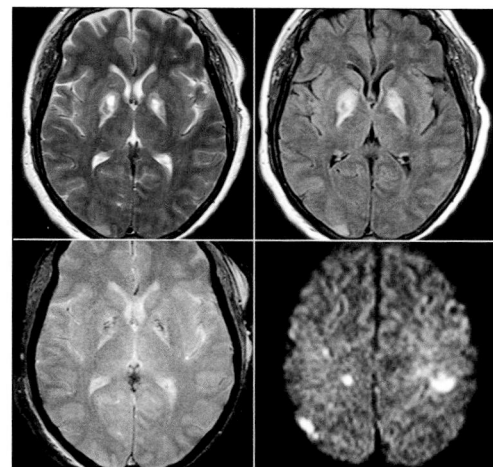

30-18. A 60-year-old depressed woman was found unconscious after overdose with benzodiazepines, opioids. Imaging shows bilateral symmetric globi pallidi lesions. *30-19.* MR scans in a 45-year-old bipolar woman with toxicology positive for opiates, benzodiazepines shows globi pallidi, cortical infarcts. She also had symmetric hemorrhagic cerebellar infarcts (not shown).

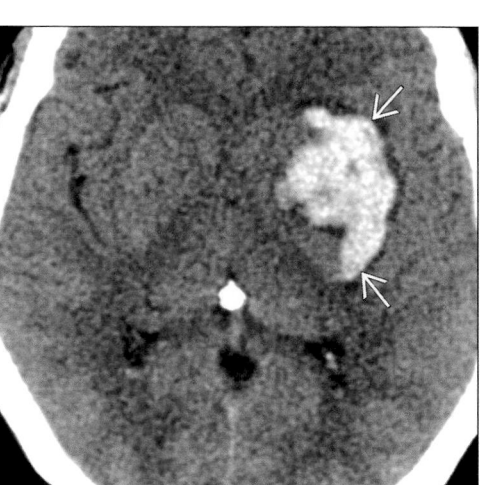
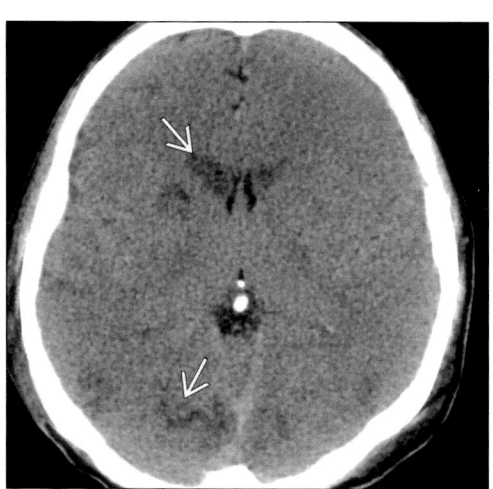

30-20. NECT shows acute hypertensive hemorrhage with putamen/external capsule hemorrhage ➡ in a patient who abused cocaine. *30-21.* NECT scan in a patient with cocaine abuse shows diffuse brain swelling, multifocal ischemic infarcts ➡.

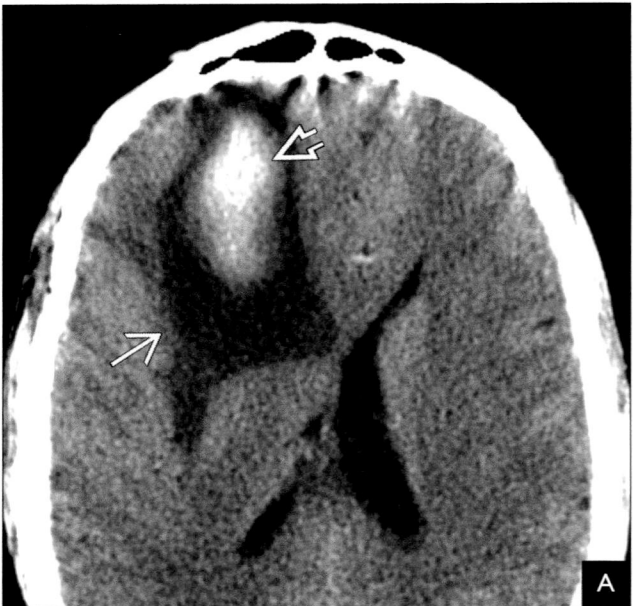

30-22A. NECT scan in a patient with cocaine abuse shows large, confluent hypodensity ➡ in the right frontal lobe with late acute hemorrhage ⇒.

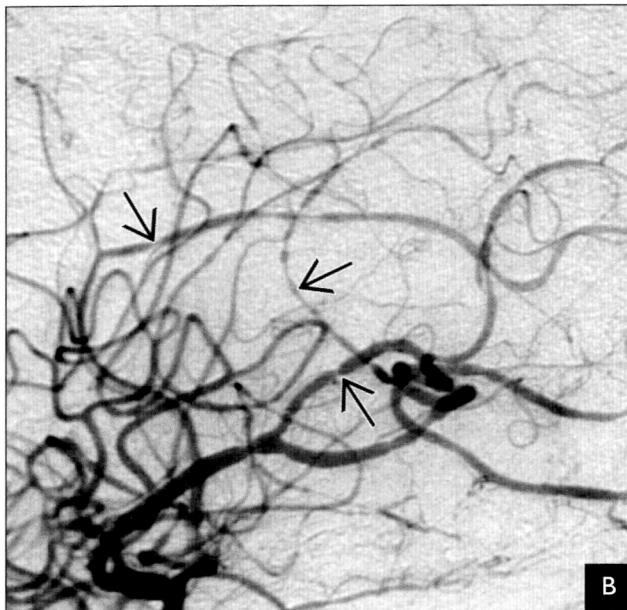

30-22B. Lateral DSA in the same patient shows multiple areas of constriction, dilatation ⇒, characteristic of drug-induced vasculitis.

Clinical Issues

EPIDEMIOLOGY. Nearly one-third of strokes in patients younger than 45 years are drug-related, with 80-90% occurring in the fourth and fifth decades. Stroke risk is highest within the first six hours after drug use.

PRESENTATION. Headache, seizure, and focal neurologic deficits are the most common symptoms.

NATURAL HISTORY. The onset of cocaine-related stroke may be immediate if hypertensive or subarachnoid hemorrhage occurs. Cocaine-induced vasculopathy with ischemic infarcts may occur up to a week after use.

Imaging

Strokes—both ischemic and hemorrhagic—are the major manifestations of cocaine-induced brain damage (30-20). The hemorrhages can be parenchymal (secondary to hypertension or vascular malformation) or subarachnoid (aneurysm rupture). Hypertensive bleeds are usually centered in the external capsule/putamen or in the thalamus.

Acute hypertensive encephalopathy with posterior reversible encephalopathy syndrome (PRES) can also occur. Vasogenic edema in the occipital lobes is the most common finding.

Ischemic strokes can be caused by vasospasm, cocaine-induced vasoconstriction, vasculitis, or thrombosis (30-21). Acute cocaine-induced strokes are positive on DWI. MRA, CTA, or DSA may show focal areas of arterial narrowing and irregularity (30-22).

Differential Diagnosis

The most common cause of spontaneous (nontraumatic) intracranial hemorrhage in children is an underlying **vascular malformation**. Unexplained parenchymal hemorrhage in young and middle-aged adults should also prompt evaluation for possible drug abuse.

Embolic infarcts from heart disease as well as **vasculitis** secondary to infection or to granulomatous, autoimmune, or collagen-vascular disease may appear identical to cocaine vasculopathy.

COCAINE AND AMPHETAMINE EFFECTS ON THE BRAIN

Amphetamines
- Methamphetamine
  - Hemorrhagic, ischemic strokes
  - Frontal atrophy
- MDMA ("ecstasy")
  - Vasospasm, infarcts
  - Location: Occipital cortex, globus pallidus
- Benzodiazepines
  - Delayed toxic leukoencephalopathy

Cocaine
- Intracranial hemorrhage
  - Hypertensive intracranial hemorrhage (50%)
  - "Unmasked" aneurysm or arteriovenous malformation (50%)
- Ischemic stroke
  - Vasospasm
  - Vasculitis
- Acute hypertensive encephalopathy
  - Posterior reversible encephalopathy syndrome (PRES)
  - Vasogenic edema (typically biooccipital)

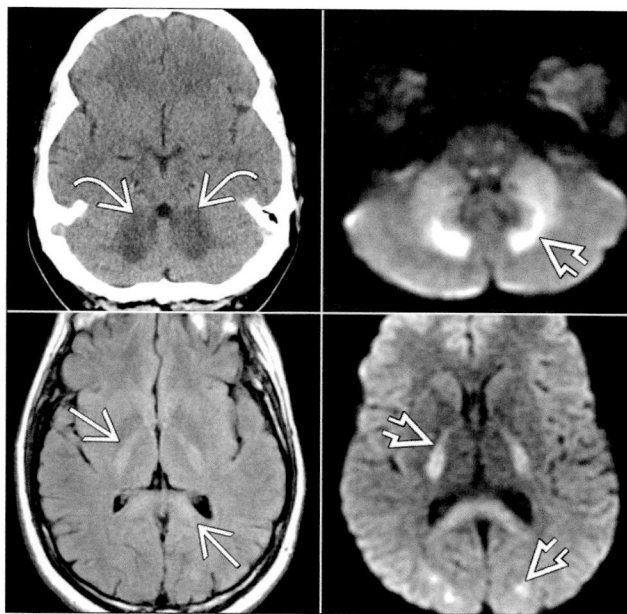

30-23. *NECT following inhaled heroin ("chasing the dragon") shows symmetric hypodensity in cerebellar WM ➔. FLAIR shows hyperintensity in corpus callosum, internal capsules ➔. Lesions restrict on DWI ➔. (Courtesy K. Nelson, MD.)*

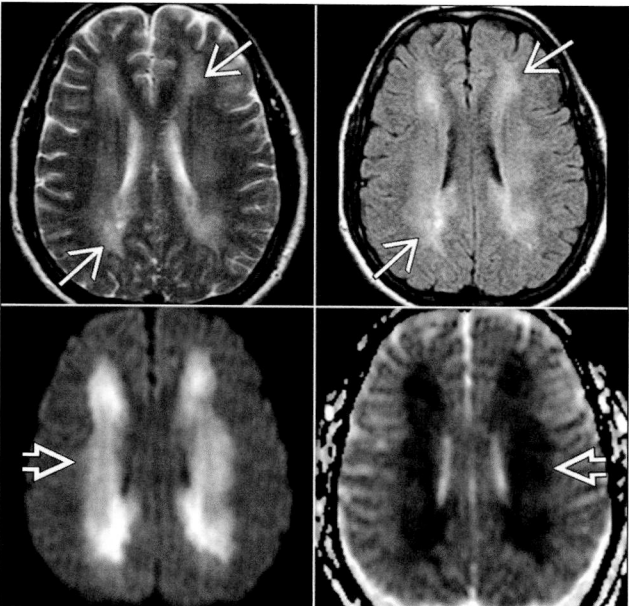

30-24. *A 57-year-old man developed acute leukoencephalopathy after "chasing the dragon." MR shows hyperintensity ➔ in the periventricular deep WM on T2/FLAIR, corresponding diffusion restriction ➔ on DWI and ADC. (Courtesy M. Michel, MD.)*

Opioids and Derivatives

Heroin is the most commonly abused opioid. Other abused drugs in this group include **morphine**, **hydrocodone**, **oxycodone**, **hydromorphone**, **codeine**, and related narcotics such as **fentanyl**, **meperidine**, **methadone**, and **opium**.

In addition to the direct effects of opioids on the brain, impurities and additives may produce systemic pathology. Hypotension and anoxia may also complicate the clinical and imaging appearance of opioid toxicity.

Heroin

Heroin is usually injected intravenously. The most common acute complication of injected heroin is stroke. Globus pallidus ischemia, very similar to that seen in carbon monoxide poisoning, is common.

The most dramatic acute effects occur with inhaled heroin. The freebase form is heated over tinfoil and the vapors inhaled (**"chasing the dragon"**). Heroin vapor inhalation causes a striking toxic leukoencephalopathy.

The most frequent secondary complication of heroin abuse is infection. Endocarditis is common and may result in septic emboli, brain abscesses, and vasculitis with mycotic aneurysm formation.

Etiology

Heroin causes both acute and chronic effects such as vasculopathy, leukoencephalopathy, and generalized brain volume loss. Stimulation of opioid receptors in vascular smooth muscle may cause reversible vasospasm. Immune-mediated response to additives in injected heroin may cause ischemia or vasculitis.

Pathology

Autopsied brains of patients with heroin-associated encephalopathy show a sponge-like appearance of the cerebral white matter. Microscopy demonstrates demyelination and white matter vacuolization. Because the cerebellum has a high density of opioid receptors, similar changes can be seen in its white matter.

Imaging

CT FINDINGS. Acute CNS toxicity from inhaled heroin ("chasing the dragon") is characterized by symmetric hypodensities in the cerebellar white matter, sometimes described as a "butterfly wing" pattern (**30-23**). The posterior cerebral white matter, posterior limb of the internal capsule, and globi pallidi are also commonly affected. The anterior limb of the internal capsule is typically spared.

MR FINDINGS. T2 and FLAIR scans in patients with early heroin-related leukoencephalopathy show symmetric hyperintensity in the cerebellar white matter with relative sparing of the dentate nuclei. There is often selective symmetric involvement of the posterior limb of the

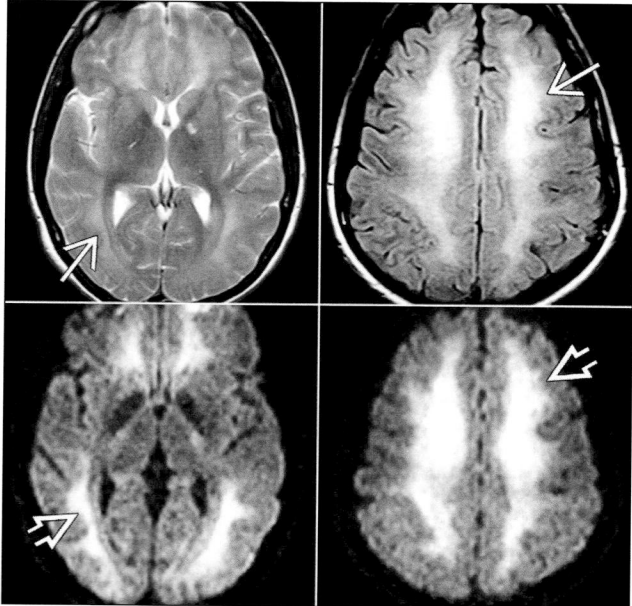

30-25. *MR scans in a 33-year-old woman who overdosed on methadone shows striking symmetric confluent hyperintensity (leukoencephalopathy) on FLAIR* ➡, *restricted diffusion on DWI* ➡.

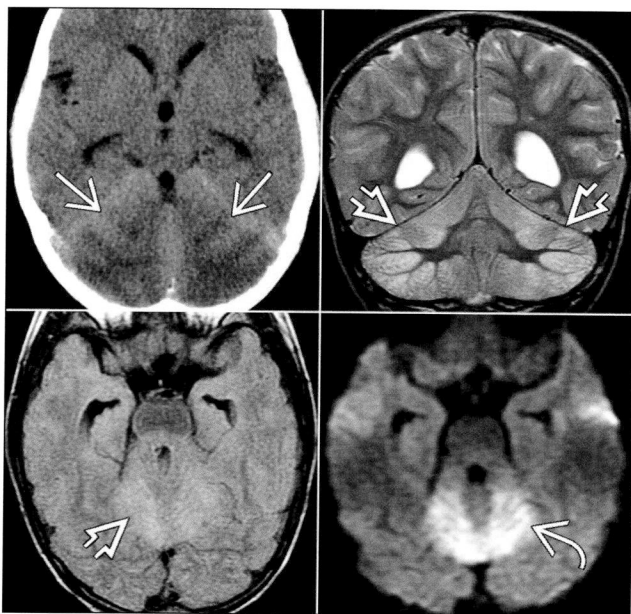

30-26. *Accidental methadone poisoning in a child shows bilateral cerebellar hypodensity on NECT* ➡, *T2/FLAIR hyperintensity* ➡, *restricted diffusion* ➡.

internal capsule, the corticospinal tract, the medial lemniscus, and the tractus solitarius (30-23).

Confluent hyperintensity in the cerebral white matter, including the corpus callosum, is common in severe cases of heroin vapor encephalopathy (30-24). DWI shows acute diffusion restriction in the affected areas; MRS shows a lactate peak in the cerebral white matter.

Chronic heroin abuse can cause microvascular disease. Scattered multifocal hyperintensities in the subcortical or periventricular white matter are common but neither as prevalent nor as severe as seen with cocaine vasculopathy.

Methadone

So-called substitute drugs such as the synthetic opioid methadone are used in the medication-assisted therapy for drug abuse/dependence as well as in the management of intractable pain. With increasing use and availability, methadone overdose is likewise growing.

A post-opioid toxic leukoencephalopathy similar to that caused by inhaled heroin has been reported with methadone. Diffuse, symmetric, confluent hyperintensity in the cerebral white matter on T2/FLAIR is seen (30-25). Sparing of the subcortical U-fibers is typical. In contrast to heroin toxicity, cerebellar and brainstem changes are subtle or absent in adults. MRS shows elevated choline, decreased NAA, and increased lactate.

Accidental ingestion of methadone has been reported to cause severe cerebellar edema with acute obstructive hydrocephalus in children (30-26).

Oxycodone

Imaging in the few reported cases of oxycodone and Oxy-Contin overdose shows restricted diffusion in the cerebellar hemispheres and globi pallidi.

OPIOID DRUGS

Heroin
- Injected
  - Most common = ischemic strokes
  - Globi pallidi, WM (resembles CO poisoning)
- Inhaled
  - "Chasing the dragon"
  - Most common = leukoencephalopathy
  - Cerebellum, cerebral WM

Methadone
- Adults
  - Toxic leukoencephalopathy
- Children
  - Usually accidental ingestion
  - Cerebellar edema

Oxycodone
- Cerebellar, globus pallidus ischemia
- Less common = toxic leukoencephalopathy

nhaled Gases and Toxins

Some drugs of abuse such as heroin have multiple potential routes of administration. Others are gases and therefore exclusively inhaled. Examples include toxins such as carbon monoxide and drugs of abuse such as nitrous oxide. Some toxins such as cyanide can be inhaled, ingested, or absorbed transdermally. Cyanides may also cause—or contribute to—deaths from smoke inhalation.

Inhaled vapors from volatile, intrinsically liquid agents include amyl nitrite ("poppers") and industrial solvents (e.g., toluene).

Carbon Monoxide Poisoning

Terminology

Carbon monoxide (CO) is a colorless, odorless, tasteless gas that is produced by the incomplete combustion of various fuels. CO poisoning is caused by deliberate or accidental inhalation.

Etiology

The toxic effects of CO result mostly from impaired oxygen transport. CO combines reversibly with hemoglobin (Hgb) with over 200 times higher the affinity than that of oxygen. If carboxyhemoglobin (CO-Hgb) levels exceed 20%, brain and cardiac damage are common.

CO-Hgb impairs erythrocyte oxygen transport, reducing cellular oxygen and causing hypoxia. In addition, lipid peroxidation leads to oxidative injury. Peroxynitrites damage the vascular endothelium.

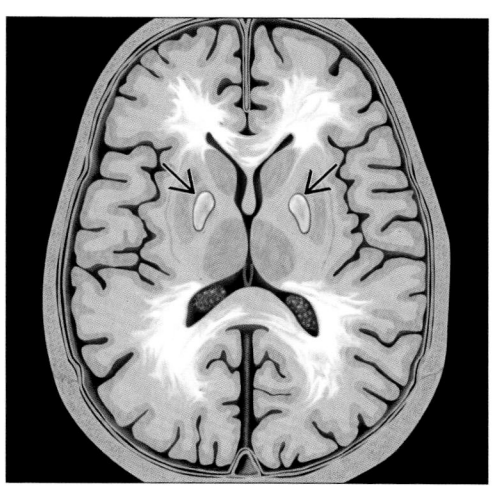

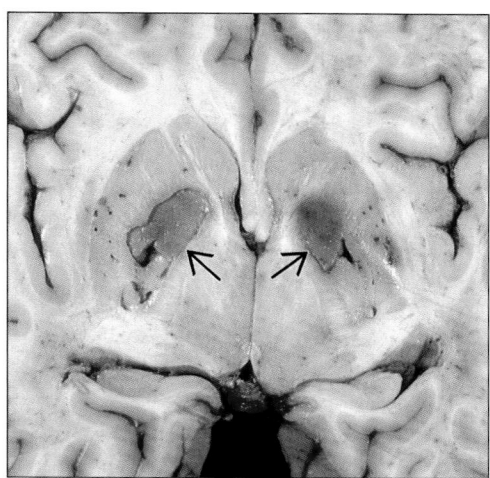

30-27. *Axial graphic shows the typical involvement of the brain by carbon monoxide poisoning. The globi pallidi (GP) ⇥ are most affected, followed by the cerebral white matter. Pathologically, there is necrosis of the GP with variable areas of necrosis and demyelination in the white matter.* 30-28. *Autopsy specimen of carbon monoxide poisoning shows symmetric coagulative (nonhemorrhagic) necrosis of both medial globi pallidi ⇥.*

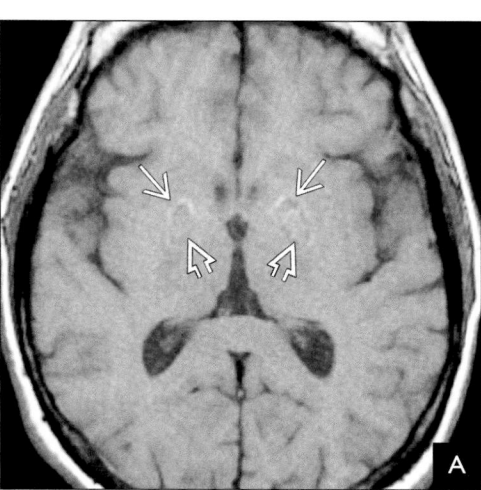

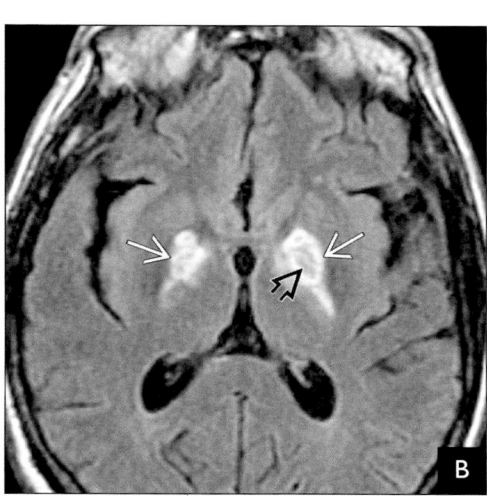

30-29A. *T1WI in a 49-year-old man with CO poisoning shows symmetric lesions in both medial globi pallidi. Note faint hyperintense rim ⇥, thin hypointense underlying rim, and central coagulative necrosis seen as mildly hyperintense lesions ⇥.* 30-29B. *FLAIR scan in the same patient shows that the lesion is mostly hyperintense ⇥ with central isointense core ⇥. The isointense parts of the lesions enhanced on T1 C+ (not shown).*

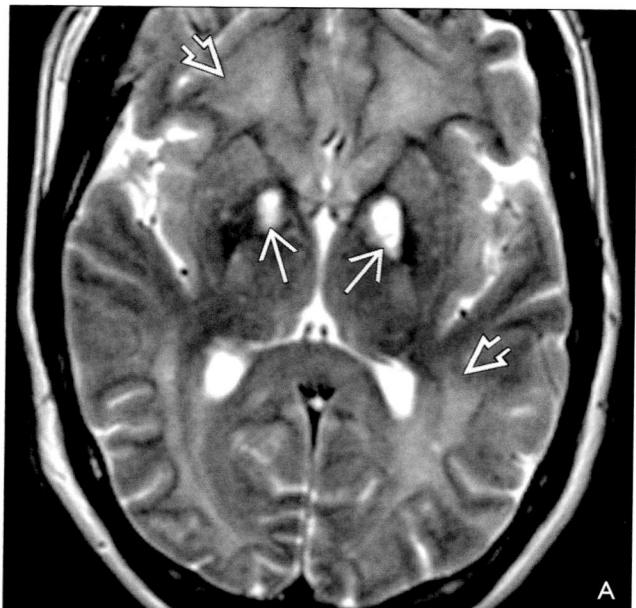

30-30A. *Axial T2WI in a patient with CO poisoning 2 weeks prior shows characteristic bilateral hyperintensities in globi pallidi* ➡. *Confluent hyperintensity now involves virtually all of the cerebral WM* ➡, *except the subcortical U-fibers.*

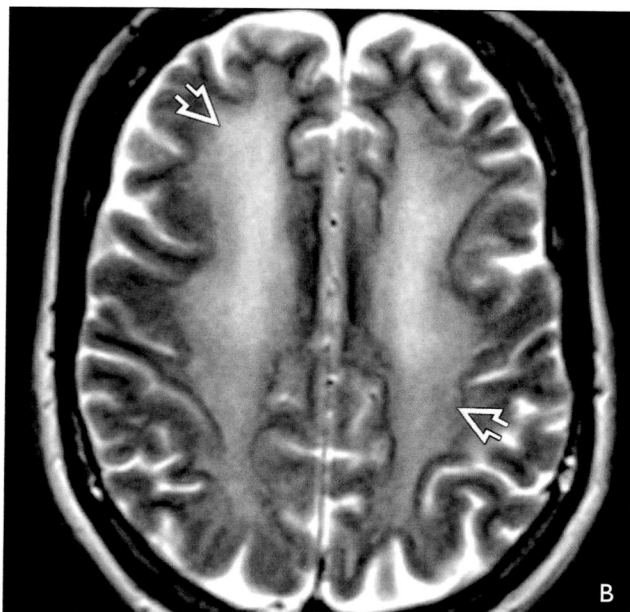

30-30B. *More cephalad T2WI shows that the hyperintensity involves most of the corona radiata* ➡, *mostly spares subcortical WM. "Interval" (subacute) form of CO poisoning with toxic demyelination.*

Pathology

LOCATION. Because the globi pallidi are exquisitely sensitive to hypoxia, the hallmark of acute CO poisoning is symmetric globus pallidi necrosis **(30-27)**, **(30-28)**. The cerebral white matter is the second most commonly affected and often shows delayed demyelination and necrosis that may appear several weeks after the initial insult.

Clinical Issues

PRESENTATION AND NATURAL HISTORY. Acute CO poisoning initially causes nausea, vomiting, headache, and impaired consciousness. Outcome depends on both duration and intensity of exposure. Seizures, coma, and death may ensue.

Patients who survive CO poisoning often develop delayed encephalopathy. Parkinson-like symptoms, memory deficits, and cognitive disturbances are common.

TREATMENT OPTIONS. Hyperbaric oxygen therapy is the treatment of choice in acute CO poisoning. Early administration of 100% inspired oxygen may help mitigate long-term neuropsychiatric sequelae.

Imaging

CT FINDINGS. Early NECT scans may be normal. Symmetric hypodensity in both Globi pallidi develops within a few hours. Gross hemorrhage is rare. Variable diffuse hypodensity in the hemispheric white matter can be seen in severe cases.

MR FINDINGS. Multiplanar MR (e.g., FLAIR, T2WI, and DWI) is the most sensitive technique for early detection of changes caused by CO poisoning. T1WI shows subtle hypointensity in the GP. A faint rim of hyperintensity caused by hemorrhage or coagulative necrosis may be present **(30-29A)**.

T2/FLAIR shows bilateral hyperintensities in the medial GP **(30-29B)**, with the putamina and caudate nuclei less commonly affected. A thin hypointense rim around the lesion may be present.

In addition to the hyperintense areas seen on T2WI, FLAIR imaging may disclose subtle involvement of the caudate nuclei, thalami, hippocampi, corpus callosum, fornices, and cerebral cortex.

DWI shows bilateral GP hyperintensities as well as foci of restricted diffusion in the subcortical white matter. ADC in the cerebral white matter increases significantly, reflecting extensive microstructural tissue damage. DTI shows FA decline in associated cortical areas.

Up to one-third of CO patients develop a delayed leukoencephalopathy with progressive white matter demyelination, the "interval" (subacute) form of CO poisoning. Extensive bilateral symmetric confluent areas of hyperintensity on T2/FLAIR are characteristic findings **(30-30)**.

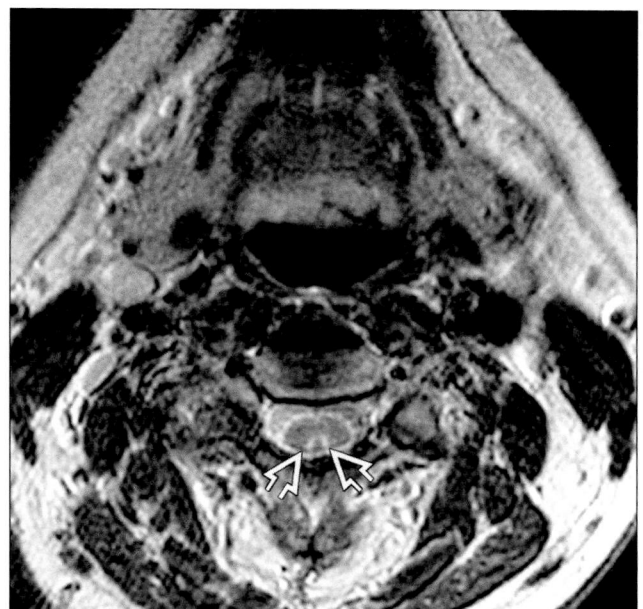

30-31. Axial T2WI in a patient with nitrous oxide abuse shows selective symmetric demyelination of the posterior columns ➔, characteristic of subacute combined degeneration. (Courtesy C. Glastonbury, MBBS.)

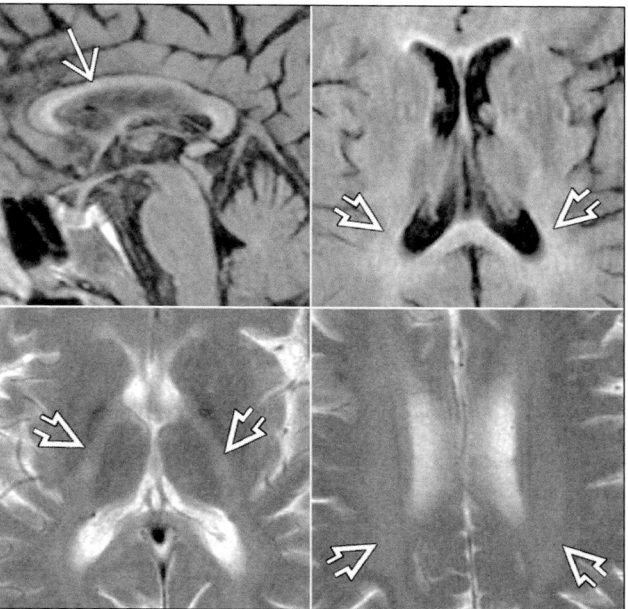

30-32. Sagittal T1WI shows thinned corpus callosum ➔, and T2/FLAIR demonstrates confluent WM hyperintensity ➔. Toluene toxicity due to chronic glue sniffing. (Courtesy S. Lincoff, MD.)

ifferential Diagnosis

The major differential diagnosis of CO poisoning is **hypoxic-ischemic encephalopathy** (HIE). As they share some common pathophysiology, imaging findings in HIE and CO poisoning overlap. HIE generally affects the entire basal ganglia and hippocampi, less often the white matter or only the GP. **Organophosphate poisoning** (accidental or suicidal exposure) can cause bilateral hemorrhagic pallidal necrosis.

Wilson disease involves the basal ganglia, mesencephalon, pons, and dentate nuclei.

Mitochondrial encephalopathies, especially **Leigh disease**, generally affect younger patients. Brainstem and putamen lesions are more common than GP involvement.

Some **viral encephalitides**, such as Japanese encephalitis, preferentially affect the basal ganglia and thalami. **Creutzfeldt-Jakob disease** (CJD) is rapidly progressive and affects the caudate nuclei, anterior basal ganglia, and cortex. Posteromedial thalamic involvement (pulvinar) is common in CJD and rare in CO poisoning.

itrous Oxide

Nitrous oxide (N_2O), commonly known as "laughing gas," is an inhaled anesthetic supplement commonly used in dentistry and oral surgery. N_2O is extremely soluble in fatty compounds and is used as an aerosol spray propellant (e.g., whipped cream canisters and cooking sprays). N_2O is sometimes inhaled for the putative euphoria.

Excess N_2O irreversibly oxidizes the cobalt ion of vitamin B12, which is necessary for methylation of myelin sheath phospholipids. Long-term nitrous oxide abuse causes progressive myelopathy and a peripheral polyneuropathy. The end result is **subacute combined degeneration of the spinal cord**. The dorsal columns and corticospinal tracts are preferentially affected **(30-31)**. Brain lesions are rare.

Toluene Abuse

The most important component of industrial solvents is toluene, so we focus our discussion on this particular solvent. Toluene, a colorless liquid found in glues, paint thinners, inks, and other industrial products, is lipid-soluble and rapidly absorbed by the CNS. Prolonged exposure through occupation or purposeful inhalation causes multifocal neurologic defects and optic neuropathy.

Terminology

Toluene, also called methylbenzene, is an aromatic hydrocarbon. Toluene poisoning results in **chronic solvent encephalopathy**.

Etiology

The common methods of solvent abuse are "sniffing" (direct inhalation from a container), "huffing" (inhalation from a soaked rag held over the nose and mouth), and "bagging" (inhalation from a plastic bag).

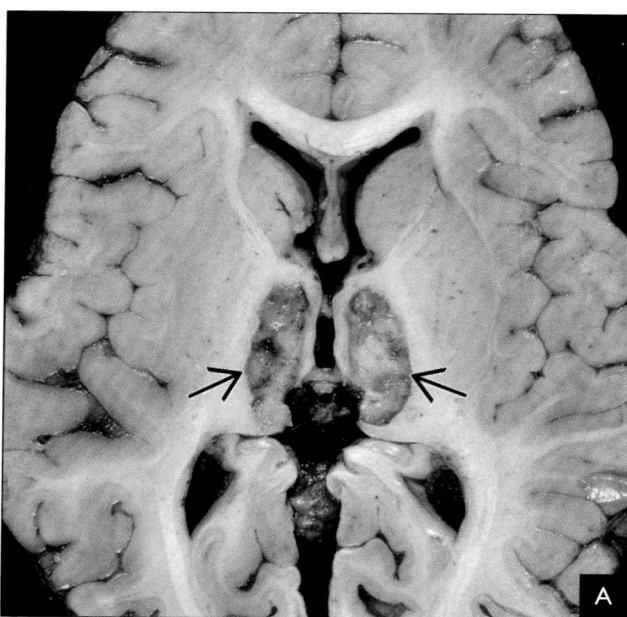

30-33A. *Autopsy specimen from a patient with smoke inhalation, possibly from burning trash with vaporized cyanide. Note bilateral thalamic necrosis* ➡.

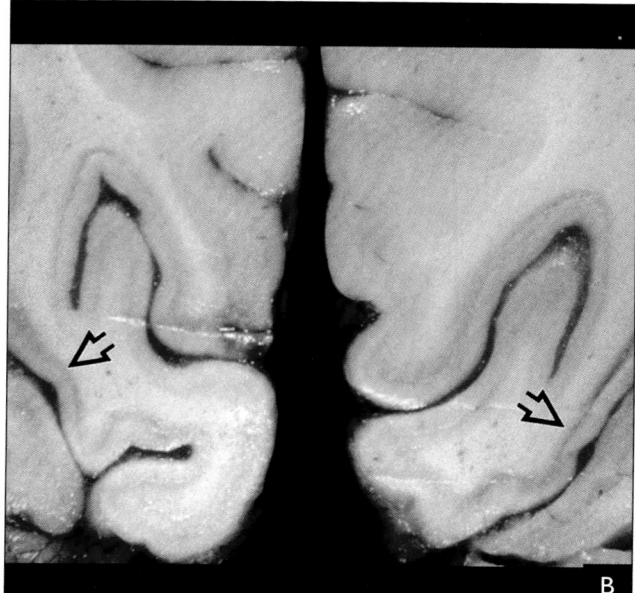

30-33B. *Coronal section through the occipital lobes shows cortical laminar necrosis* ➤. *(Courtesy R. Hewlett, MD.)*

Pathology

Toluene preferentially affects the cerebral white matter and optic nerves, causing demyelination and gliosis. Iron deposition in the thalami and basal ganglia due to demyelination and axonal loss is also common.

Clinical Issues

Solvent abuse is particularly prevalent among adolescents and young adults. Low cost and ease of access have led to increased prevalence in many countries. Regular long-term toluene abuse causes severe and irreversible cognitive impairment.

Imaging

Imaging in patients with acute toluene abuse is usually normal. Abnormalities are typically seen only after several years of chronic inhalant abuse. Diffuse white matter lesions are seen in nearly half of all patients, initially seen as T2/FLAIR hyperintensity in the deep periventricular WM with subsequent spread into the centrum semiovale and subcortical areas. The internal capsule, cerebellum, and pons are often affected **(30-32)**.

Chronic prolonged toluene exposure also causes generalized atrophy with ventricular dilatation and enlarged subarachnoid spaces. WM volume loss is seen as thinning of the corpus callosum. The extent of volume loss directly correlates with abuse duration.

Organophosphate Poisoning

Organophosphates (OPs) are common ingredients in pesticides. Because of their widespread agricultural use, ready availability, and easy accessibility, OPs are potential sources of accidental or suicidal exposure.

"Street pesticides" (illegal, unlabeled, and decanted agricultural pesticides used predominantly for urban household purposes) pose an increasing risk for significant pesticide exposures and poisonings in emerging nations.

The anticholinesterase effect of OPs causes three potential discrete neurologic syndromes. The initial acute effect is a life-threatening acute cholinergic crisis due to excessive stimulation of muscarinic receptors. The intermediate syndrome is characterized by cranial nerve palsies, proximal muscle weakness, delayed polyneuropathy, and Parkinson-like extrapyramidal symptoms. Chronic or low-dose occupational exposure may result in neurobehavioral and neuropsychiatric disorders.

Acute OP poisoning causes hemorrhagic basal ganglia necrosis with the "eye of the tiger" sign. On T2WI, a ring of marked hypointensity caused by excess iron accumulation surrounds a central hyperintense focus in the medial globus pallidus.

The differential diagnosis of OP poisoning includes other drug-induced causes of pallidal necrosis such as carbon monoxide poisoning. Hypoxic-ischemic encephalopathy and metabolic encephalopathies such as Leigh and Wilson diseases also affect the basal ganglia.

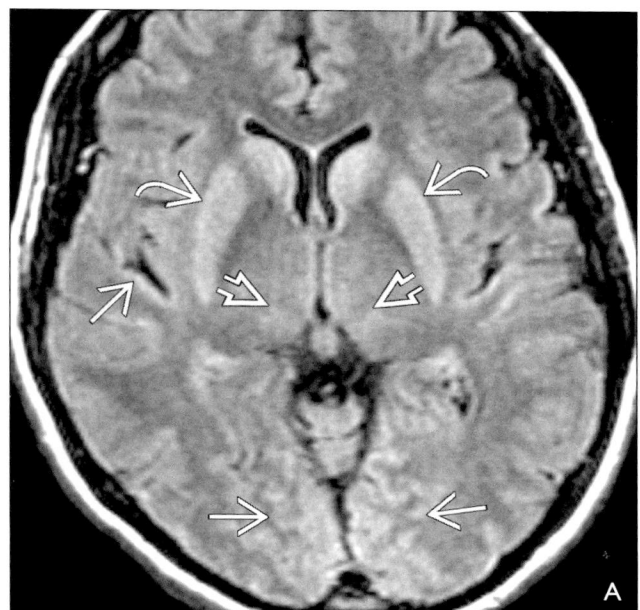

30-34A. FLAIR scan in smoke inhalation with CN poisoning from burning plastic shows symmetric hyperintensity in caudate nuclei and putamina ⇒, more subtle lesions in posteromedial thalami ⇒, curvilinear cortical hyperintensities ⇒.

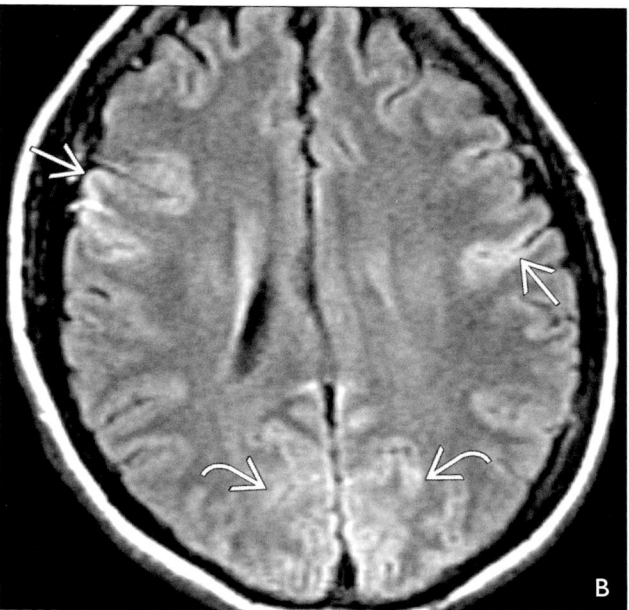

30-34B. More cephalad scan in the same patient shows the cortical hyperintensities ⇒, which are especially prominent in both occipital lobes ⇒.

Cyanide Poisoning

Terminology

Cyanide (CN) is one of the most potent and deadly of all poisons. Cyanogenic compounds may be found in household or workplace substances and deliberately or accidentally ingested.

Acute CN intoxication is also called CN poisoning and is often the result of attempted suicide or smoke inhalation. Chronic CN toxicity is usually caused by occupational exposure to substances that contain cyanogenic compounds. Chronic CN exposure results in cyanide encephalopathy.

Etiology

CN exists in gas, solid, and liquid form. CN poisoning can occur by inhalation, ingestion, or transdermal absorption. Combustion of many common materials such as some fabrics and plastics may release cyanide and cyanogenic compounds. Cyanogenic compounds are also found in some foods, including almonds, the pits of stone fruits, lima beans, and cassava root.

CN inactivates cytochrome oxidase, a key enzyme in the mitochondrial respiratory chain. Therefore, acute CN poisoning typically affects structures with high metabolic requirements. The basal ganglia and cortex are most commonly involved. Cerebral hypoxia may occur as part of the acute intoxication process, complicating both the diagnosis and treatment of CN poisoning.

Pathology

Hemorrhagic basal ganglia necrosis and laminar cortical necrosis are the pathologic hallmarks of CN poisoning **(30-33)**.

Clinical Issues

Patients with acute CN poisoning typically present with unresponsiveness, hemodynamic instability, and severe lactic acidosis. Because administered doses are usually high, acute CN poisoning is fatal in 95% of cases with death often occurring in minutes. Survivors may develop pseudo-parkinsonism with extrapyramidal symptoms.

Imaging

MR is the modality of choice to depict lesion extent. Patients who survive the initial insult show symmetric hyperintensity in the basal ganglia and linear cortical hyperintensity on T2WI and FLAIR **(30-34)**. CN poisoning usually spares the hippocampi. T1 C+ scans typically show intense enhancement in the affected areas.

In the subacute and chronic stages, hemorrhagic necrosis causes T1 hyperintensity in the basal ganglia. Laminar necrosis results in serpentine linear hyperintensity in the cortex.

Differential Diagnosis

The most important differential diagnosis of CN poisoning is **hypoxic-ischemic encephalopathy**. It may complicate CN poisoning, and their features often overlap as the basal ganglia are affected in both disorders.

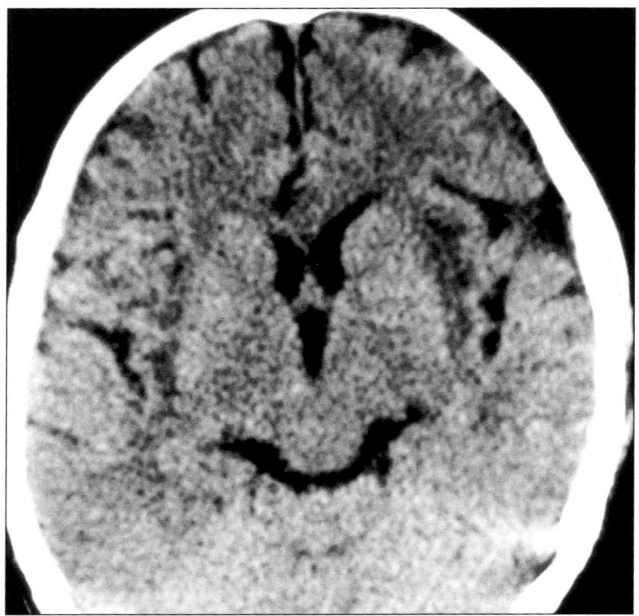

30-35. *NECT scan shows volume loss in the frontal, temporal lobes from lead poisoning. (Courtesy R. Ramakantan, MD.)*

30-36. *Autopsy case of chronic mercury poisoning shows diffuse cortical, cerebellar volume loss. The medulla, pons, and midbrain also appear shrunken. (Courtesy R. Hewlett, MD.)*

INHALED GASES AND TOXINS

Carbon Monoxide Poisoning
- Acute: Symmetric globi pallidi necrosis
- Subacute ("interval"): Confluent leukoencephalopathy

Nitrous Oxide Abuse
- Brain lesions rare
- Subacute combined degeneration of the spinal cord
  ◦ Hyperintensity in dorsal columns

Toluene (Solvent) Abuse
- Chronic, repeated use
  ◦ Atrophy
  ◦ White matter lesions
  ◦ Thalami, substantia nigra, red nuclei, dentate lesions

Organophosphate (Pesticide) Poisoning
- BG hemorrhage, necrosis
- "Eye of the tiger" sign

Cyanide Poisoning
- Suicide, smoke inhalation
- BG hemorrhage, necrosis
- Laminar cortical necrosis

Metal Poisoning and Toxicity

A variety of metals can cause serious neurologic dysfunction when deposited in excess amounts in the CNS. **Manganese** accumulation is more common in the setting of chronic liver failure (see Chapter 32) but also occurs with occupational exposure. Other environmental toxins such as **lead** and **mercury** can cause significant neurotoxicity.

Lead Poisoning

Lead (Pb) is a potent and pervasive environmental neurotoxicant that is especially harmful during childhood development. Chronic Pb poisoning occurs in three forms: (1) an **gastrointestinal form** (anorexia, vomiting, lead "colic," etc.), (2) a **neuromuscular form** (muscle weakness, myalgias, peripheral neuritis, etc.), and (3) a **cerebral** or **neuropsychiatric form** (irritability, headache, encephalopathy, seizure, etc). The cerebral form is common in children whereas neuromuscular manifestations are more common in adults. The gastrointestinal form occurs in both age groups.

Lead-containing cooking utensils and indigenous medications are common sources of Pb poisoning in developing nations. Chronic lead exposure is associated with a significant and persistent impact on white matter microstructure.

Patients with moderate to severe lead encephalopathy usually have blood lead levels that exceed 70 µg/dL. In such cases, CT or MR may reveal volume loss, especially in the frontal cortex and subcortical WM **(30-35)**.

In less severe cases, DTI may reveal subtle changes such as decreased fractional anisotropy and diffusivity in the corona radiata and corpus callosum.

Mercury Poisoning

Mercury (Hg) occurs naturally in three forms: Elemental Hg, mercury vapor, and organic/inorganic. Elemental mercury ("quicksilver") is liquid at room temperature. Liquid Hg is not absorbed through the skin, and if swallowed, passes through the GI tract without being absorbed. Mercury vaporizes easily, is highly diffusible, lipid soluble. Hg vapor is very toxic and easily absorbed.

While occupational exposures to Hg still occasionally occur in manufacturing and mining, most current cases are caused by dermal absorption from illegal skin-lightening cosmetic products or bioconcentration of inorganic methylmercury in the food chain. Seafood (fish, marine mammals) is especially susceptible to contamination. Organic mercury poisoning is known as **Minamata disease**.

Gross pathology shows widespread cortical atrophy, white matter shrinkage, and thinning of the corpus callosum (30-36). Severe spongiosis and gliosis with neuronal loss is seen on microscopic examination.

Imaging findings of Minamata disease include atrophy of the calcarine (visual) cortex, cerebellar vermis and hemispheres, and the postcentral cortex. Decreased regional blood flow in the cerebellum can be demonstrated even in the absence of cerebellar atrophy.

Treatment-related Disorders

A comprehensive treatment of all iatrogenic abnormalities in the brain is far beyond the scope of this text. Here we discuss the most common disorders with a focus on treatment effects that must be recognized on imaging studies, namely radiation, chemotherapy, and surgery.

Radiation Injury

In the United States, approximately 100,000 primary and metastatic brain tumor patients each year survive long enough (more than six months) to develop some degree of radiation-induced injury (RII) to the brain.

Many investigators divide RII into three phases: Acute injury, early delayed injury, and late delayed injury. Yet the pathophysiology and natural course of radiation therapy (XRT)-induced CNS injury are not well understood. Pathologically, radiation injury varies from mild transient vasogenic edema to frank necrosis. The damage that results from XRT depends on a number of variables including total dose, field size, number/frequency/fractionation of doses, whether chemotherapy is used in conjunction with XRT, and patient age.

Several different CNS tissues are affected by XRT. Vascular endothelial cells, oligodendrocytes, astrocytes, microglia, and neurons probably all interact in the brain's response to radiation injury.

Oligodendrocytes are especially sensitive. Vascular injury occurs in both early and late delayed injury. Once considered relatively radioresistant, neurons are now known to respond negatively to radiation and probably play a significant but as-yet-unidentified role in late radiation-induced cognitive impairment.

Acute Radiation Injury

Acute RII occurs days to weeks after irradiation and is very rarely encountered with modern XRT regimens. The major clinical manifestations of acute RII include headache and drowsiness.

Standard imaging studies are usually normal, although MRS, DTI, and fMRI may detect changes before neurocognitive symptoms or anatomic alterations emerge. Occasionally, transient white matter edema secondary to changes in capillary permeability can be seen on T2/FLAIR sequences.

Early Delayed Radiation Injury

In early delayed RII, imaging abnormalities can be detected as early as one to six months after XRT is completed. Early delayed RII is characterized pathologically by transient demyelination and clinically by somnolence, attention deficits, and short-term memory loss. Patients may have significant cognitive impairments even in the absence of detectable anatomic abnormalities.

Confluent hypodense areas on NECT and periventricular WM hyperintensity on T2/FLAIR are typical abnormalities. At this stage, RII changes are generally mild and reversible, often resolving spontaneously.

Late Delayed Radiation Injury

Late delayed RII is usually not observed until at least six months post irradiation. These late delayed injuries are viewed as progressive and largely irreversible, resulting from loss of glial and vascular endothelial cells.

Pathologically, coagulative necrosis in a "mosaic" pattern with coalescing foci produces a necrotizing leukoencephalopathy in the deep cerebral WM. The subcortical association or U-fibers and corpus callosum are typically spared (30-37). Vascular changes include fibrinoid necrosis, hyalinization, and sclerosis with thrombosis. Late delayed radiation necrosis is initially expansile and mass-like, with necrosis largely confined to WM.

Initially, late delayed RII shows mass effect and variable enhancement on imaging studies. Later, volume loss, WM spongiosis with confluent hyperintensity, and calcifications can be seen (30-37).

Long-Term Sequelae of Radiation Injury

In addition to **necrotizing leukoencephalopathy**, long-term complications of XRT include vasculopathy, mineralizing microangiopathy, microvascular glomeruloid proliferation with telangiectasis (XRT-induced vascular malformations), and the development of radiation-induced neoplasms.

Radiation-induced vasculopathy with endothelial hyperplasia results in diffusely narrowed large and medium-sized arteries. Ischemic strokes and moyamoya-like disease may result (30-38).

Mineralizing microangiopathy is usually seen in patients treated with combination XRT and chemotherapy. Mineralizing microangiopathy generally does not appear until at least two years following treatment; it is then seen as calcifications in the basal ganglia and subcortical white matter (30-39).

Radiation-induced vascular malformations (RIVMs) are primarily capillary telangiectasias or cavernous malformations, most commonly seen in children who have received whole-brain radiotherapy for acute lymphoblastic leukemia. T2* (GRE, SWI) sequences demonstrate "blooming" microhemorrhages in the majority of patients (30-40). It is uncommon to develop RIVMs less than three years following XRT. Children under 10 years of age at the time of irradiation are at higher risk.

Radiation-induced neoplasms are rare but often devastating. XRT is the single most important risk factor for developing a new primary CNS neoplasm. Approximately 70% are meningiomas, 20% malignant astrocytomas or medulloblastomas, and 10% sarcomas. Meningiomas occur an average of 17-20 years after treatment whereas gliomas occur at a mean of nine years. Sarcomas have a mean latency of seven or eight years following XRT.

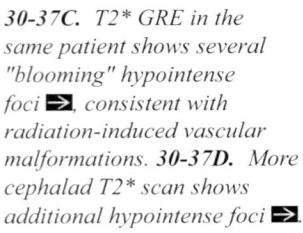
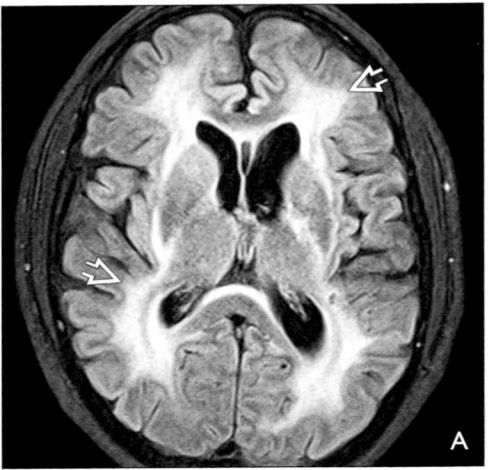
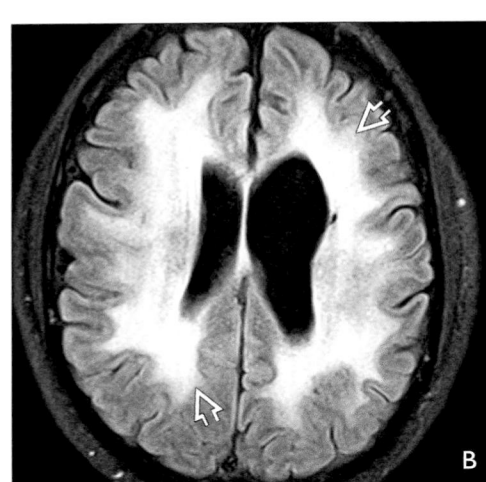

30-37A. A 47-year-old man with whole-brain XRT for leukemia developed progressive cognitive decline, functional impairment 3 years following treatment. FLAIR shows volume loss with enlarged ventricles, sulci, and confluent WM hyperintensity in the deep cerebral, periventricular WM ➡. Subcortical U-fibers are spared. 30-37B. More cephalad FLAIR scan shows confluent WM hyperintensity ➡ characteristic of necrotizing leukoencephalopathy.

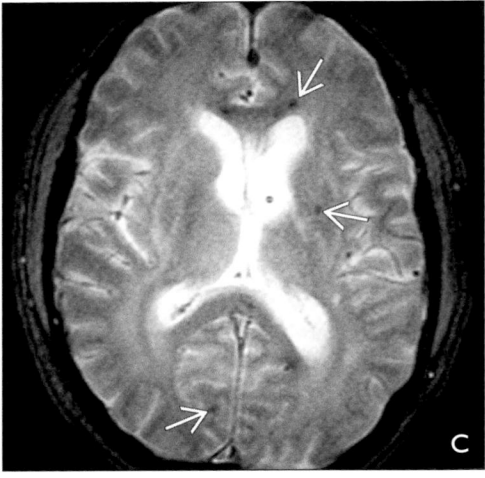
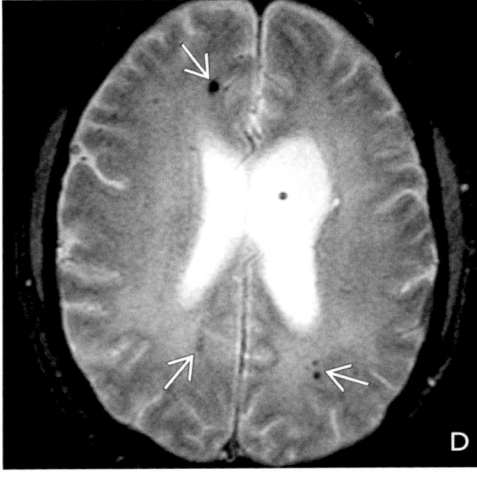

30-37C. T2 GRE in the same patient shows several "blooming" hypointense foci ➡, consistent with radiation-induced vascular malformations. 30-37D. More cephalad T2* scan shows additional hypointense foci ➡.*

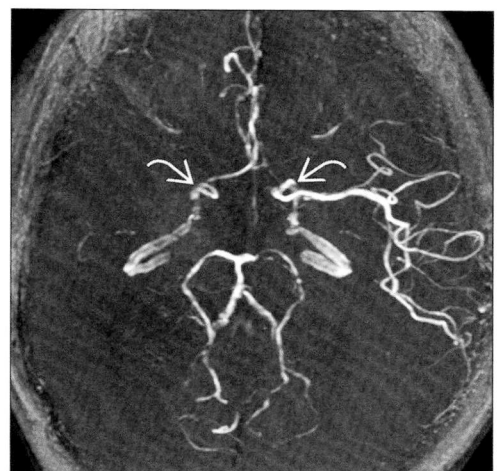

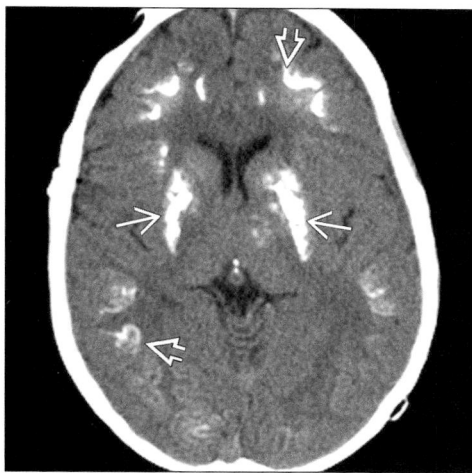

30-38. MRA in a patient with right MCA stroke years after XRT shows moyamoya pattern, post-radiation vasculopathy. High-grade stenosis of both supraclinoid ICAs ➡ is present. Right MCA is occluded. (Courtesy P. Hildenbrand, MD.) 30-39. NECT scan in a 20 yo man who had XRT and chemotherapy at age 8 for medulloblastoma. The basal ganglia ➡, subcortical WM calcifications ➡ are characteristic of mineralizing microangiopathy. (Courtesy P. Chapman, MD.)

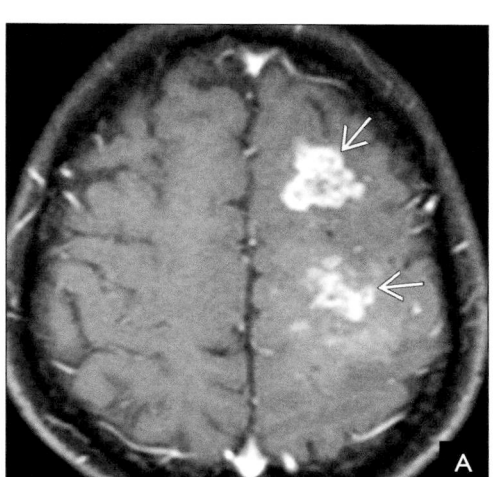

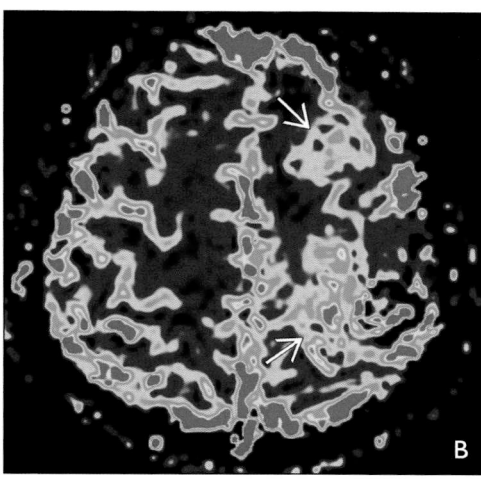

30-40A. Patient with whole-brain radiation, chemotherapy for anaplastic oligodendroglioma presented with a seizure 5 years following completion of treatment. T1 C+ FS shows multiple enhancing foci in the left hemispheric WM ➡. Delayed radiation necrosis versus tumor recurrence. 30-40B. pMR shows elevated rCBV in the enhancing areas ➡, which suggests that the enhancing foci represent recurrent tumor rather than necrotizing leukoencephalopathy.

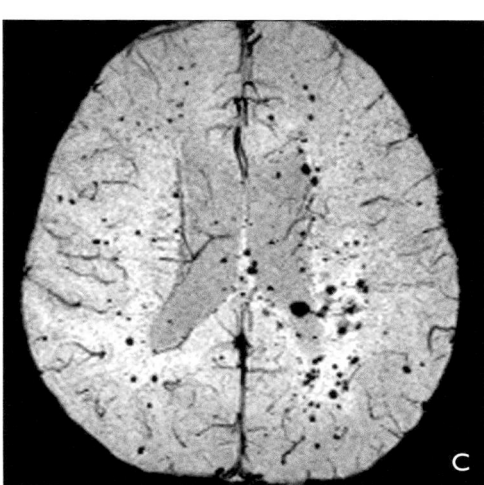

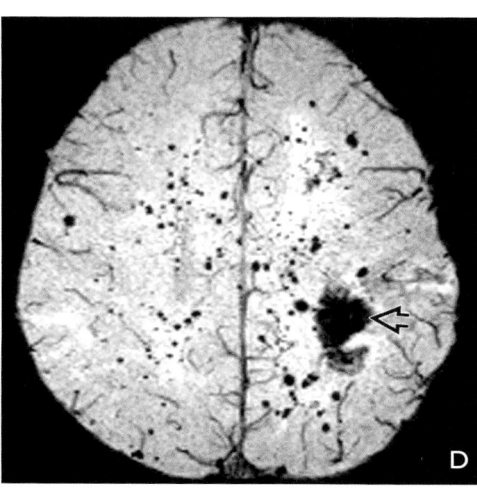

30-40C. T2* SWI scan shows innumerable "blooming" hypointense foci in the WM, consistent with radiation-induced vascular malformations. 30-40D. More cephalad T2* SWI scan in the same patient shows additional small lesions and a larger focus ➡, consistent with hemorrhage into the recurrent neoplasm. Biopsy confirmed recurrence of anaplastic oligodendroglioma (WHO grade III), capillary telangiectases.

Chemotherapy Effects

Currently, the most common chemotherapy agents implicated in CNS toxicity are methotrexate, cytarabine, vincristine, asparaginase, and corticosteroids.

Unlike radiation injury, chemotherapy-associated acute toxic CNS injury is common. The two most frequent abnormalities are posterior reversible encephalopathy syndrome and treatment-induced leukoencephalopathy.

Posterior reversible encephalopathy syndrome (PRES) is addressed in detail in Chapter 32. In chemotherapy-related PRES, imaging findings are often atypical. The occipital lobes are frequently spared whereas the cerebellum, brainstem, and basal ganglia are frequently involved. Hemorrhage, contrast enhancement, and diffusion restriction—all relatively rare in "typical" PRES—are common.

Treatment-induced leukoencephalopathy is especially common in patients treated with methotrexate. Acute neurotoxicity occurs in 5-18% of children treated for acute lymphoblastic leukemia. Bilateral, relatively symmetric, confluent areas of T2/FLAIR hyperintensity in the periventricular WM are typical **(30-41)**. Imaging abnormalities typically resolve after treatment.

Effects of Surgery

Interpreting imaging findings in the postoperative brain can be challenging. Expected findings include pneumocephalus, focal hemorrhage, retraction edema, small subdural CSF collections (hygromas), etc. We focus on just two abnormalities that are important to recognize on imaging studies: Retained surgical material ("textiloma," also discussed in Chapter 26) and sinking skin flap syndrome.

Textiloma

Textiloma—also known as muslinoma or gauzoma—is a foreign body reaction to retained surgical elements. The term has traditionally referred to reactions to surgical elements inadvertently left in the operative bed but has recently been expanded to include reactions to intentionally placed surgical elements.

30-41A. A 5-year-old girl received intrathecal methotrexate for acute lymphoblastic leukemia. Acute clinical deterioration prompted imaging. NECT scan shows confluent WM hypodensity ➡ in both hemispheres.
30-41B. T2WI in the same patient shows symmetric confluent hyperintensity in the deep cerebral WM of both hemispheres ➡. Note sparing of subcortical U-fibers.

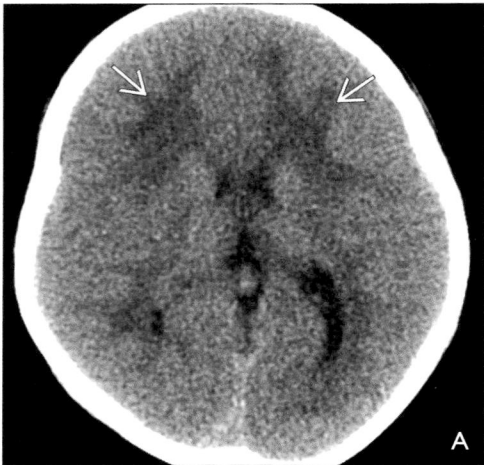
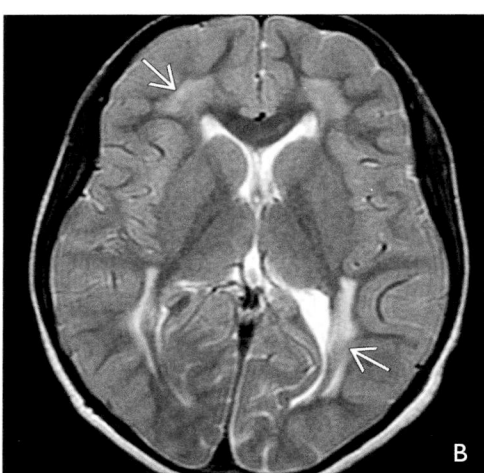

30-41C. More cephalad scan in the same patient shows the confluent WM hyperintensity ➡, spared subcortical WM.
30-41D. Coronal T2WI in the same patient 9 years later shows almost complete resolution of the WM changes.

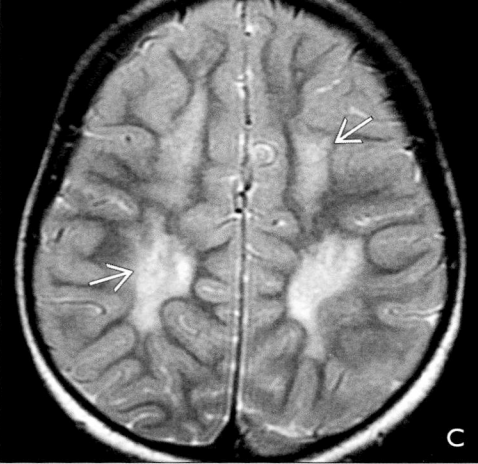
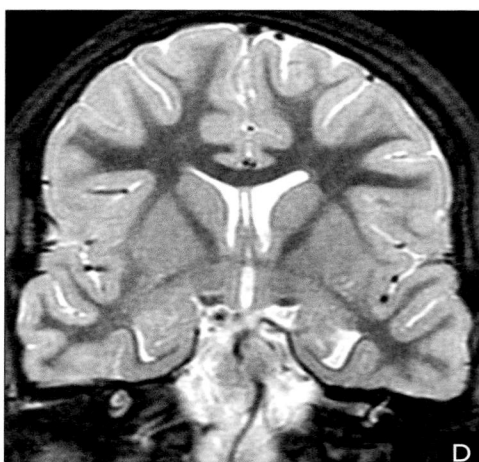

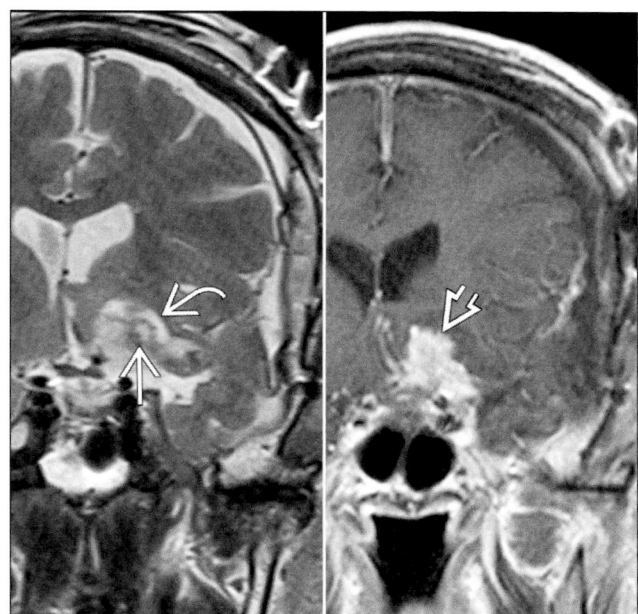

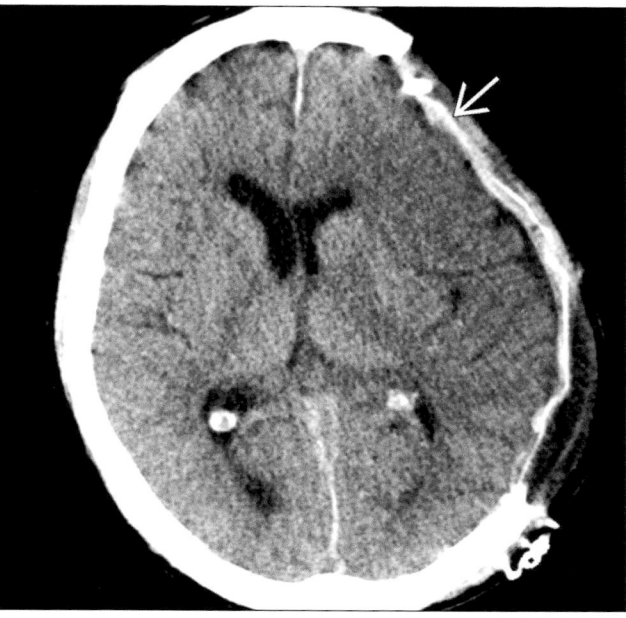

30-42. (Left) Coronal T2WI following meningioma resection shows a mixed hyper- ➘, hypointense mass ➘. (Right) The lesion ➘ enhances strongly, relatively uniformly. Surgery disclosed textiloma without recurrent or residual tumor.

30-43. Sinking skin flap syndrome 6 days following decompressive craniectomy. The skin flap ➘ has obliterated the underlying frontal sulci, caused mild left-to-right subfalcine herniation.

Textiloma incidence is 0.001-0.01% in the general surgical literature. Intracranial textilomas are rare. Both resorbable and nonresorbable hemostatic agents may be placed in the surgical bed to provide persistent hemostasis after closure.

When they occur, textilomas can be mistaken for recurrent tumor or abscesses on imaging studies. Most surgically placed materials (e.g., cotton hemostats, muslin, or polytetrafluoroethylene [Teflon]) do not have signal abnormalities on MR. They are only visualized when a foreign body reaction develops, forming a textiloma.

Nearly 40% of textilomas are hypointense on T2WI. Many "bloom" on T2* (GRE, SWI) sequences. Restriction on DWI is variable. Most enhance; both solid and ring patterns occur **(30-42)**.

inking Skin Flap Syndrome

Sinking skin flap syndrome (SSFS)—also referred to as "syndrome of the trephined"—is an unusual cause of neurologic deterioration in patients who have undergone large decompressive craniectomy for uncontrollable brain swelling (usually following trauma or "malignant" hemispheric infarction).

SSFS occurs in 20-25% of patients who survive decompressive surgery and in whom cranioplasty is delayed. It typically presents weeks to months after craniectomy and is alleviated by cranioplasty. Presenting signs and symptoms vary, but decreased consciousness and hemiparesis are the most common findings. In severe cases, SSFS

can become life-threatening, especially if exacerbated by lumbar puncture or CSF leak.

The most common imaging features of SSFS are skin flap depression and mass effect on the cortex, evidenced by sulcal obliteration and buckling of the gray-white matter interface under the skin flap. Midline shift of the interhemispheric fissure and/or septi pellucidi away from the sunken skin flap is seen in 75% of cases **(30-43)**.

Selected References

- Tamrazi B et al: Your brain on drugs: imaging of drug-related changes in the central nervous system. Radiographics. 32(3):701-19, 2012
- Sharma P et al: Toxic and acquired metabolic encephalopathies: MRI appearance. AJR Am J Roentgenol. 193(3):879-86, 2009

Alcohol and Related Disorders

- Brust JC: Ethanol and cognition: indirect effects, neurotoxicity and neuroprotection: a review. Int J Environ Res Public Health. 7(4):1540-57, 2010
- Geibprasert S et al: Alcohol-induced changes in the brain as assessed by MRI and CT. Eur Radiol. 20(6):1492-501, 2010
- Zuccoli G et al: Neuroimaging findings in alcohol-related encephalopathies. Am J Roentgenol. 195(6):1378-84, 2010
- Spampinato MV et al: Magnetic resonance imaging findings in substance abuse: alcohol and alcoholism and syndromes associated with alcohol abuse. Top Magn Reson Imaging. 16(3):223-30, 2005

Acute Alcohol Poisoning

- Kong LM et al: Acute effects of alcohol on the human brain: diffusion tensor imaging study. AJNR Am J Neuroradiol. 33(5):928-34, 2012
- Coleman LG Jr et al: Adolescent binge drinking alters adult brain neurotransmitter gene expression, behavior, brain regional volumes, and neurochemistry in mice. Alcohol Clin Exp Res. 35(4):671-88, 2011

Chronic Alcoholic Encephalopathy

- Geibprasert S et al: Alcohol-induced changes in the brain as assessed by MRI and CT. Eur Radiol. 20(6):1492-501, 2010

Wernicke Encephalopathy

- Zuccoli G et al: MR Imaging: An increasingly important tool in the early diagnosis of Wernicke encephalopathy. AJNR Am J Neuroradiol. 33(6):E92, 2012
- Geibprasert S et al: Alcohol-induced changes in the brain as assessed by MRI and CT. Eur Radiol. 20(6):1492-501, 2010

Marchiafava-Bignami Disease

- Kinno R et al: Cerebral microhemorrhage in Marchiafava-Bignami disease detected by susceptibility-weighted imaging. Neurol Sci. Epub ahead of print, 2012
- Tung CS et al: Marchiafava-Bignami disease with widespread lesions and complete recovery. Am J Neuroradiol. 31(8):1506-7, 2010
- Yoshizaki T et al: Evolution of callosal and cortical lesions on MRI in Marchiafava-Bignami disease. Case Rep Neurol. 2(1):19-23, 2010

- Zuccoli G et al: Neuroimaging findings in alcohol-related encephalopathies. Am J Roentgenol. 195(6):1378-84, 2010
- Kim MJ et al: Acute Marchiafava-Bignami disease with widespread callosal and cortical lesions. J Korean Med Sci. 22(5):908-11, 2007

Methanol Intoxication

- Sonkar SK et al: Drowsy man with breathlessness and blurred vision. Methanol toxicity. Ann Emerg Med. 59(4):255, 264, 2012
- Taheri MS et al: The value of brain CT findings in acute methanol toxicity. Eur J Radiol. 73(2):211-4, 2010
- Sefidbakht S et al: Methanol poisoning: acute MR and CT findings in nine patients. Neuroradiology. 49(5):427-35, 2007

Ethylene Glycol Poisoning

- Sharma P et al: Toxic and acquired metabolic encephalopathies: MRI appearance. Am J Roentgenol. 193(3):879-86, 2009

Amphetamines and Derivatives

- Moreno-López L et al: Neural correlates of the severity of cocaine, heroin, alcohol, MDMA and cannabis use in polysubstance abusers: a resting-PET brain metabolism study. PLoS One. 7(6):e39830, 2012
- Tamrazi B et al: Your brain on drugs: imaging of drug-related changes in the central nervous system. Radiographics. 32(3):701-19, 2012
- Geibprasert S et al: Addictive illegal drugs: structural neuroimaging. AJNR Am J Neuroradiol. 31(5):803-8, 2010

Methamphetamine

- Salo R et al: Structural, functional and spectroscopic MRI studies of methamphetamine addiction. Curr Top Behav Neurosci. 11:321-64, 2012

MDMA ("Ecstasy")

- De Smet K et al: Bilateral globus pallidus infarcts in ecstasy use. JBR-BTR. 94(2):93, 2011

Cocaine

- Dinis-Oliveira RJ et al: Clinical and forensic signs related to cocaine abuse. Curr Drug Abuse Rev. 5(1):64-83, 2012
- Polesskaya O et al: Methamphetamine causes sustained depression in cerebral blood flow. Brain Res. 1373:91-100, 2011
- Geibprasert S et al: Addictive illegal drugs: structural neuroimaging. AJNR Am J Neuroradiol. 31(5):803-8, 2010

Opioids and Derivatives

- Milroy CM et al: The histopathology of drugs of abuse. Histopathology. 59(4):579-93, 2011
- Geibprasert S et al: Addictive illegal drugs: structural neuroimaging. AJNR Am J Neuroradiol. 31(5):803-8, 2010

Heroin

- Havé L et al: [Toxic leucoencephalopathy after use of sniffed heroin, an unrecognized form of beneficial evolution.] Rev Neurol (Paris). 168(1):57-64, 2012
- Tamrazi B et al: Your brain on drugs: imaging of drug-related changes in the central nervous system. Radiographics. 32(3):701-19, 2012
- Offiah C et al: Heroin-induced leukoencephalopathy: characterization using MRI, diffusion-weighted imaging, and MR spectroscopy. Clin Radiol. 63(2):146-52, 2008
- Hagel J et al: "Chasing the dragon": imaging of heroin inhalation leukoencephalopathy. Can Assoc Radiol J. 56(4):199-203, 2005

Methadone

- Salgado RA et al: Methadone-induced toxic leukoencephalopathy: MR imaging and MR proton spectroscopy findings. AJNR Am J Neuroradiol. 31(3):565-6, 2010

Inhaled Gases and Toxins

- Borne J et al: Neuroimaging in drug and substance abuse part II: opioids and solvents. Top Magn Reson Imaging. 16(3):239-45, 2005

Carbon Monoxide Poisoning

- Lin WC et al: White matter damage in carbon monoxide intoxication assessed in vivo using diffusion tensor MR imaging. AJNR Am J Neuroradiol. 30(6):1248-55, 2009

Nitrous Oxide

- Ghobrial GM et al: Nitrous oxide myelopathy posing as spinal cord injury. J Neurosurg Spine. 16(5):489-91, 2012
- Tamrazi B et al: Your brain on drugs: imaging of drug-related changes in the central nervous system. Radiographics. 32(3):701-19, 2012

Toluene Abuse

- Spee T et al: A screening programme on chronic solvent-induced encephalopathy among Dutch painters. Neurotoxicology. 33(4):727-33, 2012
- Gupta SR et al: Toluene optic neurotoxicity: magnetic resonance imaging and pathologic features. Hum Pathol. 42(2):295-8, 2011
- Aydin K et al: Smaller gray matter volumes in frontal and parietal cortices of solvent abusers correlate with cognitive deficits. Am J Neuroradiol. 30(10):1922-8, 2009
- Aydin K et al: Cranial MR findings in chronic toluene abuse by inhalation. Am J Neuroradiol. 23(7):1173-9, 2002

Organophosphate Poisoning

- Churi S et al: Organophosphate poisoning: Prediction of severity and outcome by Glasgow Coma Scale, Poisoning Severity Score, Acute Physiology and Chronic Health Evaluation II Score, and Simplified Acute Physiology Score II. J Emerg Nurs. 38(5):493-5, 2012
- Rother HA: Improving poisoning diagnosis and surveillance of street pesticides. S Afr Med J. 102(6):485-8, 2012
- London L et al: Challenges for improving surveillance for pesticide poisoning: policy implications for developing countries. Int J Epidemiol. 30(3):564-70, 2001

Cyanide Poisoning

- Geller RJ et al: Pediatric cyanide poisoning: causes, manifestations, management, and unmet needs. Pediatrics. 118(5):2146-58, 2006
- Rachinger J et al: MR changes after acute cyanide intoxication. AJNR Am J Neuroradiol. 23(8):1398-401, 2002

Metal Poisoning and Toxicity

Lead Poisoning

- Nava-Ruiz C et al: Lead neurotoxicity: effects on brain nitric oxide synthase. J Mol Histol. Epub ahead of print, 2012
- Rolston DD: Uncommon sources and some unusual manifestations of lead poisoning in a tropical developing country. Trop Med Health. 39(4):127-32, 2011
- Brubaker CJ et al: Altered myelination and axonal integrity in adults with childhood lead exposure: a diffusion tensor imaging study. Neurotoxicology. 30(6):867-75, 2009
- Hsieh TJ et al: Subclinical white matter integrity in subjects with cumulative lead exposure. Radiology. 252(2):509-17, 2009

Mercury Poisoning

- Cooksey C: Health concerns of heavy metals and metalloids. Sci Prog. 95(Pt 1):73-88, 2012
- Chan TY: Inorganic mercury poisoning associated with skin-lightening cosmetic products. Clin Toxicol (Phila). 49(10):886-91, 2011
- Taber KH et al: Mercury exposure: effects across the lifespan. J Neuropsychiatry Clin Neurosci. 20(4):iv-389, 2008

Treatment-related Disorders

Radiation Injury

- Chowdhary A et al: Radiation associated tumors following therapeutic cranial radiation. Surg Neurol Int. 3:48, 2012
- Greene-Schloesser D et al: Radiation-induced brain injury: A review. Front Oncol. 2:73, 2012
- Li H et al: An experimental study on acute brain radiation injury: Dynamic changes in proton magnetic resonance spectroscopy and the correlation with histopathology. Eur J Radiol. Epub ahead of print, 2012
- Robbins ME et al: Imaging radiation-induced normal tissue injury. Radiat Res. 177(4):449-66, 2012
- Faraci M et al: Magnetic resonance imaging in childhood leukemia survivors treated with cranial radiotherapy: a cross sectional, single center study. Pediatr Blood Cancer. 57(2):240-6, 2011
- Sundgren PC: MR spectroscopy in radiation injury. AJNR Am J Neuroradiol. 30(8):1469-76, 2009

Chemotherapy Effects

- Vázquez E et al: Side effects of oncologic therapies in the pediatric central nervous system: update on neuroimaging findings. Radiographics. 31(4):1123-39, 2011

Effects of Surgery

- Archavlis E et al: The impact of timing of cranioplasty in patients with large cranial defects after decompressive hemicraniectomy. Acta Neurochir (Wien). 154(6):1055-62, 2012

- Gschwind M et al: Life-threatening sinking skin flap syndrome due to CSF leak after lumbar puncture - treated with epidural blood patch. Eur J Neurol. 19(5):e49, 2012

- Warren A et al: Intracranial textiloma: Meta-analysis of the world literature and four new cases. Presented at the 50th annual scientific meeting, American Society of Neuroradiology, 2012

- Chin BM et al: Sinking skin flap syndrome: Imaging characteristics of an unfamiliar yet common entity. Presented at the 49th annual scientific meeting, American Society of Neuroradiology, 2011

31

Inherited Metabolic Disorders

Inherited metabolic disorders (IMDs)—sometimes termed "inborn errors of metabolism"—are relatively uncommon diseases that pose diagnostic dilemmas for clinicians and radiologists alike. IMDs can present at virtually any age from infancy well into the fifth and sixth decades. Symptoms vary both between disorders and in the degree of severity in patients with the same disorder.

MR scans are routinely obtained in infants and children with delayed neurologic development. Familiarization with the normal evolution of white matter myelination is a prerequisite to understanding IMDs. We therefore begin this chapter with a review of how normal myelination progresses from birth to two years of age.

Once we have delineated the patterns of normal myelination as seen on MR scans, we continue with an overview and introduction to IMDs. A discussion of classification and a recommended approach to analyzing imaging abnormalities are presented.

Finally, we focus on specific IMDs. Our discussion emphasizes the inherited leukodystrophies, including those with abnormal myelin development, hypomyelination, or myelin degeneration.

Normal Myelination and White Matter Development

General Considerations

Myelination

Myelination is an orderly, highly regulated, multistep process that begins during the fifth fetal month and is largely complete by 18-24 postnatal months. Some structures (e.g., cranial nerves) myelinate relatively early in fetal development while others (e.g., optic radiations and fibers to/from association areas) often do not completely myelinate until the third or even the fourth decade of life.

Brain myelination generally progresses from **inferior to superior**, **central to peripheral**, and **posterior to anterior**. For example, the brainstem myelinates before the cerebellar hemispheres, the posterior limbs of the internal capsules myelinate before the anterior limbs, and the deep periventricular white matter (WM) myelinates before the subcortical U-fibers. The dorsal brainstem myelinates before the anterior brainstem, and—with the exception of the parietooccipital association tracts—occipital WM myelinates earlier than WM in the anterior temporal and frontal lobes.

Selected Myelination Milestones

AGE	T1 HYPERINTENSITY	T2 HYPOINTENSITY
Birth		
	Dorsal brainstem	Dorsal brainstem
	Posterior limb IC	Partial posterior limb IC
	Perirolandic gyri	Perirolandic gyri
3-4 months		
	Ventral brainstem	Posterior limb IC
	Anterior limb IC	
	CC splenium	
	Central, posterior corona radiata	
6 months		
	Cerebellar WM	Ventral brainstem
	CC genu	Anterior limb IC
	Parietal, occipital WM	CC splenium
		Occipital WM
12 months		
	Posterior fossa (≈ adult)	Most of corona radiata
	Most of corona radiata	Posterior subcortical WM
	Posterior subcortical WM	
18 months		
	All WM except temporal, frontal U-fibers	All WM except temporal, frontal U-fibers, occipital radiations
24 months		
	Anterior temporal, frontal U-fibers	Anterior temporal, frontal U-fibers

Table 31-1. CC = corpus callosum; IC = internal capsule; WM = white matter.

CT

The hemispheres of normal term infants at birth appear well-formed. The gyral pattern is mature with distinctly defined cortex and surface sulci. The lateral cerebral (sylvian) fissures may be slightly prominent but generally resemble those seen in older children. The frontal subarachnoid spaces and basal cisterns often appear prominent up to one year of age.

At birth, the WM is largely unmyelinated, so it appears quite hypodense due to its relatively high water content.

MR

Detailed anatomy of the cerebral cortex and WM is best delineated on MR. The appearance of WM maturation varies with two important factors, i.e., **patient age** and the **imaging sequence** employed.

Unmyelinated WM is hypointense relative to gray matter on T1WI. As the WM matures, it becomes hyperintense. Myelin maturation with WM hyperintensity on T1 scans is related to increasing cholesterol and galactocerebroside within myelin membranes.

Fully myelinated WM appears hypointense relative to gray matter on T2 scans. Myelin maturation results in reduced WM water content with concomitant T2 hypointensity.

During the first six to eight months of life, T1-weighted sequences are best both to evaluate gross brain structure and to assess WM maturation. Heavily weighted T2WI is the most sensitive sequence to follow WM maturation between 6 and 18 months.

As a general rule, *myelinated white matter appears hyperintense on T1 scans before hypointensity becomes apparent on T2 scans* (**Table 31-1**). At a minimum, accurate evaluation of myelination status requires both T1 and T2 scans. More advanced techniques such as DTI and magnetization transfer imaging (MTI) may provide additional information.

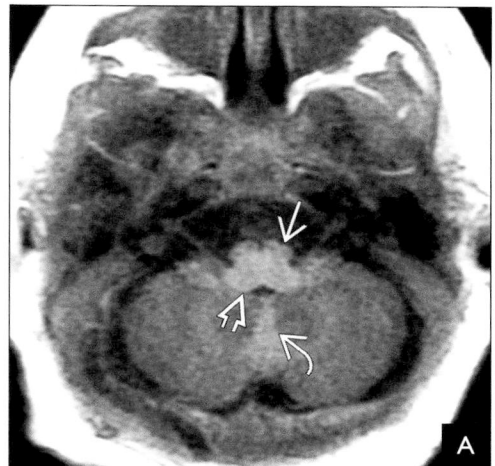

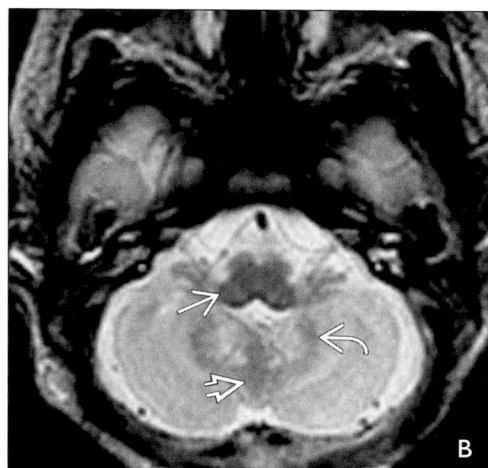

31-1A. Axial T1WI in a normal term infant at birth shows the dorsal medulla ➡, inferior cerebellar peduncles, and vermis ➡ are hyperintense and densely myelinated compared to the most ventral brainstem ➡. The cerebellar WM is unmyelinated and hypointense. 31-1B. T2WI shows the medulla and inferior cerebellar peduncles ➡ as well as the dentate nuclei ➡ and vermis ➡ are myelinated. The unmyelinated WM in the cerebellar hemispheres remains hyperintense.

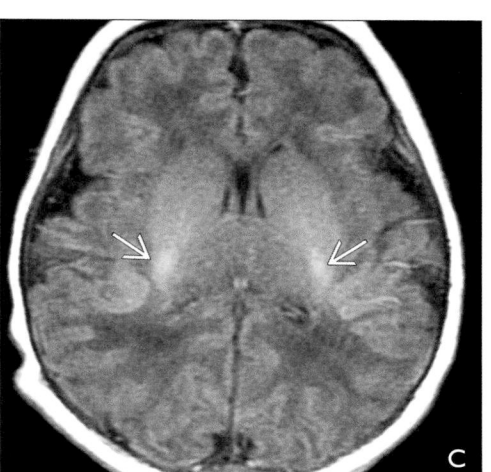

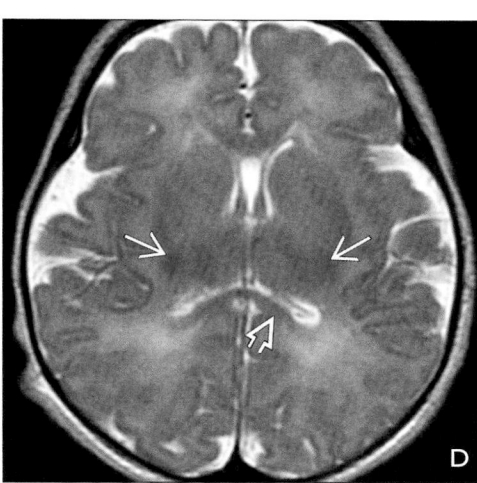

31-1C. T1WI in the same term infant shows hyperintensity of the posterior limb of the internal capsules, particularly striking in the location of the corticospinal tracts ➡. 31-1D. T2WI shows a small patch of hypointensity ➡ representing early myelination in the posterior limbs of the internal capsules. The corpus callosum splenium ➡ is unmyelinated. This is more obvious on T1WI than on T2WI.

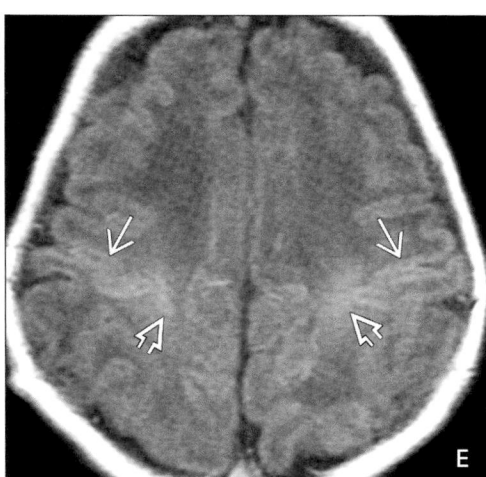

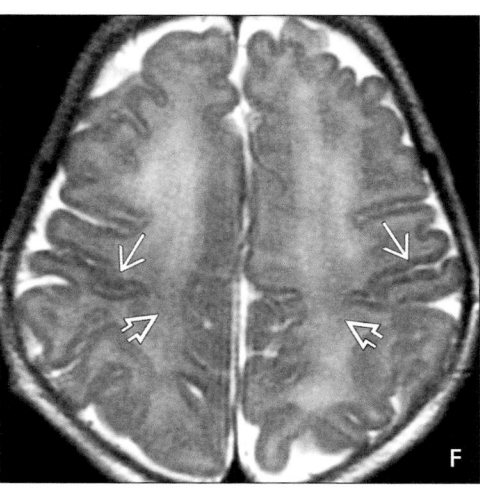

31-1E. T1WI shows hyperintensity in the rolandic and perirolandic gyri ➡ corresponding to normal early myelination in these gyri. Ill-defined hyperintensity in the WM of the corticospinal tracts ➡ represents the normal early myelination of motor tracts. 31-1F. T2WI shows predominantly hyperintense (unmyelinated) WM. Note normal hypointensity in the rolandic and perirolandic gyri ➡ and subtle "smudgy" hypointensity in the corticospinal tracts ➡.

31-2A. Axial T1WI in a normal infant at 3.5 months shows that the medulla ➔ is completely myelinated. Hyperintensity now extends into the proximal cerebellar hemispheres ➔, but the more peripheral WM remains unmyelinated and appears hypointense. *31-2B.* T2WI shows hypointensity in the dorsal brainstem ➔ and cranial nerve nuclei ➔ as well as the middle cerebellar peduncles ➔.

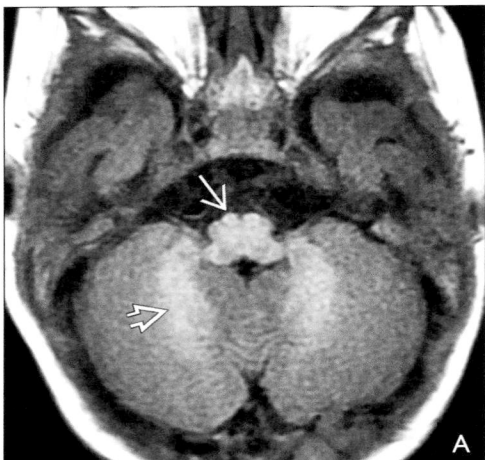
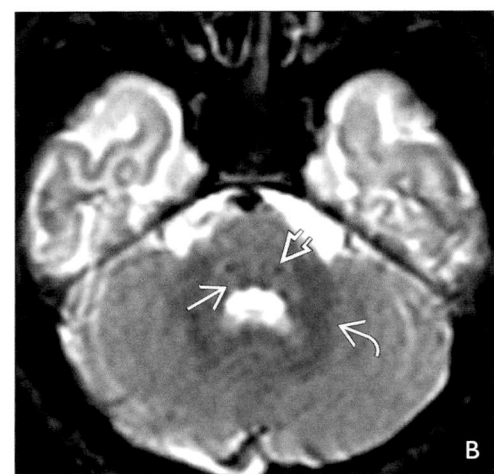

31-2C. T1WI. Note the striking hyperintensity in the posterior limbs ➔ and the subtle hyperintensity starting to appear in the anterior limbs ➔. The deep posterior occipital WM is beginning to myelinate ➔. *31-2D.* T2WI. Hypointensity is seen in the posterior limbs of the internal capsules ➔. The anterior limbs ➔ are beginning to myelinate and are not well seen between the hypointensity of the caudate and basal ganglia.

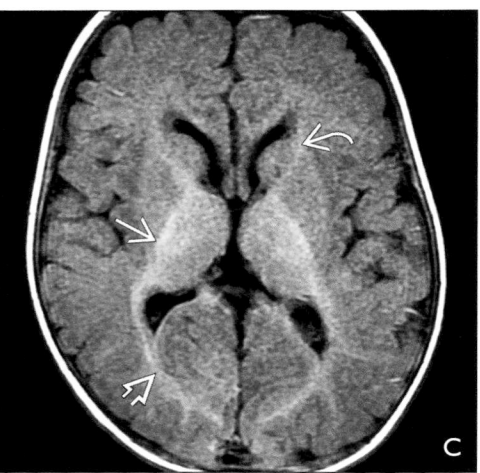
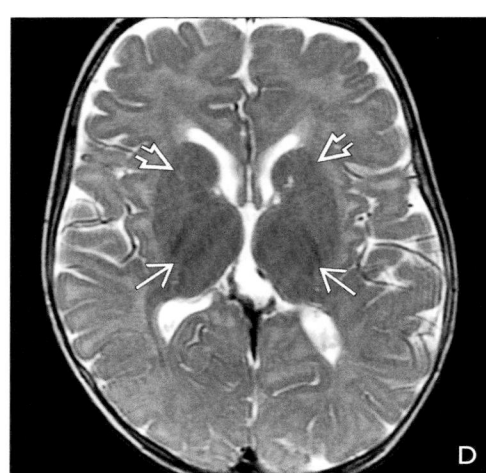

31-2E. T1WI. WM in the corona radiata remains mostly unmyelinated at 3.5 months, although some myelination in WM deep to the central sulci ➔ is present. *31-2F.* T2WI. Except for the "smudgy" areas ➔ deep to the central sulci, WM in the corona radiata remains hyperintense and unmyelinated.

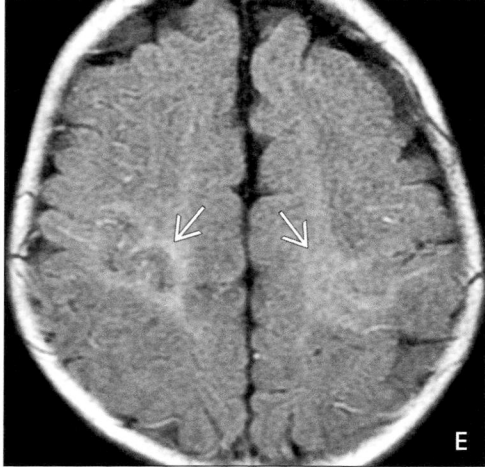
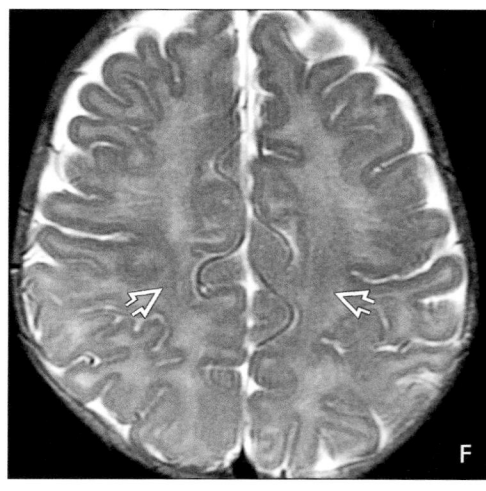

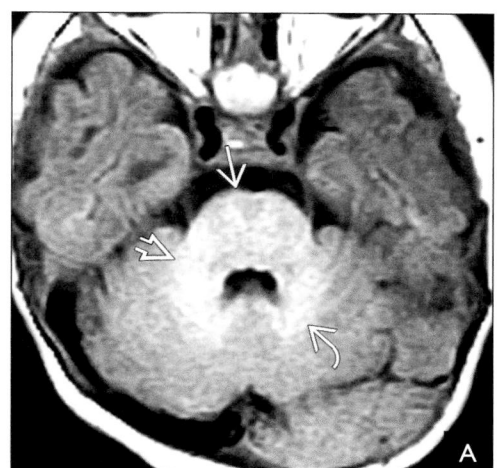

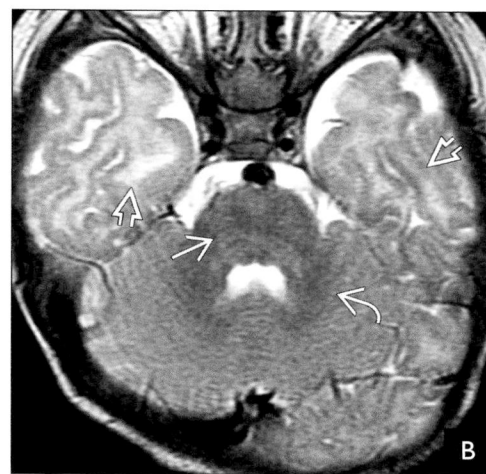

31-3A. Axial T1WI of a normal 6-month-old infant shows that the pons ➡ and middle cerebellar peduncles ➡ are completely myelinated and that hyperintensity extends further peripherally into the cerebellar hemispheres ➡. 31-3B. T2WI in the same patient shows striking contrast between the hypointense (myelinated) pons ➡ and proximal cerebellar WM ➡ compared to the unmyelinated hyperintense WM in the temporal lobes ➡.

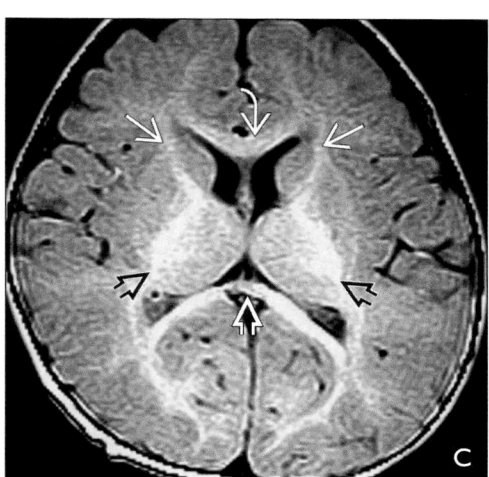

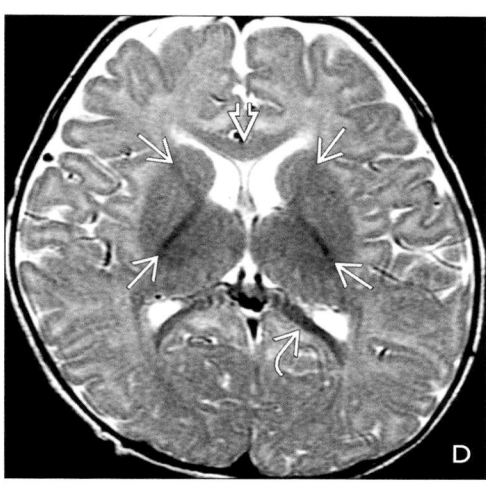

31-3C. T1WI shows hyperintensity in the posterior ➡ and anterior limbs of the internal capsule ➡ as well as the corpus callosum splenium ➡ and genu ➡. The subcortical WM is unmyelinated and isointense with cortex. 31-3D. T2WI. Both limbs ➡ of the internal capsules are myelinated and hypointense. The corpus callosum splenium ➡ is more hypointense than the genu ➡, which has just myelinated. The prominent frontal subarachnoid spaces are normal.

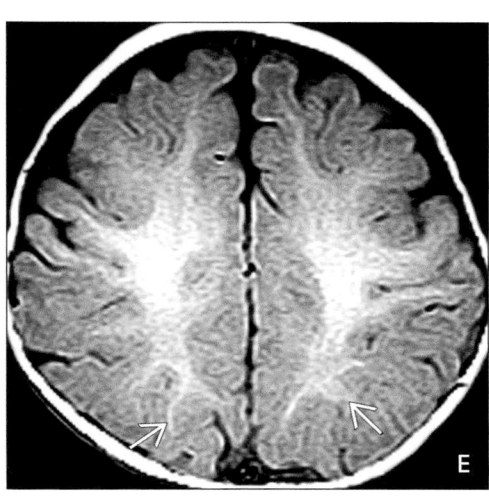

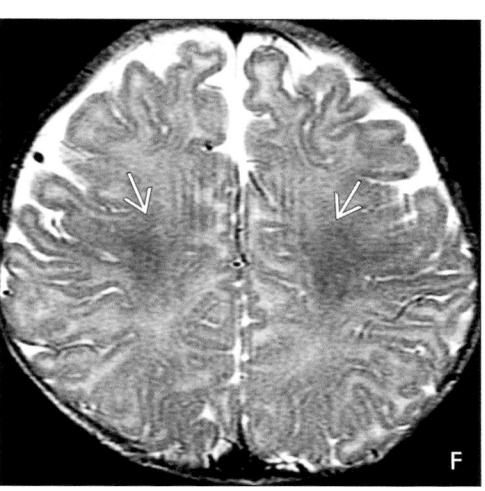

31-3E. T1WI. Myelination extends from the central WM toward the more peripheral subcortical fibers, especially in the parietal and occipital lobes ➡. 31-3F. T2WI. Hypointensity in the corona radiata ➡ is not as extensive as the hyperintensity seen on the corresponding T1WI. Indeed, myelination on T2-weighted sequences normally lags somewhat behind that seen on T1WI. Note the normal prominence of the frontal and interhemispheric subarachnoid spaces.

31-4A. *Axial T1WI in a normal 12-month-old child shows that the pons and cerebellum have a near-adult appearance. The pons* ➔ *and middle cerebellar peduncles* ➔ *are completely and densely myelinated. WM in the anterior temporal lobe* ➔ *remains largely unmyelinated.* **31-4B.** *T2WI. The cerebellar WM is hypointense and myelinated in contrast to the subcortical WM in both temporal lobes* ➔*, which is still hyperintense and unmyelinated.*

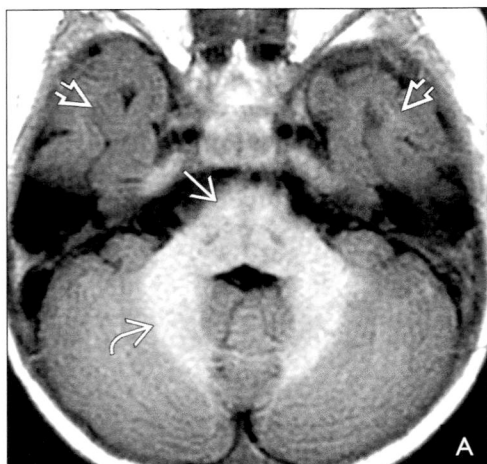
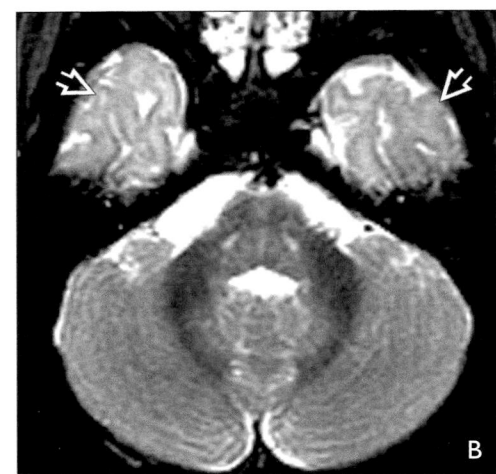

31-4C. *T1WI shows near-adult myelination. Hyperintensity extends into the subcortical fibers in the occipital* ➔ *and parietal lobes to the undersurface of the cortex. On the most anterior frontal lobe, subcortical U-fibers remain unmyelinated* ➔. **31-4D.** *T2WI shows hypointense subcortical U-fibers in the occipital* ➔, *parietal lobes but not in the temporal, frontal lobes* ➔. *Some hyperintensity lateral to the trigones, occipital horns* ➔ *is normal.*

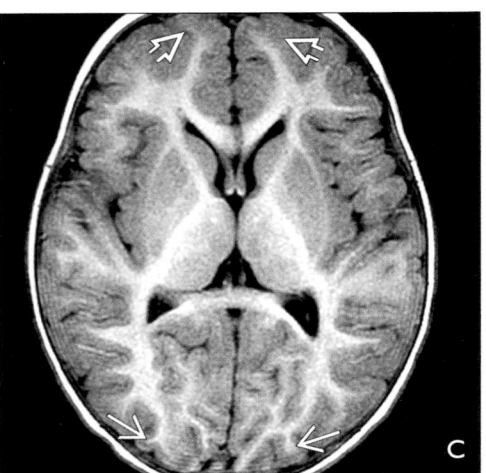
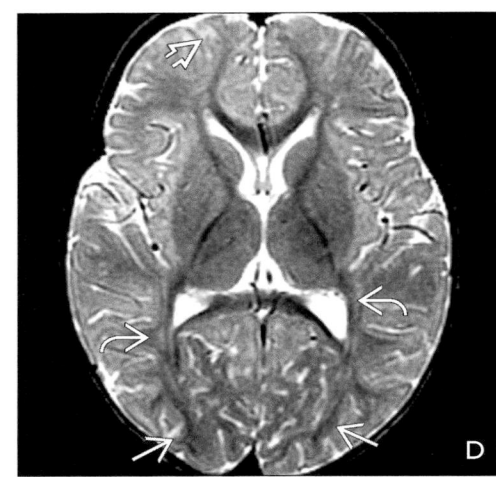

31-4E. *Myelination of corona radiata and subcortical U-fibers is almost complete on T1WI. Only the most anterior subcortical association tracts* ➔ *remain unmyelinated.* **31-4F.** *T2WI. The parietal and occipital subcortical U-fibers together with most of the central corona radiata* ➔ *appear hypointense. The frontal and most superior fibers* ➔ *remain unmyelinated. The presence of some patchy hyperintense foci lateral and posterosuperior to the lateral ventricles* ➔ *is normal.*

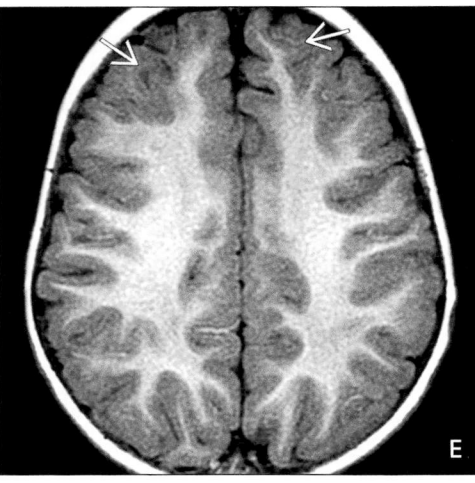
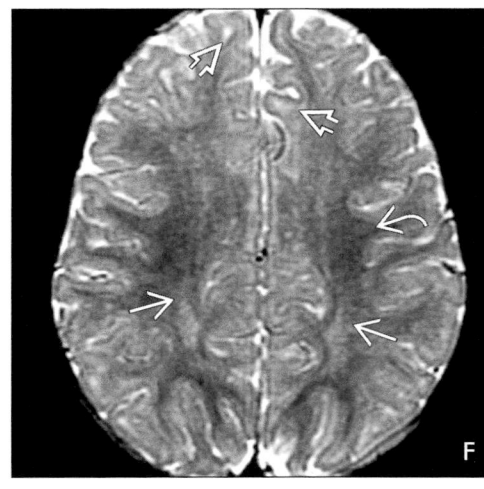

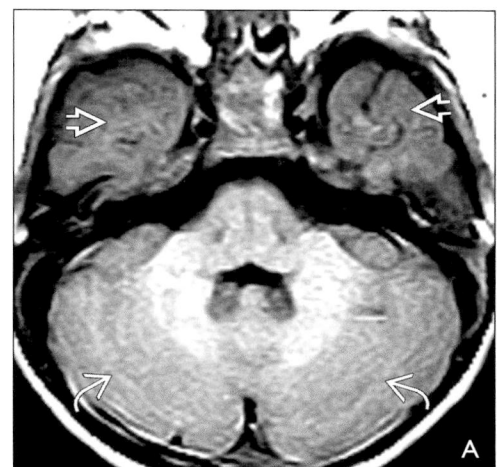

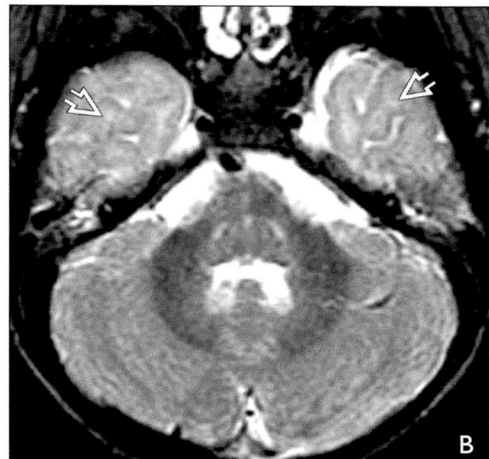

31-5A. Axial T1WI in a normal 18 month old shows that the posterior fossa structures look like those of an adult. Hyperintensity in the WM of the cerebellar folia ➜ indicates that myelination is complete. WM in the anterior temporal lobes ⊟➤ remains unmyelinated.
31-5B. T2WI. At 18 months, the posterior fossa structures are completely myelinated, but WM in the anterior temporal lobes remains unmyelinated and is still hyperintense ⊟➤.

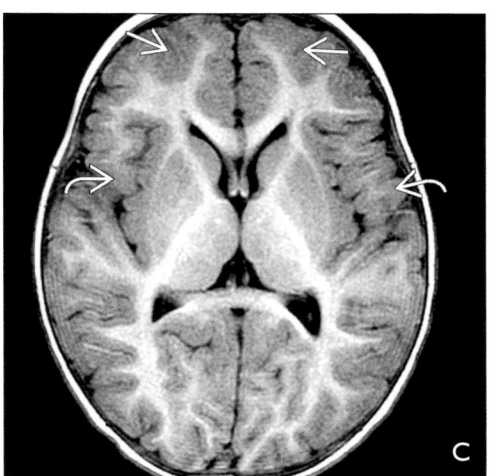

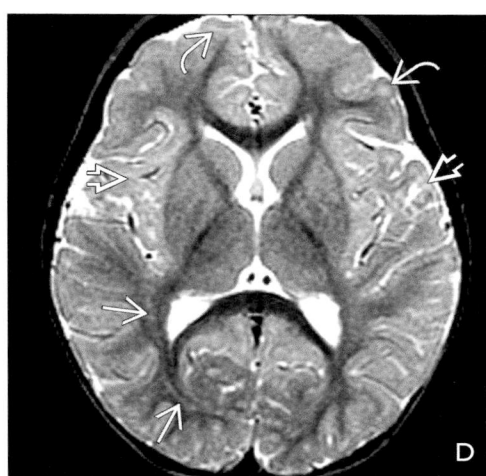

31-5C. T1WI. With the exception of the most anterior frontal ⊟➤ and superior ⊟➤ temporal lobes, the subcortical U-fibers are completely myelinated at 18 months.
31-5D. T2WI. Only the temporal ⊟➤ and frontal subcortical ➜ U-fibers remain hyperintense and unmyelinated at 18 months. Note persistent hyperintensity in the parieto-occipital association fibers ⊟➤, which often do not myelinate completely and remain hyperintense until the second or third decade.

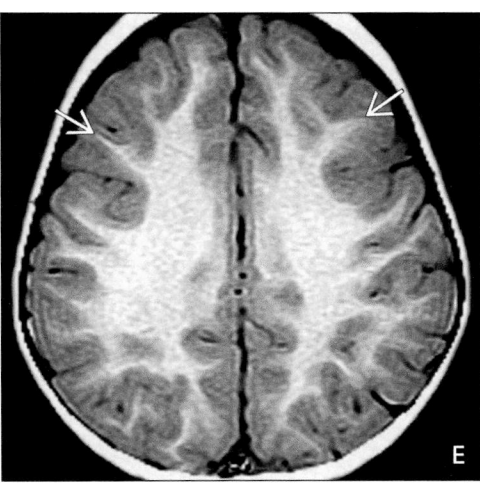

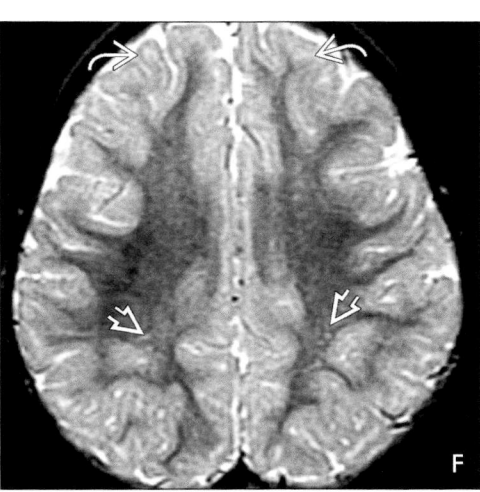

31-5E. T1WI. WM in the corona radiata now appears nearly adult-like, with hyperintensity extending into the subcortical U-fibers ⊟➤. 31-5F. T2WI. With the exception of some frontal subcortical U-fibers ➜, myelination in the corona radiata appears complete. The punctate hyperintensities in the parietal subcortical WM ⊟➤ are perivascular spaces, which are seen normally on 3.0 T MR scans in pediatric patients.

31-6A. *Axial T1WI in a normal 3 year old shows adult appearance. Cerebellar folia maturation, arborization, and myelination is complete. Note the hyperintensity in the subcortical U-fibers of the anterior temporal lobe WM ➡, indicating normal myelination.* *31-6B.* *The T2WI in this 3 year old has an adult-like appearance with myelinated (hypointense) WM in the temporal lobes ➡ and folia of the cerebellum ➡.*

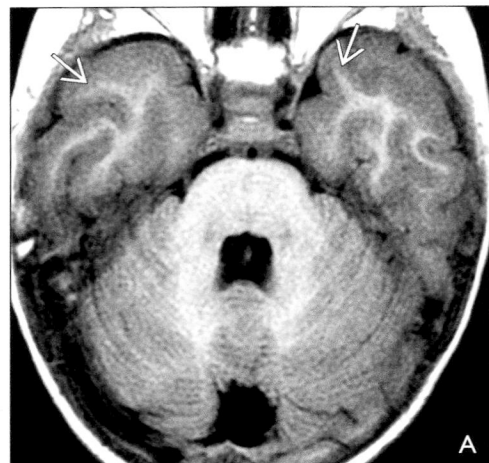

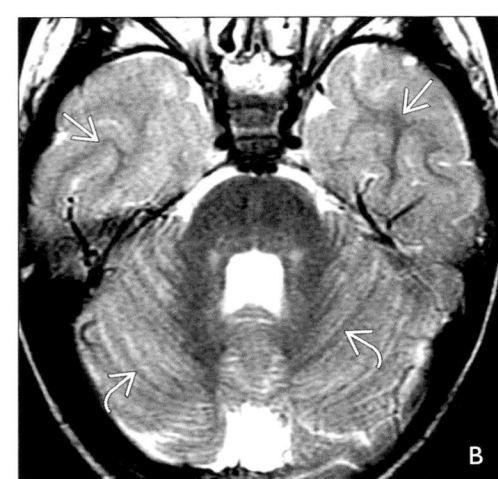

31-6C. *T1WI through the lateral ventricles shows an adult pattern of myelination extending into the frontal ➡ and temporal lobes subcortical WM ➡.* *31-6D.* *T2WI through the basal ganglia and mid-ventricular level is indistinguishable from that of an adult. Note the faint hyperintensities in the occipital radiations ➡, a normal finding.*

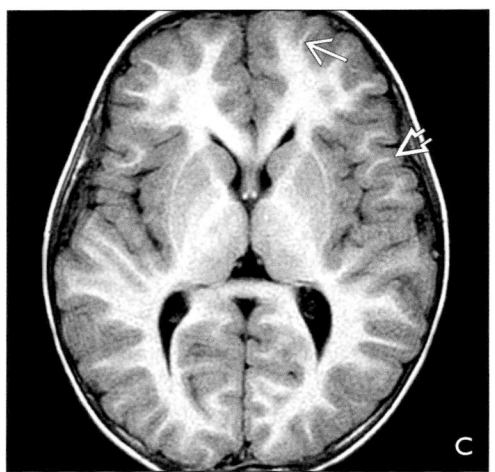

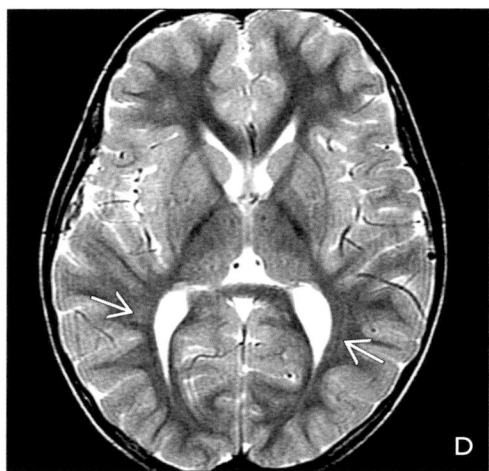

31-6E. *T1WI through the corona radiata shows that myelination is indistinguishable from that in an adult brain. Although visually complete, functional studies indicate that some degree of active myelination continues into adolescence.* *31-6F.* *T2WI. The corona radiata is hypointense except for scattered linear hyperintensities ➡ that represent interstitial fluid in the perivascular (Virchow-Robin) spaces, a normal finding.*

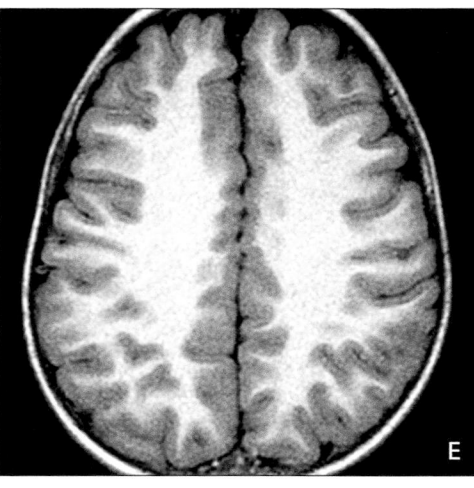

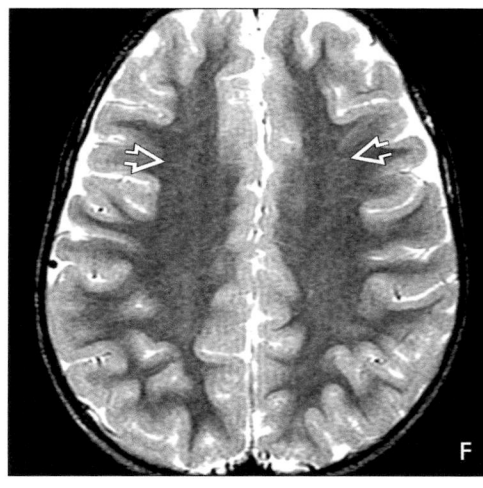

Imaging of Normal Myelination

Selected major milestones of normal myelination on T1- and T2-weighted images are summarized earlier in the chapter (Table 31-1) and discussed in greater detail here.

Birth to Three Months

T1WI. On T1-weighted sequences, the brain of a full-term infant resembles an adult's on T2WI, i.e., most of the cerebral WM has lower signal than gray matter. The dorsal brainstem, decussation of the superior cerebellar peduncles, posterior limb of the internal capsule, ventrolateral thalami, and the deep corona radiata adjacent to the lateral ventricles are the only T1 hyperintense (myelinated) structures in a normal term infant at birth (31-1).

Hyperintensity in the deep cerebellar WM starts to appear by one month and gradually extends into the folia beginning two to three months after birth.

T2WI. On T2WI, the WM of a term newborn infant resembles that of a T1 image in an adult, i.e., it has higher signal relative to gray matter. Hypointensity can be seen in the dorsal brainstem, posterior limb of the internal capsule, and ventrolateral thalamus. The dentate nuclei of the cerebellum consist of gray matter and thus also appear hypointense.

At birth, the rolandic and perirolandic gyri of the cortex appear quite hypointense. This corresponds to known early myelination of the WM within these gyri. An ill-defined "smudgy" hypointensity in the WM underlying the rolandic/perirolandic gyri also appears shortly after birth.

Three to Six Months

T1WI. The anterior limb of the internal capsule and the proximal, most central WM of the cerebellar folia become hyperintense by three postnatal months (31-2). High signal appears in the splenium of the corpus callosum (CC) by four months and can be identified in the genu at six months (31-3).

T2WI. Low signal appears in the posterior limb of the internal capsule at three months and can be seen in the CC splenium by six months. WM in the deep corona radiata extending from the motor cortex toward the lateral ventricle body myelinates early, appearing "smudgy" and slightly hypointense (31-3).

Six Months to One Year

T1WI. The WM assumes a near-adult appearance by eight months with hyperintensity extending throughout most of the cerebellum and hemispheric WM. The corona radiata is almost completely hyperintense except for its most anterior and peripheral fibers.

By 11-12 months, the WM resembles that of an adult with hyperintensity extending into most of the subcortical U-fibers. Only the anterior temporal and most peripheral frontal lobe WM remain unmyelinated, appearing isointense with the overlying cortex (31-4).

T2WI. Hypointensity appears in the corpus callosum genu by eight months and in the anterior limb of the internal capsule by 11 months. T2 hyperintensity remains in the frontal and anterior temporal subcortical WM. Low signal in the deep frontal WM appears by 14 months. Except for the most anterior temporal lobes, by 18 months, the WM assumes a near-adult appearance (31-5).

Two Years to Adulthood

T1WI. The anterior temporal lobe WM does not become completely hyperintense on T1 scans until 24-30 months (31-6). Although WM myelination is visually complete at this age, functional MR studies demonstrate that some active myelination continues well into adolescence.

T2WI. It is common to see small symmetric high signal intensity in the WM, both lateral and dorsal to the atria of the lateral ventricles. These represent "terminal zones" of incompletely myelinated brain in the parietooccipital association fibers and are considered a normal finding. These "terminal zones" often remain hyperintense on T2WI well into the second or even third decade (31-4D), (31-4F), (31-5D).

Scattered punctate and linear T2 hyperintense WM foci that suppress completely on FLAIR are also common. These are normal perivascular (Virchow-Robin) spaces and occur at all ages (31-6F).

Classification of Inherited Metabolic Disorders

Overview

The sheer number and variety of inherited metabolic disorders (IMDs) is overwhelming. New entities together with their MR findings are constantly added to the ever-growing list of these disorders. Moreover, identifying one of these elusive diseases requires not only correct interpretation of imaging features but also an understanding of clinical manifestations, genetic analysis, and specific biochemical defect(s). In some cases, brain, skin, or muscle biopsy is necessary to establish a definitive diagnosis.

An exhaustive discussion of IMDs is far beyond the scope of this book. The interested reader is referred to the superb definitive texts by A. James Barkovich. In this chapter, we consider the major as well as some of the less common but important inherited neurometabolic diseases, summarizing the pathoetiology, demographics, clinical presentation, and key imaging findings of each.

We begin by considering several approaches to classifying these unusual but fascinating disorders. One of the most common classification systems for IMDs divides these disorders according to which cellular organelle (e.g., mitochondria, lysosomes) is predominantly affected. Another characterizes them by defects in a specific metabolic pathway (e.g., disorders of carbohydrate metabolism).

We briefly discuss each of these. We then delineate—and subsequently use—an approach pioneered by A. James Barkovich that is primarily based on anatomic location and specific imaging features.

Organelle-based Approach

Three cellular organelles are primarily affected by inherited metabolic disease, i.e., the lysosomes, peroxisomes, and mitochondria. Classifying IMDs according to the affected organelle has the benefit of conceptual simplicity. However, many IMDs do not arise from disordered organelle formation or function, making this classification scheme less than comprehensive.

Lysosomal Diseases

Lysosomal disorders are characterized by abnormal lysosomes and disordered carbohydrate metabolism. The frequency of lysosomal disorders varies widely with geographic distribution. Some are far more frequent in certain locations because of the high prevalence of founder mutations.

The mucopolysaccharidoses are the classic lysosomal storage disorders. They result from deficiencies of enzymes involved in the degradation of mucopolysaccharides (glycosaminoglycans). Incompletely degraded mucopolysaccharides accumulate in the lysosomes, which often become enlarged and vacuolated. Prototypical mucopolysaccharidoses include **Hurler**, **Hunter**, **Sanfilippo**, and **Morquio** syndromes.

The gangliosidoses are rare lysosomal storage disorders characterized by deficient β-galactosidase. Abnormal oligosaccharides accumulate in the brain and viscera. Typical disorders are **GM1** and **GM2 gangliosidoses** (Tay-Sachs and Sandhoff diseases, respectively).

Peroxisomal Disorders

Peroxisomes contain multiple enzymes essential for normal growth and development. Inherited peroxisomal disorders can result in lack of organelle development or normally formed peroxisomes that nonetheless have disordered or deficient function of a single enzyme.

Deficiencies in peroxisomal formation result in syndromes such as **Zellweger syndrome**, **neonatal adrenoleukodystrophy**, and **infantile Refsum disease**. Disorders in which the peroxisomes are formed but function improperly include **X-linked adrenoleukodystrophy** and **classic Refsum disease**.

Mitochondrial Disorders

Mitochondrial disorders, also called respiratory chain disorders, are characterized by abnormal mitochondrial function. The result is impaired ATP (energy) production in affected cells.

Some mitochondrial disorders predominantly or exclusively affect striated muscle and therefore are not discussed in this text. Important mitochondrial encephalopathies include **Leigh syndrome**, **m**itochondrial **e**ncephalopathy with **l**actic **a**cidosis and **s**troke-like episodes (**MELAS**), **m**yoclonic **e**pilepsy with **r**agged **r**ed **f**ibers (**MERRF**), **Kearns-Sayre syndrome** (KSS), and **glutaric aciduria types 1 and 2**.

ORGANELLE-BASED CLASSIFICATION OF IMDs

Lysosomal Disorders
- Mucopolysaccharidoses
- Gangliosidoses
- Metachromatic leukodystrophy
- Krabbe disease
- Fabry disease

Peroxisomal Disorders
- Abnormal peroxisomal formation
  - Zellweger syndrome
  - Neonatal adrenoleukodystrophy
  - Infantile Refsum disease
- Abnormal peroxisomal function
  - X-linked adrenoleukodystrophy
  - Classic Refsum disease

Mitochondrial Disorders
- Leigh syndrome
- MELAS
- MERRF
- Kearns-Sayre
- Glutaric aciduria types 1 and 2

Metabolic Approach

Many IMDs result in accumulation of one or more abnormal metabolites such as ammonia, copper, or iron degradation products. These IMDs are summarized below and discussed in more detail later in the chapter.

Organic/Aminoacidopathies and Urea Cycle Disorders

The aminoacidopathies and urea cycle disorders result from disrupted nitrogen elimination and are characterized by hyperammonemia and elevated glutamine levels. Typical urea cycle disorders include **maple syrup urine disease**, **methylmalonic acidemia**, **ornithine transcarbamylase deficiency**, and **citrullinemia**.

Canavan disease is characterized by N-acetyl-L-aspartate (NAA) aciduria and NAA accumulation in the brain, which causes striking spongy degeneration.

Alexander disease results from mutations in the gene that encodes glial fibrillary acidic protein (GFAP). Massive accumulation of Rosenthal fibers in astrocytes results in macrocephaly and a paucity of myelin in the frontal white matter.

Disorders of Copper Metabolism

Copper is an essential trace element required by all living organisms. However, excessive amounts of copper damages cells. Disruptions to normal copper homeostasis are the hallmarks of three genetic disorders: **Wilson disease**, **Menkes disease**, and **occipital horn disease**.

Brain Iron Accumulation Disorders

Iron accumulates within the basal ganglia and dentate nuclei during normal aging. A group of genetic disorders termed **n**eurodegeneration with **b**rain **i**ron **a**ccumulation (**NBIA**) are characterized by brain iron deposition in abnormal amounts and in abnormal locations. Neuronal death results.

Imaging-based Approach

Barkovich et al. have elaborated a practical imaging-based approach to the diagnosis of IMDs derived from the seminal work of van der Knaap and Valk. This approach is based on determining whether the disease involves primarily or exclusively (1) white matter, (2) mostly gray matter, or (3) both.

In this text, we follow a classification based on these three categories of predominant imaging features. General findings for each individual category are delineated at the beginning of each section. We then discuss the major diagnostic entities in each imaging-based group.

IMDs Predominantly Affecting White Matter

The white matter (WM) disorders (leukodystrophies) are sometimes divided into two categories: (1) *dys*myelinating disorders (i.e., normal myelination does not occur) and (2) *de*myelinating disease (i.e., myelin forms nor-

mally and is deposited around axons but later breaks down or is destroyed).

A third, relatively new category of leukodystrophy consists of (3) *hypo*myelinating diseases (here the WM may partially myelinate but never myelinates completely). Hypomyelinating leukoencephalopathies are an uncommon group of genetic disorders that cause delayed myelin maturation or undermyelination.

From an imaging perspective, it can be difficult to determine whether a disorder is *dys*myelinating, *de*myelinating, or *hypo*myelinating. A more practical imaging-based approach is to determine whether the disorder primarily affects *deep* (periventricular) WM or the *subcortical* short association fibers (U-fibers). In a few diseases, both the deep and peripheral WM are affected.

Examples of leukodystrophies that exhibit *deep* WM predominance include metachromatic leukodystrophy and X-linked adrenoleukodystrophy. Leukodystrophies that involve the *subcortical* U-fibers early in the disease course include megaloencephalic leukoencephalopathy with cysts and infantile Alexander disease. Both also present with a large head.

Diseases in which virtually *all* the WM (both periventricular *and* subcortical) remains unmyelinated are rare. The imaging appearance in these disorders resembles that of a normal newborn brain with immature, almost completely unmyelinated WM. Here the entire WM—including the subcortical U-fibers—appears uniformly hyperintense on T2WI.

Periventricular White Matter Predominance

The prototypical disorder that typically begins with symmetric deep WM involvement and spares the subcortical U-fibers until late in the disease course is metachromatic leukodystrophy. Others with a similar pattern of periventricular predominance include Krabbe disease (globoid cell leukodystrophy), X-linked adrenoleukodystrophy, and vanishing white matter (VWM) disease.

MAJOR IMDs WITH PERIVENTRICULAR WM PREDOMINANCE

Common
- Metachromatic leukodystrophy
- Classic X-linked adrenoleukodystrophy

Less Common
- Globoid cell leukodystrophy (Krabbe disease)
- Vanishing white matter disease

Rare but Important
- Phenylketonuria
- Maple syrup urine disease
- Merosin-deficient congenital muscular dystrophy

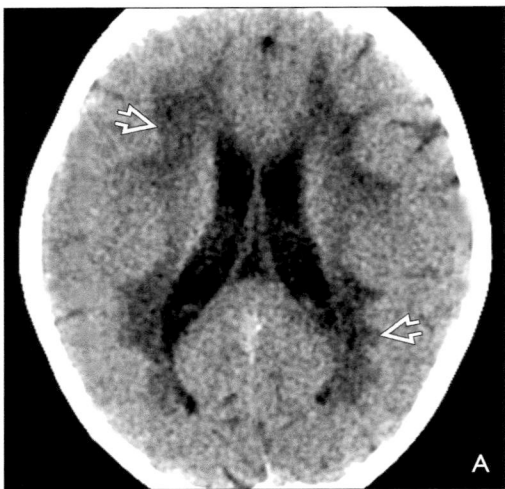

31-7A. NECT in a 6 yo boy with ALD shows symmetric periventricular WM hypodensity ➡ with noticeable sparing of the subcortical U-fibers.

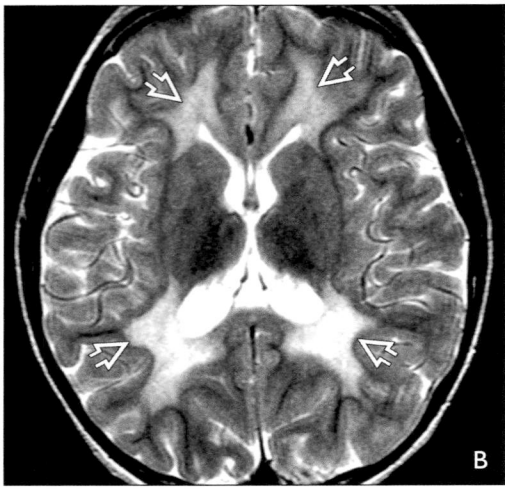

31-7B. T2WI shows the classic "butterfly" pattern of symmetric hyperintensities around the frontal horns and atria of the lateral ventricles ➡.

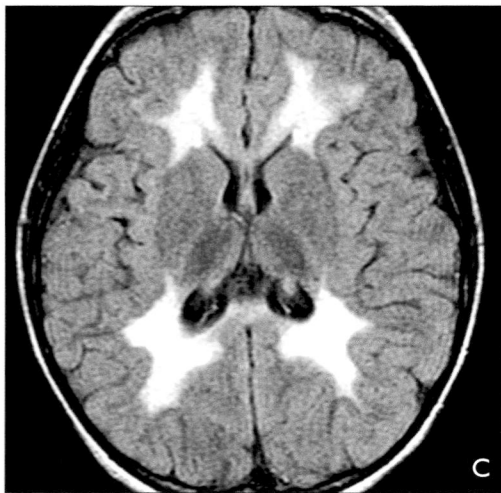

31-7C. FLAIR shows the "butterfly" pattern of MLD. The internal capsules and subcortical WM appear normal.

Metachromatic Leukodystrophy

TERMINOLOGY. Metachromatic leukodystrophy (MLD), also known as sulfatide lipoidosis, is a devastating lysosomal storage disease characterized by intralysosomal accumulation of sphingolipid sulfatide in multiple tissues.

ETIOLOGY. MLD is caused by decreased arylsulfatase A with failure of myelin breakdown and reutilization.

PATHOLOGY. Grossly, a brain affected by MLD may be normal or demonstrate mild volume loss. The periventricular WM shows a grayish discoloration with relatively normal-appearing subcortical U-fibers.

Demyelination is the main histopathological feature and affects both the central and peripheral nervous systems. Characteristic brownish metachromasia (for which the disorder is named) is seen with acidic cresyl violet stain and represents intracellular deposits of cholesterol, phospholipids, and sulfatides. Tissue assays for arylsulfatase A are positive.

CLINICAL ISSUES. MLD is one of the most common of all inherited WM disorders with a prevalence of 1:100,000 live births. MLD is most common in Habbani Jews and Navajo Indians.

The initial signs of MLD may appear at any age. Three clinical forms are currently recognized: Late infantile (onset earlier than three years), juvenile (onset earlier than 16 years), and adult MLD. The infantile form is the most common and typically presents in the second year of life with visuomotor impairment, gait disorder, and abdominal pain. Progressive decline and death within four years is typical. The juvenile form presents between 5-10 years, often with deteriorating school performance. Survival beyond 20 years is rare. The adult form may present with early-onset dementia, MS-like symptoms, and progressive cerebellar signs.

Established treatment options include hematopoietic stem cell transplantation. Therapies such as enzyme replacement and gene therapy with oligodendroglial or neural progenitor cells are still experimental.

IMAGING. The imaging hallmark of MLD is a rapidly progressive leukodystrophy. Serial CT scans show centrifugal spread of confluent hypodensity with the corpus callosum splenium and parietooccipital periventricular WM initially affected. The disease gradually extends into the frontal and then the temporal WM.

The typical MR appearance is confluent, symmetric, butterfly-shaped T2/FLAIR hyperintensity in the periventricular WM (**31-7**). The subcortical U-fibers and cerebellum are typically spared until late in the disease.

Islands of normal myelin around medullary veins in the WM may produce a striking "tiger" or "leopard" pattern with linear hypointensities in a sea of confluent hyperintensity (31-8). No enhancement is seen on T1 C+. A few cases of MLD have been reported with enlarged, enhancing cranial nerves and/or cauda equina nerve roots.

Restricted diffusion is common. MRS typically shows elevated choline with variable increase in myoinositol.

DIFFERENTIAL DIAGNOSIS. The major differential diagnosis of MLD includes other IMDs that primarily affect the periventricular WM. Globoid cell leukoencephalopathy (**Krabbe disease**) shows bithalamic hyperdensities on NECT scans, involves the cerebellum early, and often demonstrates enlarged optic nerves and chiasm.

Pelizaeus-Merzbacher disease usually presents in neonates and shows almost total lack of myelination. The cerebellum is often markedly atrophic. **Vanishing white matter disease** begins in the periventricular WM but eventually involves all the hemispheric white matter. VWM often cavitates and does not enhance.

METACHROMATIC LEUKODYSTROPHY

Etiology and Pathology
- Lysosomal storage disorder
- Decreased arylsulfatase A → sphingolipid accumulation
- Periventricular demyelination

Clinical Issues
- Most common inherited leukodystrophy
- 3 forms
  - Late infantile (most common)
  - Juvenile
  - Adult (late onset)

Imaging
- Centrifugal spread of demyelination
  - Starts in corpus callosum splenium, deep parietooccipital WM
  - Frontal, temporal WM affected later
  - Spares subcortical U-fibers, cerebellum
- Classic = "butterfly" pattern
  - Symmetric hyperintensities around frontal horns, atria
- "Tiger" pattern
  - "Stripes" of perivenular myelin sparing in WM

Differential Diagnosis
- Other disorders that predominantly affect periventricular WM
  - Globoid cell leukodystrophy (Krabbe disease)
  - Pelizaeus-Merzbacher disease
  - Vanishing white matter disease
- Destructive disorders
  - Periventricular leukomalacia

X-Linked Adrenoleukodystrophy

TERMINOLOGY. X-linked adrenoleukodystrophy (X-ALD) was called "bronze" Schilder disease and "melanodermic type leukodystrophy" before its adrenal involvement was recognized.

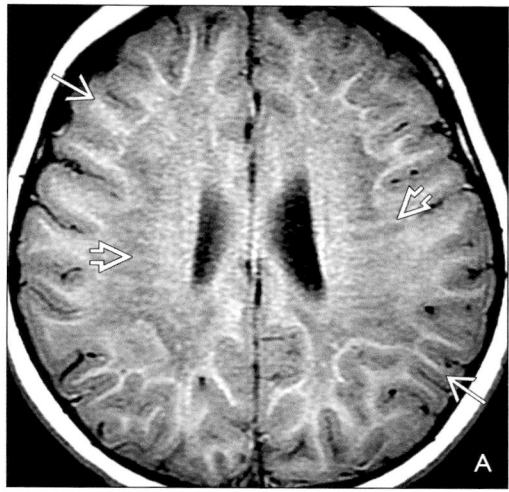

31-8A. Classic MLD in a 2 yo boy. Note sparing of subcortical U-fibers ➤, preserved islands of myelin surrounding venules ("tiger" pattern) ➤.

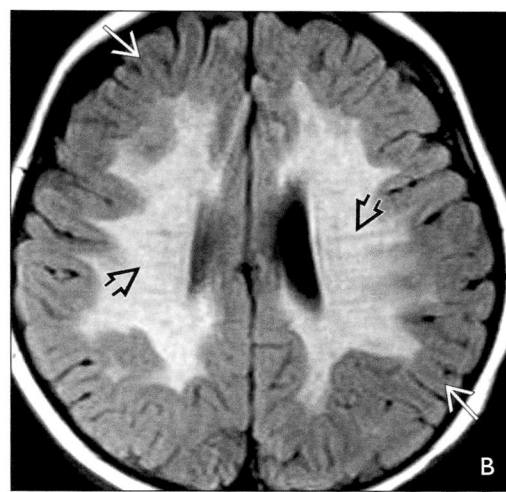

31-8B. FLAIR shows hyperintense confluent demyelination, preserved myelin ➤ ("tiger" pattern). Note sparing of subcortical U-fibers ➤.

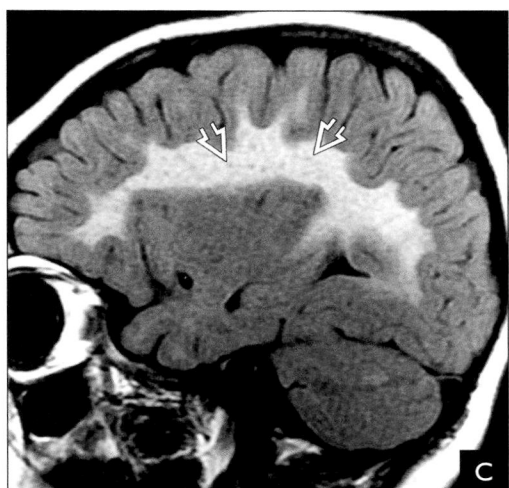

31-8C. FLAIR shows dots ("leopard" pattern) of preserved myelin ➤ within confluent deep WM demyelination that spares subcortical U-fibers.

ETIOLOGY. Adrenoleukodystrophy (ALD) is an inherited peroxisomal disorder caused by mutations in the gene *ABCD1*. Abnormal peroxisome metabolism results in impaired β-oxidation of very long chain fatty acids (VLCFAs). VLCFAs accumulate in the white matter, causing a severe inflammatory demyelination. Axonal degeneration in the posterior fossa and spinal cord are also typical of the disease.

PATHOLOGY. Three distinct zones of myelin loss are seen in ALD (31-9). The innermost zone consists of a necrotic core with astrogliosis. An intermediate zone of active demyelination and perivascular inflammation lies just outside the necrotic, "burned out" core of the lesion. The most peripheral zone consists of ongoing demyelination without inflammatory changes (31-10).

CLINICAL ISSUES. X-ALD is the most common single protein or enzyme deficiency disease to present in childhood. The estimated incidence is 1:20,000-50,000.

Several clinical forms of ALD and related disorders have been described. **Classic X-linked ALD** is the most common form (45%) and is seen almost exclusively in boys 5-12 years of age. Behavioral difficulties and deteriorating school performance are common. Approximately 10% of affected patients present acutely with seizures, adrenal crisis, acute encephalopathy, or coma.

Adrenomyeloneuropathy (AMN) is the second most common type (35%). It is another X-linked disorder that occurs primarily in males. Peak presentation is 20-35 years, later than in classic X-ALD. AMN is characterized by axonal degeneration in the brainstem and spinal cord.

Approximately 20% of X-ALD patients exhibit isolated adrenal insufficiency (**Addison disease**). Neurologic involvement is absent. Other less common forms of ALD include adolescent and adult-onset ALD and mild symptomatic disease in female carriers.

Untreated X-ALD carries a dismal prognosis. Relentless progression with spastic quadriparesis, blindness, deafness, and vegetative state is typical. Dietary intake of Lorenzo's oil (a mixture of triolein and trierucin) has helped mitigate symptoms in some patients. Early bone marrow transplantation or hematopoietic stem cell gene therapy has improved clinical outcome for others.

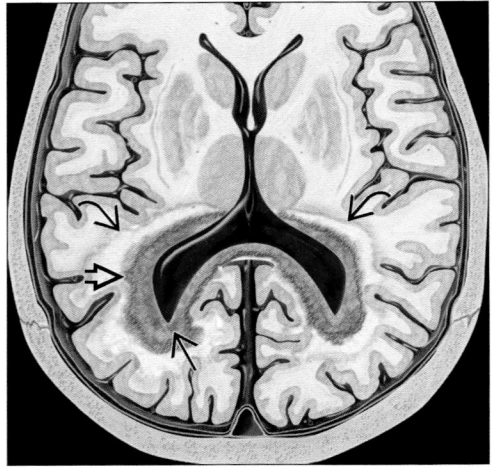
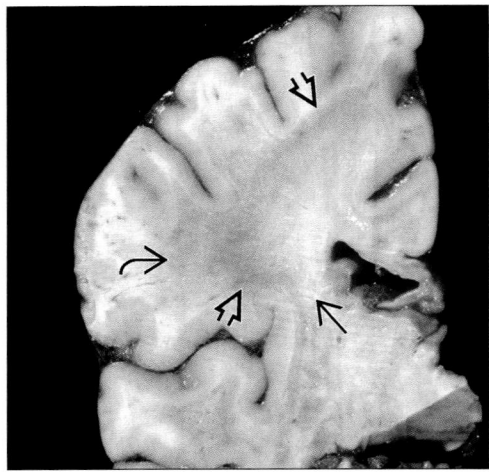
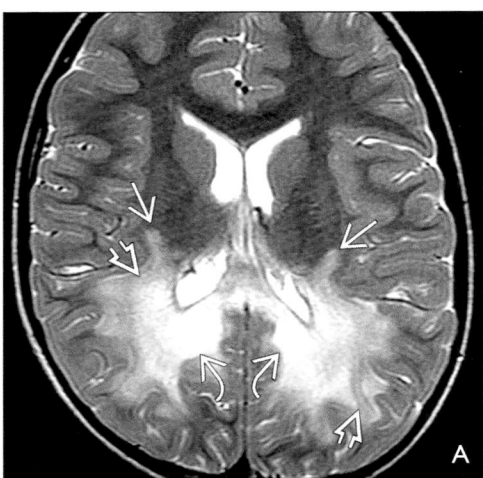
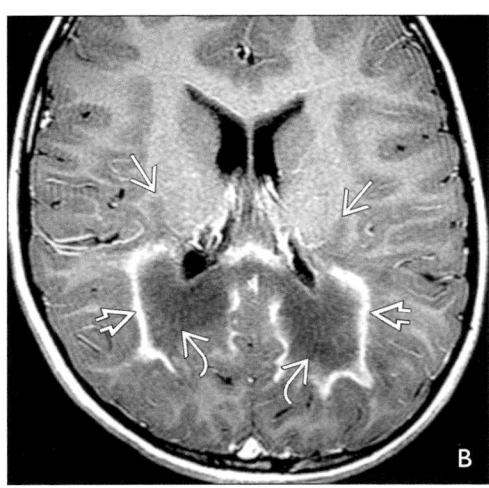

31-9. Graphic depicts distinct zones in adrenoleukodystrophy. The deepest zone is the "burned out" core ➡; the intermediate zone ⧫ shows active demyelination and inflammation; and the advancing edge ⧫ displays ongoing demyelination without inflammation. 31-10. Coronal autopsy section of X-ALD shows the 3 zones of myelin loss: "Burned out" core ➡, intermediate zone (grayish region ⧫), advancing edge (yellowish discoloration ⧫). (Courtesy AFIP Archives.)

31-11A. Classic X-ALD. Symmetric lesions surround the atria. The most hyperintense is the "burned out" core ➡. The layer of active demyelination with inflammation surrounding the core is less hyperintense ⧫. The most peripheral or leading edge zone ➡ shows ongoing demyelination without inflammatory changes. 31-11B. The intermediate zone of active demyelination enhances on T1 C+ FS ⧫, whereas the leading edge ➡ and central core ➡ do not.

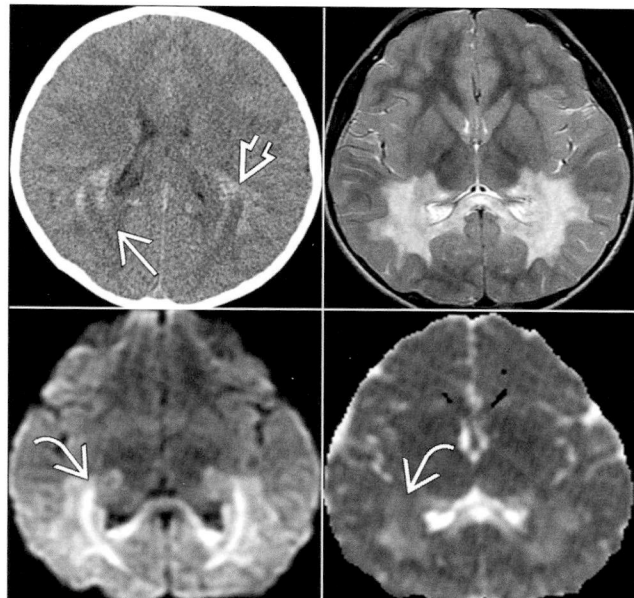

31-12. Classic ALD shows periatrial WM hypodensity ➡, calcifications ➡, and diffusion restriction ➡ in the actively demyelinating, inflammatory regions.

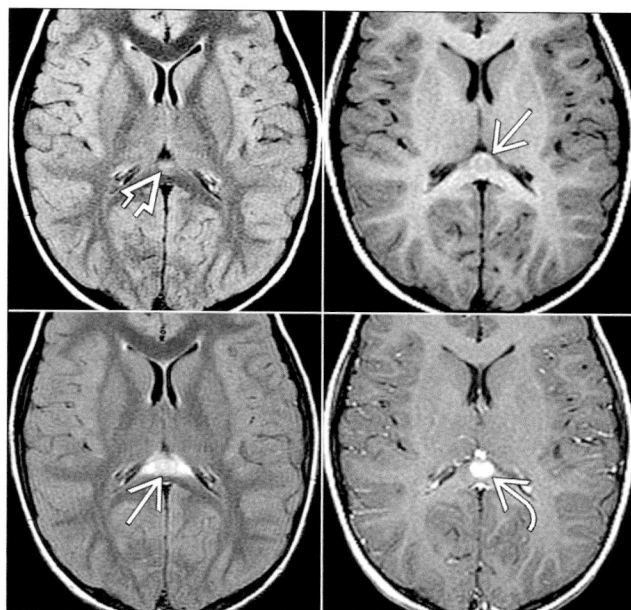

31-13. FLAIR (upper left) in a 5 yo boy with early ALD shows a small hyperintense focus in the splenium ➡. Six months later, T1WI (upper right), FLAIR (lower left) show the increasing size of the lesion ➡. T1 C+ (lower right) shows enhancement ➡.

IMAGING. The definitive diagnosis of X-ALD is established by tissue assays for increased amounts of VLCFAs. When typical, imaging findings can be strongly suggestive of the diagnosis. Although CT scans are sometimes obtained as an initial screening study in children with encephalopathy of unknown origin, MR is the procedure of choice.

CT findings. NECT scans demonstrate hypodensity in the corpus callosum splenium and WM around the atria and occipital horns of the lateral ventricles. Calcification in the affected WM is common **(31-12)**. CECT may show enhancement around the central hypodense WM.

MR findings. A *posterior-predominant* pattern is seen in 80% of patients with X-ALD **(31-11)**. The earliest finding is T2/FLAIR hyperintensity in the middle of the corpus callosum splenium **(31-13)**. As the disease progresses, hyperintensity spreads from posterior to anterior and from the center to the periphery. The peritrigonal WM, corticospinal tracts, fornix, commissural fibers, plus the visual and auditory pathways can all eventually become involved.

The leading edge of demyelination appears hyperintense on T1WI but does not enhance. The intermediate zone of active inflammatory demyelination often enhances on T1 C+.

Diffusion restriction in the intermediate zone of inflammatory demyelination may be present on DWI. MRS shows decreased NAA even in normal-appearing WM. Elevated choline, myoinositol, and lactate are common.

An MR-based visual scoring system (the Loes scale) divides the brain into nine regions with 23 subregions. Each region is scored for the presence (1) or absence (0) of atrophy, and every subregion is assessed as normal (0), unilateral abnormality (0.5), or bilateral abnormalities (1) in signal intensity.

Variant imaging patterns of X-linked ALDs are common. Approximately 10-15% of all patients with classic X-ALD have an *anterior predominant* demyelination; hyperintensity initially appears in the corpus callosum genu (not the splenium) and spreads into the frontal lobe WM **(31-14)**. Unusual reported patterns include unilateral disease, disease with both bioccipital and bifrontal lesions, and a variant that involves only the internal capsules.

Imaging findings in patients with adrenomyeloneuropathy vary from those of patients with classic X-ALD. The cerebral hemispheres are relatively spared with predominant involvement of the cerebellum, corticospinal tracts, and spinal cord **(31-15)**. Enhancement is typically absent.

DIFFERENTIAL DIAGNOSIS. When X-ALD presents in patients of classic age and gender (i.e., 5 to 12-year-old boys) and with typical posterior predominance on imaging studies, the differential diagnosis is very limited. **Leukoencephalopathy with brainstem/spinal cord involvement and high lactate (LBSL)** may resemble ALD but has a different clinical presentation and is caused by homozygous mutation in the *DARS2* gene.

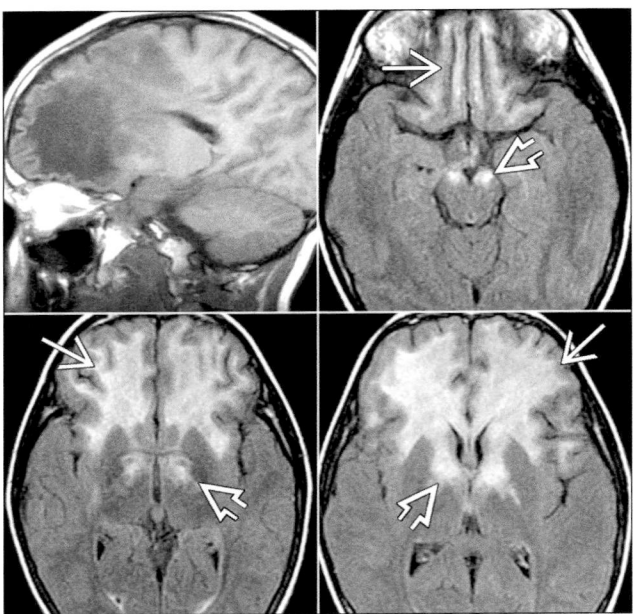

31-14. *Scans of a patient with variant ALD show symmetric confluent frontal lesions* 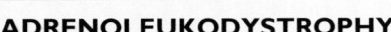 *with sparing of parietooccipital WM. Note involvement of internal capsules, cerebral peduncles* ➡.

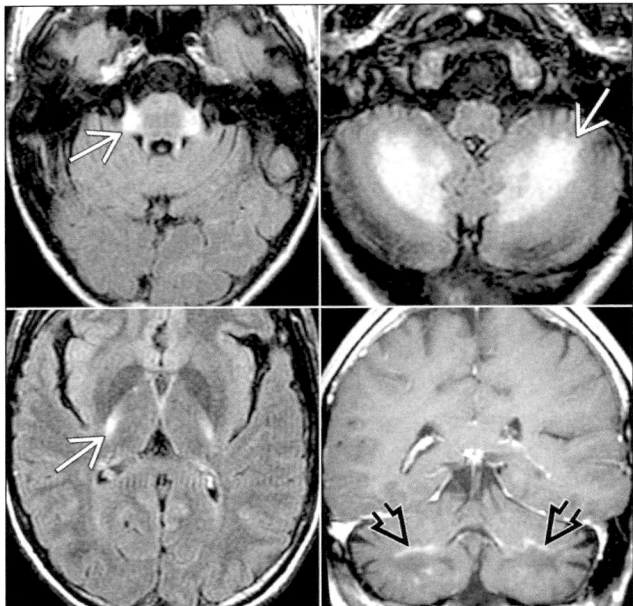

31-15. *Symmetric lesions in the cerebellar WM, lateral pons, both CNs V, superior cerebellar peduncles, internal capsules* ➡ *are seen in a 33-year-old woman with adrenomyeloneuropathy. Note peripheral enhancement of cerebellar lesions* ➡.

ADRENOLEUKODYSTROPHY

Etiology
- Peroxisomal disorder
- Impaired oxidation of VLCFAs

Pathology
- Severe inflammatory demyelination
- 3 zones
  - Necrotic "burned out" core
  - Intermediate zone of active demyelination + inflammation
  - Peripheral demyelination without inflammation

Clinical Issues
- Classic X-linked ALD
  - Most common form (45%)
  - Pre-teen males
  - Deteriorating cognition, school performance
- Adrenomyeloneuropathy (AMN)
  - Second most common form (35%)
  - Most common in males
- Addison disease without CNS involvement (20%)

Imaging
- X-linked ALD posterior predominance in 80%
  - Earliest finding: Corpus callosum splenium hyperintensity
  - Spreads posterior to anterior, center to periphery
  - Intermediate zone often enhances, restricts
- Variant patterns
  - X-linked ALD with anterior predominance (10-15%)
  - AMN involves corticospinal tracts, cerebellum, cord > hemispheric WM

Differential Diagnosis
- X-linked ALD pathognomonic if gender, age, imaging findings classic

---

Globoid Cell Leukodystrophy (Krabbe Disease)

TERMINOLOGY. Globoid cell leukodystrophy (GLD) is also commonly known as Krabbe disease. GLD is characterized by the presence of unique "globoid" cells in the demyelinating lesions.

ETIOLOGY AND PATHOLOGY. GLD is an autosomal recessive lysosomal storage disease caused by deficiency of the enzyme galactocerebroside β-galactosidase. Faulty galactose cleavage results in progressive psychosine accumulation in large ("globoid") multinucleated epithelioid cells. Because psychosine is especially toxic to oligodendrocytes, the result is severe oligodendrocyte destruction with myelin loss.

Both the central and peripheral nervous systems are affected. The brain demonstrates variable degrees of volume loss with WM thinning, dilated ventricles, and enlarged sulci. The periventricular WM shows grayish discoloration. The subcortical U-fibers are typically spared. The optic and peripheral nerves can appear enlarged and fibrotic.

Typical histopathologic findings are extensive WM demyelination and gliosis with numerous conspicuous PAS-positive multinucleated macrophages ("globoid" cells). Electron microscopy shows dense crystalloid inclusions of galactocerebroside.

CLINICAL ISSUES. GLD is a panethnic disease with an 80% female prevalence. Infantile, juvenile, and adult forms are recognized. The infantile form is the most common, typically presenting between three and six months with extreme irritability and feeding difficulties. Neonatal GLD is rapidly progressive and almost invariably fatal.

Until recently, no treatment for GLD existed. Hematopoietic stem cell transplantation has mitigated the effects of enzyme deficiency in some cases.

IMAGING. NECT scans can be helpful in the diagnosis of GLD **(31-16)**, unlike most other leukodystrophies. Bilaterally symmetric calcifications in the thalami, basal ganglia, internal capsule, corticospinal tracts, and dentate nuclei of the cerebellum can sometimes be identified even prior to the development of visible abnormalities on standard MR sequences.

Classic MR findings in GLD are corticospinal tract hyperintensity on T2/FLAIR with confluent symmetric demyelination in the deep periventricular WM. The subcortical U-fibers are typically spared. Bithalamic hypointensity on T2WI is common.

Diffusion tensor imaging (DTI) may demonstrate reduced fractional anisotropy in the corticospinal tracts before other abnormalities appear. MRS findings of elevated choline and decreased NAA in the hemispheric WM are characteristic but nonspecific.

Krabbe disease is one of the few leukodystrophies in which cerebellar findings appear early in the disease course. Alternating "halo" or ring-like hypointensities on T1WI and hyperintensities on T2WI can be identified in the cerebellar WM surrounding the dentate nuclei **(31-17)**.

Another distinctive feature of GLD is enlargement of the intracranial optic nerves and chiasm. Diffusely enlarged, enhancing cranial nerves and cauda equina nerve roots have also been reported in GLD.

DIFFERENTIAL DIAGNOSIS. While the histopathology of GLD is unique and virtually pathognomonic of the disease, the imaging differential diagnosis of GLD includes other leukodystrophies with periventricular WM predominance. The WM changes in **metachromatic leukodystrophy** and **vanishing white matter disease** may initially appear quite similar, but these disorders lack the basal ganglia/thalamic calcifications typical of GLD.

Other lysosomal storage disorders that can mimic GLD include neuronal ceroid lipofuscinosis and the GM2 gangliosidoses. **Neuronal ceroid lipofuscinosis** (also known as Batten disease) can have hyperdense thalami on NECT. "Classic" infantile **GM2 gangliosidosis** (Tay-Sachs disease) shows similar thalamic hypointensity on T2WI. Late-onset GM2 shows progressive cerebellar atrophy.

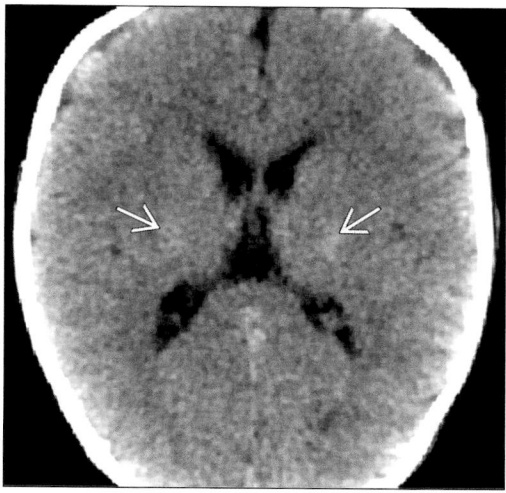

31-16. NECT in an 18 month old with infantile GLD shows symmetric hyperdensities in both thalami ➡.

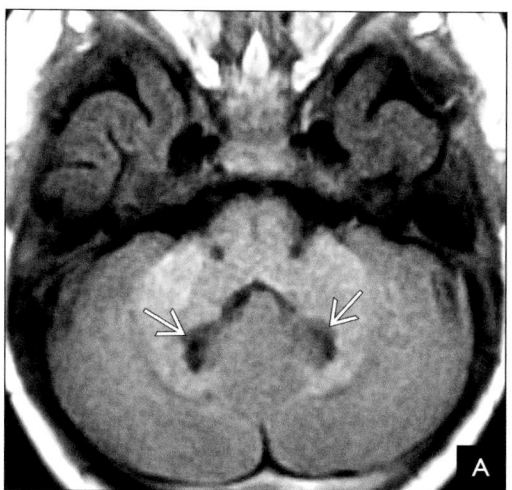

31-17A. T1WI in a 6 month old with GLD shows striking hypointensity in the dentate nuclei ➡.

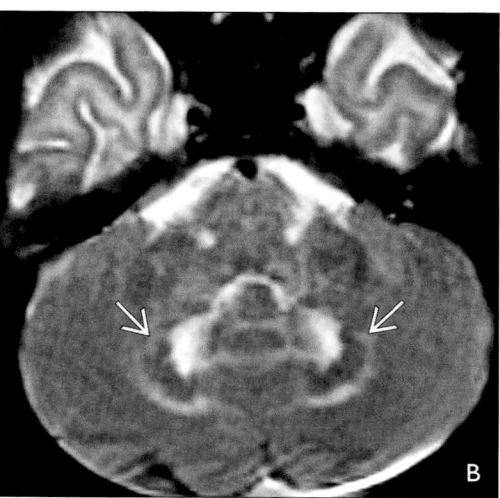

31-17B. T2WI shows the classic rings or "halos" of alternating hyper-, hypointensities ➡ *characteristic of Krabbe disease.*

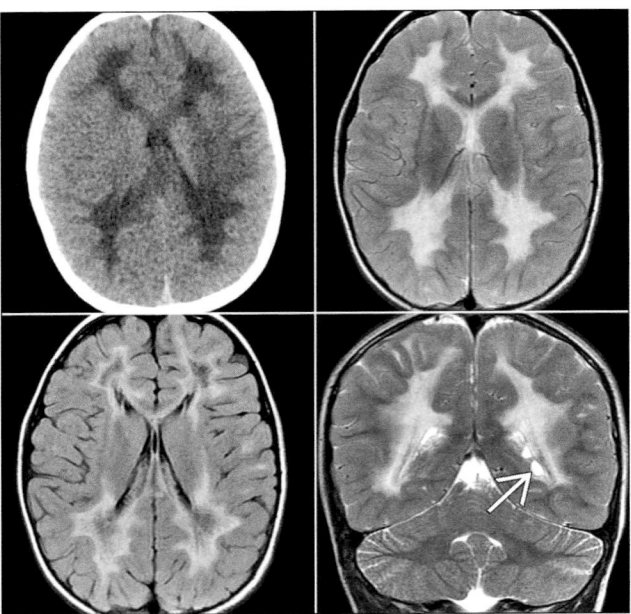

31-18. *Vanishing white matter disease in a 5-year-old boy, originally diagnosed as having MLD. Note the symmetric periventricular disease, spared U-fibers, early cyst formation* ➔. *(Courtesy S. Harder, MD.)*

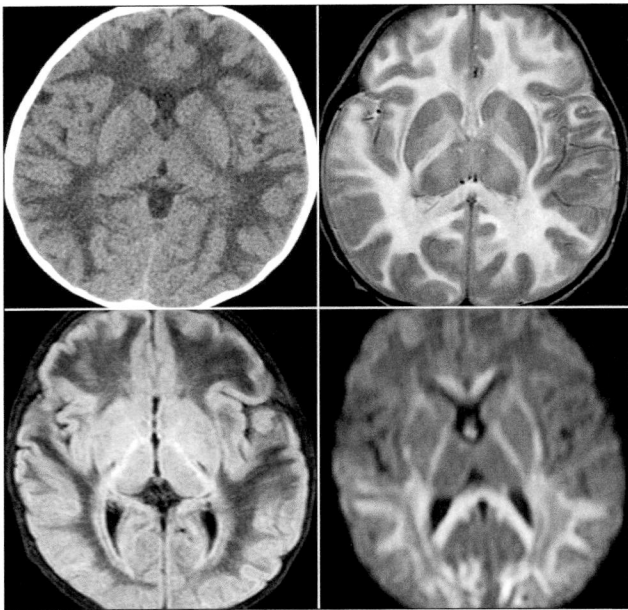

31-19. *Cree leukoencephalopathy (now recognized as a severe variant of vanishing white matter disease) in an 8 month old shows nearly complete lack of myelination.*

GLOBOID CELL LEUKODYSTROPHY (KRABBE DISEASE)

Etiology and Pathology
- Lysosomal storage disease
- Galactocerebroside β-galactosidase deficiency
- Psychosine accumulation in "globoid" cells
- Highly toxic to oligodendrocytes

Clinical Issues
- Female (80%)
- 3 forms
  - Infantile (majority)
  - Juvenile
  - Adult (rare)

Imaging
- NECT: Basal ganglia, thalamic Ca++
- MR
  - Periventricular WM, corticospinal hyperintensity
  - Subcortical U-fibers spared
  - Alternating "halos" around dentate nuclei
  - Optic nerve/chiasm enlarged ± other CNs

Differential Diagnosis
- Other disorders with periventricular WM predominance
  - Metachromatic leukodystrophy
  - Vanishing WM disease
- Other lysosomal storage diseases
  - Neuronal ceroid lipofuscinosis
  - GM2 gangliosidosis

Vanishing White Matter Disease

TERMINOLOGY. Vanishing white matter (VWM) disease, formerly termed childhood ataxia with CNS hypomyelination (CACH), is an unusual leukoencephalopathy characterized by diffusely abnormal white matter that literally "vanishes" over time. Cree leukoencephalopathy—once considered a separate entity—is now recognized as an early-onset, especially severe form of VWM.

ETIOLOGY. VWM is an autosomal recessive disorder caused by point mutations in the *eIF2B* gene, which plays an essential role in the initiation of messenger RNA translation to protein, particularly following exposure to physiological stressors (e.g., heat, trauma, infection). This results in deficient protein recycling and intracellular accumulation of denatured proteins.

PATHOLOGY. The deep frontoparietal WM is most severely affected with relatively lesser involvement of the temporal lobes. The basal ganglia, corpus callosum, anterior commissure, and internal capsules are characteristically spared. The gross appearance of the affected WM varies from grayish gelatinous discoloration to areas of cystic degeneration with frank cavitation.

VWM predominantly affects oligodendrocytes and astrocytes with relative sparing of neurons. Microscopic findings include myelin pallor, thinned myelin sheaths, vacuolation, and cystic changes. Paradoxical increase in oligodendrocytes can be seen in some areas with marked loss in others.

CLINICAL ISSUES. Classic VWM presents in children two to five years of age. Development is initially normal, but progressive motor and cognitive impairment with cerebellar and pyramidal signs follows. Death by adolescence is typical.

Cree leukoencephalopathy is an especially severe, rapidly progressive form of VWM that affects infants

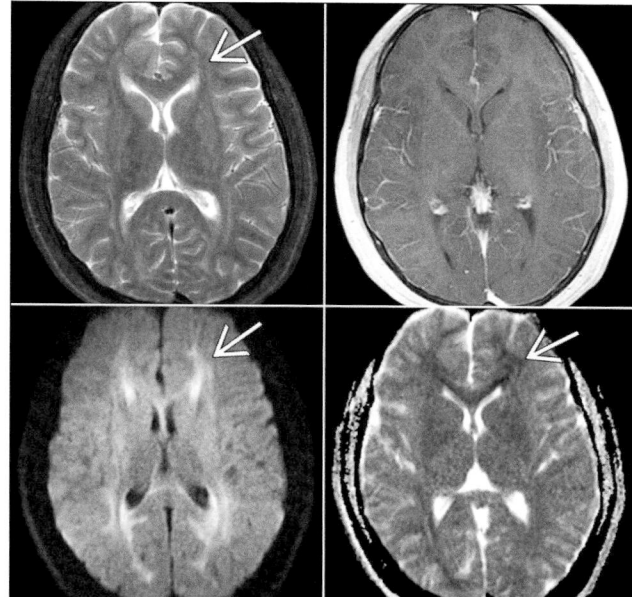

31-20. *Thirteen-year-old girl with PKU, mild cognitive impairment. Periventricular WM hyperintensity* ➡ *shows no enhancement but does restrict on DWI.*

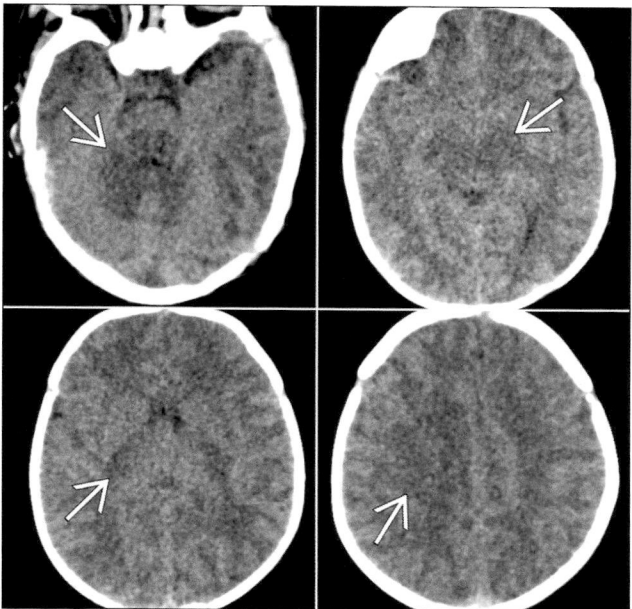

31-21. *NECT in a 13-day-old boy with MSUD shows edema* ➡ *in the dorsal midbrain and cerebellar WM, cerebral peduncles, internal capsules, hemispheres.*

between the ages of three and nine months and is invariably fatal by 21 months of age **(31-19)**.

Approximately 15% of VWM cases occur in adolescents and adults. Mean age of late-onset VWM is 30 years. Learning disabilities with insidious, protracted cognitive impairment is typical. Stress-induced rapid neurologic deterioration with death is common.

IMAGING. Extensive confluent WM T1 hypointensity with T2/FLAIR hyperintensity is typical. The disease is initially periventricular but later spreads to involve the subcortical arcuate fibers. Over time, the affected WM undergoes rarefaction. Cavitary foci of CSF-like signal intensity may develop **(31-18)**. Diffuse volume loss with enlarged ventricles and sulci is seen on serial studies. VWM does not enhance.

Decreased diffusivity in normal-appearing WM may be an early marker of brain degeneration in VWM. Decreased NAA, Cho, and Cr with normal myoinositol are seen on MRS and reflect early WM degeneration without reactive gliosis.

DIFFERENTIAL DIAGNOSIS. VWM is not the only leukoencephalopathy that causes "melting away" or "vanishing" of the cerebral WM. Alexander disease and mitochondrial encephalopathies can be associated with WM rarefaction and cystic degeneration. **Alexander disease** presents with macrocephaly. Frontal WM cysts can occur in end-stage disease. Approximately 10% of **mitochondrial encephalopathies** predominantly affect the WM and may form cavitations.

Globoid cell leukodystrophy (or **Krabbe disease**) may resemble severe VWM clinically, but the imaging findings of basal ganglia/thalamic calcifications and cerebellar "halos" help distinguish GLD from VWM.

Phenylketonuria

Phenylketonuria (PKU) is the most common inborn error of amino acid metabolism and caused by mutations in the phenylalanine hydroxylase (*PAH*) gene, which is mapped to chromosome 12q24.1. Elevated levels of phenylalanine (Phe) are toxic to the developing brain.

In the past, PKU was diagnosed by the presence of hyperphenylalaninemia and "musty-smelling" urine. Most PKU cases are now diagnosed through newborn screening programs. Untreated PKU causes severe mental retardation and global developmental delay. Dietary control mitigates the disease, and patients who are treated early may develop only minor cognitive impairment.

Imaging studies show T2/FLAIR hyperintensity in the periventricular WM, particularly in the frontal and peritrigonal regions **(31-20)**. The peripheral subcortical arcuate fibers are typically spared. PKU does not enhance following contrast administration. Mild restricted diffusion can be present on DWI. MRS typically shows a Phe peak resonating at 7.37 ppm.

Maple Syrup Urine Disease

Maple syrup urine disease (MSUD), also known as leucine encephalopathy, is an autosomal recessive disorder of branched-chain amino acid (leucine, isoleucine, valine) metabolism. Decreased activity of the branched

31-22A. *Axial T1WI in an infant who was normal at birth but developed seizures at 28 days. Note the hypodensity in the cerebellar WM ⇗, dorsal pons ➜, and paired pyramidal/ tegmental tracts ⇉. MSUD was diagnosed.* **31-22B.** *T2WI in the same patient shows well-delineated hyperintensity in the cerebellar WM and pontine tracts with sparing of the dentate nuclei gray matter ⇥.*

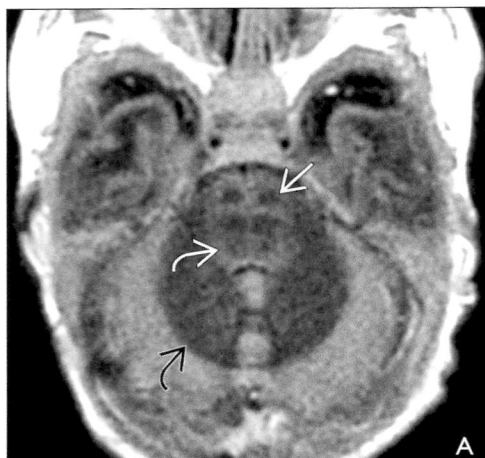

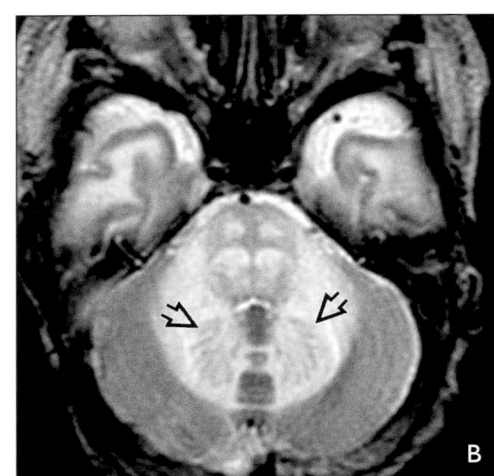

31-22C. *T2WI through the midbrain demonstrates striking edema in the cerebral peduncles ➜, clearly contrasting with the relatively normal signal intensity of the unmyelinated cerebral hemispheric WM.* **31-22D.** *The very hyperintense "MSUD edema" in the myelinated posterior limbs of the internal capsules ➜ is clearly and easily differentiated from the less hyperintense unmyelinated hemispheric WM ⇥.*

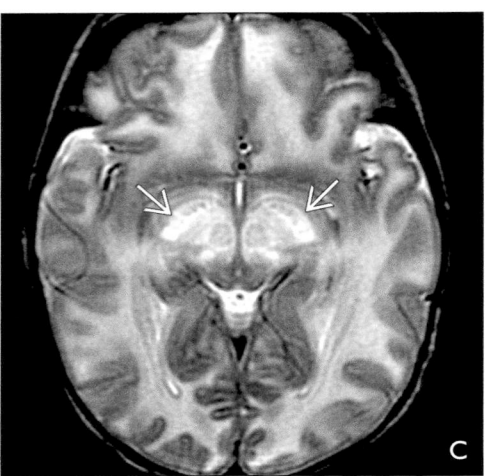

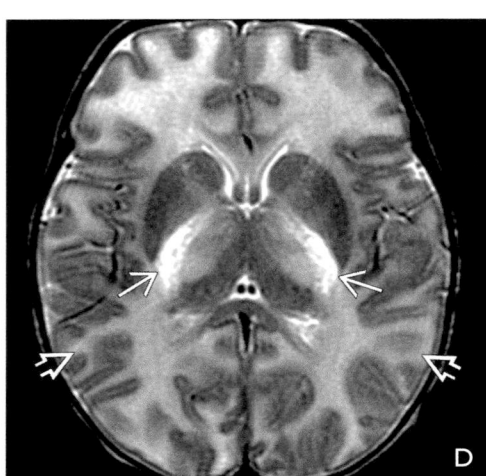

31-22E. *DWI shows striking restriction in the cerebellar WM and myelinated pontine tracts.* **31-22F.** *MRS at TE of 144 msec shows a peak at 0.9-1.0 ppm ➜ representing branched chain α-keto acids, typically seen during acute metabolic decompensation in MSUD.*

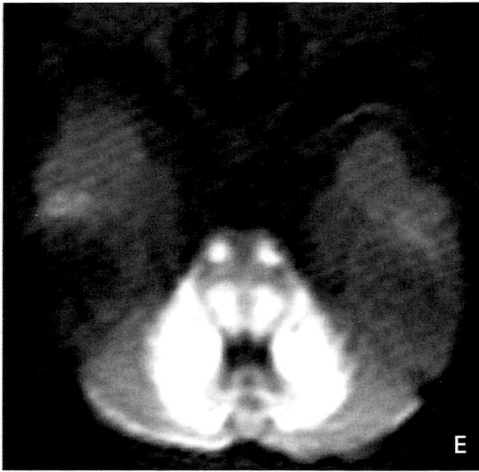

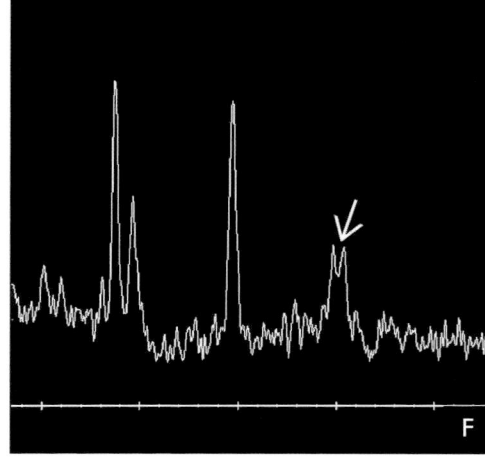

chain α-keto acid dehydrogenase complex results in elevated brain levels of leucine and other leukotoxic metabolites. In turn, these induce cytotoxic or intramyelinic edema.

Infants with classic MSUD are initially normal. Symptoms usually develop within a few days after birth and include poor feeding, lethargy, vomiting, and seizures. In severe cases, the urine smells like maple syrup or burnt sugar.

Transcranial ultrasound during the acute stage of MSUD edema shows markedly increased echogenicity in the thalami and basal ganglia.

NECT scans show profound hypodensity in the myelinated WM with vasogenic edema in the dorsal brainstem, cerebellum, cerebral peduncles, and posterior limb of the internal capsule (31-21). MR scans show striking T2/FLAIR hyperintensity with relatively crisp margins. DWI shows restricted diffusivity (31-22).

MRS shows a peak at 0.9 ppm caused by accumulation of branched-chain α-keto amino acids. Peaks are present at both short (30 msec) and intermediate (144 msec) or long TEs, distinguishing them from the normal macromolecular peak that is seen only on short TE MRS.

Hyperhomocysteinemia

Hyperhomocysteinemia (HHcy)—formerly known as homocystinuria—is a heterogeneous group of inherited disorders that affect methionine metabolism, resulting in elevated plasma homocysteine.

HHcy patients are normal at birth but develop multisystem abnormalities involving the eye, skeleton, vascular system, and CNS. Upward dislocation of the lens develops early and affects the majority of patients. Osteoporosis and kyphoscoliosis are common. Endothelial damage and hypercoagulability result in a high incidence of both arterial and venous occlusions, which occur at all ages.

The major imaging manifestations of HHcy in the brain are vascular. Stenoocclusive disease in both the arterial and venous systems is typical. Microangiopathy from premature atherosclerosis, thrombolic arterial strokes, lacunar infarcts, sinovenous occlusion, and generalized volume loss are common. An increased number of T2/FLAIR white matter hyperintensities is seen in patients

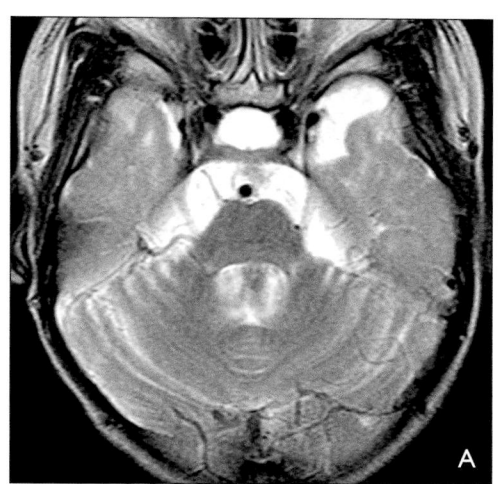

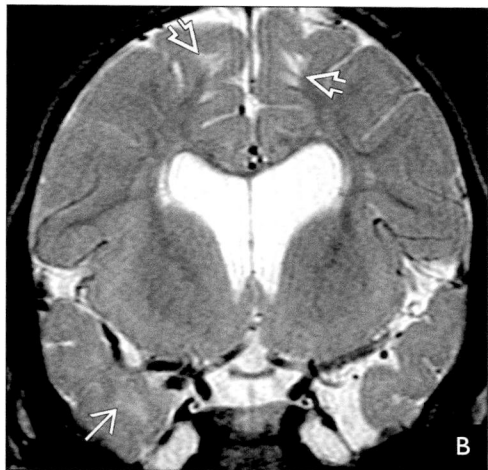

31-23A. Axial T2WI in a 4-year-old boy with hyperhomocysteinemia and a history of sinovenous occlusion as an infant shows generalized cerebellar atrophy. 31-23B. Coronal T2WI in the same patient shows atrophy, patchy WM hyperintensity in the temporal lobe ➡, and perivascular demyelinating foci ➡.

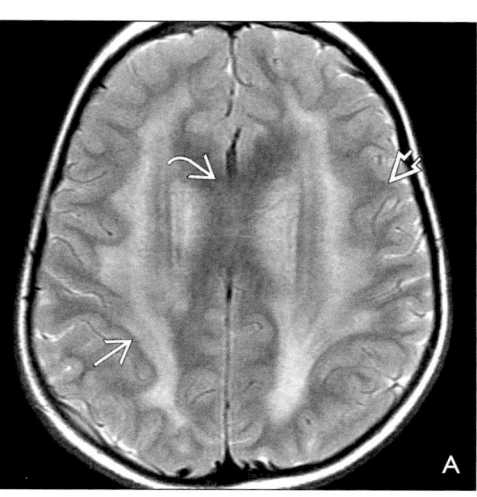

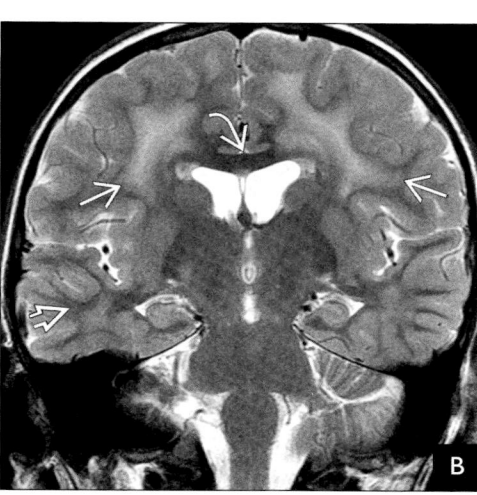

31-24A. Axial T2WI in a 10-year-old boy with merosin-deficient congenital muscular dystrophy shows confluent hyperintensity in the periventricular WM ➡. The subcortical arcuate fibers are spared ➡, as is the corpus callosum ➡. 31-24B. Coronal thin-section T2WI in the same patient shows the confluent hyperintensity in the deep WM ➡. The corpus callosum ➡ and subcortical WM ➡ are spared. No cortical malformations are seen.

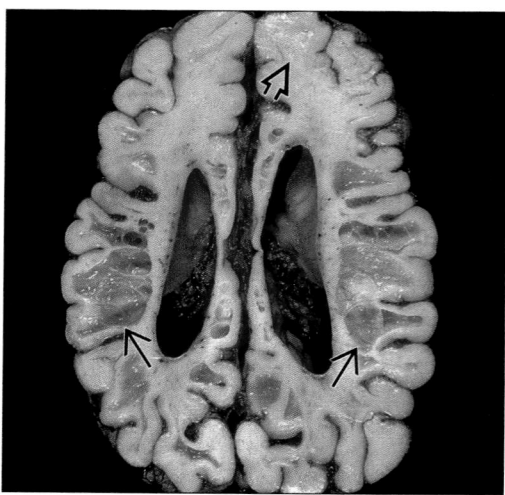

31-25. Autopsy case of MLC shows multiple subcortical cysts ➡, WM rarefaction ⊵ in the frontal subcortical WM. (R. Hewlett, MD.)

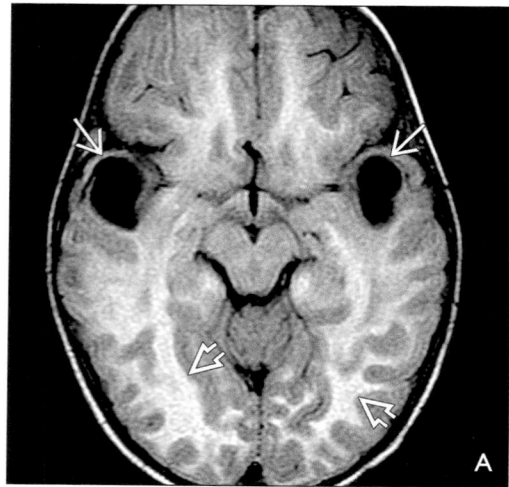

31-26A. Axial FLAIR in a 22 month old with MLC shows swollen, hyperintense, "watery" WM ⊵ and CSF-like temporal subcortical cysts ➡.

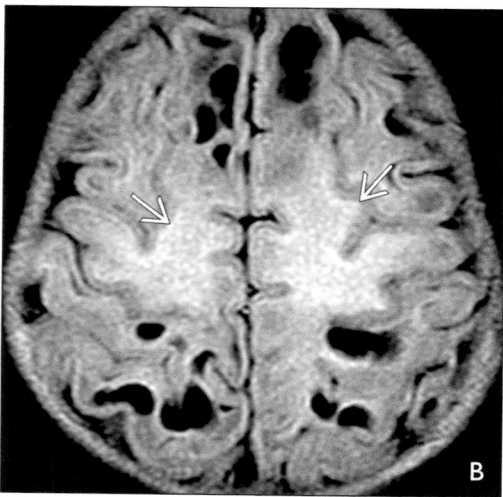

31-26B. FLAIR scan in a 2 year old with MLC shows swollen, hyperintense subcortical WM ➡. Fluid-filled cysts suppress completely.

with even mildly elevated plasma homocysteine levels **(31-23)**.

Congenital Muscular Dystrophy

The congenital muscular dystrophies (CMDs) have a variety of manifestations. Some present with hypotonia and muscle weakness without CNS symptoms. Others present with abnormal myelination and normal cortex or cortical malformations with normal myelination. The latter are considered in Chapter 37.

Most of the CMDs characterized by abnormal myelination are merosin-deficient CMDs (MD-CMDs). Muscle biopsy shows dystrophic changes with negative expression of merosin (laminin α2).

These patients are usually hypotonic at birth ("floppy infant") and exhibit severely delayed motor milestones. MR shows diffuse confluent T2/FLAIR hyperintensity in the periventricular WM. The corpus callosum, internal capsule, and subcortical U-fibers are typically spared **(31-24)**.

Subcortical White Matter Predominance

Inherited metabolic disorders (IMDs) that initially or predominantly affect the subcortical WM are much less common than those with deep periventricular involvement. The most striking IMD with preferential involvement of the subcortical WM is megaloencephalic leukoencephaly with subcortical cysts.

Megaloencephalic Leukodystrophy with Subcortical Cysts

TERMINOLOGY. Megaloencephalic leukodystrophy with subcortical cysts (MLC) is also known as vacuolating megaloencephalic leukoencephalopathy. MLC is a rare autosomal recessive disorder with characteristic MR features and a variable but mild clinical course.

ETIOLOGY. MLC is a genetically heterogeneous disorder. Approximately 75% of cases are caused by mutations in the *MLC1* gene. MLC1 is an oligomeric membrane protein located in astrocyte-astrocyte junctions. A newly described mutation in the *HEPACAM* gene that encodes for the GlialCAM protein, an IgG-like hepatic and glial cell adhesion molecule, may account for the remaining cases. Both defects lead to abnormal cell junction trafficking. Patients with *HEPACAM* mutations develop a spectrum of abnormalities ranging from benign familial macrocephaly to MLC that is indistinguishable from that caused by *MLC1* mutation.

PATHOLOGY. Gross pathology shows a swollen brain with multiple variably sized subcortical cysts **(31-25)**. The

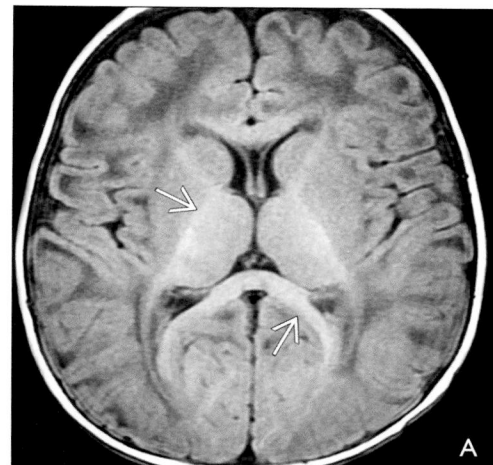

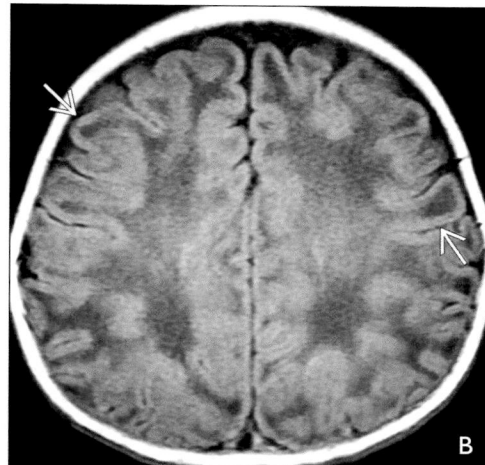

31-27A. Early findings of MLC are demonstrated in a 6-month-old boy with macrocephaly. T1WI shows normal myelination in the corpus callosum and internal capsules ➡, but the hemispheric WM is very hypointense and immature for age. 31-27B. Axial T1WI through the upper corona radiata shows striking lack of myelination. Some of the gyri appear swollen ➡ although no frank subcortical cysts are identified.

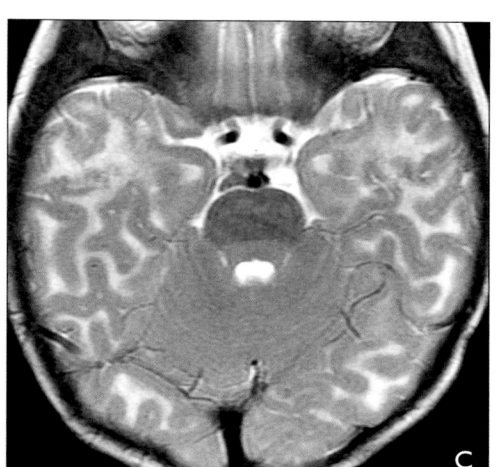

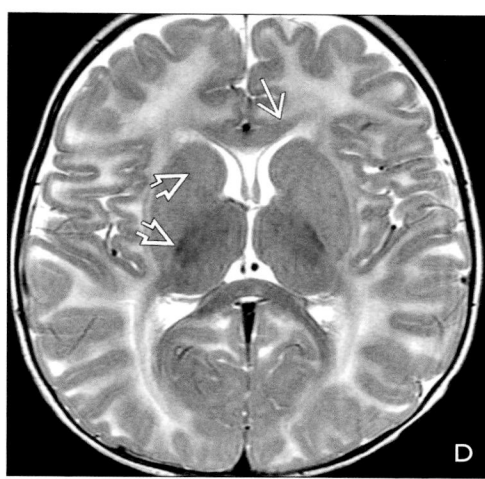

31-27C. Heavily T2-weighted scan in the same patient shows diffusely abnormal hyperintensity throughout the WM of both cerebral hemispheres, including the subcortical U-fibers. The overlying cortex appears normal. 31-27D. T2WI through the basal ganglia shows normal myelination in the corpus callosum ➡ and both limbs of the internal capsules ➡. The remainder of the hemispheric WM appears abnormally "watery" and hyperintense.

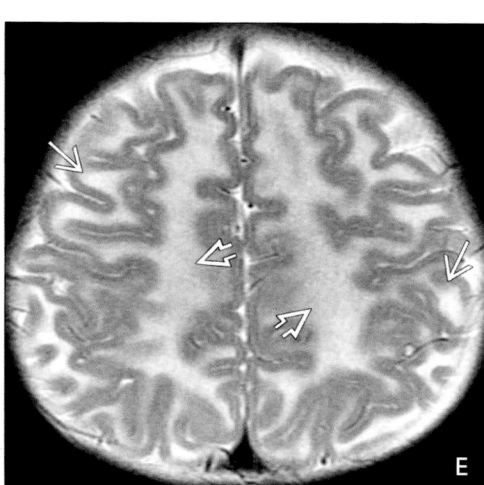

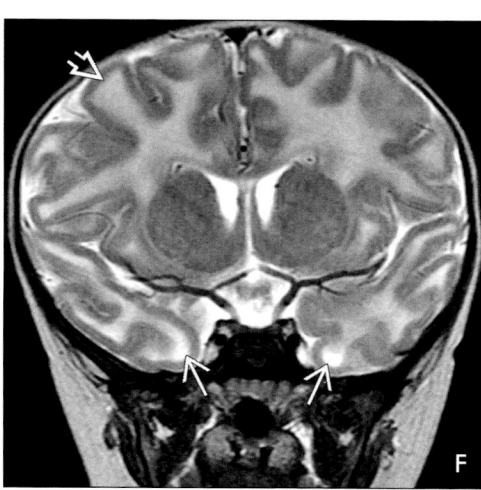

31-27E. T2WI through the upper corona radiata in the same patient shows that the subcortical WM ➡ is subtly but definitely more hyperintense than the central WM ➡, possibly indicating early cystic degeneration. 31-27F. Coronal T2WI shows that the most hyperintense WM is in the medial temporal lobes ➡ compared to the swollen convexity gyri ➡. This probably represents the earliest development of the characteristic cysts seen in MLC.

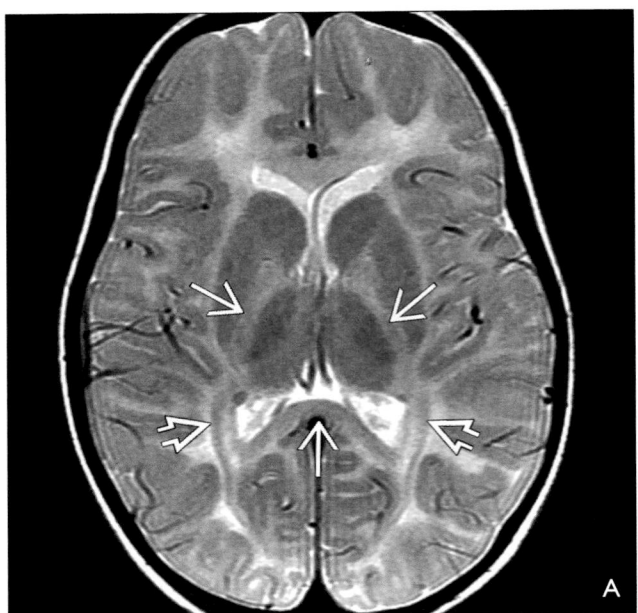

31-28A. Axial T2WI in a 3-year-old girl with 4H syndrome shows that most of the hemispheric WM is hyperintense. The T2 hypointensity in the optic tracts ⇥ and posterior limb of the internal capsules ⇥ are characteristic.

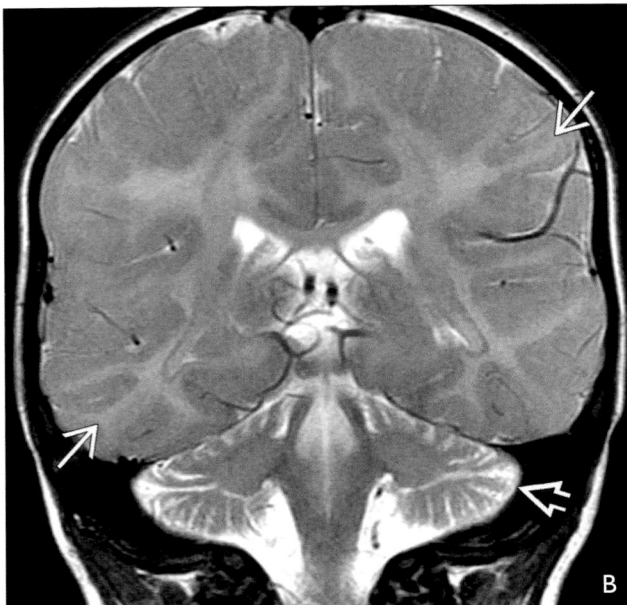

31-28B. Coronal T2WI in the same patient shows that the absent myelination also involves the subcortical U-fibers ⇥. The striking early cerebellar atrophy ⇥ is characteristic of 4H syndrome.

basal ganglia are spared. In the few reported cases of MLC with histopathology, extensive vacuolation is seen in the outer layers of myelin sheaths, accounting for the characteristic swollen appearance of the WM on MR.

CLINICAL ISSUES. MLC is distinguished clinically from other leukoencephalopathies by its remarkably slow course of neurologic deterioration. Infantile-onset macrocephaly is characteristic, but neurologic deterioration is often delayed. Age at symptom onset varies widely, ranging from birth to 25 years, with median age of six months.

Pyramidal and cerebellar signs are common. Seizures are variable. While the distribution of MLC is global, many reported patients are of northern Indian ethnicity.

IMAGING. The diagnosis of MLC is typically established by MR. A large head with diffuse confluent WM T2/FLAIR hyperintensity in the subcortical WM is typical. The affected gyri appear "watery" and swollen **(31-27)**. The basal ganglia are spared; the corpus callosum and internal capsule are usually normal. The cerebellar WM is generally normal or only mildly affected.

Characteristic CSF-like subcortical cysts develop in the anterior temporal lobes and then appear in the frontoparietal lobes. Unlike the "watery" WM, the cysts suppress completely on FLAIR **(31-26)**. The number and size of the cysts may increase over time. The abnormal WM and cysts do not enhance on T1 C+.

MRS shows mild to moderately decreased NAA and reduced NAA:Cr ratio.

DIFFERENTIAL DIAGNOSIS. MLC must be distinguished from other IMDs with macrocrania. The two major considerations are Canavan disease and Alexander disease, both of which are characterized by much greater clinical disability. **Canavan disease** almost always involves the basal ganglia, does not develop subcortical cysts, and demonstrates a large NAA peak on MRS.

Alexander disease also involves the basal ganglia, is predominantly frontal, and often enhances following contrast administration.

Hypomyelinating Disorders

A recently recognized type of rare IMDs is characterized by delayed or undermyelinated WM. Known as hypomyelinating leukoencephalopathies, these heterogeneous disorders exhibit reduced or absent myelination. *Hypo*myelinating diseases differ from other WM disorders that are characterized by abnormal myelin formation (*dys*myelinating diseases) or myelin destruction (*de*myelinating diseases).

Most of the hypomyelinating leukoencephalopathies are lysosomal storage diseases. While some have been identified and characterized, hypomyelinating disorders of unknown origin constitute the largest single category of these leukoencephalopathies.

The generally accepted imaging criterion for the diagnosis of hypomyelination is an unchanged pattern of deficient myelination on two successive MR scans obtained at least six months apart **(31-29)**. The most common find-

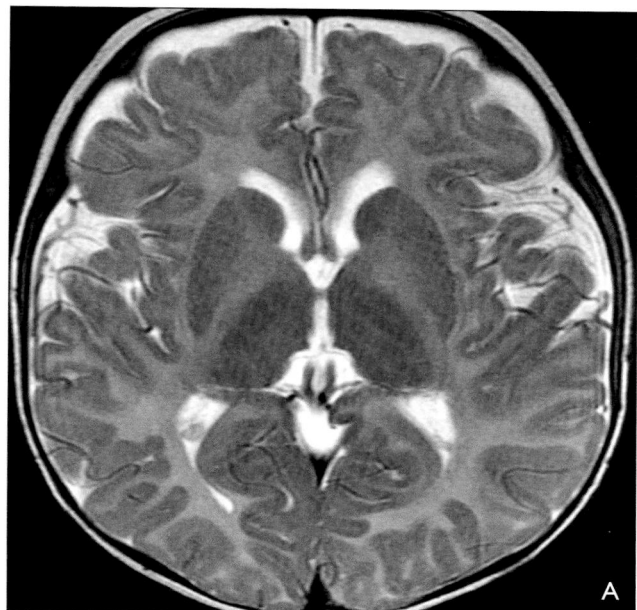

31-29A. Axial T2WI in a 6-month-old boy with delayed motor development and normal head circumference shows almost complete absence of myelination, including the subcortical U-fibers. At this age, the internal capsules should be myelinated.

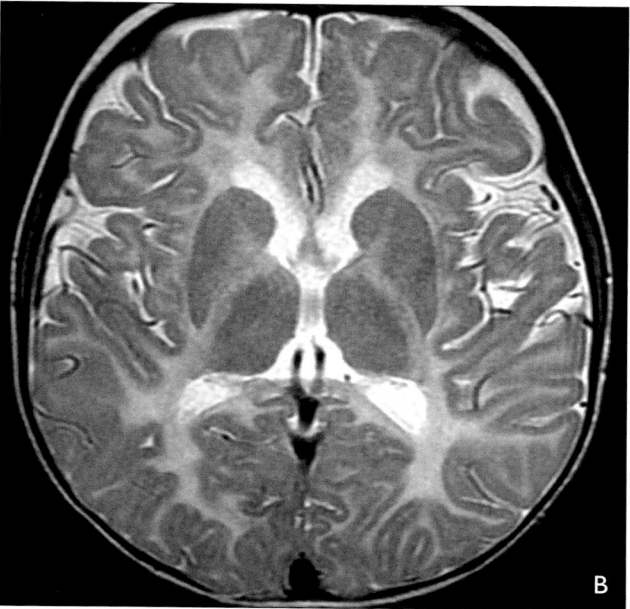

31-29B. Follow-up scan in the same patient at age 3 years shows no interval progression of myelination. Genetic analysis showed PLP1 mutation, diagnostic for PMD.

ing is mild T2 hyperintensity in much or most of the cerebral hemispheric WM. In some cases, signal intensity on T1 scans can be nearly normal.

After hypomyelination of unknown etiology, the next most commonly diagnosed inherited hypomyelinating disorder is **4H syndrome**. The best-known hypomyelination syndrome is **Pelizaeus-Merzbacher disease**. Both are caused by a mutation in the gene that encodes myelin proteolipid protein 1 (*PLP1*).

HYPOMYELINATING DISORDERS

Most Common
- Hypomyelination of unknown cause
- 4H syndrome
- Pelizaeus-Merzbacher disease
- Pelizaeus-Merzbacher-like disease

Less Common
- Hypomyelination with congenital cataract
- GM2 gangliosidosis
- Salla disease (sialuria)
- Fucosidosis
- Cockayne syndrome
- GM1 gangliosidosis
- Hypomyelination with atrophy of the basal ganglia and cerebellum

Rare
- del(18q) syndromes
- Cockayne syndrome
- Trichothiodystrophies (brittle, sulfur-deficient hair)

H Syndrome

The diagnosis of 4H syndrome is based on the combination of hypomyelination on MR, hypogonadotropic hypogonadism, and hypodontia. The hypomyelination in 4H syndrome is distinctive. T2 *hypo*intensity of the optic radiations, pyramidal tracts in the posterior limb of the internal capsule, and anterolateral thalami together with cerebellar atrophy and mild cerebellar WM hyperintensity are characteristic (**31-28**).

Pelizaeus-Merzbacher Disease

TERMINOLOGY AND ETIOLOGY. Pelizaeus-Merzbacher disease (PMD) is an X-linked disorder that results in nearly complete lack of myelination.

PMD is a hypomyelinating disorder caused by variations in *PLP1*. Two forms of PMD are recognized: Type 1 (classic) and type 2 (connatal). Classic PMD is an X-linked recessive disorder, whereas patients with the connatal form show either autosomal or X-linked recessive inheritance.

Most patients with PMD have strikingly homogeneous hyperintensity of the entire cerebral WM. Cerebellar atrophy is common.

PATHOLOGY. Grossly, the brain appears atrophic with normal cortex and shrunken, grayish, or gelatinous-appearing WM. Both the central and subcortical WM are affected. The cerebellar WM, brainstem, and spinal cord are also shrunken and gray. The optic nerves (which are brain tracts) are usually involved, but other cranial nerves (which are ensheathed with a different myelin protein called PMP 22) are normally myelinated.

Histopathology shows markedly reduced or absent oligodendrocytes with variable myelin staining. Cases of connatal PMD show almost complete lack of myelin staining whereas more slowly progressive cases demonstrate preservation of myelin islets around blood vessels in a classic "tiger" or discontinuous pattern.

CLINICAL ISSUES. Although it is one of the most common hypomyelinating disorders, PMD causes only 5-7% of all the inherited leukodystrophies. Nearly 100% of classic PMD cases occur in males. Connatal PMD can affect either gender.

PMD is typically identified in infants under one year of age and presents with nystagmus, delayed motor milestones, and spasticity. Prognosis is poor, and death occurs in early childhood.

IMAGING. The typical imaging appearance of PMD is nearly complete lack of myelination **(31-29)**. The entire cerebral WM appears strikingly and homogeneously hyperintense on T2WI. In some cases, preserved myelin around perivascular spaces gives the WM a "tiger" pattern. Hyperintensity of the pyramidal tracts or entire pons is typically present. Progressive WM and cerebellar volume loss are common. Cavitary WM changes are typically absent.

DIFFERENTIAL DIAGNOSIS. The major differential diagnosis of PMD is **other hypomyelinating disorders**. Pyramidal and pontine hyperintensity are helpful distinguishing features. Patients with **PMD-like disease** have a similar presentation but lack the *PLP1* mutation characteristic of PMD. In these cases, myelination is delayed but slowly develops after age two.

IMDs Predominantly Affecting Gray Matter

IMDs that involve the gray matter (GM) disorders without affecting the WM are also known as poliodystrophies. They can be subdivided into those that involve the cortex and those that mostly affect the deep gray nuclei. Inherited GM disorders that involve the deep gray nuclei are significantly more common than those that primarily affect the cortex.

IMDs Primarily Affecting Deep Gray Nuclei

A number of inherited disorders affect mostly the basal ganglia and thalami. Three inborn errors of metabolism with specific predilection for the deep gray nuclei are type 1 **neurodegeneration with brain iron accumulation** (also known as **pantothenate kinase-associated neuropathy** or PKAN), **creatine deficiency syndromes**, and a cytosine-adenine-guanine (CAG) repeat disorder called **Huntington disease**.

We begin this section with an overview of brain iron accumulation disorders before turning our attention specifically to PKAN, creatine deficiency syndromes, and Huntington disease. We close the section with a discussion of two inherited disorders with abnormal copper metabolism, **Wilson disease** and **Menkes disease**.

Brain Iron Accumulation Disorders

Some iron accumulation within the basal ganglia and dentate nuclei occurs as part of normal aging (see Chapter 33). Neurodegeneration with brain iron accumulation (NBIA) represents a clinically and genetically heterogeneous group of conditions characterized by progressive neurodegeneration and abnormally elevated brain iron.

Four major NBIA subtypes have been defined at the molecular genetic level: (1) pantothenate kinase-associated neurodegeneration (PKAN or NBIA type 1), (2) neuroferritinopathy (NBIA type 2), (3) infantile neuroaxonal dystrophy, and (4) aceruloplasminemia.

We focus our discussion on PKAN, the most common type of NBIA. We then briefly discuss the other three types.

PKAN.

Terminology. PKAN (pantothenate kinase-associated neuropathy) was formerly known as Hallervorden-Spatz disease.

Etiology. PKAN is a rare familial autosomal recessive disorder characterized by excessive iron deposition in the globus pallidus (GP) and substantia nigra (SN). It is caused by mutations in the pantothenate kinase gene (*PANK2*) localized to chromosome 20p12.2-13.

Pathology. Grossly, PKAN is characterized by shrinkage and rust-brown discoloration of the medial GP, the reticular zone of the SN **(31-33)**, and sometimes the dentate nuclei. The red nuclei are generally spared. Granular pigment consisting of iron, lipofuscin, and neuromelanin accumulates in axonal "spheroids" (swollen distended axons), neurons, astrocytes, and microglia, which in turn causes neuronal loss and gliosis. Immunostaining for hyperphosphorylated tau reveals numerous neurofibrillary tangles.

Clinical issues. NBIA type 1 can develop at any age. Four clinical forms are recognized: Infantile (onset in the first year of life), late-infantile (onset between two

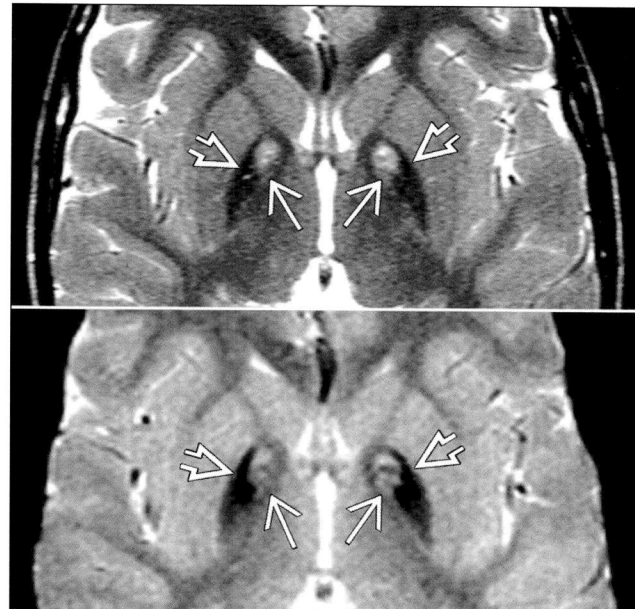

31-30. T2WI (top), GRE (bottom) in a patient with PKAN show classic "eye of the tiger" sign with bilateral hyperintense foci ➔ in the medial globi pallidi surrounded by striking hypointensity ⧉.

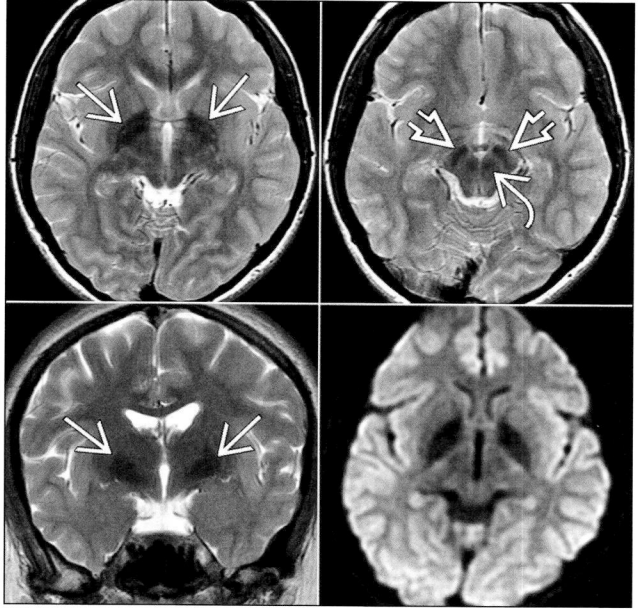

31-31. A 19-year-old woman with documented PKAN. Note the profound hypointensity in the GP ➔, SN ⧉, red nuclei ⧉ and the lack of an "eye of the tiger" sign. DWI is normal.

and five years), juvenile or "classic" (onset between 7-15 years), and adult-onset NBIA type 1.

Most cases are diagnosed in the first decade or during early adolescence. The disorder begins with slowly progressive gait disturbances and delayed psychomotor development. Hyperkinesias occur in about 50% of cases. Progressive mental deterioration finally leads to dementia. In the later stages of the disease, the dyskinesias are replaced by rigid stiffness.

PANK2 mutations are associated with younger age at onset, more rapid progression, and higher frequency of dystonia, dysarthria, intellectual impairment, and gait disturbances. Parkinsonism is seen predominantly in patients with adult-onset disease.

Imaging. Imaging findings reflect the anatomic distribution of the excessive iron accumulation. T2WI demonstrates marked hypointensity in the GP and SN. A small focus of central hyperintensity in the medial aspect of the very hypointense GP (the classic "eye of the tiger" sign) is caused by tissue gliosis and vacuolization (31-30).

It is important to note that *not all cases of PKAN demonstrate the "eye of the tiger" sign!* Striking, severe T2 shortening in the GP with "blooming" on T2* (GRE, SWI) in a child or young adult should suggest the diagnosis of an NBIA—either PKAN or infantile neuroaxonal dystrophy—even in the absence of an "eye of the tiger" sign (31-31).

PKAN does not enhance on T1 C+. Nor does it demonstrate restricted diffusion, although DTI demonstrates

significantly increased fractional anisotropy in both the GP and SN. MRS shows decreased NAA peak and reduced NAA:Cr ratio consistent with neuraxonal loss. Increased myoinositol peak and mI:Cr ratio at short TE is present, suggesting reactive glial proliferation.

Differential diagnosis. Abnormal iron deposition in the basal ganglia occurs with PKAN as well as other NBIAs. **Aceruloplasminemia** and **neuroferritinopathy** are both adult-onset disorders. Both involve the cortex, which is spared in PKAN.

Basal ganglia signal abnormalities occur in a number of other inherited metabolic disorders. **Wilson disease**, **Leigh disease**, **infantile bilateral striatal necrosis**, and **mitochondrial encephalopathies** show striatal hyperintensity (not hypointensity). They also predominantly involve the caudate and putamen, not the medial GP.

NEUROFERRITINOPATHY. Mutations in the carboxy-terminus of the ferritin light chain gene (*FTL*) interfere with its ability to transport iron. Redox active iron is deposited in neurons, causing oxidative stress with neuronal loss and gliosis. The result is **neuroferritinopathy**, an adult autosomal dominant disorder with mean age of 39 years at onset.

The predominant clinical neuroferritinopathy phenotype is an extrapyramidal disorder with choreiform movements and focal dystonia. Early cognitive and psychiatric disturbances are absent, distinguishing neuroferritinopathy from Huntington disease.

The earliest detectable imaging findings in neuroferritinopathy are T2* hypointensity in the GP and SN. T2 hypointensity in the GP and SN, red nuclei, caudate, putamen, thalamus, and cerebral cortex typically follow. In later stages, gliosis and cystic degeneration in the medial globi pallidi may produce foci of T2 hyperintensity that causes an "eye of the tiger" appearance similar to that seen in PKAN (see above).

INFANTILE NEUROAXONAL DYSTROPHY. Mutations in phospholipase A2 (*PLA2G6*) cause **infantile neuroaxonal dystrophy** (INAD), a severe psychomotor disorder characterized by progressive hypotonia, hyperreflexia, and tetraparesis. Median age at presentation is 14 months. Disease progression is usually rapid with a mean age at death of nine years.

Imaging studies in children with INAD show striking cerebellar atrophy in over 95% of cases. T2/FLAIR hyperintensity in the cerebellum secondary to gliosis is also common. Almost 50% of cases demonstrate abnormal iron deposition with T2 hypointensity in the GP and SN.

ACERULOPLASMINEMIA. Homozygous mutations in the ceruloplasmin gene cause **aceruloplasminemia**, also known as hereditary ceruloplasmin deficiency. Ceruloplasmin carries over 95% of all plasma copper and acts as a ferroxidase, thus playing an important role in mobilizing tissue iron.

Aceruloplasminemia is a disease of middle-aged adults characterized by the clinical triad of diabetes, retinopathy, and neurologic symptoms (primarily dementia, craniofacial dyskinesia, and cerebellar ataxia). T2 and T2* (GRE, SWI) demonstrate striking hypointensity in the cerebral and cerebellar cortex, globus pallidus, caudate nucleus, putamen, thalamus, red nucleus, substantia nigra, and dentate nuclei **(31-32)**.

MR is especially useful in diagnosing NBIAs. All feature iron deposition in the globi pallidi but differ in other associated findings. The distribution of T2 or T2* hypointensity can help distinguish between the different NBIA subtypes (see box below).

31-32A. Axial T2 GRE scan in a 66-year-old woman with aceruloplasminemia shows striking hypointensity in the dentate nuclei ➡ with subtle but definite linear "blooming" in the cerebellar cortex ⇒. 31-32B. Axial T2* GRE scan in the same patient shows symmetric "blooming" hypointensities in the substantia nigra ➡, red nuclei ➡, inferior putamina ➡.*

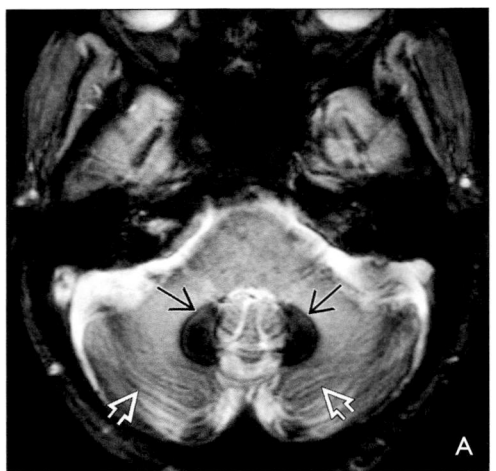
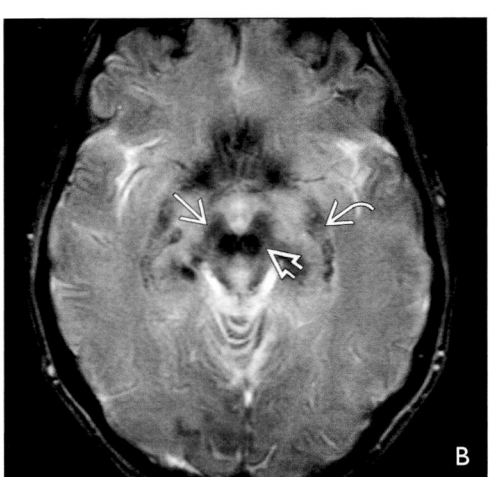

31-32C. More cephalad T2 GRE image through the lateral and third ventricles shows profound symmetric hypointensity in the caudate nuclei ➡, putamina ➡, and both thalami ⇒. Note the subtle "blooming" hypointensity in the cortex ⇒ as well. 31-32D. T2* SWI scan through the corona radiata demonstrates striking curvilinear hypointensity throughout the entire cortex of both hemispheres ⇒.*

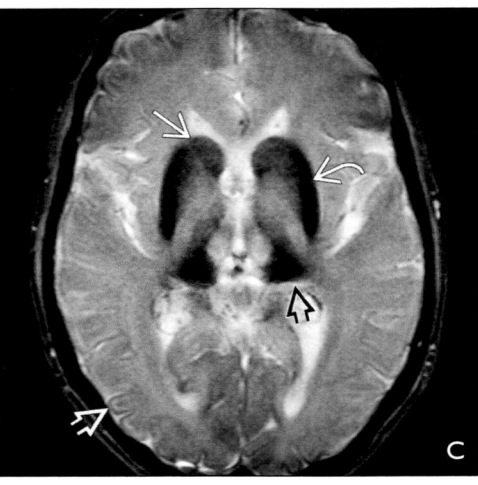
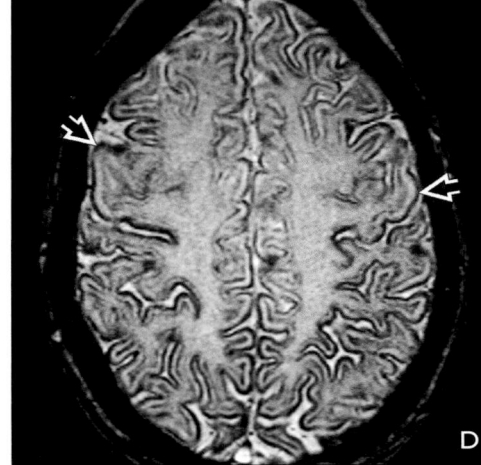

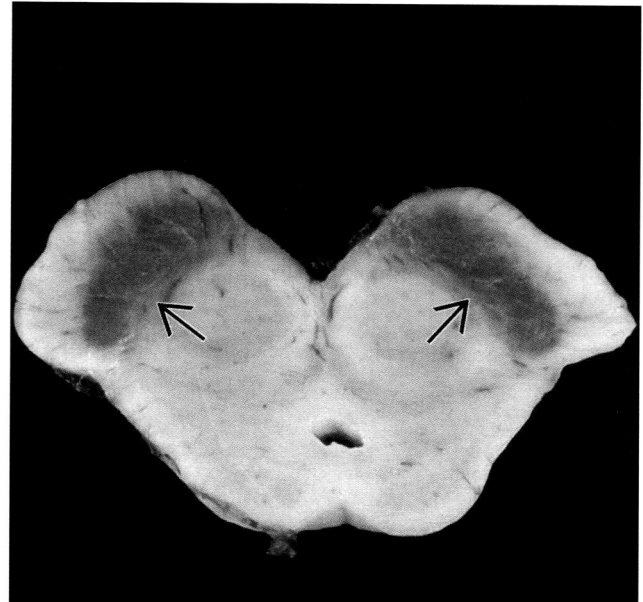

31-33. *Autopsy case of PKAN shows characteristic brownish discoloration* ➯ *caused by iron deposition in the substantia nigra. (Courtesy E. T. Hedley-Whyte, MD.)*

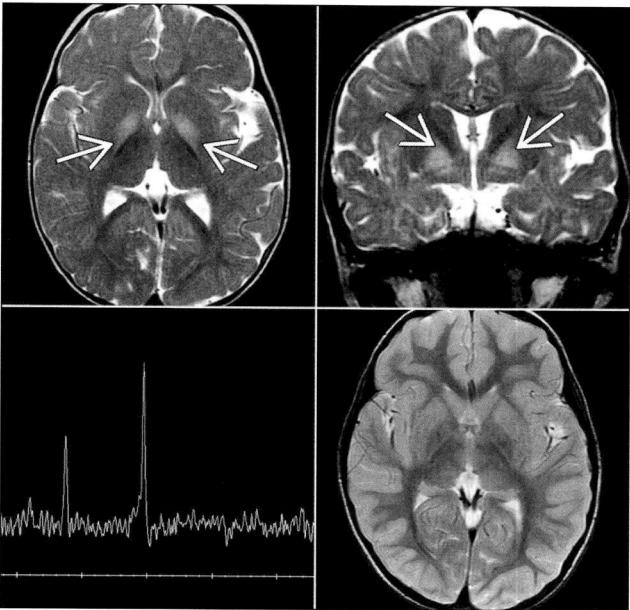

31-34. *Axial, coronal T2 scans in an 11 month old with creatine deficiency shows symmetric hyperintensity in the globi pallidi* ➯. *Long TE MRS shows absent Cr peak. With dietary supplementation, MR 3 years later is completely normal.*

NBIA T2* HYPOINTENSITY

PKAN
- GP, SN, dentate nuclei
- "Eye of tiger" sign variable
- *Spares* cortex

INAD
- Cerebellar atrophy (95%)
- T2* hypointensity in GP, SN (50%)
- *Spares* cortex

Neuroferritinopathy
- T2* hypointensity in GP, SN
- Then dentate/caudate nuclei, thalami
- *Affects* cortex

Aceruloplasminemia
- GP, caudate nuclei, putamen, thalamus
- Red nucleus, SN, dentate nuclei
- *Affects* cerebral, cerebellar cortices

Creatine Deficiency Syndromes

Creatine deficiency syndromes are autosomal recessive disorders. Creatine and creatine phosphate are essential for the storage and transmission of phosphate-bound energy in both muscle and brain. Severe creatine depletion causes hypotonia and developmental delay. Dietary supplementation can partially or completely reverse the symptoms, so making the diagnosis is crucial to patient management.

MR shows bilaterally symmetric T2/FLAIR hyperintensity in the globi pallidi. MRS is key to the diagnosis and shows a diminished or absent Cr peak on long TE studies **(31-34)**.

Huntington Disease

Until recently, Huntington disease was thought to be regionally selective, affecting only gray matter (most specifically the caudate nuclei and putamina). Although advanced imaging techniques such as DTI have demonstrated that WM is also affected, the dominant imaging features are abnormalities of the deep gray nuclei. Therefore, we include HD in this section with the other IMDs that preferentially involve the striatum.

TERMINOLOGY AND ETIOLOGY. Huntington disease (HD) is also known as Huntington chorea. HD is an autosomal dominant chronic hereditary neurodegenerative disorder with complete penetrance. The responsible genetic defect occurs on the short arm of chromosome 4 and codes for the protein huntingtin. The huntingtin gene includes a repeating CAG trinucleotide segment of variable length.

The presence of more than 38 repeats confirms the diagnosis of HD. In general, there is a progressive increase in the length of the CAG repeat sequences with successive generations.

PATHOLOGY. Aggregates of huntingtin protein accumulate in axonal terminals, which eventually leads to the death of medium spiny neurons. Autopsy shows generalized cerebral atrophy with an average of 30% reduction in brain weight. Both the cortex and hemispheric WM are affected. The most characteristic gross abnormality is volume loss with rarefaction of the caudate nucleus, putamen, and globus pallidus **(31-35)**, **(31-36)**.

Microscopically, HD features neuronal loss with huntingtin nuclear inclusions, astrocytic gliosis, and iron accumulation. The changes are most severe in the basal ganglia but can also be seen in other regions of the brain, including the cerebellum.

CLINICAL ISSUES. The incidence of HD is 4-7:100,000 in most populations. Mean age at symptom onset is 35-45 years. Only 5-10% of patients present before the age of 20 years ("juvenile-onset HD"). There is no gender predilection.

CAG repeat length and age influence both the expression and the progression of HD. Adult-onset HD is characterized by progressive loss of normal motor function, development of stereotypic choreiform movements, and deteriorating cognition. Once symptoms appear, the disease progresses relentlessly and results in death within 10-20 years.

Juvenile-onset HD is initially characterized by rigidity and dystonia, much more than by chorea. Cerebellar signs are also common.

IMAGING. Standard imaging studies (CT, MR) are normal early in the disease course. As symptoms develop and progress, NECT scans show caudate atrophy with enlarged, outwardly convex frontal horns and variable generalized diffuse atrophy (31-37).

MR shows diffuse cerebral volume loss with T2/FLAIR hyperintensity in shrunken caudate heads. Putaminal hyperintensity is common (31-38).

MR volumetric studies can demonstrate decreased basal ganglia volumes years before the onset of motor disturbances. Voxel-based morphometry, DTI, and PET have also demonstrated abnormalities in the hemispheric WM and cortex of both asymptomatic carriers and patients with "premanifest" HD.

Magnetization transfer imaging (MTI) demonstrates peak height reduction proportionate to CAG repeat length in normal-appearing GM and WM. Disturbances in MTI are apparent in early HD and are homogeneous across both GM and WM.

DIFFERENTIAL DIAGNOSIS. Some acquired neurodegenerative disorders can mimic *adult* HD. These include

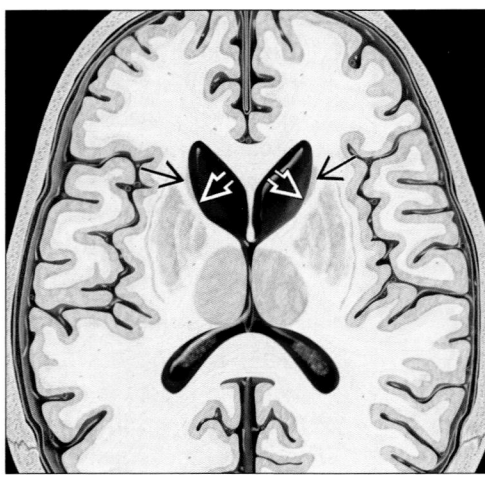
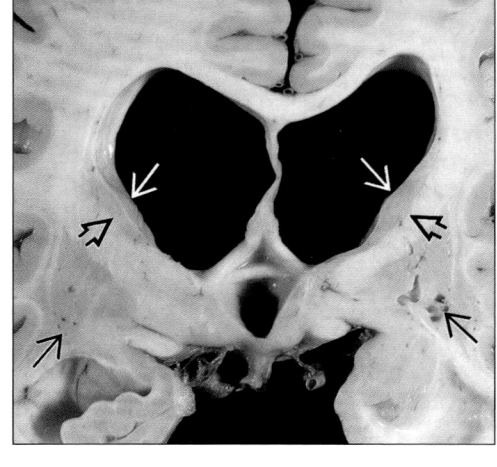

31-35. Axial graphic shows shrunken, atrophic caudate nuclei ⇗ with the outwardly convex frontal horns ⧁ that are typical of Huntington disease (HD). 31-36. Coronal autopsy of HD shows outwardly convex frontal horns ➡, severely shrunken caudate nuclei ⧁, atrophic putamina ➡. (Courtesy R. Hewlett, MD.)

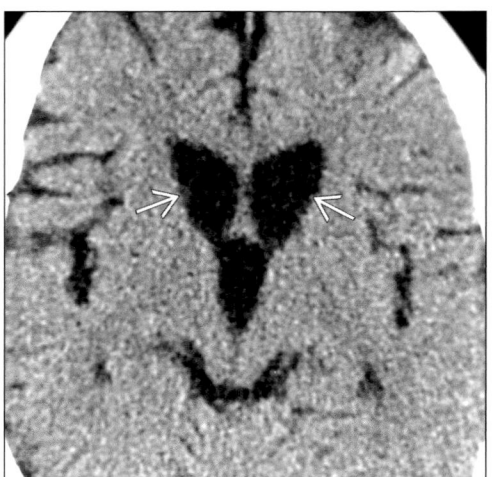
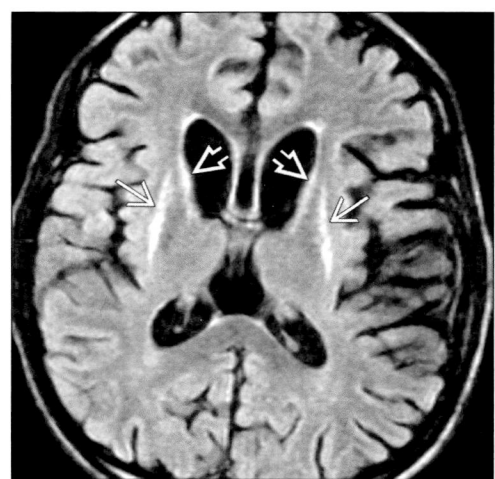

31-37. NECT of a patient with HD shows moderate generalized, severe caudate atrophy seen as outwardly convex frontal horns ➡. (Courtesy M. Huckman, MD.) 31-38. FLAIR in a patient with HD shows almost nonexistent caudate head ⧁, basal ganglia atrophy, and thinned hyperintense putamina ➡.

multiple system atrophy (MSA), **corticobasal degeneration**, and **frontotemporal lobar dementia**. All these acquired disorders are often accompanied by basal ganglia atrophy, although unlike in HD, the caudate nuclei are not disproportionately affected.

The differential diagnosis of *juvenile* HD includes late-stage **Wilson disease** with caudate and brainstem atrophy. **PKAN** with choreoathetosis and dementia can mimic the symptoms of HD. The "eye of the tiger" sign in the medial globi pallidi distinguishes PKAN from HD.

HUNTINGTON DISEASE

Etiology
- Autosomal dominant, complete penetrance
- CAG trinucleotide repeat disorder

Pathology
- Caudate nuclei, putamina, globi pallidi
  - Huntingtin protein nuclear inclusions
  - Neuronal loss, gliosis, iron accumulation

Clinical
- Adult-onset (35-45 years) = 90%
- Juvenile-onset HD (< 20 years) = 10%

Imaging
- Caudate nuclei, putamina T2/FLAIR hyperintense
- Frontal horns outwardly convex

Disorders of Copper Metabolism

Copper is essential for normal brain development. Copper-containing proteins are a critical element in a number of enzymatic systems, including iron homeostasis. Copper homeostasis is a delicate balance that requires both adequate dietary intake and proper excretion. Excess copper is neurotoxic. Two disorders of copper metabolism—Wilson disease and Menkes disease—have striking CNS manifestations.

The major manifestations of Wilson disease (WD) are found in the basal ganglia, midbrain, and dentate nucleus of the cerebellum. Therefore, WD is discussed in this section with IMDs that predominantly affect the gray matter. A brief consideration of Menkes disease follows.

WILSON DISEASE.

Etiology. WD is an uncommon autosomal recessive disorder of copper trafficking caused by mutations in the *ATP7B* gene. The mutation causes abnormal accumulation of Cu in hepatocytes, which later spills into the circulation. Copper deposition in Golgi complexes and the mitochondria results in oxidative damage primarily to the liver, brain, kidney, skeletal system, and eye.

Pathology. Selective vulnerability of the corpus striatum to mitochondrial dysfunction accounts for the predominant basal ganglia volume loss seen in WD (31-40). Gross pathologic features are nonspecific, with ventricular enlargement and widened sulci seen at autopsy in severe cases. Microscopic features include edema, necrosis, and spongiform changes in the basal ganglia. Variable gliosis and demyelination are present in the cerebral and cerebellar WM.

Clinical issues. WD most commonly affects children and young adults. The reported incidence of symptomatic WD is 1:30,000-40,000, but the frequency of asymptomatic carriers is 1:90. There is no gender predilection.

Symptoms of early-onset WD (8-16 years of age) are usually related to liver failure. Later-onset WD symptoms are primarily neurologic and are generally recognized in the second or third decade. Dysarthria, dystonia, tremors, ataxia, Parkinson-like symptoms, and behavioral disturbances are common. Copper deposition in the cornea causes the characteristic greenish yellow Kayser-Fleisher rings seen on slit-lamp examination (31-39).

Clinical symptoms generally improve, and signal abnormalities on MR may diminish with appropriate treatment. Untreated WD is always fatal.

Imaging. NECT scans may be normal, especially early in the disease course. CT grossly underestimates WD pathology. Diffuse brain atrophy, widening of the frontal horns of the lateral ventricles, and striatal or thalamic hypodensities may be seen in advanced cases.

Signal intensity on T1 scans is variable. Some cases demonstrate subtle hypointensity in the affected areas while others show T1 shortening similar to that seen in chronic hepatic encephalopathy (see Chapter 32).

The most common imaging finding of WD on MR is bilaterally symmetric T2/FLAIR hyperintensity in the putamina (70%), caudate nuclei (60%), ventrolateral thalami (55-60%), and midbrain (50%) (31-41). Hyperintensity can sometimes be seen in the pons (20%), medulla (10-15%), and cerebellum (10%). The cerebral (25%) and cerebellar WM (10%) can show focal or diffuse confluent hyperintensities.

In 10-12% of cases, diffuse tegmental (midbrain) hyperintensity with sparing of the red nuclei gives an appearance that has been termed the "face of a giant panda."

T2* (GRE, SWI) sequences show blooming in the putamina, caudate nuclei, ventrolateral thalami, and often the dentate nuclei. Contrast enhancement is typically absent although mild enhancement can occur in the acute stages.

Restricted diffusion in the corpus striatum can be seen in the early stages of WD. Elevated ADC values consistent with necrosis and spongiform degeneration are seen in chronic longstanding WD. MRS shows reduced NAA and Cho. PET shows markedly reduced glucose metabolism and diminished dopa-decarboxylase activity indicative of striatonigral dopaminergic pathway dysfunction.

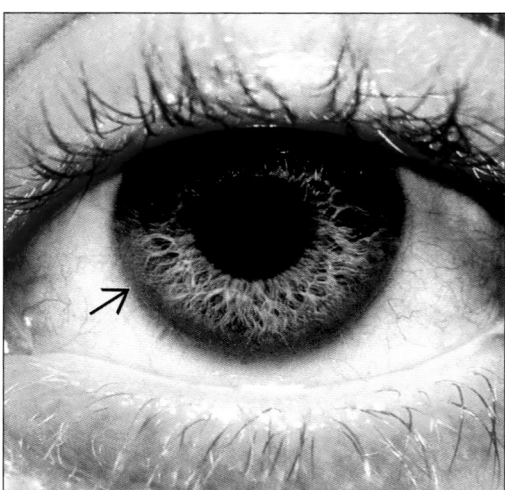

31-39. *Wilson disease with classic greenish-yellow Kayser-Fleischer ring* ➔. *(Courtesy AFIP Archives.)*

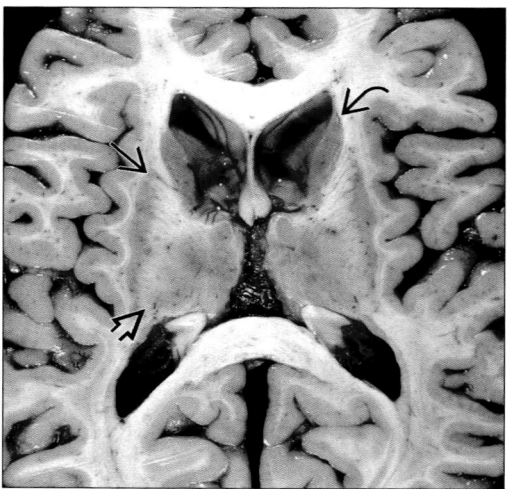

31-40. *General atrophy; thinned putamina* ➔, *caudate* ➔; *shrunken basal ganglia* ➔ *are characteristic of WD. (Courtesy R. Hewlett, MD.)*

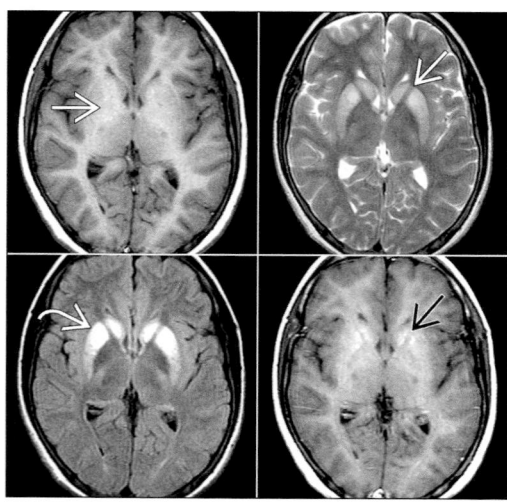

31-41. *Acute WD shows BG hyperintensity on T1-, T2WIs* ➔, *spared globi pallidi, restricted diffusion* ➔, *no enhancement* ➔. *(Courtesy M. Ayadi, MD.)*

Differential diagnosis. The differential diagnoses of WD include other inherited metabolic disorders that affect the basal ganglia, such as Leigh disease, NBIAs, and the organic acidurias. **Leigh disease** (subacute necrotizing encephalomyelopathy) shows bilateral, symmetric, spongiform and hyperintense lesions in the putamen and brainstem. The WM is often affected in Leigh disease whereas the caudate and thalamus are less commonly involved. MRS demonstrates elevated lactate levels in the basal ganglia.

Likewise, **PKAN** can resemble WD. WD predominantly affects the putamina and caudate nuclei rather than the medial globi pallidi and lacks the "eye of the tiger" sign often seen in PKAN.

MENKES DISEASE. Menkes disease (MD)—also known as kinky hair syndrome—is an X-linked, multisystemic, lethal disorder of copper metabolism caused by *ATP7A* gene mutations. Severe classic MD is characterized by progressive neurodegeneration, connective tissue abnormalities, pili torti ("kinky" hair), and death in early childhood. It accounts for 90-95% of cases.

Imaging in MD shows severe brain atrophy with subdural fluid collections and excessive tortuosity of the intracranial arteries (remember: "Kinky hair, kinky vessels") **(31-42)**.

A milder phenotype, **occipital horn syndrome** (OHS), is also called Ehlers-Danlos type 9. OHS is characterized by connective tissue manifestations (mostly skeletal abnormalities) and longer survival.

IMDs Primarily Affecting Cortex

Compared to IMDs that affect the deep gray nuclei, disorders that exclusively or primarily affect the cortical GM are rare. Two prototypical IMDs that involve the cortex are briefly discussed here: The **neuronal ceroid lipofuscinoses** and **Rett syndrome**.

Neuronal Ceroid Lipofuscinosis

The neuronal ceroid lipofuscinoses (NCLs) are a heterogeneous family of inherited neurodegenerative disorders characterized by accumulation of ceroid-lipopigment inclusions in neurons. A number of different types have been described. Previously, the NCLs were classified according to age at onset with infantile, late-infantile, juvenile (i.e., Batten disease), and adult forms (e.g., Kufs disease). The specific gene mutations that cause most forms have been identified, and the NCLs are now classified according to the eight affected genes (*CLN1-8*).

NCL is predominantly a childhood disease with an estimated incidence of 1:12,500. The diagnosis is established through clinicopathologic findings, enzymatic assay, and molecular genetic testing. Ultrastructural

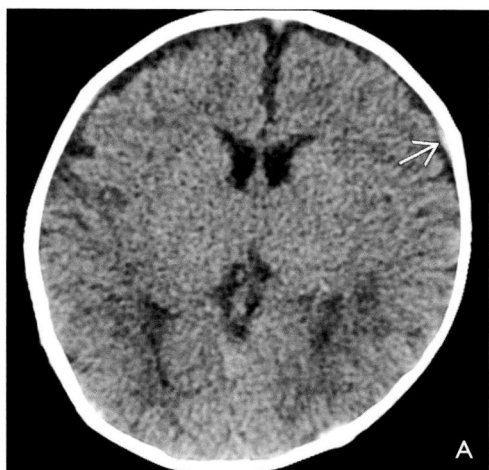

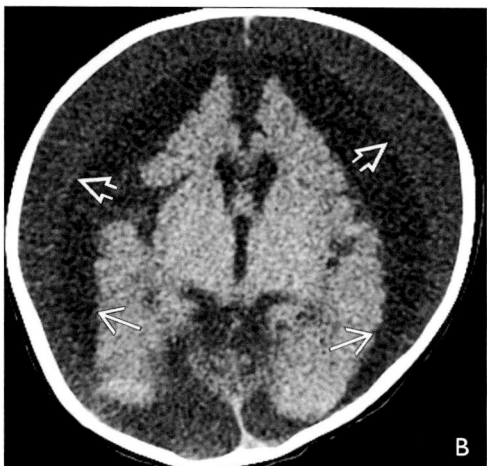

31-42A. *Case of Menkes disease shows severe progressive neurodegeneration. Axial NECT scan in a 7 month old with large head, failure to thrive appears normal except for a tiny left frontal subdural hematoma* ➡. **31-42B.** *The child was rescanned at age 16 months. Massive bilateral subdural hematomas are present* ➡. *The brain appears shrunken and severely atrophic. The overlying subarachnoid space* ➡ *is grossly enlarged.*

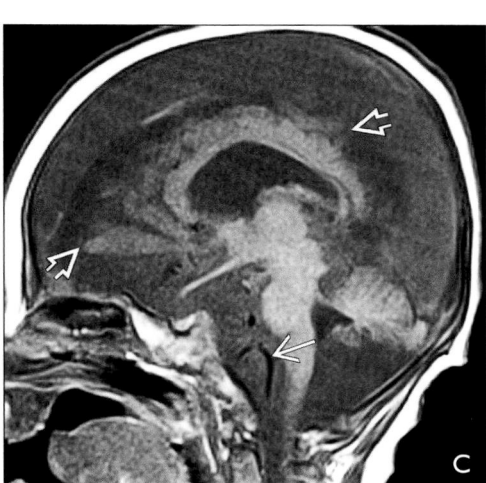

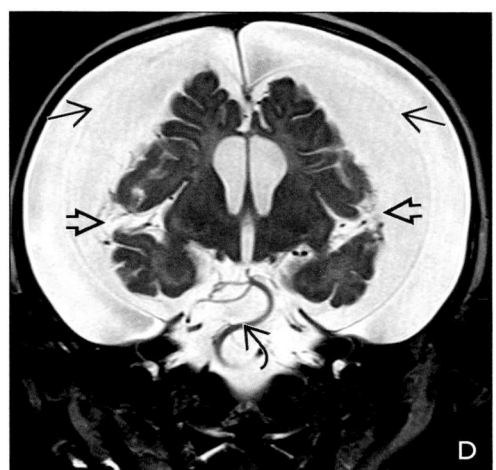

31-42C. *MR was obtained. Sagittal T1WI shows that the brain* ➡ *is extremely atrophic and the subdural hematomas are hypointense. Note the unusually tortuous "flow void" of the basilar artery* ➡. **31-42D.** *Coronal T2WI FS shows that the symmetric subdural hematomas are separated by a thin membrane* ➡. *Note the tortuous basilar artery* ➡, *cortical vessels in enlarged sylvian fissures* ➡.

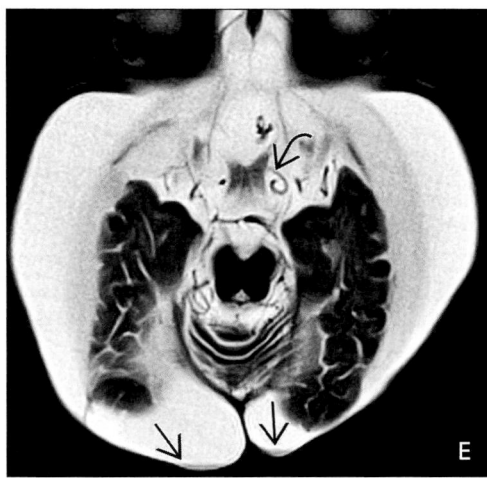

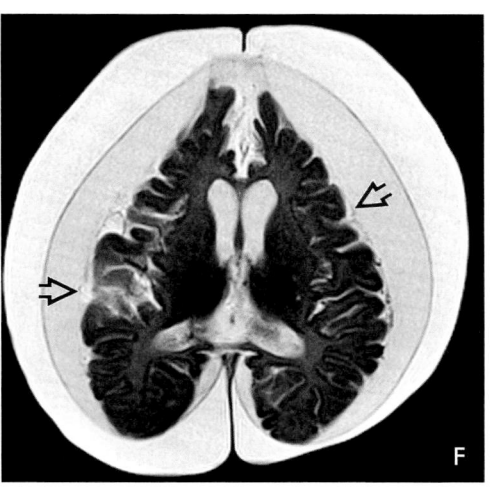

31-42E. *Axial T2WI shows tortuous vessels* ➡. *Note the dependent fluid-fluid levels* ➡ *in both subdural hematomas.* **31-42F.** *More cephalad T2WI shows the extremely atrophic brain, subdural hematomas, inwardly displaced arachnoid* ➡. *Menkes disease ("kinky hair, kinky vessels"). The severe brain atrophy, subdural fluid collections are typical, as is the excessive tortuosity of the intracranial arteries.*

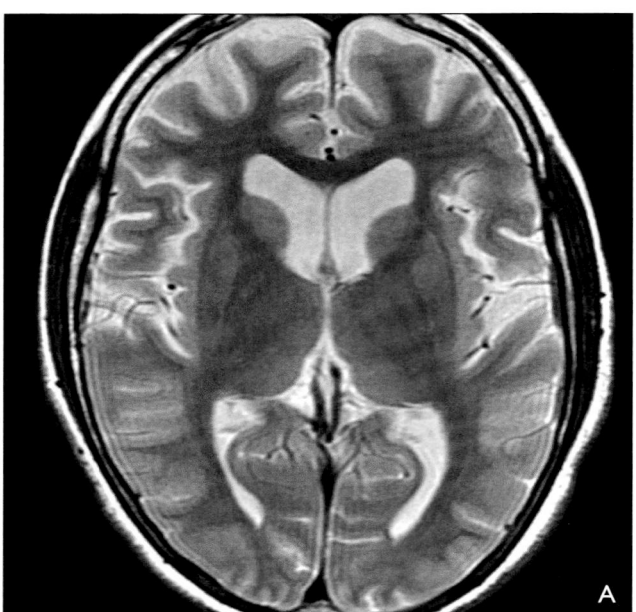

31-43A. Axial T2WI in a 7-year-old girl with Rett syndrome shows enlarged frontal horns and striking frontotemporal predominant volume loss. The hemispheric WM appears normal.

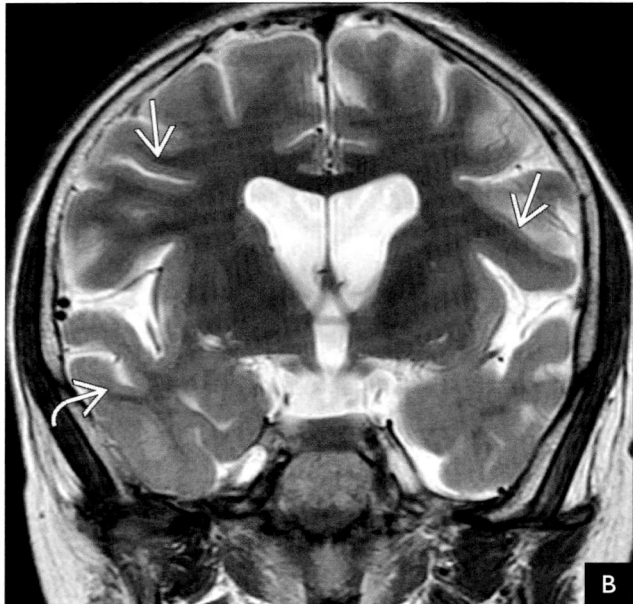

31-43B. Coronal T2WI in the same patient shows thinned cortex in the posterior frontal ⇒ *and temporal* ⇒ *lobes. Moderate volume loss with enlarged suprasellar cistern and sylvian fissures is present.*

studies—usually from skin biopsy specimens—are used to confirm the presence and nature of lysosomal storage material (i.e., specific lipopigments).

Gross pathologic findings in the childhood NCLs are striking global atrophy with no specific lobar predominance. All NCLs demonstrate similar histopathological features, i.e., abnormal accumulation of PAS- and Sudan black-positive inclusions in ballooned neurons. Cortical layers III, V, and VI are most severely affected. Progressive and selective neuronal loss and gliosis with secondary WM degeneration is universally present.

The NCLs share common but nonspecific imaging features: Variable degrees of progressive atrophy with thinned cortex, enlarged ventricles, periventricular T2/FLAIR hyperintense rims, and prominent sulci.

Rett Syndrome

Rett syndrome (RTT) is a progressive neurodevelopmental disorder that almost always affects girls. The majority of cases are sporadic, and no risk factors have been identified. A mutation in the methyl-CpG-binding protein-2 gene (*MECP2*) is identified in 80% of cases.

RTT occurs in 1:20,000 girls. Affected individuals are usually normal at birth with no obvious abnormalities. Head growth gradually decelerates after the first few months, and severe psychomotor retardation develops. Intellectual impairment, mood and behavioral changes, speech difficulty, truncal apraxia, and stereotypical hand waving develop.

Imaging studies show microcephaly with mild but diffuse reduction in both cortical and hemispheric WM volume. The most prominent loss is seen in the frontal and anterior temporal cortex (31-43). DTI shows reduced FA in the corpus callosum, internal capsule, frontal WM, and anterior cingulate gyrus with preservation or increased FA in the posterior corona radiata. MRS shows decreased NAA.

The clinical differential diagnosis of RTT includes NCL and autism. Cortical thinning in **NCL** is generalized and does not exhibit the frontotemporal pattern seen in RTT. **Autism** is excluded if the patient is *MECP2* mutation positive.

Disorders Affecting Both Gray and White Matter

In the last section of this chapter, we discuss inherited metabolic disorders that affect *both* gray and white matter. The pathoetiologies are quite variable and range from abnormal organelles to specific enzymatic dysfunctions.

Selected for discussion are the mucopolysaccharidoses, Canavan disease, Alexander disease, peroxisomal spectrum disorders, and mitochondrial disorders.

Mucopolysaccharidoses

Terminology and Etiology

The mucopolysaccharidoses (MPSs) are lysosomal storage disorders characterized by incomplete degradation and progressive accumulation of toxic glycosaminoglycan (GAG) in various organs. The MPSs were once grouped into a single entity and termed "gargoylism" for their supposedly characteristic facies.

The mucopolysaccharidoses are now designated as MPSs 1-9. Each has a specific enzyme deficiency that causes the inability to break down GAG. MPS 1H (Hurler disease) and MPS 1HS (Hurler-Scheie disease) have deficiency of α-L-iduronidase. MPS 2 (Hunter disease) is characterized by iduronate 2-sulfatase deficiency. Other MPSs include MPS 3A (Sanfilippo disease), MPS 4A (Morquio disease), and MPS 6 (Maroteaux-Lamy disease).

Pathology

Autophagy is a highly regulated process in the lysosomal pathway that degrades proteins and damaged cellular organelles. Abnormal autophagy combined with the incomplete degradation and progressive accumulation of glycosaminoglycans is the pathology that underlies the mucopolysaccharidoses.

The two distinctive gross features of the mucopolysaccharidoses are thickened meninges and dilated perivascular spaces (PVSs). The enlarged PVSs give a cribriform appearance to the brain on both pathology and imaging **(31-44)**, **(31-45)**.

Microscopically, the MPSs are characterized by dilated perivascular spaces packed with undegraded GAG **(31-46)**.

Clinical Issues

All the MPSs have different clinical phenotypes. Systemic abnormalities range from hepatosplenomegaly and skeletal dysostoses to thickened dura, coarse facies, and macrocrania. Age at presentation varies, as do gender predilection and prognosis.

Hurler (MPS 1H) and Hunter (MPS 2) diseases are two of the most common MPSs. Hurler patients appear normal at birth but soon develop CNS symptoms, including delayed development and mental retardation. Untreated Hurler disease typically results in death by age 10.

MPS 2 (Hunter disease) is an X-linked disorder and is seen only in males. Hunter disease is characterized by progressive multisystem involvement in the CNS, joints, bones, heart, skin, liver, eyes, and other organs. Patients often survive into their mid teens but usually expire from cardiac disease.

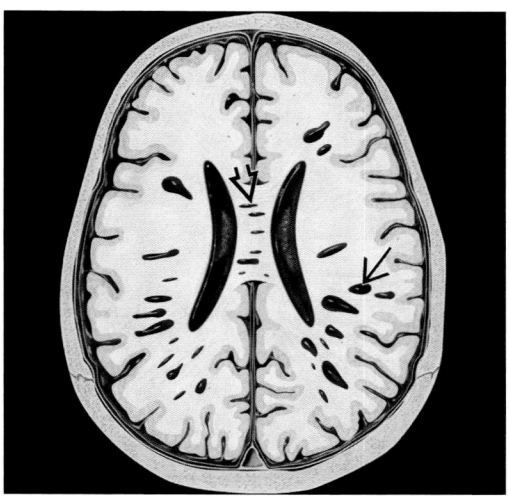

31-44. MPS with multiple dilated PVSs ⇥ radially oriented in the WM. Note posterior predominance, involvement of the corpus callosum ⇗.

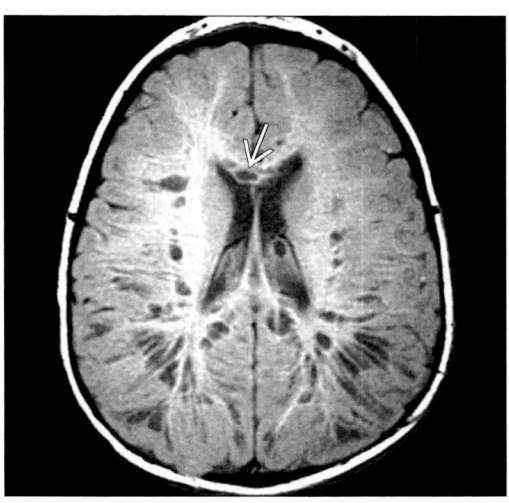

31-45. T1WI in a toddler with MPS 1H (Hurler disease) shows markedly enlarged PVSs in the WM including the corpus callosum ➡.

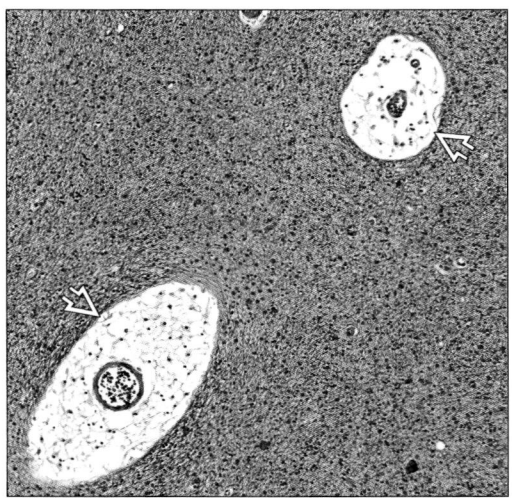

31-46. MPS 1HS (Hurler-Scheie) with myelin stain shows enlarged PVSs ➡ packed with undegraded mucopolysaccharides. (Courtesy P. Shannon, MD.)

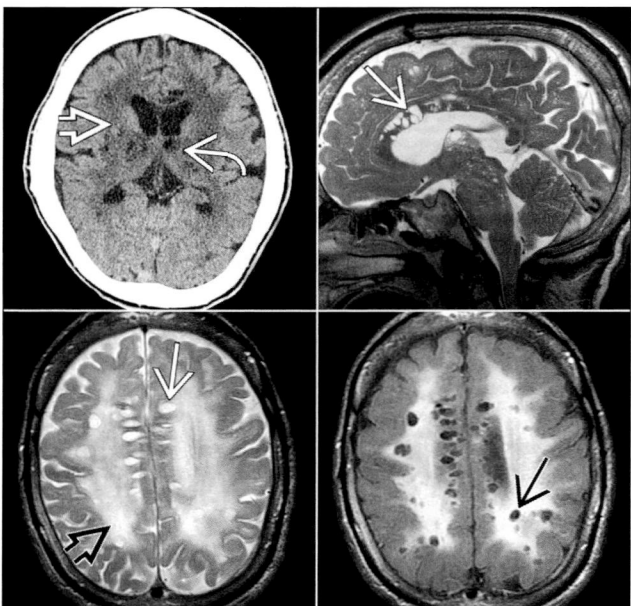

31-47. NECT of Hunter disease shows WM hypodensity ⇒ with focal basal ganglia lesions ⇒. T2WIs show enlarged PVSs in corpus callosum ⇒, confluent WM disease ⇒. Enlarged PVSs suppress on FLAIR ⇒; the WM disease remains hyperintense.

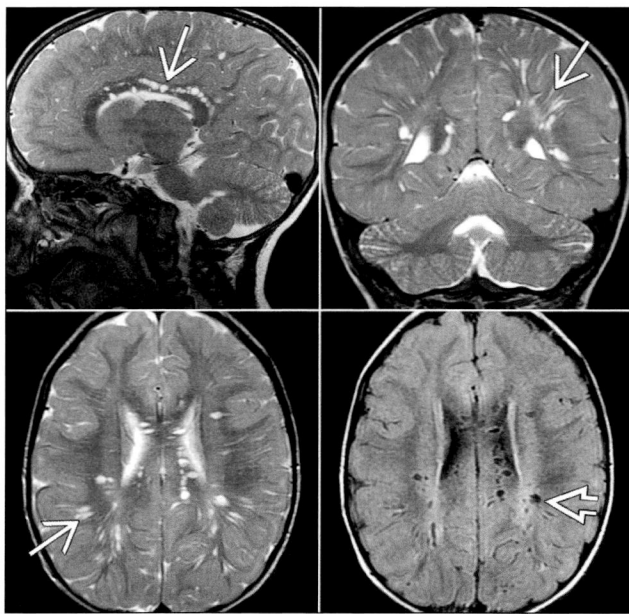

31-48. Sagittal, coronal, axial T2 scans in a 2-year-old boy with Hunter disease shows multiple enlarged PVSs ⇒. Note the posterior predominance, corpus callosum involvement. The lesions suppress on FLAIR ⇒.

Imaging

The prototypical imaging findings in MPSs are illustrated by Hurler (MPS 1H) and Hunter (MPS 2) diseases. The major features of these disorders are macrocephaly, enlarged perivascular spaces, and pachymeningopathy.

MACROCEPHALY. NECT scans show an enlarged head, often with metopic "beaking" and a scaphocephalic configuration. Progressive hydrocephalus and atrophy can be present. Sagittal MR scans also demonstrate a large head with craniofacial disproportion.

ENLARGED PERIVASCULAR SPACES. A striking sieve-like cribriform appearance in the posterior cerebral WM and corpus callosum is characteristic and is caused by numerous dilated PVSs **(31-45)**. Although sometimes called "Hurler holes," these enlarged PVSs are typical of both Hurler and Hunter diseases. They are much less common in the other MPSs.

NECT scans may show decreased density with multifocal CSF-like hypodensities in the WM and basal ganglia **(31-47)**.

T2 scans show CSF-like hyperintensity in the enlarged PVSs. The surrounding WM may show patchy or confluent hyperintensity. The PVSs themselves suppress completely on FLAIR **(31-48)**. A faint "halo" of hyperintensity often surrounds the lesions.

The enlarged PVSs do not "bloom" on T2* and do not enhance following contrast administration.

PACHYMENINGOPATHY. The meninges, especially around the craniovertebral junction (CVJ), are often thickened and appear very hypointense on T2-weighted images **(31-49)**. In severe cases, the thickened meninges can compress the medulla or upper cervical cord **(31-50)**. Odontoid dysplasia and a short C1 posterior arch—common in the MPSs—can exacerbate the craniovertebral junction stenosis, causing progressive myelopathy. A lumbar gibbus with a "beaked" L1 vertebral body is common in Hurler disease.

Differential Diagnosis

The differential diagnosis of MPS is limited. **Prominent perivascular spaces** can be normal findings in patients of any age. Although they can be seen in children and even infants, prominent PVSs are more common in middle-aged and older patients. No macrocephaly is present with this normal variant.

Dilated PVSs with a frontal predominance are a feature of **velocardiofacial syndrome**. Deviated carotid arteries in the pharynx are present, a finding not associated with the MPSs.

Canavan Disease

Canavan disease is a fatal autosomal recessive neurodegenerative disorder for which there is currently no effective treatment. Canavan disease is the only identified genetic disorder caused by a defect in a metabolite—N-acetyl-L-aspartate (NAA)—that is produced exclusively in the brain.

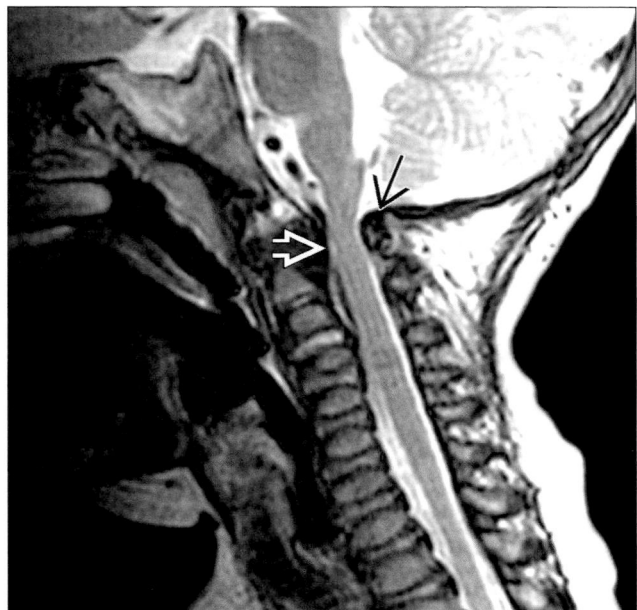

31-49. Sagittal T2WI in a patient with MPS 1H shows foramen magnum narrowing, cord compression. The CVJ narrowing is caused by a combination of a short posterior C1 arch ➡, odontoid dysplasia, thickened ligament ➡.

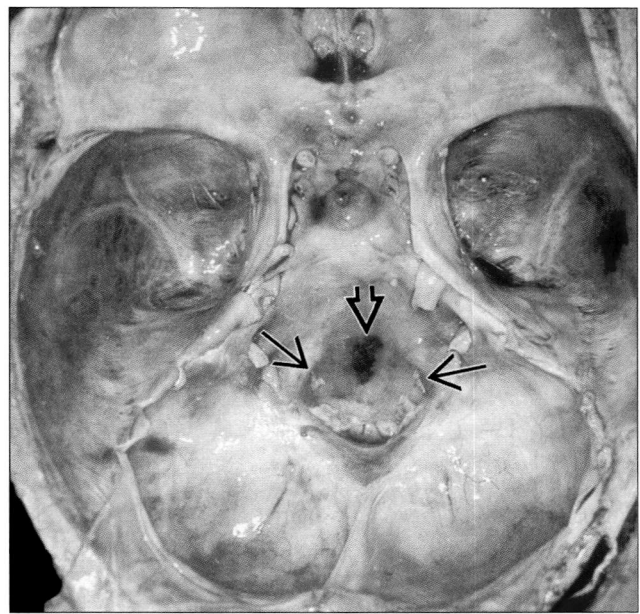

31-50. Autopsy case of MPS 1H shows remarkable dural thickening ➡ that causes exceptionally severe narrowing of the foramen magnum ➡. (Courtesy AFIP Archives.)

Terminology

Canavan disease (CD) is also known as spongiform leukodystrophy, spongy degeneration of the CNS, aspartoacyclase deficiency, and Canavan-van Bogaert-Bertrand disease.

Etiology

NAA is the second most abundant amino acid in the mammalian brain. NAA levels in the brain are normally maintained within a tightly regulated range. Aspartoacyclase—the enzyme responsible for metabolizing NAA—is a signature marker of mature oligodendrocytes. Mutations in the *aspA* gene cause abnormal NAA accumulation in the brain and result in Canavan disease.

Precisely how and why excessive NAA causes the dramatic intramyelinic edema and myelin damage associated with CD is unknown.

Pathology

The brain in CD appears grossly swollen. Microscopic analysis shows spongiform WM degeneration with swollen astrocytes in the globi pallidi and thalami.

Clinical Issues

CD is most common in Ashkenazi Jews and rare in other non-Jewish populations. One in 40 Ashkenazi Jews carries the mutated *aspA* gene. There is no gender predilection.

Three clinical variants of CD are recognized. The congenital form presents within the first few days of life and leads to profound hypotonia with poor head control. Death rapidly ensues. The most common form by far is infantile CD. Infantile CD presents between three and six months and is characterized by hypotonia, macrocephaly, and seizures. Death between one or two years is typical. Juvenile-onset CD begins between four and five years of age and is the most slowly progressive form.

Imaging

NECT shows a large head with diffuse WM hypodensity in the cerebral hemispheres and cerebellum. The globi pallidi also appear hypodense. CD does not enhance.

MR shows virtually complete absence of myelination with confluent T2/FLAIR hyperintensity throughout the WM and globi pallidi. Early in the disease course, the subcortical arcuate fibers are initially affected and the gyri may appear swollen. As the disease progresses, diffuse volume loss with ventricular and sulcal enlargement ensues. The hemispheric and cerebellar WM, basal ganglia, and cortex are all affected.

MRS is the key to the definitive diagnosis of CD. Markedly elevated NAA is seen in virtually all cases (31-51). Cr is reduced. An elevated mI peak is sometimes present.

Differential Diagnosis

The major differential diagnosis of CD is **Alexander disease**. Both CD and Alexander disease cause macrocephaly, but an elevated NAA peak on MRS distinguishes the two disorders. Furthermore, Alexander disease enhances; CD does not.

Megalencephaly with leukoencephalopathy and cysts involves the subcortical arcuate fibers, as does CD, but the basal ganglia are not affected. **Pelizaeus-Merzbacher disease** demonstrates virtually complete lack of myelination but does not cause macrocephaly and does not affect the basal ganglia.

Alexander Disease

Terminology

Alexander disease (AxD) is also known as fibrinoid leukodystrophy, a misnomer as it involves both white and gray matter.

Etiology

AxD patients have de novo heterozygous dominant mutations in the *GFAP* gene, which encodes for glial fibrillary acidic protein, an intermediate filament protein that is expressed only in astrocytes. The parents of patients with infantile- or childhood-onset AxD are neurologically normal.

GFAP mutations cause precipitation and accumulation of mutant GFAP aggregates, which begins during fetal development.

Pathology

The brains of infants with AxD have markedly increased astrocytic density and are grossly enlarged. Dramatic myelin loss in the hemispheres, brainstem, cerebellum, and spinal cord makes the WM—especially in the frontal lobes—appear very pale. In severe cases, the WM appears partially or almost entirely cystic. The subcortical arcuate fibers are relatively spared. Cortical thinning with basal ganglia and thalamic atrophy is common.

The hallmark histopathologic feature of AxD is the presence of enormous numbers of Rosenthal fibers (RFs) in astrocytes. RFs are ovoid or rod-shaped eosinophilic cytoplasmic inclusion bodies. The striking lack of nearly all myelin in AxD is considered a secondary phenome-

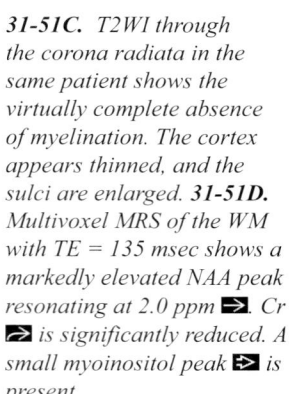

31-51A. Sagittal T1WI in a 2-year-old boy with Canavan disease shows macrocephaly with striking craniofacial disproportion. Moderate generalized volume loss is present in both the cerebral hemispheres and cerebellum. 31-51B. Axial T2WI shows diffuse WM hyperintensity throughout the brain indicating complete absence of myelination. The globi pallidi ➡ are hyperintense, so shrunken and atrophic that they have almost completely disappeared.

31-51C. T2WI through the corona radiata in the same patient shows the virtually complete absence of myelination. The cortex appears thinned, and the sulci are enlarged. 31-51D. Multivoxel MRS of the WM with TE = 135 msec shows a markedly elevated NAA peak resonating at 2.0 ppm ➡. Cr ➡ is significantly reduced. A small myoinositol peak ➡ is present.

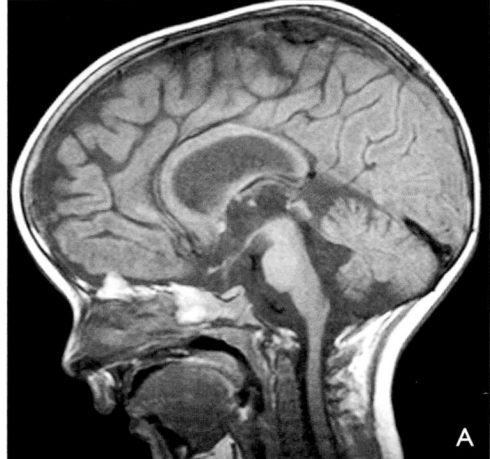

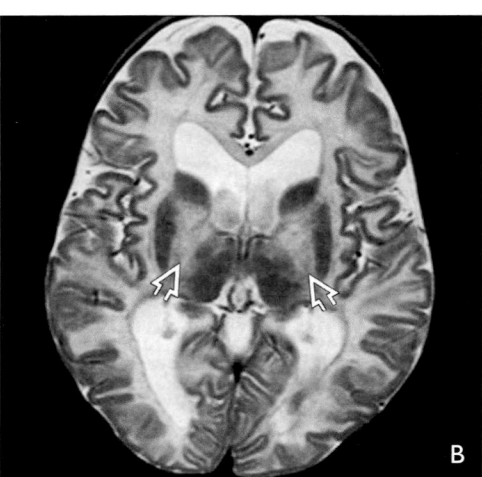

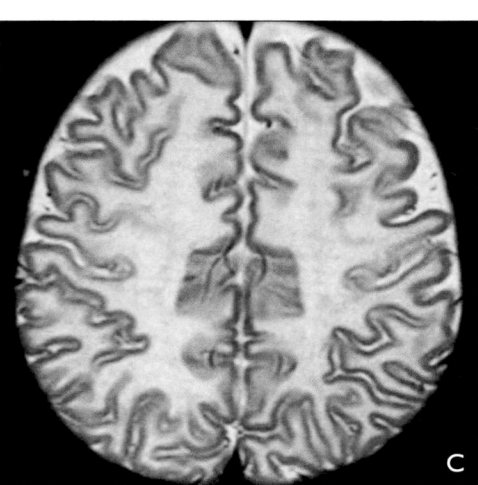

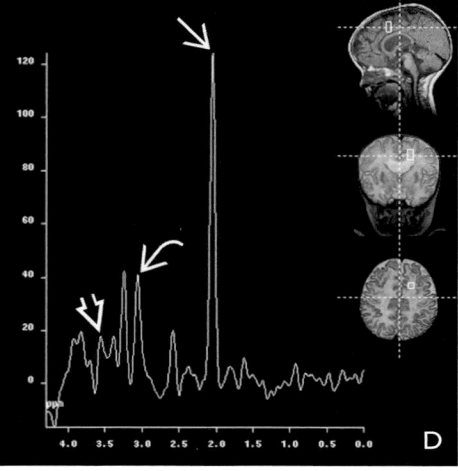

non that arises from severely disrupted astrocyte-derived myelination signaling.

Clinical Issues

AxD is rare, accounting for just 1-2% of childhood inherited leukodystrophies.

Three clinical forms are recognized: Infantile, juvenile, and adult. In the infantile form, which is the most common, patients younger than two years present with megalencephaly, progressive psychomotor retardation, and seizures. Spasticity and eventually quadriplegia often develop.

Juvenile AxD presents between ages 2-12 years and is characterized by bulbar and cerebellar signs. Patients over the age of 12 years present with a variety of signs and symptoms including ataxia, bulbar signs, and cognitive decline. Palatal myoclonus occurs in 40% of adult AxD cases.

Disease progression is variable. Patients with adult-onset AxD have a slower, more protracted course. Although imaging findings can be suggestive of the disease, the diagnosis of AxD is confirmed by increased GFAP CSF levels or *GFAP* gene analysis.

Imaging

NECT scans of infants with AxD show a large head with symmetric WM hypodensity in the frontal lobes that extends posteriorly into the caudate nuclei and internal/external capsules (31-52). AxD is one of the few inherited metabolic disorders that demonstrates enhancement following contrast administration. Intense bifrontal periventricular enhancement can be seen on CECT scans early in the disease course.

MR shows T1 hypointensity and T2/FLAIR hyperintensity in the frontal WM, caudate nuclei, and anterior putamina. Although infantile AxD involves the subcortical U-fibers early in the disease course, the periventricular WM is more severely affected in most juvenile and adults forms. A classic finding is a T1 hypointense, T2 hyperintense rim around the frontal horns. FLAIR scans may demonstrate cystic encephalomalacia in the frontal WM in more severe, protracted cases.

A unique finding in AxD is enlargement of the caudate heads and fornices, which appear swollen and hyperintense. The thalami, globi pallidi, brainstem, and cerebellum are less commonly affected.

Unlike most IMDs, AxD can demonstrate moderate to striking enhancement on T1 C+. Rims of intense enhancement can be seen around the surfaces of the swollen caudate nuclei and affected WM. In the juvenile

and adult forms, cerebellar involvement can be striking and may mimic neoplasm.

MRS shows decreased NAA, elevated myoinositol, and variably increased choline and lactate. DWI shows normal to increased diffusivity in the affected WM.

Differential Diagnosis

The major differential diagnoses of Alexander disease are other inherited leukodystrophies with macrocephaly. These primarily include **Canavan disease** and the **mucopolysaccharidoses**. While both AxD and Canavan disease show almost complete lack of myelination with T2/FLAIR WM hyperintensity, the predilection of AxD for the frontal lobes, caudate heads, and enhancement help distinguish it from Canavan disease.

The mucopolysaccharidoses, especially Hurler and Hunter diseases, display a striking "cribriform" appearance of the WM and corpus callosum caused by enlarged perivascular spaces. Deep gray involvement is absent, and the lesions do not enhance. Some of the MPSs—especially MPS-1—cause dural thickening, which is absent in AxD.

Megalencephaly with leukoencephalopathy and cysts has striking subcortical arcuate involvement early in the disease course, does not involve the basal ganglia, and does not enhance.

DIFFERENTIAL DIAGNOSIS: CHILD WITH A LARGE HEAD

Common
- Normal variant
- Benign familial macrocrania
- Benign macrocrania of infancy

Less Common
- Nonaccidental trauma with subdural hematomas

Rare but Important
- Inherited metabolic disorder
  - Canavan disease
  - Alexander disease
  - Mucopolysaccharidoses
  - Megalencephaly with leukoencephalopathy and cysts
  - Glutaric aciduria type I

Peroxisomal Biogenesis Disorders

Peroxisomes are small single-membrane-bounded organelles that contain over 50 enzymes required for normal growth, development, and cellular metabolism. Biosynthesis of plasmalogens and β-oxidation of very long chain fatty acids (VLCFAs) are among the essential functions of peroxisomes. Genetic defects that affect either peroxisomal formation or enzymatic function cause a group of diseases called peroxisomal disorders.

31-52A. NECT in 6-month-old boy with large head, documented AxD shows marked bifrontal hypodensity ➡ extending posteriorly into the basal ganglia. *31-52B.* Axial T1 C+ scan shows striking differentiation between the exceptionally hypointense frontal WM ➡ and the more normal-appearing parietooccipital WM ➡. The hypointensity extends into the external capsules. Note the characteristic hyperintense rims around the frontal horns ➡.

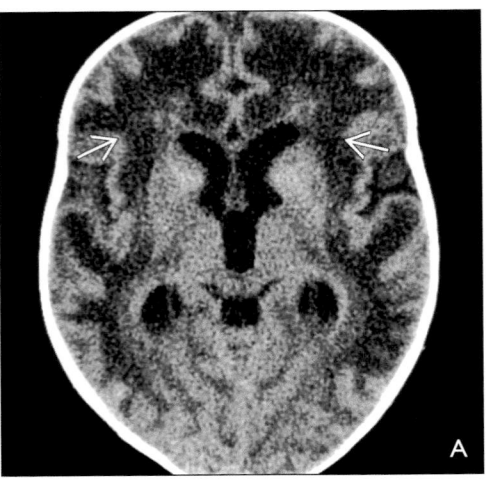

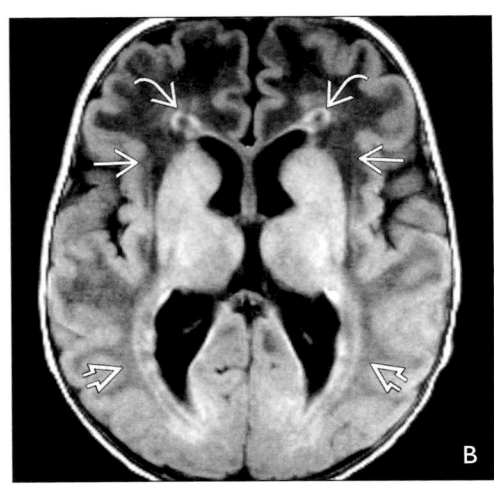

31-52C. The contrast between the swollen-appearing, hyperintense frontal WM ➡, the more normal-appearing parietooccipital WM ➡ is less striking on this T2WI. Note external capsule involvement ➡. The internal capsules are partially myelinated and thus appear less hyperintense than the frontal WM. The hypointense rim around the frontal horns ➡ is characteristic. *31-52D.* Axial T1 C+ shows enhancement in the periventricular WM ➡, basal ganglia ➡.

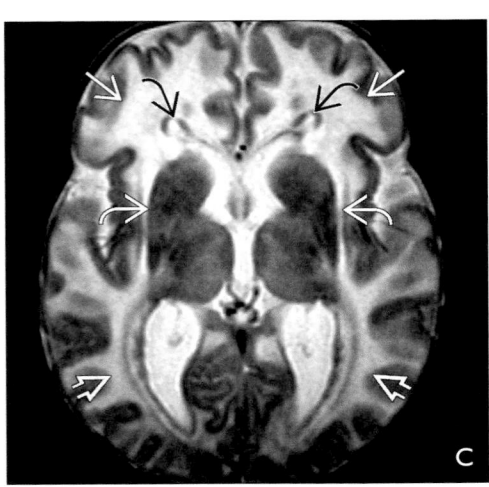

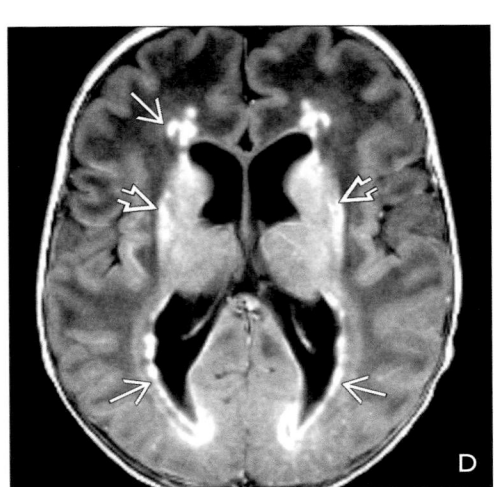

31-52E. Coronal T1 C+ scan shows striking enhancement of the deep periventricular WM ➡ and basal ganglia ➡. *31-52F.* Sagittal T1 C+ scan displays enhancement of virtually all the deep periventricular WM ➡ and striking hypointensity of the frontal and anterior parietal WM ➡ with relative sparing of the occipital lobe.

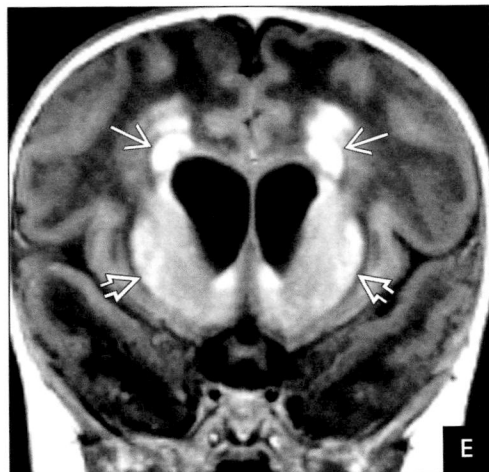

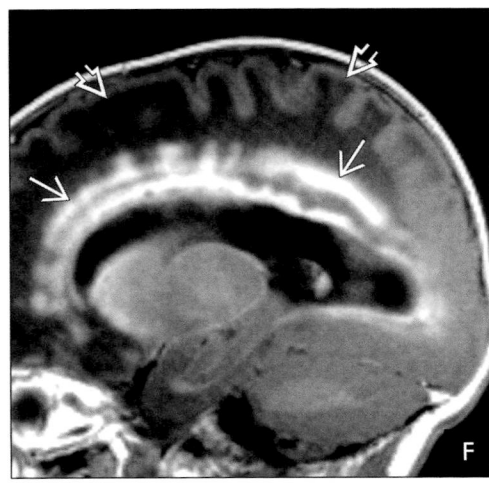

Terminology

There are two main types of peroxisomal disorders. The most common type is caused by *single protein deficiencies within intact (morphologically normal) peroxisomes*. This group includes, among others, X-linked adrenoleukodystrophy (ALD), adrenomyeloneuropathy (AMN), and classic (adult) Refsum disease. ALD and AMN affect periventricular WM and were therefore discussed earlier in the chapter with other disorders that exhibit this imaging pattern.

The second less common group of peroxisomal disorders caused by *abnormal formation of peroxisomes* and is discussed below. Disorders in which the peroxisomal organelles themselves fail to form normally are called peroxisomal biogenesis disorders (PBDs). PBDs are typically characterized by multiple (not single) enzymatic defects.

Four major PBDs are recognized: **Zellweger syndrome** (ZS, also called cerebrohepatorenal syndrome), neonatal adrenoleukodystrophy, infantile Refsum disease, and classic rhizomelic chondrodysplasia punctata. The first three disorders are grouped together and referred to as **Zellweger syndrome spectrum** (ZSS).

Etiology

PBDs are autosomal recessive disorders caused by mutations in one of 13 peroxisomal assembly (*PEX*) genes. The most severe form is ZSS, which accounts for 80% of all cases and is characterized by nearly complete absence of peroxisomes.

Pathology

PBDs are characterized pathologically by germinal matrix injury, subependymal germinolytic cysts, disordered neuronal migration, and hypomyelination.

The most common gross findings are cerebral neocortical and cerebellar abnormalities. Brain atrophy and abnormal gyration—most often pachygyria or polymicrogyria—are common in patients with severe ZSS **(31-53)**. Defective peroxisomes in oligodendroglial cells also cause abnormal WM formation and maintenance.

Clinical Issues

PBDs are less common than many other inherited metabolic disorders. The estimated incidence is 1:20,000-100,000 live births. In contrast to ALD, there is no gender predilection.

The PBDs are clinically diverse, but frequent features include dysmorphic facies with large fontanelle and sutures, high forehead, and broad nasal bridge. Hepatointestinal dysfunction, hypotonia ("floppy infant"),

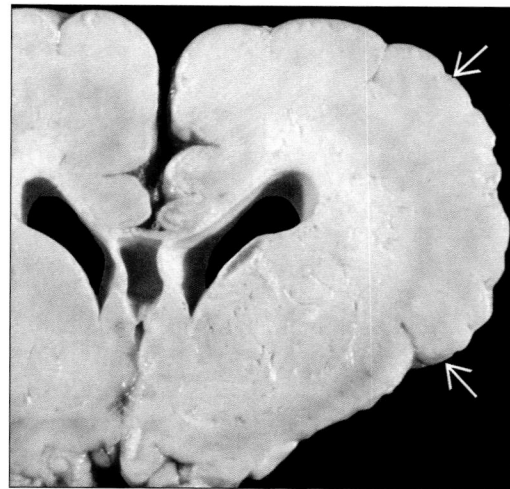

31-53. *Coronal autopsy of ZSS shows grossly abnormal gyration with pachy-, polymicrogyria ➡, poor sulcation. (Courtesy AFIP Archives.)*

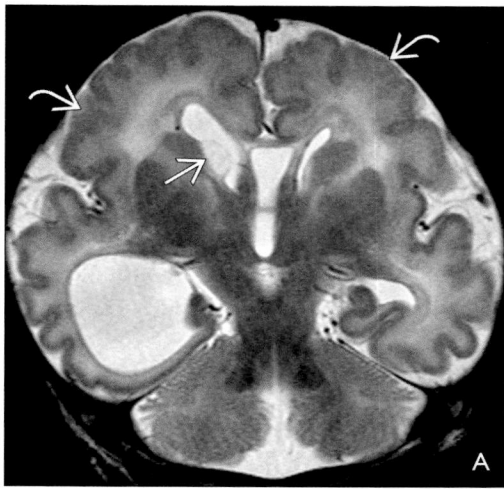

31-54A. *Coronal T2WI in newborn with ZSS shows small germinolytic cyst ➡ in the caudothalamic groove, several areas of polymicrogyria ➡.*

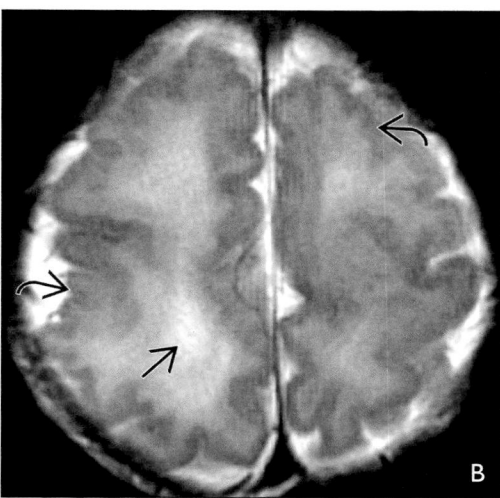

31-54B. *Axial T2WI in the same patient shows diffuse microgyria ➡ and foci of abnormal WM hyperintensity ➡.*

seizures, retinitis pigmentosa, and psychomotor retardation are common.

The disease course of different PBDs varies considerably. The most severely affected neonates with ZS typically die by six months of age whereas those with milder forms of the disease may survive more than 20 years.

Imaging

Imaging findings in the PBDs are variable, but the most common features are disordered neuronal migration and abnormal myelination. ZSS is characterized by micrgyria and pachygyria, often with bilaterally symmetric parasylvian lesions. Hypomyelinated WM is seen as confluent T2/FLAIR WM hyperintensity. Subependymal (caudothalamic) germinolytic cysts are common findings (31-54). Hyperbilirubinemia may caused increased T1 signal intensity in the globi pallidi of older patients.

Differential Diagnosis

The major differential diagnosis of ZSS is **congenital Cytomegalovirus** (CMV). Both ZSS and congenital CMV exhibit hypomyelination and cortical malformations. Calcifications are a more prominent feature of CMV, and the periventricular cysts are usually not localized to the caudothalamic groove. Isolated **neuronal migration disorders** (e.g., bilateral perisylvian polymicrogyria) occur without other clinical and imaging stigmata of ZSS.

Mitochondrial Diseases (Respiratory Chain Disorders)

The mitochondria are cellular organelles that are the "power plants" responsible for energy production. Five complexes are embedded in the inner mitochondrial membrane and are responsible for oxidative phosphorylation (OXPHOS); defects in any one result in defective oxidative phosphorylation and deficient ATP production.

Mitochondrial disorders are caused by mitochondrial DNA (mtDNA) mutations and are among the most common of all IMDs. Although virtually every organ or tissue of the body can be affected, the nervous system and skeletal muscle are especially vulnerable because of their high energy demands.

Four major encephalomyopathic syndromes have been described and are considered here: Leigh disease, Kearns-Sayre syndrome, MELAS, and MERRF. We then discuss glutaric aciduria types 1 and 2, also caused by mtDNA-mediated enzyme abnormalities. Other mitochondrial disorders—including Alpers syndrome, infantile mitochondrial myopathy, and Leber hereditary optic

neuropathy (LHON)—are rare and not examined further in this text.

Mitochondrial disorders have significant overlap and are not always easily distinguished from each other.

Leigh Disease

TERMINOLOGY AND ETIOLOGY. Leigh disease (LD) is also known as subacute necrotizing encephalopathy. LD is caused by mutations that encode for OXPHOS enzymes.

PATHOLOGY. Gross pathology of LD demonstrates brownish gray gelatinous or cavitary foci in the basal ganglia, brainstem, dentate nuclei, thalami, and spinal cord with variable WM spongiform degeneration and demyelination.

CLINICAL ISSUES. Clinical manifestations of LD are highly variable. Most patients with LD present in infancy or childhood with failure to thrive, central hypotonia, developmental regression, ataxia, bulbar dysfunction, and ophthalmoplegia. Serum and CSF lactate levels are elevated.

IMAGING. MR in LD shows bilaterally symmetric areas of T2/FLAIR hyperintensity in the basal ganglia (31-55). The putamina (especially the posterior segments) are consistently affected, as are the caudate heads. The dorsomedial thalami can also be involved whereas the globi pallidi are less commonly affected.

Mid- and lower brainstem (pons/medulla) lesions are typical in LD and in a few cases can be the *only* finding. Symmetric lesions in the cerebral peduncles are common, and the periaqueductal gray matter is frequently affected.

Acute lesions may restrict on DWI but do not enhance. MRS of the brain parenchyma and CSF typically shows a prominent lactate peak at 1.3 ppm.

DIFFERENTIAL DIAGNOSIS. As their imaging findings often overlap, the differential diagnosis of Leigh disease includes the other mitochondrial encephalomyopathies. **MELAS** typically shows stroke-like abnormalities in the cortical gray matter in a nonvascular distribution.

Metabolic and hypoxic-ischemic disease can mimic some findings of LD. **Wilson disease** (WD) shows T2/FLAIR hyperintensity in the putamina, midbrain, and thalami. The globi pallidi in WD often show T1 shortening secondary to hepatic failure. **Profound perinatal asphyxia** can affect the basal ganglia and mimic LD, but the perirolandic cortex is commonly affected.

MELAS

TERMINOLOGY AND ETIOLOGY. **M**itochondrial encephalomyopathy with **l**actic **a**cidosis and **s**troke-like episodes (MELAS) is caused by several different point mutations in mtDNA.

CLINICAL ISSUES. The clinical triad of lactic acidosis, seizures, and stroke-like episodes is the classic presentation, but other common symptoms include migraines, episodic vomiting, and alternating hemiplegia. Cardiac abnormalities, renal dysfunction, GI motility disorders, and generalized muscle weakness are also common.

MELAS is an uncommon but important cause of childhood stroke. Mean age at symptom onset is 15 years, although some patients may not become symptomatic until 40-50 years of age.

IMAGING. Imaging findings vary with disease acuity (31-56). *Acute* MELAS often shows swollen T2/FLAIR hyperintense gyri. The underlying WM is normal, and the cortical abnormalities cross vascular distribution territories, distinguishing MELAS from acute cerebral infarction (31-57). The parietal and occipital lobes are most commonly affected. Gyral enhancement on T1 C+ is typical. MRA shows no evidence of major vessel occlusion.

Chronic MELAS shows multifocal lacunar-type infarcts, symmetric basal ganglia calcifications, WM volume loss, and progressive atrophy of the parietooccipital cortex.

MRS is extremely helpful in the diagnosis of most mitochondrial encephalopathies. Nearly two-thirds of cases with MELAS show a prominent lactate "doublet" at 1.3 ppm in otherwise normal-appearing brain. Caution: One-third of cases show no evidence for elevated lactate levels in the brain parenchyma but may demonstrate a lactate peak in the ventricular CSF.

DIFFERENTIAL DIAGNOSIS. The differential diagnosis of MELAS includes major territorial **cerebral infarction**. MELAS spares the subcortical and deep WM and crosses vascular territories (often the middle and posterior cerebral distributions). **Prolonged seizures** can cause gyral swelling, hyperintensity, and enhancement that appears identical to MELAS. MRS shows no evidence of elevated lactate levels in the CSF and normal-appearing brain.

Leigh disease often involves the brainstem, which is less commonly involved in MELAS. **MERRF** shows a

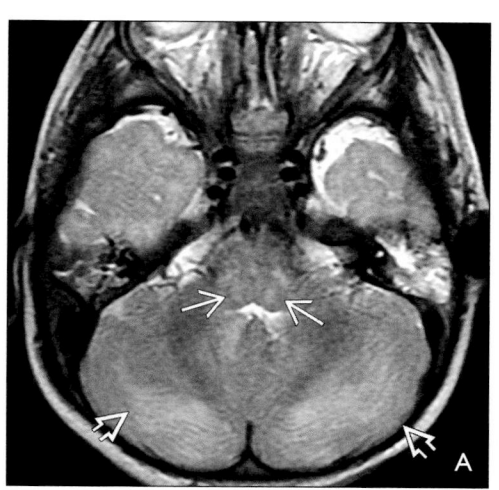 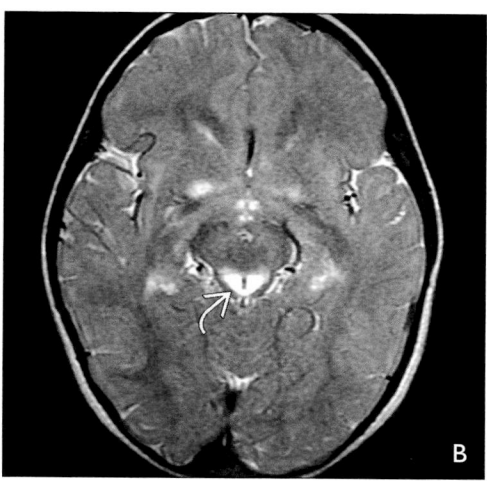

31-55A. Axial T2WI in a 19-year-old woman with Leigh disease shows bilaterally symmetric hyperintensities in the white matter of both cerebellar hemispheres, medulla. 31-55B. More cephalad T2WI in the same patient shows striking hyperintensity in the periaqueductal gray matter.

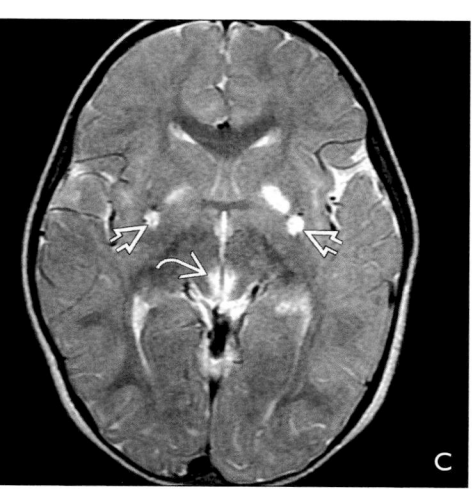 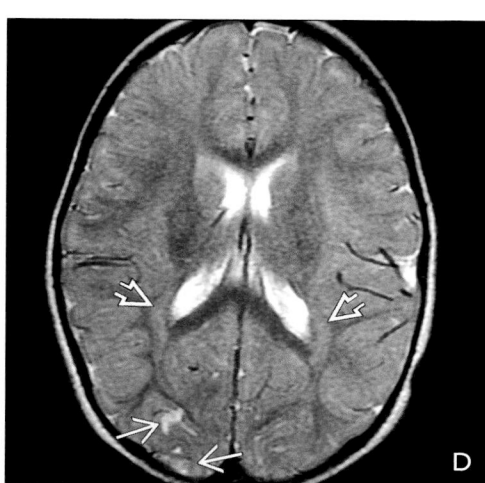

31-55C. T2WI shows symmetric hyperintensity in the upper midbrain, both basal ganglia. 31-55D. T2WI through the lateral ventricles shows focal hyperintensity in the right occipital cortex, subcortical WM consistent with infarction. Symmetric mild hyperintensity lateral and dorsal to the atria is the normal terminal zone of late myelination in parietooccipital association fibers.

propensity to involve the basal ganglia, caudate nuclei, and vascular watershed zones.

Kearns-Sayre Syndrome

TERMINOLOGY AND ETIOLOGY. Kearns-Sayre syndrome (KSS), also known as Kearns-Sayre ophthalmoplegic syndrome, is another mtDNA disorder. A number of different gene deletions have been identified in KSS patients.

PATHOLOGY. The most typical and consistent pathologic finding of KSS is spongiform WM vacuolation. The cerebral hemispheres and midbrain are most commonly affected. The cerebellum, brainstem, and spinal cord are also frequently involved whereas the corpus callosum and internal capsules are usually spared.

CLINICAL ISSUES. KSS typically presents in older children or young adults and is characterized by short stature, progressive external ophthalmoplegia, retinitis pigmentosa, sensorineural hearing loss, and ataxia.

Other organs are frequently involved in KSS. Heart block and proximal muscle weakness are common. Ragged red fibers are present on muscle biopsy.

IMAGING. CT scans show variable symmetric basal ganglia calcifications. Mild cortical and cerebellar volume loss is common.

MR shows increased signal intensity in the basal ganglia, WM, and cerebellum on T2/FLAIR. The subcortical arcuate fibers, corticospinal tracts, cerebellum, and posterior brainstem are involved early in the disease course while the periventricular WM remains relatively spared (31-58).

DWI shows reduced diffusivity in the brainstem and subcortical WM. MRS demonstrates elevated lactate.

DIFFERENTIAL DIAGNOSIS. There is significant overlap between imaging findings in KSS and other mitochondrial disorders such as **MELAS**. Early involvement of the cortex in a nonvascular distribution—particularly the parietal and occipital lobes—is characteristic of MELAS but uncommon in KSS.

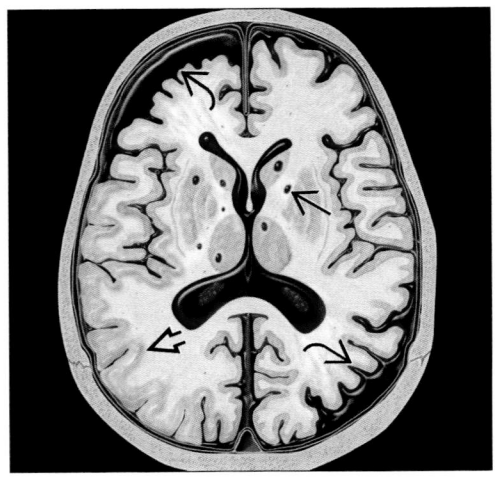
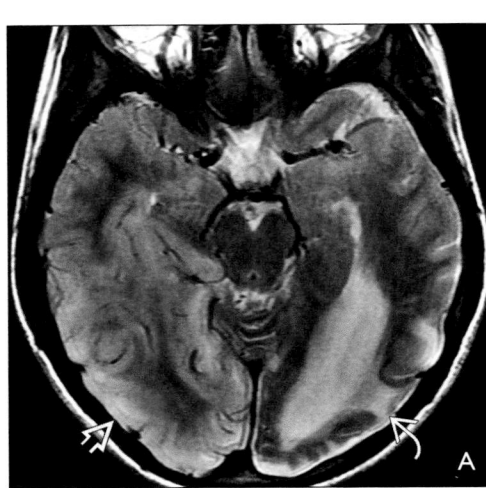
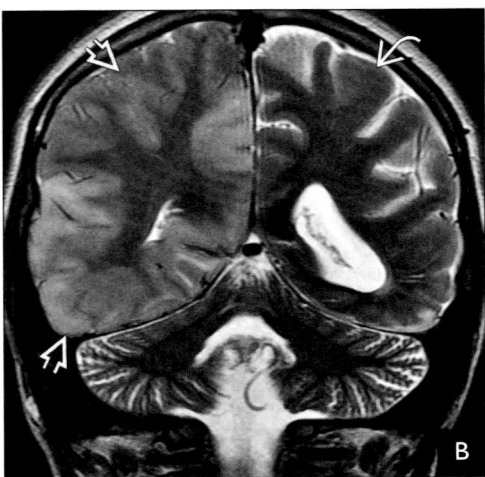
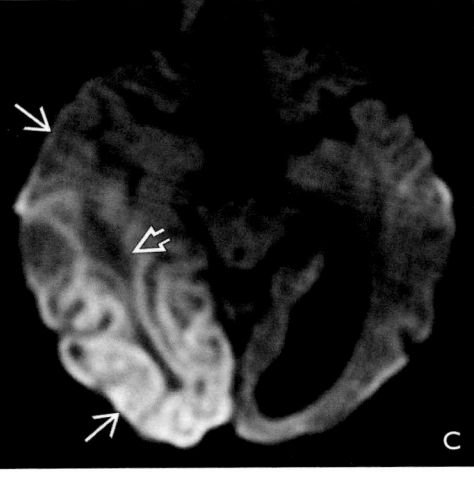

31-56. Graphic depicts changes of MELAS with evidence of both acute and chronic lesions (lacunar infarcts ➡, cortical atrophy ➘). Acute manifestation is gyral edema that crosses vascular territories ➤, spares the underlying WM. *31-57A.* T2WI in a 10-year-old girl with MELAS shows residua of remote left parietooccipital lesion ➚, acute right temporoparietal gyral swelling ➤ that spares the underlying WM.

31-57B. Coronal T2WI shows an enlarged left lateral ventricle, cortical atrophy ➡ with acute right gyral edema ➤, the "shifting spread" characteristic of MELAS. *31-57C.* DWI shows acute diffusion restriction ➡ in the swollen edematous cortex with sparing of the underlying WM ➤. MRS (not shown) demonstrated elevated lactate levels in the normal-appearing brain.

MERRF

Myoclonus **e**pilepsy with **r**agged **r**ed **f**ibers (MERRF) is another syndrome with mtDNA mutations that result in defective mitochondrial OXPHOS. MERRF is a multisystem disorder characterized by myoclonus (often the first symptom) followed by epilepsy, ataxia, weakness, cardiomyopathy, and dementia. Childhood onset is typical.

MERRF is typified pathologically by systemic degeneration involving the globus pallidus, substantia nigra, red nuclei, dentate nuclei, inferior olivary nuclei, cortex, and spinocerebellar tracts.

Imaging studies show watershed and basal ganglia infarcts. The major imaging differential diagnosis of MERRF is MELAS; the two disorders often overlap. Pathologically, the major differential diagnosis is KSS, as both can demonstrate the presence of ragged red fibers on muscle biopsy.

Glutaric Aciduria Type 1

TERMINOLOGY AND ETIOLOGY. Glutaric aciduria type 1 (GA1) is also called glutaric acidemia type 1.

ETIOLOGY. GA1 is an autosomal recessive IMD caused by deficiency of the mitochondrial enzyme glutaryl-coenzyme A dehydrogenase (GCDH). GCDH is required for metabolism of lysine, hydroxylysine, and tryptophan. GCDH deficiency leads to accumulation of glutaric acid, which impedes operculization during the third trimester of fetal development.

PATHOLOGY. Excess glutaric acid is neurotoxic. Cells in the basal ganglia and WM are especially vulnerable. Spongiform changes with neuronal loss, myelin splitting and vacuolation, and intramyelinic fluid accumulation are typical microscopic features of GA1.

CLINICAL ISSUES. The majority of infants with GA1 are initially normal. Most present during the first year of life with acute striatal necrosis, often triggered by febrile illness or immunization. Seizures, mental retardation, and dystonic-dyskinetic movements are also common.

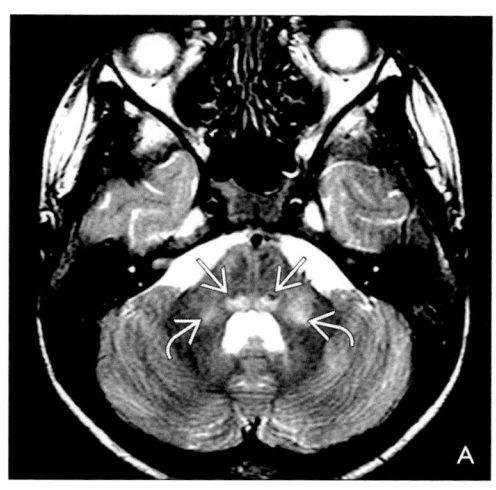

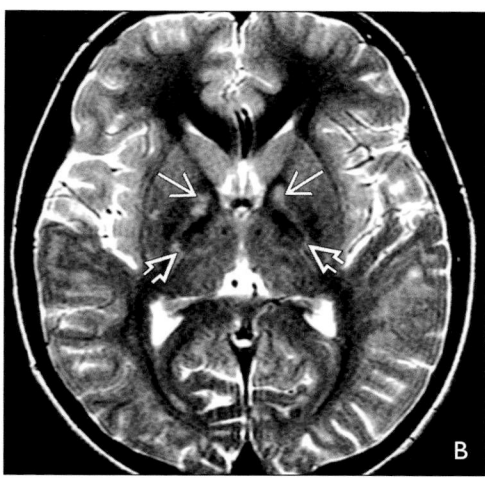

31-58A. Axial T2WI in a teenager with Kearns-Sayre syndrome demonstrates bilaterally symmetric hypointensities in the pons ➡ and middle cerebellar peduncles ➡. 31-58B. T2WI through the basal ganglia shows abnormal signal intensities within the globi pallidi ➡ and internal capsules ➡.

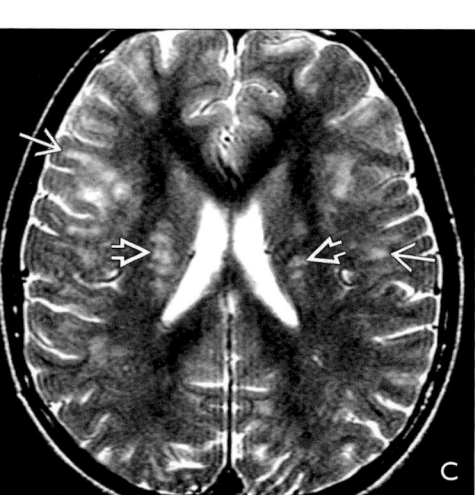

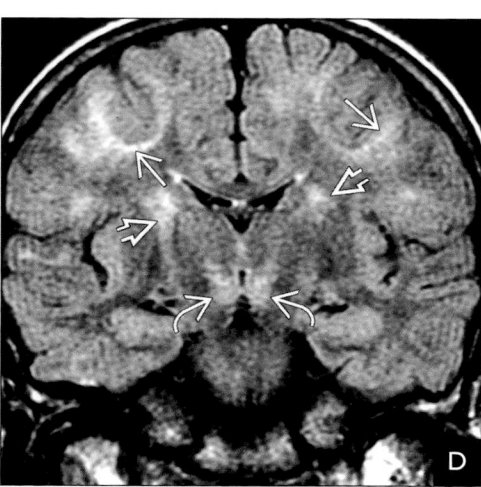

31-58C. T2WI through the lateral ventricles shows multifocal stripe-like hyperintensities in the periventricular ➡ and subcortical WM ➡. 31-58D. Coronal FLAIR in the same patient with KSS shows the involvement of the subcortical U-fibers ➡, corticospinal tracts/internal capsules ➡, and medial thalami ➡.

Patients may develop an acute Reye-like encephalopathy with ketoacidosis and vomiting. Hypoglycemia accompanied by elevated urinary organic acids is typical. Serum and urine metabolites may be completely normal between metabolic crises.

IMAGING. The three "signature" imaging findings of classic GA1 are (1) macrocrania, (2) bilateral widened ("open") sylvian fissures, and (3) bilaterally symmetric basal ganglia lesions (31-59). Severe GA1 may also cause diffuse hemispheric WM abnormalities.

GA1 infants in metabolic crisis often present with acute striatal necrosis. Bilateral diffusely swollen basal ganglia that are T2/FLAIR hyperintense and that restrict on DWI are typical (31-60).

Chronic GA1 causes enlarged CSF spaces and atrophy (31-61). The volume loss may tear bridging veins that cross from the brain surface to the dura, resulting in recurrent subdural hematomas (31-62).

GA1 does not enhance on T1 C+ scans. MRS is nonspecific with decreased NAA, increased Cho:Cr ratio, and (during crisis) elevated lactate level.

DIFFERENTIAL DIAGNOSIS. The major differential diagnosis of GA1 is **nonaccidental injury**. However, GA1 is not associated with fractures, and the subdural hematomas associated with GA1 do not occur in the absence of enlarged CSF spaces.

Other causes of macrocephaly in infants and children should be considered in the differential diagnosis. These include hydrocephalus, benign extraaxial fluid of infancy (enlarged subarachnoid spaces) in the first year of life, benign familial macrocephaly (a normal variant), and other IMDs such as the mucopolysaccharidoses, Canavan disease, and Alexander disease.

Glutaric Aciduria Type 2

Glutaric aciduria type 2 (GA2) results from a defect in the mitochondrial electron transport chain at coenzyme Q. Imaging studies show symmetric T2/FLAIR hyperintensity in the basal ganglia and hemispheric WM, but the "open" sylvian fissures characteristic of GA1 are absent.

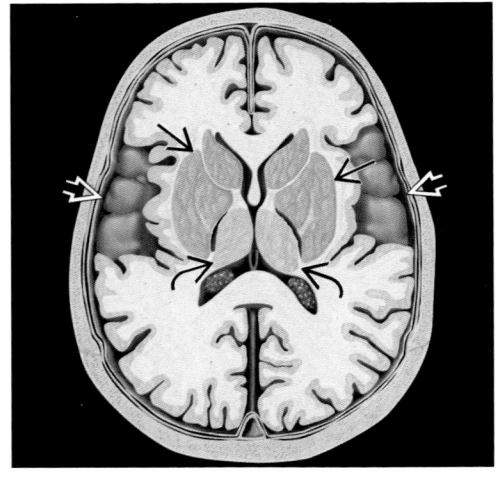
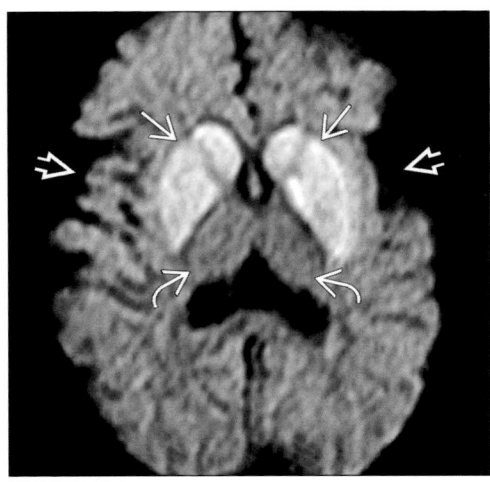

31-59. Axial graphic depicts typical findings of glutaric aciduria type 1. Note the symmetrically enlarged ⇨ basal ganglia and the bilateral "open" sylvian fissures ⇥. The thalami ⇗ appear normal.
31-60. DWI in an infant in acute metabolic crisis with acute striatal necrosis shows restricted diffusion in the basal ganglia ⇥. Note the "open" sylvian fissures ⇥, sparing of the thalami ⇗.

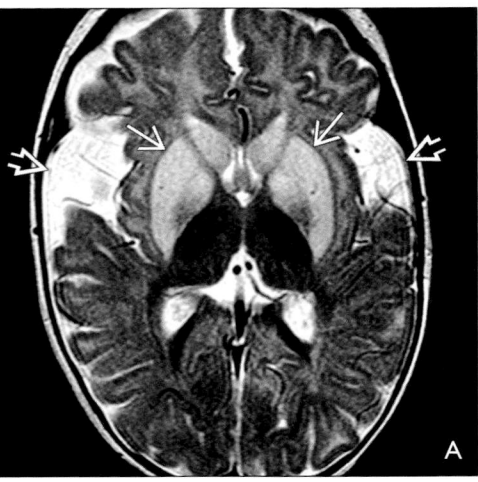
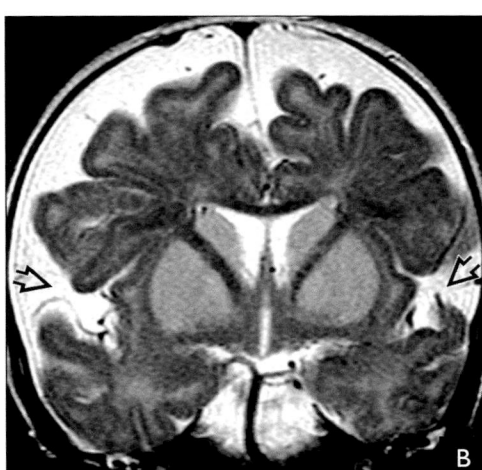

31-61A. Axial T2WI in a 7-month-old child with GA1 shows enlarged, hyperintense caudate nuclei, putamina, and globi pallidi ➡ with thalamic sparing. The sylvian fissures ⇥ are enlarged. The hemispheric WM myelination is grossly delayed. 31-61B. Coronal T2WI in the same patient shows generalized brain volume loss, swollen basal ganglia, and delayed myelination. The sylvian fissures ⇥ appear underoperculized and "open."

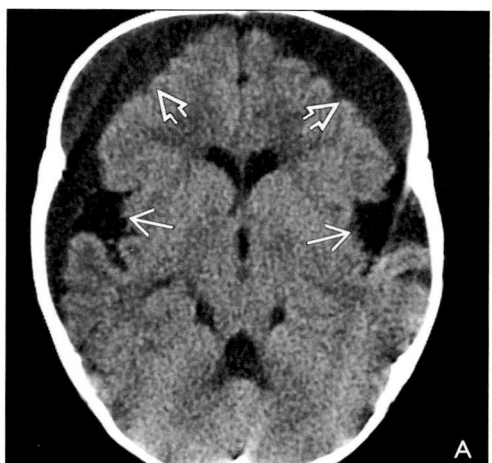

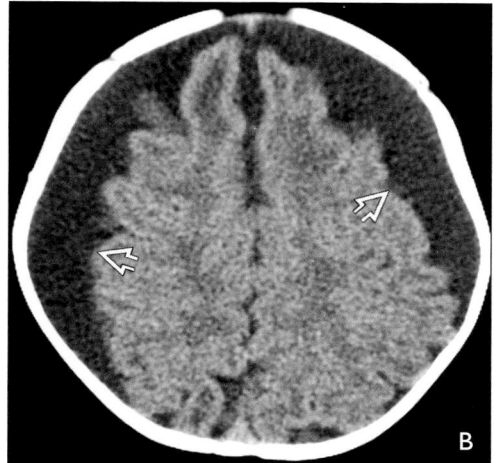

31-62A. *Classic imaging findings of GA1. Axial NECT scan in a 7 month old with a large head and delayed development shows "open" sylvian fissures* ➡️ *and large bifrontal subdural hematomas* ➡️. ***31-62B.*** *More cephalad NECT scan in the same patient demonstrates the extensive chronic-appearing bilateral subdural hematomas* ➡️.

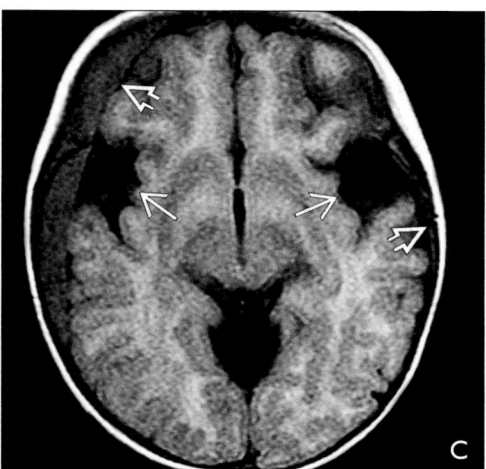

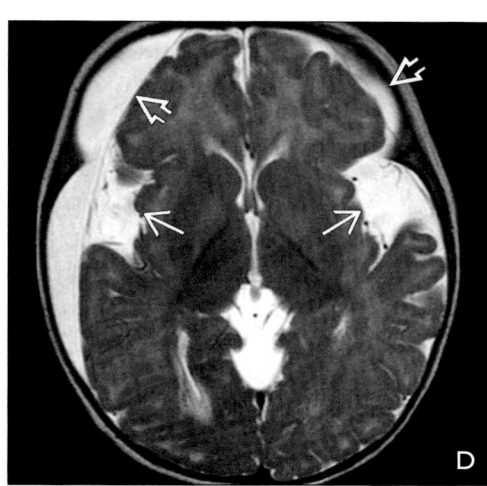

31-62C. *Axial FLAIR scan shows the "open" sylvian fissures* ➡️, *the chronic subdural hematomas* ➡️. ***31-62D.*** *T2WI shows the "open" sylvian fissures* ➡️, *subdural fluid collections* ➡️, *and significantly delayed myelination for the child's age of 7 months.*

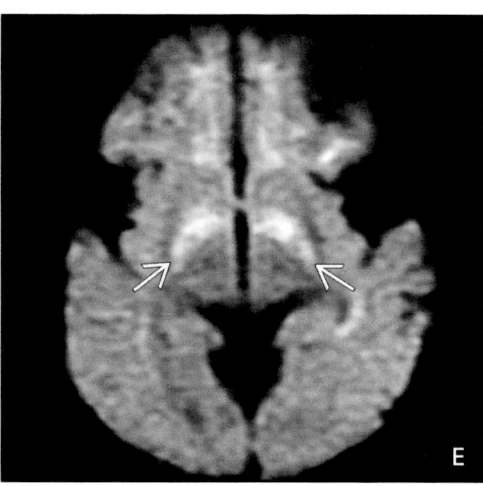

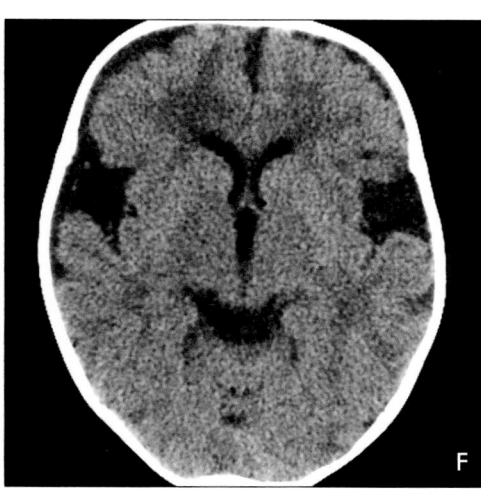

31-62E. *DWI shows mild hyperintensity in the frontal WM and internal capsules* ➡️. ***31-62F.*** *NECT scan 10 months later shows almost complete resolution of the subdural hematomas. A small residual collection is present over the right frontal and temporal lobes. The sylvian fissures still have the classic "open" appearance of GA1.*

31-63A. Axial NECT scan in a 51-year-old woman with ornithine transcarbamylase deficiency, now in acute metabolic crisis. Diffuse cerebral edema is seen. The cortex, basal ganglia, thalami are the same density as the underlying white matter. *31-63B.* More cephalad NECT scan in the same patient shows swollen, hypodense gyri with complete effacement of all surface sulci.

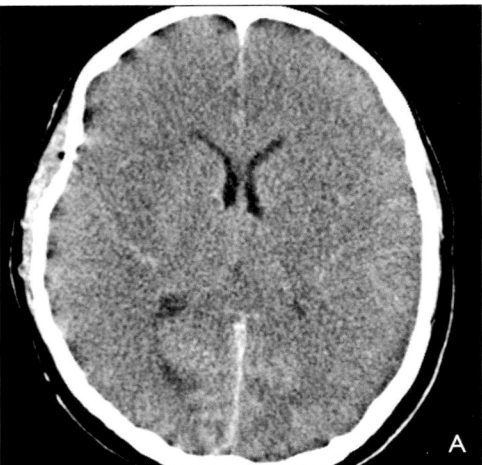
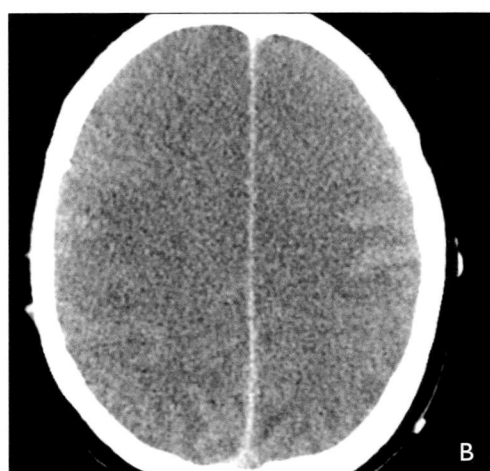

31-63C. T2WI in the same patient shows diffuse basal ganglia and cortical hyperintensity, most striking in the peri-insular and frontal cortices ➡. The occipital lobes ⇒ are relatively spared. *31-63D.* More cephalad T2WI in the same patient shows the diffusely swollen frontal, parietal cortex ➡. Again, the occipital lobes ⇒ are relatively spared, a characteristic pattern in hyperammonemia caused by ornithine transcarbamylase deficiency.

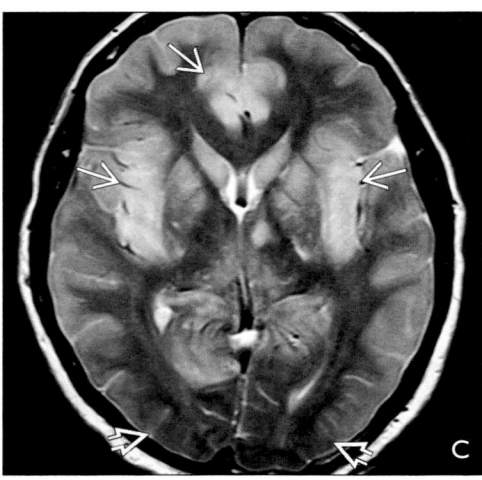
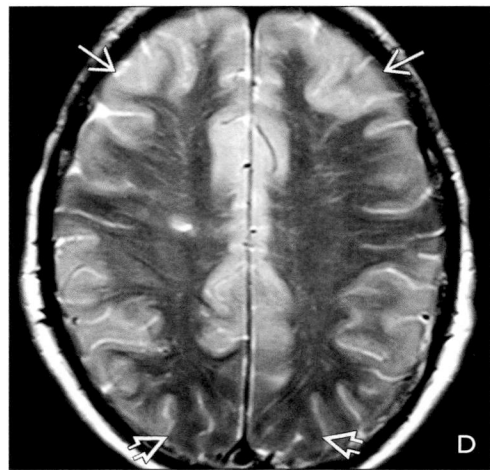

31-63E. DWI in the same patient shows restricted diffusion in the peri-insular and frontal cortices ➡ and left thalamus with less striking involvement of the corpus callosum ➡. The occipital lobes ⇒ show no evidence of restriction. *31-63F.* More cephalad DWI shows that the restriction involves the cortex, spares the underlying WM of the corona radiata.

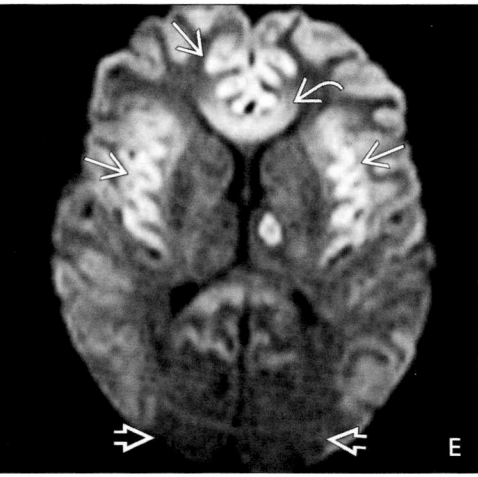
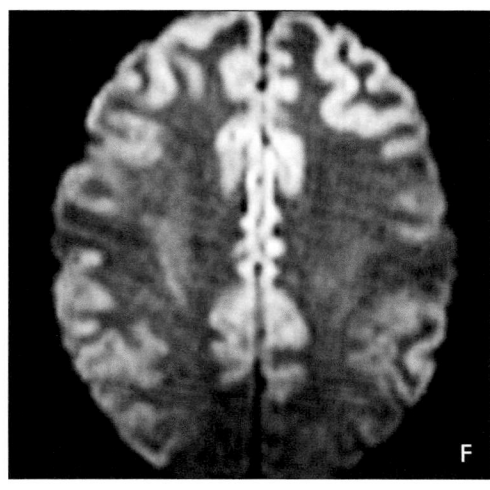

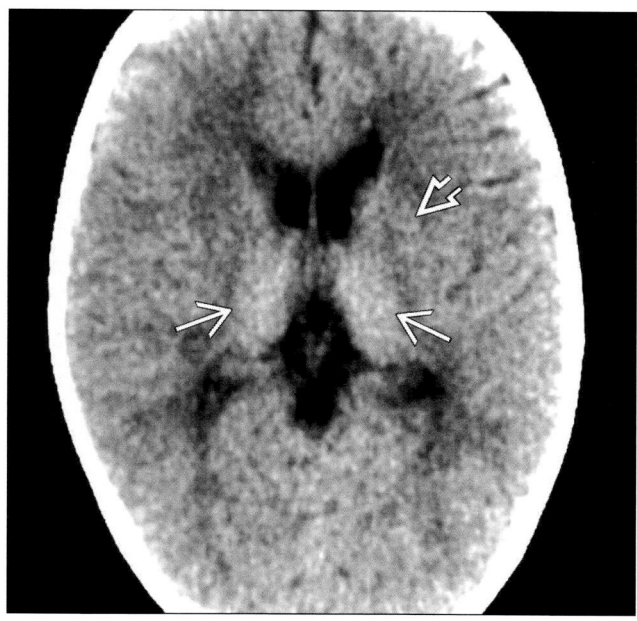

31-64. NECT scan in a developmentally delayed 1 year old with infantile GM1 (Tay-Sachs disease) shows shrunken basal ganglia ⇗, hyperdense thalami ➡.

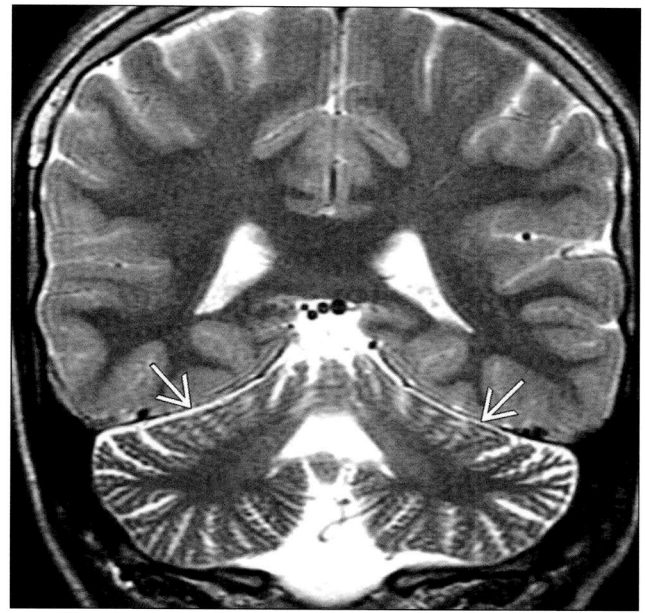

31-65. Coronal T2WI in a 15-year-old boy with juvenile onset GM2 (Sandhoff disease) shows normal cerebral hemispheres, striking cerebellar atrophy ➡.

Urea Cycle/Ammonia Disorders

Ammonia is an important source of nitrogen and is required for amino acid synthesis as well as normal acid-base balance. When present in high concentrations, ammonia is toxic.

The urea cycle normally prevents excess accumulation of toxic nitrogen products by incorporating nitrogen into urea, which is then excreted in the urine. Interruption of the urea cycle results in elevated serum ammonia, which readily crosses the blood-brain barrier and causes diffuse cerebral edema.

A number of different urea cycle disorders have been identified. Two classic disorders are **ornithine transcarbamylase deficiency** and **citrullinemia**. Both are characterized by diffuse brain swelling on NECT scans.

MR shows basal ganglia and cortical swelling with T2/FLAIR hyperintensity. The peri-insular cortex is usually affected first, with involvement then extending into the frontal, parietal, temporal, and (finally) the occipital lobes **(31-63)**. The globi pallidi, putamina, thalami are affected with prolonged hyperammonemia and may show restricted diffusion.

The major imaging differential diagnosis of acute hyperammonemia caused by urea cycle disorders is **hypoxic-ischemic encephalopathy** (HIE). Infants with HIE typically have more thalamic and perirolandic cortical abnormalities.

Methylmalonic and Propionic Acidemias

Both methylmalonic acidemia (MMA) and propionic acidemia (PPA) are autosomal recessive disorders that present clinically with episodic ketoacidosis, nausea and vomiting, progressive hypotonia, and seizures.

Imaging findings in both disorders are nonspecific. Ventricular enlargement, cortical atrophy, cerebellar volume loss, and T2/FLAIR hyperintensity in the periventricular WM are the most common abnormalities in MMA. Bilateral basal ganglia calcifications are present in 5-10% of cases. PPA generally involves the putamina and caudate nuclei and causes reduced myelination in the hemispheric WM.

Gangliosidoses

Two forms of gangliosidoses are recognized: GM1 (Tay-Sachs disease) and GM2 (Sandhoff disease). They are biochemically distinct but clinically indistinguishable.

GM1 is a rare lysosomal storage disease. Deficiency of the lysosomal enzyme β-galactosidase results in accumulation of GM1 ganglioside in the brain (especially the basal ganglia) and oligosaccharide in the abdominal viscera. GM2 is an autosomal recessive disorder of sphingolipid storage.

Both GM1 and GM2 exist in infantile, juvenile, and adult forms. Patients with infantile GM1 present between birth and six months with coarse facial features, skele-

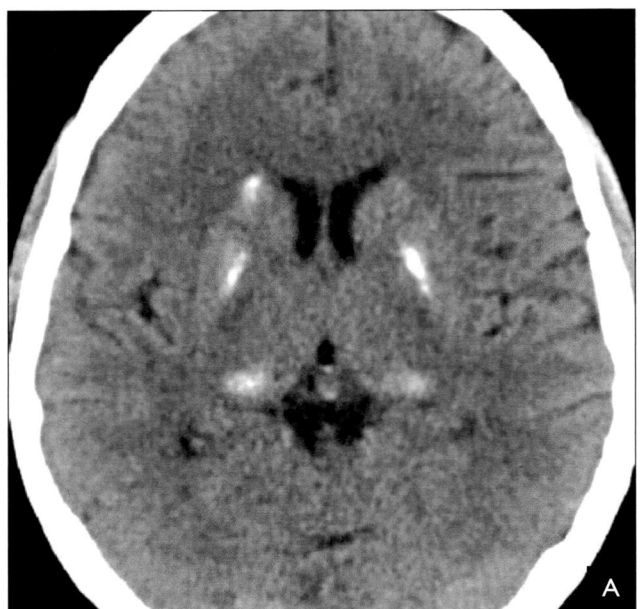

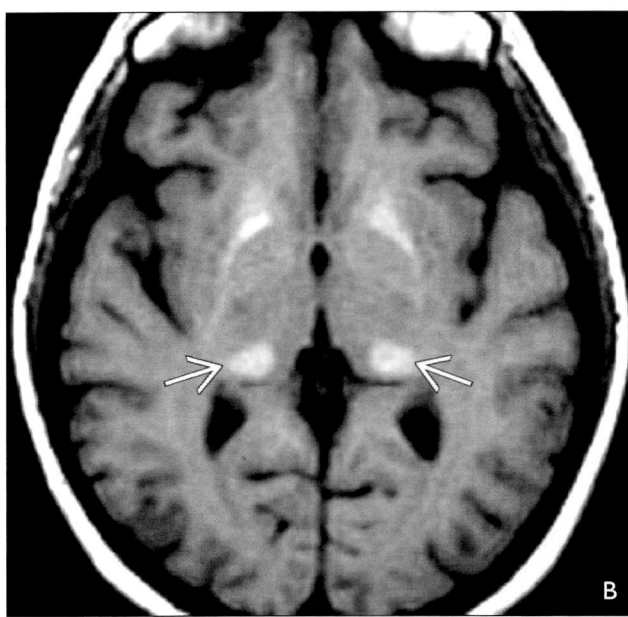

31-66A. Axial NECT scan in a patient with Fabry disease shows bilateral calcifications in the right caudate, both globi pallidi, and posterior thalami.

31-66B. T1WI in the same patient shows bright "pulvinar" sign ➔, considered virtually pathognomonic for Fabry disease.

tal dysostosis, and hepatosplenomegaly. Juvenile-onset GM1 presents with motor delay followed by mental deterioration and extrapyramidal signs. Adult-onset disease is characterized by slowly progressive dystonia and ataxia, as well as extrapyramidal signs.

Imaging findings in both GM1 and GM2 are quite similar. Patients with infantile-onset gangliosidoses show preferential involvement of the thalami, which often appear small and hyperdense on NECT scans **(31-64)**. The basal ganglia and sometimes the cerebral and cerebellar WM are often relatively hypodense. Patients with juvenile- or adult-onset disease may show only cerebellar atrophy **(31-65)**.

MR scans in infantile-onset gangliosidosis may demonstrate some T1 hyperintensity in the thalami. The globi pallidi and ventral thalami often appear profoundly shrunken and hypointense on T2WI. With the exception of the corpus callosum (which is often spared), the WM appears variably T2/FLAIR hyperintense.

Fabry Disease

Fabry disease causes 1.5-5% of unexplained strokes in young patients and is present in 4-5% of men with unexplained left ventricular hypertrophy or cryptogenic stroke. As enzyme replacement therapy is now widely available, it is important to diagnose Fabry disease before irreversible organ damage occurs.

Etiology and Pathology

Fabry disease is an X-linked lysosomal storage disorder of glycosphingolipid metabolism. Mutation in α-galactosidase leads to abnormal accumulation of glycosphingolipids in various tissues, especially in the vascular endothelium and smooth muscle cells.

Impaired endothelial function results in progressive multisystem vasculopathy. The renal, cardiac, and cerebral vessels particularly are severely affected. Cardiac emboli, large vessel arteriopathy, and microvascular disease all occur.

Clinical Issues

Infants with Fabry disease typically present with diffuse angiokeratomas, but late-onset Fabry disease is much more difficult to diagnose. Fabry-induced stroke often occurs before the definitive diagnosis has been established. While mean onset of first stroke is 39 years in males and 45 years in females, nearly 22% of patients are younger than 30 years at initial presentation.

Over 85% of strokes in Fabry disease are ischemic strokes. Hemorrhagic strokes are less common and usually occur secondary to renovascular hypertension.

Imaging

NECT scans show bilateral, often symmetric calcifications in the basal ganglia and thalami **(31-66A)**. Multifocal deep WM hypodensities consistent with lacunar infarcts can be identified in some cases. Patients with long-standing Fabry disease demonstrate volume loss with enlarged ventricles and sulci.

MR may show T1 shortening in the basal ganglia and thalami. The "pulvinar" sign (T1 hyperintensity in the posterior thalamus) is highly suggestive of Fabry disease **(31-66B)**.

Between 45-50% of adult patients with Fabry disease have patchy multifocal T2/FLAIR hyperintensities in the basal ganglia, thalami, and cerebral white matter. With time, the lesions increase in number and may become coalescent **(31-67)**.

Ten percent of patients demonstrate "blooming" hypointensities on T2* (GRE, SWI) due to microbleeds. Less common imaging findings include dolichoectasias.

Differential Diagnosis

The differential diagnosis of Fabry disease includes other disorders characterized by basal ganglia calcifications. **Fahr disease** causes bilateral, dense, thick calcifications in the basal ganglia and thalami. The cerebellum and gray-white matter interfaces are frequently affected in Fahr disease but generally not involved in Fabry disease.

Endocrinologic disorders such as hyperparathyroidism, hypoparathyroidism, pseudohypoparathyroidism, and hypothyroidism may have similar calcifications but lack the multifocal infarcts typical of Fabry disease.

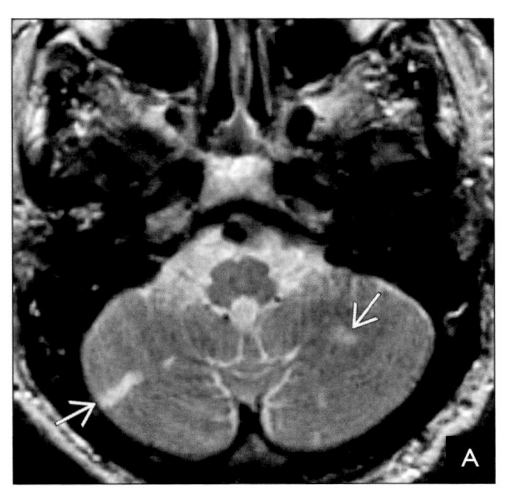

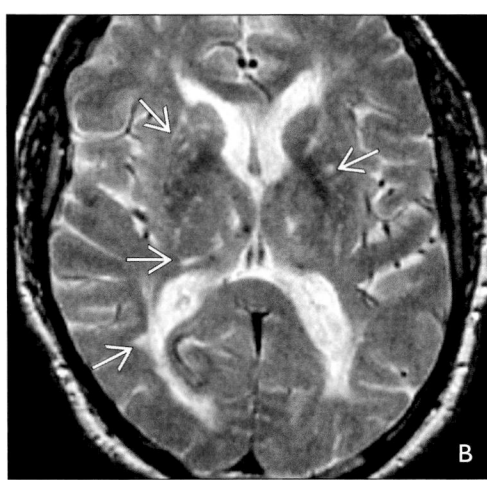

31-67A. Axial T2WI in a 42-year-old man with Fabry disease and a history of multiple strokes shows hyperintensities in both cerebellar hemispheres consistent with multifocal infarcts ➔. 31-67B. Axial T2WI in the same patient shows multifocal lacunar infarcts in the thalami, basal ganglia, and deep periventricular white matter ➔.

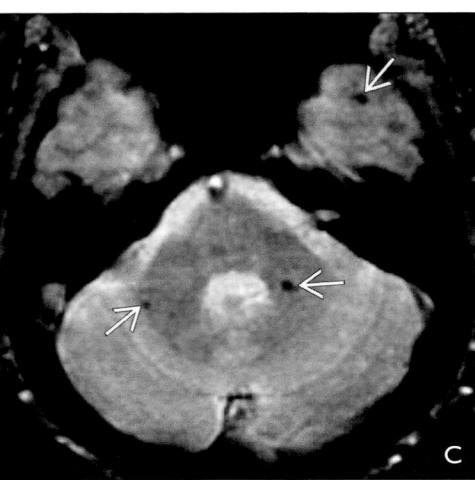

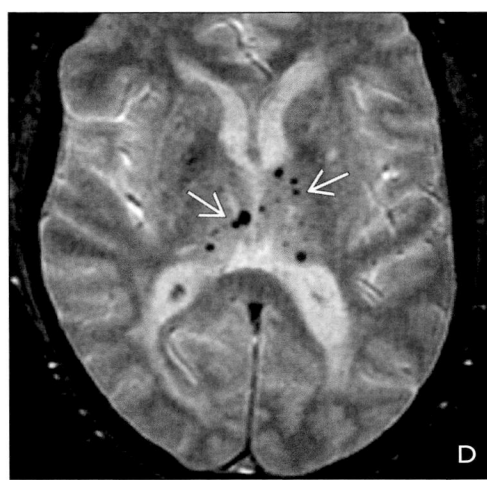

31-67C. Axial T2 GRE scan in the same patient shows multiple "blooming" hypointensities in the cerebellum and left temporal lobe ➔. 31-67D. T2* GRE scan through the lateral ventricles shows innumerable "blooming black dots" in both thalami ➔.*

Selected References

Normal Myelination and White Matter Development

General Considerations

- Welker KM et al: Assessment of normal myelination with magnetic resonance imaging. Semin Neurol. 32(1):15-28, 2012
- Deoni SC et al: Mapping infant brain myelination with magnetic resonance imaging. J Neurosci. 31(2):784-91, 2011

Imaging of Normal Myelination

- Welker KM et al: Assessment of normal myelination with magnetic resonance imaging. Semin Neurol. 32(1):15-28, 2012

Classification of Inherited Metabolic Disorders

Overview

- Barkovich AJ et al: Metabolic, toxic, and inflammatory brain disorders. In Pediatric Neuroimaging. 5th ed. Philadelphia: Lippincott Williams & Wilkins. 81-239, 2012
- Ittoop A et al: Imaging of neonatal brain emergencies: multisequence MRI analysis of pathologic spectrum including diffusion and MR spectroscopy. Emerg Radiol. 19(2):149-57, 2012
- Barkovich AJ et al: In Diagnostic Imaging: Pediatric Neuroradiology. Salt Lake City: Amirsys Publishing. I.1.40-3, 2007

Metabolic Approach

- Kodama H et al: Inherited copper transport disorders: biochemical mechanisms, diagnosis, and treatment. Curr Drug Metab. 13(3):237-50, 2012
- Mittal A et al: Pelizaeus-Merzbacher disease in siblings. J Pediatr Neurosci. 5(2):167-9, 2010

Imaging-based Approach

- Barkovich AJ et al: In Pediatric Neuroimaging. 5th ed. Philadelphia: Lippincott Williams & Wilkins. 81-239, 2012

IMDs Predominantly Affecting White Matter

- Perlman SJ et al: Leukodystrophies. Adv Exp Med Biol. 724:154-71, 2012

Periventricular White Matter Predominance

- Batzios SP et al: Developing treatment options for metachromatic leukodystrophy. Mol Genet Metab. 105(1):56-63, 2012
- Clas P et al: A semi-automatic algorithm for determining the demyelination load in metachromatic leukodystrophy. Acad Radiol. 19(1):26-34, 2012
- Ding XQ et al: Imaging evidence of early brain tissue degeneration in patients with vanishing white matter disease: a multimodal MR study. J Magn Reson Imaging. 35(4):926-32, 2012
- Kilicarslan R et al: Maple syrup urine disease: diffusion-weighted MRI findings during acute metabolic encephalopathic crisis. Jpn J Radiol. 30(6):522-5, 2012
- Moore SA et al: Leukoencephalopathy with brain stem and spinal cord involvement (and high lactate): raising the bar for diagnosis. J Neurol. Epub ahead of print, 2012
- van der Lei HD et al: Characteristics of early MRI in children and adolescents with vanishing white matter. Neuropediatrics. 43(1):22-6, 2012
- Groeschel S et al: Metachromatic leukodystrophy: natural course of cerebral MRI changes in relation to clinical course. J Inherit Metab Dis. 34(5):1095-102, 2011
- Kloppenborg RP et al: Homocysteine and cerebral small vessel disease in patients with symptomatic atherosclerotic disease: the SMART-MR study. Atherosclerosis. 216(2):461-6, 2011
- Marom L et al: A point mutation in translation initiation factor eIF2B leads to function--and time-specific changes in brain gene expression. PLoS One. 6(10):e26992, 2011
- Eichler F et al: Metachromatic leukodystrophy: a scoring system for brain MR imaging observations. AJNR Am J Neuroradiol. 30(10):1893-7, 2009

Subcortical White Matter Predominance

- Batla A et al: Megalencephalic leukoencephalopathy with subcortical cysts: a report of four cases. J Pediatr Neurosci. 6(1):74-7, 2011
- López-Hernández T et al: Molecular mechanisms of MLC1 and GLIALCAM mutations in megalencephalic leukoencephalopathy with subcortical cysts. Hum Mol Genet. 20(16):3266-77, 2011
- López-Hernández T et al: Mutant GlialCAM causes megalencephalic leukoencephalopathy with subcortical cysts, benign familial macrocephaly, and macrocephaly with retardation and autism. Am J Hum Genet. 88(4):422-32, 2011

Hypomyelinating Disorders

- Steenweg ME et al: Magnetic resonance imaging pattern recognition in hypomyelinating disorders. Brain. 133(10):2971-82, 2010

IMDs Predominantly Affecting Gray Matter

IMDs Primarily Affecting Deep Gray Nuclei

- Fermin-Delgado R et al: Involvement of globus pallidus and midbrain nuclei in pantothenate kinase-associated neurodegeneration: measurement of T2 and T2* time. Clin Neuroradiol. Epub ahead of print, 2012
- Kruer MC et al: Neuroimaging features of neurodegeneration with brain iron accumulation. AJNR Am J Neuroradiol. 33(3):407-14, 2012
- Sánchez-Castañeda C et al: Seeking Huntington disease biomarkers by multimodal, cross-sectional basal ganglia imaging. Hum Brain Mapp. Epub ahead of print, 2012
- van den Bogaard SJ et al: Magnetization transfer imaging in premanifest and manifest Huntington disease. AJNR Am J Neuroradiol. 33(5):884-9, 2012
- van den Bogaard S et al: MRI biomarkers in Huntington's disease. Front Biosci (Elite Ed). 4:1910-25, 2012
- Hegde AN et al: Differential diagnosis for bilateral abnormalities of the basal ganglia and thalamus. Radiographics. 31(1):5-30, 2011
- Hinnell C et al: Creatine deficiency syndromes: diagnostic pearls and pitfalls. Can J Neurol Sci. 38(5):765-7, 2011
- McNeill A et al: Neurodegeneration with brain iron accumulation. Handb Clin Neurol. 100:161-72, 2011
- Skjørringe T et al: Splice site mutations in the ATP7A gene. PLoS One. 6(4):e18599, 2011
- McNeill A et al: T2* and FSE MRI distinguishes four subtypes of neurodegeneration with brain iron accumulation. Neurology. 70(18):1614-9, 2008

IMDs Primarily Affecting Cortex

- Arsov T et al: Kufs disease, the major adult form of neuronal ceroid lipofuscinosis, caused by mutations in CLN6. Am J Hum Genet. 88(5):566-73, 2011
- Mahmood A et al: White matter impairment in Rett syndrome: diffusion tensor imaging study with clinical correlations. AJNR Am J Neuroradiol. 31(2):295-9, 2010
- Robertson T et al: 53-year-old man with rapid cognitive decline. Brain Pathol. 18(2):292-4, 2008

Disorders Affecting Both Gray and White Matter

Mucopolysaccharidoses

- Zafeiriou DI et al: Brain and spinal MR imaging findings in mucopolysaccharidoses: A Review. AJNR Am J Neuroradiol. Epub ahead of print, 2012
- Fan Z et al: Correlation of automated volumetric analysis of brain MR imaging with cognitive impairment in a natural history study of mucopolysaccharidosis II. AJNR Am J Neuroradiol. 31(7):1319-23, 2010

Canavan Disease

- Mersmann N et al: Aspartoacylase-lacZ knockin mice: an engineered model of Canavan disease. PLoS One. 6(5):e20336, 2011
- Le Coq J et al: Characterization of human aspartoacylase: the brain enzyme responsible for Canavan disease. Biochemistry. 45(18):5878-84, 2006
- Michel SJ et al: Case 99: Canavan disease. Radiology. 241(1):310-4, 2006

Alexander Disease

- Golden JA et al: Alexander disease. In Pathology and Genetics: Developmental Neuropathology. Basel: ISN Neuropath Press. 331-36, 2004

Peroxisomal Biogenesis Disorders

- Poll-The BT et al: Clinical diagnosis, biochemical findings and MRI spectrum of peroxisomal disorders. Biochim Biophys Acta. 1822(9):1421-9, 2012
- van der Knaap MS et al: MRI as diagnostic tool in early-onset peroxisomal disorders. Neurology. 78(17):1304-8, 2012
- Weller S et al: Cerebral MRI as a valuable diagnostic tool in Zellweger spectrum patients. J Inherit Metab Dis. 31(2):270-80, 2008

Mitochondrial Diseases (Respiratory Chain Disorders)

- Wong LJ: Mitochondrial syndromes with leukoencephalopathies. Semin Neurol. 32(1):55-61, 2012

Urea Cycle/Ammonia Disorders

- Auron A et al: Hyperammonemia in review: pathophysiology, diagnosis, and treatment. Pediatr Nephrol. 27(2):207-22, 2012
- Bireley WR et al: Urea cycle disorders: brain MRI and neurological outcome. Pediatr Radiol. 42(4):455-62, 2012

Methylmalonic and Propionic Acidemias

- Radmanesh A et al: Methylmalonic acidemia: brain imaging findings in 52 children and a review of the literature. Pediatr Radiol. 38(10):1054-61, 2008

Gangliosidoses

- De Grandis E et al: MR imaging findings in 2 cases of late infantile GM1 gangliosidosis. AJNR Am J Neuroradiol. 30(7):1325-7, 2009

Fabry Disease

- Burton JO et al: Sometimes when you hear hoof beats, it could be a zebra: consider the diagnosis of Fabry disease. BMC Nephrol. 13(1):73, 2012
- Saposnik G et al: Fabry's disease: a prospective multicenter cohort study in young adults with cryptogenic stroke. Int J Stroke. 7(3):265-73, 2012
- Reisin RC et al: Brain MRI findings in patients with Fabry disease. J Neurol Sci. 305(1-2):41-4, 2011

32

Acquired Metabolic and Systemic Disorders

The brain is highly susceptible to a number of acquired metabolic derangements. As occurs with inherited metabolic disorders and the toxic encephalopathies, the basal ganglia and cortex are especially vulnerable. While the hemispheric white matter is less often affected, some acquired diseases such as osmotic demyelination may largely spare the gray matter and present with striking WM abnormalities.

In this chapter, we focus on acquired metabolic and systemic disorders that involve the CNS. We begin with the most common—hypertension—before turning our attention to abnormalities of glucose metabolism and thyroid/parathyroid function.

We then discuss seizure disorders, as sustained ictal activity with hypermetabolism can have profound effects on the brain. We begin with a brief delineation of normal temporal lobe and limbic anatomy as a prelude to the challenging topic of epilepsy. We finish the section by exploring the puzzling phenomena of the transient corpus callosum splenium lesion and transient global amnesia.

Finally, we consider a potpourri of acquired metabolic diseases such as hepatic encephalopathy (both acute and chronic) and the osmotic demyelination syndromes.

Hypertensive Encephalopathies

If not recognized and treated, the effects of both acutely elevated blood pressure and chronic hypertension (HTN) on the brain can be devastating. We begin this section with a discussion of acute hypertensive encephalopathy, then delve into the CNS damage caused by HTN.

Acute Hypertensive Encephalopathy, Posterior Reversible Encephalopathy Syndrome

Terminology

The most common manifestation of acute hypertensive encephalopathy is **p**osterior **r**eversible **e**ncephalopathy **s**yndrome (PRES), also known as reversible posterior leukoencephalopathy syndrome (RPLS). Despite the syndrome's names, lesions are rarely limited to the "posterior" (parietooccipital) aspects of the brain (see below).

Etiology

GENERAL CONCEPTS. While the etiology of PRES is not yet completely understood, hypertension (regardless of etiology) seems to be a common factor. Failed cerebral autoregulation, hyperperfusion, blood-brain barrier disruption, and breakthrough vasogenic (*not* cytotoxic) edema is the most commonly posited explanation. In this scenario, PRES results in hydrostatic leakage with extravasation or transudation of fluid and macromolecules through arteriolar walls with damaged endothelium **(32-1)**.

An alternative theory for why PRES develops invokes vasospasm or vasculopathy with vascular endothelial dysfunction and reduced cerebral perfusion.

ASSOCIATED CONDITIONS. Initially described in association with eclampsia, immunosuppressive drugs, and acute hypertensive crisis, PRES is now recognized as a disorder that can be induced by a wide, ever-expanding number of diseases and agents. Other conditions associated with PRES include thrombotic microangiopathies (such as hemolytic-uremic syndrome [HUS]/ thrombotic thrombocytopenic purpura [TTP] and disseminated intravascular coagulation [DIC]), uremic encephalopathies (e.g., lupus nephropathy and acute glomerulonephritis), shock/sepsis syndrome, numerous drugs and chemotherapeutic agents, and tumor lysis syndromes.

Less common etiologies of PRES include ingestion of food products (such as licorice) containing substances that cause mineralocorticoid excess. The triad of hypertension, hypokalemia, and metabolic alkalosis is typical. Patients with excess mineralocorticoids also have impaired endothelium-dependent vascular reactivity, which may contribute to the development of PRES.

Rarely, PRES is associated with the so-called SMART syndrome (**s**troke-like **m**igraine **a**ttacks after **r**adiation **t**herapy).

Pathology

The pathology of PRES is largely undefined, as PRES is rarely fatal and biopsied only in exceptional circumstances. Autopsied brains from patients with complicated PRES show diffuse cerebral edema and multiple bilateral petechial microhemorrhages in the occipital lobes **(32-2)**.

Microscopic features in PRES resemble those reported in malignant hypertensive encephalopathy. The occipital

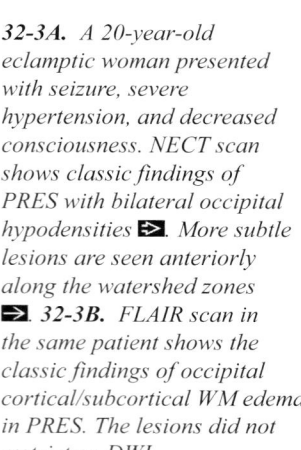
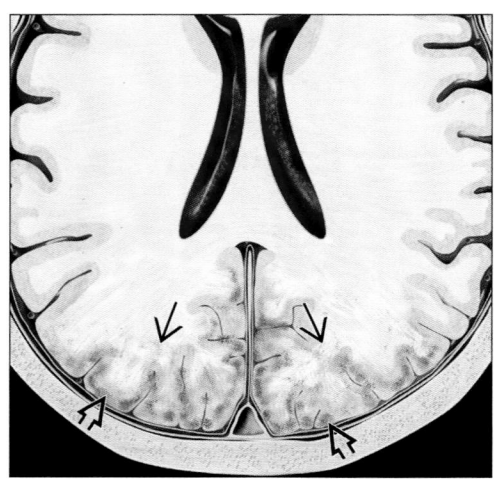
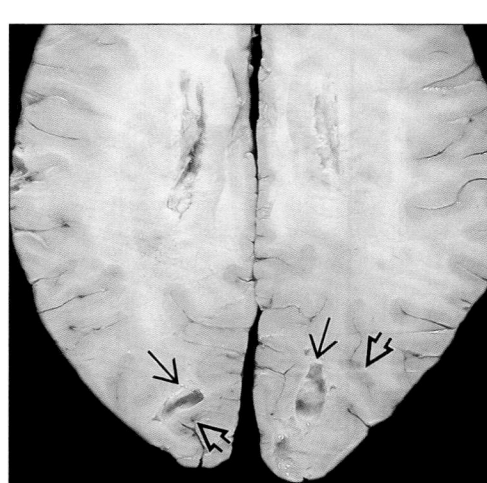

32-1. Axial graphic shows cortical/subcortical vasogenic edema ⟹ in the posterior circulation, characteristic of PRES. Petechial hemorrhage ⇗ occurs in some cases but is unusual. 32-2. Gross pathology of complicated PRES demonstrates diffuse cerebral edema with swollen gyri. Petechial hemorrhages ⇗ and foci of encephalomalacia secondary to infarction ⟹ are present. (Courtesy R. Hewlett, MD.)

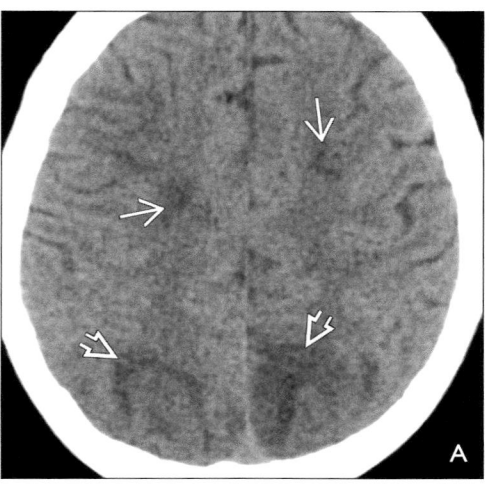
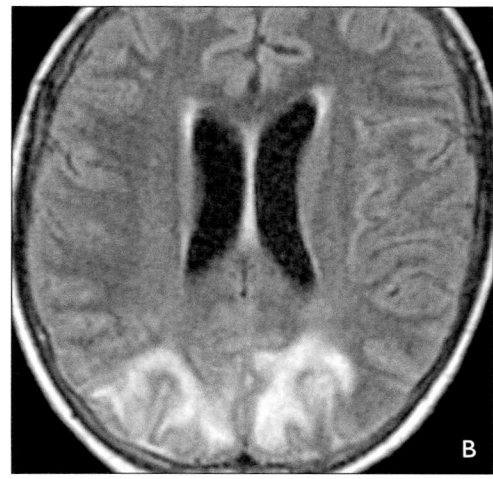

32-3A. A 20-year-old eclamptic woman presented with seizure, severe hypertension, and decreased consciousness. NECT scan shows classic findings of PRES with bilateral occipital hypodensities ⟹. More subtle lesions are seen anteriorly along the watershed zones ⟹. 32-3B. FLAIR scan in the same patient shows the classic findings of occipital cortical/subcortical WM edema in PRES. The lesions did not restrict on DWI.

cortex, subcortical white matter (WM), and cerebellum demonstrate a range of microvascular pathology, including fibrinoid arteriolar necrosis with petechial hemorrhages, proteinaceous exudates, and macrophage infiltration along the perivascular spaces. The adjacent WM is typically edematous.

Clinical Issues

EPIDEMIOLOGY AND DEMOGRAPHICS. Although the peak age of onset is 20-40 years, PRES can affect patients of all ages from infants to the elderly. There is a moderate female predominance, largely because of the strong association of PRES and preeclampsia.

Preeclampsia is the most common cause of PRES. This pregnancy-specific disorder is characterized by hypertension (blood pressure exceeding 140/90 mmHg) and proteinuria occurring after 20 weeks of gestation in a previously normotensive patient. Preeclampsia and its variants affect approximately 5% of pregnancies and remain leading causes of both maternal and fetal morbidity.

Progression from preeclampsia to eclampsia occurs in 0.5% of patients with mild and 2-3% of patients with severe preeclampsia. Eclampsia is characterized by a peak systolic pressure of 160 mmHg or greater, diastolic BO of 100 mg or greater, impaired renal function, thrombocytopenia, and/or evidence of microangiopathic hemolytic anemia, hepatocellular injury, pulmonary edema, and neurologic disturbances (primarily seizures).

PRESENTATION. While 92% of patients with PRES have acutely elevated blood pressure (mean = 200/110), *PRES can also occur in the absence of hypertension or in the presence of only mild hypertension.*

Seizure is the most common presenting clinical symptom in PRES, seen in 67-91% of cases. PRES-associated seizures are typically single, short, uncomplicated grand mal type that terminate spontaneously during the first 24 hours. Serial or recurrent seizures are uncommon.

Other frequent symptoms include headache (80%), visual disturbances (60%), and altered mental status (30%). Common comorbidities reported in recent series include

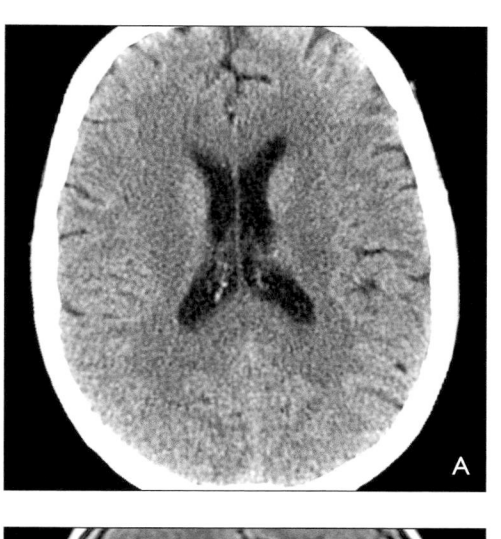

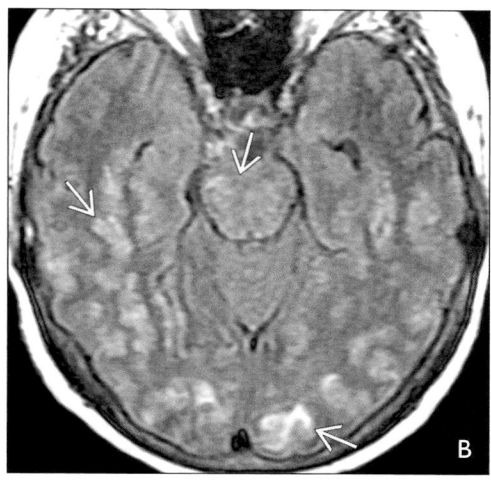

32-4A. A 63-year-old woman with end-stage renal disease had a seizure and fell. Blood pressure in the emergency department was 220/140. NECT scan performed to evaluate for intracranial hemorrhage shows normal findings. 32-4B. MR was obtained because of suspected PRES. FLAIR scan obtained 1 hour after the NECT shows multifocal patchy hyperintensities in the midbrain, posteroinferior temporal lobes, and parietooccipital cortex ➡.

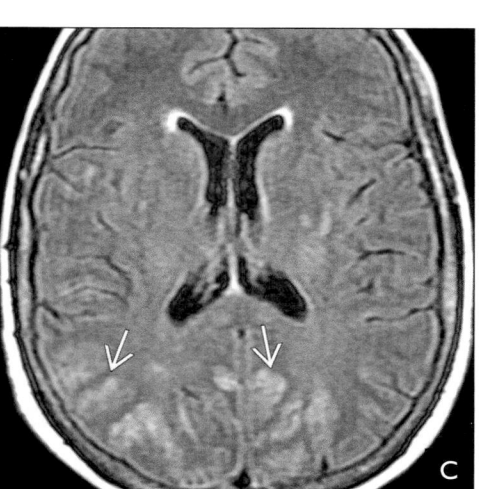

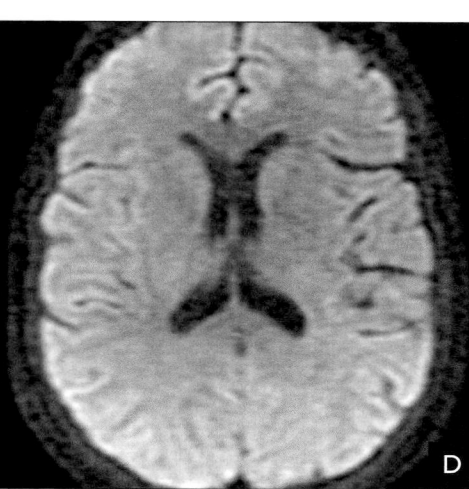

32-4C. FLAIR image through the lateral ventricles shows bilateral, relatively symmetric lesions in the parietooccipital cortex ➡. 32-4D. DWI scan in the same patient shows no evidence for diffusion restriction. DWI scans are usually (although not invariably) normal in PRES because the edema is mostly vasogenic, not cytotoxic.

32-5A. *Variant PRES is illustrated by this 23-year-old woman with lupus and severe HTN who presented in the emergency department with a grand mal seizure. T2WI through the ventricles shows bilateral parietooccipital* ➡ *and symmetric basal ganglia lesions* ➡. **32-5B.** *T2WI in the same patient through the upper corona radiata shows striking cortical/subcortical hyperintensities along the vascular watershed zones* ➡.

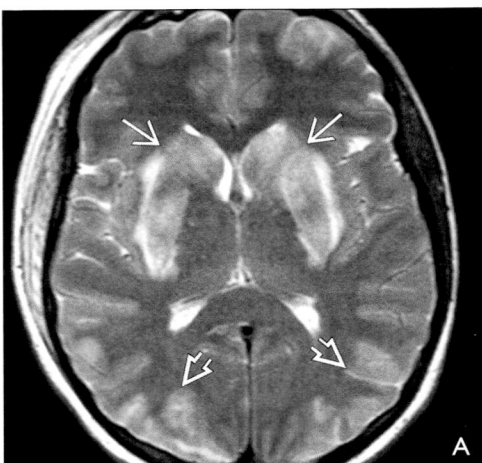
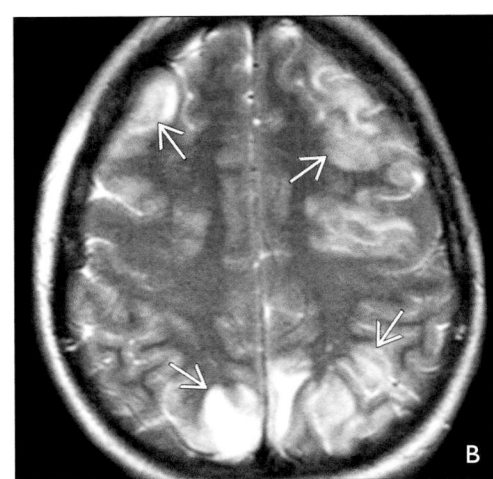

32-5C. *DWI in the same patient shows mild diffusion restriction* ➡ *in the affected areas.* **32-5D.** *Only the most severely affected gyri* ➡ *show restricted diffusion; compare with the more extensive edema seen on the T2WI above.*

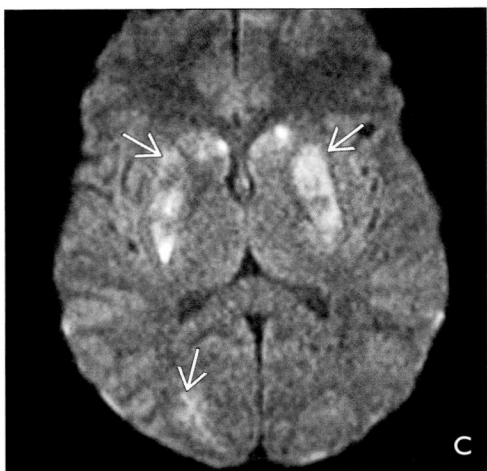
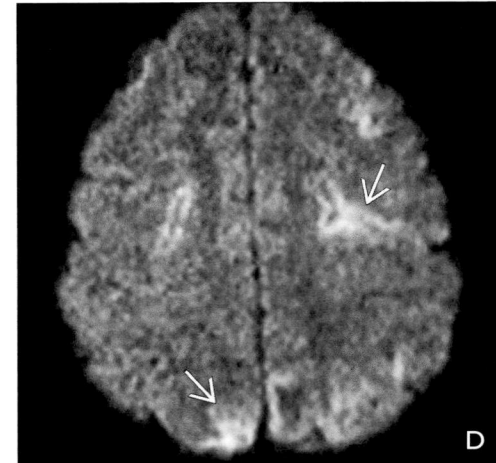

32-5E. *Axial T2WI 10 days later shows complete interval resolution of the florid lesions following blood pressure normalization. The scan shows no evidence of residual abnormalities.* **32-5F.** *DWI obtained at the same time shows no evidence of residual diffusion restriction. Even severe PRES usually resolves completely.*

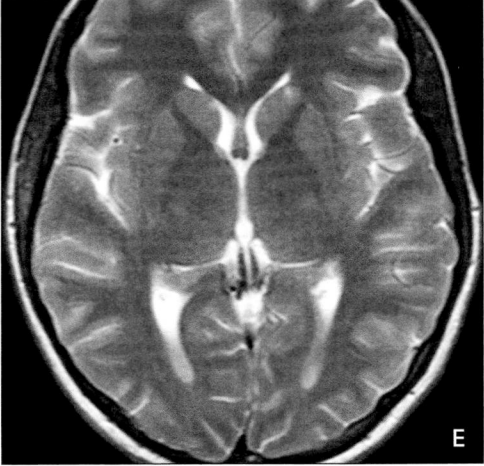
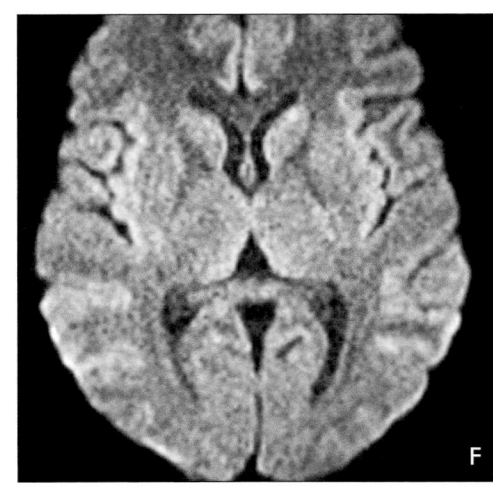

steroids or immunosuppressants (40%), systemic lupus erythematosus (30%), kidney disease (20-30%), eclampsia (20%), and miscellaneous disorders such as vasculitis.

NATURAL HISTORY AND TREATMENT OPTIONS. Severe PRES can be life-threatening. If the inciting substances or precipitating conditions are eliminated and the HTN promptly treated, PRES often resolves with minimal or no residual abnormalities. In rare cases, PRES causes permanent damage, typically hemorrhagic cortical/subcortical or basal ganglionic infarcts.

PRES: TERMINOLOGY, ETIOLOGY, AND CLINICAL ISSUES

Terminology
- Posterior reversible encephalopathy syndrome (PRES)
- Note: *Lesions often not just posterior!*

Etiology
- HTN-induced dysautoregulation vs. vasospasm, ↓ perfusion
- ↑ ↑ BP → failed autoregulation → vasogenic (not cytotoxic) edema
  ◦ Endothelial damage →"leaky" blood-brain barrier
  ◦ Fluid, macromolecules extravasate
- Causes (HTN the possible common factor)
  ◦ Preeclampsia/eclampsia
  ◦ Chemotherapy, immunosuppressive drugs
  ◦ Thrombotic microangiopathies (e.g., HUS/TTP)
  ◦ Renal failure
  ◦ Shock/sepsis
  ◦ Tumor lysis syndrome
  ◦ Food/drug-induced mineralocorticoid excess

Clinical Issues
- All ages (peak = 20-40 years)
- F > > M
- BP usually ↑ ↑ *but* can occur with normal/mildly elevated BP!
- Usually resolves completely with BP normalization

Imaging

GENERAL FEATURES. PRES is notable for its preferential involvement of the parietooccipital lobes, seen in 85-95% of cases **(32-3)**. The occipital lobes may be particularly vulnerable due to the comparatively sparse sympathetic innervation of the posterior circulation, which results in less protection against the effects of severe systemic hypertension.

The parietooccipital lobes are rarely the only affected areas in PRES! The frontal lobes are involved in 75-77% of cases, with the temporal lobes (65%) and cerebellum (50-55%) also commonly affected. Cerebellar disease is more common in patients with a history of autoimmune disease whereas patients with sepsis are more likely to demonstrate cortical involvement.

As many PRES patients present with severe headache, NECT scans are commonly obtained as a screening procedure. It is therefore extremely important to identify even subtle abnormalities that are suggestive of PRES. If the screening NECT is normal and PRES is suspected on clinical grounds, an MR scan with DWI and T2* in addition to the routine sequences (T1 and T2/FLAIR) should be obtained.

CT FINDINGS. Subtle patchy cortical/subcortical hypodensities—usually in the parietooccipital lobes, watershed zones, and/or cerebellum—may be the only initial abnormalities on NECT **(32-3)**.

PRES-associated intracranial hemorrhage is uncommon, seen in only 5-15% of cases. Three different patterns of PRES-associated intracranial hemorrhage occur in almost equal proportions: Focal parenchymal hematoma, multifocal microhemorrhages (less than five millimeters), and convexity subarachnoid hemorrhage.

CECT is usually negative although severe cases may show patchy, nonconfluent cortical/subcortical enhancing foci.

MR FINDINGS. PRES has both classic and atypical MR features. Keep in mind that PRES is rarely just posterior and not always reversible.

Classic PRES demonstrates bilateral parietooccipital cortical/subcortical hypointensities that are hypointense on T1WI and hyperintense on T2/FLAIR **(32-4)**. "Leaky" arterioles with loss of blood-brain barrier integrity may cause patchy enhancement on T1 C+ sequences.

Frank infarction is quite rare in PRES. Because most cases of PRES are caused by vasogenic—not cytotoxic—edema, DWI is usually negative. However, atypical cases (especially in children) with diffusion restriction have been reported. pMR studies have demonstrated reduced cortical rCBV in PRES.

Atypical PRES is almost as common as classic PRES. Imaging findings in atypical PRES include involvement of the frontal lobes, cortical watershed zones, basal ganglia, brainstem, and cerebellum **(32-5)**. In unusual cases, brainstem and/or cerebellar lesions may be the *only* abnormality present. The spinal cord has been reported as a rare site of PRES involvement.

Most cases of PRES resolve completely with no detectable residual abnormalities following blood pressure normalization. Irreversible lesions (e.g., infarcts, hemorrhages) are relatively uncommon, occurring in approximately 15% of cases.

ANGIOGRAPHY. Vasculopathy is a common finding on CTA, MRA, or DSA in patients with PRES. While the circle of Willis and its major trunks usually appear normal, accentuated tapering and reduced visualization of distal arterial branches—especially in the parietooccipital regions—is common. Diffuse vessel constriction or

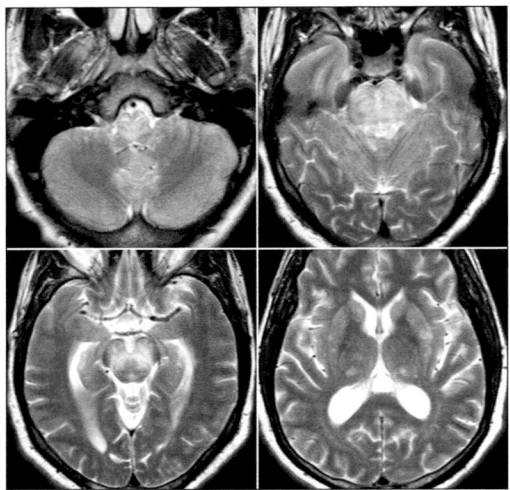

32-6. T2WIs in cocaine-induced mHTN, BP = 220/140 mmHg. Note symmetric hyperintensity from medulla to midbrain, parietooccipital sparing.

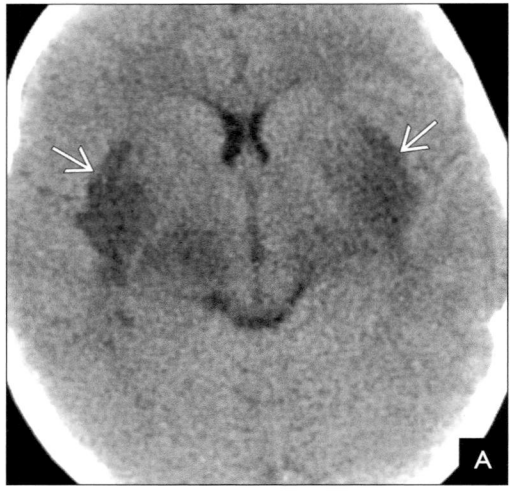

32-7A. NECT in a 4 yo boy with HUS, severe HTN, acute neurologic decline shows bilateral symmetric basal ganglia, thalamic hypodensities →*.*

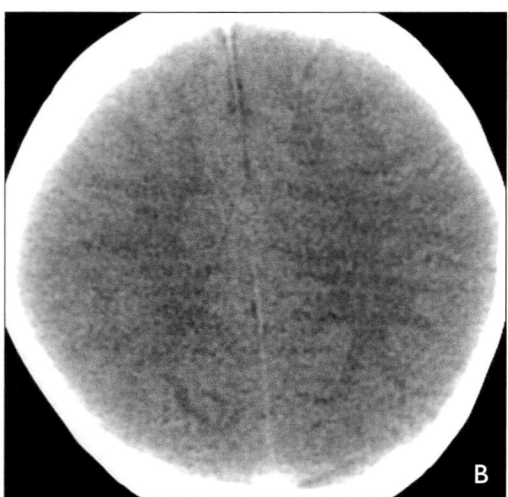

32-7B. More cephalad scan shows swollen hemispheres with sulcal effacement. Patient died 2 hours later from extreme HTN and GI hemorrhage.

narrowing, focal irregularity, and beaded appearance are typical but nonspecific findings in PRES.

Differential Diagnosis

The major differential diagnoses of PRES includes acute cerebral ischemia-infarction, vasculitis, hypoglycemia, status epilepticus, sinovenous thrombosis, reversible cerebral vasoconstriction syndrome, and the thrombotic microangiopathies.

PRES rarely involves *just* the posterior circulation, so **acute cerebral ischemia-infarction** is often easily distinguished. Bilateral PCA distribution infarcts are rare in the absence of "top of the basilar" thrombosis, which typically affects other areas such as the thalami, midbrain, and superior cerebellum.

Vasculitis can resemble PRES-induced vasculopathy at angiography. The distribution of lesions in vasculitis is much more random and less symmetric, usually does not demonstrate the parietooccipital predominance seen in PRES, and more often enhances following contrast administration.

Hypoglycemia typically affects the parietooccipital cortex and subcortical WM, so the clinical-laboratory findings (i.e., low serum glucose, lack of systemic HTN) are important differentiating features. **Status epilepticus** can cause transient gyral edema but is rarely bilateral and can affect any part of the cortex.

Less common entities that can mimic PRES include **sinovenous thrombosis** and reversible cerebral vasoconstriction syndrome. Thrombosis of the posterior (descending) aspect of the superior sagittal sinus can cause patchy bilateral parietooccipital cortical/subcortical edema. Hemorrhage is common (rare in PRES), and CTV easily demonstrates the occluded sinus. **Reversible cerebral vasoconstriction syndrome** shares some features (e.g., convexal subarachnoid hemorrhage) with PRES but is typically limited to a solitary sulcus or just a few adjacent sulci.

Thrombotic microangiopathies—HUS/TTP, DIC, malignant hypertension (mHTN)—may be difficult to differentiate from PRES solely on the basis of imaging features. HUS/TTP and DIC are clinical-laboratory diagnoses.

PRES is a common manifestation in all the thrombotic microangiopathies, although the distinction between PRES and mHTN may be largely academic. The presence of diffuse cerebral edema and multifocal microhemorrhages is more typical of mHTN. Atypical location (brainstem, cerebellum, basal ganglia), restricted diffusion, and generalized cerebral edema are all more common in mHTN.

PRES: IMAGING

Imaging
- General features
  - 85-95% parietooccipital but rarely the only sites!
  - Other sites: Frontotemporal, watershed, brainstem, cerebellum, basal ganglia
- CT
  - Can be normal or only subtly abnormal
  - Posterior cortical/subcortical hypodensities
  - Gross hemorrhage rare
- MR
  - If PRES suspected and CT normal, get MR!
  - T2/FLAIR hyperintensity (parietooccipital most common)
  - DWI usually but not invariably negative
  - Enhancement none/mild (unless severe PRES)

Differential Diagnosis
- Posterior circulation ischemia-infarction
- Vasculitis
- Status epilepticus
- Hypoglycemia
- Thrombotic microangiopathy (HUS/TTP, DIC, mHTN)
- Sinovenous thrombosis
- Reversible cerebral vasoconstriction syndrome

Malignant Hypertension

Terminology

Malignant hypertension (mHTN), sometimes termed acute hypertensive crisis, is characterized clinically by extreme blood pressure elevation and papilledema. **Accelerated HTN** is identified by the presence of severe retinopathy (exudates, hemorrhages, arteriolar narrowing, spasm, etc.) without papilledema. Both forms of HTN are associated with severe vascular injury to the kidneys and other end organs.

Hypertensive encephalopathy occurs when elevated mean arterial pressures overcome cerebral autoregulation. With the resulting loss of control of cerebral perfusion, cerebral blood flow (CBF) rises, the brain is hyperperfused, and vasogenic edema develops.

Etiology

Any form of hypertensive disorder, regardless of etiology, can precipitate a hypertensive crisis. The abruptness

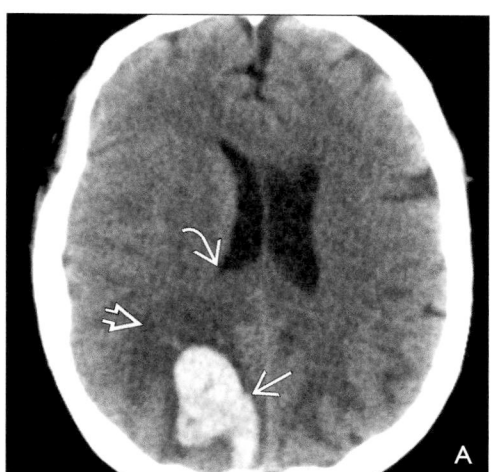
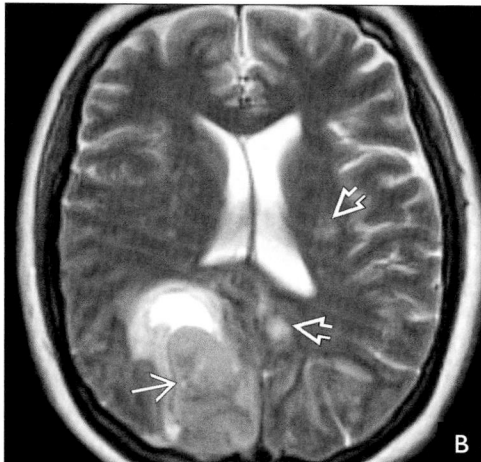

32-8A. *NECT scan in a 55-year-old woman with mHTN shows a focal right occipital lobar hematoma ➡ with surrounding edema ➡, mass effect on the adjacent lateral ventricle ➡. 32-8B. T2WI shows that the hematoma ➡ is somewhat heterogeneous but mostly isointense with cortex. Several other ill-defined hyperintensities are present in the subcortical WM ➡.*

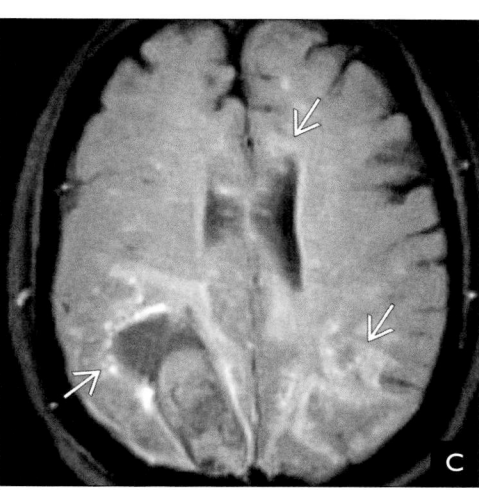
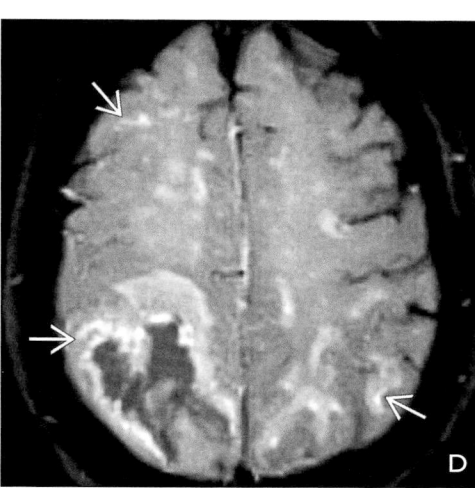

32-8C. *Axial T1 C+ FS scan in the same patient shows multiple foci of patchy and confluent contrast enhancement throughout both hemispheres ➡ secondary to widespread blood-brain barrier disruption caused by malignant hypertension. 32-8D. More cephalad T1 C+ FS scan shows innumerable enhancing foci in the cortex, subcortical, and deep WM ➡. The patient expired shortly after the scan was obtained.*

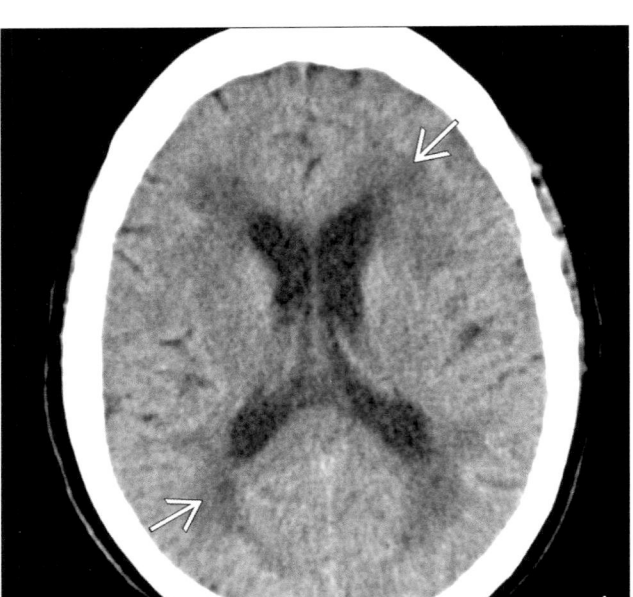

32-9A. *Axial NECT scan in a patient with longstanding chronic hypertension demonstrates bilateral frontal and periatrial WM confluent hypodensities* ➡.

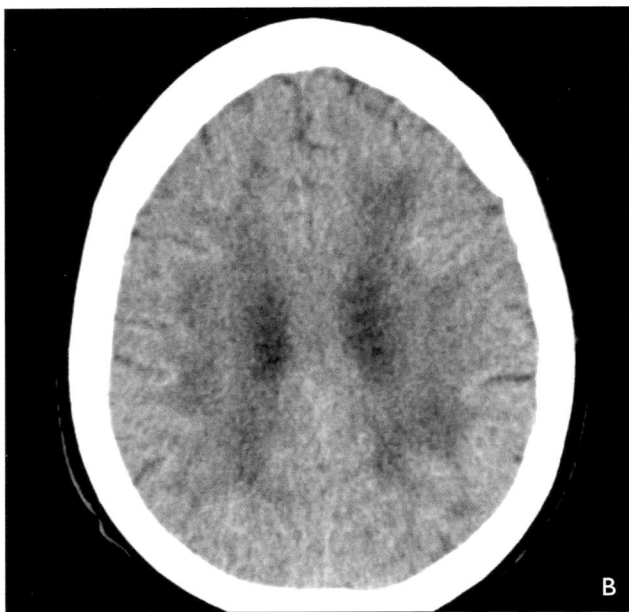

32-9B. *NECT scan through the corona radiata shows confluent subcortical and deep WM hypodensities. These lesions are sometimes called "subcortical arteriosclerotic encephalopathy" and are common in patients with HTN and hyperlipidemia.*

of blood pressure elevation seems to be more important than the absolute level of blood pressure.

mHTN in the setting of chronic hypertension is actually rare, occurring in less than 1% of all patients. Nevertheless, because the prevalence of HTN in the general population is so high, so-called essential hypertension (chronic HTN without an identifiable underlying cause) is still the most common overall condition predisposing to mHTN.

mHTN also occurs in previously normotensive individuals. Sudden onset of severe HTN can occur in children with acute glomerulonephritis, pregnant women with eclampsia, and patients of all ages with substance abuse (e.g., cocaine). Less common causes of mHTN include pheochromocytoma crisis, clonidine withdrawal syndrome, drug interactions (e.g., monoamine oxidase inhibitor + tyramine), and autonomic overactivity in patients with spinal cord disorders.

Pathology

Macroscopically, the brain appears swollen and edematous. Gross parenchymal hematomas and perivascular petechial microhemorrhages may be present. Acute microinfarcts, especially in the basal ganglia and pons, are common.

Microscopic features of mHTN include arteriolar fibrinoid necrosis and microvascular platelet/fibrin thrombi. Edema with proteinaceous exudates in the adjacent white matter is a typical associated finding.

Clinical Issues

Blood pressure in mHTN is severely elevated, with diastolic levels often exceeding 130-140 mmHg. Headache with or without coexisting encephalopathy is the most frequent symptom and is often accompanied by visual disturbances, nausea and vomiting, and altered mental status. Congestive heart failure, deteriorating renal function, and anemia are common.

The complications of acute hypertensive crisis are generally reversible if the condition is diagnosed properly and appropriate therapy instituted quickly. Rapid blood pressure reduction typically results in prompt, dramatic improvement in hypertensive encephalopathy.

Imaging

Imaging findings in mHTN range from classic PRES-like features with parietooccipital predominance to "atypical" features. "Atypical" features are more common in mHTN compared to PRES and include brainstem-dominant disease (32-6) as well as basal ganglia and/or watershed lesions (32-7). Diffuse cerebral edema may be present in especially severe cases.

Lobar and/or multifocal parenchymal microhemorrhages in the cortex, basal ganglia, pons, and cerebellum are common in mHTN and are best seen as "blooming" foci on T2* sequences (GRE, SWI). Convexal subarachnoid hemorrhage with multiple foci of short-segment arterial stenoses resembling reversible cerebral vasoconstriction syndrome (RCVS) has been reported in a few cases of mHTN.

mHTN can cause widespread blood-brain barrier disruption with striking multifocal patchy enhancement following contrast administration (32-8). Restricted diffusion on DWI is not uncommon.

Differential Diagnosis

The major differential diagnosis of mHTN is **PRES**. **TTP** with brain ischemia and microhemorrhages can appear identical on imaging studies, and the distinction is established by clinical-laboratory features, not imaging findings.

Chronic Hypertensive Encephalopathy

While the clinical and imaging manifestations of posterior reversible encephalopathy syndrome (PRES) and malignant hypertension (mHTN) can be dramatic and life-threatening, the effects of longstanding untreated or poorly treated hypertension on end-organ function can be equally devastating.

Pathology

The most consistent histopathologic feature of chronic hypertensive encephalopathy (CHtnE) is a microvasculopathy characterized by arteriolosclerosis and lipohyalinosis (see Chapter 10). Stenosis and occlusion of small arteries and arterioles from layers of hyaline collagen deposition causes decreased oligodendrocyte density, myelin pallor, gliosis, and spongiform WM volume loss. Multiple lacunar infarcts are common.

Clinical Issues

CHtnE is most common in middle-aged and elderly patients. CHtnE affects men more often than women and is especially prevalent in African-Americans. In addition to age and chronically elevated blood pressure, smoking is an independent risk factor for CHtnE. Metabolic syndrome (impaired glucose metabolism, elevated blood pressure, central obesity, and dyslipidemia) is increasingly common and contributes significantly to the worldwide burden of CHtnE.

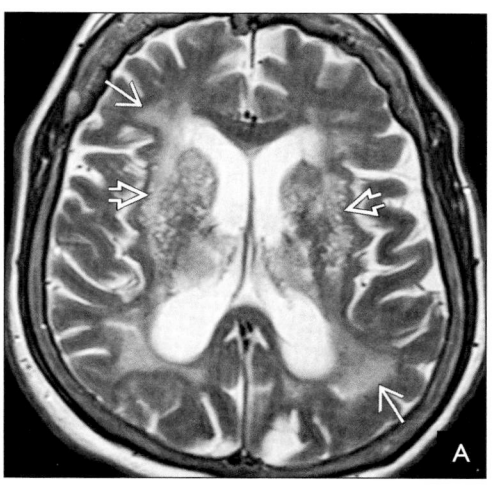 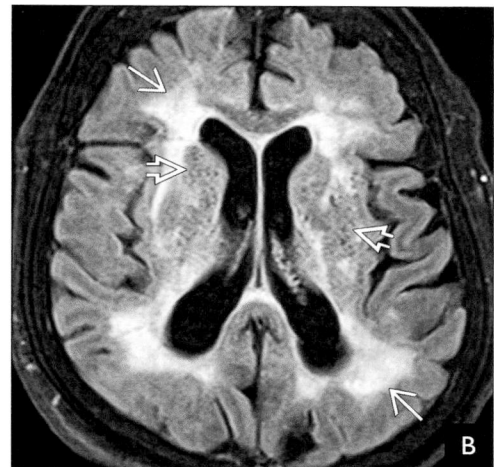
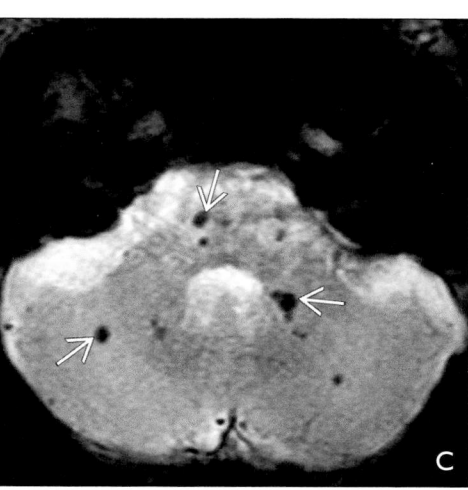 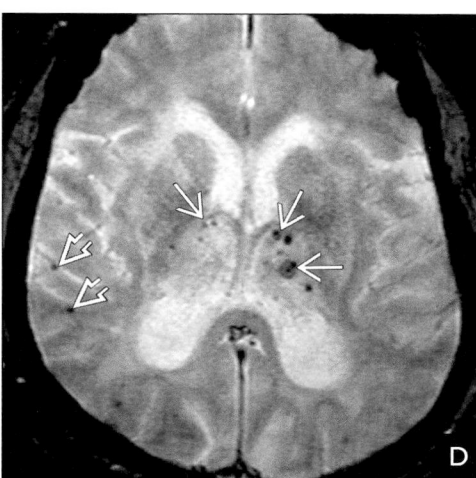

32-10A. Axial T2WI in a 74-year-old woman with poorly controlled HTN shows generalized volume loss with enlarged ventricles, sulci. Confluent hyperintensities in the deep periventricular WM together with multiple punctate cystic-appearing lesions in the basal ganglia, external capsules are present. 32-10B. FLAIR shows confluent hyperintensity in deep WM whereas the basal ganglia cysts mostly suppress and are enlarged perivascular spaces.

32-10C. T2 GRE scan through the posterior fossa shows multiple "blooming" hypointensities in the lower pons and cerebellum. 32-10D. T2* GRE scan through the lateral ventricles shows multifocal "blooming" hypointensities in the basal ganglia with only a few peripheral foci identified. Imaging is consistent with arteriolosclerosis/lipohyalinosis (the T2/FLAIR hyperintensities) and multiple hypertensive microbleeds (the "black dots").*

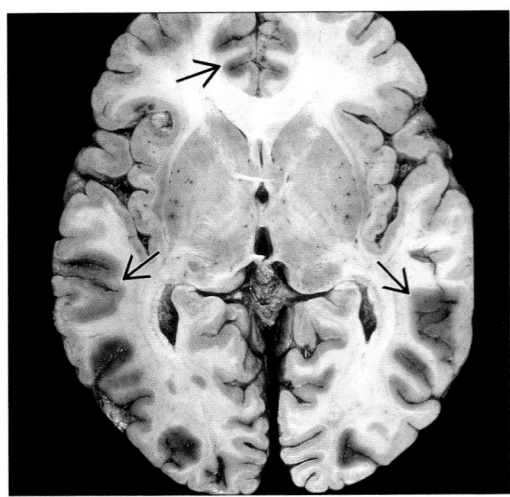

32-11. Autopsy of severe hypoglycemia shows bilateral symmetric parietooccipital, frontal cortical necrosis ➔. (Courtesy R. Hewlett, MD.)

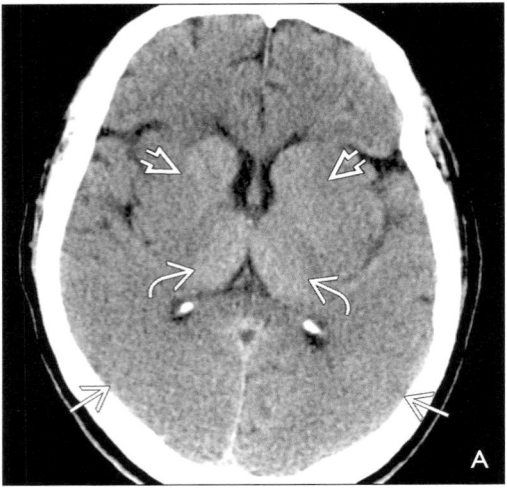

32-12A. NECT shows typical changes of hypoglycemia with parietooccipital gyral swelling ➔, putamen hypodensity ➔, spared thalami ➔.

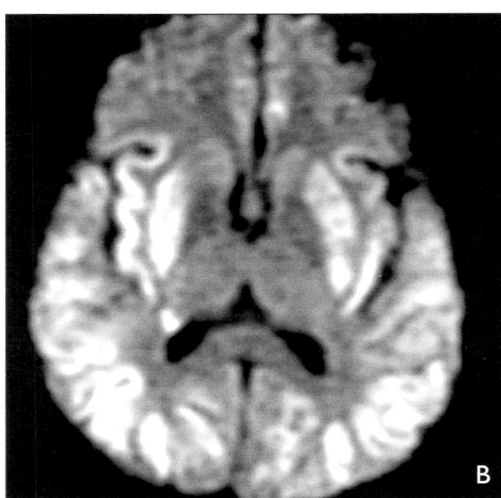

32-12B. DWI in the same case of typical AHE shows restricted diffusion in parietooccipital cortex, putamina with thalamic and WM sparing.

The most common symptom of CHtnE is nonspecific headache. Stepwise or gradual progression of cognitive dysfunction is also common and may develop into frank vascular dementia.

Imaging

The two cardinal imaging features of CHtnE are (1) diffuse patchy and/or confluent WM lesions and (2) multifocal microbleeds. The WM lesions are concentrated in the corona radiata and deep periventricular WM—especially around the atria of the lateral ventricles. The damaged WM appears hypodense on NECT scans (32-9) and hyperintense on T2/FLAIR imaging.

Multiple petechial bleeds ("microhemorrhages") are the second most common manifestation of CHtnE. These are not usually identifiable on NECT and may be invisible on standard MR sequences (FSE T2WI and FLAIR). T2* (GRE, SWI) scans show multiple "blooming" hypointensities ("black dots") that tend to be concentrated in the basal ganglia and cerebellum (32-10).

Imaging findings in CHtnE can also reflect "acute on chronic" disease. T2* scans in the majority of patients with classic basal ganglia or lobar hypertensive hemorrhages demonstrate petechial microhemorrhages. Occasionally, patients with chronic longstanding hypertension develop an acute hypertensive crisis and can demonstrate features of PRES superimposed on longstanding, chronic-appearing WM disease.

Differential Diagnosis

The major differential diagnosis of CHtnE is **cerebral amyloid angiopathy** (CAA). The WM lesions in both diseases often appear similar, and both disorders can cause hemorrhagic microangiopathy. The microbleeds of CAA are more often peripheral (e.g., cortex, leptomeninges) and rarely affect the brainstem or cerebellum. Hypertensive microhemorrhages are most common in the basal ganglia and frequently can be identified in the pons and cerebellar hemispheres.

Cerebral autosomal dominant arteriopathy without subcortical infarcts and leukoencephalopathy (CADASIL) can also mimic CHtnE. CADASIL typically presents in younger patients and causes multiple subcortical lacunar infarcts. Lesions in the anterior temporal lobes and external capsules are classic imaging findings of CADASIL.

Glucose Disorders

The brain is a glucose glutton, consuming more than half the body's total glucose. Because the brain does not store excess energy as glycogen, CNS function is highly dependent on a steady, continuous supply of blood glucose (see box below).

Blood glucose levels are tightly regulated and are normally maintained within a narrow physiologic range. Disorders of glucose metabolism—both *hypo*glycemia and *hyper*glycemia—can injure the CNS.

The neurologic manifestations of deranged glucose metabolism range from mild, reversible focal deficits to status epilepticus, coma, and death. Because the clinical and imaging manifestations differ in neonates from those of older children and adults, hypoglycemia in these two age groups is discussed separately.

The vast majority of hypoglycemia cases are acquired. A few inherited syndromes present with infantile hyperinsulinemic hypoglycemia as a secondary manifestation of systemic disease. The effects of hypoglycemia on the infant brain are identical, regardless of etiology, so they are discussed in this chapter.

Following the discussion of *hypo*glycemia, we turn our attention to *hyper*glycemia-associated disorders that affect the CNS.

GLUCOSE AND THE BRAIN

Normal Physiology
- Brain is a "glucose glutton"
  - Utilizes 100-150 g/day
- Glucose must be actively transported across blood-brain barrier
  - Glucose transport protein (GLUT-1)
- Glucose metabolism
  - Aerobic oxidation (20% of total body O_2 consumption)
  - Intracellular glucose converted to pyruvate
  - Then metabolized to ATP, phosphocreatine
- Glucose utilization linearly related to CBF
  - GM ≈ 5x WM
  - Mostly used for active ion transport, maintenance of membrane potentials
- Glucose homeostasis
  - Blood glucose concentration dynamic, tightly regulated
  - Brain monitors, "conducts" gut-CNS-endocrine axis
  - Complex interactions maintain normal glycemia

Abnormal Physiology
- Too much or too little glucose both injure brain
- Hyperglycemic > > hypoglycemic disorders

Pediatric/Adult Hypoglycemic Encephalopathy

Terminology

Hypoglycemia literally means low blood sugar and is caused by an imbalance between glucose supply and glucose utilization. Acute hypoglycemic brain injury is called hypoglycemic encephalopathy.

Etiology

Childhood hypoglycemic encephalopathy is most commonly associated with type 1 diabetes mellitus. Rarely, hypoglycemia occurs as an inherited disorder (see below) or secondary to insulin-secreting tumors.

In its most common adult setting—advanced type 2 diabetes—hypoglycemia typically results from the interplay between absolute or relative insulin excess and compromised glucose counterregulation; insulin in and of itself is not neurotoxic. Most cases of adult hypoglycemia occur as a side effect of diabetes treatment with insulin and sulfonylureas.

Factors other than absolute blood glucose levels also affect the presence and extent of hypoglycemic brain injury, including the duration and severity of hypoglycemia, presence and degree of hypoxia or other metabolic disturbances, cerebral blood flow, and CNS/cardiovascular metabolic requirements.

Pathology

Hypoglycemia has both direct and indirect effects on the brain, which is exquisitely sensitive to glucose insufficiency. Glucose insufficiency results in impaired oxygen utilization and compromised intracellular energy production. Indirect effects occur secondary to the accumulation and release of excitatory neurotransmitters, which in turn accentuates the degree of hypoglycemic brain injury.

Cortical necrosis is the most common gross finding in hypoglycemic encephalopathy. While the entire cortical ribbon can be affected, the parietooccipital regions are usually the most severely involved **(32-11)**. Other especially vulnerable areas include the basal ganglia, hippocampi, and amygdalae. The thalami, white matter, brainstem, and cerebellum are typically spared.

Clinical Issues

The typical hypoglycemic patient is an elderly diabetic on insulin replacement therapy with altered dietary glucose intake. Deliberate or accidental insulin overdose is more common in children and young or middle-aged adults.

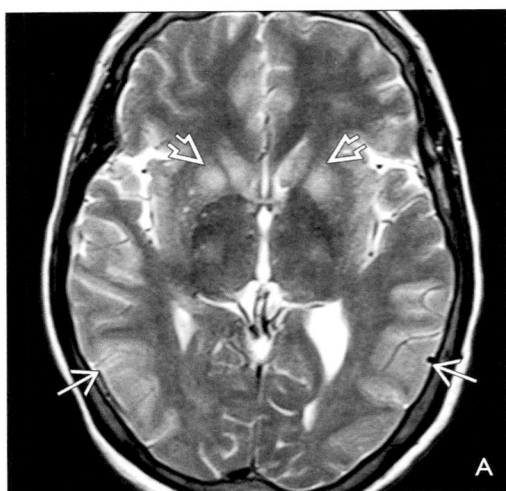

32-13A. T2WI in a 21-year-old diabetic "found down" shows bilateral parietooccipital cortical ➡, basal ganglia hyperintensity ➡.

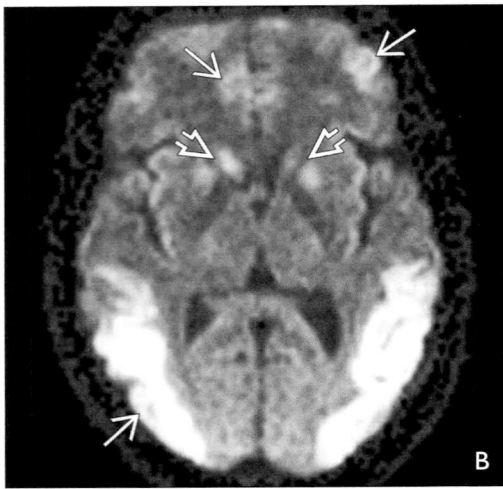

32-13B. DWI in the same patient shows diffusion restriction in the cortex ➡, basal ganglia ➡. The thalami and WM are spared.

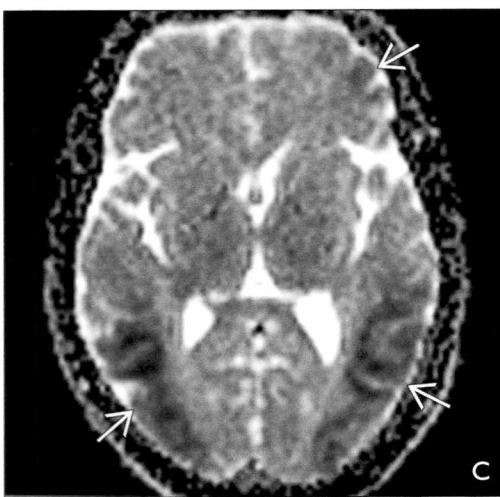

32-13C. ADC map confirms restriction in the cortex ➡.

Seizures, mental status changes, and coma are common symptoms of hypoglycemic encephalopathy. Prognosis varies with the extent of brain injury. If the basal ganglia are involved, the outcome is generally poor. If basal ganglia injury is minimal or absent, residual neurologic deficits are correlated with the severity of cortical injury.

Because of sympathoadrenergic effects, myocardial infarction and severe arrhythmias are common indirect effects of hypoglycemia and may account for the "dead in bed" syndrome.

Imaging

CT FINDINGS. NECT scans typically show symmetrically hypodense parietal and occipital lobes. The putamina frequently appear hypodense while the thalami are spared **(32-12)**. In severe cases, diffuse cerebral edema with near-total sulcal effacement and blurred gray-white matter interfaces can be seen.

MR FINDINGS. T1 scans in patients with acute hypoglycemic encephalopathy can appear normal or demonstrate only gyral swelling and sulcal effacement. In the subacute and chronic stages, curvilinear gyral hyperintensity secondary to laminar necrosis may be present.

T2/FLAIR hyperintensity in the parietooccipital cortex and basal ganglia is typical of acute hypoglycemic encephalopathy **(32-13)**. The thalami, subcortical/deep WM, and cerebellum are generally spared. T2* scans generally show minimal or no "blooming" to suggest hemorrhage.

Enhancement on T1 C+ is variable and, when present, usually mild. DWI scans show restricted diffusion **(32-12)**. MRS demonstrates reduced NAA with or without a prominent lactate peak.

Differential Diagnosis

The most important differential diagnosis of hypoglycemic encephalopathy is **hypoxic-ischemic encephalopathy** (HIE). HIE typically occurs following cardiac arrest or global hypoperfusion. In contrast to hypoglycemic encephalopathy, the thalami and cerebellum are often affected in HIE. **Acute cerebral ischemia-infarction** is wedge-shaped, involving both the cortex and underlying WM.

Acute hypertensive encephalopathy (PRES) typically affects the parietooccipital cortex but spares most of the underlying WM and rarely restricts on DWI. PRES patients present with uncontrolled hypertension, not hypoglycemia.

Neonatal/Infantile Hypoglycemia

The immature brain is relatively resistant to hypoglycemia. Unlike older children and adults, neonates have lower absolute glucose demands and can utilize other substrates such as lactate to produce energy. Nevertheless, prolonged and/or severe hypoglycemia can result in devastating brain injury in newborn infants.

Terminology

The precise clinical/laboratory definition of neonatal/infantile hypoglycemia is controversial. Between 5-15% of normal term infants have initial plasma glucose values as low as 40-45 mg/dL. Currently accepted definitions of significant hypoglycemia in the newborn are glucose levels below 30-35 mg/dL in the first 24 hours after birth and 40-45 mg/dL thereafter.

Etiology

Neonatal/infantile hypoglycemic encephalopathy is secondary to hyperinsulinemia and is most often caused by maternal diabetes with poor glycemic control. Uncontrolled maternal diabetes leads to chronic fetal hyperglycemia in utero. This results in transient neonatal hyperinsulinemia and hypoglycemia of varying severity.

Rarely, infantile hyperinsulinemic hypoglycemia is inherited. The most common types of congenital hyperinsulinism or persistent hyperinsulinemic hypoglycemia of infancy result from mutations in the genes that encode the **pancreatic β-cell ATP-sensitive potassium channel**.

Neonatal hypoglycemia may also occur in the setting of **Beckwith-Wiedemann syndrome** (BWS), an inherited disorder with macrosomia, macroglossia, visceromegaly, omphalocele, embryonal tumors, adrenocortical cytomegaly, and renal abnormalities. Most cases of BWS-associated hypoglycemia are mild and transient but can persist and—if undetected and untreated—pose significant risk for developmental sequelae.

Pathology

Transient, mild hypoglycemia generally does not injure the neonatal brain. Prolonged, severe hypoglycemia causes coagulative necrosis in the middle layers of the parietooccipital cortex and underlying WM.

Clinical Issues

Neonatal/infantile hypoglycemic encephalopathy typically presents in the first three days of life, usually within the first 24 hours. Large for gestation age babies have an increased risk of hypoglycemia even when they are not the product of diabetic pregnancies.

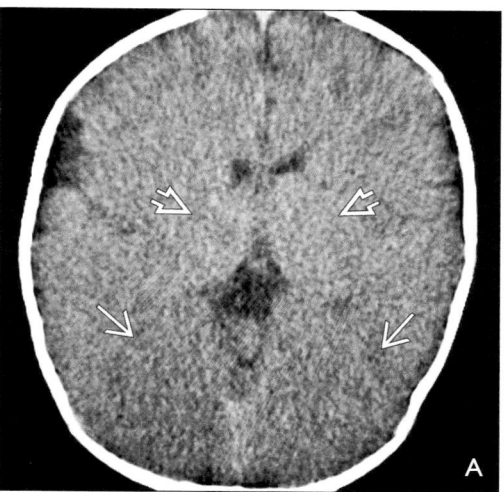

32-14A. *NECT in a 3 day old with profound hypoglycemia shows bilateral symmetric posterior hypodensity* ⇗, *ill-defined basal ganglia* ⇒.

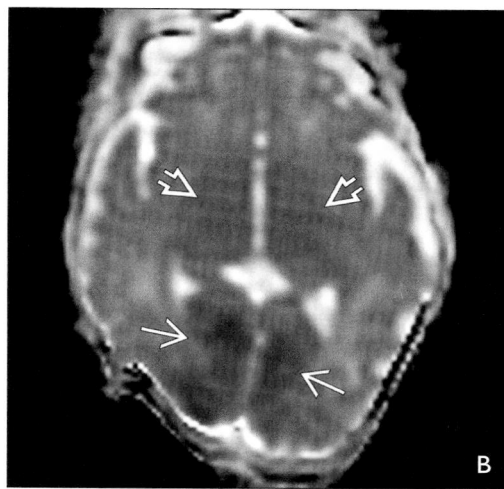

32-14B. *ADC shows restricted diffusion in the parietooccipital lobes* ⇒, *basal ganglia, and thalami* ⇒.

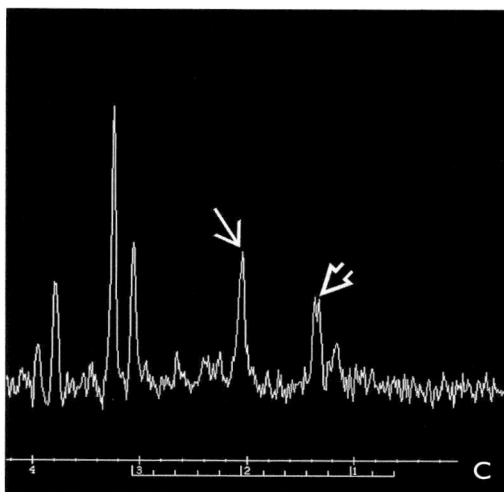

32-14C. *MRS with long TE in the same case shows decreased NAA* ⇒, *moderately elevated lactate* ⇒.

32-15A. Axial T2WI in a 5-day-old infant with hypoglycemia shows effaced GM-WM interfaces in the parietooccipital lobes ⇨ compared to the normal frontal lobes ⇨. The cortex, underlying WM ⇨, and corpus callosum splenium ⇨ are swollen and hyperintense.
32-15B. ADC map in the same patient shows profound restricted diffusion in the parietal and occipital lobes ⇨, corpus callosum splenium ⇨.

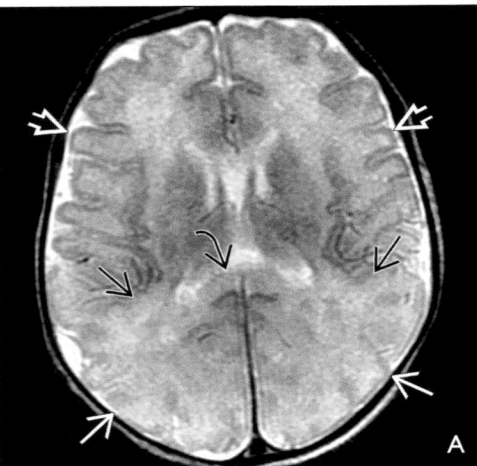

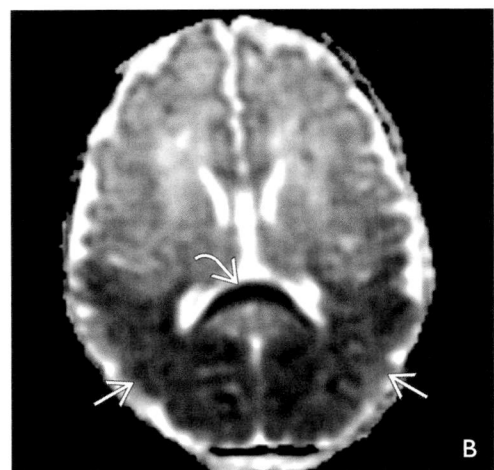

32-15C. T1WI in the same patient at 7 days shows swollen, markedly hypointense WM in the parietal, occipital lobes ⇨, hyperintense, thinned cortex ⇨, hypointense pulvinars of the thalami ⇨.
32-15D. T2WI at the same time shows thinned swollen cortex with patchy increased ⇨ and decreased ⇨ signal intensity, hyperintense pulvinars ⇨, and abnormally hyperintense internal capsules ⇨.

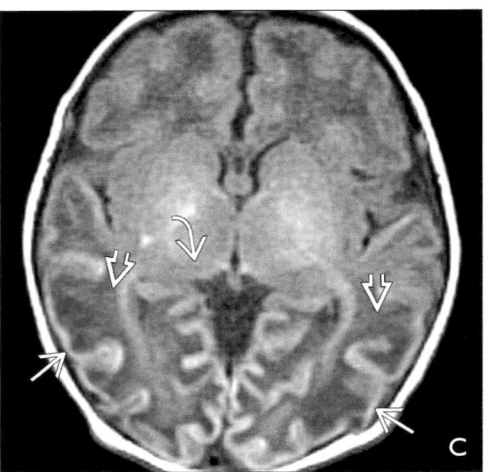

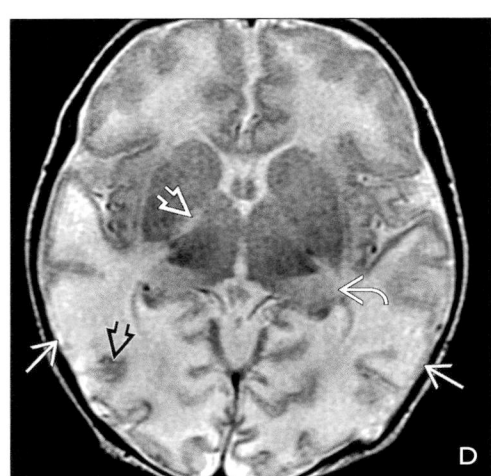

32-15E. Axial T2WI in the same infant at 1 year of age shows shrunken, hyperintense parietooccipital lobes with profound cortical loss, ulegyria, and encephalomalacic-appearing WM ⇨. *32-15F.* Coronal FLAIR scan, also performed at 1 year of age, shows extensive WM hyperintensity ⇨ and thinned, shrunken gyri with focally enlarged sulci ⇨.

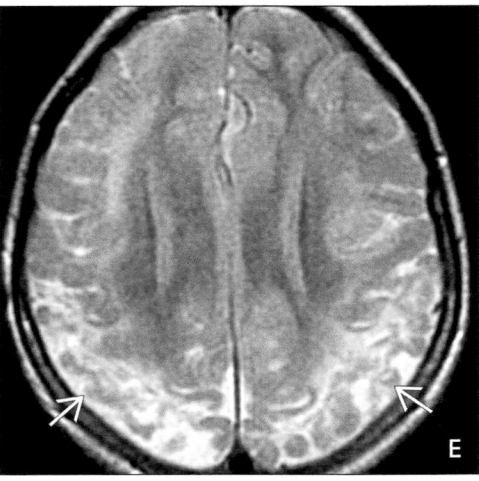

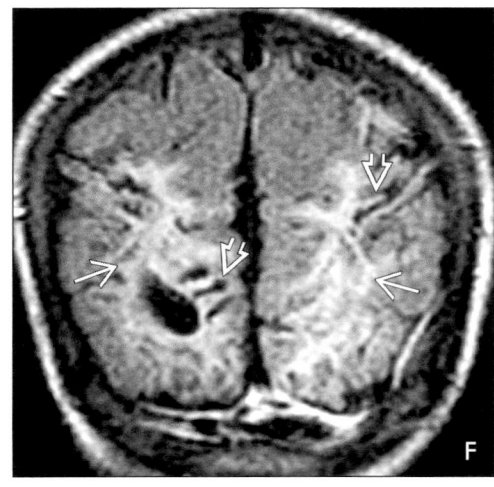

The precise level of hypoglycemia that requires treatment is controversial. Some experts recommend treating only symptomatic neonates with glucose concentrations below 45-50 mg/dL. The response to glucose therapy is typically prompt if the degree and duration of hypoglycemia is mild to moderate.

Imaging

Some imaging findings in neonatal/infantile hypoglycemia resemble those of older children and adults, i.e., predominant involvement of the parietooccipital cortex and basal ganglia. However, white matter, thalamic, and cerebellar involvement are all relatively more common in neonates compared to hypoglycemic encephalopathy in older children and adults,

NECT scans in neonates with acute hypoglycemic encephalopathy show posterior brain hypodensity with effaced gray-white matter interfaces **(32-14)**. In especially severe cases, the brain appears diffusely swollen and hypodense.

MR scans in the acute stages of neonatal hypoglycemic encephalopathy show T2/FLAIR hyperintensity and restricted diffusion in the parietooccipital cortex, subcortical WM, and corpus callosum splenium **(32-15A)**, **(32-15B)**.

In the late acute/early subacute phase, the affected areas are swollen and edematous **(32-15C)**, **(32-15D)**.

Cystic encephalomalacia may ensue. In chronic hypoglycemic encephalopathy, the parietooccipital cortices become atrophic, shrunken, and encephalomalacic **(32-15E)**, **(32-15F)**.

Differential Diagnosis

As with older children and adults, the major differential diagnosis of neonatal hypoglycemic encephalopathy is **term hypoxic-ischemic injury** (HII). Hypoglycemic encephalopathy and HII often coexist, potentiating the extent of brain injury. Imaging findings in the two disorders may be indistinguishable.

Inherited mitochondrial disorders such as **mitochondrial encephalopathy with lactic acidosis and stroke-like episodes** (MELAS) may present with cortical swelling that spares the underlying WM. MELAS is rarely bilaterally symmetric and demonstrates much more markedly elevated lactate on MRS.

HYPOGLYCEMIA

General Concepts
- Imbalance between glucose supply, utilization → hypoglycemia
- Can be mild, transient, asymptomatic
- Extent of brain injury depends on
  - Degree, duration of hypoglycemia
  - CBF, glucose utilization
  - Availability/utilization of alternative energy sources (e.g., lactate)
  - Exacerbating factors (e.g., hypoxia)
  - Recognition, prompt/appropriate treatment

Pediatric/Adult Hypoglycemia
- Etiology
  - Usually associated with diabetes
  - Absolute/relative insulin excess or glucose insufficiency
  - Energy production/O_2 utilization ↓, excitotoxic neurotransmitters ↑
- Pathology
  - Cortical necrosis
- Imaging
  - Hypodense/hyperintense parietooccipital cortex, basal ganglia
  - Restricted diffusion
  - WM, thalami, cerebellum generally spared

Neonatal/Infantile Hypoglycemia
- Etiology
  - Most common: Maternal diabetes
  - Fetal hyperglycemia → neonatal hyperinsulinemia → hypoglycemia
  - Less common: Inherited congenital hyperinsulinemia
- Clinical issues
  - Usually presents in first 3 postnatal days
  - Glucose levels variable
- Imaging
  - Often similar to adult (posterior predominance)
  - Different: Subcortical WM, thalami often involved
- Differential diagnosis
  - Term hypoxic-ischemic encephalopathy
  - Mitochondrial encephalopathy (MELAS)

Hyperglycemia-associated Disorders

While hyperglycemia can be spontaneous, it is most often associated with diabetes mellitus (DM). In this section, we briefly discuss DM itself before turning our attention specifically to hyperglycemia-induced brain injury. We first discuss the effects of *chronic* hyperglycemia on the brain, primarily seen as accelerated small vessel (microvascular) disease. We then consider two less common conditions associated with *acute* hyperglycemic changes in the CNS: Diabetic ketoacidosis and hyperglycemic hyperosmolar state (rare).

Diabetes

In **type 1 diabetes** (DM1), previously known as "juvenile diabetes," a lack of insulin results from the destruction of insulin-producing β cells in the pancreas, presumably secondary to an autoimmune-mediated process. DM1 accounts for only 5-10% of all patients with DM.

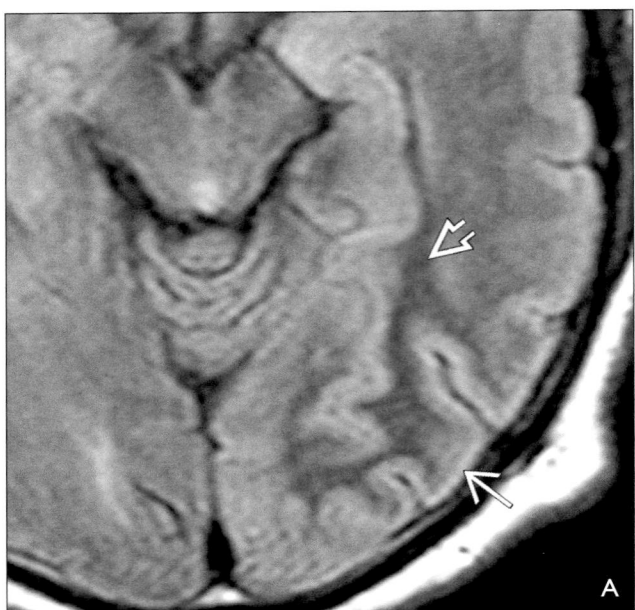

32-16A. Close-up view of an axial FLAIR scan in a patient with type 2 diabetes and hyperglycemic hyperosmolar state shows hyperintense gyri ➡, strikingly hypointense WM ➡ in the left parietooccipital lobe.

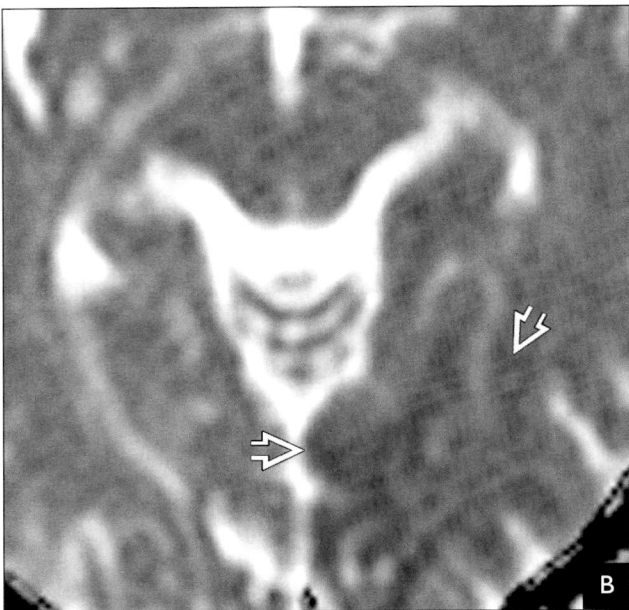

32-16B. Close-up view of the ADC map in the same patient shows restricted diffusion ➡. (Courtesy K. K. Oguz, MD.)

The vast majority of patients with diabetes have **type 2 diabetes** (DM2), previously termed "adult-onset diabetes." DM2 is also known as noninsulin-dependent diabetes and is caused by relative insulin deficiency or cellular insulin resistance. DM2 occurs in both children and adults. Risk factors include low activity level, poor diet, and excess body weight.

Chronic Hyperglycemic Brain Injury

Hyperglycemia-induced brain injury can be chronic or acute. With the worldwide rise in obesity and the soaring prevalence of DM2, the effects of chronic hyperglycemia on the brain are increasingly recognized. Patients with DM2 have accelerated arteriolosclerosis and lipohyalinosis with silent infarcts, brain volume loss, and decreased cognitive functioning.

MR shows increased numbers of T2/FLAIR subcortical and periventricular hyperintensities, especially in the frontal WM, pons, and cerebellum. DTI demonstrates loss of microstructural integrity with decreased FA.

Acute Hyperglycemic Brain Injury

Although acute brain injury in hyperglycemia is less common than in hypoglycemia, hyperglycemia can also cause major morbidity and significant mortality. Two acute conditions are associated with hyperglycemia: **Diabetic ketoacidosis** (DKA) and **hyperglycemic hyperosmolar state** (HHS). These two diseases can be considered the endpoints of a clinical-laboratory continuum from DKA with minimal symptoms and normal osmolality to HHS with minimal or no ketosis and coma.

DKA and HHS are both caused by reduction in the net effective action of circulating insulin. Intracellular starvation stimulates the release of the counterregulatory hormones glucagon, catecholamines, cortisol, and growth hormones. This leads to accelerated hepatic and renal glucose production and impaired glucose utilization in insulin-dependent peripheral tissues (e.g., muscle, liver, adipose). The result is hyperglycemia, lipolysis (with release of free fatty acids into the circulation), and hepatic fatty acid oxidation (to ketone bodies).

DKA and HHS are also associated with glycosuria, which can cause osmotic diuresis with subsequent loss of water, sodium, potassium, and other electrolytes. In severe cases, secondary changes of acute osmotic demyelination can complicate the imaging findings of both disorders.

DIABETIC KETOACIDOSIS. Although DKA can occur in patients with both DM1 and DM2, it is quite uncommon in DM2. DKA is defined as acidosis with a venous pH less than 7.3 or serum bicarbonate concentration less than 15 mmol/L in the presence of serum glucose concentration more than 11 mmol/L. DKA is characterized by glucosuria, ketonuria, and ketonemia.

DKA is often a recurrent disease. Mortality for each episode is relatively small (0.15-0.3%). Idiopathic cerebral edema accounts for at least two-thirds of fatal cases.

Imaging in patients with acute DKA is nonspecific, with vasogenic cerebral edema the most common abnormality. Younger age, severe acidosis, hypocapnia, and dehydration have all been cited as risk factors for cerebral edema.

HYPERGLYCEMIC HYPEROSMOLAR STATE. HHS occurs almost exclusively in patients with DM2. Once considered a relatively rare condition seen only in the elderly population, the emergence of childhood DM2 means HHS now occurs in patients of all ages and is becoming significantly more common.

The clinical-laboratory criteria for HHS include plasma glucose concentration > 33.3 mmol/L, serum bicarbonate concentration > 15 mmol/L, absent or minimal ketonuria and ketonemia, effective serum osmolality > 320 mOsm/kg, *and* the presence of stupor or coma. Unlike DKA, seizures are common. Glycosuria and hypernatremia from dehydration can lead to cerebral edema, osmotic demyelination, seizure, and cardiac arrest.

The most striking imaging finding in HHS is T2/FLAIR *hypo*intensity in the parietooccipital WM **(32-16)**. Patients treated for HHS with rapid correction of the hyperosmolar state may also develop osmotic demyelination with typical findings of central pontine myelinolysis (see below).

Hyperglycemia-induced Hemichorea-Hemiballismus

The syndrome called hyperglycemia-induced hemichorea-hemiballismus (HIHH) is characterized by non-patterned and involuntary unilateral movements. HIHH is a rare but potentially reversible complication of non-ketotic hyperglycemia.

HIHH usually occurs in elderly patients, more often affects females, and may be the first ("unmasking") symptom of DM2. It can resolve over days or persist for years.

MR findings are virtually pathognomonic of HIHH. Unilateral T1 basal ganglia hyperintensity with sparing of the thalamus is characteristic **(32-17)**. The signal abnormality probably represents zinc deposition, not calcium or hemorrhage.

HYPERGLYCEMIA

General Concepts
- Spontaneous (rare) or diabetes-associated (common)
- Acute (rare) or chronic (common)

Hyperglycemia
- *Chronic* diabetes-associated brain injury
  - Accelerated arteriolosclerosis, impaired cognition
  - MR: ↓ brain volume, ↑ WM hyperintensities
- *Acute* hypoglycemic brain injury
  - Diabetic ketoacidosis (DKA)
  - Hyperglycemic hyperosmolar state (HHS)
  - Hyperglycemia-induced hemichorea-hemiballismus (HIHH)
- Imaging
  - DKA: Vasogenic cerebral edema ± osmotic demyelination
  - HHS: Subcortical WM hypointensity
  - HIHH: Unilateral T1 shortening in basal ganglia

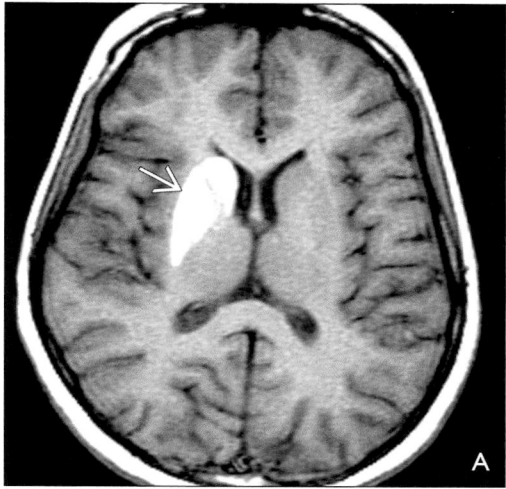

32-17A. T1WI in hyperglycemia-induced hemichorea-hemiballismus (HIHH) shows uniformly hyperintense right basal ganglia ➡.

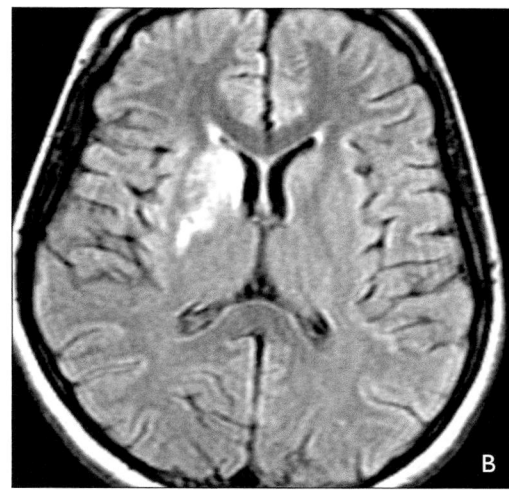

32-17B. FLAIR in the same patient shows patchy hyperintensity in the right basal ganglia. The remainder of the brain appears normal.

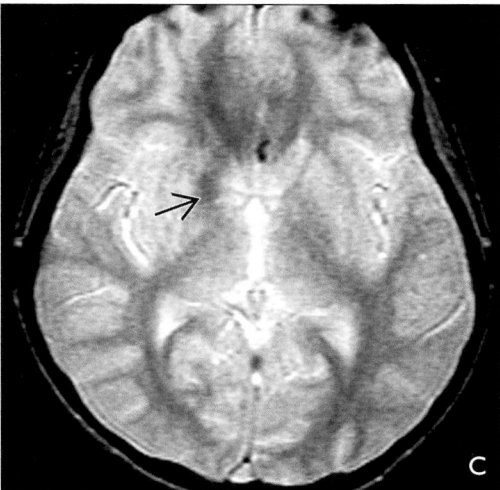

32-17C. T2* GRE shows minimal hypointensity in the globus pallidus ➡*, no significant "blooming" that would suggest hemorrhage. (K. K. Oguz, MD.)*

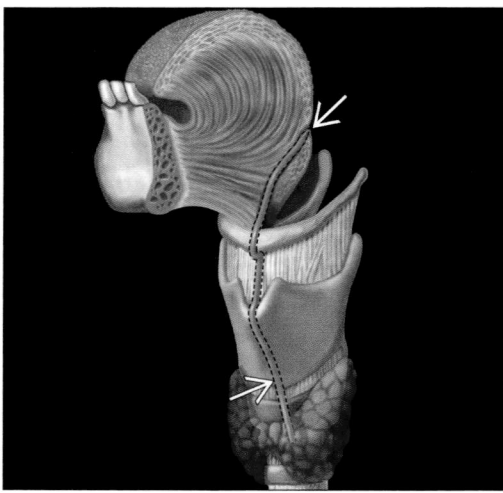

32-18. Embryonic thyroid migrates inferiorly from the tongue to the neck. Ectopic thyroid can occur anywhere along the thyroglossal duct ➡.

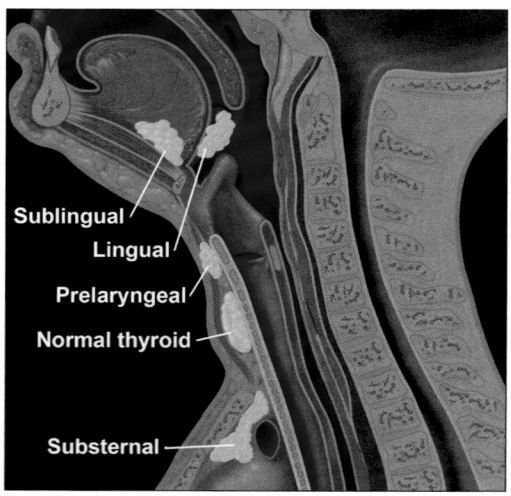

32-19. Sagittal graphic depicts possible sites of ectopic thyroid. Most occur along the thyroglossal duct but may occur elsewhere (e.g., substernal).

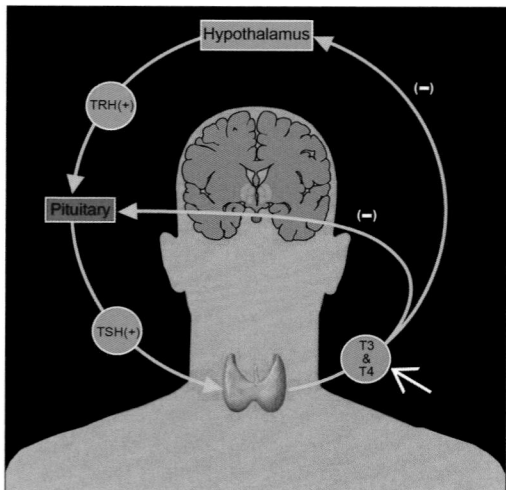

32-20. Graphic depicts hypothalamic-pituitary-thyroid axis. Note that T3 and T4 ➡ inhibit hypothalamic and pituitary stimulation of thyroid.

Thyroid Disorders

Thyroid disorders are relatively common metabolic disturbances that are usually mild and rarely affect brain function. However, several imaging findings—some of them striking—have been associated with thyroid disease. Some can be mistaken for more serious disease (e.g., hypothyroid-induced pituitary hyperplasia mimicking pituitary adenoma), and a few (e.g., Hashimoto encephalopathy) can be life-threatening.

Hypothyroidism can be congenital or acquired. We begin our discussion of thyroid disease with congenital hypothyroidism before turning our attention to acquired hypothyroid disease and its imaging manifestations. We close the section with a brief consideration of hyperthyroid disease and its effects on the CNS.

Congenital Hypothyroidism

Congenital hypothyroidism (CH) occurs in 1:2,000-4,000 newborns and is one of the most common preventable causes of mental retardation. If the diagnosis is made and treatment begun within a few weeks of birth, neurodevelopmental outcome is generally normal.

Newborns with CH normally have some initial residual thyroid function because maternal T4 crosses the placenta to the fetus. With a half-life of six days, however, maternal T4 will be almost completely metabolized and excreted by three to four weeks of age.

In developed countries with newborn screening programs, most infants with CH are diagnosed soon after birth. Serum TSH is elevated (typically more than 20-30 mU/L). In less developed countries, CH is often diagnosed later in childhood when suspicious clinical features lead to serum thyroid function testing or imaging studies. The most visible clinical feature is a facies suggestive of "cretinism," a term no longer used because of its pejorative implications.

Etiology and Presentation

CH can be caused by thyroid dysgenesis, dyshormonogenesis, or central hypothyroidism. Iodine deficiency and maternal thyroid disease can also cause hypothyroidism in neonates.

MATERNAL FACTORS. Transient CH can occur in preterm infants born in areas with endemic iodine deficiency or to families with a history of goiter.

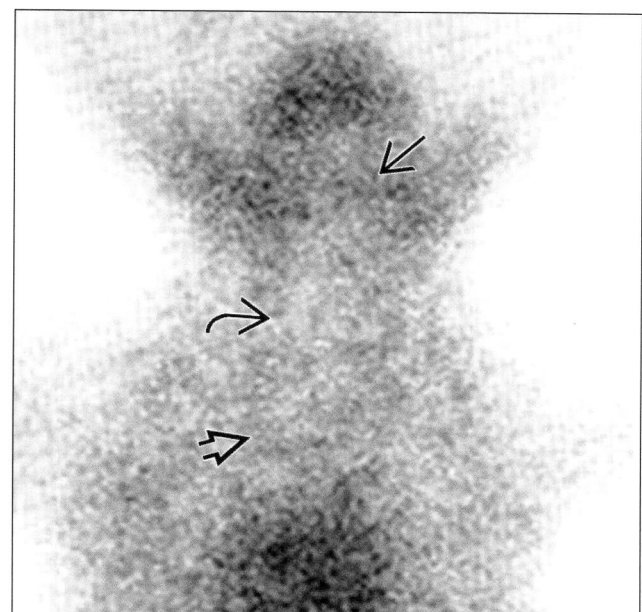

32-21. Anterior view of Tc-99m scan in an infant with congenital hypothyroidism shows no uptake in any of the possible locations for thyroid tissue, including the oropharynx/tongue base ➡, neck ➡, and mediastinum ➡. (Courtesy J. P. O'Malley, MD.)

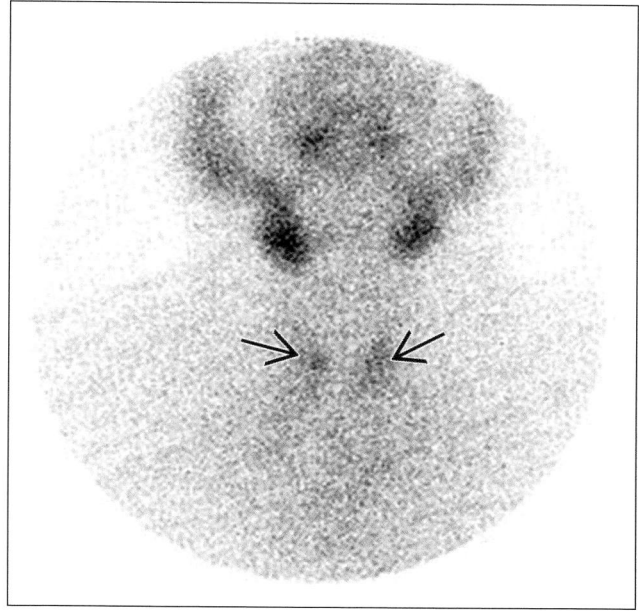

32-22. Scan in a 13 year old with worsening hypothyroidism, likely secondary to organification defect, shows a bilobed thyroid with very low uptake ➡. (Courtesy J. P. O'Malley, MD.)

In maternal autoimmune thyroiditis, IgG antibodies cross the placenta and may block fetal thyroid production. Medication or I-131 therapy for maternal hyperthyroidism or cancer can also act adversely on the fetus.

THYROID DYSGENESIS. Thyroid dysgenesis is the most common cause of CH, accounting for 70-75% of cases. Failure of normal thyroid gland development includes both abnormal gland formation and aberrant thyroid descent.

Ectopic thyroid tissue accounts for 25-50% of cases with thyroid dysgenesis. Ectopia can occur anywhere along the embryonic thyroglossal duct **(32-18)**, the path that the developing thyroid follows as it descends from the tongue base to the neck **(32-19)**. Hormone production in ectopic thyroids is low (despite the presence of functioning tissue) but not completely absent. In some cases, hormone production may be enough to delay clinical symptoms until adolescence.

Thyroid agenesis or **hypoplasia** accounts for 20-50% of CH cases and typically causes severe hypothyroidism with markedly depressed T4, elevated TSH, and undetectable levels of thyroglobulin.

DYSHORMONOGENESIS. Inborn errors of thyroid hormone biosynthesis (dyshormonogenesis) account for 5-15% of CH cases. Here defects occur in the biosynthesis, secretion, or utilization of thyroid hormone. These include enzymatic abnormalities, deficient iodide trapping due to sodium-iodide symporter defects, TSH resistance with abnormal TSH receptors on the follicular cell membranes, and peripheral thyroid hormone resistance with T3 receptor defects in peripheral cell nuclei.

CENTRAL (SECONDARY) HYPOTHYROIDISM. Pituitary or hypothalamic dysfunction causes 10-15% of CH cases. The gland is formed normally, but the hypothalamic-pituitary-thyroid axis is disrupted **(32-20)**. Most cases of secondary hypothyroidism are caused by decreased pituitary TSH and often occur in the setting of combined pituitary hormone deficiency. So-called tertiary hypothyroidism from low hypothalamic TSH is rare in children.

Imaging

Imaging studies of the face and neck demonstrate an ectopic thyroid in up to half of all CH cases. Nearly 90% occur at the tongue base, where they are seen as a well-delineated, round or ovoid, hyperdense midline mass on NECT and a T1 iso-/T2 hyperintense mass on MR. Avid uniform enhancement following contrast administration is typical.

Complete absence of the thyroid and thyroid hypoplasia account for most of the remaining cases. Nuclear medicine studies (Tc-99m pertechnetate or I-123 scans) are typically used to diagnose thyroid agenesis and demonstrate absent uptake (no activity in any of the expected sites) **(32-21)**. Inborn errors of thyroid hormone metabolism often appear as a small bilobed thyroid in the expected location **(32-22)**.

Brain MR imaging in children with CH may show mild generalized atrophy with reduced WM volume and poor differentiation of cortical layers, enlarged sylvian fissures, and T2 hypointensity in the globi pallidi and substantia nigra.

Differential Diagnosis

As the central tongue base is the most common location for an ectopic thyroid (32-23), the most important differential diagnoses are venous malformation or hemangioma, prominent/asymmetric lingual tonsil, and neoplasm (non-Hodgkin lymphoma). A lingual thyroid may expand dramatically during puberty. *In 75% of cases, a lingual thyroid is the only functioning thyroid tissue; it must not be mistaken for tumor and removed* (32-24), (32-25)!

Venous malformation exhibits prominent T2 hyperintensity. An upper airway **infantile hemangioma** is usually subglottic and asymmetric. A transglottic hemangioma involves multiple structures, not just the tongue base. **Prominent/asymmetric tonsillar tissue** has the same density/signal intensity as other lymphoid structures.

Acquired Hypothyroid Disorders

Acquired hypothyroidism is much more common than the congenital variety, affecting eight to nine million Americans and many more patients worldwide. Acquired hypothyroidism has two important imaging manifestations: Pituitary hyperplasia and Hashimoto thyroiditis/encephalopathy.

Pituitary Hyperplasia

Enlarged pituitary glands are common in young menstruating females and pregnant/lactating females. *Nonphysiologic* increase in pituitary volume—pathologic pituitary enlargement—is much less common and typically occurs in response to end-organ failure.

Hypothyroidism can result in secondary TSH cell hyperplasia, symmetrically enlarging the pituitary gland and mimicking a pituitary adenoma on imaging studies. Both physiologic and nonphysiologic pituitary hyperplasia are discussed in detail in Chapter 25. Most cases of hypothyroid-induced pituitary hyperplasia reverse with thyroid hormone replacement therapy. Caution: Any pre-

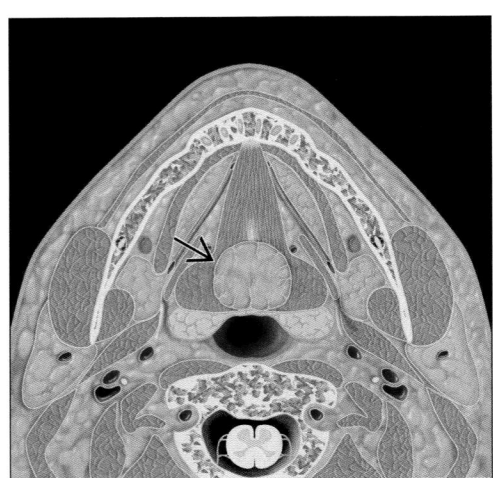

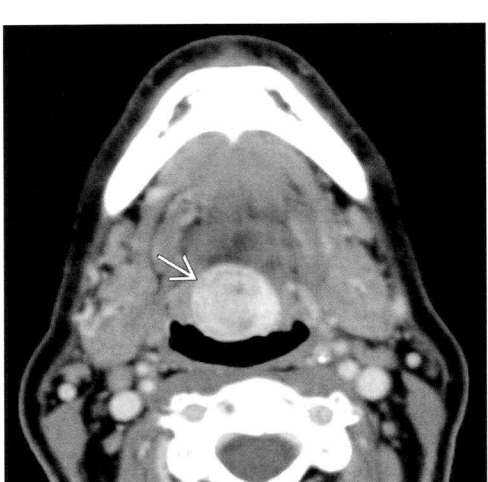

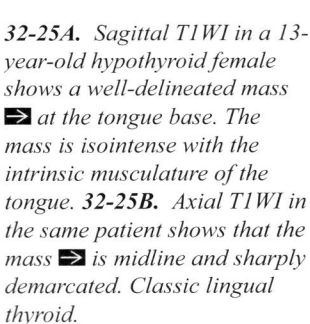

32-23. Axial graphic depicts lingual thyroid ➡ in the posterior midline of the tongue, deep to the foramen cecum. Sharply defined contour and midline location at the tongue base or floor of the mouth are typical of lingual thyroid. *32-24.* CECT scan shows classic lingual thyroid ➡, seen as a uniformly enhancing midline mass in the base of the tongue.

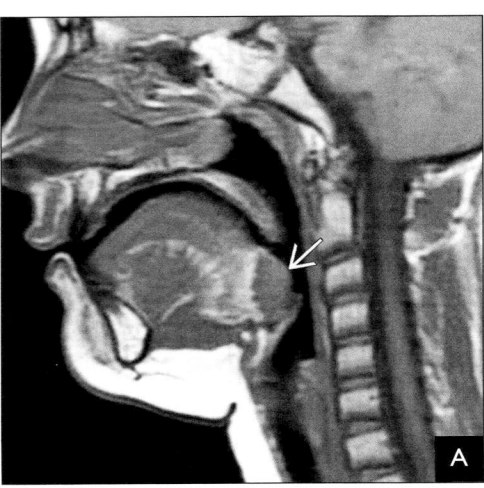

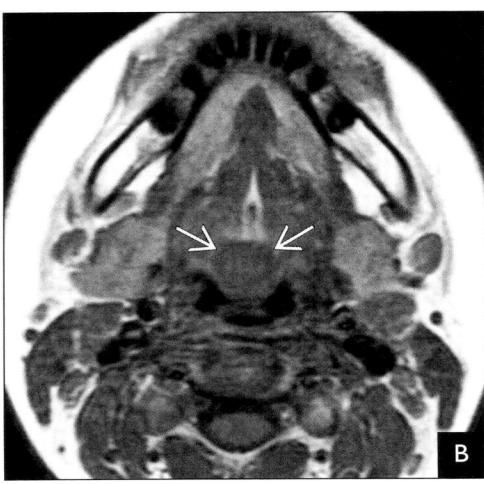

32-25A. Sagittal T1WI in a 13-year-old hypothyroid female shows a well-delineated mass ➡ at the tongue base. The mass is isointense with the intrinsic musculature of the tongue. *32-25B.* Axial T1WI in the same patient shows that the mass ➡ is midline and sharply demarcated. Classic lingual thyroid.

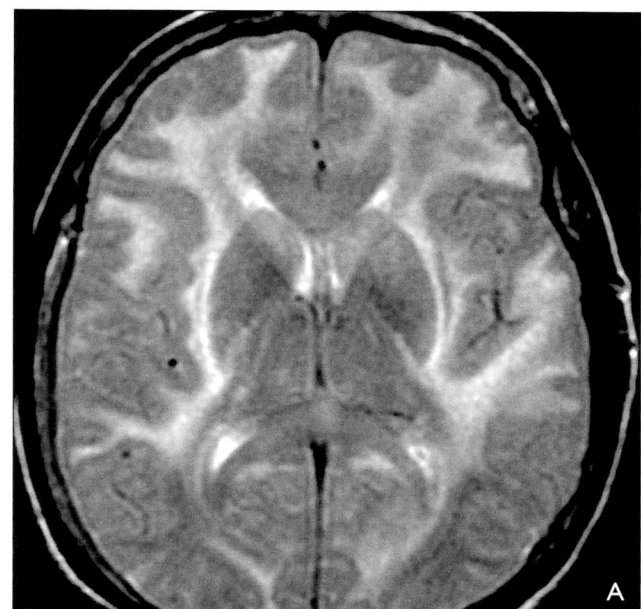

32-26A. Axial T2WI in a 58-year-old woman with acute Hashimoto encephalopathy shows confluent, symmetric hyperintensity in the subcortical, deep WM.

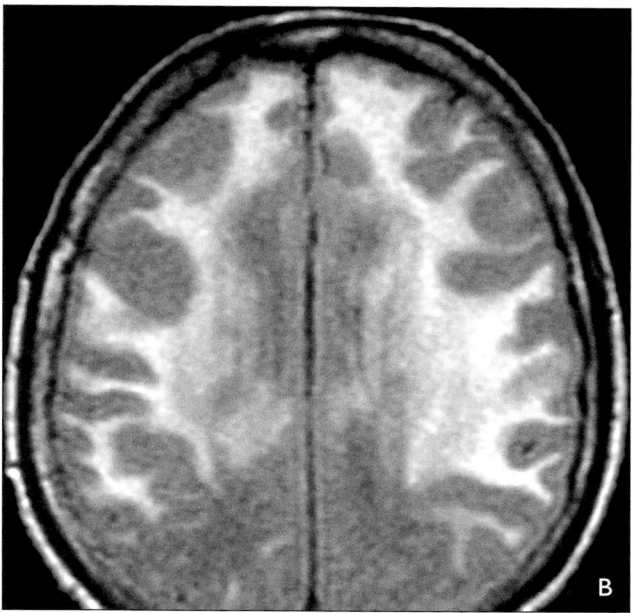

32-26B. FLAIR scan in the same patient shows involvement of the frontal subcortical WM with marked sparing of the occipital lobes.

pubescent male thought to harbor a "pituitary macroadenoma" on imaging studies should undergo comprehensive endocrine evaluation, as macroadenomas are exceptionally rare in this age group!

Hashimoto Encephalopathy

TERMINOLOGY AND ETIOLOGY. Hashimoto encephalopathy is a rare but treatable condition typically associated with Hashimoto thyroiditis (HT) and characterized by high levels of anti-thyroid antibodies. Hashimoto encephalitis is also called "steroid-responsive encephalopathy with autoimmune thyroiditis." It is a well-recognized neurologic complication of autoimmune thyroid disease and is the most common cause of acquired hypothyroidism.

Occasionally, Hashimoto encephalopathy occurs with severe "iatrogenic" hypothyroidism, typically with inadequate hormone replacement following thyroidectomy or radioactive I-131 treatment.

CLINICAL ISSUES. Hashimoto encephalopathy occurs in both children and adults. There is a moderate female predominance.

Most patients present with acute encephalopathy or severe neuropsychiatric disturbances (sometimes termed "myxedema madness"). Other common symptoms include seizures (66%), myoclonus (38%), and stroke (27%). Occasionally, patients present with more gradual cognitive decline and personality changes. These patients may be initially misdiagnosed as having "presenile" dementia.

IMAGING. Approximately half of all patients with Hashimoto encephalopathy demonstrate imaging abnormalities. The most typical MR findings are diffuse confluent or focal T2/FLAIR hyperintensities in the subcortical and deep periventricular white matter. The occipital lobes are relatively spared (32-26). Hashimoto encephalopathy typically does not enhance following contrast administration.

Hyperthyroidism

The most common manifestation of hyperthyroidism in the head and neck is thyroid ophthalmopathy (Graves disease). Brain involvement in hyperthyroidism occurs but is very rare.

Thyrotropin-secreting pituitary macroadenomas cause hyperthyroidism due to the syndrome of inappropriate TSH secretion. Hypocortisolemic states (e.g., Sheehan syndrome with peri- or postpartum pituitary necrosis) can also precipitate hyperimmunity and autoimmune hyperthyroidism.

There is an increased prevalence of psychiatric and behavioral disturbances in patients with hyperthyroidism, including apathetic hyperthyroidism and hyperthyroid dementia. Thyrotoxicosis can also cause disturbances of consciousness. Seizures, usually the generalized tonic-clonic type, occur in less than 1% of cases.

Brain imaging in hyperthyroidism is uncommon. A few cases of **acute idiopathic intracranial hyperten-**

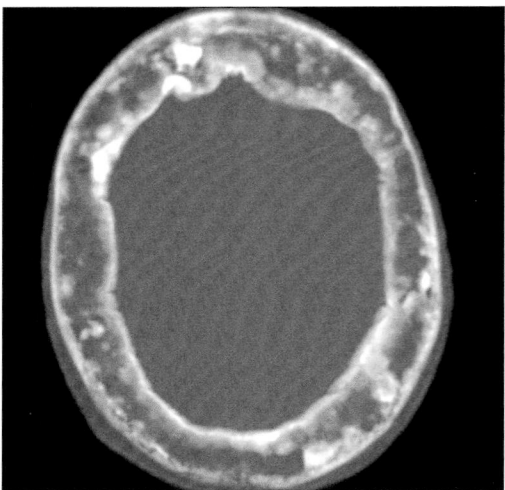

32-27. NECT scan of the skull in a patient with HPTH shows the characteristic alternating "salt and pepper" foci of resorption and sclerosis.

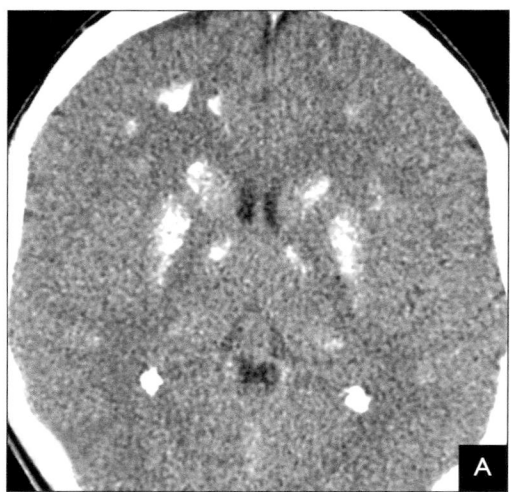

32-28A. NECT in HPTH shows bilateral symmetric Ca++ in caudate heads, putamina, globi pallidi, thalami. Some Ca++ is at the GM-WM junctions.

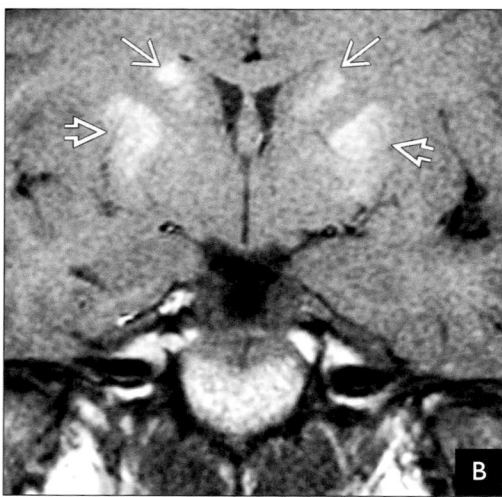

32-28B. Coronal T1WI in the same patient shows T1 shortening with symmetric hyperintensity in the caudate nuclei ➡, basal ganglia ➡.

sion ("pseudotumor cerebri") associated with hyperthyroidism have been reported.

Because of its effect on factor VIII activity, hyperthyroidism has also been reported as an independent risk factor for **dural venous sinus thrombosis**. Graves disease has been reported as a rare cause of **transient corpus callosum splenium hyperintensity** and an **MS-like multiphasic demyelinating autoimmune syndrome**.

THYROID DISORDERS

Congenital Hypothyroid Disorders
- Etiology
  - Thyroid dysgenesis, dyshormonogenesis, central hypothyroidism
- Imaging
  - Ectopic thyroid in 50% (90% at base of tongue)
  - Do not mistake for neoplasm!

Acquired Hypothyroid Disorders
- Pituitary hyperplasia
  - Prepubescent male with "fat" pituitary
- Hashimoto encephalopathy
  - WM edema (spares occipital lobes)

Hyperthyroidism
- Thyroid ophthalmopathy (Graves disease)
- Brain rarely imaged

Parathyroid Disorders

The parathyroid glands lie in the visceral space of the neck. They are normally the size and shape of kidney beans and are closely adherent to the posterior surfaces of the thyroid lobes. Ectopic parathyroid glands are found in 2% of cases, typically just below the inferior thyroid pole, although they can be found from the upper neck to the mediastinum. Most patients have four parathyroid glands, 10% have five or more, and 3% have three or fewer glands.

Metabolic abnormalities related to parathyroid hormone dysfunction include primary and secondary hyperparathyroidism as well as hypoparathyroidism, pseudohypoparathyroidism, and pseudo-pseudohypoparathyroidism.

Hyperparathyroidism

The parathyroid glands control calcium metabolism by producing parathyroid hormone (PTH). Hyperparathyroidism (HPTH) is the classic disease of bone resorption, so imaging abnormalities may be seen in both the skull and brain.

HPTH can be an acquired (common) or inherited disorder (rare). Both conditions are briefly discussed in this chapter. HPTH can also be primary, secondary, or even tertiary. Because of the increasing number of patients on dialysis, the most common type is now secondary HPTH.

Primary Hyperparathyroidism

ETIOLOGY. In primary hyperparathyroidism (1° HPTH), excessive levels of PTH result in unneeded bone resorption. The most common cause of 1° HPTH is parathyroid adenoma, responsible for 75-85% of cases. The second most common etiology is nonneoplastic parathyroid hyperplasia (10-20%). Parathyroid carcinoma is rare, accounting for just 1-5% of cases.

Sporadic 1° HPTH is much more common than hereditary HPTH. The most important inherited syndromes associated with 1° HPTH are multiple endocrine neoplasia (MEN) type 1, MEN type 2A, and familial isolated HPTH. Major features in patients with **MEN1** include parathyroid tumor (95%), pancreatic neuroendocrine tumor (40%), and pituitary neoplasm (30%). **MEN2A** is characterized by medullary thyroid carcinoma (99%), pheochromocytoma (50%), and parathyroid tumors (20-30%).

CLINICAL ISSUES. 1° HPTH is most common in middle-aged to older adults and relatively rare in children. There is a striking female predominance. 1° HPTH is characterized by hypercalcemia and hypophosphatemia (serum calcium is elevated; serum phosphorus is normal or decreased). HPTH is usually asymptomatic. General signs of symptomatic HPTH have been characterized as "stones, bones, abdominal groans, and psychic moans."

A recently described (and controversial) entity is called "normocalcemic primary hyperparathyroidism." Patients have elevated PTH levels but normal serum calcium and vitamin D levels.

IMAGING. Bone CT demonstrates diffuse patchy **"salt and pepper" lesions** in the skull. These are caused by foci of bone resorption interspersed with variable patchy sclerosis (32-27). Bilateral symmetric resorption of the lamina dura of the teeth may be present.

The most common findings in the brain are **basal ganglia calcifications** on NECT. Bilateral symmetric deposits in

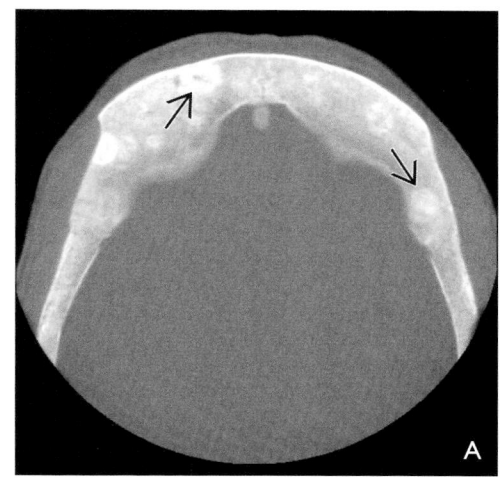

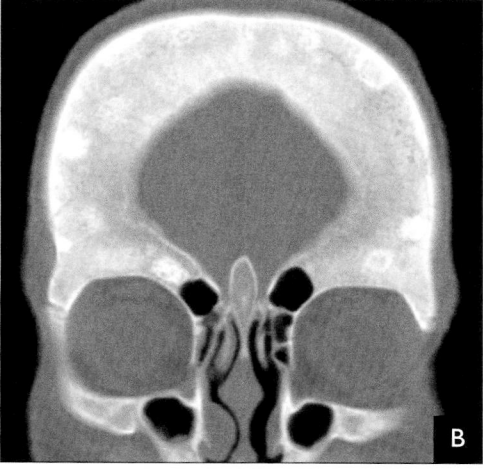

32-29A. Axial bone CT in a patient with secondary hyperparathyroidism shows uremic leontiasis ossea with marked calvarial thickening, focal sclerotic "brown tumors" ➡. 32-29B. Coronal bone CT in the same patient shows the striking calvarial thickening.

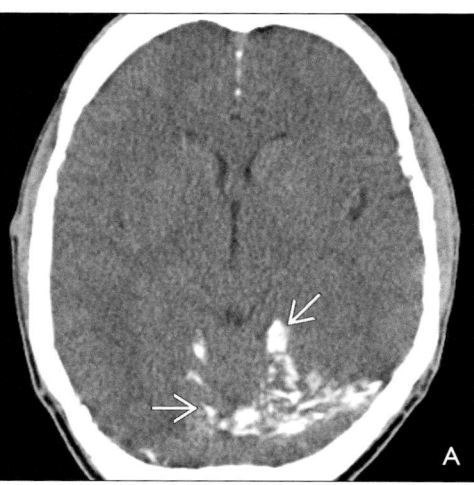

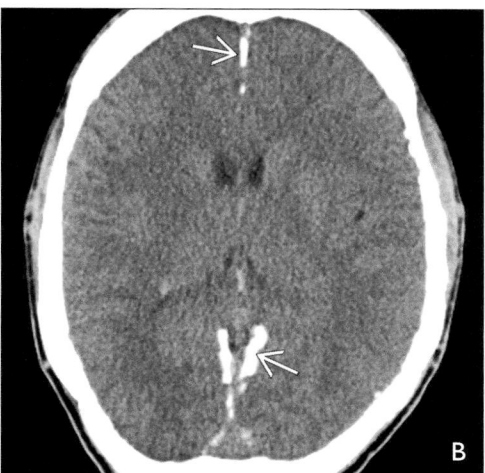

32-30A. NECT scan in a 31-year-old man with end-stage chronic renal disease and long-term dialysis shows markedly thickened, plaque-like deposits along the tentorium ➡. Note the absence of basal ganglia calcification. 32-30B. More cephalad NECT scan in the same patient shows additional foci of thick dural calcifications ➡.

32-31A. Sagittal T1WI in a 34 yo man with 25-y history of renal failure on dialysis, known secondary HPTH, and "big head disease." He developed decreasing vision and swollen optic discs. Note markedly thickened skull ➡ with multiple "brown tumors" ➡, thickened calcified pannus around the odontoid ➡. *32-31B.* Sagittal T1WI in the same patient shows thickening of the orbital wall ➡ and calvaria. Note prominent well-delineated "brown tumors" of varying signal intensity ➡.

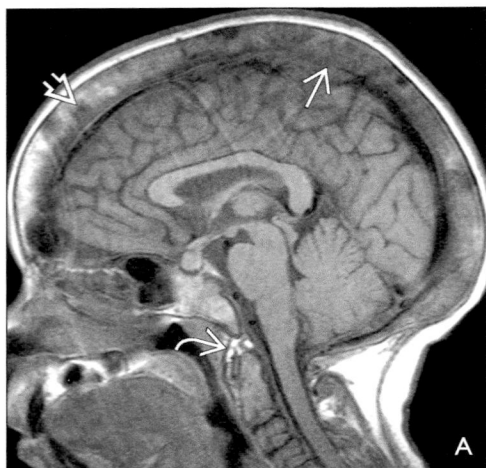

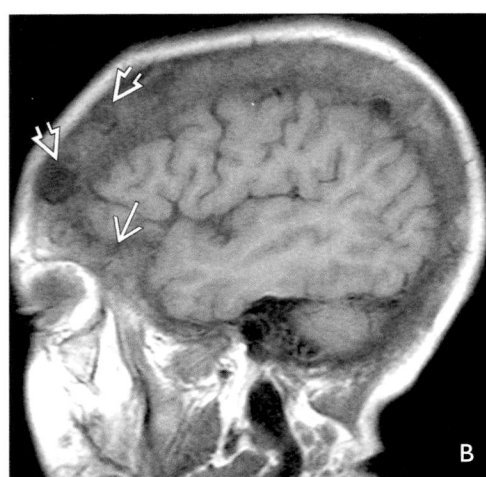

32-31C. Axial T1WI shows the markedly thickened calvaria, focal lesions. *32-31D.* T2WI shows thick calvaria ➡, multiple "brown tumors" of varying signal intensity ➡. Note that some of the more hyperintense lesions ➡ are virtually invisible on the T1WI to the left.

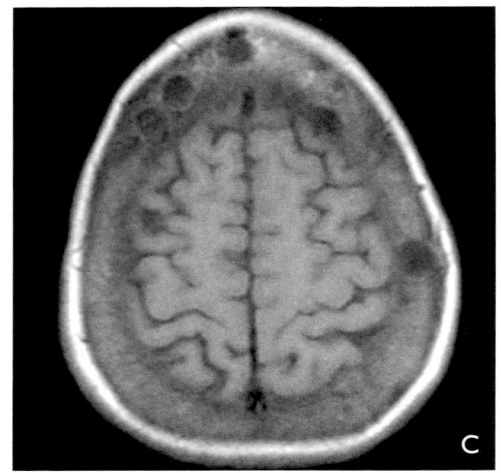

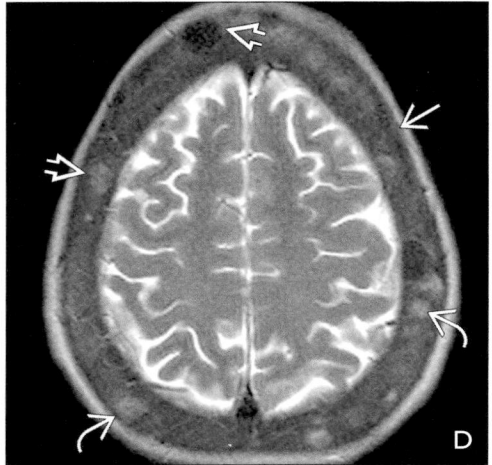

32-31E. FLAIR scan shows the thick skull, multifocal "brown tumors." The underlying brain appears normal. *32-31F.* Coronal T1 C+ FS shows that one of the "brown tumors" enhances ➡. Note thick dura ➡. The thickened bone causes significantly decreased volume of the orbits with compression of the optic nerve sheaths ➡ at the orbital apex. (Courtesy S. Chung, MD.)

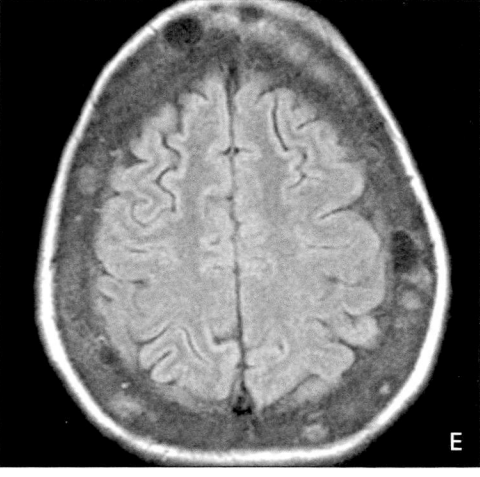

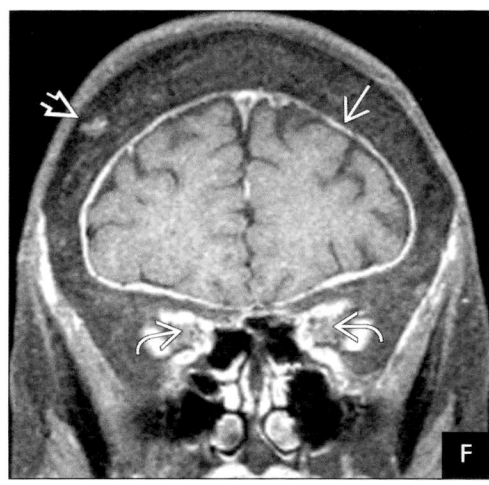

the globi pallidi, putamen, and caudate nuclei are typical. The thalami, subcortical WM, and dentate nuclei may also be affected **(32-28A)**.

MR shows symmetric T1 shortening and T2 hypointensity in the basal ganglia **(32-28B)**. Mild to moderate "blooming" on T2* (GRE, SWI) sequences is typical. **"Brown tumors"**—solitary or multiple nonneoplastic lesions in the skull—are common (see below).

Secondary Hyperparathyroidism

ETIOLOGY. Secondary hyperparathyroidism (2° HPTH) is characterized by PTH hypersecretion and parathyroid gland hyperplasia.

The most common cause of 2° HPTH is chronic renal disease (CRD). The majority of dialysis patients eventually develop 2° HPTH. Other etiologies of 2° HPTH include dietary calcium deficiency, vitamin D disorders, disrupted phosphate metabolism, and hypomagnesemia.

CLINICAL ISSUES. Most patients with 2° HPTH are older than 40 years at the time of initial diagnosis. There is no gender predilection. Serum calcium is normal or low, serum phosphorus is increased, and calcium-phosphate product is elevated. Vitamin D is low, almost always secondary to renal disease rather than dietary deficiency.

A common manifestation of CRD is renal osteodystrophy. Massive thickening of the calvaria and skull base narrows neural and vascular channels. Progressive cranial nerve involvement—most commonly compressive optic neuropathy—and carotid stenosis with ischemic symptoms are typical.

IMAGING. 2° HPTH primarily affects the skull and dura; the brain parenchyma itself is usually normal. NECT scans show markedly thickened skull and facial bones, a condition sometimes referred to as **"uremic leontiasis ossea"** or **"big head disease" (32-29)**.

"Brown tumors" can be seen in both 1° HPTH and 2° HPTH. "Brown tumors" represent a reactive—not neoplastic—process caused by osteoclastic bone resorption. Fibrous replacement, hemorrhage, and necrosis lead to formation of brownish-appearing cysts. Solitary or multiple "brown tumors" are seen on bone CT as focal expansile lytic lesions with nonsclerotic margins. Signal intensity on MR is highly variable, reflecting the age and amount of hemorrhage as well as the presence of fibrous tissue and cyst formation **(32-31)**.

The classic intracranial finding in 2° HPTH is unusually extensive, **plaque-like dural thickening (32-30)**. Longstanding CRD can also result in extensive **"pipestem" calcifications** in the internal and external carotid arteries.

Tertiary Hyperparathyroidism

Tertiary hyperparathyroidism (3° HPTH) results from longstanding 2° HPTH. Full-blown tertiary HPTH is rarely seen. The parathyroid gland becomes hyperplastic and does not respond appropriately to serum calcium levels (i.e., functions "autonomously"). Imaging findings are similar to those of 2° HPTH.

Hypoparathyroid Disorders

Three types of hypoparathyroidism are recognized: Hypoparathyroidism, pseudohypoparathyroidism, and pseudo-pseudohypoparathyroidism. All three disorders share common features on brain imaging although their clinical presentation and laboratory findings vary.

Hypoparathyroidism

Hypoparathyroidism (HP) is a childhood disorder, usually presenting around age five. It is probably an autoimmune-mediated disease with *decreased* parathyroid hormone (PTH) production. HP is characterized by hypocalcemia and hyperphosphatemia. Carpal-pedal spasm, tetany, seizures, and hyperreflexia are common presentations.

Intracranial calcifications are typical findings on NECT scans **(32-32)**. The basal ganglia are the most common site, followed by the cerebrum and cerebellum. Subcutaneous soft tissue calcifications are common in the extremities but rare in the head and neck.

The most striking extracranial findings are related to osteosclerosis. Spinal ligament calcification/ossification, osteophyte formation, and enthesopathy (especially around the pelvis) are typical.

HP in adulthood is rare and is almost always iatrogenic, occurring inadvertently after thyroidectomy. In contrast to childhood HP, adult HP has few imaging findings.

Pseudohypoparathyroidism

Pseudohypoparathyroidism (PHP) is caused by end-organ insensitivity and characterized by *elevated* PTH levels. Obesity, round face, and mental retardation are the key clinical features. Albright hereditary osteodystrophy (AHO) is a specific phenotype seen in autosomal dominant PHP and is characterized by short fourth and fifth metacarpals and short stature.

Pseudo-pseudohypoparathyroidism

Pseudo-pseudohypoparathyroidism (PPHP) is caused by incomplete expression of PHP (hence the term "pseudo-pseudo..."). Calcium and phosphate levels are normal.

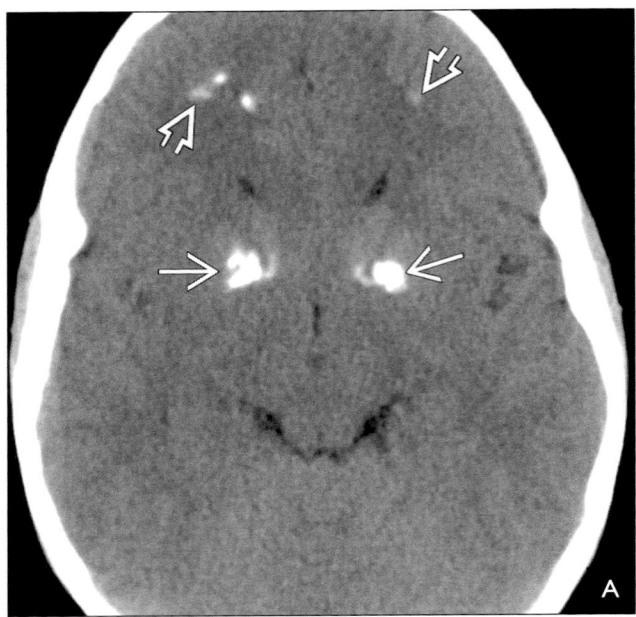

32-32A. Axial NECT scan in a 7-year-old patient with new onset of seizures and documented hypoparathyroidism shows symmetric calcifications in the globi pallidi ➡ with smaller calcific foci at the GM-WM interfaces ⇉.

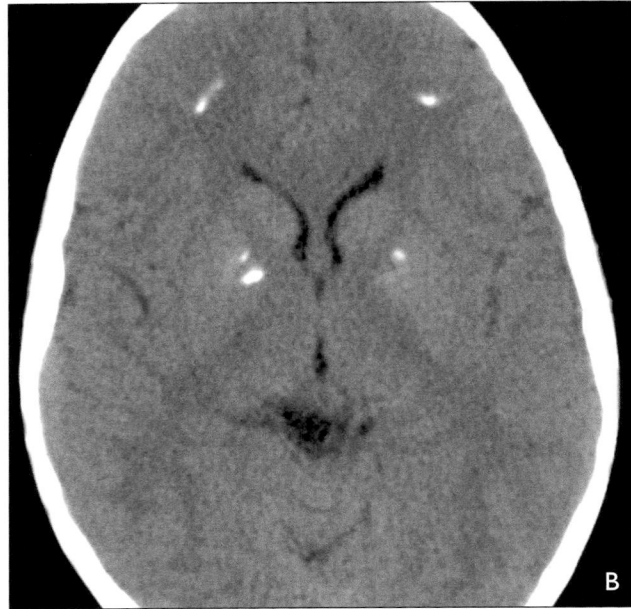

32-32B. Slightly more cephalad scan shows additional calcifications.

PARATHYROID DISORDERS

Hyperparathyroidism
- 1° hyperparathyroidism (parathyroid adenomas)
  - "Stones, bones, abdominal groans"
  - "Salt and pepper" skull (bone resorption, sclerosis)
  - "Brown tumors"
  - Basal ganglia Ca++
- 2° (chronic renal failure)
  - Renal osteodystrophy → thick skull, face ("big head" disease)
  - "Brown tumors"
  - Plaque-like dural thickening
  - "Pipestem" Ca++ in carotid arteries

Hypoparathyroid Disorders
- 3 types (distinguished by clinical, laboratory findings)
  - Hypoparathyroidism
  - Pseudohypoparathyroidism
  - Pseudo-pseudohypoparathyroidism
- All share same imaging features!
  - Ca++ in basal ganglia > cerebrum, cerebellum
  - Spinal ligament Ca++, osteophytes

Seizures and Related Disorders

Seizures can be precipitated by many infective, metabolic, toxic, developmental, neoplastic, or degenerative conditions and can affect numerous different areas of the brain. Because the temporal lobe is the most commonly affected site, we begin this section with a brief review of its normal gross and imaging anatomy. Special attention is given to the hippocampus as the site involved in mesial temporal sclerosis, an important imaging diagnosis.

We next consider the imaging manifestations of seizure activity. Two classic disorders represent the effects of chronic repeated seizures (mesial temporal sclerosis) and prolonged acute seizure activity (status epilepticus) on the brain.

We then discuss a newly described abnormality that can be seen with seizures (as well as a variety of other disorders), the "transient lesion of the corpus callosum splenium." The section concludes with a consideration of imaging findings in transient global amnesia, which specifically affects the hippocampus.

Normal Anatomy of the Temporal Lobe

Here, we briefly review general anatomy of the temporal lobe before focusing in greater detail on the hippocampus.

Gross Anatomy

TEMPORAL LOBE. The temporal lobe lies inferior to the sylvian fissure. Its lateral surface presents three gyri: The superior temporal gyrus (contains the primary auditory cortex), the middle temporal gyrus (connects with auditory, somatosensory, visual association pathways), and the inferior temporal gyrus (contains the higher visual association area).

The temporal lobe also contains major subdivisions of the limbic system (32-33). The parahippocampal gyrus lies on the medial surface of the temporal lobe and merges into the uncus (32-34).

HIPPOCAMPUS. The human hippocampus is a phylogenetically older part of the brain that plays a key role in memory. It can be affected by many common neurologic disorders, including acute ischemic stroke, transient global amnesia, epilepsy, and encephalitis.

The hippocampus is part of the limbic system, three nested C-shaped arches that surround the diencephalon and basal ganglia (32-33). The hippocampus proper is part of the middle arch, which extends from the temporal to the frontal lobes.

The hippocampus lies on the medial aspect of the temporal horn and bulges into its floor. The hippocampus has three anatomic segments: The head (pes hippocampus, the digitated anterior part), the body (cylindrical), and a posterior tail that narrows and curves around the corpus callosum splenium (32-33).

On coronal sections through the body, the hippocampus is composed of two interlocking U-shaped layers of gray matter: The Ammon horn and the dentate gyrus. The Ammon horn—the hippocampus proper—forms the more superolateral, upside-down "U" while the dentate gyrus forms the inferomedial "U" (32-35).

The Ammon horn is subdivided into four zones based on width, cell size, and cell density. These zones are designated as CA1, CA2, CA3, and CA4. CA1 (also known as the Sommer sector) is the lateral, outermost zone and consists of small pyramidal cells that are especially vulnerable to anoxia. CA2 curves superomedially from CA1 and consists of a narrow band of cells that are relatively resistant to anoxia. CA3 is a wide loose band that merges into CA4, the innermost zone. CA4 is enveloped by the dentate gyrus.

Imaging Anatomy

The superior, middle, and inferior temporal gyri are best seen on sagittal MR scans.

The hippocampus is best depicted on coronal MR scans performed perpendicular to the long axis of the hip-

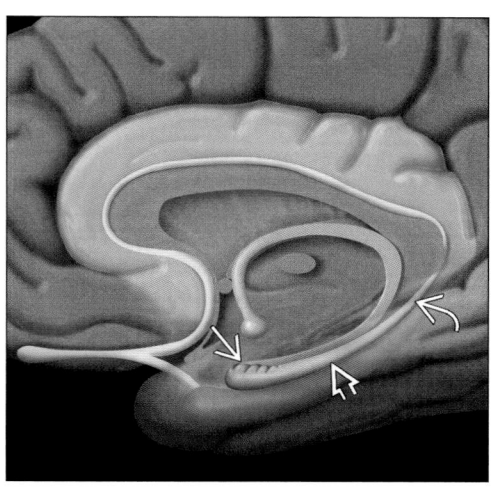

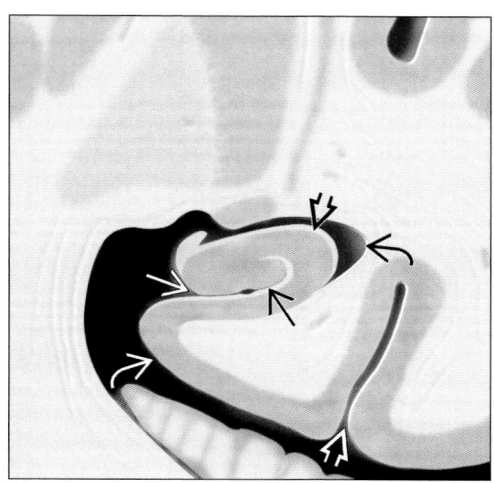

32-33. Sagittal graphic shows the 3 nested C-shaped arches of the limbic system. The hippocampus and indusium griseum are shown in yellow. The digitated anterior head ➡, body ➡, and tail ➡ of the hippocampus lie along the floor of the temporal horn of the lateral ventricle. 32-34. Coronal graphic shows dentate gyrus ➡, Ammon horn ➡, parahippocampal gyrus ➡, hippocampal sulcus ➡, collateral sulcus ➡, and temporal horn of lateral ventricle ➡.

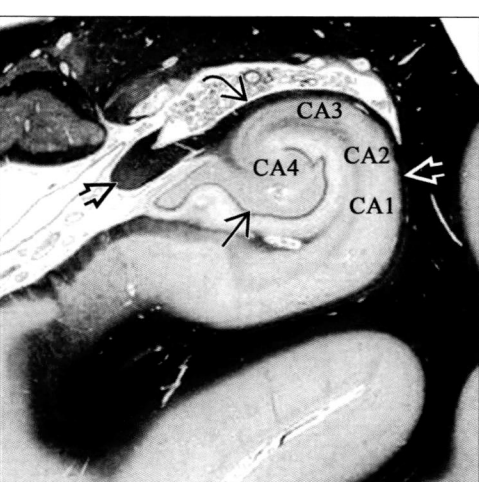

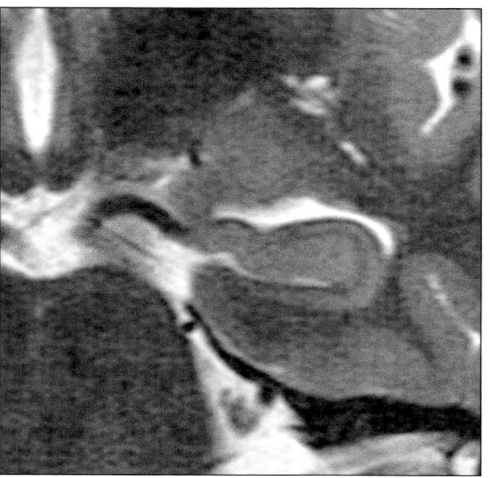

32-35. Coronal histology shows the CA1-4 zones of Ammon horn. The two U-shaped interlocking layers of gray matter formed by the dentate gyrus inside ➡ and Ammon horn outside ➡ comprise the hippocampus and are nicely seen. White matter (stained purple) of the alveus ➡ and fimbria ➡ is external to the GM of the Ammon horn. 32-36. High-resolution coronal T2WI shows normal hippocampus with distinct layers of white and gray matter.

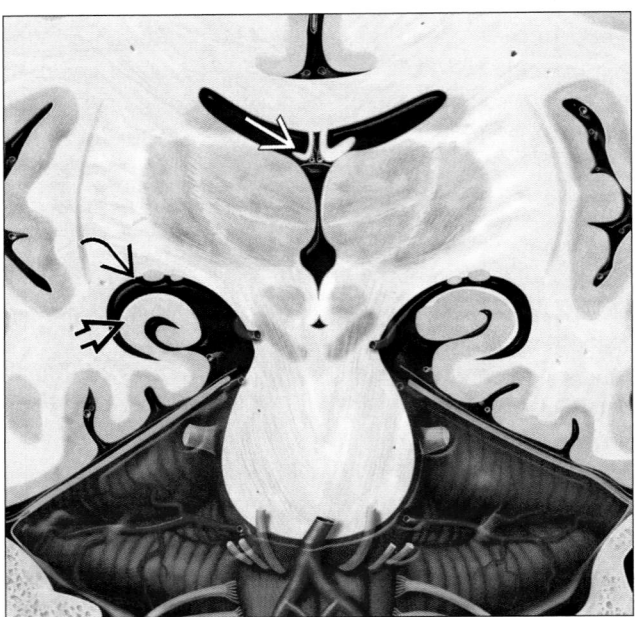

32-37. Coronal graphic depicts typical mesial temporal sclerosis. The right hippocampus ⊳ is atrophied and sclerotic with loss of normal internal architecture. The right temporal horn ⇗ is enlarged, and the ipsilateral fornix ⇒ is small.

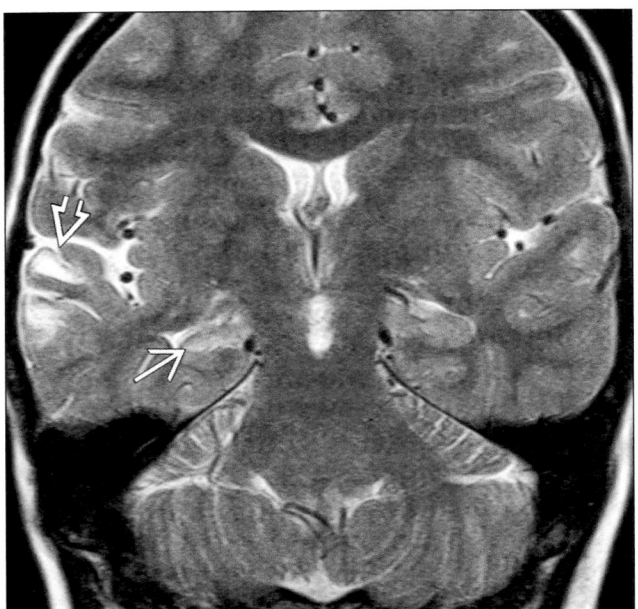

32-38. Coronal T2WI in a 27-year-old man with history of intractable epilepsy and remote closed head trauma shows temporal lobe encephalomalacia ⇒. The shrunken, hyperintense right hippocampus ⇒ is consistent with MTS.

pocampus. Thin-section true IR (or 3D T1 SPGR), high-resolution T2WI, and coronal whole brain FLAIR scans are recommended.

Coronal scans show the hippocampus as a sea-horse-shaped structure immediately below the choroid fissure and temporal horn of the lateral ventricle (32-36). The parahippocampal gyrus is separated from the dentate gyrus by the hippocampal sulcus. The collateral sulcus is an important landmark that lies just inferolateral to the parahippocampal gyrus.

Mesial Temporal Sclerosis

Temporal lobe epilepsy (TLE) is the most common form of partial complex epilepsy and can occur with or without mesial temporal sclerosis.

Terminology

Mesial temporal sclerosis (MTS) is the most common overall localization-related form of epilepsy. Its most common manifestation is complex partial seizures.

Etiology

A variety of events such as trauma or infection may precipitate intractable complex partial seizures (32-38). The end result is MTS. Although the precise pathophysiology of how and why MTS develops is unclear, inflammatory processes or prolonged seizures with hippocampal hypoxic-ischemic injury are considered the most likely candidates.

Pathology

MTS is characterized grossly by atrophy of the hippocampus and adjacent structures (32-37). The hippocampal body (85-90%) is the most commonly affected site, followed by the tail (60%) and head (50%). Approximately 15-20% of cases are bilateral but usually asymmetric.

The CA1 and CA4 areas are the most susceptible to hypoxic-ischemic damage, but all regions of the hippocampus can be affected. Neuronal loss with chronic astrogliosis is the typical histologic finding.

Clinical Issues

EPIDEMIOLOGY. Nearly 10% of all individuals experience a seizure in his/her lifetime. Two-thirds of these are nonrecurrent febrile/nonfebrile seizures. Peak prevalence is bimodal (< 1 year and > 55 years of age). One-third of patients develop repeated seizures ("epilepsy").

Approximately 20% of patients with epilepsy have complex partial seizures. Of these, 35-50% are refractory to anticonvulsant therapy.

MTS is one of the most common types of localization-related epilepsy and accounts for the majority of patients undergoing temporal lobectomy for seizure disorder.

DEMOGRAPHICS. MTS is a disease of older children and young adults. There is no gender predominance.

PRESENTATION. Most patients with MTS present with complex partial seizures lasting one to two minutes. Preceding "auras" with fear, anxiety, and associated autonomic symptoms are common.

TREATMENT OPTIONS. Anteromedial temporal lobectomy is the most common treatment for MTS with drug-resistant TLE and is successful in reducing or eliminating seizures in 70-90% of patients.

Imaging

MR FINDINGS. Imaging markers of MTS are found in 60-70% of patients with TLE. True coronal IR or 3D SPGR sequences show a shrunken hippocampus with atrophy of the ipsilateral fornix and widening of the adjacent temporal horn and/or choroid fissure (32-39). Abnormal T2/FLAIR hyperintensity with obscuration of the internal hippocampal architecture is typical. MTS typically does not enhance following contrast administration.

DWI shows increased diffusivity on ADC and hyperintensity on DWI (T2 "shine-through"). The spectroscopic hallmark of TLE is reduced NAA in the epileptogenic focus, presumably secondary to neuronal loss. Cho and Cr are typically unchanged. In MTS, NAA is reduced—and not just in the hippocampus. Widespread alterations in extrahippocampal and even extratemporal regions can be demonstrated.

NUCLEAR MEDICINE FINDINGS. FDG PET is one of the most sensitive imaging procedures for diagnosing MTS. Temporal lobe hypometabolism is the typical finding. SPECT shows hyperperfusion in the epileptogenic zone during seizure activity; hypoperfusion in the interictal period is common.

ANGIOGRAPHY. In the past, most patients with intractable TLE who were candidates for temporal lobe resection underwent a Wada test (intracarotid amobarbital test) to evaluate language lateralization and assess risk for postoperative memory disorders. With new noninvasive techniques such as resting fMRI mapping, the utilization of Wada testing is declining precipitously. It is no longer used in many epilepsy centers.

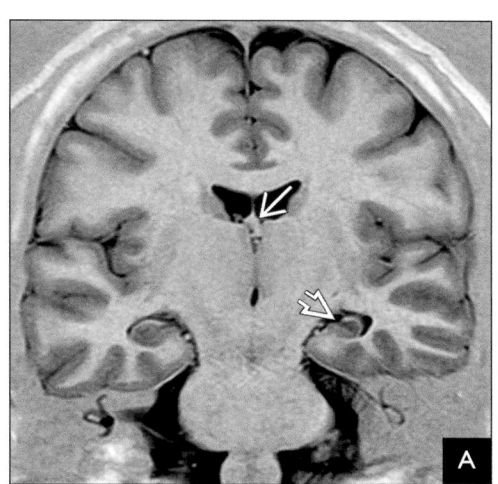

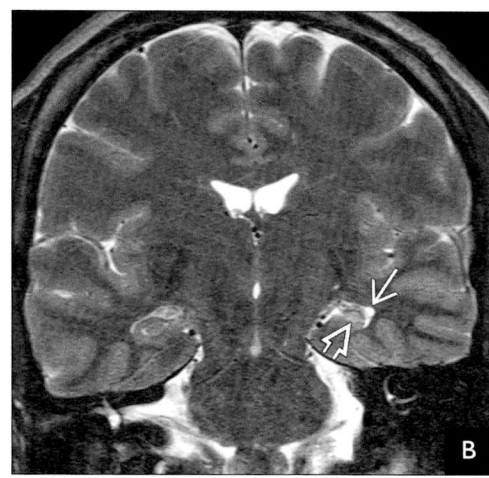

32-39A. Coronal true inversion recovery scan in a 37-year-old woman with temporal lobe epilepsy shows shrunken left hippocampus ⇥. The ipsilateral fornix ➤ is small. 32-39B. Coronal thin-section T2WI in the same patient shows that the shrunken left hippocampus is hyperintense ⇥. The temporal horn ➤ is mildly enlarged compared to the right side.

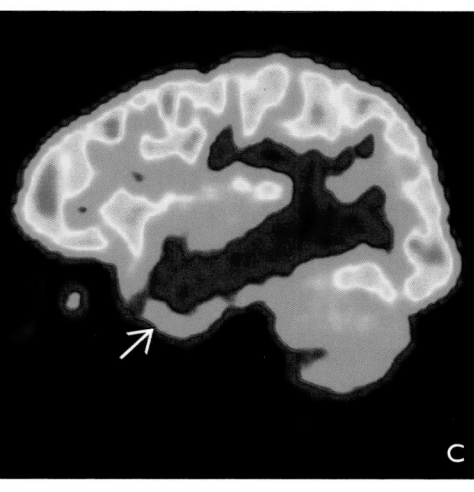

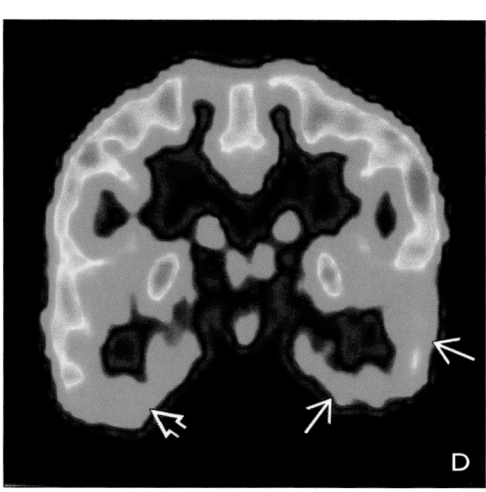

32-39C. Sagittal FDG PET shows marked hypometabolism in the affected temporal lobe ➤. 32-39D. Coronal FDG PET scan in the same patient shows that the entire left temporal lobe ➤ is markedly hypometabolic. Note reduced metabolism in the right temporal lobe ⇥, possibly reflecting chronic subclinical mirroring seizures.

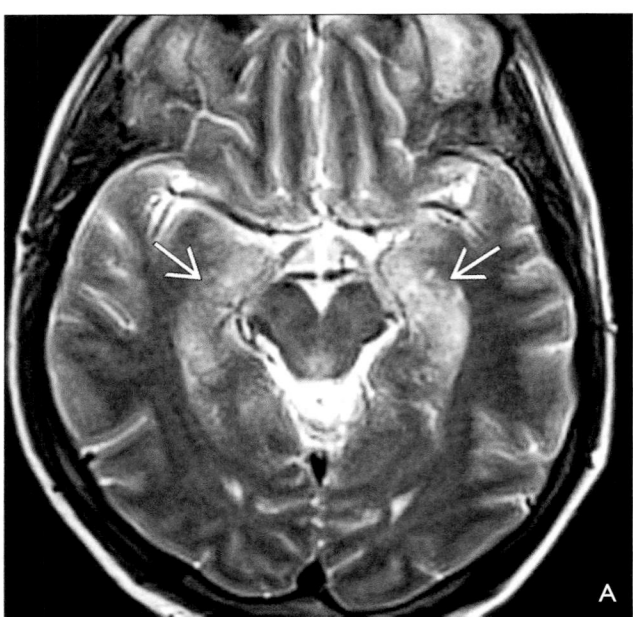

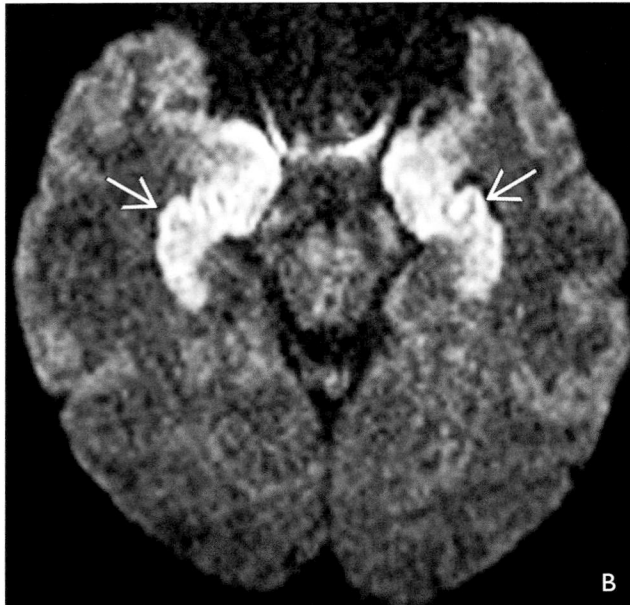

32-40A. *Axial T2WI in a 30-year-old man in status epilepticus shows that both hippocampi are swollen and hyperintense* ➡.

32-40B. *DWI in the same patient shows acute diffusion restriction in both hippocampi* ➡.

Differential Diagnosis

The major differential diagnosis of MTS is status epilepticus. **Status epilepticus** can be subclinical and may cause transient gyral edema with T2/FLAIR hyperintensity and/or enhancement in the affected cortex as well as the hippocampus.

A **low-grade glioma** (WHO grade II astrocytoma, oligodendroglioma, or oligoastrocytoma) in the temporal lobe can cause drug-resistant TLE. Gliomas are usually T2/FLAIR hyperintense and cause mass effect, not volume loss. Cortically based neoplasms associated with TLE include **dysembryoplastic neuroepithelial tumor (DNET)**. DNET typically is a well-demarcated, "bubbly" mass that is often associated with adjacent cortical dysplasia. **Cortical dysplasia** is isointense with GM but frequently causes T2 hyperintensity in the underlying temporal lobe WM.

Cystic-appearing lesions in the temporal lobe that are hyperintense on T2WI include **prominent perivascular spaces**, **hippocampal sulcus remnants**, and **choroid fissure cysts**. These "leave me alone" lesions all behave like CSF and suppress on FLAIR.

Status Epilepticus

Terminology

Status epilepticus (SE) is a prolonged (more than 30 minutes), continuously active seizure with EEG-demonstrated seizure activity. Two or more seizures without full recovery between the events is also considered status epilepticus. SE can be focal or generalized; generalized convulsive status epilepticus is potentially life-threatening if not controlled.

Etiology

Prolonged ictal activity induces hypermetabolism with increased glucose utilization. Perfusion increases but is still insufficient to match glucose demand. The result is compromised cellular energy production, cytotoxic cell swelling, and vasogenic edema. With prolonged severe seizure activity, the blood-brain barrier may become permeable, permitting leakage of fluid and macromolecules into the extracellular spaces.

Pathology

Transient vasogenic and/or cytotoxic edema causes cortical swelling that typically spares the underlying WM.

Clinical Issues

SE occurs at all ages, but the peak presentation is in young adults. There is no gender predilection.

Imaging

GENERAL FEATURES. Imaging findings in SE vary with acuity and severity. Most acute periictal abnormalities are reversible and normalize within a few days. Irreversible changes do occur, especially with generalized convulsive SE.

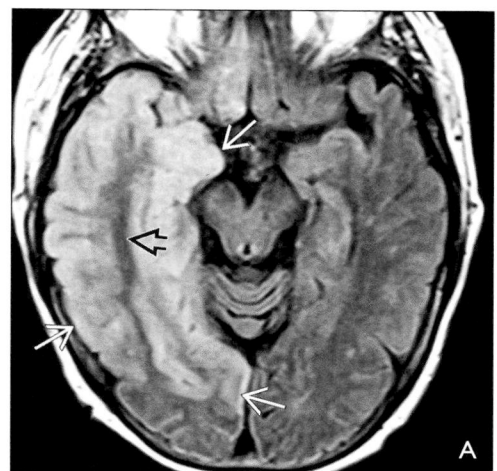

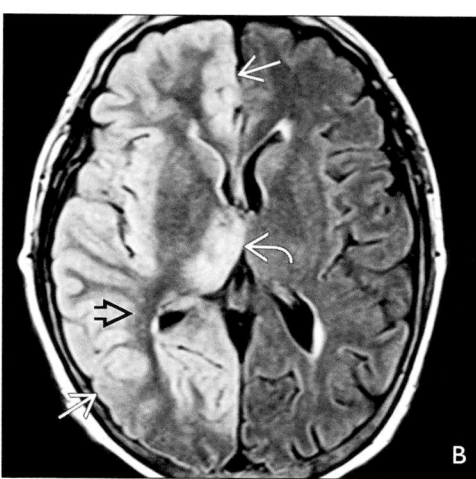

32-41A. *Axial FLAIR scan in a patient with status epilepticus for 3 days prior to imaging shows diffuse gyral edema and hyperintensity in a nonvascular distribution* ➡️. *Note relative sparing of the underlying white matter* ▷. **32-41B.** *FLAIR scan through the lateral ventricles shows that the ipsilateral thalamus is also involved* ➡️. *The cortical edema* ➡️ *spares the underlying WM* ▷. *The left hemisphere appears normal.*

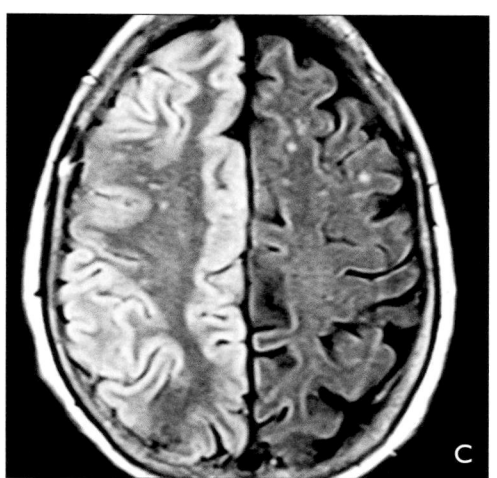

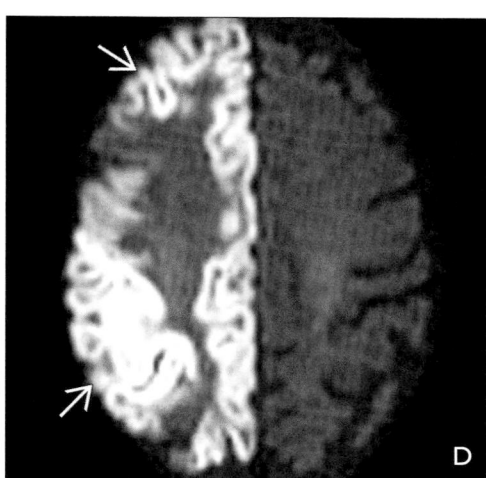

32-41C. *The gyriform hyperintensity with striking sparing of the coronal radiata is illustrated.* **32-41D.** *DWI in the same patient shows restricted diffusion in the affected cortex* ➡️. *The underlying WM and left hemisphere are spared.*

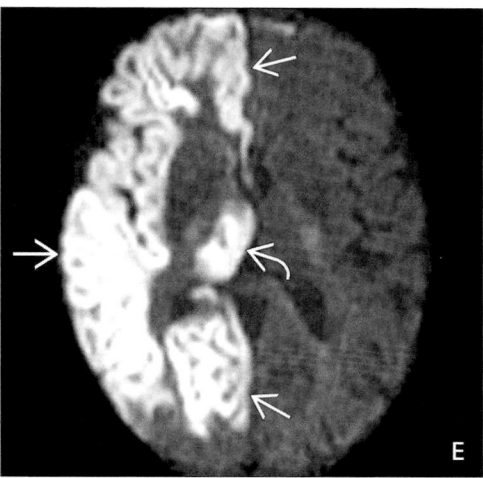

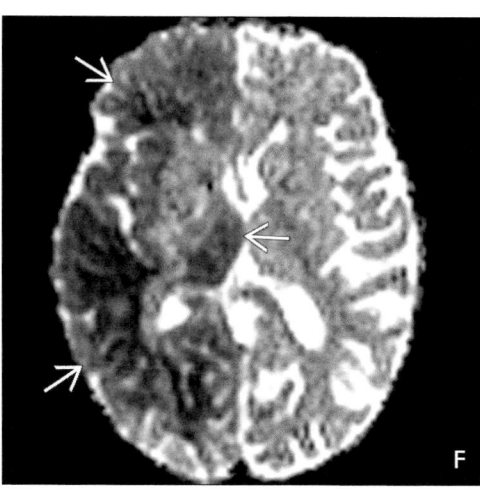

32-41E. *DWI through the lateral ventricles demonstrates gyriform diffusion restriction* ➡️ *that crosses all 3 vascular territories. Note involvement of the ipsilateral thalamus* ➡️. **32-41F.** *ADC map confirms restricted diffusion in the same areas, seen here as profound hypointensity* ➡️ *compared to the normal left hemisphere.*

CT Findings. Initial NECT scans may be normal or show gyral swelling with sulcal effacement and parenchymal hypodensity. CECT may demonstrate gyral enhancement in a nonvascular distribution.

MR Findings. Periictal MR shows T2/FLAIR hyperintensity with gyral swelling (32-40). The subcortical and deep WM is relatively spared. Crossed cerebellar diaschisis, ipsilateral thalamic involvement, and basal ganglia lesions are seen in some cases.

Gyriform enhancement on T1 C+ varies from none to striking. Diffusion restriction with uni- or bilateral hippocampal, thalamic, and cortical lesions is common (32-41). Ictal pMR and pCT studies demonstrate hyperperfusion.

Scans performed a week to several months following SE disclose structural abnormalities in approximately one-third of patients. Reported permanent abnormalities include focal brain atrophy, cortical laminar necrosis, mesial temporal sclerosis, and lower fraction anisotropy in normal-appearing WM.

Differential Diagnosis

The major differential diagnosis of periictal brain swelling is **acute cerebral ischemia-infarction**. Acute cerebral ischemia occurs in a typical vascular territorial distribution, is wedge-shaped (involving both GM, WM), and is positive on DWI *before* T2/FLAIR hyperintensity develops. In ongoing SE, DWI and T2 signal changes typically occur simultaneously.

Cerebritis may cause a T2/FLAIR hyperintense mass that restricts on DWI. Cerebritis typically involves the subcortical WM as well as the cortex. **Herpes encephalitis** is typically preceded by a viral prodrome, affects the limbic system, is frequently bilateral but asymmetric, often demonstrates petechial hemorrhage, and usually enhances.

Mitochondrial encephalopathy with lactic acidosis and stroke-like episodes (MELAS) in its initial presentation may affect the cortex in a nonvascular distribution. Symptoms are those of ischemia, not seizures. MRS in the noninvolved brain usually demonstrates a lactate peak.

32-42A. A woman in her 20s was taken off antiseizure medications 3 weeks before this scan. T2WI shows a well-delineated round hyperintense lesion ➡ in the middle of the corpus callosum splenium. *32-42B.* DWI in the same patient shows restricted diffusion ➡.

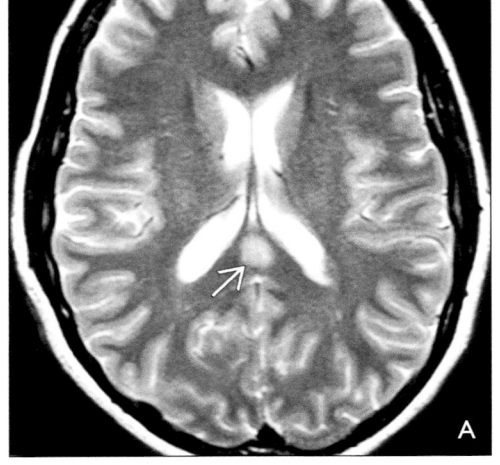
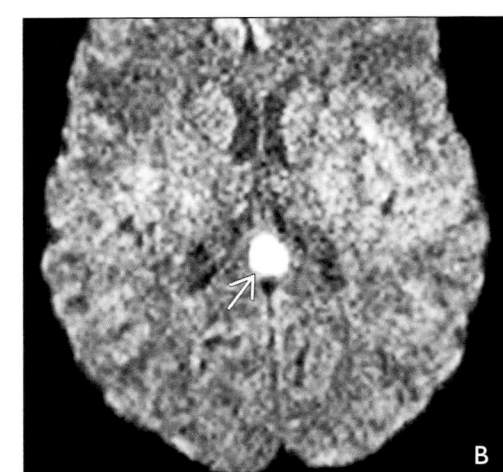

32-42C. Follow-up T2WI 3 months later shows that the lesion has resolved completely. *32-42D.* Follow-up DWI shows no abnormality. In this case, the patient was not experiencing seizures, so the transient corpus callosum splenium lesion was considered secondary to withdrawal of antiseizure medications.

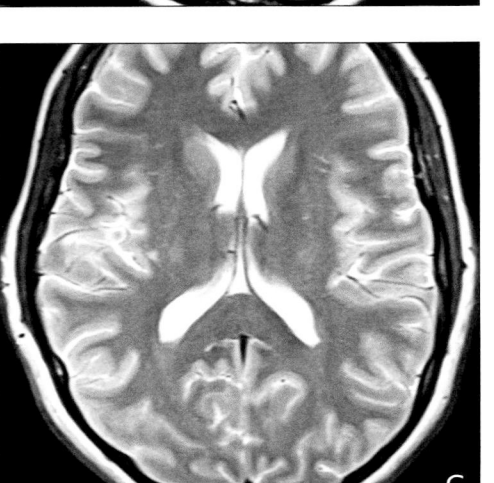
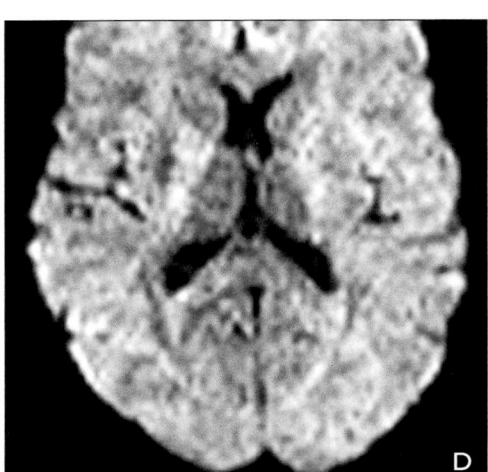

Transient global amnesia causes tiny dot-like foci of restricted diffusion in the lateral hippocampus.

Transient Lesion of the Corpus Callosum Splenium

Acquired transient splenial lesion (TSL) is an uncommon imaging finding that can be seen in a number of clinical conditions with varied etiologies.

Pathoetiology

Precisely how and why TSLs appear and then disappear is unknown. Some investigators have proposed brief, reversible failure of cellular fluid regulation. Others have suggested focal blood-brain barrier breakdown with intramyelinic edema in decussating fibers that originate in the temporal lobe. Because TSLs typically appear and disappear relatively quickly, reversible demyelination or transient osmotic myelinolysis seem less likely etiologies.

Associated Conditions

TSLs were first identified in patients with epilepsy and were initially considered a seizure- and/or therapy-related reversible abnormality. The use and withdrawal of antiepileptic drugs (AEDs) is the most commonly associated condition. At least 14 drugs have been implicated in the development of TSLs, which typically appear between 24 hours and 3 weeks after antiepileptic therapy is discontinued.

The second most common cause of TSL is infection, usually viral encephalitis. Influenza virus, rotavirus, measles, HHV-6, West Nile virus, Epstein-Barr virus, varicella-zoster virus, mumps, and adenoviruses have all been reported with TSLs. Bacterial meningoencephalitis is less commonly associated with TSL.

Metabolic derangements such as hypoglycemia and hypernatremia, acute alcohol poisoning, malnutrition, and vitamin B12 deficiency are the third most common group of TSL-associated disorders. Eclampsia and HUS have been reported as rare possible causes.

Miscellaneous reported associations include high-altitude cerebral edema, systemic lupus erythematosus, internal cerebral vein occlusion, and Charcot-Marie-Tooth disease.

A variant of TSL in which reversible pancallosal signal changes occurred in association with febrile encephalopathy has recently been described.

Imaging

On imaging studies, TSLs are round to ovoid, homogeneous, nonhemorrhagic lesions centered in the corpus callosum splenium. They are mildly hypointense on T1WI, display hyperintensity on T2/FLAIR, do not enhance, and demonstrate restricted diffusion (32-42A), (32-42B).

TSLs typically resolve completely within a few days or weeks, and follow-up imaging studies are normal (32-42C), (32-42D).

Transient Global Amnesia

Terminology

Transient global amnesia (TGA) is a unique neurologic disorder characterized by (1) sudden memory loss without other signs of cognitive or neurologic impairment and (2) complete clinical recovery within 24 hours.

As a clinical syndrome, TGA is easily recognized: The patient has isolated transient amnesia with normal consciousness and no other neurologic or cognitive disturbances.

Etiology

The underlying etiology of TGA is unknown. Paroxysmal neuronal discharges or epileptic phenomena (e.g., spreading cortical depression, seizure with delayed neuronal injury), migraine with aura, ischemic stroke or hypoxia, local nonischemic energy failures, and venous congestion have all been proposed as possible pathologic mechanisms.

Clinical Issues

Most TGA patients are between 50-70 years; TGA is rare under the age of 40. There is no gender predilection. A typical scenario is a middle-aged patient who suddenly starts forgetting conversations within minutes and tends to repeat the same questions. Anterograde amnesia with preserved alertness, attention, and personal identity are consistent features. EEGs are normal in 80-90% of cases with the remainder showing minor nonepileptiform activity. Symptoms resolve in 24 hours or less, and there are no long-term clinical sequelae.

Recurrences are relatively rare (5-10% per year). Psychometric evaluation shows no difference in cognitive performance between TGA patients and age-matched healthy subjects. There is no difference in outcome in patients with DWI-positive lesions compared to those with normal studies.

Imaging

CT scans are invariably normal, and standard MR sequences (T2/FLAIR) typically show no abnormalities.

Nearly 80% of patients with TGA develop focal hippocampal abnormalities on DWI (32-43). Thin sections

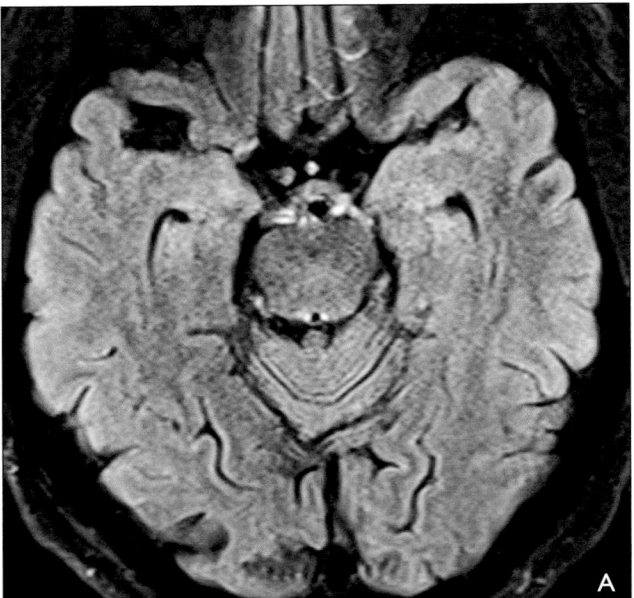

32-43A. Axial FLAIR scan in a 54-year-old man with transient global amnesia shows no abnormalities.

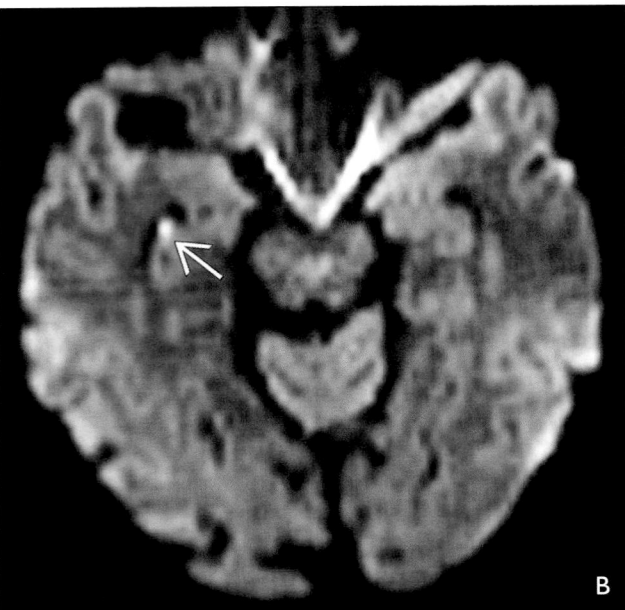

32-43B. DTI with b = 3,000 shows a single tiny focus of restricted diffusion in the right lateral hippocampus ➡, just medial to the temporal horn.

(three millimeters) obtained at high b-values (at least 2,000) and higher field strength magnets increase sensitivity.

The typical findings of TGA are one to two millimeters punctate or dot-like foci of restricted diffusion in the CA1 area of the hippocampus. These appear as hyperintensities along the lateral aspect of the hippocampus, just medial to the temporal horn. Lesions can be single (55%) or multiple (45%), unilateral (50-55%) or bilateral (45-50%). The body of the hippocampus is most commonly involved, followed by the head.

DWI abnormalities in TGA increase significantly with time following symptom onset. Between 0-6 hours, 34% show foci of restricted diffusion. This increases to 62% in patients imaged between 6-12 hours and to 67% of patients between 12-24 hours. By day three, 75% of patients demonstrate abnormalities. Follow-up scans typically show complete resolution by day 10.

A few reported cases have demonstrated both hypoperfusion and hypometabolism in the hippocampus on PET or SPECT.

Differential Diagnosis

The two major differential diagnoses of TGA are stroke and seizure. A strategic embolic stroke isolated to the mesial temporal area, thalamus, or fornix can produce isolated amnestic syndromes and mimic TGA clinically. TGA lesions are often multiple, but their exclusive location in the hippocampus mitigates against **embolic infarcts**.

Seizures can cause transient diffusion restriction but typically involve moderate to large areas of the cortex. The dot-like lesions in TGA are distinctly different from the cortical gyriform ribbons of restricted diffusion seen in **status epilepticus** and the posterior-predominant lesions seen in **hypoglycemic seizures**.

Thiamine deficiency with acute **Wernicke encephalopathy** can present as a fulminant disorder with relative preservation of consciousness. Lesions are found in the medial thalami, mammillary bodies, periaqueductal region, and tectal plate. The hippocampi are spared.

Miscellaneous Disorders

Fahr Disease

Fahr disease is an inherited disorder that results in striking basal ganglia calcifications. Once thought to be idiopathic, it is included in this chapter (rather than Chapter 31 on inherited metabolic disorders) as its imaging findings can closely resemble those seen in acquired metabolic diseases.

Terminology

Fahr disease is also known as familial idiopathic basal ganglia calcification, cerebrovascular ferrocalcinosis, and bilateral striopallidodentate calcinosis. Fahr disease

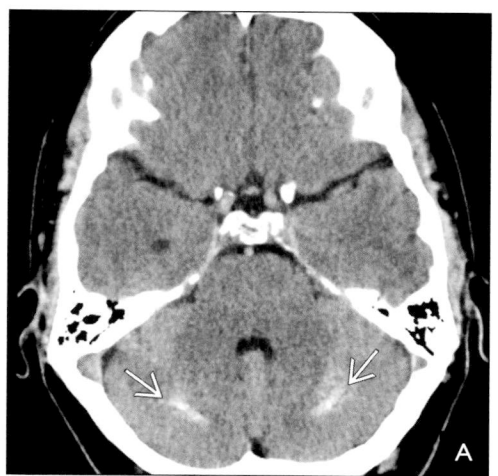

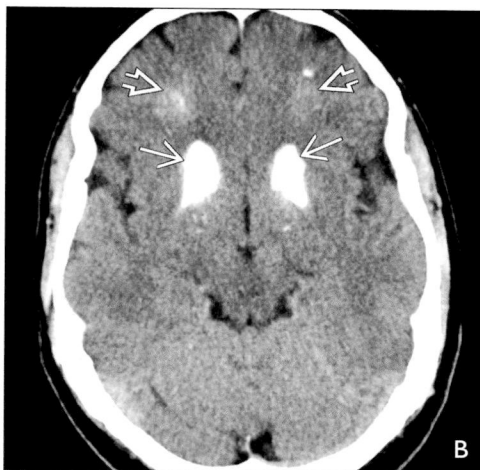

32-44A. Series of axial NECT scans in a 51-year-old man with Fahr disease shows bilaterally symmetric calcifications in the cerebellar white matter ➡. 32-44B. NECT scan shows very dense calcifications in both caudate nuclei and globi pallidi ➡, as well as more faint calcification in the frontal white matter ➡.

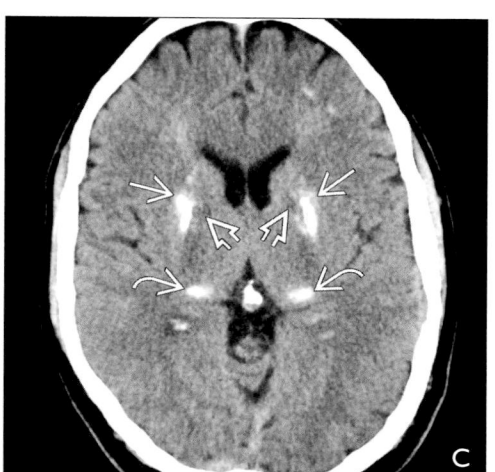

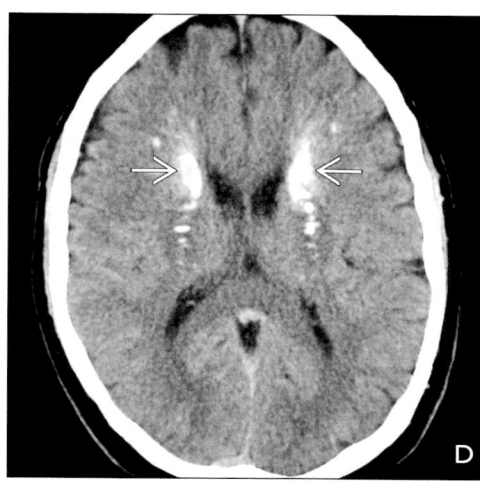

32-44C. More cephalad NECT scan in the same patient shows calcification in the putamina and lateral globi pallidi ➡, with relative sparing of the most medial GP ➡. Calcification is present in the pulvinars of both thalami ➡. Punctate calcification is seen in the cerebral WM. 32-44D. More extensive calcification is present in the caudate heads ➡ and bodies.

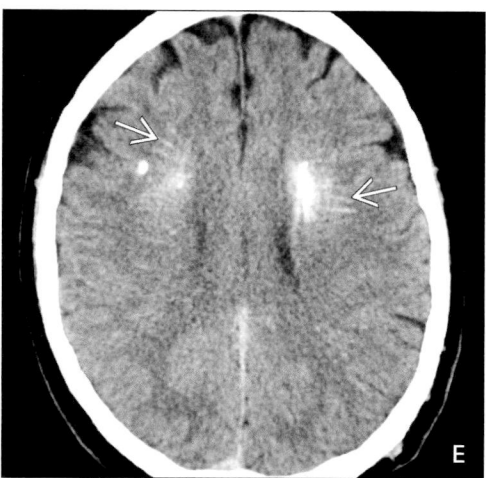

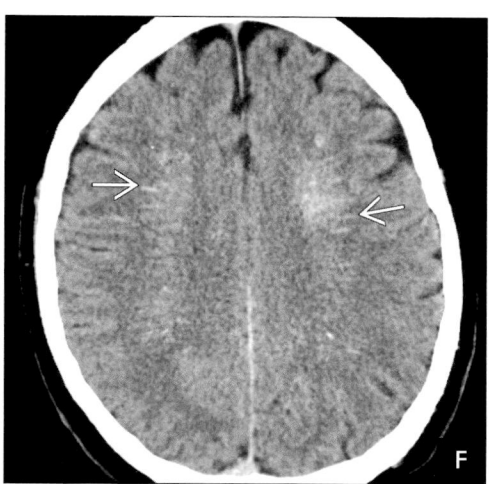

32-44E. NECT scan shows linear calcification extending perpendicularly from the caudate nuclei into the cerebral white matter ➡. 32-44F. NECT scan through the corona radiata shows innumerable faint linear calcifications extending throughout the deep cerebral WM ➡.

is characterized by basal ganglia and extraganglionic cal-cifications, parkinsonism, and neuropsychiatric symp-toms.

Etiology

The precise pathoetiology of Fahr disease is unknown. Fahr disease is a rare autosomal dominant disorder that has been linked to several different chromosomes.

Pathology

Autopsies of the few described cases of Fahr disease dis-close severe brain calcification in the basal ganglia, thal-ami, cerebellar WM, cerebral WM, and dentate nuclei. Severe cases show rows of small calcospherites along capillaries. In some cases, diffuse neurofibrillary tan-gles with Fahr-type calcification have been identified in patients with early-onset Alzheimer dementia.

Clinical Issues

Fahr disease is typically asymptomatic in the first and second decades. There is no gender predilection. Cal-

cium-phosphorus metabolism and parathyroid hormone levels are normal.

Deposition of calcium, along with other minerals, typi-cally begins in the third decade, but symptoms develop one or two decades later, usually between ages 30-60 years. Clinical findings follow a bimodal distribution: Schizophrenic-like psychosis typically presents in early adulthood with extrapyramidal symptoms, and subcorti-cal dementia predominates in patients over the age of 50.

Imaging

CT FINDINGS. NECT scan is the most sensitive imag-ing study. Extensive bilateral, relatively symmetric basal ganglia calcification is the most common finding. The lateral globus pallidus (GP) is the most severely affected with relative sparing of the medial GP. The putamen, caudate, thalami, dentate nuclei of the cerebellum, and both the cerebral and cerebellar WM (including the inter-nal capsule) are commonly affected (32-44A), (32-44B), (32-44C), (32-44D), (32-44E), (32-44F). Fahr disease does not enhance on CECT.

32-44G. Axial T1WI in the same patient as shown on the previous page shows relatively symmetric hyperintensity in the caudate heads ➡, lateral globi pallidi ⇘, and pulvinars of both thalami ➡. 32-44H. T2WI in the same patient shows no visible abnormalities.

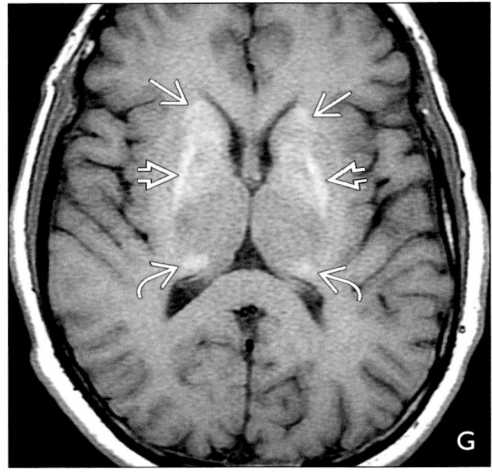

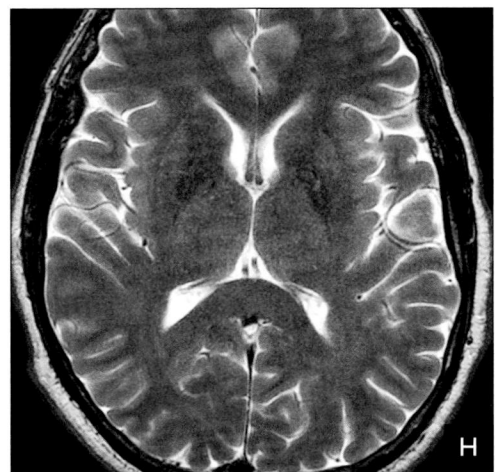

32-44I. T2* GRE scan shows striking "blooming" in the same areas (caudate heads ➡, globi pallidi ⇘, and thalamic pulvinars ➡) as the calcifications on NECT scans and corresponding hyperintensities on the T1WI above. 32-44J. T2* GRE scan shows linear "blooming" foci extending perpendicularly from the caudate nuclei into the deep periventricular white matter ➡.

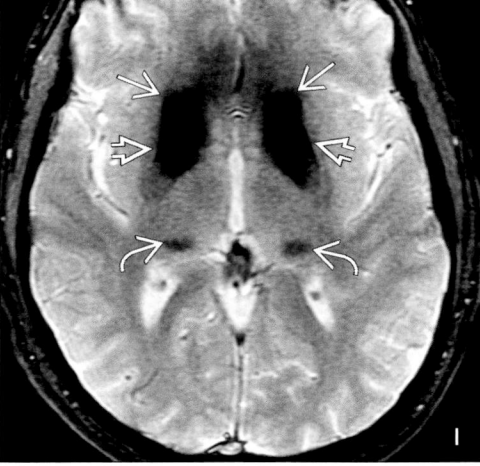

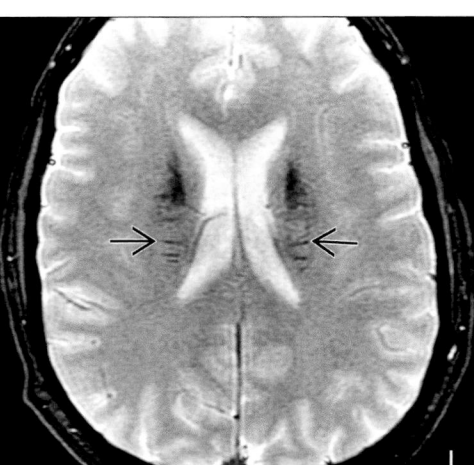

MR Findings. MR images in Fahr disease can be confusing. Signal intensity varies according to disease stage and the amount of calcification and heavy metal deposition. Calcification is typically hyperintense on T1WI but can be quite variable on T2WI **(32-44G)**, **(32-44H)**, **(32-45)**. T2/FLAIR scans may appear normal or mildly abnormal. They may also show extensive foci of T2 prolongation in the basal ganglia and cerebral WM that can be so striking as to mimic toxic/metabolic demyelination.

T2* (GRE, SWI) scans show profound susceptibility changes with "blooming" hypointensity secondary to iron deposition **(32-44I)**, **(32-44J)**. Fahr disease does not enhance on T1 C+ sequences.

Ultrasound. Transcranial sonography performed through the temporal bone acoustic windows demonstrates increased echogenicity in the basal ganglia, thalami, and substantia nigra.

Nuclear Medicine. SPECT scans have demonstrated increased uptake in the temporal lobes with decreased basal ganglia uptake. This may reflect hyperactivation with disruption of the cortical-subcortical neural circuits responsible for the psychotic episodes often associated with Fahr disease.

Differential Diagnosis

Basal ganglia calcification is nonspecific and can be physiologic or the end result of a variety of toxic, metabolic, inflammatory, and infectious insults. Specific sublocation of the calcification can be very helpful in determining its underlying etiology.

The major differential diagnosis of Fahr disease is normal **physiologic calcification of the basal ganglia**. Age-related ("senescent") calcification in the basal ganglia is common, typically localized in the *medial* GP, relatively minor, and of no clinical significance. Fahr disease has much heavier, far more extensive calcification. Fahr disease also demonstrates calcification in other locations such as the thalami, dentate nuclei, and cerebral and cerebellar WM.

Parathyroid disorders (i.e., hyperparathyroidism, hypoparathyroidism, pseudohypoparathyroidism, and pseudo-pseudohypoparathyroidism) can all have calcifi-

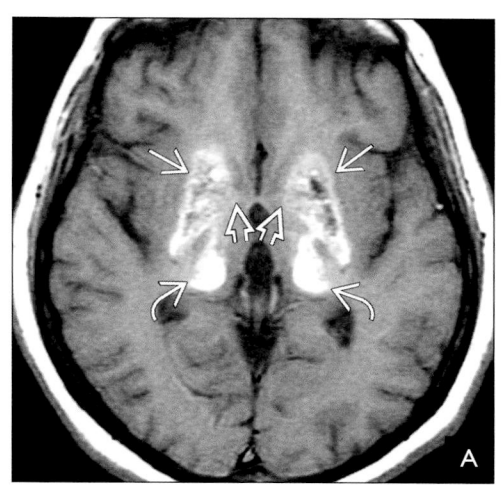

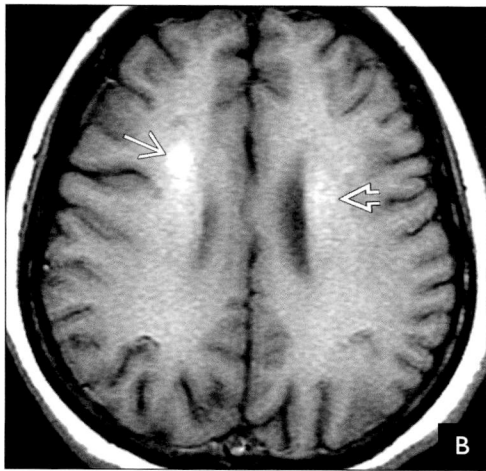

32-45A. Axial T1WI in a patient with Fahr disease shows extensive T1 shortening in the basal ganglia ➡ and thalami ➡ with relatively less involvement of the medial globi pallidi ➡. 32-45B. More cephalad T1WI in the same patient shows globular ➡ as well as more punctate and linear ➡ T1 shortening in the deep periventricular cerebral WM.

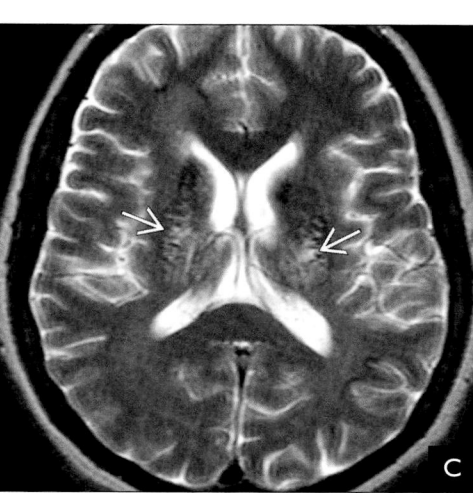

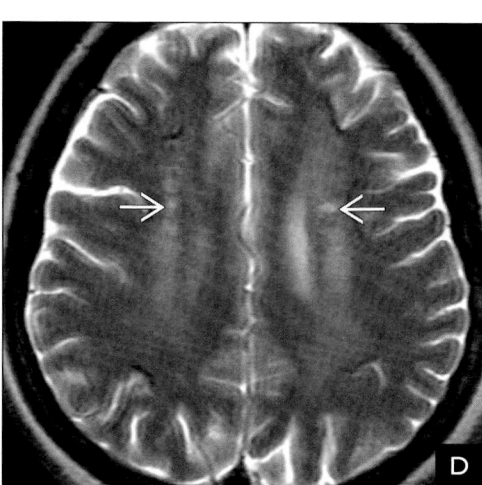

32-45C. T2WI in the same patient shows irregular punctate and linear hyperintense foci in both thalami ➡. 32-45D. More cephalad scan shows ovoid hyperintensities in the deep cerebral WM ➡ oriented perpendicularly toward the lateral ventricles. These findings of Fahr disease should not be mistaken for infarcts or multiple sclerosis plaques. (Courtesy M. Ayadi, MD.)

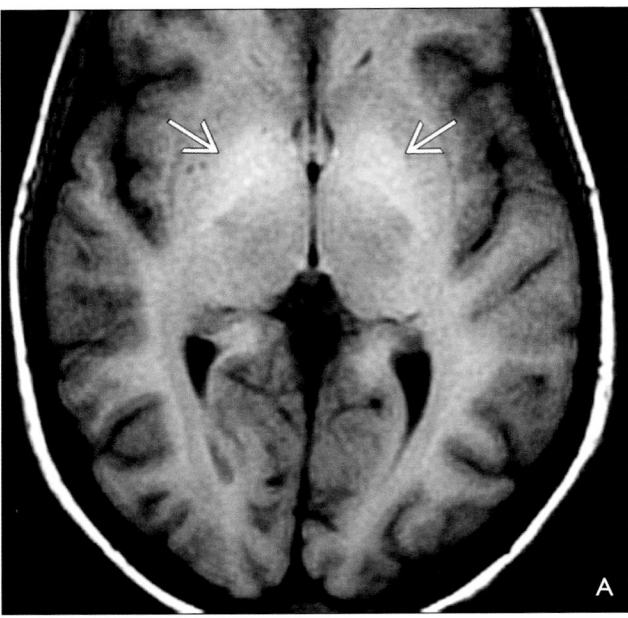

32-46A. Axial T1WI in a 31 year old with chronic liver failure shows symmetric T1 shortening in the globi pallidi ➡.

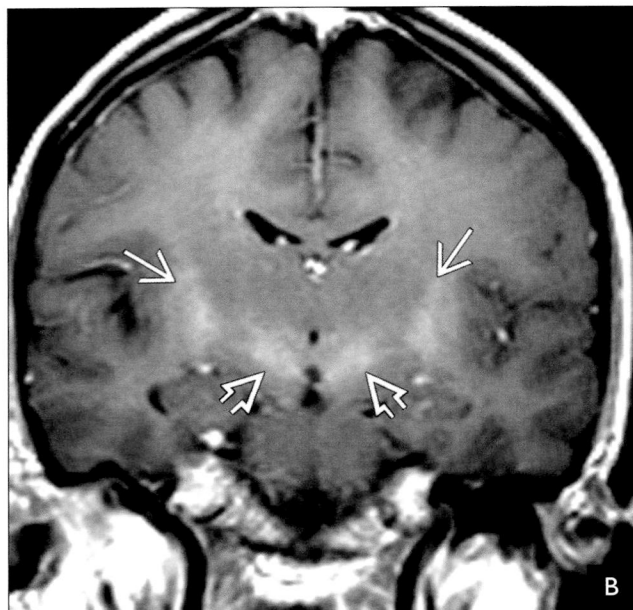

32-46B. Coronal T1 C+ scan shows the symmetric basal ganglia hyperintensity ➡ as well as hyperintensity in both cerebral peduncles and substantia nigra ➡. Findings are classic for chronic hepatic encephalopathy.

cation in a distribution similar to that of Fahr disease. Hypoparathyroidism and pseudohypoparathyroidism can be confirmed with serum calcium, phosphorus, and parathyroid hormone levels. All three are normal in both Fahr disease and asymptomatic pseudo-pseudohypoparathyroidism, which can appear identical on imaging studies.

BILATERAL SYMMETRIC BASAL GANGLIA CALCIFICATIONS

Common
- Normal (age-related; usually medial globi pallidi)
- Neurocysticercosis

Less Common
- Toxic
  ◦ Hypoxia
  ◦ CO poisoning
  ◦ XRT
  ◦ Chemotherapy
- Endocrinologic disorders
  ◦ Hypoparathyroidism spectrum
  ◦ Hypothyroidism
- Congenital infection
  ◦ CMV
  ◦ HIV
- Mitochondrial disorders

Rare but Important
- Fahr disease
- Pantothenate kinase-associated neurodegeneration (PKAN)
- Hyperparathyroidism

Hepatic Encephalopathy

Hepatic encephalopathy (HE) is an important cause of morbidity and mortality in patients with severe liver disease. HE is classified into three main groups: Minimal HE (also known as latent or subclinical HE), chronic HE, and acute HE.

Although the precise mechanisms responsible for HE remain elusive, elevated blood and brain ammonia levels have been strongly implicated in the pathogenesis of hepatic encephalopathy.

Ammonia is metabolized primarily in the liver via the urea cycle. When the metabolic capacity of the liver is severely diminished, ammonia detoxification is compromised. Nitrogenous wastes accumulate and easily cross the blood-brain barrier. Ammonia and its principal metabolite, glutamine, interfere with brain mitochondrial metabolism and energy production. Increased osmolarity in the astrocytes causes swelling, loss of autoregulation, and results in cerebral edema.

We first discuss chronic HE, then focus on the acute manifestations of liver failure and its most fulminant manifestation, hyperammonemic encephalopathy.

Chronic Hepatic Encephalopathy

Chronic hepatic encephalopathy (CHE) is a potentially reversible clinical syndrome that occurs in the setting of chronic severe liver dysfunction. Both children and adults are affected. Most patients have a longstanding history of cirrhosis, often accompanied by portal hypertension and portosystemic shunting.

NECT scans typically are normal or show mild volume loss. In the vast majority of cases, MR scans show bilateral symmetric hyperintensity in the globi pallidi and substantia nigra on T1WI, probably secondary to manganese deposition (32-46). T1 hyperintensity has also been reported in the pituitary gland and hypothalamus but is less common. The T1 hyperintensity in the striatopallidal system may decrease or even disappear completely after liver transplantation.

Acute Hepatic Encephalopathy and Hyperammonemia

TERMINOLOGY. Acute hepatic encephalopathy (AHE) is caused by hyperammonemia, which can be both hepatic *and* nonhepatic.

ETIOLOGY. While acute hepatic decompensation is the most common cause of hyperammonemia in adults, drug toxicity is also an important consideration. Valproate, asparaginase, acetaminophen, and chemotherapy have all been implicated in the development of hyperammonemic encephalopathy. Other important nonhepatic causes of hyperammonemia include hematologic disease, parenteral nutrition, bone marrow transplantation, urinary tract infection, and fulminant viral hepatitis.

Inherited urea cycle abnormalities or organic acidemias such as citrullinemia and ornithine transcarbamylase deficiency are other potential causes of acute hyperammonemic encephalopathy (see Chapter 31).

Many patients with AHE have multiple systemic and metabolic abnormalities. Hypoxic injury, seizures, and hypoglycemia all exacerbate the acute toxic effects of ammonia on the brain.

PATHOLOGY. AHE is characterized grossly by laminar necrosis of the cerebral cortex. Severe cytotoxic edema in astrocytes with anoxic neuronal damage is the typical histologic appearance of AHE.

CLINICAL ISSUES. Early clinical manifestations of hyperammonemia can be seen with plasma ammonia levels of 55-60 µmol/L. Irritability, lethargy, vomiting, and somnolence are typical. Progressively decreasing consciousness, seizures, and coma are the principal manifestations of severe AHE and are usually seen when ammonia levels are at least four times the normal range.

AHE is a life-threatening disorder with high morbidity and mortality. Recognition and aggressive treatment are critical to patient outcome. Traditional management strategies have focused on reducing ammonia generation from the bowel, although only 15% of ammonia originates in the colon. Recent studies have shown that admin-

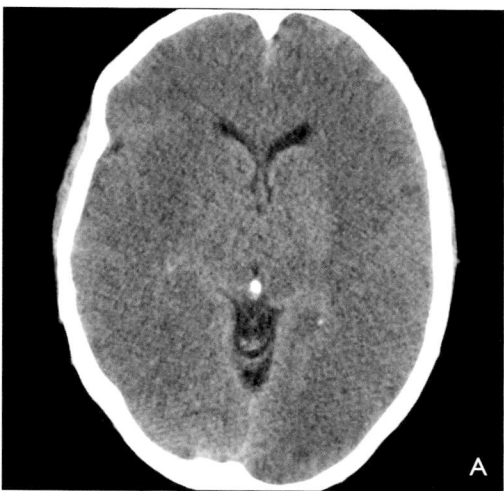

32-47A. NECT scan in a 50 yo woman with acute hyperammonemia shows diffuse cerebral edema with effaced sulci, loss of GM-WM interfaces.

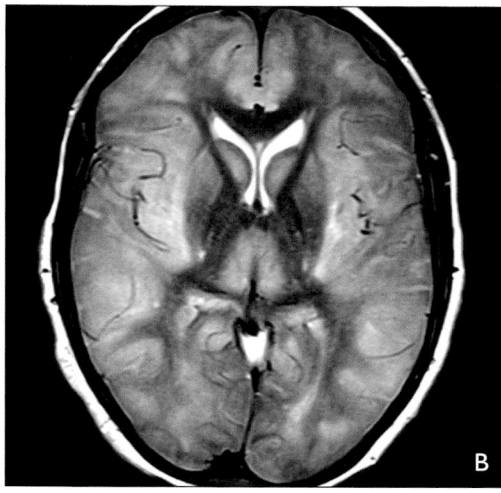

32-47B. T2WI shows diffusely swollen, hyperintense cortex, basal ganglia, and medial thalami.

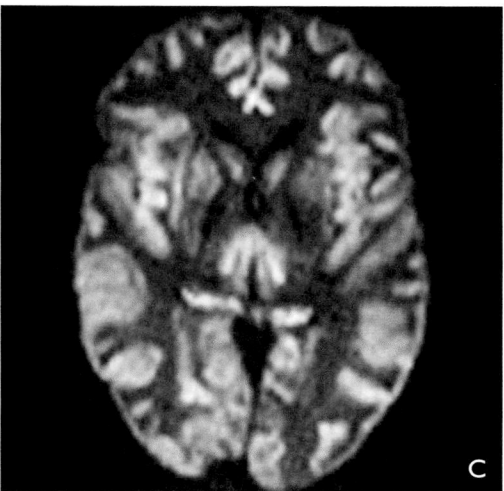

32-47C. DWI shows restricted diffusion in the same structures. Note sparing of subcortical, deep WM.

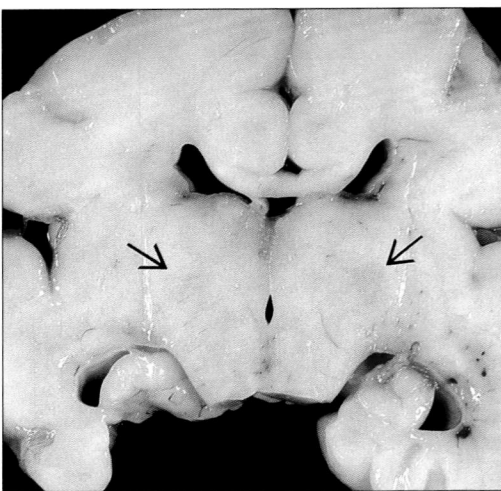

32-48. *Coronal autopsy specimen of bilirubin encephalopathy shows obvious yellow staining of the globi pallidi* ➔. *(Courtesy R. Hewlett, MD.)*

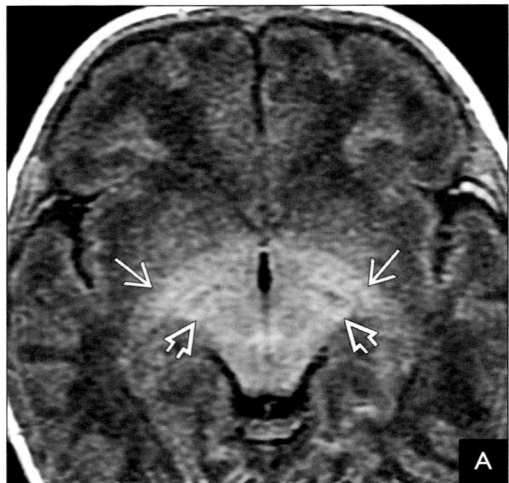

32-49A. *Axial T1WI in a 5-day-old girl with bilirubin encephalopathy shows hyperintensity in the subthalamic nuclei* ➔, *substantia nigra* ➔.

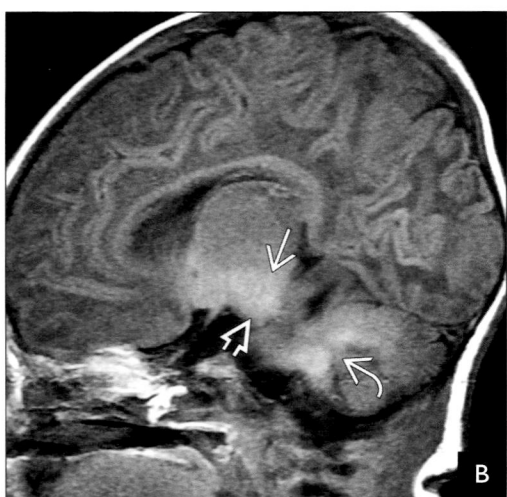

32-49B. *Sagittal T1WI in the same patient shows the hyperintensity in the subthalamic nuclei* ➔, *midbrain* ➔, *and dentate nuclei* ➔.

istration of L-ornithine L-aspartate (LOLA) improves mental status and decreases CSF ammonia levels.

IMAGING. Initially, NECT scans may show only minimal cerebral edema with mild sulcal effacement. As the brain swelling increases, the gray-white matter interfaces are "blurred," the hemispheres become diffusely hypodense, and complete central brain descending herniation ensues **(32-47A)**.

On T1WI, the gyri appear swollen and hypointense. The CSF spaces are compressed. Bilaterally symmetric T2/FLAIR hyperintensity in the insular cortex, cingulate gyri, and basal ganglia is typical, as is relative sparing of the perirolandic and occipital regions **(32-47B)**. More diffuse cortical injury with involvement of the thalami and brainstem is also common. The hemispheric white matter is typically spared, although some involvement of the subcortical association fibers can be seen in children and occasionally adults.

AHE restricts strongly on DWI **(32-47C)**. MRS may show a glutamate-glutamine peak at short echo times.

DIFFERENTIAL DIAGNOSIS. The major differential diagnoses of AHE/hyperammonemia are hypoglycemia, hypoxic-ischemic encephalopathy, and status epilepticus. **Hypoglycemia** is a common comorbidity in patients with chronic HE. Acute hypoglycemia typically affects the parietooccipital cortex. Serum glucose is low, and ammonia is normal.

Hypoxic-ischemic encephalopathy may be difficult to distinguish from AHE on imaging alone. Nevertheless, symmetric involvement of the insular cortex and cingulate gyri should suggest AHE. **Status epilepticus** is usually unilateral, and the basal ganglia are generally spared.

ACUTE vs. CHRONIC HEPATIC ENCEPHALOPATHY

Chronic Hepatic Encephalopathy
- More common
- Etiology
  - Chronic severe liver disease (cirrhosis)
- Imaging
  - T1 hyperintense globi pallidi, substantia nigra
  - Probably due to manganese deposition

Acute Hepatic Encephalopathy
- Rare
- Etiology
  - Usually associated with hyperammonemia
  - Acute liver decompensation (viral hepatitis, etc.)
  - Drug toxicity (acetaminophen, valproate, etc.)
  - Parenteral nutrition, infection
- Imaging findings = those of hyperammonemia
  - Bilateral swollen T2/FLAIR hyperintense gyri
  - Most severe: Insular cortex, cingulate gyri
  - ± basal ganglia, thalami
  - DWI 4+
  - MRS may show glutamate-glutamine peak

Bilirubin Encephalopathy

Terminology

Bilirubin encephalopathy (BRE), also known as kernicterus, is caused by hyperbilirubinemia. A milder form of chronic BRE is termed bilirubin-induced neurologic dysfunction (BIND).

Etiology

In kernicterus, the liver is basically unable to conjugate insoluble bilirubin into water-soluble bilirubin diglucuronide.

It is unclear how bilirubin gets into the brain. Neonatal hyperbilirubinemia results in unconjugated bilirubin passing across an immature or compromised blood-brain barrier.

Hyperbilirubinemia is associated with a number of predisposing conditions, including prematurity, hemolytic disorders (especially blood group incompatibility), breast feeding, significant loss of birth weight, polycythemia, and dehydration. Inherited or acquired defects of bilirubin conjugation, glucose metabolism, GI transit disorders, and drugs that compete with bilirubin for albumin binding are other factors that increase the risk of BRE.

Pathology

The cardinal gross pathologic feature is yellow discoloration of the globi pallidi, mammillary bodies, substantia nigra, subthalamic nuclei, hippocampi, dentate nuclei, and spinal cord (32-48). The major histologic feature of acute BRE is neuronal necrosis with little or no inflammatory reaction. Demonstration of bilirubin pigment within the neurons is uncommon.

Clinical Issues

Although neonatal jaundice is common, kernicterus is rare in developed countries. The estimated incidence in the United States is approximately five cases per year.

Not all infants with kernicterus exhibit symptoms. Neonates with overt hyperbilirubinemia present in the first few days of life. Jaundice, stupor, hypotonia, and poor sucking are followed by opisthotonus and hyperreflexia.

Findings in children with classic chronic kernicterus vary in severity. Most show some type of movement disorder, most commonly athetosis. Other abnormalities include auditory disturbances, oculomotor impairments (particularly upward gaze), and teeth with dysplastic enamel. Frank mental retardation is relatively uncommon.

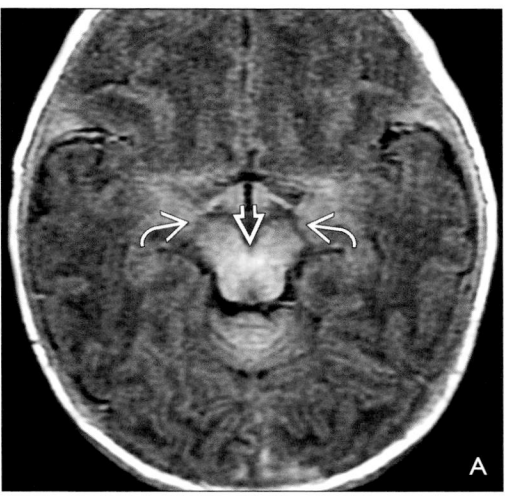

32-50A. Axial T1WI shows hyperintensity in the midbrain ➡, hippocampi ➡.

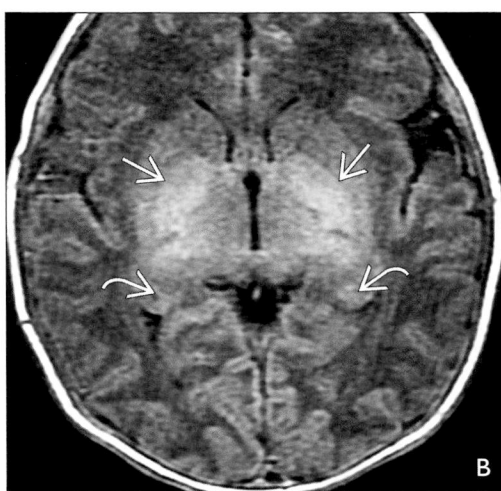

32-50B. T1WI shows striking hyperintensity in the globi pallidi ➡, lesser hyperintensity in the tails of the hippocampi ➡.

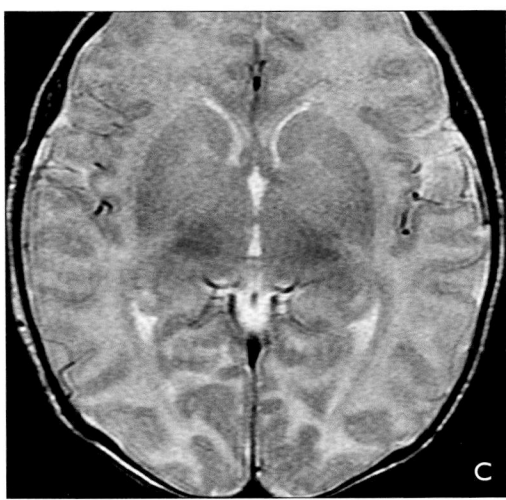

32-50C. Axial T2WI at the same level shows no evidence of signal abnormality in the globi pallidi, as typical for acute bilirubin encephalopathy.

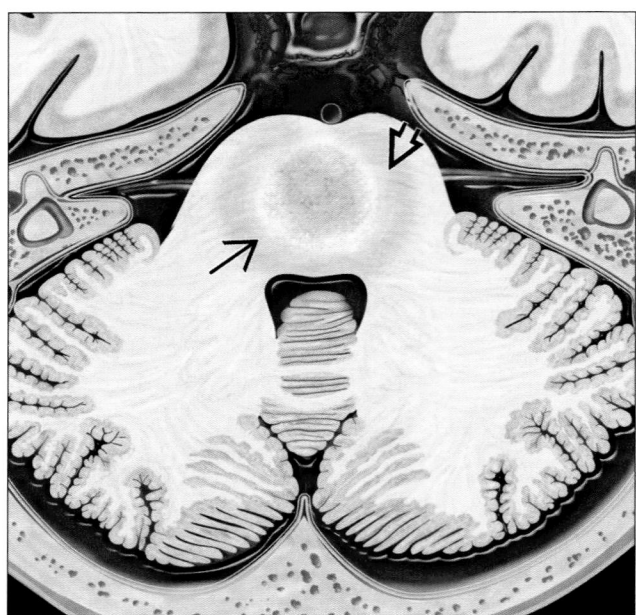

32-51. *Axial graphic shows acute osmotic demyelination* ➡ *affecting the central pons. Note sparing of peripheral WM, traversing corticospinal tracts* ⊳.

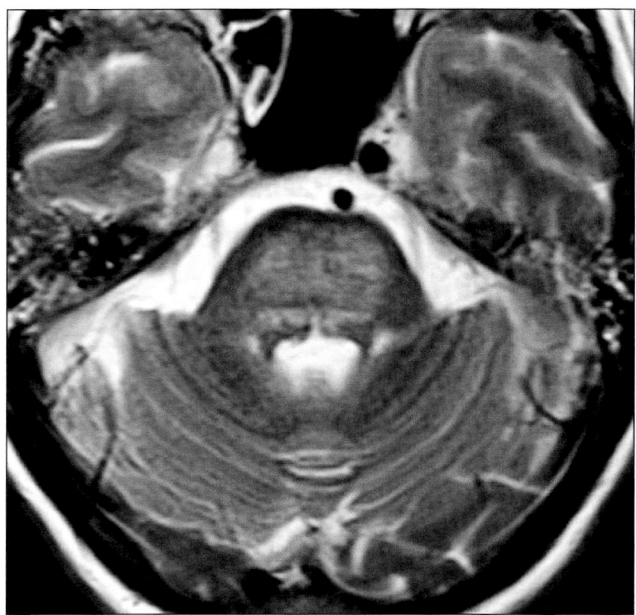

32-52. *Axial T2WI shows classic osmotic demyelination. The peripheral pons is spared as are the corticospinal tracts and transverse pontine fibers.*

Patients with BIND may show subtle neurodevelopmental disabilities without the classic clinical findings of kernicterus.

Imaging

MR is the procedure of choice as CT is almost always normal. T1 scans during the *acute* stages of BRE show bilaterally symmetric hyperintensities in the globi pallidi (GP), subthalamic nuclei, substantia nigra, hippocampi, and dentate nuclei **(32-49)**. The thalami and cortex are typically spared. T2 scans are typically normal in the acute stage **(32-50)**.

Chronic BRE may show T2/FLAIR hyperintensity in the typical areas. Bilateral hippocampal sclerosis with volume loss and T2 hyperintensity is common.

DWI is normal in both acute and chronic BRE. MRS shows decreased NAA:Cho and NAA:Cr ratios. Preterm infants with BRE may demonstrate increased glutamate-glutamine.

Differential Diagnosis

The major imaging differential diagnoses of BRE are the other disorders that cause GP abnormalities. The GP is an area of especially high metabolic activity with significant glucose and oxygen demands, which is thus vulnerable to a number of metabolic and systemic diseases.

In term neonates with suspected BRE, the major differential diagnosis is acute **hypoxic-ischemic injury** (HII). In term HII, the putamen is the most commonly affected site. T2/FLAIR hyperintensity and restricted diffusion are typical in HII but absent in BRE.

Bilaterally symmetric T1 hyperintense GP are seen in **chronic liver failure**, **hyperalimentation**, and **nonketotic hyperglycemia**. **Neurofibromatosis type 1** can also cause mild T1 shortening in the GP. Late sequelae of **carbon monoxide poisoning** can cause T1 shortening and T2 hyperintensity in the medial GP.

Osmotic Demyelination Syndrome

Acute electrolyte and osmolality disorders can cause alarming alterations in mental status. Extreme hyperosmolality is rare; hypoosmolar states are much more common. The most common hypoosmolar state is hyponatremia.

Terminology

Osmotic demyelination syndrome (ODS) was formerly called **central pontine myelinolysis** and/or **extrapontine myelinolysis**.

Etiology

ODS classically occurs when wide fluxes in serum sodium levels are induced by too-rapid correction of hyponatremia Exactly how this results in myelin loss is unknown.

Oligodendrocytes, which form the myelin sheaths, are particularly vulnerable to osmotic changes. Myelin sheaths can rupture and split if the osmotic stress on oligodendrocytes is severe.

In hyponatremia/hypoosmolar states, extracellular water moves into cells with higher solute content, leading to cellular edema. Glial cells selectively swell after hypotonic stress whereas neurons do not. Dysfunction of glia-specific water channels—aquaporin-4 and -1—results in cerebral edema and increased intracranial pressure.

Pathology

LOCATION. ODS is traditionally considered primarily a pontine lesion (32-51), (32-52). However, multifocal involvement is not only common but typical. Only 50% of ODS cases have isolated pontine lesions. In 30% of cases, myelinolytic foci occur both outside and inside the pons. The basal ganglia and hemispheric are common sites. WM demyelination is exclusively extrapontine in 20-25% of cases.

Other parts of the CNS that can be involved in ODS include the cerebellum (especially the middle cerebellar peduncles), basal ganglia, thalami, lateral geniculate body, and hemispheric WM. Some ODS cases involve the cortex.

GROSS PATHOLOGY. Grossly, the central pons is abnormally soft and exhibits a rhomboid or trident-shaped area of grayish tan discoloration. The peripheral pons is spared.

Laminar cortical necrosis can occur in ODS, either primarily or in association with hypoxia or anoxia. In such cases, the affected cortex appears soft and pale.

MICROSCOPIC FEATURES. Microscopically, ODS is characterized by myelin loss with relative sparing of axons and neurons. Active demyelination without evidence of significant inflammation is typical. The presence of reactive astrocytes and abundant foamy, lipid-laden macrophages is characteristic.

Clinical Issues

EPIDEMIOLOGY AND DEMOGRAPHICS. ODS is a rare disorder, and its exact prevalence is unknown. It can occur at any age but is most common in middle-aged patients (peak = 30-60 years). There is a moderate male

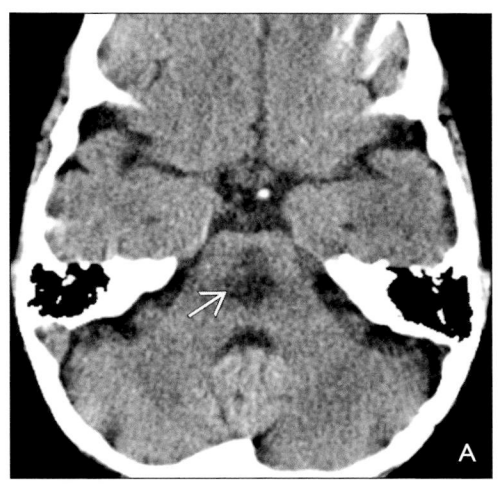

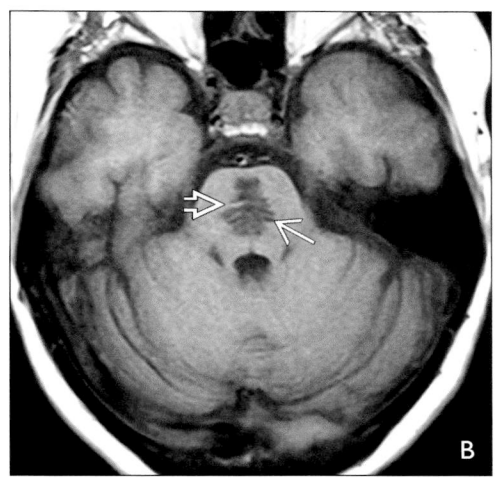

32-53A. NECT scan in a 37-year-old woman with osmotic demyelination syndrome shows a triangular central pontine hypodensity ➡. 32-53B. T1WI in the same patient shows that the lesion is hypointense ➡. The transverse pontine fibers are spared and are seen here as lines of preserved brain ➡ passing from one side to the other.

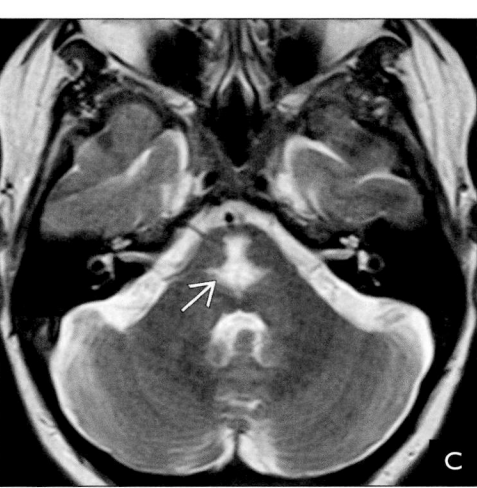

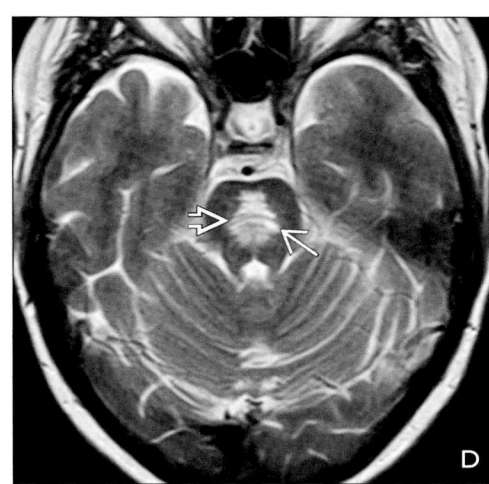

32-53C. T2WI shows the symmetric "trident" or "bat wing" shape of pontine myelinolysis ➡. The peripheral pons is spared. 32-53D. More cephalad T2WI through the upper pons shows the lesion ➡ with "stripes" of preserved myelinated transverse pontine tracts ➡ seen crossing the lesion.

predominance. Pediatric patients with ODS typically have diabetes or anorexia.

The most common causes of ODS are rapid correction of hyponatremia, alcoholism, liver transplantation, and malnutrition.

Comorbid conditions that predispose to developing ODS include renal, adrenal, pituitary, and paraneoplastic disease. Prolonged vomiting (e.g., hyperemesis gravidarum), severe burns, transplants, and prolonged diuretic use may all contribute to the development of ODS.

PRESENTATION. The most common presenting symptoms of ODS are altered mental status and seizures. A biphasic clinical course is common. As normonatremia is restored, mental status improves but can then rapidly deteriorate. Other findings include pseudobulbar palsy, dysarthria, and dysphagia. Movement disorders are common when myelinolysis involves the basal ganglia.

NATURAL HISTORY. The outcome of ODS varies significantly, ranging from complete recovery to coma and death. Some patients survive with minimal or no residual deficits. In severe cases, the patient may become quadriparetic and "locked in."

TREATMENT OPTIONS. Initial serum sodium in ODS is usually under 115-120 mmol/L and serum osmolality less than 275 mOsm/kg. Although there is no consensus regarding the optimal correction rates for hyponatremia, correction of more than 12 mmol/L/day seems to increase the risk of ODS.

ODS may also occur (1) in normonatremic patients and (2) independent of changes in serum sodium!

Imaging

GENERAL FEATURES. Imaging findings in ODS typically lag one or two weeks behind clinical symptoms.

CT FINDINGS. NECT scans can be normal or show hypodensity in the affected areas, particularly the central pons (32-53A).

MR FINDINGS. Standard MR sequences may be normal in the first several days. Eventually, ODS becomes hypointense on T1WI and hyperintense on T2/FLAIR.

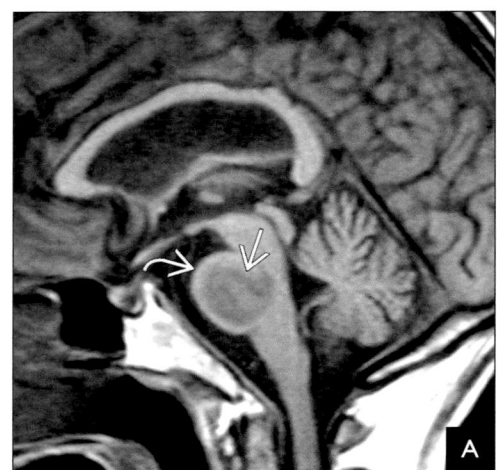
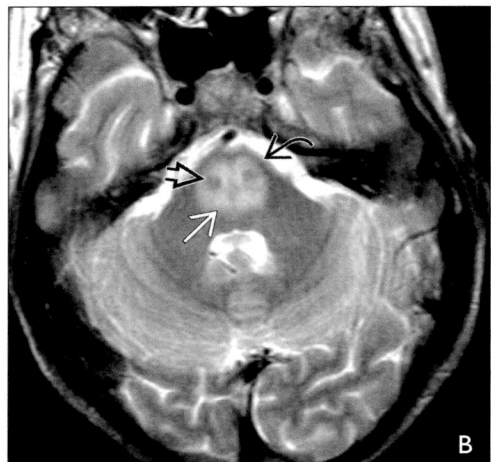

32-54A. Sagittal T1WI in a 44-year-old male alcoholic with vomiting, seizures, and acutely altered mental status. The central pons is slightly swollen and hypointense ➡️, whereas the peripheral pons ➡️ is spared. 32-54B. T2WI in the same patient shows symmetric central hyperintensity ➡️ with sparing of the peripheral pons ➡️ and corticospinal tracts ➡️.

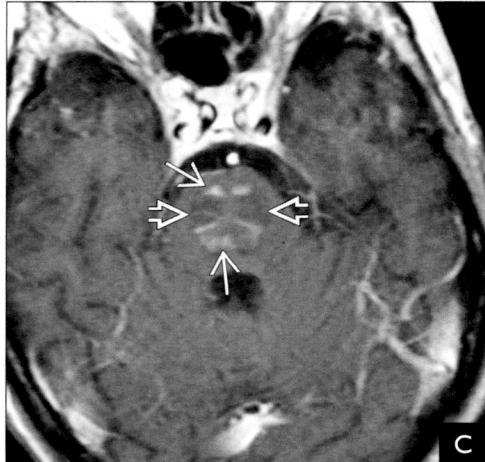
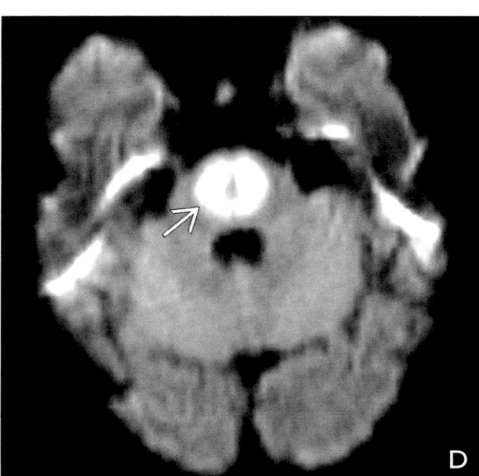

32-54C. Axial T1 C+ scan in the same patient shows patchy but symmetric enhancement in the affected WM ➡️ with sparing of the corticospinal tracts ➡️. 32-54D. DWI in the same patient shows acutely restricted diffusion ➡️. ODS with acute demyelination can both enhance and restrict.

The lesions are typically well-demarcated and symmetric. Pontine ODS is round, triangular, or "bat wing"-shaped. The peripheral pons as well as the corticospinal tracts and transverse pontine fibers is spared **(32-53B)**, **(32-53C)**, **(32-53D)**. Involvement of the basal ganglia and hemispheric WM is seen in at least half of all cases.

T2* (GRE, SWI) shows no evidence of hemorrhage. Late acute or subacute ODS lesions may demonstrate moderate confluent enhancement on T1 C+ **(32-54)**.

DWI is the most sensitive sequence for acute ODS and can demonstrate restricted diffusion when other sequences are normal **(32-55)**, **(32-56)**. DTI shows disruption of central pontine WM with sparing of peripheral, transverse tracts **(32-57)**.

Differential Diagnosis

The major differential diagnosis of "central" ODS is pontine ischemia-infarction. **Basilar perforating artery infarcts** involve the surface of the pons and are usually asymmetric.

Demyelinating disease can involve the pons but is rarely symmetric. Sagittal FLAIR scans usually demonstrate lesions elsewhere, especially along the callososeptal interface.

Neoplasm rarely mimics ODS. Pontine gliomas can expand the pons and appear hyperintense on T2/FLAIR scans. They are neoplasms of children and young adults. Metastatic disease in the posterior fossa is typically in the cerebellum, not the pons.

The major differential diagnosis of extrapontine ODS with basal ganglia and/or cortical involvement is metabolic disease. **Hypertensive encephalopathy** (PRES) can involve the pons but does not spare the peripheral WM tracts. The basal ganglia are affected in both **Wilson disease** and **mitochondrial disorders**, but the pons is less commonly involved.

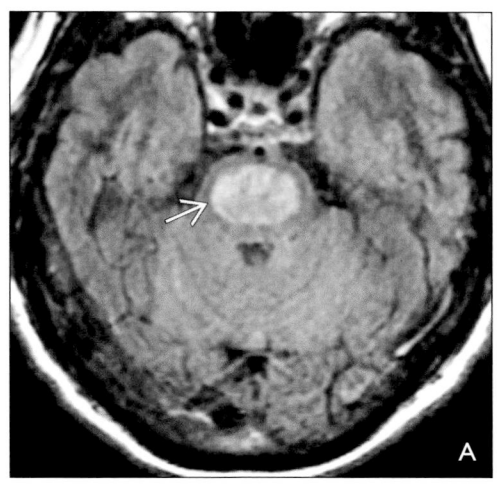

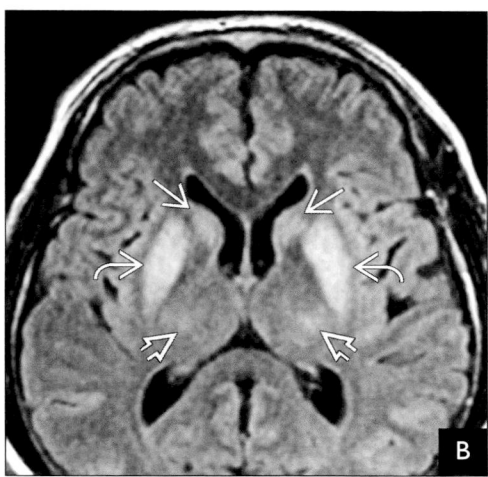

32-55A. Axial FLAIR scan in a 45-year-old man shows hyperintensity in the central pons ➔. The peripheral pons is spared, a classic finding in ODS. 32-55B. FLAIR scan in the same patient shows symmetric hyperintensity in the caudate nuclei ➔ and putamina ➔ with faint hyperintensity in the thalami ➔. ODS commonly involves both the pons and extrapontine sites.

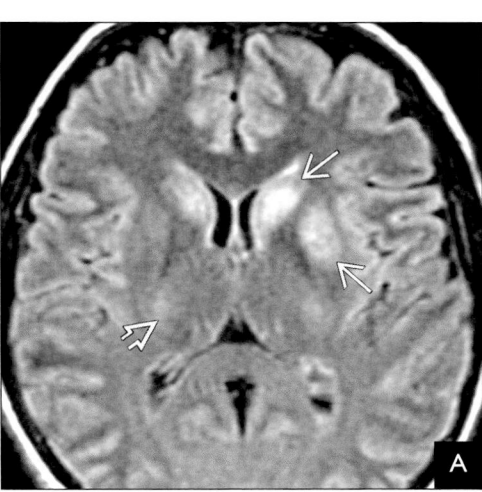

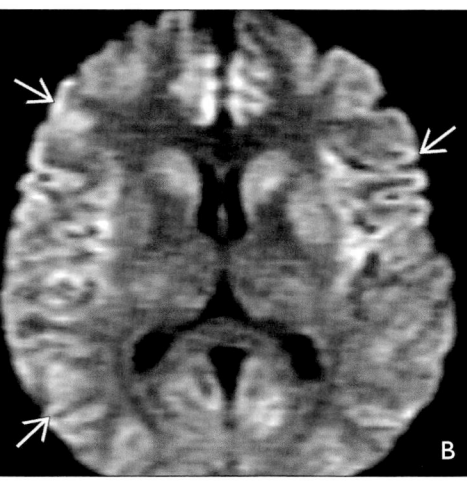

32-56A. A variant case of ODS is illustrated by this axial FLAIR scan in a 56-year-old man with confusion after rapid correction of hyponatremia. Note hyperintensity in the basal ganglia ➔, both thalami ➔. 32-56B. DWI shows that the cortex is also diffusely but somewhat asymmetrically affected ➔. Cortical laminar necrosis can sometimes be seen in ODS.

32-57A. *Variant ODS with both pontine, extrapontine myelinolysis is illustrated by this case of a 46-year-old male alcoholic who became severely hyponatremic following surgery, then was rapidly corrected. Sagittal T1WI shows a band of hypointensity in the central pons ➡ with peripheral sparing.* **32-57B.** *T2WI shows central pontine hyperintensity ➡ with symmetric lesions in both major cerebellar peduncles ⧎.*

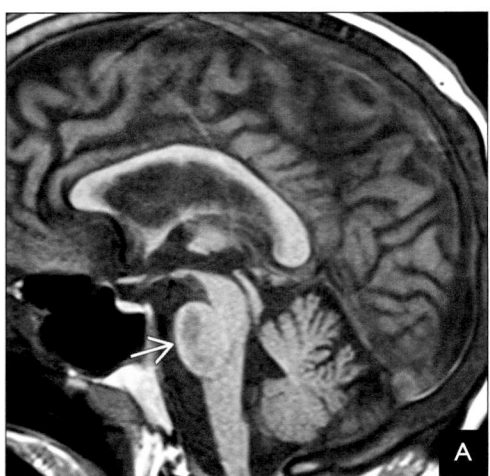

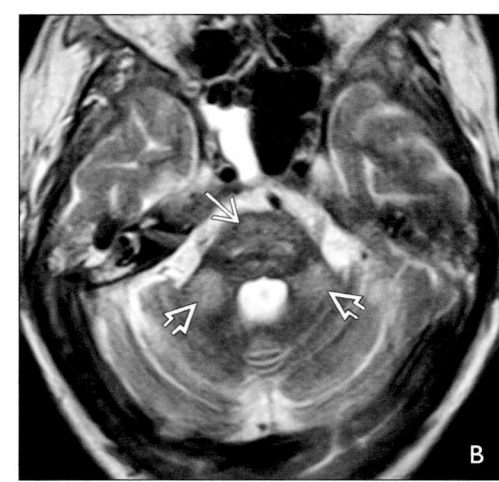

32-57C. *DTI with b = 3,000 shows a cruciform area of restricted diffusion in the central pons ➡ together with large ovoid areas of restricted diffusion in both major cerebellar peduncles ⧎.* **32-57D.** *More cephalad DTI shows restricted diffusion in both lateral geniculate bodies ➡ and the subthalamic nuclei ⧎.*

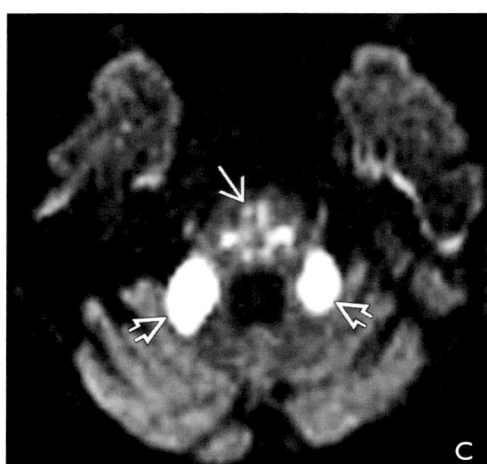

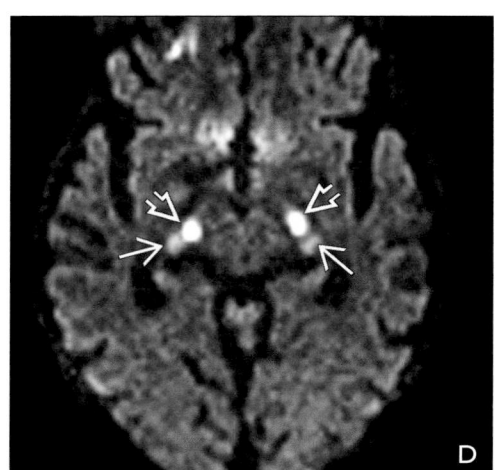

32-57E. *DTI through the lateral ventricles shows symmetric restriction in the posterior limbs of both internal capsules ➡ and thalami ⧎.* **32-57F.** *Color DTI map shows preserved peripheral pontine fibers in green ➡ with disruption of the central pontine WM ⧎. The transverse pontine tracts (in red) are preserved ➡.*

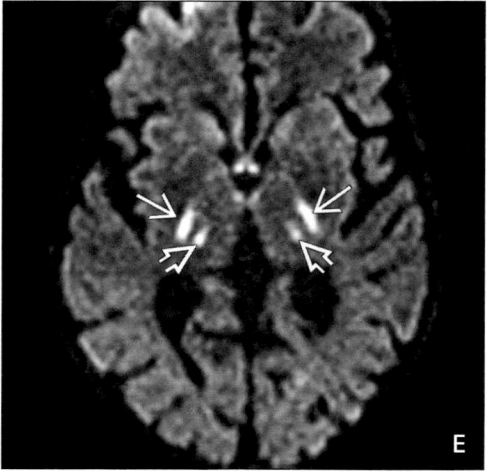

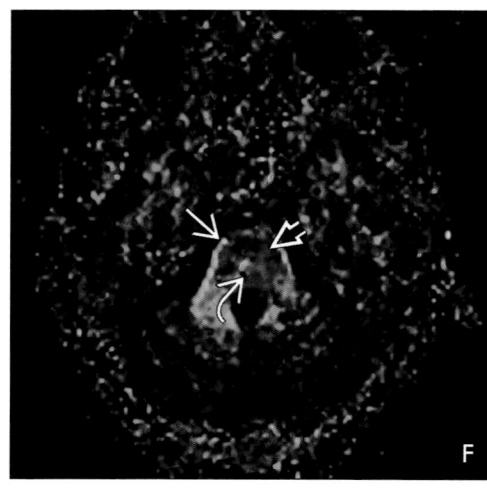

OSMOTIC DEMYELINATION SYNDROMES

Terminology
- ODS (formerly pontine, extrapontine myelinolysis)

Etiology
- Hypoosmolar state (hyponatremia)
- Too-rapid correction → wide fluxes in serum sodium
- Oligodendrocytes especially vulnerable to osmotic stress

Pathology
- Isolated pontine (50%)
  - Spares periphery, transverse pontine tracts
- Pons + extrapontine (30%)
  - Basal ganglia, thalami, hemispheric WM
- Exclusively extrapontine (20-25%)
- ± cortical laminar necrosis

Clinical Issues
- Any age; peak = 30-60 years
- Can occur without serum sodium disturbances!

Imaging
- Can be initially normal
- Hypodense on NECT
- Hypointense on T1, hyperintense on T2
- May restrict on DWI, enhance

Iron Overload Disorders

Iron is vital for normal neuronal metabolism and plays a key role in brain oxygen transport, electron transfer, neurotransmitter synthesis, and myelin production.

Brain iron deposition occurs as a part of normal aging. However, excessive iron is neurotoxic. Ferritin, a protein that contains iron nanoparticles, induces reactive oxygen species formation and inhibits glutamate uptake from synaptic junctions, potentially leading to neurodegeneration.

Iron overload disorders encompass a broad spectrum of both inherited and acquired etiologies. Inherited disorders of iron metabolism are discussed in Chapter 31. Acquired iron overload disorders are addressed here.

Terminology

Acquired brain iron overload is called **siderosis**. When iron deposition occurs along cranial nerves or the pial surface of the brain, it is termed **superficial siderosis**. **Hemochromatosis** is the pathologic accumulation of intracellular iron in parenchymal tissues.

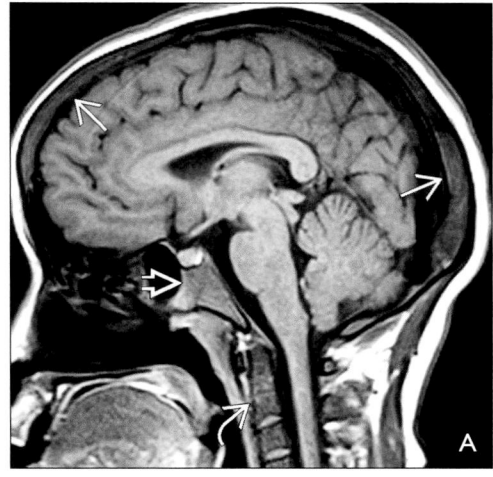

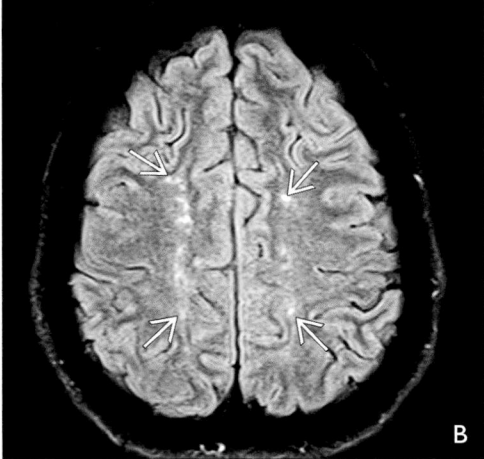

32-58A. Sagittal T1WI in a 29-year-old woman with sickle cell disease and hemochromatosis shows very hypointense marrow in the skull ⇥, clivus ⇥, and cervical spine ⇥ (with "bright disc" sign). 32-58B. Axial FLAIR scan shows thick, hypointense skull and multifocal hyperintensities along the deep watershed zone of the corona radiata ⇥, common findings in sickle cell disease.

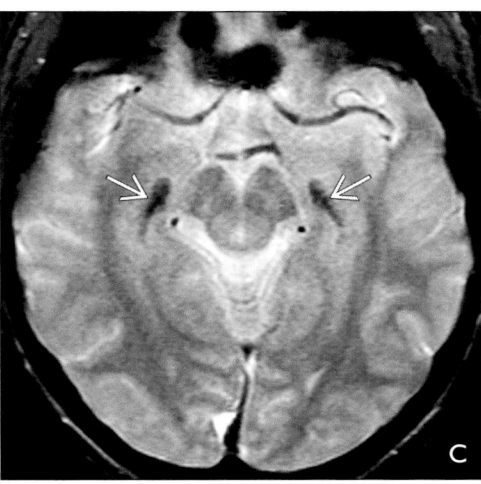

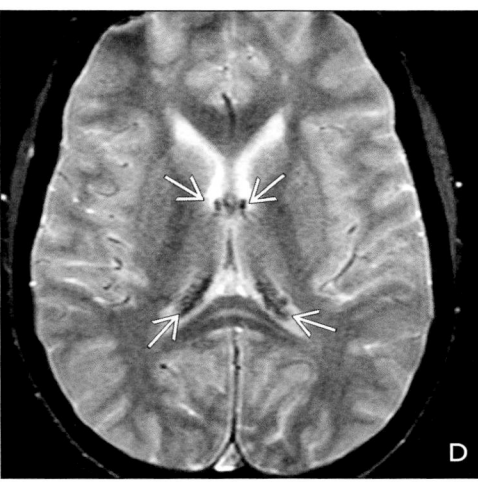

32-58C. T2* GRE in the same patient shows marked hypointensity with "blooming" of the choroid plexuses ⇥ in both temporal horns of the lateral ventricles. 32-58D. More cephalad T2* GRE scan in the same patient shows extensive siderosis of both choroid plexuses ⇥.

Etiology

Systemic iron overload can be caused by inherited or acquired blood dyscrasias (e.g., thalassemia major, sickle cell disease, aplastic or refractory anemia, myelodysplastic disorders) or by upregulated intestinal iron absorption.

Abnormal iron deposition also occurs as a feature of many degenerative disorders. Parkinson and Alzheimer disease as well as amyotrophic lateral sclerosis and chronic progressive multiple sclerosis are all associated with increased iron deposition in the basal ganglia.

In the brain, superficial siderosis is more common than iron accumulation within the cortex itself (i.e., hemochromatosis). Superficial siderosis is usually caused by trauma, tumor, prior surgery, or repeated subarachnoid hemorrhage from an arteriovenous malformation or aneurysm. Amyloid angiopathy is a common cause of siderosis in elderly patients.

Imaging

The **pituitary gland**—especially the anterior lobe—is very sensitive to early toxic effects from iron overload. Progressive iron deposition causes profound pituitary hypointensity on T2WI.

Iron deposition in the **choroid plexus** occurs in the setting of hematologic dyscrasias such as sickle cell disease. NECT scans are typically normal, but T2* (GRE, SWI) MR shows symmetric "blooming" hypointensity in the choroid plexus **(32-58)**.

Superficial siderosis along the **brain surfaces** and **cranial nerves** is usually associated with repeated subarachnoid hemorrhages and not uniformly distributed. T2* scans show "blooming" along the pia (gyral surfaces).

Iron deposition within the **cortex** and **basal ganglia** is less common and is associated with neuroferritinopathies and brain degeneration syndromes. Diffuse symmetric serpentine hypointensities and very hypointense deep gray nuclei are seen on T2* sequences.

Selected References

Hypertensive Encephalopathies

Acute Hypertensive Encephalopathy, Posterior Reversible Encephalopathy Syndrome

- Hugonnet E et al: Posterior reversible encephalopathy syndrome (PRES): Features on CT and MR imaging. Diagn Interv Imaging. Epub ahead of print, 2012
- Ishikura K et al: Children with posterior reversible encephalopathy syndrome associated with atypical diffusion-weighted imaging and apparent diffusion coefficient. Clin Exp Nephrol. 15(2):275-80, 2011
- Ni J et al: The clinical and radiological spectrum of posterior reversible encephalopathy syndrome: a retrospective series of 24 patients. J Neuroimaging. 21(3):219-24, 2011
- Wagner SJ et al: Posterior reversible encephalopathy syndrome and eclampsia: pressing the case for more aggressive blood pressure control. Mayo Clin Proc. 86(9):851-6, 2011
- Fugate JE et al: Posterior reversible encephalopathy syndrome: associated clinical and radiologic findings. Mayo Clin Proc. 85(5):427-32, 2010
- Kheir JN et al: Neuropathology of a fatal case of posterior reversible encephalopathy syndrome. Pediatr Dev Pathol. 13(5):397-403, 2010
- Bartynski WS et al: Catheter angiography, MR angiography, and MR perfusion in posterior reversible encephalopathy syndrome. Am J Neuroradiol. 29(3):447-55, 2008

Malignant Hypertension

- Tuncel M et al: Hypertensive emergencies: etiology and management. Am J Cardiovasc Drugs. 3(1):21-31, 2003

Chronic Hypertensive Encephalopathy

- Prasad H et al: Metabolic syndrome: definition and therapeutic implications. Postgrad Med. 124(1):21-30, 2012
- Ito S et al: Chronic hypertensive encephalopathy showing only headache: report of a case with longstanding brain MR abnormalities suggesting extensive vasogenic edema. Eur Neurol. 53(4):220-2, 2005

Glucose Disorders

- Scheen AJ: Central nervous system: a conductor orchestrating metabolic regulations harmed by both hyperglycaemia and hypoglycaemia. Diabetes Metab. 36 Suppl 3:S31-8, 2010

Pediatric/Adult Hypoglycemic Encephalopathy

- Scheen AJ: Central nervous system: a conductor orchestrating metabolic regulations harmed by both hyperglycaemia and hypoglycaemia. Diabetes Metab. 36 Suppl 3:S31-8, 2010

Neonatal/Infantile Hypoglycemia

- McCrimmon RJ: Update in the CNS response to hypoglycemia. J Clin Endocrinol Metab. 97(1):1-8, 2012
- Straussman S et al: Neonatal hypoglycemia. Curr Opin Endocrinol Diabetes Obes. 17(1):20-4, 2010

Hyperglycemia-associated Disorders

- Hsu JL et al: Microstructural white matter abnormalities in type 2 diabetes mellitus: a diffusion tensor imaging study. Neuroimage. 59(2):1098-105, 2012
- Ondo WG: Hyperglycemic nonketotic states and other metabolic imbalances. Handb Clin Neurol. 100:287-91, 2011
- Umemura T et al: Endothelial and inflammatory markers in relation to progression of ischaemic cerebral small-vessel disease and cognitive impairment: a 6-year longitudinal study in patients with type 2 diabetes mellitus. J Neurol Neurosurg Psychiatry. 82(11):1186-94, 2011

Thyroid Disorders

Congenital Hypothyroidism

- LaFranchi SH: Approach to the diagnosis and treatment of neonatal hypothyroidism. J Clin Endocrinol Metab. 96(10):2959-67, 2011
- Rastogi MV et al: Congenital hypothyroidism. Orphanet J Rare Dis. 5:17, 2010

Acquired Hypothyroid Disorders

- Zimmermann P et al: Steroid-responsive encephalopathy associated with Hashimoto thyroiditis. Pediatr Radiol. 42(7):891-3, 2012
- Chang T et al: Hashimoto encephalopathy: clinical and MRI improvement following high-dose corticosteroid therapy. Neurologist. 16(6):394-6, 2010

Hyperthyroidism

- Sharma D et al: Addison's disease presenting with idiopathic intracranial hypertension in 24-year-old woman: a case report. J Med Case Reports. 4:60, 2010
- Song TJ et al: The prevalence of thyrotoxicosis-related seizures. Thyroid. 20(9):955-8, 2010
- Kurne A et al: White matter alteration in a patient with Graves' disease. J Child Neurol. 22(9):1128-31, 2007
- Herwig U et al: Hyperthyroidism mimicking increased intracranial pressure. Headache. 39(3):228-30, 1999

Parathyroid Disorders

Hyperparathyroidism

- Macdonald DS et al: Calcification of the external carotid arteries and their branches. Dentomaxillofac Radiol. 41(7):615-8, 2012
- Shlapack MA et al: Normocalcemic primary hyperparathyroidism-characteristics and clinical significance of an emerging entity. Am J Med Sci. 343(2):163-6, 2012
- Mackenzie-Feder J et al: Primary hyperparathyroidism: an overview. Int J Endocrinol. 2011:251410, 2011
- Petersilge CA: Introduction to metabolic bone disease. In Manaster BJ et al: Diagnostic Imaging: Musculoskeletal: Non-Traumatic Disease. Salt Lake City: Amirsys Publishing. 11.2-7, 2010
- Abid F et al: Cranial nerve palsies in renal osteodystrophy. Pediatr Neurol. 36(1):64-5, 2007

Hypoparathyroid Disorders

- Bhadada SK et al: Spectrum of neurological manifestations of idiopathic hypoparathyroidism and pseudohypoparathyroidism. Neurol India. 59(4):586-9, 2011
- Petersilge CA: Hypoparathyroidism, pseudo- and pseudopseudohypoparathyroidism. In Manaster BJ et al: Diagnostic Imaging: Musculoskeletal: Non-Traumatic Disease. Salt Lake City: Amirsys Publishing. 11.26-7, 2010

Seizures and Related Disorders

Normal Anatomy of the Temporal Lobe

- Huntgeburth SC et al: Morphological patterns of the collateral sulcus in the human brain. Eur J Neurosci. 35(8):1295-311, 2012
- Salzman KL: Limbic system. In Harnsberger HR et al: Diagnostic and Surgical Imaging Anatomy: Brain, Head and Neck, Spine. Salt Lake City: Amirsys Publishing. I.76-85, 2006

Mesial Temporal Sclerosis

- Lopinto-Khoury C et al: Surgical outcome in PET-positive, MRI-negative patients with temporal lobe epilepsy. Epilepsia. 53(2):342-8, 2012
- Mueller SG et al: Widespread extrahippocampal NAA/(Cr + Cho) abnormalities in TLE with and without mesial temporal sclerosis. J Neurol. 258(4):603-12, 2011

Status Epilepticus

- Förster A et al: Diffusion-weighted imaging for the differential diagnosis of disorders affecting the hippocampus. Cerebrovasc Dis. 33(2):104-15, 2012
- Yoong M et al: The role of magnetic resonance imaging in the follow-up of children with convulsive status epilepticus. Dev Med Child Neurol. 54(4):328-33, 2012
- Huang YC et al: Periictal magnetic resonance imaging in status epilepticus. Epilepsy Res. 86(1):72-81, 2009

Transient Lesion of the Corpus Callosum Splenium

- Ito S et al: Transient splenial lesion of the corpus callosum in H1N1 influenza virus-associated encephalitis/encephalopathy. Intern Med. 50(8):915-8, 2011
- Sreedharan SE et al: Reversible pancallosal signal changes in febrile encephalopathy: report of 2 cases. AJNR Am J Neuroradiol. 32(9):E172-4, 2011

Transient Global Amnesia

- Uttner I et al: Long-term outcome in transient global amnesia patients with and without focal hyperintensities in the CA1 region of the hippocampus. Eur Neurol. 67(3):155-160, 2012
- Hunter G: Transient global amnesia. Neurol Clin. 29(4):1045-54, 2011
- Weon YC et al: Optimal diffusion-weighted imaging protocol for lesion detection in transient global amnesia. Am J Neuroradiol. 29(7):1324-8, 2008

Miscellaneous Disorders

Fahr Disease

- Hegde AN et al: Differential diagnosis for bilateral abnormalities of the basal ganglia and thalamus. Radiographics. 31(1):5-30, 2011
- Acou M et al: Fahr disease. JBR-BTR. 91(1):19, 2008
- Shoyama M et al: Evaluation of regional cerebral blood flow in fahr disease with schizophrenia-like psychosis: a case report. AJNR Am J Neuroradiol. 26(10):2527-9, 2005

Hepatic Encephalopathy

- Chopra A et al: Valproate-induced hyperammonemic encephalopathy: an update on risk factors, clinical correlates and management. Gen Hosp Psychiatry. 34(3):290-8, 2012
- U-King-Im JM et al: Acute hyperammonemic encephalopathy in adults: imaging findings. Am J Neuroradiol. 32(2):413-8, 2011
- Blanco Vela CI et al: Efficacy of oral L-ornithine L-aspartate in cirrhotic patients with hyperammonemic hepatic encephalopathy. Ann Hepatol. 10 Suppl 2:S55-9, 2011

Bilirubin Encephalopathy

- Kamei A et al: Proton magnetic resonance spectroscopic images in preterm infants with bilirubin encephalopathy. J Pediatr. 160(2):342-4, 2012
- Shapiro SM: Chronic bilirubin encephalopathy: diagnosis and outcome. Semin Fetal Neonatal Med. 15(3):157-63, 2010
- Wang X et al: Studying neonatal bilirubin encephalopathy with conventional MRI, MRS, and DWI. Neuroradiology. 50(10):885-93, 2008
- Rorke LB: Kernicterus. In Golden JA et al: Pathology and Genetics: Developmental Neuropathology. Basel: ISN Neuropath Press. 206-08, 2004

Osmotic Demyelination Syndrome

- de Souza A et al: More often striatal myelinolysis than pontine? A consecutive series of patients with osmotic demyelination syndrome. Neurol Res. 34(3):262-71, 2012
- Gankam Kengne F et al: Astrocytes are an early target in osmotic demyelination syndrome. J Am Soc Nephrol. 22(10):1834-45, 2011
- King JD et al: Osmotic demyelination syndrome. Am J Med Sci. 339(6):561-7, 2010
- Howard SA et al: Best cases from the AFIP: osmotic demyelination syndrome. Radiographics. 29(3):933-8, 2009

Iron Overload Disorders

- Sondag MJ et al: Case 179: Hereditary hemochromatosis. Radiology. 262(3):1037-41, 2012
- Haacke EM et al: Imaging iron stores in the brain using magnetic resonance imaging. Magn Reson Imaging. 23(1):1-25, 2005

33

Dementias and
Brain Degenerations

Worldwide public health efforts to improve living conditions, prevent disease, and enhance medical treatment have resulted in a burgeoning elderly population. Individuals over 65 years of age now represent 13% of the population and by 2030 will account for nearly 20%.

As the world's population ages, the number of patients with chronic debilitating diseases and brain degeneration will also increase. The prevalence and incidence of dementia increase dramatically between the ages of 65 and 85 years. Dementia is already one of most challenging public health issues of the twenty-first century and will reach near-epidemic levels in the next several decades.

Understanding the biology and imaging of normal aging is a prerequisite to understanding the pathobiology of degenerative brain diseases. Therefore, we first delineate normal age-related changes in brain structure and function.

We then turn our attention to dementias and brain degenerative disorders. **Dementia** is a loss of brain function that affects memory, thinking, language, judgment, and behavior. Dementia has many causes but most often

occurs secondary to degenerative processes in the brain. Most dementing illnesses are irreversible.

Neurodegeneration occurs when neurons in specific parts of the brain, spinal cord, or peripheral nerves die. While dementia always involves brain degeneration, not all neurodegenerative disorders are dementing illnesses. Some neurodegenerative disorders (e.g., Parkinson disease) can have associated dementia, but most do not.

The Normal Aging Brain

Introduction to the Normal Aging Brain

Terminology

Age-related changes take place in virtually all parts of the brain. The term **"normal aging brain"** as used in this chapter refers to the spectrum of age-related neuroimaging findings delineated by the Rotterdam Scan Study (RSS), a continuing population-based longitudinal study that began in the 1990s. The RSS now includes advanced MR imaging sequences and has been expanded to persons 45 years and older who are scanned every three to four years.

The term **"successfully aging brain"** refers to patients whose imaging studies do not demonstrate markers of small vessel ("microvascular") disease such as white matter hyperintensities with arteriolosclerosis and lipohyalinosis, silent lacunar infarcts, and microbleeds.

Individuals 65-85 years old are considered "elderly," and the cohort of "oldest-old" patients are those over the age of 90.

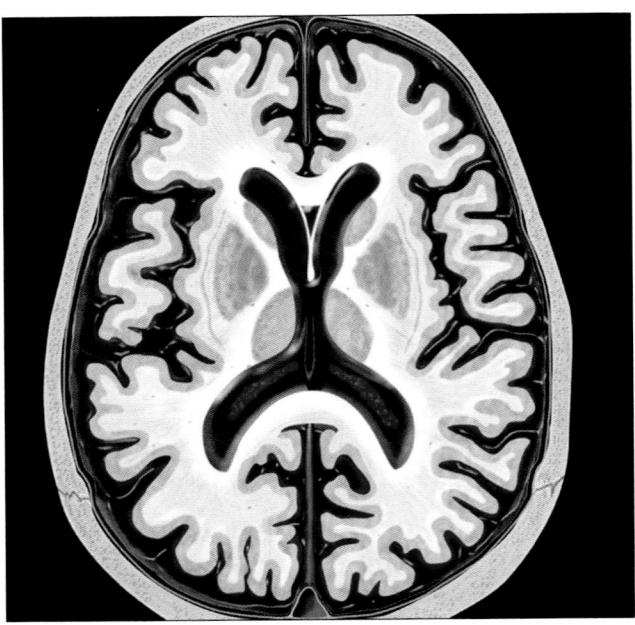

33-1. Axial graphic depicts a normally aging brain in an 80-year-old patient. Note the widening of sulci and ventricles in the absence of any parenchymal abnormalities.

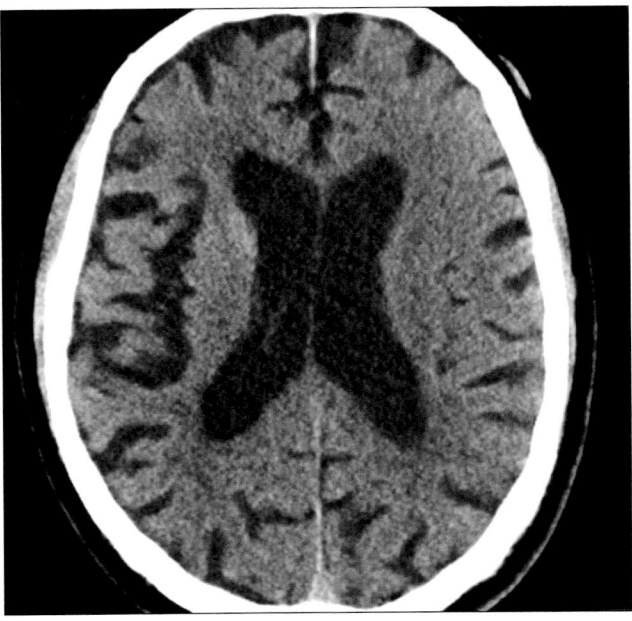

33-2. NECT scan in a 100-year-old, independent, cognitively normal man who had a ground level fall shows mildly enlarged ventricles and sulci with no evidence of white matter lesions.

Genetics

Genetic factors clearly affect brain aging and age-related cognitive decline. Apolipoprotein E (ApoE) and six novel risk-associated single nucleotide polymorphisms (SNPs) on chromosome 17q25 are genetic variants that are robustly associated with brain pathology on MR.

Pathology

GROSS PATHOLOGY. Overall brain volume decreases with advancing age and is indicated by a relative increase in the size of the CSF spaces. Widened sulci with proportionate enlargement of the ventricles is common (33-1). While minor thinning of the cortical mantle occurs with aging, the predominant neuroanatomic changes occur in the subcortical white matter.

MICROSCOPIC FEATURES. Physiologic brain aging is accompanied by ubiquitous degeneration of neurons and oligodendrocytes. Neuronal dysfunction—rather than frank neuronal loss—seems to predominate with a reduction in cell size (rather than number). Dendritic pruning and loss of synapses occur in selected areas (e.g., the hippocampus) but not globally.

The subcortical white matter (WM) demonstrates decreased numbers of myelinated fibers, increased extracellular space, and gliosis. Perivascular (Virchow-Robin) spaces in the subcortical WM and basal ganglia enlarge.

Three histologic markers are associated with dementias: Senile plaques, neurofibrillary tangles, and Lewy bodies. All can be identified to some extent in normal aging brains, so the border between normal and "preclinical" dementia is unclear.

Senile plaques (SPs) are extracellular amyloid deposits that accumulate in cerebral gray matter. Nearly half of cognitively intact older individuals demonstrate moderate or frequent SP density.

Neurofibrillary tangles (NFTs) are caused by tau aggregations within neurons. The Braak pathoanatomic staging divides Alzheimer disease into six distinct stages based on the topographical distribution of NFTs. Braak stage 5 or 6 NFTs are found in 6% of cognitively normal cases.

Lewy bodies are intraneuronal clumps of α-synuclein and ubiquitin proteins. They are found in 5-10% of cognitively intact individuals.

Many investigators believe that most cognitively normal elderly people with these histologic markers of AD pathology will eventually develop symptomatic AD. The differences among cognitively normal individuals, older patients with very subtle cognitive decline, and those with "preclinical" or presymptomatic Alzheimer disease are difficult to determine (see below). Decades may elapse between initial cortical accumulations of NFTs and SPs and the development of overt cognitive changes.

Clinical Issues

EPIDEMIOLOGY AND DEMOGRAPHICS. Brain maturation continues well into the third decade of life, after which brain aging predominates. While the incidence of dementias increases dramatically with aging, nearly two-thirds of patients over 85 years of age remain neurologically intact and cognitively normal.

PRESENTATION. The distinction between normal aging and early ("preclinical") dementia is unclear. The term minimal cognitive impairment is used to designate a transitional state between the expected cognitive changes of normal aging and frank dementia.

Most older people with memory loss *do not* have dementia. As we age, we all experience memory deficits. As one writer put it, "To forget where we placed our keys is a memory deficit, but to forget what a key is used for is dementia."

Imaging the Normal Aging Brain

Because age-associated brain pathology begins long before clinical symptoms develop, imaging plays an increasingly central role in evaluating older patients for early signs of dementia. Just as imaging findings reflect the dramatic changes in brain morphology that occur with

fetal and postnatal development, others mirror normal alterations in the aging brain.

CT Findings

The normal aging brain demonstrates mildly enlarged ventricles and widened sulci on NECT scans **(33-2)**. Punctate calcifications in the medial basal ganglia are physiologic.

Curvilinear calcifications in the cavernous carotid arteries and vertebrobasilar system are common. The significance of macrovascular calcification as a marker of microvascular disease is debated.

A few scattered patchy WM hypodensities are common, but confluent subcortical hypointensities, especially around the atria of the lateral ventricles, are a marker of arteriolosclerosis.

CECT scans demonstrate no foci of parenchymal enhancement in normal aging brains.

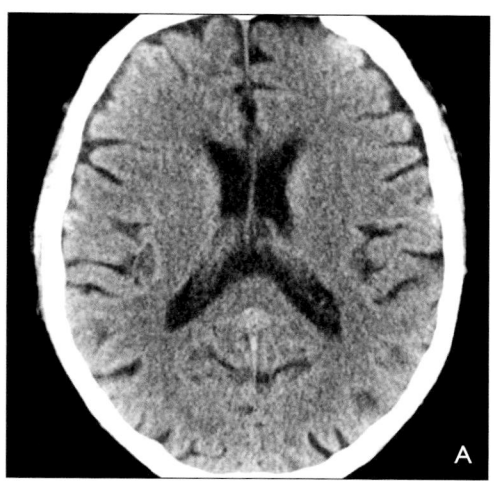

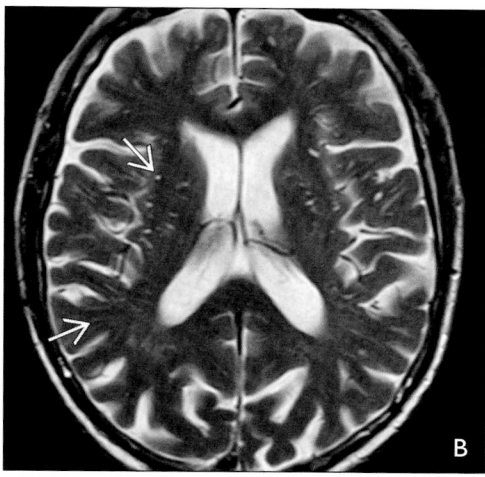

33-3A. NECT scan in a 71-year-old, neurologically normal man with a squamous cell carcinoma of the pinna shows mildly enlarged ventricles and sulci with normal-appearing white matter. 33-3B. T2WI in the same patient shows multifocal round and linear hyperintensities ➡ that probably represent prominent but normal perivascular spaces.

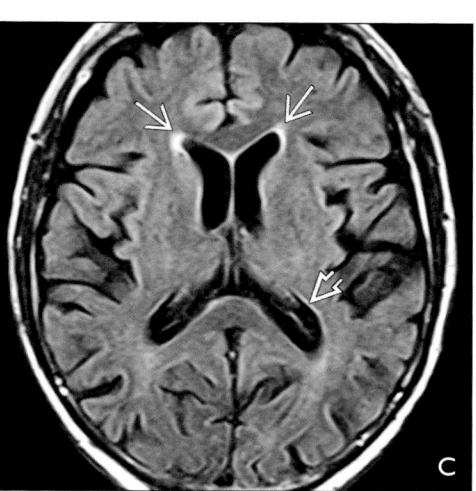

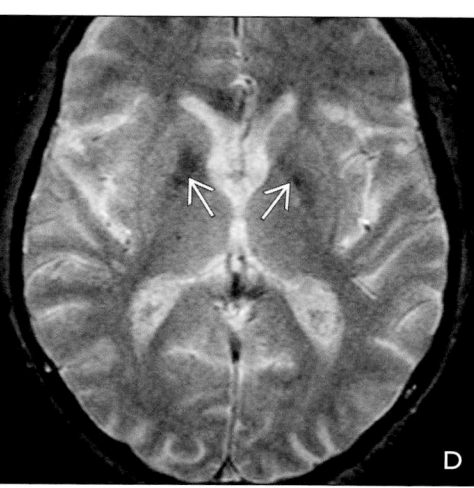

33-3C. FLAIR scan in the same patient shows frontal periventricular "caps" ➡ and a thin hyperintense rim around the lateral ventricles ➡. 33-3D. T2 GRE scan in the same patient shows hypointensity in the globi pallidi ➡ but not in the putamina or thalami. No microbleeds are present. Normal "successfully" aging brain.*

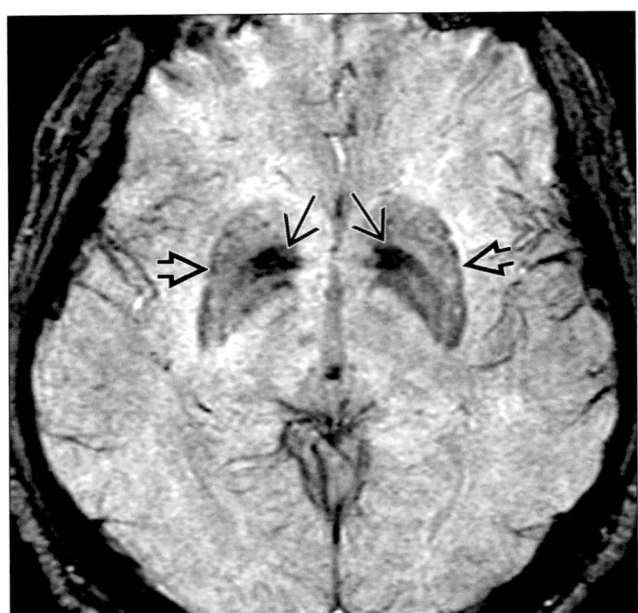

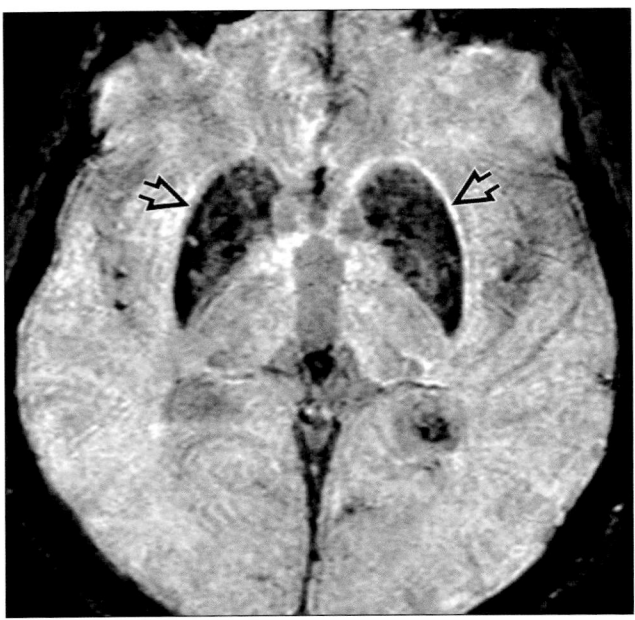

33-4. Axial 3.0 T SWI scan in a normal 65-year-old man shows striking hypointensity in the medial globi pallidi ⇥ with less prominent hypointensity in the putamina ⇗.

33-5. 3.0 T SWI in a normal 82-year-old woman shows moderate enlargement of third, lateral ventricles. BG are profoundly hypointense. Iron deposition in the putamina ⇗ is equal to that in the globi pallidi. Note absence of hypointensity in thalami.

MR Findings

T1WI. T1-weighted images show mild but symmetric ventricular enlargement and proportionate prominence of the subarachnoid spaces **(33-3)**. The corpus callosum may appear mildly thinned on sagittal T1 scans. Prominent perivascular spaces are a normal finding. They are filled with interstitial fluid (not CSF) but behave like CSF on all imaging sequences.

T2/FLAIR. White matter hyperintensities (WMHs) and lacunar infarcts on T2/FLAIR scans are highly prevalent in the elderly. They are associated with cardiovascular risk factors such as diabetes and hyperlipidemia. "Successfully" aging brains may demonstrate a few scattered nonconfluent WMHs (a reasonable number is one WMH per decade).

Perivascular spaces increase in prevalence and size with aging and are seen on T2WI as well-delineated round, ovoid, or linear CSF-like collections in the basal ganglia, subcortical WM, midbrain, etc. (see Chapter 28). PVSs suppress completely on FLAIR. Between 25-30% may display a thin, smooth, hyperintense rim. Lacunar infarcts typically demonstrate an irregular hyperintense rim around the lesions.

FLAIR scans in normal older patients demonstrate a smooth, thin, periventricular hyperintense rim around the lateral ventricles that probably represents increased extracellular interstitial fluid in the subependymal WM. A "cap" of hyperintensity around the frontal horns is common and normal.

T2* (GRE, SWI). Brain iron is not present at birth but gradually accumulates as part of normal development. Iron accumulation is greatest in the pars reticulata of the substantia nigra (SN), followed by the globus pallidus (GP), where iron deposition progresses from medial to lateral. The red nucleus and putamen are other common sites where ferritin normally accumulates. Iron deposition in the GP and SN plateaus in early adulthood, but iron storage in the putamen continues well past 80 years of age.

Ferric iron deposition is best demonstrated on T2* sequences. Susceptibility-weighted images (SWI) are more sensitive than gradient-refocussed (GRE) images. As field heterogeneity and magnetic susceptibility effects are proportional to field strength, hypointensity increases on 3.0 T images.

Hypointensity on T2* scans is normal in the medial globi pallidi **(33-4)**. Putaminal hypointensity is typically less prominent until the eighth decade. The caudate nucleus shows a scarce iron load at any age. The thalamus does not normally exhibit any hypointensity on T2* sequences **(33-5)**.

Microbleeds on T2* scans are common in the aging brain. GRE, SWI sequences demonstrate cerebral microbleeds in 20% of patients over age 60 years and one-third of patients aged 80 years and older. While common and therefore *statistically* "normal," microbleeds are not characteristic of *successful* brain aging. Basal ganglia and cerebellar microbleeds are usually indicative of chronic hypertensive encephalopathy. Lobar and cortical microbleeds are typical of amyloid angiopathy and are associated with worse cognitive performance.

DTI. The deleterious effect of WM changes on cognition depends on lesion burden, volume loss, and characteristics such as WM integrity that may not be apparent on standard imaging sequences. Even "normal-appearing white matter" may demonstrate loss of fractional anisotropy on DTI imaging.

MRS. MRS shows a gradual decrease in NAA in the cortex, cerebral WM, and temporal lobes with concomitant increases in both Cho and Cr.

FDG PET/pMR

FDG PET studies show a gradual decrease in rCBF with aging, particularly in the frontal lobes. Patients with low total brain perfusion on pMR studies have more WMHs, but the precise relationship to cognitive performance is unclear.

Differential Diagnosis

The correlation between cognitive performance and brain imaging is complex and difficult to determine. Therefore, the major differential diagnosis of a normal aging brain is **mild cognitive impairment** and early "preclinical" **Alzheimer disease**. WMHs are markers of microvascular disease, so there is considerable overlap between normal brains and those with **subcortical arteriosclerotic encephalopathy**.

ROTTERDAM IMAGING PARAMETERS OF BRAIN AGING
- Brain tissue volumes
  - Cortex
  - White matter
  - Sublocations (e.g., hippocampi)
- Volume of CSF-containing structures
  - Ventricles
  - Sulci
- White matter hyperintensities
- Infarcts
  - Lacunar
  - Cortical
- Iron deposition
  - Globus pallidus
  - Red nucleus
  - Substantia nigra
- Microbleeds
- White matter integrity and connectivity
- Cerebral blood flow
- Cerebral metabolism

Dementias

Dementia is an acquired impairment in intellectual abilities that affects multiple cognitive domains including memory, language, and visuospatial skills. Emotional lability, behavioral alterations, and deteriorating ability to execute the activities of daily living are common. Dementia is one of the greatest fears people have about aging.

The three most common dementias are **Alzheimer disease**, **dementia with Lewy bodies**, and **vascular dementia**. Together they account for the vast majority of all dementia cases. Less frequent causes include **frontotemporal lobar degeneration** (formerly known as Pick disease) and **corticobasal degeneration**. It can be difficult to distinguish between the various dementia syndromes, as clinical features frequently overlap and so-called mixed dementias are common.

As new disease-modifying agents enter clinical practice, correctly diagnosing dementia type is becoming increasingly important. Assessment of patients with a potential dementing illness requires a detailed clinical history and careful physical examination as well as evaluation of cognition, behavior, and functional and social capacity.

Currently there is no single behavioral marker that can reliably discriminate Alzheimer disease—by far the most common dementing disorder—from other major dementia syndromes. As imaging plays a growing role in the diagnosis of dementias, we discuss each major type. Where possible, we point out features and new imaging modalities that help distinguish the different types from potentially reversible nondementing disorders.

Alzheimer Disease

Terminology

Alzheimer disease (AD) is a progressive neurodegenerative condition that leads to cognitive decline, impaired ability to perform the activities of daily living, and a range of behavioral and psychological conditions.

AD is also known as senile dementia of Alzheimer type. There is increasing evidence that AD is not a single, all-encompassing disorder but instead a continuum of severity. The pathogenic process of AD is prolonged and may extend over several decades. A prodromal **preclinical/asymptomatic disease** (i.e., pathology is present but cognition remains intact) may exist for years before evidence of **mild cognitive impairment** (MCI) develops.

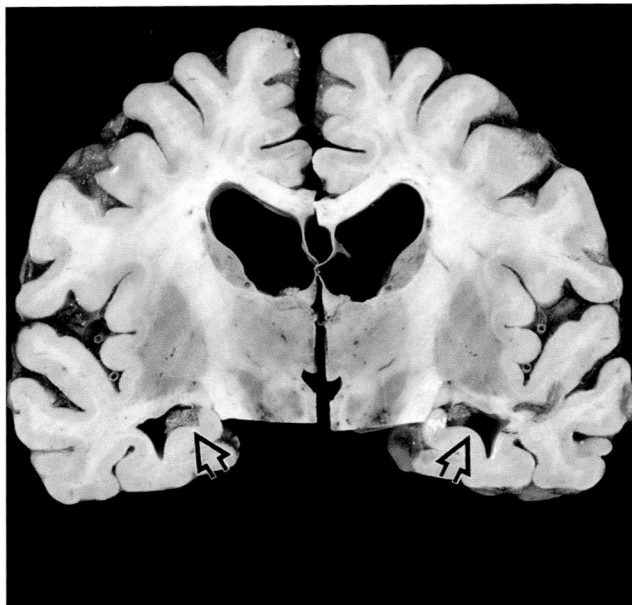

33-6. Coronal autopsy specimen from a patient with histologically proven early Alzheimer disease shows enlarged lateral ventricles. The temporal horns are proportionally enlarged, and the hippocampi ⊵ appear mildly atrophic.

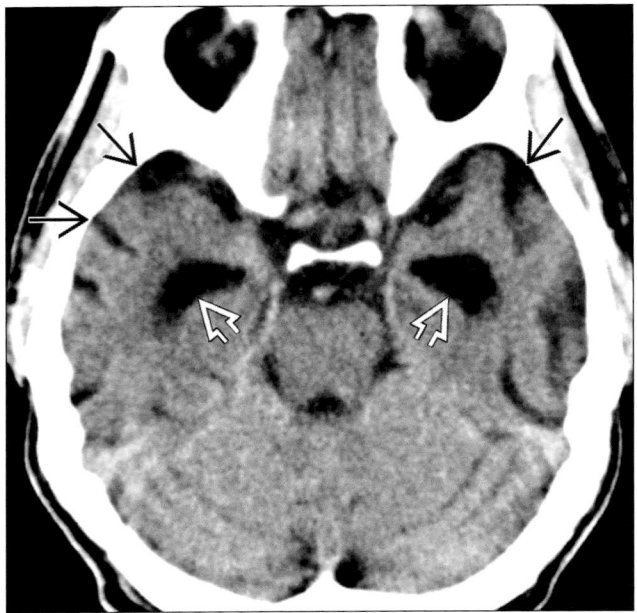

33-7. Axial NECT scan in a 54-year-old woman with severe early onset Alzheimer disease shows markedly enlarged temporal horns ➤, sulci ⇒.

Etiology

GENERAL CONCEPTS. AD is characterized pathophysiologically by an "amyloid cascade." Reduced clearance of the protein aggregate amyloid-β (Aβ) results in its abnormal accumulation in neurons. The Aβ42 residue is both insoluble and highly neurotoxic. Aβ42 clumps form **senile plaques** in the cortical gray matter. Aβ42 deposits also thicken the walls of cortical and leptomeningeal arterioles, causing **amyloid angiopathy**.

Another key feature of AD is **tauopathy**. Abnormal phosphorylation of a microtubule-associated protein known as "tau" eventually leads to the development of **neurofibrillary tangles** and **neuronal death**. CSF tau levels are almost tripled in patients with AD.

GENETICS. Approximately 10% of cases have a strong family history of AD. Almost all familial gene variation in AD points to *APP* (amyloid precursor protein), presenilin (*PSEN1*, *PSEN2*), and *APOE*E4* gene polymorphisms as the strongest inherited risk factors for AD.

Pathology

GROSS PATHOLOGY. Grossly, brains affected by AD show generalized atrophy with shrunken gyri, widened sulci, and enlarged lateral ventricles (especially the temporal horns). Changes are most marked in the medial temporal and parietal lobes (33-6). The frontal lobe is commonly involved, while the occipital lobe and motor cortex are relatively spared.

AD has distinct clinicopathological subtypes. The hippocampus is severely affected in 75% of cases. Relative hippocampal sparing is seen in 10%, and limbic-predominance accounts for 15% of AD cases.

MICROSCOPIC FEATURES. The three characteristic histologic hallmarks of AD are senile plaques, neurofibrillary tangles, and exaggerated neuronal loss. All are characteristic of—but none is specific for—AD.

AD also often coexists with other pathologies such as cerebrovascular disease or Lewy bodies. Variable amounts of amyloid deposition in arterioles of the cortex and leptomeninges (amyloid angiopathy) are present in over 90% of AD cases. There is compelling evidence that vascular pathology and AD pathology are additive and that patients with a combination of both have clinically more severe dementia.

STAGING, GRADING, AND CLASSIFICATION. There are several scales for the histologic staging of Alzheimer pathology. One of the most widely used—the Braak and Braak system—is based on the topographic distribution of neurofibrillary tangles and neuropil threads, with grades from 1 to 6. The CERAD (Consortium to Establish a Registry for Alzheimer Disease) scale is based on the quantity of neocortical neuritic plaques in relation to age.

A third system (the Poly Pathology AD Assessment 9 or PPAD9) is based not just on NFTs and neuritic plaques but a combination of other factors, including the extent of neuronal degeneration, microvacuolization, cytoarchi-

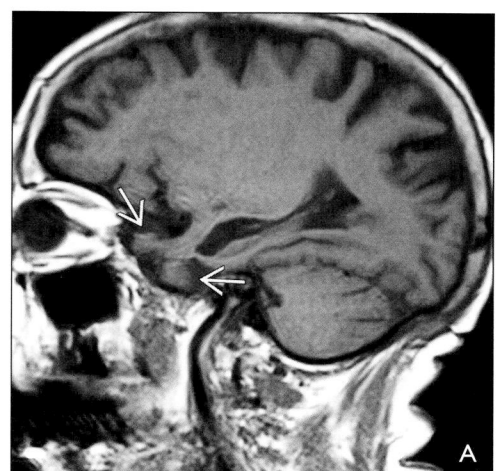

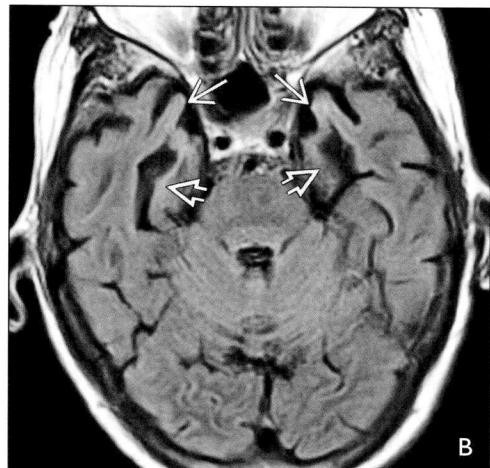

33-8A. *Sagittal T1WI in a 67-year-old woman with clinically definite AD shows markedly atrophic temporal lobe* ➡. ***33-8B.*** *Axial FLAIR in the same patient shows severely shrunken, hyperintense hippocampi* ➡ *and medial temporal lobes* ➡.

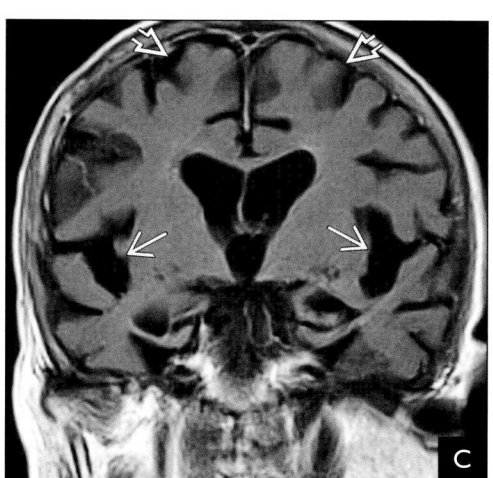

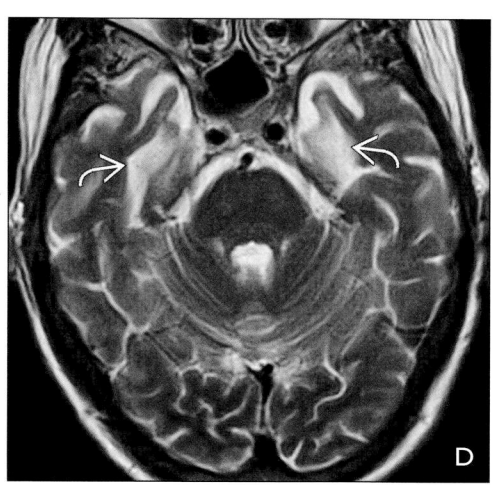

33-8C. *Coronal FLAIR shows the striking temporal lobe atrophy with enlarged sylvian fissures* ➡, *relative preservation of frontal lobe volume* ➡. ***33-8D.*** *T2WI shows that the temporal horns of the lateral ventricles are markedly enlarged* ➡.

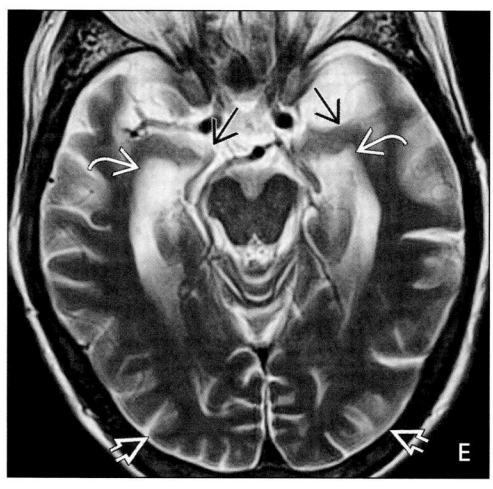

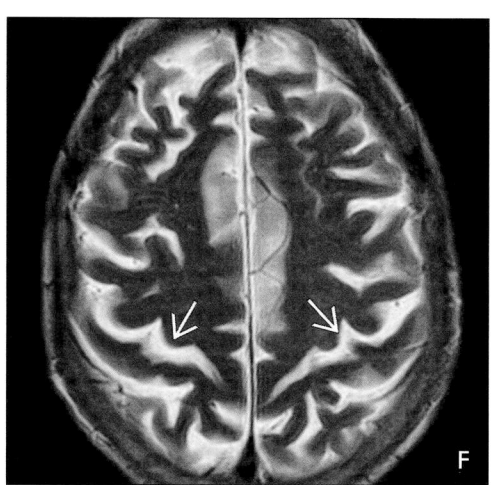

33-8E. *More cephalad T2WI in the same patient shows enlarged temporal horns* ➡, *disproportionate volume loss in the temporal lobes* ➡ *compared to the normal-appearing occipital lobes* ➡. ***33-8F.*** *Scan through the upper cerebral hemispheres shows symmetric parietal lobe atrophy* ➡.

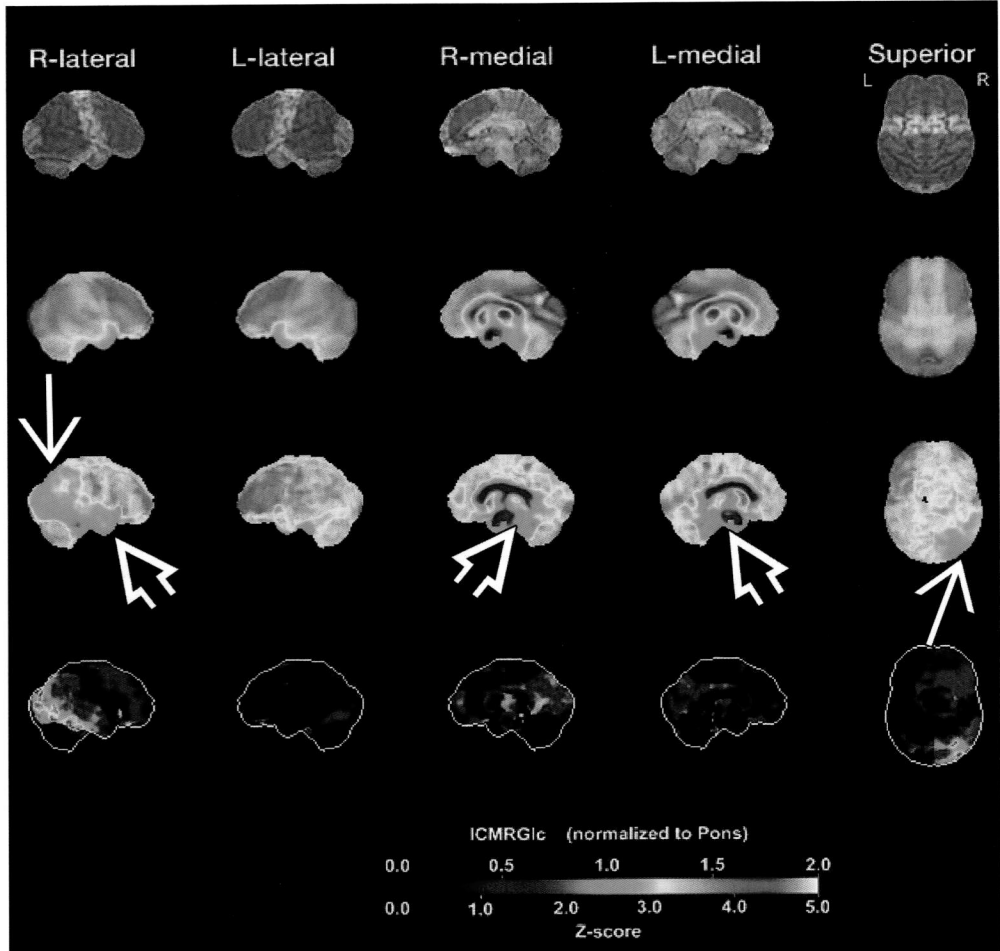

33-9. *Sagittal FDG PET with stereotactic surface projections in a 70-year-old woman with possible AD. Standard MR had disclosed no visible abnormalities. Top row = reference map. Second row = glucose metabolism in normal elderly control group. Third row = patient's glucose metabolism map. Note striking decrease in the medial temporal ⧉ and parietal lobes ⧉ with sparing of the frontal, occipital lobes. Bottom row = Z-score map. (Courtesy N. Foster, MD.)*

tectural disorder, and gliosis. Each finding is calculated for nine different regions of the brain.

To date, correlation between these major staging systems is suboptimal. Choice of staging system affects the evaluation of AD pathology and therefore the final diagnosis.

Clinical Issues

EPIDEMIOLOGY AND DEMOGRAPHICS. AD is the most common cause of dementia, accounting for approximately 50-60% of all cases and affecting more than 35 million people worldwide. The World Alzheimer Report predicts that this number will almost double by 2030 and will exceed 100 million by 2050.

Age is the biggest risk factor for developing AD. The prevalence of AD is 1-2% at age 65 and increases by 15-25% each decade. In the "oldest-old" patients (more than 90 years), mixed pathologies—typically AD plus vascular dementia—predominate.

DIAGNOSIS. Historically, the *definitive* diagnosis of AD was made only by biopsy or autopsy. The *clinical* diagnosis of AD using NINCDS-ADRA (National Institute of Neurological Disorders and Stroke-Alzheimer Disease and Related Disorders) criteria defines three levels of certainty: Possible, probable, and definite AD. The diagnosis of definite AD currently requires the clinical diagnosis of probable AD *plus* neuropathological confirmation.

The Alzheimer Disease Neuroimaging Initiative (ADNI) is an ongoing longitudinal, multicenter study designed to identify clinical, imaging, genetic, and biochemical biomarkers for the early detection and tracking of AD. ADNI research protocols have identified new imaging modalities and CSF biomarkers that may eventually help differentiate healthy from pathological aging.

PRESENTATION. Minimal cognitive impairment causes a slight but noticeable (and measurable) decline in cognitive abilities. The mildest MCI is a single cognitive domain (amnestic) form that is characterized by memory loss beyond that expected for age and education. Here global cognitive function is maintained and the capacity to perform activities of daily living is preserved.

Individuals with MCI do not meet the diagnostic guidelines for dementia but are nevertheless at increased risk of eventually developing AD or another type of dementia.

Patients with very early AD show impaired short-term memory. As the disease progresses, memory deficits increase and are associated with neuropsychiatric changes, difficulties in word-finding, spatial cognition, and reduced executive functioning. Motor, sensory, and gait disturbances are uncommon until relatively late in the disease.

NATURAL HISTORY AND TREATMENT OPTIONS. AD is a chronic disease. Progression is gradual, and patients live an average of 8-10 years after diagnosis. Between 5-10% of patients with MCI progress to probable AD each year.

There are no established treatments to prevent or reverse AD. Many current disease-modifying drugs focus on reducing Aβ amyloidosis. Treating MCI patients with cholinesterase inhibitors or NMDA receptor antagonists may transiently improve cognitive functioning but does not delay conversion from MCI to AD.

Imaging

GENERAL FEATURES. One of the most important goals of routine CT and MR imaging is to identify specific abnormalities that could support the clinical diagnosis of AD. The other major role is to exclude alternative etiologies that can mimic AD clinically, i.e., "causes of reversible dementia" (see below).

The introduction of radiotracers for the noninvasive in vivo quantification of Aβ burden in the brain has revolutionized the approach to the imaging evaluation of AD.

CT FINDINGS. NECT is a helpful screening procedure that may exclude potentially reversible or treatable causes of dementia such as subdural hematoma and normal pressure hydrocephalus. Otherwise, CT scans are generally uninformative, especially in the early stages of AD.

Medial temporal lobe atrophy is generally the earliest identifiable finding on CT **(33-7)**. Late findings include generalized cortical atrophy.

MR FINDINGS. The current role of conventional MR in the evaluation of patients with dementing disorders is to (1) exclude other causes of dementia, (2) identify region-specific patterns of brain volume loss (e.g., "lobar-predominant" atrophy), and (3) identify imaging markers of comorbid vascular disease such as amyloid angiopathy.

The most common morphologic changes on standard MR are thinned gyri, widened sulci, and enlarged lateral ven-

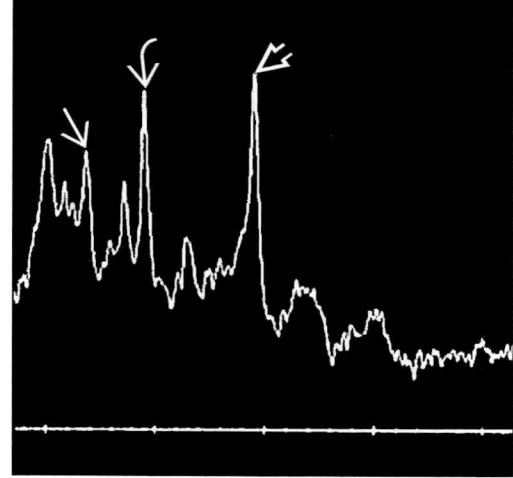

33-10. MRS in AD shows elevated myoinositol (mI) peak ➡. The NAA ➡ to mI ratio is decreased; creatine (Cr) peak ➡ is decreased.

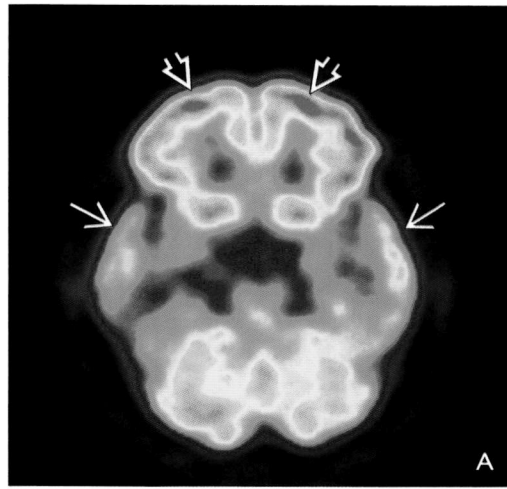

33-11A. 18F FDG PET in AD shows markedly reduced metabolism in both temporal lobes ➡ with comparatively normal frontal lobes ➡.

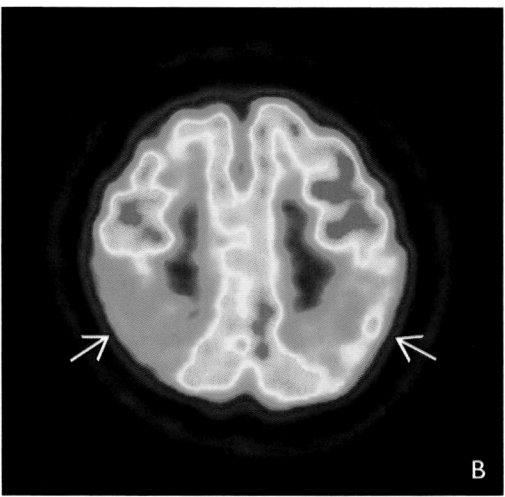

33-11B. Parietal hypometabolism ➡ on cephalad scan. Temporal/parietal hypometabolism, preserved frontal activity is characteristic of AD.

tricles. The medial temporal lobe—particularly the hippocampus and entorhinal cortex—are often disproportionately affected **(33-8)**. High-resolution imaging (T1-weighted MP-RAGE or SPGR sequences) with multiplanar reconstructions are ADNI-recommended sequences. Automated or semiautomated computer-assisted volumetric analysis of the hippocampi and parahippocampal gyri may help distinguish patients with MCI from the normal elderly.

T2* (GRE, SWI) sequences are much more sensitive than standard FSE in detecting cortical microhemorrhages that may suggest amyloid angiopathy.

MRS shows decreased NAA and increased mI in patients with AD, even during the early stages of the disease **(33-10)**. The NAA:mI ratio is relatively sensitive and highly specific in differentiating AD patients from the normal elderly. NAA:Cr ratio in the posterior cingulate gyri and left occipital cortex predicts conversion from MCI to probable AD with relatively high sensitivity and good specificity.

DTI in patients with AD shows decreased FA in multiple regions, especially the superior longitudinal fasciculus and corpus callosum splenium. Reduced FA reflects early microstructural WM changes.

FUNCTIONAL NEUROIMAGING. Morphologic brain pathology is often present years before clinical onset and can only be visualized using special imaging studies. fMRI shows decrease in intensity and/or extent of activation in the frontal and temporal regions in cognitive tasks, especially those that require semantic or phonological decisions.

pMR may demonstrate subtly reduced rCBV in the temporal and parietal lobes in patients with MCI.

NUCLEAR MEDICINE. 18F FDG PET demonstrates areas of regional hypometabolism and helps distinguish AD from other lobar-predominant dementias (e.g., frontotemporal lobar degeneration) **(33-9)**, **(33-11)**.

PET using amyloid-binding radiotracers such as 11C PiB (Pittsburgh compound B) has emerged as one of the best techniques for early AD diagnosis. As new therapies enter clinical trials, the importance of in vivo Aβ imaging is becoming increasingly crucial.

Aβ burden as measured by PET matches histopathological reports of Aβ distribution in aging and dementia. It appears more accurate than 18F FDG PET and is an excellent tool in differentiating AD from frontotemporal lobar degeneration (FTLD).

Although Aβ burden as assessed by PET does not correlate strongly with cognitive impairment in AD, it does correlate with memory impairment and risk of cog-

nitive decline in aging patients. The correlation with memory impairment—one of the earliest symptoms of AD—suggests that Aβ deposition is not part of normal aging. Aβ deposition occurs well before symptom onset and likely represents preclinical AD in asymptomatic individuals and prodromal AD in patients with MCI.

Differential Diagnosis

Distinguishing between **normal age-related degenerative processes** and early "preclinical" AD is difficult. There is no generally available way to distinguish between the two, although FDG PET is helpful.

"Mixed dementias" are common, especially in patients over the age of 90 years. **Vascular dementia** (VaD) is the most common dementia associated with AD. Lacunar and cortical infarcts are typical findings in VaD. **Cerebral amyloid angiopathy** often coexists with AD. **Lewy bodies** are sometimes found in AD patients ("Lewy body variant of AD").

Frontotemporal lobar degeneration shows frontal and/or anterior temporal atrophy and hypometabolism; the parietal lobes are generally spared. **Dementia with Lewy bodies** typically demonstrates generalized, nonfocal hypometabolism. Patients with **corticobasal degeneration** have prominent extrapyramidal symptoms.

Causes of reversible dementia that can be identified on imaging studies include mass lesions such as chronic subdural hematoma or neoplasm, vitamin deficiencies (thiamine, B12), endocrinopathy (e.g., hypothyroidism), and normal pressure hydrocephalus.

ALZHEIMER DISEASE

Pathoetiology
- Neurotoxic "amyloid cascade"
  - Aβ42 accumulation → senile plaques, amyloid angiopathy
- Tauopathy → neurofibrillary tangles, neuronal death

Clinical Issues
- Most common dementia (50-60% of all cases)
- Prevalence increases 15-25% per decade after 65 years

Imaging
- Frontoparietal dominant lobar atrophy
  - Hippocampus, entorhinal cortex
  - FDG PET shows hypometabolism
  - Amyloid-binding radiotracers (11C PiB)
- Amyloid angiopathy → T2* "blooming black dots"

Differential Diagnosis
- Exclude reversible dementias!
- Normal aging, vascular dementia, frontotemporal lobar degeneration

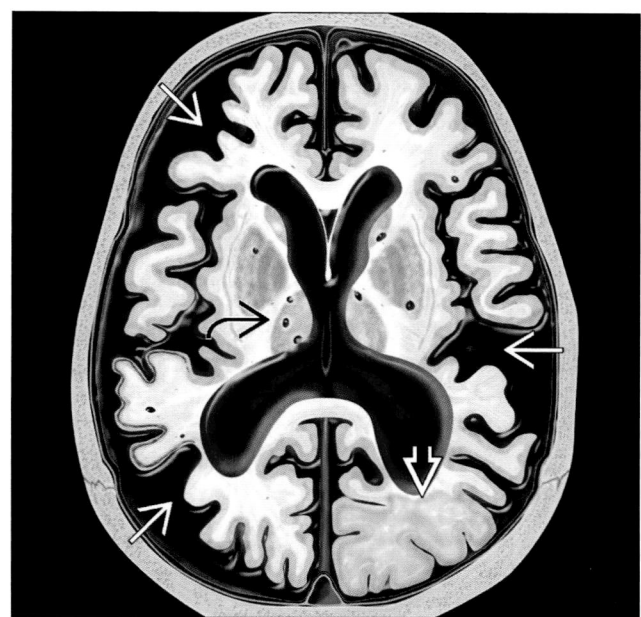

33-12. Axial graphic of vascular dementia shows diffuse cerebral atrophy, focal volume loss due to multiple chronic infarcts ➡, an acute left occipital lobe infarct ➡, and small lacunar infarcts in the basal ganglia/thalami ➡.

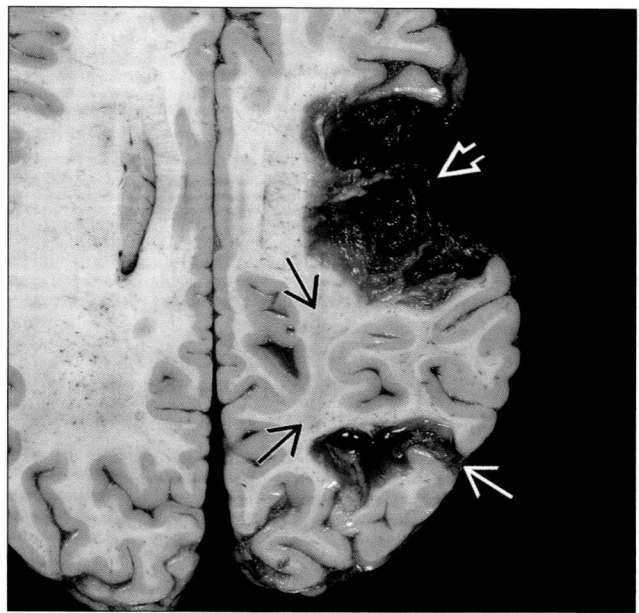

33-13. Autopsy specimen shows large territorial ➡ and smaller cortical ➡ infarcts, as well as WM lesions ➡ in the left hemisphere. Large infarcts are a less common cause of VaD than diffuse small vessel disease. (Courtesy R. Hewlett, MD.)

Vascular Dementia

Cerebrovascular disease is a common cause of cognitive decline. The burden of "silent" microvascular disease and its long-term deleterious effect on cognition is becoming increasingly well-recognized.

Terminology

Vascular dementia (VaD) is sometimes also called multi-infarct dementia, vascular cognitive disorder, vascular cognitive impairment, subcortical ischemic vascular dementia, and post-stroke dementia. All are broadly encompassing terms for cognitive dysfunction associated with—and presumed to be caused by—vascular brain damage.

Etiology

VaD is usually an acquired disease caused by the cumulative burden of cerebrovascular lesions. While any vessel—small or large—can be affected, the majority of cases are microvascular angiopathies (see below).

Rarely, VaD is caused by an inherited disorder such as **c**erebral **a**utosomal **d**ominant **a**rteriopathy with **s**ubcortical **i**nfarcts and **l**eukoencephalopathy (CADASIL) or mitochondrial encephalopathy. CADASIL is the most common hereditary stroke disorder and is caused by *NOTCH3* mutations on chromosome 19.

Pathology

GROSS PATHOLOGY. The most common readily identifiable gross finding in VaD is multiple infarcts with focal atrophy (33-12), (33-13). Cortical branch occlusions and large territorial infarcts are less common than multiple subcortical lacunar infarcts or widespread white matter ischemia.

MICROSCOPIC FEATURES. Vessel wall modifications are the most common and presumably the earliest identifiable changes associated with VaD. **Arteriolosclerosis** and **amyloid angiopathy** are the major underlying pathologies in small vessel vascular disease. Myelin loss and modifications in perivascular spaces are the next most common vascular findings in dementia.

So-called **microinfarcts**—minute foci of neuronal loss, gliosis, pallor, or frank cystic degeneration—and other cerebrovascular lesions are seen at autopsy in nearly two-thirds of patients with VaD and more than half of all cases with other dementing disorders (e.g., Alzheimer disease [AD], dementia with Lewy bodies). Lesions are found in all brain regions and are especially common in the cortex, subcortical WM, and basal ganglia.

Clinical Issues

EPIDEMIOLOGY AND DEMOGRAPHICS. Vascular dementia is the second most common cause of dementia (after AD) and accounts for approximately 10% of all dementia cases in developed countries. VaD is a common component of "mixed" dementias and is especially prevalent in patients with Alzheimer disease.

The incidence of VaD increases with age. Risk factors include hypertension, diabetes, dyslipidemia, and smoking. There is a moderate male predominance.

PRESENTATION. A history of multiple stroke-like episodes with focal neurologic deficits is characteristic of patients with VaD. Mood and behavioral changes are more typical than memory loss.

NATURAL HISTORY. Progressive, episodic, stepwise neurologic deterioration interspersed with intervals of relative clinical stabilization is the typical pattern of VaD.

Imaging

GENERAL FEATURES. The general imaging features of VaD are those of multifocal infarcts and WM ischemia.

CT FINDINGS. NECT scans often show generalized volume loss with multiple cortical, subcortical, and basal ganglia infarcts. Patchy or confluent hypodensities in the subcortical and deep periventricular WM, especially around the atria of the lateral ventricles, are typical.

MR FINDINGS. T1WI often shows greater than expected generalized volume loss. Multiple hypointensities in the basal ganglia and deep WM are typical. Focal cortical and large territorial infarcts with encephalomalacia can be identified in many cases.

T2/FLAIR scans show multifocal diffuse and confluent hyperintensities in the basal ganglia and cerebral WM. The cortex and subcortical WM are commonly affected **(33-14A)**, **(33-14B)**, **(33-14C)**. T2* sequences may demonstrate multiple "blooming" hypointensities in the cortex and along the pial surface of the hemispheres **(33-15)**, **(33-16)**.

DTI may demonstrate decreased FA and increased ADC values in otherwise normal-appearing or minimally abnormal WM. Multiple regions are affected, especially the inferior-frontal-occipital fascicles, corpus callosum, and superior longitudinal fasciculus.

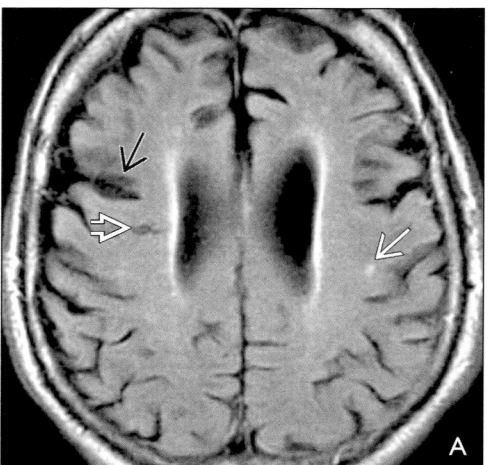
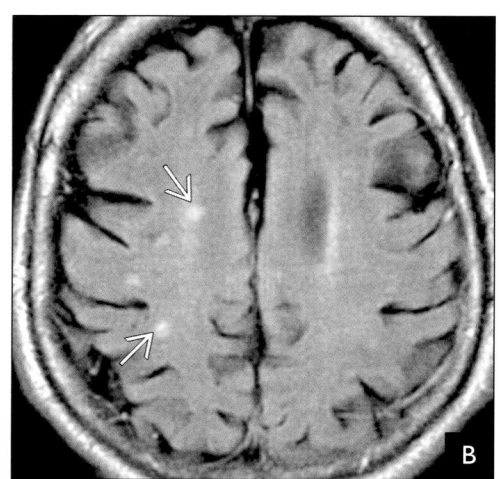

33-14A. Axial FLAIR in an 82-year-old woman with VaD shows a small lacunar infarct ➡, a focal cortical infarct ➡, subcortical WM hyperintensities ➡. 33-14B. More cephalad FLAIR scan in the same patient shows additional WM hyperintensities ➡.

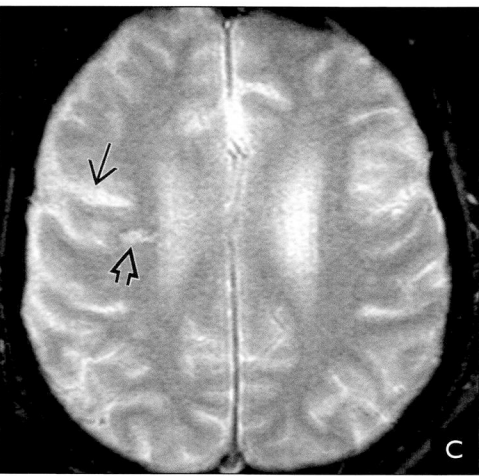
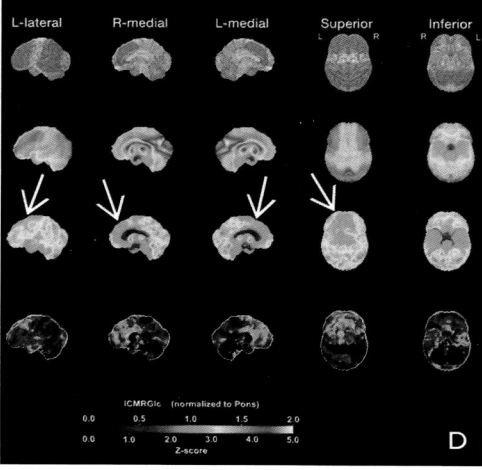

33-14C. T2 GRE sequence in the same patient shows the lacunar ➡ and cortical ➡ infarcts but no "blooming" hypointensities suggestive of amyloid angiopathy. 33-14D. PET scan shows normal age-matched controls (second row) and the patient's scan (third row). Note multifocal cortical areas of decreased glucose metabolism ➡. Z-score map (bottom) shows severely affected areas in green. (Courtesy N. Foster, MD.)*

NUCLEAR MEDICINE. FDG PET shows multiple diffusely distributed areas of hypometabolism, generally without specific lobar predominance **(33-14D)**, **(33-15D)**.

Differential Diagnosis

The major differential diagnosis of VaD is **Alzheimer disease**. The two disorders overlap and often coexist. AD typically shows striking and selective volume loss in the temporal lobes, especially the hippocampi. The basal ganglia are typically spared in AD, whereas they are often affected in VaD.

CADASIL is the most common *inherited* cause of VaD. Onset is typically earlier than in *sporadic* VaD. Large territorial infarcts are less common in CADASIL compared to VaD; anterior temporal and external capsule lesions are highly suggestive of CADASIL.

Frontotemporal lobar degeneration is characterized by early onset of behavior changes while visuospatial skills remain relatively unaffected. Frontotemporal atrophy with knife-like gyri is typical.

Dementia with Lewy bodies (DLB) may be difficult to distinguish from VaD without biopsy. The entire brain is hypometabolic, and atrophy is generally minimal or absent. DLB typically occurs without infarcts.

Cerebral amyloid angiopathy commonly coexists with both Alzheimer disease and VaD and may be indistinguishable without biopsy.

Alcoholic encephalopathy is the third most common cause of dementia worldwide. Generalized volume loss with focal involvement of the superior vermis is typical.

Vitamin B12 levels in the subclinical low-normal range (less than 250 ρmol/L) are associated with AD, VaD, and Parkinson disease. This small subset of dementias is reversible with vitamin B12 therapy, which is inexpensive and safe.

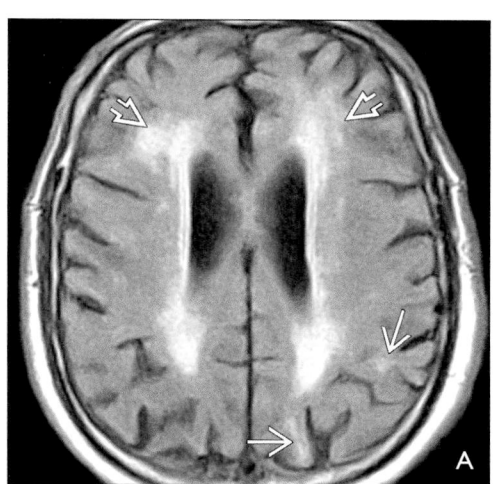

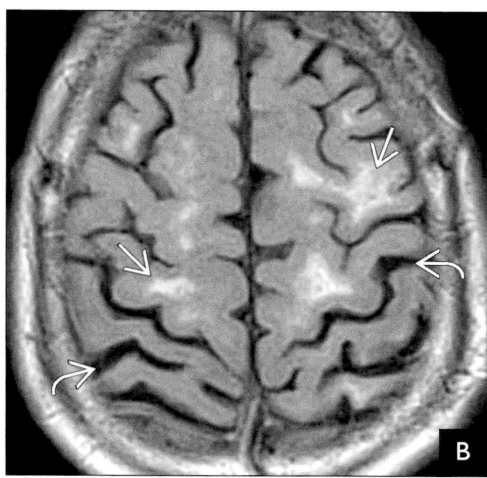

33-15A. *FLAIR scan in a 76-year-old normotensive demented man shows multifocal confluent hyperintensities in the subcortical* ➡️, *deep periventricular WM* ➡️.
33-15B. *More cephalad FLAIR scan in the same patient shows significant lesion burden in the subcortical WM* ➡️. *Note enlarged parietal sulci* ➡️.

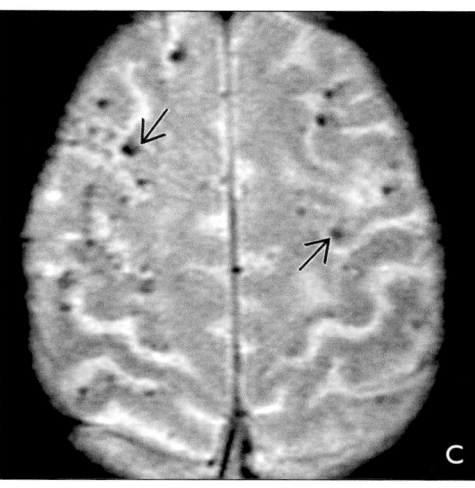

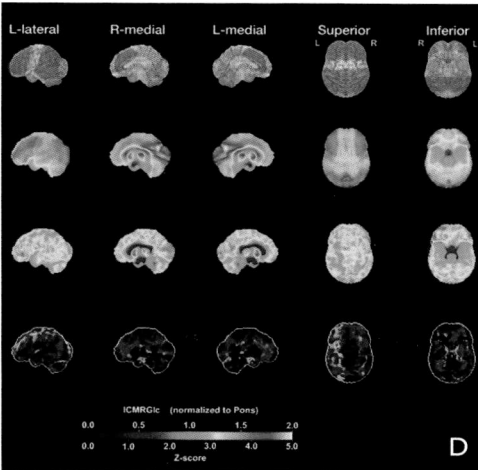

33-15C. *T2* GRE scan in the same patient shows multifocal cortical "blooming" hypointensities* ➡️ *characteristic of cerebral amyloid angiopathy.* *33-15D.* *PET scan in the same patient shows multifocal areas of decreased glucose metabolism (third row) compared to age-matched normal controls (second row). Z-score map (bottom row) shows the diffuse nature of the lesions seen in VaD. (Courtesy N. Foster, MD.)*

VASCULAR DEMENTIA

Pathoetiology
- Multiple ischemic episodes
- Can be small, large vessel
- Atherosclerosis, arteriolosclerosis, amyloid angiopathy

Clinical Issues
- Second most common dementia (10%)
- Commonly mixed with other dementias (e.g., AD)
- Multiple strokes; episodic step-like deterioration

Imaging
- Multifocal infarcts (lacunae, cortical > large territorial)
- WM ischemia
- T2* "blooming black dots" (amyloid or hypertension-associated)

Differential Diagnosis
- Alzheimer disease
- CADASIL (most common *inherited* VaD)
- Frontotemporal lobar degeneration
- Dementia with Lewy bodies
- Nutrition-related dementias

Frontotemporal Dementias

Terminology

The frontotemporal dementias are a heterogeneous family of disorders characterized by selective involvement of the frontal and temporal lobes. They were formerly lumped together and known collectively as Pick disease. The term **Pick disease** is now reserved for cases with widespread presence of so-called Pick bodies, round silver-staining intraneuronal inclusions that contain several proteins including tau (a complex protein that regulates microtubule dynamics).

The term **frontotemporal lobar degeneration** (FTLD) is a gross anatomical description for the relatively selective atrophy of the frontal and temporal lobes that characterizes most—but by no means all—frontotemporal dementias. This characteristic atrophy is caused by pathologic processes that vary in their microscopic and molecular features (see below).

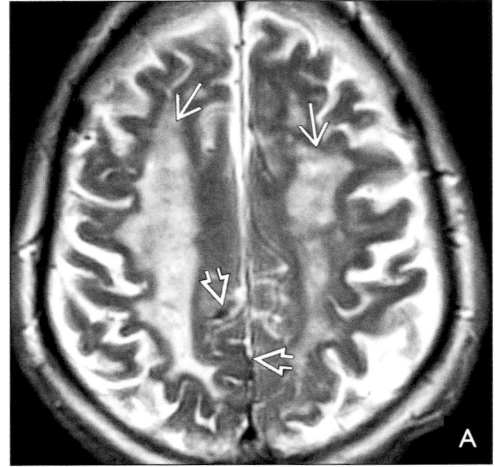
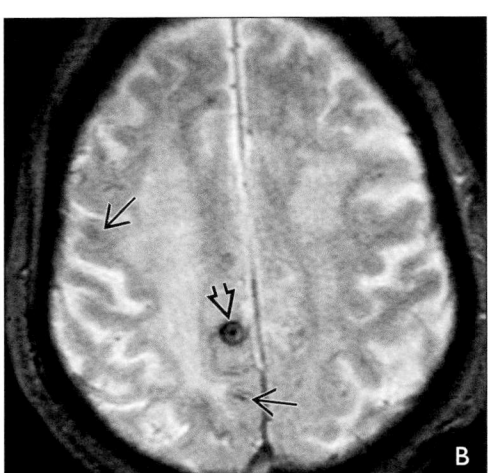

33-16A. Axial T2WI in a 76-year-old woman with a history of multiple strokes and clinical diagnosis of VaD shows generalized volume loss with confluent subcortical WM hyperintensity ➡. Insensitivity of FSE scans to hemorrhage is demonstrated by this case; only faint hypointensities ➡ can be identified. 33-16B. T2* GRE shows a round, focal "blooming" lesion ➡ with several faint linear hypointensities ➡.

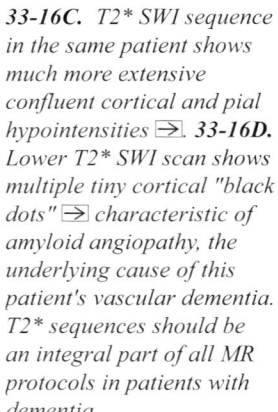
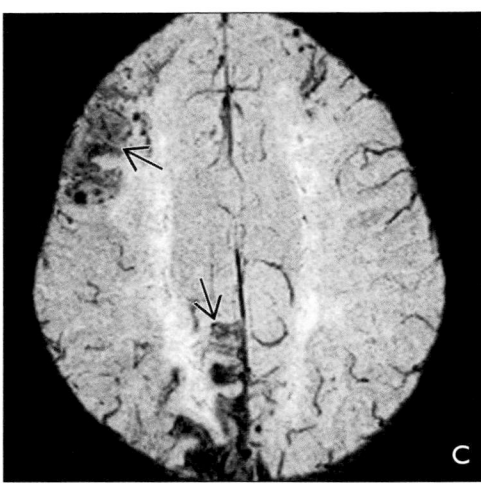
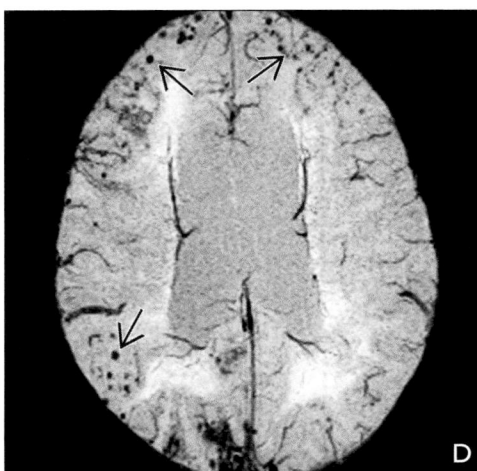

33-16C. T2* SWI sequence in the same patient shows much more extensive confluent cortical and pial hypointensities ➡. 33-16D. Lower T2* SWI scan shows multiple tiny cortical "black dots" ➡ characteristic of amyloid angiopathy, the underlying cause of this patient's vascular dementia. T2* sequences should be an integral part of all MR protocols in patients with dementia.

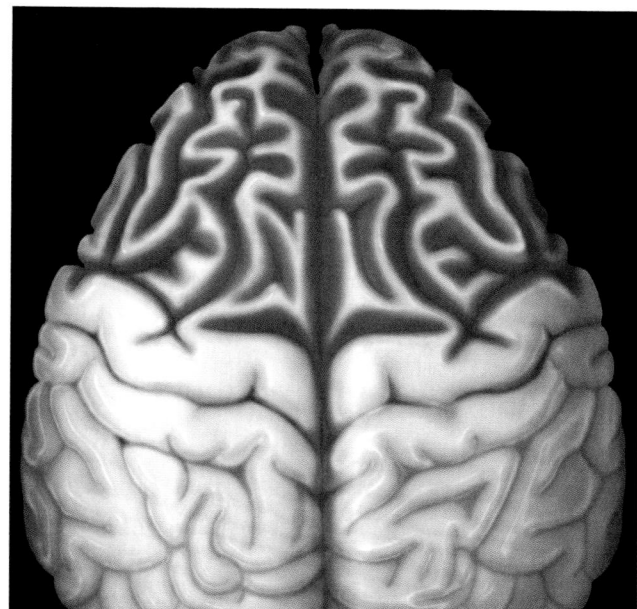

33-17. Graphic depicts the classic disproportionate frontal lobe atrophy of late-stage frontotemporal dementia. The sulci are widened, and the gyri are knife-like. Parietooccipital lobes are spared. Gyri around the central sulcus are normal.

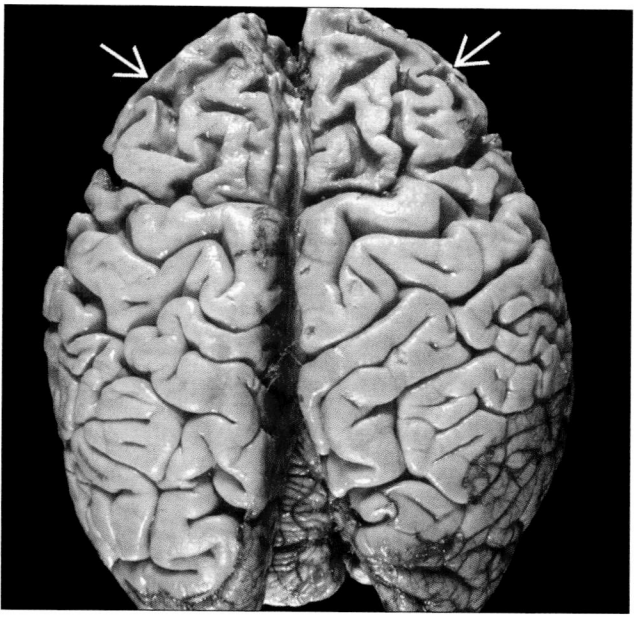

33-18. Autopsy specimen of frontotemporal lobar degeneration shows striking atrophy of the frontal gyri ➡ with normal-appearing parietal, occipital lobes. (Courtesy R. Hewlett, MD.)

Etiology

GENERAL CONCEPTS. While there are a number of entities included in the frontotemporal dementias, one of the most frequent is tau-positive **frontotemporal lobar degeneration** (FTLD-TAU). Some less common sporadic tauopathies overlap with FTLD clinically, neuropathologically, and genetically and are now recognized as forming a single disease spectrum.

Corticobasal degeneration, **progressive supranuclear palsy**, and **amyotrophic lateral sclerosis parkinsonism-dementia complex** are all part of the expanded family of frontotemporal dementias. As their imaging findings are quite different from those of classic FTLD, these disorders are considered separately below under "Miscellaneous Degenerations."

GENETICS. The normal brain contains six isoforms of tau, with either three (3R-) or four (4R-) microtubule-binding repeats. Mutations lead to abnormal accumulations in neurons and/or glia. Most sporadic tauopathies (including corticobasal degeneration and progressive supranuclear palsy) have predominant 4R-tau deposition, although Pick bodies contain predominantly or exclusively 3R-tau.

Most cases of FTLD are sporadic. However, 20-30% are familial and exhibit an autosomal dominant pattern of inheritance. Approximately 10% are caused by mutations in the microtubule-associated protein tau gene (*MAPT*), and 10% have mutations in the progranulin gene (*GRN*). A highly penetrant repeat hexanucleotide expansion on chromosome 9p21 (*C9ORF72*) has been associated with both FTLD and ALS.

Pathology

GROSS PATHOLOGY. FTLDs are characterized by severe frontotemporal atrophy with neuronal loss, gliosis, and spongiosis of the superficial cortical layers (33-17). The affected gyri are thinned and narrowed, causing the typical appearance of knife-like gyri. The posterior brain regions, especially the occipital poles, are relatively spared until very late in the disease process (33-18).

MICROSCOPIC FEATURES. FTLD-related tauopathies are classified according to both the morphologic features and the biochemical composition of tau inclusions. Pick disease—the prototypical FTLD tauopathy—is characterized by the presence of Pick bodies, round or oval argyrophilic (silver-staining) inclusions in the cytoplasm of neurons. Pick bodies are most commonly found in the dentate gyrus, amygdala, and frontal and temporal neocortex.

STAGING, GRADING, AND CLASSIFICATION. A new *histopathologic* classification of FTLD defines four major categories based on the presence or absence of specific cellular inclusion bodies: (1) FTLD with tau inclusions (FTLD-TAU), (2) FTLD with tau-negative and TDP-43-positive inclusions (FTLD-TDP), (3) FTLD with tau/TDP-negative and fused-in sarcoma (FUS)-positive inclusions (FTLD-FUS), and (4) FTLD with positive immunohistochemistry against proteins of the ubiquitin proteasome system (FTLD-UPS).

Clinical Issues

EPIDEMIOLOGY AND DEMOGRAPHICS. FTLD is the second most common cause of "presenile dementia," accounting for 20% of all cases in patients under the age of 65 years. Excluding alcoholic encephalopathy, it is the third most common overall cause of dementia. FTLD constitutes 10-25% of all dementia cases. The estimated prevalence varies between 5-15 cases/100,000.

PRESENTATION. Mean age of onset is younger than seen in AD and other neurodegenerative dementias. FTLD occurs between the third and ninth decades, but the peak incidence is between 45 and 65 years of age.

Three different *clinical* subtypes of frontotemporal dementia (FTD) are recognized. The most common is **behavioral-variant frontotemporal dementia** (bvFTD), which is characterized by changes in personality and social conduct. In contrast to AD, visuospatial functions are initially well-preserved.

The other two FTLD syndromes are language-variant types. **Progressive nonfluent aphasia** (PNFA) is a dis-

order of language output that may occur in the absence of impairment in other cognitive domains. Patients with **semantic dementia** (SD) exhibit behavioral changes and difficulties with language comprehension while speech itself remains relatively fluent.

The correlation between histopathology and clinical syndromes varies. bvFTD is histopathologically heterogeneous while SD is usually associated with TDP pathology and PNFA with tau pathology.

NATURAL HISTORY. Median survival for patients with FTLD is 6-11 years following symptom onset.

Imaging

GENERAL FEATURES. Neuroimaging features of the frontotemporal dementias should be assessed according to whether they produce focal temporal or extratemporal (e.g., frontal) atrophy, whether the pattern is relatively symmetric or strongly asymmetric, and which side (left versus right) is most severely affected.

CT FINDINGS. Abnormalities on CT represent late-stage FTLD. Severe symmetric atrophy of the frontal lobes

33-19A. NECT scan in a 59-year-old man with FTLD shows striking frontal atrophy with knife-like gyri ➡. Note temporal lobe atrophy ➡ with markedly enlarged sylvian fissures. The parietal, occipital lobes appear normal. 33-19B. More cephalad scan in the same patient shows the frontal-predominant atrophy ➡ especially well. The parietal sulci are also moderately prominent for a patient of this age.

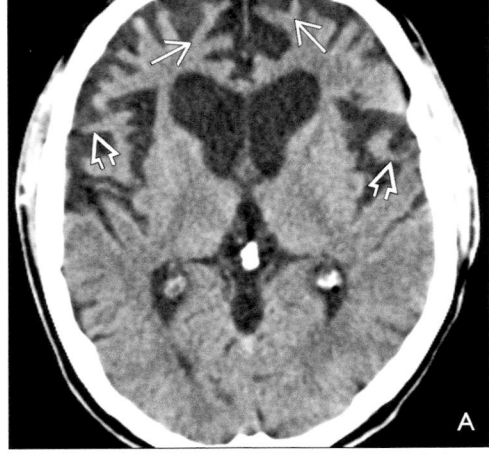 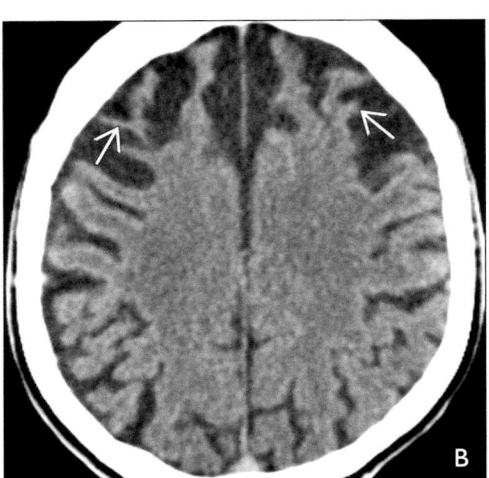

33-19C. FDG PET in the same patient shows markedly decreased glucose metabolism in both frontal lobes ➡. The temporal lobes ➡ are somewhat less severely affected. The occipital lobes both appear normal. 33-19D. More cephalad scan in the same patient shows striking frontal hypometabolism ➡, but the parietal lobes also show moderately reduced glucose utilization.

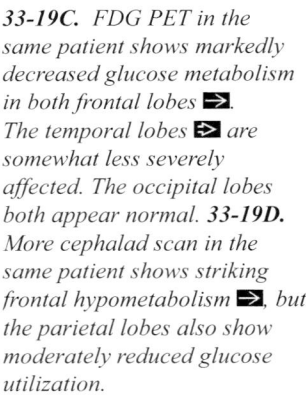 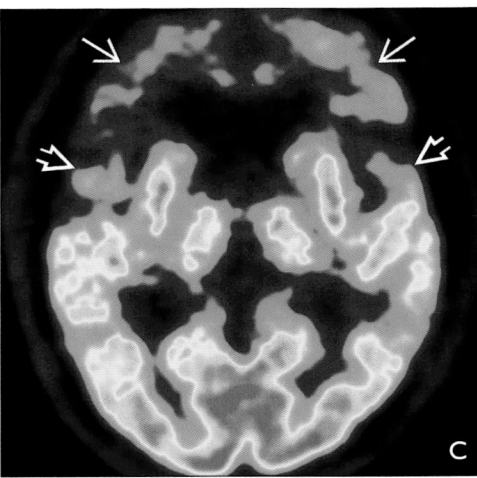 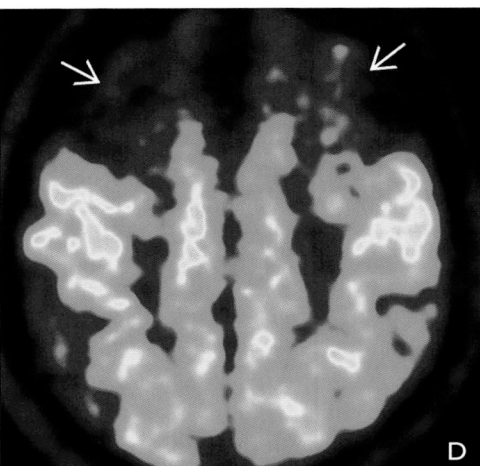

with lesser volume loss in the temporal lobes is the most common finding **(33-19)**.

MR FINDINGS. While standard T1 scans may show generalized frontotemporal volume loss, voxel-based morphometry can discriminate between various *pathologic* subtypes. Pick disease (FTLD-TAU) is associated with strongly asymmetric atrophy involving the temporal and/ or extratemporal (i.e., frontal) regions. FTLD-TDP disease shows asymmetric, relatively localized temporal lobe atrophy.

Some genetic mutations in FTLD also exhibit different patterns of volume loss. *C9ORF72* is associated with symmetric frontal lobe atrophy with additional volume loss in anterior temporal lobes, parietal lobes, occipital lobes and cerebellum **(33-21)**. In contrast, striking anteromedial temporal atrophy is associated with tau mutations and temporoparietal atrophy was associated with progranulin mutations.

Clinical FTLD subtypes also correlate with frontal-versus-temporal and left-versus-right atrophy predominance. The SD subtype shows bilateral temporal volume loss but little or no frontal atrophy **(33-20)**. bvFTD and PNFA both demonstrate bilateral frontal and temporal volume loss, but the right hemisphere is most affected in bvFTD while left-sided volume loss dominates in PNFA.

WM damage also occurs in FTLD and is probably secondary to damage in the overlying cortex. DWI shows elevated mean diffusivity in the superior frontal gyri, orbitofrontal gyri, and anterior temporal lobes.

DTI with reduced FA in the superior longitudinal fasciculus is common in bvFTD and correlates with behavior disturbances whereas the inferior longitudinal fasciculus is more affected in the SD variant.

MRS shows decreased NAA and elevated mI in the frontal lobes.

NUCLEAR MEDICINE FINDINGS. FDG PET scans show hypoperfusion and hypometabolism in the frontal and temporal lobes.

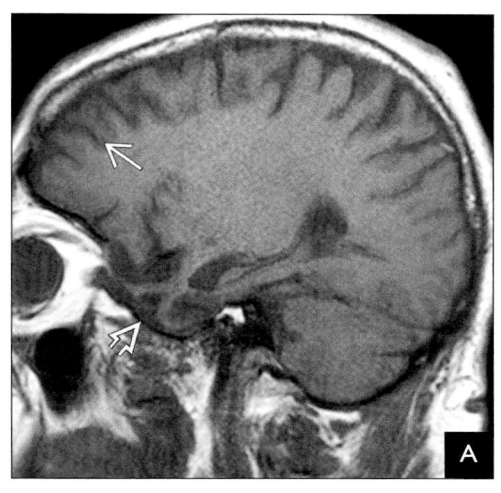
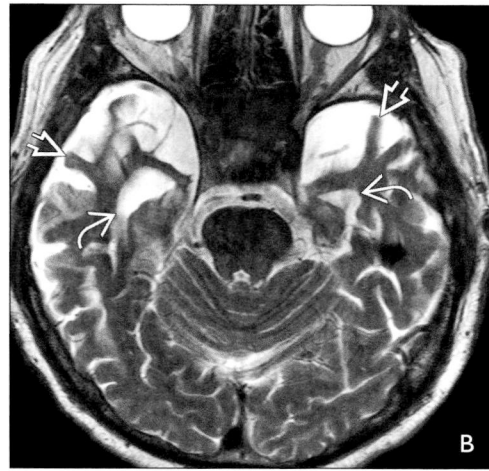

33-20A. Series of images in a 63-year-old man with FTLD shows the utility of detailing cerebral atrophy patterns. Note striking temporal lobe volume loss ➡ with relatively well-preserved frontal gyri ➡. 33-20B. Axial T2WI in the same patient shows striking, relatively symmetric temporal lobe atrophy with knife-like gyri ➡ and markedly enlarged temporal horns of the lateral ventricles ➡.

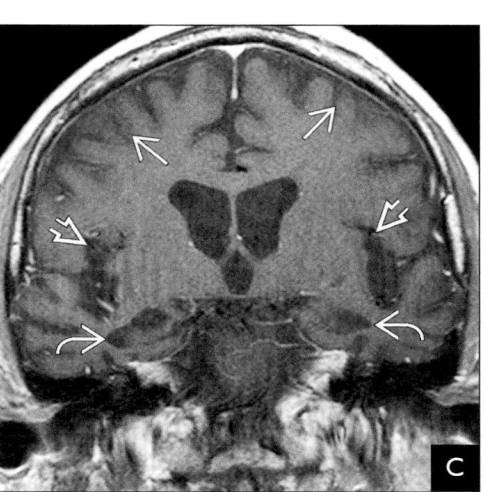
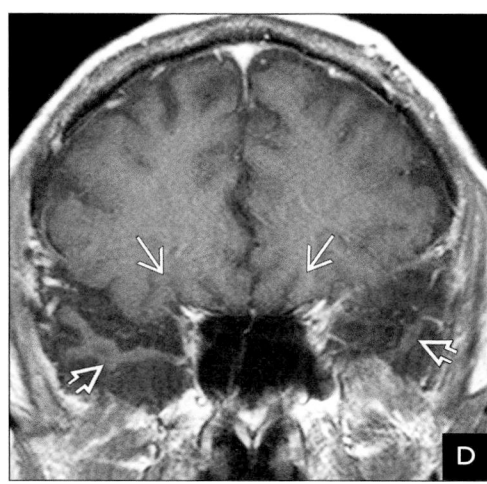

33-20C. Coronal T1 C+ scan in the same patient shows symmetrically enlarged sylvian fissures ➡ and temporal horns ➡ indicating temporal lobe volume loss. The posterior frontal gyri ➡ appear normal. 33-20D. More anterior coronal scan shows shrunken, knife-like temporal lobe gyri ➡, normal frontal gyri ➡. The relatively symmetric, predominantly temporal lobe atrophy is most consistent with the SD FTLD subtype.

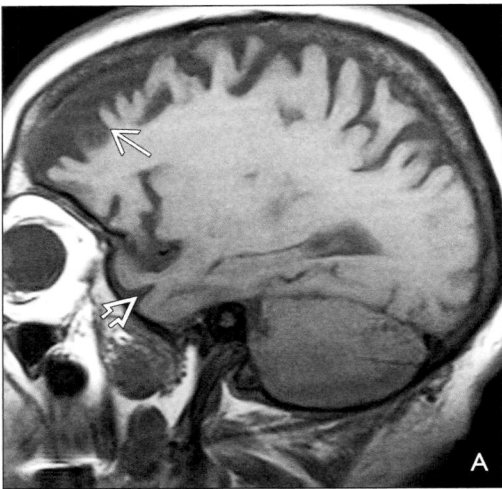

33-21A. Sagittal T1WI through the middle cranial fossa shows striking frontal ➡, moderate temporal lobe ⧰ volume loss.

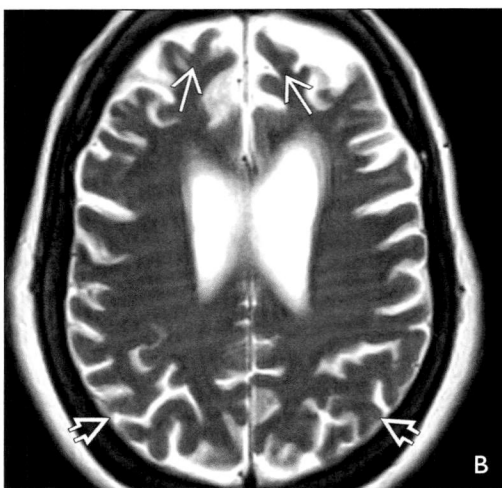

33-21B. Axial T2WI shows relatively symmetric, severe frontal ➡ and moderate parietal lobe ⧰ volume loss for the patient's age of 65 years.

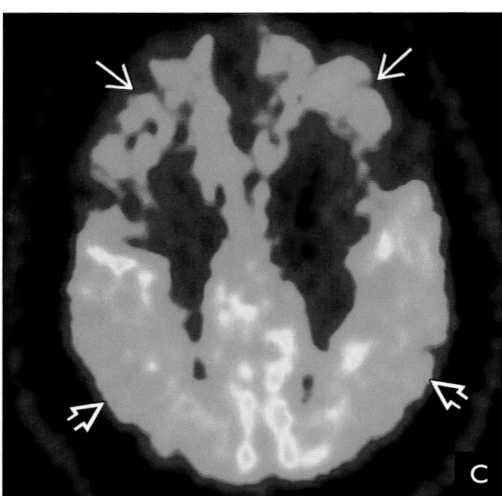

33-21C. Hypometabolism in frontal lobes ➡, but parietal lobes ⧰ are moderately hypometabolic on PET. Possible FTLD with C9ORF72 mutation.

Differential Diagnosis

The major differential diagnosis of FTLD is **Alzheimer disease**, in which the atrophy is predominantly temporal and parietal with disproportionate volume loss in the hippocampi. Atrophy in the anterior cingulated, orbitofrontal, and frontoinsular cortex are more characteristic of FTLD.

Vascular dementia is characterized by multifocal cortical or territorial infarcts, WM ischemia, and basal ganglia lacunae.

FRONTOTEMPORAL LOBAR DEGENERATION

Pathoetiology
- Classified according to cellular inclusions
  - FTLD with tau inclusions
  - FTLD with tau(-), TDP(+) inclusions
  - FTLD with tau/TDP(-), fused-in sarcoma (+)
  - FTLD with ubiquitin proteasome system (+)

Clinical Issues
- Second most common cause of "presenile" dementia
- Accounts for 20% of all cases < 65 years of age
- Clinical subtypes
  - Behavioral variant (bvFTD)
  - Progressive nonfluent aphasia (PNFA)
  - Semantic dementia (SD)

Imaging
- Classify atrophy (volumetric MR best)
  - Temporal vs. extratemporal (frontal) predominance
  - Symmetric or asymmetric
- 18F FDG PET
  - Frontotemporal hypometabolism

Differential Diagnosis
- Alzheimer disease
  - Parietal, temporal > frontotemporal
- Vascular dementia
  - Multifocal infarcts
  - WM ischemic changes

Dementia with Lewy Bodies

Terminology

Dementia with Lewy bodies (DLB) is also termed diffuse Lewy body disease (DLBD). Other diseases with LBs include **Parkinson disease** (PD), **Parkinson disease dementia** (PDD), and the so-called **Lewy body variant** (LBV) **of Alzheimer disease** (AD). All three diseases overlap DLB and comprise an expanding group of clinical phenotypes that ranges from the relatively pure motor difficulties in PDD to the cognitive and behavioral disturbances that predominate in DLB. Collectively these diseases are grouped under the umbrella term **Lewy body disorders** (LBDs).

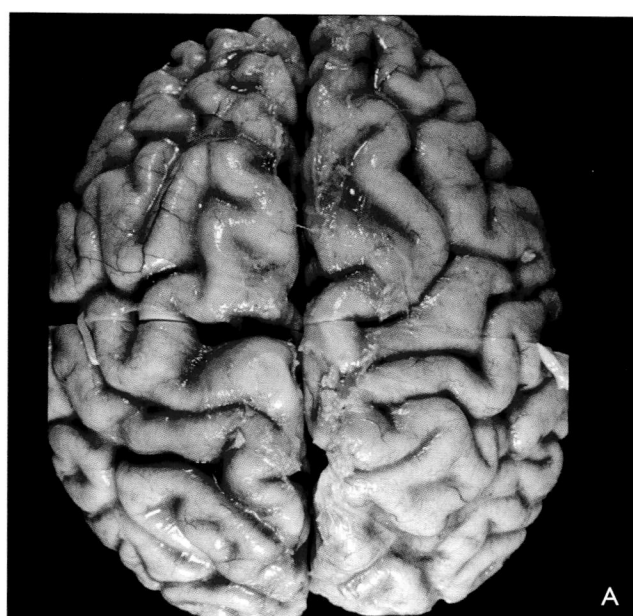

33-22A. Autopsy case of dementia with diffuse Lewy bodies shows mild generalized volume loss without specific lobar predominance.

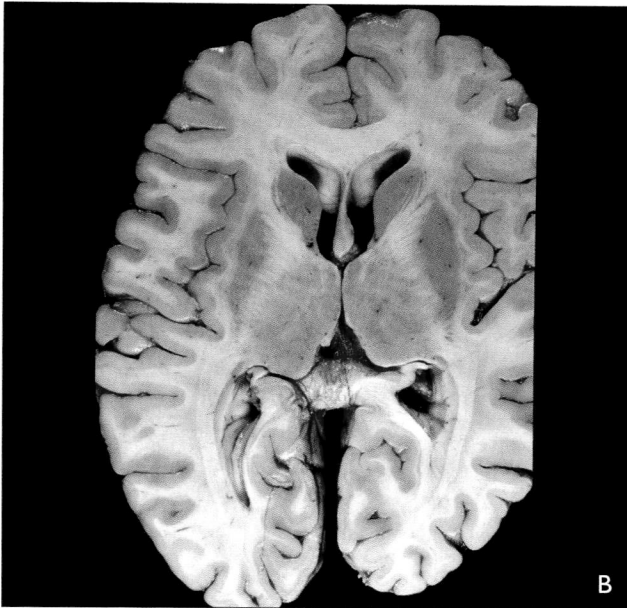

33-22B. Axial section shows mildly enlarged ventricles with no other definite abnormalities identified. The occipital lobes appear normal. (Courtesy R. Hewlett, MD.)

Etiology

Lewy bodies (LBs) are spherical intraneuronal protein aggregates that consist primarily of α-synuclein (α-syn), a presynaptic microtubule-associated misfolded protein similar to tau. DLB is therefore considered a **synucleinopathy**, a group of disorders with α-synuclein gene mutations that also includes PD, PDD, multisystem atrophy, pure autonomic failure, and REM sleep behavior disorder.

Pathology

GROSS PATHOLOGY. The gross appearance of DLB resembles early AD. Frontotemporal and parietal atrophy is generally mild to moderate, while the hippocampi and occipital lobes are typically spared **(33-22)**. The substantia nigra and locus ceruleus often appear pale.

MICROSCOPIC FEATURES. The histopathologic hallmark of DLB is the presence of Lewy body inclusions in the cortex and brainstem, especially the substantia nigra and dorsal mesopontine GM. Some pathologic hallmarks of AD, viz., amyloid plaques and neurofibrillary tangles, can be found in many patients with DLB. In turn, Lewy body inclusions have also been identified in some Alzheimer patients (Lewy body variant of AD).

Clinical Issues

EPIDEMIOLOGY AND DEMOGRAPHICS. DLB is now recognized as the second most common neurodegenerative dementia, accounting for approximately 15-20% of all cases.

PRESENTATION AND DIAGNOSIS. Because DLB symptoms can resemble other more commonly recognized dementias (AD, PD), it is widely underrecognized as a cause of progressive cognitive decline.

Three core diagnostic features of DLB have been defined: (1) recurrent visual hallucinations and visuospatial disturbances, (2) spontaneous parkinsonism, and (3) fluctuating cognition with variations in attention and alertness. The presence of two of these three features is considered evidence of probable DLB.

NATURAL HISTORY. Patients with pure DLB have annual rates of atrophy and ventricular enlargement that are comparable to those of age-matched controls and less marked than those of patients with AD.

Imaging

GENERAL FEATURES. Despite the prominent visual symptoms that often characterize DLB, major occipital volume loss is not a typical finding. Standard anatomic imaging studies are often normal or show only mild generalized volume loss. The combination of MR volumetry and PET or SPECT seems to be most helpful.

MR FINDINGS. T1 scans show only mild generalized atrophy without lobar predominance **(33-23)**. T2/FLAIR may demonstrate nonspecific WM hyperintensities that are similar to those found in cognitively normal aging patients.

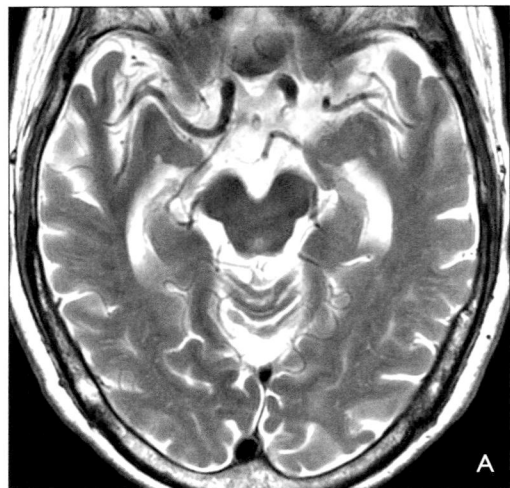

33-23A. T2WI in a patient with cognitive decline and visual hallucinations shows mild diffuse atrophy. Occipital lobes appear relatively normal.

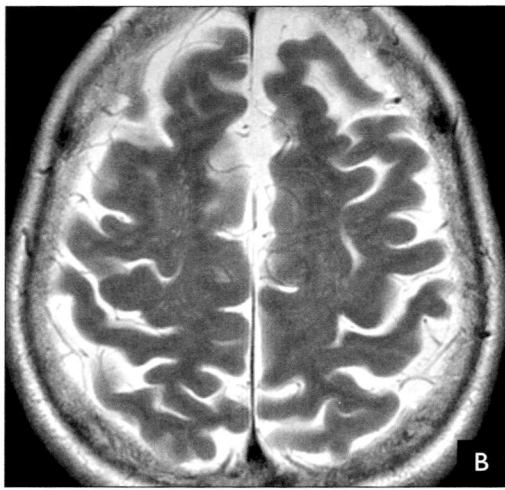

33-23B. More cephalad scan in the same patient shows mild symmetric and diffuse volume loss. Clinical diagnosis was probable DLB.

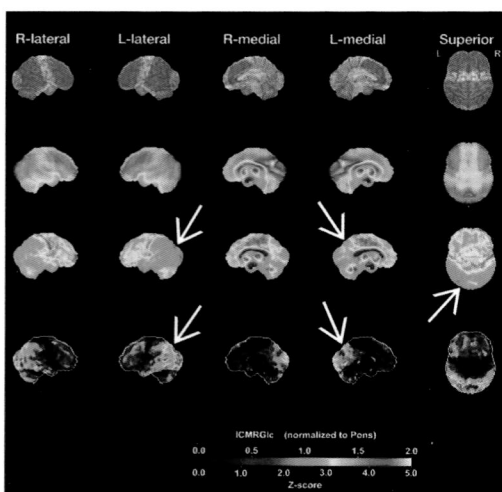

33-24. FDG PET scan in another patient with DLB shows occipital hypometabolism ➤. *(Courtesy N. Foster, MD.)*

Volumetric studies generally show relatively little cortical atrophy. Reduced volume in the hypothalamus, basal forebrain, and midbrain may be seen in some cases. There is usually more putaminal and relatively less medial temporal lobe atrophy in DLB compared to AD.

DTI demonstrates increased mean diffusivity in the amygdala and decreased FA in the inferior longitudinal and inferior occipitofrontal fasciculi. MRS shows relatively normal NAA:Cr ratios.

NUCLEAR MEDICINE. Occipital hypometabolism on FDG PET and reduced cerebral blood flow on SPECT-HMPAO or pMR are typical of DLB **(33-24)**. The primary visual cortex is especially affected.

Presynaptic dopamine transporter imaging with the FP-CIT ligand shows almost absent uptake in the putamen and markedly reduced uptake in the caudate. Cholinergic radioligands may help identify the profound cholinergic neuronal loss that occurs in DLB and PDD.

Decreased sympathetic innervation to the heart occurs across the entire Lewy body disease spectrum and can be measured with I-123 MIBG, a noradrenaline analogue, and may prove very helpful in distinguishing DLB from AD.

Differential Diagnosis

Because movement abnormalities are a core feature of DLB, the major differential diagnosis is **Parkinson disease with dementia**. Between 20-40% of Parkinson disease patients eventually develop a progressive dementing disorder, so it is often difficult to distinguish the two disorders purely on clinicopathologic features.

The second most important differential diagnosis is **Alzheimer disease**. Clinical and histopathologic features of these two disorders also often overlap. Patients with DLB have decreased glucose metabolism and hypoperfusion in the occipital lobes with variable basal ganglia volume loss. Hippocampal hypometabolism and volume loss are more common in AD.

Posterior cortical atrophy (see below) is a newly described disorder that can mimic DLB but generally occurs in younger patients.

Miscellaneous Dementias

Corticobasal Degeneration

TERMINOLOGY AND ETIOLOGY. Corticobasal degeneration (CBD) is an uncommon sporadic neurodegenerative and dementing disorder whose characterization continues to evolve. Once thought to represent a distinct clinicopathologic entity, CBD has multiple clinical phenotypes and different associated syndromes. The umbrella terms

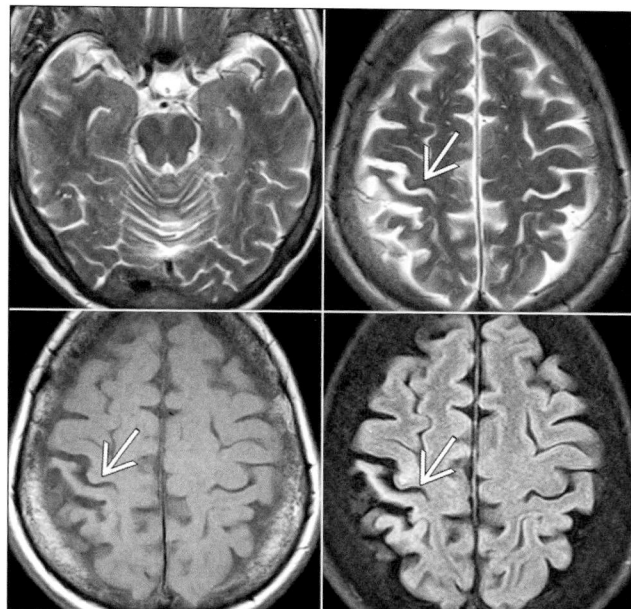

33-25. Cortical basal degeneration in a 61-year-old woman with spastic left arm. The temporal and occipital lobes appear normal. Note asymmetric atrophy, thin cortex, hyperintense WM in right perirolandic region ➡.

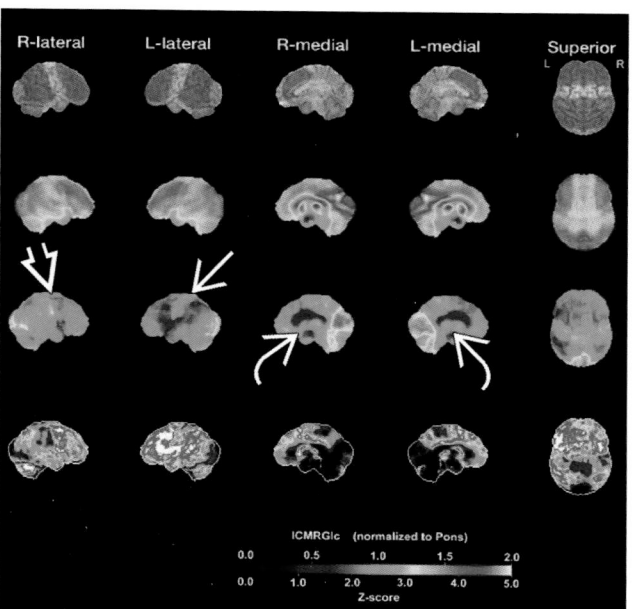

33-26. FDG PET scan in CBD (third row) shows marked hypometabolism in the frontoparietal lobes and basal ganglia ➡ *compared to normal (second row). Left hemisphere* ➡ *is more severely affected than right* ➡. *(Courtesy N. Foster, MD.)*

corticobasal syndrome (CBS) and CBS/CBD have been used to acknowledge the clinicopathologic heterogeneity of CBD.

CBD is classified as a **tauopathy** as it demonstrates abnormal tau accumulations in neurons and glia.

PATHOLOGY. The most common gross features of CBD are asymmetric frontoparietal atrophy, especially in the motor and sensory areas. The temporal and occipital cortex are relatively spared. Striatonigral degeneration is seen with striking atrophy and discoloration of the substantia nigra. The putamen, pallidum, thalamus, and hypothalamus are affected to a lesser degree.

Microscopically, CBD is characterized by neuronal achromasia (pale ballooned neurons) and tau-positive cytoplasmic inclusions in astrocytes within the atrophic cortex.

CLINICAL ISSUES. CBD typically affects patients 50-70 years of age. Its onset is both insidious and progressive. CBD can be associated with a broad variety of motor, sensory, behavioral, and cognitive disturbances. Levodopa-resistant, asymmetric, akinetic-rigid parkinsonism and limb dystonia (usually affecting an arm) are classic findings. Rigidity is followed by bradykinesia, gait disorder, and tremor. "Alien limb phenomenon" occurs in 50% of cases.

Variable cortical features of CBD include cognitive decline with impaired language production (nonfluent aphasia) and symptoms that mimic progressive supranu-

clear palsy or posterior cortical atrophy. Learning and memory are relatively preserved.

IMAGING AND DIFFERENTIAL DIAGNOSIS. Conventional imaging studies show moderate but asymmetric frontoparietal atrophy, contralateral to the side that is more severely affected clinically. The dorsal prefrontal and perirolandic cortex, striatum, and midbrain tegmentum are the most severely involved regions **(33-25)**. FLAIR scans may show patchy or confluent hyperintensity in the rolandic subcortical WM.

SPECT and PET demonstrate asymmetric frontoparietal and basal ganglia/thalamic hypometabolism **(33-26)**. Studies using striatal dopamine transporter imaging are sometimes helpful in differentiating CBD from other neurodegenerative disorders such as Parkinson disease.

The differential diagnosis of CBD includes **idiopathic** and **atypical parkinsonian syndromes** (e.g., progressive supranuclear palsy and multiple system atrophy). In patients with cognitive dysfunction, symptoms can mimic **dementia with Lewy bodies** or one of the **frontotemporal lobar degeneration syndromes**.

Creutzfeldt-Jakob Disease

Transmissible spongiform encephalopathies (TSEs), also known as **prion diseases**, are a group of neurodegenerative disorders that includes **Creutzfeldt-Jakob disease** (CJD), **kuru**, **Gerstmann-Sträussler-Schenker** syndrome, and **fatal familial insomnia**. Animal TSEs include scrapie (from sheep and goats), chronic wasting disease (from mule deer and elk), bovine spongi-

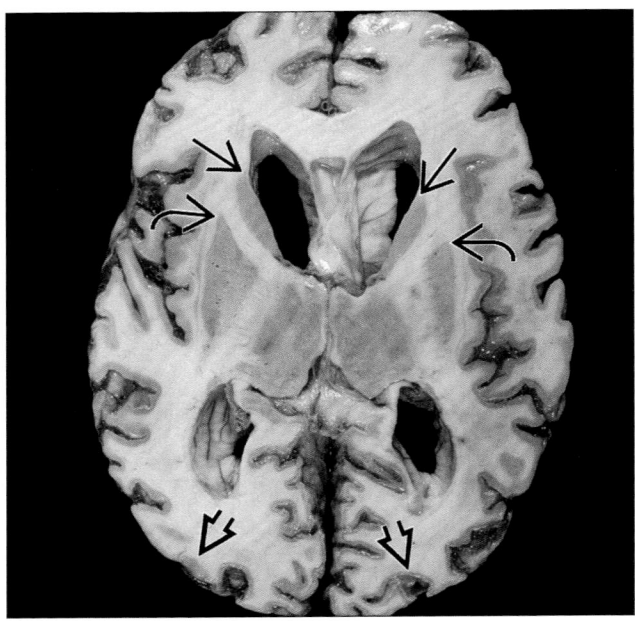

33-27. Autopsy of sporadic CJD shows marked atrophy of the caudate nuclei ➡ and anterior basal ganglia ➡. The cerebral cortex is severely thinned, especially in the occipital lobes ➡, where it is almost inapparent. (Courtesy R. Hewlett, MD.)

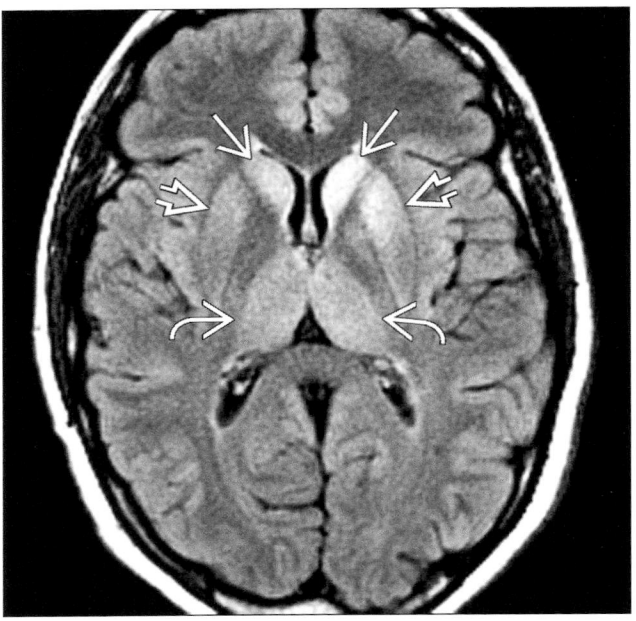

33-28. Axial FLAIR shows classic findings of sCJD with hyperintense caudate nuclei ➡, anterior putamina ➡, thalami ➡.

form encephalopathy ("mad cow disease"), and feline encephalopathy (from domestic cats).

Kuru was the first recognized human TSE, occurring in the Fore population of Papua New Guinea. Kuru is a uniformly fatal cerebellar ataxic syndrome; it has now almost disappeared with the discontinuation of cannibalism, the only source of human-to-human transmission.

CJD is the most common human TSE and has a worldwide distribution. CJD is unique, as it is both an infectious and neurogenetic dementing disorder. CJD is the archetypical human TSE and is detailed in the following discussion.

ETIOLOGY. CJD is a rapidly progressive neurodegenerative disorder caused by proteinaceous infectious particles ("prions") that are devoid of DNA and RNA. The abnormal prion protein, PrP(Sc), is a misfolded isoform (a β-pleated sheet) of the normal host prion protein, PrP(C). The abnormal form propagates itself by recruiting the normal isoform and imposing its conformation on the homologous host cell protein. *The conformational conversion of PrP(C) to PrP(Sc) is the fundamental event underlying all prion diseases.*

Four types of CJD are recognized: **Sporadic** (sCJD), **familial** or **genetic**, **iatrogenic**, and **variant** (vCJD). sCJD is the most common type. Genetic CJD is caused by diverse mutations in the *PRNP* gene. Iatrogenic CJD is caused by prion-contaminated materials (e.g., surgical instruments, dura mater grafts, cadaveric corneal transplants, and pituitary-derived human growth hormone).

vCJD typically results from the transmission of bovine spongiform encephalopathy from cattle to humans. vCJD is also known as "new variant" CJD.

PATHOLOGY. Gross pathology shows ventricular enlargement, caudate atrophy, and cortical volume loss that varies from minimal to striking (33-27). The white matter is relatively spared.

The classic triad of histopathologic findings in CJD is marked neuronal loss, spongiform change, and striking astrogliosis. The cerebral and cerebellar cortex are often most severely affected, although the basal ganglia and thalami are also frequently involved. Amyloid plaques can be identified in 10% of cases.

Various deposits of PrP(Sc) are present, and PrP(Sc) immunoreactivity is the gold standard for the neuropathologic diagnosis of human prion diseases.

EPIDEMIOLOGY AND DEMOGRAPHICS. CJD now accounts for more than 90% of all prion diseases in humans. Approximately 85% of CJD cases are sporadic (sCJD) with an annual worldwide incidence of one to two cases per million. Peak age of onset is 55-75 years. There is no gender predilection. Genetic CJD causes most of the remaining cases (15%). vCJD and iatrogenic CJD together now account for less than 1%.

Variant CJD typically presents in younger patients between 15 and 40 years. Psychiatric symptoms predominate. Approximately 220 vCJD cases have been reported with most—but not all—occurring in the United Kingdom. The incidence of vCJD has declined in recent years, but small numbers of new cases are still identified.

CLINICAL ISSUES. Five clinicopathologic subtypes of sCJD have been identified. Three subtypes prominently affect cognitive functions, and the other two impair cerebellar motor activities. In the most common subtype, rapidly worsening dementia is followed by myoclonic jerks and akinetic mutism. In two-thirds of sCJD cases, EEG shows a characteristic pattern of periodic bi- or triphasic complexes.

Two less common but important presentations of sCJD are the so-called Brownell-Oppenheimer variant (a pure cerebellar syndrome) and the Heidenhain variant (pure visual impairment leading to cortical blindness).

CJD is a progressive and fatal illness. Median survival is approximately four months, although vCJD progresses more slowly. While the definitive diagnosis of sCJD requires autopsy or brain biopsy, the clinical pattern plus imaging studies allow the diagnosis of probable sCJD. vCJD can sometimes be diagnosed by tonsil biopsy.

IMAGING. CJD primarily involves the gray matter structures of the brain. WM disease is much less common and is usually a late finding.

CT scans are typically normal, especially in the early stages of disease. Serial studies may show progressive ventricular dilatation and sulcal enlargement.

MR with DWI is the imaging procedure of choice. T1 scans are are often normal. T2/FLAIR hyperintensity in the basal ganglia, thalami, and cerebral cortex is the most common initial abnormality in classic sCJD. The anterior caudate and putamen are more affected than the globus pallidus **(33-28)**. Cortical involvement—especially involving the frontal, temporal, and parietal lobes—is common but often appears asymmetric. Occipital lobe involvement predominates in the Heidenhain variant **(33-29)**, whereas the cerebellum is primarily affected in the Brownell-Oppenheimer variant.

T2/FLAIR hyperintensity in the posterior thalamus ("pulvinar" sign) or posteromedial thalamus ("hockey stick" sign) is seen in 90% of vCJD cases but can also occur in sCJD **(33-30)**.

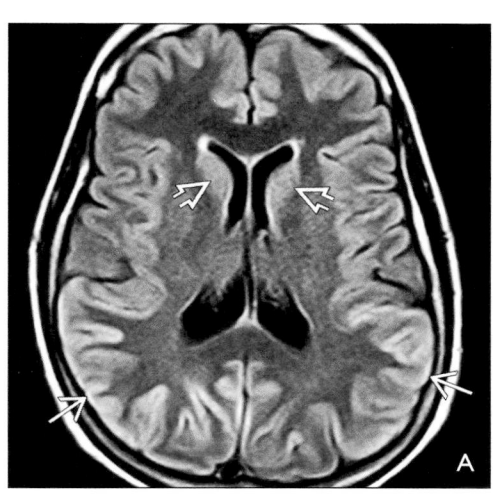

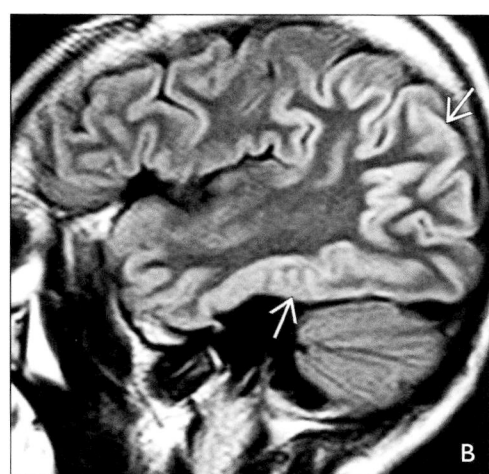

33-29A. Series of images demonstrates classic findings of the Heidenhain variant of sCJD. Axial FLAIR scan shows bilateral cortical hyperintensity in both occipital lobes ➡. While the anterior caudate nuclei ➡ appear mildly hyperintense, the basal ganglia are generally spared. 33-29B. Sagittal FLAIR scan demonstrates occipital, posterior temporal hyperintensity ➡. The frontal and anterior parietal lobes are spared.

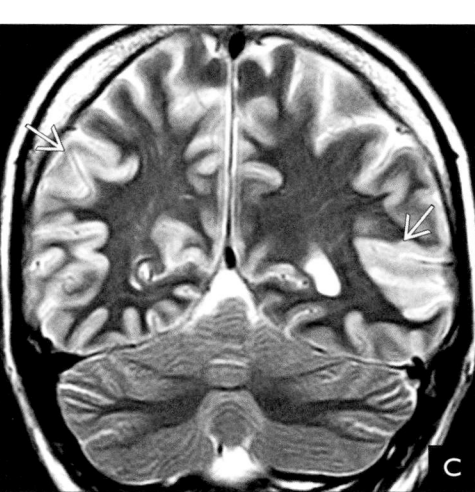

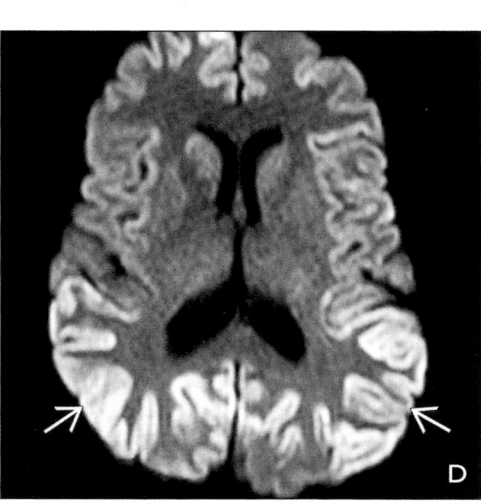

33-29C. Coronal T2WI in the same patient shows striking hyperintensity in both occipital cortices ➡. 33-29D. DWI shows striking diffusion restriction in the cortex of both occipital lobes ➡. The underlying WM is spared.

DWI shows hyperintensity in the striatum and thalami (33-31). Gyriform diffusion restriction in the cerebral cortex is common. CJD does not enhance on T1 C+.

DIFFERENTIAL DIAGNOSIS. CJD must be distinguished from other causes of dementia such as **Alzheimer disease** and **frontotemporal lobar degeneration**. The basal ganglia involvement in CJD is a helpful differentiating feature. Unlike most dementing diseases, CJD shows striking diffusion restriction.

Gerstmann-Sträussler-Schenker disease (GSS) and **fatal familial insomnia** (FFI) can be distinguished clinically from sCJD. GSS presents as cerebellar ataxia with late-onset cognitive decline. FFI begins with autonomic and sleep disturbances.

CREUTZFELDT-JAKOB DISEASE

Pathology and Etiology
- Most common human transmissible spongiform encephalopathy
- CJD is a prion disease
  - Proteinaceous particles without DNA, RNA
  - Misfolded isoform PrP(Sc) of normal host PrP(C)
  - Propagated by conformational conversion of PrP(C) to PrP(Sc)
- 4 CJD types recognized
  - Sporadic (sCJD) (85%)
  - Genetic/familial (15%)
  - Iatrogenic (< 1%)
  - Variant ("mad cow" disease, vCJD) (< 1%)

Clinical Issues
- Peak age = 55-75 years
- Rapidly progressive dementia, death in sCJD within 4 months

Imaging
- T2/FLAIR hyperintensity
  - Basal ganglia, thalami, cortex
  - "Pulvinar" sign: Posterior thalami
  - "Hockey stick" sign: Posteromedial thalami
  - Occipital cortex in Heidenhain variant
- Restricted diffusion

33-30A. Axial DWI in a patient with sCJD shows the classic "hockey stick" sign in the posteromedial thalami ➡. The anterior caudate nuclei ➡ and both putamina ➡ are also involved. 33-30B. DWI in the same patient with sCJD shows corresponding strong diffusion restriction in the posteromedial thalami ➡, caudate nuclei ➡, and putamina ➡.

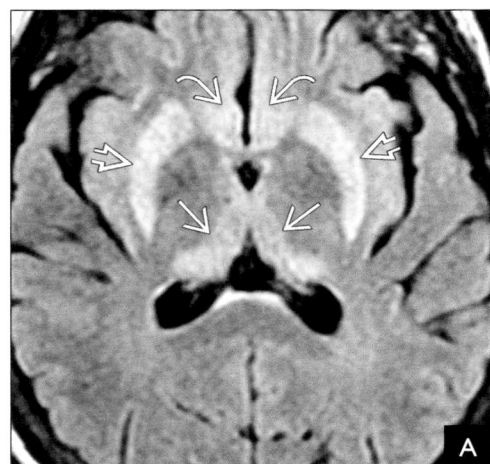
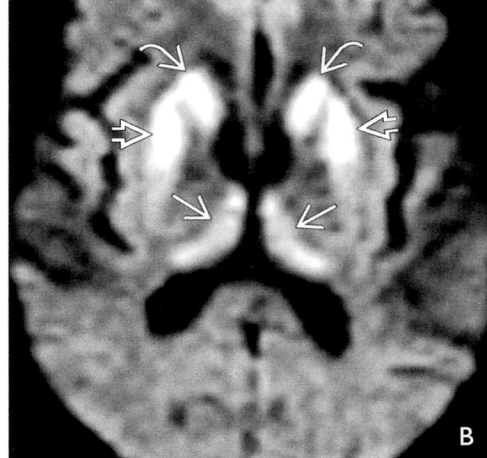

33-31A. Axial FLAIR scan in a patient with vCJD shows classic "pulvinar" sign with symmetric hyperintensity in the posterior thalami ➡. 33-31B. DWI in the same patient shows focal restricted diffusion in both posterior thalami ➡ corresponding to the "pulvinar" sign seen on FLAIR.

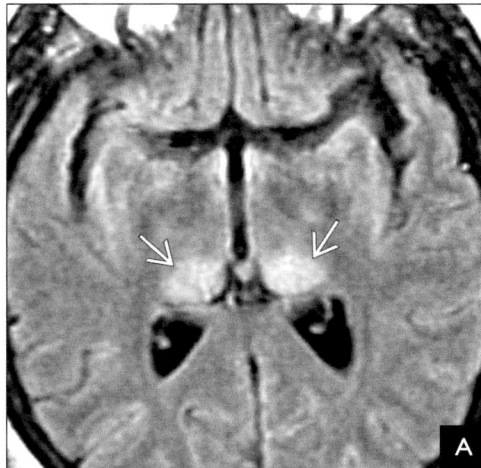
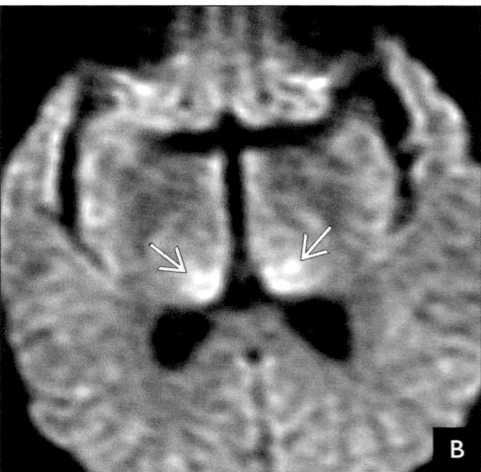

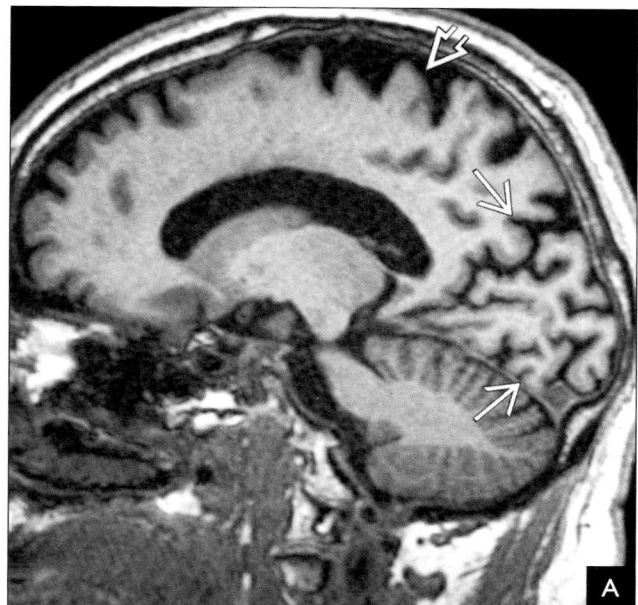

33-32A. Sagittal MP-RAGE in a patient with gradually worsening visuoperceptual skills and the clinical diagnosis of posterior cortical atrophy shows severe occipital ➡, moderate parietal ➡ volume loss.

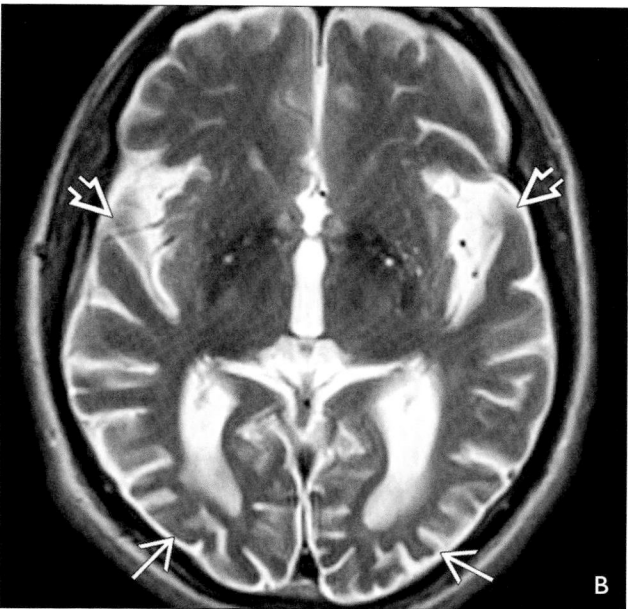

33-32B. T2WI in the same patient shows enlarged occipital horns, markedly diminished WM, severe cortical atrophy in both occipital lobes ➡, and moderate superior temporal volume loss with enlargement of both sylvian fissures ➡.

Posterior Cortical Atrophy

Posterior cortical atrophy (PCA) is a rare neurodegenerative syndrome characterized by insidious onset and selective, gradual decline in visuospatial and visuoperceptual skills. Memory and verbal fluency are relatively well-preserved. Age at symptom onset is typically 50-65 years.

PCA primarily affects the parietal, occipital, and occipitotemporal cortex with relative sparing of the frontal and inferomedial temporal lobes. In contrast to AD, the highest density of NFTs and senile plaques is found in the parietooccipital regions while the frontal lobes are less involved.

Posterior-predominant atrophy on imaging studies is typical **(33-32)**, *although not all patients with PCA demonstrate volume loss*. Asymmetric involvement, especially in the occipital lobes, is common. Limited data from DTI studies suggest that PCA adversely affects WM tract integrity in the posterior brain regions. FDG PET shows hypometabolism in the parietooccipital lobes and both frontal eye fields.

The major differential diagnosis of PCA is the **occipital (Heidenhain) variant of CJD**. While the clinical and histopathologic features of both diseases overlap, PCA demonstrates greater right parietal with less left medial temporal and hippocampal atrophy. Other diagnostic considerations include **dementia with Lewy bodies** and **corticobasal degeneration**.

Degenerative Disorders

In this section, we consider a range of brain degenerations. Although some (such as Parkinson disease) can be associated with dementia, most are not. Because Parkinson disease (PD) occurs more often as a movement disorder than a dementing illness, it is discussed with other degenerative diseases.

The use of deep brain stimulators (DBSs) in treating patients with disabling akinetic-rigid PD is increasingly common, so a brief review of the dopaminergic striatonigral system and its relevant anatomy will be helpful before we discuss PD.

Dopaminergic Striatonigral System

Dopaminergic neurons are found throughout the brain, but by far the largest collections lie in the midbrain. Here dopaminergic neurons are located in three specific areas: The ventral tegmental area (VTA), the pars compacta of the substantia nigra (SNPc), and the retrobulbar field. Neurons in the VTA project to the frontal cortex and ventral striatum while SNPc neurons project to the putamen and caudate nuclei.

Mesencephalic dopaminergic neurons help regulate voluntary movement and influence reward behavior.

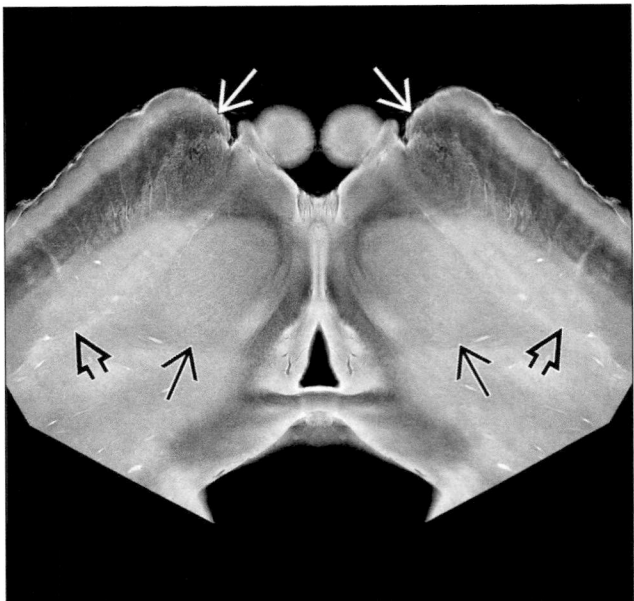

33-33. Axial 9.0 T MR scan through midbrain shows lens-shaped subthalamic nuclei ⊳ positioned between rostral poles of red nuclei medially ➔, substantia nigra ➔ laterally. (Courtesy T. P. Naidich, MD, B. N. Delman, MD).

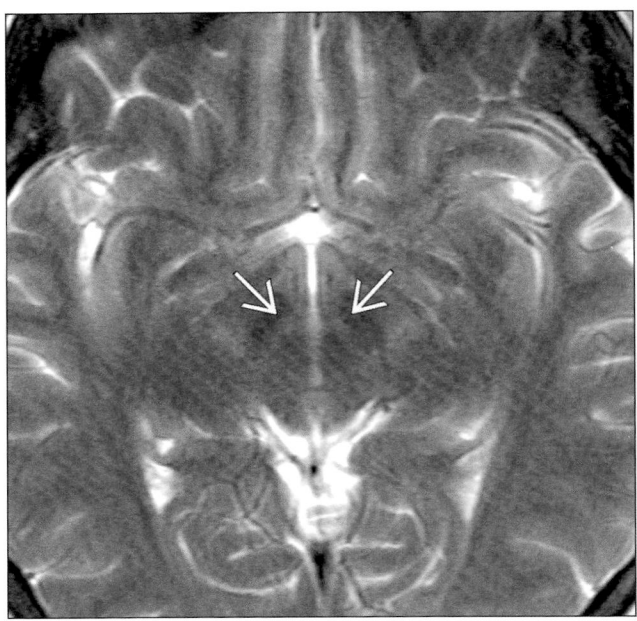

33-34. T2WI of upper midbrain shows approximate position of hypointense subthalamic nuclei ➔, located medial to cerebral peduncles and enveloped by anteromedial substantia nigra. STN is separated from RN by a thin hyperintense band.

Relevant Gross Anatomy

The striatonigral system consists of the basal ganglia (caudate nucleus, putamen, and globus pallidus), the substantia nigra, and the subthalamic nucleus. The gross and imaging anatomy of the basal ganglia are discussed in Chapter 32.

The **substantia nigra** (SN) lies in the midbrain tegmentum between the cerebral peduncles and red nuclei. The SN consists of pigmented gray matter that extends through the midbrain from the pons to the subthalamic region. The SN has two parts: The **pars compacta** (which contains *dopaminergic* cells) and the **pars reticularis** (which contains *GABAergic* cells). The **red nucleus** (RN) is a round gray matter formation that lies medial to the SN and serves as a relay station between the cerebellum, globus pallidus, and cortex **(33-33)**.

The **subthalamic nucleus** (STN) is a small lens-shaped structure that measures approximately 100-125 mm³ in total volume. The SN envelopes the anterior and inferior borders of the STN. The STN lies just inside the internal capsule, one to two millimeters from the anterolateral edge of the red nucleus.

The *superior* border of the STN is formed by the lenticular fasciculus while the *lateral* aspect of the STN abuts the internal capsule. The *medial* border of the STN is formed by a band of subthalamic white matter—the zona incerta (ZI)—that lies between it and the red nucleus.

The subthalamic nucleus is currently the preferred target for both direct (imaging-based) and indirect (atlas-based) stereotactic DBS electrode placement in the treatment of movement disorders.

Imaging Anatomy

On thin-section 1.5 or 3.0 T2-weighted MR scans, the STNs are seen as hypointense almond-shaped structures that are obliquely oriented in all three standard planes. In the axial plane, the STN lies between the SN anterosuperiorly and the RN posteromedially. The hypointensity of the STN blends imperceptibly into that of the SN **(33-34)**, but medially the white matter of the ZI separates the STN from the RN.

The midpoint of the STN lies between 9.7-9.9 mm lateral to the midline. Its position (and the correct location of the tip of a DBS) can thus be estimated on CT scans by finding the upper cerebral peduncles and measuring 9-10 mm from the midline.

Parkinson Disease

Terminology

Parkinson disease (PD) is a multisystem neurodegenerative disorder that affects diverse neural pathways and several neurotransmitter circuits. The constellation of resting tremor, bradykinesia, and rigidity is often termed **parkinsonism**. When PD is accompanied by dementia, it is referred to as **Parkinson disease dementia** (PDD). When PD is combined with other clinical signs, it is called "**Parkinson plus**," an overarching term

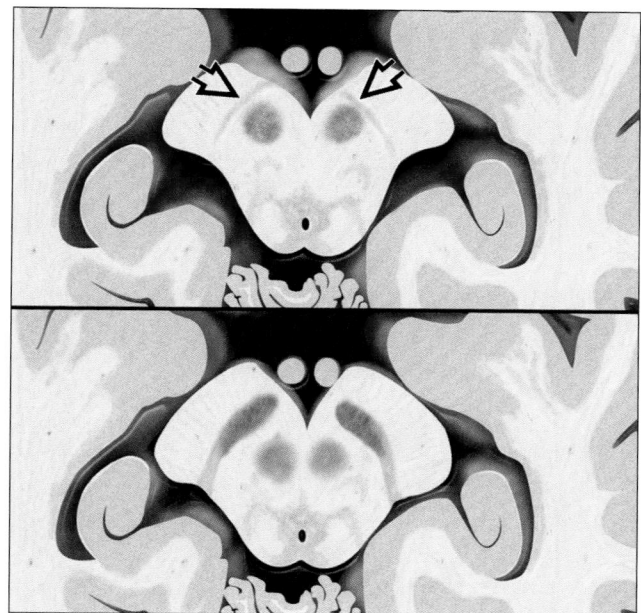

33-35. Axial diagram shows midbrain atrophy with narrowing and depigmentation of the substantia nigra (SN) ⧯ in Parkinson disease (top) relative to normal anatomy (bottom). Note narrowing of pars compacta between red nuclei, SN.

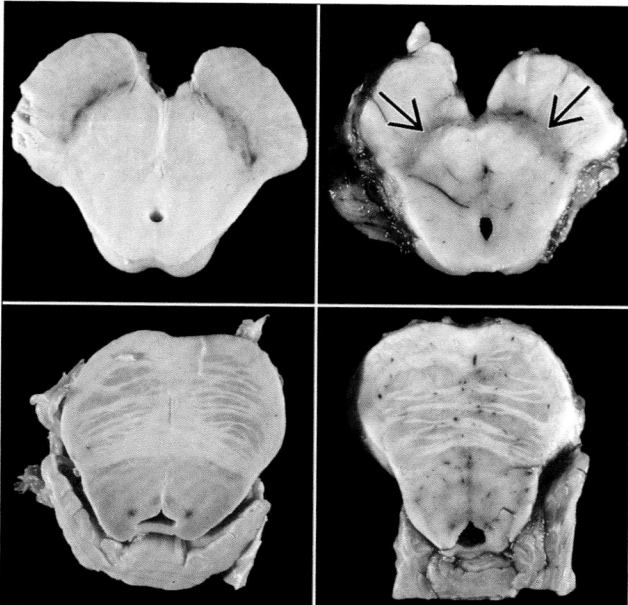

33-36. Autopsied sections compare normal midbrain (left) to one affected by Parkinson disease (right). Note midbrain volume loss in PD, abnormal pallor of the substantia nigra ⧯. (Courtesy R. Hewlett, MD.)

that includes **multiple system atrophy** and **progressive supranuclear palsy** (see below).

PD is classified clinically as a neurodegenerative disorder, histopathologically as a **Lewy body disease**, and immunohistochemically as a **synucleinopathy**.

Etiology

GENERAL CONCEPTS. While a number of environmental factors have been implicated, aging is the most significant known risk factor for PD.

In PD, degeneration of dopaminergic neurons in the SNPc reduces dopaminergic input to the striatum. Neuronal degeneration is relatively advanced histopathologically before it becomes apparent clinically. By the time clinical symptoms develop, over 60% of dopaminergic neurons are lost and 80% of striatal dopamine is already depleted.

The death of dopaminergic neurons in PD is regional and very selective with neuronal loss centered mainly in the SNPc. The precise mechanisms underlying the susceptibility of dopaminergic neurons and regional propensity for cell death in the SNPc are poorly understood.

GENETICS. Most cases of PD are sporadic and idiopathic. Between 10-20% are familial. Eleven genetic loci, including glucocerebrosidase (*GBA*) mutations, have recently been identified as risk factors for PD.

Pathology

GROSS PATHOLOGY. The midbrain may appear mildly atrophic with a splayed or "butterfly" configuration of the cerebral peduncles **(33-35)**. Depigmentation of the substantia nigra is a common pathologic feature of PD and is related to loss of neuromelanin **(33-36)**.

MICROSCOPIC FEATURES. The most devastating effects of PD are seen in the dopaminergic striatonigral system. The two histopathologic hallmarks of PD are (1) severe depletion of dopaminergic neurons in the SNPc and (2) the presence of Lewy bodies (LBs) in the surviving neurons. Immunohistochemistry shows the LBs stain positively for ubiquitin and α-synuclein.

STAGING, GRADING, AND CLASSIFICATION. Braak et al have divided PD into six stages, which correlate clinical symptoms with the distribution of Lewy bodies. Lewy bodies begin to accumulate well before diagnosis. The disease process in the brainstem generally pursues an ascending course.

Stage 1 and 2 are preclinical. In stage 1, the LBs are confined to the medulla and the olfactory system. As the disease progresses, LBs spread into the upper brainstem and forebrain. At Braak stage 3, numerous LBs are present in the SN, loss of dopaminergic neurons is evident, the forebrain cholinergic system is involved, and the first clinical symptoms begin to emerge.

In Braak stage 4, the limbic system becomes involved. In the most advanced stages (Braak stages 5 and 6), LBs are distributed throughout the entire neocortex.

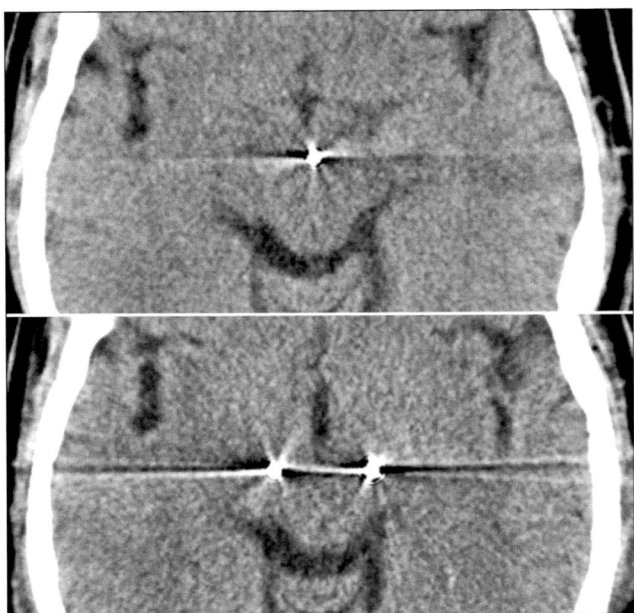

33-37. Axial NECT scan in a patient with incorrect placement of left DBS (top) shows the tip lying above and medial to the subthalamic nucleus. Repositioned left DBS and a new right DBS (bottom) are in the correct anatomic position in the STN.

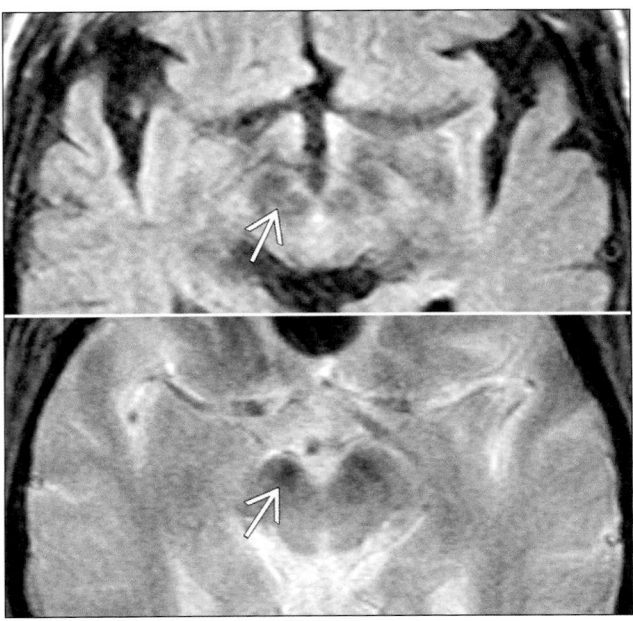

33-38. Axial FLAIR (top) and T2* GRE (bottom) in a 61-year-old man show mild midbrain volume loss with narrowed SNPc, especially on the right side ➜ where it is difficult to delineate the border between the substantia nigra and red nucleus.

Clinical Issues

EPIDEMIOLOGY AND DEMOGRAPHICS. PD is both the most common movement disorder and the most common of the Lewy body diseases. Its distribution is worldwide, and the estimated overall prevalence is 150-200:100,000. There is a slight male predominance.

Peak age at onset is 60 years; PD onset under 40 years is uncommon. Rarely, PD occurs as a juvenile-onset autosomal dominant dystonia.

PRESENTATION. PD diagnosis depends on a constellation of symptoms. The three cardinal clinical features of PD are resting tremor, rigidity, and bradykinesia (slowness in executing movements). An expressionless face, sometimes termed "masked" or "stone" face, is a common manifestation of bradykinesia.

Other classic symptoms are "pill-rolling" tremor, "cogwheel" or "lead pipe" rigidity, and postural instability with shuffling gait. Rigidity occurs in both agonist and antagonist muscles, affects movements in both directions, and can be elicited at very low speeds of passive movement.

Dementia eventually develops in 40% of PD patients. Other less common features of PD include autonomic dysfunction, behavioral abnormalities, depression, and sleep disturbances.

NATURAL HISTORY. PD typically follows a slowly progressive course with an overall mean duration of 13 years. Falls and "gait freezing" eventually become a major cause of disability.

TREATMENT OPTIONS.

Medical treatment. A number of medications are available to control PD symptoms. Levodopa was introduced more than 40 years ago and remains the most efficacious treatment, especially in young patients.

As SNPc dopamine-secreting neurons are lost, striatal dopamine levels become increasingly dependent on peripherally administered levodopa. In turn, this nonphysiologic stimulation further disrupts an already unstable striatum and fluctuations in motor symptoms increase. Motor complications of levodopa such as "wearing off," dyskinesias, and "on-off" phenomena are common. In fact, they develop in nearly half of all patients who have received the drug for more than five years, in 80% treated for 10 years, and in nearly all patients with early-onset disease.

Emerging disease-modifying therapies such as adenosine A2A antagonists, MAO-b inhibitors, and dopamine agonists are under consideration, as is gene therapy to enhance in vivo dopamine production.

Surgical options. High-frequency stimulation of deep brain structures is now preferred to ablative/lesional therapy. Deep brain stimulation (DBS) has become the preferred technique for treating a gamut of advanced PD-related symptoms.

The STN is considered one of the most optimal DBS targets. Electrodes are inserted via burr holes 25-30 mm lateral to the sagittal sutures, 20-30 mm anterior to the coronal sutures, and angled approximately 60% from the horizontal plane of the anterior-posterior commissure (AC-PC) line. Electrode positions are determined from preoperative MR or by using standard computerized atlases.

The distance of the STN from the midline varies somewhat from individual to individual. As the STN is often difficult to identify on standard MR, many neurosurgeons identify the red nucleus and position the DBSs slightly anterolateral to it. Recent studies indicate that some patients—those with a so-called dominant STN—may do as well with one DBS as with bilateral electrodes.

Imaging

CT FINDINGS. CT is used primarily following DBS placement to evaluate electrode position and to check for surgical complications. Correct positioning in the STN is seen when the tips of the electrodes are approximately nine millimeters from the midline and located just inside the upper margin of the cerebral peduncles **(33-37)**.

MR FINDINGS. Standard MR is often disappointing in the imaging diagnosis of PD. Mild midbrain volume loss with a "butterfly" configuration can be seen at 1.5 T in some advanced cases. Findings that may support the diagnosis of PD include thinning of the pars compacta (with "touching" RNs, SNs) and loss of normal SN hyperintensity on T1WI **(33-38)**.

The STNs are difficult to identify on standard 1.5 and 3.0 T MR scans as their hypointensity blends in with the hypointensity of the SN. At 7.0 T the shapes and boundaries of the SN on susceptibility-weighted sequences, which normally appear smooth and arch-like, may become irregular ("serrated" or "lumpy-bumpy") and blurred in PD patients.

NUCLEAR MEDICINE. The dopamine transporter (DAT) is responsible for clearing dopamine from synaptic clefts after its release. DAT imaging with SPECT or PET is used to assess integrity of presynaptic dopaminergic nerve cells in patients with movement disorders. Decreased uptake of radioligands such as I-123 FP-CIT and 6-F18 fluoro-L-dihydroxyphenylalanine is considered highly suggestive of PD.

Differential Diagnosis

When dementia is present, the major differential diagnosis of PDD is **dementia with Lewy bodies**. The clinical features overlap and are distinguished by whether parkinsonism precedes dementia by more than a year. If so, the diagnosis is PDD rather than LBD. Parkinsonism is a prominent clinical feature in **multiple system atrophy** (see below).

PARKINSON DISEASE

Etiology and Pathology
- Degeneration of dopaminergic neurons in SNPc
  - Reduced dopaminergic input to striatum
  - 60% of SNPc neurons lost, 80% striatal dopamine depleted before clinical PD develops
- Substantia nigra becomes depigmented
- Pars compacta thins
- Lewy bodies develop
  - PD is most common Lewy body disease

Clinical Issues
- Peak age = 60 years
- 3 cardinal features
  - Resting tremor
  - Rigidity
  - Bradykinesia

Treatment Options
- Medical
  - Levodopa (L-dopa), other drugs
- Surgical
  - Deep brain stimulation (DBS)
  - Electrodes implanted into subthalamic nuclei

Imaging
- Difficult to diagnose on standard MR
  - ± midbrain atrophy
  - ± thinned, irregular substantia nigra
  - ± "touching" SN, red nuclei
- Dopamine transporter (DAT) imaging
  - PET or SPECT can show decreased uptake

Multiple System Atrophy

Terminology

Multiple system atrophy (MSA) is an adult-onset sporadic neurodegenerative disorder that is one of the more common **Parkinson-plus** syndromes. Parkinson-plus syndromes exhibit the classic dyskinetic features of PD plus additional deficits that are not present in simple idiopathic PD. Parkinson-plus syndromes include MSA, progressive supranuclear palsy, and corticobasal degeneration. Each will be discussed in turn.

MSA includes three disorders that were previously regarded as separate entities: **Striatonigral degeneration**, **olivopontocerebellar atrophy**, and **Shy-Drager syndrome**. These disorders are now recognized as clinical MSA subtypes. The subtypes are identified by dominant symptomatology and have been renamed MSA-P, MSA-C, and MSA-A, respectively.

When parkinsonian (extrapyramidal) symptoms predominate, the disease is designated **MSA-P**. If cerebellar symptoms such as ataxia predominate, the disorder is designated **MSA-C**. When signs of autonomic failure such as orthostatic hypotension, global anhydrosis, or urogenital dysfunction predominate, the condition is designated **MSA-A**.

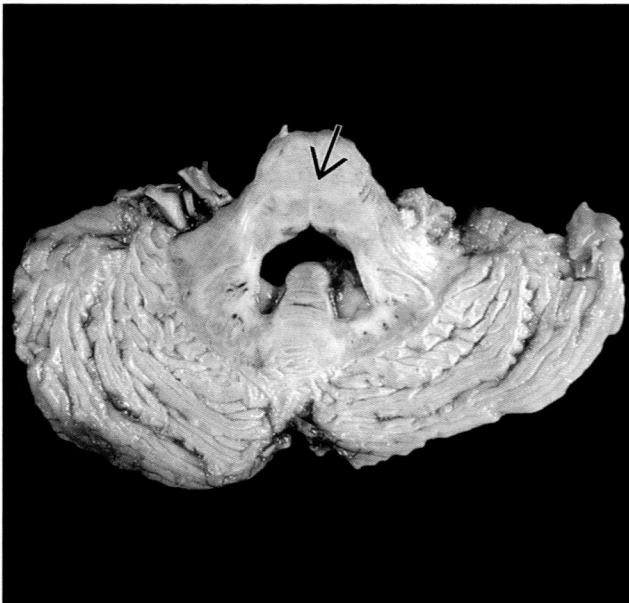

33-39. *Autopsy case of MSA-C shows cerebellar atrophy, shrunken middle cerebellar peduncles, small pons with "hot cross bun" sign* ➔. *(Courtesy J. Townsend, MD.)*

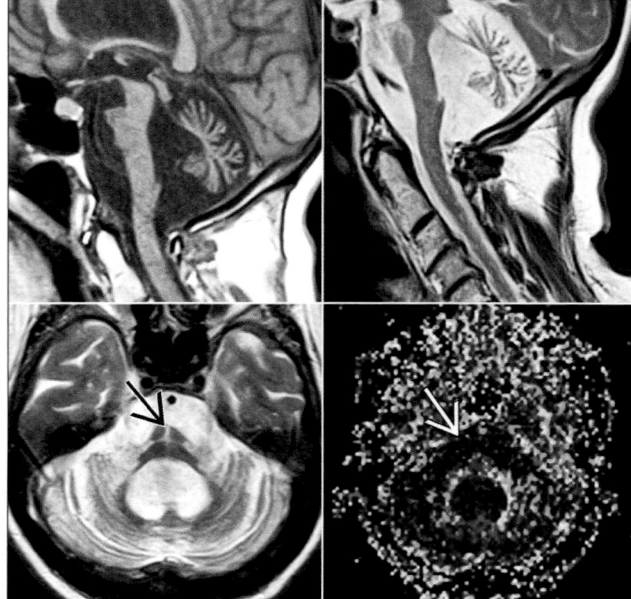

33-40. *Severe MSA-C with markedly atrophic pons, cerebellum, grossly enlarged fourth ventricle, "hot cross bun" sign* ➔. *DTI shows almost no normal pontine, MCP WM tracts* ➔.

Etiology and Pathology

The etiology of MSA is unknown.

Gross pathology shows two distinct atrophy patterns. MSA-P shows depigmentation and pallor of the substantia nigra. The putamen may be atrophic and show a grayish discoloration secondary to lipofuscin pigment accumulation. In MSA-C, marked volume loss in the cerebellum, pons, middle cerebellar peduncles (MCPs), and medulla gives the pons a "beaked" appearance **(33-39)**. MSA-A may demonstrate a combination of these patterns.

Microscopically, MSA is characterized by glial cytoplasmic inclusions that are immunopositive for α-synuclein and ubiquitin.

Clinical Issues

Mean age of onset is 58 years; mean disease duration is 5.8 years.

Parkinson-like features are present in 85-90% of all MSA patients, regardless of subtype. Other symptoms such as dysautonomia, cerebellar ataxia, and pyramidal signs can occur in any combination. Nearly two-thirds of MSA cases are classified as parkinsonian type (MSA-P) and 32% as MSA-C. Some degree of symptomatic dysautonomia is present in almost all patients but is rarely the dominant feature. Less than 5% of MSA patients have MSA-A.

MULTIPLE SYSTEM ATROPHY: TERMINOLOGY, PATHOLOGY, AND CLINICAL ISSUES

Terminology
- Parkinson-plus syndrome
- 3 disorders now considered part of MSA
  - Striatonigral degeneration
  - Olivopontocerebellar atrophy
  - Shy-Drager syndrome

Pathology
- MSA-P
  - Substantia nigra depigmented
  - Putamen atrophic, grayish discoloration
- MSA-C
  - "Flat" atrophic pons
  - "Beaked" appearance
  - Cerebellar peduncles/hemispheres atrophic
- Microscopic features
  - Glial cytoplasmic inclusions
  - Immunohistochemistry (+) for synuclein, ubiquitin

Clinical Issues
- Divided into subtypes by dominant symptoms
  - Parkinsonian → MSA-P
  - Cerebellar → MSA-C
  - Autonomic → MSA-A
- Parkinsonian features in 85-90% of all MSA patients
- Mean onset = 58 years, duration = 5.8 years

Imaging

GENERAL FEATURES. Although there can be some overlap, the imaging findings for the two most common MSA subtypes (MSA-C and MSA-P) are somewhat different.

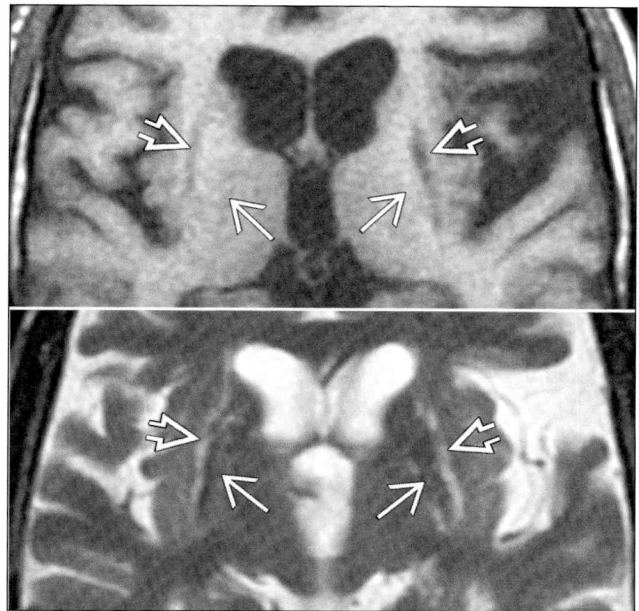

33-41. *Axial T1WI (top) and T2WI (bottom) show changes of MSA-P. Note large ventricles/sulci and thinned, atrophic putamina* ➡ *with an irregular lateral rim of hypo- and hyperintensity* ➡.

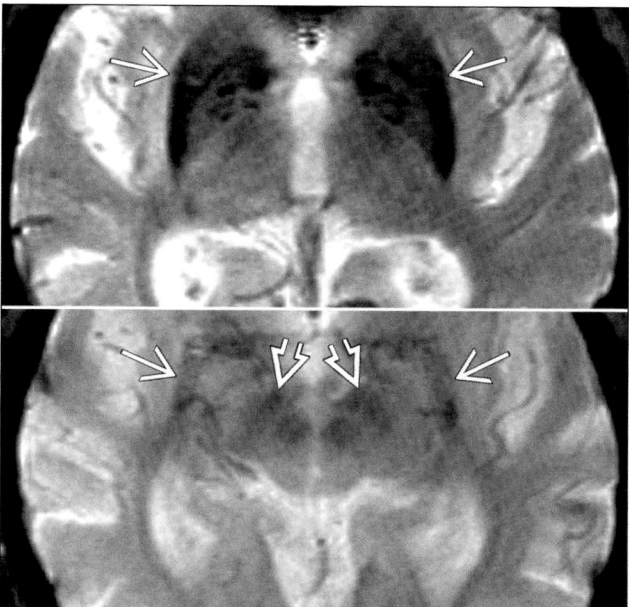

33-42. *Axial T2* GRE scans in a patient with MSA-P show abnormal putamen hypointensity* ➡, *unusually prominent hypointensity in the substantia nigra* ➡.

CT FINDINGS. NECT scans in MSA-C show cerebellar atrophy with the hemispheres more severely affected than the vermis. A small flattened pons and an enlarged fourth ventricle are common associated findings. Cortical atrophy—especially involving the frontal and parietal lobes—may be present. Findings in MSA-P are less obvious; NECT may demonstrate shrunken putamina with flattened lateral margins.

MR FINDINGS.

MSA-C. T1 scans in MSA-C show a shrunken pons and medulla, symmetric cerebellar atrophy, small concave-appearing MCPs, and an enlarged fourth ventricle.

T2/FLAIR scans demonstrate a cruciform hyperintensity in the pons termed the **"hot cross bun"** sign **(33-40)**. The "hot cross bun" sign results from selective loss of myelinated transverse pontocerebellar fibers and neurons in the pontine raphe.

DWI shows elevated ADC in the pons, middle cerebellar peduncles, cerebellar WM, and dentate nuclei.

DTI demonstrates decreased volume of fiber bundles and reduced FA in the degenerated transverse pontocerebellar fibers. Corticospinal tract involvement is often inapparent on standard T2WI but can be demonstrated clearly with DTI.

MSA-P. In patients with MSA-P, the putamina appear small and hypointense on T2WI and often have a somewhat irregular high signal intensity rim along their lateral borders on 1.5 T scans (**"hyperintense putaminal rim"**

sign) **(33-41)**. Caution: A thin, smooth, slit-like hyperintense line along the lateral putamina is a normal finding at 3.0 T.

T2* (GRE, SWI) scans show significantly higher iron deposition in the putamen compared to both age-matched controls and patients with PD **(33-42)**.

NUCLEAR MEDICINE. MSA is a preganglionic disorder so PET scanning with postganglionic adrenergic markers such as I-123 MIBG is normal.

Differential Diagnosis

The major differential diagnosis of MSA is **Parkinson disease**. Clinical findings often overlap. Imaging shows that the width of the middle cerebellar peduncles is diminished in MSA but not PD. Putaminal iron deposition appears earlier and is more prominent in MSA-P compared to PD. DAT imaging shows markedly reduced or absent uptake in PD but is normal in MSA.

Atypical parkinsonian syndromes (e.g., **progressive supranuclear palsy** and **corticobasal degeneration**) can also be difficult to distinguish clinically from MSA, but regional ADC values and MCP widths are normal.

Spinocerebellar ataxia can look identical to MSA-C, demonstrating atrophic, hyperintense middle cerebellar peduncles and a "hot cross bun" sign. **Hypoglycemia** can cause transient hyperintensity and acutely restricted diffusion in the MCPs and pyramidal tracts.

MULTIPLE SYSTEM ATROPHY: IMAGING

Imaging
- MSA-P
  - Small hypointense putamina with T2/FLAIR hyperintense lateral rim
  - ↑ putaminal iron deposition on T2*
- MSA-C
  - Cerebellar atrophy
  - Small, concave middle cerebellar peduncles
  - Shrunken "beaked" pons, "hot cross bun" sign
  - Reduced FA in transverse pontocerebellar, corticospinal tracts
- MSA-A
  - No distinctive imaging findings

Differential Diagnosis
- Parkinson disease
- Atypical parkinsonian syndromes (progressive supranuclear palsy, corticobasal degeneration)
- Spinocerebellar ataxia
- Hypoglycemia (transient MCP hyperintensity)

Progressive Supranuclear Palsy

Terminology

Progressive supranuclear palsy (PSP)—also known as Steele-Richardson-Olszewski syndrome—is a neurodegenerative disease characterized by supranuclear gaze palsy, postural instability, and mild dementia.

Etiology and Pathology

Unlike Lewy body disease, Parkinson disease (PD), and multiple system atrophy (which are synucleinopathies), PSP is a **tauopathy**. When tau protein fibrilized, it becomes less soluble and its microtubule-stabilizing properties are reduced. PSP shares many clinical, pathological, and genetic features with other tau-related diseases such as corticobasal degeneration and tau-positive frontotemporal lobar degeneration (FTLD).

The major gross pathologic findings are substantia nigra and locus ceruleus depigmentation with midbrain atrophy. Variable atrophy of the pallidum, thalamus, and subthalamic nucleus together with mild symmetric frontal volume loss may also be present **(33-43)**, **(33-44)**.

Pathological heterogeneity is common in PSP. Histologic findings consistent with other coexisting neurodegenerative diseases such as Alzheimer disease or diffuse Lewy body disease are present in the majority of cases.

PSP is characterized histopathologically by neuronal loss and astrocytic gliosis. Tau-immunoreactive cellular inclusions accumulate within both neurons and glia (in "tufted" or star-shaped astrocytes). The distribution of tau inclusions is predominantly subcortical with the globus pallidus, STN, substantia nigra, and brainstem most severely affected. Cortical involvement is common.

Clinical Issues

EPIDEMIOLOGY AND DEMOGRAPHICS. PSP is the second most common form of parkinsonism (after idiopathic PD) and is the most common of the so-called Parkinson-plus syndromes.

The prevalence of PSP is age-dependent and estimated at 6-10% that of PD.

PRESENTATION AND NATURAL HISTORY. PSP symptom onset is insidious, typically beginning in the sixth or seventh decade. Peak onset is 63 years, and no cases have been reported in patients under the age of 40.

Two PSP phenotypes are recognized: Richardson syndrome (PSP-RS) and parkinsonian-type PSP (PSP-P). PSP-RS is the classic, more common presentation with lurching gait, axial dystonia, and early ocular symptoms. Vertical supranuclear gaze palsy is the definitive diagnostic feature but typically develops years after disease onset.

One-third of patients exhibit the PSP-P phenotype. Parkinsonism dominates the early clinical picture with bradykinesia, rigidity, normal eye movements, and transient response to levodopa.

Although disease course is variable, PSP is a progressive neurodegenerative process. Neuropsychiatric symptoms develop in over half the patients within two years of disease onset. In 15-30% of cases, cognitive decline and behavioral changes are the presenting complaints and can remain the only clinical feature throughout the disease course.

Imaging

CT FINDINGS. NECT scans show variable midbrain volume loss with prominent interpeduncular and ambient cisterns. Mild to moderate ventricular enlargement is common.

MR FINDINGS. Sagittal T1- and T2-weighted images show midbrain atrophy with a concave upper surface (the **"penguin"** or **"hummingbird" sign) (33-45)**. Volumetric calculations show that the sagittal midbrain is less than 70 mm³ and that the midbrain to pons ratio is less than 0.15, only half that of normal controls. Axial scans show a widened interpeduncular angle and abnormal concavity of the midbrain tegmentum.

In addition to a small midbrain, enlarged third ventricle, and prominent perimesencephalic cisterns, the *superior* cerebellar peduncles also appear atrophic and the quadrigeminal plate is often thinned.

DTI indices (FA, mean diffusivity, etc.) demonstrate widespread WM abnormalities that are often mild or inapparent on T2/FLAIR. WM changes are more severe in PSP-RS.

NUCLEAR MEDICINE. FDG PET shows glucose hypometabolism in the midbrain and along medial frontal regions. Dopamine transporter (DAT) radioligands show uniformly decreased dopamine nerve terminals in both the caudate nuclei and putamen.

Differential Diagnosis

The major differential diagnosis of includes **other tauopathies** such as **corticobasal degeneration** and some forms of **FTLD**. All share common molecular mechanisms and are therefore probably part of the same disease spectrum. **Alzheimer disease**, **PD**, and **MSA-P** usually do not exhibit the severe midbrain volume loss or atrophy of the superior colliculi that is seen with PSP.

PROGRESSIVE SUPRANUCLEAR PALSY

Etiology and Pathology
- Abnormal tau protein ("tauopathy")
- Substantia nigra depigmented
- Prominent midbrain atrophy

Clinical Issues
- Second most common cause of parkinsonism
- Insidious onset (sixth, seventh decades)
- Neuropsychiatric symptoms develop in 50%

Imaging
- Midbrain volume loss
  - "Penguin" or "hummingbird" sign on sagittal T1WI
  - Quadrigeminal plate thinned (especially superior colliculi)
  - Adjacent cisterns ↑
- Midbrain, medial frontal hypometabolism

Differential Diagnosis
- Other tauopathies
  - Corticobasal degeneration
  - Some forms of FTLD
- Alzheimer, PD, MSA-P
  - No disproportionate atrophy of midbrain, superior colliculi

---

Amyotrophic Lateral Sclerosis

Terminology

Amyotrophic lateral sclerosis (ALS) is also known as motor neuron disease (ALS/MND) or Lou Gehrig disease.

Etiology

GENERAL CONCEPTS. Upper motor neurons (UMNs) in the primary motor cortex send axons inferiorly along the corticospinal tract (CST) to pass through the brainstem, decussate at the cervicomedullary junction, and travel into the spinal cord. There, they synapse with anterior horn cells (lower motor neurons [LMNs]).

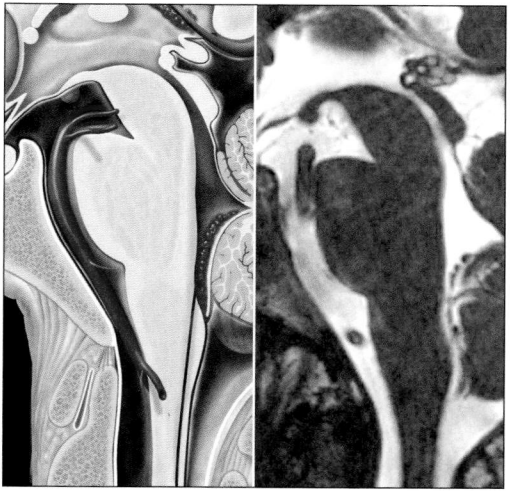

33-43. *Sagittal graphic (left) and high-resolution T2WI (right) show normal midbrain, pons.*

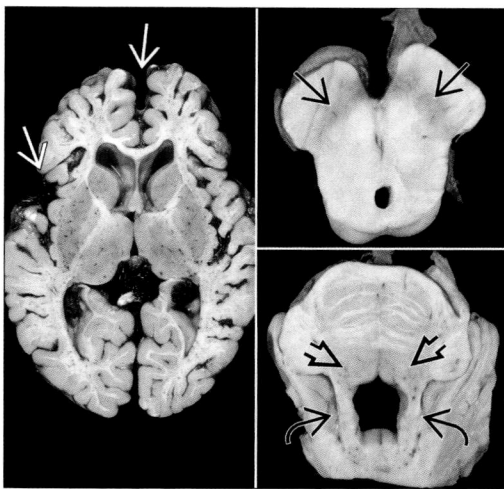

33-44. *PSP with frontotemporal atrophy ➡, depigmented substantia nigra ➡, locus ceruleus ➡, small superior cerebellar peduncles ➡.*

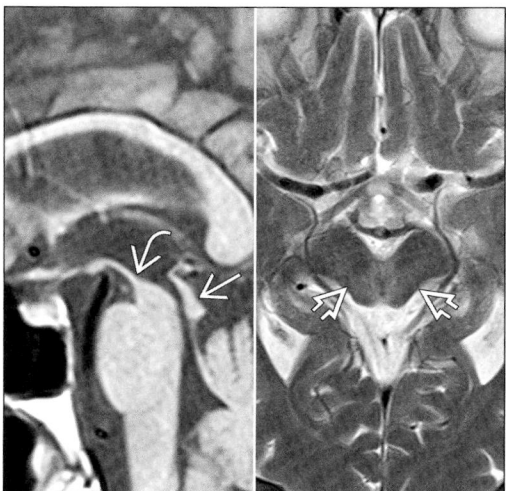

33-45. *PSP shows small midbrain with upper concavity and "penguin" or "hummingbird" sign ➡, tectal atrophy ➡, concave midbrain ➡.*

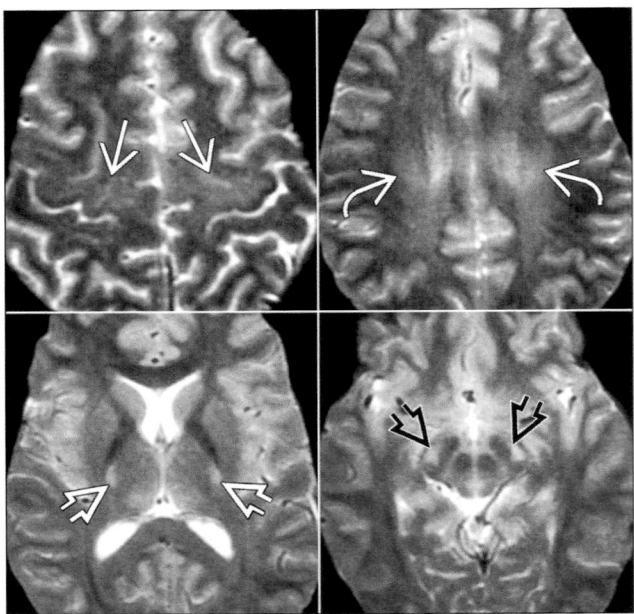

33-46. Axial T2 scans in a 19 year old with ALS show striking bilateral CST hyperintensity extending from the subcortical WM in motor cortex ➡ through corona radiata ➡ into posterior limbs of internal capsules ➡ and cerebral peduncles ➡.

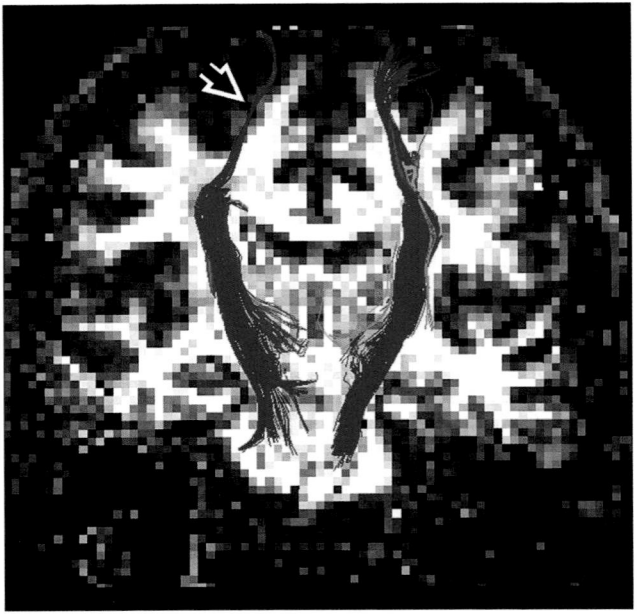

33-47. Coronal tractography in a patient with ALS shows that the upper right CST ➡ is significantly smaller than the relatively more normal-appearing left side. (Courtesy N. Agarwal, MD.)

ALS is characterized by progressive degeneration of motor neurons in both the brain and spinal cord. Whether the degeneration is a neuronopathy (i.e., begins in the cell body and proceeds in an anterograde fashion) or an axonopathy with retrograde degeneration is unknown.

GENETICS. A hexanucleotide repeat expansion in the gene *C9ORF72* has been associated with both ALS and FTLD. The mutation occurs in sporadic as well as familial cases.

Pathology

GROSS PATHOLOGY. Evidence of widespread muscle atrophy affecting limb and intercostal muscles and the diaphragm is typical at autopsy. Macroscopically, the brain is generally unremarkable, but mild focal atrophy of the precentral gyrus can be seen in some cases.

MICROSCOPIC FEATURES. The major histopathologic change in ALS is loss of motor neurons in the motor cortex, brainstem, and anterior horns of the spinal cord. Demyelination, axonal degeneration, and astrocytosis are typical features.

An RNA-mediated proteinopathy with mutated TDP-43 and FUS occurs in both FTLD and ALS. Immunohisto-chemistry demonstrates the presence of TDP-43 ubiquitinated cytoplasmic inclusion bodies in motor neurons. Extramotor pathology is also commonly found in the frontal cortex and CA4 neurons of the hippocampus.

Clinical Issues

EPIDEMIOLOGY AND DEMOGRAPHICS. ALS has an incidence of 1-2 per 100,000 per year and is the most common motor neuron disease, representing approximately 85% of all cases.

ALS is mostly sporadic; 10-15% of cases are familial. The average age of onset in familial ALS is 10 years earlier than in sporadic ALS.

PRESENTATION. Signs of *both* UMN and LMN disease are generally required for the clinical diagnosis of ALS. Evidence of UMN degeneration includes hypertonicity, hyperreflexia, and pathologic reflexes. LMN disease results in muscle fasciculations, atrophy, and weakness.

While ALS shares the same genetic spectrum with FTLD, muscle weakness is its dominant feature and dementia rarely—if ever—occurs. Disease onset is typically insidious, as at least 30% of anterior horn cells are lost before weakness becomes clinically apparent.

NATURAL HISTORY. Although median survival from diagnosis to death is between three and four years, 10% of patients survive beyond 10 years. Death is generally from respiratory failure due to diaphragm weakness.

Imaging

MR FINDINGS. Macroscopic atrophy on T1WI is uncommon in ALS. Voxel-based morphometry may demonstrate subtle gray matter atrophy in the precentral gyri.

Patients with ALS/FTLD exhibit a more pronounced frontotemporal volume loss.

The CST and subcortical WM appear normal in the majority of ALS patients with predominant UMN signs!

A small percentage demonstrate CST hyperintensity on PD- and T2-weighted or FLAIR sequences. The hyperintensity can occur anywhere from the subcortical WM to the cerebral peduncles and pons. Changes are usually most prominent in the posterior limbs of the internal capsules and cerebral peduncles (33-46). As the CST is normally slightly hyperintense, this finding lacks both sensitivity and specificity as an imaging "biomarker" for ALS.

No matter the intensity of the CST, DTI shows reduced FA in the internal capsules of ALS patients, indicating loss of microanatomical integrity. The extramotor WM also often shows decreased FA. Tractography demonstrates subcortical truncation of the CST in patients with demonstrable hyperintensity on PD- or T2-weighted sequences (33-47).

MRS is generally nonspecific with decreased NAA:Cr in the precentral cortex.

Differential Diagnosis

The major differential diagnosis of ALS is the **normal hyperintensity of compact, fully myelinated WM tracts**. The CST is typically slightly hyperintense on T2 scans, especially at 3.0 T.

Another diagnostic consideration is **primary lateral sclerosis** (PLS). PLS is a juvenile-onset autosomal recessive motor neuron disease that affects only upper motor neurons. **Wallerian degeneration** can cause T2/FLAIR hyperintensity along the CST but is unilateral.

Other disorders that may demonstrate T2 hyperintensity along the CSTs include **demyelinating** and **inflammatory diseases**, metabolic disorders such as **acute hypoglycemic coma**, and **infiltrating neoplasms** (most commonly high-grade astrocytomas).

AMYOTROPHIC LATERAL SCLEROSIS

Terminology and Etiology
- Lou Gehrig disease
- Progressive motor neuron atrophy in brain, spinal cord

Pathology
- Brain macroscopically normal
- Loss of motor neurons

Clinical Issues
- Sporadic > familial ALS
- Insidious onset
- Both UMN, LMN symptoms
- Death from respiratory failure

Imaging
- T2/FLAIR often normal
  - CST hyperintensity occurs but uncommon
  - Posterior limb IC, cerebral peduncles
- DTI shows reduced FA
  - Tractography shows thinning of one or both subcortical CSTs

Differential Diagnosis
- Most common: Normal!
  - CST normally slightly hyperintense
  - Especially in posterior limb of IC, peduncles
- Less common
  - Wallerian degeneration (unilateral)
  - Primary lateral sclerosis
  - Demyelinating disease
  - Tumor infiltration

Wallerian Degeneration

Terminology

Wallerian degeneration (WaD) is an intrinsic anterograde degeneration of distal axons and their myelin sheaths caused by detachment from—or injury to—their proximal axons or cell bodies.

Etiology

In the brain, WaD most often occurs after trauma, infarction, demyelinating disease, or surgical resection. Descending WM tracts ipsilateral to the injured neurons degenerate—but not immediately. Axons may stay morphologically stable for the first 24-72 hours. The distal part of the axon then undergoes progressive fragmentation that proceeds directionally along the axon stump.

Most forms of acute axonal degeneration involve a stepwise "cascade" of events. Compromise of the blood-nerve barrier causes rapid calcium influx from the extracellular space into the axonal cytoplasm, activation of the calcium-sensitive protease calpain, and impaired axonal transport. Mitochondria are damaged and vacuoles accumulate, leading to axonal swelling and beading.

The ubiquitin/proteasome degradation pathway is activated, and axons eventually undergo autophagy with degradation of intracellular proteins and organelles.

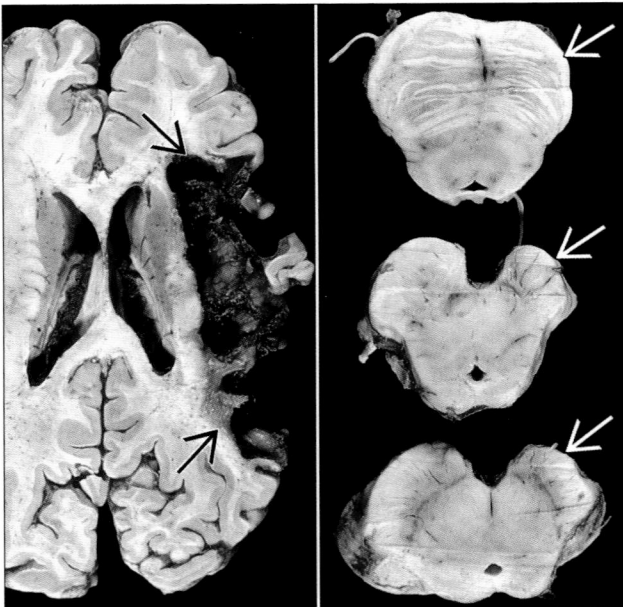

33-48. Autopsy specimen from a patient with chronic WaD following large left MCA infarct ➡ shows volume loss in the left cerebral peduncle and upper pons ➡. (Courtesy R. Hewlett, MD.)

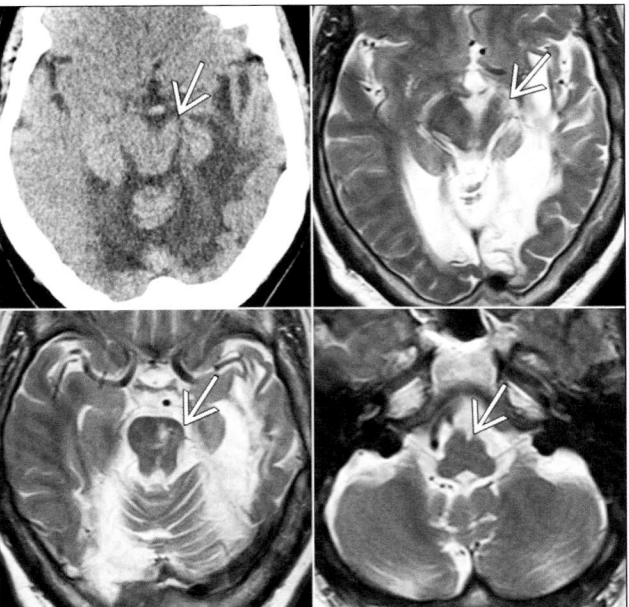

33-49. NECT (upper left) and a series of T2 scans demonstrate changes of chronic WaD following major territorial infarction. Note atrophy of the left cerebral peduncle, upper pons, midbrain ➡.

Macrophage infiltration exacerbates cell damage by releasing toxic proinflammatory mediators. The final result is granular disintegration of the cytoskeleton and volume loss in the affected WM tracts or nerves.

Pathology

Virtually any WM tract or nerve in the brain, spinal cord, or peripheral nervous system can exhibit changes of WaD. The caudally directed motor fiber pathways of the descending corticospinal tract (CST) are the most common sites of visible brain involvement. Other affected locations include the corpus callosum, optic radiations, fornices, and cerebellar peduncles.

In chronic WaD, midbrain and pons volume loss ipsilateral to a destructive lesion (e.g., a large territorial infarct) are grossly visible (33-48). Microscopic findings include early changes of myelin disintegration and axon breakdown.

Clinical Issues

Imaging abnormalities in WaD (see below) seem to correlate with motor deficits and poor outcome.

Imaging

CT FINDINGS. NECT scans are insensitive in the acute-subacute stages of WaD. Atrophy of the ipsilateral cerebral peduncle is the most common finding in chronic WaD (33-49).

MR FINDINGS. The development of visible WaD following stroke, trauma, or surgery is unpredictable. Fewer than half of all patients with motor deficits following acute cerebral infarction demonstrate T2/FLAIR hyperintensities or diffusion restriction in the CST that might herald WaD (33-50).

When it does develop, T2/FLAIR hyperintensity along the CST ipsilateral to the damaged cortex may occur as early as three days after major stroke onset but more typically becomes visible between three to four weeks later. The hyperintensity may be transient or permanent. Chronic changes include foci of frank encephalomalacia with volume loss of the ipsilateral peduncle, rostral pons, and medullary pyramid. Chronic WaD does not enhance on T1 C+, but acute degeneration may show transient mild enhancement.

Transient restricted diffusion in the CST may develop in acute ischemic stroke within 48-72 hours. Decreased ADC and FA are characteristic findings.

Microstructural changes in WM tracts are especially well-demonstrated with DTI (33-51), (33-52). Chronic hemispheric infarction shows decreased mean diffusivity (MD) and fractional anisotropy (FA) with absence of color in the CST.

Differential Diagnosis

The major differential diagnosis of WaD is primary neurodegenerative disease. The T2/FLAIR hyperintensity sometimes seen in **amyotrophic lateral sclerosis** is bilateral and extends from the subcortical WM adjacent to

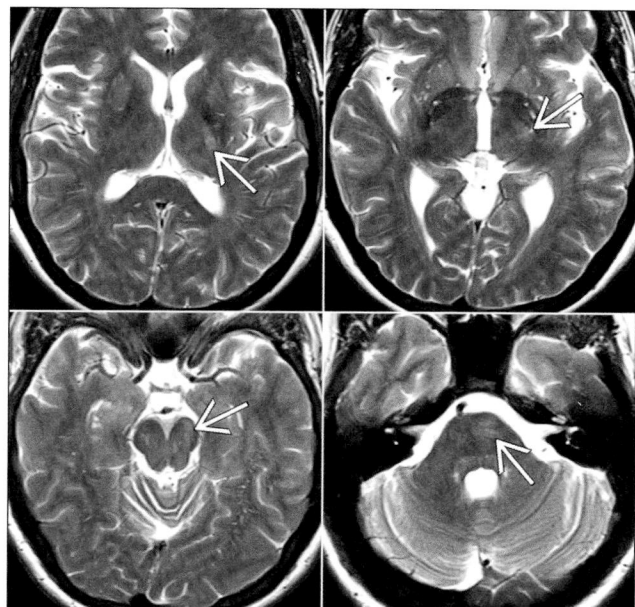

33-50. A patient with acute WaD was imaged 3 weeks following left hemisphere tumor resection. MR scans show CST hyperintensity ➡ without volume loss.

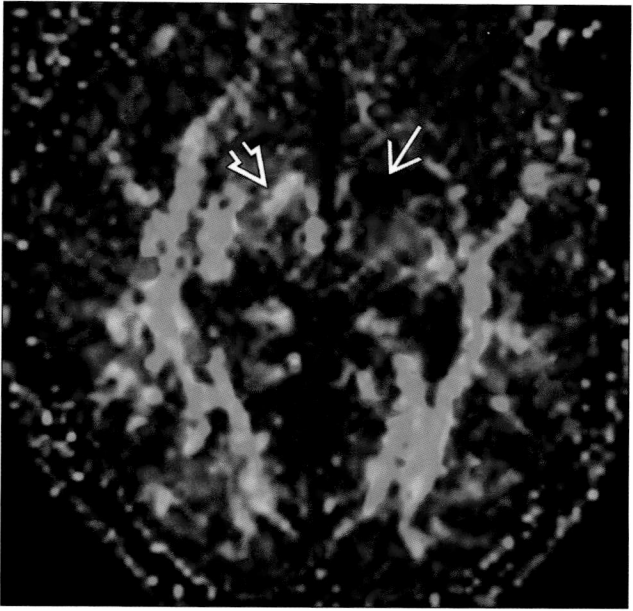

33-51. DTI in a patient with WaD shows the absence of blue color (descending fibers) ➡ in the left cerebral peduncle (corticospinal tract) compared to the normal right CST ➡.

the motor cortex into the brainstem. High-grade infiltrating primary brain tumors (typically **anaplastic astrocytoma** or **glioblastoma multiforme**) infiltrate along compact WM tracts but cause expansion, not atrophy.

Hypertrophic Olivary Degeneration

In order to understand the imaging findings in hypertrophic olivary degeneration, it is necessary first to understand the underlying anatomy of the medulla and the functional connections between the olives, red nuclei, and cerebellum.

Anatomy of the Medulla and Guillain-Mollaret Triangle

Two prominent ventral bulges are present on the anterior surface of the medulla: The pyramids and olives. The **pyramids** are paired structures, separated in the midline by the ventral median fissure of the medulla. The pyramids contain the ipsilateral corticospinal tracts above their decussation.

The **olives** are a crenelated complex of gray nuclei that are lateral to the pyramids and separated from them by the ventrolateral (preolivary) sulcus **(33-53)**.

The **Guillain-Mollaret triangle** consists of the **ipsilateral inferior olivary nucleus** (ION), **contralateral dentate nucleus** (DN), and **ipsilateral red nucleus** (RN) together with their three connecting neural pathways, i.e., the **olivocerebellar tract**, **dentatorubral tract**, and **central tegmental tract**.

Olivocerebellar fibers from the ipsilateral ION cross the midline through the inferior cerebellar peduncle, connecting it with the contralateral DN and cerebellar cortex. Dentatorubral fibers then enter the superior cerebellar peduncle (brachium conjunctivum) and decussate in the midbrain to connect to the opposite RN. The ipsilateral central tegmental tract then descends from the RN to the ipsilateral ION, completing the Guillain-Mollaret triangle **(33-54)**.

Terminology

Hypertrophic olivary degeneration (HOD) is a secondary degeneration of the ION caused by injury to the dentato-rubro-olivary pathway. Interruption of the dentato-rubro-olivary pathway at any point can cause HOD.

Etiology

Unlike other degenerations, in hypertrophic olivary degeneration, the degenerating structure (the olive) becomes hypertrophic rather than atrophic. Cerebellar symptoms and olivary hypertrophy typically develop many months after the inciting event. Understanding the clinical and pathologic underpinnings of HOD as well as its imaging manifestations will help avoid potential misinterpretation of this unusual lesion as an ischemic event, neoplasm, or focus of tumefactive demyelination.

HOD is a trans-synaptic degeneration caused by lesions in the Guillain-Mollaret triangle. Lesions in the dentatorubral or central tegmental (rubroolivary) tracts func-

33-52A. Axial T2WI in a patient with biopsy-proven acute wallerian degeneration shows a mass-like hyperintense lesion in the deep left cerebral white matter ➡. 33-52B. Hyperintensity in continuity with the hemispheric WM lesion is seen in the left corticospinal tract ➡. Compare with mild, normal hyperintensity in the right cerebral peduncle ➡.

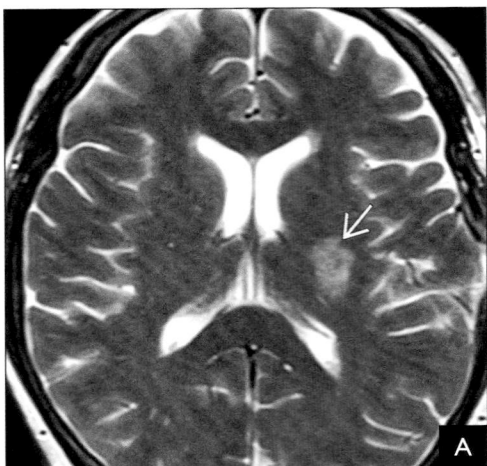

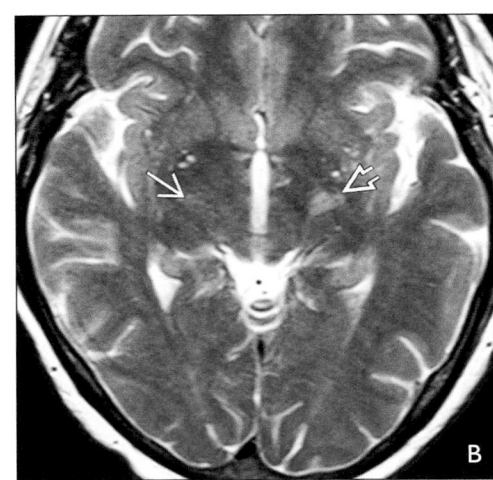

33-52C. Coronal T2WI shows hyperintensity in continuity from the deep WM lesion ➡ all the way along the internal capsule ➡, through the pons ➡, and down into the medulla ➡. 33-52D. Coronal T1 C+ FS shows enhancement along the cephalad internal capsule ➡.

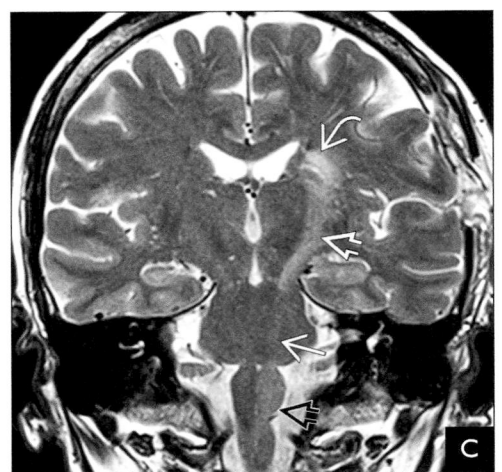

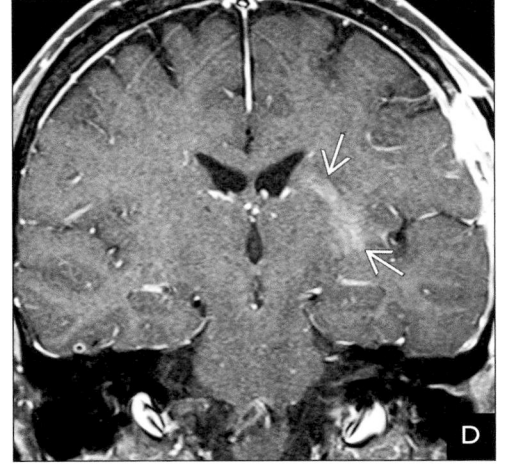

33-52E. Coronal DWI shows diffusion restriction in the left corticospinal tract ➡. 33-52F. Color DTI shows some reduction in the blue (superior to inferior) fiber tracts in the left internal capsule ➡.

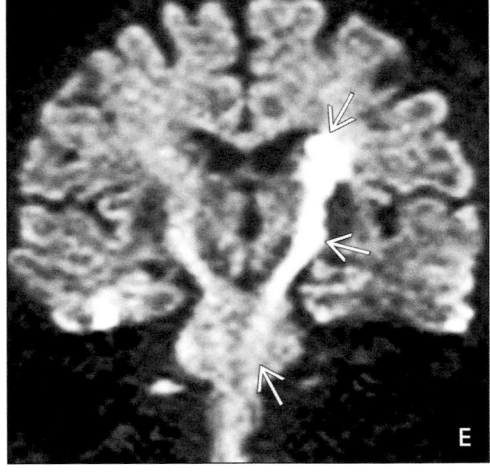

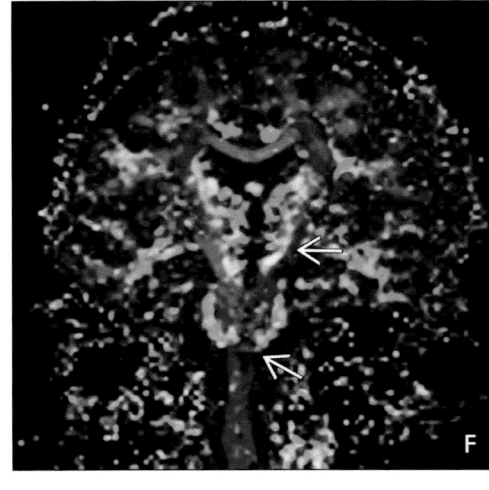

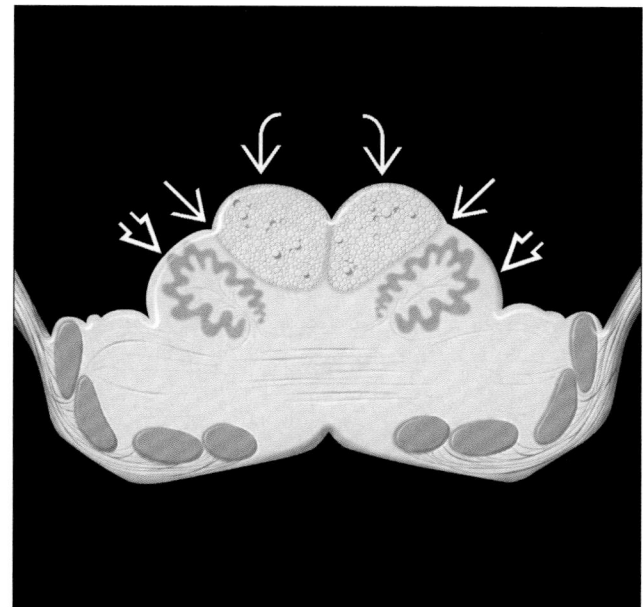

33-53. Axial graphic of the upper medulla shows the medullary pyramids ➡ on each side of the ventral median fissure. The olives ➡ lie just posterior to the preolivary sulci ➡.

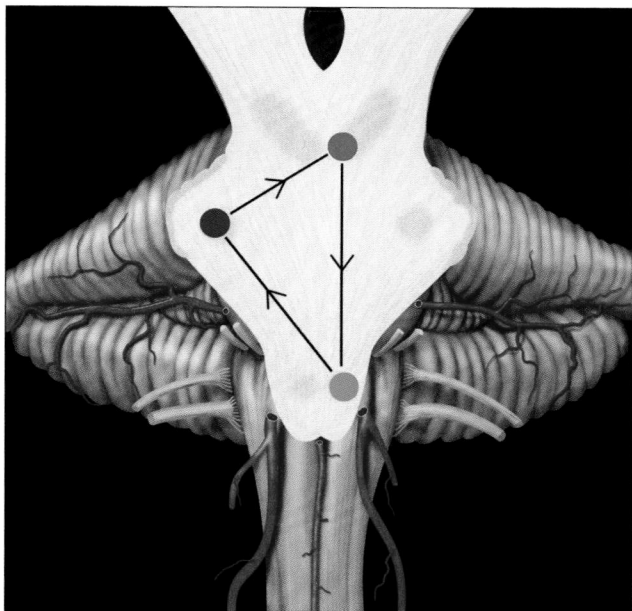

33-54. Coronal graphic depicts the Guillain-Mollaret triangle. The triangle is composed of the ipsilateral inferior olivary nucleus (green), the dentate nucleus (blue) of the contralateral cerebellum, and the ipsilateral red nucleus (red).

tionally deafferent the olive and cause HOD more often than lesions located in the olivocerebellar pathway.

The primary lesion in HOD is often hemorrhage, either from hypertension, surgery, vascular malformation, or trauma. Pontomesencephalic stroke also occasionally causes HOD.

Some cases of mitochondrial disorders with *POLG* and *SURF1* mutations have been described as causing HOD. Occasionally, no inciting lesion can be identified.

Pathology

LOCATION. Three distinct patterns develop, all related to the location of the inciting lesion. In **ipsilateral HOD**, the primary lesion is limited to the central tegmental tract of the brainstem. In **contralateral HOD**, the primary lesion is located within the cerebellum (either the DN or the superior cerebellar peduncle). In **bilateral HOD**, the lesion involves both the central tegmental tract and the superior cerebellar peduncle.

Approximately 75% of HOD cases are unilateral and 25% bilateral.

GROSS PATHOLOGY. Olivary hypertrophy is seen grossly as asymmetric enlargement of the anterior medulla. The contralateral RN often appears pale. In chronic HOD, the ipsilateral ION and contralateral cerebellar cortex may be shrunken and atrophic.

MICROSCOPIC FEATURES. Interruption of the Guillain-Mollaret triangle functionally deafferents the olive. The result is vacuolar cytoplasmic degeneration, neu-

ronal enlargement, and proliferation of gemistocytic astrocytes. The enlarged neurons and proliferating astrocytes cause the initial hypertrophy. Over time, the affected olive atrophies.

Clinical Issues

EPIDEMIOLOGY AND DEMOGRAPHICS. HOD is rare. It has been reported in patients of all ages, from young children to the elderly. There is no gender predilection.

PRESENTATION AND NATURAL HISTORY. The classic clinical presentation of HOD is palatal myoclonus, typically developing 4-12 months following the brain insult. Palatal myoclonus is seen as involuntary rhythmic movements of the soft palate, uvula, pharynx, and larynx. A dentatorubral tremor ("Holmes tremor") may occur before the onset of palatal myoclonus.

Imaging

GENERAL FEATURES. The development of HOD is a delayed process. While changes can sometimes be detected within three or four weeks after the initial insult, maximum hypertrophy occurs between 5 and 15 months. The hypertrophy typically resolves in one to three years, and the ION eventually becomes atrophic.

CT FINDINGS. While NECT scans may demonstrate the primary inciting lesion (e.g., hemorrhage), the HOD is generally not depicted.

MR FINDINGS. T1 scans are usually normal or show mild enlargement of the ION. T2/FLAIR hyperintensity with-

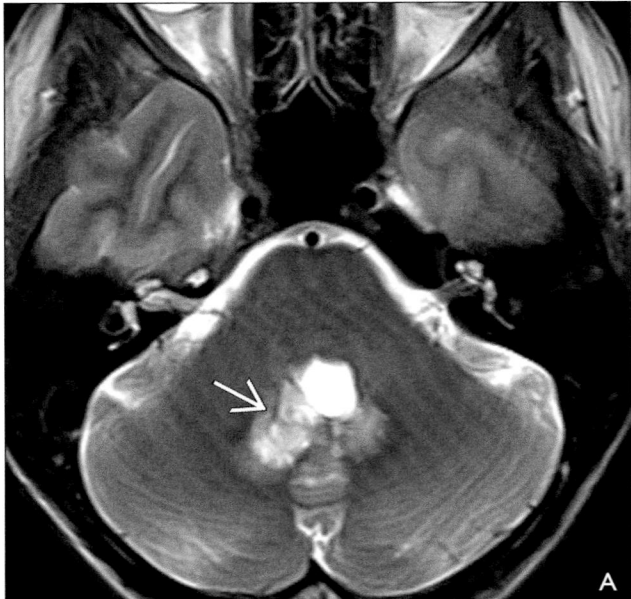

33-55A. *Axial T2WI in a patient who developed palatal myoclonus 6 months after medulloblastoma resection shows surgical changes in the right dentate nucleus* ➡.

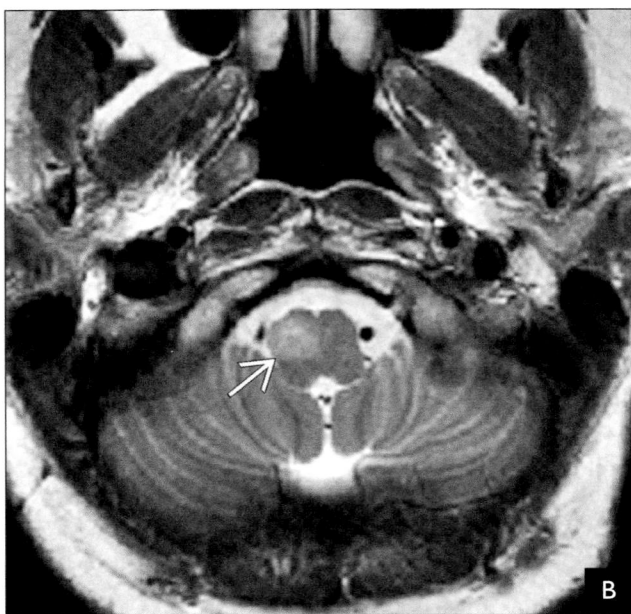

33-55B. *Axial T2WI through the medulla in the same patient shows unilateral HOD* ➡.

out enlargement of the ION occurs in four to six months but may be detectable as early as three weeks after the initial insult. Between six months and several years later, the ION appears both hyperintense and hypertrophied **(33-55)**, **(33-56)**. While the hypertrophy typically resolves and atrophy eventually ensues, the hyperintensity may persist indefinitely.

HOD does not enhance on T1 C+.

T2* SWI imaging may detect degeneration of the red nucleus, seen as loss of the normal RN hypointensity; the signal should be similar to that of the substantia nigra.

NUCLEAR MEDICINE. PET shows increased metabolic activity in the early stages of HOD while SPECT may demonstrate hyperperfusion.

Differential Diagnosis

The major differential diagnosis of HOD is the variety of other lesions that cause T2/FLAIR hyperintensity in the anterior medulla. These include **demyelinating disease**, **neoplasm**, and **perforating artery infarction**. The presence of an inciting lesion in the Guillain-Mollaret triangle (e.g., hemorrhage) establishes the olivary abnormality as HOD.

A rare mimic of bilateral HOD is caused by a nitroimidazole antibiotic called metronidazole. **Metronidazole neurotoxicity** is a drug-induced encephalopathy with T2/FLAIR hyperintense lesions in the corpus callosum splenium and red nuclei as well as the caudate, lentiform, oli-

vary, and dentate nuclei. Lesions are usually bilateral and symmetric.

HYPERTROPHIC OLIVARY DEGENERATION

Etiology
- Interruption of Guillain-Mollaret triangle
  ○ Causes trans-synaptic degeneration
- Usually secondary to midbrain lesion
  ○ Cavernous malformation, neoplasm

Pathology
- Inferior olivary hypertrophies
  ○ Can be uni- or bilateral
- Variable location
  ○ Ipsi- or contralateral to primary lesion

Clinical Issues
- Rare
- Can occur at any age
- Delayed onset
  ○ Usually occurs 4-12 months after insult
- Palatal myoclonus, dentatorubral tumor

Imaging
- Maximum hypertrophy at 5-15 months
  ○ Usually resolves in 1-3 years
  ○ Then ION atrophies
- ION T2/FLAIR hyperintensity
- Does not enhance

Differential Diagnosis
- Common
  ○ MS, neoplasm
  ○ Perforating artery infarct
- Rare but important
  ○ Metronidazole neurotoxicity

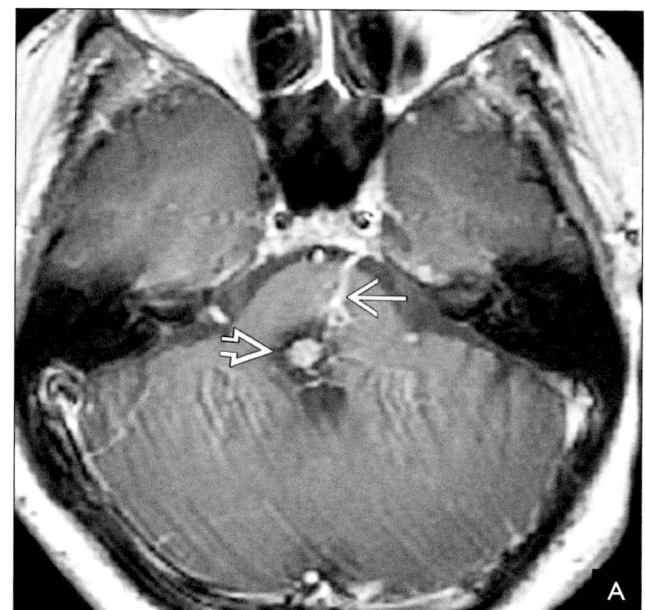

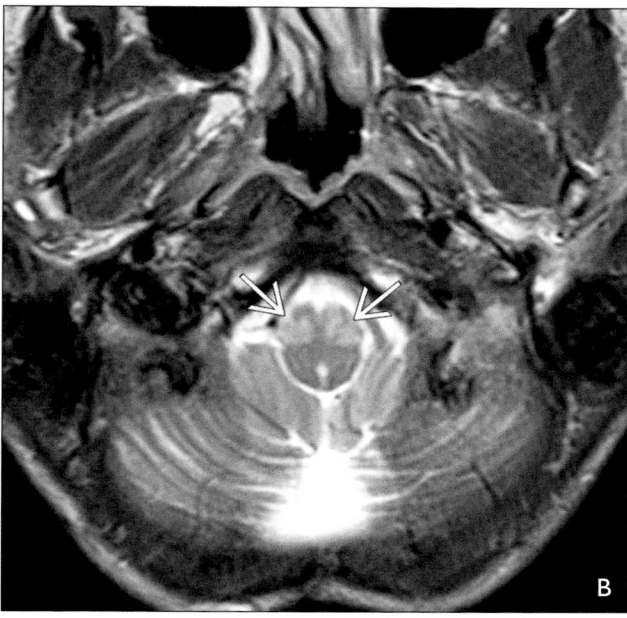

33-56A. Axial T1 C+ scan in a 46-year-old woman who developed palatal myoclonus 18 months following brainstem hemorrhage secondary to a mixed cavernous ⇒ and venous ⇒ malformation.

33-56B. T2WI in the same patient shows bilateral HOD ⇒.

Cerebral Hemiatrophy (Dyke-Davidoff-Masson)

Terminology and Etiology

Dyke-Davidoff-Masson syndrome (DDMS), also known as cerebral hemiatrophy, is typically caused by an in utero or early childhood cerebral insult such as an infarct, trauma, or (less commonly) infection.

Lack of ipsilateral brain growth causes the calvaria and diploic space to thicken, while the paranasal sinuses and mastoids become enlarged and hyperaerated (33-57).

Clinical Issues

Patients typically present with contralateral hemiplegia or hemiparesis. Seizures and mental retardation are common.

Imaging

GENERAL FEATURES. The affected hemisphere demonstrates diffuse volume loss with encephalomalacia and gliosis. Left-sided hemiatrophy is more common (70%) than right-sided hemiatrophy.

CT FINDINGS. NECT scans show an atrophic hemisphere with enlarged sulci and dilatation of the ipsilateral ventricle. The superior sagittal sinus and interhemispheric fissure are often displaced across the midline (33-58).

Bone CT shows variable degrees of calvarial thickening, elevation of the sphenoid wing and petrous temporal bone, and expanded sinuses and mastoids.

MR FINDINGS. T1WI shows hemispheric volume loss with prominent sulci and cisterns. T2/FLAIR scans demonstrate encephalomalacia with shrunken hyperintense gyri and subcortical WM (33-59). The ipsilateral cerebral peduncle is usually small. Atrophy of the contralateral cerebellum is common, secondary to crossed cerebellar diaschisis.

DDMS neither enhances on T1 C+ nor demonstrates restricted diffusion.

Differential Diagnosis

The major differential diagnosis is **Sturge-Weber syndrome** (SWS). DDMS lacks the enhancing pial angioma, enlarged choroid plexus, and typical dystrophic cortical calcifications of SWS. **Rasmussen encephalitis** lacks the calvarial changes typical of DDMS and demonstrates more focal encephalomalacia, typically in the medial temporal lobe and around the sylvian fissure.

In **hemimegaloencephaly**, the abnormal hemisphere is enlarged (not small as in DDMS) and has dysplastic-appearing features caused by hamartomatous overgrowth. **Large territorial MCA infarcts** that occur after the age of two or three years do not cause the calvarial changes that typify DDMS.

33-57. *Axial graphic depicts Dyke-Davidoff-Masson syndrome with shrunken, atrophic left hemisphere, thickened calvaria* ➡️, *off-midline insertion of the falx* ➡️ *and superior sagittal sinus* ▷. **33-58.** *NECT scan shows the typical findings of Dyke-Davidoff-Masson with significant atrophy, dystrophic calcification in the left hemisphere. The falx inserts off the midline* ➡️, *and the overlying calvaria is thickened* ➡️.

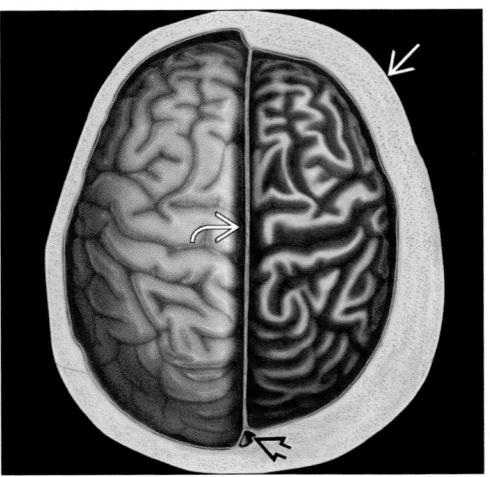
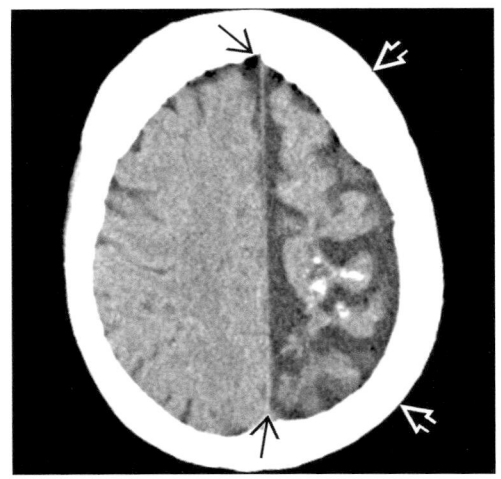

33-59A. *Axial T1WI in a 13 year old with longstanding seizures and left hemiparesis shows striking right cerebral hemiatrophy with enlarged lateral ventricle* ➡️, *off-midline falx and interhemispheric fissure* ➡️, *thickened calvaria* ➡️. **33-59B.** *More cephalad T2WI in the same patient shows that CSF fills the space above the atrophic right hemisphere. Compare the thickened calvaria* ➡️ *with the normal-appearing left side.*

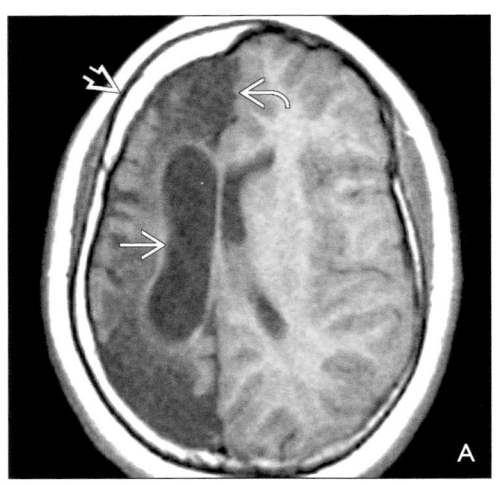
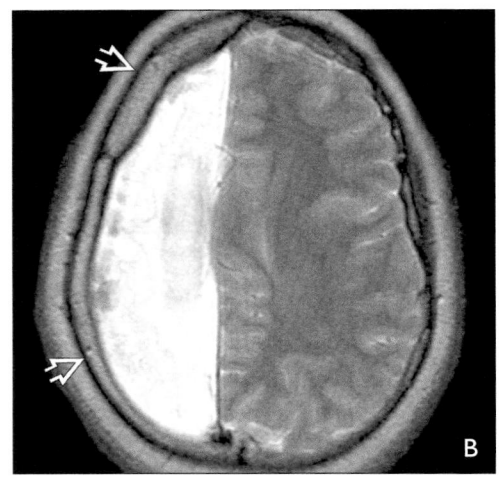

33-59C. *FLAIR scan in the same patient shows cortical atrophy with extensive WM gliosis* ➡️, *shrunken basal ganglia* ➡️, *and prominent right frontal sinus* ➡️. **33-59D.** *Coronal T1 C+ FS scan in the same patient shows elevation, hyperaeration of the right temporal bone* ➡️, *off-midline insertion of the falx and superior sagittal sinus* ➡️. *(Courtesy M. Edwards-Brown, MD.)*

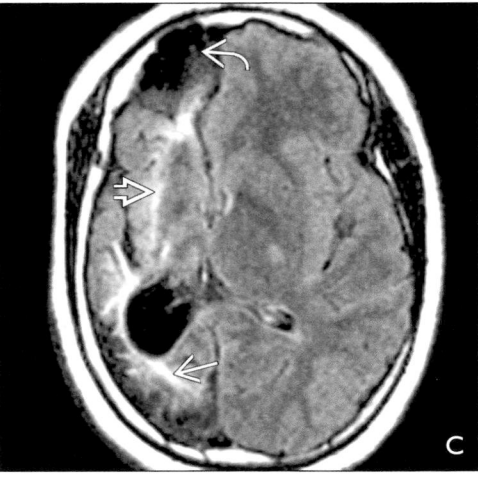
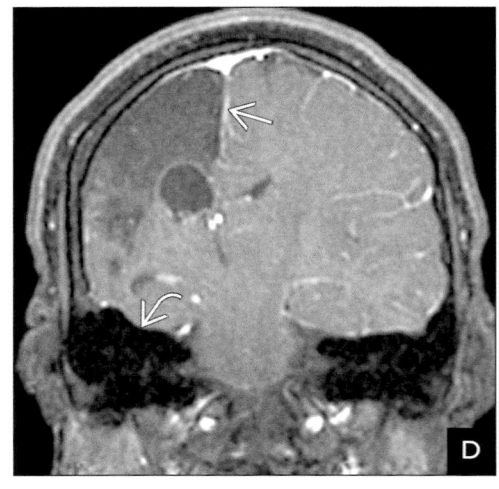

Selected References

The Normal Aging Brain

Introduction to the Normal Aging Brain

- Flicker LA et al: Memory loss. Med J Aust. 196:114-7, 2012
- Ikram MA et al: The Rotterdam Scan Study: design and update up to 2012. Eur J Epidemiol. 26(10):811-24, 2011
- Shim YS et al: Biomarkers predicting Alzheimer's disease in cognitively normal aging. J Clin Neurol. 7(2):60-8, 2011
- Sonnen JA et al: Ecology of the aging human brain. Arch Neurol. 68(8):1049-56, 2011

Imaging the Normal Aging Brain

- Ikram MA et al: The Rotterdam Scan Study: design and update up to 2012. Eur J Epidemiol. 26(10):811-24, 2011
- Aquino D et al: Age-related iron deposition in the basal ganglia: quantitative analysis in healthy subjects. Radiology. 252(1):165-72, 2009

Dementias

- Almeida OP: Dementia: What is it all about? The Neuroradiology Journal. 19(4): 433-440, 2006

Alzheimer Disease

- Fayed N et al: Magnetic resonance imaging based clinical research in Alzheimer's disease. J Alzheimers Dis. 31(0):S5-S18, 2012
- Shoji M: Molecular approaches to the treatment, prophylaxis, and diagnosis of Alzheimer's disease:clinical molecular and genetic studies on Alzheimer's disease. J Pharmacol Sci. 118(3):345-9, 2012
- Villemagne VL et al: Long night's journey into the day: amyloid-β imaging in Alzheimer's disease. J Alzheimers Dis. Epub ahead of print, 2012
- Brunnström H et al: Comparison of four neuropathological scales for Alzheimer's disease. Clin Neuropathol. 30(2):56-69, 2011
- Dawe RJ et al: Neuropathologic correlates of hippocampal atrophy in the elderly: a clinical, pathologic, postmortem MRI study. PLoS One. 6(10):e26286, 2011
- Karantzoulis S et al: Distinguishing Alzheimer's disease from other major forms of dementia. Expert Rev Neurother. 11(11):1579-91, 2011

Vascular Dementia

- Brundel M et al: Cerebral microinfarcts: a systematic review of neuropathological studies. J Cereb Blood Flow Metab. 32(3):425-36, 2012
- Deramecourt V et al: Staging and natural history of cerebrovascular pathology in dementia. Neurology. 78(14):1043-50, 2012
- Fu JL et al: The value of diffusion tensor imaging in the differential diagnosis of subcortical ischemic vascular dementia and Alzheimer's disease in patients with only mild white matter alterations on T2-weighted images. Acta Radiol. 53(3):312-7, 2012
- Nichtweiß M et al: White matter lesions and vascular cognitive impairment : part 1: typical and unusual causes. Clin Neuroradiol. 22(3):193-210, 2012

Frontotemporal Dementias

- Borroni B et al: Is long-term prognosis of frontotemporal lobar degeneration predictable by neuroimaging? Evidence from a single-subject functional brain study. J Alzheimers Dis. 29(4):883-90, 2012
- Fecto F et al: What is repeated in ALS and FTLD. Lancet Neurol. 11(1):25-7, 2012
- Premi E et al: Frontotemporal lobar degeneration. Adv Exp Med Biol. 724:114-27, 2012
- Whitwell JL et al: Neuroimaging signatures of frontotemporal dementia genetics: C9ORF72, tau, progranulin and sporadics. Brain. 135(Pt 3):794-806, 2012
- Rohrer JD et al: Clinical and neuroanatomical signatures of tissue pathology in frontotemporal lobar degeneration. Brain. 134(Pt 9):2565-81, 2011
- Rollinson S et al: Frontotemporal lobar degeneration genome wide association study replication confirms a risk locus shared with amyotrophic lateral sclerosis. Neurobiol Aging. 32(4):758, 2011
- Lindberg O et al: Cortical morphometric subclassification of frontotemporal lobar degeneration. AJNR Am J Neuroradiol. 30(6):1233-9, 2009

Dementia with Lewy Bodies

- Kantarci K et al: Focal atrophy on MRI and neuropathologic classification of dementia with Lewy bodies. Neurology. 79(6):553-60, 2012
- Taylor JP et al: Neuroimaging of dementia with Lewy bodies. Neuroimaging Clin N Am. 22(1):67-81, viii, 2012
- Goto H et al: Differential diagnosis of dementia with Lewy bodies and Alzheimer disease using combined MR imaging and brain perfusion single-photon emission tomography. AJNR Am J Neuroradiol. 31(4):720-5, 2010

Miscellaneous Dementias

- Crutch SJ et al: Posterior cortical atrophy. Lancet Neurol. 11(2):170-8, 2012
- Liberski PP et al: Kuru: genes, cannibals and neuropathology. J Neuropathol Exp Neurol. 71(2):92-103, 2012
- Puoti G et al: Sporadic human prion diseases: molecular insights and diagnosis. Lancet Neurol. 11(7):618-28, 2012
- Sikorska B et al: Creutzfeldt-Jakob disease. Adv Exp Med Biol. 724:76-90, 2012
- Boeve BF: The multiple phenotypes of corticobasal syndrome and corticobasal degeneration: implications for further study. J Mol Neurosci. 45(3):350-3, 2011

- Cilia R et al: Dopamine transporter SPECT imaging in corticobasal syndrome. PLoS One. 6(5):e18301, 2011
- Colby DW et al: Prions. Cold Spring Harb Perspect Biol. 3(1):a006833, 2011
- Lee SE et al: Clinicopathological correlations in corticobasal degeneration. Ann Neurol. 70(2):327-40, 2011
- Mastrolilli F et al: An unusual cause of dementia: essential diagnostic elements of corticobasal degeneration-a case report and review of the literature. Int J Alzheimers Dis. 2011: Article ID 536141, 2011
- Rajagopalan V et al: Diffusion tensor imaging evaluation of corticospinal tract hyperintensity in upper motor neuron-predominant ALS patients. J Aging Res. 2011:481745, 2011
- Tokumaru AM et al: Imaging-pathologic correlation in corticobasal degeneration. AJNR Am J Neuroradiol. 30(10):1884-92, 2009

Degenerative Disorders

- Massey LA et al: High resolution MR anatomy of the subthalamic nucleus: imaging at 9.4 T with histological validation. Neuroimage. 59(3):2035-44, 2012
- Hodaie M et al: The dopaminergic nigrostriatal system and Parkinson's disease: molecular events in development, disease, and cell death, and new therapeutic strategies. Neurosurgery. 60(1):17-28; discussion 28-30, 2007
- Slavin KV et al: Direct visualization of the human subthalamic nucleus with 3T MR imaging. AJNR Am J Neuroradiol. 27(1):80-4, 2006

Parkinson Disease

- Anheim M et al: Penetrance of Parkinson disease in glucocerebrosidase gene mutation carriers. Neurology. 78(6):417-20, 2012
- Brooks DJ: Parkinson's disease: diagnosis. Parkinsonism Relat Disord. 18 Suppl 1:S31-3, 2012
- Kumar KR et al: Genetics of Parkinson disease and other movement disorders. Curr Opin Neurol. 25(4):466-74, 2012
- Massey LA et al: High resolution MR anatomy of the subthalamic nucleus: imaging at 9.4 T with histological validation. Neuroimage. 59(3):2035-44, 2012
- Castrioto A et al: The dominant-STN phenomenon in bilateral STN DBS for Parkinson's disease. Neurobiol Dis. 41(1):131-7, 2011
- Cho ZH et al: Direct visualization of Parkinson's disease by in vivo human brain imaging using 7.0T magnetic resonance imaging. Mov Disord. 26(4):713-8, 2011
- Hickey P et al: Available and emerging treatments for Parkinson's disease: a review. Drug Des Devel Ther. 5:241-54, 2011
- Schwarz ST et al: T1-weighted MRI shows stage-dependent substantia nigra signal loss in Parkinson's disease. Mov Disord. 26(9):1633-8, 2011

Multiple System Atrophy

- Iodice V et al: Autopsy confirmed multiple system atrophy cases: Mayo experience and role of autonomic function tests. J Neurol Neurosurg Psychiatry. 83(4):453-9, 2012
- Massey LA et al: Conventional magnetic resonance imaging in confirmed progressive supranuclear palsy and multiple system atrophy. Mov Disord. Epub ahead of print, 2012
- Tsukamoto K et al: Significance of apparent diffusion coefficient measurement for the differential diagnosis of multiple system atrophy, progressive supranuclear palsy, and Parkinson's disease: evaluation by 3.0-T MR imaging. Neuroradiology. 54(9):947-55, 2012
- Köllensperger M et al: Presentation, diagnosis, and management of multiple system atrophy in Europe: final analysis of the European multiple system atrophy registry. Mov Disord. 25(15):2604-12, 2010
- Matsusue E et al: Putaminal lesion in multiple system atrophy: postmortem MR-pathological correlations. Neuroradiology. 50(7):559-67, 2008
- Naka H et al: Characteristic MRI findings in multiple system atrophy: comparison of the three subtypes. Neuroradiology. 44(3):204-9, 2002

Progressive Supranuclear Palsy

- Massey LA et al: Conventional magnetic resonance imaging in confirmed progressive supranuclear palsy and multiple system atrophy. Mov Disord. Epub ahead of print, 2012
- Saini J et al: In vivo evaluation of white matter pathology in patients of progressive supranuclear palsy using TBSS. Neuroradiology. 54(7):771-80, 2012
- Morelli M et al: Accuracy of magnetic resonance parkinsonism index for differentiation of progressive supranuclear palsy from probable or possible Parkinson disease. Mov Disord. 26(3):527-33, 2011
- Bouchard M et al: Tauopathies: one disease or many? Can J Neurol Sci. 38(4):547-56, 2011
- Barsottini OG et al: Progressive supranuclear palsy: new concepts. Arq Neuropsiquiatr. 68(6):938-46, 2010

Amyotrophic Lateral Sclerosis

- Cooper-Knock J et al: Clinico-pathological features in amyotrophic lateral sclerosis with expansions in C9ORF72. Brain. 135(Pt 3):751-64, 2012
- Kassubek J et al: Neuroimaging of motor neuron diseases. Ther Adv Neurol Disord. 5(2):119-27, 2012
- Langenhove TV et al: The molecular basis of the frontotemporal lobar degeneration-amyotrophic lateral sclerosis spectrum. Ann Med. Epub ahead of print, 2012
- Whitwell JL et al: Neuroimaging signatures of frontotemporal dementia genetics: C9ORF72, tau, progranulin and sporadics. Brain. 135(Pt 3):794-806, 2012
- Rajagopalan V et al: Diffusion tensor imaging evaluation of corticospinal tract hyperintensity in upper motor neuron-predominant ALS patients. J Aging Res. 2011:481745, 2011
- Turner MR et al: Advances in the application of MRI to amyotrophic lateral sclerosis. Expert Opin Med Diagn. 4(6):483-496, 2010

Wallerian Degeneration

- Lingor P et al: Axonal degeneration as a therapeutic target in the CNS. Cell Tissue Res. 349(1):289-311, 2012

- Liu X et al: Hyperintensity on diffusion weighted image along ipsilateral cortical spinal tract after cerebral ischemic stroke: a diffusion tensor analysis. Eur J Radiol. 81(2):292-7, 2012
- Gaudet AD et al: Wallerian degeneration: gaining perspective on inflammatory events after peripheral nerve injury. J Neuroinflammation. 8:110, 2011
- Jason E et al: Diffusion tensor imaging of chronic right cerebral hemisphere infarctions. J Neuroimaging. 21(4):325-31, 2011
- Puig J et al: Wallerian degeneration in the corticospinal tract evaluated by diffusion tensor imaging correlates with motor deficit 30 days after middle cerebral artery ischemic stroke. AJNR Am J Neuroradiol. 31(7):1324-30, 2010
- Domi T et al: Corticospinal tract pre-wallerian degeneration: a novel outcome predictor for pediatric stroke on acute MRI. Stroke. 40(3):780-7, 2009

Hypertrophic Olivary Degeneration

- Bruno MK et al: Hypertrophic olivary degeneration. Arch Neurol. 69(2):274-5, 2012
- Kinghorn KJ et al: Hypertrophic olivary degeneration on magnetic resonance imaging in mitochondrial syndromes associated with POLG and SURF1 mutations. J Neurol. Epub ahead of print, 2012
- Sanverdi SE et al: Hypertrophic olivary degeneration in children: four new cases and a review of the literature with an emphasis on the MRI findings. Br J Radiol. 85(1013):511-6, 2012
- Vossough A et al: Red nucleus degeneration in hypertrophic olivary degeneration after pediatric posterior fossa tumor resection: use of susceptibility-weighted imaging (SWI). Pediatr Radiol. 42(4):481-5, 2012
- Kim E et al: MR imaging of metronidazole-induced encephalopathy: lesion distribution and diffusion-weighted imaging findings. AJNR Am J Neuroradiol. 28(9):1652-8, 2007

Cerebral Hemiatrophy (Dyke-Davidoff-Masson)

- Chand G et al: Dyke-Davidoff-Masson syndrome. Arch Neurol. 67(8):1026, 2010
- Singh P et al: Dyke-Davidoff-Masson syndrome: Classical imaging findings. J Pediatr Neurosci. 5(2):124-5, 2010
- Atalar MH et al: Cerebral hemiatrophy (Dyke-Davidoff-Masson syndrome) in childhood: clinicoradiological analysis of 19 cases. Pediatr Int. 49(1):70-5, 2007

34

Hydrocephalus and CSF Disorders

The brain CSF spaces include the ventricular system—a series of interconnected, CSF-filled cavities—and the subarachnoid space. Understanding the normal anatomy of these CSF spaces and their variants is a prerequisite to deciphering their pathology. We therefore begin this chapter with a brief discussion of the normal development of the ventricles and CSF spaces, then delineate their normal gross and imaging anatomy.

We next describe normal variants, which should not be mistaken for disease, then turn our attention to hydrocephalus and the manifestations of elevated CSF pressure, including idiopathic intracranial hypertension ("pseudotumor cerebri"). We close the chapter with a discussion of CSF leaks and intracranial hypotension.

Normal Development of the Ventricles and Cisterns

Ventricles

The embryonic ventricular system is a series of interconnected fluid-filled chambers that arise as expansions from the central cavity of the embryonic neural tube. As the developing brain bends and expands, it forms forebrain, midbrain, and hindbrain vesicles. The forebrain cavity divides into two lateral ventricles, which develop as outpouchings from the rostral third ventricle and are connected to it by the interventricular foramen (foramen of Monro) (34-1).

The cerebral aqueduct develops from the midbrain vesicle. The fourth ventricle develops from the hindbrain cavity and merges proximally with the aqueduct and caudally with the central canal of the spinal cord. In the coronal plane, the developing lateral and third ventricles form a central H-shaped monoventricle that continues inferiorly into the aqueduct and then connects to the fourth ventricle.

At the eleventh or twelfth gestational week, the inferomedial aspect of the fourth ventricular roof thins and opens, creating the foramen of Magendie. The foramina of Luschka open shortly thereafter, establishing communication between the developing ventricular system and subarachnoid space.

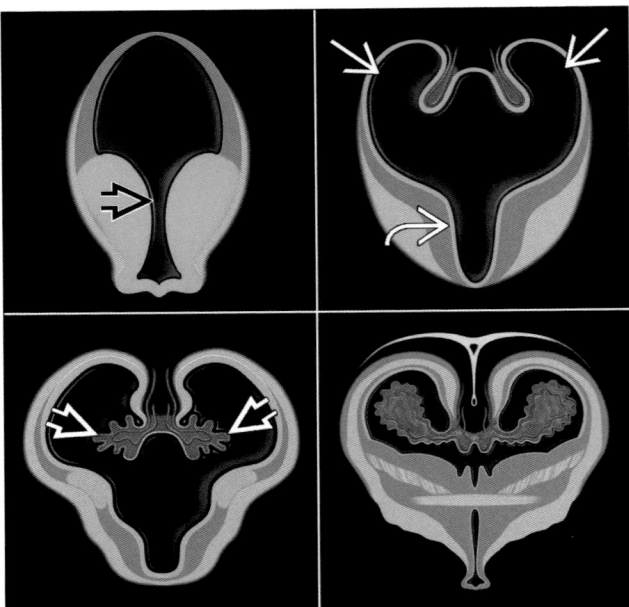

34-1. Embryology of forebrain, ventricles, choroid plexus. Central cavity of neural tube ⊵ *develops outpouchings* ➔ *from rostral third ventricle* ⤴*, forming H-shaped monoventricle. Choroid plexus* ⧨ *develops along choroid fissure.*

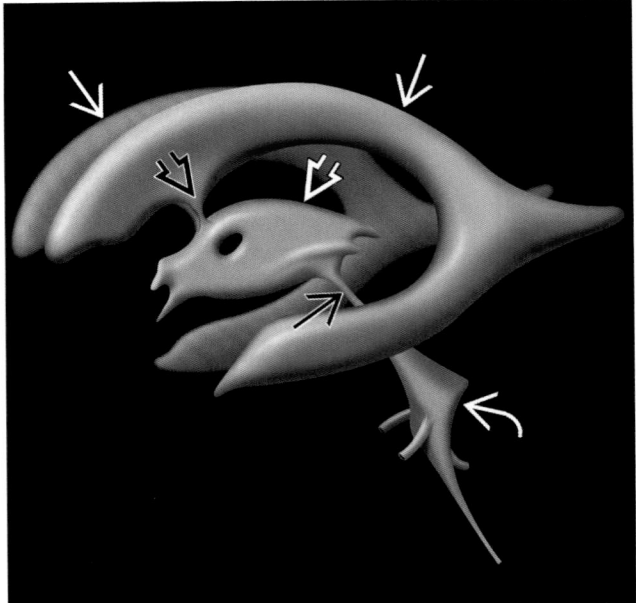

34-2. Graphic depicts the paired lateral ventricles ➔*, foramen of Monro* ⊵*, third ventricle* ⧨*, aqueduct* ⤳*, fourth ventricle* ⧨ *with its 3-outlet foramina and inferiorly directed obex.*

Choroid Plexus

The embryonic choroid plexus forms where infolded meningeal mesenchyme—the tela choroidea—contacts the ependymal lining of the ventricles. The invagination occurs along the entire choroidal fissure, a narrow cleft that lies in the medial lateral ventricle between the fornix and the thalamus.

Initially, the fetal choroid plexus is large relative to the size of the lateral ventricles, occupying nearly three-quarters of the ventricular lumen (34-1). As the brain and ventricular system grow, the choroid plexus gradually diminishes in relative volume.

Subarachnoid Spaces

The leptomeninges are derived from a gelatinous layer of paraxial mesoderm—the primary meninx or "meninx primitiva"—that envelops the neural tube. At day 32, the innermost zone of the primary meninx systematically degenerates, forming irregular spaces on the ventral aspect of the rhombencephalon. These spaces then extend caudally and dorsally, eventually coalescing to form the fluid-filled leptomeninges.

Normal Anatomy of the Ventricles and Cisterns

Ventricular System

The ventricular system is composed of four interconnected ependyma-lined cavities that lie deep within the brain (34-2). The paired lateral ventricles communicate with the third ventricle via the Y-shaped foramen of Monro. The third ventricle communicates with the fourth ventricle via the cerebral aqueduct (of Sylvius). In turn, the fourth ventricle communicates with the subarachnoid space.

Lateral Ventricles

Each lateral ventricle is a C-shaped structure with a body, atrium, and three projections ("horns"). We consider each part of the lateral ventricle from front to back.

The **frontal horn** is the most anterior segment of the lateral ventricle. Its roof is formed by the corpus callosum genu, and it is bordered inferolaterally by the head of the caudate nucleus. The septi pellucidi is a thin bilayered membrane that extends from the corpus callosum to the foramen of Monro, forming the medial borders of both frontal horns.

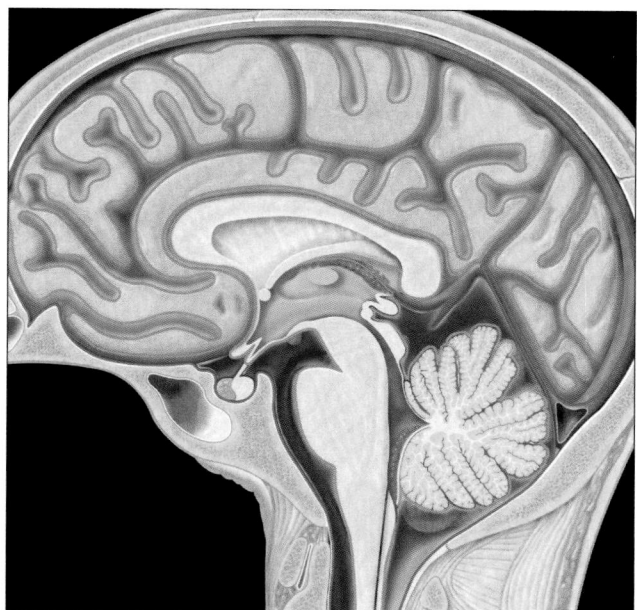

34-3. Sagittal graphic depicts subarachnoid spaces with CSF (blue) between arachnoid (purple), pia (orange). The pia is closely adherent to the brain while the arachnoid loosely adheres to the dura.

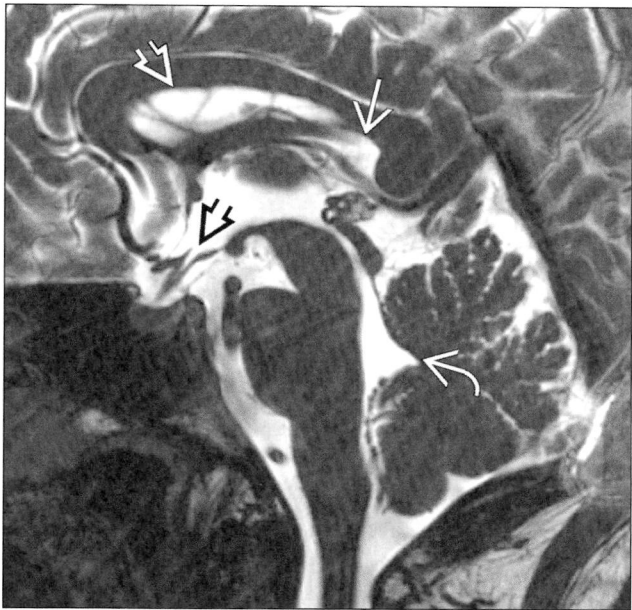

34-4. Sagittal T2WI shows lateral ventricle ⊡, velum interpositum ⊡, "pointed" recesses of the anterior third ventricle ⊡, fastigium of fourth ventricle ⊡.

The **body** of the lateral ventricle passes posteriorly under the corpus callosum. Its floor is formed by the dorsal thalamus, and its medial wall is bordered by the fornix. Laterally, it curves around the body and tail of the caudate nucleus.

The **atrium** contains the choroid plexus glomus and is formed by the convergence of the body with the temporal and occipital horns. The **temporal horn** extends anteroinferiorly from the atrium and is bordered on its floor and medial wall by the hippocampus. The **occipital horn** is surrounded entirely by white matter tracts, principally the geniculocalcarine tract and the forceps major of the corpus callosum.

Foramen of Monro

The foramen of Monro (interventricular foramen) is a Y-shaped structure with two long arms extending toward each lateral ventricle and a short inferior common stem that connects with the roof of the third ventricle. The anterior borders of the foramen on Monro are formed by the pillars (bodies) of the fornices. The posterior border is formed by the choroid plexus.

Third Ventricle

The third ventricle is a single, slit-like, midline, vertically oriented cavity that lies between the thalami. Its roof is formed by the tela choroidea, a double layer of invaginated pia. The anterior commissure lies along the anterior border of the third ventricle. The floor of the third ventricle is formed by the optic chiasm, hypothalamus, mammillary bodies, and roof of the midbrain tegmentum.

The third ventricle has two inferiorly located projections, the slightly rounded **optic recess** and the more pointed **infundibular recess**. Two small recesses, the **suprapineal** and **pineal recesses**, form the posterior border of the third ventricle. A variably sized interthalamic adhesion (the massa intermedia) lies between the lateral walls of the third ventricle.

Cerebral Aqueduct

The cerebral aqueduct is an elongated tubular conduit that lies between the midbrain tegmentum and the quadrigeminal plate. It connects the third ventricle with the fourth ventricle.

Fourth Ventricle

The fourth ventricle—sometimes called the rhomboid fossa—is a diamond-shaped cavity that lies between the dorsal pons and the vermis (34-3), (34-4). The fourth ventricle has five distinct recesses. The **fastigium** is a prominent triangular dorsal midline outpouching that points toward the vermis. The **posterior superior recesses** are paired, slender, CSF-filled pouches that curve over the cerebellar tonsils. The **lateral recesses** curve anterolaterally from the fourth ventricle, passing under the major cerebellar peduncles into the lower cerebellopontine angle cisterns (34-5).

The fourth ventricle gradually narrows as it courses inferiorly, forming the **obex**. Near the cervicomedullary junction, the obex becomes continuous with the central canal of the spinal cord. The junction between the obex and

34-5A. These 3.0 T T2 scans demonstrate normal ventricular anatomy. Inferior fourth ventricle ➡ contains small "dots" of choroid plexus. The posterolateral recesses ➡ and foramina of Luschka ➡ are indicated. *34-5B.* The body of the fourth ventricle resembles a kidney bean on its side. Note indentations caused by the facial colliculi ➡. The posterior superior recesses ➡ cap the cerebellar tonsils.

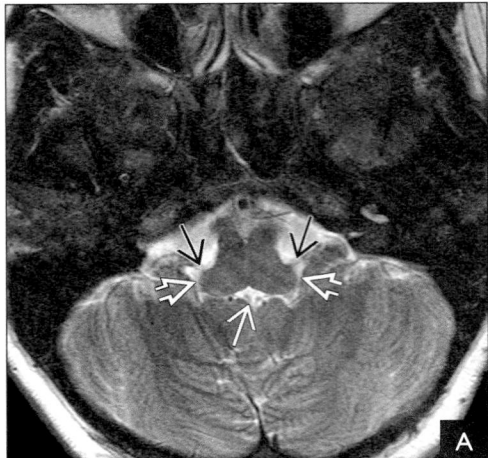

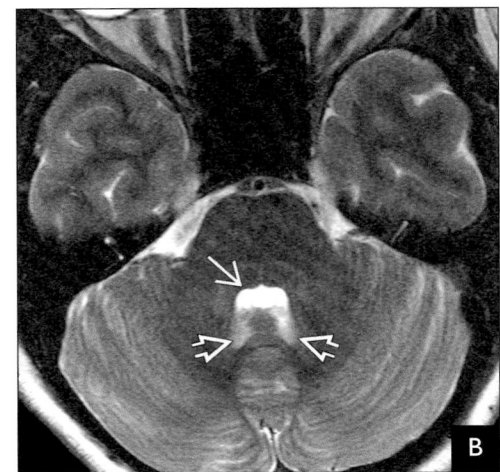

34-5C. The suprasellar cistern with the hypothalamus and infundibular recess of the third ventricle ➡, mammillary bodies bodies ➡ are clearly seen. The cerebral aqueduct is small and triangular ➡. Quadrigeminal cisterns ➡ contain choroidal arteries, basal vein of Rosenthal, and the trochlear nerves. *34-5D.* Frontal horns of the lateral ventricles are separated by the septi pellucidi. A tiny CSP is present ➡. Note foramen of Monro with its 2 connections ➡.

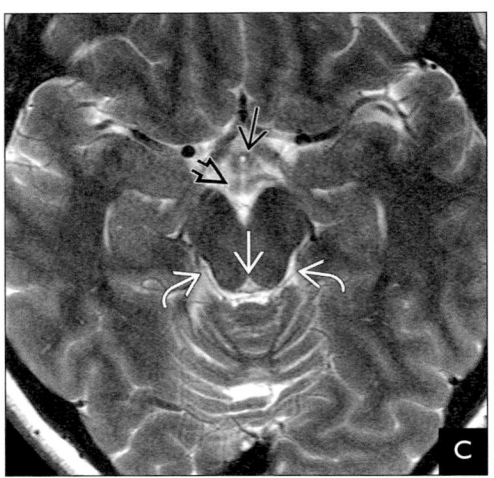

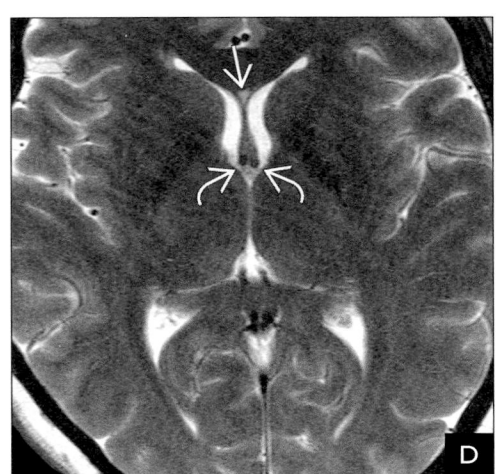

34-5E. Choroid plexus ➡, vessels course anteromedially toward the foramen of Monro (seen on the lower section). Surface sulci ➡ are small but well-delineated in this normal scan. *34-5F.* Coronal scan shows the velum interpositum ➡ lying below the fornices ➡. The rhomboid fourth ventricle joins the aqueduct above ➡. Midline foramen of Magendie ➡, posterosuperior recesses ➡ capping the cerebellar tonsils are shown.

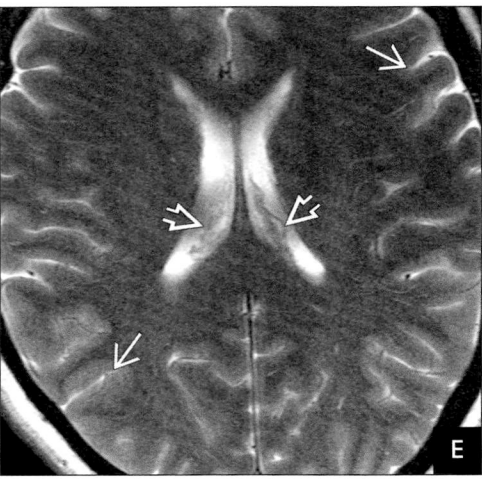

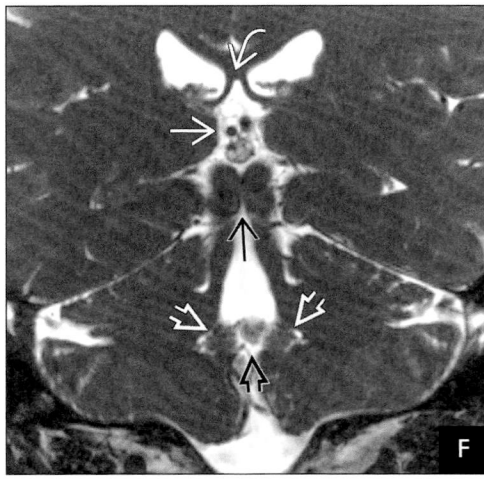

central canal is demarcated by a prominent dorsal "bump" formed by the nucleus gracilis.

Choroid Plexus and the CSF

The CSF space is a dynamic pressure system with a hydrostatic balance between CSF production and absorption. CSF pressure determines intracranial pressure, and normal values range from 3-4 mmHg before one year of age to 10-15 mmHg in adults.

Anatomy

The choroid plexus (CP) is composed of numerous highly vascular papillary or frond-like excrescences. These papillae consist of a central connective tissue core covered by ependyma-derived secretory epithelium.

The largest mass of CP is the **glomus**, which is located in the atrium of the lateral ventricles. The choroid plexus extends anterosuperiorly along the floor of the lateral ventricle, lying between the fornix and the thalamus. The CP extends anteroinferiorly from the glomus into the temporal horn, where it fills the choroidal fissure and lies superomedial to the hippocampus.

Function

The choroid plexus has two major functions: CSF production and maintenance of the blood-CSF barrier. In adult humans, the choroid plexus epithelium forms CSF at the rate of about 0.4 mL per minute or about 500 mL every 24 hours. CSF is turned over about four times a day, allowing for the removal of waste products.

The CP is not the only source of CSF. Brain interstitial fluid is a significant extrachoroidal source of CSF. Smaller potential sources of CSF production include the ventricular ependyma and brain capillaries.

The total CSF volume in neonates is 10-60 mL and approximately 150 mL in adults. The ventricles contain just 25 mL of CSF, and the vast bulk (125 mL) resides in the craniospinal subarachnoid spaces.

The CP maintains the blood-CSF barrier via tight junctions between epithelial cells. Protein transfer across the blood-CSF barrier is highly regulated. Specialized subpopulations of CP epithelial cells are responsible for the transfer of plasma proteins from blood to the CSF via the albumin-binding protein SPARC.

CSF was once thought a simple fluid envelope whose only function was to protect the CNS. It is now recognized that CSF plays an essential role in the maintenance of brain interstitial fluid homeostasis and regulation of neuronal functioning.

CSF Circulation

Normally, CSF circulates freely between the two intracranial reservoirs—the ventricles and CSF cisterns—and the spinal subarachnoid space. CSF flow in the ventricular cavities is unidirectional and rostrocaudal. CSF exits the fourth ventricle through the medial foramen (of Magendie) and the two lateral foramina (of Luschka) into the cerebellopontine angle cisterns. The only natural communication between the ventricles and subarachnoid spaces (SASs) is via the fourth ventricle.

In contrast to the unidirectional flow in the ventricles, CSF flow in the SASs is multidirectional. CSF circulates rostrally to the arachnoid villi and caudally into the spinal subarachnoid spaces.

CSF absorption occurs via two routes. The primary drainage is through the arachnoid villi into the dural venous sinuses. Experimental evidence indicates that a smaller but substantial amount exits the brain via connections between the perivascular spaces, cranial and spinal nerve sheaths, and lymphatics of the head and neck.

Exactly how the CSF circulates is controversial. Two mechanisms have been posited: Bulk flow or pulsatile flow. In **bulk flow**, it is the arachnoid membrane and granulations that are considered primarily responsible for maintaining CSF homeostasis and regulating intracranial pressure. A slight hydrostatic pressure gradient exists between the sites where CSF is produced (the choroid plexus) and absorbed (arachnoid granulations), allowing for bulk flow. Villous CSF absorption then adapts its filtration rate to CSF pressure.

In **pulsatile flow**, CSF movement is thought to be propelled by pressure waves generated by the cardiac cycle. When the choroid plexus and cerebral arteries expand with systole, the CSF is passively mixed and moved. Pressure waves are also transmitted to the brain parenchyma and need to be dampened. The brain is encased in the rigid unyielding cranium, so it is thought that pressure is modulated by expansion of the venous sinuses and the elastic thecal sac of the spine.

CSF circulation may reflect combinations of both bulk and pulsatile flow.

Subarachnoid Spaces/Cisterns

The **subarachnoid spaces** (SASs) lie between the pia and arachnoid **(34-3)**. The **sulci** are small, thin SASs that are interposed between the gyral folds. Focal expansions of the SASs form the brain CSF cisterns. Numerous pial-covered septa cross the SASs from the brain to the arachnoid, which is loosely attached to the inner layer of the dura.

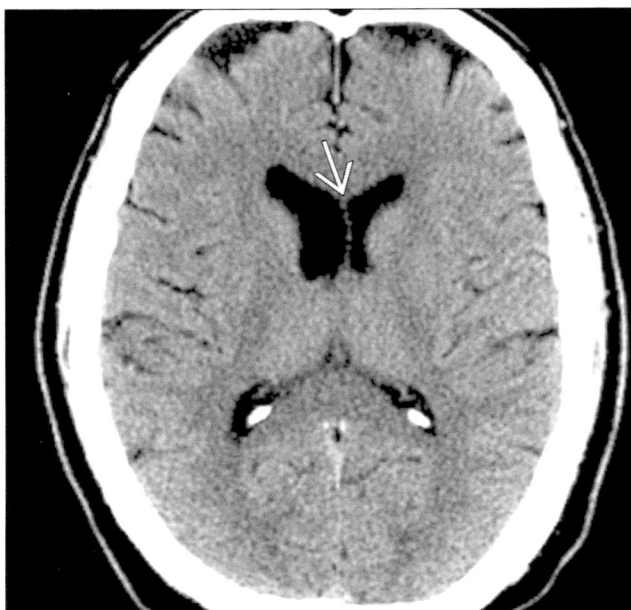

34-6. Axial NECT scan shows normal asymmetry of the lateral ventricles. The septi pellucidi ➔ are slightly bowed and displaced across the midline. There is no periventricular interstitial fluid or evidence of mass effect.

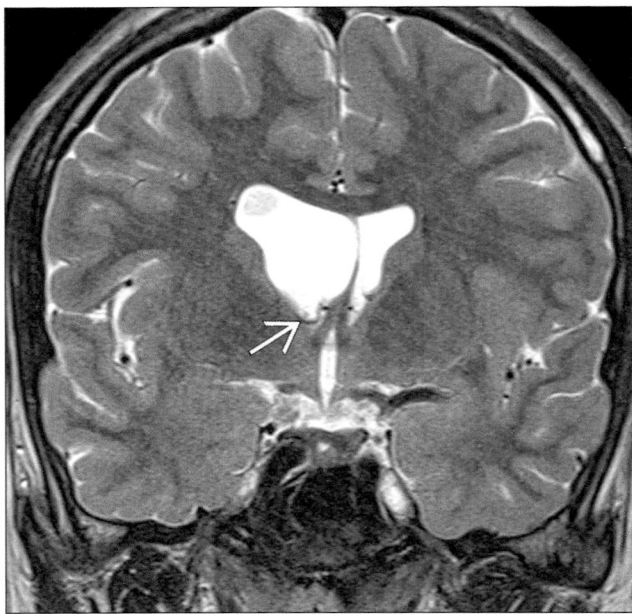

34-7. High-resolution thin-section coronal T2WI shows unilateral obstructive hydrocephalus. The right lateral ventricle is enlarged secondary to a web ➔ that obstructs outflow near the foramen of Monro.

The major cisterns are found at the base of the brain above the sella turcica, around the brainstem, at the tentorial apex, adjacent to the cerebellopontine angles, and above/below the foramen magnum. All SASs normally communicate freely with each other and the ventricular system, providing natural pathways for disease dissemination.

Normal Variants

Asymmetric Lateral Ventricles

Asymmetric lateral ventricles can be identified on imaging studies in approximately 5-10% of normal patients. The asymmetry is typically mild to moderate (34-6). Bowing, deviation, or displacement of the septi pellucidi across the midline is common; by itself, it neither indicates pathology nor implicates an etiology for nonspecific headache.

Severe degrees of asymmetry, diffuse nonfocal ventricular enlargement, or evidence of transependymal CSF migration should prompt a search for possible accompanying disorders.

The major differential diagnosis for asymmetric lateral ventricles is **unilateral obstructive hydrocephalus**. Unilateral obstructive hydrocephalus is rare, occurring

when only one arm of the foramen of Monro becomes occluded (34-7). Membranous obstruction of the foramen of Monro can be overlooked and is best differentiated from benign ventricular asymmetry using special MR imaging techniques (see below).

Cavum Septi Pellucidi and Vergae

Terminology

A **cavum septi pellucidi** (CSP) is a CSF-filled cavity that lies between the frontal horns of the lateral ventricles. A **cavum vergae** (CV) is an elongated finger-like posterior extension from the CSP that lies between the fornices (34-8).

A CSP may occur in isolation, but a CV occurs only in combination with a CSP. When the two occur together, the correct Latin terminology is "cavum septi pellucidi et vergae." In common usage, the combination is often referred to simply as a CSP.

Etiology

The septa pellucida are two paired triangular membranes ("leaves") that develop at about 12 weeks' gestation. The embryonic septa pellucida are unfused, and the cavity between them is filled with CSF. This single cavity between the two leaves has two different names. Anterior to the foramen of Monro it is called the **cavum septi pellucidi** (CSP). Its posterior continuation between the fornices is designated the **cavum vergae** (CV).

Normally the two septa pellucida eventually fuse, and the cavity between them is obliterated. The fused membranes then become the **septum pellucidum**.

Clinical Issues

CSP prevalence decreases with increasing age. By three to six months of age, the CSP is closed in 80-85% of infants. A CSP persists into adulthood in 15-20%.

A CSP is usually asymptomatic and is typically a "leave-me-alone" lesion found incidentally at imaging studies.

Imaging

CT AND MR. The appearance of CSPs and CVs on both CT and MR varies from an almost inapparent, slit-like cavity (34-9) to a prominent collection measuring several millimeters in diameter (34-10). A CSP is isodense with CSF on NECT and follows CSF signal intensity exactly on MR. It suppresses completely on FLAIR.

In rare cases, an unusually large CSP/CV creates significant mass effect, splaying the fornices and leaves of the septi pellucidi laterally.

ULTRASOUND. A CSP is present in 100% of fetuses and is therefore always identified during obstetric sonography. The CSP increases in size between 19-27 gestational weeks, plateaus at 28 weeks, and then gradually closes from back to front. By term, the posterior part is usually fused, and in 85% of cases, the CSP is completely closed by three to six postnatal months. A CSP may persist into adulthood as a normal variant.

Differential Diagnosis

The location and appearance of a CSP with or without a CV is virtually pathognomonic and should not be confused with a **cavum velum interpositum** (CVI). A CVI is a thin, triangular CSF space that overlies the thalami and third ventricle. A CVI typically occurs *without* a CSP.

An **absent septi pellucidi** lacks septal leaves, and the frontal horns appear as a single squared-off or "box-like" CSF cavity. An **asymmetric lateral ventricle** has a fused septi pellucidi that may be displaced across the midline. **Ependymal cysts** in the frontal horn are rare. When present, they focally displace the septi pellucidi rather than splaying its leaves apart.

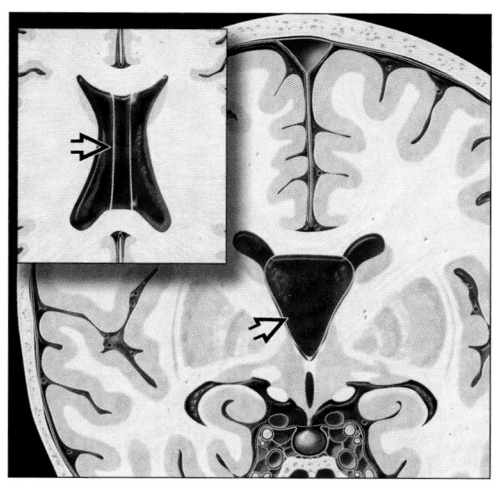

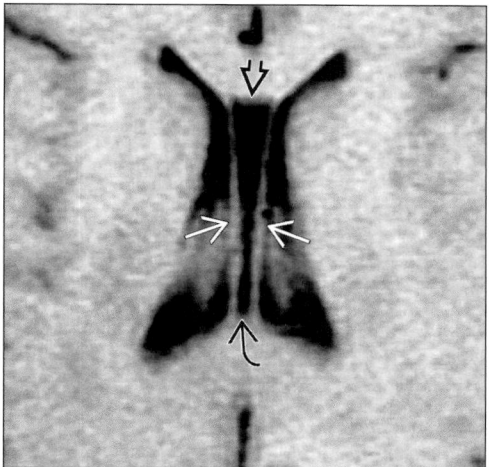

34-8. Coronal graphic with axial inset shows classic cavum septi pellucidi (CSP) with cavum vergae (CV) ⧎. The CSP appears triangular on the coronal image but finger-like on the axial view. 34-9. Close-up view of a T1WI shows a very small CSP with CV, seen as a finger-like CSF collection lying between the fornices ➡. Note that the cavity is continuous between the CSP ⧎ and the CV ⧉.

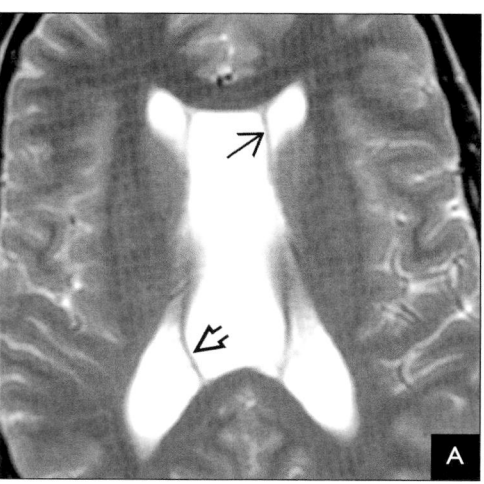

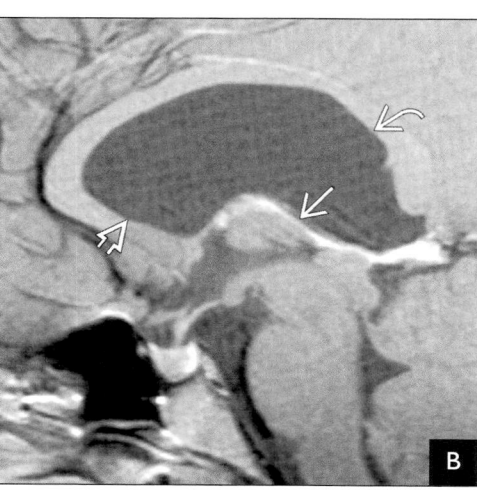

34-10A. Variant form of CSP with CV is illustrated by this axial T2WI. Note that the large CSF collection between the lateral ventricles bows the leaves of the septi pellucidi ➡ and the bodies of the fornices ⧎ outward. 34-10B. Sagittal T1 C+ FS in the same case shows that the CSF-filled space is continuous from the CSP anteriorly ➡ to the CV posteriorly ➡. The internal cerebral vein is displaced inferiorly ➡.

Cavum Velum Interpositum

Terminology

The velum interpositum (VI) is a thin translucent membrane formed by two infolded layers of pia-arachnoid. The VI is adherent to the undersurface of the fornices and extends laterally over the thalami to become continuous with the choroid plexus of the lateral ventricles. Together with the fornices, the VI forms the roof of the third ventricle (see Chapter 20).

The VI is often CSF-filled and open posteriorly, communicating directly with the quadrigeminal cistern. In such cases, it is called a cavum velum interpositum (CVI) (34-11). A CVI is considered a normal anatomic variant.

Clinical Issues

CVIs can be found at any age. They are usually asymptomatic and discovered incidentally on imaging studies. Mild nonspecific and nonfocal headache is the most common reported symptom.

Imaging

On imaging studies, a CVI appears as a triangular CSF space that curves over the thalami between the lateral ventricles. Its apex points toward the foramen of Monro (34-12).

CVI size varies from an almost inapparent slit-like cavity to a round or ovoid cyst-like mass that elevates and splays the fornices superiorly (34-13), (34-14) while flattening and displacing the internal cerebral veins inferiorly.

A CVI is isodense with CSF on NECT and isointense on all MR sequences. It suppresses completely on FLAIR, does not enhance, and does not restrict on DWI.

Differential Diagnosis

The major differential diagnosis of CVI is epidermoid cyst. An **epidermoid cyst** of the VI can occur but is rare. An epidermoid cyst shows some diffusion restriction and does not suppress completely on FLAIR. A large CVI may be impossible to distinguish from an **arachnoid cyst** in the VI on the basis of imaging studies alone.

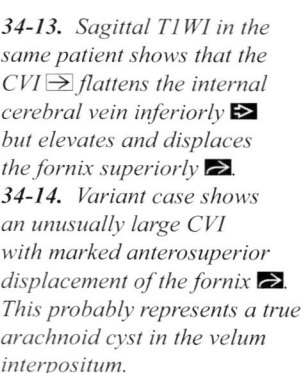

34-11. Sagittal graphic with axial inset shows a cavum vellum interpositum. Note the elevation and splaying of the fornices ➡. Also noted is the inferior displacement of the internal cerebral veins and third ventricle ➡. 34-12. Axial T2WI shows a CVI. The triangular shape with the apex ➡ pointed anteriorly and the fornices ➡ displaced laterally is the classic appearance of a CVI.

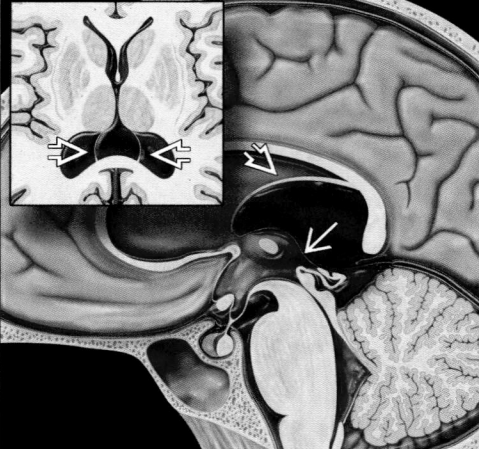

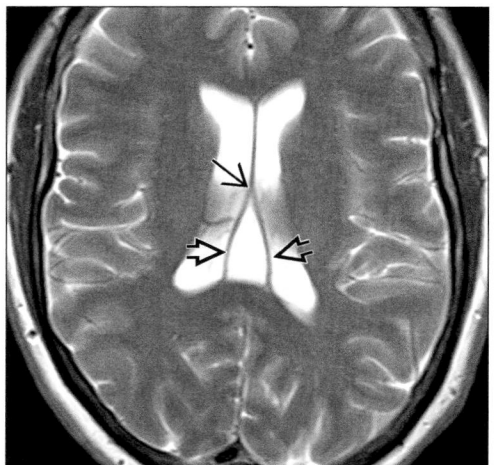

34-13. Sagittal T1WI in the same patient shows that the CVI ➡ flattens the internal cerebral vein inferiorly ➡ but elevates and displaces the fornix superiorly ➡. 34-14. Variant case shows an unusually large CVI with marked anterosuperior displacement of the fornix ➡. This probably represents a true arachnoid cyst in the velum interpositum.

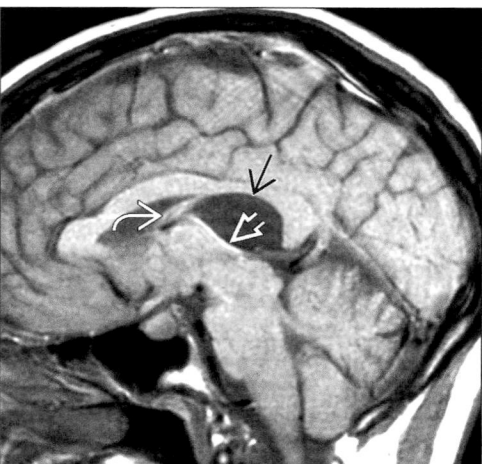

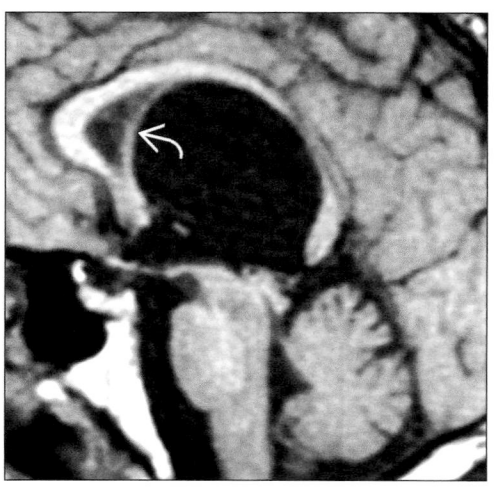

A **cavum septi pellucidi with cavum vergae** is elongated and finger-shaped, not triangular.

Enlarged Subarachnoid Spaces

Enlarged subarachnoid spaces occur in three conditions: Communicating hydrocephalus, brain atrophy, and benign enlargement of the subarachnoid spaces. Communicating hydrocephalus (both the intra- and extraventricular types) is discussed below. Brain atrophy—sometimes inappropriately called "hydrocephalus ex vacuo"—is discussed in Chapter 33 as a manifestation of aging and brain degeneration. In this section, we discuss benign physiologic enlargement of the subarachnoid space.

Terminology

Idiopathic enlargement of the subarachnoid spaces (SASs) with normal to slightly increased ventricular size is common in infants. Large CSF spaces in developmentally and neurologically normal children with or without macrocephaly may be called benign subarachnoid space enlargement, benign idiopathic external hydrocephalus, and benign extracerebral fluid collections of infancy. The preferred term is **benign enlargement of the subarachnoid spaces**.

Etiology

The precise etiology of benign enlarged SASs in infants is unknown but probably related to immature CSF drainage pathways. Pacchionian granulations do not fully mature until 12-18 postnatal months, by which time the benign SAS enlargement generally resolves.

There is no known genetic predisposition, although 80% of infants with benign enlarged SASs have a family history of macrocephaly.

Pathology

Grossly, the SASs appear deep and unusually prominent but otherwise normal (34-15). There are no subdural membranes present that would suggest chronic subdural hematomas or effusions.

Clinical Issues

Epidemiology and Demographics. The incidence of benign enlargement of the SASs is difficult to ascertain. It is reported on 2-65% of imaging studies for macrocrania in children under one year of age.

Benign enlarged SASs typically present between three and eight months. There is a 4:1 M:F predominance.

Presentation. Occipitofrontal head circumference (OFC) tends to be in the high-normal range at birth and increases rapidly within the first few months. Macrocra-

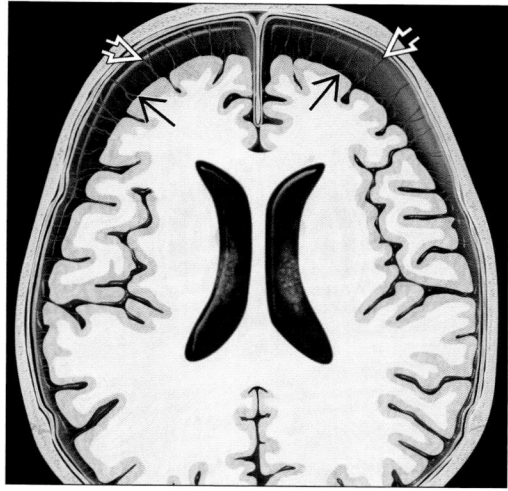

34-15. Graphic depicts benign enlarged frontal SASs ➡. Posterior SASs are normal. Note cortical veins crossing the prominent SASs ➡.

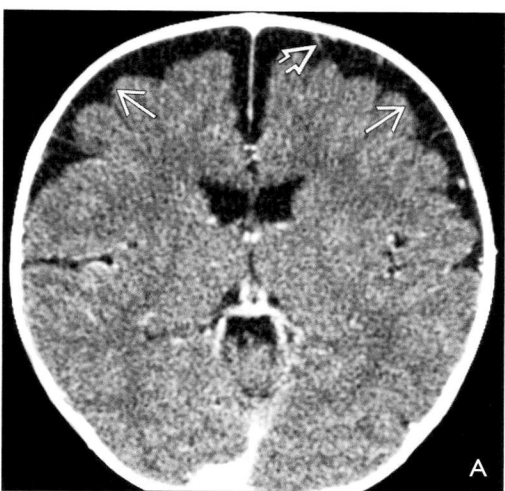

34-16A. CECT scan in a 7-month-old infant shows prominent bifrontal, interhemispheric subarachnoid spaces ➡, bridging veins ➡.

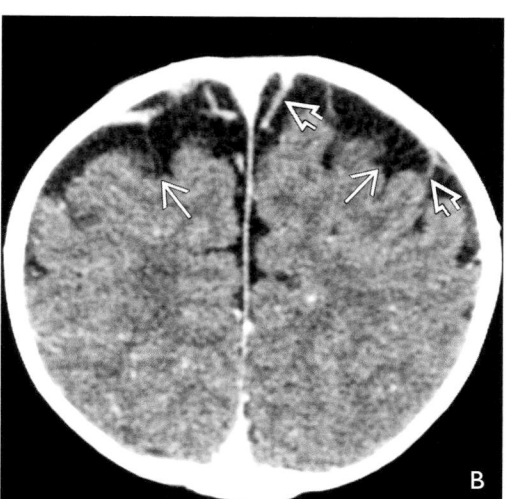

34-16B. More cephalad CECT in the same patient shows fluid collections ➡, bridging veins ➡. Benign enlarged SASs of infancy.

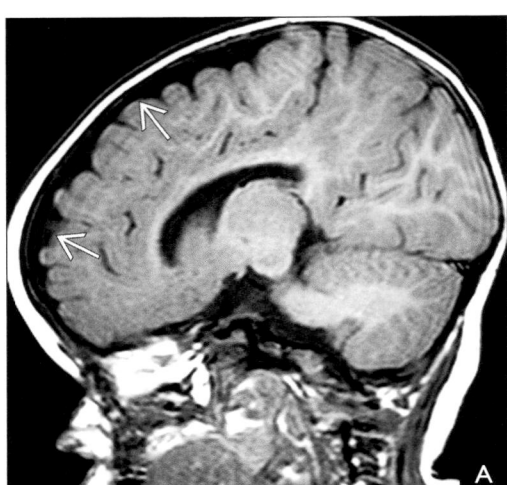

34-17A. Sagittal T1WI in a developmentally normal 7 month old with a large head shows macrocrania, enlarged frontal subarachnoid spaces ➡.

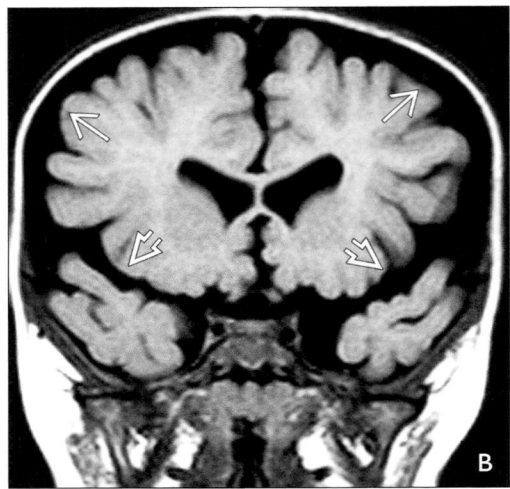

34-17B. Coronal T1WI in the same patient shows prominent SASs ➡, *sylvian fissures* ➡.

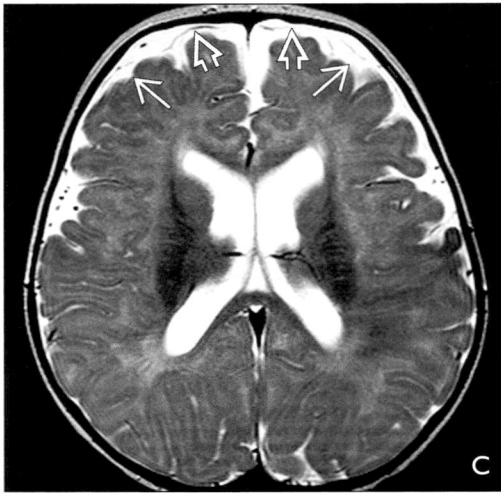

34-17C. Axial T2WI shows prominent frontal, interhemispheric subarachnoid spaces ➡, *bridging veins* ➡.

nia with OFC above the 95th percentile is typical at presentation.

There are no findings indicative of elevated intracranial pressure or nonaccidental trauma. Mildly delayed development is present in about half of all cases, but normal milestones are eventually reached.

NATURAL HISTORY. Benign enlarged SASs are a self-limited phenomenon that typically resolve by 12-24 months without intervention. The associated macrocephaly may resolve by two years, but it often levels off, remaining at the 98th percentile.

TREATMENT OPTIONS. No treatment is generally required.

Imaging

The frontal SASs in infants can normally appear somewhat prominent, reaching maximum size at about seven months. The presence of prominent SASs in and of itself does not establish the diagnosis of benign enlarged SASs; head circumference should be at or above the 95th percentile.

CT FINDINGS. Typical NECT findings in infants with benign enlarged SASs are prominent bifrontal and anterior interhemispheric SASs larger than five millimeters in diameter, enlarged suprasellar/chiasmatic cisterns, prominent sylvian fissures, and mildly enlarged lateral and third ventricles. The posterior and convexity sulci appear normal.

CECT scans demonstrate bridging veins traversing the SAS **(34-16)**. There is *no* evidence of thickened enhancing membranes to suggest subdural hematoma or hygroma.

MR FINDINGS. Fluid in the enlarged frontal SASs exactly parallels CSF because it *is* CSF **(34-17)**. The fluid suppresses completely on FLAIR, and there is no evidence of "blooming" on T2* (GRE, SWI). Enhancing veins can be seen traversing the SASs on T1 C+. DWI is normal.

ULTRASOUND. Ultrasound shows increased craniocortical width with linear echogenic foci caused by bridging veins that can be seen coursing directly into the superior sagittal sinus. Color Doppler demonstrates venous structures traversing the prominent SASs.

Differential Diagnosis

The major differential diagnoses of benign enlarged SASs are atrophy, extraventricular obstructive hydrocephalus, and nonaccidental trauma. In **atrophy**, the OFC is normal to small. In **extraventricular obstructive hydrocephalus** secondary to infection or trauma, the fourth ventricle is frequently enlarged, and the CSF in the extraaxial spaces does not parallel that of CSF in density or signal intensity.

Occasionally, infants with benign enlarged SASs have minor superimposed hemorrhagic subdural collections, similar to those sometimes observed with arachnoid cysts. In such infants, **nonaccidental trauma** must be a consideration until careful screening discloses no substantiating evidence of inflicted injury.

CSF Flow Artifacts

Normal CSF has long T1 and T2 relaxation times, causing the familiar dark and bright signal, respectively. CSF-related artifacts in the brain and spine are common on MR scans, primarily due to the to-and-fro pulsatile nature of CSF motion. Although a complete discussion of CSF flow-related phenomena is beyond the scope of this text, we briefly describe three examples of major CSF artifacts that can mimic pathology on MR imaging.

CSF flow-related phenomena are caused by time-of-flight (TOF) effects, turbulent flow, and patient motion.

Time-of-Flight Effects

TOF effects can result in **signal loss** (dark CSF signal) or flow-related enhancement, which produces bright CSF signal. TOF signal loss is directly related to CSF velocity and most prominent where flow is accelerated through narrow confines. Typical locations for TOF signal loss are around the foramen of Monro and in the third and fourth ventricles **(34-18)**.

Incomplete CSF nulling on FLAIR scans causes sulcal-cisternal CSF to appear spuriously bright, mimicking subarachnoid hemorrhage, infection, or metastatic disease **(34-19)**.

Entry-slice phenomena are most striking on T1 scans **(34-20)**. Bright signal is caused by inflow of unsaturated spins that have full longitudinal magnetization. The first slices of the imaging volume show the most prominent flow-related enhancement effects, which are most pronounced in the lower posterior fossa on axial sequences and around the foramen of Monro on coronal images. These entry-slice phenomena create artifacts that can mimic masses.

Turbulent Flow

Turbulent flow causes varied flow velocities and different directions with signal loss secondary to intravoxel spin dephasing. In the brain, turbulent flow with signal loss is common in the cerebral aqueduct, the fourth ventricle, and around pulsating vessels. This effect is especially pronounced around the basilar artery, where it can mimic aneurysmal dilatation.

Motion Artifacts

The most problematic artifact on MR imaging is voluntary patient motion. Voluntary patient motion can be minimized with verbal reminders or mild sedation. Some patient motion is both intrinsic and involuntary, caused by pulsating arteries or CSF.

Pulsation artifacts along the phase-encoding direction cause propagation of "ghosting" artifacts in a straight linear band across the entire imaged plane. Phase-encoding artifacts are often seen as alternating foci of bright and dark signal **(34-21)**.

Hydrocephalus

Hydrocephalus is the most common disorder requiring neurosurgical intervention in children. Its treatment consumes a disproportionate share of healthcare dollars, approaching nearly a billion dollars a year in the United States alone. Once considered predominantly a disease of childhood, hydrocephalus is increasingly recognized as a less common but still-important cause of neurologic disability in adults.

There is much that we still don't (but should) know about hydrocephalus. Here, we briefly consider the some of the major controversies surrounding hydrocephalus, focusing primarily on its imaging manifestations and complications.

Terminology

A rigorous definition of hydrocephalus is surprisingly difficult. Its terminology and classification are a matter of continuing debate. We follow the common approach of subclassifying hydrocephalus by the presumed site of CSF obstruction, i.e., inside (**intraventricular obstructive hydrocephalus** [IVOH]) or outside the ventricles (**extraventricular obstructive hydrocephalus** [EVOH]). The distinction is important, as treatment for IVOH (CSF diversion) differs from that of EVOH (membrane fenestration).

The outdated term "ex vacuo hydrocephalus" referred to ventricular and cisternal enlargement caused by parenchymal volume loss is no longer used.

Etiology

Hydrocephalus is a heterogeneous disease with disparate causes. The presence of enlarged ventricles combined with elevated intracranial pressure is only one presentation along a spectrum that ranges from idiopathic intracranial hypertension ("pseudotumor cerebri") to the

34-18A. Axial T2WI shows spin dephasing (gray areas ➡) in the CSF of the prepontine cistern caused by basilar artery pulsations. *34-18B.* Axial T2WI shows hypointense CSF in the upper third ventricle ➡ caused by pulsatile CSF flow through the foramen of Monro.

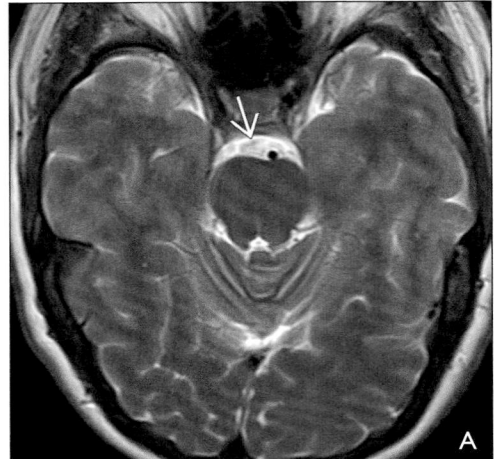

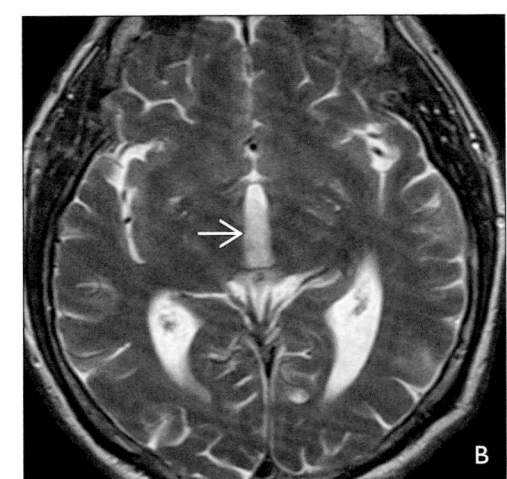

34-19. FLAIR shows fully suppressed CSF in ventricles ➡, superior vermian cistern ➡ while CSF in prepontine cistern remains bright ➡. *34-20.* First slice of a coronal T1WI shows artifactually bright signal in the third ventricle ➡ caused by flow-related enhancement. Turbulent flow with spin dephasing around the foramen of Monro causes hyperintensities ➡ in both lateral ventricles. Note "ghosting" artifacts across the image in the phase-encoding direction ➡.

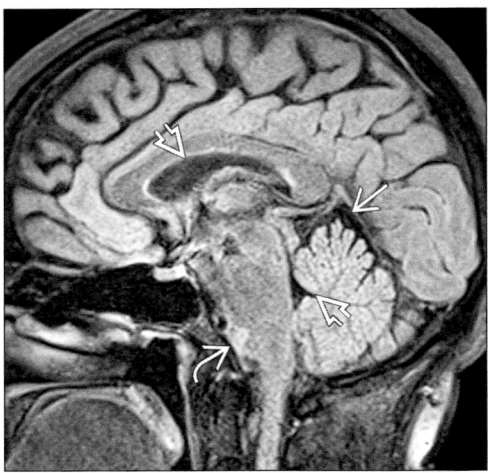

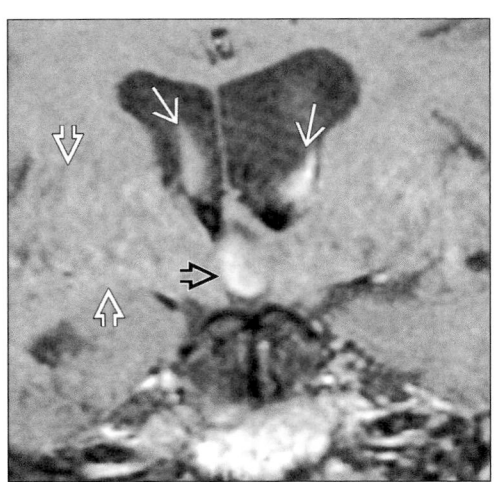

34-21A. Axial FLAIR scan shows prominent round hyperintense focus in the fourth ventricle ➡ caused by CSF pulsation artifact. Note propagation in a linear band in the phase-encoding direction ➡. *34-21B.* Phase-encoding artifact propagates horizontally across ventricles, parenchyma ➡.

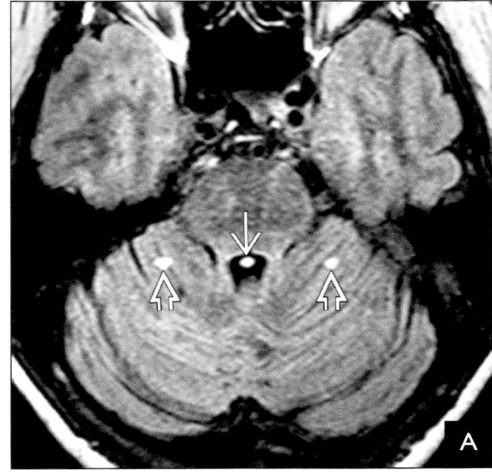

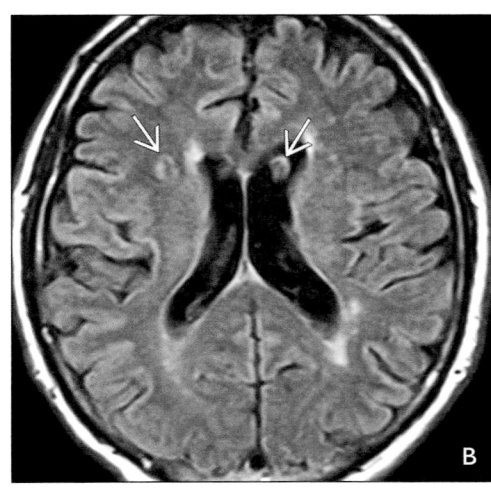

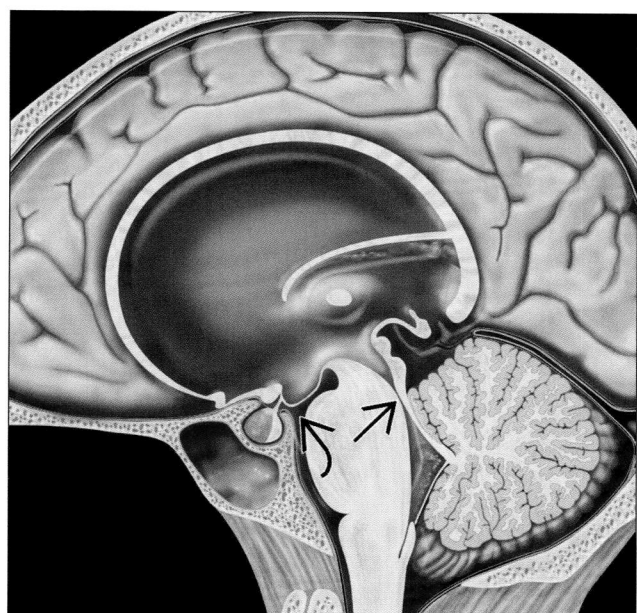

34-22. *Triventricular IVOH with markedly enlarged lateral, third ventricles, stretched corpus callosum, funnel-shaped cerebral aqueduct* → *with distal obstruction. Note normal size of fourth ventricle, bulging floor of third ventricle* →.

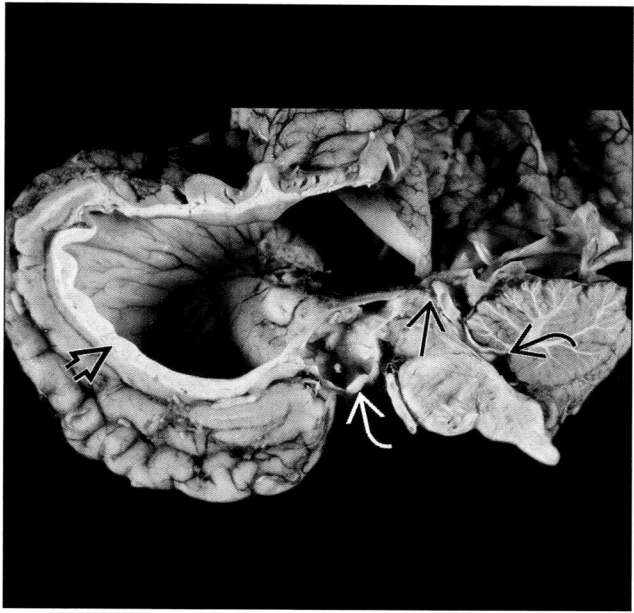

34-23. *Sagittal autopsy case with aqueduct stenosis* →, *massively enlarged lateral ventricle* →, *ballooned third ventricle* →, *normal fourth* →. (Courtesy Rubinstein Collection, AFIP Archives.)

recently recognized, enigmatic syndrome of low-pressure hydrocephalus.

Three different theories have been invoked to explain the development of hydrocephalus.

Longstanding traditional thinking about the etiology of hydrocephalus (literally "water on the brain") supposes that it results from an imbalance between CSF production and absorption. As CSF production remains relatively constant and does not decrease significantly until intracranial pressure approaches systolic pressure, hydrocephalus is thought to result from impaired absorption. True CSF overproduction is rare (occurring only in the setting of choroid plexus neoplasms and villous hyperplasia).

In this conventional model, CSF circulation and absorption occurs mostly via bulk flow. Bulk flow is a largely passive mechanism that depends on a slight pressure gradient between the SASs and venous sinuses. When CSF absorption is compromised, the ventricles enlarge and hydrocephalus results. Absorption can be blocked at any level within the ventricular system, the cisterna magna, basilar cisterns, or cerebral convexities. Connections between the perivascular spaces, cranial and spinal nerve sheaths, and lymphatics of the head and neck have been postulated as alternative CSF drainage pathways but are inadequate.

An alternative model uses altered CSF flow dynamics to explain the development of hydrocephalus. In this scenario, altered compliance of the spinal dural sac, abnormal dampening of the vascular bed, or increased pressure waves from pulsating arteries and the choroid plexus exert abnormal pressure on the brain parenchyma. The delicate balance of the system is compromised, resulting in hydrocephalus.

In this approach, hydrocephalus is divided into two main groups, acute hydrocephalus and chronic hydrocephalus. Acute hydrocephalus is caused by an intraventricular obstruction. Chronic hydrocephalus consists of two subtypes, communicating hydrocephalus and chronic obstructive hydrocephalus. Altered hydrodynamics—not faulty absorption—is considered the origin of both types of chronic hydrocephalus.

Aquaporins (AQPs)—and their role in water movement at brain-fluid interfaces—are invoked in the newest attempt to explain the development of hydrocephalus. Animal studies show that, with increased intracranial pressure and ventricular fluid accumulation, AQP1 is initially downregulated and then AQP1 ion channels are subsequently activated.

Intraventricular Obstructive Hydrocephalus

Terminology

The terms intraventricular obstructive hydrocephalus (IVOH) and noncommunicating hydrocephalus are both used to designate physical obstruction at or proximal to the fourth ventricular outlet foramina.

Etiology

GENERAL CONCEPTS. IVOH can be **congenital** or **acquired**, **acute** (aIVOH) or **chronic** (cIVOH). Congenital IVOH occurs with disorders such as aqueductal stenosis.

Although acute IVOH can occur suddenly (e.g., foramen of Monro obstruction by a colloid cyst), it usually develops over a period of weeks or even months. Any gradually expanding intraventricular mass (such as a neoplasm or cyst) can cause IVOH, as can an extraventricular mass of sufficient size to occlude a critical structure (e.g., the cerebral aqueduct).

When the ventricles become obstructed, CSF outflow is impeded. As CSF production continues, the ventricles expand. As the ventricles expand, increased pressure is exerted on the adjacent brain parenchyma. Increased intraparenchymal pressure compromises cerebral blood flow, reducing brain perfusion. The increased pressure also compresses the subependymal veins, which reduces absorption of brain interstitial fluid via the deep medullary veins and perivascular spaces. The

result is **periventricular interstitial edema**. Whether CSF is extruded across the ventricular ependyma (**"transependymal CSF flow"**) is unknown.

In chronic "compensated" IVOH, the ventricles expand slowly enough that CSF homeostasis is relatively maintained. Periventricular interstitial edema is absent.

PATHOETIOLOGY. The general causes of obstructive hydrocephalus range from developmental/genetic abnormalities to trauma, infection, intracranial hemorrhage, neoplasms, and cysts.

The most common cause of acquired IVOH ("noncommunicating" hydrocephalus) is intraventricular inflammatory or posthemorrhagic membranous obstruction. The most common sites of obstructing membranes are, in order, the foramina of Luschka, the cerebral aqueduct, and the foramen of Magendie. The foramen of Monro is a relatively rare location.

Intraventricular masses are the next most common cause of acquired IVOH. The prevalence of specific pathologies varies with location. Colloid cyst is the most common mass found at the foramen of Monro, followed by

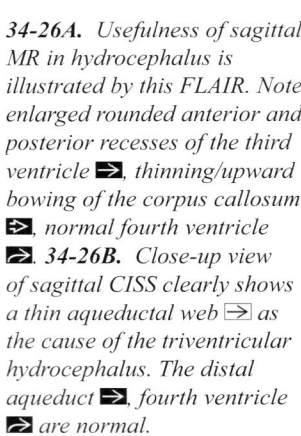

34-24. General signs of obstructive hydrocephalus shown on this NECT include enlarged temporal horns ➡ relative to the size of the basal cisterns. The third ventricle appears ovoid ➡ instead of slit-like. 34-25. NECT in another patient with IVOH shows enlarged rounded, frontal horns, large third ventricle, "blurred" margins of the lateral ventricles ➡ from periventricular interstitial edema, and effaced superficial sulci.

34-26A. Usefulness of sagittal MR in hydrocephalus is illustrated by this FLAIR. Note enlarged rounded anterior and posterior recesses of the third ventricle ➡, thinning/upward bowing of the corpus callosum ➡, normal fourth ventricle ➡. 34-26B. Close-up view of sagittal CISS clearly shows a thin aqueductal web ➡ as the cause of the triventricular hydrocephalus. The distal aqueduct ➡, fourth ventricle ➡ are normal.

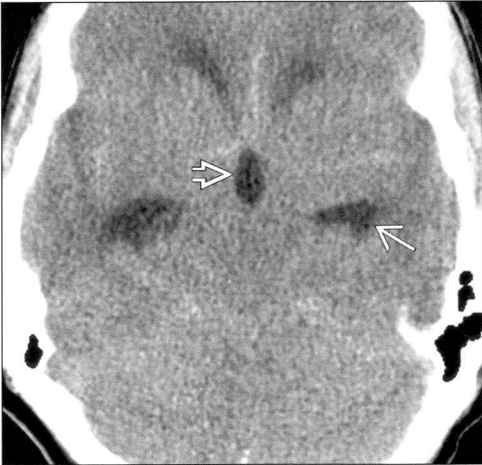
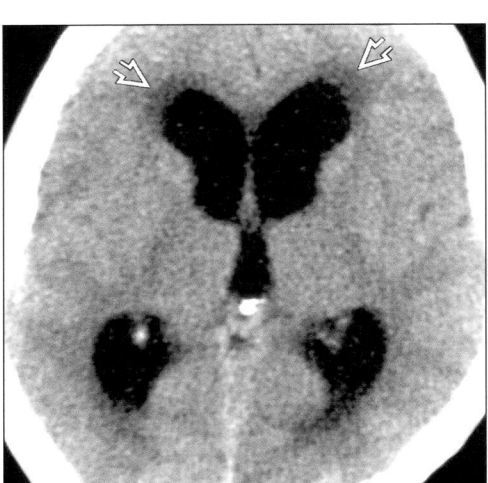
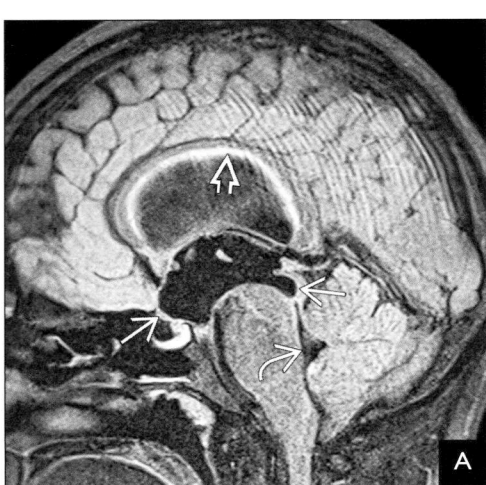
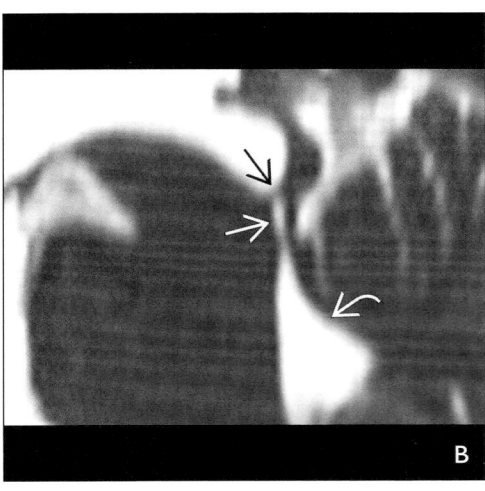

tuberous sclerosis (subependymal nodules and giant cell astrocytoma). After benign (membranous) obstruction, the most common lesions to obstruct the aqueduct of Sylvius are tectal plate glioma and pineal region neoplasms.

The fourth ventricle is a common site for neoplasms that can cause obstructive hydrocephalus. In children, medulloblastoma is the most common tumor that causes IVOH, followed by ependymoma, pilocytic astrocytoma, diffusely infiltrating astrocytoma, and atypical teratoid/rhabdoid tumor (AT/RT).

In adults, metastases, hemangioblastoma, epidermoid cyst, and choroid plexus papilloma are fourth ventricular lesions that may cause hydrocephalus. Inflammatory cysts (e.g., neurocysticercosis) occur throughout the ventricular system and in patients of all ages.

GENETICS. Congenital hydrocephalus can be syndromic or nonsyndromic. To date, only one gene—the neural cell adhesion molecule L1 (*L1CAM*)—has been recognized as a cause of congenital hydrocephalus. X-linked

hydrocephalus (hereditary aqueduct stenosis) is caused by mutation in the *L1CAM* gene.

Pathology

Grossly, the ventricles proximal to the obstruction appear ballooned (34-22), (34-23). The ependyma is thinned and may be focally disrupted or even absent. The corpus callosum is thinned and displaced superiorly against the rigid, unyielding falx cerebri. Focal encephalomalacic changes are common in the CC body.

Microscopic examination shows that the ependymal lining is discontinuous or inapparent. The periventricular extracellular space is increased, and the surrounding WM is rarefied and pale-staining. The cortex is relatively well-preserved.

Clinical Issues

EPIDEMIOLOGY AND DEMOGRAPHICS. IVOH can affect people at any age, from the fetus (in utero congenital hydrocephalus) to the elderly. There is no gender predilection except for primary congenital hydrocephalus, in which the M:F ratio is 2.6:1.

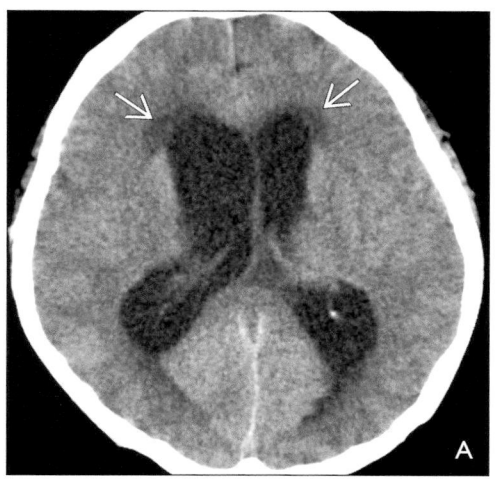
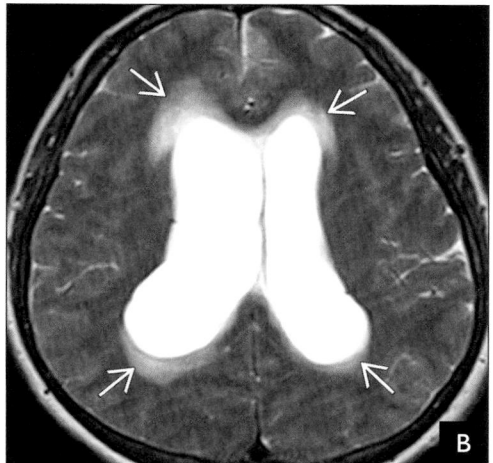

34-27A. NECT demonstrates classic findings of acute intraventricular obstructive hydrocephalus. Markedly enlarged lateral ventricles with "blurred" margins and periventricular hypodensity ➡ indicate interstitial edema. The surface sulci are compressed and not well seen. 34-27B. T2WI in the same patient shows the enlarged lateral ventricles, hyperintense fluid in the deep periventricular WM ➡.

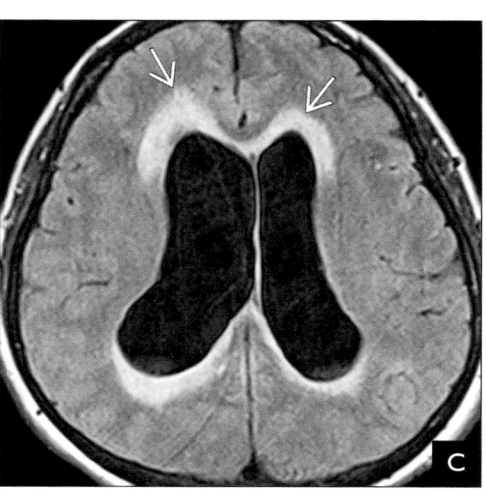
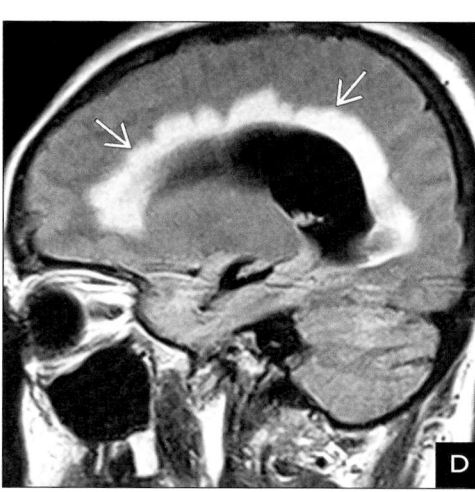

34-27C. FLAIR scan shows a hyperintense rim of interstitial fluid ➡ around the acutely enlarged lateral ventricles. 34-27D. Sagittal FLAIR in the same patient shows hyperintense "fingers" ➡ extending outward along the entire margin of the lateral ventricle. This probably represents compromised absorption of interstitial fluid rather than transependymal CSF migration from the ventricle into the WM.

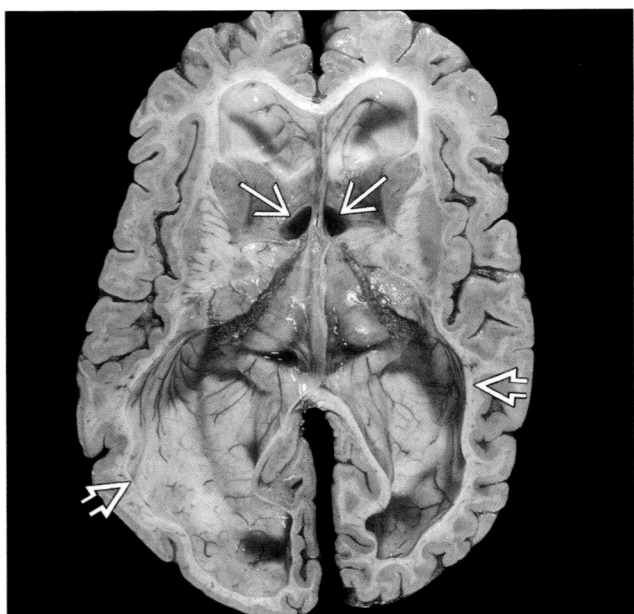

34-28. Longstanding "compensated" IVOH from aqueductal stenosis shows symmetrically enlarged lateral ventricles, dilated foramen of Monro ➡. WM ⮕ is severely reduced in volume, but cortex appears normal. (Courtesy R. Hewlett, MD.)

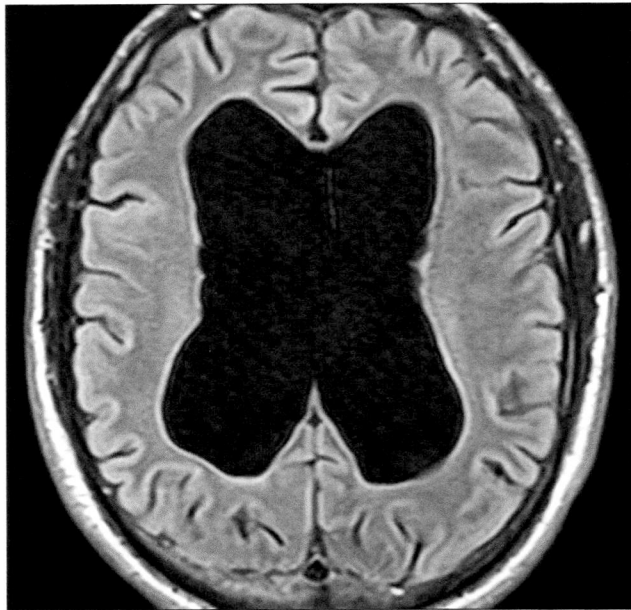

34-29. FLAIR scan in longstanding aqueductal stenosis illustrates "compensated" obstructive hydrocephalus. The ventricles are markedly enlarged, but there is no "halo" of periventricular interstitial edema around the ventricles.

PRESENTATION. The presentation of IVOH varies with acuity and severity. Headache is the most common overall symptom, and papilledema is the most common sign. Nausea, vomiting, and CN VI palsy are also common with acute IVOH.

NATURAL HISTORY. The natural history of IVOH varies. Most cases are typically progressive unless treated. Untreated severe aIVOH can result in coma and even death. Some patients with slowly developing compensated IVOH may not present until late in adult life (e.g., the recently recognized syndrome of late-onset aqueductal stenosis).

TREATMENT OPTIONS. CSF diversion (shunt, ventriculostomy, endoscopic fenestration of the third ventricle floor) is common, often performed as a first step before definitive treatment of the obstruction (e.g., removal of a colloid cyst or resection of an intraventricular neoplasm).

Imaging

GENERAL FEATURES. A number of measurements have been devised to quantify hydrocephalus. These include indices such as diameter of the frontal horns in relation to the inner table of the skull ("ventricular or 'Evans' index"), frontal horn radius, and ventricular angle. The utility of such two-dimensional measurements versus visual judgment is uncertain. Computer-generated volume measurements have been proposed as providing better normative standards but are time-consuming and difficult to obtain.

Despite its acknowledged inaccuracies, subjective neuroradiologic evaluation remains the most common method of assessing ventricular size. Hydrocephalus is usually diagnosed when the ventricles appear disproportionately enlarged relative to the subarachnoid spaces.

While NECT scans are often used as an emergent screening procedure in patients with headache and signs of increased intracranial pressure, MR is the procedure of choice. Multiplanar MR best delineates the hydrocephalus and often permits identification of its etiology.

On axial studies, helpful general imaging findings include enlarged temporal horns of the lateral ventricles (out of proportion to the basal subarachnoid spaces) **(34-24)**. The frontal horns assume a "rounded" appearance. The third ventricle—which usually appears slit-like on axial views—expands, losing its normal tapered appearance **(34-25)**. The walls first become parallel, then expand outward so that the third ventricle appears oblong or ovoid. As the ventricles continue to enlarge, the subarachnoid cisterns and convexity sulci may become compressed and gyri appear flattened against the calvaria.

Sagittal views show that the corpus callosum is thinned, stretched, bowed upward, and, in severe cases, even impacted against the falx cerebri. The anterior recesses of the third ventricle enlarge, losing their normal "pointed" appearance **(34-26A)**.

In cases of chronic IVOH, pulsating CSF in the third ventricle pounds the central skull base relentlessly. The bony sella turcica gradually enlarges and assumes an "open" configuration. In severe cases, the anterior third ventricle may protrude into the sella itself.

If both lateral and third ventricles are enlarged but the fourth ventricle remains normal (e.g., as occurs with aqueductal stenosis), the condition is termed **triventricular hydrocephalus**. If all four chambers of the ventricular system are enlarged, it is called **quadriventricular hydrocephalus**. Quadriventricular hydrocephalus is caused by a mass in the fourth ventricle or obstruction of the outlet foramina (typically infection or subarachnoid hemorrhage).

In approximately 0.5-1% of IVOH cases, just one lateral ventricle is enlarged (**"unilateral hydrocephalus"**). Most cases are acquired, associated with intraventricular neurocysticercosis or the presence of a membranous web at the junction of the inferior frontal horn with the foramen of Monro.

CT FINDINGS. Imaging findings vary with acuity and severity. NECT scans in aIVOH demonstrate enlarged lateral and third ventricles, while the size of the fourth ventricle varies. The temporal horns are prominent, the frontal horns are "rounded," and the margins of the ventricles appear indistinct or "blurred." Periventricular fluid—whether from compromised drainage of interstitial fluid or transependymal CSF migration—causes a "halo" of low density in the adjacent WM **(34-27A)**. The sulci and basal cisterns appear compressed or indistinct.

MR FINDINGS. Axial T1WI shows that both lateral ventricles are symmetrically enlarged. On sagittal views, the corpus callosum appears thinned and stretched superiorly, whereas the fornices and internal cerebral veins are displaced inferiorly.

In aIVOH, T2 scans may demonstrate "fingers" of CSF-like hyperintensity extending outward from the lateral ventricles into the surrounding WM. Fluid in the periventricular "halo" does not suppress on FLAIR **(34-27B)**, **(34-27C)**, **(34-27D)**. In longstanding chronic "compensated" hydrocephalus, the ventricles appear enlarged and the WM attenuated but without periventricular "halo" **(34-28)**, **(34-29)**.

High-resolution thin-section T2WI, FIESTA, or CISS sequences exquisitely delineate the CSF spaces and may demonstrate subtle abnormalities not detected on standard sequences **(34-26B)**. 2D cine phase contrast imaging is helpful to depict CSF dynamics in the aqueduct and around the foramen magnum.

COMPLICATIONS OF HYDROCEPHALUS. In severe cases of IVOH, the CC becomes compressed against the free inferior margin of the falx **(34-30)**, **(34-31)**. This can cause pressure necrosis and loss of callosal axons, the so-called **corpus callosum impingement syndrome** (CCIS). In

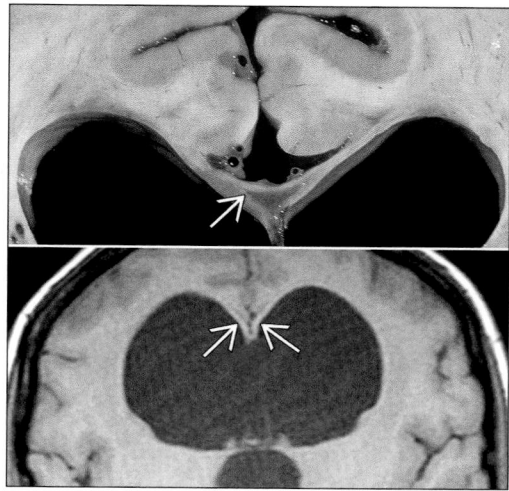

34-30. (Top) IVOH with thin encephalomalacic corpus callosum ➡ *caused by falx impingement. (Bottom) T1WI shows CC impingement* ➡.

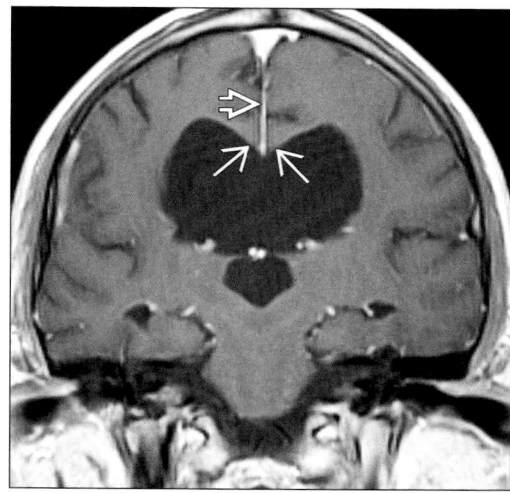

34-31. Coronal T1 C+ of longstanding IVOH shows the lateral ventricles ➡, *corpus callosum are forced upward against the falx cerebri* ➡.

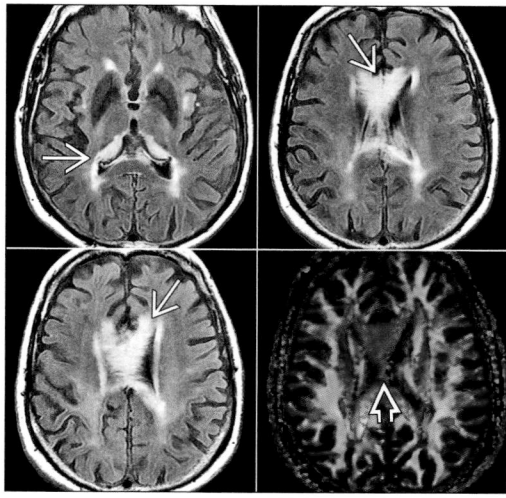

34-32. CCIS with decompression, post-shunt FLAIR shows hyperintensity in CC, periventricular WM ➡, *disrupted fibers on DTI* ➡.

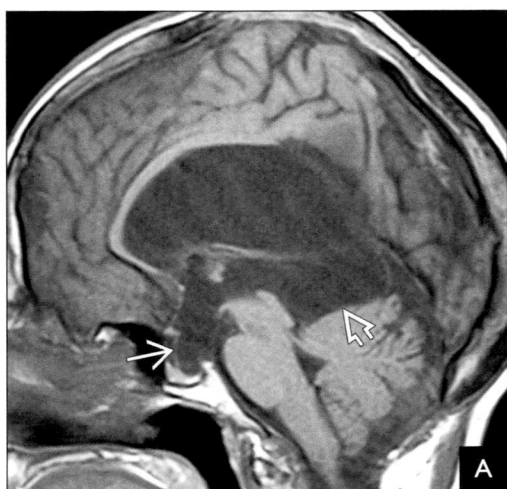

34-33A. *Triventricular hydrocephalus with intrasellar herniation of third ventricle* ➡️, *CSF collection compressing/displacing the vermis* ⏩.

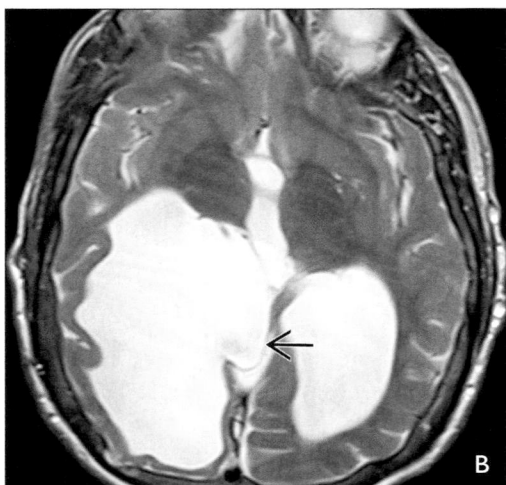

34-33B. *T2WI in the same patient shows enlarged lateral ventricles with right medial atrial diverticulum, thinned intact ventricular wall* ⏩.

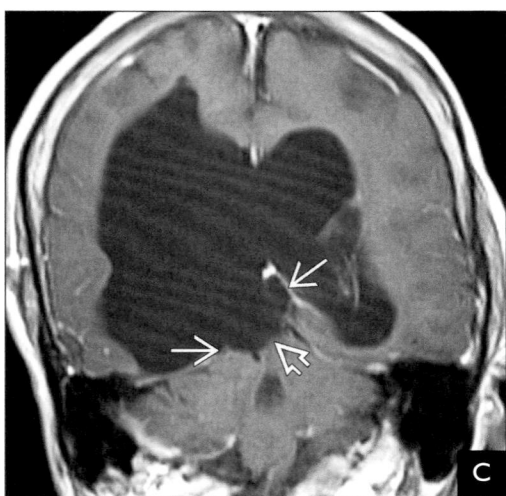

34-33C. *Coronal T1 C+ nicely shows the medial atrial diverticulum* ➡️ *herniating through the tentorial incisura, compressing the vermis* ⏩.

acute CCIS, the CC may initially appear swollen and hyperintense on T2WI and FLAIR. Subacute and chronic changes are seen as encephalomalacic foci in a shrunken, atrophic-appearing CC. In 15% of treated IVOH cases, the CC shows T2/FLAIR hyperintensity after decompression. In rare cases, the hyperintensity extends beyond the CC itself into the periventricular WM (34-32).

Massive ventricular enlargement may weaken the medial wall of the lateral ventricle enough that a pulsion-type diverticulum of CSF extrudes through the inferomedial wall of the atrium. Such **medial atrial diverticula** may cause significant mass effect on the posterior third ventricle, tectal plate, and aqueduct. Large atrial diverticula can herniate inferiorly through the tentorial incisura into the posterior fossa, compressing the vermis and fourth ventricle (34-33).

In rare cases, the ependyma may actually rupture and spill CSF into the adjacent WM (**"ventricular disruption"**), creating a fluid-filled cleft in the hemisphere.

Differential Diagnosis

The major differential diagnosis of IVOH is **extraventricular obstructive hydrocephalus** (see below). Patients often have a history of aneurysmal subarachnoid hemorrhage or meningitis. The lateral, third, and fourth ventricles are symmetrically and proportionately enlarged.

Parenchymal volume loss causes secondary dilatation of the ventricles with proportional enlargement of the surface sulci and cisterns. In infants with large ventricles, measuring head size is a critical component of the total evaluation. The finding of large ventricles in a large head favors hydrocephalus; seeing large ventricles with a normal to small head is more common with congenital anomalies or volume loss (atrophy).

A helpful feature to distinguish obstructive hydrocephalus from atrophy is the appearance of the temporal horns. In obstructive hydrocephalus, they appear rounded and moderately to strikingly enlarged. If the IVOH is acute, a periventricular "halo" is often present.

Even with relatively severe volume loss, the temporal horns retain their normal kidney-bean shape and are only minimally to moderately enlarged. The lateral ventricle margins remain sharply defined. Periventricular hypodensity appears patchy and is caused by chronic microvascular ischemia, not interstitial edema or transependymal CSF migration.

Normal pressure hydrocephalus is typically a disorder of older adults and is typified clinically by progressive dementia, gait disturbance, and incontinence (see below). The ventricles often appear disproportionately enlarged relative to the sulci and cisterns.

Overproduction hydrocephalus is rare, associated with choroid plexus papilloma and the even rarer villous hyperplasia. The choroid plexus glomus is enlarged and avidly enhancing.

Extraventricular Obstructive Hydrocephalus

Terminology

Extraventricular obstructive hydrocephalus (EVOH) is sometimes called communicating hydrocephalus to indicate that the obstruction is located somewhere outside the ventricular system.

Etiology

The obstruction causing EVOH can be located at any level from the fourth ventricular outlet foramina to the arachnoid granulations. Subarachnoid hemorrhage, whether traumatic or aneurysmal, is the most frequent cause. Other common etiologies include purulent meningitis, granulomatous meningitis, and disseminated CSF metastases.

Pathology

Gross pathology demonstrates generalized ventricular dilatation. The basal cisterns and convexity sulci may be filled with acute or chronic exudates **(34-34)**, meningeal fibrosis, or arachnoid adhesions from chronic siderosis.

Clinical Issues

As with IVOH, the presentation of EVOH varies with acuity and severity. The most common symptom is headache, followed by signs of increased intracranial pressure such as papilledema, nausea, vomiting, and diplopia.

Imaging

CT FINDINGS. The classic appearance of EVOH on NECT scans is that of symmetric, proportionally enlarged lateral, third, and fourth ventricles. The basal subarachnoid spaces are hyperdense in acute subarachnoid hemorrhage and may appear isointense and effaced in pyogenic or neoplastic meningitis. CECT scans may demonstrate enhancement in cases of EVOH secondary to infection or neoplasm.

MR FINDINGS. The same imaging sequences used in IVOH apply to the evaluation of EVOH. If the hydrocephalus is caused by acute subarachnoid hemorrhage or meningitis, the CSF appears "dirty" on T1WI and hyperintense on FLAIR. T1 C+ scans may demonstrate sulcal-cisternal enhancement **(34-35)**.

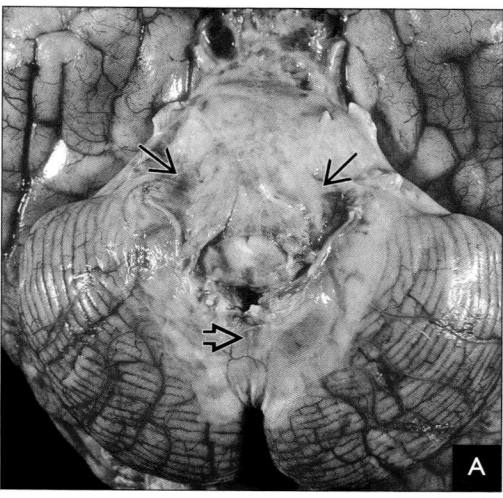

34-34A. Extensive tuberculous meningitis with thick exudate in the basal cisterns occludes the foramina of Magendie ⊵ and Luschka ➔.

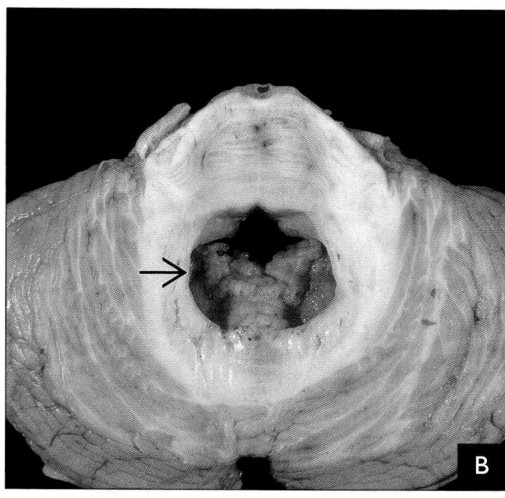

34-34B. Axial section through the cerebellum shows that the fourth ventricle ➔ is markedly enlarged and rounded ("ballooned").

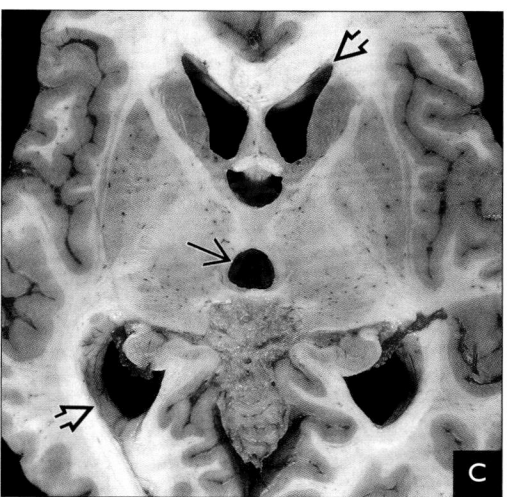

34-34C. Third ➔, both lateral ventricles ⊵ are enlarged. Extraventricular "communicating" hydrocephalus. (Courtesy R. Hewlett, MD.)

In contrast to IVOH, more than half the cases of EVOH have no discernible cause for the obstruction on standard MR sequences. In such cases, it is especially important to identify subtle thin membranes that may be causing the extraventricular obstruction.

The CSF cisterns, ventricles, and outlet foramina are best demonstrated by special pulse sequences such as 3D constructive interference in the steady state (3D-CISS).

Using high-resolution 3D-CISS, thin membranous obstruction can be demonstrated in nearly 20% of patients with unexplained hydrocephalus. Even if the membrane is not visualized directly, differences in CSF signal intensity proximal and distal to the culprit membrane are helpful in localizing the obstruction.

Differential Diagnosis

The major differential diagnosis of EVOH is **IVOH**. In some cases—even with special sequences such 3D-CISS—it may be difficult, if not impossible, to localize the level of the obstruction.

OBSTRUCTIVE HYDROCEPHALUS
Intraventricular Obstructive Hydrocephalus
- a.k.a. noncommunicating hydrocephalus
  ○ Obstruction at/proximal to 4th v. foramina
- Congenital or acquired, acute or chronic
  ○ Post-inflammation/post-hemorrhage membranes
  ○ Obstructing intraventricular mass
- Acute IVOH
  ○ Ventricles proximal to obstruction are ballooned
  ○ Periventricular interstitial edema
  ○ "Blurred" margins of ventricles
  ○ "Halo" ± "fingers" of fluid around ventricles
  ○ T2 hyperintense, does not suppress on FLAIR
- Chronic compensated IVOH
  ○ Large ventricles
  ○ No periventricular fluid, hyperintensity
- Complications of IVOH
  ○ Corpus callosum impingement syndrome
  ○ Atrial diverticula

Extraventricular Obstructive Hydrocephalus
- a.k.a. "communicating" hydrocephalus
- Obstruction outside ventricular system
  ○ 4th v. foramina to arachnoid granulations
- Imaging
  ○ > 50% show no discernible etiology
  ○ Use CISS to look for obstructing membranes

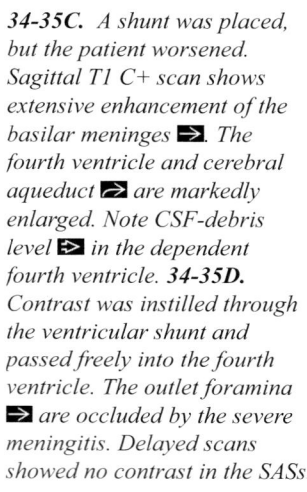

34-35A. FLAIR scan in a patient with cryptococcal meningitis and deteriorating mental status shows an enlarged fourth ventricle ➡ surrounded by striking "fingers" of periventricular interstitial fluid ➡. 34-35B. FLAIR scan in the same patient shows "caps" of hyperintense interstitial fluid surrounding symmetrically enlarged lateral ventricles ➡. The sulci are severely compressed and inapparent.

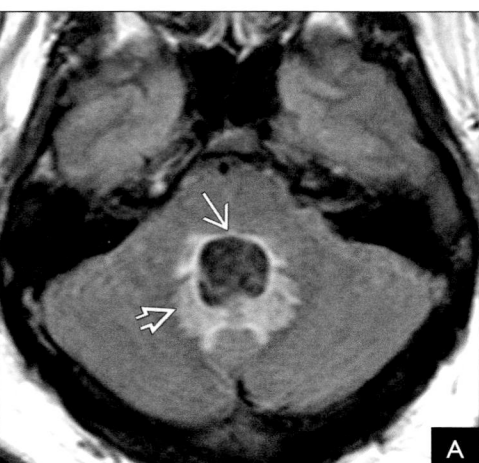
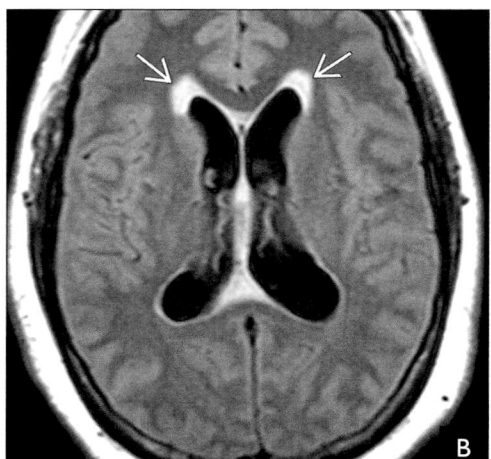

34-35C. A shunt was placed, but the patient worsened. Sagittal T1 C+ scan shows extensive enhancement of the basilar meninges ➡. The fourth ventricle and cerebral aqueduct ➡ are markedly enlarged. Note CSF-debris level ➡ in the dependent fourth ventricle. 34-35D. Contrast was instilled through the ventricular shunt and passed freely into the fourth ventricle. The outlet foramina ➡ are occluded by the severe meningitis. Delayed scans showed no contrast in the SASs.

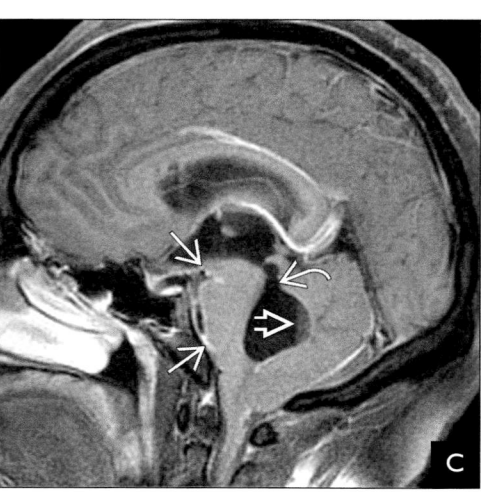
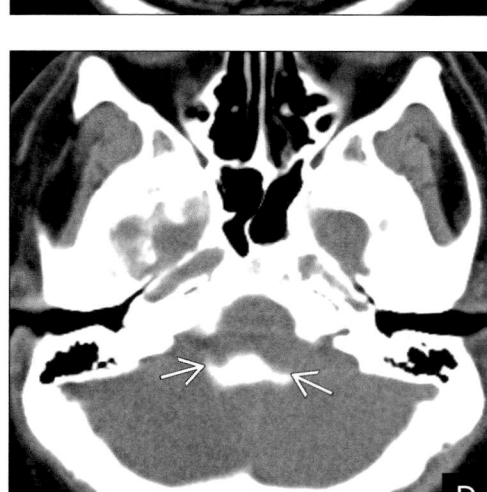

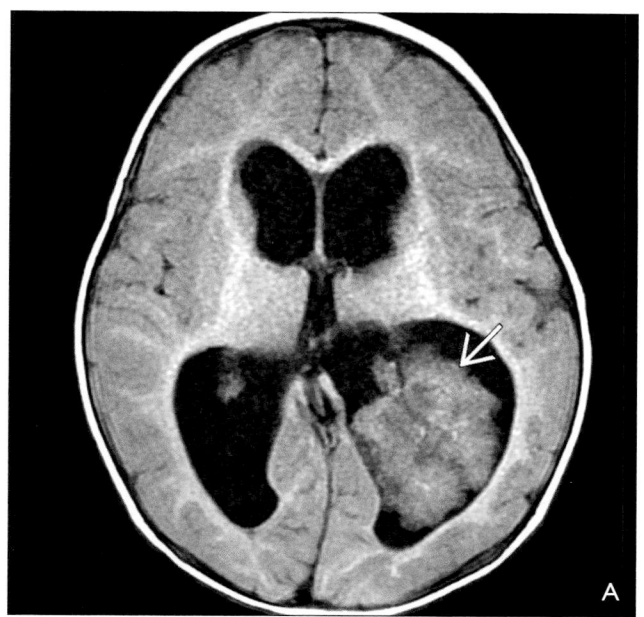

34-36A. *Axial T1WI in an 18-month-old child with macrocrania shows symmetrically enlarged lateral and third ventricles. The papillary mass* ➔ *is seen in the atrium of the left lateral ventricle.*

34-36B. *T1 C+ scan in the same patient shows that the mass enhances intensely. Overproduction hydrocephalus caused by choroid plexus papilloma.*

Overproduction Hydrocephalus

Overproduction hydrocephalus is uncommon and results from excessive CSF formation. Panventricular enlargement is the most common imaging finding in overproduction hydrocephalus but is not invariably present.

Choroid plexus papillomas (CPPs) are the most common cause of overproduction hydrocephalus **(34-36)**. CPPs account for 2-4% of childhood neoplasms and typically occur in children younger than five years. Some CPPs produce enormous amounts of CSF, overwhelming the capacity of the arachnoid villi and other structures to absorb the excess fluid. **Choroid plexus carcinomas** (CPCas) can also cause overproduction hydrocephalus but are only a tenth as common as CPPs. Imaging findings of both CPP and CPCa are delineated in Chapter 18.

Diffuse villous hyperplasia of the choroid plexus (DVHCP) is a rare cause of overproduction hydrocephalus. CSF production in DVHCP can exceed three liters per day. DVHCP is histologically normal with little to no pleomorphism or hyperchromasia.

Imaging studies in DVHCP show severe hydrocephalus with massive enlargement of the entire choroid plexus. The diffusely enlarged choroid plexus enhances strongly and often contains multiple nonenhancing cysts of varying sizes. DVHCP can be difficult to distinguish from rare bilateral CPPs, which typically cause focal—not diffuse—enlargement of the choroid plexus.

Normal Pressure Hydrocephalus

There are no currently accepted evidence-based guidelines for either the diagnosis or treatment of normal pressure hydrocephalus. In this section, we briefly review the syndrome and summarize the spectrum of imaging findings that—in conjunction with clinical history and neurologic examination—may suggest the diagnosis.

Terminology

Normal pressure hydrocephalus (NPH) was first described by Hakim and Addams as "symptomatic occult hydrocephalus with 'normal' CSF pressure." NPH has sometimes been called idiopathic adult hydrocephalus syndrome. **Primary** or **idiopathic NPH** (iNPH) is distinguished from **secondary NPH**, in which there is a known antecedent such as subarachnoid hemorrhage, traumatic brain injury, or meningitis.

Etiology

NPH is characterized by ventriculomegaly with normal CSF pressure and altered CSF hydrodynamics. Its pathogenesis is poorly understood and controversial. Some investigators have posited that altered viscoelastic properties of the ventricular walls and adjacent parenchyma cause a "water hammer" effect of the CSF pulsations. Intermittent high pressure "B" waves together with altered compliance of the venous system and craniospinal subarachnoid space are other proposed etiologies. Decreased regional cerebral blood flow and accelerated microvascular disease probably contribute to the parenchymal degeneration that typically accompanies NPH.

Pathology

The ventricles appear grossly enlarged. The periventricular WM often appears abnormal without frank infarction. Neurofibrillary tangles and other microscopic changes typically found in Alzheimer disease are seen in 20% of cases.

Clinical Issues

EPIDEMIOLOGY AND DEMOGRAPHICS. NPH accounts for approximately 5-6% of all dementias. The incidence of NPH is estimated at 1-5 new cases per 100,000 per year. While it is most common in patients older than 60 years, NPH also occasionally occurs in children following intraventricular hemorrhage or meningitis. There is a moderate male predominance.

NPH is designated as "possible" or "probable" based on the combination of clinical findings, imaging studies, and response to high volume lumbar tap.

PRESENTATION. The nature and severity of symptoms as well as the disease course vary in NPH. Impaired gait and balance are the typical initial symptoms. The classic "Hakim" triad of dementia, gait apraxia, and urinary incontinence is present in a minority of patients and typically represents advanced disease. While gait disturbances are seen in most cases, not all patients exhibit impaired cognition.

NATURAL HISTORY. The natural history of NPH has not been well characterized nor is the tempo of progression uniform. Many patients experience continuing cognitive and motor decline.

TREATMENT OPTIONS. Some patients initially respond dramatically to ventricular shunting ("shunt-responsive" NPH). The favorable response to shunting varies from about 35-40% in patients with clinically "possible" NPH to 65% in patients diagnosed with "probable" NPH.

Long-term outcome is more problematic. While early gait improvement is common, only one-third of patients experience continued improvement three years after

34-37A. Sagittal T1WI in a 62-year-old man with dementia, mild gait disturbance shows large lateral ventricle ➡, normal-appearing sulci. Evidence of hyperdynamic CSF is seen as exaggerated "flow voids" in the fourth ventricle ➡. 34-37B. Axial FLAIR scan in the same patient shows symmetrically enlarged lateral, third ventricles with normal to small sulci. Note mild periventricular "halo" ➡.

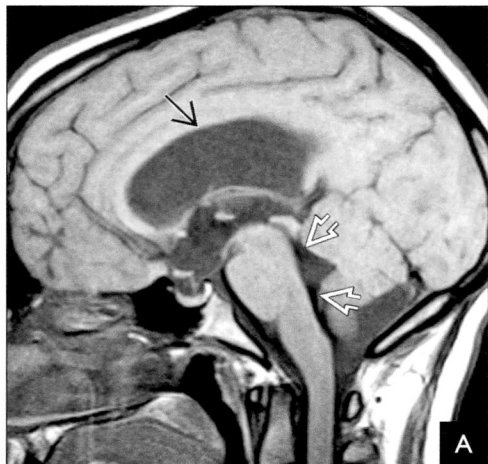
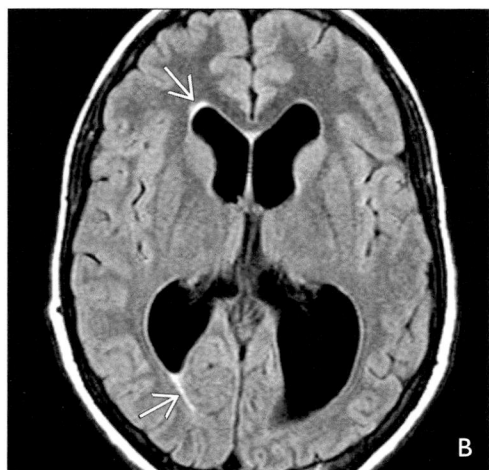

34-37C. T2WI shows an enlarged aqueduct with an unusually prominent "flow void" ➡. Again, note disproportionately enlarged lateral, third ventricles compared to the normal sylvian fissures, surface sulci. 34-37D. 2D PC MR shows enlarged aqueduct with hyperdynamic CSF flow ➡. The diagnosis of probable iNPH was made, and the patient underwent ventriculoperitoneal shunting.

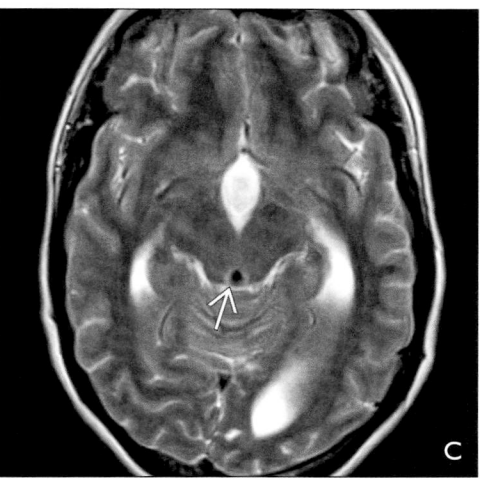
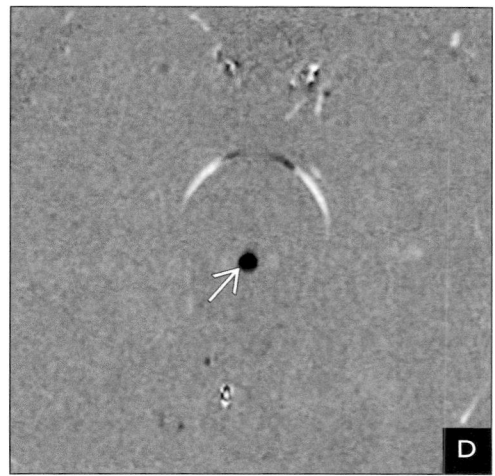

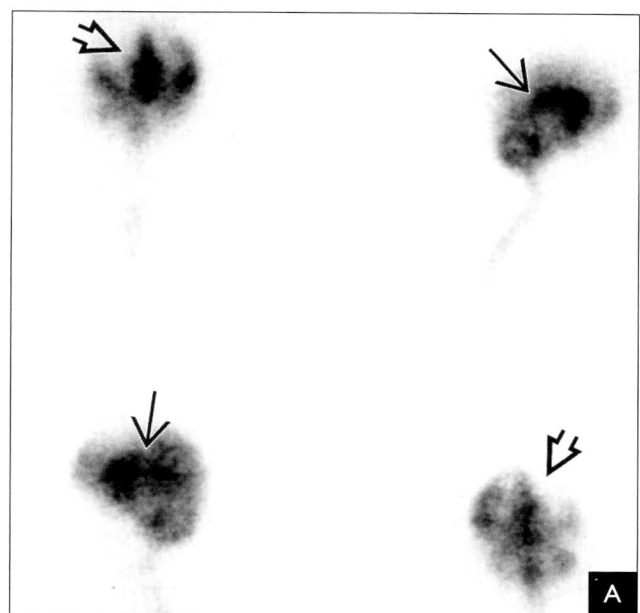

34-38A. In this patient with NPH, 24-hour multiplanar In-111 DTPA cisternography shows tracer in lateral ventricles ➡, lack of activity over convexity ▷. (Courtesy K. Morton, MD.)

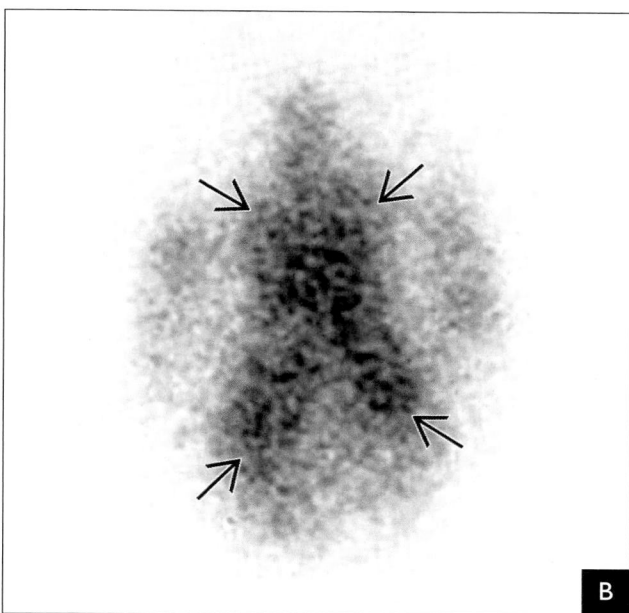

34-38B. Planar vertex view of top of head in the same patient, also at 24 hours, shows clear activity in the lateral ventricles ➡, confirming diagnosis of probable iNPH. (Courtesy K. Morton, MD.)

shunting. Cognition and urinary incontinence are even less responsive.

Imaging

GENERAL FEATURES. Imaging studies in suspected NPH are necessary but insufficient to establish the definitive diagnosis of NPH. The goal of identifying patients who are likely to improve following ventriculoperitoneal shunting likewise remains elusive.

The most common general imaging feature of NPH is a degree of ventriculomegaly (Evans index of at least 0.3) that appears out of proportion to sulcal enlargement ("ventriculosulcal disproportion") (34-37).

CT FINDINGS. NECT scans show enlarged lateral ventricles with rounded frontal horns. The third ventricle is moderately enlarged while the fourth ventricle appears relatively normal.

The basal cisterns and sylvian fissures may be somewhat prominent,- but compared to the degree of ventriculomegaly, generalized sulcal enlargement is mild. Periventricular hypodensity is common and often represents a combination of increased interstitial fluid and WM rarefaction secondary to microvascular disease.

MR FINDINGS. T1 scans show large lateral ventricles. A prominent, exaggerated aqueductal "flow void" may be present. The corpus callosum is usually thinned. Most patients have a mild to moderate periventricular "halo" on T2/FLAIR (34-37B).

DTI is a good marker of WM pathology and shows increased FA in the posterior limb of the internal capsule.

Either 2D or 3D phase-contrast flow studies may show hypermotile flow and markedly elevated aqueductal stroke volume.

NUCLEAR MEDICINE. Prominent ventricular activity at 24 hours on In-111 DTPA cisternography is considered a relatively good indicator of NPH (34-38). 18F FDG PET shows decreased regional cerebral metabolism.

Differential Diagnosis

The major difficulty in diagnosing iNPH is distinguishing it from other neurodegenerative disorders. Up to 75% of patients with NPH have another neurodegenerative disorder, most commonly **Alzheimer disease** and **vascular dementia**. In **age-related atrophy**, both the ventricles and the subarachnoid spaces are proportionately enlarged.

Syndrome of Inappropriately Low-Pressure Acute Hydrocephalus

Most patients with acute obstructive hydrocephalus have ventriculomegaly and elevated intracranial pressure (ICP). However, a small subset of patients with acute obstructive hydrocephalus have ventriculomegaly with inappropriately *low* ICP.

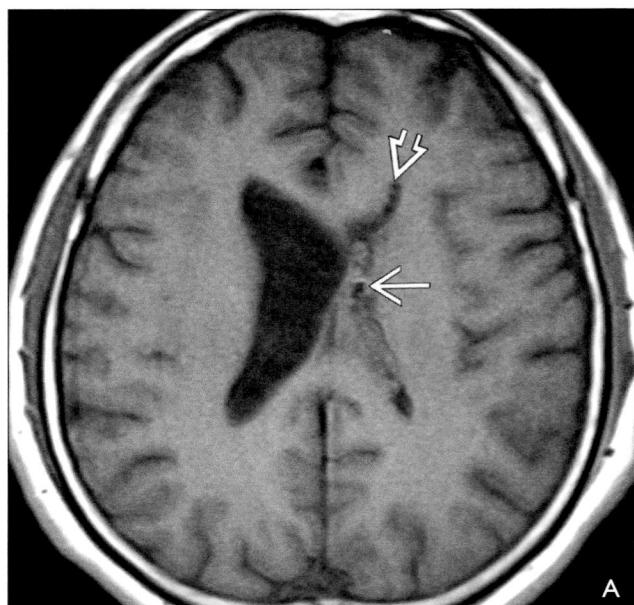

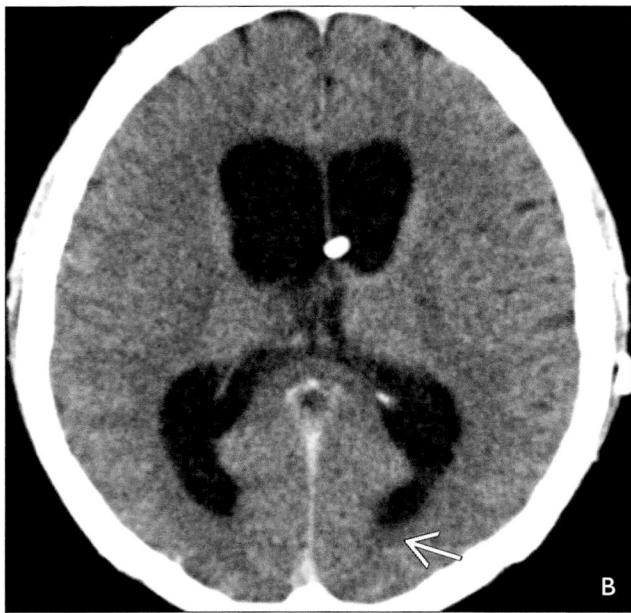

34-39A. Axial T1WI in a patient with ventriculoperitoneal shunt and headache shows shunt catheter ▶ in a collapsed, slit-like left lateral ventricle ▶. The right lateral ventricle is moderately enlarged; the sulci appear normal.

34-39B. The shunt was replaced. The patient had acute neurologic deterioration 10 days later. NECT shows "ballooned" ventricles, periventricular edema ▶, small sulci. EVD showed unexpectedly low pressure, consistent with SILPAH.

Terminology

The syndrome of inappropriately low-pressure acute hydrocephalus (SILPAH) has sometimes been called "negative-pressure hydrocephalus." As opening pressures are not always "negative" (i.e., subzero), the terms SILPAH or "very low-pressure hydrocephalus" are more accurate.

Etiology

Once thought to occur only in patients with a preexisting ventriculoperitoneal shunt, SILPAH is now known to occur in other patients, too. The common factor is isolation of the ventricular system from a subarachnoid space that leaks (or is drained of) CSF, resulting in low brain turgor and decreased ICP. CSF production continues, builds up, and expands the ventricles.

Clinical Issues

SILPAH is both uncommon and—because of its enigmatic and counterintuitive nature—often unrecognized.

Patients with SILPAH present with progressive neurological deterioration, *acute* progressive ventriculomegaly, and ICP that is inappropriately low when an external ventricular drain (EVD) is inserted (34-39). SILPAH affects patients of all ages; 20% are children.

Shunted patients with SILPAH typically have opening pressures < 0 mmH$_2$O. Patients without a shunt typically have much lower than expected pressures that rapidly

become even lower. In both scenarios, ICP is too low to allow CSF drainage with normal EVD protocols.

Treatment by neck wrapping with a tensor bandage and/or lowering the EVD to negative levels typically results in clinical improvement and resolution of the ventriculomegaly. Reestablishing communication between the ventricular system and the SAS may be required to correct ICP dynamics.

Imaging

Imaging findings are identical to those of acute severe obstructive hydrocephalus. "Quadriventricular" enlargement, "halos" of periventricular interstitial edema, and small—sometimes almost inapparent—subarachnoid spaces are present.

Differential Diagnosis

The major differential diagnosis of SILPAH is the much more common syndrome of **acute obstructive hydrocephalus** with elevated intracranial pressures. Imaging findings are identical, so the definitive diagnosis is established only when EVD discloses unexpectedly low ICP.

SILPAH must be differentiated from **idiopathic intracranial hypotension**, a disorder also characterized by low ICP (see below). Intracranial hypotension is characterized by downward displacement of the central core brain structures, midbrain sagging, tonsillar descent, and dural thickening/enhancement.

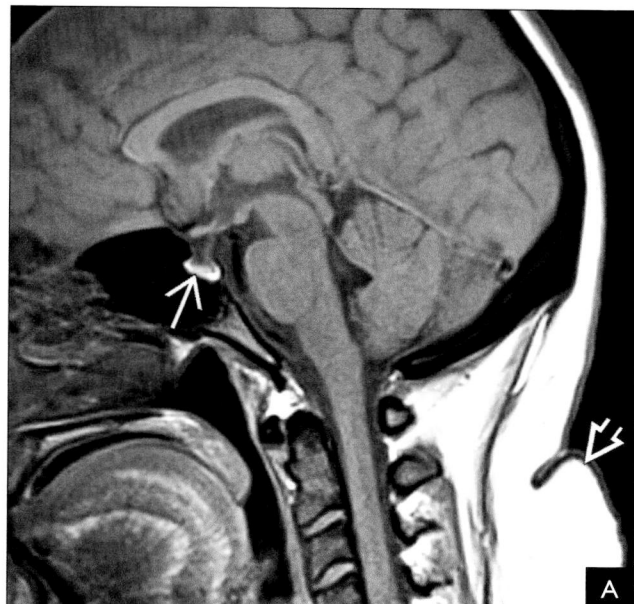

34-40A. Sagittal T1WI in a 33-year-old obese woman shows excessive subcutaneous fat ⇉ and a partial empty sella ⇥.

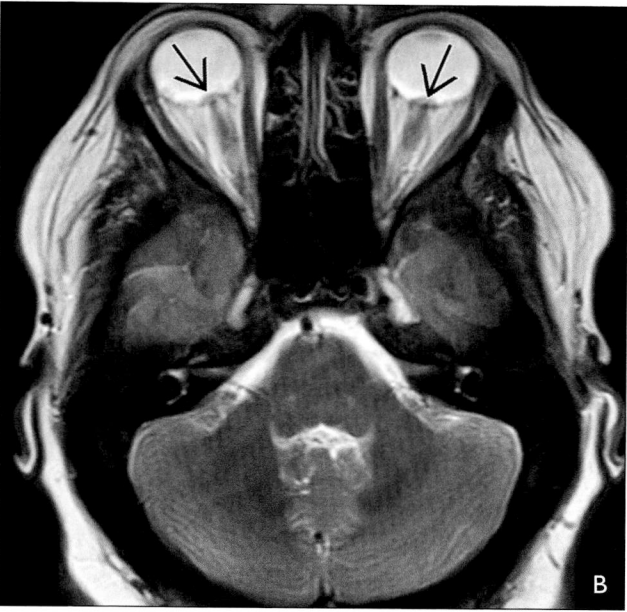

34-40B. Axial T2WI in the same patient shows posterior flattening of the globes with intraocular protrusion of the optic nerve heads ⇥. Opening pressure on LP was 440 mmH₂O, consistent with moderately severe IIH.

Critical post-craniotomy CSF hypovolemia can cause marked cerebral hypotension with dramatic downward migration of intracranial structures. In both idiopathic intracranial hypotension and post-craniotomy CSF hypovolemia, the ventricles are usually small, not large.

OTHER HYDROCEPHALUS

Overproduction Hydrocephalus
- Rare
- Results from CSF overproduction
  - Choroid plexus tumor > > hyperplasia
- Imaging shows panventricular enlargement

Normal Pressure Hydrocephalus
- Ventriculomegaly with normal CSF pressure, altered fluid dynamics
- Accounts for ≈ 5% of dementias
- Dementia, gait apraxia, incontinence (minority)
- Imaging diagnosis difficult
  - Disproportionately enlarged ventricles vs. sulci
  - MR may show exaggerated aqueductal "flow void," elevated stroke volume
  - In-111 DTPA cisternography: Intraventricular tracer at 24 hours

Syndrome of Inappropriately Low-Pressure Acute Hydrocephalus
- Progressive neurological deterioration
  - Acute progressive obstructive hydrocephalus
  - CSF opening pressure very low or negative
- Imaging
  - Like acute obstructive hydrocephalus with ↑ ICP
  - Quadriventricular enlargement
  - Small/inapparent sulci common
- Differential diagnosis
  - Acute obstructive hydrocephalus with ↑ ICP
  - Idiopathic intracranial hypotension
  - Critical post-craniotomy CSF hypovolemia

Idiopathic Intracranial Hypertension

Terminology

Idiopathic intracranial hypertension (IIH) is also known as **benign intracranial hypertension** and **pseudotumor cerebri**.

Etiology, Pathology

IIH is characterized by elevated intracranial pressure (ICP) without an identifiable cause from among the many entities such as hydrocephalus, mass lesion, CSF abnormality, or dural sinus thrombosis.

Clinical Issues

EPIDEMIOLOGY AND DEMOGRAPHICS. IIH is rare. Classically, IIH presents in overweight females who are 20-45 years of age.

PRESENTATION. Headache is the most common symptom (90-95%), followed by tinnitus and visual disturbances. Papilledema is the most common sign on neurologic examination.

NATURAL HISTORY. IIH can cause progressive visual impairment and even blindness.

TREATMENT OPTIONS. The optimal treatment for IIH is controversial. Diuretics and dieting are effective in many patients, but the relapse rate is high (25-30%).

Stent placement in patients who have transverse sinus stenosis with significant pressure differentials across the

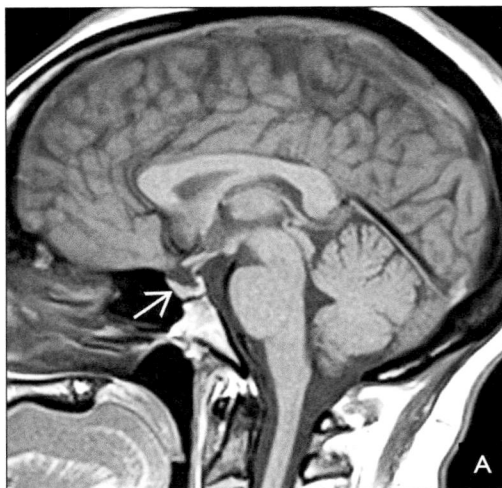

34-41A. *Midline sagittal T1WI in a pregnant female with severe headaches and visual changes, papilledema shows partial empty sella* ➡️.

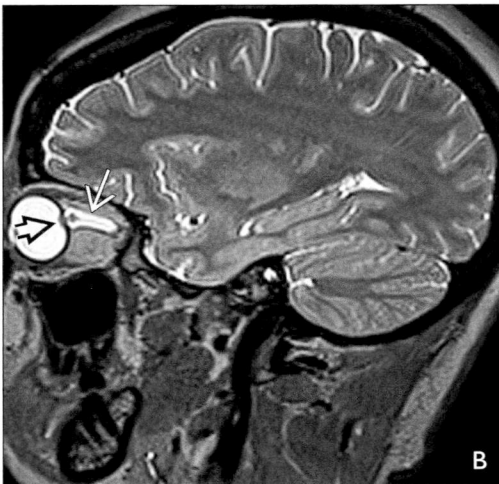

34-41B. *Sagittal T2FS through the globe shows markedly enlarged optic nerve sheath, compressed optic nerve* ➡️. *Optic head bulges into globe* ⊳.

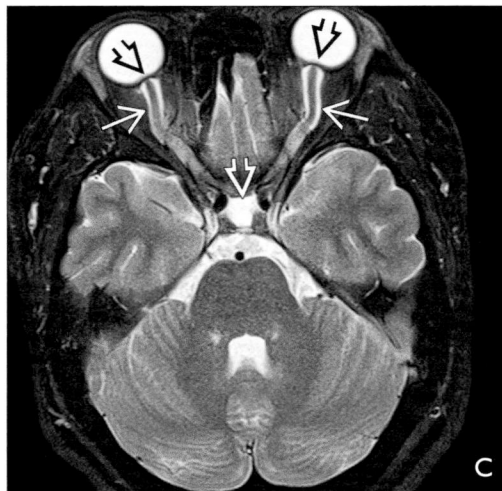

34-41C. *T2WI shows empty sella* ➡️, *dilated optic nerve sheaths* ➡️, *optic nerve head protrusion* ⊳. *Intracranial hypertension.*

lesion has been successful in improving symptoms and reducing papilledema **(34-42D)**, **(34-42E)**. High-volume lumbar puncture and optic nerve fenestration are options in patients with severe IIH.

Imaging

Neuroimaging is used to (1) exclude identifiable causes of increased ICP (e.g., neoplasm or obstructive hydrocephalus) and (2) detect findings associated with IIH.

The most significant imaging findings of IIH include **flattening of the posterior globes**, **intraocular optic nerve protrusion**, **partial empty sella**, and **venous sinus stenosis (34-42)**. The presence of one or a combination of these signs significantly increases the odds of IIH. Their absence does not rule out IIH. The definitive diagnosis of IIH is established by lumbar puncture, which demonstrates elevated ICP (higher than 200 mmH$_2$O) with otherwise normal CSF.

MR FINDINGS. Sagittal scans show a partial empty sella **(34-40)**. Here the pituitary gland occupies less than 50% of the pituitary fossa, and its superior surface appears concave. The posterior globe is flattened or concave, and intraocular protrusion of the optic nerve may be visible **(34-41)**. The prevalence of other reported findings such as slit-like or "pinched" ventricles, "tight" subarachnoid spaces (small sulci and cisterns), inferiorly displaced tonsils, and dilated/tortuous optic nerve sheaths does not differ significantly from the prevalence in normal controls.

CTV/MRV. MRV often shows transverse sinus stenosis and "flow gaps." Whether this is the cause or consequence of raised ICP is controversial. CTV is helpful in differentiating a hypoplastic sinus segment from thrombosis.

Differential Diagnosis

The most important differential diagnosis in patients with suspected IIH is **secondary intracranial hypertension** (i.e., increased ICP with an identifiable cause). While dilated optic nerve sheaths ("hydrops") and flattened posterior globes indicate elevated ICP, they can be seen in both secondary and idiopathic intracranial hypertension. Ventriculomegaly is more common in secondary intracranial hypertension whereas the ventricles are usually normal to small in IIH.

Dural sinus thrombosis (DST) is another important consideration. T2* (GRE, SWI) shows "blooming" thrombus in the affected sinuses. MRV and CTV demonstrate a cigar-shaped, long-segment clot.

CSF Shunts and Complications

Although endoscopic third ventriculostomy is gaining acceptance, the standard treatment for all types of

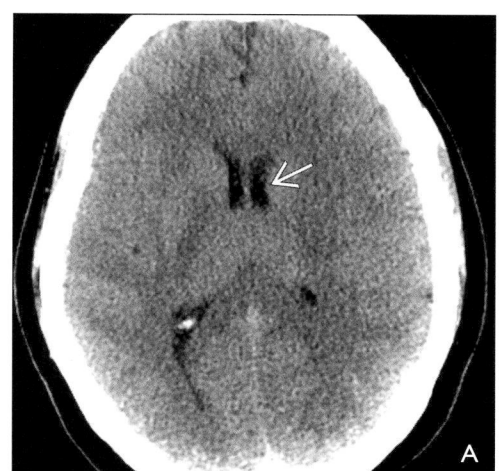

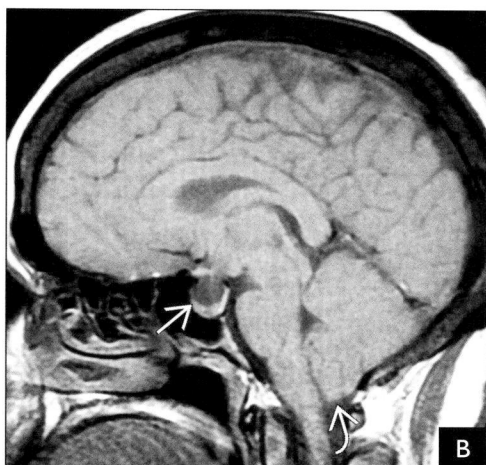

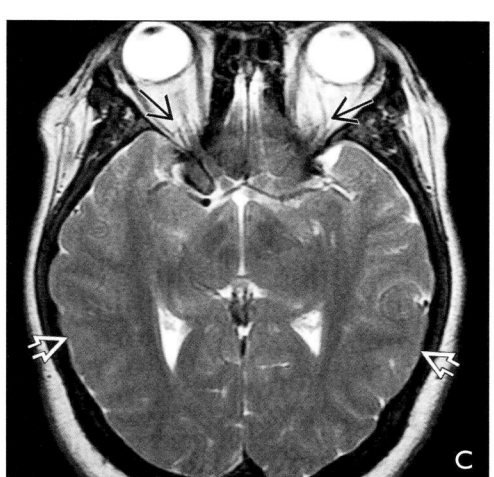

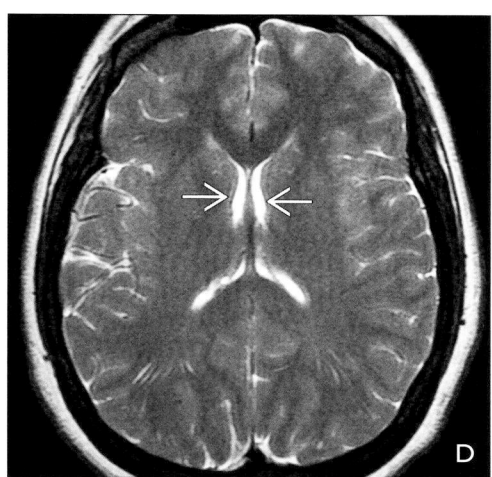

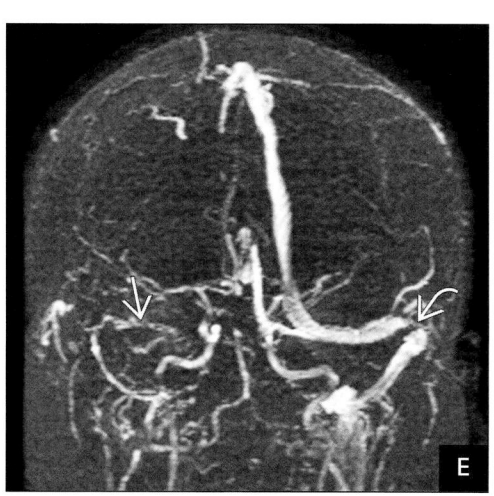

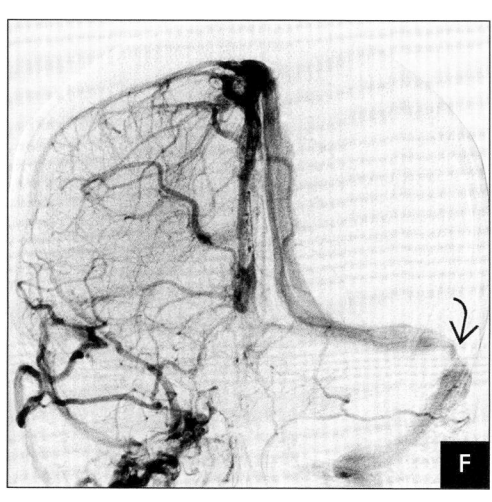

34-42A. Axial NECT scan in a 29-year-old woman with severe intractable headaches shows small lateral ventricles ➡, almost inapparent sulci over the surfaces of the hemispheres. 34-42B. Sagittal T1WI in the same patient shows partially empty sella ➡, mild tonsillar descent ➡ without significant midbrain "slumping" or dural engorgement.

34-42C. T2WI shows subtle dilatation of optic nerve sheaths ➡, relative lack of CSF-filled sulci over brain surfaces ➡. The globes appear normal. 34-42D. More cephalad T2WI shows that both lateral ventricles appear small ➡.

34-42E. MRV shows a hypoplastic right transverse sinus ➡, dominant left transverse sinus with an apparent high-grade stenosis ➡. 34-42F. AP DSA confirms the left transverse stenosis ➡. Pressure gradient across the stenosis was 10 mmHg. A stent was placed across the stenosis with resolution of the patient's headaches. Venous sinus stenosis or web causing intracranial hypertension is a rare but potentially remediable cause of IIH.

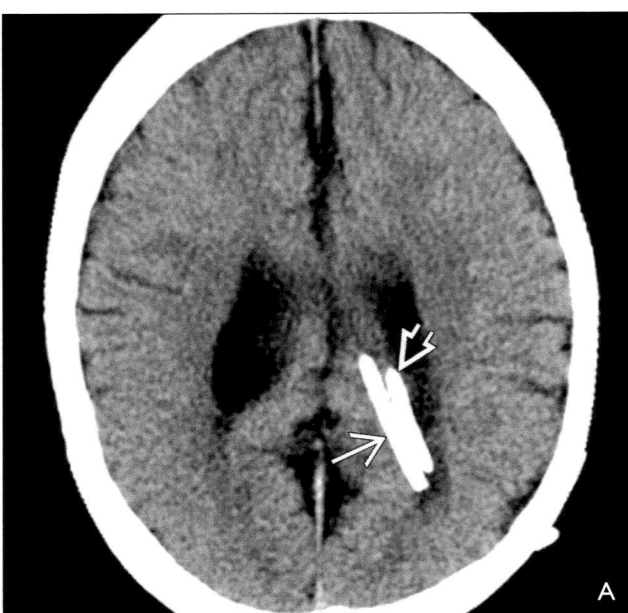

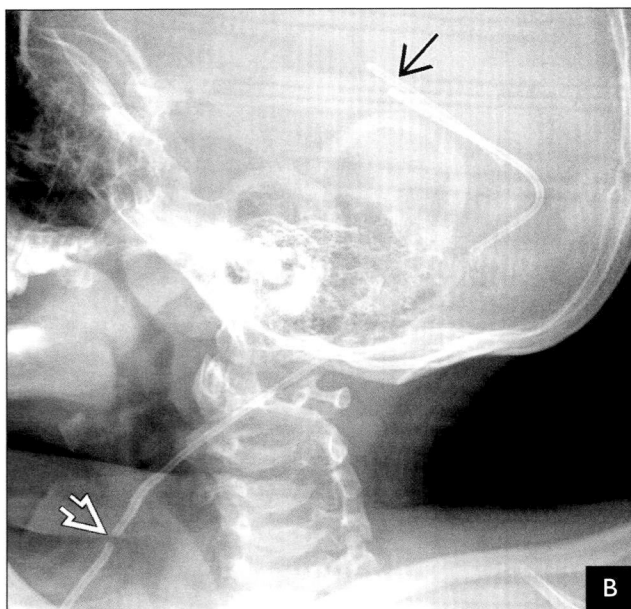

34-43A. *Axial NECT in a patient with multiple shunt revisions shows an abandoned catheter* ⇱ *and a second "active" catheter* ⇱ *in the left lateral ventricle. Both ventricles were moderately enlarged compared to prior studies (not shown).*

34-43B. *Image from a shunt series shows the abandoned catheter fragment* ⇱. *The cervical segment of the "active" catheter has fractured* ⇱. *(Courtesy S. Blaser, MD.)*

obstructive hydrocephalus remains placement of a shunt for CSF diversion.

Placement of ventricular shunts are one of the most common of all neurosurgical procedures. Multiple surgeries are the rule, not the exception; approximately 50% of ventricular shunts in children fail in the first two years and the vast majority have failed by 10 years after insertion.

The costs and lifelong morbidity associated with shunt placement to treat both childhood and adult hydrocephalus are substantial. More than half of all pediatric and adult patients require shunt revision. Almost 55% of children have four or more shunt revisions, and nearly 10% experience three or more shunt infections. Direct treatment-related costs for patients of all ages with hydrocephalus exceed $1 billion annually in the USA alone.

Imaging is a key component in evaluating patients with CSF diversions. Shunt failure can result in either enlarging or collapsing ventricles. The most common imaging manifestation of shunt failure is enlarging ventricles. CT is generally the preferred technique to assess patients with intracranial shunt catheters. Alternative modalities include transfontanelle ultrasound and new rapid MR techniques such as fast steady-state gradient-recalled-echo (SS-GRE) sequences.

We now briefly examine some of the most common causes of shunt malfunction.

Mechanical Failure

Mechanical failures represent nearly 75% of shunt malfunctions. Disconnection or fracture account for another 15% or so **(34-43)**.

Most ventriculoperitoneal shunts have several components. The commonly used systems consist of three pieces: (1) a ventricular catheter connected to (2) an inline valve and (3) a distal peritoneal catheter. Shunt discontinuity can occur at any site, but disconnection is most common at the junctions of the various components.

The most common imaging modality to assess mechanical failure is a shunt series. While some evidence suggests only a small number (less than 1%) of shunt series help in surgical decision-making, shunt series are still frequently requested studies.

Standard shunt series are composed of skull (two views), neck, chest, and abdomen/pelvis radiographs to track shunt trajectory and integrity. Accurate diagnosis of shunt fractures and disconnections is complicated by three factors: (1) the wide variety of systems used, (2) the accumulation of residual "abandoned" catheter fragments in patients who have undergone multiple shunt revisions, and (3) nonradiopaque shunt segments. Careful comparison of current and prior studies is essential to determine whether the "active" shunt system is intact.

Programmable Valve Failures

Many neurosurgeons now use a programmable rather than a fixed-pressure valve for the treatment of hydro-

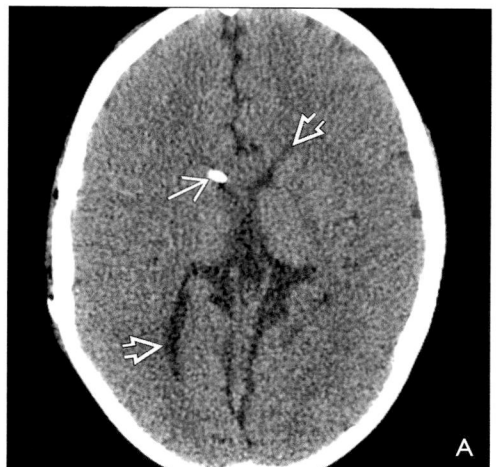

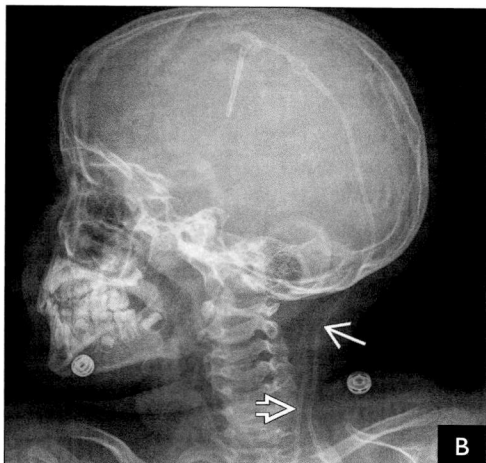

34-44A. NECT scan in an infant with shunted hydrocephalus shows shunt ➡, slit-like lateral ventricles ⇒. Despite the shunt failure, the patient was asymptomatic. 34-44B. Skull radiograph obtained at the same time shows contiguity of the active shunt ➡. An abandoned shunt fragment in the neck is present ⇒.

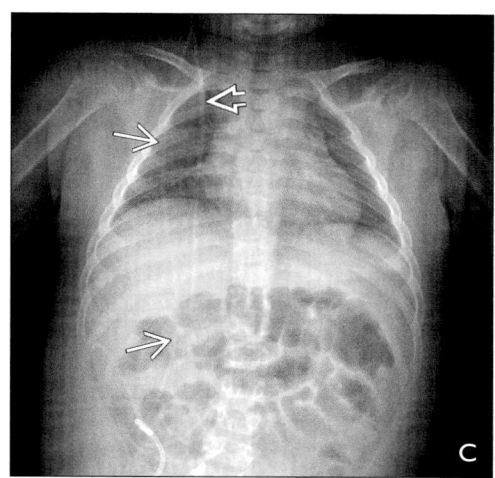

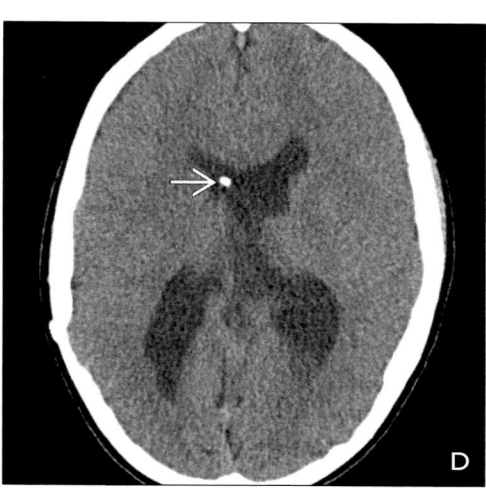

34-44C. Chest radiograph obtained as part of the shunt series confirms contiguity of the actively functioning shunt ➡ and shows the distal aspect of the abandoned shunt fragment ⇒. 34-44D. Several years later, the child developed severe headaches. NECT scan shows that the ventricular catheter segment ➡ has not changed in position. However, the lateral ventricles now appear moderately enlarged compared to the prior baseline examination.

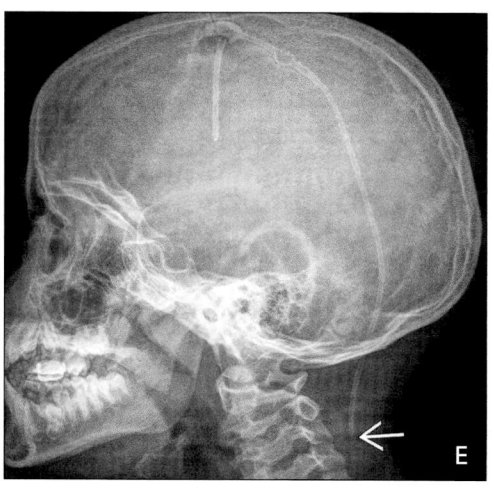

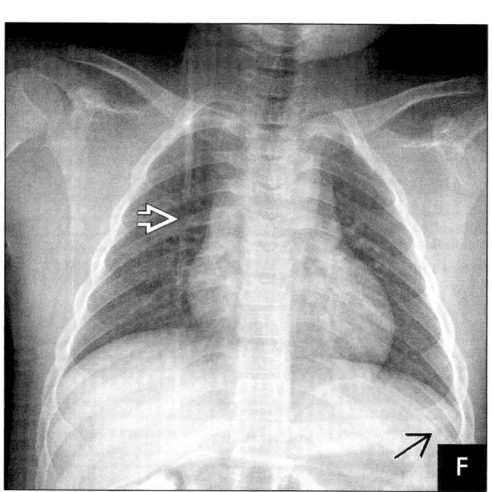

34-44E. Compared to the lateral skull radiograph from the prior shunt series (Figure 34-44B), the active catheter now abruptly terminates in the neck ➡. 34-44F. Chest radiograph shows a second discontinuity in the catheter ⇒. The distal segment is coiled in the left upper quadrant ⇒, a suboptimal position. (Courtesy K. Moore, MD.)

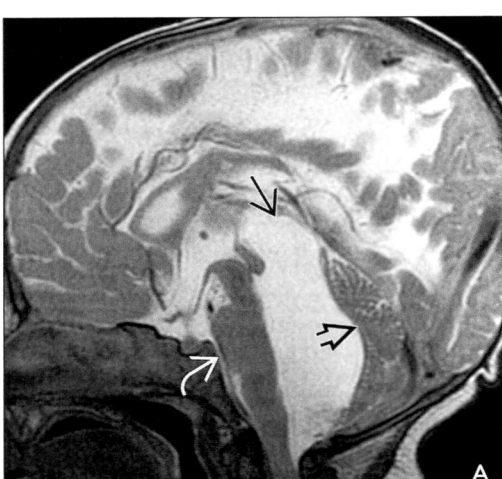

34-45A. *T2WI following shunting shows large "isolated" fourth ventricle ➤ flattening pons against clivus ➤, compressing vermis ➤.*

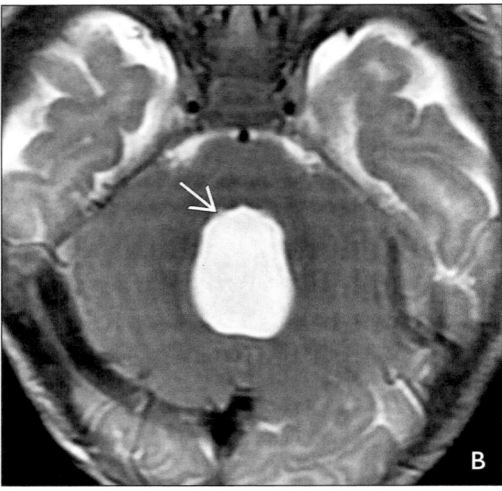

34-45B. *Axial T2WI shows that the markedly enlarged, trapped fourth ventricle ➤ has lost its normal "kidney bean on its side" appearance.*

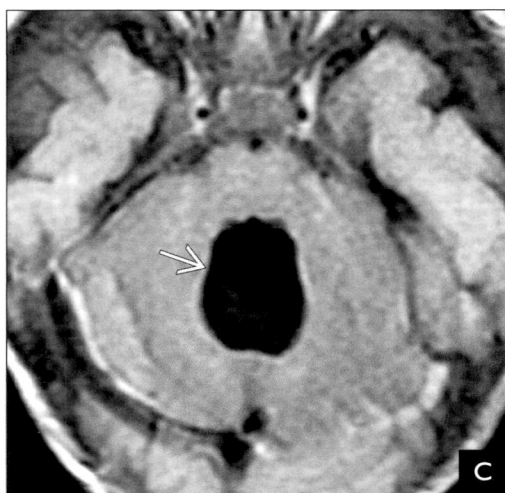

34-45C. *FLAIR scan shows no evidence of periventricular interstitial fluid around the encysted fourth ventricle ➤. (Courtesy K. Moore, MD.)*

cephalus. Such devices allow noninvasive adjustment of valve pressure settings. (In up to 50% of cases, the opening pressure of an implanted valve has to be changed, sometimes months or even years later.)

Imaging is often performed to assess valve settings. Interested readers are referred to the comprehensive guide to valves and their radiographic appearances by Lollis et al.

Slit Ventricle Syndrome

Some shunted hydrocephalus patients exhibit clinical signs of shunt failure without evidence of ventricular enlargement, a condition called slit ventricle syndrome (SVS) **(34-44)**.

The etiology of SVS is controversial. Some patients have scarred ventricular walls with decreased compliance and reduced tolerance for the normal fluctuations in intracranial pressure. Others may have low pressure with collapsed ventricles secondary to overdrainage or CSF leak. Intermittent or partial shunt obstruction may be a contributory factor.

Comparison to prior imaging studies is essential. NECT scans show that one or both lateral ventricles are small or slit-like. Functional studies show that the shunt may fill slowly but still functions, although flow is often reduced.

Miscellaneous Complications

Decompression of longstanding hydrocephalus and CSF overdrainage both increase the risk of **subdural hematoma**. Intraventricular scarring and adhesions can block CSF flow from one compartment to another, causing an **encysted "trapped" (isolated) ventricle (34-45)**. Continued CSF production can result in massive enlargement of the affected ventricle. Infection is a relatively uncommon complication but can result in meningitis, ventriculitis, and pyocephalus.

Abdominal complications from ventriculoperitoneal shunts include loculated CSF collections ("pseudocysts"), ascites, and bowel perforations. Distal shunt obstruction can cause shunt failure and hydrocephalus.

CSF Leaks and Sequelae

CSF Leaks

Terminology

CSF anywhere outside the subarachnoid space of the brain and spine is abnormal. CSF leaks are named by loca-

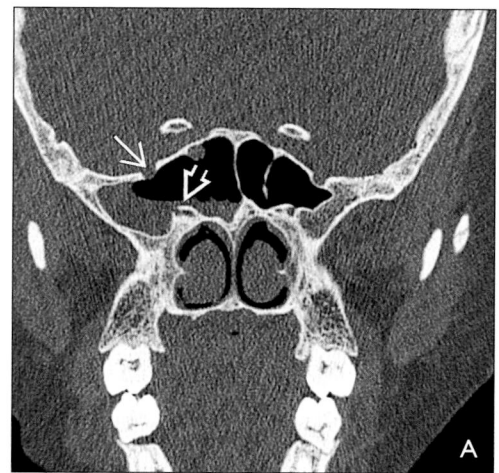

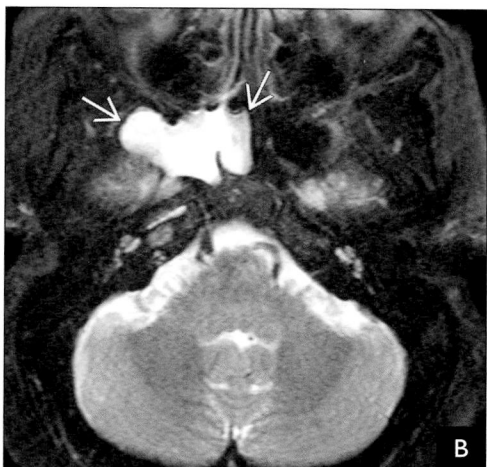

34-46A. Bone CT in a patient with a spontaneous CSF leak shows a defect in the right sphenoid wing ➡, sphenoid sinus air-fluid level ➡. **34-46B.** T2 FS scan in the same patient shows fluid filling the right sphenoid sinus ➡. The left sphenoid is normally aerated. In-111 DTPA cisternogram (not shown) demonstrated activity in nose, sphenoid sinus, confirming CSF leak. (Courtesy H. R. Harnsberger, MD.)

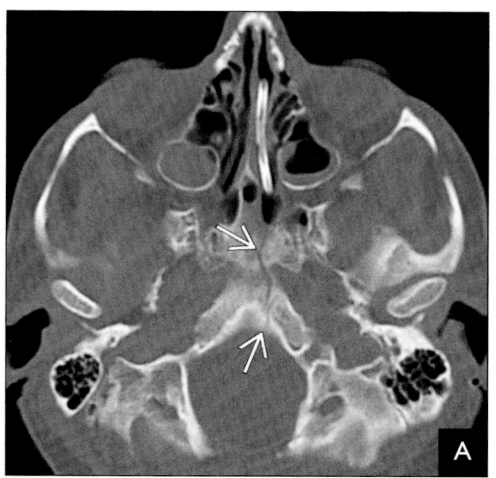

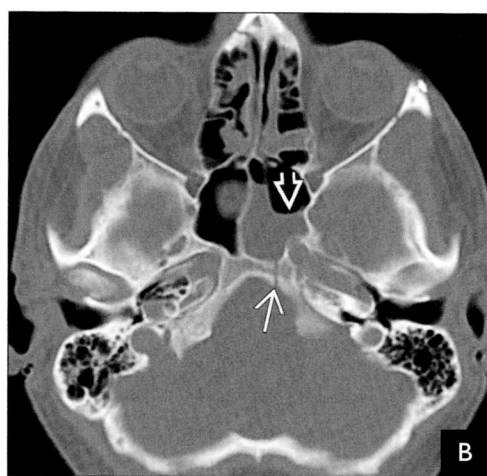

34-47A. Axial bone CT in a patient with left-sided CSF rhinorrhea following severe head trauma shows a linear fracture extending through the clivus ➡. **34-47B.** More cephalad scan in the same patient shows that the fracture ➡ extends into the sphenoid sinus. Note air-fluid level ➡ consistent with CSF leak. (Courtesy H. R. Harnsberger, MD.)

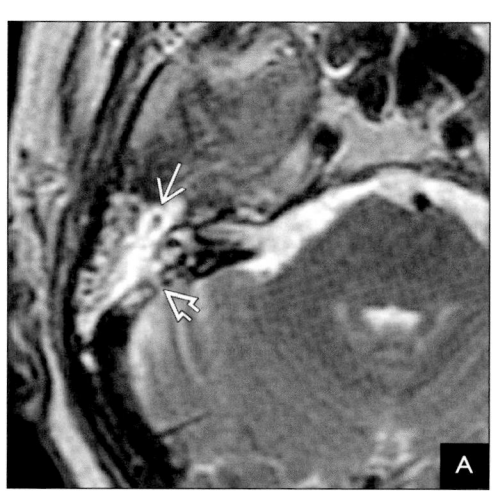

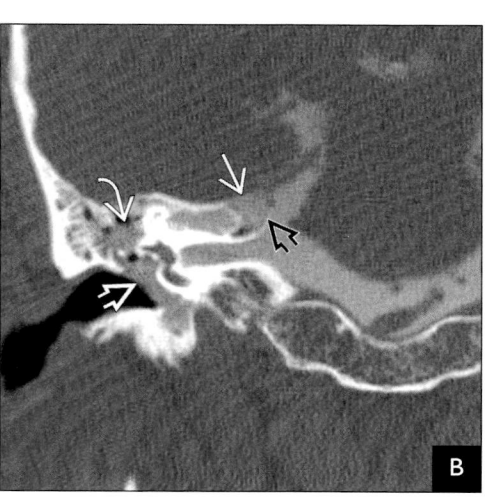

34-48A. Axial T2WI in a patient with severe headaches, recurrent meningitis shows fluid filling the right mastoid ➡, filling defect in temporal bone ➡. **34-48B.** Coronal CT cisternogram in the same patient shows contrast in the CPA cistern entering the petrous temporal bone ➡ through a defect caused by a giant arachnoid granulation ➡, then filling the mastoid ➡ and middle ear ➡. (Courtesy H. R. Harnsberger, MD.)

tion, e.g., CSF rhinorrhea (nasopharynx), CSF otorrhea (temporal bone).

Etiology

CSF leaks can be congenital or acquired. Congenital CSF leaks can occur with a cephalocele, persistent craniopharyngeal canal, or cribriform plate defect.

Acquired CSF leaks can be spontaneous, post-traumatic, or iatrogenic. Spontaneous intracranial CSF leaks are most commonly associated with arachnoid granulations in the lateral sphenoid sinus. Post-traumatic CSF leaks typically occur with fractures of the sphenoid sinus, cribriform plate, or ethmoid roof. Iatrogenic CSF leaks are seen with skull base surgery or following functional endoscopic sinus surgery.

Clinical Issues

EPIDEMIOLOGY AND DEMOGRAPHICS. CSF leaks can occur in patients of all ages. Trauma, prior skull base operation, and sinonasal surgery are common antecedents. Spontaneous CSF leaks usually develop in middle-aged obese women with idiopathic intracranial hypertension.

PRESENTATION. The most common symptoms are CSF rhinorrhea, especially if the nasal discharge increases with Valsalva or head-down maneuvers.

Imaging

CT FINDINGS. Bone CT with multiplanar reformations is the procedure of choice and may obviate the need for invasive CT cisternography. A bone defect, with or without an air-fluid level in the adjacent sinus, is the typical finding (34-46), (34-47). Defects under three or four millimeters may be difficult to detect, especially in areas where the bone is normally very thin.

CT cisternography is indicated if standard bone CT is negative or shows more than one potential leakage site (34-48).

MR FINDINGS. MR is generally used only if CT is negative or the presence of brain parenchyma within a cephalocele is suspected. T2 scans disclose an osseous defect with fluid in the adjacent sinus cavity.

34-49. Intracranial hypotension with distended dural sinuses ➡, enlarged pituitary ⧫, herniated tonsils ➡. Central brain descent causes midbrain "slumping," inferiorly displaced pons, "closed" pons-midbrain angle ⇗, splenium depressing ICV/VofG junction ➡. 34-50A. Sagittal T1WI shows tonsillar herniation ➡, prominent venous "flow voids" ⧫, "sagging" midbrain with decreased pons-midbrain angle ➡, "fat" pituitary ⧫, optic chiasm draped over sella ➡.

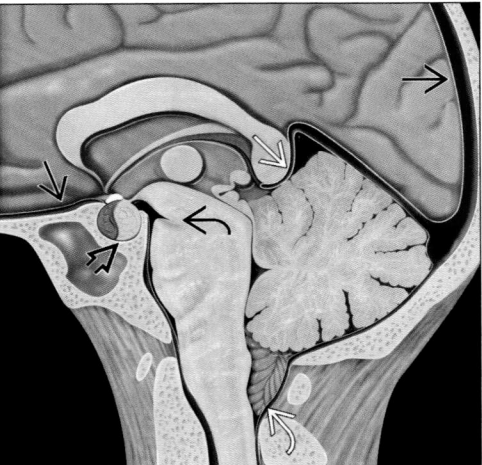

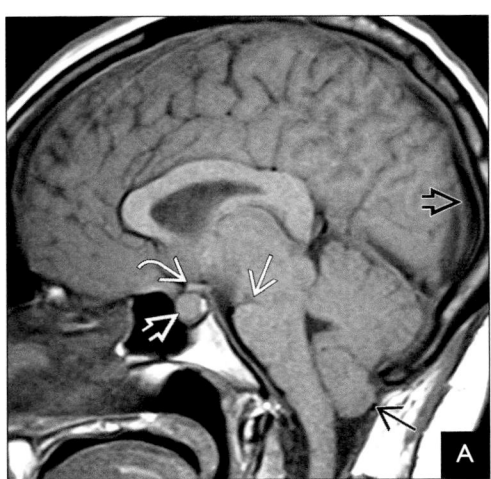

34-50B. T1 C+ FS in the same patient shows dural enhancement ➡ and very prominent, distended transverse sinuses ⧫. 34-50C. Coronal T1 C+ SPGR shows diffuse dural enhancement ➡ extending into internal auditory canals ⧫. Ventricular angle is 111° (≥ 120° is normal) consistent with downward traction of core central brain structures. Classic intracranial hypotension.

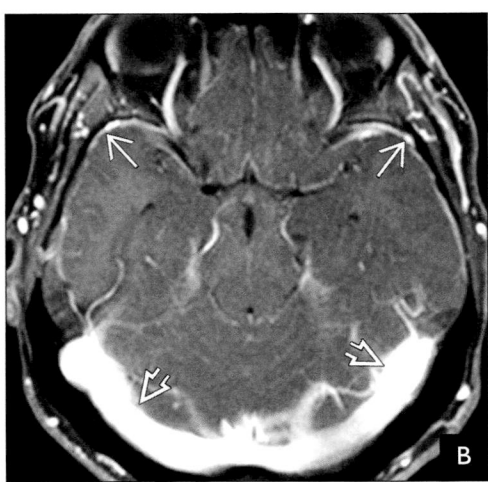

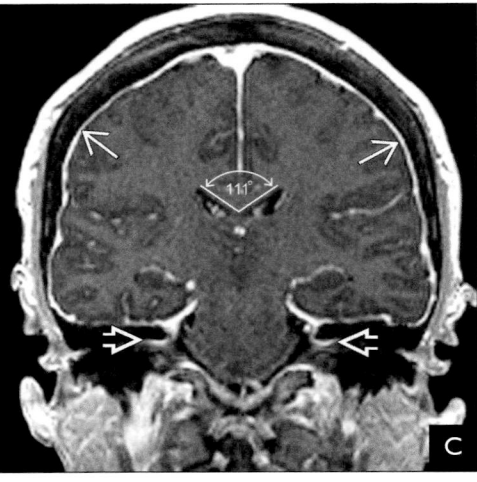

NUCLEAR MEDICINE. In isotope cisternography, CSF is labeled with intrathecal Tc-99m or In-111 DTPA and the activity over the head and spine scanned. Pledgets can be packed into the nose or ear and then counted, usually one to two hours after tracer injection. Pledget counts should be at least 1.5 times the serum count.

Differential Diagnosis

The major differential diagnosis of a cranial CSF leak is a **skull base defect without CSF leak**. Some areas of the skull base—such as the cribriform plate, olfactory recesses, and petrous ridges—are often very thin.

Intracranial Hypotension

Intracranial hypotension is a poorly understood, frequently misdiagnosed entity that can present with a wide variety of symptoms. Imaging is key to the diagnosis, sometimes providing the first insight into the cause of often puzzling symptoms.

Terminology

Intracranial hypotension is also known as **CSF hypovolemia syndrome**.

Etiology

Intracranial hypotension can be spontaneous or acquired. Common antecedent causes include lumbar puncture, spinal surgery, and trauma. Spinal arachnoid diverticula can rupture suddenly and may be responsible for many cases of "spontaneous" intracranial hypotension.

Vigorous coughing, exercise, and severe dehydration are other reported causes of spontaneous intracranial hypotension (SIH). Patients with Marfan and Ehlers-Danlos syndromes have abnormal connective tissue and an increased risk of CSF rupture through the weakened dura. Occasionally, CSF leaks occur through a dural breach from degenerative cervical spine pathology. Skull base CSF leaks rarely cause SIH.

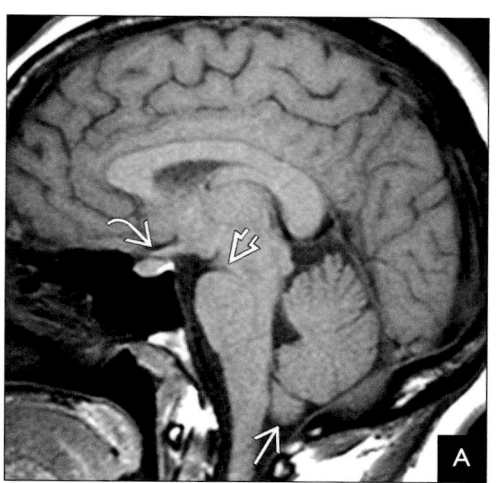

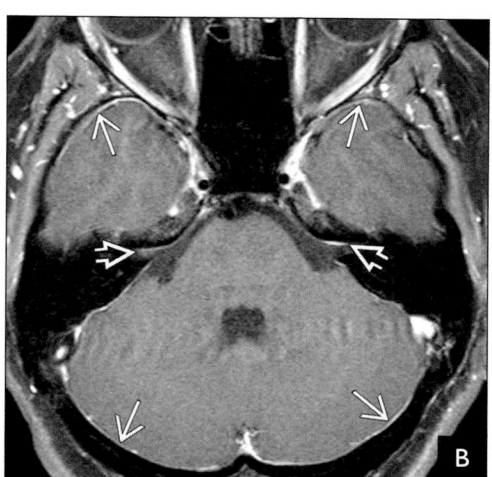

34-51A. Mild intracranial hypotension is illustrated by this case of a 32-year-old woman with postural headaches 10 days following lumbar puncture. Sagittal T1WI demonstrates normal tonsillar position, configuration ➡. There is slight midbrain "slumping" ➡, and the optic chiasm is draped over the sella ➡. 34-51B. Axial T1 C+ FS scan reveals subtle dural enhancement ➡ that also extends into both internal auditory canals ➡.

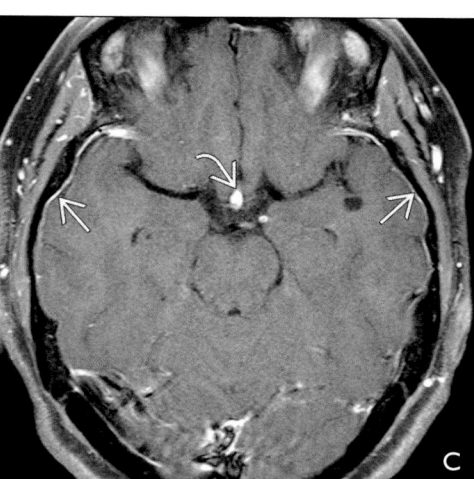

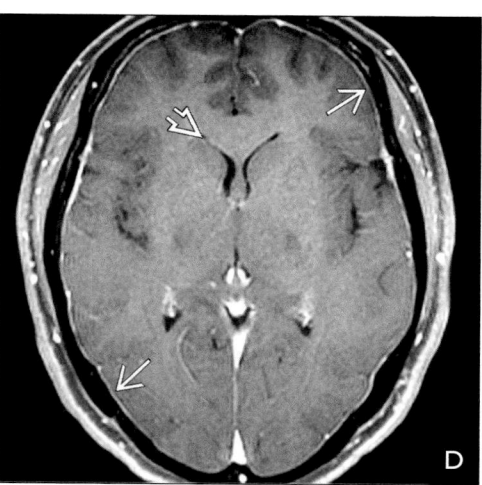

34-51C. T1 C+ FS shows slightly "fat" infundibular stalk ➡, mild dural thickening and enhancement ➡. 34-51D. T1 C+ FS shows small lateral ventricles ➡, mild diffuse dural enhancement ➡. The patient's symptoms resolved completely after epidural blood patch.

34-52A. *Sagittal T1WI in a 30-year-old man with severe headache, decreasing consciousness illustrates the findings of moderately severe intracranial hypotension. Note tonsillar descent* ➡, *"sagging" midbrain with "closed" midbrain-pontine angle* ➡, *reduced suprasellar subarachnoid space with anterior recesses of third ventricle draped over sella* ➡. **34-52B.** *T1WI in the same patient shows a "fat" pons* ➡, *convex margins of transverse sinuses* ➡.

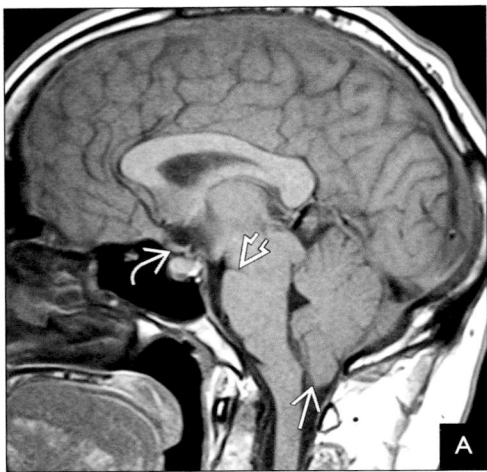

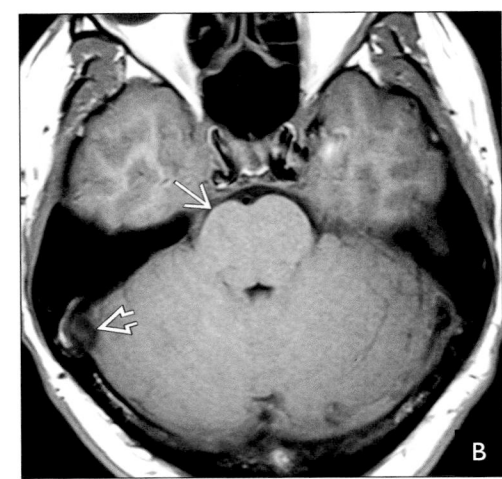

34-52C. *T1WI shows complete obliteration of the basal cisterns and surface sulci. The third ventricle* ➡ *is inferiorly displaced, the temporal lobes herniate medially* ➡, *and the midbrain appears severely compressed with concave posterior margins* ➡. **34-52D.** *T2WI at the same level shows the downwardly displaced third ventricle* ➡, *obliterated sulci and cisterns. The midbrain* ➡ *appears compressed and elongated in the axial plane.*

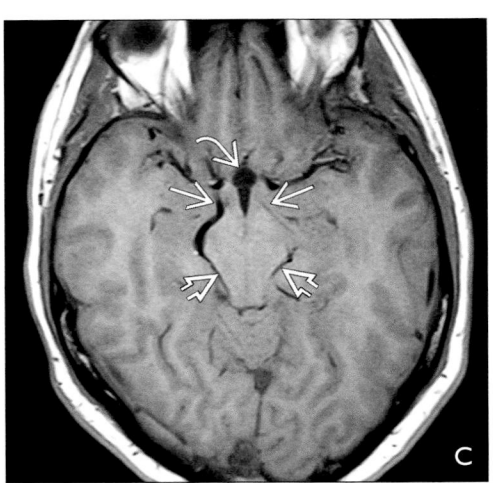

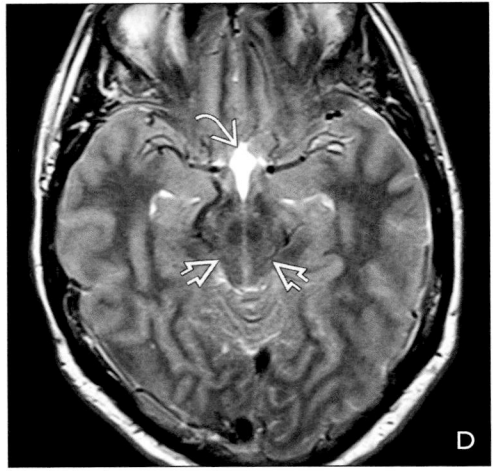

34-52E. *Axial T1 C+ FS shows mild diffuse dural enhancement* ➡. **34-52F.** *Coronal T1 C+ SPGR scan confirms the diffuse dural enhancement* ➡.

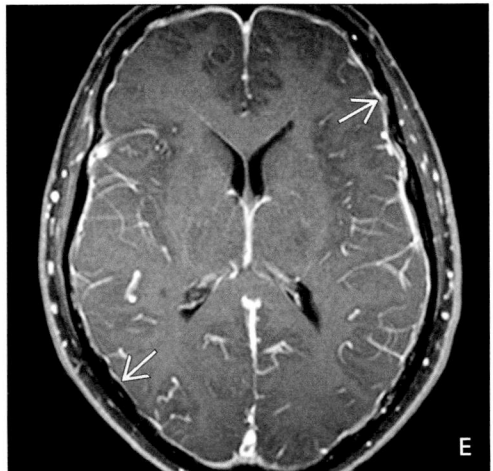

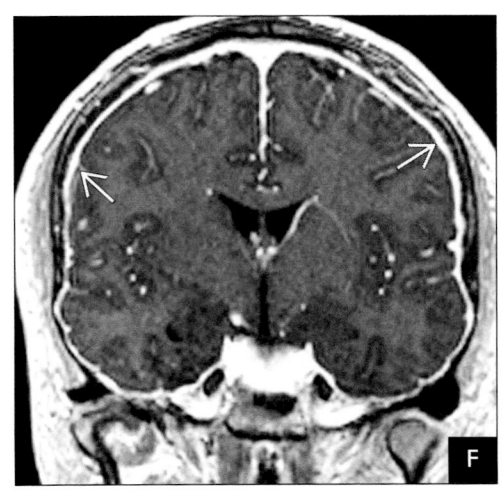

Pathology

CSF hypovolemia and hypotension (< 60 mmH$_2$O) result in venous engorgement and brain descent ("sagging") (34-49). The dura typically appears normal without evidence of neoplasia or inflammation. Longstanding cases of SIH may have dura-arachnoid fibrosis with nests of prominent meningothelial cells; these should not be mistaken for meningioma.

Clinical Issues

EPIDEMIOLOGY AND DEMOGRAPHICS. The true incidence of SIH is unknown. Estimated prevalence is 1:50,000 per year. While SIH can occur at any age, peak prevalence is in the third and fourth decades. There is a moderate female predominance.

PRESENTATION. Symptoms range widely, from mild headache to coma. The classic presentation of SIH is a severe orthostatic headache that is relieved by lying down. (Loss of approximately 10% of the total CSF volume is required to induce orthostatic headache.) Nonorthostatic headache, nuchal rigidity, and visual disturbances are less common. Severe cases may present with progressive encephalopathy.

NATURAL HISTORY. Most cases of SIH resolve spontaneously. In rare cases, severe unrelieved brain descent can result in coma or even death.

TREATMENT OPTIONS. Treatment is aimed at restoring CSF volume. Fluid replacement and bed rest can be sufficient in many cases. In others, epidural blood patch or surgical repair may be required. Emergent intrathecal saline infusion may be lifesaving in obtunded, severely encephalopathic patients.

Epidural blood patch is often performed on the basis of clinical and brain imaging findings alone. If low- and high-volume patches are unsuccessful, further studies may be necessary to localize precisely the level of the CSF leak.

Imaging

While CT is often obtained as an initial screening study in patients with severe or intractable headache, MR is the procedure of choice to evaluate possible SIH. A spectrum

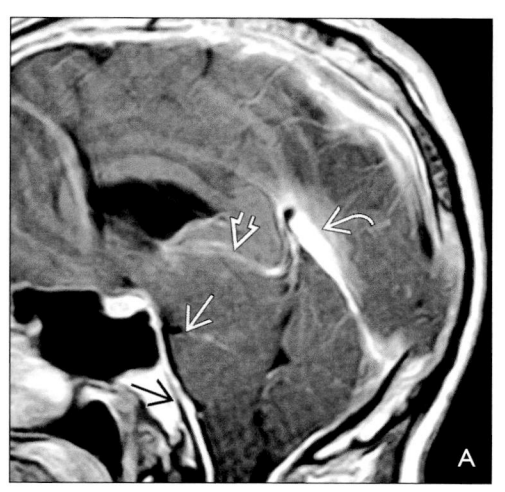
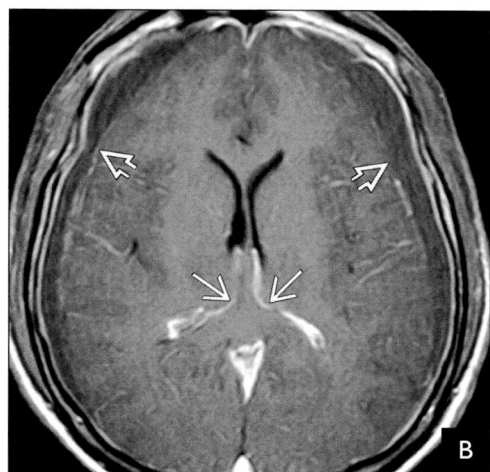
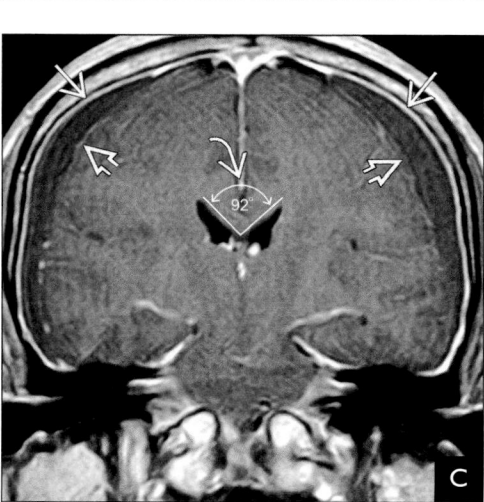
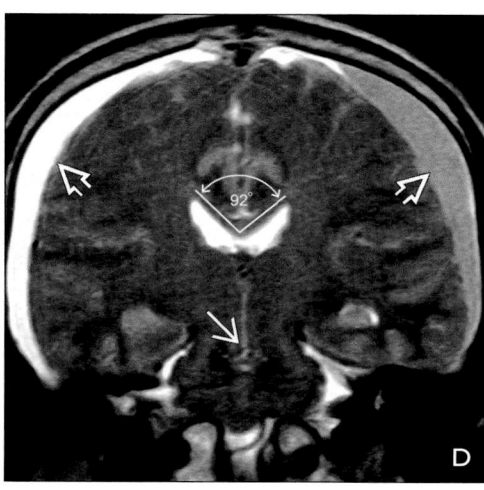

34-53A. Intracranial hypotension can be life-threatening if downward herniation becomes severe or large subdural hematomas (SDHs) develop, as happened in this case. Sagittal T1 C+ scan shows severe midbrain "slumping" and downward compression of the pons ➤, flattened internal cerebral veins ➤, thick dural enhancement ➤, venous distension ➤. 34-53B. T1 C+ FS scan demonstrates medially displaced ICVs and ventricles ➤, bilateral SDHs ➤.

34-53C. Coronal T1 C+ shows the SDHs ➤, diffuse dural enhancement ➤, markedly decreased ("closed") ventricular angle ➤ from downward traction on the central core structures of the brain. 34-53D. Coronal T2WI in the same patient shows downward displacement of the slit-like third ventricle ➤ through the tentorial incisura, SDHs of different ages ➤, and "closed" ventricular angle.

34-54A. *CT findings in intracranial hypotension can be subtle, as illustrated by this case. Note absence of suprasellar cisterns, CSF spaces with tight-appearing brain. The temporal lobes ➡ are displaced medially over the tentorium.* **34-54B.** *NECT in the same patient has some motion artifact ⇢ but shows small ventricles, complete lack of surface sulci, medially displaced atria ➡.*

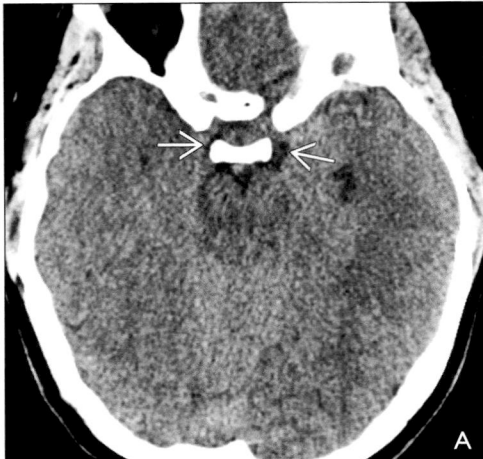
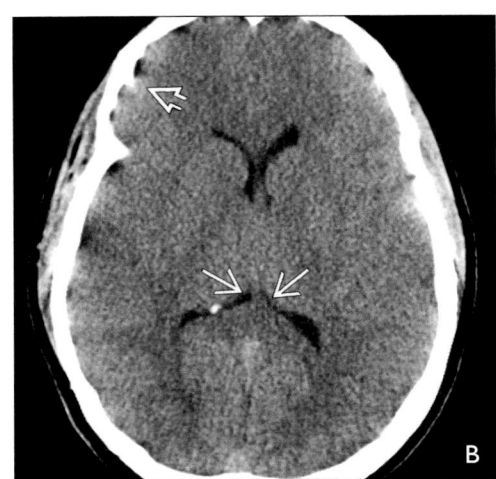

34-54C. *NECT through the vertex shows bilateral hypodense extraaxial fluid collections ⇢ with a more acute-appearing subdural hematoma ➡.* **34-54D.** *MR was obtained because of suspected intracranial hypotension. Sagittal T1WI shows mild tonsillar descent ➡, "slumping" midbrain with "closed" midbrain-pons angle ➡. Suprasellar cistern is almost nonexistent, and the optic chiasm ➡ is draped over the sella.*

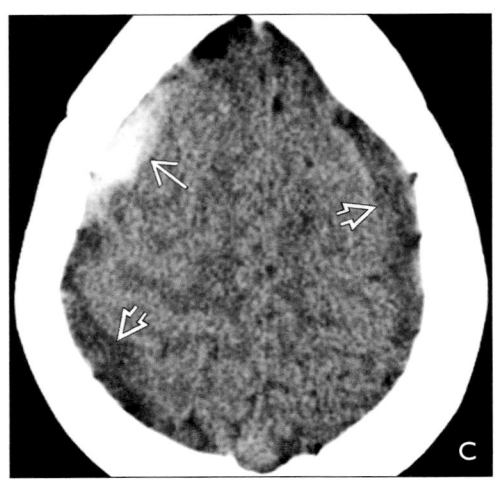
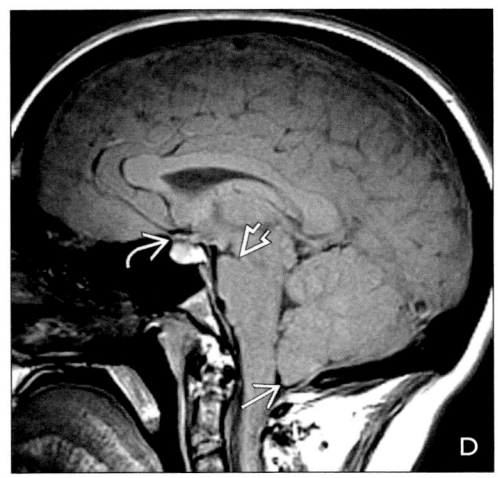

34-54E. *T2WI shows appearance of a "tight" brain with reduced sulci. A slit-like third ventricle is superimposed over the midbrain ➡, suggesting inferior displacement. Small bilateral hyperintense extraaxial fluid collections are present ➡.* **34-54F.** *More cephalad T2WI in the same patient shows mixed signal intensity of the subdural hematomas ➡.*

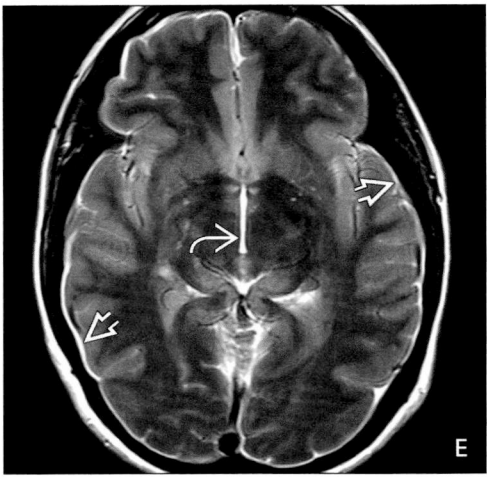
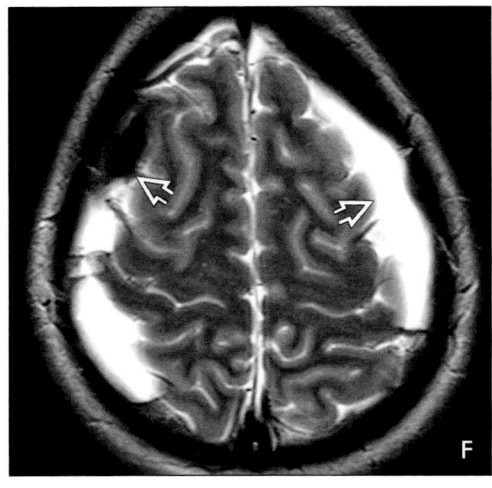

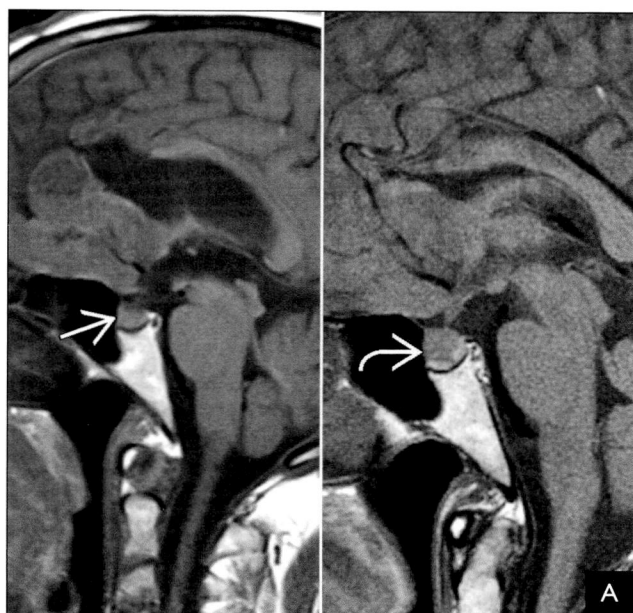

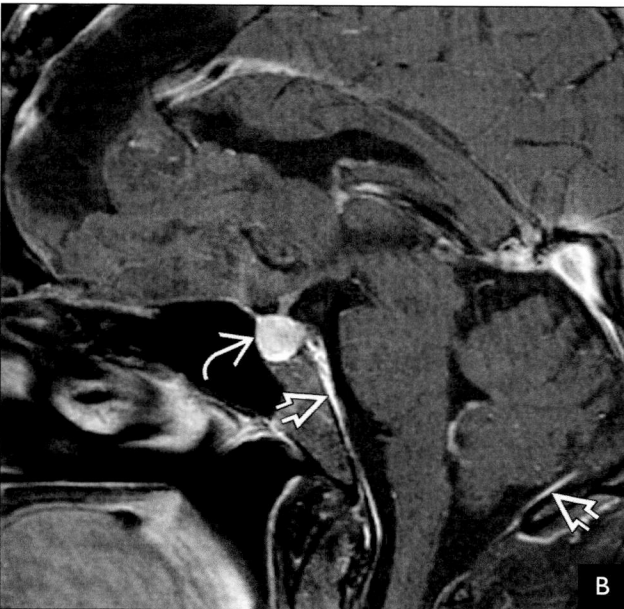

34-55A. (Left) Sagittal T1WI prior to reoperation for recurrent oligodendroglioma shows normal pituitary gland ➡. (Right) Postoperatively, the patient developed worsening headaches. Note interval enlargement of pituitary gland ➡.

34-55B. Sagittal T1 C+ FS shows the rounded, enhancing pituitary gland ➡ together with dural engorgement ➡. One of the most reliable imaging finding in postoperative intracranial hypotension is interval enlargement of the pituitary gland.

of findings occurs with SIH; only rarely are *all* imaging signs present in the same patient!

CT FINDINGS. The most obvious findings on NECT scans are subdural fluid collections, although they are present in only 15% of cases. Subtle CT clues to the presence of SIH include effacement of the basal cisterns (especially the suprasellar subarachnoid space), medial herniation of the temporal lobes into the tentorial incisura, small ventricles with medial deviation of the atria of the lateral ventricles, and a "fat" pons.

MR FINDINGS.

T1WI. Sagittal T1 scans show brain descent in approximately half of all cases. Midbrain "sagging" with the midbrain displaced below the level of the dorsum sellae, the angle between the peduncles and pons decreased below 90°, and flattening of the pons against the clivus are typical findings. Caudal displacement of the tonsils is common but not invariably present.

The optic chiasm and hypothalamus are often draped over the sella, effacing the suprasellar cistern. The pituitary gland appears enlarged in at least 50% of all cases **(34-50A)**, **(34-51)**, **(34-55)**.

Axial scans show the basal cisterns are effaced. The midbrain and pons often appear elongated ("fat pons" sign), and the temporal lobes are displaced medially over the tentorium into the incisura. The lateral ventricles are usually small and distorted as they are pulled medially and inferiorly by the brain "sagging" **(34-53)**.

In cases with severe brain descent, coronal scans show that the angle between the roof of the lateral ventricles progressively decreases (< 120°) **(34-50B)**.

The dural sinuses often appear distended with outwardly convex margins and exaggerated "flow voids" **(34-50C)**. Subdural fluid collections (hygromas > hematomas) are variable **(34-53)**, **(34-54)**.

T2/FLAIR. The slit-like third ventricle is displaced downward and on axial scans appears almost superimposed on the midbrain **(34-52)**.

T1 C+. One of the most consistent findings in SIH, diffuse dural thickening with intense enhancement is seen in 85% of cases. Linear dural thickening may extend into the internal auditory canals, down the clivus, and through the foramen magnum into the upper cervical canal **(34-51)**.

SPINE IMAGING. Engorged enhancing cervical venous plexuses may appear like a "draped curtain," narrowing the canal. Thickened dura may mimic sarcoid or metastatic disease.

MR imaging of the entire spine can be helpful in detecting extraarachnoid CSF. When the precise localization of the spinal leak becomes important in managing CSF hypovolemia, dynamic CT myelography (CTM) can be helpful. MR myelography with intrathecal gadolinium (currently an off-label use) may detect leaks in selected patients in whom conventional CTM does not demonstrate a leak.

NUCLEAR MEDICINE. In-111 DTPA intrathecal radionuclide cisternography can help detect CSF leaks. Extradural egress of tracer, typically into the paraspinal space, is readily detected. SPECT/CT fusion imaging is very helpful to determine the precise spinal level responsible for the CSF leak.

Differential Diagnosis

The major differential diagnosis of intracranial hypotension is **Chiari 1 malformation**. The only intracranial abnormality in Chiari 1 is displaced tonsils, which appear peg-like with vertically oriented folia. *Mistaking SIH for Chiari 1 on imaging studies can lead to decompressive surgery, worsening CSF hypovolemia, and clinical deterioration!*

Other causes of dura-arachnoid thickening (infection, metastases, etc.) do not have the spectrum of findings associated with SIH. **Idiopathic hypertrophic pachymeningitis** is generally not as diffuse as the dural thickening seen in SIH. Bone invasion (temporal bone, orbits) may be present but is not a feature of SIH.

Dural sinus thrombosis may cause engorged sinuses secondary to collateral venous drainage. T2* (GRE, SWI) sequences demonstrate "blooming" clot in the affected sinuses and slow flow in distended medullary (white matter) veins if clot extends into the internal cerebral veins.

INTRACRANIAL HYPOTENSION

Etiology and Pathology
- CSF hypovolemia → brain "sags," dural/venous sinuses ↑
- Can be spontaneous (idiopathic) or acquired

Clinical Issues
- Orthostatic headache
- Severe intracranial hypotension may cause coma, even death

MR Findings
- Common
  - Midbrain "sags" down
  - Angle between midbrain, pons decreases (< 90°)
  - Optic chiasm/hypothalamus draped over sella
  - Diffusely thickened enhancing dura
- Less common
  - Pons, midbrain may appear "fat"
  - ± tonsils displaced downward
  - Effaced cisterns/sulci
  - Small lateral ventricles ± atria "tugged" inferomedially
  - Ventricular angle < 120°
  - ± subdural collections (hygromas > frank hematomas)
  - Enlarged dural sinuses with outwardly bulging (convex) margins

---

Selected References

Normal Development of the Ventricles and Cisterns

Subarachnoid Spaces

- Sakka L et al: Anatomy and physiology of cerebrospinal fluid. Eur Ann Otorhinolaryngol Head Neck Dis. 128(6):309-16, 2011
- Lowery LA et al: Totally tubular: the mystery behind function and origin of the brain ventricular system. Bioessays. 31(4):446-58, 2009

Normal Anatomy of the Ventricles and Cisterns

Choroid Plexus and the CSF

- Sakka L et al: Anatomy and physiology of cerebrospinal fluid. Eur Ann Otorhinolaryngol Head Neck Dis. 128(6):309-16, 2011

Normal Variants

Asymmetric Lateral Ventricles

- Kiroğlu Y et al: Cerebral lateral ventricular asymmetry on CT: how much asymmetry is representing pathology? Surg Radiol Anat. 30(3):249-55, 2008

Cavum Septi Pellucidi and Vergae

- Tubbs RS et al: Cavum velum interpositum, cavum septum pellucidum, and cavum vergae: a review. Childs Nerv Syst. 27(11):1927-30, 2011
- Winter TC et al: The cavum septi pellucidi: why is it important? J Ultrasound Med. 29(3):427-44, 2010

Cavum Velum Interpositum

- Tubbs RS et al: Cavum velum interpositum, cavum septum pellucidum, and cavum vergae: a review. Childs Nerv Syst. 27(11):1927-30, 2011
- Tubbs RS et al: The velum interpositum revisited and redefined. Surg Radiol Anat. 30(2):131-5, 2008

Enlarged Subarachnoid Spaces

- Zahl SM et al: Benign external hydrocephalus: a review, with emphasis on management. Neurosurg Rev. 34(4):417-32, 2011
- Hellbusch LC: Benign extracerebral fluid collections in infancy: clinical presentation and long-term follow-up. J Neurosurg. 107(2 Suppl):119-25, 2007

CSF Flow Artifacts

- Lisanti C et al: Normal MRI appearance and motion-related phenomena of CSF. AJR Am J Roentgenol. 188(3):716-25, 2007

Hydrocephalus

- Harris CA et al: What we should know about the cellular and tissue response causing catheter obstruction in the treatment of hydrocephalus. Neurosurgery. 70(6):1589-601; discussion 1601-2, 2012
- Raybaud C et al: Hydrocephalus. In Barkovich AJ et al: Pediatric Neuroimaging. 5th ed. Philadelphia: Lippincott Williams and Wilkins. 808-56, 2012
- Paul L et al: Expression of aquaporin 1 and 4 in a congenital hydrocephalus rat model. Neurosurgery. 68(2):462-73, 2011
- Bergsneider M et al: What we don't (but should) know about hydrocephalus. J Neurosurg. 104(3 Suppl):157-9, 2006
- Greitz D: Radiological assessment of hydrocephalus: new theories and implications for therapy. Neurosurg Rev. 27(3):145-65; discussion 166-7, 2004

Intraventricular Obstructive Hydrocephalus

- Vaz-Guimarães Filho FA et al: Neuroendoscopic surgery for unilateral hydrocephalus due to inflammatory obstruction of the Monro foramen. Arq Neuropsiquiatr. 69(2A):227-31, 2011
- Ambarki K et al: Brain ventricular size in healthy elderly: comparison between Evans index and volume measurement. Neurosurgery. 67(1):94-9; discussion 99, 2010
- Aukland SM et al: Assessing ventricular size: is subjective evaluation accurate enough? New MRI-based normative standards for 19-year-olds. Neuroradiology. 50(12):1005-11, 2008
- Naidich TP et al: Atrial diverticula in severe hydrocephalus. AJNR Am J Neuroradiol. 3(3):257-66, 1982

Extraventricular Obstructive Hydrocephalus

- Dinçer A et al: Is all "communicating" hydrocephalus really communicating? Prospective study on the value of 3D-constructive interference in steady state sequence at 3T. AJNR Am J Neuroradiol. 30(10):1898-906, 2009

Overproduction Hydrocephalus

- Anei R et al: Hydrocephalus due to diffuse villous hyperplasia of the choroid plexus. Neurol Med Chir (Tokyo). 51(6):437-41, 2011
- Cataltepe O et al: Diffuse villous hyperplasia of the choroid plexus and its surgical management. J Neurosurg Pediatr. 5(5):518-22, 2010

Normal Pressure Hydrocephalus

- Leinonen V et al: Cortical brain biopsy in long-term prognostication of 468 patients with possible normal pressure hydrocephalus. Neurodegener Dis. 10(1-4):166-9, 2012

- Rosenbaum RB: Normal pressure hydrocephalus: how often does the diagnosis hold water? Neurology. 78(2):152; author reply 152, 2012
- Stadlbauer A et al: Magnetic resonance velocity mapping of 3D cerebrospinal fluid flow dynamics in hydrocephalus: preliminary results. Eur Radiol. 22(1):232-42, 2012
- Dinçer A et al: Radiologic evaluation of pediatric hydrocephalus. Childs Nerv Syst. 27(10):1543-62, 2011
- Kim MJ et al: Differential diagnosis of idiopathic normal pressure hydrocephalus from other dementias using diffusion tensor imaging. AJNR Am J Neuroradiol. 32(8):1496-503, 2011
- Klassen BT et al: Normal pressure hydrocephalus: how often does the diagnosis hold water? Neurology. 77(12):1119-25, 2011
- Dinçer A et al: Is all "communicating" hydrocephalus really communicating? Prospective study on the value of 3D-constructive interference in steady state sequence at 3T. AJNR Am J Neuroradiol. 30(10):1898-906, 2009

Syndrome of Inappropriately Low-Pressure Acute Hydrocephalus

- Hamilton MG et al: Syndrome of inappropriately low-pressure acute hydrocephalus (SILPAH). Acta Neurochir Suppl. 113:155-9, 2012
- Clarke MJ et al: Very low pressure hydrocephalus. Report of two cases. J Neurosurg. 105(3):475-8, 2006

Idiopathic Intracranial Hypertension

- Maralani PJ et al: Accuracy of brain imaging in the diagnosis of idiopathic intracranial hypertension. Clin Radiol. 67(7):656-63, 2012
- Ahmed RM et al: Transverse sinus stenting for idiopathic intracranial hypertension: a review of 52 patients and of model predictions. AJNR Am J Neuroradiol. 32(8):1408-14, 2011
- Rohr AC et al: MR imaging findings in patients with secondary intracranial hypertension. AJNR Am J Neuroradiol. 32(6):1021-9, 2011

CSF Shunts and Complications

- Lollis SS et al: Programmable CSF shunt valves: radiographic identification and interpretation. AJNR Am J Neuroradiol. 31(7):1343-6, 2010
- Miller JH et al: Improved delineation of ventricular shunt catheters using fast steady-state gradient recalled-echo sequences in a rapid brain MR imaging protocol in nonsedated pediatric patients. AJNR Am J Neuroradiol. 31(3):430-5, 2010
- Rughani AI et al: Radiographic assessment of snap-shunt failure: report of 2 cases. J Neurosurg Pediatr. 6(3):299-302, 2010
- Vassilyadi M et al: The necessity of shunt series. J Neurosurg Pediatr. 6(5):468-73, 2010
- Gupta N et al: Long-term outcomes in patients with treated childhood hydrocephalus. J Neurosurg. 106(5 Suppl):334-9, 2007

CSF Leaks and Sequelae

CSF Leaks

- Schievink WI et al: Lack of causal association between spontaneous intracranial hypotension and cranial cerebrospinal fluid leaks. J Neurosurg. 116(4):749-54, 2012
- Daele JJ et al: Traumatic, iatrogenic, and spontaneous cerebrospinal fluid (CSF) leak: endoscopic repair. B-ENT. 7 Suppl 17:47-60, 2011

Intracranial Hypotension

- Akbar JJ et al: The role of MR myelography with intrathecal gadolinium in localization of spinal CSF leaks in patients with spontaneous intracranial hypotension. AJNR Am J Neuroradiol. 33(3):535-40, 2012
- Kranz PG et al: CT-guided epidural blood patching of directly observed or potential leak sites for the targeted treatment of spontaneous intracranial hypotension. AJNR Am J Neuroradiol. 32(5):832-8, 2011
- Taguchi Y et al: SPECT/CT fusion imaging by radionuclide cisternography in intracranial hypotension. Intern Med. 50(20):2433-4, 2011

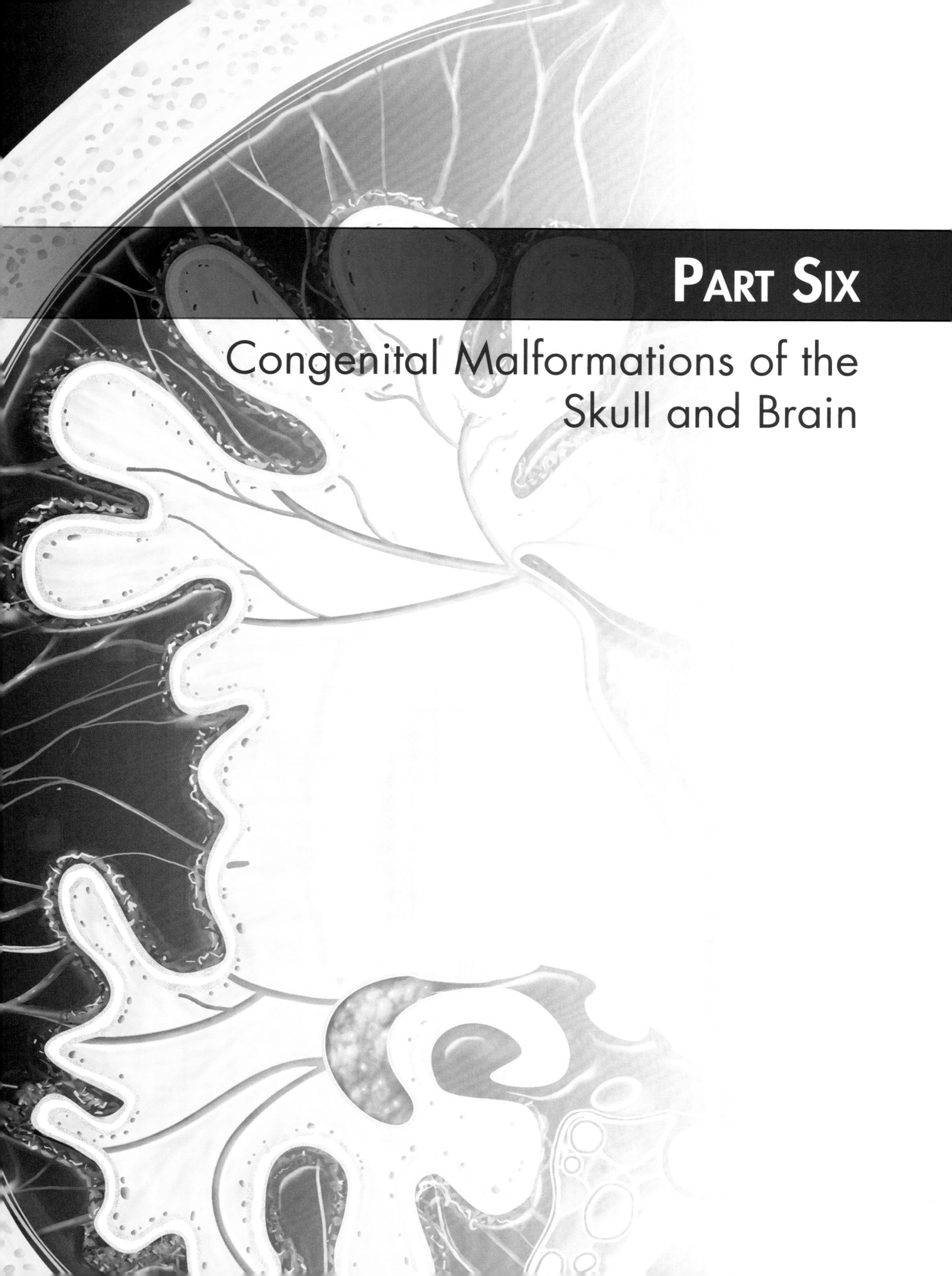

PART SIX

Congenital Malformations of the Skull and Brain

35

Embryology and Approach to Congenital Malformations

A basic knowledge of normal brain development and maturation provides the essential foundation for understanding congenital malformations, the subject of the final part of this book.

This text approaches embryology step by step, discussing different aspects of CNS development with their relevant pathology. Some concepts have already been elucidated in previous chapters. Myelination maturation from birth to age three was discussed in Chapter 31 with inherited metabolic disorders, and development of the ventricles and choroid plexus was presented in conjunction with the discussion of hydrocephalus and CSF disorders in Chapter 34.

Here we briefly consider normal development of the cerebral hemispheres and cerebellum. We first focus on the basics of neurulation and neural tube closure, then turn our attention to how the neural tube flexes, bends, and evolves into the forebrain, midbrain, and hindbrain. Developmental errors and the resulting malformations that may occur at each stage are briefly summarized. (They are discussed in detail in subsequent chapters.)

Growth of the cerebral hemispheres with their elaboration into lobes, the development of sulci and gyri, patterns of gray matter migration and layering of the neocortex are all succinctly delineated. Development of the three major brain commissures (corpus callosum, anterior commissure, and hippocampal commissure) is

detailed in Chapter 37 as a prelude to our consideration of callosal anomalies.

We then touch lightly on the complex choreography required for proper development of the midbrain and hindbrain structures (pons, cerebellum, medulla). We include a brief discussion of how the midbrain and cerebellum develop. The final section of this chapter suggests an approach to analyzing brain malformations.

Cerebral Hemisphere Formation

The major embryologic events in brain development begin with neurulation, neuronal proliferation, and neuronal migration. The processes of operculization, gyral and sulcal development, and the earliest steps in myelination all take place later, between gestational weeks 11 and birth.

Neurulation

Neural Tube and Brain Vesicles

The earliest step in brain development occurs during the third fetal week when the three layers of the trilaminar germ disc emerge. The **neural plate** develops at the cranial end of the embryo as a thickening of ectoderm on either side of the midline.

During the fourth fetal week, the neural plate indents and thickens laterally, forming the **neural folds**. The neural folds bend upward, meet in the midline, and then fuse to form the **neural tube**. The primitive **notochord** lies ventral to the neural tube, and the **neural crest** cells are extruded and migrate laterally. The neural tube forms the brain and spinal cord whereas the neural crest gives rise to peripheral nerves, roots, and ganglia of the autonomic nervous system (**35-1**).

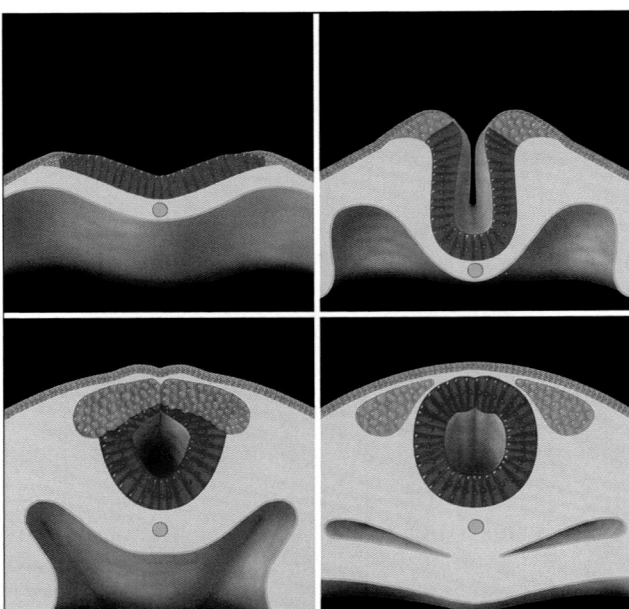

35-1. Graphic shows the formation, closure of the neural tube. The neural plate (red) forms, folds, and fuses in the midline. The neural and cutaneous ectoderm then separate. Notochord (green), neural crest (blue) are shown.

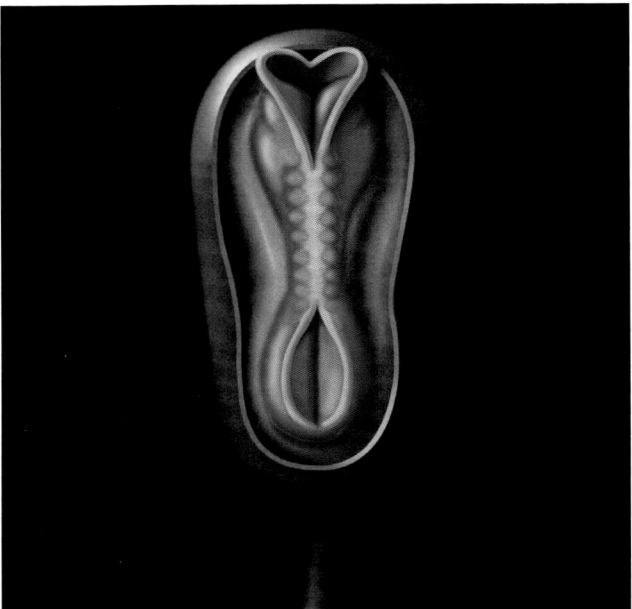

35-2. The neural tube closes in a bidirectional zipper-like manner, starting in the middle and proceeding toward both ends.

As the neural tube closes, the neuroectoderm (which will form the CNS) separates from the cutaneous ectoderm in a process known as disjunction. Neural tube closure probably begins at two or three levels in the middle of the embryo (35-2). Closure proceeds bidirectionally in a zipper-like fashion along the length of embryo. The cephalic and caudal ends of the neural tube (the so-called anterior and posterior neuropores) do not fuse until the twenty-fifth and twenty-seventh gestational days, respectively.

Three primary brain vesicles—the **prosencephalon** (forebrain), **mesencephalon** (midbrain), and **rhomben-cephalon** (hindbrain)—also form during the fourth week. The embryonic brain grows rapidly and begins to bend, forming several flexures (35-3).

During the fifth week, the forebrain further divides into two vesicles, forming the **telencephalon** and the **diencephalon**. The hindbrain divides into the **meten-cephalon** and **myelencephalon**. Together with the mes-encephalon, the brain now has five definitive or "sec-ondary" vesicles (35-4).

Neurulation Errors

Errors in neurulation result in a spectrum of congenital anomalies. The most severe is **anencephaly**—essentially complete absence of the cerebral hemispheres—which is caused by failure of the anterior neuropore to close (see Chapter 38). Various types of **cephaloceles** also result from abnormalities of neurulation.

Incomplete closure of the posterior neuropore results in **spina bifida**. If the neuroectoderm fails to separate com-

pletely from the cutaneous ectoderm, **myelomeningocele** results. Abnormal neurulation of the hindbrain leads to a **Chiari 2 malformation** (see Chapter 36).

Neuronal Proliferation

Embryonic Stem Cells

*Pluri*potent embryonic stem cells are derived from the inner cell mass of the four- to five-day blastocyst. These cells are able to proliferate and differentiate into all three germ layers (ectoderm, mesoderm, endoderm). MicroR-NAs seem to play an important role as genetic regula-tors of stem cell development, differentiation, growth, and neurogenesis.

Histogenesis of Neurons and Glia

As the cerebral vesicles develop and expand, layers of stem cells arise around the primitive ventricular ependyma, forming the germinal matrix. These neural stem cells (NSCs) are *multi*potent cells that generate the main CNS phenotypes, i.e., neurons, astrocytes, and oligodendrocytes. NSCs are found primarily in the ger-minal zones (see Chapter 16).

*Pluri*potent NSCs in the specialized subventricular zone of the germinal matrix give rise to neuroblasts ("prim-itive" or "young" **neurons**) that migrate through the developing telencephalon to form the cortical man-tle zone, the precursor of the definitive cortex. Axons from the migrating neurons form an intermediate zone between the germinal matrix and cortical mantle that will eventually become the cerebral white matter.

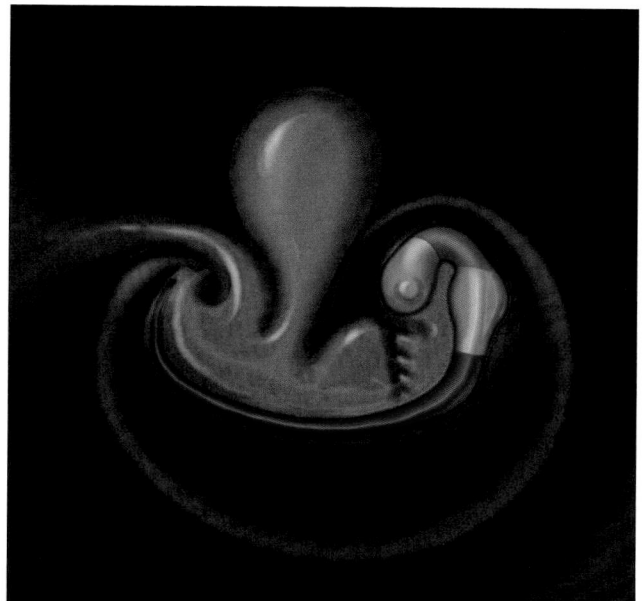

35-3. Development of primary vesicles is depicted. The prosencephalon (green) gives rise to the forebrain, the mesencephalon (purple) to the midbrain, and the rhombencephalon (light blue) to the hindbrain.

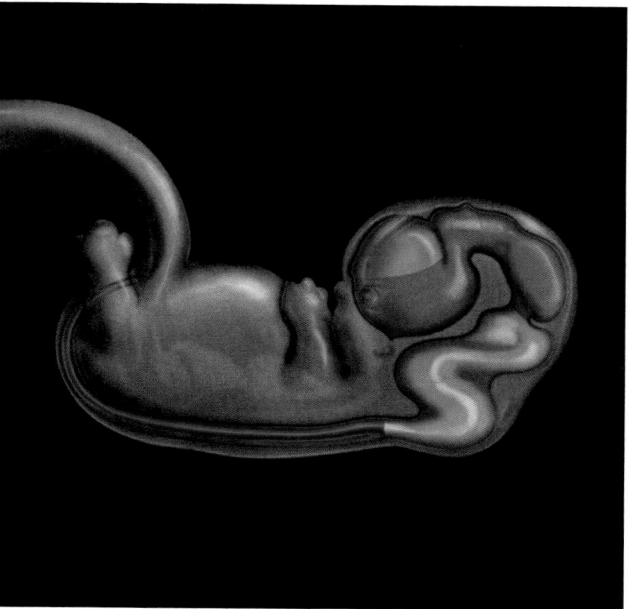

35-4. The brain develops flexures as prosencephalon gives rise to telencephalon (green), diencephalon (red). Mesencephalon (purple) elongates while rhombencephalon gives rise to metencephalon (yellow), myelencephalon (light blue).

Some NSCs become specialized **radial glial cells** (RGCs) that will eventually span the entire hemisphere from the ventricular ependyma to the pia. RGCs are also stem cells and can give rise to both neurons and glia. Elongated cell bodies of the RGCs serve as a "rope ladder" that guides migrating neurons from the germinal matrix to the cortex.

Astrocytes arise from two sources: Glial progenitor cells in the ventricular zone and RGCs in the intermediate zone. **Oligodendrocytes** arise from oligodendrocyte precursor cells in the ventricular and subventricular zones. Before differentiating into myelinating oligodendrocytes, these precursor cells proliferate, migrate, and then spread throughout the CNS.

Errors in Histogenesis

Errors in histogenesis and differentiation result in a number of embryonal neoplasms, including medulloblastoma and primitive neuroectodermal tumors. Problems with NSC proliferation and differentiation also contribute to malformations of cortical development (see below).

Neuronal Migration

Genesis of Cortical Neurons

Neurogenesis occurs in a predictable manner with sequential generation of specific neural subtypes from designated areas in the germinal matrix. For example, glutamatergic cerebral cortical neurons arise in dorsal ventricular zones whereas GABAergic neurons destined for the striatum originate in the more ventral zones.

Once the "young" neurons have been generated in the germinal matrix and dorsal ventricular zones, they must leave their "home" to reach their final destination (the cortex). The definitive cerebral cortex develops through a highly ordered process of neuronal proliferation, migration, and differentiation. The neocortex of the cerebral hemispheres has six cell layers, each with its own distinctive pattern of organization and connections.

Neuronal Migration

Migration of newly proliferated neurons occurs along scaffolding provided by the RGCs. Neurons travel from the germinal zone to the cortical mantle in a generally "inside-out" sequence. Cells initially form the deepest layer of the cortex with each successive migration ascending farther outward and progressively forming more superficial layers. Each migrating group passes through layers already laid down by the earlier-arriving cells.

Peak neuronal migration occurs between 11-15 fetal weeks although migration continues up to 35 weeks.

Errors in Neuronal Migration and Cortical Organization

The primary result of errors at these stages are **malformations of cortical development**. Problems with NSC proliferation or differentiation, migration, and cortical organization can all result in developmental anomalies of the neocortex. Examples include **microcephaly**, **megalencephaly**, **heterotopias**, **cortical dysplasias**, and **lissencephaly**.

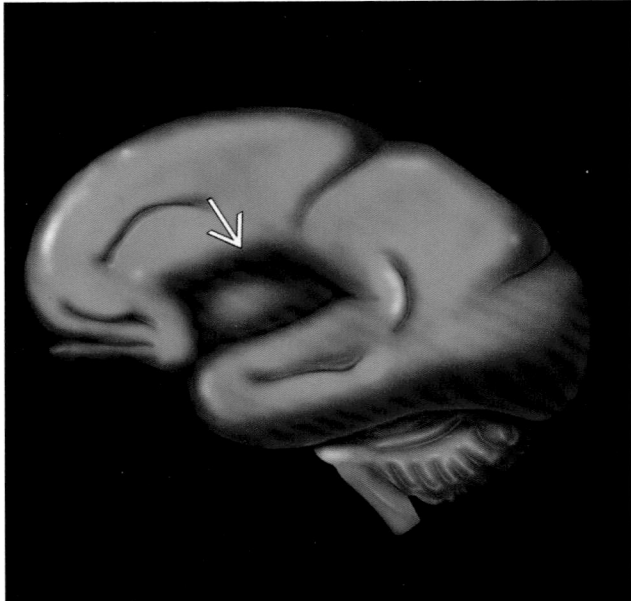

35-5. Embryonic brain at 22 weeks is mostly agyric with shallow sylvian fissures ➡. Prosencephalon (green), metencephalon (yellow), and myelencephalon (light blue) are shown. Mesencephalic, midbrain structures are not visible.

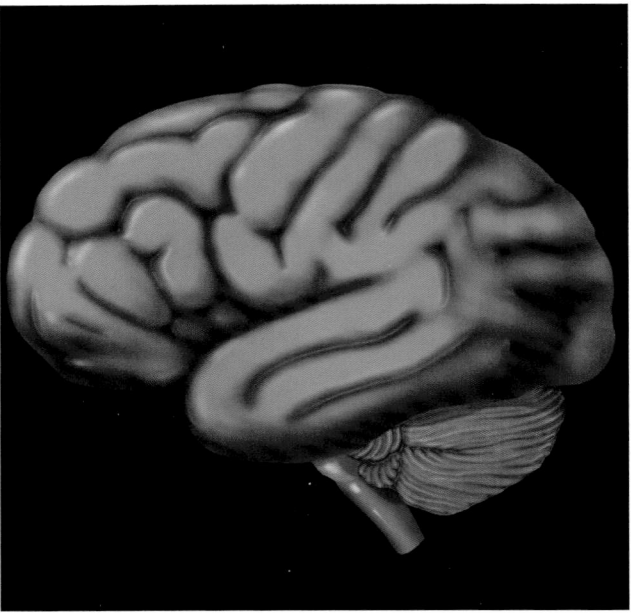

35-6. With advancing gestational age, multiple secondary and tertiary gyri develop, and the number and complexity of the cerebellar folia increase.

Operculization, Sulcation, and Gyration

Lobulation and Operculization

The cerebral hemispheres first appear as outpouchings of the embryonic telencephalon. The hemispheres are initially almost featureless; the cortex is thin and smooth. The fetal cerebral vasculature covers the brain surface in a basket-like network of thin-walled, undifferentiated vessels.

The cerebral hemispheres expand, first covering the diencephalon and then the midbrain and hindbrain. The roofs of the hemispheres grow more rapidly than the floors. As the hemispheres elongate and rotate, they assume a "C" shape with the caudal ends turning ventrally to form the temporal lobes.

Sulcation and Gyration

Sulcation and gyration—the **progressive folding** of the telencephalon into a complex pattern of lobes and gyri—occurs relatively late in embryonic development. Shallow triangular surface indentations along the sides of the hemisphere—the beginnings of the sylvian (lateral) fissures—first appear between the fourth and fifth fetal months **(35-5)**.

As the forebrain enlarges, the emerging frontal, parietal, and temporal lobes begin to overhang the lateral fissures, forming the opercula. As the opercula develop and the lateral indentations deepen, cortex that was once on the brain surface becomes completely covered **(35-6)**. This tissue—now buried in the depths of the sylvian fissures—forms the insula ("island of Reil"). The sylvian fissures gradually lose their "open" fetal configuration and assume their narrow slit-like adult configuration.

The definitive middle cerebral arteries follow the indented surfaces of the insulae, first dipping into and then out of the sylvian fissures to ramify over the lateral surfaces of the frontal, parietal, and temporal lobes.

After the sylvian fissures form **(35-7)**, the next groups of surface indentations to appear are the calcarine and parietooccipital sulci **(35-8)**, followed by the central sulci **(35-9)**. Gyral development occurs most rapidly around the sensorimotor and visual pathways.

Anomalies in Sulcation and Gyration

Developmental errors in operculization, sulcation, and gyration are relatively uncommon. **Microcephaly** with simplified gyral pattern and **microlissencephaly** are representative anomalies that have too few gyri and abnormally shallow sulci.

Myelination

Myelination occurs in an orderly, predictable manner and can be detected as early as 20 fetal weeks. Normal brain myelination patterns as well as abnormalities in myelin formation and maintenance are discussed in greater detail in Chapter 31. In general, myelination proceeds from **inferior to superior**, from **back to front**, and from **central to peripheral**.

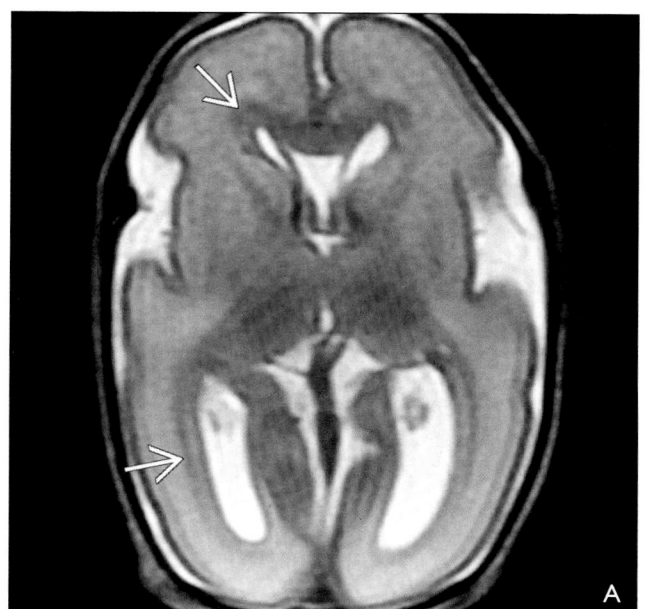

35-7A. *Axial T2WI in a 26-week, 5-day premature infant. The sylvian fissures are just beginning to form. The hypointensity around the ventricles* ➡ *is mostly in the germinal matrix.*

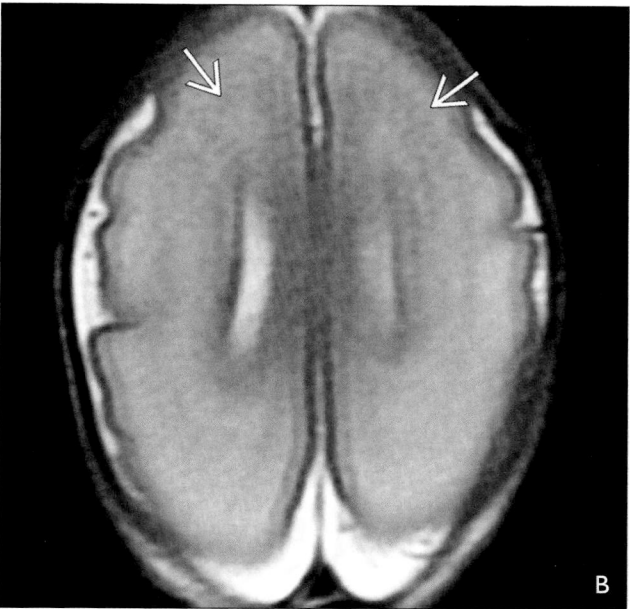

35-7B. *Image through the corona radiata shows that the brain is almost completely smooth with only a few shallow sulci. Waves of hypointense migrating neurons* ➡ *give the WM a layered and "smudgy" appearance.*

Midbrain and Hindbrain Development

We now summarize the major embryologic events involved in forming the midbrain and hindbrain. A description of the consequences of errors in their development follows.

Major Embryologic Events

The mesencephalon gives rise to the brainstem, and the rhombencephalon elaborates into the medulla, pons, and cerebellum. Each is "patterned" along both the rostral-caudal and dorsal-ventral axes. The mesencephalon is divided into ventral (tegmentum) and dorsal (tectum) regions. Likewise, the metencephalon is divided into ventral (pons) and dorsal (cerebellum) regions.

The pons is formed by a proliferation of cells and fiber tracts along the ventral metencephalon. The alar plates of the rhombencephalon ("rhombencephalic lips") thicken to form cerebellar plates, which in turn proliferate and eventually form the two cerebellar hemispheres and midline vermis. Embryologically, the cerebellum is an extension of the midline and thus part of the dorsal pons.

The rhombencephalic lips fuse, forming the cerebellar commissures in the roof of the fourth ventricle. Each hemisphere subsequently fuses and fissures in a cranial-to-caudal direction.

Formation of the fourth ventricle is a complex process. A ridge of developing choroid plexus divides the emerging fourth ventricle into anterior and posterior membranous areas. Normally, the anterior membrane is incorporated into the developing choroid plexus while the posterior membranous area persists and eventually cavitates, forming the midline foramen of Magendie. Precisely how and when the lateral foramina open is unknown.

Midbrain-Hindbrain Anomalies

A number of different classifications of midbrain and hindbrain malformations have been proposed. Barkovich et al use an approach that categorizes lesions according to developmental and genetic considerations. Such a system makes consummate sense and certainly aids understanding the pathogenesis of these fascinating anomalies. However, the more traditional morphologic-based approach in which malformations are grouped according to imaging findings is the simplest for radiologists to follow. The interested reader is referred to the publications cited at the end of this chapter.

35-8A. *Axial T2WI in a normal 30-week premature infant shows hyperintensity (myelination) in the dorsal brainstem ➡. The ventral brainstem ➡ and cerebellar WM ➡ are hypointense and unmyelinated.* **35-8B.** *T2WI in the same patient shows that the dorsal brainstem ➡ is myelinated and appears hypointense in comparison to the hyperintense (unmyelinated) ventral pons ➡ and cerebellar WM ➡.*

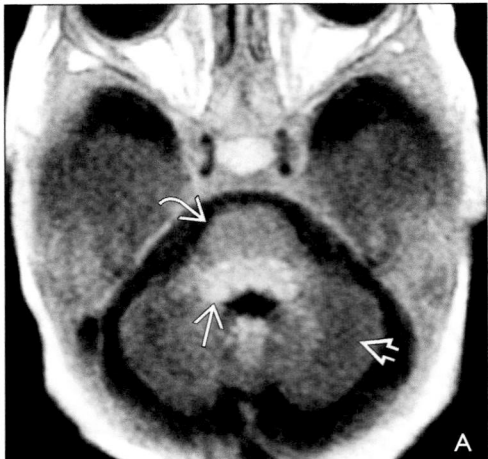

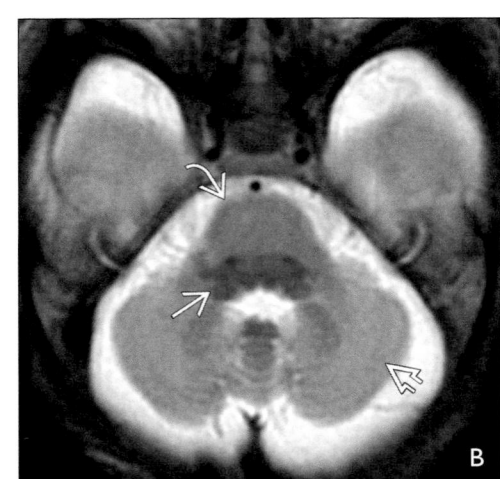

35-8C. *T1WI in the same patient shows that the posterior limbs of the internal capsules ➡ are unmyelinated. The cerebral WM is completely unmyelinated and shows relative lack of gyration and sulci. Note the shallow, open-appearing sylvian fissures ➡.* **35-8D.** *T2WI shows layers of hypointensity ➡ that represent migrating neurons and germinal matrix residua ➡. The thin cortex ➡ and shallow, incompletely formed sulci are normal for such a premature infant.*

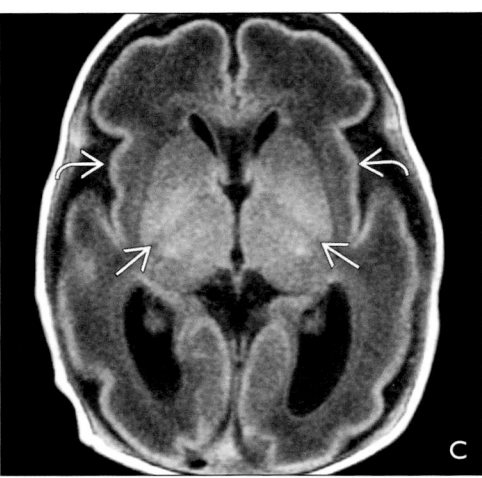

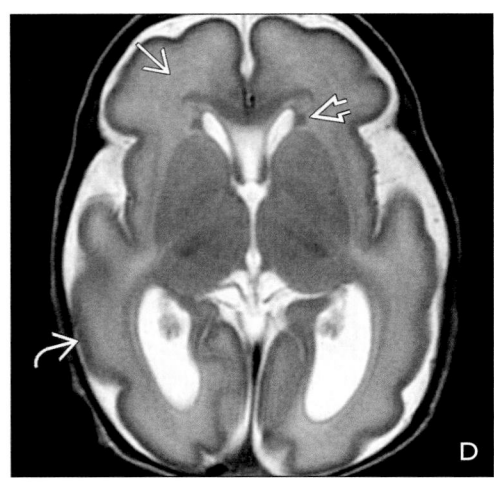

35-8E. *T1WI through the corona radiata shows that the WM is hypointense and completely unmyelinated. The sulci are primitive-appearing and very shallow, related to immaturity. The cortical gray matter is thin ➡.* **35-8F.** *T2WI shows that the WM is hyperintense compared to the hypointensity of the thin but normal cerebral cortex. This early in development, the brain essentially looks like a "water bag" of unmyelinated WM covered by a thin, incomplete shell of gray matter.*

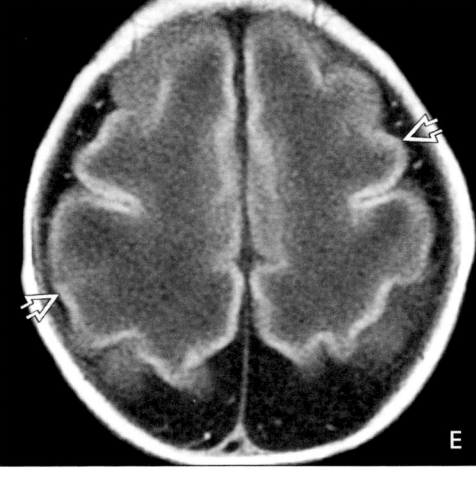

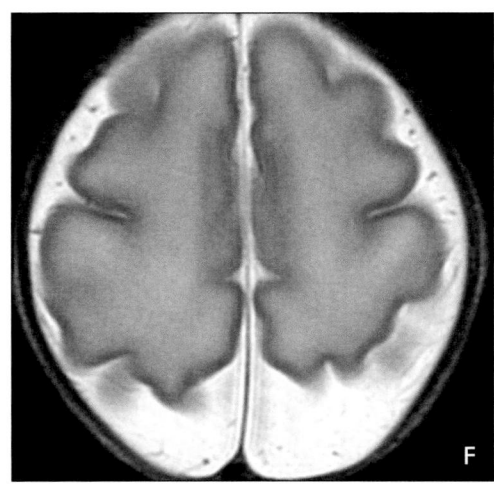

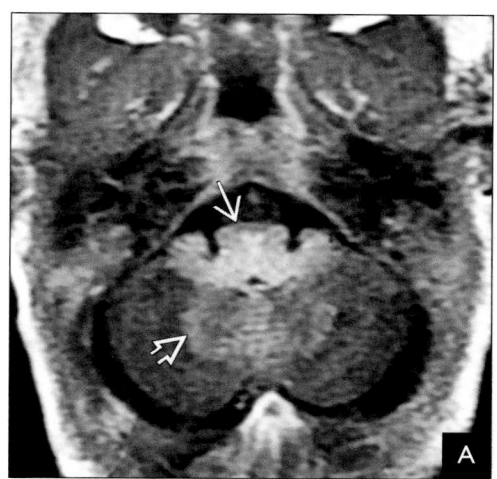

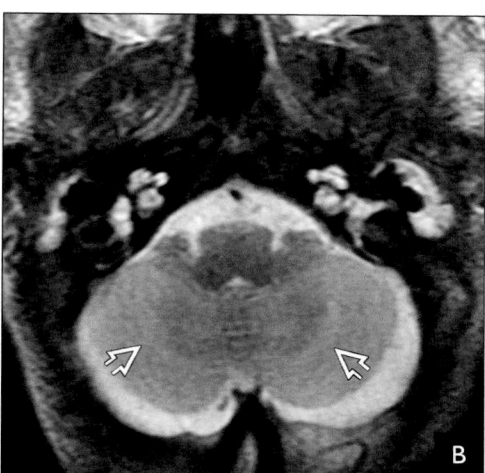

35-9A. Axial T1WI in a normal 33-week, 3-day gestation premature infant. The medulla ➡ has myelinated and increased in signal intensity, as have the flocculi and dentate nuclei ➡. 35-9B. Axial T2WI shows that the medulla, flocculi, and dentate nuclei are hypointense, but the cerebellar hemisphere WM ➡ remains unmyelinated and hyperintense.

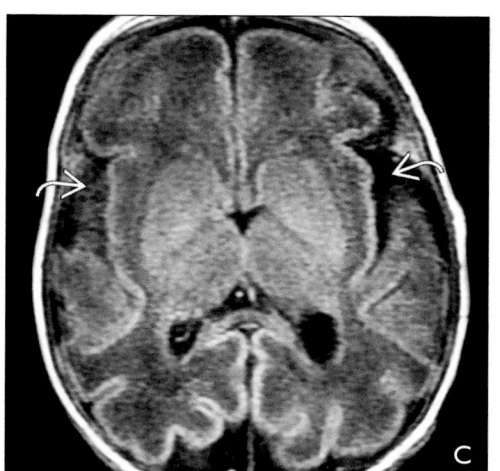

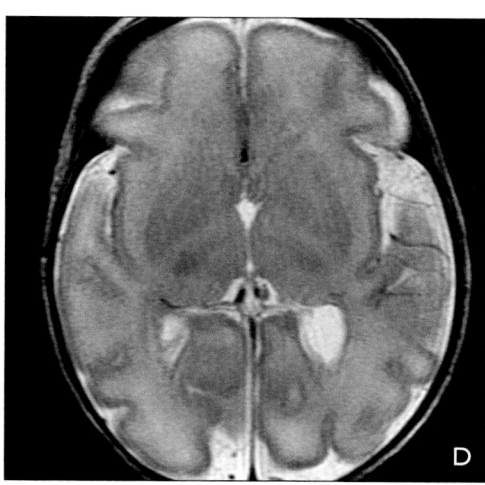

35-9C. As the opercula continue developing, the sylvian fissures ➡ appear less prominent. 35-9D. T2WI shows that the WM of the cerebral hemispheres remains unmyelinated and hyperintense.

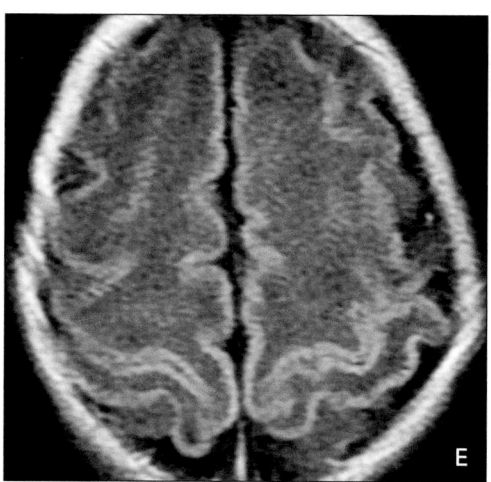

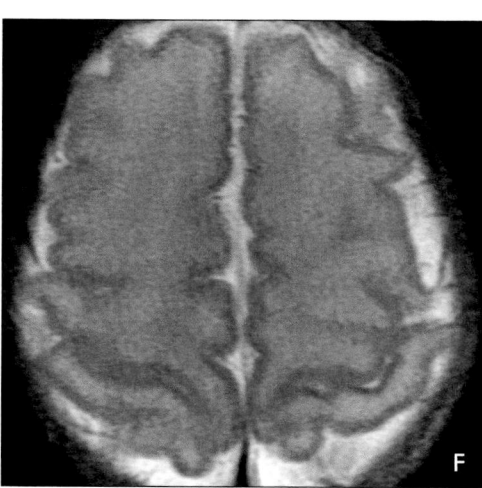

35-9E. More surface sulci and gyri are now apparent, especially in the parietal and occipital lobes. The cortex appears thicker. Compare to scans of the 30-week premature infant on Figure 35-8. The increased sulcation and gyration of both hemispheres is quite striking. 35-9F. At 33 weeks, the WM of the corona radiate is completely unmyelinated.

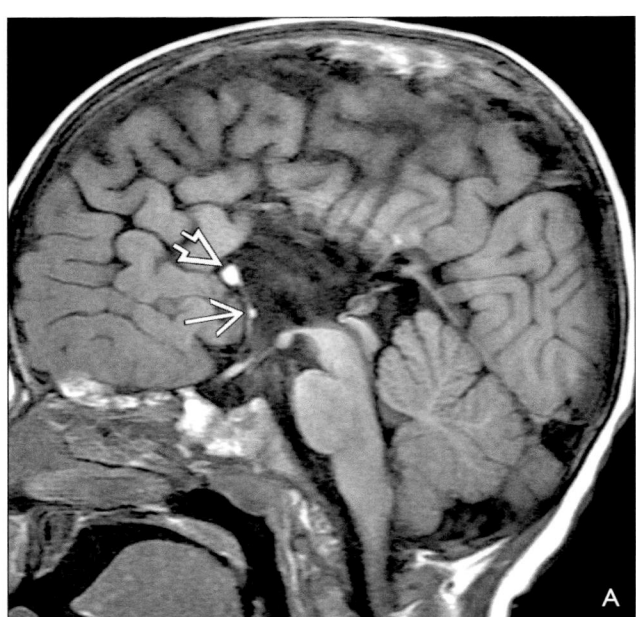

35-10A. Sagittal midline T1WI shows classic callosal agenesis. The anterior commissure ➡ is present, as is a tiny remnant of the genu ➡.

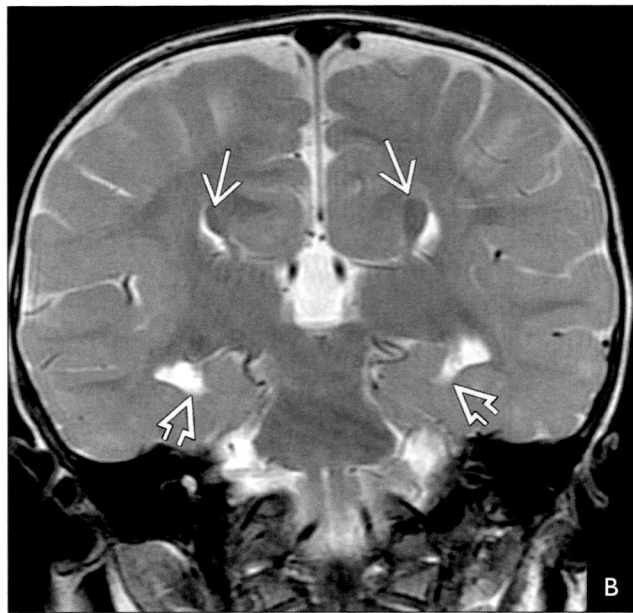

35-10B. Coronal T2WI in the same patient shows classic "Viking helmet" appearance of the lateral/third ventricles. Note the Probst bundles ➡, vertically oriented hippocampi ➡.

Imaging Approach to Brain Malformations

Technical Considerations

CT

Clinicians sometimes order NECT scans as an initial screening procedure in a patient with seizures or suspected brain malformation. Although parenchymal calcifications, ventricular size/configuration, and major abnormalities can be identified, subtle abnormalities such as cortical dysplasia are difficult to detect and easy to overlook.

Bone CT is helpful in depicting midline facial defects and synostoses.

MR

MR is the procedure of choice. The two most important factors are gray-white matter differentiation and high spatial resolution. Many pediatric neuroradiologists recommend a sagittal T1 or T1 FLAIR sequence, volumetric T1 sequences (e.g., MP-RAGE), and sagittal and coronal heavily T2-weighted sequences with very long TR/TEs.

A T2* sequence (GRE, SWI) can be a helpful addition if abnormal mineralization or vascular anomaly is suspected. DTI tractography is valuable when commissural anomalies are identified on initial sequences.

Contrast-enhanced T1 and FLAIR sequences are generally optional as they add little useful information in most congenital malformations. However, they can be very helpful in delineating associated vascular anomalies. DWI and MRS are useful in evaluating mass lesions and inborn errors of metabolism.

Image Analysis

The following approach to analyzing imaging studies is modified and adapted from A. James Barkovich's guidelines on imaging evaluation of the pediatric brain.

Sagittal Images

Begin with the midline section, and examine the craniofacial proportion. At birth, the ratio of calvaria to face should be 5:1 or 6:1. At two years, it should be 2.5:1. In adults and children over the age of 10 years, it should be approximately 1.5:1.

The most common of all brain malformations are anomalies of the cerebral commissures (especially the corpus callosum), which can be readily identified on sagittal T1 scans (35-10A). Commissural anomalies are also the most common malformation associated with other anomalies and syndromes, so if you see one, keep looking! Look for abnormalities of the pituitary gland and hypothalamus. Evaluate the size and shape of the third ventricle, especially its anterior recesses.

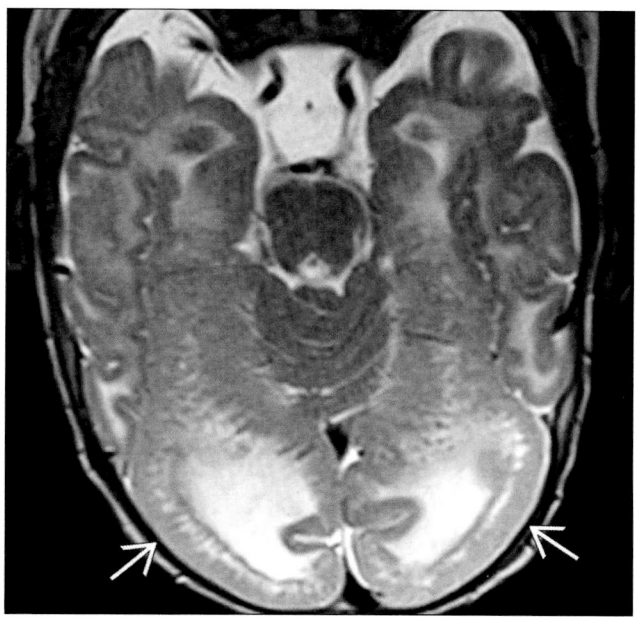

35-11. Axial T2WI shows "cobblestone" lissencephaly in both occipital poles ➡. *(Courtesy M. Warmuth-Metz, MD).*

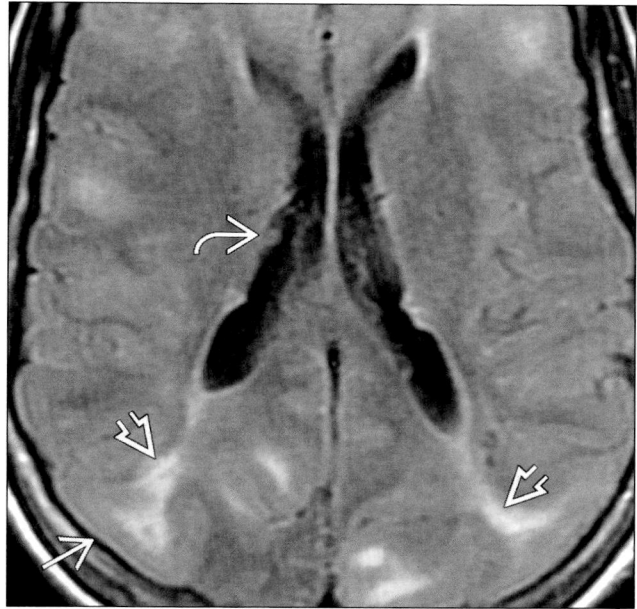

35-12. FLAIR scan shows subependymal nodules ➡, *cortical tubers* ➡ *with the typical flame-shaped subcortical hyperintensities* ➡ *of tuberous sclerosis complex.*

Look for other lesions such as lipomas and cysts. These are often midline or paramidline and can be readily identified. The midline sagittal scan also permits a very nice evaluation of the posterior fossa structures. Does the fourth ventricle appear normal? Can you find its dorsally pointing fastigium? Evaluate the position of the tonsils and the craniovertebral junction for anomalies.

If the lateral and third ventricles are large and the fourth ventricle appears normal, look for a funnel-shaped aqueduct indicating aqueductal stenosis. If you see aqueductal stenosis, look at the quadrigeminal plate carefully to see if the cause might be a low-grade tectal glioma.

Sagittal images are also especially useful in evaluating the cerebral cortex. Is the cortex too thick? too thin? irregular? "lumpy-bumpy"? Anomalies of cortical development such as pachygyria and cortical dysplasia associated with brain clefting ("schizencephaly") are often most easily identified on sagittal images.

Coronal Images

Cortical dysplasias are often bilateral and most frequently cluster around the sylvian fissure. Coronal scans make side-to-side comparison relatively easy. Follow the interhemispheric fissure (IHF) all the way from front to back. If the hemispheres are in contiguity across the midline, holoprosencephaly is present. If the IHF appears irregular and the gyri "interdigitate" across the midline, the patient almost certainly has a Chiari 2 malformation.

Evaluate the size, shape, and position of the ventricles. If the third ventricle appears "high riding" and the frontal horns of the lateral ventricles look like a "Viking helmet," corpus callosum dysgenesis is present (35-10B). If the frontal horns appear squared-off or box-like, look carefully for an absent cavum septi pellucidi. Absent cavum septi pellucidi is seen in septooptic dysplasia and is often seen with callosal dysplasia or schizencephaly.

Carefully evaluate the temporal horns and hippocampi to make sure that they are normally folded and oriented horizontally (not vertically, as often occurs with holoprosencephaly, lissencephaly, callosal anomalies, and malformations of cortical development).

Axial Images

The combination of a true T1WI together with a long TR/TE T2WI is necessary in evaluating all cases of delayed development to assess myelin maturation. The thickness and configuration of the cortical mantle are well seen (35-11). The size, shape, and configuration of the ventricles is easily evaluated on these sequences.

FLAIR sequences are especially useful in evaluating abnormalities such as focal or Taylor cortical dysplasia and the flame-shaped subcortical WM hyperintensities seen in tuberous sclerosis complex (35-12).

Don't forget the posterior fossa! The fourth ventricle in axial plane is normally shaped like a kidney bean on its side. If the vermis is absent and the cerebellar hemispheres appear continuous from side to side, rhombencephalosynapsis is present (35-13). If the fourth ventricle and superior cerebellar peduncles resemble a molar tooth, then a molar tooth malformation is present (35-14).

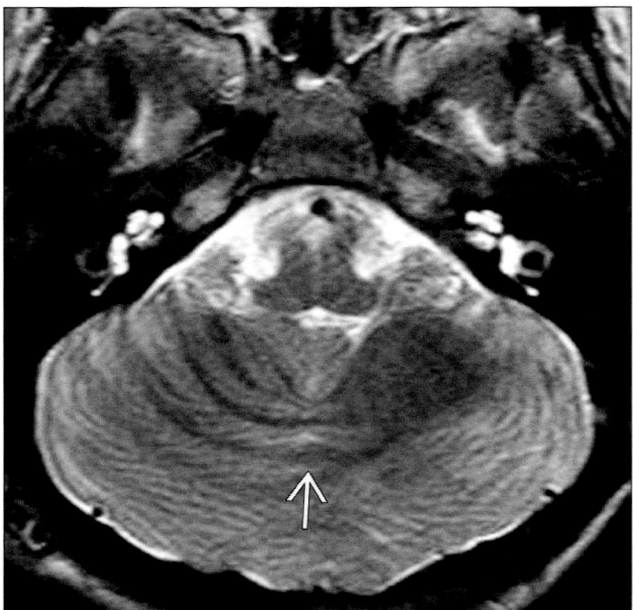

35-13. Axial T2WI in a patient with rhombencephalosynapsis shows absent vermis with continuity of both cerebellar hemispheres across the midline ➡. (Courtesy M. Warmuth-Metz, MD.)

35-14. Axial T2WI shows classic "molar tooth" anomaly with elongated upper fourth ventricle ➡, thickened superior cerebellar peduncles ➡, "split" vermis ➡.

Selected References

Cerebral Hemisphere Formation

Neuronal Proliferation

- Barkovich AJ et al: Congenital malformations of the brain and skull. In Pediatric Neuroradiology. 5th ed. Philadelphia: Lippincott Williams & Wilkins. 367-75, 2012

Neuronal Migration

- Aronica E et al: Malformations of cortical development. Brain Pathol. 22(3):380-401, 2012
- Barkovich AJ et al: A developmental and genetic classification for malformations of cortical development: update 2012. Brain. 135(Pt 5):1348-69, 2012
- Glenn OA et al: Malformations of cortical development: diagnostic accuracy of fetal MR imaging. Radiology. 263(3):843-55, 2012
- Swartling FJ et al: Distinct neural stem cell populations give rise to disparate brain tumors in response to N-MYC. Cancer Cell. 21(5):601-13, 2012

Midbrain and Hindbrain Development

Midbrain-Hindbrain Anomalies

- Barkovich AJ et al: A developmental and genetic classification for midbrain-hindbrain malformations. Brain. 132(Pt 12):3199-230, 2009

Imaging Approach to Brain Malformations

Image Analysis

- Vedolin L et al: Inherited cerebellar ataxia in childhood: a pattern- recognition approach using brain MRI. AJNR Am J Neuroradiol. Epub ahead of print, 2012
- Barkovich AJ: Congenital malformations overview. In Osborn AG et al: Diagnostic Imaging: Brain. 2nd ed. Salt Lake City: Amirsys Publishing. I.1.2-5, 2010

36

Posterior Fossa Malformations

The cerebellum is one of the earliest cerebral structures to develop. Its development is also unusually protracted as cellular proliferation, migration, and maturation extend into the first few postnatal months. It is therefore particularly vulnerable to development mishaps.

Neural structures in the posterior fossa are derived from the embryonic hindbrain (rhombencephalon) whereas the mesencephalon gives rise to midbrain structures. Mesodermal elements give rise to the meninges and bone that surround and protect the neural structures. Developmental errors in either give rise to the spectrum of midbrain and hindbrain malformations that we will discuss in this chapter. A summary of the imaging findings of these malformations is presented at the end of this chapter **(Table 36-1)**.

We begin our discussion of posterior fossa malformations with the anomalies known as Chiari malformations. Moving to the hindbrain, we consider the Dandy-Walker spectrum and a group of miscellaneous malformations.

We review the normal posterior fossa anatomy as the foundation for understanding these lesions. Some structures (e.g., the fourth ventricle, arteries, dural venous sinuses, cranial nerves) have been discussed in detail in previous chapters. Here, we summarize the major anatomic features specifically as they relate to the posterior fossa itself.

Posterior Fossa Anatomy

Gross Anatomy

The posterior fossa (PF) is the largest and deepest of all the cranial fossae. It is a bowl-shaped, relatively protected space that lies below the tentorium. The PF contains the *hindbrain* with the brainstem (pons, medulla) anteriorly, the vermis, and the cerebellar hemispheres posterolaterally.

The *midbrain* lies within the tentorial incisura. The midbrain represents the transition between the cerebral hemispheres above and the pons and cerebellar hemispheres below the tentorium.

PF CSF-containing spaces include part of the cerebral aqueduct, the fourth ventricle, and CSF cisterns that surround the brainstem and cerebellum.

Bone and Dura

The dorsum sellae of the sphenoid body and **clivus** of the basioccipital bone form the anterior wall of the PF. Laterally, the PF is bordered by the petrous temporal bone. The occipital squamae form most of its concave floor, and the tent-shaped tentorium cerebelli covers the PF superiorly. The PF communicates superiorly with the supratentorial compartment through the U-shaped **tentorial incisura** and inferiorly with the cervical subarachnoid space through the ovoid **foramen magnum**.

A layer of dura with a loosely adherent arachnoid membrane lines the bony part of the PF. The cranial dura has two layers, an inner (meningeal) and an outer (endosteal) layer, that are fused together except where they separate to enclose the dural venous sinuses.

The meningeal layer of the dura covers the PF with two prominent crescentic infoldings, the leaves of the **tentorium cerebelli**, that separate the infra- from the supraten-

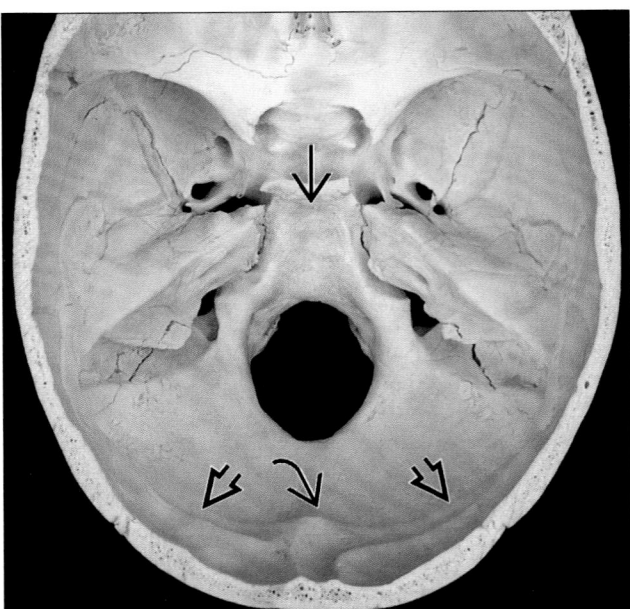

36-1. Bony posterior fossa (PF) as seen from above. Pons nestles in the gently curved clivus ➔. Occipital squamae form most of the PF floor. Grooves for the torcular ➔, transverse sinuses ➤ are clearly seen. (Courtesy M. Nielsen, MS.)

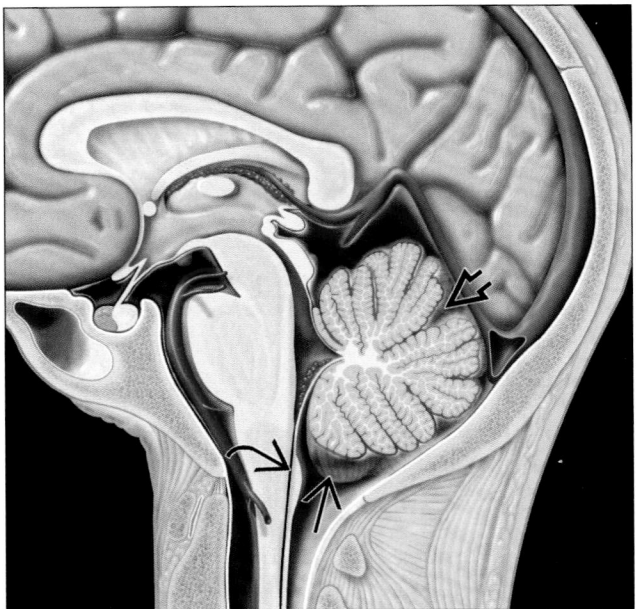

36-2. Sagittal graphic of normal PF. Note rounded bottom of tonsil ➔. Nucleus gracilis ➔, junction between fourth ventricle obex and central canal lie above the foramen magnum. The primary fissure of the vermis ➤ lies along the tentorial surface.

torial compartments. A large U-shaped central opening, the **tentorial incisura**, contains the midbrain. Variable amounts of the upper cerebellar hemispheres and vermis project into the tentorial hiatus behind the midbrain.

The convex outer margins of the dura split posteriorly along the occipital squamae to contain the sinus confluence (torcular herophili) and transverse sinuses, attaching laterally to the temporal bones and posteriorly to the occipital bone. The **falx cerebelli** consists of one or more small crescentic folds of dura that project into the cisterna magna and attach superiorly to the undersurface of the tentorium.

The dura divides into two distinct layers as it passes inferiorly through the foramen magnum into the upper cervical canal. The endosteal layer becomes the periosteum of the vertebral canal, and the meningeal layer becomes the dura of the thecal sac. In the spine, the two layers are separated by fat, the epidural venous plexus, and loose connective tissue.

Brainstem

The brainstem has three anatomic divisions: The midbrain, pons, and medulla. The **midbrain** (mesencephalon) lies partly above and partly below the tentorium. It courses through the tentorial incisura, connecting the pons and cerebellum with the basal forebrain structures and cerebral hemispheres.

The bulb-shaped **pons** nestles into the gentle curve of the clivus (36-1). Its ventral aspect contains both transverse pontine fibers and the large descending white mat-

ter (WM) tracts that are continuous with the cerebral peduncles superiorly and the medullary pyramids inferiorly. Its dorsal part—the tegmentum—is common to all three brainstem structures (midbrain, pons, medulla) and contains the reticular formation and multiple cranial nerve nuclei.

The **medulla** is the most caudal brainstem segment and represents the transition from the brain to the spinal cord. Its ventral (anterior) segment contains the olives and pyramidal tracts. An important imaging landmark is the prominent "bump" along the dorsal medulla created by the nucleus gracilis. This demarcates the junction between the fourth ventricle (obex) and central canal of the spinal cord. The nucleus gracilis normally lies above the foramen magnum.

Cerebellum

The cerebellum is a bilobed structure located posterior to the brainstem and fourth ventricle. It consists of two hemispheres and the midline vermis.

Each cerebellar hemisphere has three surfaces: Superior (tentorial), inferior (suboccipital), and anterior (petrosal). The superior surface abuts the undersurface of the tentorium. The inferior surface is mostly bordered by the occipital squamae, and the anterior surface lies along the posterior wall of the petrous temporal bone.

Fissures divide the cerebellum into lobes and lobules. The most prominent is the large **horizontal fissure**. This deep cleft wraps around the cerebellum and separates its superior from the inferior surfaces. The obliquely ori-

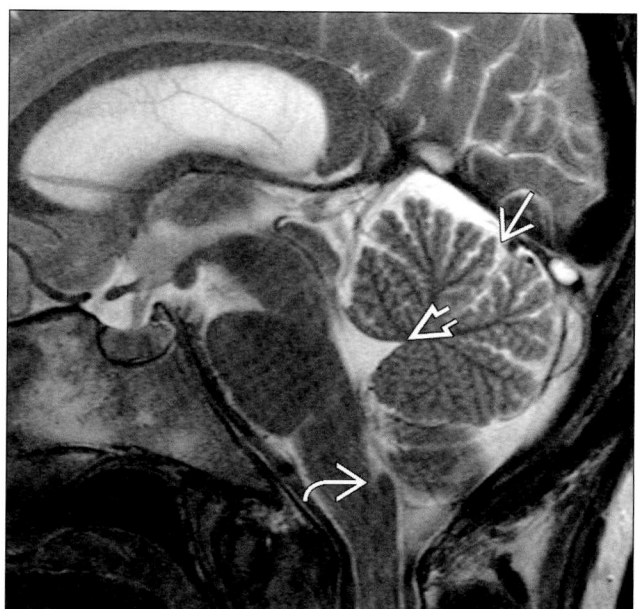 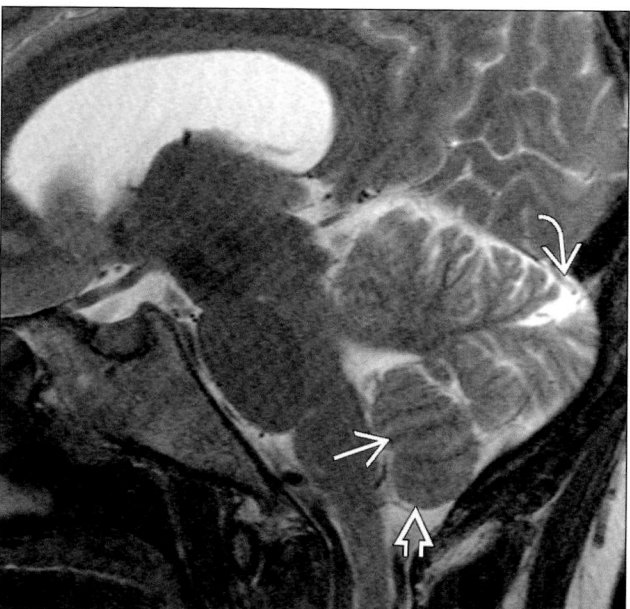

36-3. Sagittal T2WI shows normal PF imaging landmarks: Nucleus gracilis with junction of the fourth ventricle and central canal of the spinal cord ➡, fastigium of the fourth ventricle ➡, and primary fissure of the vermis ➡.

36-4. Slightly more lateral scan shows the horizontally oriented folia ➡, rounded bottom of the tonsil ➡, the horizontal fissure ➡.

ented **primary fissure** divides the cerebellum into anterior and posterior lobes. Smaller fissures subdivide the lobes into lobules.

Prominent superficial landmarks of the cerebellar hemispheres include the cerebellar **tonsils**, which extend inferomedially from the biventral lobules (36-2). A small nubbin of tissue, the **flocculus**, lies below each middle cerebellar peduncle and projects anteriorly into the cerebellopontine angle cistern.

Three paired peduncles attach the cerebellar hemispheres to the brainstem. The **superior cerebellar peduncles** (brachium conjunctivum) connect the cerebellum to the cerebral hemispheres via the midbrain. The superior cerebellar peduncles contain efferents to the red nucleus and thalamus.

The **middle cerebellar peduncles** (brachium pontis) connect the cerebellum to the pons and represent the continuation of the corticopontine tracts. The **inferior cerebellar peduncles** (also known as the restiform bodies) connect the cerebellum to the medulla and contain spinocerebellar tracts and tracts to the vestibular nuclei.

The **vermis** lies between both cerebellar hemispheres, behind the fourth ventricle. Its lobules are (moving clockwise from the fourth ventricle roof) the lingula, central lobule, culmen, declive, folium, tuber, pyramid, uvula, and nodulus. The prominent **primary fissure** continues across the vermis from the cerebellar hemispheres and separates the culmen from the declive. With the exception of the lingula, each vermian lobule is also in direct con-

tiguity with an adjoining lobule of the cerebellar hemisphere.

The cerebellar cortex is a continuous sheet of tissue that is folded in accordion-like fashion to form a series of prominent ridges. The cortex has three main layers. The **molecular layer** is the most superficial and is a relatively neuron-sparse layer. The **Purkinje cell layer** primarily contains Purkinje cells, which are arranged in a single row between the more superficial molecular layer and the deeper granular layer. The **granular layer** is the most complex and most cellular, containing the bodies and axons of granular neurons.

Fourth Ventricle and Cisterns

Anatomy of the fourth ventricle is delineated in more detail in Chapter 34.

The **fourth ventricle** is a complex diamond-shaped space that runs along the dorsal pons and upper medulla. Important anatomic landmarks are the dorsally pointed **fastigium**, the paired **lateral recesses** that empty into the cerebellopontine angle cisterns via the **foramina of Luschka**, and the midline **foramen of Magendie** (the outlet from the fourth ventricle into the cisterna magna).

The **posterior superior recesses** are thin, blind-ending, ear-like outpouchings that curve over the tops of the cerebellar tonsils. The **obex** is the inferior extension of the fourth ventricle and communicates directly with the central canal of the cervical spinal cord.

The major PF cisterns are the prepontine cistern, the cerebellopontine angle cistern, and the variably sized cisterna magna. Part of the cisterna magna (the **vallecula**) extends superiorly between the two cerebellar tonsils and is connected to the fourth ventricle via the foramen of Magendie.

Arteries, Veins, and Dural Sinuses

The arteries of the PF are detailed in Chapter 8; the veins and dural venous sinuses are discussed in Chapter 9.

Cranial Nerves

The cranial nerves—together with the cisterns through which they course and the bony foramina through which they enter or leave the cranial cavity—are discussed in detail in Chapter 23.

Imaging Anatomy

Sagittal Plane

Midline images show the smooth floor of the fourth ventricle extending from the cerebral aqueduct above to the obex below. The junction of the obex and central canal is marked by a dorsal bump, the nucleus gracilis (36-3). The

nucleus gracilis normally lies above a line drawn between the tip of the clivus anteriorly and the rim of the foramen magnum posteriorly ("basion-opisthion line").

The sharply pointed fastigium forms a triangle of CSF whose apex points toward the vermis. The primary fissure of the vermis is a well-demarcated cleft that faces the tentorium and divides the culmen from the declive.

Just slightly lateral to the midline, the cerebellar tonsils can be identified as ovoid structures lying between the vermis and inferior fourth ventricle. Normal tonsils display horizontally oriented folia and a gently rounded bottom (36-4). More lateral sections through the hemispheres show the dentate nuclei, the brachium pontis, and the primary fissure of the cerebellum.

Axial Plane

Images through the upper posterior fossa (PF) show the vermis and superior surfaces of the cerebellar hemispheres lying behind the pons and midbrain, just inside the tentorial incisura. Slightly farther down, the superior cerebellar peduncles are seen as thin white matter bands lying along either side of the upper fourth ventricle (36-5).

36-5. Axial T2WI shows normal superior cerebellar peduncles ➡, vermis ➡, horizontal fissures ➡ of the cerebellum. 36-6. Axial scan through the body of the fourth ventricle shows CSF-filled posterior superior recesses ➡ capping the tops of the cerebellar tonsils ➡. Dentate nuclei ➡ are mineralized, hypointense.

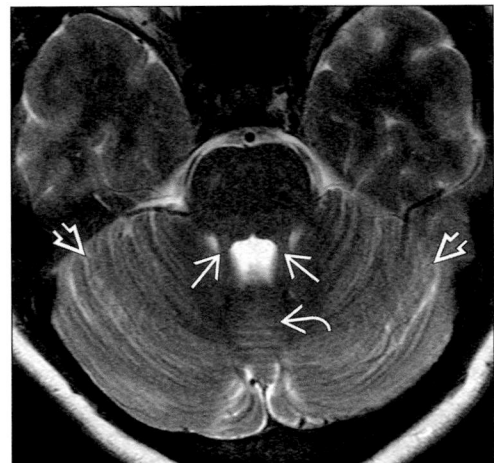
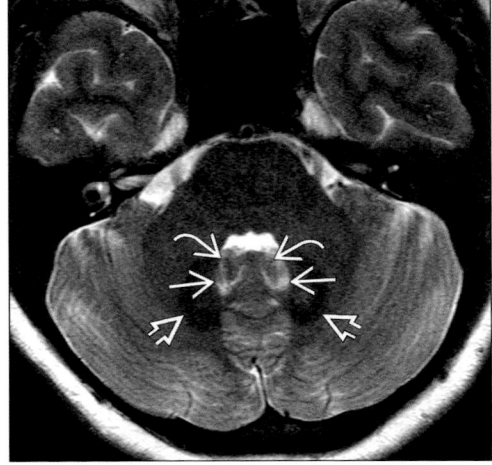

36-7. More inferior scan through the bottom of the fourth ventricle shows the midline foramen of Magendie ➡, lateral recesses ➡, tonsils ➡, floccular lobes of the cerebellum ➡ projecting into cerebellopontine angle cisterns. 36-8. T2WI through the foramen magnum shows the medulla ➡, cerebellar tonsils ➡, vallecula lying between the tonsils at the bottom of the cisterna magna ➡.

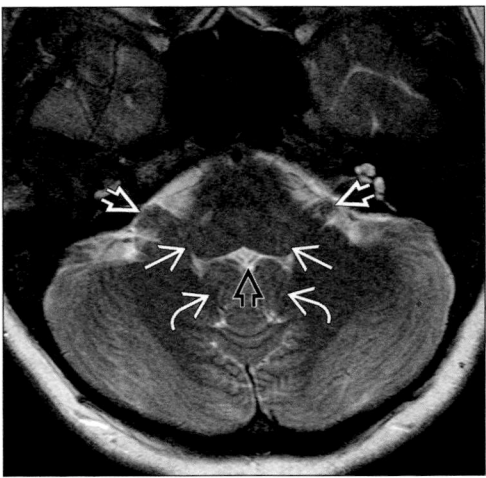
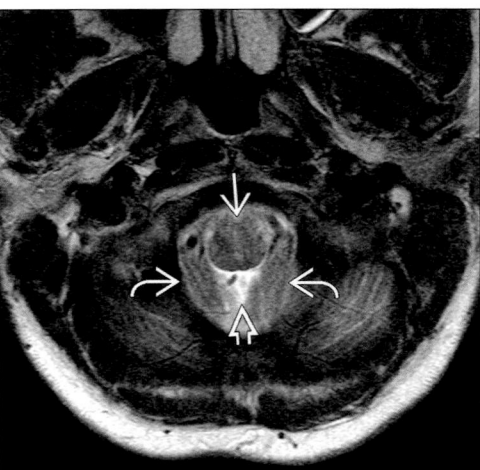

At the level of the middle cerebellar peduncles, the body of the fourth ventricle resembles a kidney bean on its side. The two bumps along its anterior aspect are the facial colliculi, and the midline posterior bump is the nodulus of the vermis. Sometimes, the thin posterior superior recesses can be seen capping the tops of the cerebellar tonsils (36-6). Anterolaterally, a flocculus projects from each hemisphere into the cerebellopontine angle cistern.

Moving inferiorly, the lateral recesses of the fourth ventricle pass anterolaterally under the middle cerebellar peduncles (36-7). Tufts of choroid plexus pass through the lateral recesses and the foramina of Luschka into the inferior cerebellopontine angle cisterns just medial to the flocculi.

The cerebellar tonsils can be identified just above or at the foramen magnum. The vallecula—part of the cisterna magna that receives the midline foramen of Magendie—is the CSF space that lies between the tonsils (36-8). The medulla lies just in front of (and medial to) the cerebellar tonsils. The anterior medulla is marked by paired "bumps" of tissue: The pyramids and the olives.

Coronal Plane

Images through the anterior "belly" of the pons show the large biventral lobules of the inferior cerebellar hemispheres with the cerebellar tonsils projecting inferomedially (36-9), (36-10). The flocculi lie just in front of the horizontal fissure (36-9).

Moving posteriorly, the rhomboid or diamond shape of the fourth ventricle can be appreciated. Thin caps of CSF, the posterior superior recesses, cover the tops of the cerebellar tonsils (36-11). Inferiorly, the fourth ventricle opens into the cisterna magna via the foramen of Magendie. The large middle cerebellar peduncles are seen along the sides of the fourth ventricle. More posteriorly, the vermis can be seen lying between the two hemispheres (36-12).

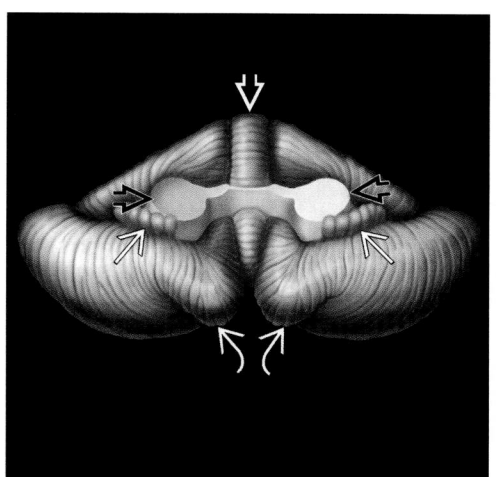

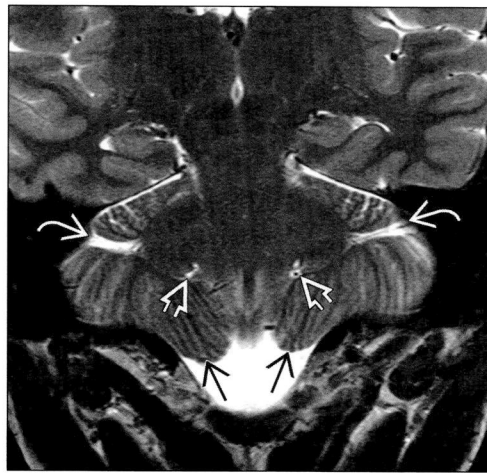

36-9. Coronal graphic shows brachium pontis (middle cerebellar peduncles) ⇗, vermis ⇗, flocculi ⇗, tonsils ⇗ projecting inferiorly from the biventral lobules. 36-10. Coronal T2WI shows tonsils ⇗, foramina of Luschka ⇗, horizontal fissures ⇗.

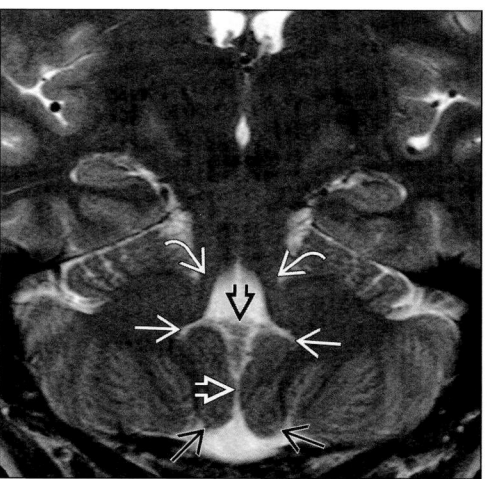

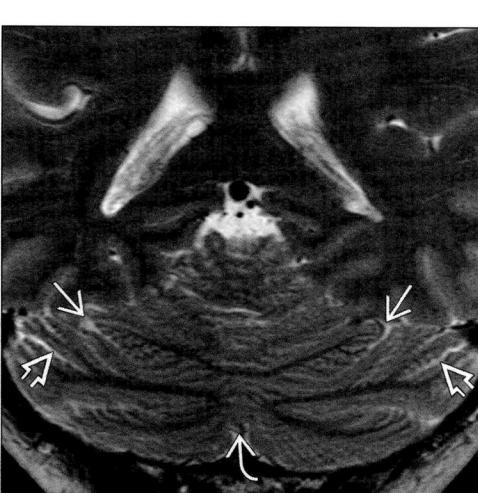

36-11. More posterior coronal image shows foramen of Magendie ⇗, vermis ⇗, superior cerebellar peduncles ⇗, posterior superior recesses ⇗ capping tonsils ⇗. 36-12. More posterior T2WI shows the primary fissures ⇗, horizontal fissures ⇗, midline vermis ⇗.

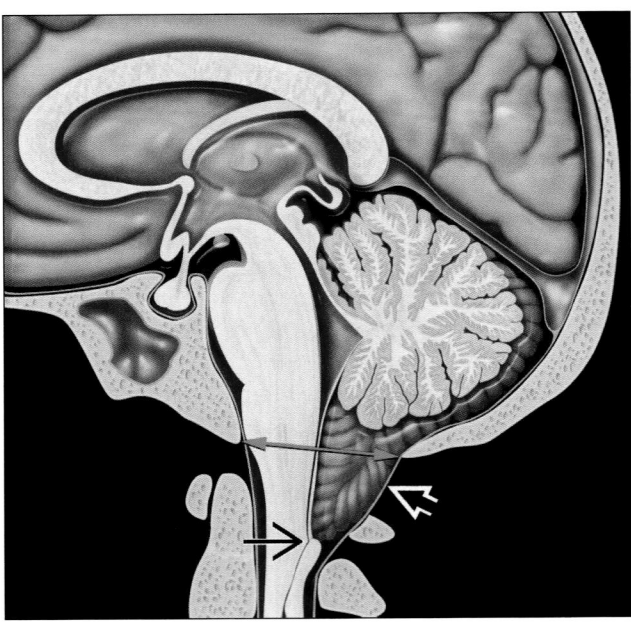

36-13. *Chiari 1 malformation with the basion-opisthion line shown in green. Note the low-lying, pointed tonsil with vertically oriented folia* ⇉*. The nucleus gracilis* ⇒ *is inferiorly displaced.*

36-14. *Semi-axial view of autopsy case shows Chiari 1 malformation. Note inferiorly displaced tonsils with vertically oriented folia* ⇉*. (Courtesy E. T. Hedley-Whyte, MD.)*

Chiari Malformations

Introduction to Chiari Malformations

Chiari malformations were first described in the late nineteenth century by the Austrian pathologist Hans Chiari. He described what seemed to be a related group of hindbrain malformations associated with hydrocephalus and divided them into three types: Chiari 1-3.

Chiari 1 and 2 are pathogenetically distinct disorders. **Chiari 1** involves inferior dislocation of the cerebellar tonsils **(36-13)**; **Chiari 2** is always associated with myelodysplasia and involves herniation of the medulla and vermis. **Chiari 3** is classically characterized as herniation of posterior fossa contents through a low occipitocervical bony defect.

"Chiari 4 malformation" was originally used to designate what is now recognized as primary cerebellar agenesis, not a hindbrain herniation. The term has been abandoned.

Some authors have expanded the Chiari spectrum to include variants such as **Chiari 0** (syrinx without frank tonsillar herniation), **Chiari 1.5** (caudal protrusion of brainstem in addition to the tonsils), and **Chiari 5** (Chiari 2 plus occipital or high cervical myelomeningocele).

These variants are controversial and are briefly discussed at the end of this section.

Chiari 1

Overview

Type 1 Chiari malformation (CM1) is defined as caudal cerebellar tonsillar ectopia. However, the precise distance of the tonsils below the foramen magnum required to diagnose CM1 is not agreed upon. Some investigators consider tonsillar ectopia measuring five millimeters or more as sufficient to establish the diagnosis of CM1. However, other investigators insist additional abnormalities such as tonsillar deformity, obliterated retrotonsillar CSF spaces, or altered CSF flow dynamics should also be present.

Abnormalities of the cervical spinal cord are common in CM1. A complex CSF-filled cavity with multiple septations of spongy glial tissue is typical. *Glia*-lined cord cavitations are generally referred to as **syringomyelia**. The term **hydromyelia** refers to an *ependyma*-lined expansion of the central canal. In CM1, extensive areas of ependymal denuding and astrocytic scarring make it difficult to distinguish between hydro- and syringomyelia even on histologic examination. Therefore, these nonneoplastic, septated, paracentral, fluid-containing cavitations are often referred to as **hydrosyringomyelia** or simply syrinx.

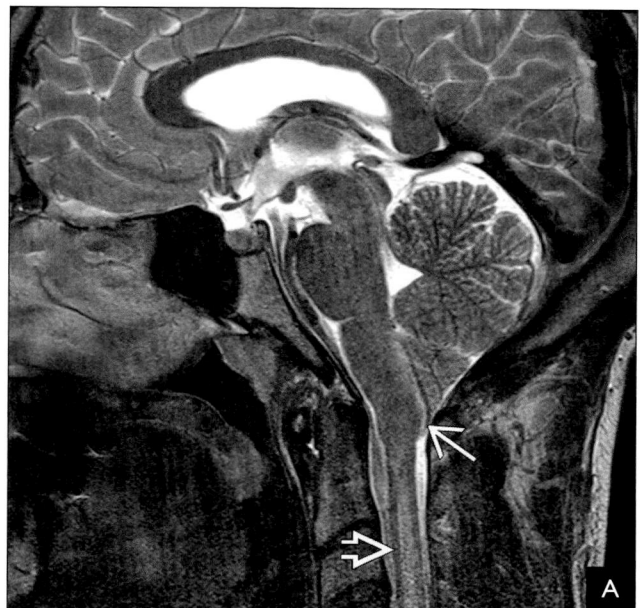

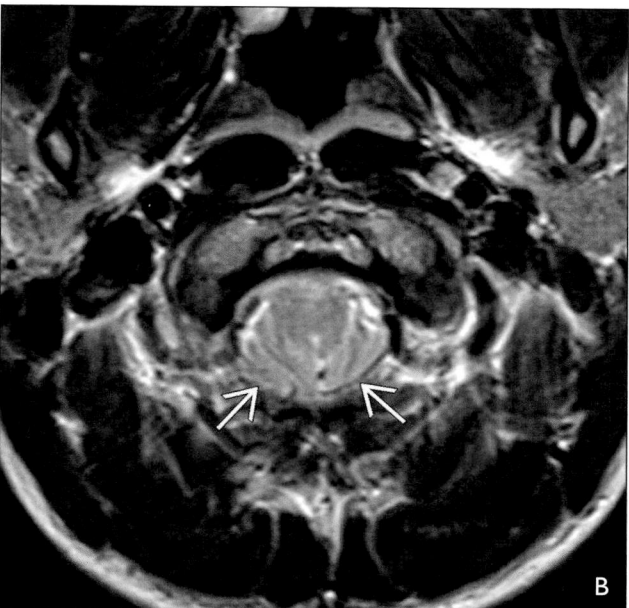

36-15A. Sagittal T2WI in a 23-year-old man with classic Chiari 1 malformation shows a low-lying, pointed tonsil ➡, *normal-sized posterior fossa. Cord T2 hyperintensity* ➡ *represents "pre-syrinx" state.*

36-15B. Axial T2WI in the same patient shows "crowded" foramen magnum with obliterated retrocerebellar CSF spaces ➡.

Etiology

GENERAL CONCEPTS. The pathogenesis of CM1 is incompletely understood and remains controversial. Genetic, nongenetic, and epigenetic factors have all been proposed.

Primary paraxial mesodermal insufficiency with under-developed occipital somites has also been invoked to explain the development of CM1. Other theories suggest that disorders of neural crest-derived elements could lead to hyper- or hypoossification of the basi-chondro-cranium, resulting in morphometric changes in the posterior fossa.

A combination of altered bony anatomy and abnormal CSF hydrodynamics is the most widely accepted concept.

ABNORMAL POSTERIOR FOSSA. Many—but by no means all—patients with CM1 demonstrate abnormal geometry of the bony posterior fossa (*"normal-sized hindbrain housed in a too-small bony envelope"*). Various combinations of congenitally reduced clival length, shortened basiocciput, and craniovertebral junction (CVJ) fusion anomalies may all result in diminished posterior cranial fossa depth and/or an abnormally small posterior fossa volume.

ALTERED CSF DYNAMICS. Syringomyelia is present in 40-80% of individuals with symptomatic CM1. Its etiology is also a controversial subject. Tonsillar impaction and posterior arachnoid adhesions cause increased resistance to CSF flow between the intracranial and spinal subarachnoid spaces. Systolic piston-like descent of the impacted tonsils may create abnormal intraspinal CSF pressure waves, which in turn could result in the development of hydrosyringomyelia in the upper cervical cord.

Altered CSF hydrodynamics with accelerated flow velocity and increased pressure gradients may also cause or contribute to the displacement of brain tissue out of the cranium and into the upper cervical canal.

GENETICS. Familial aggregation studies, twin studies, the cosegregation of CM1 with known genetic conditions such as achondroplasia and Klippel-Feil syndrome, and recent genome-wide analyses all provide strong evidence for a genetic component of CM1.

While the specific genetic causes of CM1 are not yet fully elucidated, chromosomes 9q 21 and 15q21 (also the site of the fibrillin-1 gene, the major cause of Marfan syndrome) have been implicated in some studies.

Pathology

Grossly, the herniated tonsils in CM1 are inferiorly displaced and grooved by impaction against the opisthion (36-14). They often appear firm and sclerotic. Arachnoid thickening and adhesions around the CVJ are common. Microscopically, degenerative changes with Purkinje and granular cell loss may be present.

Clinical Issues

EPIDEMIOLOGY AND DEMOGRAPHICS. CM1 is the most common of the Chiari malformations and can be identified in patients of all ages. Its estimated prevalence in

36-16A. *Sagittal T1WI shows "crowded" foramen magnum, tonsillar ectopia with the "pointed" appearance* ➡ *that is typical of Chiari 1. Note syrinx in the upper cervical cord* ➡. **36-16B.** *Sagittal T2WI shows "pointed" tonsil* ➡, *obliquely oriented tonsillar folia* ➡. *Multiple septations in the syrinx cavity are clearly seen* ➡. *The inferior fourth ventricle is somewhat elongated, and the nucleus gracilis* ➡ *is slightly low-lying.*

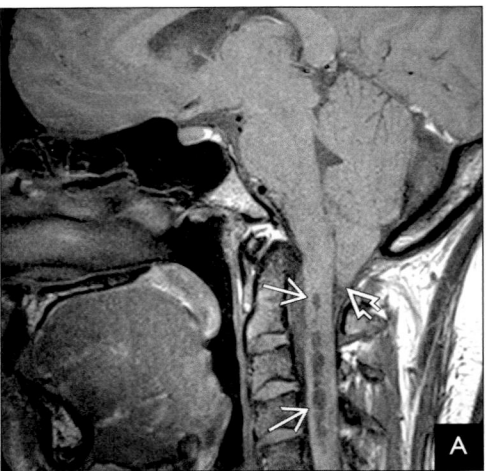

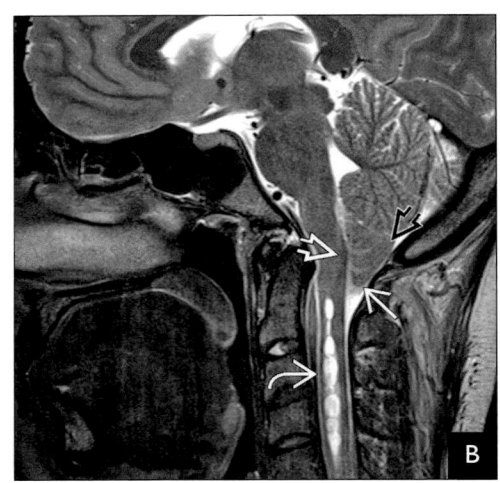

36-16C. *Sagittal T1 C+ FS shows that the syrinx* ➡ *does not enhance.* **36-16D.** *Axial T2WI shows a well-demarcated CSF cavity* ➡ *in the middle of the central cervical spinal cord. It is not possible by imaging to distinguish between ependyma-lined dilatation of the central canal (hydromyelia) and glia-lined paracentral cord cavitations (syringomyelia), so the term hydrosyringomyelia is generally used to designate this CM1-associated finding.*

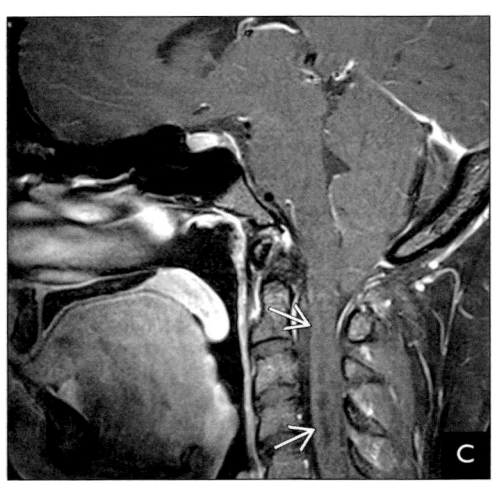

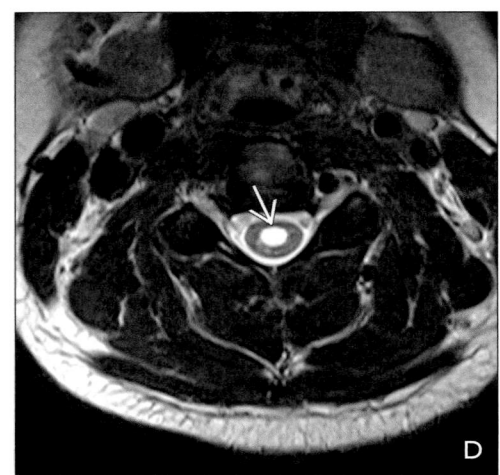

36-16E. *T2WI in the same patient shows tonsils* ➡, *a compressed and slightly deformed medulla* ➡, *giving the appearance of the "crowded" foramen magnum typical of CM1.* **36-16F.** *Sagittal phase-contrast CSF flow study in systole (left), diastole (right) shows normal CSF flow* ➡ *in front of the cervicomedullary junction, no posterior flow in the foramen magnum* ➡. *Tonsillar "crowding," adhesions prevent normal CSF circulation.*

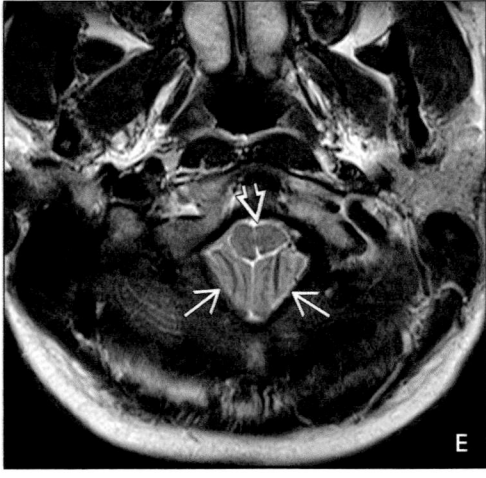

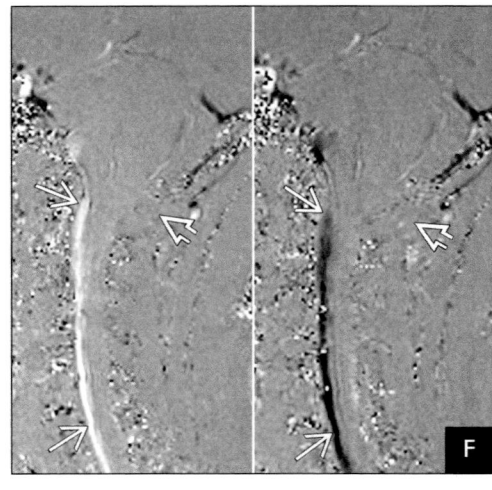

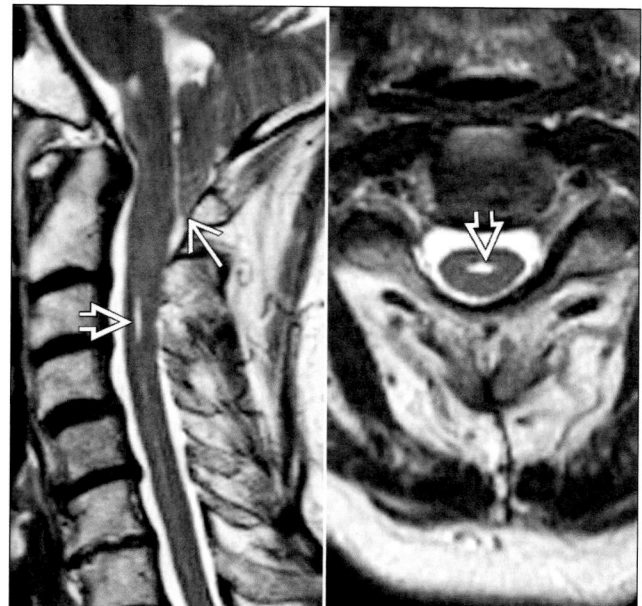

36-17. Sagittal (left) and axial (right) T2-weighted images show tonsillar ectopia ⮕ and syrinx ⮘ in a patient with CM1.

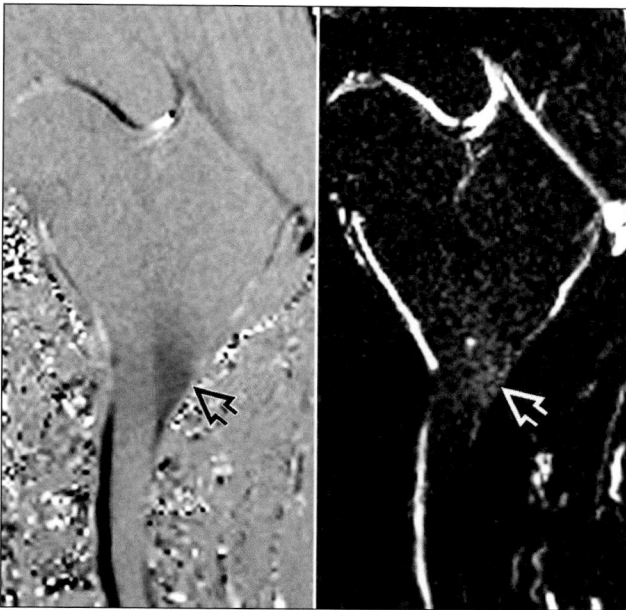

36-18. 2D PC cine CSF flow study shows change in signal from dark ⮘ to bright ⮘ behind the cervical spinal cord, consistent with "pistoning" tonsillar pulsations.

the general population is 0.6-1%, but recent studies have found a Chiari 1 malformation in 3.6% of children undergoing routine brain or cervical spine MR. There is no gender predilection.

A CM1-associated syrinx is rare in infants under one year, but the incidence rises with age. This age-related increase is most pronounced in the first five years of life.

PRESENTATION. Between one-third and one-half of all patients with imaging findings consistent with CM1 are asymptomatic at the time of diagnosis.

Presentation of symptomatic CM1 differs with age. Children who are two years and younger most commonly present with oropharyngeal dysfunction (nearly 80%). Those between three and five years present with headache (57%) or symptoms related to syringomyelia (86%) and scoliosis (38%). Uncommon presentations include hypersomnolence and sleep apnea. Valsalva-induced suboccipital headache (i.e., with coughing or sneezing), neck pain, and syncope are common in adults.

NATURAL HISTORY. The natural history of CM1 varies. Many patients remain asymptomatic. Some investigators believe that the degree of tonsillar ectopia in CM1 gradually increases with time and is associated with a greater likelihood of becoming symptomatic.

Outcomes of CM1-associated syringomyelia are likewise uncertain. Longitudinal studies show that a syrinx remains stable or decreases in size in nearly 90% of pediatric patients who have minimal neurological symptoms.

Others develop progressive scoliosis, spinal cord symptoms, or bulbar deficits. Such deficits are sometimes precipitated or exacerbated by relatively minor head or neck injury.

TREATMENT OPTIONS. Like almost everything else about CM1, management is controversial. Asymptomatic tonsillar ectopia in the absence of an associated syrinx or scoliosis is usually not treated. Periodic surveillance of patients with documented hydrosyringomyelia is generally recommended, as 12% of syringes show increase in size and may require craniocervical decompression if symptoms worsen.

Treatment of symptomatic CM1 attempts to restore normal CSF fluid dynamics at the foramen magnum (FM). A suboccipital/posterior C1 decompression with or without partial tonsillar resection is the most common procedure.

Imaging

GENERAL FEATURES. The basion-opisthion line (BOL) is a line drawn from the tip of the clivus to the posterior rim of the FM (36-13). Measuring the distance from this line to the inferior margin of the cerebellar tonsils on sagittal MR imaging defines tonsillar position.

Tonsillar descent five millimeters or more below the BOL—often considered diagnostic of Chiari 1—is by itself a poor criterion for definitive diagnosis. Tonsils six millimeters below the FM are common during the first decade of life. Almost 15% of normal patients have tonsils that lie one to four millimeters below the FM, and

0.5-1% have tonsils that project five millimeters into the upper cervical canal.

Great caution should be exercised in establishing a diagnosis of CM1, especially on the basis of borderline tonsillar ectopia alone. Unless (1) the tonsils appear compressed and pointed (peg-like) instead of gently rounded **(36-15A)**, (2) the tonsillar folia are angled obliquely or inferiorly (instead of horizontally), and (3) the retrocerebellar CSF spaces at the FM/C1 level are effaced **(36-15B)**, the diagnosis may not be warranted. Low-lying tonsils that retain their rounded shapes and are surrounded by normal-appearing CSF spaces are usually asymptomatic and of no diagnostic significance.

CT FINDINGS. NECT scans may reveal a "crowded" FM and effaced retrotonsillar CSF space. Bone CT often demonstrates a combination of undersized, shallow posterior cranial fossa, short clivus, and CVJ assimilation anomalies. Look carefully for calvarial anomalies as nearly 10% of patients with nonsyndromic single suture craniosynostosis have CM1.

MR FINDINGS. Sagittal T1 and T2 scans show "pointed" tonsils with more vertically oriented folia, obliterated retrocerebellar and premedullary subarachnoid spaces, and a "crowded" FM. The posterior fossa may appear normal or somewhat small with a short clivus and steeply angled straight sinus. In contrast to Chiari 2 (see below), the fourth ventricle usually displays a normal fastigium (dorsal point). In some cases, the inferior fourth ventricle is mildly elongated, and the nucleus gracilis—which demarcates the end of the obex and beginning of the central canal—can appear slightly low-lying **(36-16)**.

The proximal cervical spinal cord should be carefully examined for the presence of hydrosyringomyelia **(36-17)**. T2/FLAIR parenchymal hyperintensity without frank cyst formation may indicate a "pre-syrinx" state.

The diameter of the central canal relative to the cord normally decreases significantly during the first few years of life. A CSF-like central cord cavity three millimeters or larger on axial scans is abnormal in older children and adults and should be considered a syrinx. Mean syrinx size in a large series of CM1 patients was nearly eight millimeters in width and averaged nine vertebral levels in length.

Sagittal phase-contrast CSF flow studies show diminished or absent alternating bright (systolic) and dark (diastolic) signals behind the cervicomedullary junction. Any change in signal intensity of the cerebellar tonsils in cine mode suggests tonsillar pulsations **(36-18)**. Both altered CSF flow at the FM and abnormal tonsillar pulsations are usually associated with peg-like tonsillar morphology.

ASSOCIATED ABNORMALITIES. Complete imaging evaluation in CM1 includes the brain, CVJ, and entire spine. Mild to moderate hydrocephalus is present in 10% of patients with CM1. Callosal dysgenesis is seen in 3% and absent septi pellucidi in 2.4% of cases. Other supratentorial anomalies are uncommon.

Hydrosyringomyelia is present in 10-20% of asymptomatic patients and 40-80% of symptomatic CM1 patients. Associated skeletal anomalies include a retroverted dens, Klippel-Feil anomaly, basilar invagination, platybasia, CVJ fusion anomalies, kyphosis, and/or scoliosis.

Differential Diagnosis

Congenital tonsillar descent (CM1) must be distinguished from **normal variants** (mild uncomplicated tonsillar ectopia). The most important pathological differential diagnosis is *acquired* tonsillar herniation caused by increased intracranial pressure **or** intracranial hypotension.

Increased intracranial pressure due to supratentorial mass effect with transmission of the pressure cone through the tentorial incisura can be easily distinguished from CM1. Signs of descending transtentorial herniation are present along with downward midbrain displacement. Tonsillar herniation in such cases is a secondary effect and should *not* be termed "acquired Chiari 1."

Intracranial hypotension shows a constellation of other findings besides inferiorly displaced tonsils. "Slumping" midbrain, enlarged pituitary gland, draping of the optic chiasm and hypothalamus over the dorsum sellae, subdural hematoma, engorged venous sinuses, and dura-arachnoid thickening and enhancement are typical abnormalities. *Mistaking intracranial hypotension for CM1 can have disastrous consequences, as surgical decompression may exacerbate brainstem "slumping."*

Approximately 20% of patients with **idiopathic intracranial hypertension** ("pseudotumor cerebri") exhibit cerebellar tonsillar ectopia ≥ 5 mm. Half of these patients exhibit a peg-like tonsil configuration, and many have a low-lying obex. Looking for other signs of idiopathic intracranial hypertension (e.g., optic nerve head protrusion into the globe) is essential to avoid misdiagnosis as Chiari 1.

Other conditions that reduce posterior cranial fossa volume can also displace the tonsils below the foramen. Such causes of **cranial constriction** include craniosynostosis, achondroplasia, acromegaly, and Paget disease. Cranial "settling" from rheumatoid arthritis, osteogenesis imperfecta, hereditary connective tissue disorders, and occipitoatlantoaxial joint instability can also force the tonsils below the FM.

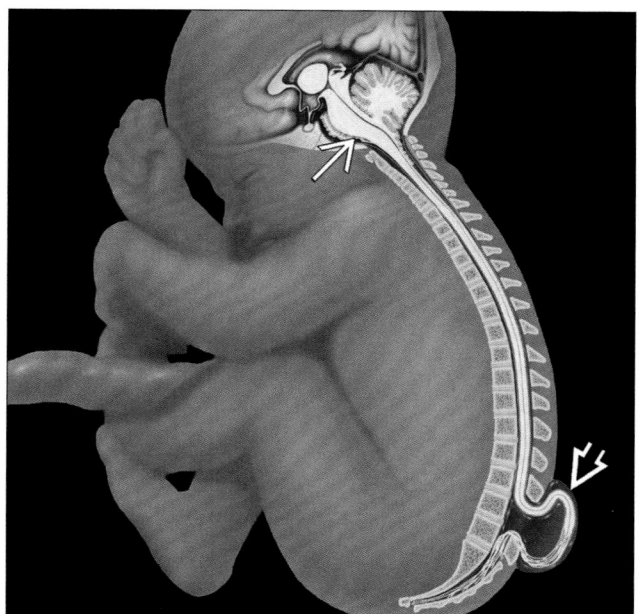

36-19. Graphic depicts a fetus with Chiari 2 malformation ➡, spinal cord tethered into a myelomeningocele ➡.

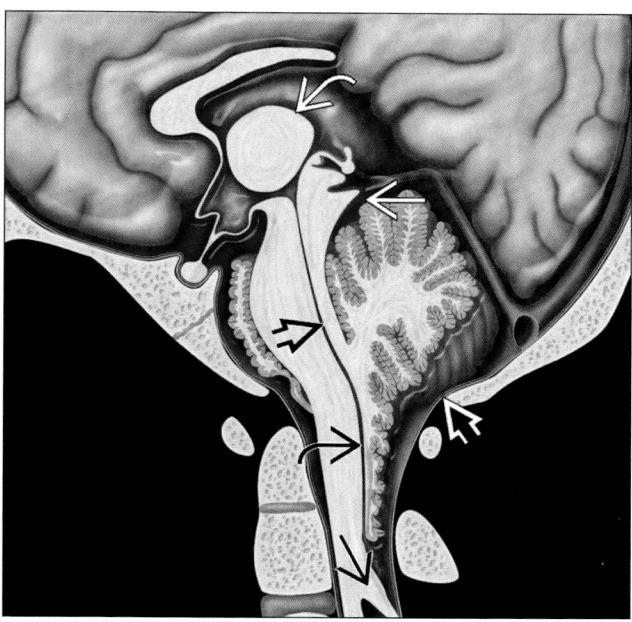

36-20. Graphic depicts CM2 with small posterior fossa ⧁, large massa intermedia ➡, "beaked" tectum ➡, callosal dysgenesis, elongated fourth ventricle ⧁ with "cascade" of inferiorly displaced nodulus ⧁ and choroid plexus, medullary spur ➡.

Chiari 2

Terminology and Definition

Chiari 2 malformation (CM2) is a complex hindbrain malformation that is almost always associated with myelodysplasia (myelomeningocele) (36-19).

Etiology

GENERAL CONCEPTS. CM2 is a disorder of neural tube closure but also involves paraxial mesodermal abnormalities of the skull and spine. A number of steps are required for proper neural tube closure and formation of the focal expansions that subsequently form the cerebral vesicles and ventricles. Skeletal elements of both the skull and vertebral column become "modeled" around the neural tube.

Only if the posterior neuropore closes will the developing ventricles expand sufficiently for a normal-sized posterior fossa to form around the hindbrain. If this does not happen, the cerebellum develops in a small posterior fossa with abnormally low tentorial attachments. The growing cerebellum is squeezed cephalad through the tentorial incisura and stretched inferiorly through the foramen magnum (FM).

GENETICS. Nearly half of all neural tube closure anomalies have mutations on the methylene-tetra-hydrofolate reductase gene (*MTHFR*). Maternal folate deficiency and teratogens such as anticonvulsants have been linked to increased risk of CM2.

Pathology

Grossly, a broad spectrum of findings can be present in CM2. Myelomeningocele and a small posterior fossa with concave clivus and petrous pyramids are virtually always present (36-20). The cerebellar vermis (typically the nodulus) is displaced inferiorly along the dorsal aspect of the cervical spinal cord. The fourth ventricle, pons, and medulla are elongated and partially dislocated into the cervical spinal canal. The lower medulla may be kinked.

Unlike Chiari 1, supratentorial abnormalities are the rule in CM2, not the exception. Hydrocephalus is present in the majority of cases, and aqueductal stenosis is common. Corpus callosum dysgenesis and gray matter anomalies such as polymicrogyria and heterotopias are frequent (36-21), (36-22), (36-23), (36-24), (36-25), (36-26).

Clinical Issues

EPIDEMIOLOGY AND DEMOGRAPHICS. The overall prevalence of CM2 is 0.44 in 1,000 live births but has been decreasing with prophylactic maternal folate therapy. A dose of four milligrams per day reduces the risk of CM2 by at least 70%.

PRESENTATION. CM2 is identified in utero with ultrasound or fetal screening for elevated α-fetoprotein. At birth, coexistent myelomeningocele and hydrocephalus are dominant clinical features in over 90% of cases. Lower cranial nerve deficits, apneic spells, and bulbar

36-21. (Left) CM2 shows medullary spur ➡, "cascade" ➱ of nodulus, choroid plexus behind medulla, elongated "soda straw" fourth ventricle ➱, "beaked" tectum ➡, large massa intermedia ➘. (Courtesy T. P. Naidich, MD.) (Right) CM2 with stenogyria ➡, heterotopic GM ➱, "pointed" lateral ventricles ➘. (Courtesy E. T. Hedley-Whyte, MD.) *36-22.* CM2 shows medullary spur ➡, "cascade" of nodulus, choroid plexus ➱, elongated "straw-like" fourth ventricle ➱. (R. Hewlett, MD.)

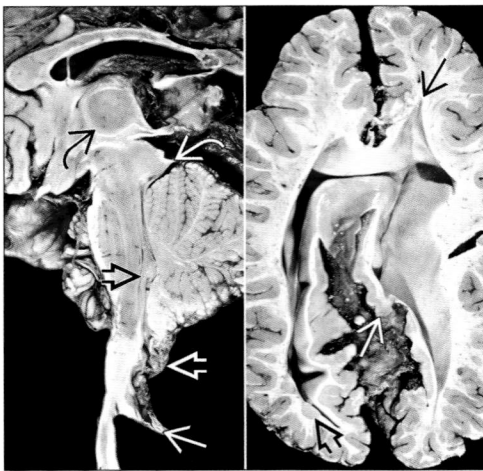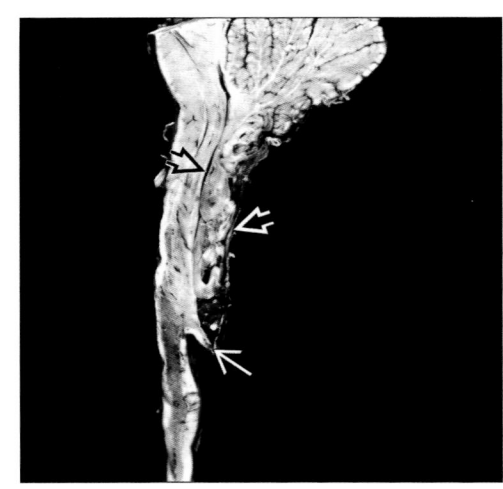

36-23. Autopsy specimen from a patient with CM2 shows a very small posterior fossa ➡, cerebellar hemispheres "creeping" anteriorly ➱ around the medulla. (Courtesy R. Hewlett, MD.) *36-24.* Autopsy specimen of CM2 shows a very small posterior fossa ➡, huge massa intermedia ➱, corpus callosum dysgenesis with radiating gyri converging on a "high-riding" third ventricle ➡ that is open dorsally to the interhemispheric fissure. (Courtesy R. Hewlett, MD.)

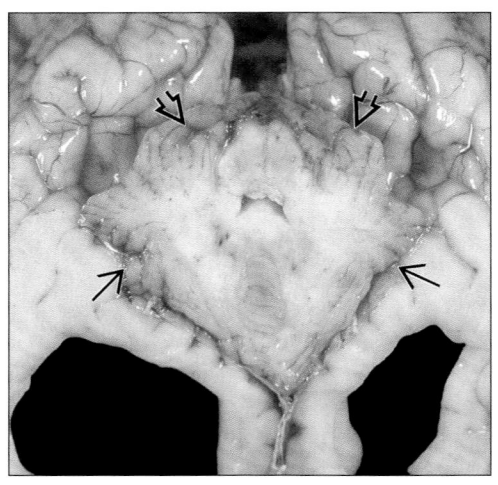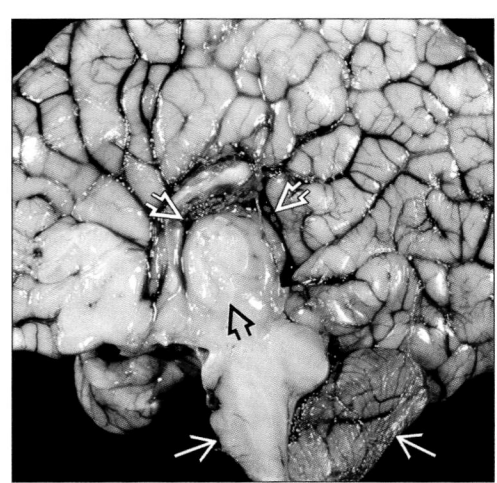

36-25. Coronal autopsy specimen of CM2 shows corpus callosum agenesis with "Viking helmet" or "moose head" appearance to third, lateral ventricles ➡. Note interdigitating gyri ➱ creating an irregular, "serrated" appearance to the interhemispheric fissure ➡. (Courtesy J. Townsend, MD.) *36-26.* Axial view of autopsied spine from a patient with CM2. Note wide dorsal dysraphism ➡, myelomeningocele ➡ with exposed neural placode ➡. (Courtesy R. Hewlett, MD.)

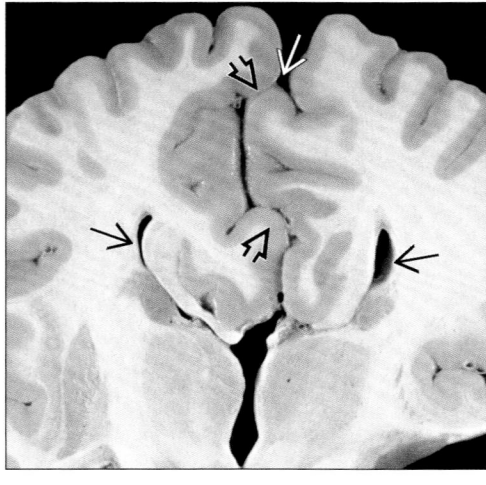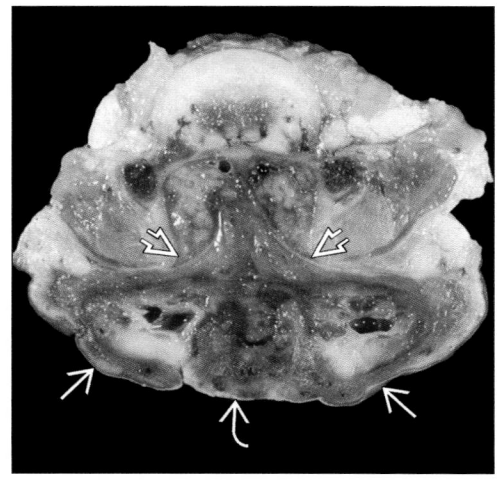

signs may be present. Lower extremity paralysis, sphincter dysfunction, and spasticity often develop later.

TREATMENT OPTIONS. Fetal repair of myelomeningocele is increasingly common and may reduce subsequent symptoms. Surgical repair within 72 hours following delivery reduces mortality and morbidity from the open dysraphism.

Imaging

CM2 affects many regions of the skull, brain, and spine, so a variety of imaging abnormalities may be seen.

SKULL AND DURA. The calvarial vault forms from membranous bone. With failure of neural tube closure and absence of fetal brain distension, normal induction of the calvarial membranous plates does not occur. Disorganized collections of collagen fibers and deficient radial growth of the developing calvaria ensue. The result is a striking anomaly called **lacunar skull** (i.e., Lückenschädel) **(36-27)**. Lacunar skull is caused by the mesenchymal abnormality and is *not* a consequence of increased intracranial pressure.

Focal calvarial thinning and a "scooped-out" appearance are typical imaging findings of lacunar skull. The calvaria appears thinned with numerous circular or oval lucent defects and shallow depressions. Changes diminish with age and are mostly resolved by six months, although some scalloping of the inner table often persists into adulthood.

A **small, shallow, bony posterior fossa** with low-lying transverse sinuses is almost always present in CM2. A **large, "gaping" foramen magnum** is common. **Concave petrous temporal bones** and a **short concave clivus** are often present **(36-28)**.

Dural abnormalities are common. A widened, open, **heart-shaped tentorial incisura** and **thinned, hypoplastic, or fenestrated falx** are frequent findings. The fenestrated falx allows gyri to cross the midline. Interdigitating gyri and the deficient falx result in the appearance of an **irregular interhemispheric fissure** on imaging studies **(36-28C)**, **(36-29C)**.

MIDBRAIN, HINDBRAIN, AND CEREBELLUM. Hindbrain and cerebellum anomalies are a constant in CM2.

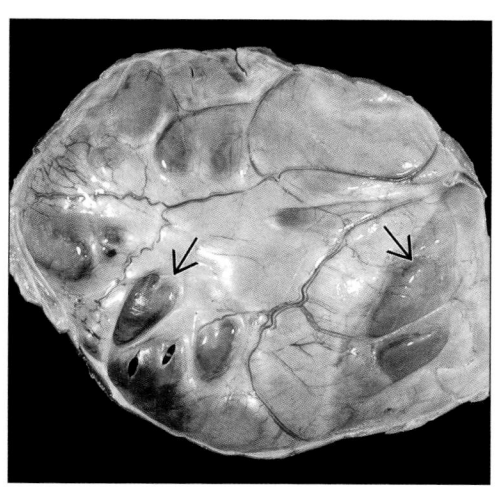

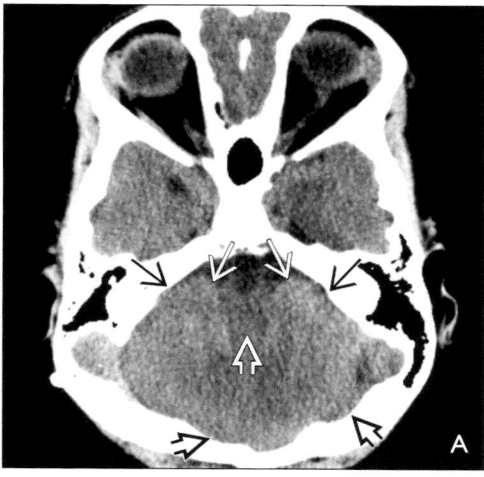

36-27. Autopsy case of lacunar (Lückenschädel) skull in CM2 shows multiple "scooped" out foci of thinned, almost translucent bone ➡. (Courtesy R. Hewlett, MD.) 36-28A. NECT scan of a patient with CM2 shows a small posterior fossa with concave petrous ridges ➡, scalloped inner table ➡, no visible fourth ventricle, and "creeping" cerebellar hemispheres ➡ almost enveloping an elongated, inferiorly stretched medulla ➡.

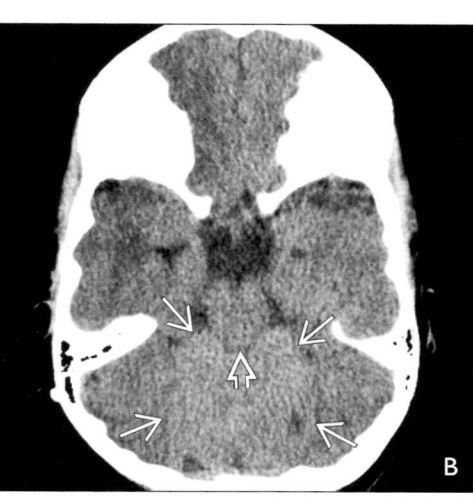

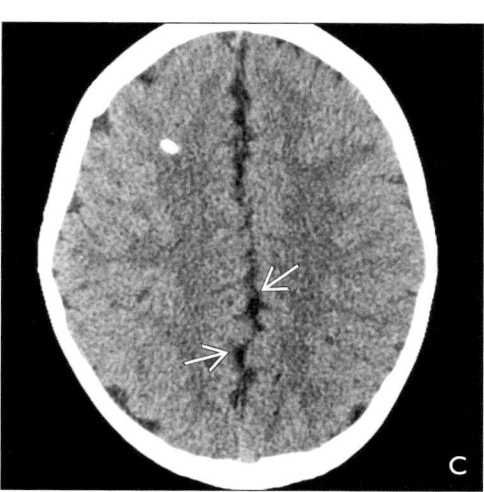

36-28B. NECT scan in the same patient shows widely gaping, heart-shaped incisura with "towering" cerebellum protruding superiorly ➡, mild "beaking" of the tectum ➡. 36-28C. More cephalad scan in the same patient shows the typical "serrated" appearance of the interhemispheric fissure ➡ due to the interdigitating gyri typically seen in CM2.

The medulla and cerebellar vermis (*not* the tonsils!) are displaced downward into the upper cervical canal for a variable distance. The **inferiorly displaced cerebellar tissue** is typically the **nodulus**, with variable contributions from the uvula and pyramid. A **cervicomedullary "kink"** with a **"medullary spur"** is common in the upper cervical canal but may lie as low as T1-4 in severe cases.

On sagittal T1 and T2 scans, the inferiorly displaced vermis, medulla, and choroid plexus form a **"cascade" of tissue** that protrudes downward through the gaping FM to lie behind the spinal cord. The superiorly herniated cerebellum may compress and deform the quadrigeminal plate, giving the appearance of a **"beaked" tectum** (36-29A), (36-29B).

In addition to the cephalocaudal displacement of posterior fossa contents, the cerebellar hemispheres often curve anteromedially around the brainstem. In severe cases, the pons and medulla appear nearly engulfed by the "creeping" cerebellum on axial imaging studies.

The cerebellar hemispheres and vermis are pushed upward through the incisura, giving the appearance of a **"towering" cerebellum** on coronal T1 and T2 scans (36-29D).

VENTRICLES. Abnormalities of the ventricles are present in over 90% of CM2 patients. The fourth ventricle is caudally displaced, typically lacks a fastigium (dorsal point), and appears thin and elongated (**"soda straw" fourth ventricle**). The third ventricle is often large and has a very **prominent massa intermedia** (36-29A).

The lateral ventricles vary in size and configuration. Hydrocephalus is almost always present at birth. The atria and occipital horns are often disproportionately enlarged (**"colpocephaly"**), suggesting the presence of callosal dysgenesis. Following shunting, the lateral ventricles frequently retain a **serrated** or **scalloped appearance**. A large CSF space between the occipital lobes often persists.

CEREBRAL HEMISPHERES. Malformations of cortical development such as **polymicrogyria**, contracted narrow gyri (**"stenogyria"**) (36-29B), and **heterotopic gray mat-**

36-29A. Sagittal image in a 13 year old demonstrates many features of Chiari 2, including small posterior fossa, elongated "soda straw" fourth ventricle ➦, "cascade" of vermis/choroid plexus behind the medulla ➔, "beaked" tectum ➘, large massa intermedia ➦, and multiple gyral malformations ("stenogyria") ➶. 36-29B. Axial T2WI shows "beaked" tectum ➘, stenogyria ➶, scalloped calvaria ➦.

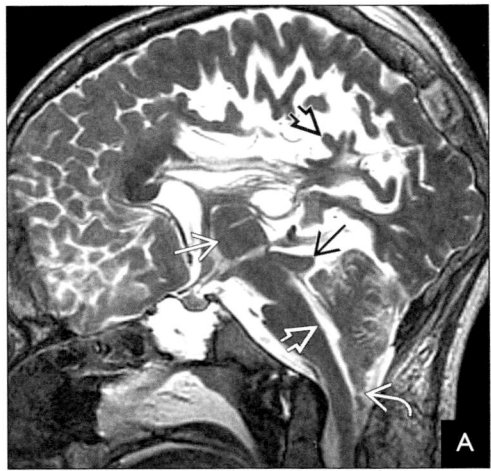
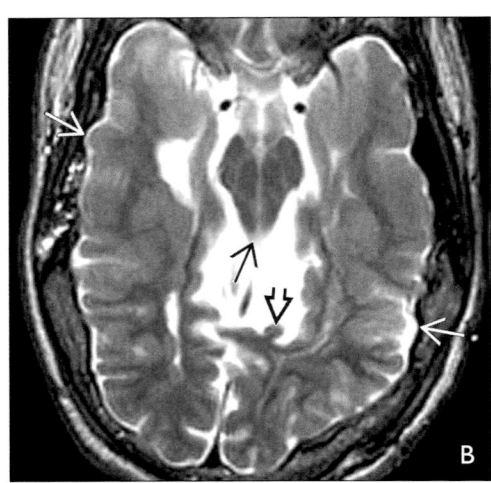

36-29C. Axial T2WI shows fenestrated falx with shortened interdigitating gyri ➶, irregular "serrated" appearance to interhemispheric fissure. 36-29D. Coronal T2WI shows low-lying transverse sinuses ➦ with a very small posterior fossa, "towering" cerebellum ➚ that protrudes upward through the tentorial incisura, interdigitating gyri ➶ giving a "serrated" appearance to the interhemispheric fissure.

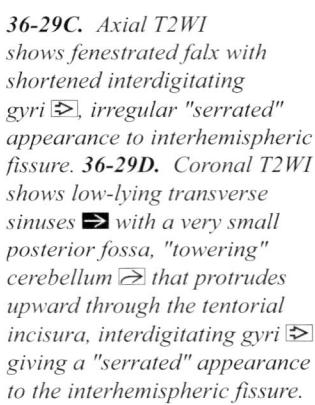
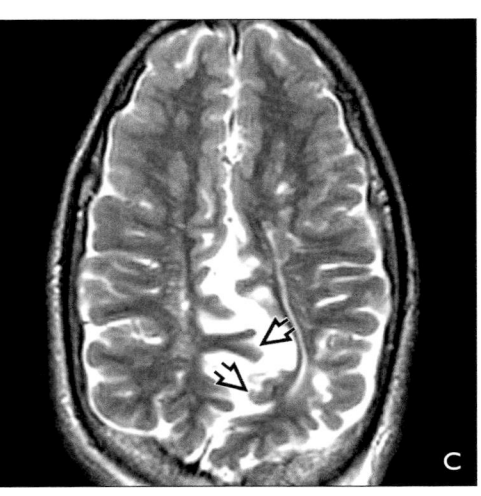
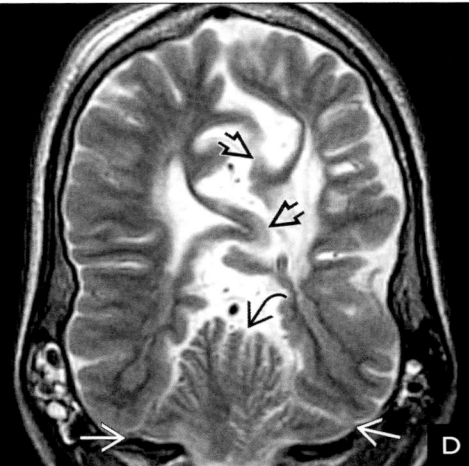

ter are frequent associated findings. **Callosal dysgenesis** is found in nearly two-thirds of all cases, and **abnormalities of the fornices** are also common.

SPINE AND SPINAL CORD. Open spinal dysraphism with **myelomeningocele** is present in almost all cases of CM2. **Hydrosyringomyelia** is seen in 50%.

Differential Diagnosis

The major differential diagnosis of CM2 is other Chiari malformations. In **Chiari 1**, it is the tonsils (not the vermis) that are herniated inferiorly. Myelomeningocele is absent, and other than being somewhat small, the posterior fossa and its contents appear relatively normal. If findings of CM2 plus a low occipital or high cervical cephalocele are present, the diagnosis is **Chiari 3**.

A few cases of posteriorly angled odontoid, brainstem descent, and tonsillar ectopia without myelodysplasia have been described and are considered by some investigators as **Chiari 1.5** (see below).

Severe chronic shunted congenital hydrocephalus may cause cerebellar herniation upward through the ten-

torial incisura, but brainstem descent and myelomeningocele are absent.

Chiari 3

Terminology

Chiari 3 malformation (CM3) is the rarest of the Chiari malformations. CM3 consists of a small posterior fossa with a caudally displaced brainstem and variable herniation of meninges/posterior fossa contents through a low occipital or upper cervical bony defect.

Pathology

The cephalocele contains meninges together with variable amounts of brain tissue, vessels, and CSF spaces. The brain is often featureless, dysplastic-appearing, and disorganized with extensive gliosis and gray matter heterotopias.

Clinical Issues

The cephalocele in CM3 generally appears as a large skin-covered, sac-like suboccipital mass protruding pos-

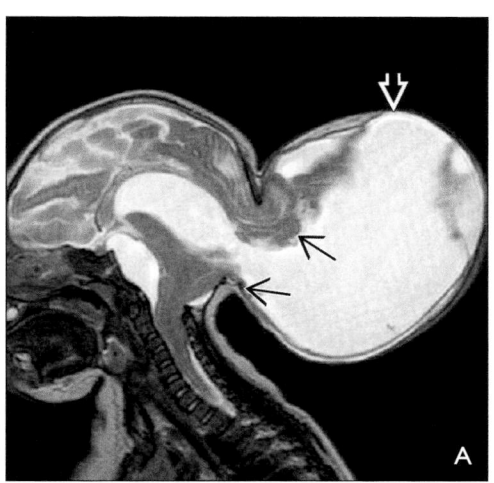

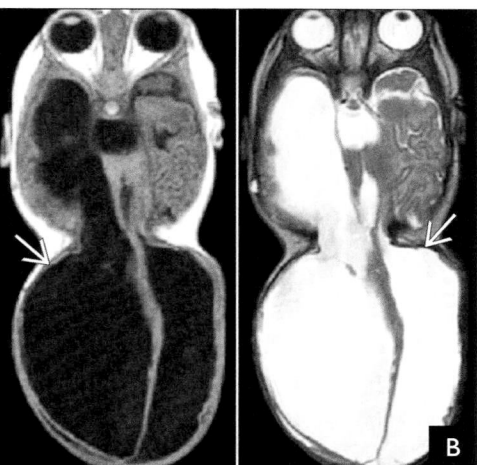

36-30A. Sagittal T2WI in a 3-day-old infant shows Chiari 3 with a cephalocele ➡ that contains herniated dysplastic brain ➡, CSF in continuity with a lateral ventricle. 36-30B. Axial T1WI (left), T2WI (right) in the same patient show extension of the lateral ventricles ➡ into the cephalocele. (Courtesy G. Hedlund, MD.)

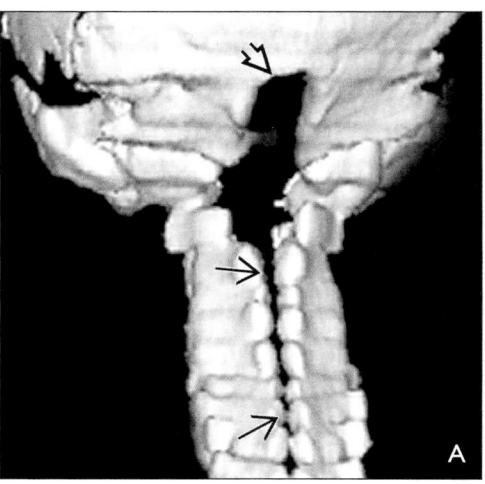

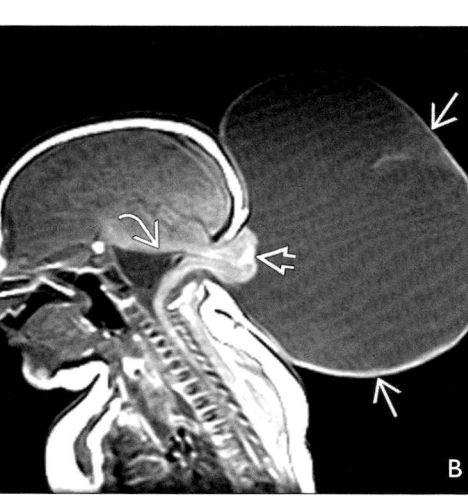

36-31A. Chiari 3 with extensive cranium bifidum extending from the occipital bone ➡ through the entire cervical spine ➡. 36-31B. Sagittal T2WI in the same patient with cranium bifidum and Chiari 3 shows an enormous meningocele sac ➡ with herniated, dysplastic-appearing brain ➡. The fourth ventricle ➡ is enlarged, elongated, and "tugged" toward the cephalocele. (Courtesy A. Illner, MD.)

teroinferiorly from the craniovertebral junction. Microcephaly is common, and in extreme cases, the cephalocele exceeds the cranium in size **(36-30)**.

Some cases are diagnosed with antenatal ultrasound. Other patients present at birth with bulbar and long tract signs, seizures, and developmental delay. Surgical mortality is high, and prognosis is generally poor as survivors usually have severe residual neurologic deficits.

Imaging

NECT scans show bony features similar to those seen in CM2, i.e., a small posterior cranial fossa, short scalloped clivus, lacunar skull, a defect in the ventral chondral portion of the supraoccipital bone, and low cranium bifidum that may extend inferiorly to involve much of the cervical spine **(36-31)**.

MR best delineates sac contents, which often include dysplastic-appearing cerebellum and/or brainstem as well as distorted CSF spaces and vessels. A deformed fourth and sometimes third ventricle can be partially found within the mass of herniated brain and meninges. Veins, dural sinuses, and even the basilar artery are sometimes "pulled" into the defect.

Differential Diagnosis

The differential diagnosis of CM3 includes isolated occipital cephalocele, iniencephaly, and syndromic occipital cephaloceles. **Isolated occipital cephalocele** lacks the typical intracranial features of CM2 and is not associated with cervical dysraphism.

Iniencephaly is an occipital cephalocele with extensive spinal dysraphism and fixed retroflexion of the neck ("stargazer" fetus). **Syndromic occipital cephalocele** occurs with other specific features (e.g., in Meckel-Gruber and Goldenhar-Gorlin syndromes).

CHIARI MALFORMATIONS

Chiari 1
- Etiology (controversial)
  ○ Paraxial mesodermal insufficiency?
  ○ Small bony posterior fossa?
  ○ Altered CSF dynamics?
- Clinical issues
  ○ Most common Chiari malformation
  ○ Found in 3-4% of children on routine brain imaging
  ○ Up to 50% asymptomatic
  ○ Valsalva-induced suboccipital headache, neck pain
- Imaging
  ○ Caudal tonsillar ectopia (≥ 5 mm below FM)
  ○ Pointed, peg-like tonsils with angled folia
  ○ "Crowded" foramen magnum with effaced CSF spaces
  ○ Diminished/absent CSF flow at posterior FM
  ○ Syrinx in 10-20% asymptomatic, 40-80% symptomatic patients
- Differential diagnosis
  ○ Normal "low-lying" tonsils (rounded, no disturbed CSF flow)
  ○ Acquired herniation (↑ ICP, intracranial hypotension)

Chiari 2
- Terminology
  ○ Complex hindbrain malformation with myelomeningocele
- Etiology
  ○ Posterior neuropore closure disorder
  ○ Developing vesicles fail to expand
  ○ Paraxial mesodermal abnormalities (skull, spine)
  ○ "Too small" bony posterior fossa
- Clinical issues
  ○ Prevalence ↓ with maternal folate
  ○ Myelomeningocele, hydrocephalus dominate clinical picture at birth
- Imaging
  ○ Myelomeningocele (almost always)
  ○ Lacunar skull
  ○ Small posterior fossa
  ○ Abnormal dura (gaping FM, heart-shaped incisura, fenestrated falx)
  ○ Inferiorly displaced medulla, vermis → "cascade" of tissue
  ○ Cervicomedullary "kink," medullary "spur"
  ○ "Towering" and "creeping" cerebellum
  ○ "Soda straw" fourth ventricle
  ○ Prominent massa intermedia
  ○ Hydrocephalus, shunted ventricles appear scalloped
  ○ Callosal dysgenesis
  ○ Stenogyria, gray matter heterotopias

Chiari 3
- Pathology
  ○ Small posterior fossa
  ○ Caudally displaced brainstem
  ○ Low occipital or upper cervical bony defect
  ○ Cephalocele with herniation of meninges, dysplastic brain, ventricles
- Sac may contain
  ○ Meninges
  ○ Dysplastic brain
  ○ Deformed ventricle(s)
  ○ Blood vessels (venous sinuses, arteries)

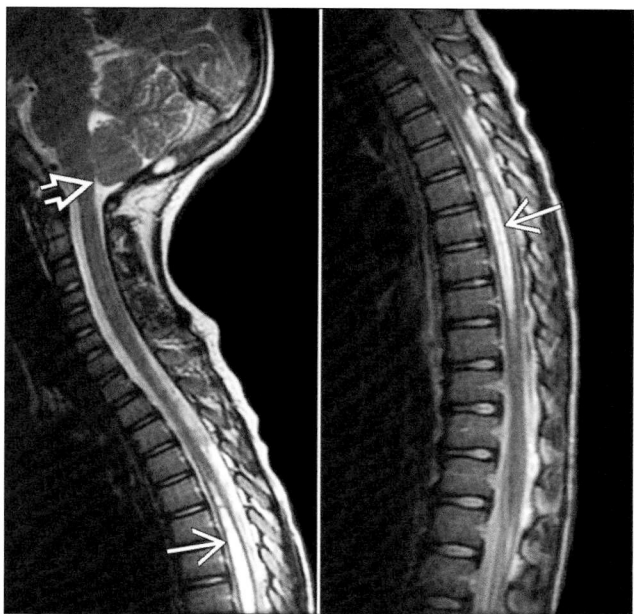

36-32. Sagittal T2 scans show Chiari 0 malformation with thoracic syrinx ➡️*. The cerebellar tonsil* ➡️ *is rounded and in normal position, but the FM appears "crowded" posteriorly.*

36-33. Sagittal T2WI in a 6-year-old girl with Chiari 1.5 malformation shows retroflexed odontoid ➡️*, tonsillar herniation* ➡️*, crowded FM, and low-lying nucleus gracilis* ➡️*.*

Chiari Variants

Some additions to the original Chiari classification have been proposed by neurosurgeons to account for hindbrain herniations that do not conform to the classic Chiari 1-3 definitions. Although these additions have not been universally adopted, radiologists should at least be familiar with these newly described entities.

Chiari 0 Malformation

This variant consists of hydrosyringomyelia and foramen magnum (FM) "crowding." Chiari 0 differs from Chiari 1 as *the cerebellar tonsils are normally positioned* (i.e., either above or less than three millimeters below the FM) **(36-32)**. Chiari 0 patients are typically symptomatic (usually because of the syrinx).

Chiari 1.5 Malformation

TERMINOLOGY. The term Chiari 1.5 malformation (CM1.5) has been coined by neurosurgeons to designate a "complex Chiari" malformation in which cerebellar tonsillar herniation is complicated by other abnormalities (e.g., caudally displaced brainstem and fourth ventricle and/or cervicomedullary "kink"). CM1.5 differs from classic Chiari 1 (CM1) as *caudal descent of the brainstem is present in addition to tonsillar ectopia.* CM 1.5 differs from Chiari 2 (CM2) as *myelomeningocele is absent.*

CLINICAL ISSUES. The exact prevalence of CM1.5 is unknown. Recent large series show that cases fulfilling the imaging criteria for CM1.5 represent approximately 22% of all patients 16 years or younger referred for surgical management of Chiari-related malformations.

No single sign or symptom is peculiar to CM1.5. The most frequent symptom is headache (often Valsalva-induced). Progressive scoliosis and syrinx-related symptoms such as extremity paresthesias are common.

Management strategies for CM1.5 differ significantly from those for CM1 and CM2. Symptomatic patients with "classic" CM1 often require only suboccipital decompression (with or without duraplasty). Patients with "complex" CM1.5 abnormalities require other additional interventions such as transoral odontoid resection and occipitocervical fusion. Patients with CM2 require myelomeningocele repair.

IMAGING. In addition to tonsillar ectopia (see above), patients with CM1.5 demonstrate a several other significant imaging abnormalities. The major finding that differentiates CM1.5 from CM1 is the presence of brainstem herniation through the FM (hence the term "Chiari 1.5 malformation"). Elongation/caudal displacement of the brainstem and fourth ventricle and displacement of the obex below the FM are common **(36-33)**. FM "crowding" with a medullary "kink" or "bulb" is often present in addition to the inferiorly displaced tonsils.

Bony abnormalities are common in CM1.5. These include a "retroflexed" odontoid, abnormal clival-cervical angle, occipitalization of the atlas, basilar invagination with odontoid compression of the brainstem, and

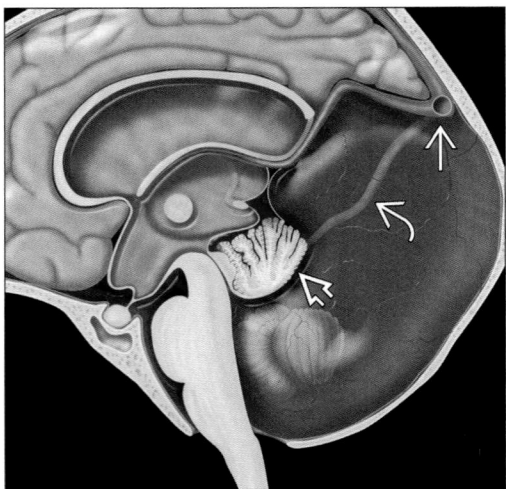

36-34. DWM. Transverse sinus, elevated torcular ➡, steeply angled TS ➡, superiorly rotated hypoplastic cerebellar vermis ➡, hydrocephalus.

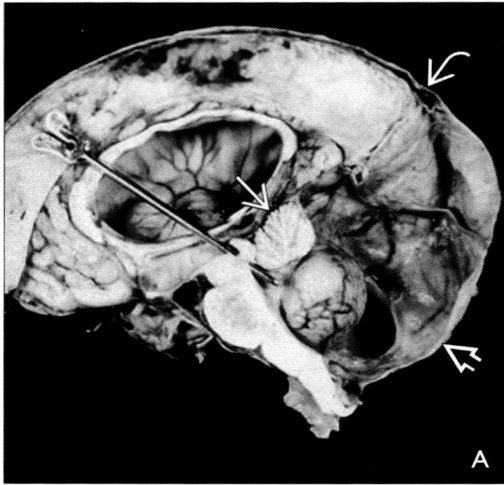

36-35A. Autopsy specimen of DWM shows large PF with cyst ➡, hypoplastic rotated vermis ➡, high-inserting torcular ➡. Probe is in aqueduct.

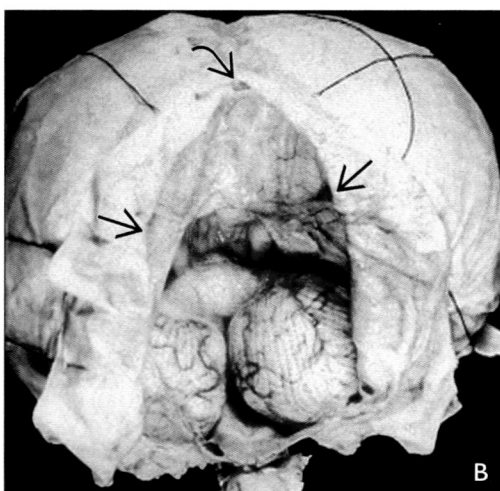

36-35B. Posterior view with dura opened shows a large PF cyst, high-inserting torcular ➡, steeply angled transverse sinuses ➡. (E. Ross, MD.)

scoliosis. Syringomyelia is present in 50% of cases, but spina bifida and myelodysplasia are absent.

DIFFERENTIAL DIAGNOSIS. The major differential diagnosis of CM1.5 is **CM1**. As management strategies differ, the distinction is important. While both CM1.5 and CM1 share common features such as tonsillar descent and bony anomalies, caudal brainstem descent distinguishes the two malformations.

Chiari 4 and Chiari 5 Malformations

The terms "primary cerebellar agenesis" or "severe cerebellar hypoplasia" should be used instead of "Chiari 4 malformation." The posterior fossa is normal in size and mostly filled with CSF. The pons is small and appears flat. There is no myelomeningocele, and the intracranial features of Chiari 2 are absent.

A case in which the cerebellum was absent and the occipital lobe herniated through the foramen magnum into the upper cervical spinal canal was dubbed a "Chiari 5 malformation."

Hindbrain Malformations

Dandy-Walker Spectrum

Dandy-Walker (DW) spectrum is a controversial subject. Some authors include related disorders such as mega cisterna magna—which others regard as a normal variant—and the so-called Dandy-Walker variant as mild abnormalities within the DW spectrum. In this section, we use an expanded definition of DW spectrum and include abnormalities from mega cisterna magna to classic Dandy-Walker malformation.

Terminology

Dandy-Walker spectrum (DWS) is a generalized disorder of mesenchymal development that affects both the cerebellum and overlying meninges.

Dandy-Walker malformation (DWM) consists of a large posterior fossa (PF) with a high-inserting venous sinus confluence, large PF cyst extending dorsally from the fourth ventricle, and varying degrees of vermian and cerebellar hemispheric hypoplasia **(36-34)**.

Dandy-Walker variant (DWV) is an older term used to designate a *hypoplastic rotated vermis* with or without accompanying fourth ventricle enlargement. DWV is now considered a mild form of DWS.

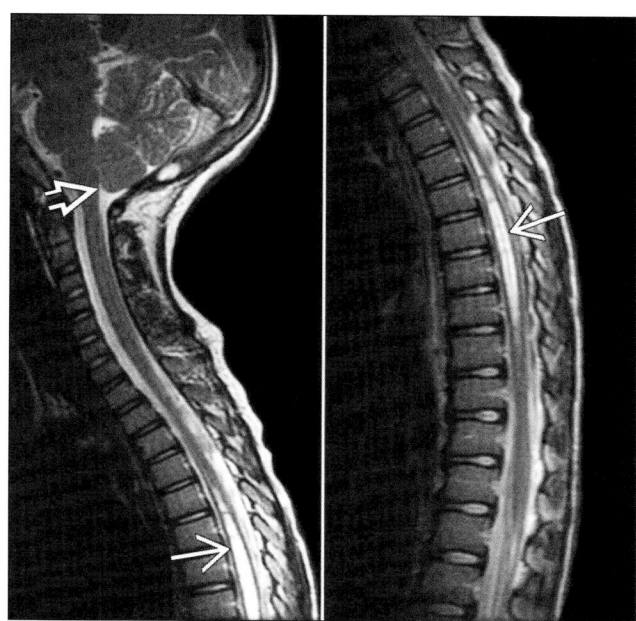

36-32. Sagittal T2 scans show Chiari 0 malformation with thoracic syrinx ➡. The cerebellar tonsil ➡ is rounded and in normal position, but the FM appears "crowded" posteriorly.

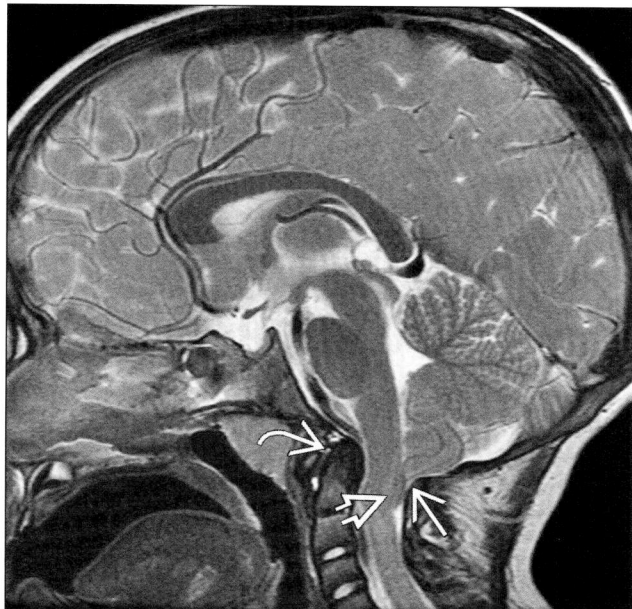

36-33. Sagittal T2WI in a 6-year-old girl with Chiari 1.5 malformation shows retroflexed odontoid ➡, tonsillar herniation ➡, crowded FM, and low-lying nucleus gracilis ➡.

Chiari Variants

Some additions to the original Chiari classification have been proposed by neurosurgeons to account for hindbrain herniations that do not conform to the classic Chiari 1-3 definitions. Although these additions have not been universally adopted, radiologists should at least be familiar with these newly described entities.

Chiari 0 Malformation

This variant consists of hydrosyringomyelia and foramen magnum (FM) "crowding." Chiari 0 differs from Chiari 1 as *the cerebellar tonsils are normally positioned* (i.e., either above or less than three millimeters below the FM) **(36-32)**. Chiari 0 patients are typically symptomatic (usually because of the syrinx).

Chiari 1.5 Malformation

TERMINOLOGY. The term Chiari 1.5 malformation (CM1.5) has been coined by neurosurgeons to designate a "complex Chiari" malformation in which cerebellar tonsillar herniation is complicated by other abnormalities (e.g., caudally displaced brainstem and fourth ventricle and/or cervicomedullary "kink"). CM1.5 differs from classic Chiari 1 (CM1) as *caudal descent of the brainstem is present in addition to tonsillar ectopia.* CM 1.5 differs from Chiari 2 (CM2) as *myelomeningocele is absent.*

CLINICAL ISSUES. The exact prevalence of CM1.5 is unknown. Recent large series show that cases fulfilling the imaging criteria for CM1.5 represent approximately 22% of all patients 16 years or younger referred for surgical management of Chiari-related malformations.

No single sign or symptom is peculiar to CM1.5. The most frequent symptom is headache (often Valsalva-induced). Progressive scoliosis and syrinx-related symptoms such as extremity paresthesias are common.

Management strategies for CM1.5 differ significantly from those for CM1 and CM2. Symptomatic patients with "classic" CM1 often require only suboccipital decompression (with or without duraplasty). Patients with "complex" CM1.5 abnormalities require other additional interventions such as transoral odontoid resection and occipitocervical fusion. Patients with CM2 require myelomeningocele repair.

IMAGING. In addition to tonsillar ectopia (see above), patients with CM1.5 demonstrate a several other significant imaging abnormalities. The major finding that differentiates CM1.5 from CM1 is the presence of brainstem herniation through the FM (hence the term "Chiari 1.5 malformation"). Elongation/caudal displacement of the brainstem and fourth ventricle and displacement of the obex below the FM are common **(36-33)**. FM "crowding" with a medullary "kink" or "bulb" is often present in addition to the inferiorly displaced tonsils.

Bony abnormalities are common in CM1.5. These include a "retroflexed" odontoid, abnormal clival-cervical angle, occipitalization of the atlas, basilar invagination with odontoid compression of the brainstem, and

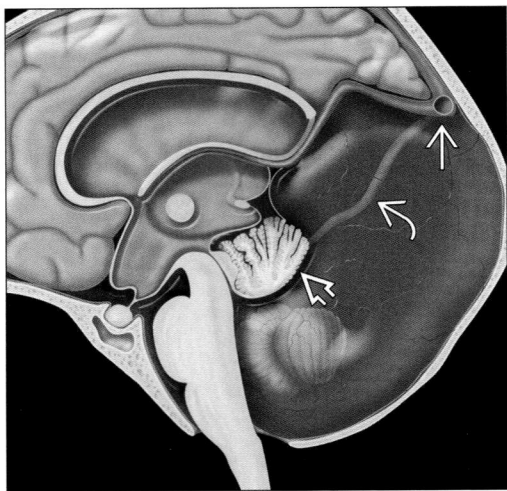

36-34. DWM. Transverse sinus, elevated torcular ➡️, steeply angled TS ➡️, superiorly rotated hypoplastic cerebellar vermis ➡️, hydrocephalus.

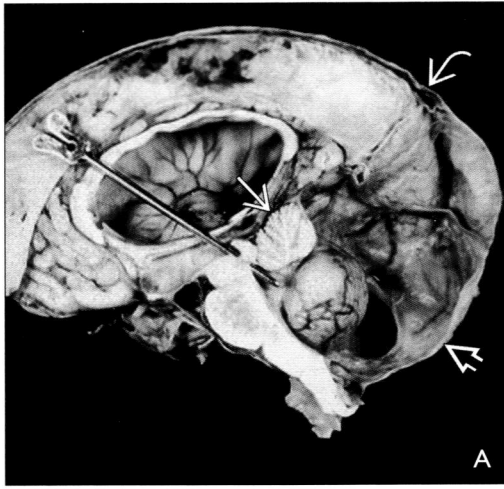

36-35A. Autopsy specimen of DWM shows large PF with cyst ➡️, hypoplastic rotated vermis ➡️, high-inserting torcular ➡️. Probe is in aqueduct.

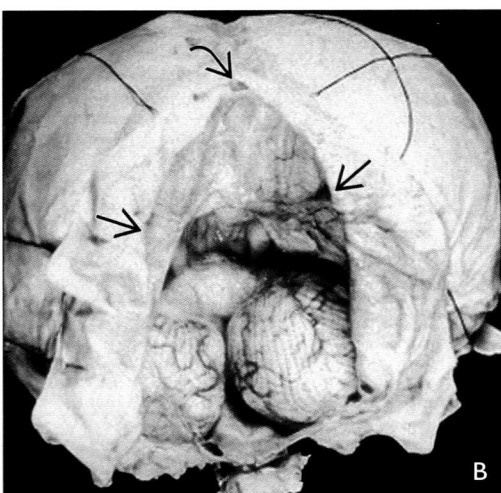

36-35B. Posterior view with dura opened shows a large PF cyst, high-inserting torcular ➡️, steeply angled transverse sinuses ➡️. (E. Ross, MD.)

scoliosis. Syringomyelia is present in 50% of cases, but spina bifida and myelodysplasia are absent.

DIFFERENTIAL DIAGNOSIS. The major differential diagnosis of CM1.5 is **CM1**. As management strategies differ, the distinction is important. While both CM1.5 and CM1 share common features such as tonsillar descent and bony anomalies, caudal brainstem descent distinguishes the two malformations.

Chiari 4 and Chiari 5 Malformations

The terms "primary cerebellar agenesis" or "severe cerebellar hypoplasia" should be used instead of "Chiari 4 malformation." The posterior fossa is normal in size and mostly filled with CSF. The pons is small and appears flat. There is no myelomeningocele, and the intracranial features of Chiari 2 are absent.

A case in which the cerebellum was absent and the occipital lobe herniated through the foramen magnum into the upper cervical spinal canal was dubbed a "Chiari 5 malformation."

Hindbrain Malformations

Dandy-Walker Spectrum

Dandy-Walker (DW) spectrum is a controversial subject. Some authors include related disorders such as mega cisterna magna—which others regard as a normal variant—and the so-called Dandy-Walker variant as mild abnormalities within the DW spectrum. In this section, we use an expanded definition of DW spectrum and include abnormalities from mega cisterna magna to classic Dandy-Walker malformation.

Terminology

Dandy-Walker spectrum (DWS) is a generalized disorder of mesenchymal development that affects both the cerebellum and overlying meninges.

Dandy-Walker malformation (DWM) consists of a large posterior fossa (PF) with a high-inserting venous sinus confluence, large PF cyst extending dorsally from the fourth ventricle, and varying degrees of vermian and cerebellar hemispheric hypoplasia (36-34).

Dandy-Walker variant (DWV) is an older term used to designate a *hypoplastic rotated vermis* with or without accompanying fourth ventricle enlargement. DWV is now considered a mild form of DWS.

A **persistent Blake pouch cyst** is an ependyma-lined protrusion of the fourth ventricle through the foramen of Magendie into the retrovermian cistern. The fourth ventricle choroid plexus is displaced, and the tegmentovermian angle is increased, but the *vermis is normal* in size and configuration.

A **mega cisterna magna** (MCM) consists of a large PF with an enlarged cisterna magna. The fourth ventricle, vermis, and supratentorial brain are normal. MCM represents the mildest end of the DWS.

Etiology

EMBRYOLOGY. If the anterior membranous area of the embryonic fourth ventricle fails to incorporate properly into the choroid plexus or if there is delayed opening of the foramen of Magendie, the fourth ventricle roof balloons posteriorly and forms the CSF-filled cisterna magna cyst characteristic of DWM.

GENETICS. Three DWM causative genes have been identified: *FOXC1* on chromosome 6p25 and the linked *ZIC1* and *ZIC4* genes on chromosome 3q24. Each member of the *ZIC* gene family encodes a highly related zinc-finger (ZF) transcription factor that is broadly expressed throughout cerebellar development. Both *ZIC1* and *ZIC4* have key roles in the regulation of both cerebellar size and normal cerebellar foliation. Zic proteins compete or interact with Gli proteins to regulate Shh signaling, which is crucial for normal cerebellar development.

Mice with heterozygous deletions of the linked genes *ZIC1* and *ZIC4* model human DWM, although the developmental basis of this phenotype remains unknown.

Pathology

GROSS PATHOLOGY. The most striking gross findings in DWM are (1) an enlarged PF with (2) upward displacement of the tentorium and accompanying venous sinuses and (3) cystic dilatation of the fourth ventricle **(36-35)**. Vermian abnormalities range from complete absence to varying degrees of hypoplasia.

DWM is frequently associated with other CNS anomalies. Almost two-thirds of patients have gyral abnormalities (e.g., pachy- or polymicrogyria, heterotopic GM). Callosal dysgenesis is common. Craniofacial, cardiac, and urinary tract anomalies are frequent.

MICROSCOPIC FEATURES. The PF cyst in DWM is typically lined by two layers: An outer layer of pia-arachnoid and an inner layer of ependyma. Occasionally, microscopic remnants of cerebellar tissue are present in the cyst wall.

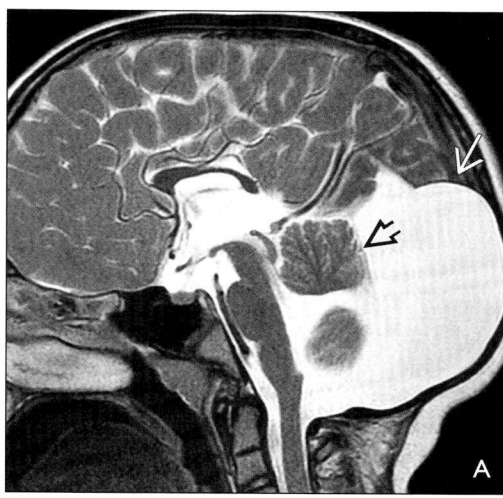

36-36A. Classic DWM with large PF cyst elevating torcular ➡, *superiorly rotated vermian remnant* ⧫, *small pons, dysgenetic corpus callosum.*

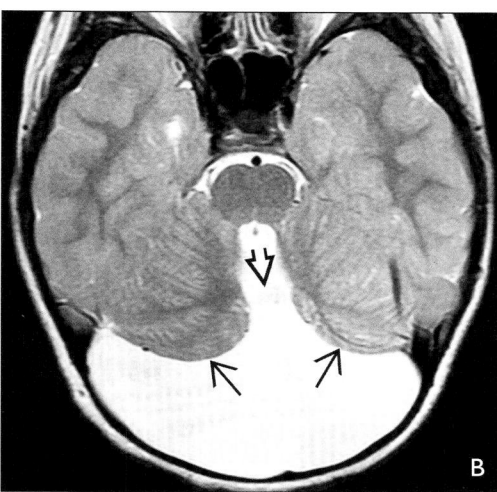

36-36B. Axial T2WI shows fourth ventricle open dorsally ⧫ *to the large PF cyst. Cerebellar hemispheres are small, "winged" anteriorly* ➡.

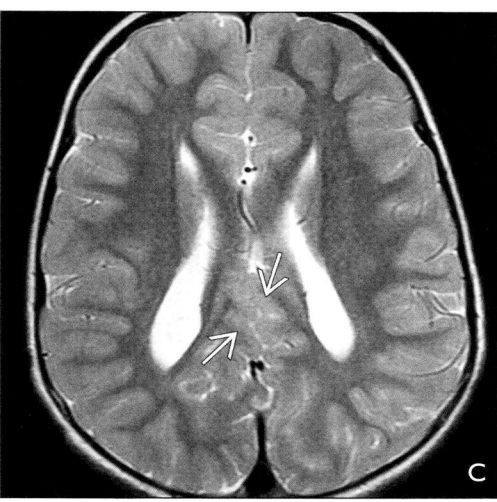

36-36C. Axial T2WI shows callosal dysgenesis with polymicrogyria ➡.

Clinical Issues

EPIDEMIOLOGY AND DEMOGRAPHICS. DWM is the most common congenital cerebellar malformation with an estimated prevalence of 1:5,000 live births. There is a slight female predominance (F:M = 1.5-2:1).

PRESENTATION. The most common presentation of DWM is increased intracranial pressure secondary to hydrocephalus. Despite the extensive cerebellar abnormalities, cerebellar signs are relatively uncommon.

NATURAL HISTORY. Early death is common in classic DWM. If DWM is relatively mild and uncomplicated by other CNS anomalies, intelligence can be normal and neurologic deficits minimal.

TREATMENT OPTIONS. CSF diversion, usually ventriculoperitoneal shunting with or without cyst shunting or marsupialization, is the standard treatment for DWM-related hydrocephalus.

Imaging

The spectrum of imaging abnormalities in DW is broad, affecting—to varying degrees—the skull and dura, ventricles and CSF spaces, and brain.

SKULL AND DURA, VENOUS SINUSES. In contrast to Chiari 2 (CM2), in which the PF is abnormally small, the PF in DWM is strikingly enlarged. The straight sinus, sinus confluence, and tentorial apex are elevated above the lambdoid suture ("lambdoid-torcular inversion"). The transverse sinuses descend at a steep angle from the torcular herophili toward the sigmoid sinuses **(36-36)**.

The occipital bone may appear scalloped, focally thinned, and remodeled with *all* DWS types, including MCM. The straight sinus descends at a normal angle in MCM, but the torcular is often slightly elevated. MCM often demonstrates partially infolded dura-arachnoid (falx cerebelli) on axial T2 scans.

VENTRICLES AND CISTERNS. The floor of the fourth ventricle is present and appears normal in DWM. The anterior medullary velum and fastigium are absent. The

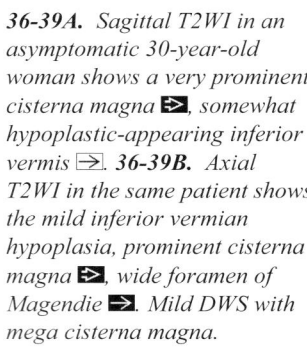

36-37. NECT scan in an 11-year-old girl with mild DWS shows the "keyhole" appearance of the fourth ventricle ➡ opening into the prominent foramen magnum ➡ via an enlarged foramen of Magendie ➡. 36-38. Axial NECT scan in a 10-day-old infant shows a more pronounced "keyhole" deformity of mild DWS with inferior vermian hypoplasia, large fourth ventricle ➡ opening into the cisterna magna ➡ via a gaping foramen of Magendie ➡.

36-39A. Sagittal T2WI in an asymptomatic 30-year-old woman shows a very prominent cisterna magna ➡, somewhat hypoplastic-appearing inferior vermis ➡. 36-39B. Axial T2WI in the same patient shows the mild inferior vermian hypoplasia, prominent cisterna magna ➡, wide foramen of Magendie ➡. Mild DWS with mega cisterna magna.

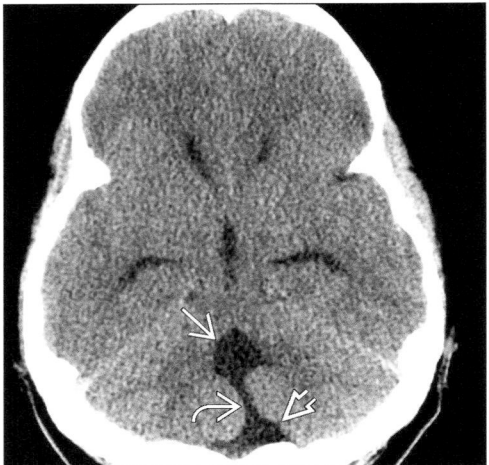

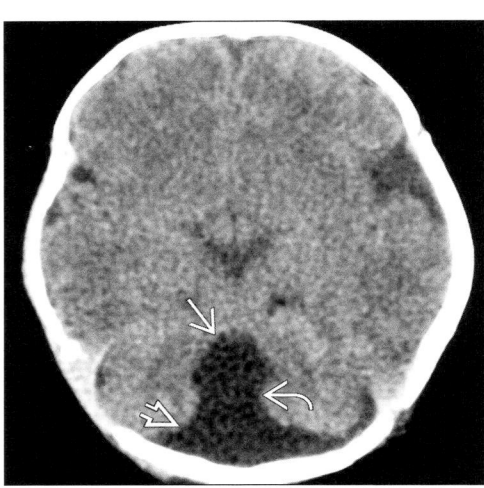

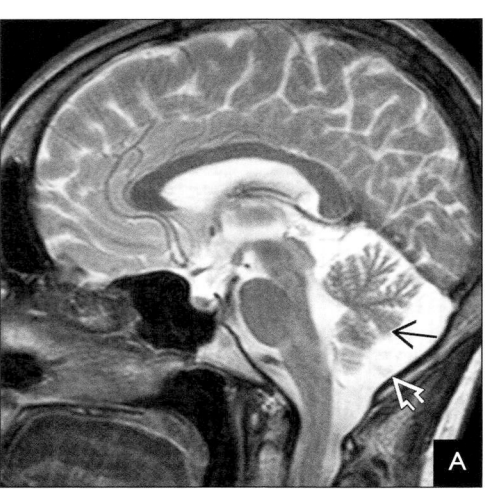

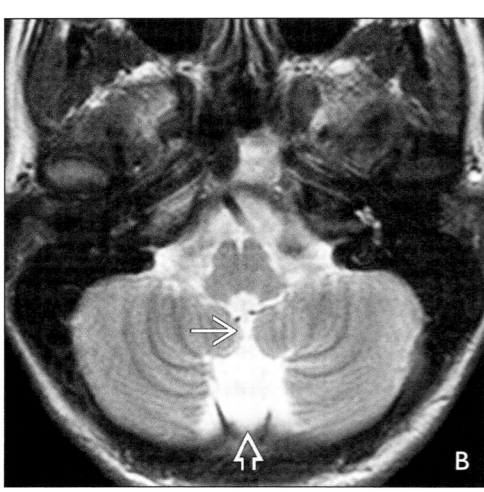

fourth ventricle opens dorsally to a variably sized CSF-containing cyst that balloons posteriorly behind and between the cerebellar hemisphere remnants.

Generalized obstructive hydrocephalus is present in over 80% of neonates with DWM at birth. If callosal dysgenesis is present, the lateral ventricles are widely separated and may have unusually prominent occipital horns (colpocephaly).

The fourth ventricle is normal in MCM and shows a normal fastigium (dorsal point) on sagittal MR scans. In mild DWS (previously called Dandy Walker "variant"), the fourth ventricle has a "keyhole" configuration on axial imaging caused by a widely patent vallecula that communicates with a prominent cisterna magna **(36-37)**, **(36-38)**.

A Blake pouch cyst is an ependyma-lined protrusion from the fourth ventricle that exhibits an increased tegmentovermian angle.

BRAINSTEM, CEREBELLUM, AND VERMIS. The brainstem appears normal in mild forms of DWM but often appears somewhat small in moderate to more severe DWM.

The vermis is normal in MCM, the mildest of all DWMs. Varying degrees of vermian hypoplasia are seen in the remainder of the DW spectrum disorders **(36-39)**, **(36-40)**. The inferior lobules are often hypoplastic in mild DWM. In classic DWM, the vermian remnant appears rotated and elevated above the large PF cyst.

The cerebellar hemispheres also demonstrate varying degrees of hypoplasia. They appear normal or nearly normal in MCM and DWV but are hypoplastic in DWM. In severe cases of DWM, the cerebellar remnants appear "winged" outward and displaced anterolaterally.

ASSOCIATED ABNORMALITIES. Other CNS abnormalities are present in 70% of DWM. The most common finding is callosal agenesis or dysgenesis. A dorsal interhemispheric cyst may be present. Gray matter abnormalities (e.g., heterotopias, clefts, pachy- and polymicrogyria) are common associated abnormalities.

Differential Diagnosis

Because Dandy-Walker really is a spectrum, there are many "in between" cases. From a clinical perspective, it may be meaningless to distinguish a **hypoplastic rotated vermis** from a mild Dandy-Walker malformation. A Blake pouch cyst may likewise be indistinguishable from mild DWS.

A **retrocerebellar arachnoid cyst** is considered by some investigators as part of the DWS. Here a midline arachnoid-lined cyst is located behind the vermis and fourth ventricle but does not communicate with the latter. There

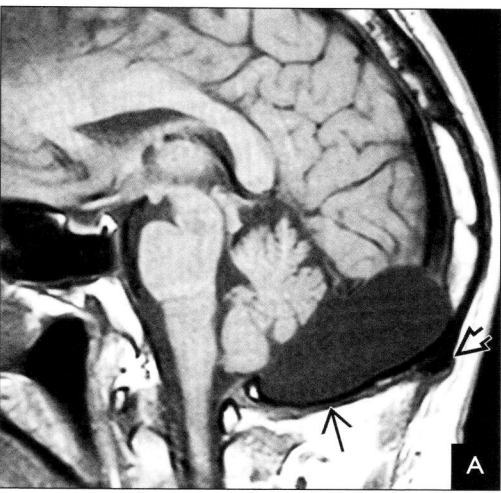

36-40A. Sagittal T1WI shows mild DWS (mega cisterna magna). Note thinned ⇥*, scalloped* ⇲ *occipital bone. Pons, fourth v., vermis are normal.*

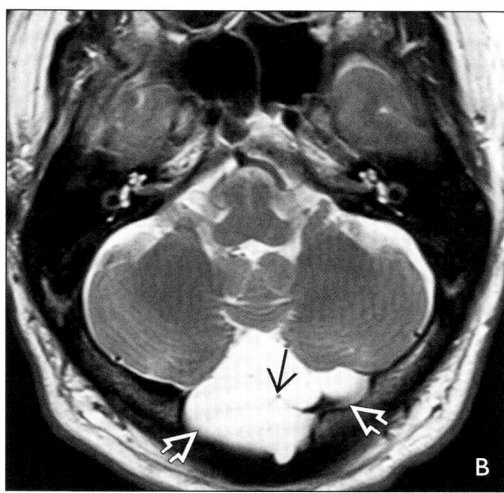

36-40B. Axial T2WI in the same patient shows bone "scalloping" ⇥*, partially infolded dura-arachnoid of falx cerebelli* ⇥*.*

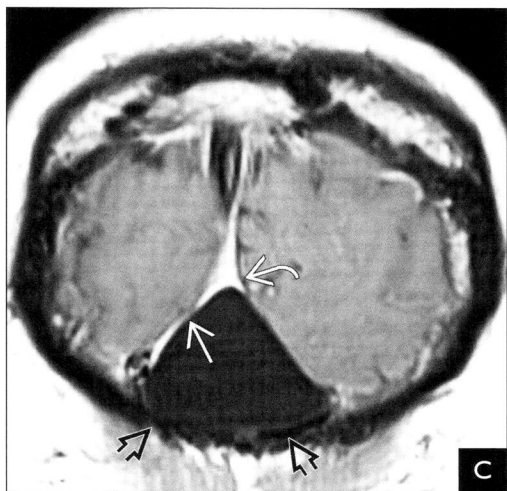

36-40C. Coronal T1 C+ shows that mega cisterna magna ⇲ *elevates the posterior tentorium* ⇥*, torcular* ⇥*.*

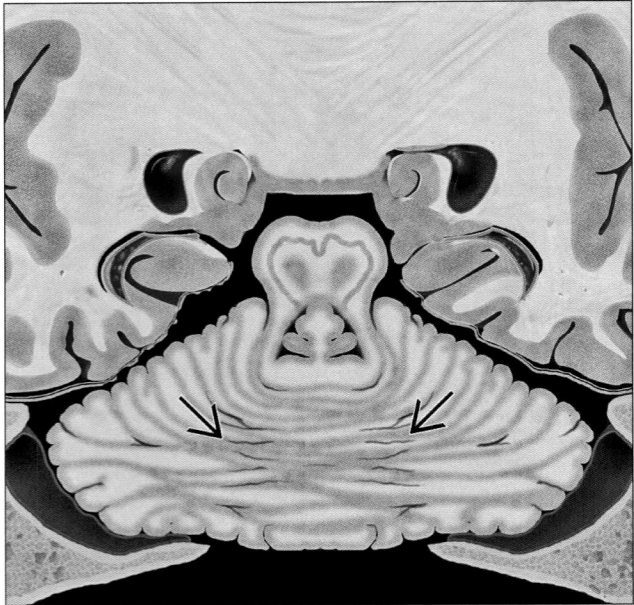

36-41. Coronal graphic of rhombencephalosynapsis shows that no vermis is present in the midline of the cerebellum. Instead, the folia, interfoliate sulci, and cerebellar white matter ➡ are continuous across the cerebellar midline.

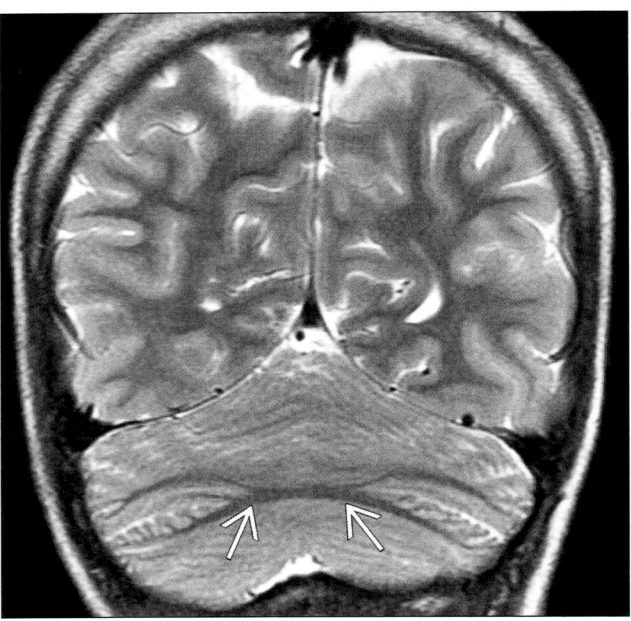

36-42. Coronal T2WI shows classic rhombencephalosynapsis. Note absent vermis, transversely oriented folia, continuity of cerebellar white matter across the midline ➡.

is no associated hydrocephalus or cerebellar dysgenesis. In contrast to MCM, veins and falx cerebelli do not traverse the CSF collection.

DANDY-WALKER SPECTRUM

Dandy-Walker Malformation
- Large posterior fossa (PF)
- Cyst extending posteriorly from fourth ventricle
- Variable vermian, cerebellar hypoplasia
- High-inserting venous confluence

Hypoplastic Rotated Vermis
- Old term = Dandy-Walker variant
- PF normal size
- "Keyhole" opening of fourth ventricle

Blake Pouch Cyst
- Ependyma-lined protrusion from fourth ventricle
- Increased tegmentovermian angle
- May be difficult to distinguish from DWM

Mega Cisterna Magna
- Large PF
- Enlarged cisterna magna
- May scallop, remodel occiput
- Crossed by veins, falx cerebelli
- Fourth ventricle, vermis normal
- No supratentorial abnormalities

Miscellaneous Malformations

A number of less common PF malformations occur. We now discuss several of those in which the abnormalities are largely defined by imaging features: Rhombencephalosynapsis, Joubert syndrome, and cerebellar hypoplasias and unclassified dysplasias.

Rhombencephalosynapsis

TERMINOLOGY. Rhombencephalosynapsis is a midline brain malformation characterized by (1) a "missing" cerebellar vermis and (2) apparent fusion of the cerebellar hemispheres (36-41).

PATHOLOGY. Severity ranges from mild (partial absence of the nodulus, anterior and posterior vermis) to complete (the entire vermis, including the nodulus, is absent). Dorsal midline continuity of the cerebellar hemispheres is characteristic. The tonsils, dentate nuclei, and superior cerebellar peduncles are usually fused.

CLINICAL ISSUES. Rhombencephalosynapsis can be seen in patients with **VACTERL** (**v**ertebral anomalies, **a**nal atresia, **c**ardiovascular anomalies, **t**racheoesophageal fistulas, **r**enal anomalies, and **l**imb defects).

IMAGING. Sagittal MR scans show an upwardly rounded fastigial recess of the fourth ventricle and lack of the normal midline foliar pattern of the vermis. Coronal images show transverse folia and continuity of the cerebellar white matter across the midline (36-42). Axial scans confirm absence of the vermis. Images through the rostral fourth ventricle may demonstrate a diamond or pointed shape (36-43).

Aqueductal stenosis and hydrocephalus are common. Absent cavum septi pellucidi is seen in half of all cases. The thalami, fornices, and tectum may be partially or completely fused. Other forebrain anomalies include absent olfactory bulbs and corpus callosum dysgenesis.

Joubert Syndrome and Related Disorders

TERMINOLOGY AND CLASSIFICATION. Joubert syndrome (JS) and related disorders (JSRD) are a group of syndromes in which the obligatory hallmark is the "molar tooth" sign, a complex mid- and hindbrain malformation that resembles a molar tooth on axial MR scans.

Anomalies of the kidneys, eyes, extremities, liver, and bile ducts are common in the JSRD spectrum. Six major JSRD phenotypic subgroups are recognized: Pure JS, JS with ocular defect, JS with renal defect, JS with oculo-renal defects, JS with hepatic defect, and JS with oro-facio-digital defects.

Classic JS is the "pure" syndrome. The oculo-renal form is termed CORS (**c**erebello-**o**culo-**r**enal **s**yndrome). JS with preaxial or mesoaxial polydactyly and orofacial defects is known as type 6 **o**ro-**f**acial-**d**igital syndrome (OFD-6). COACH syndrome consists of **c**erebellar vermis hypoplasia, **o**ligophrenia, **a**taxia, ocular **c**oloboma, and **h**epatic fibrosis.

ETIOLOGY. With the exception of rare X-linked recessive cases, JSRD follows autosomal recessive inheritance. At least 10 affected genes that help regulate normal axon growth and decussation have been identified in JSRD.

JSRD is genetically heterogeneous. Molar tooth disorders are, at least in part, "ciliopathies" with mutations of ciliary/centrosomal proteins that affect cell migration.

PATHOLOGY. JSRD is characterized grossly by a dysmorphic vermis with sagittal clefting, nondecussating enlarged superior cerebellar peduncles, and an elongated rounded fastigium of the fourth ventricle **(36-44)**, **(36-45)**. The anteroposterior diameter of the midbrain is reduced. Microscopically, dysplasias and heterotopias of the cerebellar nuclei are common.

CLINICAL ISSUES. The estimated incidence of JSRD is 1:80,000-100,000 live births. There is no gender predilection.

JSRD typically presents in infancy and childhood. The classic clinical presentation is a child with developmental delay, ataxia, and oculomotor and respiratory abnormal-

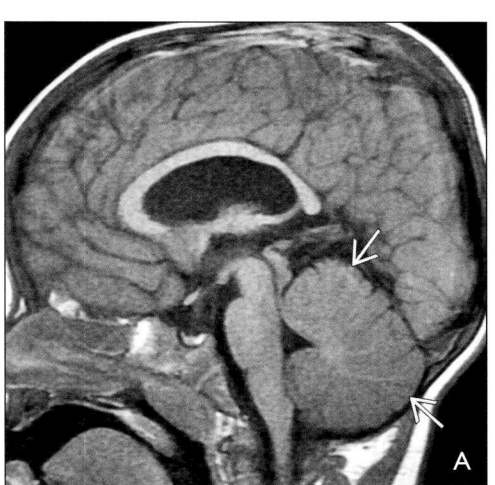
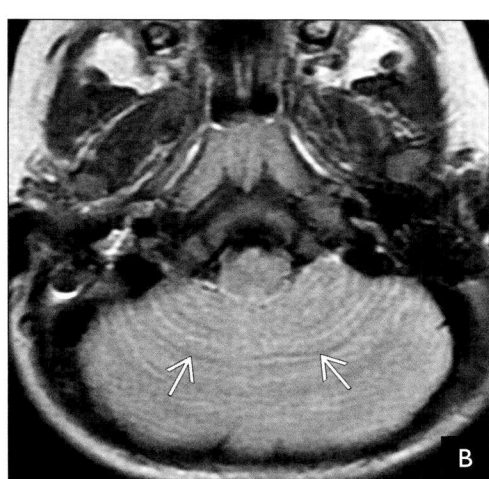

36-43A. *Sagittal T1WI in a patient with rhombencephalosynapsis shows abnormal foliation of what appears to be the vermis* ➡. **36-43B.** *Axial T2WI in the same patient shows absent vermis, white matter continuity across the midline* ➡.

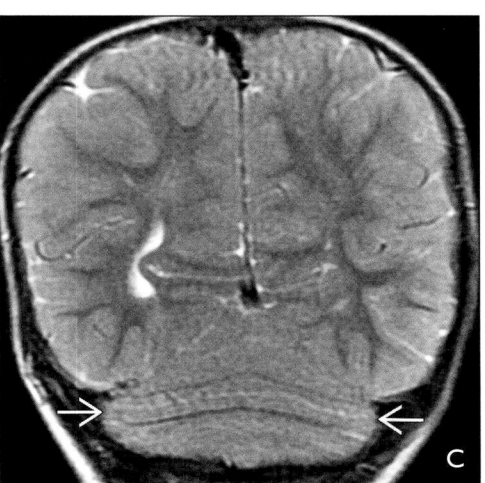
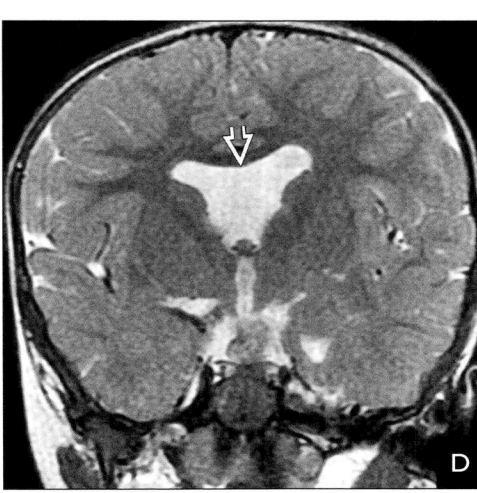

36-43C. *Coronal T2WI nicely shows absent vermis, transversely oriented cerebellar folia* ➡. **36-43D.** *Coronal T2WI in the same patient demonstrates septooptic dysplasia with absent cavum septi pellucidi* ➡, *an abnormality commonly associated with rhombencephalosynapsis.*

ities. Neonates may exhibit nystagmus, alternating apnea and hyperpnea, and seizures.

IMAGING. Axial NECT scans demonstrate vermian clefting and an oddly shaped fourth ventricle with a "bat wing" configuration.

MR imaging is the cornerstone in establishing a diagnosis of JSRD. Midline sagittal scans show a small dysmorphic vermis. The fourth ventricle appears deformed with a thin upwardly convex roof and loss of the normal pointed fastigium (**36-46A**).

Axial scans demonstrate the classic "molar tooth" appearance with foreshortened midbrain, narrow isthmus, deep interpeduncular fossa, and thickened superior cerebellar peduncles surrounding an oblong or diamond-shaped fourth ventricle. The superior vermis is clefted, and the cisterna magna may appear enlarged (**36-46B**).

DTI shows that fibers of the superior cerebellar peduncles do not decussate in the mesencephalon and that the corticospinal tracts fail to cross in the caudal medulla.

DIFFERENTIAL DIAGNOSIS. The major imaging differential diagnosis of JSRD is **vermian and pontocerebellar hypoplasia**, in which the vermis is small but is not clefted. In **rhombencephalosynapsis**, the cerebellar hemispheres and dentate nuclei are fused across the midline, not split.

Multiple syndromes exhibit "molar tooth" posterior fossa malformations. Many pediatric neurologists therefore consider the "molar tooth" sign nonspecific, instead requiring both imaging *and* clinical evidence of JSRD. Developmental delay and hypotonia should be present along with either abnormal breathing episodes or abnormal eye movements.

Genetic analysis may be required to distinguish among the different JSRD subtypes.

Cerebellar Hypoplasia

Cerebellar hypoplasia (once called Chiari 4 malformation) shows a spectrum of findings. In severe cases, the posterior fossa appears virtually empty. The cerebellar hemispheres and vermis are almost completely absent. The pons is hypoplastic (**36-47**).

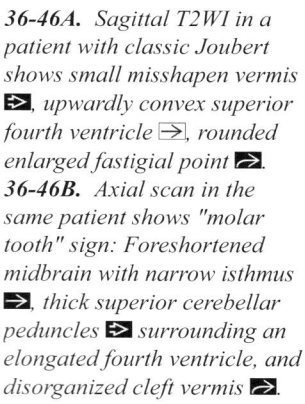

36-44. Axial graphic depicts Joubert malformation. Thickened superior cerebellar peduncles ⇨ around an elongated fourth ventricle form the classic "molar tooth" sign. Note cleft cerebellar vermis ⇨. 36-45. Autopsy specimen of JSRD shows foreshortened midbrain with narrowed isthmus ⇨, thick superior cerebellar peduncles ⇗, "bat wing" fourth ventricle ⇘, clefted superior vermis ⇨. (Courtesy R. Hewlett, MD.)

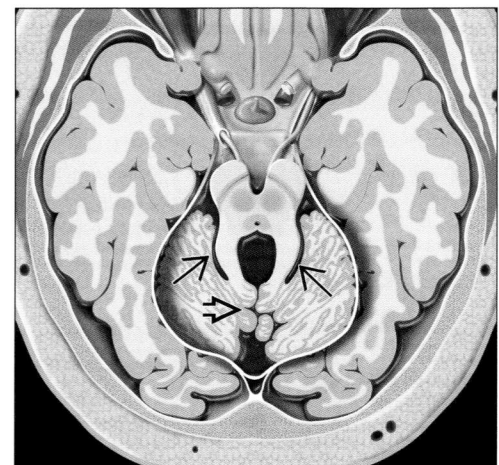 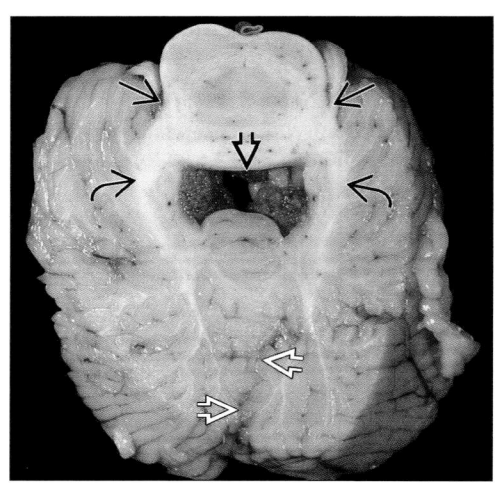

36-46A. Sagittal T2WI in a patient with classic Joubert shows small misshapen vermis ⇨, upwardly convex superior fourth ventricle ⇨, rounded enlarged fastigial point ⇗. 36-46B. Axial scan in the same patient shows "molar tooth" sign: Foreshortened midbrain with narrow isthmus ⇨, thick superior cerebellar peduncles ⇨ surrounding an elongated fourth ventricle, and disorganized cleft vermis ⇗.

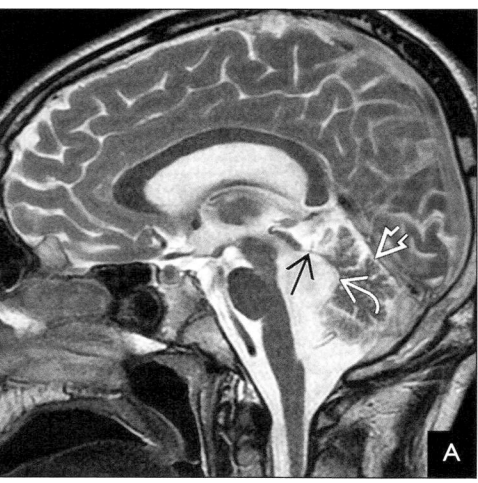 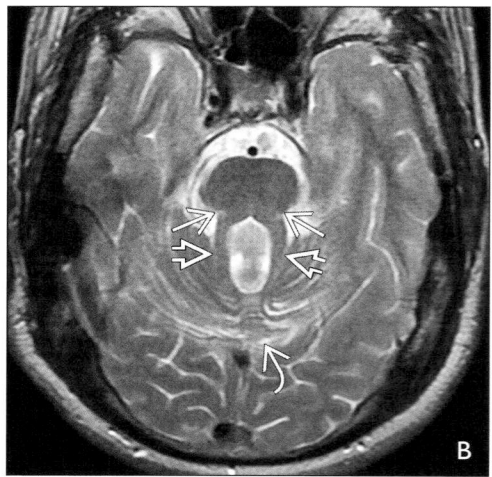

Hindbrain Malformations: Imaging

	Vermis Position	Vermis Size	Torcular Position	Cerebellar Hemispheres	Fourth Ventricle
Mega cisterna magna	N	N	N	N	N
Blake pouch cyst	Rotated	N	N	N	"Enlarged"; communicates with posterior fossa via valleculae
Arachnoid cyst	May be displaced	N or compressed	N	N or compressed	N or compressed
Vermian dysgenesis	May be rotated	Small or absent	N	N	Abnormal shape; lacks normal fastigial point
Dandy-Walker malformation	Rotated	Small or absent	Elevated	Often small	Dilated, enlarged; lacks normal fastigial point
Cerebellar hypoplasia	N	Small	N	Small	N or small
Pontocerebellar hypoplasia	N	Small	N	Small	Pontine bulge missing
Cerebellar disruption	N	N or small	N	Asymmetric; one smaller, abnormal structure	Variable depending on part of cerebellum disrupted
Rhombencephalo-synapsis		Absent	N	Fused with continuous horizontal folia	Small; lacks normal fastigial point
Joubert syndrome		Small or absent	N	Small	Large (associated with elongated superior cerebellar peduncles and "molar tooth" sign)

Table 36-1. *N = normal.*

Unclassified Cerebellar Dysplasias

A group of unclassified focal or diffuse dysplasias that involves the cerebellar hemispheres and/or vermis. These are not associated with other known malformations or syndromes such as molar tooth malformation, Dandy-Walker spectrum, congenital muscular dystrophy, or rhombencephalosynapsis.

These unclassified cerebellar dysplasias demonstrate asymmetry or focal disruption of cerebellar folia and sulcal morphology. A variety of findings are seen on imaging studies. Enlarged, vertically oriented fissures or clefts **(36-48)**, disordered or primitive foliation, lack of normal white matter arborization, gray matter heterotopias, and small cyst-like cavities in the subcortical white matter are some of the many abnormalities seen in such cases **(36-49)**.

Selected References

Posterior Fossa Anatomy

Gross Anatomy

- Carrasco CR: Brainstem and cerebellum overview. In Harnsberger HR: Diagnostic and Surgical Imaging Anatomy: Brain, Head and Neck, Spine. Salt Lake City: Amirsys Publishing. I.104-13, 2006

Chiari Malformations

Chiari 1

- Aiken AH et al: Incidence of cerebellar tonsillar ectopia in idiopathic intracranial hypertension: a mimic of the Chiari I malformation. AJNR Am J Neuroradiol. Epub ahead of print, 2012

- Bunck AC et al: Magnetic resonance 4D flow analysis of cerebrospinal fluid dynamics in Chiari I malformation with and without syringomyelia. Eur Radiol. 22(9):1860-70, 2012

- Di Rocco C et al: Hydrocephalus and Chiari type I malformation. Childs Nerv Syst. 27(10):1653-64, 2011

- Loukas M et al: Associated disorders of Chiari type I malformations: a review. Neurosurg Focus. 31(3):E3, 2011

- Massimi L et al: Chiari type I malformation in children. Adv Tech Stand Neurosurg. 37:143-211, 2011

- Sekula RF Jr et al: The pathogenesis of Chiari I malformation and syringomyelia. Neurol Res. 33(3):232-9, 2011

- Singhal A et al: Natural history of untreated syringomyelia in pediatric patients. Neurosurg Focus. 31(6):E13, 2011

- Strahle J et al: Chiari malformation type I and syrinx in children undergoing magnetic resonance imaging. J Neurosurg Pediatr. 8(2):205-13, 2011

- Albert GW et al: Chiari malformation type I in children younger than age 6 years: presentation and surgical outcome. J Neurosurg Pediatr. 5(6):554-61, 2010

Chiari 2

- Geerdink N et al: Essential features of Chiari II malformation in MR imaging: an interobserver reliability study-part 1. Childs Nerv Syst. 28(7):977-85, 2012

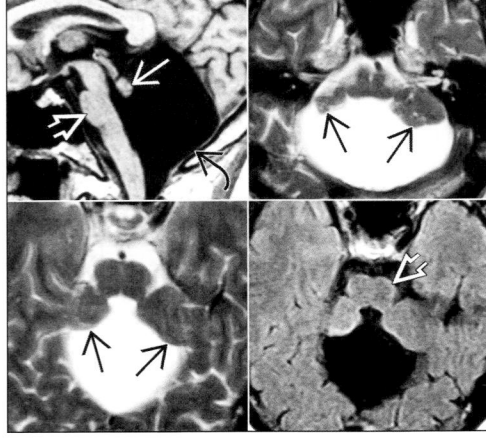
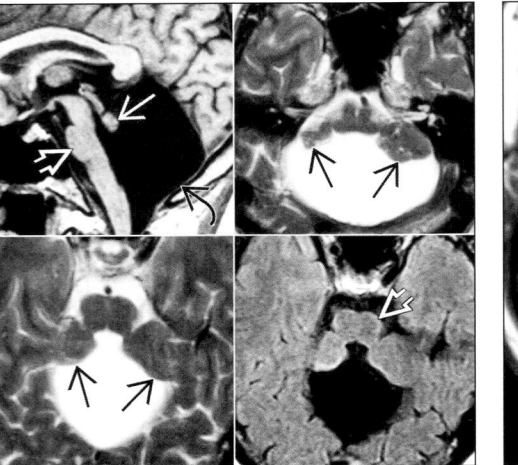
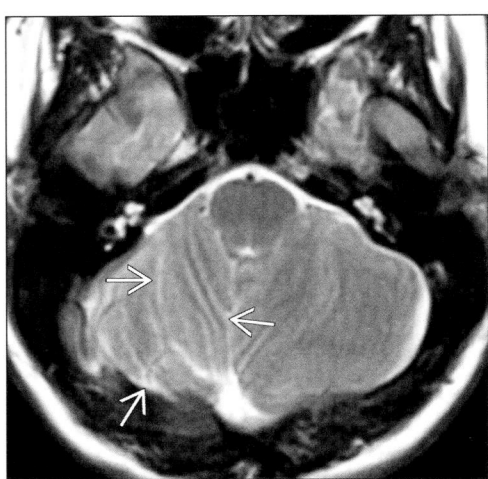

36-47. Extreme cerebellar hypoplasia with small brainstem ➡, nearly "empty" appearing but normal-sized PF ➡, tiny nubbins of vermian ➡, cerebellar remnants ➡. 36-48. Axial T2WI of a patient with unclassified cerebellar dysplasia shows several clefts ➡ with abnormal-appearing and misaligned folia.

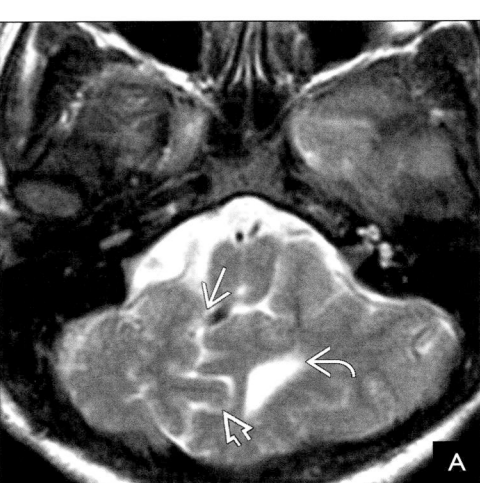
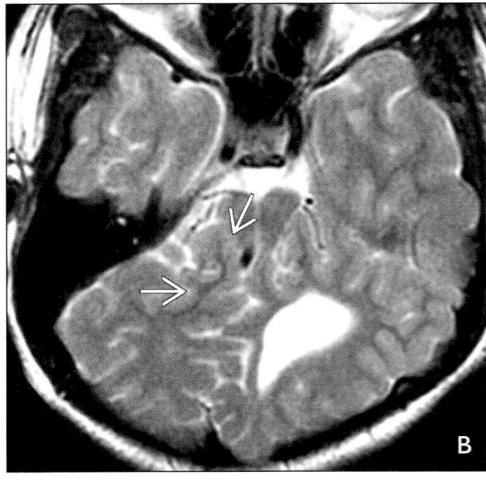

36-49A. Unclassified cerebellar dysplasia with cleft ➡, interdigitating dysplastic folia ➡, hemispheric cyst ➡. 36-49B. More cephalad scan in the same patient shows the cyst, cleft, and appearance of polymicrogyria ➡ in the grossly abnormal folia.

- Chiapparini L et al: Neuroradiological diagnosis of Chiari malformations. Neurol Sci. 32 Suppl 3:S283-6, 2011

Chiari Variants

- Tubbs RS et al: A new form of herniation: the Chiari V malformation. Childs Nerv Syst. 28(2):305-7, 2012
- Markunas CA et al: Clinical, radiological, and genetic similarities between patients with Chiari type I and type 0 malformations. J Neurosurg Pediatr. 9(4):372-8, 2012
- Brockmeyer DL: The complex Chiari: issues and management strategies. Neurol Sci. 32 Suppl 3:S345-7, 2011

Hindbrain Malformations

Dandy-Walker Spectrum

- Blank MC et al: Multiple developmental programs are altered by loss of Zic1 and Zic4 to cause Dandy-Walker malformation cerebellar pathogenesis. Development. 138(6):1207-16, 2011
- Garel C et al: The fetal cerebellum: development and common malformations. J Child Neurol. 26(12):1483-92, 2011
- Judkins AR: Dandy-Walker malformation. In Golden JA et al: Pathology and Genetics: Developmental Neuropathology. Basel: ISN Neuropath Press. 95-9, 2004

Miscellaneous Malformations

- Ishak GE et al: Rhombencephalosynapsis: a hindbrain malformation associated with incomplete separation of midbrain and forebrain, hydrocephalus and a broad spectrum of severity. Brain. 135(Pt 5):1370-86, 2012
- Garel C et al: The fetal cerebellum: development and common malformations. J Child Neurol. 26(12):1483-92, 2011
- Brancati F et al: Joubert Syndrome and related disorders. Orphanet J Rare Dis. 5:20, 2010
- Saleem SN et al: Role of MR imaging in prenatal diagnosis of pregnancies at risk for Joubert syndrome and related cerebellar disorders. Am J Neuroradiol. 31(3):424-9, 2010
- Poretti A et al: Diffusion tensor imaging in Joubert syndrome. AJNR Am J Neuroradiol. 28(10):1929-33, 2007

37

Commissural and Cortical Maldevelopment

Corpus callosum dysgenesis and malformations of cortical development (MCDs) are two of the most important congenital brain anomalies. Anomalies of the cerebral commissures are the most common of all congenital brain malformations, and corpus callosum dysgenesis is the single most common malformation that accompanies other developmental brain anomalies.

Although they affect very different parts of the forebrain, commissural and cortical malformations share a very important feature: They arise when migrating precursor cells fail to reach their target destinations.

We begin this chapter with a brief consideration of normal development and anatomy of the cerebral commissures, then focus on callosal dysgenesis as the most important anomaly that affects these white matter (WM) tracts.

We devote the second half of the chapter to malformations of cortical development. MCDs are intrinsically epileptogenic and may be responsible for 25-40% of all medically refractory childhood epilepsies. Prior to the development of high-resolution MR imaging techniques, many complex partial epilepsies were considered cryptogenic. Their imaging detection, localization, and characterization has become increasingly important in patient management.

Normal Development and Anatomy of the Cerebral Commissures

In this section, we briefly review normal development of the commissures and then delineate their gross and imaging anatomy.

Normal Development

The telencephalon has three major commissural tracts: The corpus callosum (CC), which is the largest and most prominent, the anterior commissure, and the hippocampal (posterior) commissure. Coordinated transfer of information between the cerebral hemispheres is essential for normal brain function and occurs via these three axonal commissures.

Commissural development is a carefully choreographed process in which axons from cortical neurons are actively guided across the midline to reach their targets in the contralateral hemisphere. A set of genetically mediated steering mechanisms are used by these axons to locate and innervate their targets.

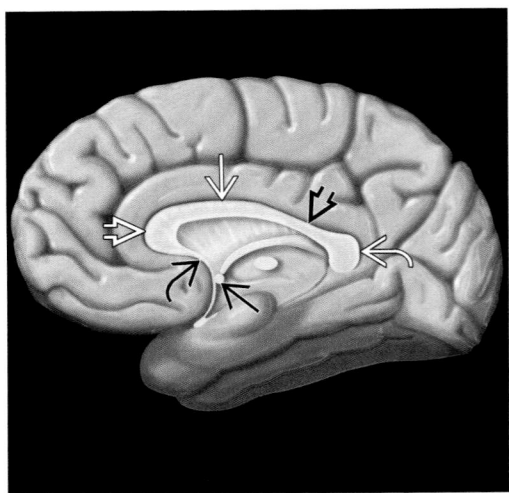

37-1. Sagittal graphic of the anterior commissure ⇨ and corpus callosum segments: Rostrum ↗, genu ⇛, body ⇛, isthmus ⇗, splenium ↗.

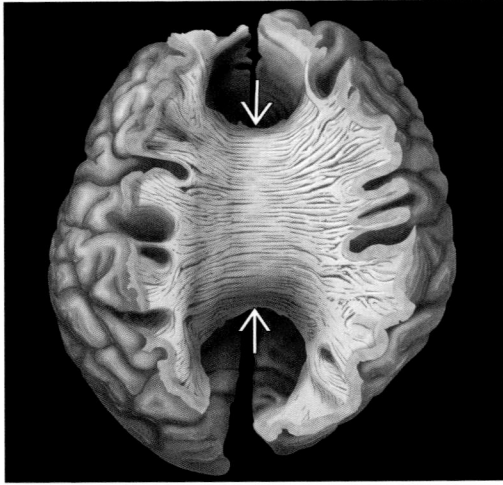

37-2. Graphic depicts fibers from corona radiata converging into and crossing transversely through the corpus callosum ⇛.

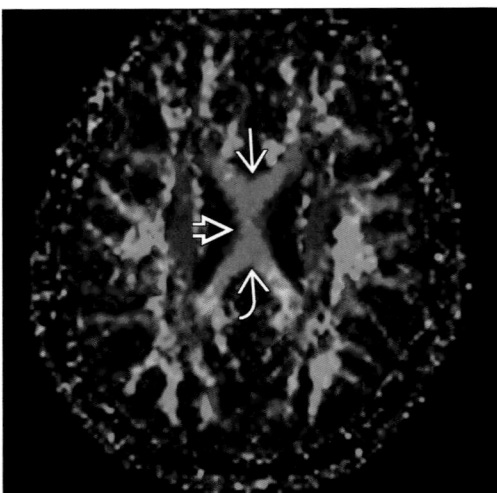

37-3. DTI shows the normal red X-shaped corpus callosum formed by the genu ⇛ with forceps minor, body ⇛, splenium ⇛ with forceps major.

The anterior commissure is the first forebrain commissure to develop (eighth fetal week). The hippocampal commissure forms posteriorly around week 11 and is followed by axons that eventually become the posterior body and splenium of the CC.

The CC forms in two separate segments. Between 13-14 fetal weeks, anterior axons cross a guiding structure called the glial sling while others follow the hippocampal commissure posteriorly. The genu, rostrum, and body appear in rapid succession; the splenium does not form until 18-19 weeks. Fiber bundles in the anterior and posterior callosum eventually unite to form a single continuous structure, the definitive corpus callosum.

At birth, the CC is very thin and relatively flat in gross appearance. It continues to grow for several postnatal months. As myelination proceeds, the genu and splenium thicken noticeably. Both the length and thickness of the CC also increase. By 10 months of age, the overall appearance resembles that of a normal adult.

Normal Gross and Imaging Anatomy

Corpus Callosum

The CC is the largest and most important of the forebrain commissures. It is composed of five parts. From front to back these are the rostrum, genu, body, isthmus, and splenium. The **rostrum** is the smallest segment and connects the orbital surfaces of the frontal lobes. A prominent anterior "knee"—the **genu**—connects the lateral and medial frontal lobes **(37-1)**. White matter fibers curve anterolaterally from the genu into the frontal lobes as the forceps minor.

The longest CC segment is the **body**. Its fibers pass laterally and intersect with projection fibers of the corona radiata **(37-2)**. The body connects broad regions of each hemispheric cortex together and forms a red *X* on axial DTI scans **(37-3)**.

The **isthmus** is a shorter, slightly narrower area that lies between the posterior body and splenium. The isthmus connects the pre- and postcentral gyri and auditory cortex with their counterparts in the contralateral hemisphere. The **splenium** is the expanded, rounded termination of the CC. Most of its fibers curve posterolaterally into the occipital lobes as the **forceps major**.

Sagittal T1 and T2 scans demonstrate the rostrum as a thin WM tract that curves posteroinferiorly from the genu. The dorsal CC surface is typically not straight but has a slightly "wavy" appearance with a distinct posterior narrowing—the isthmus—just before the the CC widens again into the splenium **(37-4)**.

Coronal scans show the CC curving from side to side across the midline. Anteriorly, the genu is seen as a continuous band of WM connecting the frontal lobes. More posteriorly, the CC lies above the fornices. Bands of WM fibers fan outward from the splenium into the forceps major.

Anterior Commissure

The anterior commissure (AC) is a transversely oriented bundle of compact, heavily myelinated fibers that crosses the midline anterior to the fornix. It is much smaller than the CC but is a crucial anatomic landmark for stereotactic neurosurgery.

The AC lies in the anterior wall of the third ventricle **(37-5)**. From the midline, it curves laterally in the basal forebrain and splits into two fascicles. The smaller more anterior bundle courses toward the orbitofrontal cortex and olfactory tract. The much larger posterior bundle splays out into the temporal lobe. The AC connects the anterior parts of the temporal lobes **(37-6)** and lies antero-superior to the temporal horn of the lateral ventricle.

On sagittal T1 scans, the AC is seen as a hyperintense ovoid structure lying midway up the anterior wall of the third ventricle. On axial T2 scans, the AC can be identified as a compact well-defined hypointense band of tissue lying just in front of the third ventricle. As it courses laterally, both sides of the AC curve slightly anteriorly to resemble an archer's bow on axial MR scans.

Hippocampal Commissure

The hippocampal commissure (HC) is the smallest of the three major commissures. It is a transversely oriented fiber bundle that crosses the midline in the posterior pineal lamina.

In contrast to the CC and AC, the HC is less easily distinguished on MR scans. In the midline sagittal plane, its myelinated fibers blend imperceptibly with those of the inferomedial WM in the CC splenium. On coronal scans through the lateral ventricle atria, the HC can be seen lying below the CC where its fibers blend in with those of the fornices.

Commissural Anomalies

Any one of or combination of the three forebrain commissures can be affected by developmental failures. Recognizing the surprisingly broad spectrum of commissural malformations and delineating any associated abnormalities is essential for accurate and complete diagnosis.

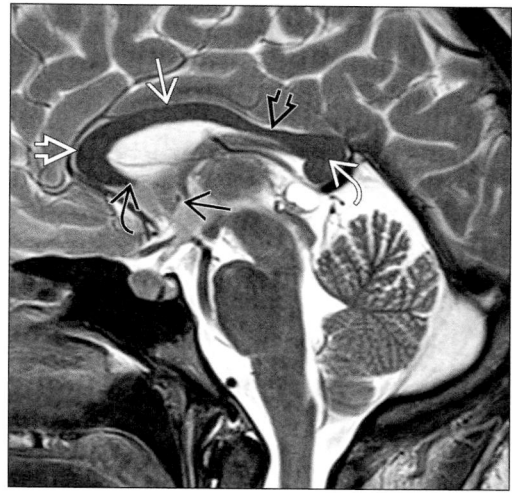

37-4. Sagittal T2WI shows AC ⇥ as well as the rostrum ⇗, genu ⇥, body ⇥, isthmus ⇥, and splenium ⇗ of the CC.

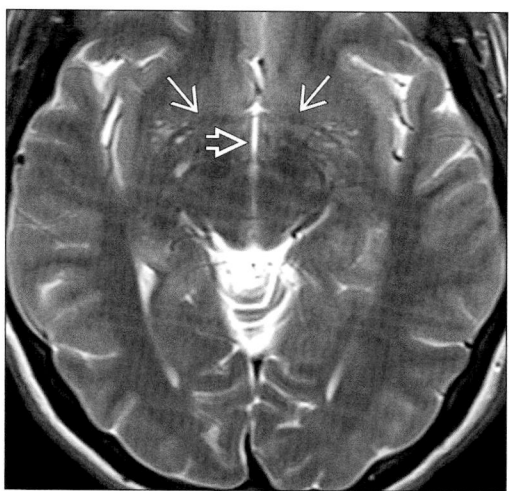

37-5. Axial T2WI shows the compact, hypointense, bow-shaped anterior commissure ⇥ passing in front of the third ventricle ⇥.

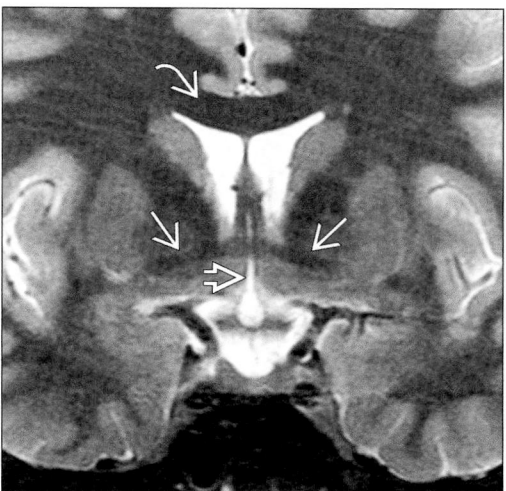

37-6. Coronal T2WI shows the anterior commissure ⇥, third ventricle ⇥, body of the corpus callosum ⇗.

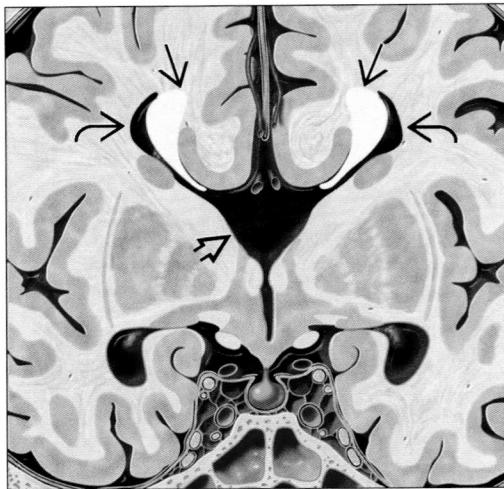

37-7. CC agenesis shows "Viking helmet" appearance with "high-riding" third ventricle ⊵, pointed lateral ventricles ⇗, Probst bundles ➡.

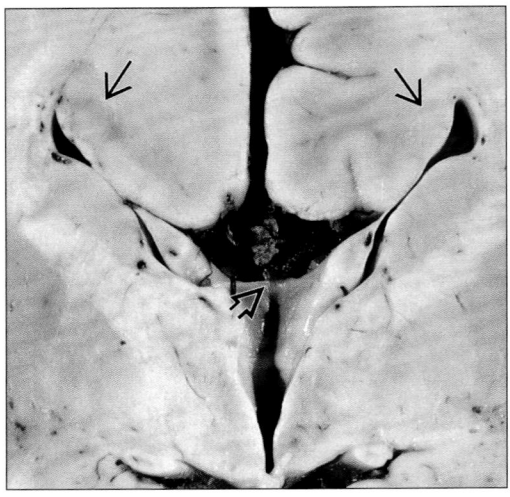

37-8. Coronal autopsy of coronal agenesis shows thin third ventricle roof ⊵, Probst bundles ➡. (Courtesy J. Townsend, MD.)

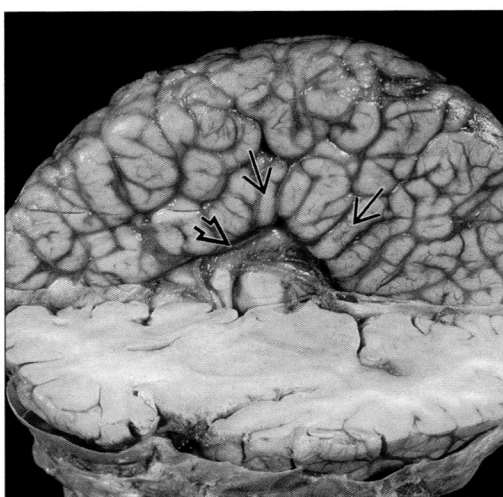

37-9. CC agenesis shows absent cingulate gyrus, "radiating" gyri ⇗ converging on "high-riding" third ventricle ⊵. (Courtesy R. Hewlett, MD.)

We now discuss corpus callosum malformations together with some representative syndromes and associated lesions.

Callosal Dysgenesis Spectrum

Terminology

The corpus callosum (CC) can be completely absent (agenesis) **(37-7)**, **(37-8)** or partially formed (hypogenesis). **Complete CC agenesis** is almost always accompanied by the absence of the hippocampal commissure (HC); the anterior commissure (AC) is usually present and normal. If the CC is hypogenetic, the posterior segments and the inferior genu and rostrum are usually absent.

Pathology

In *complete* CC agenesis, all five segments are missing. The **cingulate gyrus** is absent on sagittal sections while the hemispheres demonstrate a radiating **"spoke-wheel" gyral pattern** extending perpendicularly to the roof of the third ventricle **(37-9)**.

On coronal sections, the **"high-riding" third ventricle** looks as if it opens directly into the interhemispheric fissure. It is actually covered by a thin membranous roof that bulges into the interhemispheric fissure, displacing the fornices laterally. The lateral ventricles have upturned, pointed corners **(37-8)**.

A prominent longitudinal WM tract called the **Probst bundle** is situated just inside the apex of each ventricle **(37-7)**. These bundles consist of the misdirected commissural fibers, which should have crossed the midline but instead course from front to back, indenting the medial walls of the lateral ventricles.

The septi pellucidi often appear absent but actually have widely separated leaves that course laterally—not vertically—from the fornices to the Probst bundles.

Axial sections show that the lateral ventricles are parallel and nonconverging. The occipital horns are often disproportionately dilated, a condition termed colpocephaly.

The gross pathology of CC *hypogenesis* varies according to which segments are missing. The splenium is usually small or absent.

Clinical Issues

Epidemiology and Demographics. CC dysgenesis is the most common CNS malformation and is found in 3-5% of individuals with neurodevelopmental disorders. It has a prevalence of at least 1:4,000 live births. Nonsyndromic CC dysgenesis is found in patients of all ages.

PRESENTATION. Minor CC dysgenesis/hypogenesis is often discovered incidentally on imaging studies or at autopsy. Major commissural malformations are associated with seizures, developmental delay, and symptoms secondary to disruptions of the hypothalamic-pituitary axis.

Imaging

CT FINDINGS. Axial NECT scans show parallel, nonconverging, widely separated lateral ventricles. Disproportionate enlargement of the occipital horns is common.

MR FINDINGS. Sagittal T1 and T2 scans best demonstrate complete CC absence or partial dysgenesis.

Complete corpus callosum agenesis. With complete agenesis, the third ventricle appears continuous with the interhemispheric fissure and is surrounded dorsally by fingers of radiating gyri that "point" toward the third ventricle **(37-10)**.

A midline interhemispheric cyst may be present above the third ventricle. Such cysts can be ventricular outpouchings or separate structures that do not communicate with the ventricular system.

An azygous anterior cerebral artery (ACA) can be seen "wandering" upward in the interhemispheric fissure. Look for associated malformations of the eyes, hindbrain, and hypothalamic-pituitary axis.

Axial scans demonstrate the parallel lateral ventricles especially well. The prominent myelinated tracts of the Probst bundles can appear quite prominent **(37-14)**.

Coronal scans show a "Viking helmet" or "moose head" appearance caused by the curved, upwardly pointed lateral ventricles and "high-riding" third ventricle that expands into the interhemispheric fissure. The Probst bundles are seen as densely myelinated tracts lying just inside the lateral ventricle bodies. The hippocampi appear abnormally rounded and vertically oriented. Moderately enlarged temporal horns are common. Look for malformations such as heterotopic gray matter **(37-13)**.

DTI is especially helpful in depicting CC agenesis. The normal red (right-to-left encoded) color of the corpus callosum is absent. Instead, prominent front-to-back (green) tracts of the Probst bundles are seen **(37-15)**.

Corpus callosum hypogenesis. In partial agenesis, the rostrum and splenium are usually absent **(37-11)**, and the remaining genu and body often have a "blocky," thickened appearance **(37-12)**. The hippocampal commissure is typically absent, but the AC is generally preserved and often appears quite normal or even larger than usual.

ANGIOGRAPHY. In complete CC agenesis, CTA, DSA, and MRA demonstrate an azygous ACA that courses

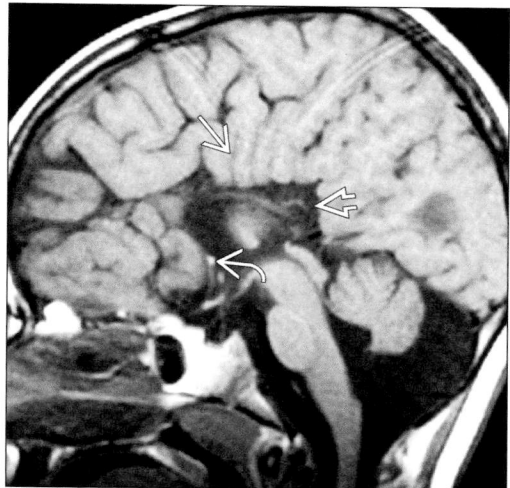

37-10. "Spoke-wheel" gyri ➡ *converge on third ventricle* ➡. *Anterior commissure is normal* ➡. *Hippocampal commissure is absent. CC agenesis.*

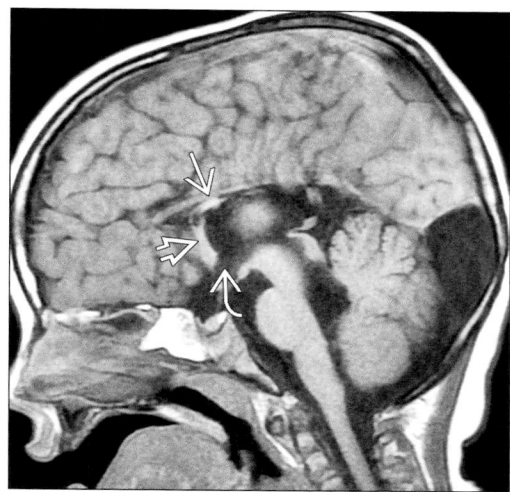

37-11. Genu ➡, *remnant of body* ➡ *are present. Rostrum* ➡, *splenium are absent. CC hypogenesis.*

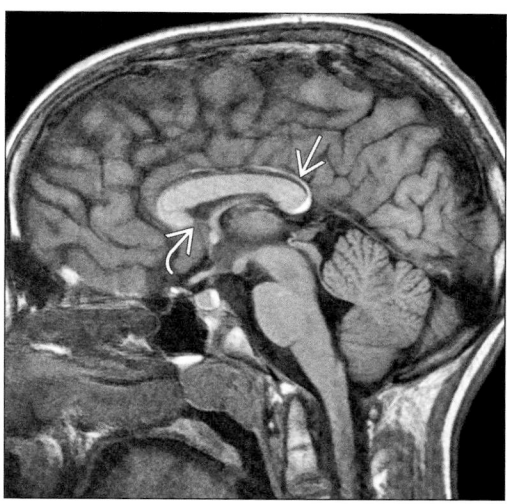

37-12. CC appears short and "blocky" with absent rostrum ➡, *tapered splenium with curvilinear lipoma* ➡. *Mild callosal hypogenesis.*

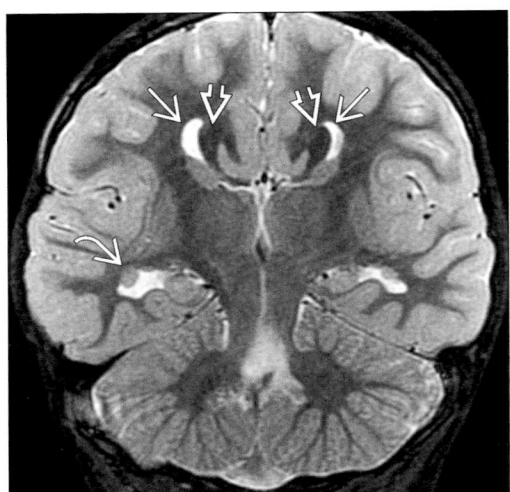

37-13. Coronal T2WI shows "Viking helmet" of CC agenesis with curving, upturned lateral ventricles ➡, *Probst bundles* ➡, *heterotopic GM* ➡.

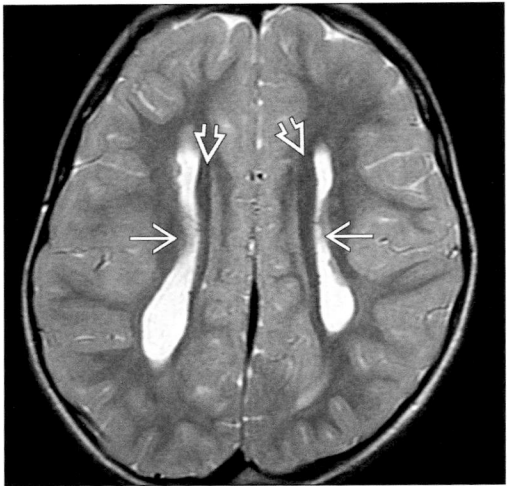

37-14. Axial scan shows parallel, "nonconverging" lateral ventricles ➡, *Probst bundles* ➡.

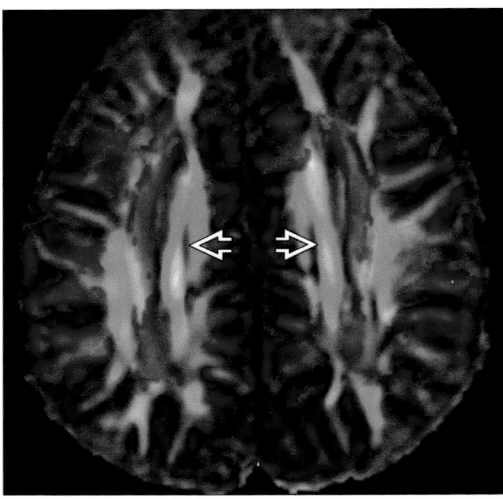

37-15. Axial DTI shows absence of normal red X-shaped corpus callosum. Probst bundles ➡ *are green, indicating anterior-to-posterior course.*

directly upward within the interhemispheric fissure **(37-17)**.

Differential Diagnosis

The major differential diagnosis of CC dysgenesis is destruction caused by **trauma**, **surgery (callosotomy)**, or **ischemia**. Occasionally, if the **hippocampal commissure** forms but the CC is absent, the HC may mimic a remnant portion of the CC on sagittal images. Coronal views show that the HC connects the fornices, not the hemispheres.

Associated Anomalies and Syndromes

The corpus callosum (CC) forms at the same time as the cerebral hemispheres and cerebellum are undergoing rapid changes. Neuronal migration also peaks during the same period. Although CC dysgenesis can occur as an isolated phenomenon, it is not surprising that—of all the malformations—CC anomalies are the single most common malformation associated with other CNS anomalies and syndromes.

Malformations Associated with Callosal Dysgenesis

Chiari 2 malformation, **Dandy-Walker spectrum**, **frontonasal dysplasia**, **median cleft face** syndromes, syndromic **craniosynostoses**, **hypothalamic-pituitary** anomalies, **cerebellar hypoplasia/dysplasia**, and **malformations of cortical development** all have an increased prevalence of CC anomalies. Corpus callosum agenesis and regional increases in cortical thickness are the most common brain morphologic defects in **fetal alcohol syndrome**.

Genetic Conditions with Callosal Involvement

Anomalies of the cerebral commissures have been described in nearly 200 different syndromes! A few of the more striking examples are included here.

AICARDI SYNDROME. Aicardi syndrome is an X-linked neurodevelopmental disorder associated with severe cognitive and motor impairment. It occurs almost exclusively in females and is defined by the diagnostic triad of corpus callosum dysgenesis, chorioretinal lacunae, and infantile spasms. Other common associated abnormalities are polymicrogyria, periventricular and subcortical heterotopic gray matter, and choroid plexus papillomas.

Callosal agenesis or hypogenesis—often with interhemispheric cysts—is the most common anatomic abnormality in Aicardi syndrome **(37-16)**. DTI in patients with Aicardi syndrome shows gross deficits in white matter organization, with absence of multiple major corticocortical association WM tracts such as the left arcuate fasciculus.

APERT SYNDROME. Apert syndrome is also called acrocephalosyndactylia type 1. Apert syndrome is characterized by craniostenosis, mid-face hypoplasia, and symmetric syndactylia of the hands and feet. Associated CNS malformations are frequent; the most common are CC or septi pellucidi hypoplasias.

CRASH SYNDROME. CRASH syndrome—also known as **X-linked hydrocephalus** and hereditary stenosis of the aqueduct of Sylvius—is a rare inherited disorder characterized by **c**orpus callosum hypoplasia, mental **r**etardation, **a**dducted thumbs, **s**pastic paraplegia, and **h**ydrocephalus. CRASH is caused by mutation in the gene (*L1CAM*) that regulates the L1 cell adhesion molecule, which plays an essential role in normal development of the CNS.

22Q11.2 DELETION SYNDROME. The 22q11.2 deletion syndrome (22qDS) is also known as **DiGeorge syndrome**. Atypical facial morphometry, obsessive-compulsive disorder, autistic spectrum disorder, and other psy-

chological disturbances are common in patients with 22qDS. Many patients have an abnormally large, misshapen CC.

WILLIAMS SYNDROME. Williams syndrome (WS) is caused by a microdeletion of genes on locus 7q11.23, which is crucial for neuronal migration and maturation. Overall brain size is reduced, and some degree of CC dysgenesis is typical. The CC in WS is smaller or shorter than normal with a less concave shape.

FRAGILE X SYNDROME. Fragile X syndrome is an X-linked disorder caused by the expansion of a single trinucleotide gene sequence (CGG) on the X chromosome and the most common inherited cause of mental retardation in boys. The CC is generally thinned but present.

MORNING GLORY SYNDROME. Morning glory syndrome is a rare optic disc anomaly named for its characteristic appearance on funduscopic examination. A wide funnel-shaped excavation of the optic disc with whitish central gliosis is surrounded by retinal vessels that emerge from the disc periphery. CNS findings include retinal coloboma, scleral staphyloma, optic nerve

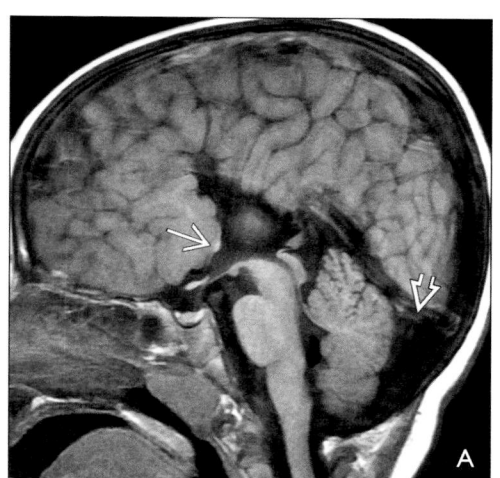

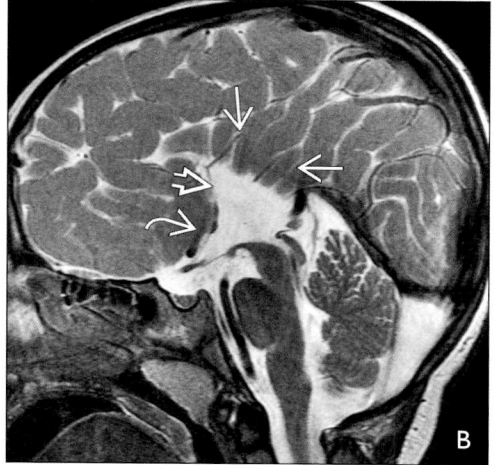

37-16A. Sagittal T1WI in a 3-year-old girl with Aicardi syndrome shows complete agenesis of the corpus callosum and hippocampal commissure. The anterior commissure ➡ is present but small. Note mild Dandy-Walker malformation with mega cisterna magna ➡. 37-16B. Sagittal T2WI shows complete CC agenesis, absent cingulate gyrus, "high-riding" third ventricle ➡, radiating gyri ➡, azygous ACA ➡.

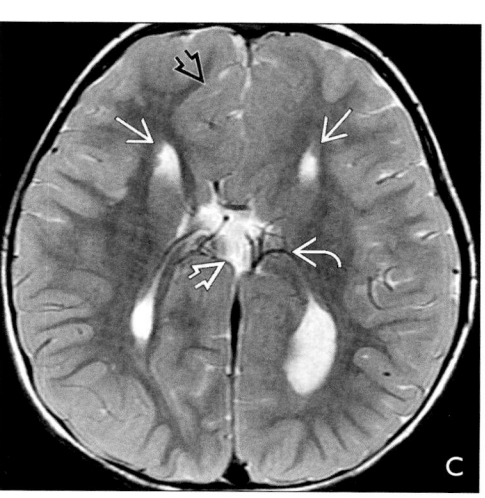

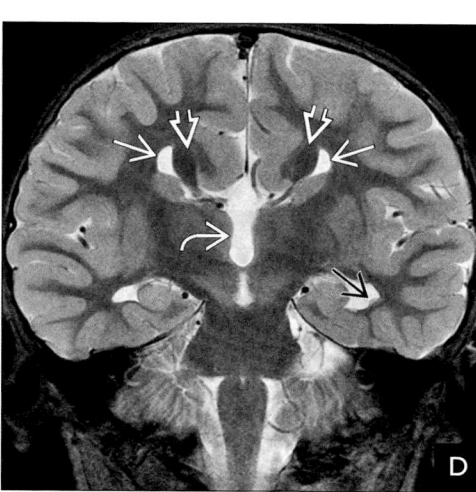

37-16C. Axial T2WI in the same patient shows a small interhemispheric cyst ➡, branches of azygous ACA ➡, parallel lateral ventricles, heterotopic GM ➡, pachygyria ➡. 37-16D. Coronal T2WI shows classic "moose head" with "high-riding" third ventricle ➡ ("face" of the moose), pointed lateral ventricles ➡ ("horns" of the moose), prominent Probst bundles ➡, small nodule of heterotopic GM ➡.

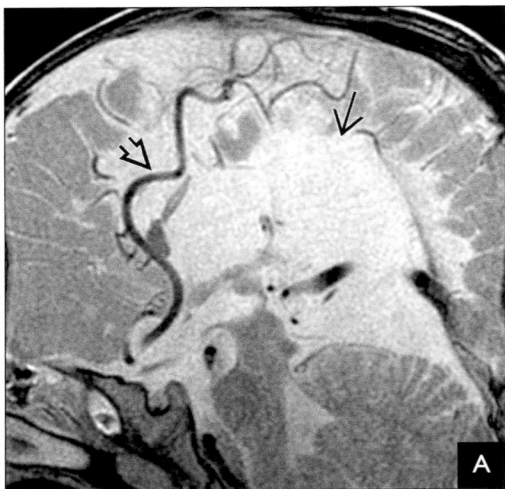

37-17A. Sagittal T2WI shows CC agenesis, interhemispheric cyst ➡, azygous ACA ⊳.

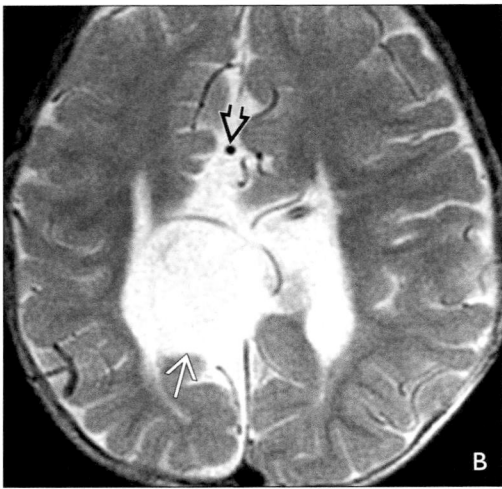

37-17B. Axial T2WI in the same patient shows parallel lateral ventricles, large interhemispheric cyst ➡, azygous ACA ⊳.

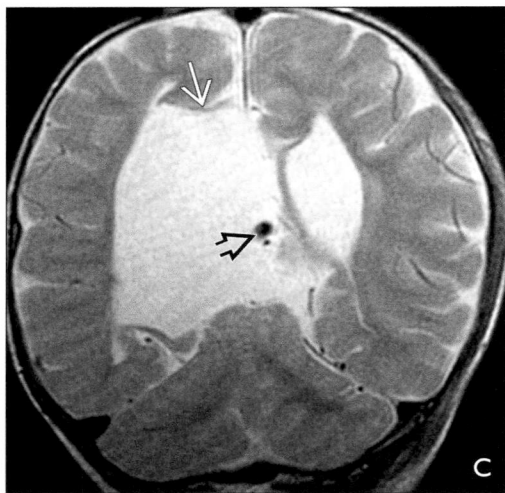

37-17C. Coronal T2WI shows the interhemispheric cyst ➡, azygous artery ⊳.

cyst, and midline disorders such as CC dysgenesis, basal encephalocele, and frontonasal dysplasia.

CALLOSAL DYSGENESIS SPECTRUM

Terminology
- Complete absence of corpus callosum (CC) = agenesis
  - Hippocampal commissure (HC) absent
  - Anterior commissure (AC) often present
  - All 3 absent = tricommissural agenesis
- Hypogenetic, dysgenetic CC
  - Rostrum, splenium often absent in partial agenesis
  - Partial posterior agenesis = HC, splenium, ± posterior body

Etiology and Pathology
- Embryonic guiding mechanisms fail
  - Axons may fail to form
  - Molecular guidance fails
  - Glial sling and/or HC fail to develop normally
  - Failure to guide axons across midline
- Multiple genes implicated

Clinical Issues
- Most common CNS malformation
- Found in 3-5% of neurodevelopmental disorders

Imaging
- Sagittal
  - Partial or complete CC agenesis
  - Third ventricle appears "open" to interhemispheric fissure
  - Cingulate gyrus absent → gyri "radiate" outward from third ventricle
- Axial
  - Lateral ventricles parallel, nonconverging, widely separated
- Coronal
  - "Viking helmet" or "moose head" appearance
  - "High-riding" third ventricle
  - Pointed, upcurving lateral ventricles
  - Probst bundles

Associated Anomalies and Syndromes
- Malformations
  - Chiari 2
  - Dandy-Walker
  - Frontonasal dysplasia, clefts
  - Cerebellar hypoplasia/dysplasia
  - Hypothalamic-pituitary axis malformations
  - Malformations of cortical development
- Nearly 200 inherited syndromes
  - Aicardi syndrome
  - Apert syndrome
  - CRASH syndrome
  - 22q11.2 deletion syndrome (DiGeorge)
  - Morning glory syndrome

Malformations of Cortical Development Overview

Malformations of cortical development (MCDs) represent a broad spectrum of cortical lesions resulting from deranged developmental processes and formation of the cortical mantle. These malformations were once defined as "neuronal migration disorders." It is now recognized that not all cortical abnormalities are caused by deranged migration. The umbrella term MCD is used to denote a heterogeneous group of focal or diffuse lesions that develop during cortical ontogenesis.

The three major stages of cortical development are **proliferation**, **neuronal migration**, and **postmigrational development**. These stages have some overlap: Proliferation continues after neuronal migration starts, and postmigrational development (e.g., process of cortical organization) begins before neuronal migration ends. In addition, cells resulting from abnormal proliferation often neither migrate nor organize properly.

Barkovich et al suggest classifying MCDs according to which of the three development stages is primarily affected. Group I consists of **abnormalities of neuronal and glial proliferation or apoptosis** (resulting in either too many or too few cells). Three subcategories reflect malformations due to (A) reduced proliferation or accelerated apoptosis (congenital microcephalies), (B) increased proliferation or decreased apoptosis (megaloencephalies), and (C) abnormal proliferation (focal and diffuse dysgenesis and dysplasia).

Group II represents **abnormalities of neuronal migration** and has been divided into four subgroups: (A) abnormalities in the neuroependyma during initiation of migration cause periventricular nodular heterotopia; (B) lissencephalies are caused by *generalized* abnormalities of transmantle migration; (C) *localized* abnormalities of transmantle migration result in subcortical heterotopia; and (D) terminal migration anomalies and defects in the pial limiting membranes result in the cobblestone malformations.

Abnormalities of **postmigrational development** comprise group III. These result from injury to the cortex during later stages and are associated with prenatal and perinatal insults.

A simplified version of the new classification together with representative malformations in each group and subgroup is summarized in the following box.

MALFORMATIONS OF CORTICAL DEVELOPMENT

I. Malformations Secondary to Glial/Neuronal Proliferation or Apoptosis
- A. Microcephaly
- B. Megalencephaly
  - Polymicrogyria and megalencephaly
- C. Cortical dysgeneses with abnormal cell proliferation
  - Cortical tubers
  - Focal cortical dysplasia (FCD IIb, Taylor type)
  - Hemimegaloencephaly

II. Malformations Secondary to Abnormalities of Neuronal Migration
- A. Heterotopia
  - Periventricular nodular heterotopia
- B. Lissencephaly spectrum
  - Agyria
  - Pachygyria
  - Subcortical band heterotopia
- C. Subcortical heterotopia and sublobar dysplasia
  - Large focal collections of neurons in deep WM
- D. Cobblestone malformations
  - Congenital muscular dystrophies

III. Abnormalities of Postmigrational Development
- A. Polymicrogyria
- B. Schizencephaly
- C. Focal cortical dysplasia (types I and III)
- D. Postmigrational microcephaly

Malformations with Abnormal Cell Numbers/Types

Microcephalies

Microcephaly (MCPH), which literally means "small head," can be primary (genetic) or secondary (nongenetic).

Primary MCPH is a congenital malformation caused by a defect in brain development. Secondary MCPH is an *acquired* disorder resulting from an insult that affects fetal, neonatal, or infantile brain growth. Ischemia, infection, maternal diabetes, and trauma are the most common causes. A few examples of MCPH microcephaly induced by intrauterine infection are illustrated in Chapter 12. In this section, we focus on primary (congenital) microcephaly.

Terminology and Classification

Microcephaly is defined as a head circumference more than three standard deviations below the mean for age and sex. In primary MCPH, there is no evidence of other

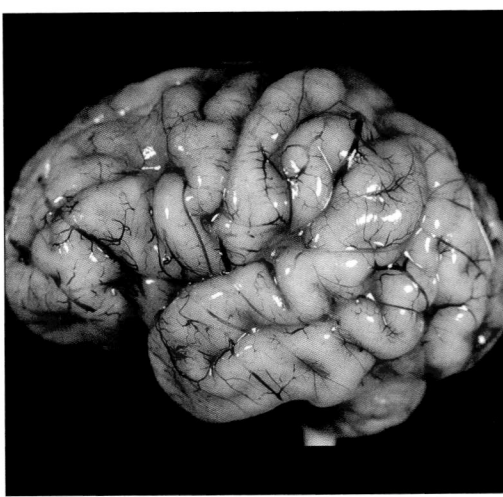

37-18. *Autopsy shows microcephaly with simplified gyral pattern. The gyri appear less convoluted than normal. (Courtesy R. Hewlett, MD.)*

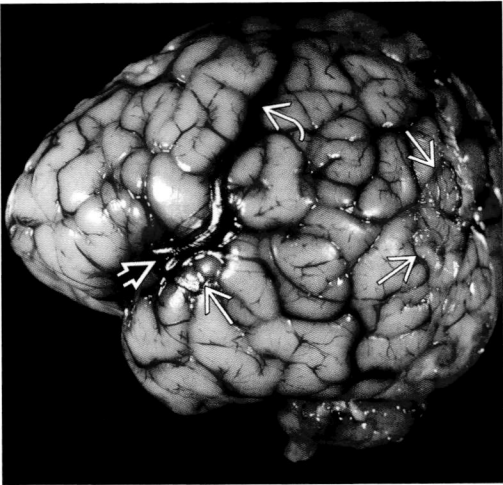

37-19. *Microcephaly with polymicrogyria* ➡, *abnormal veins in sylvian fissure* ➡, *large vein of Trolard* ➘. *(Courtesy R. Hewlett, MD.)*

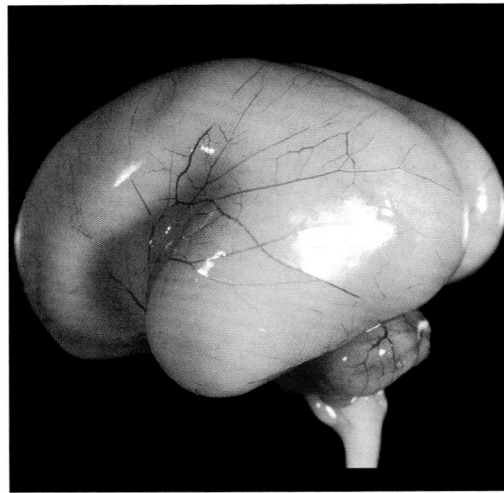

37-20. *Microcephaly with lissencephaly looks that of a 24-week fetus with smooth surface, shallow sylvian fissure. (Courtesy R. Hewlett, MD.)*

causes of small brain such as craniostenosis, perinatal infection, or trauma.

Barkovich et al. classify primary MCPH on the basis of morphologic characteristics such as gyral patterns, cortical thickness, the presence of heterotopias or other malformations, and normal versus delayed myelination. The gyral pattern can be normal, "simplified," microgyric, or pachygyric.

Three types of primary microcephaly are recognized. **Microcephaly with simplified gyral pattern** (MSG) is the most common and the mildest form **(37-18)**. Simplified gyri and abnormally shallow sulci are the hallmarks of MSG. The cortex is normal or thinned, not thickened. The gyri are also reduced in number and demonstrate a "simplified" pattern. Various MSG subtypes are described with normal or delayed myelination, heterotopias, and arachnoid cysts.

Microlissencephaly is characterized by severe microcephaly and abnormal sulcation. The brain is extremely small, and the sulcation pattern appears greatly simplified or almost completely smooth **(37-20)**. The cortex is thickened, usually measuring more than three millimeters. In **microcephaly with extensive polymicrogyria**, the brain is small, and polymicrogyria is the predominant gyral pattern **(37-19)**.

Etiology and Pathology

Glioneuronal proliferation and apoptosis both play key roles in determining brain size, so abnormalities in either can result in microcephaly. Familial primary microcephaly is an autosomal recessive disorder with a single clinical phenotype and genetic heterogeneity.

Several chromosomal syndromes are characterized by mental retardation and microcephaly. These include trisomy 21 (Down), trisomy 18 (Edward), cri-du-chat ("cat cry," 5p syndrome), Cornelia de Lange, and Rubinstein-Taybi syndromes.

Clinical Issues

EPIDEMIOLOGY AND DEMOGRAPHICS. The incidence of primary MCPH ranges from 1:10,000-30,000. Most cases of primary (genetic) microcephaly are detected in utero or shortly after birth.

PRESENTATION AND NATURAL HISTORY. Mental retardation, developmental delay, and seizures are the most common clinical symptoms. Prognosis is variable.

Imaging

GENERAL FEATURES. The craniofacial ratio is decreased (usually ≤ 1.5:1). The forehead is often slanted, and the calvarial sutures may appear overriding.

CT FINDINGS. Bone CT shows a small cranial vault, often with closely apposed and overlapping sutures. In older children, the skull is thickened and the sinuses appear overpneumatized.

The cortical surface can be normal, simplified, microlissencephalic, or polymicrogyric. The ventricles may appear normal or moderately enlarged.

MR FINDINGS. Sagittal T1WI demonstrates slanted frontal bones and a marked decrease in cranial-to-facial proportions **(37-21)**. The brain can appear small but relatively normal, small with simplified gyral pattern, or microlissencephalic.

In microcephaly with simplified gyral pattern, the gyri are fewer in number and appear simplified. The sulci are shallow (25-50% of normal depth). Delayed myelin milestones may be present. Associated anomalies such as callosal dysgenesis and cephaloceles are common.

T2* (GRE, SWI) sequences are helpful to delineate secondary insults with hemorrhagic residua.

Differential Diagnosis

The major diagnostic dilemma is differentiating primary from **secondary microcephaly**. Calcifications, cysts, gliosis, and encephalomalacia are more common in microcephaly secondary to TORCH infection, trauma, or ischemic encephalopathy.

Focal Cortical Dysplasias

The distinctive histological features of focal cortical dysplasia (FCD) were first characterized by Taylor et al. It is now recognized that FCD is a common cause of medically refractory epilepsy in both children and adults. Surgical resection is an increasingly important treatment option, so recognition and accurate delineation of FCD on imaging studies are key to successful patient management.

Terminology and Classification

Focal cortical dysplasias—sometimes called **Taylor cortical dysplasia**—are localized regions of nonneoplastic malformed gray matter.

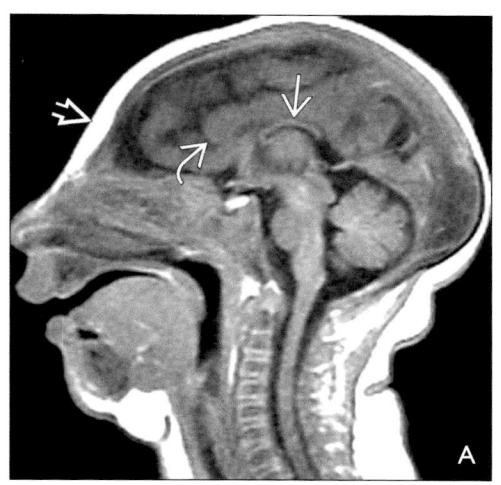

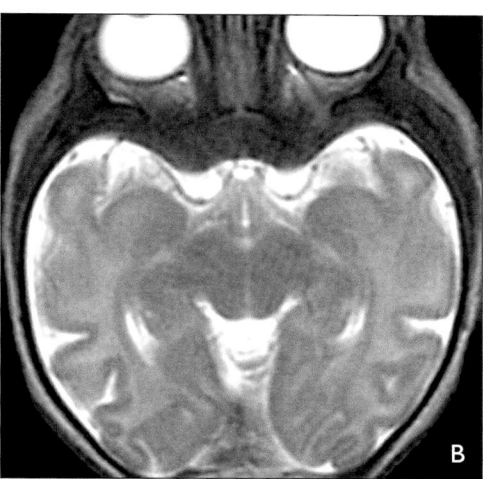

37-21A. Sagittal T1WI in a patient with primary microcephaly shows craniofacial disproportion with a 1.5:1 ratio, sloping forehead ⇨. Note the thin dysplastic corpus callosum ⇥, simplified gyral pattern ⇗. 37-21B. T2WI in the same patient shows the simplified gyral pattern with too few gyri, shallow-appearing sulci. The eyes are disproportionately large.

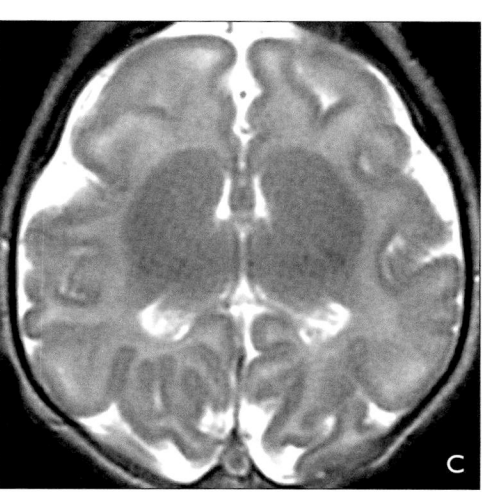

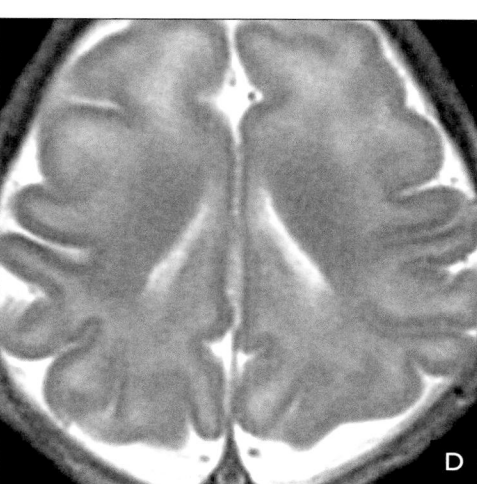

37-21C. T2WI through the ventricles shows the simplified gyral pattern with numerous shallow sulci. Cortical thickness appears normal, but myelination is delayed. 37-21D. T2WI in the same patient again shows the simplified gyral pattern. Compare Figure 37-18.

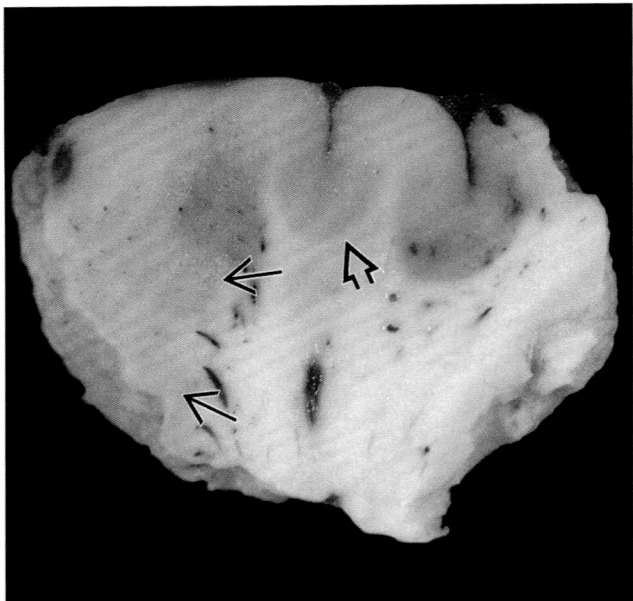

37-22. Resected surgical specimen from a patient with intractable epilepsy shows a funnel-shaped area of thickened cortex, blurred gray-white interface ➡. Contrast with adjacent normal sulcus, gyrus ⬦.

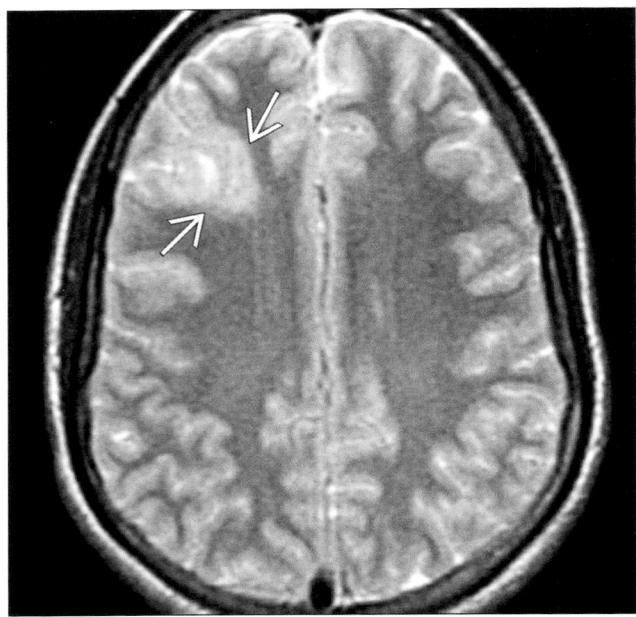

37-23. T2WI in a 17-year-old female with seizures shows a right frontal wedge-shaped area of malformed cortex ➡. Biopsy disclosed focal cortical dysplasia IIb. This is a classic Taylor FCD, the most common type.

The International League Against Epilepsy (ILAE) Task Force has recently proposed a three-tiered classification of FCD based on clinical, imaging, and neuropathologic findings. **FCD type I** is an isolated malformation with abnormal cortical layering that demonstrates either vertical (radial) persistence of developmental microcolumns (FCD type Ia) or loss of the horizontal hexalaminar structure (FCD type Ib) in one or multiple lobes. FCD type Ic is characterized by both patterns of abnormal cortical layering.

FCD type II is an isolated lesion characterized by altered cortical layering and dysmorphic neurons without (type IIa) or with **balloon** (type IIb) **cells**. Type II is the most common type of FCD.

A third type of FCD, **FCD type III**, was recently recognized as a postmigrational disorder secondary to ischemia, infection, trauma, etc. In such cases, cytoarchitectural abnormalities occur together with hippocampal sclerosis (FCD type IIIa), epilepsy-associated tumors (FCD type IIIb), vascular malformations (FCD type IIIc), or—in the case of FCD type IIId—other epileptogenic lesions acquired in early life.

Etiology

The molecular pathology and genetics of FCD are intensely investigated but incompletely understood. Most cases appear to be sporadic.

Aberrant phosphorylation of mammalian target of rapamycin (mTOR) substrates seems to be a biomarker for type II FCD. In addition, FCD type IIb specimens typ-

ically have sequence alterations in the *TSC1* (hamartin) gene and resemble the cortical tubers in tuberous sclerosis complex (TSC).

Alterations in a double cortin-like protein that is critically involved in neuronal division and radial migration may affect early corticogenesis in both FCD and TSC.

Pathology

GROSS PATHOLOGY. Surgical specimens often appear grossly normal. Mildly thickened, slightly firm cortex with poor demarcation from the underlying white matter may be present **(37-22)**.

MICROSCOPIC FEATURES. The histopathologic hallmarks of FCD are disorganized cytoarchitecture and neurons with abnormal shape, size, and orientation.

FCD type II has pronounced cytoarchitectural disturbances. Dysmorphic neurons with increased diameter of their cell bodies and nuclei are found in both types IIa and IIb. Cortical thickness is increased, and the gray-white matter interface is blurred in both subtypes.

Prominent balloon cells together with lack of myelin and oligodendrocytes are typical of type IIb. These balloon cells are histologically identical to giant cells in the tubers from TSC patients.

Clinical Issues

EPIDEMIOLOGY AND DEMOGRAPHICS. As a group, FCDs are the single most common cause of severe therapy-refractory epilepsy in children and young adults.

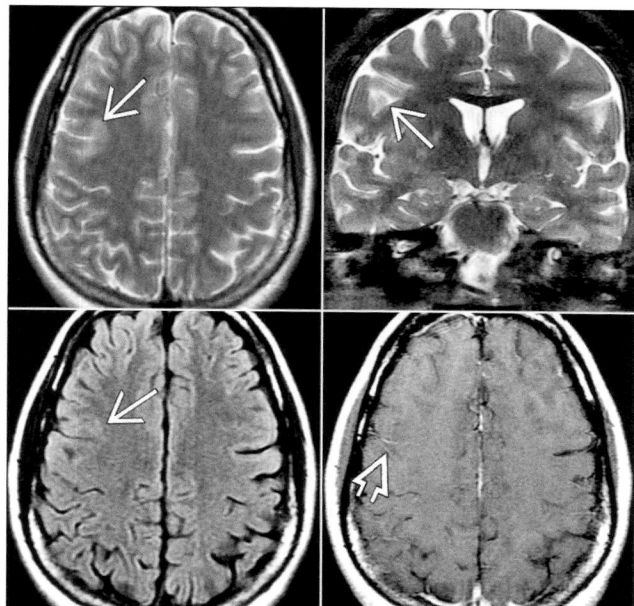

37-24. *Images show subtle findings of FCD ➡. Signal intensity is similar to GM on both T2/FLAIR. T1 C+ shows enhancement of "primitive" cortical veins ➡ over the focal dysplasia. (Courtesy P. Hildenbrand, MD.)*

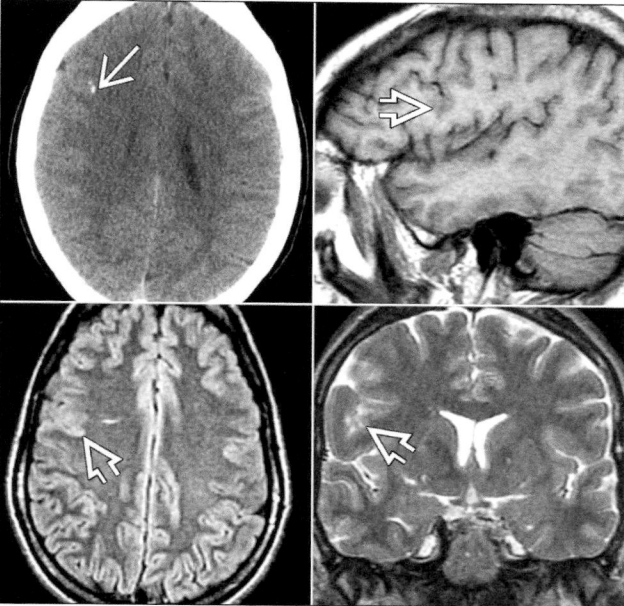

37-25. *Images in a different patient show very subtle findings of FCD ➡, including a tiny focus of calcification ➡ on NECT. Biopsy-proven FCD. (Courtesy P. Hildenbrand, MD.)*

FCD type II is found in 15-20% of patients undergoing epilepsy surgery. There is no gender predilection.

PRESENTATION AND NATURAL HISTORY. FCD-associated seizures usually begin in the first decade but can present in adolescence or even adulthood. Patients with FCD type Ia are typically young with early seizure onset and severe psychomotor retardation.

TREATMENT OPTIONS. Medically resistant chronic epilepsy secondary to FCD may be treated by surgical resection. Outcome varies with FCD subtype; excellent seizure control is reported in 70-100% of patients with FCD type IIb.

Imaging

GENERAL FEATURES. Imaging findings of FCD are often subtle. Most foci are smaller than two centimeters in diameter and can be difficult to detect, especially on standard imaging studies **(37-24)**. Larger lesions can mimic neoplasm or focal demyelination.

CT FINDINGS. CT scans are usually normal unless the lesion is unusually large. A few patients with calcified FCD type IIb lesions have been reported **(37-25)**.

MR FINDINGS. MR findings in FCD depend on lesion size and type. For example, FCD type Ia causes only mild hemispheric hypoplasia without other visible lesions.

FCD type IIb shows a localized area of increased cortical thickness and a funnel-shaped area of blurred gray-white interface at the bottom of a sulcus, the **"transman-**tle MR" sign** (37-23)**. Signal intensity varies with age. In neonates and infants, FCD type IIb appears hyperintense on T1WI and mildly hypointense on T2WI. In older patients, FCD appears as a wedge-shaped area of T2/FLAIR hyperintensity extending from the bottom of a sulcus into the subcortical and deep WM.

A subcortical linear or curvilinear focus of T2/FLAIR hyperintensity sometimes extends toward the superolateral margin of the lateral ventricle.

FCD type IIb does not enhance on T1 C+. It shows increased diffusivity and decreased FA on DWI. MRS shows decreased NAA:Cr and elevated mI. Perfusion MR shows normal or reduced rCBV.

The recently defined FCD type III is primarily encountered in patients with hippocampal sclerosis (FCD IIIa). Anterior temporal lobe volume loss with abnormal WM hyperintensity on T2/FLAIR with otherwise normal-appearing cortex is characteristic.

Voxel-based morphometry, statistical parametrical mapping, and texture analysis are advanced techniques that may increase detection of epileptogenic lesions in patients with negative standard MR scans.

FUNCTIONAL IMAGING. Ictal SPECT, PET, and magnetoencephalography (MEG) can be beneficial tools in patients with normal MRs who are suspected of harboring FCD. Fused images have been used to guide intraoperative lesionectomy. Functional imaging has also been used in conjunction with subdural and depth electrodes to localize the ictal zone.

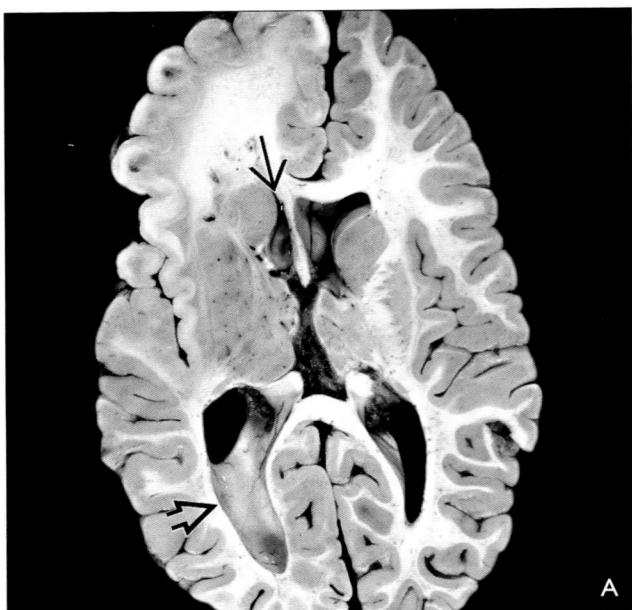

37-26A. Hemimegaloencephaly shows enlarged right hemisphere with "overgrown" WM. Note pointed frontal horn ➡, enlarged occipital horn ➡.

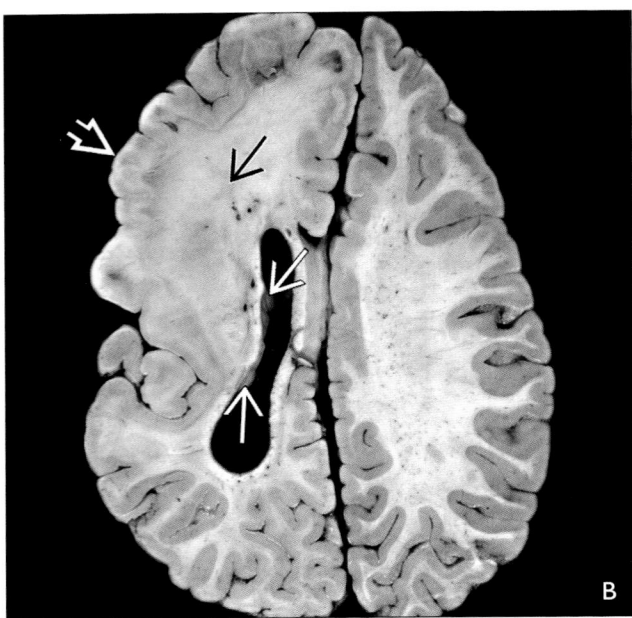

37-26B. More cephalad image shows large hemisphere/ventricle with subependymal heterotopic GM ➡, polymicrogyria ➡, "overgrown" WM with abnormal myelination ➡. (Courtesy B. Horten, MD.)

Differential Diagnosis

The major differential diagnosis of FCD (especially type IIb) includes neoplasm, tuberous sclerosis, and demyelinating disease. The most common **cortically based neoplasms** associated with longstanding epilepsy include dysembryoplastic neuroepithelial tumor (DNET), ganglioglioma, oligodendroglioma, and low-grade diffusely infiltrating astrocytoma (WHO grade II). It may be difficult (if not impossible) to distinguish between FCD and neoplasm on the basis of imaging findings alone.

The cortical lesions in **tuberous sclerosis complex** can look very similar to FCD type IIb. Both can calcify; both are funnel- or flame-shaped and involve the cortex and subcortical WM. TSC usually demonstrates other imaging stigmata such as subependymal nodules.

A solitary **demyelinating lesion** can mimic FCD. The myelin and oligodendrocyte loss in FCD results in similar signal intensity changes, i.e., T2/FLAIR hyperintensity. "Tumefactive" demyelination often has an incomplete enhancing rim whereas FCD does not enhance.

Hemimegaloencephaly

Terminology

Hemimegaloencephaly (HMEG)—also called unilateral megalencephaly—is a rare malformation characterized by enlargement and cytoarchitectural abnormalities of one cerebral hemisphere.

Etiology

The precise etiology of HMEG is unknown. It is thought to represent abnormally increased proliferation of progenitor cells together with failure of normal post-neurogenesis apoptosis. Aberrant mTOR signaling may play a role in the development of HMEG and other malformations of cortical development ("TORopathies").

HMEG can occur as an isolated malformation, but approximately 30% of cases are syndromic. Associations with Proteus, Klippel-Weber-Trenaunay, and epidermal nevus syndromes, neurofibromatosis type 1, and hypomelanosis of Ito have been reported.

Pathology

GROSS PATHOLOGY. The affected hemisphere appears enlarged with abnormal gyral pattern, thickened cortex, and areas of dysplastic hamartomatous overgrowth. The gray-white matter junction is blurred (37-26).

MICROSCOPIC FEATURES. Severe cortical dyslamination, hypertrophic and dysmorphic neurons, and parenchymal and leptomeningeal glioneuronal heterotopias are typical histologic features of HMEG. Balloon cells are identified in half of all cases.

The white matter is often grossly abnormal and poorly myelinated. Gray matter heterotopias and clusters of hypertrophic astrocytes are frequent findings. Gliosis, WM vacuolation, and cystic changes are common.

Clinical Issues

EPIDEMIOLOGY AND DEMOGRAPHICS. HMEG is rare, representing less than 5% of MCDs diagnosed on imaging studies.

PRESENTATION, NATURAL HISTORY, AND TREATMENT OPTIONS. HMEG usually presents in infancy and is characterized by macrocrania, developmental delay, and seizures. Extracranial hemihypertrophy of part or all of the ipsilateral body may be present.

Prognosis is poor, as seizures are usually intractable and developmental delay is severe. HMEG-associated seizures are usually resistant to anticonvulsants. Anatomic or functional hemispherectomy has had variable success as *abnormalities in the contralateral "normal" hemisphere are common.*

Imaging

GENERAL FEATURES. HMEG is characterized by an enlarged, dysplastic-appearing hemisphere with abnormal gyration, thickened cortex, and white matter abnormalities. The lateral ventricle usually appears enlarged and deformed. In rare cases, the dysplastic changes involve only part of one hemisphere ("focal," "localized," or "lobar" hemimegaloencephaly).

CT FINDINGS. NECT shows an enlarged hemisphere and hemicranium. The posterior falx often appears displaced across the midline (37-27). Abnormal white matter myelination may increase in attenuation, making the contralateral "normal" WM appear unusually hypodense. Dystrophic calcifications are common.

CECT may disclose abnormal, "uncondensed," primitive-appearing superficial veins over regions of severely dysplastic cortex.

MR FINDINGS. The cortex often appears thickened and "lumpy-bumpy" on T1 scans. Myelination is disordered and accelerated with shortened T1. Neuronal heterotopias are common. The ipsilateral ventricle is usually enlarged and deformed. In severe cases, almost no normal hemispheric architecture can be discerned.

T2 scans show areas of pachy- and polymicrogyria with indistinct borders between gray and white matter (37-28). White matter signal intensity on T2/FLAIR is often het-

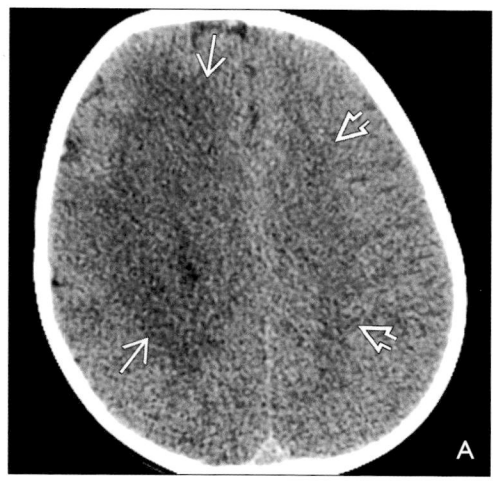

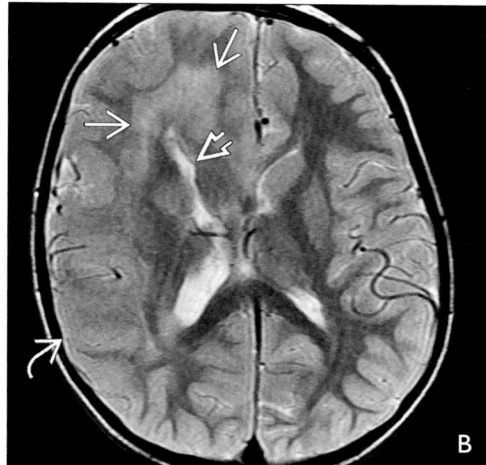

37-27A. NECT in a 4-year-old girl with hemimegaloencephaly, intractable seizures shows enlarged right hemisphere, hemicranium with enlarged WM in the corona radiata ➡. Compare this to the normal-appearing WM of the left hemisphere ➡. 37-27B. T2WI in the same patient shows enlarged hemisphere, hyperintense WM ➡, enlarged deformed lateral ventricle ➡, thickened dysplastic cortex ➡. Again compare to the normal left side.

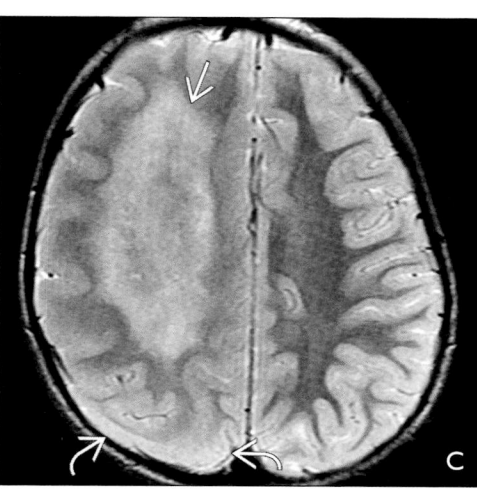

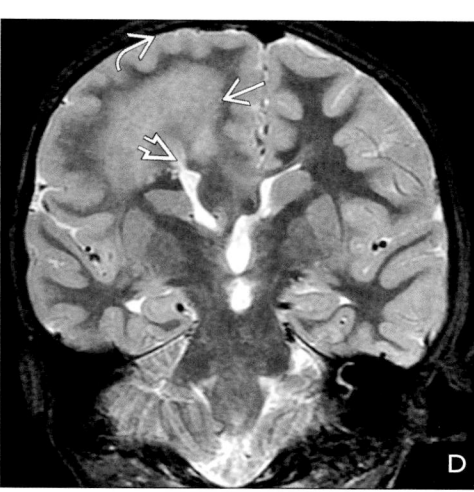

37-27C. T2WI through the corona radiata in the same patient shows hypertrophied heterogeneously hyperintense WM ➡, pachygyria ➡. 37-27D. Coronal T2WI in the same patient shows the hyperplastic, hyperintense WM ➡, deformed pointed lateral ventricle ➡, polymicrogyria ➡.

erogeneous with cysts and gliosis-like hyperintensity (37-27).

Differential Diagnosis

The major differential diagnosis of HMEG is **focal MCD**. While the entire hemisphere is usually involved in HMEG, cases of "focal" or "lobar" megalencephaly are difficult to distinguish. They show identical histologic features. The presence of associated extracerebral abnormalities (hemihypertrophy) may be a helpful differentiating feature.

Tuberous sclerosis complex with widespread cortical dysplasia does not enlarge the hemisphere and exhibits other imaging stigmata such as subependymal nodules.

Cases of severe HMEG with almost no identifiable normal anatomic landmarks can be mistaken for neoplasm, typically **gangliocytoma**.

Abnormalities of Neuronal Migration

Abnormalities of neuronal migration are divided into four main subgroups as discussed above. We begin with the heterotopias and then turn to lissencephaly spectrum disorders. The section concludes with a brief discussion of subcortical heterotopias, sublobar dysplasias, and cobblestone complex.

Heterotopias

Arrest of normal neuronal migration along the radial glial cells can result in grossly visible masses of "heterotopic" gray matter. These collections come in many shapes and sizes and can be found virtually anywhere between the ventricles and the pia. They can be solitary or multifocal

37-28A. NECT scan in a 35-week premature infant shows enlarged right hemisphere, lateral ventricle ➡. The right hemispheric WM appears less hypodense than the left. 37-28B. More cephalad scan in the same patient shows the enlarged right hemisphere, lateral ventricle ➡, off-midline insertion of the falx ➡. Initial diagnosis was left MCA stroke.

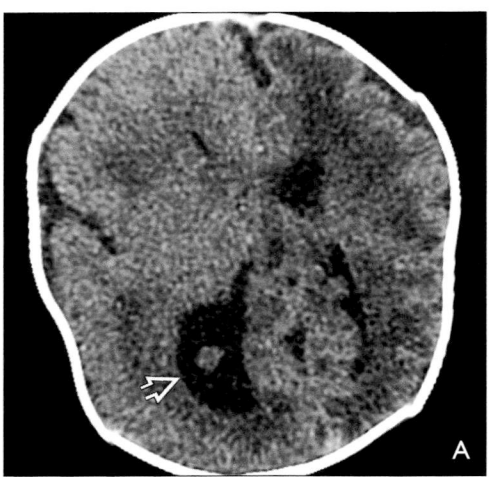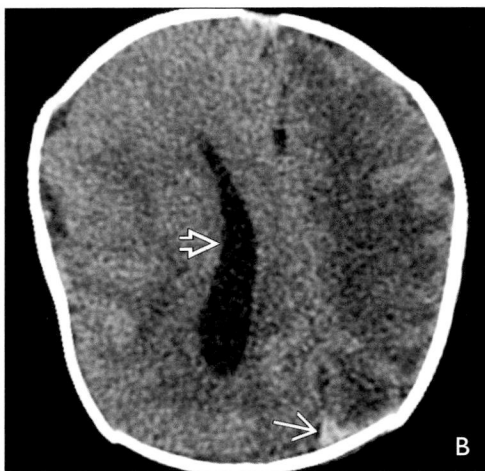

37-28C. T2WI in the same patient shows expanded right hemispheric WM that appears "dirty" ➡ (i.e., less hyperintense than the unmyelinated left WM). Note the markedly enlarged fornices ➡. 37-28D. More cephalad T2WI shows that corona radiata WM is less hyperintense than normal ➡, and there is extensive cortical thickening with polymicrogyria ➡. Note the prominent, primitive-appearing veins ➡.

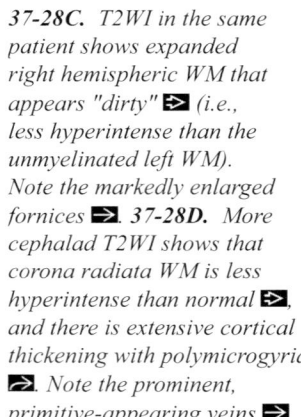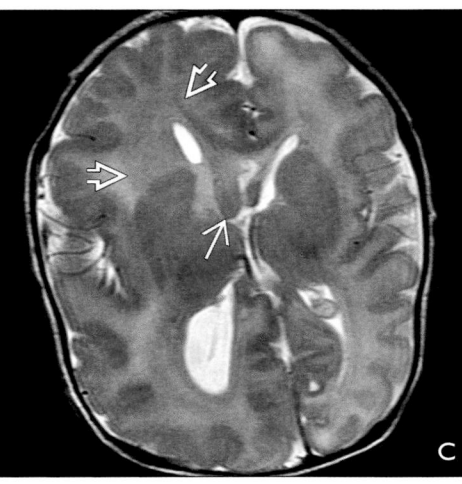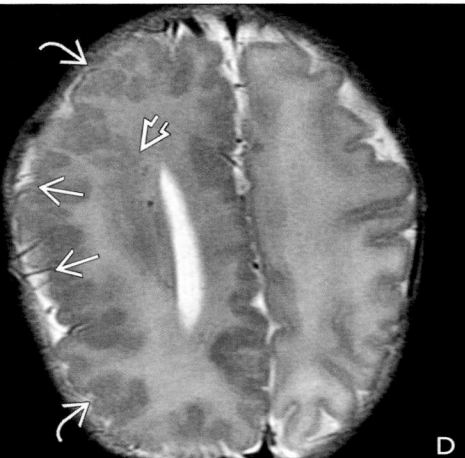

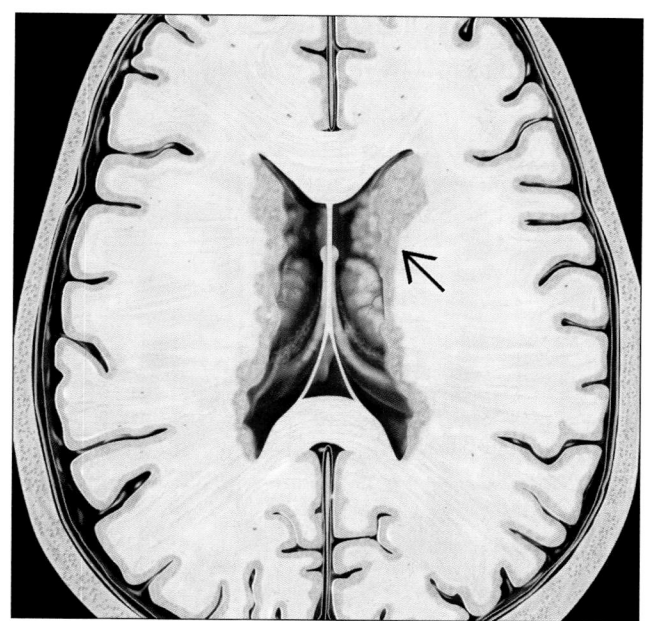

37-29. *Axial graphic shows extensive bilateral subependymal heterotopia ⇒ lining the lateral ventricles. The gray matter cortical ribbon is thin, and the sulci are shallow.*

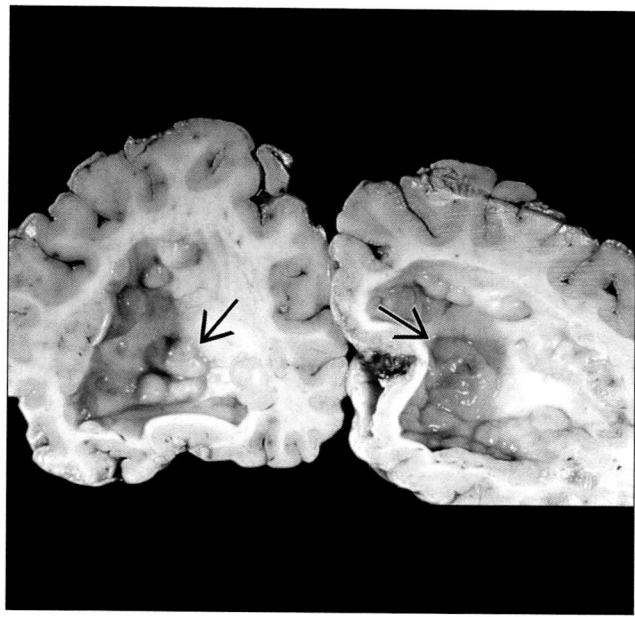

37-30. *Autopsy specimen shows nodules of subependymal heterotopic gray matter ⇒. Ventricles are enlarged and the overlying cortex thin. (Courtesy J. Ardyn, MD.)*

and exist either as an isolated phenomenon or in association with other malformations.

Periventricular nodular heterotopia (PVNH) is the most common form of cortical malformation in adults. Here one or more subependymal nodules of gray matter (GM) line the lateral walls of the ventricles **(37-29)**, **(37-30)**. Nodules of PVNH follow GM in density/signal intensity and do not enhance following contrast administration **(37-31)**.

PVNH commonly occurs with other abnormalities (e.g., Dandy-Walker and Chiari 2 malformations) and is most often asymmetric with one or more focal nodules along the temporal and occipital horns. *FLNA* mutations, when present in the X-linked dominant form, cause bilateral ectopic GM nodules, which are perinatal lethal in males.

Less commonly, PVNH lines most or even all of the lateral ventricular walls. Collections of round or ovoid nodules indent the lateral walls of the ventricles, giving them a distinctive "lumpy-bumpy" appearance. They follow GM on all sequences, do not enhance, and—unlike the subependymal nodules of tuberous sclerosis—do not calcify. The overlying cortex often appears thinned, but sulcation and gyration are typically normal.

The major differential diagnosis of GM heterotopias is neoplasm, most specifically **gangliocytoma**. Because the histologic features of GM heterotopia are so similar to those of gangliocytoma, recognizing that the imaging findings are characteristic of a PVNH is essential to avoid misdiagnosis.

Lissencephaly Spectrum

Malformations due to widespread abnormal transmantle migration include **agyria, pachygyria**, and **band heterotopia**. All are part of the **lissencephaly spectrum**.

Terminology

The term lissencephaly (LIS) literally means "smooth brain." In classic lissencephaly (cLIS), the brain surface lacks normal sulcation and gyration. **Classic lissencephaly** is also called **type 1 lissencephaly, four-layer lissencephaly**, or **agyria-pachygyria complex**. Agyria is defined as a thick cortex with absence of surface gyri (**"complete" lissencephaly**).

True agyria with complete loss of all gyri is relatively uncommon. Most cases of classic lissencephaly show parietooccipital agyria with some areas of broad, flat gyri ("pachygyria") and shallow sulci along the inferior frontal and temporal lobes (**"incomplete" lissencephaly**).

Some rare forms of LIS are associated with a disproportionately small cerebellum and are referred to as **lissencephaly with cerebellar hypoplasia**.

Variant lissencephaly (vLIS) consists of thick cortex and reduced sulcation without a cell-sparse zone. Examples include X-linked lissencephaly with callosal agenesis and ambiguous genitalia and lissencephaly with Reelin signaling pathway mutations.

Band heterotopia is also called **"double cortex" syndrome** and is the mildest form of classic lissencephaly **(37-32)**.

Etiology

GENETICS. Neuronal genes have layer-specific identities that are selectively expressed by cortical progenitor cells. Other genes regulate the migration of postmitotic neurons from the ventricular and subventricular zones to the cortex. Disturbances in the latter result in lissencephaly.

A majority of patients with cLIS have a defect of the *LIS1* gene on chromosome 17p. *LIS1* is deleted in all patients with Miller-Dieker syndrome.

Another 10-15% of patients with cLIS have double cortex gene (*DCX*) mutations.

Genes that regulate microtubule-associated proteins are especially important in neuronal migration. Tubulin (*TUB*) mutations have been specifically associated with lissencephaly. Mutations of *TUBA1A* are responsible for 1-4% of classic lissencephalies and 30% of cases with lissencephaly with cerebellar hypoplasia. *TUBA1A* missense mutations usually result in complete agyria.

A third gene, *RELN* ("reelin," also known as *LIS2*), encodes an extracellular matrix protein that controls cell-cell interactions critical for proper cell positioning and neuronal migration. *RELN* mutations are associated with autosomal recessive lissencephaly with cerebellar hypoplasia.

Pathology

GROSS PATHOLOGY. In cLIS, the external surface of the brain shows a marked lack of gyri and sulci. In the most severe forms, the cerebral hemispheres are smooth with poor operculization and underdeveloped sylvian fissures. Coronal sections demonstrate a markedly thickened cerebral cortex with broad gyri and reduced volume of the underlying white matter **(37-33)**.

MICROSCOPIC FEATURES. In cLIS, the normal six-layer cortex is replaced by a thick four-layer cortex. From the outermost to the innermost, these layers are (1) a thin subpial molecular layer, (2) a thin outer cortex composed of

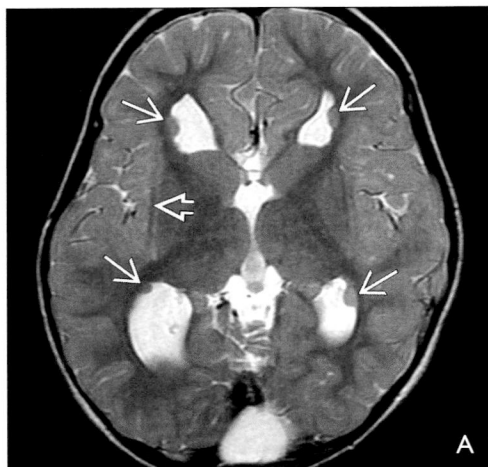
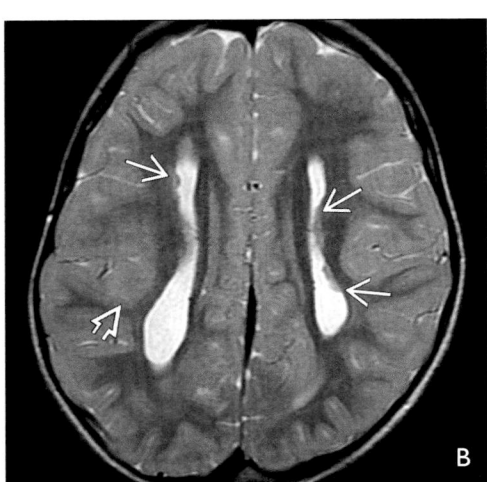

37-31A. Axial T2WI in a patient with corpus callosum agenesis shows multiple nodules of subependymal heterotopic gray matter ➡. Cortex shows perisylvian areas of pachy- and polymicrogyria ➡. 37-31B. More cephalad image in the same patient shows additional foci of subependymal heterotopic GM ➡ and cortical dysplasia ➡.

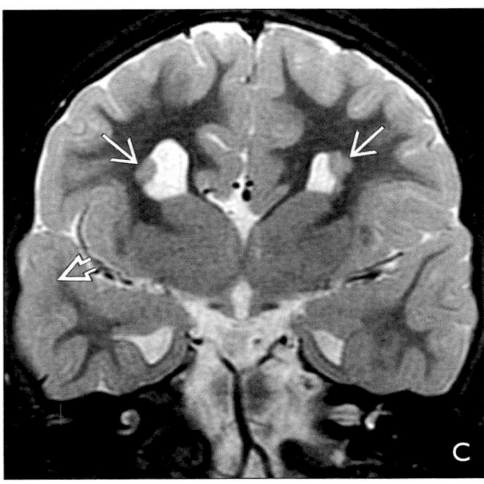
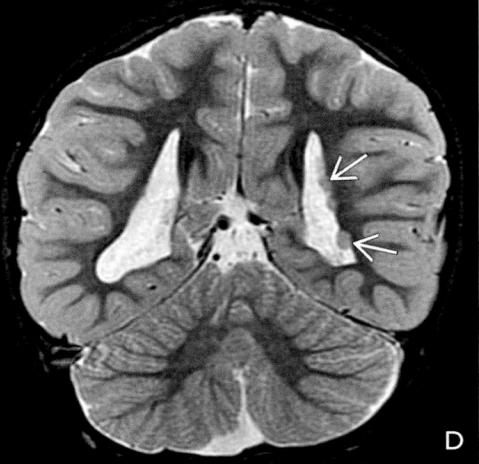

37-31C. Coronal T2WI in the same patient nicely demonstrates the subependymal heterotopias ➡, pachy- and polymicrogyria ➡. 37-31D. T2WI through the atria of the lateral ventricles shows the subependymal heterotopias ➡. The heterotopias followed gray matter signal intensity on all sequences.

disorganized large pyramidal neurons, (3) a "cell-sparse" zone that consists mostly of axons (myelinated after the age of two years), and (4) a broad inner band of disorganized neurons. The white matter is severely reduced in volume and often contains foci of heterotopic neurons.

Clinical Issues

EPIDEMIOLOGY AND DEMOGRAPHICS. Lissencephaly occurs in 1-4:100,000 live births. Patients with band heterotopia are almost always female.

PRESENTATION. Patients with cLIS typically exhibit moderate to severe developmental delay, impaired neuromotor functions, variable mental retardation, and seizures. Microcephaly and mildly dysmorphic facies are frequent. Patients with band heterotopia typically present with developmental delay and a milder seizure disorder.

Patients with cLIS and severe facial deformities are diagnosed with **Miller-Dieker syndrome** (MDS). Frontal bossing, hypertelorism, upturned nose, small jaw, and prominent upper lip with thin vermilion border are characteristic features of MDS.

Imaging

GENERAL FEATURES. Imaging in patients with complete cLIS (agyria) shows a smooth, featureless brain surface with shallow sylvian fissures and large ventricles. The cortex is thickened, and the WM is diminished in volume. The normal finger-like interdigitations between the cortical GM and subcortical WM are absent. In some cases, the cerebellum appears hypoplastic.

CT FINDINGS. Axial NECT scans in cLIS show an "hourglass" or "figure-eight" appearance caused by the flat brain surface and shallow, wide sylvian fissures. A thick band of relatively well-delineated dense cortex surrounds a thinner, smooth band of white matter (37-34A).

CECT scans show prominent "primitive-appearing" veins running in the shallow sylvian fissures and coursing over the thickened cortices.

MR FINDINGS.

Classic lissencephaly. In **cLIS**, T1 scans show a smooth cortical surface, a thick band of deep gray matter that is sharply demarcated from the underlying WM, and

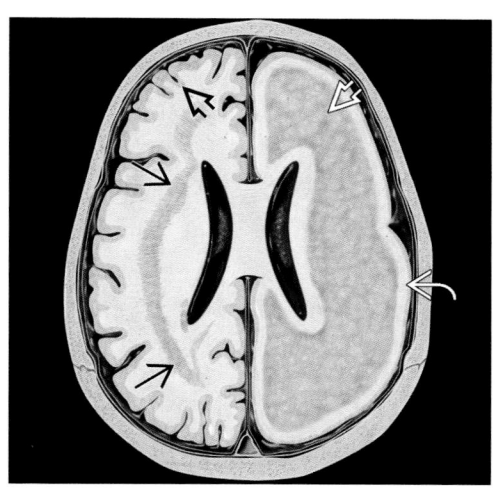

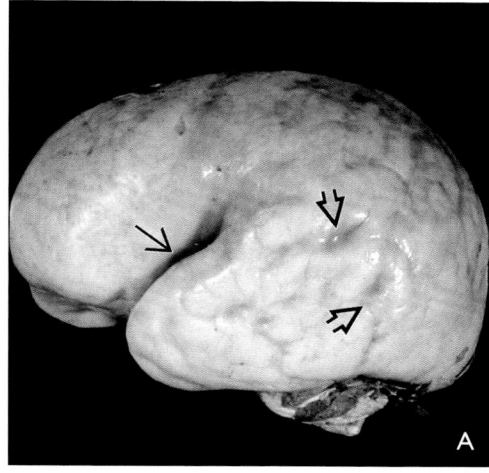

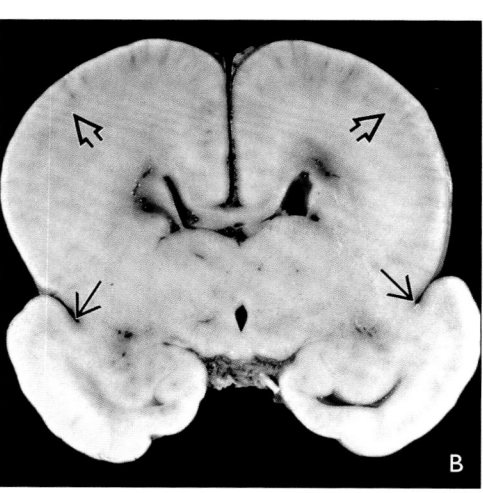

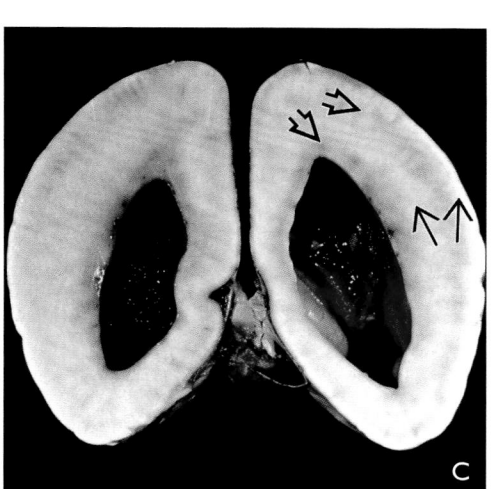

37-32. Axial graphic composite shows classic lissencephaly in the left hemisphere with thick subcortical gray matter band, thin cortex, and "cell-sparse" zone. The right hemisphere demonstrates milder lissencephaly with band heterotopia ("double cortex" syndrome), thin outer cortex. 37-33A. Lissencephaly shows shallow sylvian fissure, near-complete lack of sulcation. A few shallow surface indentations are present.

37-33B. Coronal section shows "hourglass" configuration with shallow sylvian fissures, absent sulci, thick incompletely layered cortex. 37-33C. Posterior coronal section shows occipital horn dilatation ("colpocephaly"), alternating bands of GM, WM.

large ventricles. T2 sequences are best to distinguish the separate cortical layers. A thin outer cellular layer that is isointense with GM covers a hyperintense "cell-sparse" layer. The WM layer is smooth and reduced in volume. A deeper, thick layer of arrested migrating neurons is common and may mimic band heterotopia **(37-34B)**, **(37-34C)**.

Callosal anomalies are common in cLIS. The predominant abnormality is callosal hypogenesis. The corpus callosum has a thin flat body with a more vertically oriented splenium. DTI shows marked "pruning," rarefaction, and disorganization of subcortical association ("U") fibers. FA and axial diffusivity are decreased, and radial diffusivity is increased. The main WM tracts also appear aberrant and heterotopic **(37-34D)**.

Variant lissencephaly. In **vLIS**, sulcation is reduced, and the cortex appears thick (although not as thick as in cLIS). There is no "cell-sparse" layer.

Band heterotopia or "double cortex" syndrome. In **band heterotopia**, a band of smooth GM is separated from a relatively thicker, more gyriform cortex by a layer of normal-appearing white matter.

MR scans show a more normal gyral pattern with relatively thicker cortex. The distinguishing feature of band heterotopia is its "double cortex," a homogeneous layer of gray matter separated from the ventricles and cerebral cortex by layers of normal-appearing WM **(37-35)**.

Differential Diagnosis

Extremely premature brain is smooth at 24-26 gestational weeks and normally has a "lissencephalic" appearance (see Chapter 35). Full sulcation and gyration do not develop completely until approximately 40 weeks.

In **microcephaly with simplified gyral pattern**, the head circumference is at least three standard deviations below normal. Too few gyri, abnormally shallow sulci, and a normal or thin (not thick) cortex are present.

cLIS should also be distinguished from the so-called **cobblestone lissencephalies** (type 2 lissencephaly or LIS2). Here the brain surface appears "pebbly" instead of smooth. LIS2 is typically associated with congenital muscular dystrophies (see below).

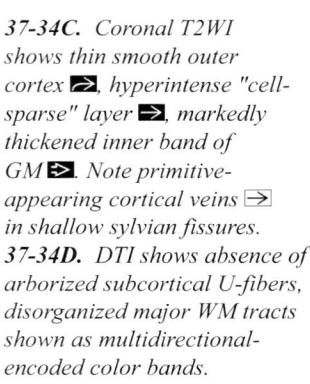

37-34A. NECT scan in a 4-month-old girl with classic lissencephaly shows smooth, nearly agyric surface with shallow sylvian fissures ➡ and "hourglass" configuration. The cortex is thick ➡, and the white matter ➡ is reduced. The ventricles are moderately enlarged. 37-34B. T1WI shows a few shallow sulci, broad flat gyri. Thin outer, thick inner layers of GM are separated by a hypointense "cell-sparse" layer ➡. WM volume ➡ is reduced.

37-34C. Coronal T2WI shows thin smooth outer cortex ➡, hyperintense "cell-sparse" layer ➡, markedly thickened inner band of GM ➡. Note primitive-appearing cortical veins ➡ in shallow sylvian fissures. 37-34D. DTI shows absence of arborized subcortical U-fibers, disorganized major WM tracts shown as multidirectional-encoded color bands.

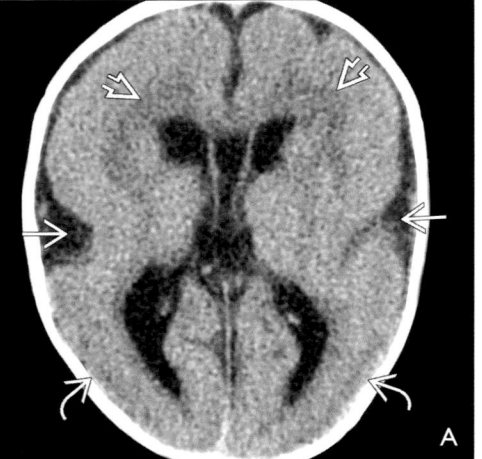
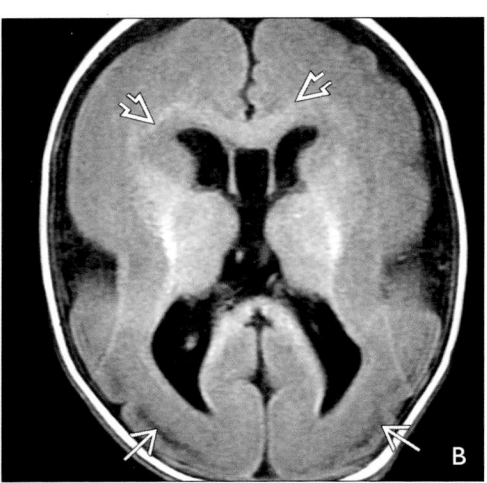
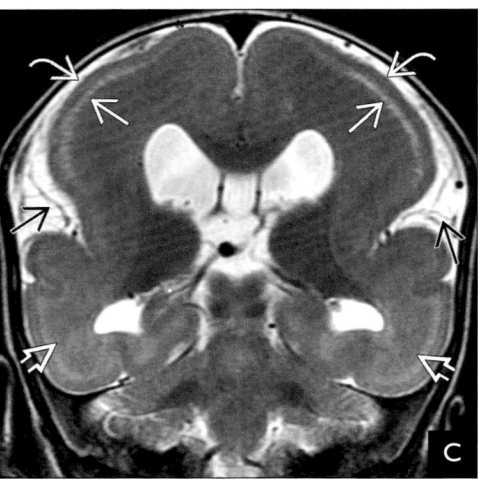
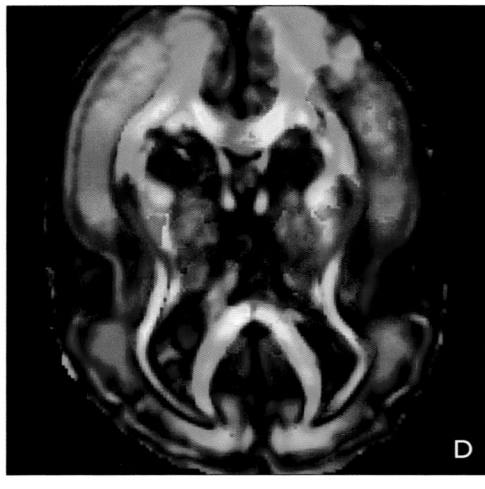

Pachygyria histologically resembles cLIS but is more localized, often multifocal, and usually asymmetric. In contrast to cLIS, the gray-white junction along the thickened cortex is indistinct.

Cytomegalovirus-associated lissencephaly may demonstrate periventricular calcifications.

LISSENCEPHALY SPECTRUM

Classic Lissencephaly (cLIS)
- Pathology: Thick, 4-layer cortex
  - Thin subpial layer
  - Thin outer cortex
  - "Cell-sparse" zone
  - Broad inner band of disorganized neurons
- Clinical issues
  - cLIS + severe facial anomalies = Miller-Dieker
- Imaging
  - Smooth, "hourglass" brain
  - Flat surface, shallow "open" sylvian fissures

Band Heterotopia ("Double Cortex")
- Clinical issues
  - Almost always in females
- Imaging: Looks like "double cortex"
  - Thin, gyriform cortex
  - Normal-appearing WM under cortex
  - Smooth inner band of GM
  - Normal-appearing periventricular WM

Differential Diagnosis
- Extremely premature brain
  - cLIS looks like 20-24 week fetal brain
- Microcephaly with simplified gyral pattern
  - Brain ≥ 3 standard deviations below normal
- Cobblestone lissencephalies (type 2 lissencephaly)
  - Associated with congenital muscular dystrophies
  - "Pebbly" (cobblestone) surface, not smooth
- Pachygyria
  - More localized, often multifocal
  - GM-WM interface indistinct
- Congenital CMV
  - Often microcephalic
  - Smooth brain, periventricular Ca++

Subcortical Heterotopias and Lobar Dysplasias

Subcortical Heterotopias

Subcortical heterotopias are malformations in which large, focal, mass-like collections of neurons are found in the deep cerebral white matter anywhere from the ependyma to the cortex **(37-36)**. The involved portion of the affected hemisphere is abnormally small, and the overlying cortex appears thin and sometimes dysplastic.

In other forms of heterotopia, focal masses of ectopic GM occur in linear or swirling curved columns of neurons that extend through normal-appearing white matter from the ependyma to the pia. The overlying cortex is thin, and the underlying ventricle often appears distorted. The masses

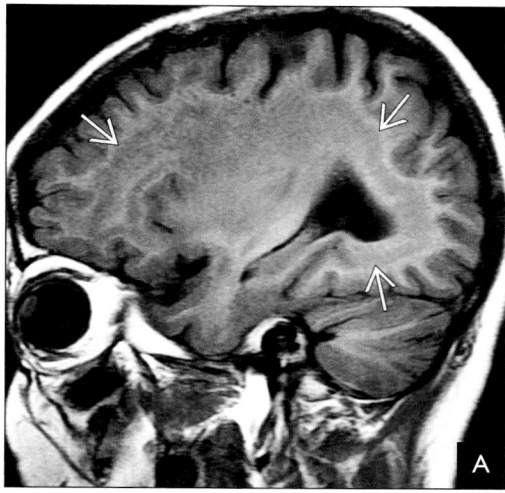

37-35A. *Sagittal T1WI shows band heterotopia with thin outer cortex, myelinated WM, band of GM ➡, periventricular WM ("double cortex").*

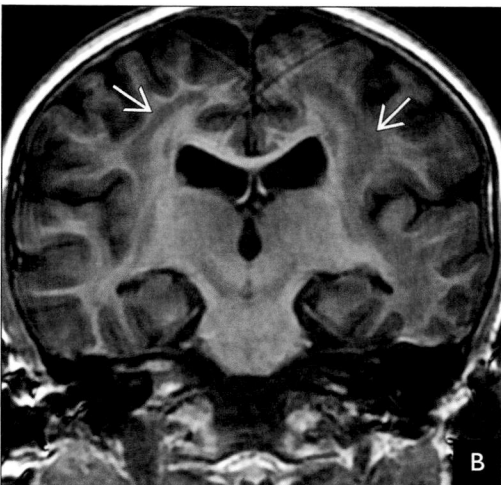

37-35B. *Coronal SPGR in the same patient nicely demonstrates bilateral homogeneous-appearing bands of subcortical heterotopic gray matter ➡.*

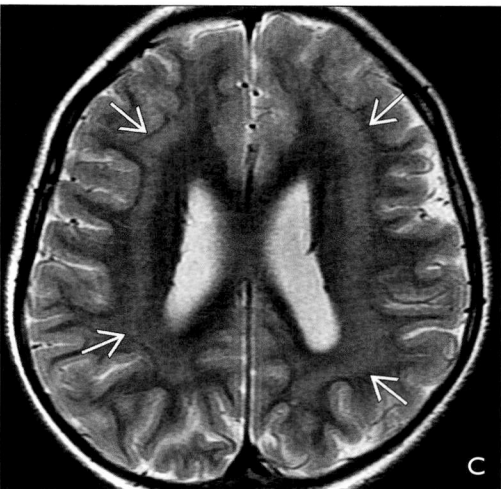

37-35C. *Axial T2WI in the same patient shows that the subcortical bands ➡ follow GM signal intensity. The overlying cortex is thin.*

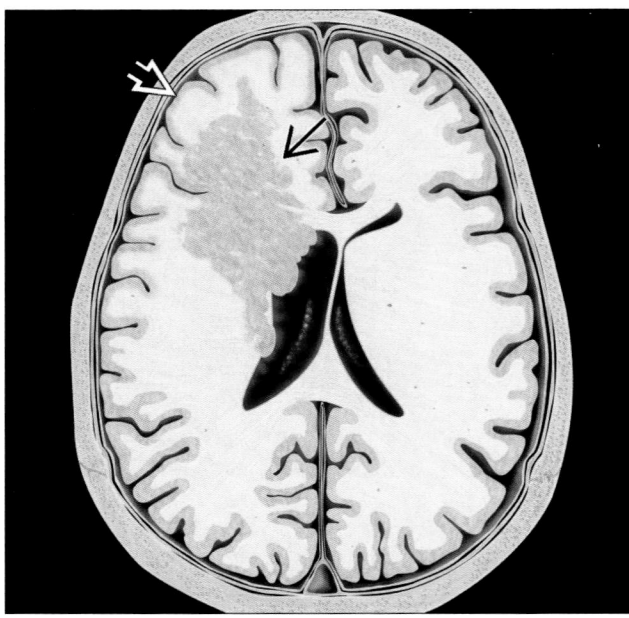

37-36. Graphic depicts subcortical heterotopia. The large, focal, mass-like collection of gray matter ⇥, thin overlying cortex ⇥ are typical.

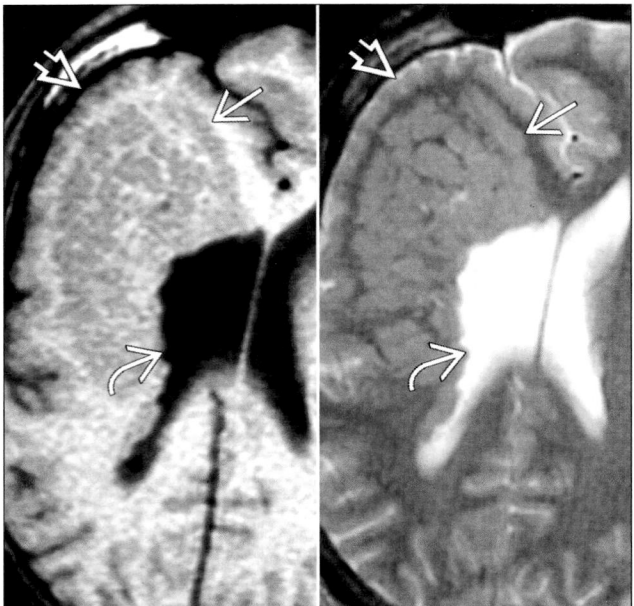

37-37. T1WI (L), T2WI (R) show a focal subcortical mass of heterotopic gray matter ⇥, thin overlying cortex ⇥. Note deformity of underlying ventricle ⇥. Heterotopic GM can mimic neoplasm on both imaging, histopathology (gangliocytoma).

follow GM on all sequences, do not demonstrate edema, and do not enhance **(37-37)**.

The differential diagnosis of subcortical heterotopia is neoplasm, especially **gangliocytoma**. Heterotopic collections of GM can be mass-like and deform the adjacent ventricle. However, they follow gray matter on all imaging sequences and do not enhance following contrast administration.

Lobar Dysplasias

Sublobar dysplasia is a very rare malformation characterized clinically by epilepsy in an otherwise developmentally normal patient. Pathologically, sublobar dysplasia is a region of dysmorphic brain within an otherwise normal-appearing hemisphere. A deep infolding of dysplastic cortex with irregular and indistinct GM-WM interfaces is characteristic on imaging studies.

Cobblestone Malformations and the Congenital Muscular Dystrophies

Cobblestone lissencephaly is also known as type 2 lissencephaly and is genetically, embryologically, and pathologically distinct from type 1 ("classic") lissencephaly.

Terminology

Cobblestone lissencephaly is also called **cobblestone complex** (CBSC) and is characterized by an uneven, nodular, "pebbly" brain surface that resembles a cobblestone street. Almost all cases of cobblestone

lissencephaly are associated with ocular anomalies and occur as a part of a congenital muscular dystrophy (CMD).

CBSC includes three CMD phenotypes: **Walker-Warburg syndrome** (WWS), **muscle-eye-brain disease** (MEB), and **Fukuyama congenital muscular dystrophy** (FCMD).

Etiology

Cobblestone cortex results from abnormalities caused by defects in the limiting pial basement membrane. These create a "leakage" that allows overmigration of neuroblasts and glial cells beyond the external glial-pial limitans. Overmigration results in an extracortical layer of aberrant gray matter nodules—the "cobblestones"—on the brain surfaces.

All the disorders associated with type 2 lissencephaly exhibit autosomal recessive inheritance. The common molecular mechanism that links the brain, eye, and muscle disorders is a defect in O-mannosylation of α-dystroglycan. Most CBSCs are **α-dystroglycanopathies**. Multiple genes have been implicated in their development.

Pathology

GROSS PATHOLOGY. Grossly, the brain is usually small. Broadened gyri and loss of sulci give the brain its lissencephalic appearance. The affected areas exhibit a "lumpy-bumpy" appearance **(37-38)**. In WWS, the entire brain is often involved whereas patients with MEB and

FCMD show variable amounts of affected cortex, usually the posterolateral parietal and occipital lobes.

The cerebral WM volume is reduced, and the cortex appears irregularly thickened. The GM-WM junction can have an irregular and nodular appearance.

The brainstem is almost always small. The cerebellum is often small, and its folia are frequently fused and disorganized. From 15-20% of patients with WWS also have a Dandy-Walker malformation.

MICROSCOPIC FEATURES. The histopathology of type 2 lissencephaly shares many features with polymicrogyria. The cortex is unlayered and highly disorganized. Unlike type 1 ("classic") lissencephaly, no recognizable laminations are identified. There are numerous areas in which a breach in the pial-glial limitans has occurred, possibly providing a migratory route for aberrant neurons.

Histopathology of skeletal muscle shows classic features of CMD, i.e., degenerating and regenerating muscle fibers with marked fibrosis.

Clinical Issues

EPIDEMIOLOGY AND DEMOGRAPHICS. All the CMDs are rare. Walker-Warburg syndrome is the most severe form and is found worldwide. Muscle-eye-brain disease is intermediate in severity and is found primarily in Finland. Fukuyama congenital muscular dystrophy—the mildest form—occurs almost exclusively in Japan and in patients of Japanese descent.

PRESENTATION AND NATURAL HISTORY. The hallmark of all type 2 lissencephalies is the combination of congenital muscular dystrophy with CNS involvement. Most patients present during the first year of life, but the relative degree of weakness varies.

WWS is characterized by the triad of CMD, brain anomalies (primarily cobblestone cortex), and ocular abnormalities. Infants with WWS have profound hypotonia ("floppy baby"), ocular abnormalities (such as colobomas and persistent hypoplastic primary vitreous), severe developmental delay, and seizures. Most affected individuals do not survive beyond one or two years.

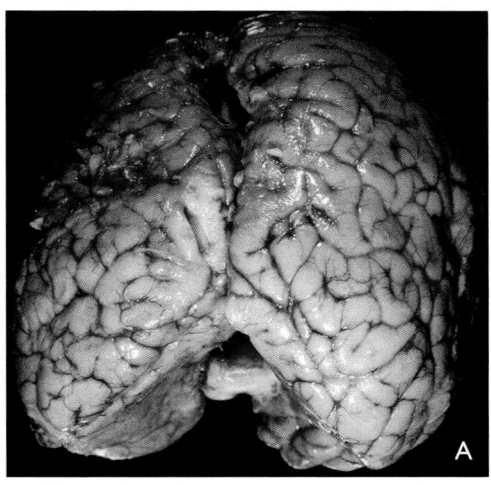

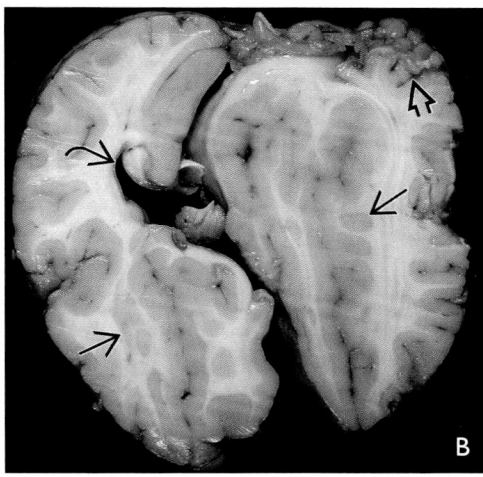

37-38A. Cobblestone lissencephaly is named for the nodular, "pebbly" appearance of brain surface, which resembles the surface of a cobblestone street. 37-38B. Coronal section shows cobblestone cortex ▷, multiple lines, columns, swirls, and nodules of subcortical heterotopic gray matter ▨. The right lateral ventricle ▨ is grossly malformed with nodules of subependymal heterotopic GM.

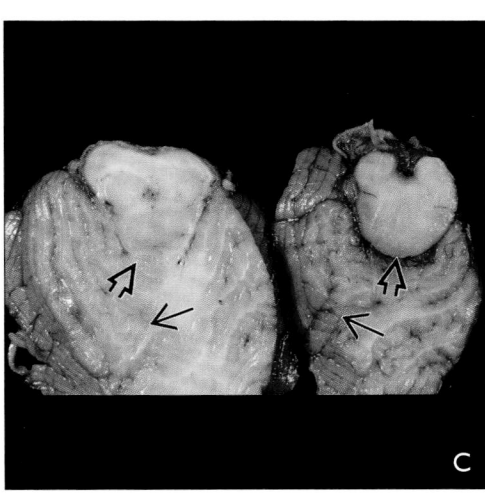

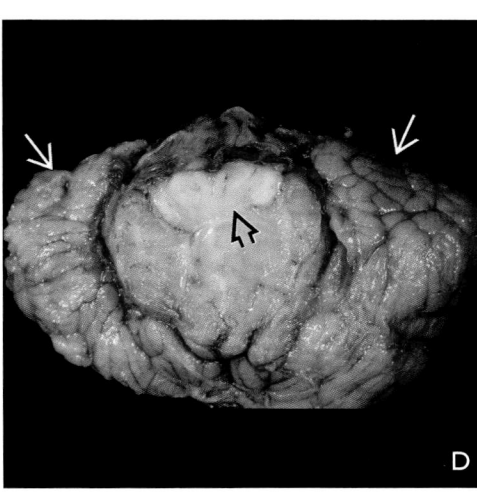

37-38C. Sections through the midbrain and cerebellum show thick fused colliculi ▷, bizarre dysplastic cerebellar folia ▨. 37-38D. More inferior section shows a small medulla ▷, distinct "pebbly" appearance to the cerebellar hemispheres and vermis ▨. (Courtesy R. Hewlett, MD.)

MEB patients are hypotonic and have impaired vision, seizures, and mental retardation. The eye findings are usually present at birth and motor retardation often presents earlier than symptoms caused by brain involvement.

Infants with FCMD present with hypotonia, developmental delay, and seizures. The eye abnormalities are less severe than those of WWS or MEB.

Imaging

WALKER-WARBURG SYNDROME. WWS has a distinctive appearance on MR. Part or all of the cortex is grossly thickened with nodules of disorganized neurons on the surface (accounting for the cobblestone appearance) and linear bundles of GM that project into the underlying WM. Hydrocephalus is common. The brainstem is usually hypoplastic and appears "kinked"; the tectum is enlarged; and the cerebellum appears small and dysmorphic with abnormal foliation.

Multiple tiny cerebellar cysts are typical of WWS. They are best demonstrated on thin-section, high-resolution T2WI and suppress completely with FLAIR.

MUSCLE-EYE-BRAIN DISEASE. Retinal detachment with microphthalmia is typical with MEB. Cortical dysplasia, polymicrogyria, and hypoplasia of the inferior vermis are typical (37-39) although the cortical dysplasia may not be apparent on MR until several postnatal months.

FUKUYAMA CONGENITAL MUSCULAR DYSTROPHY. Patients with FCMD have temporooccipital cobblestone cortex. The brainstem is small, and the collicular plate appears enlarged and fused. The cerebellum is grossly dysmorphic with disorganized folia and subcortical T2/FLAIR hyperintense cysts.

Differential Diagnosis

The major differential diagnosis of type 2 lissencephaly with CMD includes type 1 ("classic") lissencephaly and polymicrogyria. CMD is not a feature of **type 1 lissencephaly**. In **polymicrogyria**, the absence of eye

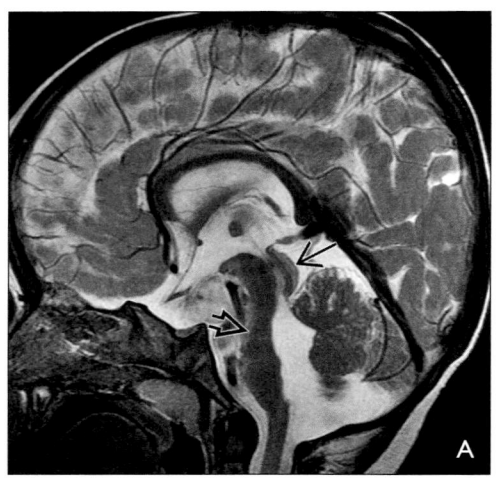
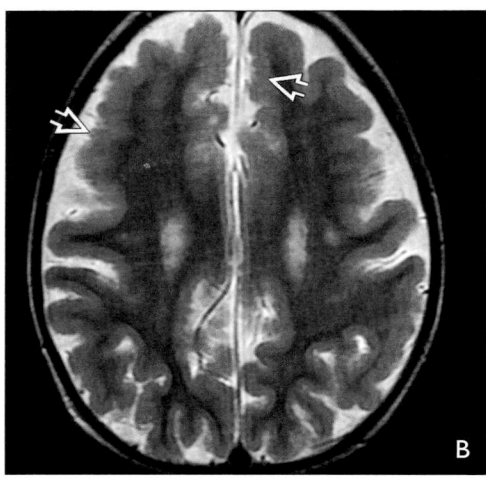

37-39A. Sagittal T2WI in a patient with cobblestone lissencephaly associated with muscle-eye-brain disease. Note enlarged, fused collicular plate ➡, small pons ⇗ with "kinked" appearance to the midbrain, thin upwardly arched corpus callosum. 37-39B. Axial T2WI in the same patient shows frontal-predominant cobblestone lissencephaly ⇗.

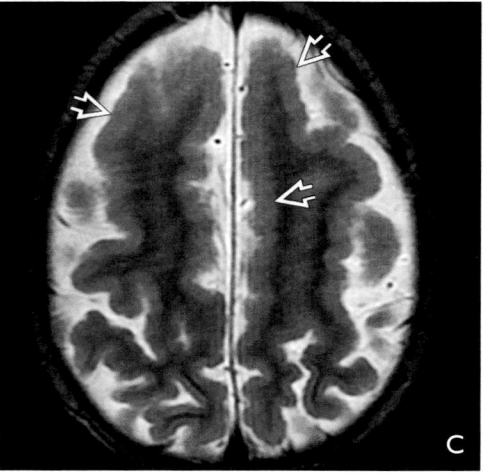
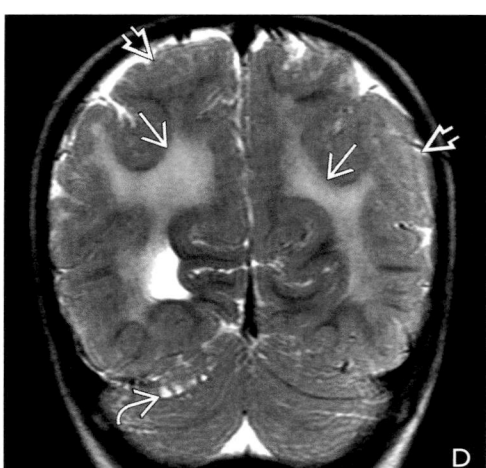

37-39C. More cephalad scan in the same patient nicely demonstrates the distinctive cobblestone appearance of the thickened frontal gyri ⇗. 37-39D. Coronal T2WI in the same patient shows delayed myelination ➡, cobblestone cortex ⇗, cerebellar cysts ➚.

anomalies and muscle weakness are helpful distinguishing features.

Malformations Secondary to Abnormal Postmigrational Development

According to Barkovich et al., the third group of cortical malformations is secondary to abnormal postmigrational development and typically reflects infectious or ischemic insults. This group was formerly designated "abnormalities of cortical organization." It is currently divided into four subtypes of polymicrogyria according to whether clefts (schizencephaly) are present and whether they occur as part of a recognized multiple malformation syndrome or an inherited metabolic disorder.

Polymicrogyria

Terminology and Etiology

The signature feature of polymicrogyria (PMG) is an irregular cortex with numerous small convolutions and shallow or obliterated sulci. The appearance is that of tiny miniature gyri piled on top of other disorganized gyri **(37-40)**.

There is evidence of both genetic and nongenetic causes of PMG. Many cases occur with other malformations (e.g., Zellweger syndrome). A number of associated genetic anomalies such as mutations in the homeobox gene *PAX6* have recently been identified.

Encephaloclastic insults such as infection (e.g., TORCH), intrauterine vascular accident (e.g., middle cerebral artery occlusion), trauma, and metabolic disorders have also been implicated in the development of PMG.

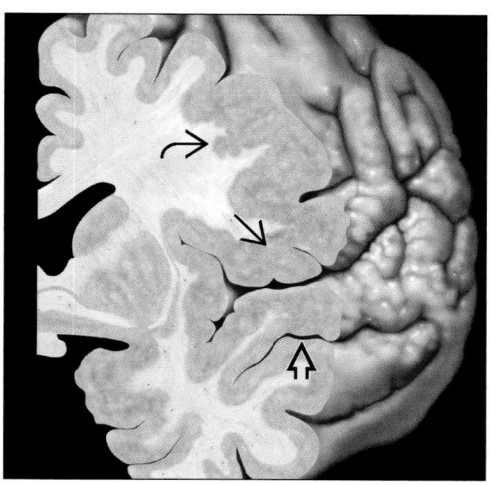

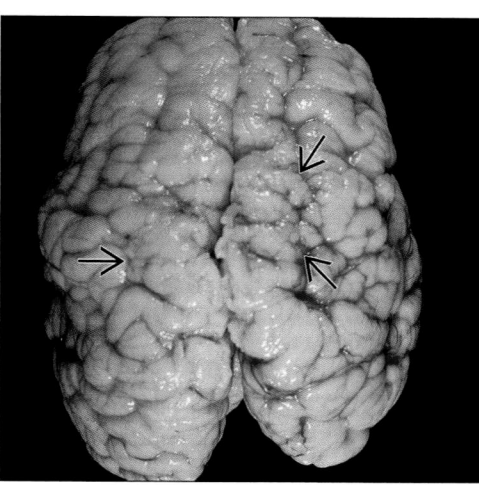

37-40. Coronal oblique graphic shows the thickened "pebbly" gyri of polymicrogyria involving the frontal ⇨ and temporal ⇨ opercula. Note abnormal sulcation and the irregular cortical-white matter interface ⇨ in the affected regions. 37-41. Autopsy specimen shows both pachy- and polymicrogyria. Note several foci of tiny nodules ("gyri piled on top of gyri") ⇨ giving the brain surface an irregular "pebbly" appearance.

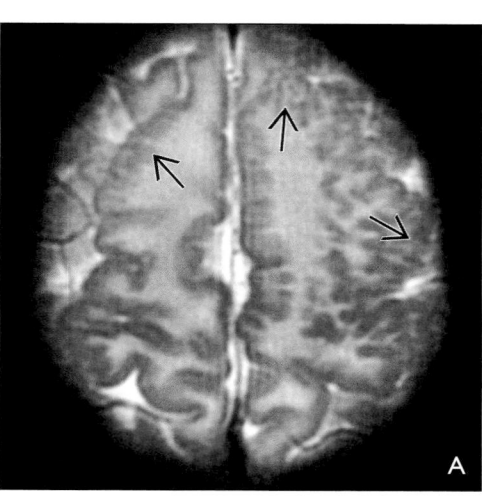

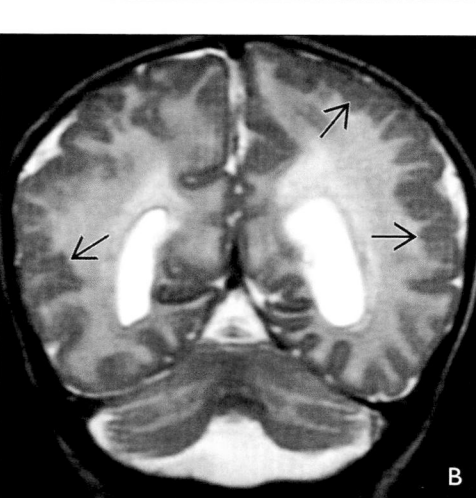

37-42A. Axial T2WI in a 2-week-old infant with seizures shows multiple foci of polymicrogyria ⇨. The left hemisphere is much more severely affected than the right. 37-42B. Coronal T2WI in the same patient also shows the polymicrogyria ⇨. The appearance of multiple tiny nodules of gray matter piled on top of gyri is characteristic.

Pathology

LOCATION. Bilateral perisylvian PMG is the most common location (61% of cases). Generalized (13%), frontal (5%), and parasagittal parietooccipital (3%) sites are less common. Associated periventricular GM heterotopias are found in 11% of cases, and other anomalies such as schizencephaly are common.

GROSS PATHOLOGY. The gross findings of PMG vary widely. PMG can involve a single gyrus or most of an entire cerebral hemisphere. It can be uni- or bilateral, symmetric or asymmetric, and focal or diffuse.

Part or all of the brain surface is covered by innumerable heaped up and fused tiny gyri, giving it a "lumpy-bumpy" appearance that has been likened to the look and feel of morocco leather **(37-41)**. Bilateral disease—especially in the perisylvian regions—is present in the majority of cases.

MICROSCOPIC FEATURES. Microscopically, the cortical ribbon appears thin and excessively folded. Two main histological types of PMG—unlayered and four-layered forms—occur. In the unlayered form, a continuous molecular layer is present without any discernible laminar organization. In four-layered PMG, the cortex shows complex folding, fusion, and branching. A laminar structure composed of a molecular layer, outer neuronal layer, nerve fiber layer, and inner neuronal layer is present.

Clinical Issues

PMG can present at any age. Some types of PMG are more common in males, suggesting the involvement of X-linked genes.

Symptoms depend on the location and extent of PMG, ranging from global developmental delay to focal neurologic deficit(s) and seizures.

Imaging

MR is the procedure of choice. Multiplanar imaging with high-resolution thin sections is required for complete delineation and detection of subtle lesions. Thickened or overfolded cortex with nodular surfaces and irregular "stippled" gray-white matter interfaces are the most characteristic findings **(37-42)**.

37-43. Coronal oblique graphic shows an "open lip" schizencephaly in the frontal lobe. Note irregular gray-white interface of the cortex lining the cleft ➡, indicating its dysplastic nature. 37-44. Autopsy shows bilateral schizencephalic clefts. Note that the thick, abnormal cortex curves over the "lips" of the clefts ➡ and follows them all the way medially to the ventricular ependyma. (Courtesy R. Hewlett, MD.)

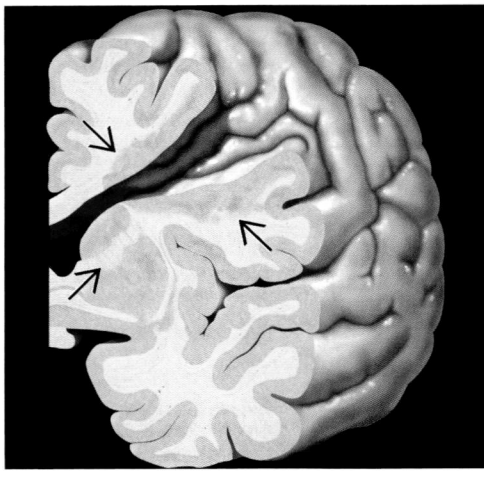

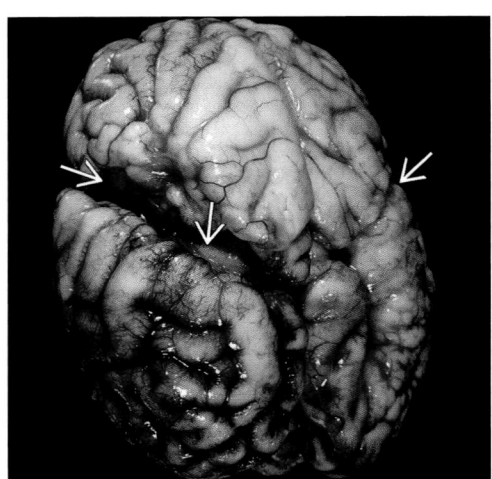

37-45A. NECT in a 19-year-old man following minor head trauma shows the classic findings of unilateral schizencephaly. A nipple-like outpouching of CSF from the lateral ventricle ➡ is continuous with a thin "seam" of CSF ➡ that extends to the surface of the hemisphere. The cleft is lined with dysplastic-appearing GM ➡ 37-45B. More cephalad scan shows cleft ➡, dysplastic GM ➡ extending to ventricular ependyma ➡.

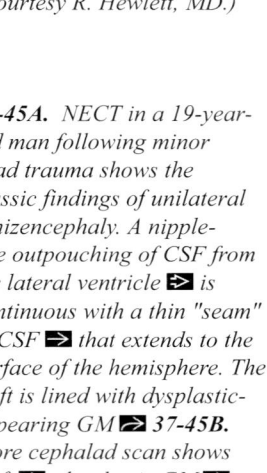

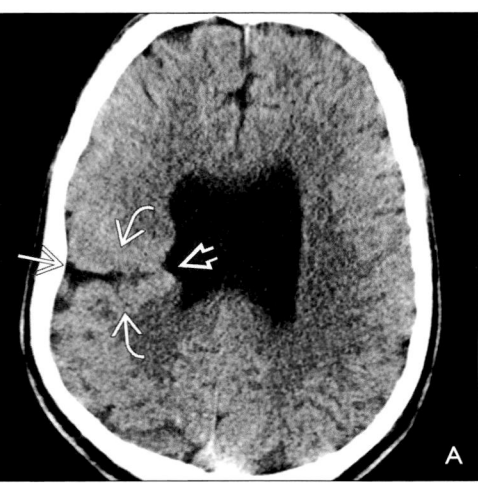

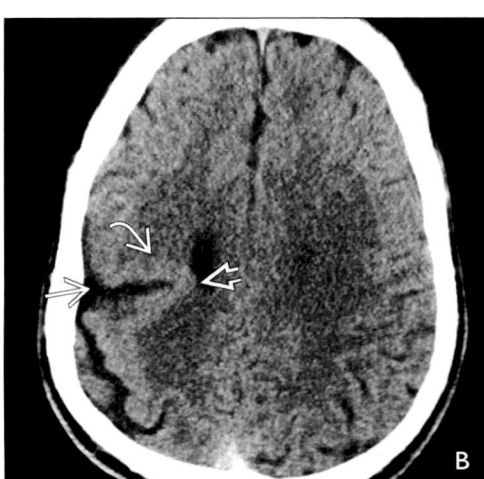

Differential Diagnosis

The major differential diagnosis of polymicrogyria is **type 2 lissencephaly** (cobblestone malformation). The absence of congenital muscular dystrophy is a helpful clinical distinction.

Sometimes **pachygyria** can be confused with PMG. The cortex in PMG is thin, nodular, and excessively folded. In **focal cortical dysplasia**, the gray matter is thickened, and the GM-WM interface is blurred.

Schizencephaly

Terminology

Schizencephaly (literally meaning "split brain") is a gray-matter-lined cleft that extends from the ventricular ependyma to the pial surface of the cortex. The cleft spans the full thickness of the affected hemisphere **(37-43)**.

Etiology

Once thought to represent an early malformation of cortical development, schizencephaly is now regarded as a disorder with heterogeneous causes. Destructive vascular lesions (e.g., MCA occlusion) and infections (e.g., TORCH) occurring before 28 fetal weeks are considered likely etiologies. Focal destruction of radial glial fibers with impaired neuronal migration has been invoked as the potential consequence of these early vascular or infectious insults.

The majority of schizencephaly cases are sporadic, but some instances of familial schizencephaly have been described.

One-third of all cases have an associated non-CNS abnormality secondary to vascular disruption (e.g., amniotic band syndrome or gastroschisis).

Pathology

Grossly, the brain exhibits a deep cleft that extends from its surface to the ventricle. The cleft is surrounded and lined by disorganized, dysmorphic-appearing cortex **(37-44)**. The "lips" of the cleft can be fused or closely apposed ("closed lip" schizencephaly) or appear widely separated ("open lip" schizencephaly). Clefts may be

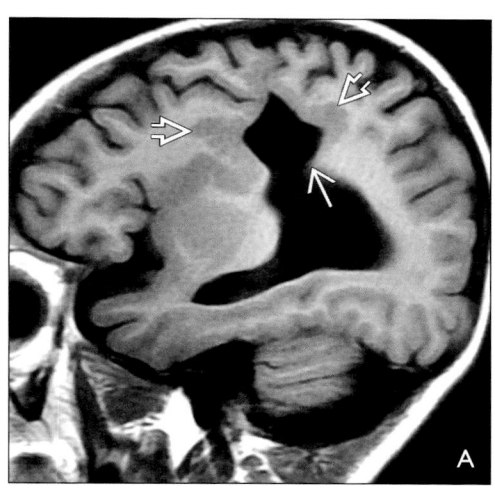

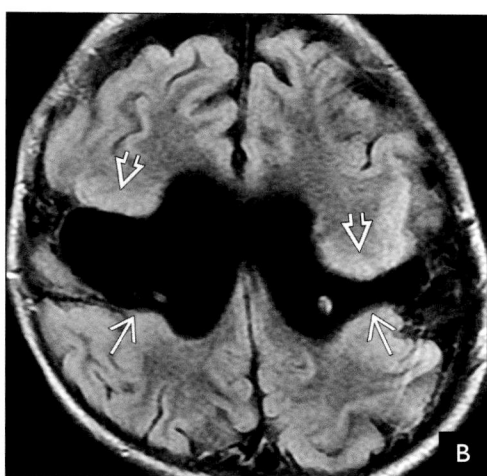

37-46A. Sagittal T1WI shows a large CSF-filled cleft ➡ extending superiorly from the lateral ventricle. The cleft is lined with dysplastic-appearing gray matter ➡. 37-46B. FLAIR scan in the same patient shows bilateral schizencephalic clefts ➡ that are lined by dysplastic GM ➡. The clefts suppress completely.

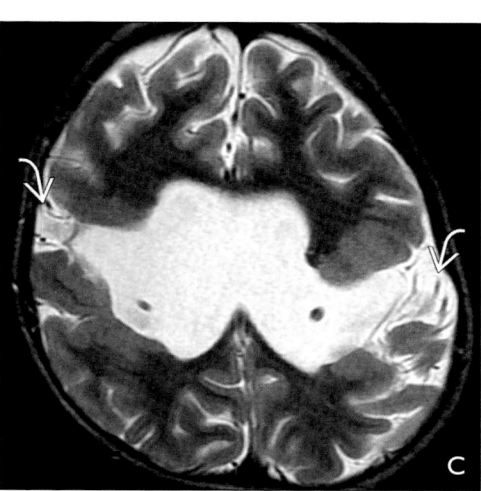

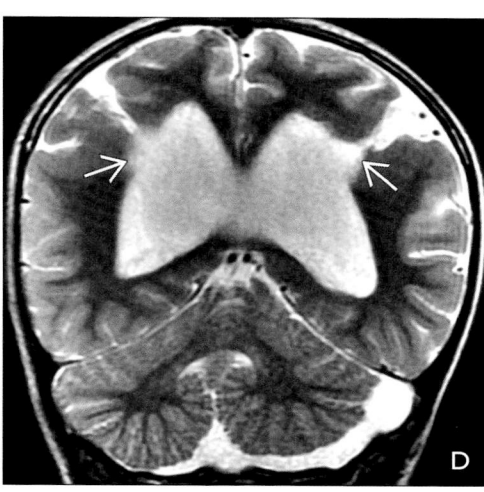

37-46C. Axial T2WI shows that the open "lips" of both clefts contain prominent "flow voids" ➡ consistent with the primitive, "uncondensed" cortical veins that commonly accompany schizencephaly. 37-46D. Coronal T2WI show the pointed "nipples" ➡ of CSF that extend outward from the ventricles into the schizencephalic clefts.

associated with a range of other macroscopic abnormalities involving the septi pellucidi, corpus callosum, optic chiasm, and hippocampus.

Microscopically, the gray matter that lines the cleft is disorganized and does not exhibit normal cortical layers.

Clinical Issues

EPIDEMIOLOGY AND DEMOGRAPHICS. Schizencephaly is rare. The estimated prevalence is approximately 1-2:100,000 population. There is no gender predilection.

PRESENTATION AND NATURAL HISTORY. The most common clinical manifestations of schizencephaly are drug-resistant epilepsy, developmental delay, and motor impairment. The severity of the motor and mental deficits correlates with the extent of the anatomic defect. "Open lip" clefts usually result in the most significant impairment. A unilateral "closed lip" cleft may cause only seizures. A few cases are discovered incidentally.

Imaging

The key imaging features of schizencephaly are (1) a CSF-filled defect extending from the ventricle wall to the pial surface and (2) dysplastic gray matter lining the cleft.

NECT scans typically show a focal V-shaped outpouching or "dimple" of CSF extending outward from the lateral ventricle. The clefts can be uni- (60%) or bilateral (40%) with prominent ("open lip") or barely visible ("closed lip") **(37-45)**. The cortex lining the cleft is hyperdense relative to white matter and interrupts the relatively uniform appearance of the corona radiata.

Common associated abnormalities are absent septi pellucidi (70% of cases) and a focally thinned or dysgenetic corpus callosum.

MR is more sensitive than CT, especially in delineating associated abnormalities such as cortical dysplasia (polymicrogyria, pachygyria) and heterotopic gray matter. The cleft follows CSF signal intensity on all sequences **(37-46)**, **(37-47)**, **(37-48)**.

37-47A. Axial T1WI shows severe "open lip" schizencephalic clefts ➡ in both hemispheres. 37-47B. T2WI shows the thalami ➡, some brain remnants ➢ in the frontal, occipital poles.

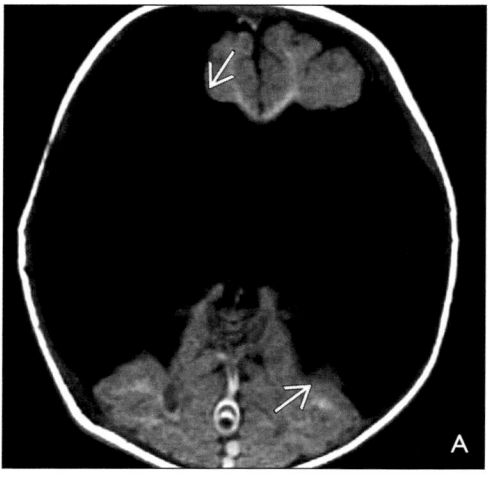
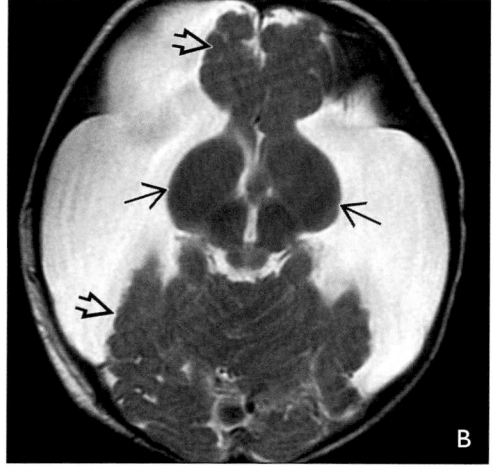

37-47C. More cephalad scan shows the presence of a falx and interhemispheric fissure ➢ distinguishing this extreme case of schizencephaly from holoprosencephaly. The remnant anterior, posterior "nubbins" of brain are different from the thin rim of cortex around the maximally enlarged lateral ventricles in severe hydrocephalus. 37-47D. Coronal T2WI shows that there is no cortex external to the huge "open" schizencephalic clefts.

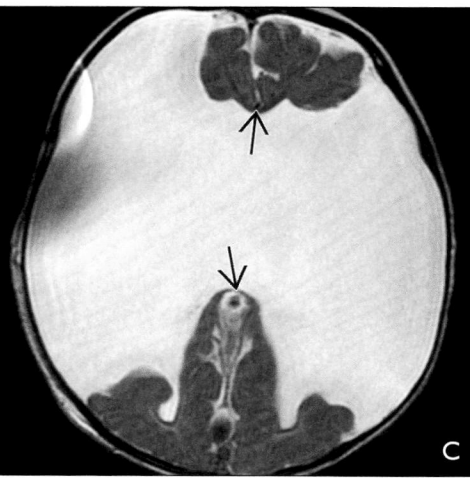
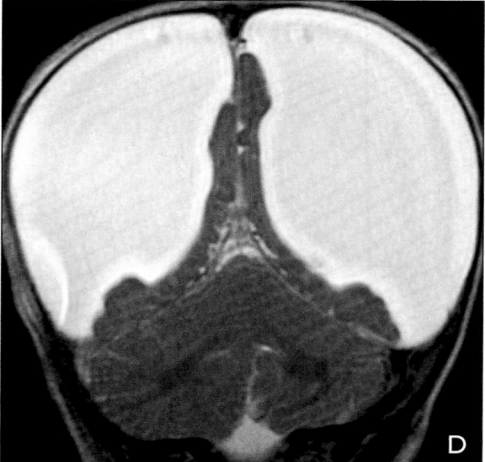

DSA or CTA/MRA have demonstrated occlusion or absence of the middle cerebral artery in some cases.

Differential Diagnosis

The differential diagnosis of CSF-filled brain defects includes both developmental and destructive lesions. The major differential diagnosis of schizencephaly is **porencephaly**. In porencephaly, the cleft is lined by gliotic white matter, not dysplastic gray matter.

A large **arachnoid cyst** can mimic "open lip" schizencephaly. An arachnoid cyst displaces the adjacent cortex, which is otherwise normal in appearance.

Transmantle **heterotopia** or deeply infolded **polymicrogyria** may be difficult to distinguish from schizencephaly with closed, nearly fused "lips." Multiple imaging planes with high-resolution T2WI or thin-section T1-weighted sequences with 3D reformatting and shaded surface displays are helpful in differentiating these entities.

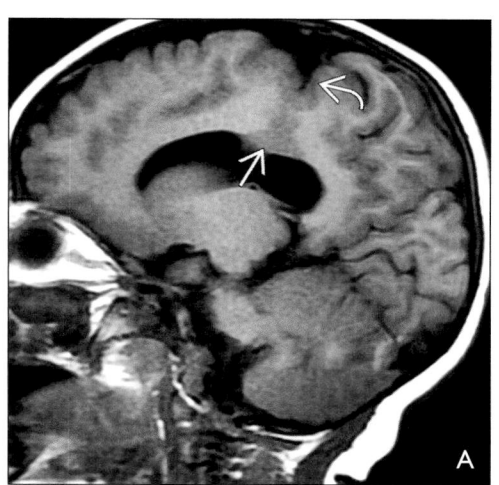
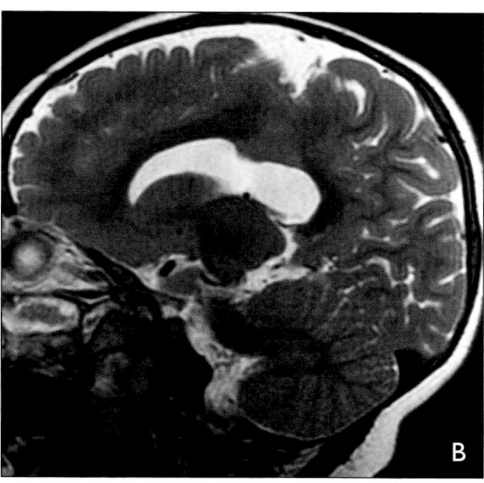

37-48A. Unilateral "closed lip" schizencephaly is illustrated by this case. Note gray matter extending from the ventricle ➡ to the pial surface of the brain ➡. 37-48B. Sagittal T2WI shows that the GM lining the cleft is the same signal intensity as the cortex.

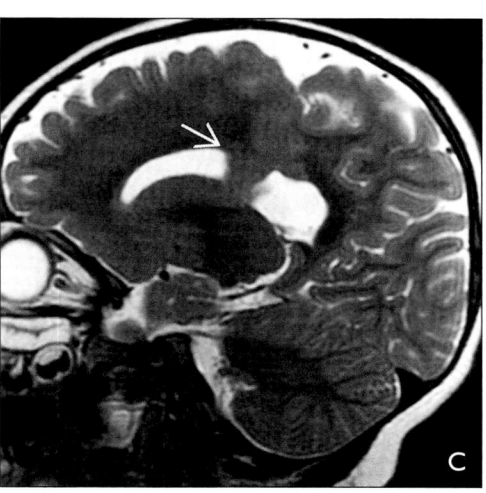
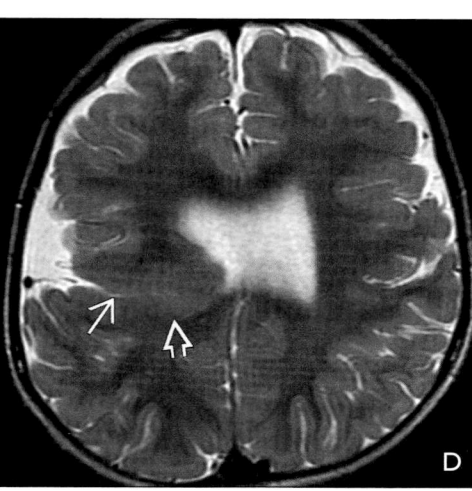

37-48C. Sagittal T2WI shows that the heterotopic GM around the cleft bulges into the lateral ventricle body ➡. 37-48D. Axial T2WI shows the heterotopic GM ➡ surrounding the cleft ➡, which is difficult to discern as it is so thin.

Selected References

Normal Development and Anatomy of the Cerebral Commissures

Normal Development

- Barkovich AJ et al: Congenital malformations of the brain and skull. In Pediatric Neuroimaging. 5th ed. Philadelphia: Lippincott Williams & Wilkins. 368-83, 2012
- Raybaud C: The corpus callosum, the other great forebrain commissures, and the septum pellucidum: anatomy, development, and malformation. Neuroradiology. 52(6):447-77, 2010

Normal Gross and Imaging Anatomy

- Peltier J et al: Microsurgical anatomy of the anterior commissure: correlations with diffusion tensor imaging fiber tracking and clinical relevance. Neurosurgery. 69(2 Suppl Operative):241-6; discussion 246-7, 2011
- Wang F et al: Microsurgical and tractographic anatomical study of insular and transsylvian transinsular approach. Neurol Sci. 32(5):865-74, 2011
- Patel MD et al: Distribution and fibre field similarity mapping of the human anterior commissure fibres by diffusion tensor imaging. MAGMA. 23(5-6):399-408, 2010

Commissural Anomalies

- Barkovich AJ: Congenital malformations overview. In Osborn AG et al: Diagnostic Imaging: Brain. 2nd ed. Salt Lake City: Amirsys Publishing. I.1.2-5, 2010
- Ren T et al: Imaging, anatomical, and molecular analysis of callosal formation in the developing human fetal brain. Anat Rec A Discov Mol Cell Evol Biol. 288(2):191-204, 2006

Callosal Dysgenesis Spectrum

- Paul LK: Developmental malformation of the corpus callosum: a review of typical callosal development and examples of developmental disorders with callosal involvement. J Neurodev Disord. 3(1):3-27, 2011

Associated Anomalies and Syndromes

- Wahl M et al: Diffusion tensor imaging of Aicardi syndrome. Pediatr Neurol. 43(2):87-91, 2010
- Yacubian-Fernandes A et al: Apert syndrome: analysis of associated brain malformations and conformational changes determined by surgical treatment. J Neuroradiol. 31(2):116-22, 2004
- Brunberg JA et al: Fragile X premutation carriers: characteristic MR imaging findings of adult male patients with progressive cerebellar and cognitive dysfunction. AJNR Am J Neuroradiol. 23(10):1757-66, 2002

Malformations of Cortical Development Overview

- Barkovich AJ et al: A developmental and genetic classification for malformations of cortical development: update 2012. Brain. 135(Pt 5):1348-69, 2012
- Aronica E et al: Malformations of cortical development. Brain Pathol. 22(3):380-401, 2012
- Barkovich AJ et al: Malformations of cerebral cortical development. In Pediatric Neuroimaging. 5th ed. Philadelphia: Lippincott Williams & Wilkins. 383-444, 2012
- Abdel Razek AA et al: Disorders of cortical formation: MR imaging features. AJNR Am J Neuroradiol. 30(1):4-11, 2009

Malformations with Abnormal Cell Numbers/Types

Microcephalies

- Poulton CJ et al: Microcephaly with simplified gyration, epilepsy, and infantile diabetes linked to inappropriate apoptosis of neural progenitors. Am J Hum Genet. 89(2):265-76, 2011

Focal Cortical Dysplasias

- Aronica E et al: Malformations of cortical development. Brain Pathol. 22(3):380-401, 2012
- Barkovich AJ et al: A developmental and genetic classification for malformations of cortical development: update 2012. Brain. 135(Pt 5):1348-69, 2012
- Chassoux F et al: Type II focal cortical dysplasia: electroclinical phenotype and surgical outcome related to imaging. Epilepsia. 53(2):349-58, 2012
- Fellah S et al: Epileptogenic brain lesions in children: the added-value of combined diffusion imaging and proton MR spectroscopy to the presurgical differential diagnosis. Childs Nerv Syst. 28(2):273-82, 2012
- Mühlebner A et al: Neuropathologic measurements in focal cortical dysplasias: validation of the ILAE 2011 classification system and diagnostic implications for MRI. Acta Neuropathol. 123(2):259-72, 2012
- Blümcke I et al: The clinicopathologic spectrum of focal cortical dysplasias: a consensus classification proposed by an ad hoc task force of the ILAE Diagnostic Methods Commission. Epilepsia. 52(1):158-74, 2011
- Chern JJ et al: Surgical outcome for focal cortical dysplasia: an analysis of recent surgical series. J Neurosurg Pediatr. 6(5):452-8, 2010
- Thom M: Epilepsy part I: cortical dysplasia. In Golden JA et al: Pathology and Genetics: Developmental Neuropathology. Basel: ISN Neuropath Press. 61-66, 2004
- Taylor DC et al: Focal dysplasia of the cerebral cortex in epilepsy. J Neurol Neurosurg Psychiatry. 34(4):369-87, 1971

Hemimegaloencephaly

- Aronica E et al: Malformations of cortical development. Brain Pathol. 22(3):380-401, 2012

- Barkovich AJ et al: A developmental and genetic classification for malformations of cortical development: update 2012. Brain. 135(Pt 5):1348-69, 2012
- Broumandi DD et al: Best cases from the AFIP: hemimegalencephaly. Radiographics. 24(3):843-8, 2004

Abnormalities of Neuronal Migration

- Barkovich AJ et al: A developmental and genetic classification for malformations of cortical development: update 2012. Brain. 135(Pt 5):1348-69, 2012

Heterotopias

- Barkovich AJ et al: A developmental and genetic classification for malformations of cortical development: update 2012. Brain. 135(Pt 5):1348-69, 2012
- Clapham KR et al: FLNA genomic rearrangements cause periventricular nodular heterotopia. Neurology. 78(4):269-78, 2012

Lissencephaly Spectrum

- Barkovich AJ et al: A developmental and genetic classification for malformations of cortical development: update 2012. Brain. 135(Pt 5):1348-69, 2012
- Friocourt G et al: Role of cytoskeletal abnormalities in the neuropathology and pathophysiology of type I lissencephaly. Acta Neuropathol. 121(2):149-70, 2011
- Iannetti P et al: Fiber tractography assessment in double cortex syndrome. Childs Nerv Syst. 27(8):1197-202, 2011

Subcortical Heterotopias and Lobar Dysplasias

- Barkovich AJ et al: A developmental and genetic classification for malformations of cortical development: update 2012. Brain. 135(Pt 5):1348-69, 2012
- Tuxhorn I et al: Sublobar dysplasia--A clinicopathologic report after successful epilepsy surgery. Epilepsia. 50(12):2652-7, 2009

Cobblestone Malformations and the Congenital Muscular Dystrophies

- Rathod SB et al: Walker- Warburg syndrome: demonstration of cerebellar cysts with CISS sequence. Magn Reson Med Sci. 11(2):137-40, 2012
- Longman C et al: Antenatal and postnatal brain magnetic resonance imaging in muscle-eye-brain disease. Arch Neurol. 61(8):1301-6, 2004

Malformations Secondary to Abnormal Postmigrational Development

- Barkovich AJ et al: A developmental and genetic classification for malformations of cortical development: update 2012. Brain. 135(Pt 5):1348-69, 2012
- Devisme L et al: Cobblestone lissencephaly: neuropathological subtypes and correlations with genes of dystroglycanopathies. Brain. 135(Pt 2):469-82, 2012

- Rathod SB et al: Walker- Warburg syndrome: Demonstration of cerebellar cysts with CISS sequence. Magn Reson Med Sci. 11(2):137-40, 2012

Polymicrogyria

- Mavili E et al: Polymicrogyria: correlation of magnetic resonance imaging and clinical findings. Childs Nerv Syst. 28(6):905-9, 2012
- Leventer RJ et al: Clinical and imaging heterogeneity of polymicrogyria: a study of 328 patients. Brain. 133(Pt 5):1415-27, 2010

38

Holoprosencephalies, Related Disorders, and Mimics

In this chapter, we discuss the holoprosencephalies and related disorders. Holoprosencephalies and variants such as syntelencephaly are classified as anomalies of ventral prosencephalon development. Other anomalies of the ventral prosencephalon include septooptic dysplasia (with or without anomalies of the hypothalamic-pituitary axis) and arrhinencephaly, both of which are discussed in this chapter.

We also consider two midline facial anomalies—solitary median maxillary central incisor syndrome and congenital pyriform aperture stenosis/choanal atresia spectrum—that are often present in holoprosencephaly or arrhinencephaly.

Finally, we conclude the chapter with a brief discussion of hydranencephaly, an in utero acquired destruction of the cerebral hemispheres that can sometimes be confused with alobar holoprosencephaly or severe "open lip" schizencephaly.

Anencephaly

Anencephaly (literally meaning "no brain") occurs when the cephalic end of the neural tube fails to close, resulting in absence of the forebrain, skull, and scalp. The remaining brain—usually only the brainstem—is not covered by bone or skin. Most anencephalic fetuses are aborted or die shortly after birth **(38-1)**.

Two rare lethal malformations—**aprosencephaly** and **atelencephaly** (AP/AT)—are intermediate in the continuum between anencephaly and holoprosencephaly. AP/AT is now considered the most severe end of the holoprosencephaly spectrum. These three extreme malformations are usually diagnosed at fetal MR, sonography, or postmortem examination **(38-2)**.

Holoprosencephaly

Holoprosencephaly spans a continuum from alobar to lobar forms. While each is delineated separately, keep in mind that the holoprosencephalies are really a spectrum with no clear boundaries that reliably distinguish one type from another.

Terminology

In holoprosencephaly (HPE), the fetal forebrain fails to bifurcate into two hemispheres. "Holoprosencephaly" literally means a single ("holo") ventricle involving the embryonic prosencephalon ("pros") of the brain ("encephaly").

Holoprosencephaly is a continuum that ranges from the most severe type (alobar HPE) to milder lobar forms. An

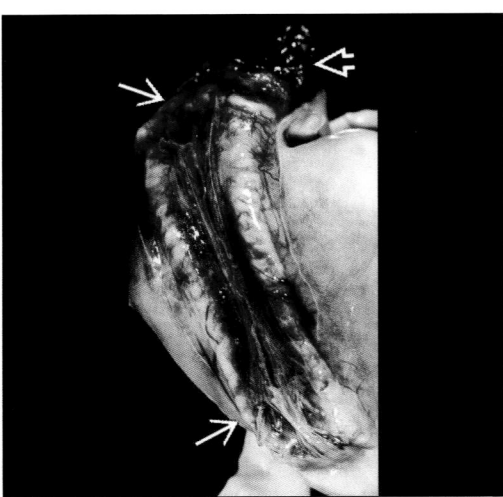

38-1. *Autopsy specimen shows total failure of neural tube closure with complete spine dysraphism* ➡, *anencephaly* ➡. *(Courtesy R. Hewlett, MD.)*

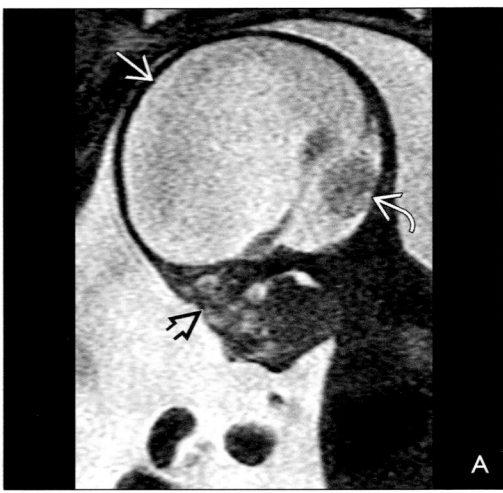

38-2A. *Fetal sagittal T2WI in aprosencephaly shows no supratentorial brain* ➡, *absent nose* ➡, *small remnant of cerebellum* ➡.

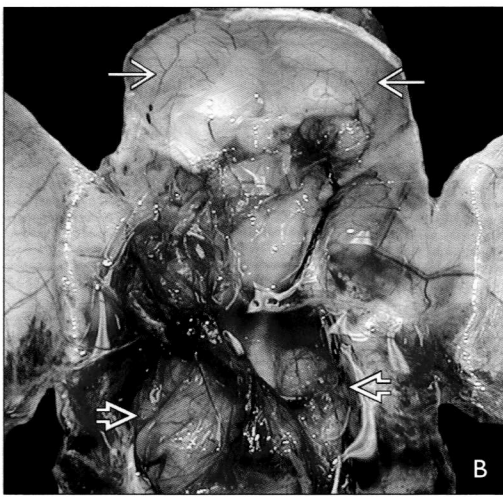

38-2B. *Autopsy of the same case, viewed from above, shows no supratentorial tissue* ➡. *Only cerebellum is present* ➡.

intermediate type, semilobar HPE, is more severe than alobar HPE but not nearly as well differentiated as the lobar variety. The distinction between these three forms is based primarily on the presence or absence of a midline fissure separating the hemispheres.

Etiology

EMBRYOLOGY. In normal embryologic development, the fetal forebrain starts as a featureless, fluid-filled, frontal sac; evolves through a series of folds, flexures, and out-pouchings; and becomes the definitive cerebral ventri-cles and hemispheres. In the earliest stages, bilateral out-pouchings from the neural tube initially form a single cen-tral fluid-filled cavity ("monoventricle") that will even-tually develop into the lateral and third ventricles (see Chapter 34). The separation into two hemispheres is nor-mally completed by the fifth gestational week.

The holoprosencephalies are characterized by failure of normal dorsal-ventral induction and lack of rostral forebrain cleavage. In the most severe forms, dien-cephalic-derived structures such as the basal ganglia also remain fused in the midline. As ventral induction is closely related to facial development, HPE is also associ-ated with a number of characteristic facial anomalies.

GENERAL CONCEPTS. Between one-quarter and one-half of HPE patients have a recognized syndrome (e.g., Pallis-ter-Hall) or a single gene defect. Nonsyndromic HPE has previously been associated with a number of environmen-tal teratogens (e.g., retinoic acid and alcohol) and mater-nal factors such as pre-pregnancy diabetes, smoking, and substance abuse. However, recent studies have cast doubt on these assertions.

GENETICS. At least 12 regions on 11 separate chromo-somes have been identified as playing a role in familial HPE. Mutations in four main HPE genes (*SHH, ZIC2, SIX3, TGIF*) are identified in 25% of cases. The most severe forms of HPE are associated with *SIX3* and *ZIC2* mutations.

Clinical Issues

EPIDEMIOLOGY AND DEMOGRAPHICS. Holoprosen-cephaly is the most common human forebrain malfor-mation. The overall incidence of HPE varies from 1:250 aborted conceptuses to 1:10,000-20,000 live births.

PRESENTATION. Presentation and prognosis in HPE both vary widely. There is a broad range of brain and associated midface anomalies. Craniofacial malforma-tions such as cyclopia or single proboscis, hypotelorism, nasal anomalies, and facial clefts occur in approximately 75-80% of cases. The statement "the face predicts the brain" means that the most severe facial defects generally (although not invariably) are found with the most severe intracranial anomalies **(38-3A)**.

Yet functional abnormalities range further. Nearly three-quarters of HPE patients have endocrinopathies; severity generally correlates with the degree of hypothalamic nonseparation.

NATURAL HISTORY. Fetuses with severe alobar HPE are often spontaneously aborted, and severely affected children frequently die as neonates. Surviving individuals usually exhibit variable mental retardation and seizures. Pituitary insufficiency and congenital anosmia with absent CN I ("arrhinencephaly") are other common clinical features of HPE.

Imaging

Imaging findings range from a pancake-like holosphere with central monoventricle (alobar HPE) to well-differentiated, almost completely separated hemispheres with minimal abnormalities (lobar HPE).

Alobar Holoprosencephaly

Terminology and Pathology

Alobar holoprosencephaly (aHPE) is the most severe form of HPE. No midline fissure divides the brain into two separate cerebral hemispheres, and no identifiable lobes are seen **(38-3B)**. The basal ganglia are usually present but fused. The falx and sagittal sinus are absent, as are the olfactory bulbs and tracts. The optic nerves can be normal, fused, or absent.

The brain itself is often smaller than normal. Its configuration varies from flat ("pancake") to cup- or ball-shaped. The sylvian fissures are unformed, and the brain surface often appears completely agyric or minimally sulcated with shallow sulci and flat, disordered gyri.

Cut sections demonstrate a single crescent-shaped monoventricle that opens dorsally into a large CSF-filled dorsal cyst **(38-4)**.

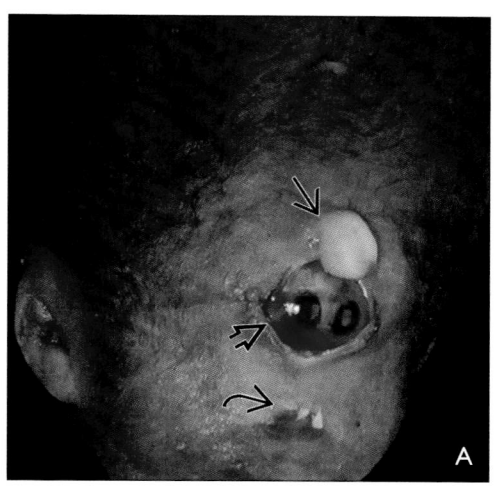

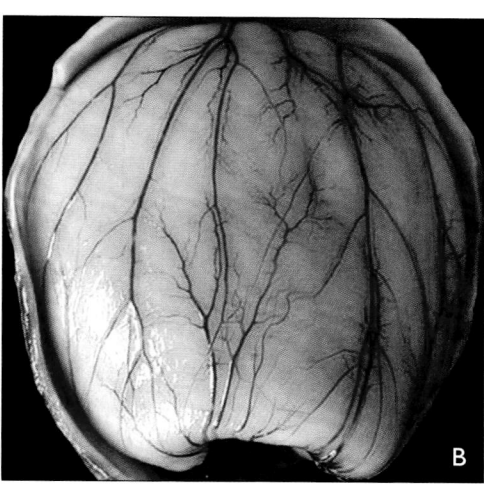

38-3A. *Clinical photograph of aborted fetus with alobar holoprosencephaly shows extreme facial anomalies with central proboscis ➡, cyclops ⊒, slit-like oral cavity ➡.* **38-3B.** *View of autopsied brain in the same case shows completely smooth, featureless brain with no evidence of sulcation, gyration, or midline structures such as the falx or interhemispheric fissure. (Courtesy R. Hewlett, MD.)*

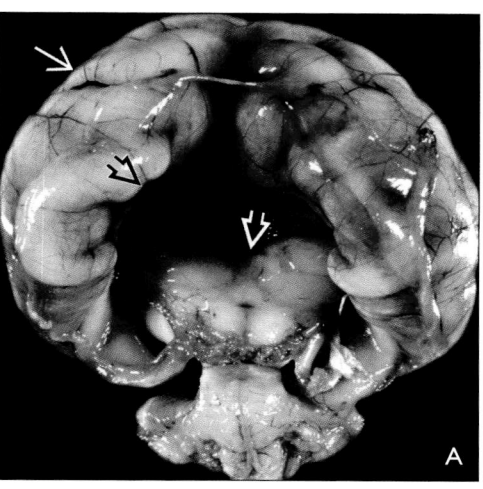

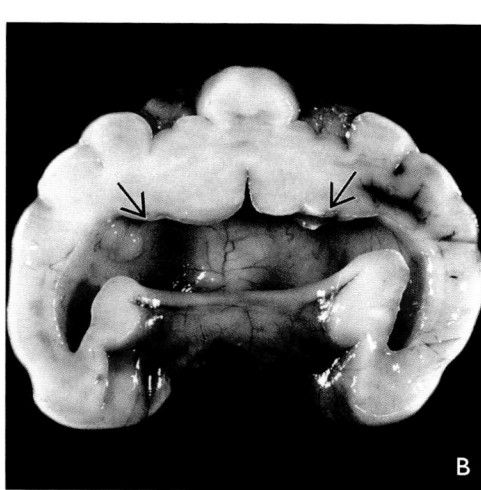

38-4A. *Autopsy of alobar holoprosencephaly shows large dorsal cyst ⊒, fused thalami ➡, rudimentary hemispheres ➡ with minimal sulcation, gyration.* **38-4B.** *Coronal cut section in the same case demonstrates no evidence of midline fissure with fusion of the rudimentary hemispheres across the midline. The central monoventricle ➡ has a "horseshoe" shape. (Courtesy J. Townsend, MD.)*

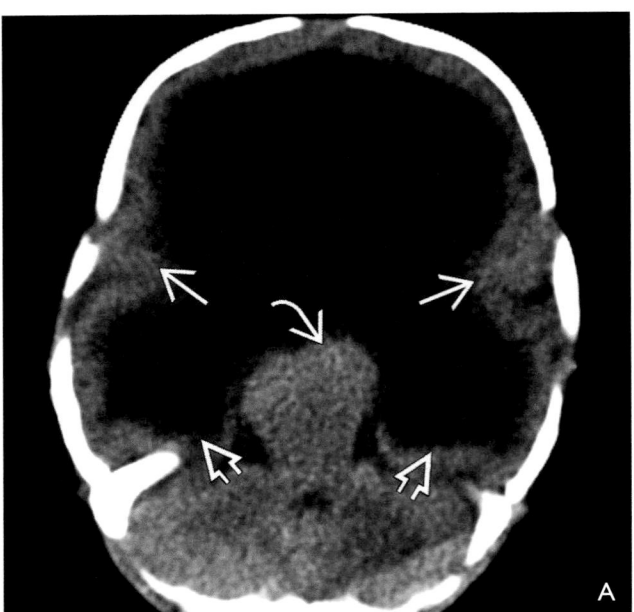

38-5A. NECT scan shows holoprosencephaly. Small rim of cortex ➡ surrounds "horseshoe" central monoventricle ➡. Thalami are fused ➡.

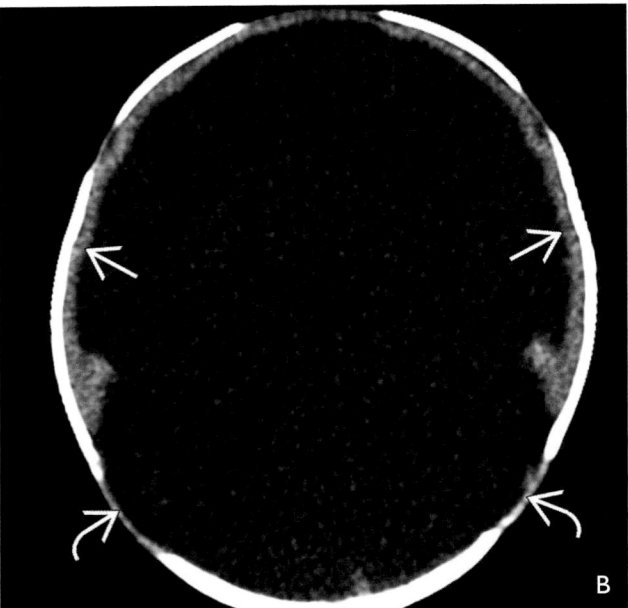

38-5B. More cephalad scan in the same patient shows a large dorsal cyst ➡, central monoventricle with thin rim of surrounding brain ➡. No falx or interhemispheric fissure is present.

Clinical Issues

Alobar HPE has a high intrauterine lethality and still birth rate. It is found in 1:250 terminated pregnancies and approximately 1:15,000 live births. In utero demise and stillbirths are common.

With severe facial deformities such as cyclopia and proboscis, survival is often less than one week. Prognosis in surviving infants is poor. At least half of all patients with aHPE die in less than five months, and 80% die before one year of age.

Imaging

No normal ventricles can be identified. NECT scans show a CSF-filled horseshoe-shaped cavity that is usually continuous posteriorly with a large dorsal cyst (38-5).

Sagittal T1 scans show a thin anteroinferior pancake of tissue with poor gyration and no discernible midline fissure. Most of the calvaria appears CSF-filled and virtually featureless. In contrast, the brainstem and cerebellum often seem relatively normal.

Coronal scans best demonstrate the central monoventricle. The septi pellucidi and third ventricle are absent, as are the falx cerebri and interhemispheric fissure. The cerebral mantle is fused across the midline anteriorly. The brain appears thin and almost agyric, although a few shallow sulci may be present. The basal ganglia are small and fused across the midline. There are no discernible commissures.

Axial scans show that the brain is completely fused across the midline without evidence of an anterior interhemispheric fissure. The monoventricle opens dorsally into a large CSF-filled cyst.

Differential Diagnosis

The major differential diagnosis of aHPE is **hydranencephaly**. In hydranencephaly, the face is normal. A falx is present, but most of the cerebral tissue has been destroyed, usually by an intrauterine vascular accident or infection.

Semilobar Holoprosencephaly

Terminology and Pathology

Semilobar holoprosencephaly (sHPE) is intermediate in severity between alobar HPE and lobar HPE. A gradation of findings is present. The most severe sHPE shows a rudimentary interhemispheric fissure and incomplete falx (38-6), (38-7). The temporal horns of the lateral ventricle may be partially formed, but the septi pellucidi are absent. A dorsal cyst is often present.

Imaging

With progressively better-differentiated sHPE, more of the interhemispheric fissure appears formed. The deep nuclei exhibit various degrees of separation. If a rudimentary third ventricle is present, the thalami may be partially separated. The basal ganglia and hypothalami are still largely fused. The caudate heads are continuous across the midline (38-8).

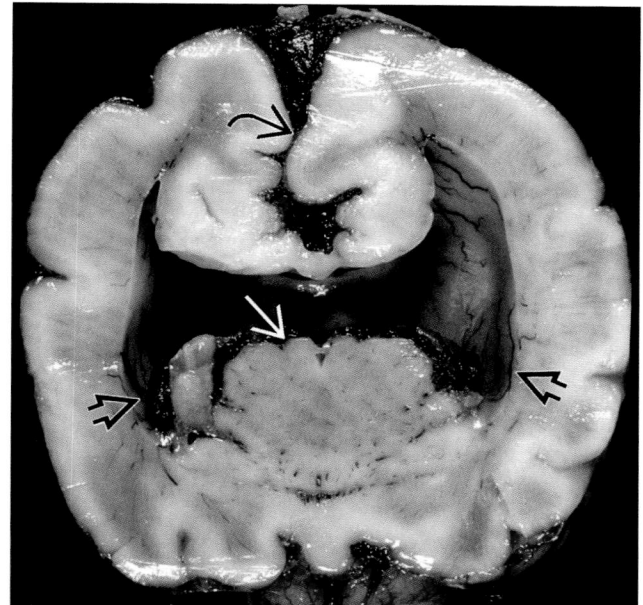

38-6. Coronal autopsy case of severe semilobar HPE shows H-shaped central ventricle with primitive-appearing temporal horns ⊵, fused basal ganglia ➡, rudimentary interhemispheric fissure ➘. (Courtesy R. Hewlett, MD.)

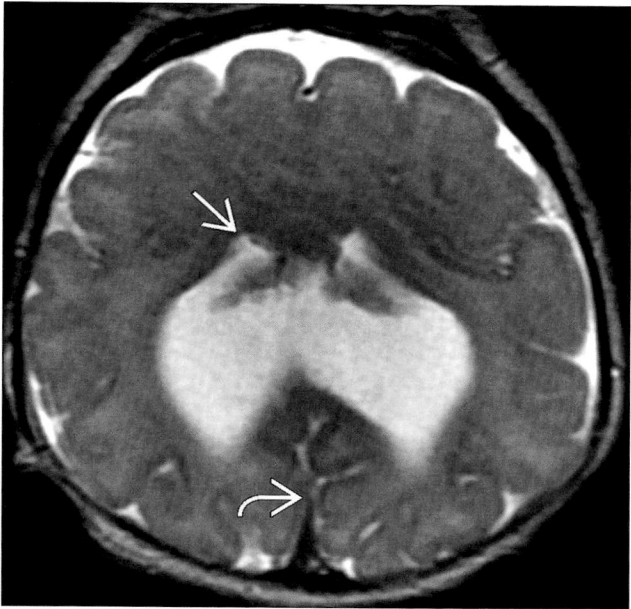

38-7. Axial T2WI shows severe sHPE with rudimentary posterior interhemispheric fissure ➘, primitive ventricular horns ➡, anterior midline fusion.

A corpus callosum splenium is present, but the body and genu are absent. Barkovich points out that (1) holoprosencephaly is the only malformation in which the posterior corpus callosum forms while the anterior aspects are absent and (2) the farther anteriorly the corpus forms, the better the brain is developed.

Differential Diagnosis

The major differential diagnoses of semilobar HPE are **alobar HPE and lobar HPE**, depending on the severity of the sHPE.

Lobar Holoprosencephaly

Terminology and Pathology

Lobar HPE is the best-differentiated of the holoprosencephalies. The interhemispheric fissure and falx are clearly developed, although their most anterior aspects are often somewhat shallow and dysplastic-appearing.

The third ventricle and lateral ventricular horns are generally well-formed, although the septi pellucidi are absent and the frontal horns almost always appear dysmorphic. The hippocampi are present but often more vertically oriented than normal.

Clinical Issues

Patients with lobar holoprosencephaly are less severely affected compared to individuals with sHPE. Mild developmental delay, hypothalamic-pituitary dysfunction, and visual disturbances are the most common symptoms.

Imaging

In lobar HPE, the cerebral hemispheres—including the thalami and most of the basal ganglia—are mostly separated. At least some of the most rostral and ventral portions of the frontal lobes are continuous across the midline (38-9). The thalami and basal ganglia are separated, although the caudate heads may remain fused.

The frontal horns of the lateral ventricles are present but dysplastic-appearing. The temporal and occipital horns are better-defined, and the third ventricle generally appears normal. There are no septi pellucidi.

The corpus callosum is present and can be normal, incomplete, or hypoplastic. The splenium and most of the body can usually be identified, although the genu and rostrum are often absent. In contrast to isolated or syndromic corpus callosum dysgenesis, there are no Probst bundles in any of the HPEs.

The walls of the hypothalamus remain unseparated, and the optic chiasm is often smaller than normal. The olfactory bulbs are present in well-differentiated lobar HPE. The pituitary gland can be flattened, hypoplastic, or ectopic.

Differential Diagnosis

The major differential diagnosis of lobar HPE is **septooptic dysplasia** (SOD). Some authors consider SOD the best-differentiated of the HPE spectrum. In contrast to lobar HPE, the frontal horns are well-formed in

38-8A. *Sagittal T1WI shows semilobar HPE with partial differentiation of third ventricle ➡, occipital horns ➘. The midbrain, pons, and cerebellum are comparatively normal.* **38-8B.** *Axial T2WI in the same patient shows mild hypotelorism with no other midface anomalies. Rudimentary temporal ➡ and occipital ➡ horns are present. The third ventricle ➡ is partially formed. The thalami ➡ are separated, but the hypothalamus ➘ remains fused.*

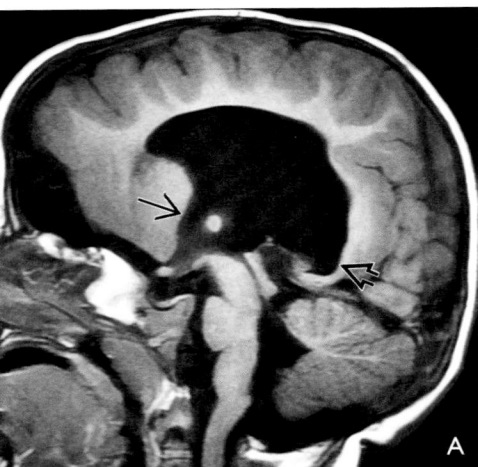

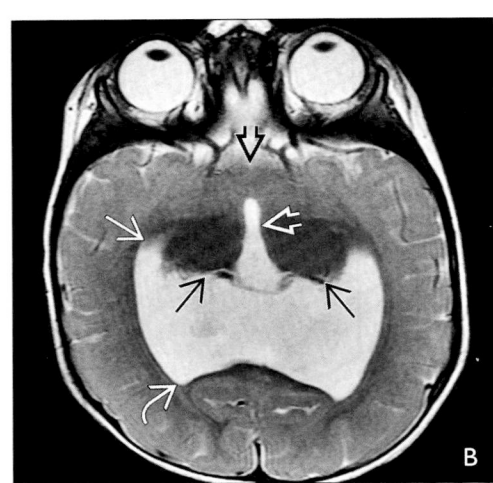

38-8C. *More cephalad T2WI in the same patient shows fused basal ganglia ➡, rudimentary posterior interhemispheric fissure ➡, absence of anterior interhemispheric fissure with the brain fused across the midline ➘.* **38-8D.** *More cephalad scan shows the upper aspect of a poorly differentiated central monoventricle. The corpus callosum and all normal midline structures are absent.*

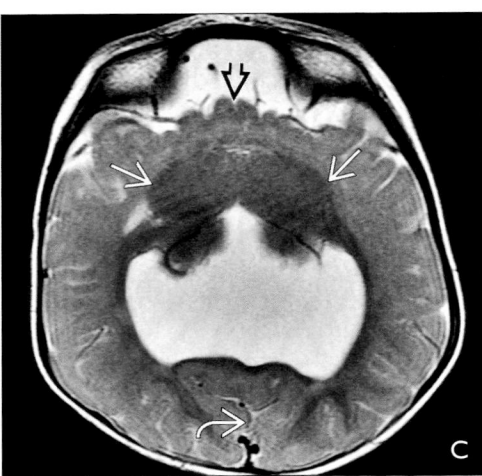

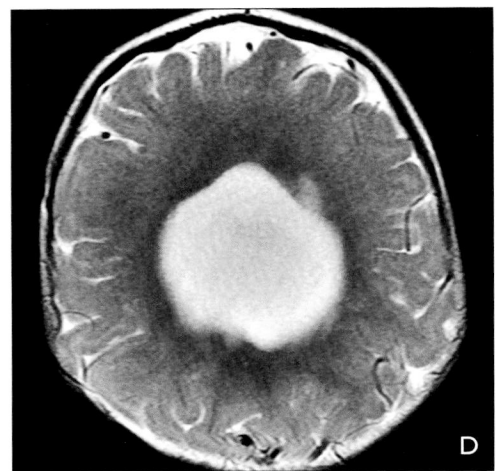

38-8E. *Coronal T2WI shows the monoventricle with rudimentary temporal horns ➡. A partially formed third ventricle ➡ separates the thalami ➡. The interhemispheric fissure is absent.* **38-8F.** *Color DTI shows the central monoventricle surrounded by unidentifiable disorganized, chaotic white matter tracts.*

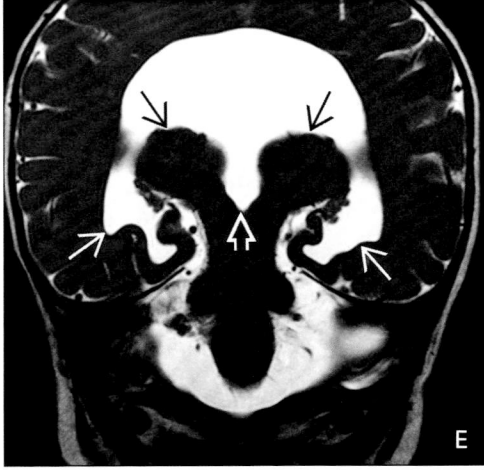

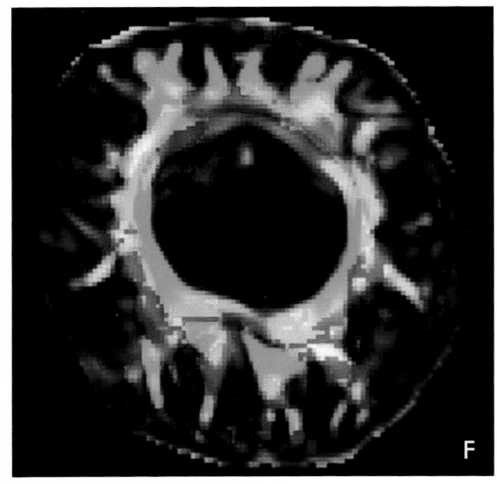

SOD. **Arrhinencephaly** may resemble lobar HPE, but the olfactory bulbs are usually present in lobar HPE.

In **syntelencephaly** (the middle interhemispheric variant of HPE), the corpus callosum genu and splenium are formed, but the body is missing and the posterior frontal lobes are continuous across the midline.

HOLOPROSENCEPHALY

Alobar Holoprosencephaly
- Most severe; high intrauterine lethality
- "Pancake" brain with central monoventricle
- BG fused; no falx, no interhemispheric fissure (IHF)

Semilobar Holoprosencephaly
- Rudimentary falx, posterior IHF
- Primitive ventricular horns, third ventricle
- Thalami often separated, but BG fused

Lobar Holoprosencephaly
- Best-differentiated form of HPE
- BG separated, falx/IHF present except anteroinferiorly
- Ventral frontal lobes remain fused across midline

Holoprosencephaly Variants

Several HPE variants have been identified, including syntelencephaly and septopreoptic holoprosencephalies. Arrhinencephaly, which some authors consider a variant of HPE, is considered together with septooptic dysplasia later in the chapter.

Syntelencephaly

Syntelencephaly is also called the **middle interhemispheric variant of HPE** (mivHPE). Here the anterior and posterior hemispheres are separated by the falx and interhemispheric fissure, but their midsections are fused across the midline **(38-10)**. In contrast to classic HPE, the ventral aspects of the basal forebrain are largely spared so the basal ganglia and olfactory sulci appear normal.

Imaging findings in mivHPE are diagnostic. Sagittal T1 and T2 scans show that the corpus callosum splenium and genu are present but that the body is absent. The posterior frontal lobes are continuous across the midline on coronal images. The lateral ventricle bodies appear narrow and fused. A characteristic nodule of gray matter is perched along the dorsal aspect of the fused lateral ventricles. The third ventricle is well-formed, but the septi pellucidi are absent.

Axial scans show the anterior and posterior parts of the interhemispheric fissure and the absence of the mid-section. The falx also narrows and disappears in both the

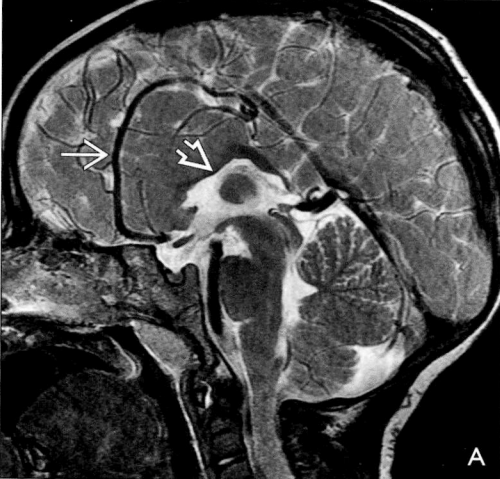

38-9A. Sagittal T2WI of lobar HPE shows well-differentiated brain, nearly normal-appearing third ventricle ➡, azygous ACA ➡.

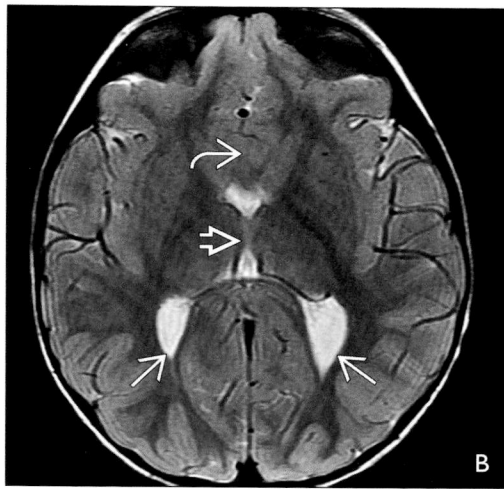

38-9B. Axial T2WI shows well-developed occipital horns ➡, third ventricle ➡, poorly seen frontal horns with minimal anterior midline fusion ➡.

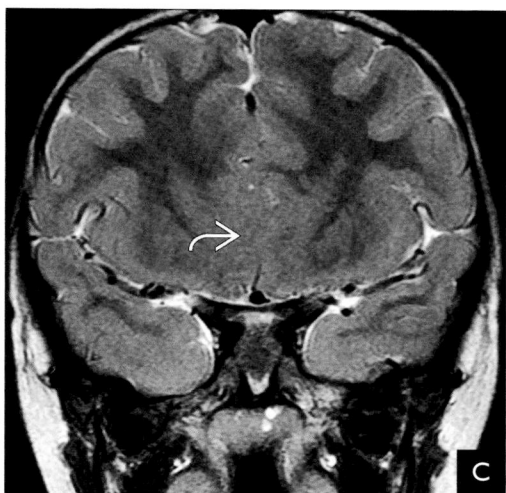

38-9C. Coronal T2WI shows that the anteroinferior frontal cortex is fused across the midline ➡.

38-10. *Axial graphic depicts syntelencephaly with absent midsection of the interhemispheric fissure, upward extension of an anomalous sylvian fissure across the midline* ⇨*, and foci of both gray and white matter* ⧑ *that bridge the hemispheres.* **38-11A.** *Axial NECT scan in a patient with syntelencephaly shows that the mid-portions of the hemispheres appear fused across the midline with bridges of both white* ➡ *and gray matter* ⇨*.*

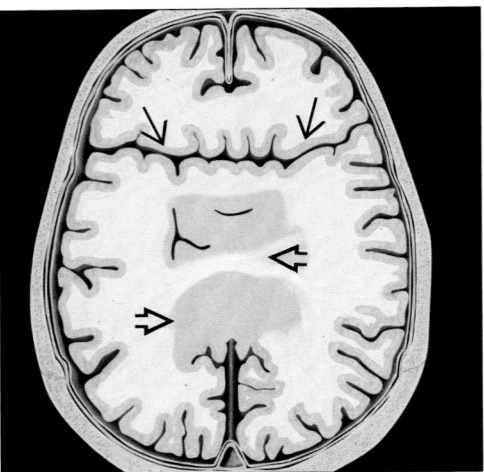
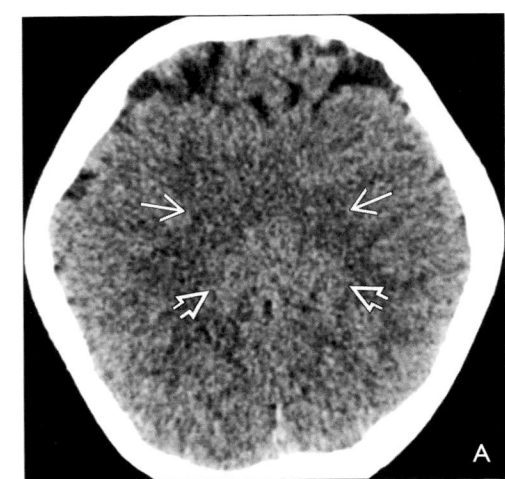

38-11B. *Sagittal T1WI in the same patient shows classic findings of syntelencephaly. The corpus callosum genu* ➡ *and splenium* ⧑ *are present without an intervening body. Note abnormal-appearing gray matter* ⧑ *that deforms the lateral ventricle.* **38-11C.** *Coronal T2WI shows narrow, nonseparated lateral ventricles* ➡ *with a nodule of gray matter* ⧑ *perched on top of the fused lateral ventricle. The posterior frontal lobes are continuous across the midline* ➡ *without an interhemispheric fissure.*

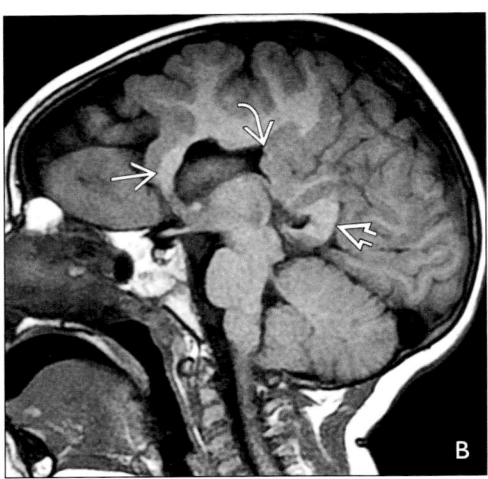
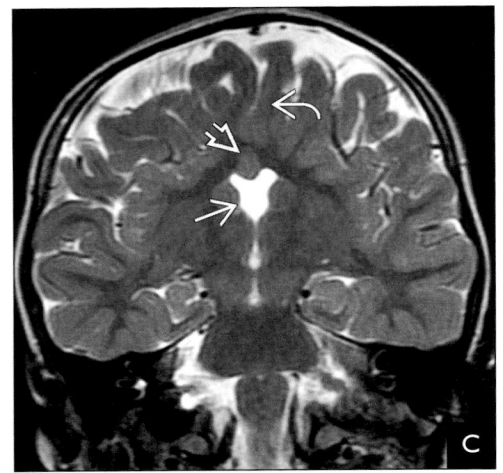

38-11D. *Axial T2WI shows that abnormal sylvian fissures* ➡ *continue superiorly, meeting over the cerebral convexities and crossing the midline* ⧑*.* **38-11E.** *Axial DTI in the same patient shows WM tracts in the posterosuperior frontal lobes meeting and crossing in the midline* ➡*.*

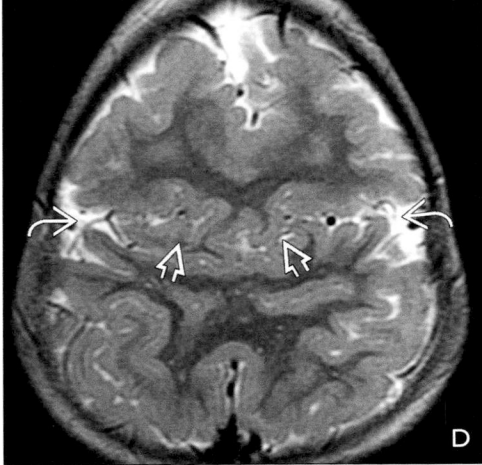
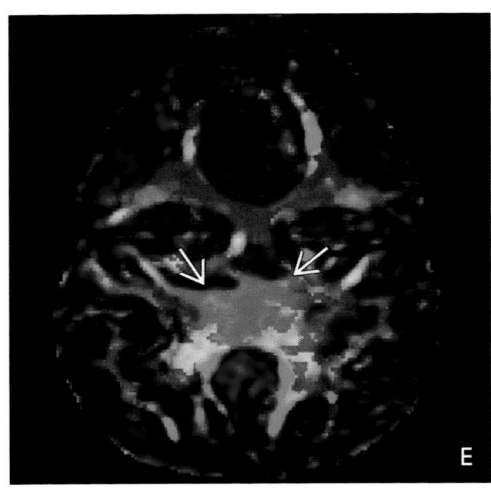

posterior frontal and anterior parietal regions. In 85% of cases, the sylvian fissures course superiorly and meet in a coronally oriented, cortically lined fissure that is continuous across the midline **(38-11A)**, **(38-11B)**, **(38-11C)**, **(38-11D)**.

DTI demonstrates the horizontal white matter tracts that cross the midline just under the fused cortex **(38-11E)**.

Septopreoptic Holoprosencephaly

Recently, several very mild forms of HPE have been described in which the failure of hemispheric separation is restricted to the septal (subcallosal) and/or preoptic regions or both. Patients with these types of HPE—termed septopreoptic holoprosencephaly—often present with mild midline craniofacial malformations. These variants include **solitary median maxillary central incisor** (SMMCI) and **congenital nasal pyriform aperture stenosis** (CNPAS). Both are briefly discussed here.

Solitary Median Maxillary Central Incisor Syndrome

Solitary median maxillary central incisor syndrome is a rare malformation that consists of multiple (mainly midline) defects. Most authors suggest that SMMCI is a holoprosencephaly variant, although others consider it a distinct entity.

Neonates with SMMCI often present with breathing difficulties secondary to nasal obstruction. Neurodevelopmental delay and endocrine abnormalities such as short stature and precocious puberty are common associated findings.

Imaging findings in SMMCI range from isolated dental abnormalities with a single maxillary incisor and V-shaped palate to more complex abnormalities that involve the brain **(38-12)**. Anomalies of the fornix, septi pellucidi, and anterior corpus callosum are often present. An azygous anterior cerebral artery is common. Pituitary stalk hypoplasia occurs in some cases.

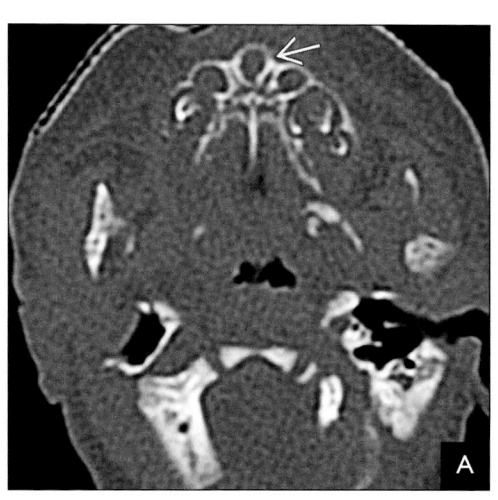

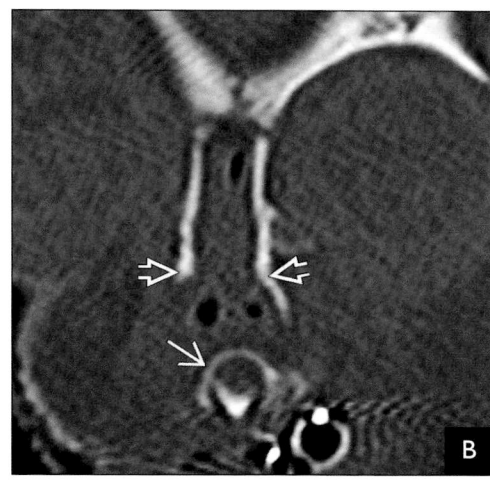

38-12A. *Axial bone CT in a 3-day-old infant with breathing difficulty shows a single midline maxillary incisor* ➡. **38-12B.** *Coronal bone CT in the same patient shows the central incisor* ➡ *and narrowed pyriform aperture stenosis* ➡.

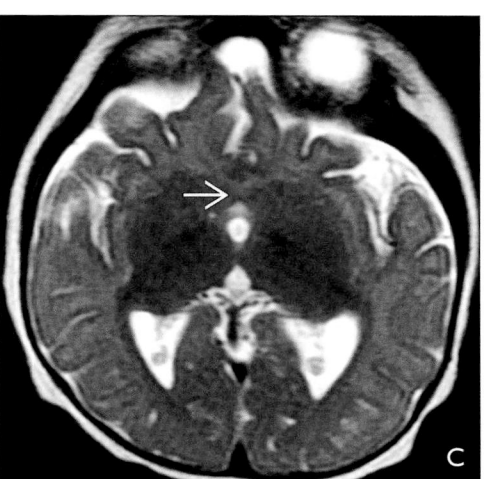

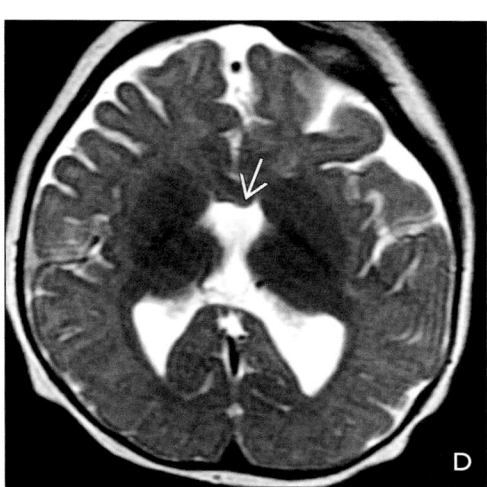

38-12C. *Axial T2WI in the same patient at age 7 months shows lobar HPE with mild hypotelorism, fusion across the ventral frontal lobes* ➡. **38-12D.** *More cephalad scan shows absent septi pellucidi, thickened dysplastic-appearing fornices* ➡.

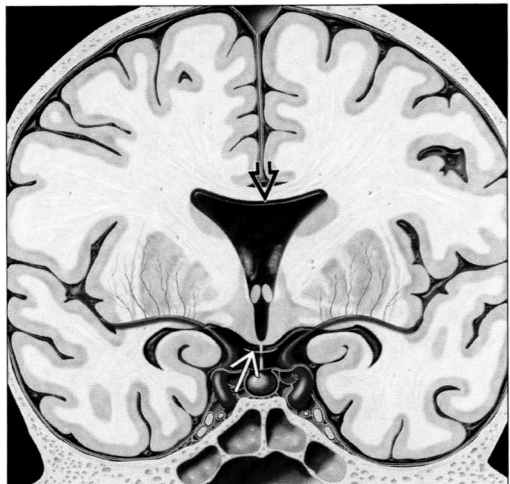

38-13. *Coronal graphic shows SOD with absent cavum septi pellucidi with flat-roofed anterior horns ➡, small optic chiasm ➡.*

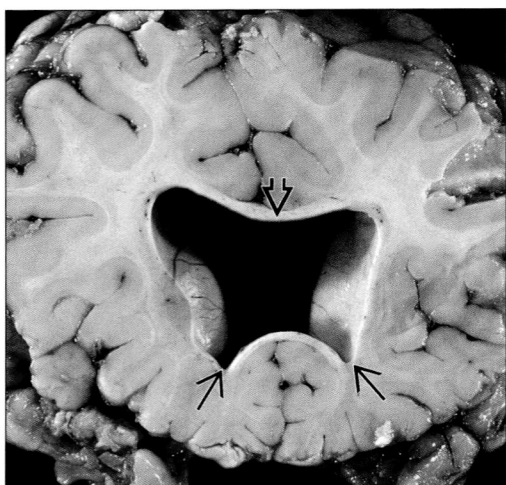

38-14. *Absent cavum septi pellucidi ➡, box-like lateral ventricles with inferiorly pointed frontal horns ➡. (Courtesy J. Townsend, MD.)*

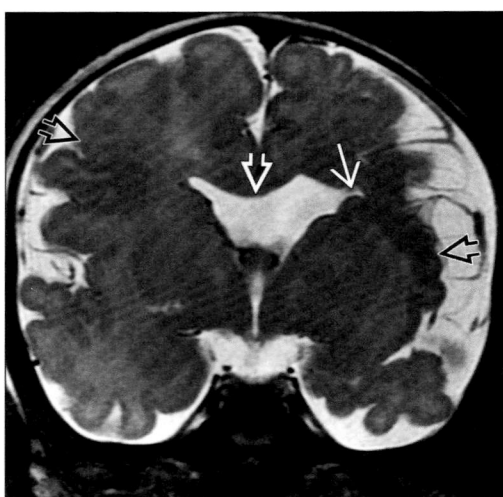

38-15. *Coronal T2WI in a newborn shows absent cavum septi pellucidi ➡, schizencephaly ➡, extensive polymicrogyria ➡.*

Congenital Nasal Pyriform Aperture Stenosis

Congenital nasal pyriform aperture stenosis (CNPAS) can exist as an isolated abnormality with choanal atresia, midnasal stenosis, or pyriform aperture stenosis. CNPAS may also coexist with SMMCI. CNPAS is associated with a high incidence of hypothalamic-pituitary-adrenal axis dysfunction.

HOLOPROSENCEPHALY VARIANTS

Syntelencephaly
- Also known as middle interhemispheric variant of HPE
- CC genu, splenium present; middle absent
  - Only brain malformation with that morphology
- Mid-sections of falx, interhemispheric fissure absent
- Posterior frontal gray/white matter fused across midline

Solitary Median Maxillary Central Incisor Syndrome
- Single midline incisor
- Often coexists with nasal anomalies
- Brain anomalies of fornix, septi pellucidi, CC common

Congenital Nasal Pyriform Aperture Stenosis
- Choanal atresia, mid-nasal stenosis, pyriform aperture stenosis
- Often coexists with SMMCI
- Hypothalamic-pituitary-adrenal axis dysfunction common

Related Midline Disorders

Septooptic Dysplasia

Some authors consider septooptic dysplasia simply a very well-differentiated form of lobar holoprosencephaly. However, the lack of ventral midline fusion and the heterogeneous nature of the disorder are more consistent with a separate but related midline malformation.

Terminology and Pathology

Septooptic dysplasia (SOD) is also known as de Morsier syndrome. Two cardinal pathologic features define SOD: (1) absence of the septi pellucidi and (2) optic nerve hypoplasia **(38-13)**, **(38-14)**.

When SOD occurs with other anomalies such as schizencephaly or callosal dysgenesis, the syndrome is sometimes called SOD plus **(38-15)**.

Etiology

Most SOD cases are sporadic. Mutation of the homeobox gene *HESX1* has been identified in some cases. Anomalies of the *SOX* genes—transcription factors involved in pituitary development—have been seen in others.

Clinical Issues

The most common clinical feature of SOD is visual impairment. Nearly two-thirds of SOD patients also develop endocrine abnormalities from hypothalamic-pituitary insufficiency. Symptomatic hypoglycemia and diabetes insipidus are common in infants; growth retardation may become apparent later.

Imaging

Imaging findings in SOD are diagnostic. Thin-section coronal T1- and T2-weighted images show absent or hypoplastic septi pellucidi. The frontal horns appear "squared-off" or box-like with distinct inferior pointing. The optic chiasm and one or both optic nerves appear small in about half of all cases.

Sagittal images show that the septi pellucidi are absent and the fornices are low-lying, giving the lateral ventricles an "empty" appearance (38-16).

Isolated absence of the septi pellucidi relatively rare, so look carefully for other abnormalities. One subset of patients with SOD has malformations of cortical development (e.g., heterotopias, schizencephaly, and polymicrogyria) in addition to optic nerve hypoplasia. Another subset demonstrates a small pituitary gland with thin or absent stalk and an ectopic neurohypophysis, typically seen as a "spot" or "dot" of T1 hyperintensity along the median eminence of the hypothalamus (see Chapter 25).

Differential Diagnosis

The major differential diagnosis of SOD is well-differentiated **lobar HPE**. The olfactory bulbs are present in lobar HPE but are frequently absent in SOD. The cerebral hemispheres and basal ganglia are completely separated in SOD.

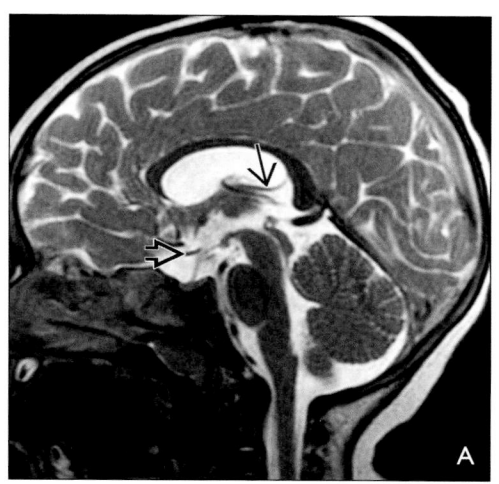

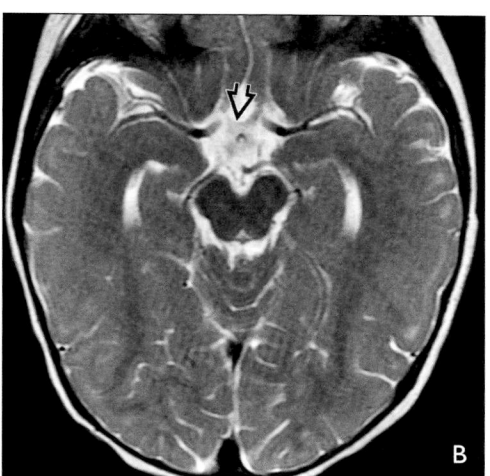

38-16A. *Sagittal T2WI in a 13-month-old boy with septooptic dysplasia shows an empty-appearing lateral ventricle with low-lying fornix ➡. The optic chiasm ⧨ appears small.* **38-16B.** *Axial T2WI in the same patient shows that the optic chiasm ⧨ appears tiny.*

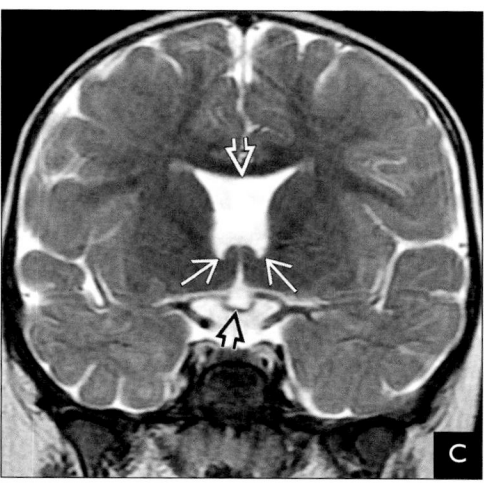

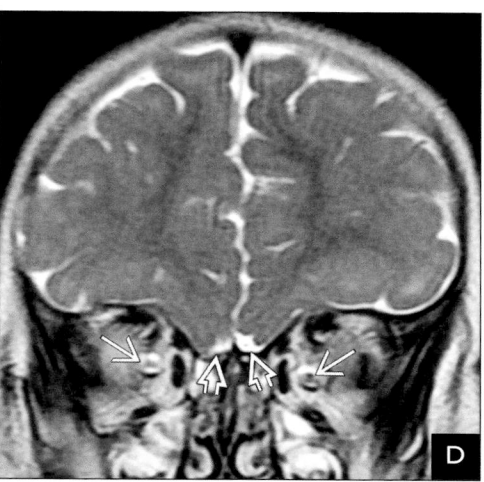

38-16C. *Coronal T2WI shows the hypoplastic optic chiasm ⧨, absent septi pellucidi ➡, and the peculiar box-like or "squared-off" appearance of the frontal horns. The inferior pointing ➡ of both frontal horns is also characteristic of SOD.* **38-16D.** *Both optic nerves ➡ are very small. The olfactory bulbs should be easily identified on coronal T2 scans through the olfactory recesses, but they are absent ⧨.*

Arrhinencephaly

Arrhinencephaly (ARR) is a congenital malformation in which the olfactory bulb and tracts are absent **(38-17)**, **(38-18)**, **(38-19)**, **(38-20)**. While ARR can exist in isolation, most cases occur with multiple other midline facial anomalies such as cleft palate, cleft lip, nasal and/or ocular malformations.

Common associated intracranial abnormalities include abnormalities of the hypothalamic-pituitary axis, callosal dysgenesis, alobar and semilobar HPE.

When olfactory aplasia/hypoplasia occurs with hypogonadotropic hypogonadism, it is termed Kallmann syndrome. Olfactory agenesis occurs in approximately 25% of patients with CHARGE (**c**oloboma, **h**eart malformations, choanal **a**tresia, developmental **r**etardation, **g**enital anomalies, **e**ar anomalies) syndrome.

Holoprosencephaly Mimics

Hydranencephaly

While some authors consider hydranencephaly a congenital malformation, it is actually the consequence of severe brain destruction in utero. We discuss it here, as it is important to recognize and distinguish hydranencephaly from other disorders such as alobar holoprosencephaly or maximal hydrocephalus.

Terminology

The term hydranencephaly is a contraction of "hydro-anencéphalie" and literally means water without the brain.

In rare instances, only one hemisphere is destroyed. This condition is termed **hemihydranencephaly**.

38-17. Submentovertex graphic depicts the normal olfactory bulbs ➡️*, trigones* ➡️*, and lateral olfactory stria* ➡️ *passing into the temporal lobes. 38-18. Coronal T2WI in a newborn shows olfactory bulbs* ➡️*, normal olfactory sulci* ➡️*.*

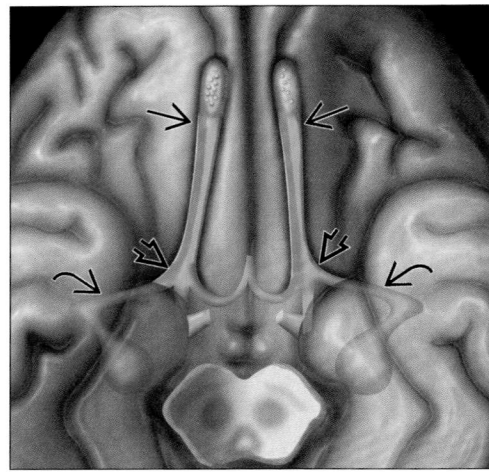
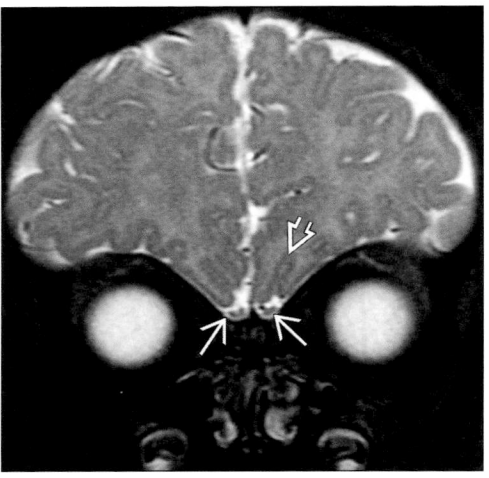

38-19. Autopsy case of arrhinencephaly shows absent olfactory bulbs and shallow, deformed olfactory sulci ➡️*. (Courtesy R. Hewlett, MD.) 38-20. Coronal T2WI in a newborn with multiple congenital anomalies demonstrates arrhinencephaly with absent olfactory bulbs* ➡️*, no olfactory sulci* ➡️*. (Courtesy S. Blaser, MD.)*

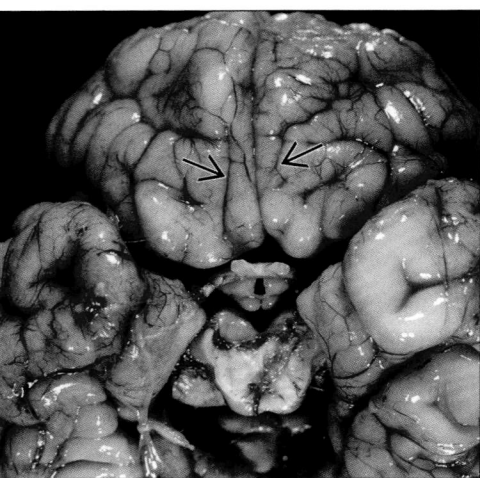
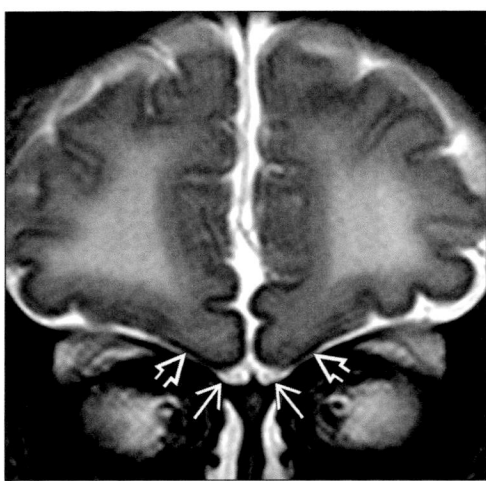

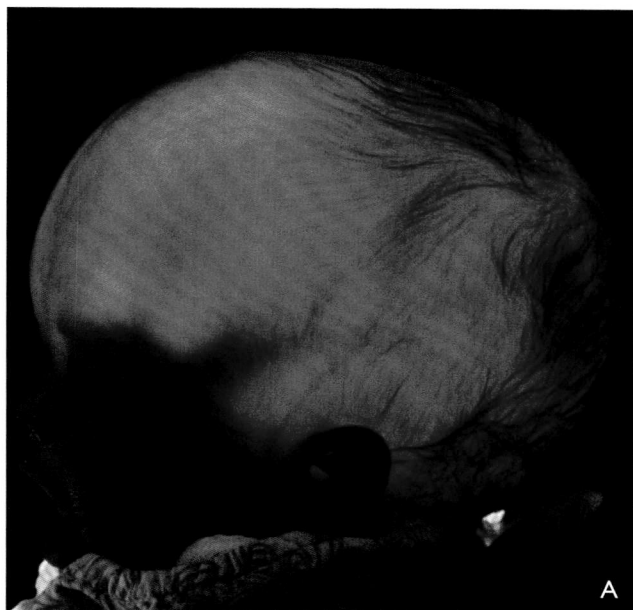

38-21A. Autopsy case of hydranencephaly demonstrates a large head with striking transillumination indicating that most of the cranium is water-filled.

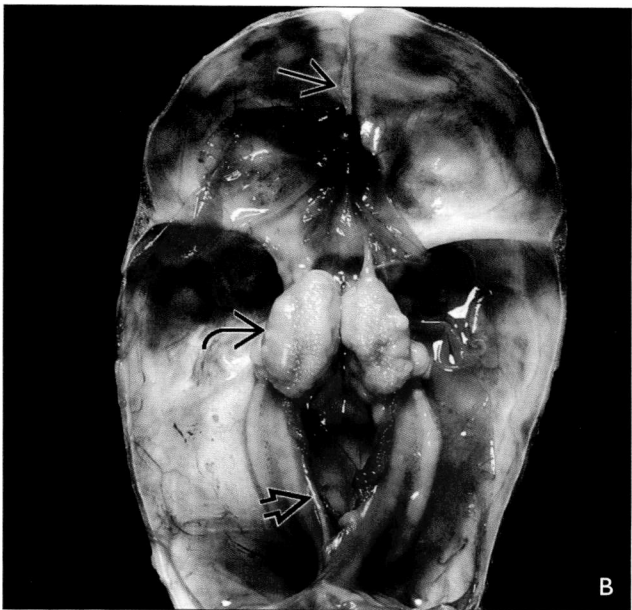

38-21B. The water-filled calvaria is enlarged, and the cerebral hemispheres are absent. A falx cerebri ⇨ and tentorium ⧊ are present, as are the basal ganglia ⤳, which appear normally separated.

Etiology and Pathology

The precise etiology of hydranencephaly is unknown, but most investigators believe compromise of the internal carotid artery circulation before 16 gestational weeks followed by diffuse liquefactive necrosis of the cerebral mantle is responsible. Maternal trauma, toxins, twin-twin transfusion syndrome, massive hemorrhage, and infection have all been cited as possible contributory factors.

In hydranencephaly, most of the cerebral hemispheres have been destroyed and are totally or partially replaced by translucent thin-walled sacs of CSF that fill most of the supratentorial space (38-21). The outer layer consists of leptomeninges, and the inner layer is glial tissue without demonstrable ependymal elements.

The falx is intact. The medial temporal lobes, brainstem, cerebellum, and parts of the thalami—all supplied by the posterior circulation—are often relatively preserved. As some of the choroid plexus is also supplied by the posterior circulation, CSF continues to be elaborated but not normally resorbed. This distends the fluid-filled sacs that are the dominant pathologic feature of hydranencephaly.

Hydranencephaly usually occurs sporadically without other associated malformations. Fowler syndrome is a rare autosomal recessive disorder in which hydranencephaly is accompanied by glomeruloid vasculopathy of the CNS vessels and neurogenic muscular atrophy.

Clinical Issues

Hydranencephaly occurs in 1-2 per 10,000 live births and represents 0.6% of CNS malformations in perinatal/neonatal autopsy series.

Prognosis is poor. Half of liveborn infants with hydranencephaly die within the first postnatal month, and 85% die by the end of the first year. Occasional long-term survivors have been reported. The major management problem is controlling the macrocephaly that usually accompanies hydranencephaly. Patients with hemihydranencephaly have a better prognosis and may experience long-term survival.

Imaging

GENERAL FEATURES. A normal or large head with fluid-filled cranial vault ("water bag" brain) and small nubbins of remnant brain with a normal falx cerebri and posterior fossa are the typical findings (38-22).

CT FINDINGS. NECT scans show that CSF almost completely fills the supratentorial space. The falx cerebri is generally intact and appears to "float" in the water-filled cranial vault (38-23). The basal ganglia are present and separated but may appear moderately atrophic. Small remnants of the medial frontal and parietooccipital lobes can be present.

MR FINDINGS. MR demonstrates a largely absent cerebral mantle. The falx is easily identified. The fluid-filled spaces follow CSF on all sequences, although some signal heterogeneity is often present secondary to CSF pulsations (38-24).

In hemihydranencephaly, one hemisphere appears absent and the CSF-filled space often displaces the falx across the midline (38-25).

Differential Diagnosis

The most important differential diagnosis of hydranencephaly is severe **obstructive hydrocephalus** (OH). In severe OH (e.g., secondary to aqueductal stenosis), a thin cortex can be seen compressed against the dura and inner table of the calvaria.

In **alobar holoprosencephaly**, the falx and interhemispheric fissure are absent. The basal ganglia are fused. Severe **bilateral "open lip" schizencephaly** has large transmantle CSF clefts that are lined with dysplastic-appearing cortex. Severe **cystic encephalomalacia** shows large ventricles with multiple parenchymal CSF-filled cavities.

38-22. Graphic depicts hydranencephaly. The head is large, the thalami are separated in midline ⬇, a falx ⬧ is present. The supratentorial compartments are almost completely filled with CSF. There is no brain surrounding the CSF-filled cavities; only dura-arachnoid ⬇ is present. *38-23.* NECT shows hydranencephaly. Both hemispheres are replaced by CSF. The basal ganglia/thalami are separated ⬧, a falx present ⬧. There is no brain visible over the CSF-filled cavities ⬈.

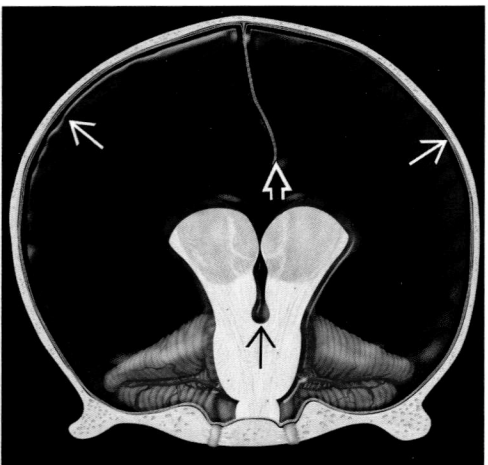

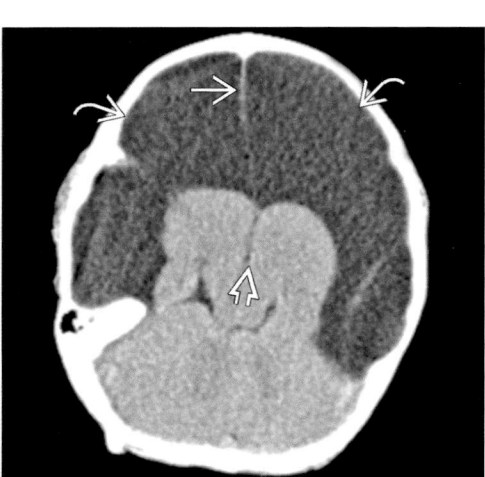

38-24A. Sagittal T1WI shows hydranencephaly with macrocephaly; CSF fills virtually all of the supratentorial spaces. Brainstem, cerebellum are normal. *38-24B.* Coronal T1WI in the same case shows expanded, CSF-filled cranial vault, tiny remnants of brain ⬧. A falx is present ⬧. (Courtesy A. Illner, MD.)

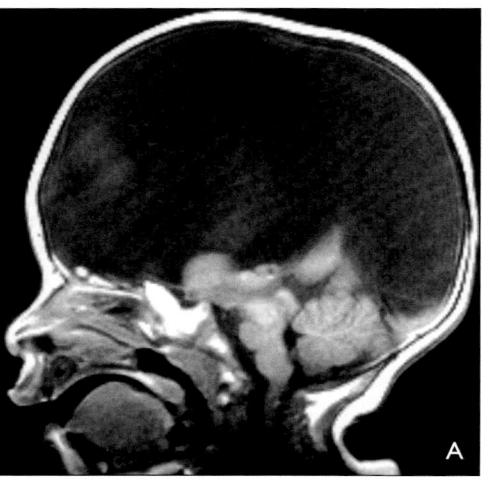

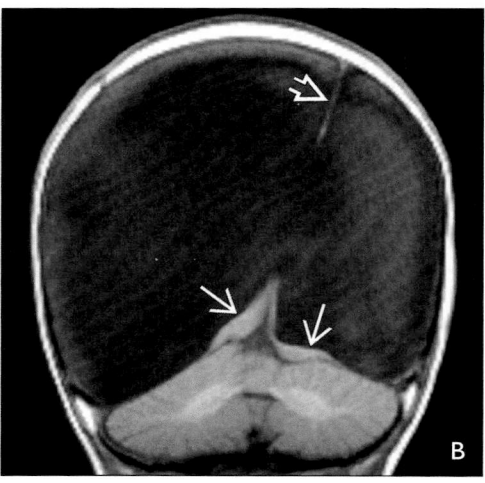

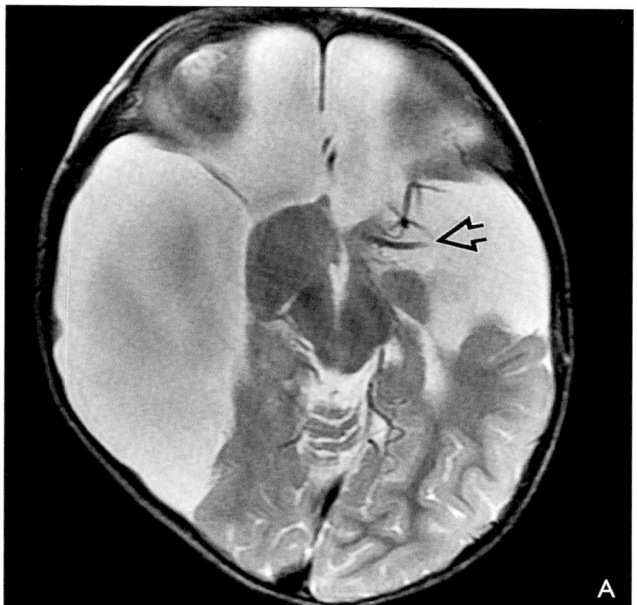

38-25A. *Axial T2WI shows that the right frontal, temporal lobes are absent in this 2-year-old boy with hemihydranencephaly. The right occipital lobe and most of the left hemisphere are present. Note "flow voids" of left ICA branches ⊵.*

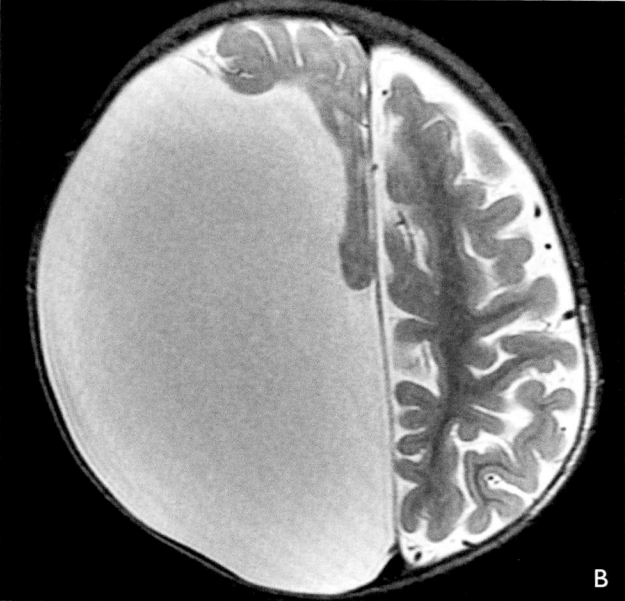

38-25B. *More cephalad T2WI in the same patient shows that the right hemicalvaria is enlarged and CSF-filled. Small frontal remnant is present. The left hemisphere is largely intact.*

Selected References

Holoprosencephaly

- Vaz SS et al: Risk factors for nonsyndromic holoprosencephaly: A Manitoba case-control study. Am J Med Genet A. 158A(4):751-8, 2012
- Mercier S et al: New findings for phenotype-genotype correlations in a large European series of holoprosencephaly cases. J Med Genet. 48(11):752-60, 2011
- Hahn JS et al: Neuroimaging advances in holoprosencephaly: Refining the spectrum of the midline malformation. Am J Med Genet C Semin Med Genet. 154C(1):120-32, 2010
- Roessler E et al: The molecular genetics of holoprosencephaly. Am J Med Genet C Semin Med Genet. 154C(1):52-61, 2010
- Solomon BD et al: Holoprosencephaly overview. GeneReviews [Internet]. Updated 2011 Nov 03, 2000

Alobar Holoprosencephaly

- Kanekar S et al: Malformations of ventral induction. Semin Ultrasound CT MR. 32(3):200-10, 2011
- Marcorelles P et al: Neuropathology of holoprosencephaly. Am J Med Genet C Semin Med Genet. 154C(1):109-19, 2010

Semilobar Holoprosencephaly

- Barkovich AJ: Anomalies of ventral prosencephalon development. In Pediatric Neuroradiology. Philadelphia: Lippincott Williams & Wilkins. 445-57, 2012

Lobar Holoprosencephaly

- Barkovich AJ: Anomalies of ventral prosencephalon development. In Pediatric Neuroradiology. Philadelphia: Lippincott Williams & Wilkins. 445-57, 2012
- Cohen MM Jr: Holoprosencephaly: clinical, anatomic, and molecular dimensions. Birth Defects Res A Clin Mol Teratol. 76(9):658-73, 2006

Holoprosencephaly Variants

Syntelencephaly

- Merrow AC et al: Syntelencephaly: postnatal sonographic detection of a subtle case. Pediatr Radiol. 40 Suppl 1:S160, 2010
- Simon EM et al: The middle interhemispheric variant of holoprosencephaly. AJNR Am J Neuroradiol. 23(1):151-6, 2002

Septopreoptic Holoprosencephaly

- Szakszon K et al: Endocrine and anatomical findings in a case of solitary median maxillary central incisor syndrome. Eur J Med Genet. 55(2):109-11, 2012
- Hahn JS et al: Septopreoptic holoprosencephaly: a mild subtype associated with midline craniofacial anomalies. AJNR Am J Neuroradiol. 31(9):1596-601, 2010

Related Midline Disorders

Septooptic Dysplasia

- Trabacca A et al: Septo-optic dysplasia-plus and dyskinetic cerebral palsy in a child. Neurol Sci. 33(1):159-63, 2012

- Ferran K et al: Septo-optic dysplasia. Arq Neuropsiquiatr. 68(3):400-5, 2010

Arrhinencephaly

- Hahn JS et al: Neuroimaging advances in holoprosencephaly: Refining the spectrum of the midline malformation. Am J Med Genet C Semin Med Genet. 154C(1):120-32, 2010

Holoprosencephaly Mimics

Hydranencephaly

- Hassanein SM et al: Hemihydranencephaly syndrome: case report and review. Dev Neurorehabil. 14(5):323-9, 2011

39

Neurocutaneous Syndromes

The term **neurocutaneous syndromes** denotes a group of CNS disorders that are characterized by brain malformations or neoplasms and skin/eye lesions. These disorders have also been called the **phakomatoses**. The term is derived from the Greek root *phako*, which refers to the lens; phakomatosis thus means a tumor-like condition of the eye (lens).

Most—but not all—neurocutaneous syndromes are inherited. Most—but not all—are associated with a distinct predilection to develop CNS neoplasms; these have also been called **inherited cancer syndromes**. Most—but again not all—of these also have characteristic cutaneous lesions. Many—but not all—also have prominent visceral and connective tissue abnormalities.

More recently, the term **cancer predisposition syndrome** has been advocated to describe familial cancers in which a clear mode of inheritance can be established.

The molecular bases of most cancer predisposition syndromes with CNS manifestations are now well-delineated. Although the definitive diagnosis is established by genetic analysis, clinical findings and imaging features sometimes provide the first suggestions that a patient may have an inherited cancer syndrome.

In this chapter, we consider familial tumor syndromes that involve the nervous system, beginning with the neurofibromatoses and schwannomatosis. Major attention is also directed to tuberous sclerosis complex and von Hippel-Lindau syndrome. We close with a brief discussion of some rare but intriguing neurocutaneous syndromes.

Neurofibromatosis and Schwannomatosis

"Neurofibromatosis" is not a single entity but a group of genetically and clinically distinct disorders with few overlapping features. While they are the most common CNS tumor predisposition syndromes, neurofibromatoses are multisystem disorders with both neoplastic and nonneoplastic manifestations.

Two types of neurofibromatosis are widely recognized: Neurofibromatosis type 1 (NF1) and neurofibromatosis type 2 (NF2).

A third related disorder—schwannomatosis—is a rare non-NF1/NF2 syndrome characterized by multiple nonvestibular schwannomas. Together, these three inherited disorders affect approximately 100,000 persons in the United States alone.

Neurofibromatosis Type 1

Terminology

Neurofibromatosis type 1 (NF1) was formerly known as **von Recklinghausen disease** or "peripheral neurofibromatosis." Because NF1 often has central lesions, the term "peripheral neurofibromatosis" should not be used. When

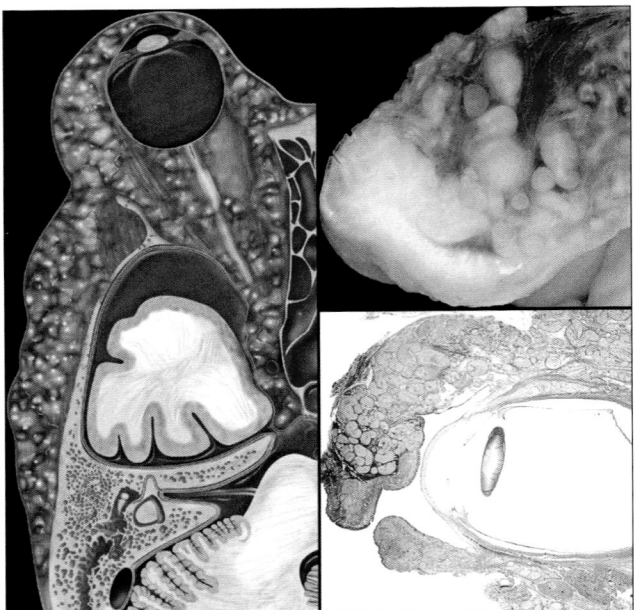

39-1. *Graphic (left) and surgical specimens (right) depict NF1 with typical plexiform neurofibroma of orbit, eyelid, scalp.*

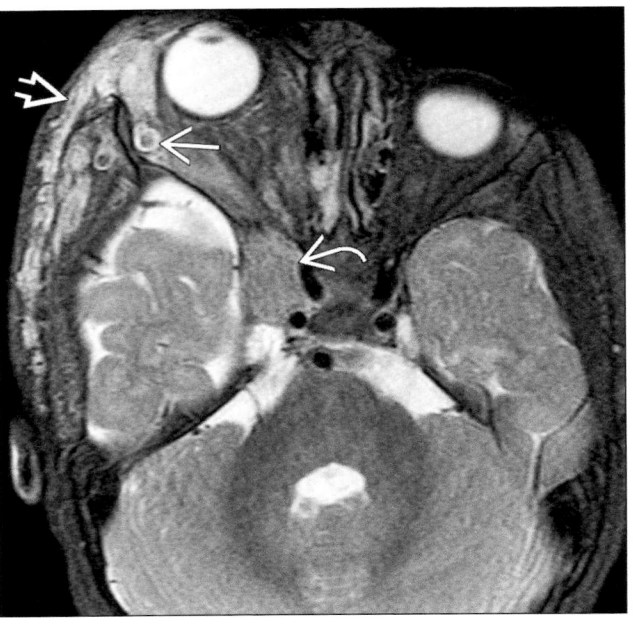

39-2. *T2WI shows plexiform NF infiltrating orbit, masticator space* ➡, *cavernous sinus* ➡. *Lesion is hyperintense with typical "target" appearance* ➡.

extreme, NF1 can be highly disfiguring and is sometimes dubbed "elephantiasis neuromatosa" or "elephant man disease."

An uncommon form, **segmental NF1** (formerly called neurofibromatosis type 5), affects one region of the body (e.g., a limb) or sometimes just a single dermatome. Segmental NF1 is a mosaicism in which localized disease results from a postzygotic *NF1* gene mutation.

An even more uncommon NF1 type is **localized NF1**. Localized NF1 is isolated to a small area and is caused by a sporadic *somatic* (not germline) mutation.

Etiology

GENERAL CONCEPTS. NF1 is an autosomal dominant disorder with variable expression, a high rate of new mutations, and virtually complete penetrance by age 20.

GENETICS. NF1 is caused by mutation of the *NF1* gene on chromosome 17q11.2. This large gene has one of the highest rates of spontaneous mutation in the entire human genome. Mutations vary from complete gene deletions to insertions, stop and splicing mutations, as well as amino acid substitutions and chromosomal rearrangements.

Mutations inactivate the gene that encodes the protein product **neurofibromin**. Neurofibromin is a cytoplasmic protein that functions as a tumor suppressor protein through negative regulation of the *RAS* oncogene. The Ras/MAPK signaling pathway is critical for control of cellular growth and differentiation.

Neurofibromin also acts as a regulator of neural stem cell proliferation and differentiation; it is required for normal glial and neuronal development. The oligodendrocyte myelin glycoprotein—a major myelin protein—is also embedded in the *NF1* gene and is often also mutated.

Neurofibromin is expressed at low levels in all cells with higher levels expressed in the CNS (astrocytes and oligodendrocytes as well as neurons, Schwann cells) and skin (melanocytes).

Approximately half of all NF1 cases are familial. Nearly 50% are sporadic ("de novo") and represent new mutations. NF1 patients already harboring a heterozygous germline *NF1* mutation develop neurofibromas upon somatic mutation of the second (wild-type) *NF1* allele. About 10% of NF1 patients display somatic mosaicism.

Pathology

CNS lesions are found in 15-20% of patients. A variety of nonneoplastic lesions as well as benign and malignant tumors are associated with NF1. An increased risk of non-CNS malignancies also occurs in NF1 patients.

NONNEOPLASTIC CNS LESIONS. Multiple waxing and waning **dysplastic white matter lesions** on T2/FLAIR are commonly identified in patients with NF1 (see below). Histopathologically, these lesions represent myelin vacuolization and dysgenesis, not hamartomas.

Uncommon nonneoplastic CNS lesions include macrocephaly and subependymal glial nodules. Hydrocephalus occurs in 10-15% of cases. **Dural ectasia** may cause

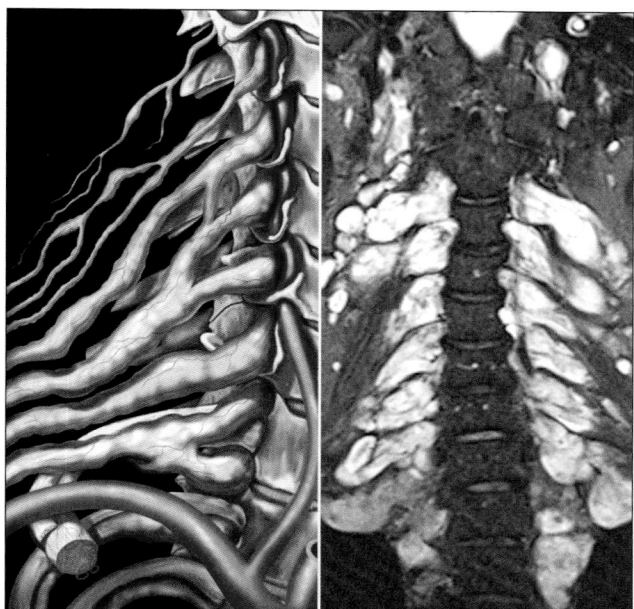

39-3. Plexiform NF involving cervical nerve roots is depicted in graphic (left), on coronal STIR scan (right).

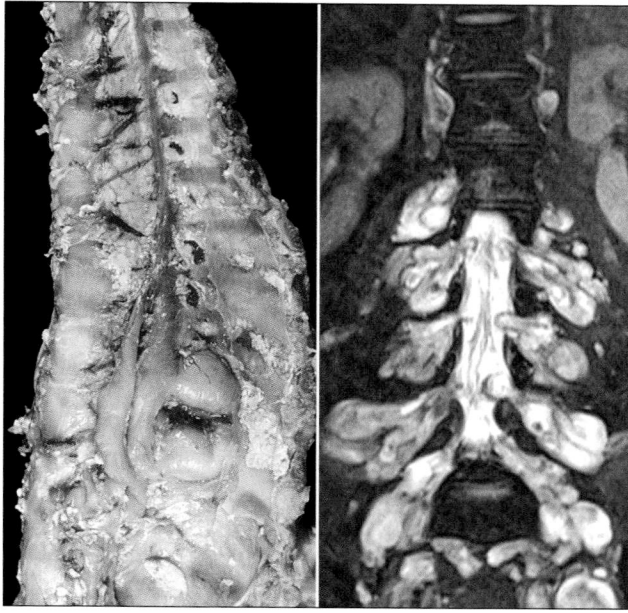

39-4. Coronal autopsy specimen (left) and coronal STIR (right) show plexiform NF of thoracolumbar nerve roots. (Autopsy courtesy R. Hewlett, MD.)

dilatation of the optic nerve sheaths, Meckel cave, or internal auditory canals.

Arteriopathy occurs in at least 6% of cases. The most common manifestation is progressive intimal fibrosis of the supraclinoid internal carotid arteries, resulting in moyamoya. Both intra- and extracranial aneurysms and arteriovenous fistulas occur in NF1 but are relatively rare. The vertebral arteries are more commonly affected than the carotid arteries.

CNS NEOPLASMS. A variety of both benign and malignant tumors occurs in NF1. All involve tumorigenesis of neural crest-derived cells and can be found in both the central and peripheral nervous systems. Benign NF1-related neoplasms include neurofibromas and schwannomas. Malignant tumors include malignant peripheral nerve sheath tumors and gliomas.

Neurofibromas. A spectrum of NF1-associated neurofibromas (NFs) occurs. Tumors derived from skin sensory nerves are designated dermal or **cutaneous neurofibromas (39-5)**. The prevalence of cutaneous neurofibromas increases with age, so more than 95% of adults with NF1 have at least one lesion. Cutaneous NFs are benign tumors that are mostly composed of Schwann cells and fibroblasts. Most are localized, well-circumscribed, and discrete but unencapsulated tumors restricted to a single nerve ending.

Less commonly, a tumor within a larger nerve appears as a more diffuse mass within the dermis (**"diffuse" cutaneous neurofibroma**).

Plexiform neurofibromas (PNFs) are virtually pathognomonic of NF1. PNFs are generally large bulky tumors usually associated with major nerve trunks and plexuses. PNFs are found in 30-50% of patients with NF1. PNFs are rope-like, diffusely infiltrating, noncircumscribed lesions that resemble a "bag of worms" **(39-1)**, **(39-2)**.

The scalp and orbit are common sites for PNFs. Spinal neurofibromas and PNFs are found in approximately 40% of patients with NF1 **(39-3)**, **(39-4)**.

Malignant peripheral nerve sheath tumors. While most PNFs remain benign, 10-15% become malignant. Deep-seated PNFs are at particular risk for development into malignant peripheral nerve sheath tumors (**MPNSTs**). MicroRNA misregulation appears to be a critical event in the malignant transformation of PNFs.

MPNSTs that occur in the setting of NF1 tend to present at a younger age and may also include rhabdomyoblastic and other heterologous elements. These histologically mixed neoplasms—referred to as **malignant Triton tumors**—are very characteristic of NF1.

Gliomas. The overwhelming majority of CNS neoplasms in NF1 are optic pathway **pilocytic astrocytomas**. Optic pathway "gliomas" (OPGs) occur in 15-20% of patients with NF1 and can be uni- or bilateral **(39-6)**. Some OPGs involve the optic chiasm and optic tracts. In comparison to most sporadic diffusely infiltrating pontine gliomas, NF1-associated gliomas of the medulla, tectum, and pons are typically more benign.

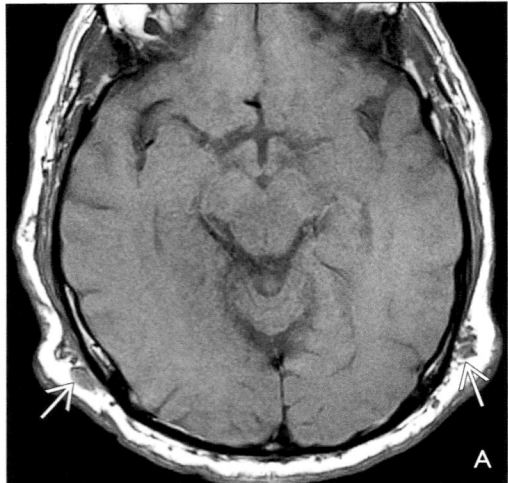

39-5A. *Axial T1WI shows multiple small cutaneous NFs* ➡ *in an adult with NF1.*

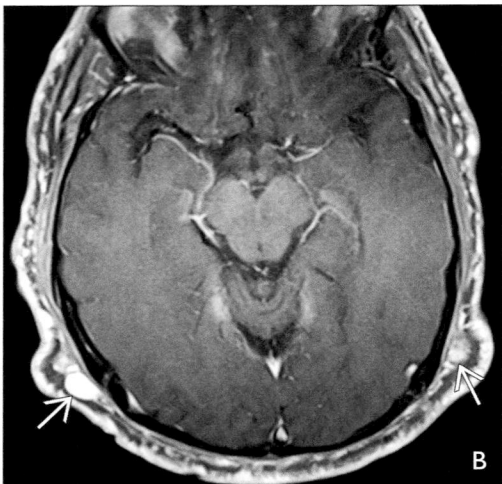

39-5B. *T1 C+ FS scan in the same patient shows that the cutaneous NFs enhance strongly* ➡.

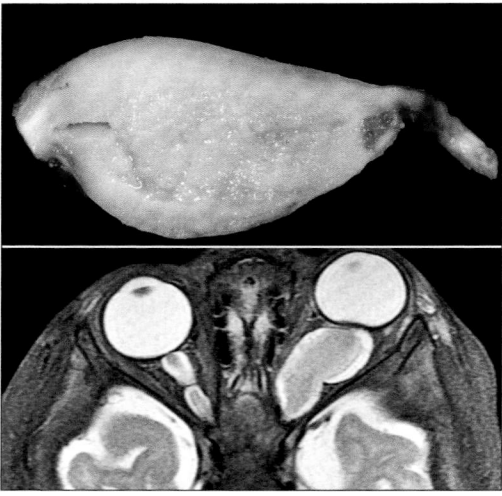

39-6. *Optic nerve glioma in NF1 (top), axial T2WI (bottom) show fusiform enlargement of the optic nerve. Nerve sheaths are moderately patulous.*

Approximately 20% of NF1-associated gliomas are malignant (WHO grades II-IV). These include **diffusely infiltrating ("low-grade") fibrillary astrocytoma**, **anaplastic astrocytoma**, and **glioblastoma multiforme**.

NON-CNS NEOPLASMS. NF1 is associated with an increased risk of leukemia (especially juvenile myelomonocytic leukemia and myelodysplastic syndromes), gastrointestinal stromal tumors (6%), and adrenal or extraadrenal pheochromocytoma (0.1-5%).

Rare NF1-associated systemic neoplasms include rhabdomyosarcoma, juvenile xanthogranuloma, melanoma, thyroid medullary carcinoma, and glomus tumors.

NF1-ASSOCIATED NEOPLASMS

Common
- Cutaneous neurofibromas (95% of adults)
- Plexiform neurofibromas (30%)
- Spinal neurofibromas

Less Common
- Optic pathway glioma (15-20%)
  - Pilocytic astrocytoma (80%)
- Other astrocytomas (20%)
  - Diffusely infiltrating fibrillary astrocytoma
  - Anaplastic astrocytoma
  - Glioblastoma multiforme

Rare but Important
- Malignant peripheral nerve sheath tumors
  - Develop in 10-15% of PNFs
- Juvenile chronic myeloid leukemia
- Gastrointestinal stromal tumor
- Pheochromocytoma
- Rhabdomyosarcoma
- Juvenile xanthogranuloma
- Melanoma
- Thyroid medullary carcinoma
- Glomus tumors

Clinical Issues

EPIDEMIOLOGY AND DEMOGRAPHICS. NF1 is one of the most common CNS single-gene disorders, affecting 1:3,000 live births. There is no gender predilection.

PRESENTATION. The clinical manifestations of NF1 are quite heterogeneous, and intrafamilial variation is common. Although absence of visible stigmata does not exclude the diagnosis of NF1, most patients exhibit characteristic cutaneous lesions **(39-7)**. Most are diagnosed as children or young adults.

Characteristic features include cutaneous neurofibromas (present in almost all adults with NF1), hyperpigmentary skin abnormalities with café au lait macules (95%) **(39-8)**, inguinal/axillary freckling (65-85%), and iris hamartomas or Lisch nodules **(39-9)**. Funduscopic examination using near-infrared reflectance demonstrates bright patchy choroidal nodules in 70% of pediatric patients and 80% of adults.

Other less common NF1-associated features include distinctive skeletal abnormalities such as sphenoid dysplasia, long bone cortex thinning, pseudarthroses, and progressive kyphoscoliosis. Cardiovascular anomalies can result in renovascular hypertension and strokes.

Cognitive impairment is common in NF1 and manifests primarily as learning difficulties and attention deficit disorder.

General surveillance recommendations in children with NF1 include annual physical examination (including ophthalmologic examination up to age five years), developmental assessment, and regular blood pressure monitoring. Additional specialist evaluations depend on associated CNS, skeletal, or cardiovascular manifestations.

Clinical Diagnosis. Molecular diagnostic testing distinguishes NF1 from other disorders that share similar phenotypic features. With the exception of plexiform neurofibroma, most clinical stigmata of NF1 also occur in other disorders (e.g., multiple café au lait macules in McCune-Albright syndrome). Consensus criteria for the clinical diagnosis of NF1 are summarized in the box below.

NF1: DIAGNOSTIC CLINICAL FEATURES (AT LEAST TWO REQUIRED)

Cutaneous Lesions
- ≥ 6 café au lait spots (earliest manifestation)
  - Prepubertal: ≥ 0.5 cm
  - Postpubertal: ≥ 1.5 cm
- Freckling of armpits or groin
- ≥ 2 neurofibromas (any type)
- 1 plexiform neurofibroma

Eye Abnormalities
- ≥ 2 Lisch nodules (pigmented iris hamartomas)
- Optic pathway pilocytic astrocytoma

Distinctive Bone Lesion
- Sphenoid dysplasia/absence
- Long bone cortex dysplasia/thinning

Family History
- First-degree relative with NF1

Natural History. Prognosis in NF1 is variable and relates to its specific manifestations. Median age at death for all NF1 patients is 59 years. Increased mortality is related to MPNST, glioma, cardiovascular disease, and organ compression by neurofibromas.

The foci of myelin vacuolization increase in number and size over the first decade, then regress and eventually disappear. They are rarely identified in adults, and their relationship to intellectual impairment is uncertain.

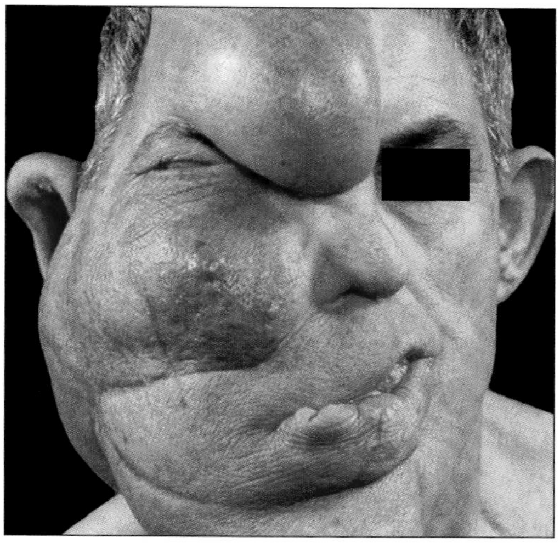

39-7. *Clinical photo shows extensive facial plexiform NF. (Courtesy A. Ersen, MD.)*

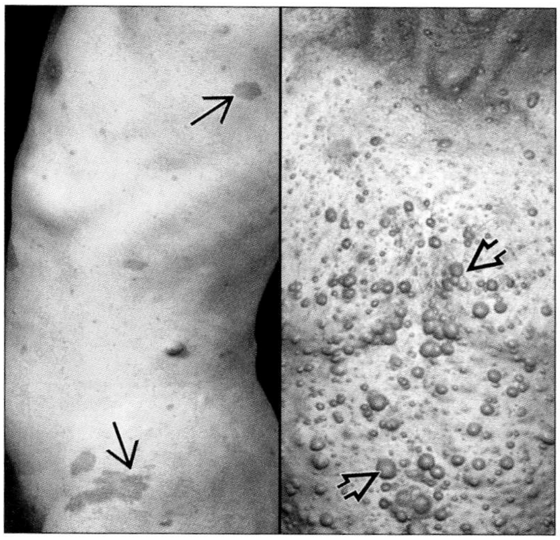

39-8. *Photographs show multiple café au lait spots (left) →, cutaneous neurofibromas ⇨ (right) in NF1. (Courtesy A. Ersen, MD.)*

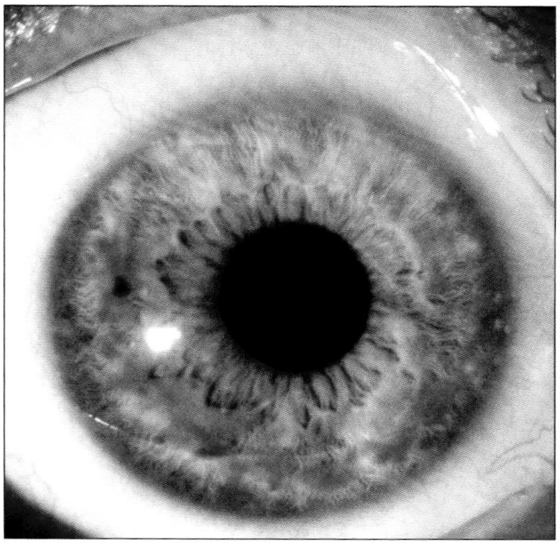

39-9. *Clinical photo shows multiple Lisch nodules in a patient with NF1. (Courtesy A. Ersen, MD.)*

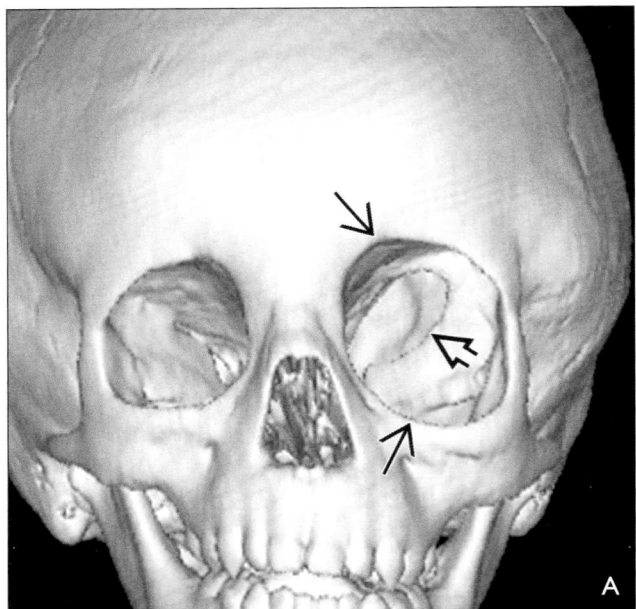

39-10A. 3D bone CT in a patient with NF1 and sphenoid dysplasia shows enlarged left orbit ⊒, widened superior orbital fissure ⊵.

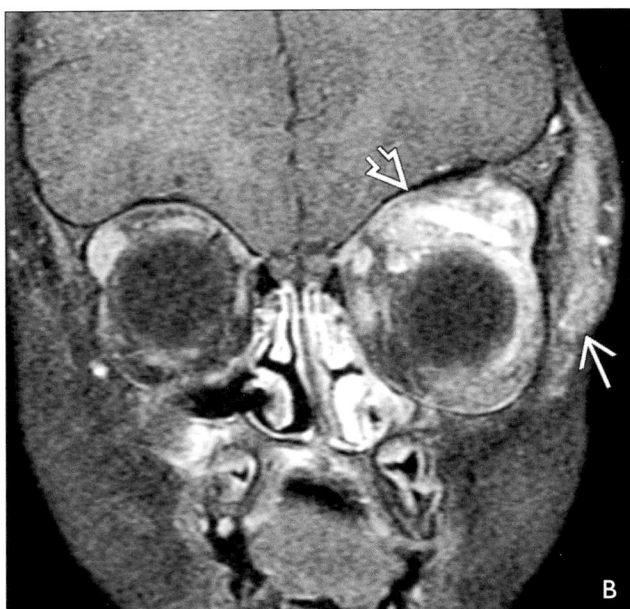

39-10B. Coronal T1 C+ FS scan in the same patient shows enhancing plexiform NF infiltrating the orbit ⊐, high deep masticator space ⊐.

TREATMENT OPTIONS. Foci of myelin vacuolization do not undergo neoplastic transformation and do not require treatment.

Imaging

Imaging features vary with the specific type of NF1-related abnormalities.

NONNEOPLASTIC CNS LESIONS. Bone dysplasias occur in both the skull and spine. NECT scans may demonstrate a hypoplastic sphenoid wing **(39-10A)** and enlarged middle cranial fossa, with or without an associated arachnoid cyst. Protrusion of the anterior temporal lobe may result in ipsilateral proptosis. The globe is frequently enlarged ("buphthalmos"), and a plexiform neurofibroma is often present **(39-2)**.

Dural dysplasias are also common. Enlarged, patulous optic nerve sheaths, internal auditory canals, and Meckel caves can occur **(39-11)**.

Dysplastic white matter lesions are seen as multifocal hyperintensities on T2/FLAIR imaging. These foci of abnormal signal (FASIs) are seen in 70% of children with NF1. They generally increase in size and number until approximately 10 years of age but then wane and resolve **(39-15)**. FASIs are rarely seen in adults.

The most common sites are the globi pallidi (GP), centrum semiovale, cerebellar WM and dentate nuclei, thalamus, and brainstem **(39-14)**. Most are smaller than two centimeters in diameter **(39-15)**. They generally exhibit little or no mass effect, although the corpus callosum may

appear thickened in severe cases. Confluent midbrain, tectum, brainstem, and hypothalamic lesions with unusually extensive myelin vacuolization can occasionally cause mass effect and even obstructive hydrocephalus.

Most FASIs are iso- or minimally hypointense on T1WI although GP lesions are often mildly hyperintense. FASIs do not enhance following contrast administration and demonstrate increased ADC values on DWI.

Most NF1-associated **vascular lesions** are extracranial and range from renal artery stenosis to aortic coarctation and aneurysmal dilatations of the great vessels.

Relentless endothelial hyperplasia can cause progressive stenosis of the intracranial internal carotid arteries, resulting in a moyamoya pattern. Careful scrutiny of the intracranial vasculature demonstrates attenuation of the middle cerebral artery "flow voids" **(39-12)**.

CNS NEOPLASMS.

Neurofibromas. Patients with **cutaneous neurofibromas** often demonstrate solitary or multifocal discrete round or ovoid scalp lesions that are hypointense to brain on T1WI and hyperintense on T2WI. A "target" sign with a hyperintense rim and relatively hypointense center is common. Strong but heterogeneous enhancement following contrast administration is typical **(39-5)**.

Plexiform NFs are most common in the orbit, where they are seen as poorly marginated serpentine masses that infiltrate the orbit, extraocular muscles, and eyelids **(39-2)**, **(39-10B)**. They often extend inferiorly into the pterygopalatine fossa and buccal spaces as well as superiorly into the adjacent scalp and masticator spaces. Transspatial extension into the neck is common. PNFs enhance strongly and resemble a "bag of worms."

Malignant peripheral nerve sheath tumors. **MPNSTs** arising within a PNF can be difficult to detect and to differentiate from the parent tumor. MPNSTs tend to be more heterogeneous in signal intensity, often exhibiting intratumoral cysts, perilesional edema, and peripheral enhancement.

Gliomas. The most common glioma in NF1 is **pilocytic astrocytoma**. Optic pathway glioma (OPG) is the most common lesion and is seen as diffuse fusiform enlargement of one or both optic nerves **(39-6)**. Tumor may extend posteriorly into the optic chiasm, superiorly into the hypothalamus, fornices, and cavum septi pellucidi, laterally into the temporal lobes, posteriorly into the optic tracts and lateral geniculate bodies, and posteroinferiorly into the cerebral peduncles and brainstem **(39-13)**.

Signal intensity is variable. Most OPGs are isointense with brain on T1WI and iso- to moderately hyperintense on T2WI. Enhancement on T1 C+ FS scans varies from none to striking.

MRS is generally not helpful, as pilocytic astrocytomas often demonstrate a malignant-appearing spectrum with elevated choline and increased Cho:Cr ratio. Neither extent of signal intensity nor enhancement indicates malignancy, so interval surveillance is necessary. NF1-associated OPGs can be stable for many years or involute spontaneously.

NF1-associated **low-grade fibrillary astrocytomas** can be difficult to distinguish from FASIs. They are usually moderately hypointense on T1WI and hyperintense on T2WI and show progression on follow-up imaging.

Anaplastic astrocytoma and **glioblastoma multiforme** are more aggressive, more heterogeneous tumors that demonstrate relentless progression. A progressively enlarging mass that enhances following contrast administration in a child with NF1 should raise suspicion of malignant neoplasm.

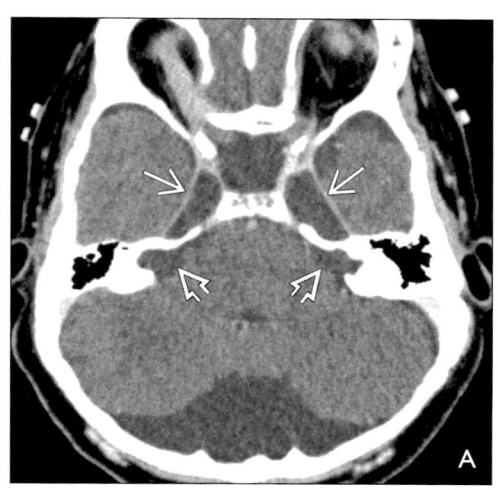
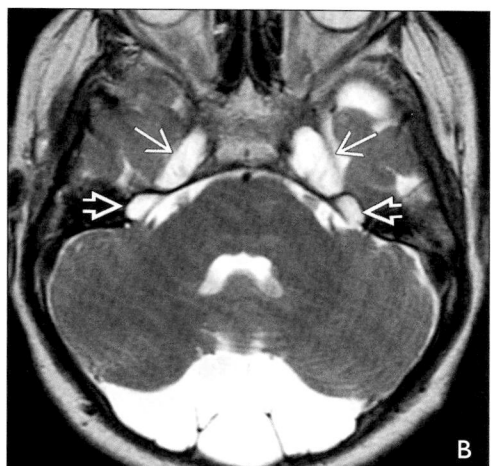

39-11A. *Axial CECT scan in a patient with NF1 shows findings of intracranial dural ectasia with bilateral patulous Meckel caves* ➡, *expanded CSF-filled internal auditory canals* ➡. **39-11B.** *T2WI in the same patient demonstrates that the patulous Meckel caves* ➡, *internal auditory canals* ➡ *are filled with CSF, not schwannoma (which would be characteristic of NF2, not NF1).*

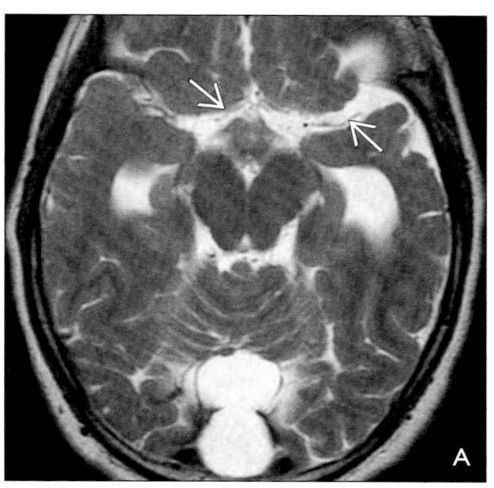
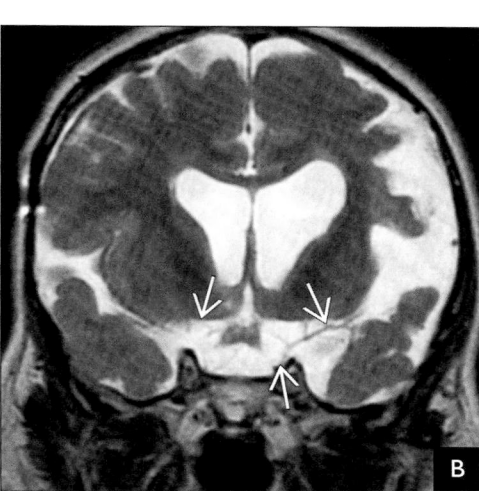

39-12A. *Axial T2WI in a teenager with NF1 shows extremely attenuated anterior and middle cerebral arteries* ➡, *a vascular manifestation of NF1.* **39-12B.** *Coronal T2WI in the same patient shows the typical appearance of "moyamoya" in NF1 with markedly attenuated supraclinoid internal carotid, anterior cerebral, and middle cerebral arteries* ➡.

39-13A. Axial T2WI in a patient with NF1 shows an enlarged hyperintense left optic nerve ➡, a prosthetic globe ➡, and a hyperintense mass ➡ in the pons. 39-13B. More cephalad T2WI shows enlarged optic chiasm ➡, mass extending into right midbrain ➡, foci of abnormal signal intensity in both medial temporal lobes and left midbrain ➡.

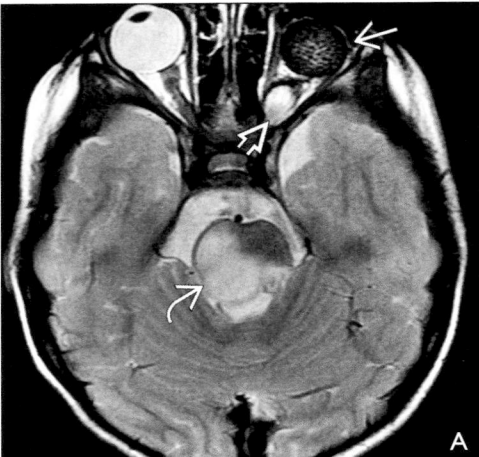
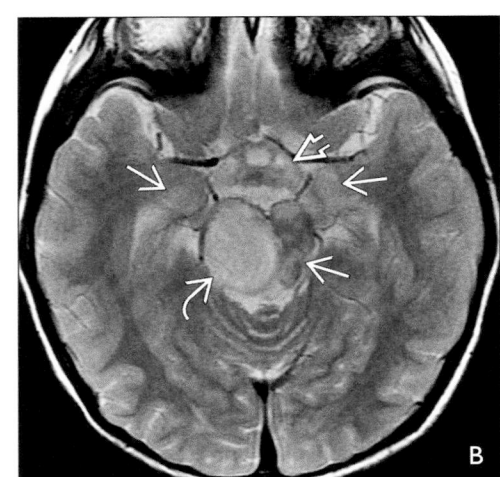

39-13C. T1 C+ FS scan shows intense enhancement in the enlarged optic chiasm ➡, medial temporal lobes ➡, and midbrain ➡. 39-13D. More cephalad scan shows that the enhancement extends posteriorly along both optic radiations ➡.

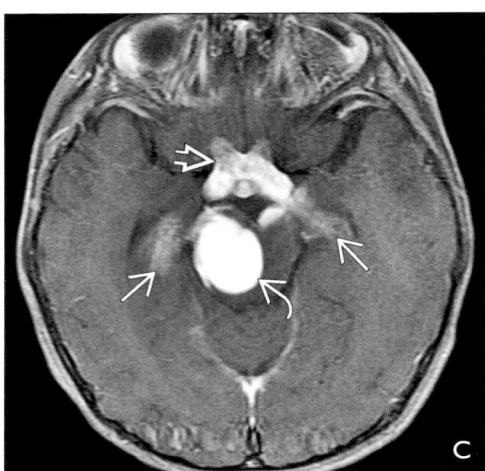
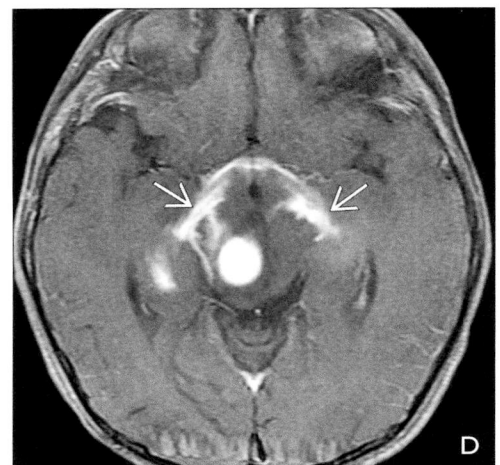

39-13E. DTI in the same patient shows disturbed anisotropy in the midbrain ➡. 39-13F. Perfusion MR shows significantly elevated rCBV in the upper pons ➡. Biopsy demonstrated pilocytic astrocytoma (WHO grade I) without evidence of malignant degeneration.

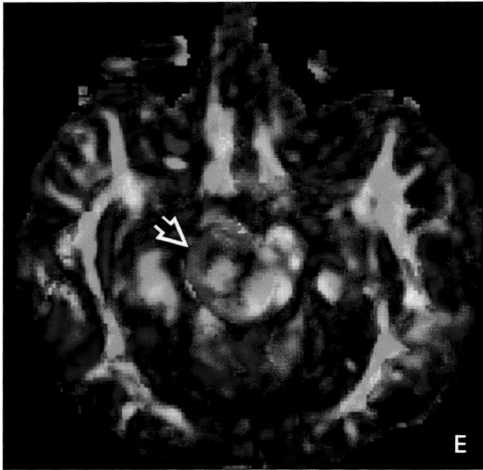
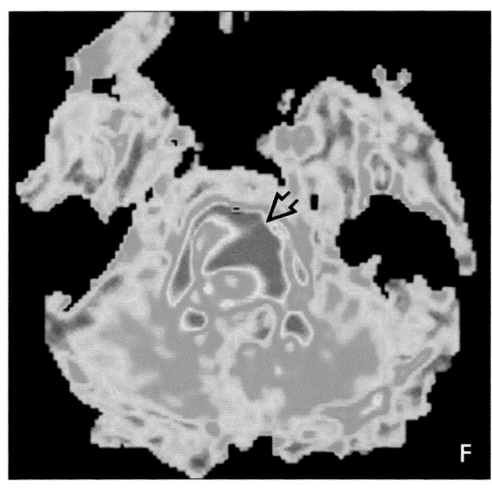

NF1: IMAGING

Scalp/Skull, Meninges, and Orbit
- Cutaneous scalp, plexiform NFs
  - Solitary/multifocal scalp nodules
  - PNFs infiltrate, may extend into cavernous sinus
- Sphenoid wing dysplasia
  - Hypoplasia → enlarged orbital fissure
  - Enlarged middle fossa ± arachnoid cyst
  - Temporal lobe may protrude into orbit
- Dural ectasia
  - Tortuous optic nerve sheath
  - Patulous Meckel caves
  - Enlarged IACs

Brain
- Hyperintense T2/FLAIR WM foci
  - Wax in first decade, then wane
  - Rare in adults
- Astrocytomas
  - Most common: Pilocytic
  - Optic pathway, hypothalamus > brainstem
  - Malignant astrocytoma (anaplastic astrocytoma, glioblastoma multiforme) less common

Arteries
- Progressive ICA stenosis → moyamoya
- Fusiform ectasias, AVFs
  - Vertebral > carotid

Differential Diagnosis

In combination with appropriate clinical findings (see above), the presence of FASIs on MR with or without OPG is diagnostic of NF1. In and of themselves, multifocal T2/FLAIR hyperintensities are nonspecific and can be seen in a variety of nonneoplastic disorders including **demyelinating disease** and **viral encephalitis**.

Unusually extensive, confluent FASIs can mimic **neoplasm** (i.e., pilocytic astrocytoma, diffusely infiltrating low-grade astrocytoma, anaplastic astrocytoma, glioblastoma multiforme, or gliomatosis cerebri). Both FASIs and gliomas are part of the NF1 spectrum, so follow-up imaging may be necessary.

A recently described disorder parallels NF1 in some ways—multiple café au lait macules, axillary freckling, and macrocephaly—but the causative gene (*SPRED1*) is different. This disorder has been termed **NF1-like syndrome**. Patients lack cutaneous or plexiform neurofibromas, typical NF1 bone lesions, and optic pathway gliomas.

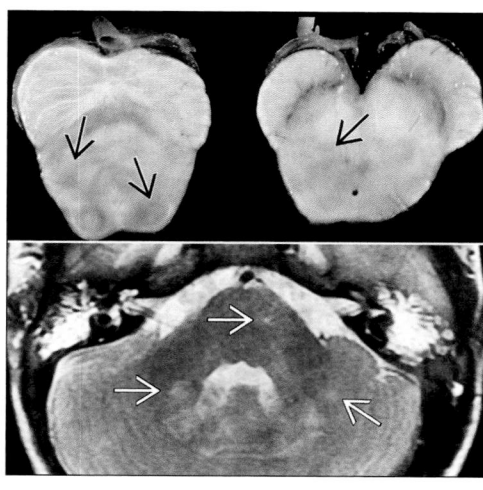

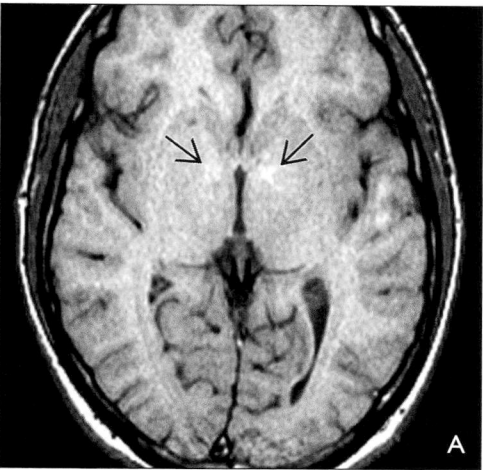

39-14. *Autopsy specimens from a patient with NF1 (top) show multiple foci of discolored white matter in the midbrain* →, *mild mass effect with expansion of the brainstem tegmentum. (Courtesy AFIP Archives.) Axial T2WI (bottom) in another case shows typical hyperintense lesions* → *of NF1 seen in the pons, cerebellum.* **39-15A.** *T1WI in a child with NF1 shows bilateral hyperintense foci in the medial basal ganglia* →.

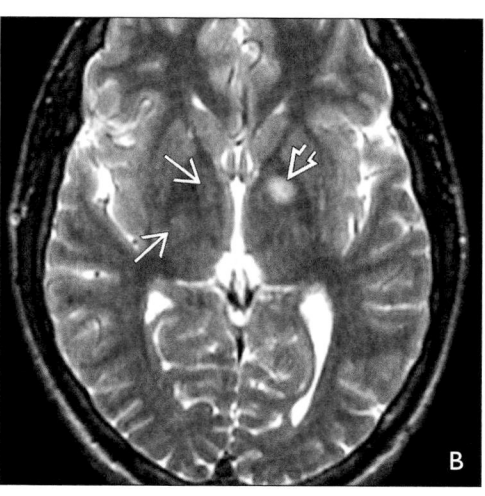

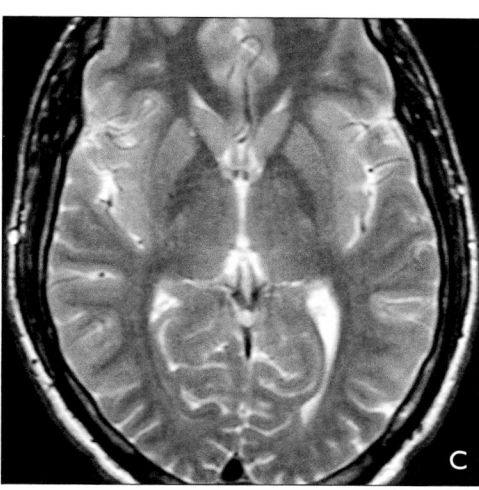

39-15B. *T2WI in the same patient shows foci of abnormal signal intensity (FASIs) in right* →, *left basal ganglia* →. **39-15C.** *Six years later, the FASIs have resolved completely without residual abnormality. These T2/FLAIR hyperintense lesions seen in children with NF1 represent foci of myelin vacuolization, increasing in number and size until approximately age 10, then waning and disappearing. They are rare in adults with NF1.*

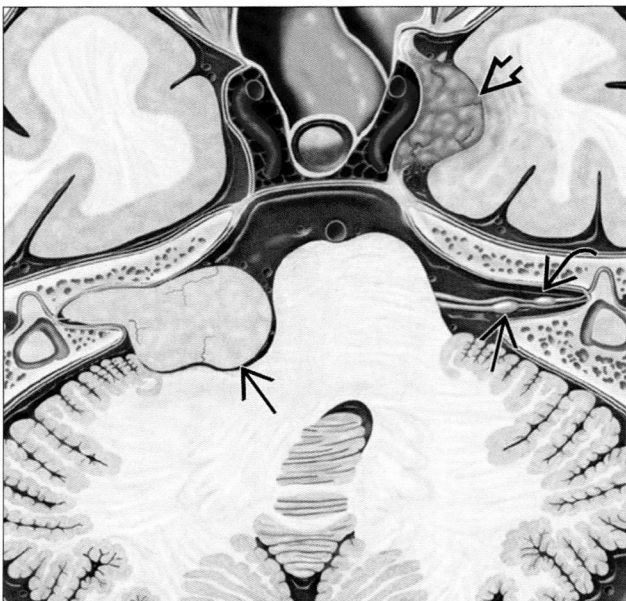

39-16. Graphic depicts classic NF2 with bilateral vestibular schwannomas ⇥, facial schwannoma ⇗, and cavernous sinus meningioma ⇥.

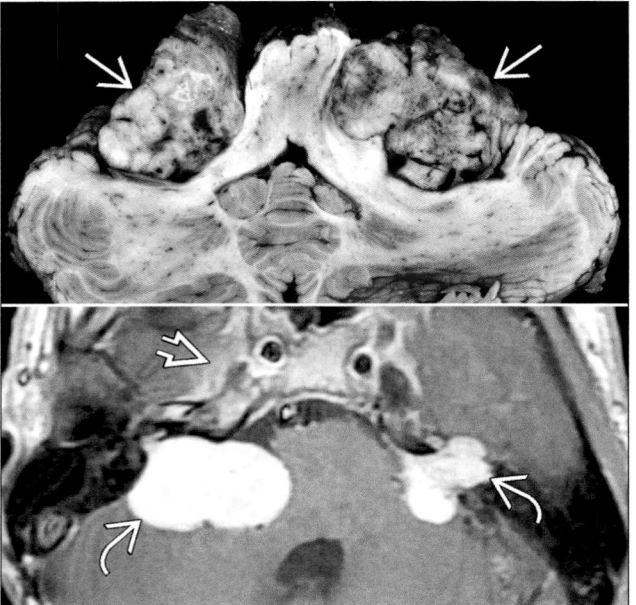

39-17. Autopsy specimen (top) demonstrates bilateral vestibular schwannomas ⇥ in NF2. (Courtesy A. Ersen, MD.) Typical T1 C+ scan (bottom) shows bilateral vestibular schwannomas ⇥, right cavernous sinus meningioma ⇥.

Neurofibromatosis Type 2

Though historically grouped with NF1, neurofibromatosis type 2 (NF2) is a distinct syndrome with totally different mutations, clinical features, and imaging findings. Neurofibromas characterize NF1 and are composed of Schwann cells plus fibroblasts. Schwannomas (especially bilateral vestibular schwannomas) are the major feature of NF2 and contain only Schwann cells.

The associated neoplasms are also different from those in NF1. Astrocytomas are found in NF1 while ependymomas and meningiomas are the predominant tumors in NF2.

There is only one similarity between NF1 and NF2: They both predispose affected individuals to develop benign Schwann cell tumors.

Terminology

NF2 is also known as neurofibromatosis with bilateral vestibular ("acoustic") schwannomas. Historically, NF2 was termed central neurofibromatosis (to distinguish it from so-called peripheral neurofibromatosis, i.e., NF1). The term "von Recklinghausen neurofibromatosis" is associated only with NF1 and should not be used for neurofibromatosis type 2.

Etiology

GENERAL CONCEPTS. Like NF1, NF2 is an autosomal dominant disorder. About half of all cases occur in individuals with no family history of NF2 and are caused by newly acquired germline mutations. Approximately 30% of these patients have mosaic genetic alterations.

GENETICS. NF2 is caused by mutations of the *NF2* gene on chromosome 22q12. The *NF2* gene encodes the protein Merlin (**m**oesin-**e**rzin-**r**adixin-like prote**in**), which is also known as schwannomin. Merlin is implicated in the regulation of membrane organization and cytoskeleton-based cellular processes such as adhesion, migration, cell-cell contact, and signaling.

Merlin functions as a growth inhibitor and tumor suppressor and regulates antiangiogenic factors. Inactivating mutations of the *NF2* gene result in loss of contact-dependent inhibition of proliferation and cause predominantly benign neoplasms (schwannomas and meningiomas). Biallelic *NF2* inactivation is detected in the majority of sporadic meningiomas and nearly all schwannomas.

Pathology

LOCATION. CNS lesions are present in virtually all patients with NF2.

The most common NF2-related schwannomas are vestibular schwannomas (VSs) **(39-16)**. Approximately 50% of patients have nonvestibular schwannomas (NVSs). The most common locations for NVSs are the trigeminal and oculomotor nerves. NF2-associated schwannomas of the trochlear and lower cranial nerves occur but are relatively rare.

Meningiomas occur in approximately half of all patients with NF2 and can be found anywhere in the skull and

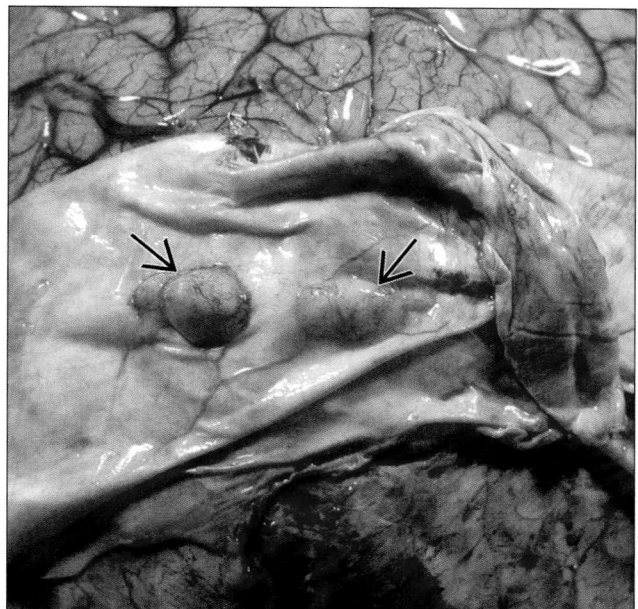

39-18. *Autopsy specimen demonstrates multiple small asymptomatic meningiomas ➡, a common finding in NF2. (Courtesy R. Hewlett, MD.)*

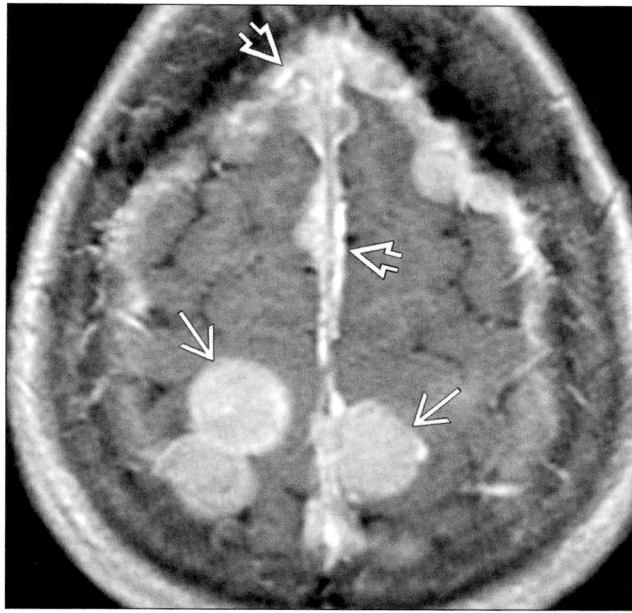

39-19. *T1 C+ scan in a patient with NF2 shows multiple globular meningiomas ➡ and diffuse "en plaque" dural thickening ➡.*

spine. The most frequent sites are along the falx and cerebral convexities.

Intracranial ependymomas are rare in NF2. Most are found in the spinal cord, especially within the cervical cord or at the cervicomedullary junction.

SIZE AND NUMBER. NF2-related schwannomas, meningiomas, and ependymomas are often multiple. The presence of bilateral VSs is pathognomonic of NF2; adult patients with NF2 have an average of three meningiomas.

Size varies from tiny to several centimeters. Innumerable tiny schwannomas ("tumorlets") throughout the cauda equina are seen in the majority of patients. Intramedullary ependymomas are often small; multiple tumors are present in nearly 60% of patients.

GROSS PATHOLOGY. NF2 is characterized by multiple schwannomas, meningiomas, and ependymomas. Virtually all patients have bilateral vestibular schwannomas, considered the hallmark of NF2 **(39-17)**. Most schwannomas are well-delineated round or ovoid encapsulated masses that are attached to—but do not infiltrate—their parent nerves.

Multiple meningiomas are the second pathologic hallmark of NF2. They are found in approximately 50% of patients and may be the presenting feature (especially in children). Meningiomas appear as unencapsulated but sharply demarcated masses **(39-18)**.

MICROSCOPIC FEATURES. Schwannomas are composed of neoplastic Schwann cells. Areas of alternating high

and low cellularity (Antoni A pattern) are admixed with foci that exhibit microcysts and myxoid changes (Antoni B pattern). Schwann cells are strongly immunoreactive for S100 and usually do not express Merlin.

STAGING, GRADING, AND CLASSIFICATION. Although NF2-associated schwannomas often have higher proliferative activity than sporadic tumors, they are not necessarily more aggressive. They are considered WHO grade I tumors.

Most NF2-associated meningiomas are WHO grade I neoplasms. Among symptomatic resected meningiomas, grades II and III tumors are found in 29% and 6% of cases, respectively.

NF2-associated ependymomas are very low grade (dubbed "grade 1/2").

Clinical Issues

EPIDEMIOLOGY AND DEMOGRAPHICS. NF2 is much less common than NF1, with an estimated prevalence of 1:25,000 births. There is no geographic, ethnic, or gender predilection.

PRESENTATION. Unlike NF1 patients, individuals with NF2 generally do not become symptomatic until the second to fourth decades; symptoms often precede definitive diagnosis by five to eight years. Average age at initial diagnosis is 17-24 years; less than 20% of patients with NF2 present under the age of 15.

Unlike NF1, most of the clinical features of NF2 involve the nervous system. Cutaneous schwannomas and/or

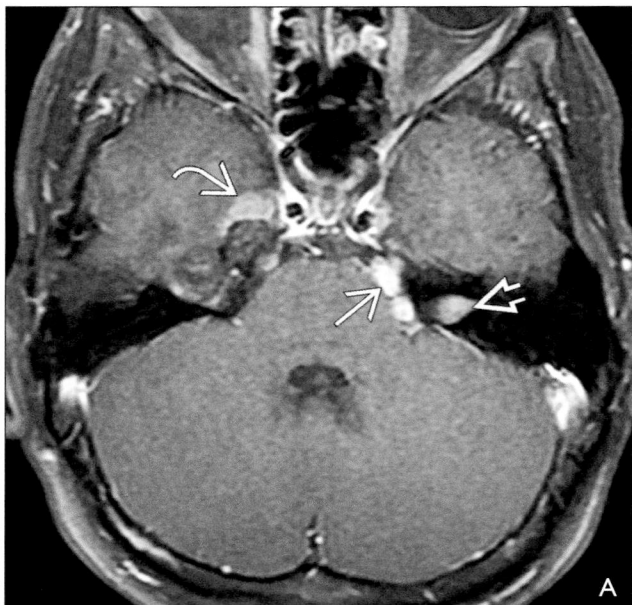

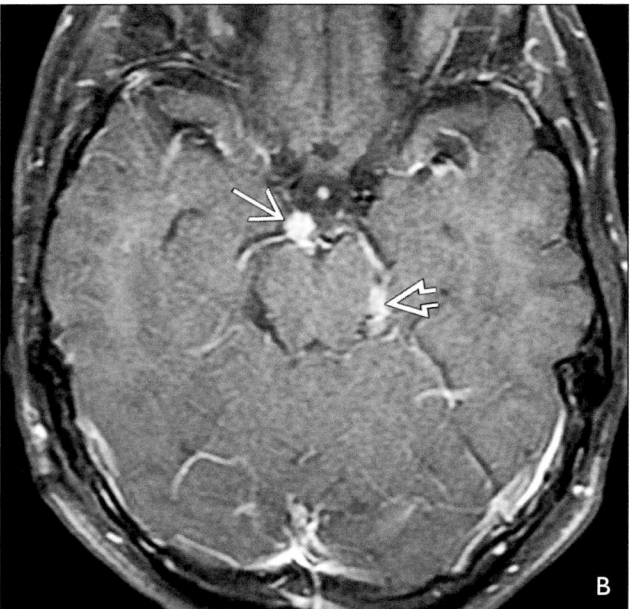

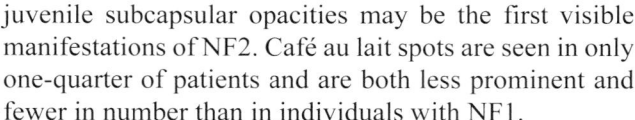

39-20A. Axial T1 C+ FS scan in a patient with documented NF2 shows schwannomas of left CNs V ➔ and VIII ➔, plus a right cavernous sinus meningioma ➔.

39-20B. More cephalad scan in the same patient shows schwannomas of the right CN III ➔ and left CN IV ➔.

juvenile subcapsular opacities may be the first visible manifestations of NF2. Café au lait spots are seen in only one-quarter of patients and are both less prominent and fewer in number than in individuals with NF1.

Most adult patients exhibit CN VIII dysfunction with progressive sensorineural hearing loss, tinnitus, and difficulties with balance. Other common symptoms include facial pain and/or paralysis, vertigo, and seizures. Hearing loss is relatively uncommon in children. Subcapsular cataracts, seizures, facial nerve palsy, and other cranial neuropathies are common.

Many NF2-related meningiomas are asymptomatic and discovered incidentally on imaging studies; if symptoms appear, seizures or focal neurologic deficits are the most common. Spinal cord ependymomas are asymptomatic in 75% of patients.

CLINICAL DIAGNOSIS. The definitive diagnosis of NF2 is established genetically. Similar to NF1, consensus criteria have been developed for the clinical diagnosis and are summarized in the box below. Findings are divided into those of "definite" and "probable" NF2.

NF2: DIAGNOSTIC CLINICAL FEATURES

Definite NF2
- Bilateral vestibular schwannomas (VSs)
- First-degree relative with NF2 *and* unilateral VS younger than 30 years of age
- *Or* first-degree relative with NF2 *and* 2 of the following
  ◦ Meningioma
  ◦ Glioma
  ◦ Schwannoma
  ◦ Juvenile posterior subcapsular lenticular opacities or cataracts

Probable NF2
- Unilateral VS younger than 30 years of age *and* 1 of the following
  ◦ Meningioma
  ◦ Glioma
  ◦ Schwannoma
  ◦ Juvenile posterior subcapsular lenticular opacities or cataracts
- ≥ 2 meningiomas *and* 1 of the following
  ◦ 1 VS younger than 30 years of age
  ◦ 1 meningioma, glioma, schwannoma, or lens opacity

NATURAL HISTORY. Actuarial survival for NF2 patients after diagnosis is 85% at 5 years, 67% at 10 years, and 38% at 20 years. While NF2-associated meningiomas have a mean annual growth rate of 1.5 mm, de novo and meningiomas with brain edema may require active treatment.

NF2-associated intracranial neoplasms often demonstrate a "saltatory" growth pattern characterized by alternating periods of growth and quiescence. Resection may be best reserved for symptom-producing tumors. How-

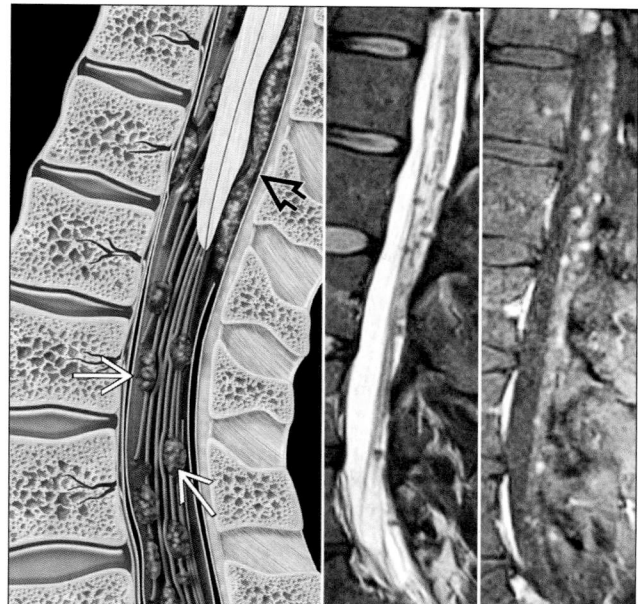

39-21. Graphic (left) depicts multiple spinal "tumorlets" ➡, *meningioma* ⊵ *in NF2. Sagittal T2WI (middle) and T1 C+ (right) show multiple tiny enhancing cauda equina schwannomas.*

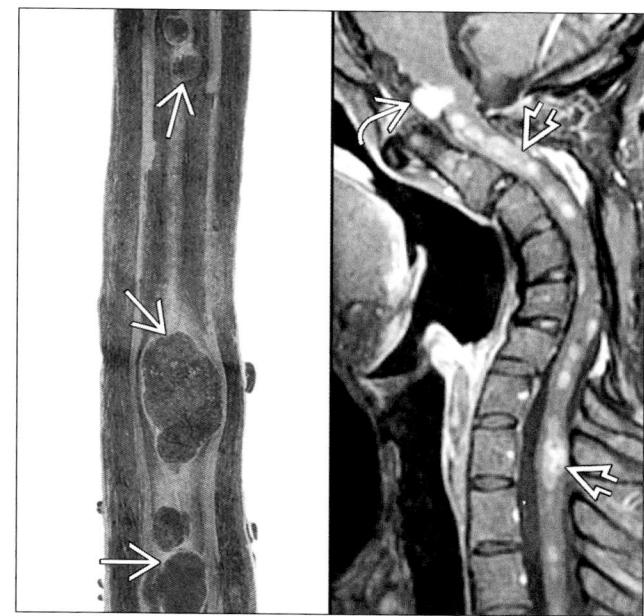

39-22. Autopsy (left) shows multiple intramedullary ependymomas ➡ *in NF2. (Courtesy A. Ersen, MD.) Sagittal T1 C+ (right) shows multiple ependymomas* ➡, *foramen magnum meningioma* ➡.

ever, as new tumors can develop and radiographic progression and symptom development are unpredictable, continued surveillance is necessary.

TREATMENT OPTIONS. Surgery is the standard treatment for NF2-related tumors. Complete resection of VSs is desirable. However, excision of all lesions is often not possible or even advisable. Subtotal microsurgical resection with cochlear nerve preservation in the last hearing ear is common.

Imaging

GENERAL FEATURES. The cardinal imaging feature of NF2 is bilateral vestibular schwannomas.

CT FINDINGS. NECT scans typically demonstrate a mass in one or both cerebellopontine angle (CPA) cisterns. Both schwannomas and meningiomas are typically iso- to slightly hyperdense on NECT and exhibit strong enhancement following contrast administration.

Nonneoplastic choroid plexus calcifications in atypical locations (e.g., temporal horn) are a rare manifestation of NF2 but can be striking. Cerebral and cerebellar parenchymal calcification have been reported in a few cases.

Bone CT typically shows that one or both internal auditory canals are widened. Schwannomas of other cranial nerves may demonstrate enlargement and remodeling of their exit foramina (e.g., enlarged foramen ovale with trigeminal schwannoma).

MR FINDINGS. MR findings of NF2-related schwannomas and meningiomas are similar to those of their sporadic counterparts **(39-19)**, **(39-20)**. If NF2 is suspected on the basis of brain imaging, the entire spine and spinal cord should be screened. High-resolution T2WI and contrast-enhanced sequences disclose asymptomatic tiny schwannomas **(39-21)** and intramedullary ependymomas **(39-22)** in at least half of all individuals with NF2.

Differential Diagnosis

The major differential diagnosis of NF2 is **schwannomatosis**. Schwannomatosis lacks cutaneous stigmata, is characterized by multiple nonvestibular schwannomas, is not associated with meningiomas, and has a different genetic mutation (see below).

Multiple meningiomatosis is characterized by multifocal globose and en plaque meningiomas without schwannomas.

NF1 vs. NF2

Neurofibromatosis Type 1
- Common (90% of all NF cases)
- Chromosome 17 mutations
- Almost always diagnosed by age 10
- Cutaneous/eye lesions common (> 95%)
  - Café au lait spots
  - Lisch nodules
  - Cutaneous NFs (often multiple)
  - Plexiform NFs (pathognomonic)
- CNS lesions less common (15-20%)
  - T2/FLAIR hyperintensities (myelin vacuolization; lesions wax, then wane)
  - Astrocytomas (optic pathway gliomas—usually pilocytic—other gliomas)
  - Sphenoid wing, dural dysplasias
  - Moyamoya
  - Neurofibromas of spinal nerve roots

Neurofibromatosis Type 2
- Much less common (10% of all NF cases)
- Chromosome 22 mutations
- Usually diagnosed in second to fourth decades
- Cutaneous, eye lesions less prominent
  - Mild/few café au lait spots
  - Juvenile subcapsular opacities
- CNS lesions in 100%
  - Bilateral vestibular schwannomas (almost all)
  - Nonvestibular schwannomas (50%)
  - Meningiomas (50%)
  - Cord ependymomas (often multiple)
  - Schwannomas of spinal nerve roots

Schwannomatosis

Terminology

Schwannomatosis, which is the third major form of neurofibromatosis, is a rare hereditary cancer syndrome in which patients develop multiple **nonvestibular nonintradermal schwannomas**.

Etiology and Pathology

Schwannomatosis is caused by missense mutations in the chromatin remodeling gene *SMARCB1* (also known as *INI1* and *hSNF5*). Unlike NF1 and NF2, most cases of schwannomatosis arise de novo, as less than 15% appear to be familial. The rate of transmission to offspring is low, likely due to the high rate of genetic mosaicism in founder mutations.

Multiple schwannomas of the spine (75%), subcutaneous tissues (15%), and nonvestibular cranial nerves (10%) are characteristic. While these schwannomas vary from multiple discrete nodules to plexiform lesions, histologic features are those of typical schwannoma.

Recent evidence indicates that schwannomatosis patients with *SMARCB1* mutations are at risk to develop multiple cranial meningiomas. Nearly two-thirds of meningiomas in patients with this tumor predisposition syndrome are located at the falx cerebri.

Clinical Issues

Schwannomatosis affects 1:40,000 births. Symptoms vary, but pain is the most common presentation. Prognosis is excellent, as anaplastic transformation is very rare.

Imaging and Differential Diagnosis

Multiple enhancing nodules occur along the cauda equina and peripheral nerves. Cranial NVSs are common and resemble both sporadic and NF2-associated schwannomas. Meningiomas are less frequent; when present, they exhibit a distinct affinity for the cerebral convexities and falx.

The major differential diagnosis of schwannomatosis is **NF2**. By definition, schwannomatosis lacks the bilateral VSs characteristic of NF2. Enhancing lesions along the spinal nerve roots and cauda equina that resemble schwannomatosis can be caused by **leptomeningeal "drop metastases."**

Other Common Familial Tumor Syndromes

Tuberous Sclerosis Complex

Tuberous sclerosis complex is a neurocutaneous syndrome characterized by the formation of nonmalignant hamartomas and neoplastic lesions in the brain, heart, skin, kidney, lung, and other organs. It is associated with autism, seizures, and neurocognitive and behavioral disabilities. Because its clinical manifestations vary widely, establishing the diagnosis of tuberous sclerosis complex was particularly challenging prior to the advent of modern neuroimaging and genetic phenotyping.

Terminology

Tuberous sclerosis complex (TSC) has also been called Bourneville or Bourneville-Pringle disease. The classic clinical triad of TSC consists of facial lesions ("adenomata sebaceum"), seizures, and mental retardation.

Etiology

GENERAL CONCEPTS. Approximately 50% of TSC cases are inherited and follow an autosomal dominant pattern. The other half represents de novo mutations and germline mosaicism.

GENETICS. Two separate genes are mutated or deleted in TSC: *TSC1* and *TSC2*. *TSC2* mutations are approximately five times as frequent as those affecting *TSC1*.

The *TSC1* gene is located on chromosome 9q34 and encodes a protein called **hamartin**. The *TSC2* gene is localized to chromosome 16p13.3 and encodes the **tuberin** protein. Mutations in either gene are identified in 75-85% of patients with TSC.

The TSC1/TSC2 protein dimer complex functions as a tumor suppressor. Hamartin/tuberin inhibits the complex signaling pathway called mammalian target of rapamycin (mTOR). Mammals possess only a single *mTOR* gene. The mTOR protein product is a component of two complexes, mTORC1 and mTORC2. Activation of either mTORC regulates protein synthesis and cell growth.

Mutations that lead to increased mTOR activation promote cellular disorganization, overgrowth, and abnormal differentiation that may result in tumorigenesis.

Pathology

The four major pathologic features of TSC in the brain are cortical tubers, subependymal nodules, white matter lesions, and subependymal giant cell astrocytoma **(39-23)**, **(39-24)**.

CORTICAL TUBERS. Cortical tubers are firm, whitish, pyramid-shaped, elevated areas of smooth gyral thickening, with or without central depressions, that grossly resemble potatoes ("tubers").

Microscopically, cortical tubers consist of giant cells and dysmorphic neurons with foci of gliosis, disrupted lamination, and disordered myelin. Balloon cells similar to those seen in Taylor-type focal cortical dysplasia (FCD IIb) are also commonly found in tubers. Tubers do not undergo malignant transformation.

SUBEPENDYMAL NODULES. Subependymal nodules (SENs) are located immediately beneath the ependymal lining of the lateral ventricles, along the course of the caudate nucleus.

SENs appear as elevated, rounded, hamartomatous lesions that grossly resemble candle guttering or drippings. They often calcify with increasing age. SENs along the caudothalamic groove adjacent to the foramen of Monro may undergo neoplastic transformation into subependymal giant cell astrocytoma.

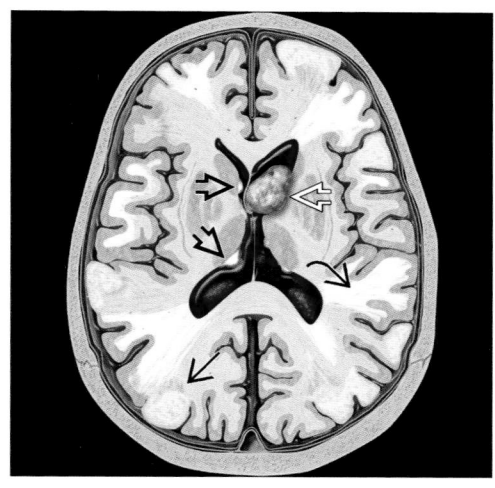

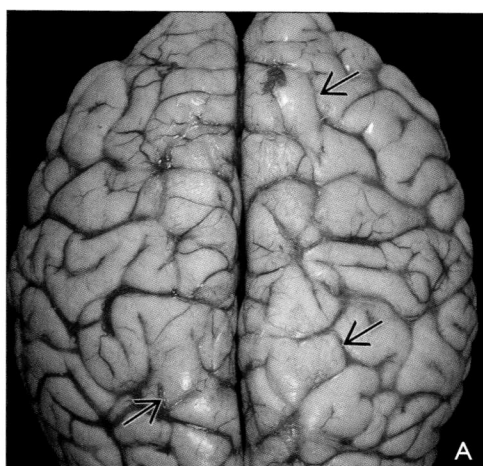

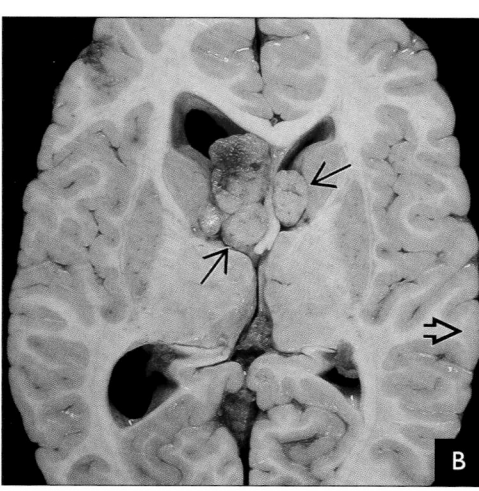

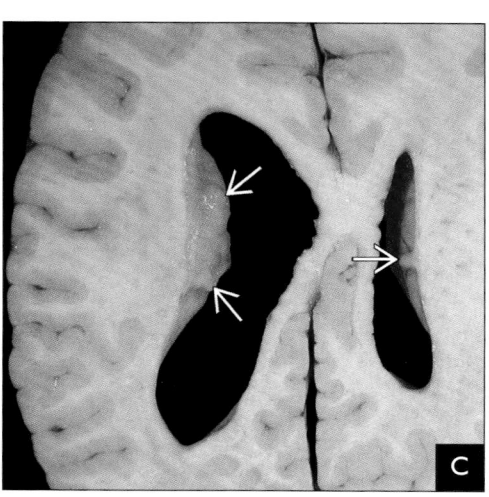

39-23. Axial graphic of typical brain involvement in tuberous sclerosis complex shows a giant cell astrocytoma ⇒ in the left foramen of Monro, subependymal nodules ⇒, radial migration lines ⇗, and cortical/subcortical tubers ⇒. *39-24A.* Autopsy specimen from a patient with TSC shows multiple expanded gyri with the potato-like appearance characteristic of cortical tubers ⇒.

39-24B. Axial cut section from the same case shows bilateral subependymal giant cell astrocytomas ⇒, cortical tubers ⇒. *39-24C.* Axial section from the same case through the lateral ventricles shows the "heaped-up" appearance of subependymal nodules along the striothalamic groove ⇒. (Courtesy R. Hewlett, MD.)

WHITE MATTER LESIONS. White matter (WM) lesions are almost universal in patients with TSC. They appear as foci of bizarre dysmorphic neurons and balloon cells in the subcortical WM and/or fine radial lines extending outward from the lateral ventricles.

SUBEPENDYMAL GIANT CELL ASTROCYTOMA. Subependymal giant cell astrocytoma (SEGA)—also known as subependymal giant cell tumor—is seen almost exclusively in the setting of TSC. Grossly, SEGAs appear as well-circumscribed solid intraventricular masses located near the foramen of Monro. SEGAs are WHO grade I tumors that often cause obstructive hydrocephalus but do not invade adjacent brain. While most SEGAs are unilateral, bilateral tumors occur in 10-15% of cases.

Typical microscopic features are large (not truly giant), plump cells that resemble astrocytes and/or ganglion cells in a fibrillar background. Tumor cell GFAP positivity varies, but most SEGAs are positive for neurofilament protein, neuron-specific enolase, and synaptophysin on immunohistochemistry.

Intratumoral calcifications are relatively common, but necrosis is rare. Mitoses are few, and the MIB-1 index is generally low.

Clinical Issues

EPIDEMIOLOGY AND DEMOGRAPHICS. TSC is one of the most common inherited tumor syndromes with a prevalence of approximately 1:6,000 live births. Almost 80% of cases are diagnosed before the age of 10 years. Between 20-30% are diagnosed during the first year of life when infantile spasms are observed in the patients with a positive family history. Patients with *TSC2* mutations are diagnosed an average of nine years earlier than patients with a *TSC1* mutation.

PRESENTATION. TSC patients generally present within the first two decades of life. The most common skin lesions are hypomelanotic macules, which are ovoid depigmented areas with irregular margins that are best visualized by ultraviolet light (Woods lamp). These "ash leaf" spots are seen in over 90% of cases and may be the first visible manifestation of TSC (39-26). Other common cutaneous findings such as forehead plaques, sha-

39-25. Clinical photo shows the typical facial "adenomata sebaceum" seen in tuberous sclerosis complex. (Courtesy B. Krafchik, MD.) 39-26. Clinical photo shows an "ash leaf" spot ▷, characteristic of TSC. Other macules show areas of hypopigmentation ➔. (Courtesy B. Krafchik, MD.)

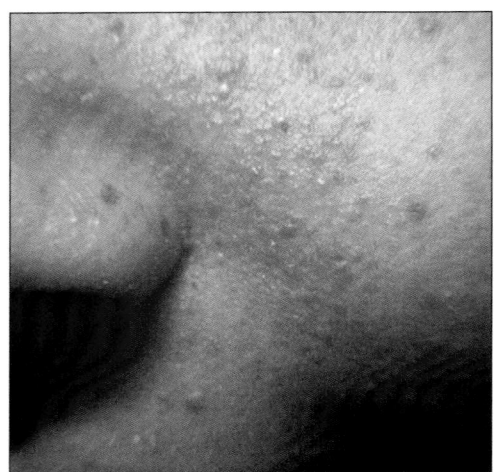

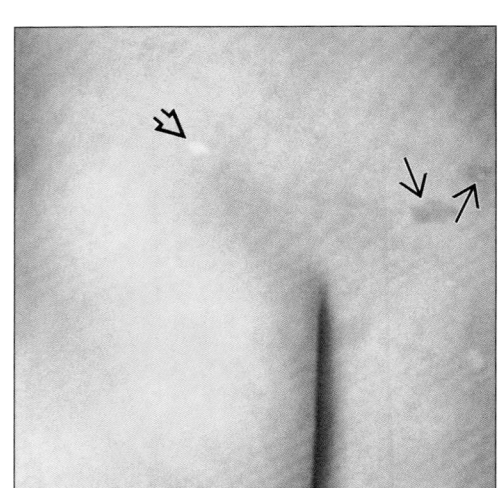

39-27. Clinical photo shows shagreen patches, a typical finding in TSC. (Courtesy B. Krafchik, MD.) 39-28. Periungual fibromas are common in the toes and fingernails in patients with TSC. (Courtesy B. Krafchik, MD.)

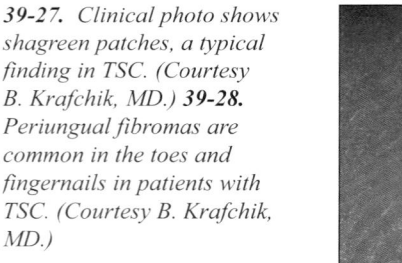

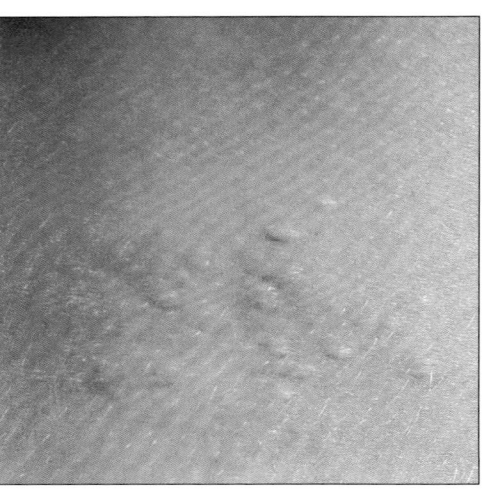

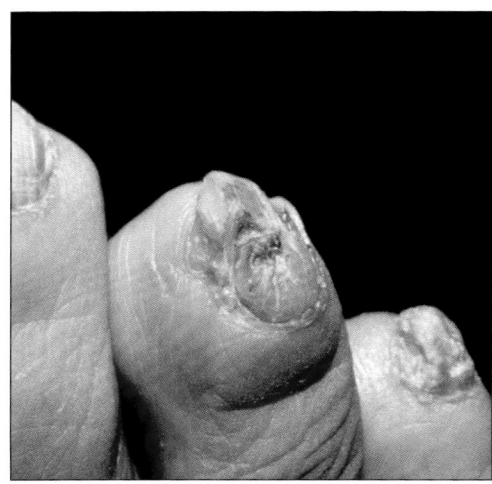

green patches **(39-27)**, facial angiofibromas ("adenoma sebaceum"), and periungual fibromas **(39-28)** usually do not appear until after puberty.

CLINICAL DIAGNOSIS. The clinical diagnosis of TSC is problematic because all cutaneous features are age-dependent and may not become apparent until later in childhood. The classic triad of facial "adenomata sebaceum" **(39-25)**, seizures, and mental retardation is seen in only 30% of patients.

The various clinical features of TSC are designated as either major or minor features. Based on these features, the diagnosis is divided into definite, probable, and possible TSC (see box below). While DNA testing is useful for diagnosis and determining the causative mutation, approximately 30% of patients with definite TSC have negative results for *TSC1* and *TSC2* mutations.

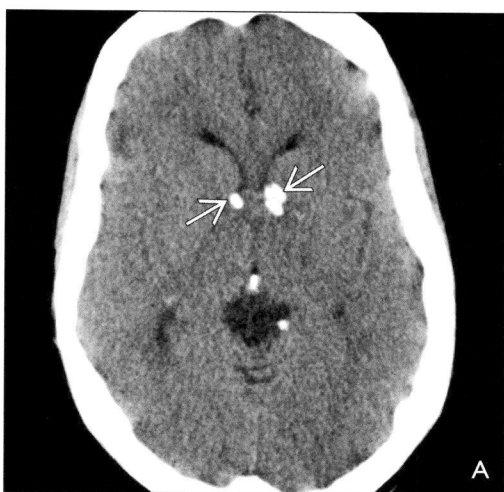

39-29A. NECT in a 22-year-old woman with TSC demonstrates typical calcifications ➡ seen in subependymal nodules.

TSC: DIAGNOSTIC CLINICAL FEATURES

Diagnosis
- Definite TSC
  - 2 major features *or* 1 major + 2 minor
- Probable TSC
  - 1 major + 1 minor feature
- Possible TSC
  - 1 major *or* ≥ 2 minor features

Major Features
- Identified clinically
  - ≥ 3 hypomelanotic ("ash leaf") macules (97%)
  - Facial angiofibromas (75%) or forehead plaque (15-20%)
  - Shagreen patch (45-50%)
  - Ungual/periungual fibroma (15%)
  - Multiple retinal hamartomas (15%)
- Identified on imaging
  - Subependymal nodules (98%)
  - Cortical tubers (95%)
  - Cardiac rhabdomyoma (50%)
  - Renal angiomyolipoma (50%)
  - Subependymal giant cell astrocytoma (15%)
  - Lymphangioleiomyomatosis (1-3%)

Minor Features
- Identified clinically
  - Gingival fibromas (70%)
  - Affected first-degree relative (50%)
  - Pitting of dental enamel (30%)
  - Retinal achromic patch (35%)
  - Confetti-like skin macules (2-3%)
- Identified on imaging
  - WM hamartomas, radial migration lines (100%)
  - Hamartomatous rectal polyps (70-80%)
  - Nonrenal hamartomas (40-50%)
  - Bone cysts (40%)
  - Renal cysts (10-20%)

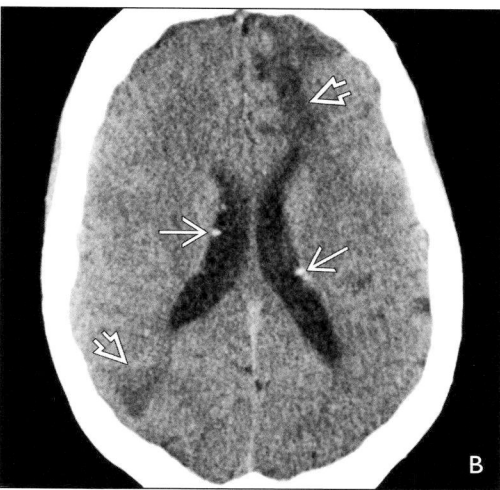

39-29B. NECT scan shows additional calcified SENs ➡, wedge-shaped hypodensities ⇉ characteristic of the WM lesions in TSC.

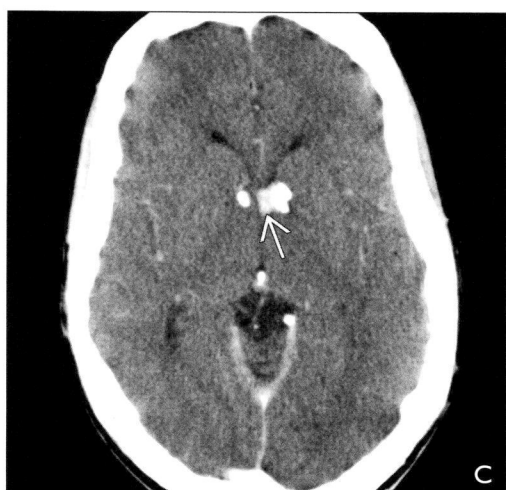

39-29C. CECT scan shows enhancement ➡ adjacent to the foramen of Monro, suspicious for subependymal giant cell astrocytoma.

NATURAL HISTORY. TSC is characterized by wide phenotypic variation in disease severity and natural course. Neurologic manifestations—primarily intractable seizures from brain hamartomas and obstructive hydrocephalus secondary to SEGA—are the leading cause of morbidity and mortality.

TREATMENT OPTIONS. Until recently, few treatment options other than surgery for SEGA existed. Rapamycin inhibitors such as everolimus and sirolimus are currently in clinical trials in patients with TSC. When growing cells are treated with rapamycin, both mTORC1 and mTORC2 are depleted. Downregulation of general protein synthesis, upregulation of macroautophagy, and activation of stress-responsive anabolic proteins occurs.

Imaging

GENERAL FEATURES. Imaging studies in TSC are abnormal in over 98% of all patients.

CT FINDINGS.

Cortical tubers. Neonatal and infantile cortical tubers are initially seen as hypodense cortical/subcortical masses within broadened and expanded gyri **(39-29B)**. The lucency decreases with age; tubers in older children and adults are mostly isodense with cortex.

Calcifications in cortical tubers progressively increase with age. By 10 years, 50% of affected children demonstrate one or more globular or gyriform cortical calcifica-

tions. Between 15-25% of all TSC patients demonstrate focal cerebellar calcifications.

Subependymal nodules. Subependymal nodules (SENs) are a near-universal finding in TSC. Most are found along the caudothalamic groove. The walls of the atria and temporal horns of the lateral ventricles are less common sites.

SENs are rarely calcified in the first year of life. Calcification in SENs increases with age. Eventually, 50% demonstrate some degree of globular calcification **(39-29A)**. SENs typically do not enhance on CECT scans. An enhancing or enlarging SEN—especially if located near the foramen of Monro—is suspicious for SEGA **(39-29C)**.

White matter lesions. Most WM lesions are relatively small and difficult to detect on CT scans.

Subependymal giant cell astrocytoma. SEGAs show mixed density on NECT scans and frequently demonstrate focal calcification. Frank hemorrhage is rare. Moderate enhancement on CECT is typical.

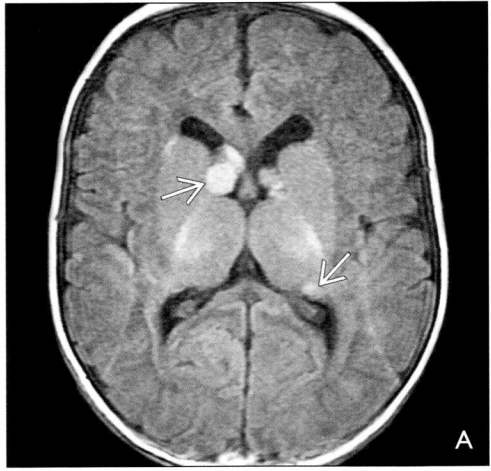

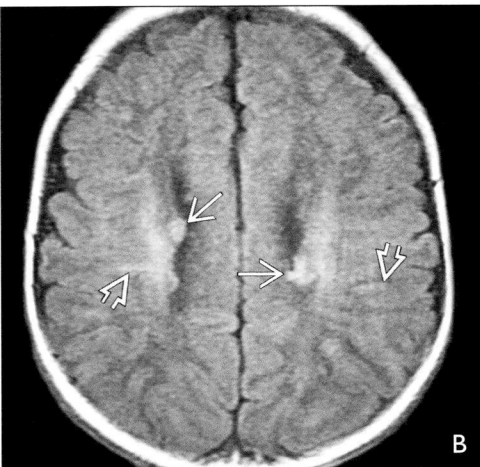

39-30A. Axial T1WI in an 8-week-old male with TSC shows multiple hyperintense noncalcified subependymal nodules ➡. 39-30B. More cephalad scan shows additional hyperintense subependymal nodules ➡ as well as multiple hyperintense radial bands ⇨ extending outward from the lateral ventricles.

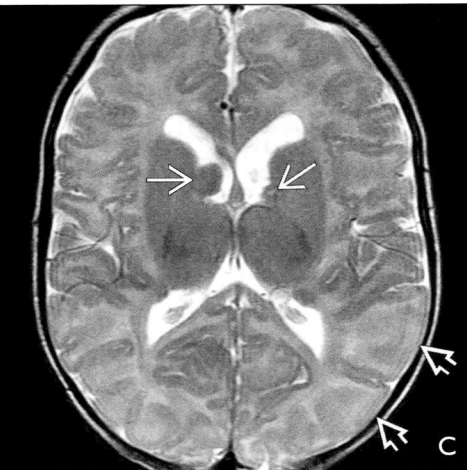

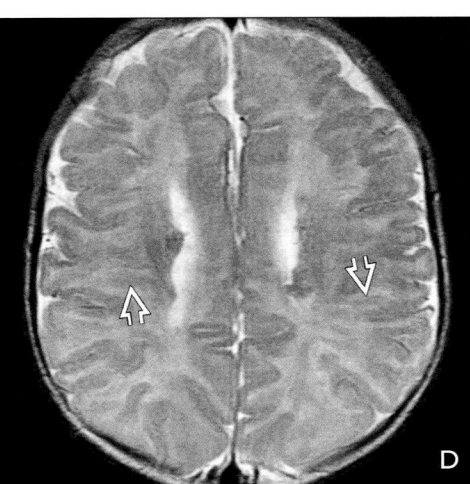

39-30C. T2WI shows that the WM is largely unmyelinated. The SENs ➡ are isointense with gray matter. Cortical tubers ⇨ have poor GM-WM delineation. 39-30D. More cephalad T2WI shows that the thickened radial bands ⇨ are hypointense relative to the unmyelinated white matter.

MR FINDINGS. In general, MR is much more sensitive than CT in depicting parenchymal abnormalities in TSC. Findings vary with lesion histopathology, patient age, and imaging sequence.

Cortical tubers. In infants, tubers appear as thickened hyperintense cortex compared to the underlying unmyelinated WM on T1WI and become moderately hypointense on T2WI. "Streaky" linear or wedge-shaped T2/FLAIR hyperintense bands may extend from the tuber all the way through the WM to the ventricular ependyma **(39-30A)**, **(39-30B)**, **(39-30C)**, **(39-30D)**.

Signal intensity changes after myelin maturation. Tubers gradually become more isointense relative to cortex on T1WI (unless calcification is present and causes T1 shortening) **(39-30E)**, **(39-30F)**, **(39-30G)**, **(39-30H)**. Occasionally the outer margin of a tuber is mildly hyperintense to GM, while the subcortical component appears hypointense relative to WM.

Tubers in older children and adults demonstrate mixed signal intensity on T2/FLAIR. The periphery of the expanded gyrus is isointense with cortex while the deeper component is strikingly hyperintense. Between 3-5% of cortical tubers show mild enhancement on T1 C+ imaging.

Subependymal nodules. SENs are seen as small (generally < 1.3 cm) nodular "bumps" that protrude from the walls of the lateral ventricles. In the unmyelinated brain, SENs appear hyperintense on T1WI and hypointense on T2WI. With progressive myelination, the SENs gradually become isointense with WM. Calcified SENs appear variably hypointense on T2WI and are especially easy to detect on T2* sequences (GRE, SWI).

Enhancement of SENs following contrast administration is variable. About half of all SENs show moderate or even striking enhancement, which—in contrast to enhancement on CECT—does not indicate malignancy per se. As SENs near the foramen of Monro may become malignant, close interval follow-up is essential. It is the interval change in size seen on serial examinations—not the degree of enhancement—that is significant.

White matter lesions. WM lesions are seen in 100% of cases. Even though they are considered a "minor"

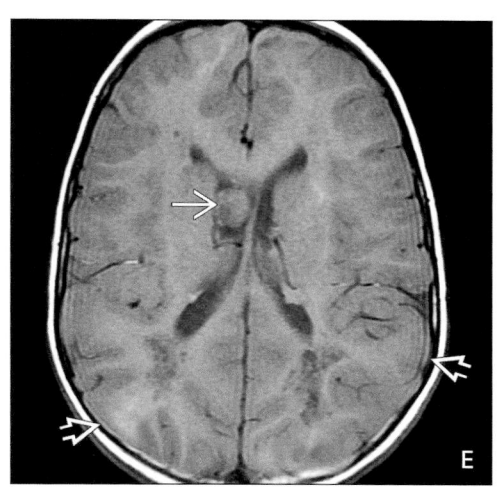
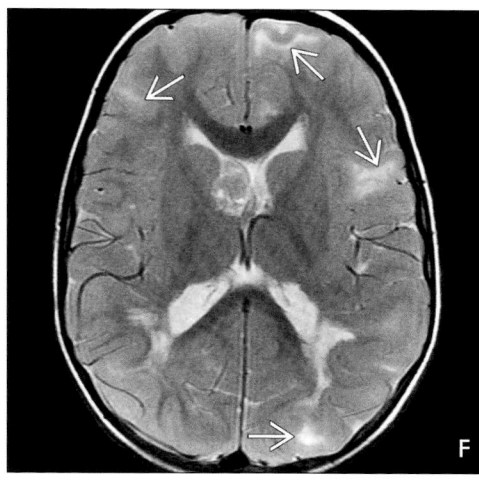
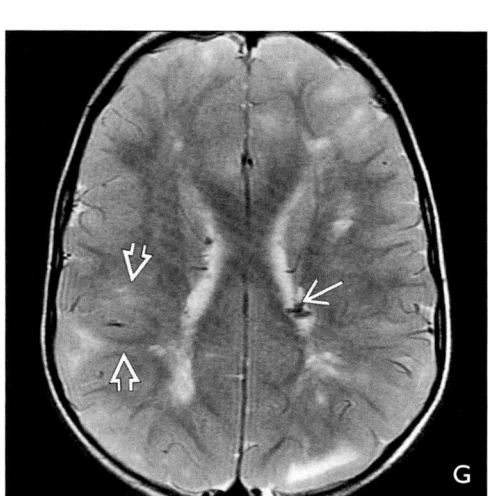
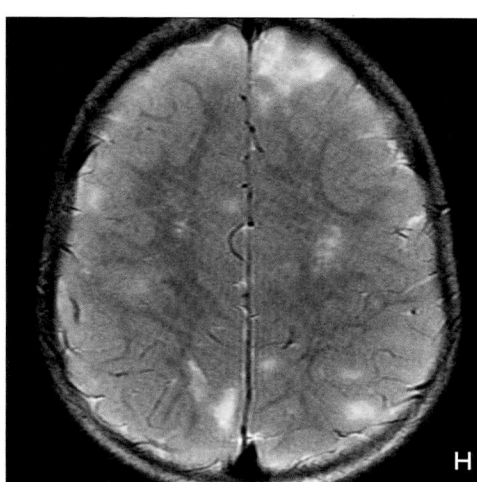

39-30E. Follow-up MR in the same patient as shown on the opposite page was obtained at 3 years of age and shows interval development of a subependymal giant cell astrocytoma ➡ in the right frontal horn. Expanded gyri characteristic of cortical tubers ⧉ are now well seen. 39-30F. T2WI shows the characteristic linear and flame-shaped WM hyperintensities ➡ under the cortical tubers.

39-30G. More cephalad scan demonstrates multiple radial hyperintensities ⧉ extending outward from the ventricles through the corona radiata. The SENs ➡ are now calcified and appear hypointense relative to brain. 39-30H. Scan through the upper corona radiata demonstrates multiple cortical tubers with isointense peripheries, deep hyperintensities in the subcortical WM.

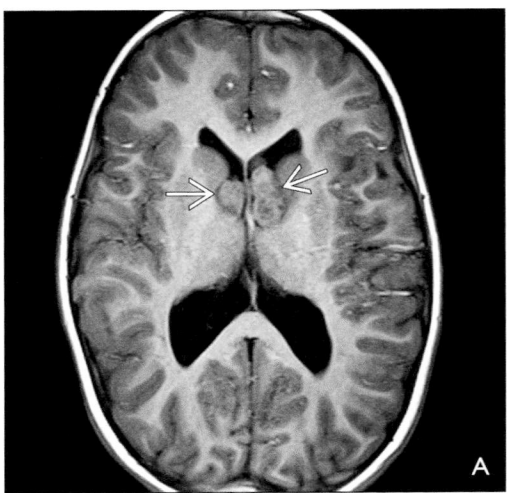

39-31A. Axial T1WI in TSC shows classic appearance and location of subependymal giant cell astrocytomas ➡ near the foramen of Monro.

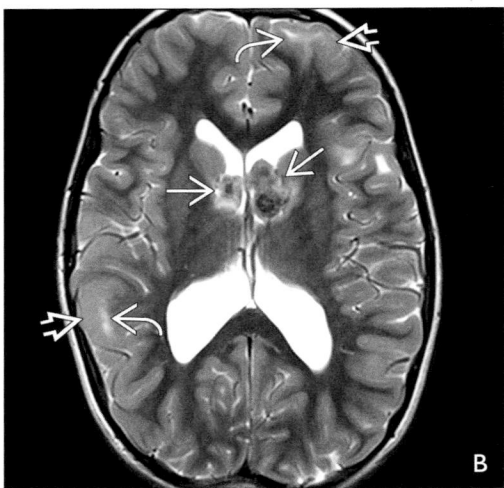

39-31B. T2WI shows that the SEGAs ➡ are mixed iso- and hypointense. Note typical cortical tubers ➡, characteristic WM lesions ➡.

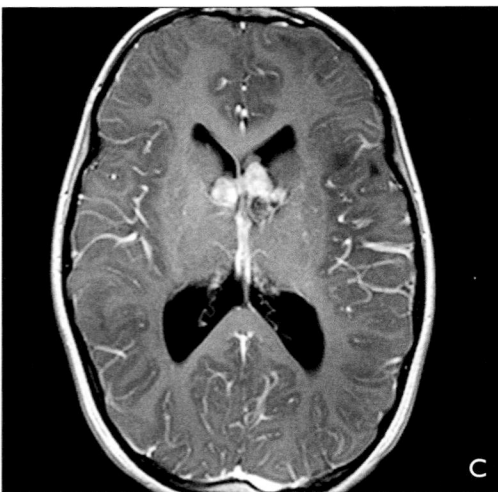

39-31C. T1 C+ scan shows the SEGAs enhancing intensely.

criterion for TSC, their appearance is highly characteristic of the disease. Streaky linear or wedge-shaped lesions extend along radial bands from the ventricles to the undersurfaces of cortical tubers. In the unmyelinated brain, these linear foci appear mildly hyperintense to WM on T1WI. In older children and adults, they are hyperintense on T2/FLAIR.

Subependymal giant cell astrocytoma. While SEGAs can occur anywhere along the ventricular ependyma, the vast majority are found near the foramen of Monro. SEGAs are mixed signal intensity on both T1- and T2WI. Virtually all enhance moderately strongly on T1 C+ scans **(39-31)**.

SEGAs become symptomatic when they obstruct the foramen of Monro and cause hydrocephalus. Even large SEGAs rarely invade brain.

TSC: IMAGING

Cortical Tubers
- Broad, expanded gyrus
- CT: Initially hypodense; Ca++ ↑ with age
  - 50% of patients eventually develop ≥ 1 calcified tuber(s)
- MR: Periphery isointense, subcortical portion T2/FLAIR hyperintense

Subependymal Nodules
- CT: Ca++ rare in first year; ↑ with age
  - 50% eventually calcify
  - Don't enhance
- MR: T1 hyper-, T2 hypointense; 50% enhance

White Matter Lesions
- T2/FLAIR hyperintense radial lines/wedges

Subependymal Giant Cell Astrocytoma
- CT: Mixed-density mass at foramen of Monro, moderate enhancement
- MR: Heterogeneous signal, strong enhancement

Differential Diagnosis

The major differential diagnosis of TSC is **Taylor focal cortical dysplasia** (FCD type IIb). FCD is solitary; the imaging and histopathologic features may be indistinguishable from those of a single cortical tuber. Multiple tubers are present in TSC.

von Hippel-Lindau Disease

Terminology

von Hippel-Lindau disease (VHL) is also known as von Hippel-Lindau syndrome and familial cerebello-retinal angiomatosis. VHL is characterized by retinal and CNS hemangioblastomas **(39-32)**, endolymphatic sac tumors (ELSTs) **(39-33)**, abdominal neoplasms (adrenal pheochromocytomas, clear cell renal carcinomas), and pancreatic and renal cysts **(39-34)**.

Etiology

GENERAL CONCEPTS. VHL is an autosomal dominant familial tumor syndrome with marked phenotypic variability and age-dependent penetrance. Approximately 20% of cases are due to new germline mutations.

GENETICS. Mutations in the *VHL* tumor suppressor gene on chromosome 3p25.3 cause inactivation of the VHL protein (pVHL). pVHL combines with other proteins involved in the ubiquitin-dependent proteolysis of hypoxia inducible factor. Dysregulation of this VHL-associated function causes increased expression of erythropoietin, PDGF, VEGF, and TGF. In turn, upregulation of these factors leads to angiogenesis and tumorigenesis.

Two VHL phenotypes are recognized and distinguished by the presence or absence of associated pheochromocytoma; each is caused by different mutations. Type 1 VHL has a *low risk* of pheochromocytoma and is caused by truncating and exon deletion mutations of the *VHL* gene.

Type 2 VHL is caused by missense mutations and has a *high risk* of developing pheochromocytoma. Type 2 VHL is subdivided into type 2A (low risk of renal cell carcinoma [RCC]), 2B (high risk of RCC), and 2C (familial pheochromocytoma without either hemangioblastoma or RCC).

VHL: GENETICS

Type I VHL
- Truncating/exon deletion mutations of *VHL*
- *Low* risk of pheochromocytoma

Type 2 VHL
- Missense *VHL* mutations
- *High* risk of pheochromocytoma
- Subtypes
  - Type 2A (low risk of renal cell carcinoma)
  - Type 2B (high risk of renal cell carcinoma)
  - Type 2C (familial pheochromocytoma, no hemangioblastoma, no renal cell carcinoma)

Pathology

The great majority of VHL patients harbor significant CNS disease. The two most common VHL-related CNS neoplasms are craniospinal **hemangioblastomas** (HGBLs, found in 60-80% of all VHL cases) and **endolymphatic sac tumors** (seen in 10-15% of patients).

HEMANGIOBLASTOMAS. HGBLs are well-circumscribed red or yellowish masses that usually abut a pial surface. The vast majority of intracranial HGBLs are infratentorial; the dorsal half of the cerebellum is the most common site, followed by the medulla.

Approximately 10% are supratentorial; the most common site is the pituitary stalk (30% of all supratentorial HGBLs and 3% of those in patients with VHL). Less common

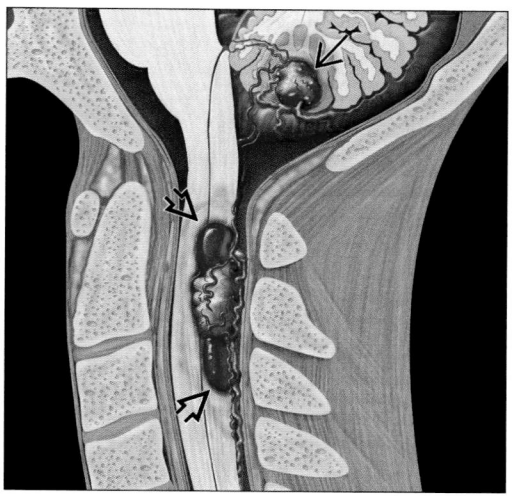

39-32. Two HGBLs in VHL. Spinal cord tumor has associated cyst ▷ that would cause myelopathy. Small cerebellar HGBL ⇨ would be asymptomatic.

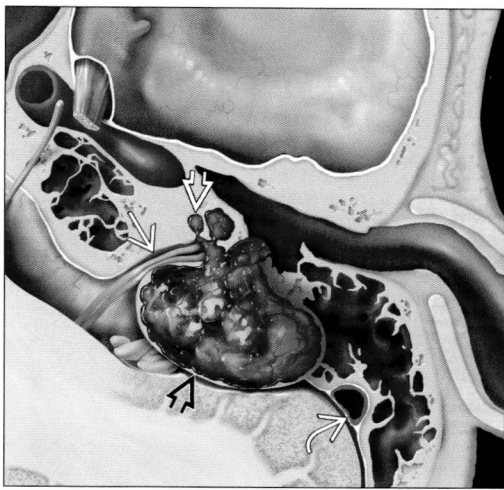

39-33. ELST ▷ is a lytic, vascular, hemorrhagic mass between IAC ➡, sigmoid sinus ➡. Note tendency to fistulize inner ear ➡.

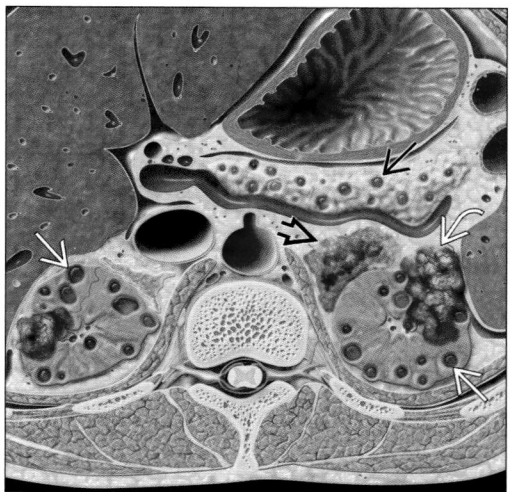

39-34. Abdominal VHL lesions include bilateral renal cysts ➡, carcinomas ➡, pancreatic cysts ➡, adrenal pheochromocytoma ▷.

locations are along the optic pathways and in the cerebral hemispheres.

Nearly half of all VHL-associated HGBLs occur in the spinal cord. Intraspinal HGBLs are often multiple and are frequently associated with a syrinx.

Between one-quarter and one-third of HGBLs are solid; two-thirds are at least partially cystic and contain amber-colored fluid. One or more cysts together with a variably sized mural tumor nodule is the typical appearance. HGBLs are highly vascular with large arteries and prominent draining veins.

Two microscopic features dominate HGBLs and are identical in both sporadic and VHL-associated cases: A rich capillary network and large, vacuolated, variably lipid-laden stromal cells with clear cytoplasm. The cyst wall is nonneoplastic compressed brain with prominent piloid gliosis and Rosenthal fibers.

HGBLs often demonstrate nuclear pleomorphism and hyperchromasia with scattered large, dark nuclei. Mitoses are absent or few, and MIB-1 is generally low. HGBLs are designated as WHO grade I neoplasms.

RETINAL HEMANGIOBLASTOMAS ("ANGIOMAS"). Retinal capillary angiomas are the typical ocular lesions of VHL and are seen in half of all cases. Retinal angiomas are small but often multifocal and frequently bilateral. They are identical in histopathology to CNS HGBLs; the differing terminology reflects ophthalmological tradition, not histopathological diagnosis.

ENDOLYMPHATIC SAC TUMORS. ELSTs are slow-growing, benign but locally aggressive papillary cystadenomatous tumors of the endolymphatic sac. Sporadic ELSTs are more common than VHL-associated tumors. Approximately 10-15% of VHL patients develop an ELST; of these, 30% are bilateral.

Grossly, ELSTs appear as vascular "heaped up" tumors along the posterior aspect of the petrous temporal bone. Microscopically, ELSTs demonstrate interdigitating papillary processes embedded in sheets of dense fibrous tissue. Cystic foci and evidence of old and recent hemorrhage are common.

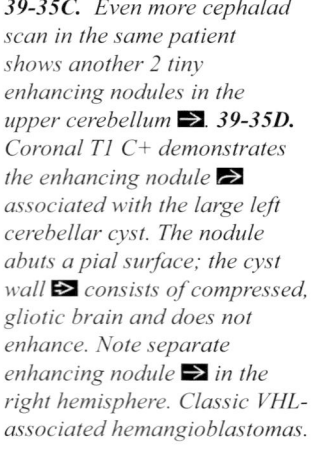

39-35A. Axial T1 C+ FS scan in an asymptomatic 26-year-old man with pancreatic cysts and a strong family history of VHL shows a large cystic mass in the left cerebellar hemisphere ➡ and a smaller cyst ➡ with enhancing nodule ➡ in the right hemisphere. 39-35B. More cephalad scan in the same case shows 2 tiny enhancing nodules ➡.

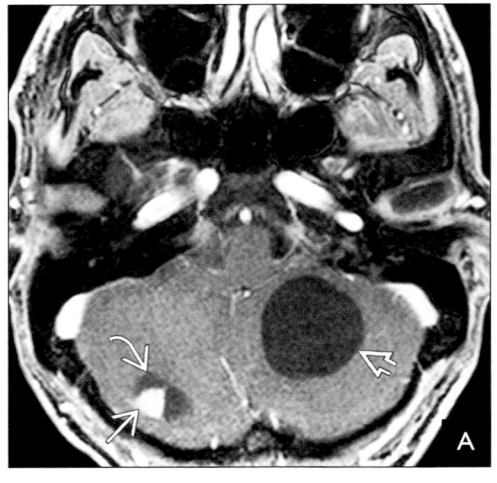

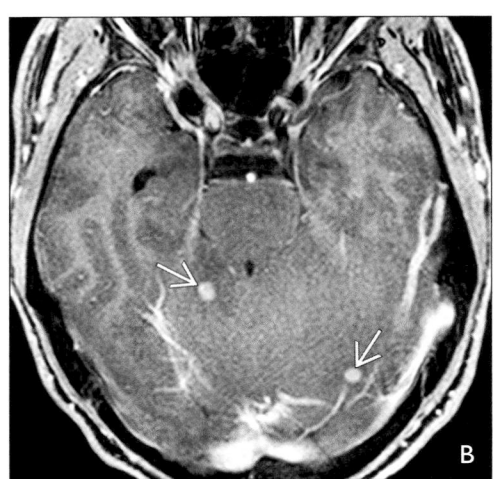

39-35C. Even more cephalad scan in the same patient shows another 2 tiny enhancing nodules in the upper cerebellum ➡. 39-35D. Coronal T1 C+ demonstrates the enhancing nodule ➡ associated with the large left cerebellar cyst. The nodule abuts a pial surface; the cyst wall ➡ consists of compressed, gliotic brain and does not enhance. Note separate enhancing nodule ➡ in the right hemisphere. Classic VHL-associated hemangioblastomas.

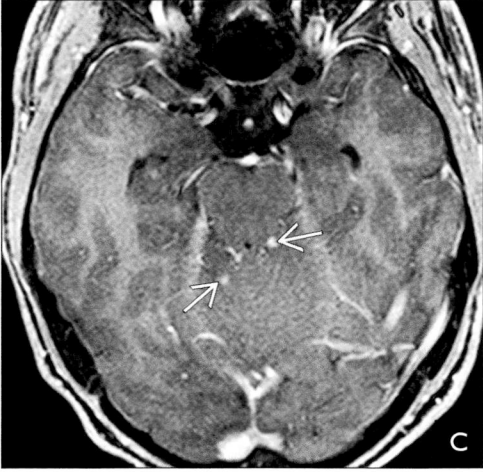

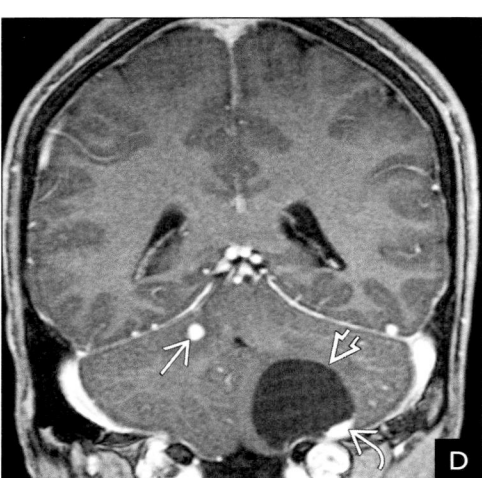

VHL: PATHOLOGY

CNS Neoplasms
- Hemangioblastomas (60-80%)
  - Retinal HGBLs ("angiomas") (50%)
- Endolymphatic sac tumors (10-15%)

Visceral Lesions
- Renal lesions (2/3 of all VHL patients)
  - Cysts (50-75%)
  - Clear cell renal carcinomas (25-45%)
- Adrenal pheochromocytoma (10-20%)
  - Hallmark of type 2 VHL
- Pancreatic cysts (35-70%), nonsecretory islet cell tumors (5-10%)
- Epididymal cysts, cystadenomas (60% of males, often bilateral)
- Broad ligament cystadenomas (females, rare)

Clinical Issues

EPIDEMIOLOGY AND DEMOGRAPHICS. VHL is uncommon; estimated incidence is 1:35,000-50,000 live births.

PRESENTATION AND CLINICAL DIAGNOSIS. Because all VHL-associated lesions can occur as sporadic (i.e., non-familial) events, a clinical diagnosis of VHL disease in a patient without a positive family history requires the presence of at least two tumors (see box below).

Age at diagnosis varies. Although VHL can present in children and even infants, most patients become symptomatic as young adults. Painless visual loss from retinal angioma-induced hemorrhage is often the first symptom (mean: 25 years).

Hemangioblastomas, pheochromocytomas, and endolymphatic tumors typically present in the 30s, while RCCs tend to present somewhat later. Mean age at diagnosis of symptomatic RCCs is 40 years, but asymptomatic tumors are frequently detected earlier on screening abdominal CT.

VHL: DIAGNOSTIC CLINICAL FEATURES

No Family History of VHL
- ≥ 2 CNS hemangioblastomas *or*
- 1 CNS HGBL + visceral tumor

Positive Family History of VHL
- 1 CNS HGBL *or*
- Pheochromocytoma *or*
- Clear cell renal carcinoma

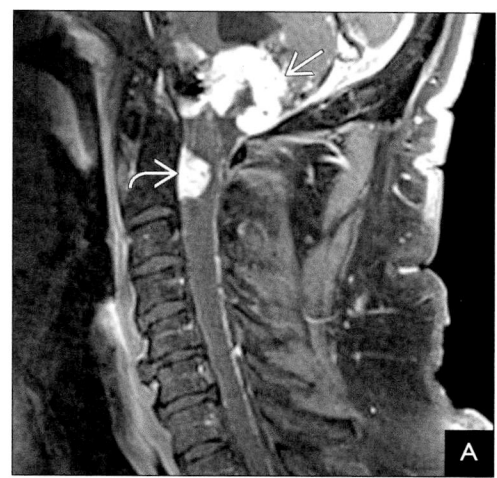

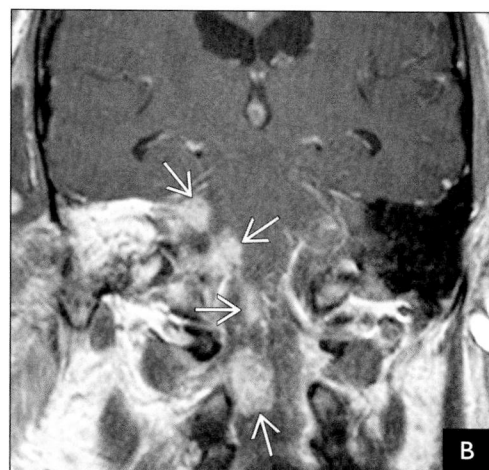

39-36A. *Sagittal T1 C+ scan in a 38-year-old man with VHL shows multiple HGBLs in the cerebellum* ➡ *and cervical spinal cord* ↗. **39-36B.** *Coronal T1 C+ scan shows at least 4 separate HGBLs* ➡.

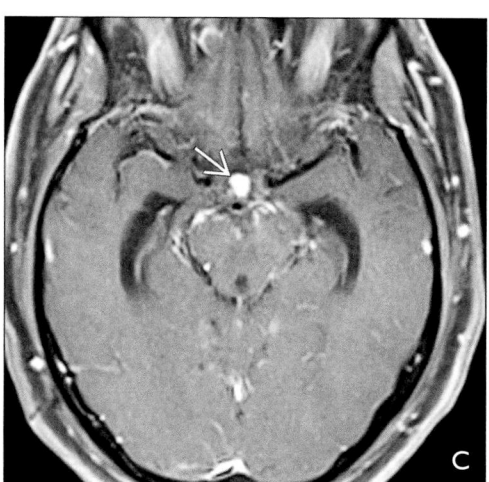

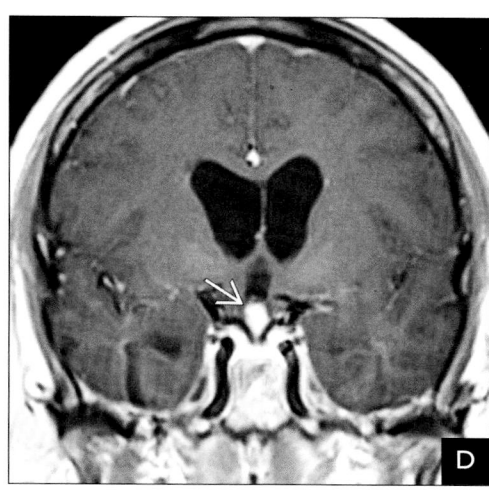

39-36C. *Axial T1 C+ FS scan in the same patient demonstrates an enlarged enhancing pituitary stalk* ➡. **39-36D.** *Coronal T1 C+ scan shows that the pituitary stalk is enlarged and enhances intensely* ➡. *The patient's endocrine status was normal. The pituitary infundibulum is the most common site for supratentorial HGBLs in VHL.*

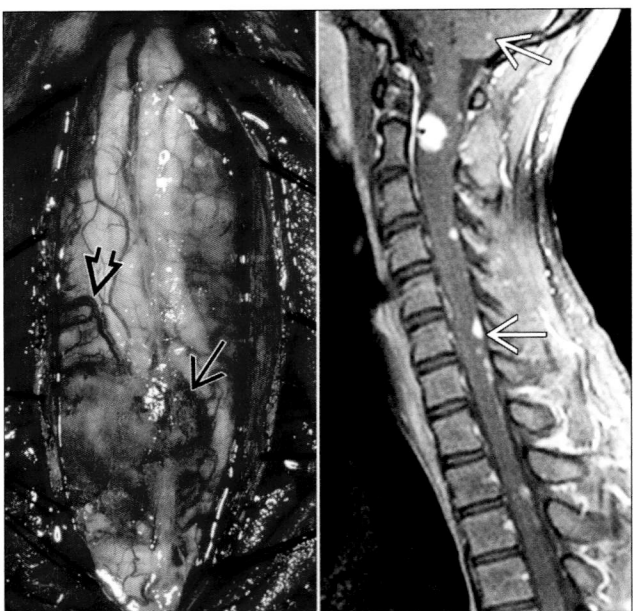

39-37. *(Left) Intraoperative photograph shows typical dorsal subpial location of HGBL nodule ⇥, prominent vessels ⇥. (Right) Sagittal T1 C+ shows multiple HGBLs ⇥.*

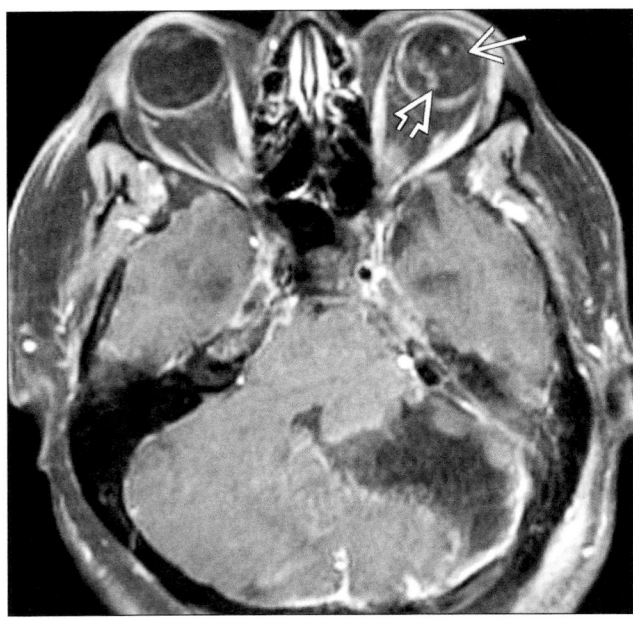

39-38. *Postoperative T1 C+ scan in a 43-year-old man blind in the left eye shows enhancing angioma ⇥, retinal detachment ⇥.*

NATURAL HISTORY. VHL-associated hemangioblastomas demonstrate a "saltatory" growth pattern characterized by quiescent periods (averaging slightly over two years) interspersed with periods of growth. Nearly half of all patients develop de novo lesions after the initial diagnosis of VHL.

The two major causes of death in VHL patients are RCC (50%) and CNS neoplasms. Overall median life expectancy is 49 years.

SURVEILLANCE RECOMMENDATIONS. Patients with a family history of VHL should undergo annual screening (ophthalmoscopy, physical/neurological examination) beginning in infancy or early childhood. Brain MR scans are recommended every one to three years starting in adolescence. Abdominal MR or ultrasound screening for RCC and pancreatic tumors is recommended annually, beginning at age 16.

Methods for pheochromocytoma screening vary. Blood pressure should be monitored and 24-hour urine catecholamines obtained annually. More intense surveillance beginning at age eight years should be considered in families at high-risk for pheochromocytoma (i.e., type 2 VHL).

TREATMENT OPTIONS. Laser treatment for angioma-induced retinal hemorrhages is common. Surgical resection of HGBLs is generally based on symptoms, not evidence of radiologic progression.

Imaging

GENERAL FEATURES. The best imaging clue for VHL is the presence of two or more CNS HGBLs **(39-35)** or one HGBL plus a visceral lesion or the presence of retinal hemorrhage (highly suggestive of intraocular HGBL).

HEMANGIOBLASTOMAS. Approximately two-thirds of HGBLs are cystic; one-third are solid or mixed solid/cystic lesions. NECT scans typically demonstrate a hypodense cyst with isodense mural nodule that abuts the pial surface of the cerebellum. The tumor nodule enhances intensely on CECT.

MR shows that the cyst is slightly to moderately hyperintense to CSF on T1WI and iso- to hyperintense on T2/FLAIR. Signal intensity of the nodule is variable; large lesions may show prominent "flow voids." Hemorrhage is common, and peritumoral edema varies.

Tumor nodules enhance strongly on T1 C+ **(39-36)**. Enhanced scans often demonstrate several tiny nodules in the cerebellum and/or spinal cord **(39-37)**. Less commonly, HGBLs are identified in the pituitary stalk (the most common supratentorial site) **(39-36C)**, **(39-36D)**, optic tracts, or cerebral hemispheres. An uncommon manifestation of recurrent VHL-associated HGBL, disseminated leptomeningeal hemangioblastomatosis, is seen as multiple tumor nodules with diffuse pial enhancement of the spinal cord and/or brain.

DSA demonstrates one or more intensely vascular masses with prolonged tumor "blush" and variable arteriovenous shunting.

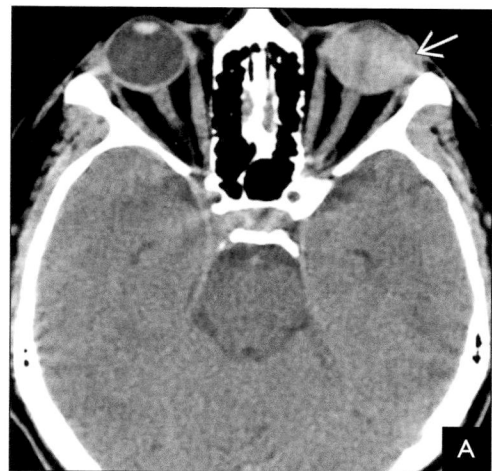

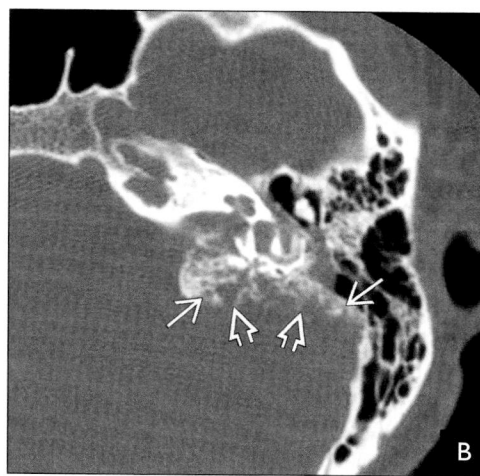

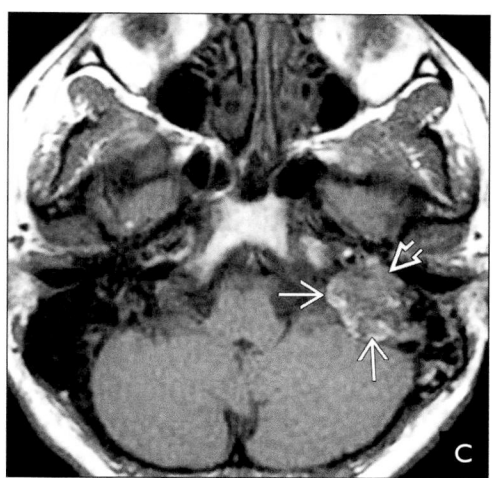

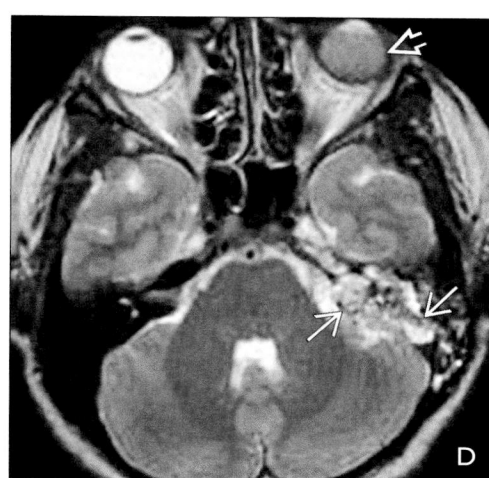

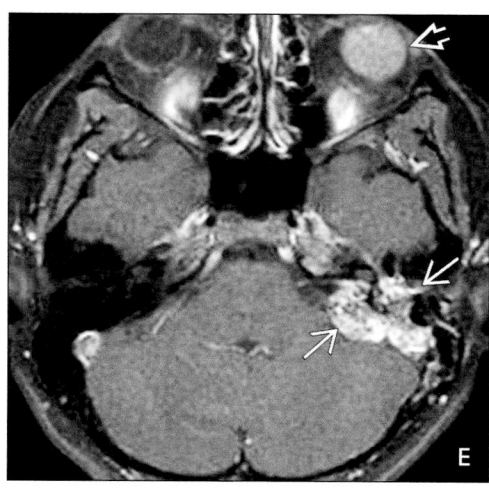

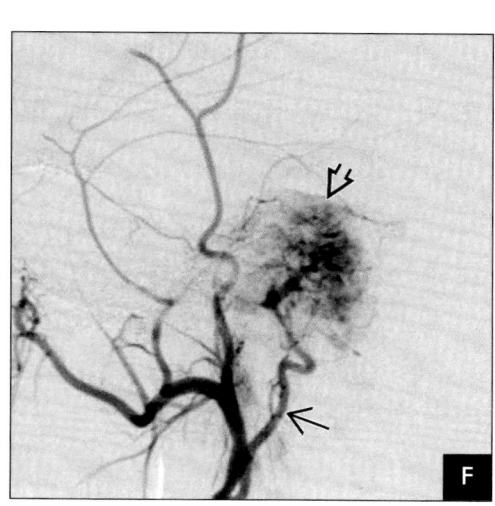

39-39A. Axial NECT in a 51-year-old woman with known VHL and sensorineural hearing loss shows a classic feature of VHL, i.e., a hyperdense V-shaped hemorrhagic retinal detachment ➡ caused by an underlying "angioma" (retinal HGBL). *39-39B.* Temporal bone CT in the same patient shows a lytic infiltrative lesion ➡ along the left posterior petrous temporal bone. Note preserved "spicules" of bone ➡ within the lesion. Location between the IAC, sigmoid sinus is characteristic for ELST.

39-39C. Axial T1WI in the same patient shows that the lesion is mixed iso- ➡ and hyperintense ➡ relative to brain. *39-39D.* The lesion ➡ is heterogeneously hyperintense on T2WI. Note that the left vitreous body ➡ is hypointense compared to the normal right side.

39-39E. Axial T1 C+ FS scan in the same patient shows that the lesion ➡ enhances intensely but heterogeneously. Note hyperintense retinal hemorrhage ➡. *39-39F.* Lateral selective external carotid angiogram shows that the enlarged posterior auricular artery ➡ supplies the highly vascular tumor ➡. Classic endolymphatic sac tumor in VHL. (Courtesy D. Shatzkes, MD.)

RETINAL HEMANGIOBLASTOMAS ("ANGIOMAS"). Retinal angiomas (actually small capillary HGBLs) are usually visualized as hemorrhagic retinal detachments that are hyperdense compared to normal vitreous on NECT. Tiny enhancing nodules can sometimes be identified on T1 C+ MR **(39-38)**.

ENDOLYMPHATIC SAC TUMORS. ELSTs are located along the posterior petrous temporal bone between the internal auditory canal and the sigmoid sinus. The imaging hallmark of ELST is that of a retrolabyrinthine mass associated with osseous erosion. Bone CT shows an infiltrative, poorly circumscribed, lytic lesion with central intratumoral bone spicules **(39-39)**.

MR demonstrates T1 hyperintense foci in 80% of cases. Signal intensity is mixed hyper- and hypointense on T2WI. Heterogeneous enhancement is seen following contrast administration. ELSTs are vascular lesions that may demonstrate prominent "flow voids" on MR and prolonged tumor "blush" on DSA.

VHL: IMAGING

Multiple Hemangioblastomas
- 2/3 cystic, 1/3 solid
- Nodule abuts pia
- 50% in cord (dorsal > ventral surface)

Retinal Angiomas
- Hemorrhagic retinal detachment
- ± enhancing "dots" (tiny HGBLs)

Uni- or Bilateral Endolymphatic Sac Tumors
- Dorsal T-bone between IAC, sigmoid sinus
- Infiltrative, lytic, intratumoral bone spicules
- T1 iso/hyper; T2 hyper; strong enhancement

Differential Diagnosis

The major differential diagnosis of VHL in the brain is **sporadic non-VHL-associated hemangioblastoma**. Between 60-80% of HGBLs are sporadic tumors *not* associated with VHL. Multiple HGBLs and/or supratentorial lesions are highly suggestive of VHL.

A **pilocytic astrocytoma** with cyst and mural tumor nodule can resemble a solitary HGBL. PAs are solitary tumors of children, whereas HGBLs are rarely seen in patients younger than 15 years. In contrast to HGBL, the tumor nodule in pilocytic astrocytoma typically does not abut a pial surface.

Vascular metastases can mimic multiple HGBLs but are rarely isolated to the cerebellum and/or spinal cord.

Rare Neurocutaneous Syndromes

A number of other neurocutaneous syndromes have been identified in recent years.

As with the more common inherited cancer syndromes discussed above, the neoplasms associated with these disorders do not differ much—if at all—from their sporadic counterparts. They are histopathologically identical and often feature the same genetic mutations. What sets them apart is the *constellation* of clinical features—often skin lesions—combined with systemic and CNS neoplasms.

We close the chapter with a brief consideration of these interesting syndromes.

Li-Fraumeni Syndrome

Terminology

Li-Fraumeni syndrome (LFS) is also known as the sarcoma family syndrome of Li and Fraumeni. LFS is an autosomal dominant familial tumor syndrome characterized by a spectrum of malignant neoplasms.

Etiology

Nearly three-quarters of all patients have loss-of-function *TP53* germline mutations. To date, the etiology of the other 25% of LFS cases remains unknown.

Pathology

CNS TUMORS. Nearly half of all CNS neoplasms in LFS are astrocytomas, primarily the diffusely infiltrating fibrillary type (WHO grades II-IV), and gliosarcoma **(39-42)**, **(39-40)**.

Choroid plexus tumors (15%) **(39-41)** and medulloblastoma/primitive neuroectodermal tumor (PNET) (10-12%) are the next most common types. Ependymoma, oligodendroglioma, and meningioma together account for less than 5% of LFS-associated neoplasms. Histologically, LFS-associated neoplasms are indistinguishable from their sporadic counterparts.

EXTRANEURAL MANIFESTATIONS. Together with brain tumors, breast cancer and sarcomas (osteosarcomas and soft tissue tumors) account for almost 75% of LFS-associated neoplasms. Other reported LFS-associated neoplasms with *TP53* mutations include hematopoietic and lymphoid tumors, lung cancer, skin cancers, stomach cancer, and ovarian cancer.

Clinical Issues

The revised diagnostic clinical criteria for LFS are shown in the accompanying box.

Prognosis is poor; almost half of all patients develop an invasive cancer by age 30 and have a lifelong increased risk of osteosarcoma, soft tissue sarcoma, leukemia, breast cancer, brain tumors, melanoma, and adrenal cortical tumors. Age at tumor onset in LFS patients is significantly younger compared to their sporadic counterparts.

Individuals with LFS have a 50% chance of developing cancer by age 40 and a 90% chance by age 60. As breast cancer is the most common LFS-associated malignancy, females—particularly those with *TP53* and *BRAC1* germline mutations—have an increased risk compared to males. Adrenocortical carcinoma associated with *TP53* germline mutation develops almost exclusively in children.

LI-FRAUMENI SYNDROME: DIAGNOSTIC CLINICAL FEATURES

Proband With
- Sarcoma diagnosed < 45 years of age *and*
- First or second degree relative with
  ○ Any cancer diagnosed < 45 years *or*
  ○ Any sarcoma at any age

Or Proband With
- Multiple tumors (exception = breast)
  ○ 2 of which are known LFS-associated neoplasms *and*
  ○ The first of which occurred < age 45 years *or*
  ○ Adrenocortical carcinoma or choroid plexus tumor

Imaging

Brain imaging in LFS patients with CNS symptoms varies with tumor type. Imaging findings and differential diagnoses in LFS-associated CNS neoplasms are similar to those of their sporadic counterparts.

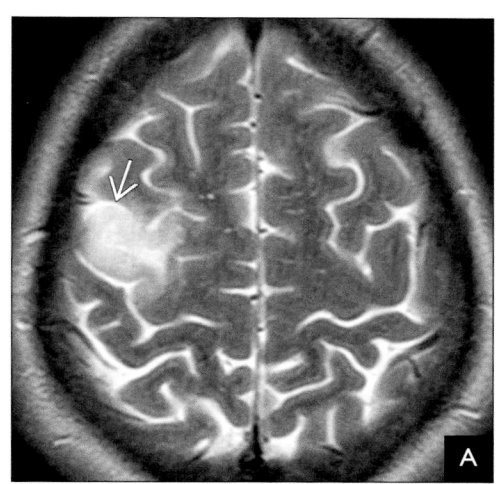
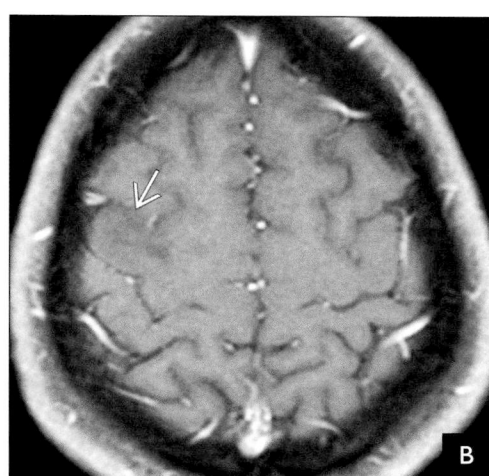

39-40A. *T2WI in a 26-year-old man with seizures and Li-Fraumeni syndrome shows a hyperintense mass ➡ in the right posterior frontal cortex and subcortical white matter.* **39-40B.** *T1 C+ FS scan in the same patient shows that the lesion ➡ does not enhance. Biopsy showed diffusely infiltrating fibrillary astrocytoma, WHO grade II.*

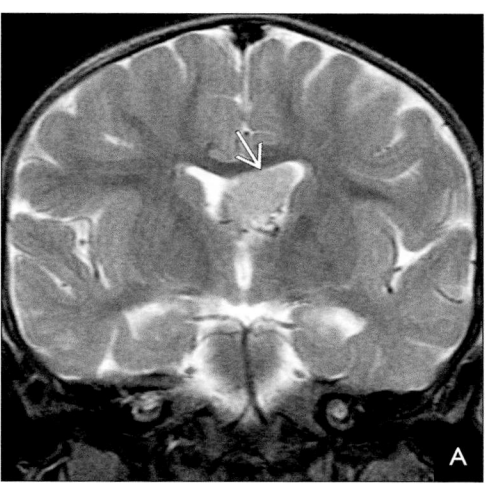
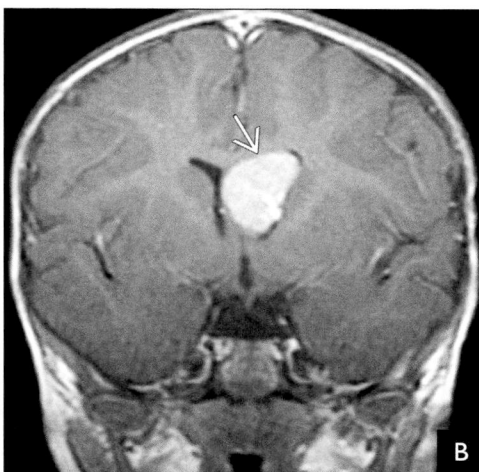

39-41A. *Coronal T2WI in a child with Li-Fraumeni syndrome shows a mass ➡ filling and slightly expanding the body of the left lateral ventricle.* **39-41B.** *Coronal T1 C+ scan in the same patient shows that the mass ➡ enhances intensely and quite uniformly. Final histopathologic diagnosis was choroid plexus carcinoma.*

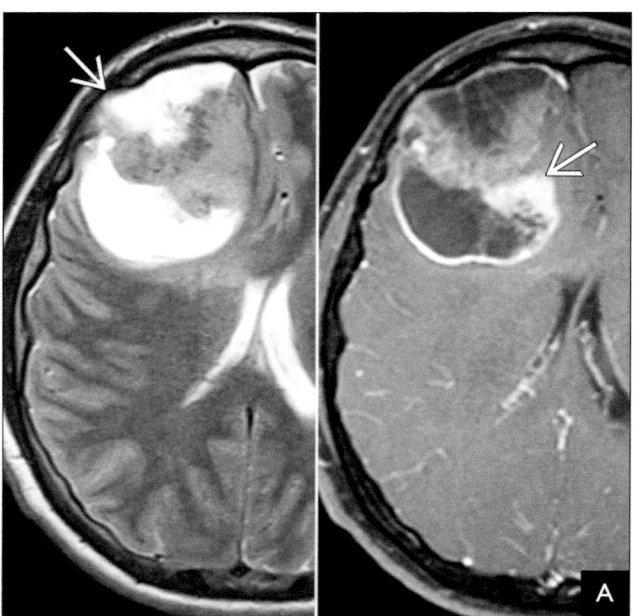

39-42A. (Left) Axial T2WI and (right) T1 C+ scans in a 22-year-old man with Li-Fraumeni shows surgically proven glioblastoma multiforme ➡.

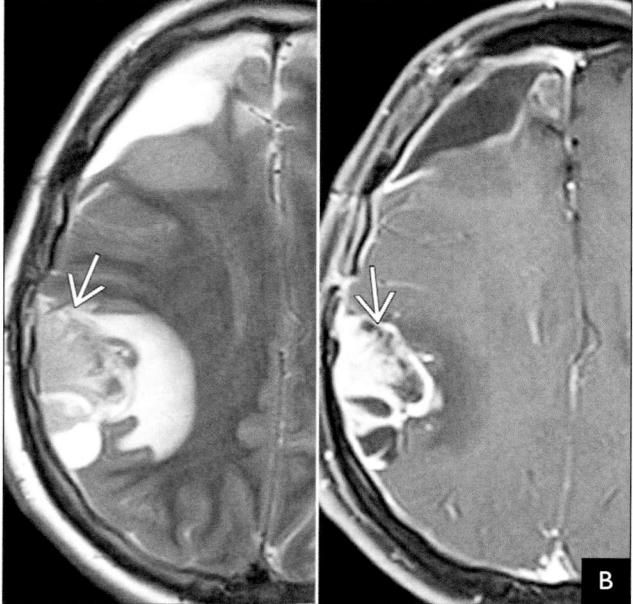

39-42B. Six months following resection, a new dura-based lesion ➡—*a gliosarcoma—has developed.*

Differential Diagnosis

The differential diagnosis of LFS is sporadic neoplasms. Imaging findings are similar, so definitive diagnosis requires clinical correlation.

Cowden Syndrome

Terminology

Cowden syndrome (CS) is also known as **multiple hamartoma-neoplasia syndrome**. It is the most common phenotype of the **PTEN hamartoma tumor syndrome**.

CS involves hamartomatous overgrowth of tissues of all three embryonic origins. The characteristic hamartomas of CS are noncancerous lesions of the skin, mucous membranes, and gastrointestinal tract. The classic brain hamartoma is dysplastic gangliocytoma of the cerebellum, also known as **Lhermitte-Duclos disease** (LDD). If CS and LDD occur together, the disorder is known as **COLD** (**Co**wden-**L**hermitte-**D**uclos syndrome). COLD is considered a new phakomatosis.

Etiology

CS is an autosomal dominant disorder with variable expression and age-related penetrance. Over 80% of patients have identifiable *PTEN* mutations.

Pathology

The most common brain imaging finding is nonspecific macrocephaly, with or without foci of heterotopic GM (39-43), (39-44).

The most characteristic associated lesion is dysplastic cerebellar gangliocytoma (39-45) (see Chapter 19). Grossly, marked enlargement of the cerebellar hemisphere/vermis is present. The folia are enlarged and distorted but not obliterated. Macrocephaly with heterotopic GM foci is common.

Microscopic features include accumulation of abnormal ganglion cells in the inner granule cell layer, loss of Purkinje cells in the middle layer, and thickening with hypermyelination of the outer (molecular) layer.

Clinical Issues

EPIDEMIOLOGY AND DEMOGRAPHICS. CS is uncommon; its estimated incidence is 1:200,000-250,000. Age at onset is variable. Most cases have been identified in adults, but LDD can occur in infants.

PRESENTATION. In addition to multiple tumors and hamartomas, CS patients may have megalencephaly, heterotopic GM, hydrocephalus, mental retardation, and seizures. Other features include gastrointestinal polyps and characteristic mucocutaneous lesions (trichilemmomas, acral keratoses, papillomatous lesions) as well as benign breast, thyroid, and uterine lesions.

CLINICAL DIAGNOSIS. CS is diagnosed clinically by the presence of pathognomonic lesions or a combination of major and minor criteria (see box below). The pathognomonic criteria are those features most likely to be associated with CS whereas the major and minor criteria are not as specific.

COWDEN SYNDROME:
DIAGNOSTIC CLINICAL FEATURES

Pathognomonic Criteria
- Dysplastic cerebellar gangliocytoma (Lhermitte-Duclos disease) *and*
- Characteristic mucocutaneous lesions
  - Papillomatous lesions
  - Facial trichilemmomas
  - Acral keratoses

Major Criteria
- Breast cancer
- Thyroid cancer (especially follicular)
- Endometrial cancer
- Macrocephaly
  - Occipitofrontal circumference > 97th percentile

Minor Criteria
- Other thyroid lesions
- Mental retardation
- GI polyps
- Fibrocystic breast disease
- Lipomas
- Fibromas
- GU tumors (especially renal cell carcinoma)
- Genitourinary structural malformations
- Uterine fibroids

NATURAL HISTORY. CS carries a significantly increased lifetime risk of developing malignancies. For example, women with CS have a 50% lifetime risk of developing breast cancer, 10% risk for follicular thyroid cancer, and 5-10% risk of developing endometrial cancer. The risk is even higher for patients with germline *PTEN* mutations and now extends to renal and colorectal cancers as well as melanoma.

Imaging

Imaging findings of dysplastic cerebellar gangliocytoma in the setting of CS/PTEN hamartoma tumor syndrome are identical to those of LDD. An enlarged cerebellar hemisphere with thickened folia in a gyriform or striated appearance is typical.

Differential Diagnosis

LDD plus CS is diagnostic of COLD. Patients with LDD should be screened for Cowden syndrome and vice versa. A dysplastic cerebellar gangliocytoma without a characteristic mucocutaneous lesion or other criteria (e.g., breast cancer, thyroid lesions) is simply **Lhermitte-Duclos disease.**

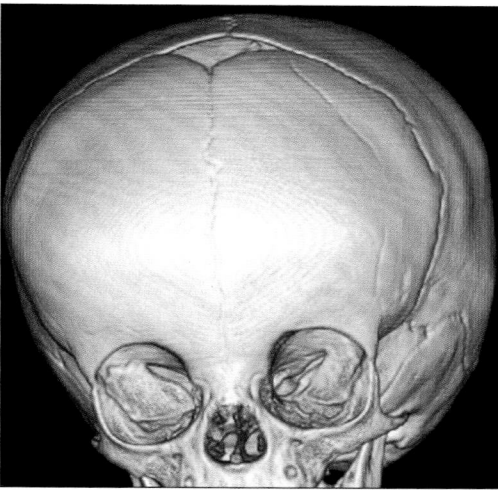

39-43. 3D CT in a 16-month-old boy with skin lesions characteristic of Cowden disease and PTEN mutation shows gross macrocephaly.

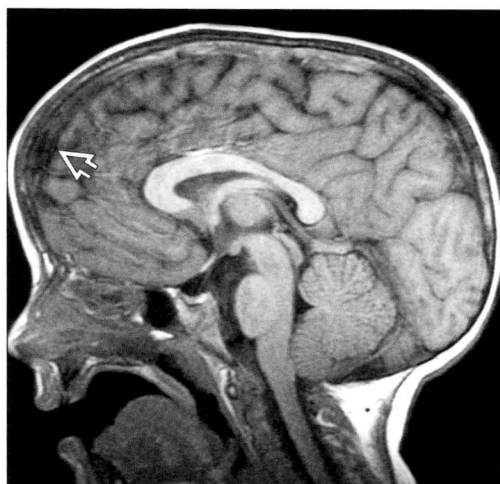

39-44. Sagittal T1WI in a 6-year-old boy with CS and macrocephaly shows increased craniofacial proportion and prominent frontal bossing ➡.

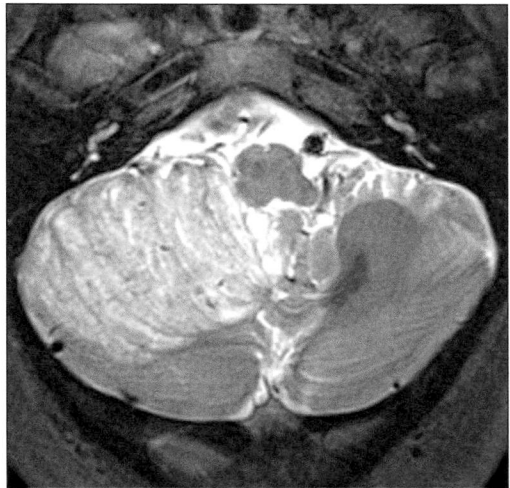

39-45. Axial T2WI shows dysplastic cerebellar gangliocytoma (Lhermitte-Duclos disease) with thickened, striated cerebellar folia.

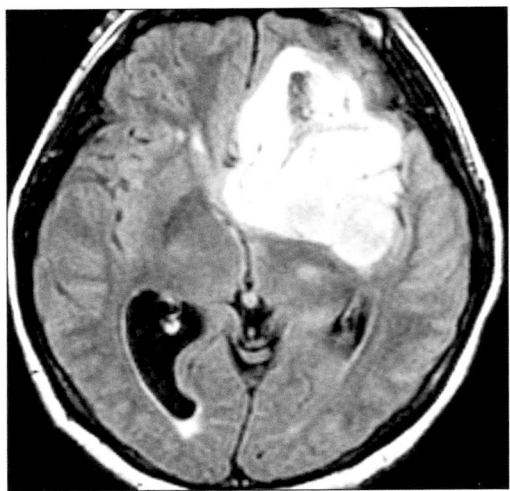

39-46. *FLAIR scan in type 1 Turcot shows heterogeneously hyperintense left frontal mass. Anaplastic astrocytoma. (Courtesy T. Tihan, MD.)*

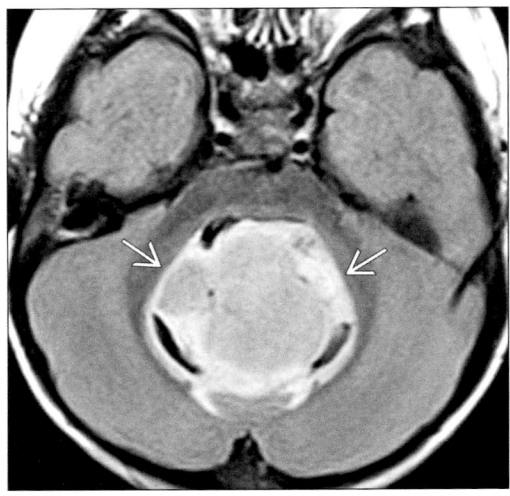

39-47. *FLAIR scan in type 2 Turcot shows typical appearance of medulloblastoma ➡. (Courtesy T. Tihan, MD.)*

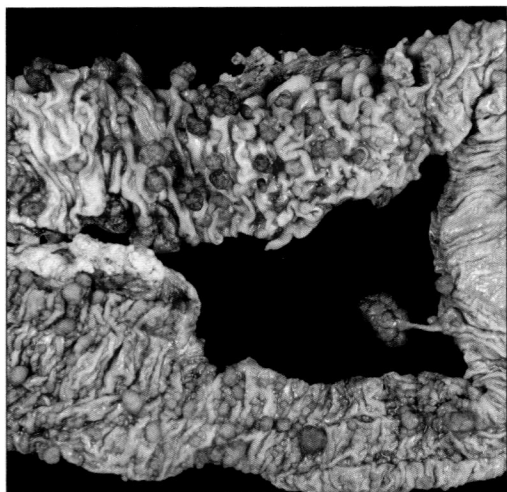

39-48. *Surgical colon specimen from a patient with type 2 Turcot shows innumerable small polyps. (Courtesy T. Tihan, MD.)*

Turcot Syndrome

Terminology

Turcot syndrome (TS) is a rare autosomal dominant disorder characterized by gastrointestinal and CNS neoplasms.

Two types of TS are recognized. In type 1 Turcot (also known as **hereditary nonpolyposis colorectal cancer**), colorectal, endometrial, gastric, pancreaticobiliary, and genitourinary tumors occur together with malignant astrocytomas.

In type 2 Turcot, colorectal tumors (**familial adenomatous polyposis**) and skin lesions (such as epidermoid cysts) occur together with medulloblastoma and craniofacial exostosis (39-46), (39-47), (39-48).

Etiology

TS is associated with biallelic DNA mismatch repair mutations. Type 1 Turcot is caused by germline mutations of mismatch repair genes. In type 2 Turcot, mutations in the *APC* gene are present.

Pathology

Three CNS neoplasms—medulloblastoma, anaplastic astrocytoma, and glioblastoma multiforme—account for 95% of all Turcot-associated brain tumors. The histologic features of these tumors are indistinguishable from those of their sporadic counterparts.

Clinical Issues

Patients with type 1 Turcot-associated anaplastic astrocytoma or glioblastoma multiforme present *earlier* than those with nonsyndromic tumors. Median age at onset is 18 years. Family history of polyposis is absent.

Patients with type 2 Turcot-associated medulloblastoma present *later* than patients in the general PNET population. Median age is 15 years. Patients with type 2 Turcot frequently have a family history of polyposis.

Imaging

Imaging findings in Turcot-related CNS neoplasms are identical to those of their nonsyndromic counterparts.

Basal Cell Nevus Syndrome

Terminology

Basal cell nevus syndrome (BCNS) is also known as **nevoid basal cell carcinoma syndrome** and **Gorlin (or Gorlin-Goltz) syndrome**. Patients with BCNS exhibit a broad spectrum of neurodevelopmental disorders and are predisposed to develop multiorgan benign and malignant neoplasms.

Etiology

BCNS is an autosomal dominant disease with full penetrance but variable clinical phenotypes. BCNS is caused by germline mutations of the *PTCH* gene on chromosome 9q22. Approximately 5% of patients with germline *PTCH* mutations develop medulloblastoma; about 1-2% of medulloblastoma patients have *PTCH* germline mutations.

Pathology

Systemic BCNS-associated lesions include **basal cell carcinomas** and **epidermal cysts**, **multiple keratocystic odontogenic tumors** (KOTs) **(39-49)**, and **skeletal anomalies** (e.g., bifid ribs).

The CNS neoplasm most commonly associated with BCNS is **medulloblastoma**, predominantly the desmoplastic type (often associated with pathological hedgehog pathway activation) or medulloblastoma with extensive nodularity.

Clinical Issues

EPIDEMIOLOGY AND DEMOGRAPHICS. BCNS has a prevalence of 1:57,000 in population-based studies.

PRESENTATION. Patients with BCNS are usually diagnosed by age 5-10 years. Basal cell carcinomas are the most common initial presentation and may appear as early as two years of age. Multiple enlarging jaw masses are frequent and can be asymptomatic or painful.

Medulloblastomas develop in 4-20% of patients with BCNS and generally present within the first two years of life with symptoms of obstructive hydrocephalus.

NATURAL HISTORY. The major morbidity and mortality in BCNS is caused by its associated neoplasms. Basal carcinomas often become more aggressive after puberty and may exhibit distant metastases. KOTs eventually develop in 80% of patients and have a high recurrence rate.

Imaging

Typical brain/head and neck abnormalities seen in BCNS are multiple jaw cysts, macrocephaly, dense lamellar dural calcifications, and medulloblastoma.

KERATOCYSTIC ODONTOGENIC TUMORS. KOTs are seen as multiple expansile, well-corticated cysts in the mandible and maxilla on bone CT. They can be uni- or multilocular and often exhibit scalloped borders **(39-50)**. They typically do not enhance on CECT scans.

KOTs exhibit low to intermediate signal intensity on T1WI and appear heterogeneously hyperintense on T2WI.

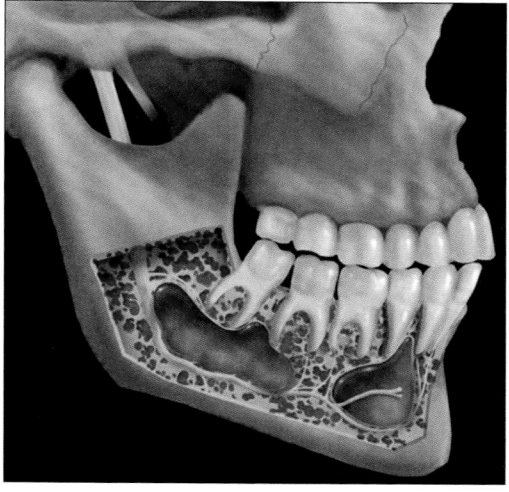

39-49. *Lateral graphic of BCNS shows classic appearance of multiple odontogenic keratocysts. Lesions tend to splay teeth roots, displace nerves.*

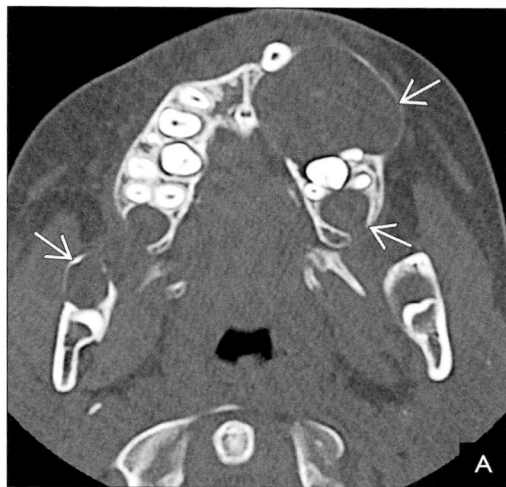

39-50A. *Axial bone CT in a 9 yo boy with BCNS shows multiple biaxial lytic lesions in the maxilla and mandible* ➔. *Typical odontogenic keratocysts.*

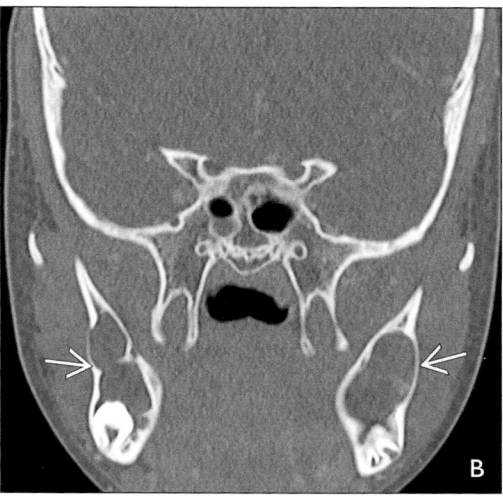

39-50B. *Coronal bone CT in the same patient nicely demonstrates the expansile, lobulated nature of the cysts* ➔.

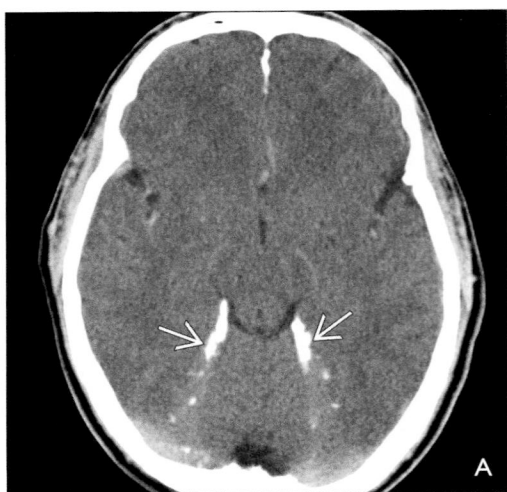

39-51A. *Axial NECT scan in a patient with BCNS demonstrates dense lamellar calcifications ➔ along the tentorium cerebelli.*

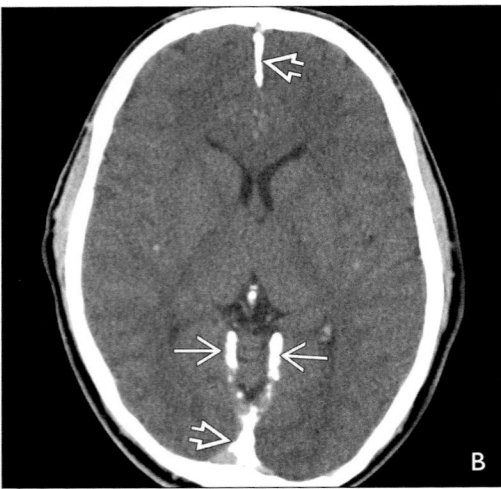

39-51B. *More cephalad NECT in the same patient shows dense calcification at the tentorial apex ➔ and along the falx cerebri ⏩.*

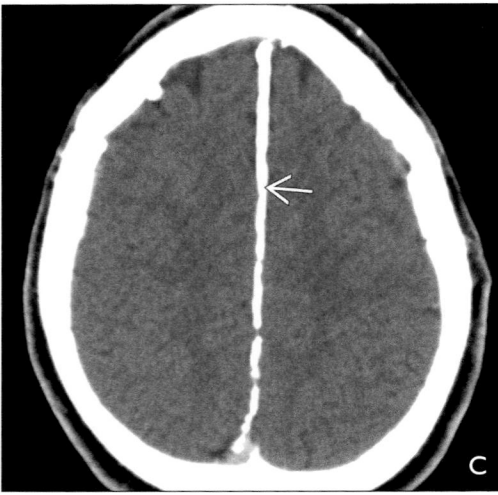

39-51C. *Scan through the corona radiata shows that the falx is thickly and densely calcified ➔.*

DURAL CALCIFICATIONS. Abnormal dural calcification eventually develops in 80% of patients older than 20 years (39-51). Subtle flecks of calcium deposition along the falx can occur in very young children and—together with the unusually early appearance of medulloblastoma—should suggest the diagnosis of BCNS.

Thick, slightly irregular lamellar calcifications along the falx, tentorium, petroclinoid ligaments, and diaphragma sellae are typical findings in teenagers and adults with BCNS.

MEDULLOBLASTOMA. The imaging appearance of BCNS-associated medulloblastoma is identical to that of nonsyndromic tumors.

Differential Diagnosis

The major differential diagnosis of the abnormal calcifications in BCNS is **physiologic** or **metabolic-related dural calcifications** (e.g., as occurs with secondary hyperparathyroidism). Physiologic calcification is much less striking and is rarely seen in young children. Thick dural calcifications can be seen in patients with chronic renal failure and long-term hemodialysis.

The differential diagnosis of KOTs includes **periapical (radicular) cysts**—usually unilocular and associated with dental caries—and **dentigerous (follicular) cysts**. Dentigerous cysts are seen as a single unilocular cyst surrounding the crown of an unerupted tooth.

The differential diagnosis of BCNS-related medulloblastoma is **sporadic (nonsyndromic) posterior fossa PNET**. As imaging findings of the tumors are identical, look for other differentiating features such as atypical dural calcifications and jaw cysts.

Rhabdoid Tumor Predisposition Syndrome

Rhabdoid tumor predisposition syndrome (RTPS) is characterized by markedly increased risk of developing malignant rhabdoid tumors. Most cases are caused by biallelic germline mutations with inactivation of the *hSFN5/INI1* tumor suppressor gene on chromosome 22q11.

The most common CNS tumor in RTPS is **atypical teratoid/rhabdoid tumor** (AT/RT). AT/RT is composed of poorly differentiated neuroectodermal and mesenchymal elements (39-52). The rhabdoid component can be subtle, making the diagnosis difficult.

Approximately 60% of AT/RTs are found in the posterior fossa. Tumors tend to be large bulky masses with mixed cystic and solid components that demonstrate variable

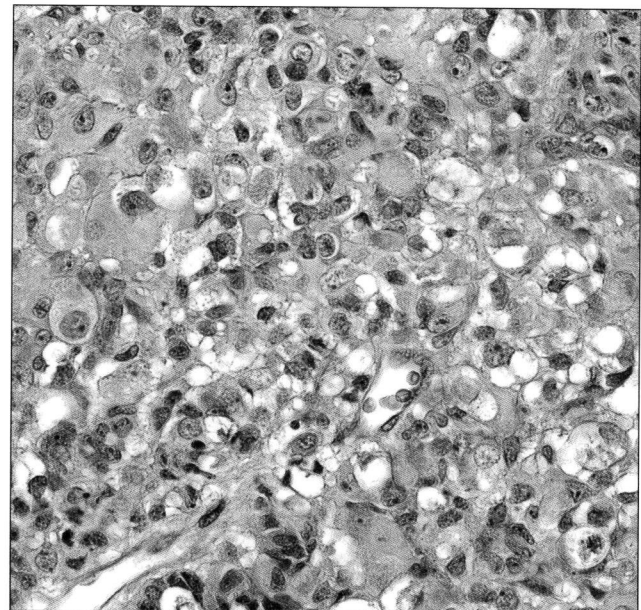

39-52. *As in this microscopic image from an AT/RT biopsy specimen, most AT/RTs are not overtly rhabdoid, if at all. Large pale jumbled cells are more characteristic. (Courtesy P. Burger, MD.)*

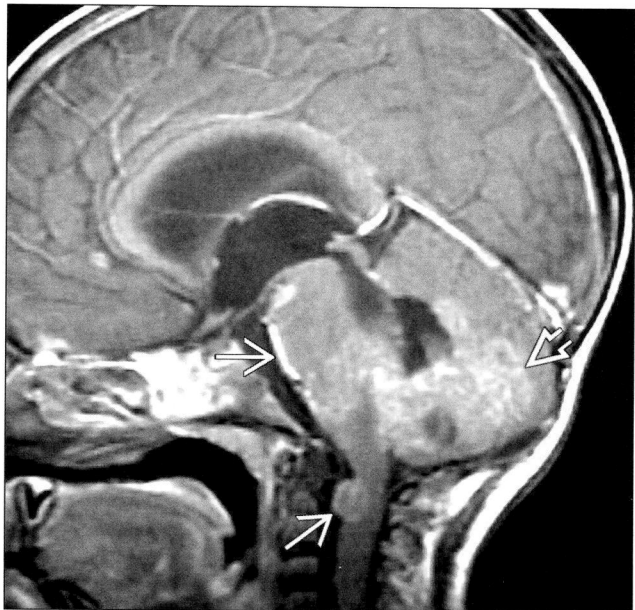

39-53. *Sagittal T1 C+ scan in a patient with AT/RT shows a large, heterogeneously enhancing posterior fossa mass* ⧉ *with disseminated tumor* ⧉.

enhancement following contrast administration. Dissemination at the time of initial diagnosis is common **(39-53)**.

Other familial CNS tumors associated with RTPS include **choroid plexus carcinoma**, which has the same inactivating mutation of *hSFN5/INI1*.

The most common non-CNS neoplasm in RTPS is malignant rhabdoid tumor (MRT) of the kidney. Prognosis is poor; MRTs are highly aggressive cancers that occur in young children and are generally lethal within months or a few years.

Meningioangiomatosis

Terminology

Meningioangiomatosis (MA) is a rare neurocutaneous syndrome characterized by a focal hamartomatous lesion that involves the pia and underlying cerebral cortex.

Etiology and Pathology

While its precise etiology is unknown, MA is a benign, slow-growing lesion of presumed hamartomatous or developmental origin. MA can occur as a solitary or multifocal lesion.

Grossly, MA appears as a reddish gyriform mass that infiltrates the pia and underlying brain **(39-54)**. MA can occur without or with an accompanying neoplasm (most commonly meningioma).

Microscopic features are those of a plaque-like intracortical and leptomeningeal proliferation consisting of small

blood vessels, meningothelial cells, and fibroblasts. The adjacent cortex may show dense gliosis and neurofibrillary tangles. MIB-1 index is low.

Clinical Issues

MA can occur sporadically or as a *forme fruste* of neurofibromatosis type 2 (NF2). Sporadic MA usually occurs as a single lesion in a child or young adult who presents with seizures or persistent headaches.

Imaging

NECT scans typically demonstrate an iso- to slightly hyperdense cortically based lesion with nodular, linear, or gyriform calcification **(39-55)**. The frontal or temporal lobes are the most common sites. Mass effect is minimal or absent. Little or no enhancement is seen on CECT.

MA is iso- to hypointense on T1WI. Although signal intensity on T2WI varies, most MAs are moderately hypointense to adjacent brain with variable amounts of associated edema or gliosis **(39-56)**.

T1 C+ shows mild to moderate serpentine enhancement extending over the surface of adjacent gyri and into adjacent sulci. In some cases, cortical infiltration along the penetrating perivascular spaces thickens the cortex and obliterates the normal gray-white matter interface **(39-55)**.

A few cases of MA with associated focal cortical dysplasia have been reported.

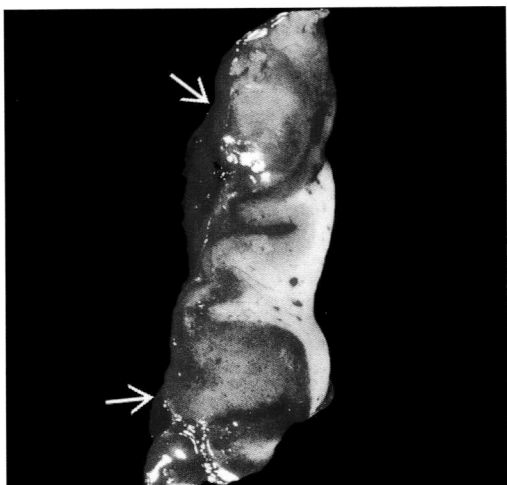

39-54. *Specimen shows characteristic gross findings of MA. Thickened cortex is invaded by vascular-appearing tissue ➡. (AFIP Archives.)*

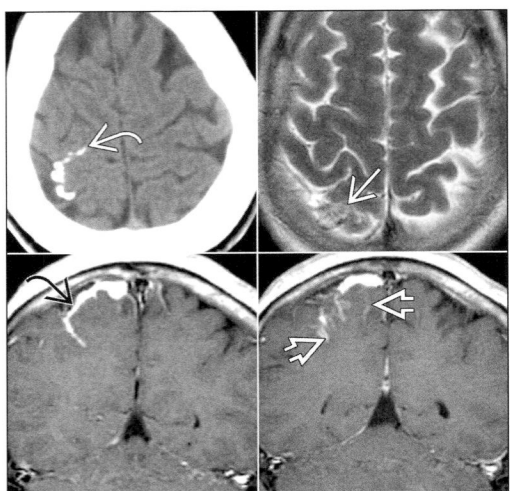

39-55. *Scans in a patient with MA show gyriform calcification ➡, thickened cortex ➡, curvilinear enhancement ↗, parenchymal infiltration ➡.*

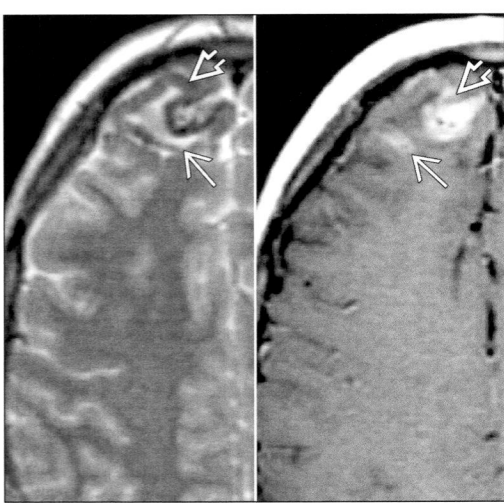

39-56. *(Left) T2WI in MA shows serpentine hypointense infiltration ➡, gliosis ➡. (Right) Globular ➡, gyriform enhancement ➡.*

Differential Diagnosis

The most important differential diagnosis of MA is **neoplasm**. Imaging findings are not pathognomonic, so the definitive diagnosis is generally a pathologic one. *It is extremely important that the neuropathologist does not mistake MA for an invasive atypical or malignant meningioma!* MA does not recur after complete resection and does not require radiation or adjuvant chemotherapy.

MENINGIOANGIOMATOSIS

Pathology
- Benign mass of proliferating meningothelial cells, small vessels
- Curvilinear plaque-like lesion
- May show focal brain invasion

Clinical Issues
- *Forme fruste* of NF2

Imaging
- Iso-/hypointense on T1WI; usually hypointense on T2WI
- Serpentine enhancement ± PVS invasion
- DDx: Invasive neoplasm

Neurocutaneous Melanosis

Terminology

Neurocutaneous melanosis (NCM) is a rare nonfamilial syndrome characterized by giant and/or multiple congenital melanocytic nevi, excessive proliferation of melanin-containing cells in the leptomeninges, and benign and malignant tumors of the CNS **(39-57)**.

Etiology

Scattered melanocytes are normally present in the pia over the convexities and around the base of the brain, ventral brainstem, and parts of the spinal cord. Focal or diffuse proliferation of these melanin-producing cells in the skin and meninges results in NCM.

Melanocytes are derived from neural crest cells (NCCs). Around 8-10 weeks of gestation, NCC-derived pluripotent precursors migrate to the fetal epidermis via the paraspinal ganglia and peripheral nerve sheath, ultimately generating differentiated melanocytes.

NCM is thought to be a neurocristopathy caused by neural crest aberration during early embryonic development. Some abnormalities in neural tube-derived cells also occur, possibly resulting in NCM-associated brain malformation (e.g., Dandy-Walker malformation) **(39-59)**.

Pathology

CNS disease can be parenchymal or leptomeningeal, benign or malignant. **Melanosis** consists of focal collections of histologically benign melanotic cells. A malignant **melanoma** consists of proliferating anaplastic melanotic cells. The estimated prevalence of malignant melanoma in the setting of NCM is 40-60%.

Grossly, leptomeningeal melanosis appears as superficial dark gray or black pigmentation in the pia **(39-59)**. The most common locations for parenchymal melanotic deposits are the amygdala and cerebellum, followed by the pons, thalami, and inferior frontal lobes.

Clinical Issues

Many patients are asymptomatic. Seizures and signs of elevated intracranial pressure can occur with leptomeningeal melanosis and malignant melanoma. The prognosis in symptomatic NCM is extremely poor.

Imaging

Bilateral round or ovoid T1 hyperintensities in the anterior temporal lobes are the most characteristic findings **(39-60)**. Focal or diffuse T1 shortening in the leptomeninges with serpentine enhancement on T1 C+ scans is much less common and is generally seen only in cases

in which melanotic deposits have undergone malignant transformation **(39-58)**.

Hydrocephalus is common. Cortical invasion along the penetrating perivascular spaces may cause significant mass effect and edema.

Between 8-10% of patients with NCM harbor an associated Dandy-Walker malformation.

NEUROCUTANEOUS MELANOSIS

Pathology
- Black or grayish deposits
- Leptomeninges, amygdala, cerebellum
- Benign or malignant melanotic cells

Imaging
- T1 hyperintensities
- Round/ovoid deposits in amygdala
- Serpentine pial lesions, PVS invasion in malignant
- Variable enhancement

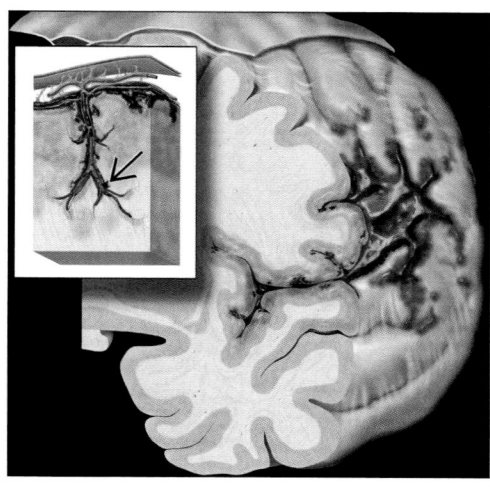

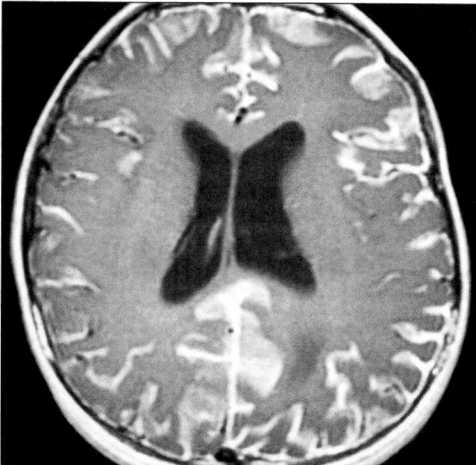

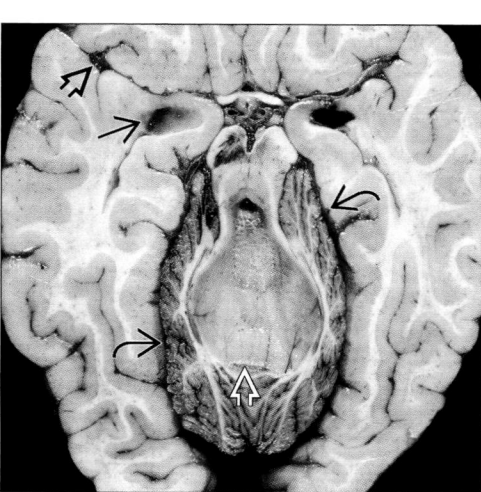

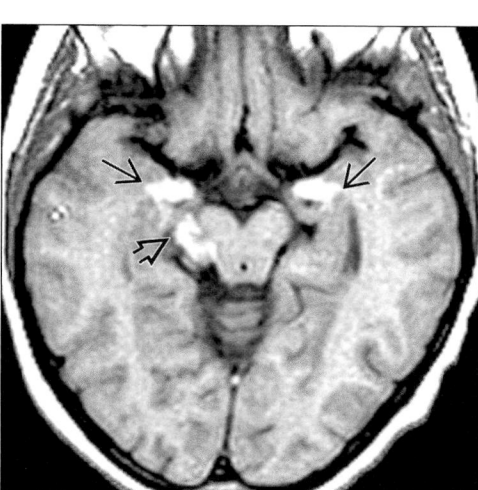

39-57. Graphic shows localized dark (melanotic) pigmentation of the leptomeninges. Inset demonstrates extension of melanosis into the brain substance along the Virchow-Robin spaces ⇨. 39-58. Axial T1 C+ MR in a patient with extensive neurocutaneous melanosis shows diffuse pia-subarachnoid space enhancement. (Courtesy M. Martin, MD.)

39-59. Autopsy specimen of NCM shows ovoid melanotic deposits in the amygdalae of both anterior temporal lobes ⇨. Black discoloration in the sylvian fissures ⇨ and over the cerebellum ⇗ represents diffuse leptomeningeal melanin deposits. Note the cerebellar cyst ⇨. Dandy-Walker malformation has a strong association with NCM. (Courtesy R. Hewlett, MD.) 39-60. Axial T1WI shows T1 shortening in the amygdalae ⇨ and leptomeninges ⇨. (Courtesy S. Blaser, MD.)

Encephalocraniocutaneous Lipomatosis

Encephalocraniocutaneous lipomatosis (ECCL), also known as Haberland syndrome, is a rare neurocutaneous disorder whose hallmark CNS lesions are benign lipomas of the brain and spinal cord.

ECCL is a mesenchymal disorder that affects neural crest derivatives.

ECCL is characterized clinically by ocular choristomas (typically lipodermoids), a smooth hairless scalp lipoma called a nevus psiloliparus (39-61), and subcutaneous cervicofacial fatty soft tissue masses. Approximately one-half of all patients have seizures, and one-third demonstrate mild or moderate mental retardation.

Most patients with ECCL have one or more CNS lipomas. ECCL-associated lipomas have a predilection for the posterior fossa and spine. They are generally stable but may increase with age (39-62), becoming moderately large and extending over multiple spinal segments. Other congenital anomalies of the meninges such as arachnoid cysts and meningioangiomatosis are common.

Epidermal Nevus Syndrome

Epidermal nevus syndrome consists of an epidermal nevus (EN)—a benign congenital skin hamartoma—with developmental abnormalities of the skin, eyes, and CNS with variable involvement of the skeletal, cardiovascular, and urogenital systems (39-63).

Several different types of nevi are included as part of "epidermal nevus syndrome"—some pigmented hairy nevi, nevus comedonicus, inflammatory linear verrucous epidermal nevus, and linear sebaceous nevi.

ENs are caused by genetic mosaicism (represented by two or more different but coexisting clones of the same cell line). Embryonic epidermal cells appear early in fetal development. They proliferate and then migrate from their origin in neural crest to their destinations along so-called Blaschko lines. Mutated cells are phenotypically manifested along this pathway, resulting in the characteristic distribution of ENs.

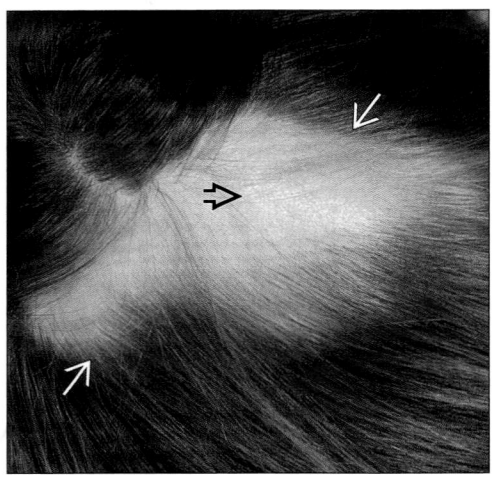
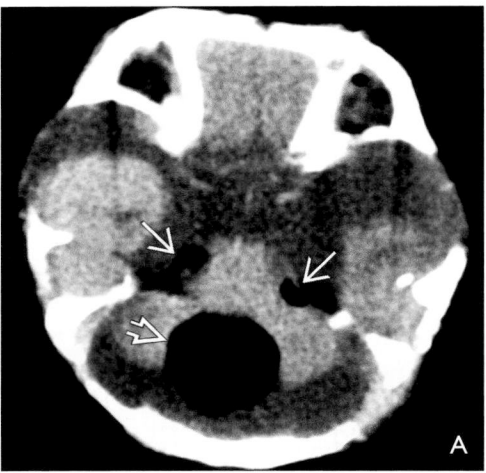

39-61. Clinical photograph demonstrates a nevus psiloliparus, the dermatologic token of ECCL. A focal area of alopecia ➜ (hair loss) covers an underlying scalp lipoma ⊳, seen here as a rubbery, slightly elevated mass. (Courtesy A. Illner, MD.) **39-62A.** NECT scan in a 2-year-old child with ECCL shows focal lipomas in both cerebellopontine angle (CPA) cisterns ➜ and the cisterna magna ➜.

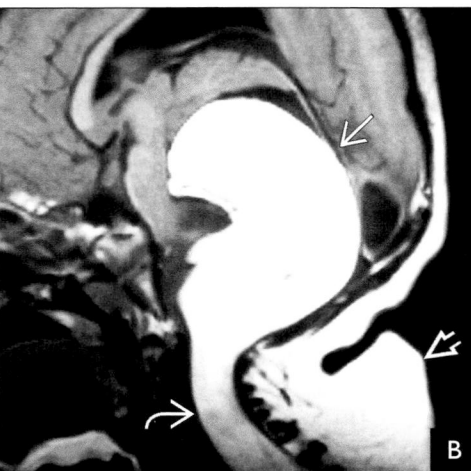
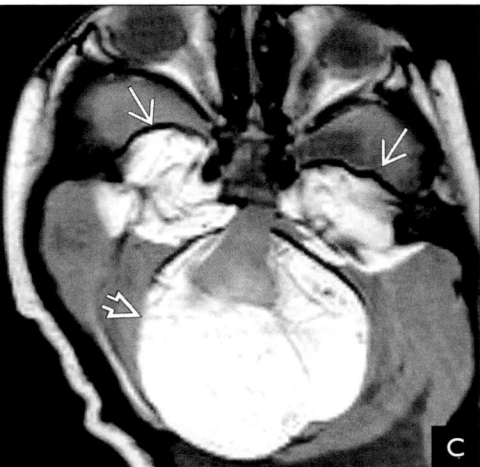

39-62B. Three years later, sagittal T1WI shows a very large suboccipital lipoma ➜. The cisterna magna lipoma has massively increased in size. It now occupies almost the entire posterior fossa ➜ and extends inferiorly into the upper cervical spinal canal ➜. **39-62C.** Axial PD shows the large posterior fossa lipoma ➜. The CPA lipomas have also increased in size, now extending into both Meckel caves ➜.

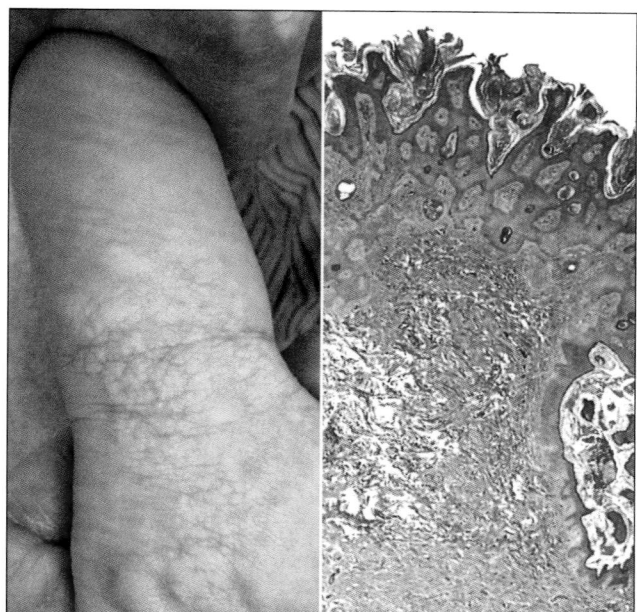

39-63. (Left) Epidermal nevus is a warty band of hypopigmented growth. (Courtesy University of Utah Department of Dermatology.) (Right) EN shows hyperkeratosis, papillomatosis, acanthosis. (Courtesy J. Comstock, MD.)

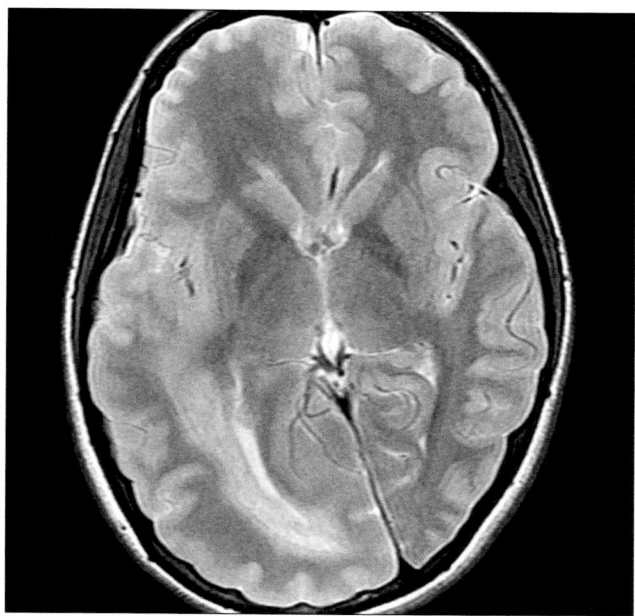

39-64. Axial T2WI shows right hemisphere hemimegaloencephaly, the most common CNS malformation seen in epidermal nevus syndrome.

ENs are present at birth or develop during the first few years of life. Clinically, an epidermal nevus is seen as a linear or zosteriform warty plaque that may exhibit scaly discoloration. Most are found on the neck, trunk, and extremities.

CNS malformations are present in the majority of patients with EN syndrome. The most common are malformations of cortical development (hemimegaloencephaly, pachygyria-polymicrogyria) **(39-64)**. Eye lesions are present in 40-70% of patients and include ocular colobomas, choristomas (epibulbar dermoids and lipodermoids), and optic nerve dysplasia.

A new variant of EN syndrome with papular epidermal nevi and "skyline" basal cell layer (PENS) has recently been described. Patients develop psychomotor retardation and epilepsy during the first year of life. To date, no specific imaging abnormalities have been described in PENS.

Proteus Syndrome

Proteus syndrome is a rare hamartomatous disorder with multiple and diverse somatic manifestations. PS is characterized by localized, progressive, postnatal limb overgrowth with bony distortion, dysregulated adipose tissue, epidermal nevi, and CNS malformations. Hemimegaloencephaly, pachygyria-polymicrogyria, and heterotopic gray matter are common associated abnormalities.

The major differential diagnosis of Proteus is a newly described syndrome called **CLOVE** (**c**ongenital **l**ipo-matous **o**vergrowth, **v**ascular malformations, **e**pidermal nevi). CLOVE has large truncal vascular malformations, manifests limb overgrowth at birth, and lacks the progressive, distorted bony overgrowth of Proteus syndrome. Other disorders with asymmetric overgrowth include **Klippel-Trenaunay-Weber syndrome**, **Ollier disease**, **Maffucci syndrome**, and **encephalocraniocutaneous lipomatosis**.

Selected References

Neurofibromatosis and Schwannomatosis

- Monsalve J et al: Imaging of cancer predisposition syndromes in children. Radiographics. 31(1):263-80, 2011
- Shinagare AB et al: Hereditary cancer syndromes: a radiologist's perspective. AJR Am J Roentgenol. 197(6):W1001-7, 2011
- Lu-Emerson C et al: The neurofibromatoses. Part 1: NF1. Rev Neurol Dis. 6(2):E47-53, 2009
- Lu-Emerson C et al: The neurofibromatoses. Part 2: NF2 and schwannomatosis. Rev Neurol Dis. 6(3):E81-6, 2009

Neurofibromatosis Type 1

- Kaas B et al: Spectrum and prevalence of vasculopathy in pediatric neurofibromatosis type 1. J Child Neurol. Epub ahead of print, 2012
- Vizina V et al: The phakomatoses. In Barkovich AJ et al: Pediatric Neuroimaging. Philadelphia: Lippincott Williams & Wilkins. 569-636, 2012
- Plotkin SR et al: Quantitative assessment of whole-body tumor burden in adult patients with neurofibromatosis. PLoS One. 7(4):e35711, 2012
- Adigun CG et al: Segmental neurofibromatosis. Dermatol Online J. 17(10):25, 2011
- Laycock-van Spyk S et al: Neurofibromatosis type 1-associated tumours: their somatic mutational spectrum and pathogenesis. Hum Genomics. 5(6):623-90, 2011
- Messiaen L et al: Mosaic type-1 NF1 microdeletions as a cause of both generalized and segmental neurofibromatosis type-1 (NF1). Hum Mutat. 32(2):213-9, 2011
- Monsalve J et al: Imaging of cancer predisposition syndromes in children. Radiographics. 31(1):263-80, 2011
- Wasa J et al: MRI features in the differentiation of malignant peripheral nerve sheath tumors and neurofibromas. AJR Am J Roentgenol. 194(6):1568-74, 2010
- Boyd KP et al: Neurofibromatosis type 1. J Am Acad Dermatol. 61(1):1-14; quiz 15-6, 2009
- Lu-Emerson C et al: The Neurofibromatoses. Part 1: NF1. Rev Neurol Dis. 6(2):E47-53, 2009
- Messiaen L et al: Clinical and mutational spectrum of neurofibromatosis type 1-like syndrome. JAMA. 302(19):2111-8, 2009
- Rea D et al: Cerebral arteriopathy in children with neurofibromatosis type 1. Pediatrics. 124(3):e476-83, 2009
- Lopes Ferraz Filho JR et al: Unidentified bright objects on brain MRI in children as a diagnostic criterion for neurofibromatosis type 1. Pediatr Radiol. 38(3):305-10, 2008

Neurofibromatosis Type 2

- Carroll SL: Molecular mechanisms promoting the pathogenesis of Schwann cell neoplasms. Acta Neuropathol. 123(3):321-48, 2012
- Dirks MS et al: Long-term natural history of neurofibromatosis Type 2-associated intracranial tumors. J Neurosurg. 117(1):109-17, 2012
- Goutagny S et al: Long-term follow-up of 287 meningiomas in neurofibromatosis type 2 patients: clinical, radiological, and molecular features. Neuro Oncol. 14(8):1090-6, 2012
- Hoa M et al: Neurofibromatosis 2. Otolaryngol Clin North Am. 45(2):315-32, viii, 2012
- Kalamarides M et al: Neurofibromatosis 2011: a report of the Children's Tumor Foundation annual meeting. Acta Neuropathol. 123(3):369-80, 2012
- Plotkin SR et al: Quantitative assessment of whole-body tumor burden in adult patients with neurofibromatosis. PLoS One. 7(4):e35711, 2012
- Uhlmann EJ et al: Neurofibromatoses. Adv Exp Med Biol. 724:266-77, 2012
- Wong HK et al: Merlin/NF2 regulates angiogenesis in schwannomas through a Rac1/semaphorin 3F-dependent mechanism. Neoplasia. 14(2):84-94, 2012
- Goutagny S et al: Meningiomas and neurofibromatosis. J Neurooncol. 99(3):341-7, 2010
- Lu-Emerson C et al: The neurofibromatoses. Part 2: NF2 and schwannomatosis. Rev Neurol Dis. 6(3):E81-6, 2009
- Fisher LM et al: Distribution of nonvestibular cranial nerve schwannomas in neurofibromatosis 2. Otol Neurotol. 28(8):1083-90, 2007

Schwannomatosis

- Smith MJ et al: Frequency of SMARCB1 mutations in familial and sporadic schwannomatosis. Neurogenetics. 13(2):141-5, 2012
- van den Munckhof P et al: Germline SMARCB1 mutation predisposes to multiple meningiomas and schwannomas with preferential location of cranial meningiomas at the falx cerebri. Neurogenetics. 13(1):1-7, 2012
- Plotkin SR et al: Spinal ependymomas in neurofibromatosis type 2: a retrospective analysis of 55 patients. J Neurosurg Spine. 14(4):543-7, 2011
- Lu-Emerson C et al: The neurofibromatoses. Part 2: NF2 and schwannomatosis. Rev Neurol Dis. 6(3):E81-6, 2009

Other Common Familial Tumor Syndromes

Tuberous Sclerosis Complex

- Katz JS et al: Intraventricular lesions in tuberous sclerosis complex: a possible association with the caudate nucleus. J Neurosurg Pediatr. 9(4):406-13, 2012
- Dobashi Y et al: Mammalian target of rapamycin: a central node of complex signaling cascades. Int J Clin Exp Pathol. 4(5):476-95, 2011

- Hake S: Cutaneous manifestations of tuberous sclerosis. Ochsner J. 10(3):200-4, 2010

von Hippel-Lindau Disease

- Mills SA et al: Supratentorial hemangioblastoma: clinical features, prognosis, and predictive value of location for von Hippel- Lindau disease. Neuro Oncol. 14(8):1097-104, 2012
- Sun YH et al: Endolymphatic sac tumor: case report and review of the literature. Diagn Pathol. 7(1):36, 2012
- Zhang Q et al: Von Hippel-Lindau disease manifesting disseminated leptomeningeal hemangioblastomatosis: surgery or medication? Acta Neurochir (Wien). 153(1):48-52, 2011
- Wind JJ et al: Management of von Hippel-Lindau disease-associated CNS lesions. Expert Rev Neurother. 11(10):1433-41, 2011
- Maher ER et al: von Hippel-Lindau disease: a clinical and scientific review. Eur J Hum Genet. 19(6):617-23, 2011
- Lonser RR et al: Pituitary stalk hemangioblastomas in von Hippel-Lindau disease. J Neurosurg. 110(2):350-3, 2009

Rare Neurocutaneous Syndromes

Li-Fraumeni Syndrome

- Gonçalves A et al: Li-Fraumeni-like syndrome associated with a large BRCA1 intragenic deletion. BMC Cancer. 12(1):237, 2012
- Monsalve J et al: Imaging of cancer predisposition syndromes in children. Radiographics. 31(1):263-80, 2011
- Shinagare AB et al: Hereditary cancer syndromes: a radiologist's perspective. AJR Am J Roentgenol. 197(6):W1001-7, 2011
- Ohgaki H et al: Li-Fraumeni syndrome and TP53 germline mutations. In Louis DN et al: WHO Classification of Tumours of the Central Nervous System. Lyon, France: IARC Press. 222-5, 2007

Cowden Syndrome

- Eberhart CG et al: Cowden disease and dysplastic gangliocytoma of the cerebellum/Lhermitte-Duclos disease. In Louis DN et al: WHO Classification of Tumours of the Central Nervous System. Lyon, France: IARC Press. 226-8, 2007

Turcot Syndrome

- Tihan T: Turcot syndrome. In Burger P et al: Diagnostic Pathology: Neuropathology. Salt Lake City: Amirsys Publishing. I.5.12-13, 2012
- Chung KH et al: Metachronous multifocal desmoid-type fibromatoses along the neuraxis with adenomatous polyposis syndrome. J Neurosurg Pediatr. 6(4):372-6, 2010
- Koontz NA et al: AJR teaching file: brain tumor in a patient with familial adenomatous polyposis. AJR Am J Roentgenol. 195(3 Suppl):S25-8, 2010
- Cavenee WK et al: Turcot syndrome. In Louis DN et al: WHO Classification of Tumours of the Central Nervous System. Lyon, France: IARC Press. 229-31, 2007

Basal Cell Nevus Syndrome

- Varan A et al: Primitive neuroectodermal tumors of the central nervous system associated with genetic and metabolic defects. J Neurosurg Sci. 56(1):49-53, 2012
- Koch B: Basal cell nevus syndrome. In Harnsberger HR: Diagnostic Imaging: Head and Neck. 2nd ed. Salt Lake City: Amirsys Publishing. III.2.2-3, 2011
- Kimonis VE et al: Radiological features in 82 patients with nevoid basal cell carcinoma (NBCC or Gorlin) syndrome. Genet Med. 6(6):495-502, 2004

Rhabdoid Tumor Predisposition Syndrome

- Harris TJ et al: Case 168: rhabdoid predisposition syndrome-- familial cancer syndromes in children. Radiology. 259(1):298-302, 2011
- Wesseling P et al: Rhabdoid tumor predisposition syndrome. In Louis DN et al: WHO Classification of Tumours of the Central Nervous System. Lyon, France: IARC Press. 234-5, 2007

Meningioangiomatosis

- Batra A et al: Meningioangiomatosis associated with focal cortical dysplasia and neurofibrillary tangles. Clin Neuropathol. Epub ahead of print, 2012
- Arcos A et al: Meningioangiomatosis: clinical-radiological features and surgical outcome. Neurocirugia (Astur). 21(6):461-6, 2010
- Perry A et al: Insights into meningioangiomatosis with and without meningioma: a clinicopathologic and genetic series of 24 cases with review of the literature. Brain Pathol. 15(1):55-65, 2005

Neurocutaneous Melanosis

- Ginat DT et al: Intracranial lesions with high signal intensity on T1-weighted MR images: differential diagnosis. Radiographics. 32(2):499-516, 2012
- Kinsler VA et al: Neuropathology of neurocutaneous melanosis: histological foci of melanotic neurones and glia may be undetectable on MRI. Acta Neuropathol. PubMed Central PMCID: PMC3282914, 2012
- Ramaswamy V et al: Spectrum of central nervous system abnormalities in neurocutaneous melanocytosis. Dev Med Child Neurol. 54(6):563-8, 2012
- Marnet D et al: Neurocutaneous melanosis and the Dandy-Walker complex: an uncommon but not so insignificant association. Childs Nerv Syst. 25(12):1533-9, 2009

Encephalocraniocutaneous Lipomatosis

- Lee RK et al: Encephalocraniocutaneous lipomatosis: a rare case with development of diffuse leptomeningeal lipomatosis during childhood. Pediatr Radiol. 42(1):129-33, 2012
- Ayer RE et al: Encephalocraniocutaneous lipomatosis: a review of its clinical pathology and neurosurgical indications. J Neurosurg Pediatr. 8(3):316-20, 2011

- Svoronos A et al: Imaging findings in encephalocraniocutaneous lipomatosis. Neurology. 77(7):694, 2011
- Gucev ZS et al: Congenital lipomatous overgrowth, vascular malformations, and epidermal nevi (CLOVE) syndrome: CNS malformations and seizures may be a component of this disorder. Am J Med Genet A. 146A(20):2688-90, 2008

Epidermal Nevus Syndrome

- Tadini G et al: PENS syndrome: a new neurocutaneous phenotype. Dermatology. 224(1):24-30, 2012
- Amato C et al: Schimmelpenning syndrome: a kind of craniofacial epidermal nevus associated with cerebral and ocular MR imaging abnormalities. AJNR Am J Neuroradiol. 31(5):E47-8, 2010

Proteus Syndrome

- Biesecker L: The challenges of Proteus syndrome: diagnosis and management. Eur J Hum Genet. 14(11):1151-7, 2006

40

Vascular Phakomatoses

A number of syndromes with prominent cutaneous manifestations occur *without* associated neoplasms. Many of these are disorders in which both cutaneous and intracranial vascular lesions are the predominant features. These so-called **vascular phakomatoses**—also known as **vascular metameric syndromes**—demonstrate the developmental association between skin lesions and intracranial malformations in the same embryonic metamere.

Some vascular phakomatoses, such as Sturge-Weber syndrome, are present at birth (i.e., congenital) but *not* inherited. Others, including hereditary hemorrhagic telangiectasia, have specific gene mutations and known inheritance patterns. We delineate these and other pertinent features of the major vascular neurocutaneous syndromes here.

Sturge-Weber Syndrome

Sturge-Weber syndrome (SWS) is noteworthy among neurocutaneous syndromes: It is one of the very few syndromes that is sporadic, i.e., not inherited. It is also one of the most disfiguring syndromes, as a prominent nevus flammeus or port-wine stain is seen in the vast majority of cases.

Over the past decade, the number of published reports dealing with has increased significantly, reflecting progress in the diagnosis and understanding of neurological involvement in this disorder. A number of centers and advocacy groups have arisen, both to care for SWS patients and to stimulate research.

Imaging has always played a central role in the diagnosis and management of SWS. With the advent of functional imaging, we are gaining new insights into the clinical manifestations and pathophysiology of this disorder.

Terminology

Sturge-Weber syndrome is also known as **encephalotrigeminal angiomatosis**. Its hallmarks are variable combinations of (1) a capillary malformation of the skin (port-wine birthmark) in the distribution of the trigeminal nerve, (2) retinal choroidal angioma (either with or without glaucoma), and (3) a cerebral capillary-venous leptomeningeal angioma **(40-1)**.

Etiology

The origin and pathophysiology of SWS remain poorly understood. At four or five weeks of gestation, the visual cortex is juxtaposed to the optic vesicle and the upper part of the embryonic face. During this period, a primordial venous plexus surrounds the neural tube and invades the adjacent fetal brain, skin, and eye. A spontaneous somatic mutation could prevent normal maturation with persistent primitive thin-walled vessels. This could result in a paucity of normal cortical draining veins, which in turn causes thrombosis and stasis with venous ischemia of the underlying cortex.

Pathology

A tangle of thin-walled vessels—multiple capillaries and venous channels—forms the characteristic leptomeningeal (pial) angioma. The angioma covers the brain surface, dipping into the enlarged sulci between shrunken apposing gyri **(40-2)**.

The most common location is the parietooccipital region, followed by the frontal and temporal lobes. Part or all of one hemisphere can be affected. SWS is unilateral in 80% of cases and is typically ipsilateral to the facial angioma. Bilateral involvement is seen in 20% of cases. Infratentorial lesions are seen in 11% of cases.

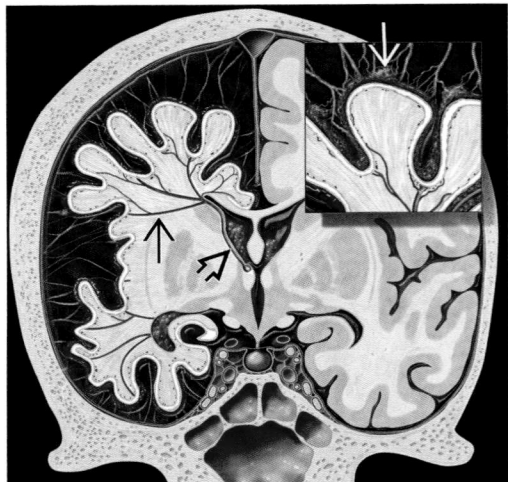

40-1. SWS shows pial angiomatosis ➡️, *deep medullary collaterals* ➡️, *enlarged choroid plexus* ➡️, *atrophy of the right cerebral hemisphere.*

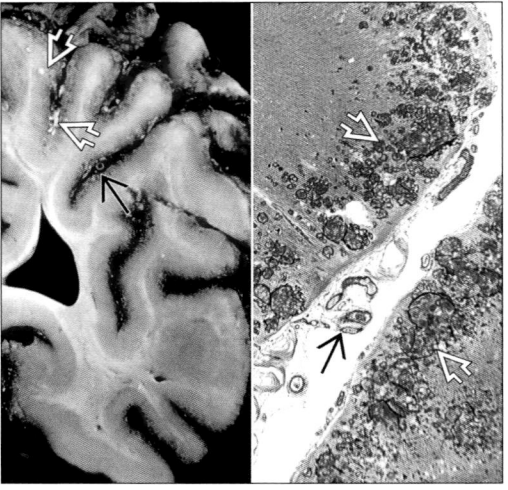

40-2. Gross (left), photomicrograph (right) of SWS show cortical atrophy, calcifications ➡️, *pial angioma* ➡️ *within sulci. (AFIP Archives.)*

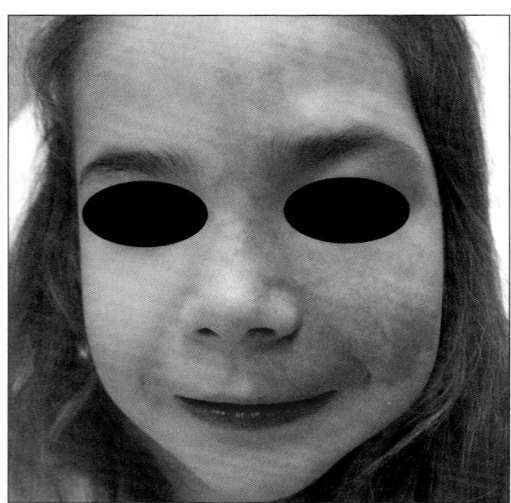

40-3. Photograph shows the classic CN V_1-V_2 nevus flammeus characteristic of SWS.

Dystrophic laminar cortical calcifications are typical. Frank hemorrhage and large territorial infarcts are rare.

Clinical Issues

EPIDEMIOLOGY AND DEMOGRAPHICS. SWS is rare with an estimated prevalence of 1:40,000-50,000 live births. There is no gender predilection.

PRESENTATION. The vast majority of SWS patients exhibit a nevus flammeus—formerly termed a facial "angioma" or "port-wine stain"—that is plainly visible at birth. It can be uni- (63%) or bilateral (31%) and is distributed over the skin innervated by one or more sensory branches of the trigeminal nerve. CN V_1 (forehead and/or eyelid) or a combination of CN V_1-V_2 (plus cheek) are the most common sites **(40-3)**. All three trigeminal divisions are involved in 13% of cases. *No facial nevus flammeus is present in 5% of cases,* so lack of a port-wine nevus does not rule out SWS!

Similarly, presence of a port-wine birthmark (PWB) is *not* sufficient in and of itself for the definitive diagnosis of SWS. Patients with PWBs in the CN V_1 distribution have only a 10-20% risk of SWS, although the risk increases with size, extent, and bilaterality of the nevus flammeus.

Seizures developing in the first year of life (75-90%), glaucoma (70%), hemiparesis (30-65%), and migraine-like headaches are other common manifestations of SWS.

Occasionally, children with SWS also have extensive cutaneous capillary malformations, limb hypertrophy, and vascular and/or lymphatic malformations. These children are diagnosed as having **Klippel-Trenaunay-Weber syndrome** (KTWS), which is also known as angioosteohypertrophy or hemangiectatic hypertrophy. Whether SWS and KTWS are overlapping or distinct syndromes is unknown.

Endocrine disorders are a newly recognized aspect of SWS. Patients with SWS have a significantly increased risk of growth hormone deficiency and central hypothyroidism.

NATURAL HISTORY. SWS-related seizures are often medically refractory and worsen with time. Progressive hemiparesis and stroke-like episodes with focal neurologic deficits are common. Most patients are mentally retarded.

TREATMENT OPTIONS. Despite adequate treatment with antiepileptic drugs, seizure control is achieved in less than half of all cases. Early lobectomy or hemispherectomy in infants with drug-resistant epilepsy and widespread hemispheric angioma may be an option in severe cases.

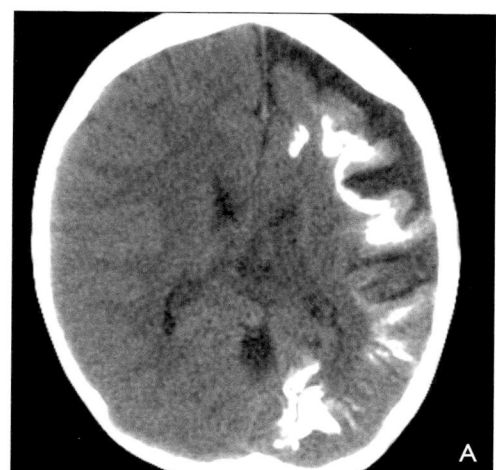
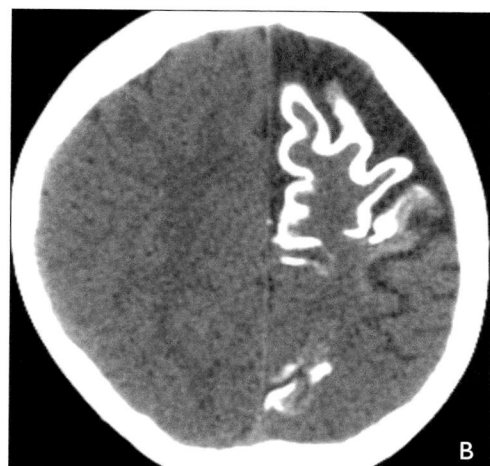

40-4A. NECT in an 8-year-old girl with SWS shows striking cortical atrophy, extensive calcifications in the cortex and subcortical WM throughout most of the left cerebral hemisphere. 40-4B. More cephalad NECT in the same patient shows the typical serpentine gyral calcifications together with significant volume loss.

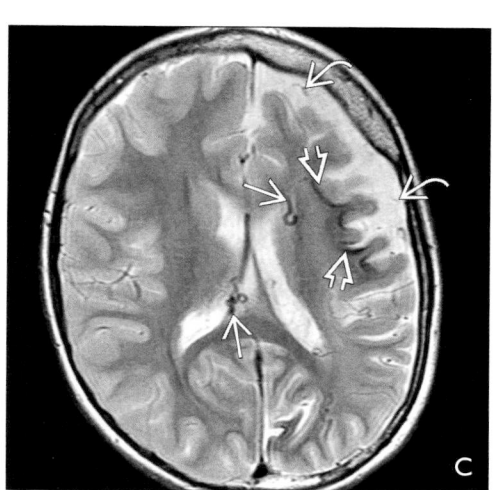
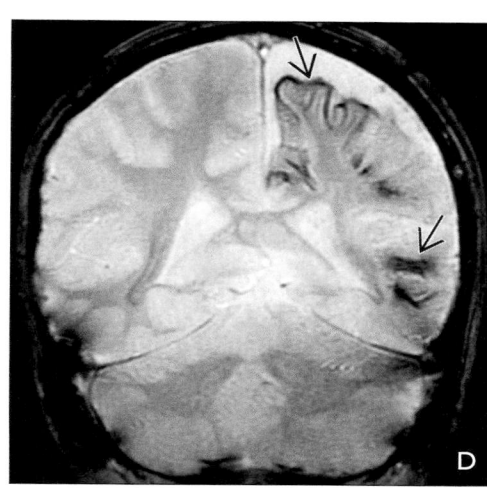

40-4C. T2WI in the same patient shows atrophy with thinned cortex, extensive curvilinear hypointensity in the GM-WM interface ➡. Note the prominent "flow voids" in the subependymal veins ➡. The CSF in the enlarged subarachnoid space appears somewhat "dirty" with enlarged traversing trabeculae and veins ➡. 40-4D. Coronal T2* GRE scan shows "blooming" of the extensive cortical/subcortical calcifications ➡.

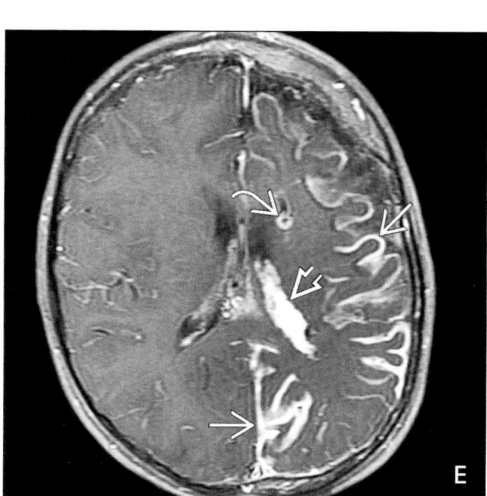
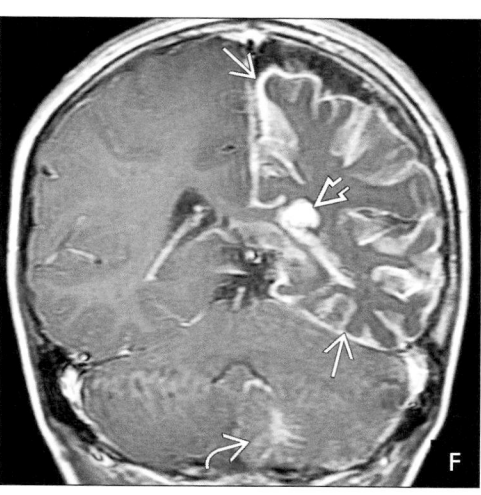

40-4E. Axial T1 C+ FS scan shows serpentine enhancement covering the gyri and filling the sulci ➡ over the entire hemisphere. The pial angioma is most prominent in the parietal, occipital regions. Note the enlargement, enhancement of the ipsilateral choroid plexus ➡ and draining subependymal vein ➡. 40-4F. Coronal T1 C+ scan nicely shows the pial angioma ➡ and enlarged choroid plexus ➡. A developmental venous anomaly is seen in the left cerebellar hemisphere ➡.

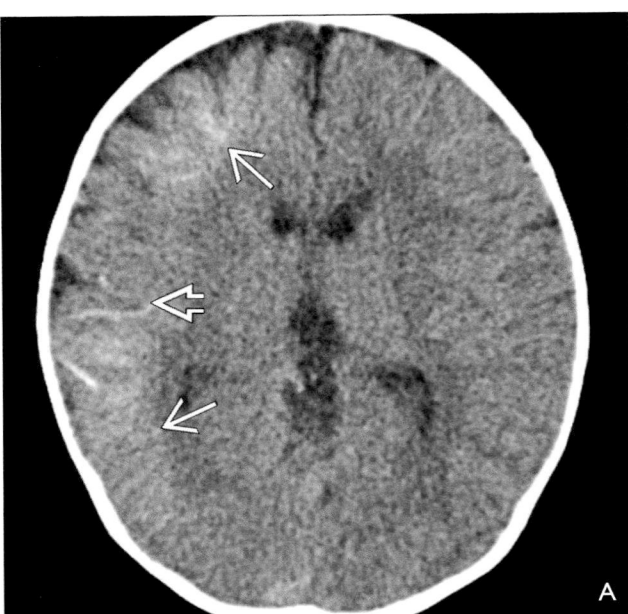

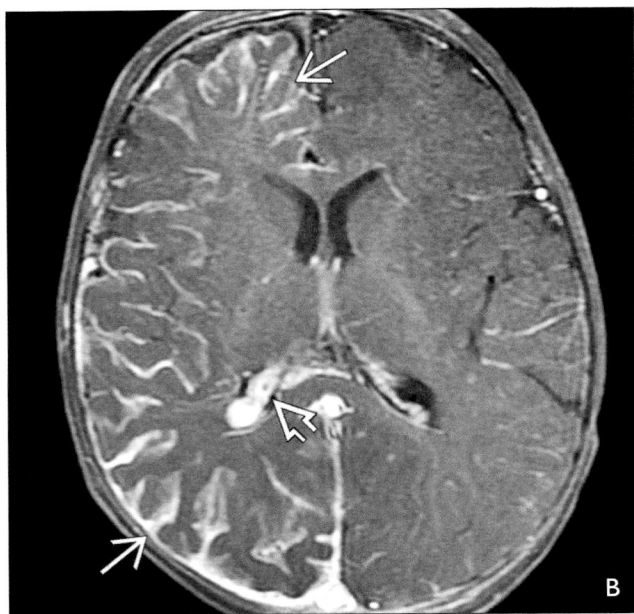

40-5A. NECT scan in a 5-month-old child with SWS shows curvilinear Ca++ ➡ and faint hyperdensity in the right hemisphere ➡. The sulci are minimally enlarged compared to the normal left side.

40-5B. T1 C+ FS scan in the same patient shows that an extensive pial angioma ➡ covers the entire right hemisphere. Note the enlargement of the ipsilateral choroid plexus ➡.

Imaging

GENERAL FEATURES. Neuroimaging is used to identify the intracranial pial angioma and the sequelae of long-standing venous ischemia. This enables the radiologist to (1) establish or confirm the diagnosis of SWS and (2) evaluate the extent and severity of intracranial involvement.

Sequential examinations of SWS patients show progressive cerebral cortical-subcortical atrophy, especially during the first years of life. *Findings may be minimal or absent in newborn infants, so serial imaging is necessary in suspected cases.*

CT FINDINGS. NECT is especially useful to depict the dystrophic cortical/subcortical calcifications that are one of the imaging hallmarks of SWS **(40-4)**, **(40-5)**, **(40-7)**. (Note that the calcifications are in the underlying brain, not the pial angioma). Cortical calcification, atrophy, and enlargement of the ipsilateral choroid plexus are typical findings in older children and adults with SWS.

Heavily calcified cortex correlates with decreased perfusion in the underlying WM and is also associated with more severe epilepsy.

Bone CT shows thickening of the diploë and enlargement with hyperpneumatization of the ipsilateral frontal sinuses secondary to longstanding volume loss in the underlying brain. Dense cortical calcifications may obscure enhancement of the pial angioma on CECT, but an enlarged enhancing choroid plexus can usually be identified.

MR FINDINGS. T1 and T2 scans show volume loss in the affected cortex with enlargement of the adjacent subarachnoid spaces **(40-4C)**. Prominent trabeculae and enlarged veins often cross the subarachnoid space, making the CSF appear somewhat grayish or "dirty" **(40-6)**.

Dystrophic cortical/subcortical calcifications are seen as linear hypointensities on T2WI that "bloom" on T2* (GRE, SWI) **(40-4D)**. SWI scans often demonstrate linear susceptibility in enlarged medullary veins **(40-6E)**. Frank hemorrhagic foci are uncommon.

FLAIR scans may demonstrate serpentine hyperintensities in the sulci, the "ivy" sign **(40-6A)**. DWI is usually negative unless acute ischemia is present.

Post-contrast T1WI or FLAIR sequences best demonstrate the pial angioma. Serpentine enhancement covers the underlying gyri, extending deep into the sulci and sometimes almost filling the subarachnoid space **(40-4E)**, **(40-4F)**, **(40-5B)**. Enlarged medullary veins—sources of compensatory collateral venous drainage—can sometimes be identified as linear enhancing foci extending deep into the hemispheric white matter **(40-6D)**. The ipsilateral choroid plexus is almost always enlarged and enhances intensely **(40-4F)**, **(40-5B)**.

FUNCTIONAL IMAGING. Both pMR and PET/CT are useful techniques to depict progressive deficits in cerebral perfusion and metabolism that correspond to the patterns of neurological deterioration. Ictal SPECT may demonstrate impaired autoregulation of blood flow to meet metabolic demand during seizures.

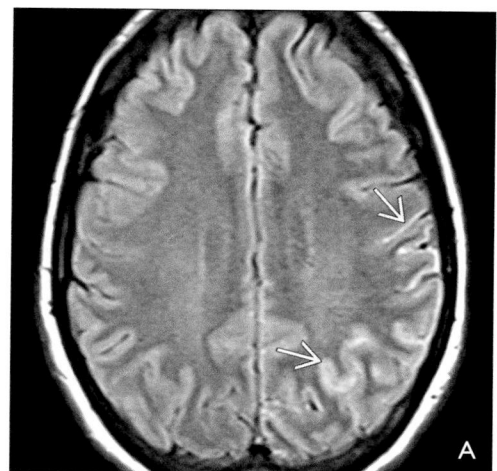

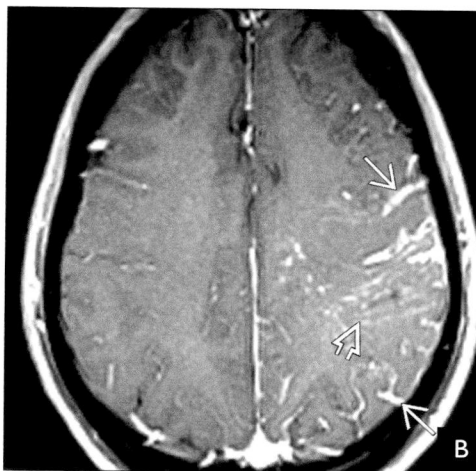

40-6A. *Axial FLAIR scan in a 25-year-old woman with seizures and SWS shows left parietooccipital sulcal hyperintensity ("ivy" sign)* ➡. **40-6B.** *T1 C+ FS scan in the same patient shows that the enhancing pial angioma fills the affected sulci* ➡. *Note the linear enhancing foci caused by enlarged medullary veins* ⇨ *that provide collateral venous drainage into the subependymal veins and galenic system.*

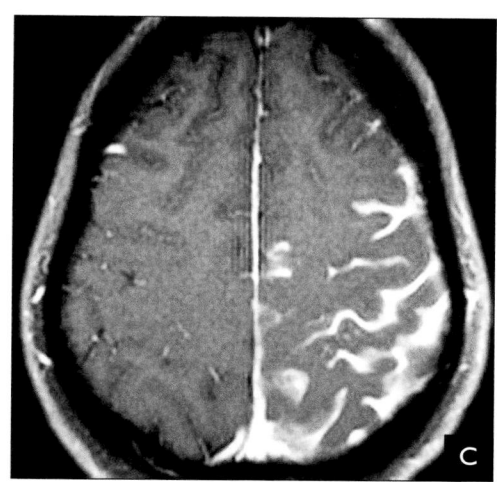

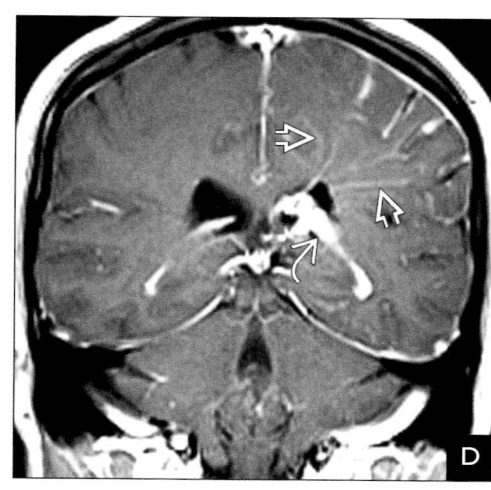

40-6C. *More cephalad T1 C+ scan in the same patient shows that the sulci and subarachnoid spaces are enlarged, completely filled by the enhancing pial angioma.* **40-6D.** *Coronal T1 C+ scan nicely demonstrates the prominent enhancing medullary veins* ⇨ *as they drain through the hemispheric white matter to converge on the subependymal veins that line the lateral ventricles. The ipsilateral choroid plexus* ➡ *is markedly enlarged.*

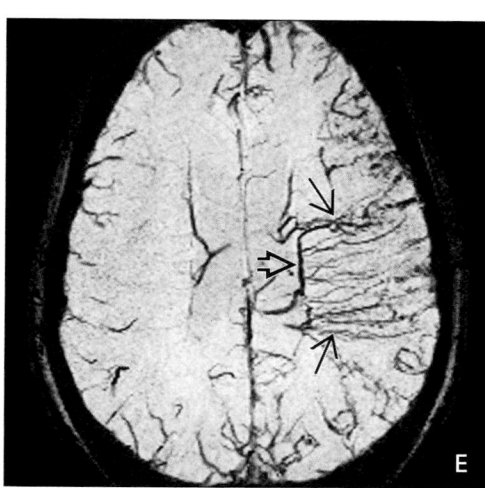

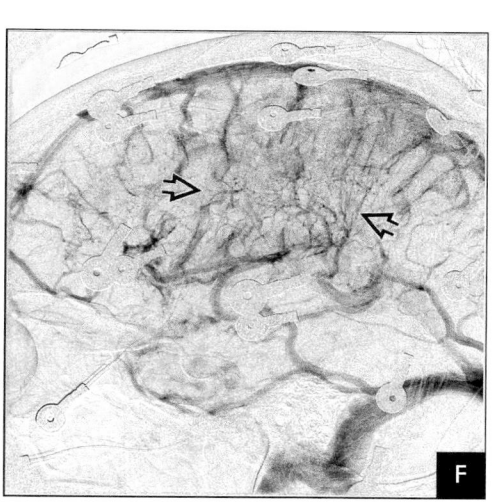

40-6E. *Axial T2* susceptibility-weighted image (SWI) beautifully demonstrates deoxyhemoglobin in the enlarged, tortuous medullary veins* ➡ *that are slowly draining the adjacent brain into enlarged subependymal veins* ➡. **40-6F.** *Venous phase DSA in the same patient performed as part of a Wada test for language localization shows a paucity of normal cortical veins with a prolonged vascular "blush" caused by contrast stasis in multiple enlarged medullary veins* ➡.

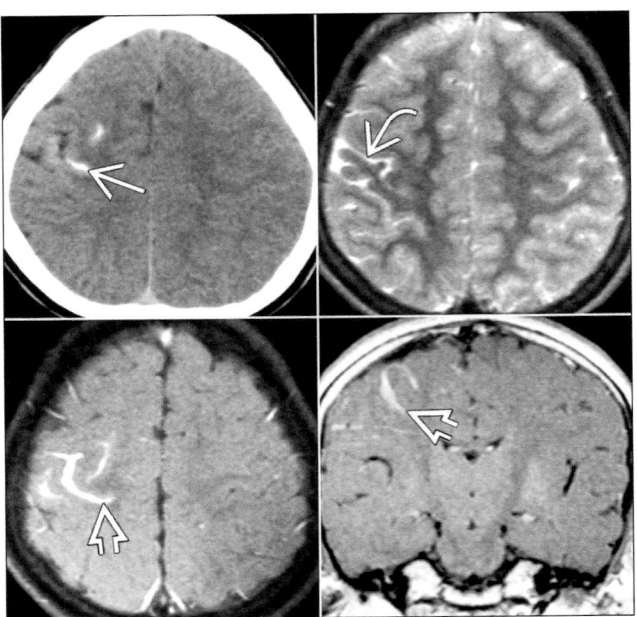

40-7. *Variant SWS case shows focal Ca++* ➡, *atrophy* ➡, *and a very localized enhancing pial angioma that fills just a few adjacent sulci* ➡.

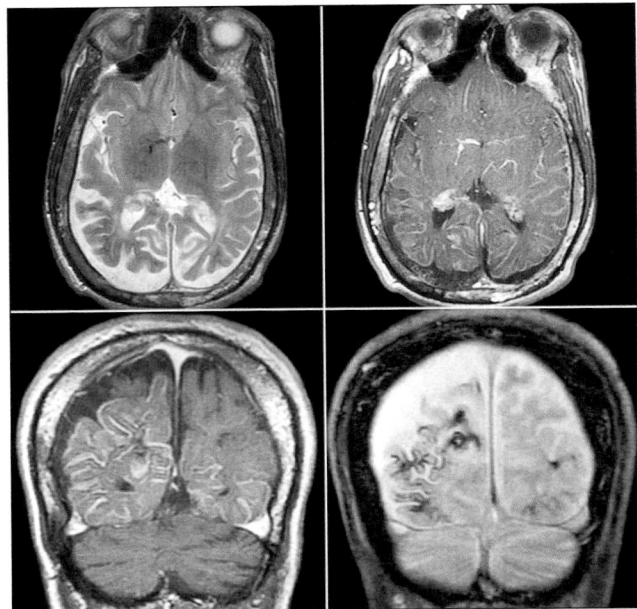

40-8. *Series of images from a patient with Klippel-Trenaunay-Weber syndrome shows bilateral pial angiomas.*

ANGIOGRAPHY. DSA typically demonstrates a lack of superficial cortical veins with corresponding dilatation of deep medullary and subependymal veins **(40-6F)**. The arterial phase is normal.

Differential Diagnosis

The major differential diagnoses of SWS are other vascular neurocutaneous syndromes. Patients with **meningioangiomatosis** (MA) typically lack the facial nevus flammeus seen in SWS. The meningeal angioma of MA often extends into the adjacent brain along the perivascular spaces.

Klippel-Trenaunay-Weber syndrome shares some CNS features of SWS (i.e., pial angiomas) **(40-8)**. KTWS is characterized by osseous/soft tissue hemihypertrophy (95% involve the legs), cutaneous capillary malformations (usually in the enlarged limb), and extremity vascular malformations (varicose veins or venous malformations).

Patients with **PHACES** (**p**osterior fossa malformations, **h**emangioma, **a**rterial cerebrovascular anomalies, **c**oarctation of the aorta and cardiac defects, **e**ye abnormalities, and **s**ternal clefting or supraumbilical raphe) have posterior fossa malformations plus cardiac and vascular anomalies (see below). Cutaneous or ophthalmoscopic findings help differentiate other vascular neurocutaneous syndromes such as **blue rubber bleb nevus syndrome** (bluish venous blebs) and **Wyburn-Mason syndrome** (multiple retinal, cerebral, and facial arteriovenous malformations) from SWS.

A recently described syndrome called **renal lymphangiomatosis and interrupted inferior vena cava** features persistent primitive hepatic venous plexus, hemihypertrophy, and meningeal angiomas similar to those seen in SWS and KTWS. This syndrome and **cutis marmorata telangiectasia congenita** may be overlapping entities within a spectrum of vascular neurocutaneous syndromes.

STURGE-WEBER SYNDROME

Etiology
- Congenital but sporadic, not inherited
- Visual cortex, optic vesicle, upper face juxtaposed in early embryo
- Somatic mutation results in persistence of primitive veins, lack of definitive cortical veins?

Pathology
- Pial ("leptomeningeal") angioma
- Cortical venous ischemia, atrophy
- Parietooccipital > frontal

Clinical Issues
- Unilateral facial nevus flammeus ("port-wine stain")
- Usual cutaneous distribution = CN V I$_1$, V$_2$ > V$_3$

Imaging
- CT: Atrophic cortex
  ◦ Ipsilateral calvaria thick, sinuses enlarged
  ◦ Cortical Ca++ (*not* in angioma!) ↑ with age
- MR: Cortical/subcortical hypointensity on T2
  ◦ Ca++ "blooms" on T2*
  ◦ Pial angioma enhances
  ◦ Ipsilateral choroid plexus enlarged

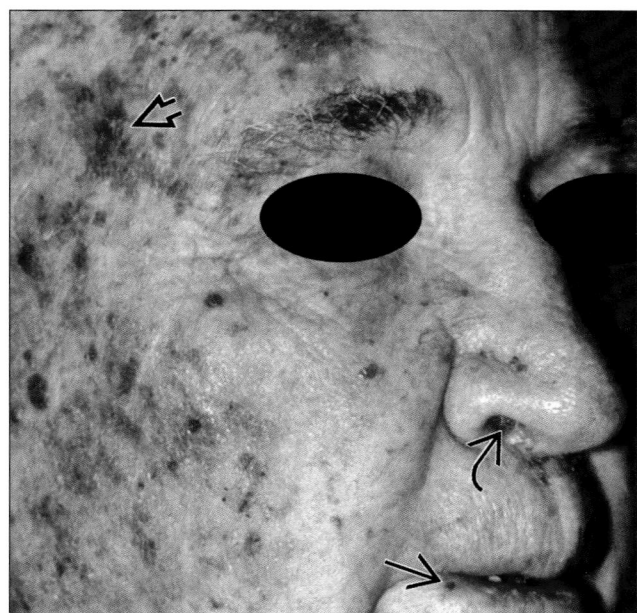

40-9. *Clinical photograph of a patient with HHT and multiple episodes of severe epistaxis shows multiple mucocutaneous telangiectasias of the scalp* ⊃*, nose* ⊃*, lips* ⊃*.*

40-10. *ECA (top), ICA (bottom) angiograms in patient with HHT and epistaxis shows tiny capillary telangiectases* ⊃ *in the nasal, orbital mucosa.*

Other Vascular Phakomatoses

Hereditary Hemorrhagic Telangiectasia

Terminology

Hereditary hemorrhagic telangiectasia (HHT) is also known as Osler-Weber-Rendu or Rendu-Osler-Weber syndrome. HHT is an autosomal dominant monogenetic disorder characterized by widely distributed, multisystem angiodysplastic lesions.

Etiology

Mutations in at least five genes can result in HHT. Mutations in three (*ENG*, *ACVRL1/ALK1*, and *SMAD4*) cause approximately 85% of cases. *ENG* (endoglin) gene mutations cause **type 1 HHT** and are associated with mucocutaneous telangiectases, early onset of epistaxis, pulmonary arteriovenous fistulas (AVFs), and brain arteriovenous malformations (AVMs). *ACVRL1/ALK1* mutation causes **type 2 HHT**, is associated with lower penetrance and milder disease, and presents primarily as GI bleeds and pulmonary arterial hypertension. *SMAD4* mutations cause **HHT/juvenile polyposis combined syndrome**.

Pathology

Multiple brain AVMs are found in 10-40% of patients with HHT and are highly predictive of the diagnosis. Capillary telangiectasias are common in the skin and mucous membranes of patients with HHT but are relatively rare in the brain.

Paradoxical emboli can pass through pulmonary AVFs and result in TIAs, strokes, and cerebral abscesses.

Clinical Issues

EPIDEMIOLOGY AND DEMOGRAPHICS. HHT is a rare but probably underdiagnosed disease, with a prevalence of 1-2:10,000. There is no gender predilection.

PRESENTATION. The most common features of HHT are nosebleeds and telangiectases on the lips, hands, and oral mucosa **(40-9)**. Epistaxis typically begins by age 10, and 80-90% have nosebleeds by age 21 **(40-10)**. The onset of visible telangiectases is generally 5-30 years later than for epistaxis. Almost 95% of affected individuals eventually develop mucocutaneous telangiectases.

NATURAL HISTORY. HHT displays age-related penetrance with increasing manifestations developing over a lifetime; penetrance approaches 100% by age 40. Epistaxis increases in frequency and severity and, in some cases, can require multiple transfusions or even become life-threatening. Approximately 25% of adults with HHT eventually develop gastrointestinal bleeding.

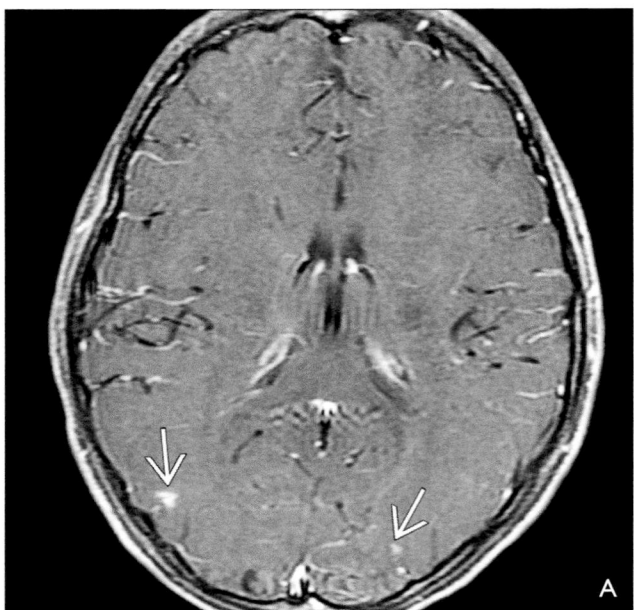

40-11A. Axial T1 C+ FS scan in an 11-year-old girl with HHT shows 2 small enhancing foci ➡.

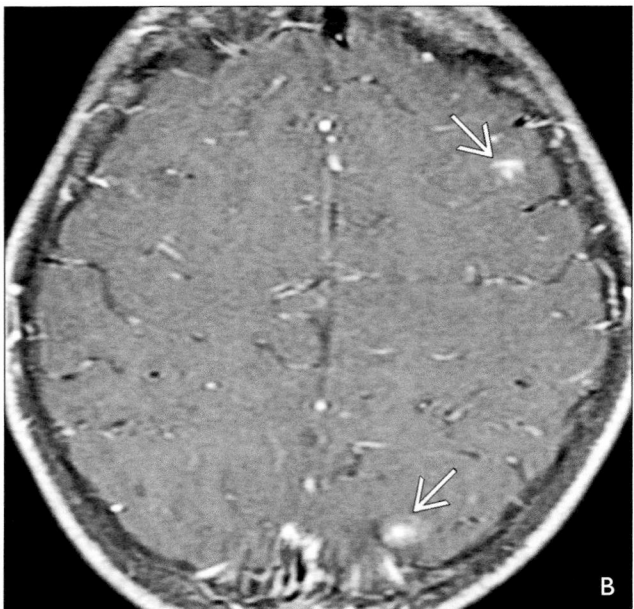

40-11B. T1 C+ FS scan through the corona radiata demonstrates 2 additional enhancing lesions ➡. Presumed multiple "micro" AVMs.

TREATMENT OPTIONS. Laser coagulation of mucosal telangiectases can be effective. Cerebral AVMs > 1.0 cm in diameter are usually treated with surgery, embolotherapy, and/or stereotactic radiosurgery.

Imaging

Brain MR without and with contrast enhancement is the recommended screening procedure for patients diagnosed with HHT and, when possible, should be obtained within the first six months of life. Molecular diagnostics may obviate further imaging. In adults, if no AVMs are detected on initial MR scans, further screening for cerebral AVMs is unnecessary.

AVMs are the most common intracranial vascular malformations. Although some HHT-associated AVMs are large, the majority are small (Spetzler-Martin grade 1 or 2) or even "micro" AVMs **(40-12)**. Large lesions can demonstrate prominent "flow voids" on T2WI; small lesions are seen as punctate enhancing foci on T1 C+ studies **(40-11)**.

Other reported imaging findings in HHT are pallidal (globus pallidus, cerebral peduncles) hyperintensities on T1WI, possibly caused by manganese overload. Less common HHT-associated cerebrovascular malformations include developmental venous anomalies and cavernous malformations.

HEREDITARY HEMORRHAGIC TELANGIECTASIA

Terminology
- Also known as Rendu-Osler-Weber syndrome
- Multisystem angiodysplastic disorder

Etiology
- Type 1 HHT: Endoglin (*ENG*) mutation
  - Mucocutaneous telangiectases, epistaxis, pulmonary AVFs/brain AVMs
- Type 2 HHT: *ACVRL1/ALK1* mutation
  - Milder; predominantly GI bleeds

Pathology
- Multiple brain AVMs (10-40%)
- Capillary telangiectases (mucocutaneous; rare in brain)

Clinical Issues
- Epistaxis: 80-90% by age 21
- Visible telangiectases 5-30 years later
- Manifestations increase with age

Imaging
- Multiple AVMs
  - Most are Spetzler grades 1, 2; often "micro"
  - Best demonstrated on MR without/with contrast
- Other vascular malformations less common

PHACES Syndrome

Terminology

PHACES syndrome is an acronym for **p**osterior fossa malformations, **h**emangioma, **a**rterial cerebrovascular anomalies, **c**oarctation of the aorta and cardiac defects, **e**ye abnormalities, and **s**ternal clefting or supraumbilical raphe. PHACES is diagnosed when a **craniofacial**

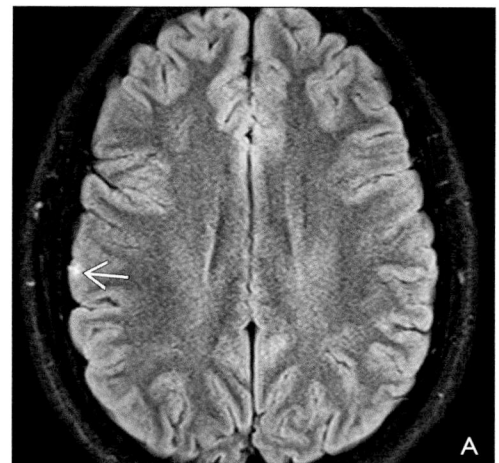

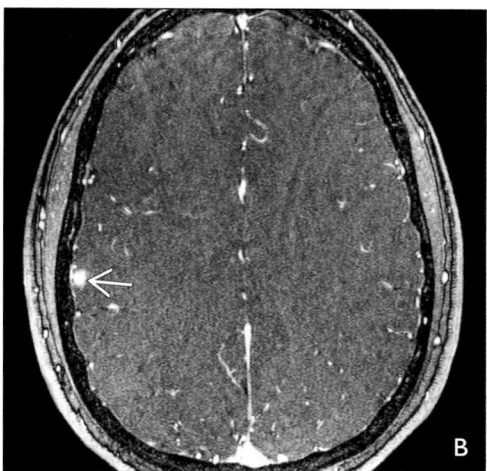

40-12A. FLAIR scan in a 17-year-old asymptomatic male with a family history of HHT is normal except for a tiny hyperintensity ➔ located in the cortex of the right hemisphere. 40-12B. Source image from the contrast-enhanced MRA performed as part of the screening study shows that the lesion ➔ enhances intensely, uniformly.

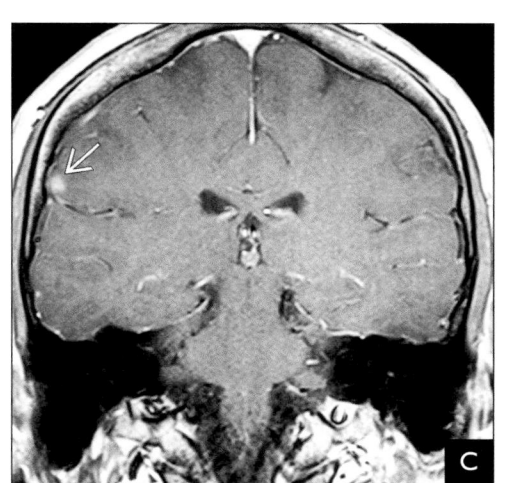

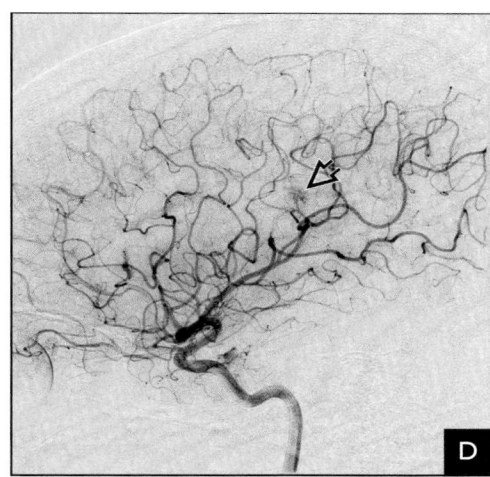

40-12C. Standard coronal T1 C+ scan shows that the lesion ➔ has faint brush-like borders. 40-12D. Right internal carotid angiogram, arterial phase, lateral view in the same patient shows a tiny "tangle" of abnormal vessels ➔ in the anterior parietal lobe.

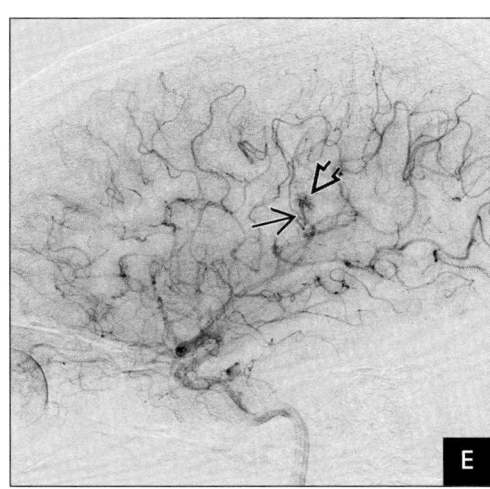

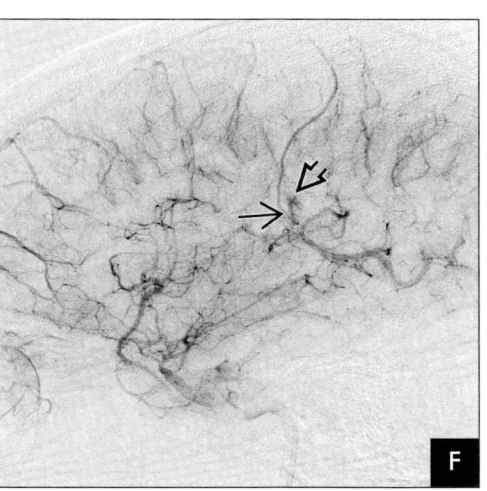

40-12E. Late arterial-early capillary phase image in the same patient shows a linear focus of enhancement ➔ extending inferiorly from the lesion ➔ consistent with an "early draining" vein. 40-12F. Late capillary-early venous phase study shows contrast persisting in the lesion ➔ and "early draining" vein ➔. Classic "micro" AVM of HHT.

hemangioma is present together with one or more of these characteristic extracutaneous anomalies.

Etiology

The precise etiology of PHACES is unknown. The infantile hemangioma and cerebral vasculopathy appear to be linked by an insult occurring early in embryogenesis, probably during the fifth fetal week or even earlier. Segmental neural crest cell disturbances could result in the formation of facial and intracranial hemangiomas in the same embryonic metamere. Neural crest cells also contribute to formation of the optic vesicles, possibly explaining the eye malformations that often occur as part of the PHACES syndrome.

Pathology

Hemangiomas are—by definition—found in 100% of PHACES patients. Hemangiomas are the most common benign tumor of infancy, occurring in 2-3% of neonates and 10-12% of children under one year of age. Hemangiomas are true vascular neoplasms. The majority are sporadic nonsyndromic lesions; approximately 20% meet the other diagnostic criteria for PHACES.

CUTANEOUS HEMANGIOMAS. The topographic distribution of PHACES-associated hemangiomas is significant. Patients with lesions in the upper half of the face typically have structural brain, cerebrovascular, and ocular abnormalities **(40-13)** whereas hemangiomas in a mandibular or beard-like distribution are associated with ventral developmental defects such as sternal abnormalities and supraumbilical raphe.

The hemangiomas in PHACES can be single (70%) or multiple (30%). Trans- and multispatial lesions are common.

EXTRACUTANEOUS HEMANGIOMAS. Extracutaneous hemangiomas occur in 20-25% of patients. The subglottis is the most common site and can cause potentially life-threatening airway obstruction.

Ophthalmologic findings are present in 30% of cases. Choroidal hemangiomas, colobomas, microphthalmos, and optic atrophy are common eye lesions in PHACES.

40-13. Clinical photograph of a patient with PHACES shows a typical facial infantile hemangioma. (Courtesy S. Yashar, MD.) 40-14A. T2WI in an infant with PHACES shows a hemangioma filling the right orbit ➡, extending posteriorly into the cavernous sinus ⬌ and cerebellopontine angle ⬅. Note hypoplasia of the ipsilateral cerebellar hemisphere ⬆.

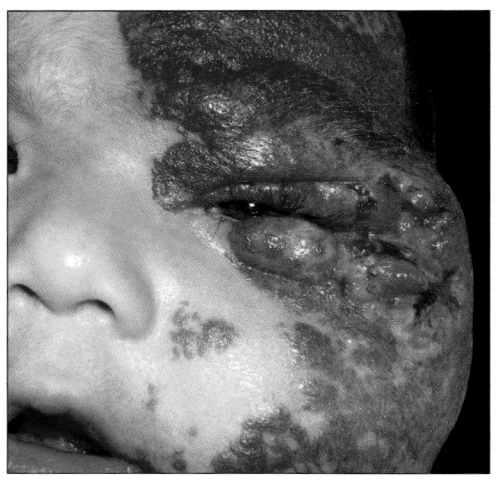
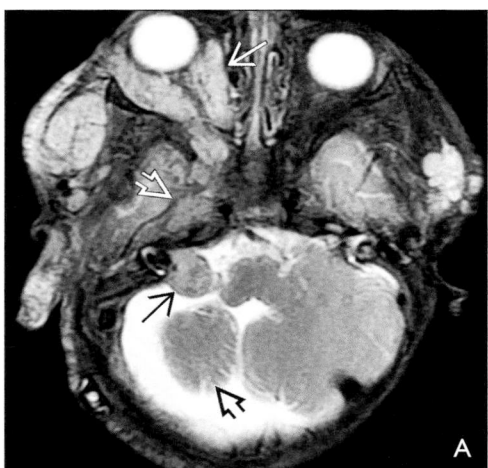

40-14B. Axial T1 C+ FS in the same patient shows intensely enhancing hemangiomas in massively enlarged parotid glands ➡ and right ear ➡. Hemangioma also infiltrates the scalp ➡ and posterior cervical space. 40-14C. More cephalad T1 C+ FS scan shows the intracranial extension of the hemangioma into the cavernous sinus ➡ and CPA cistern ➡.

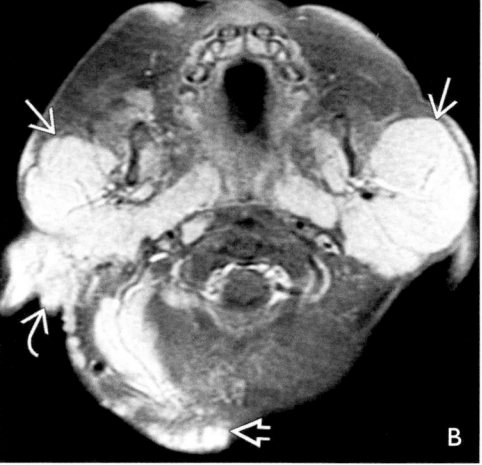
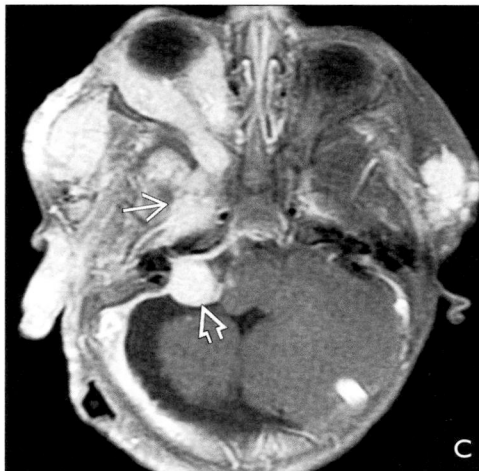

Although not included in the acronym PHACES, otologic abnormalities are also common. These include middle ear atelectasis, tympanic membrane hemangiomas with conductive hearing loss, skin and cartilage ulcerations, and dysphagia.

INTRACRANIAL HEMANGIOMAS. Intracranial hemangiomas are relatively uncommon. When present, they exhibit a predilection for the cavernous sinus and cerebellopontine angle cistern and are generally ipsilateral to the facial hemangioma.

OTHER INTRACRANIAL MALFORMATIONS. Nonvascular intracranial malformations are present in half of all PHACES patients. Posterior fossa malformations are identified in 50-75% of these cases, most commonly ipsilateral cerebellar hypoplasia. Other associated anomalies include Dandy-Walker spectrum malformations, corpus callosum dysgenesis, septi pellucidi anomalies, polymicrogyria, gray matter heterotopias, and arachnoid cysts.

NONCUTANEOUS SYSTEMIC MANIFESTATIONS. Over 90% of PHACES patients have more than one extracutaneous finding. Ventral developmental defects such as sternal clefting and supraumbilical raphe are common. Two-thirds of all patients have vasculopathy or exhibit cardiac anomalies.

PHACES-related vasculopathy includes a number of congenital and progressive large vessel lesions. Arterial anomalies of the craniocervical vasculature are seen in over 75% of patients. Aortic coarctation (35%), arterial occlusions (21%), progressive stenoses (18%), and saccular aneurysms (13%) are the most common potentially symptomatic anomalies. Persistent embryonic arteries (most often a persistent trigeminal artery) are seen in 17% of cases. Aberrant course or origin, dolichoectasia, and dysgenesis/agenesis of the internal carotid and/or vertebral arteries and circle of Willis are also frequent anomalies.

Clinical Issues

EPIDEMIOLOGY AND DEMOGRAPHICS. PHACES is a rare syndrome, but the exact incidence is unknown. The F:M ratio is 9:1.

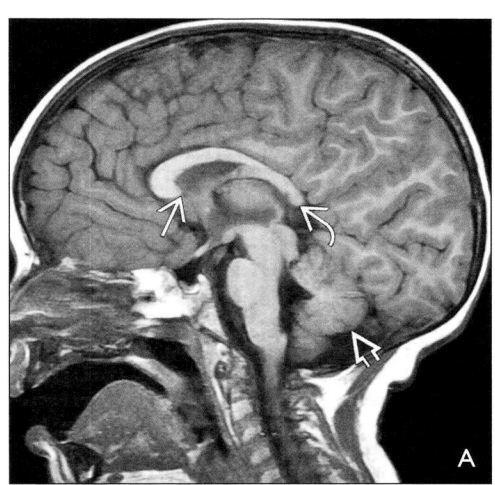

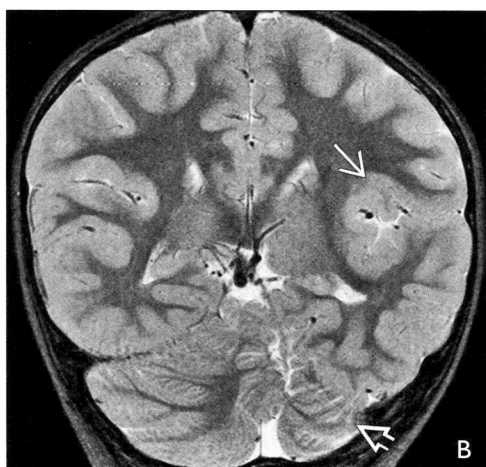

40-15A. Sagittal T1WI in a 3-year-old boy with known PHACES and a prominent facial hemangioma at birth shows cerebellar hypoplasia ➡, corpus callosum dysgenesis with absent rostrum ➡, and truncated hypoplastic splenium ➡. 40-15B. Coronal T2WI shows the hypoplastic, malformed left cerebellar hemisphere ➡ and thickened, dysplastic perisylvian gray matter ➡.

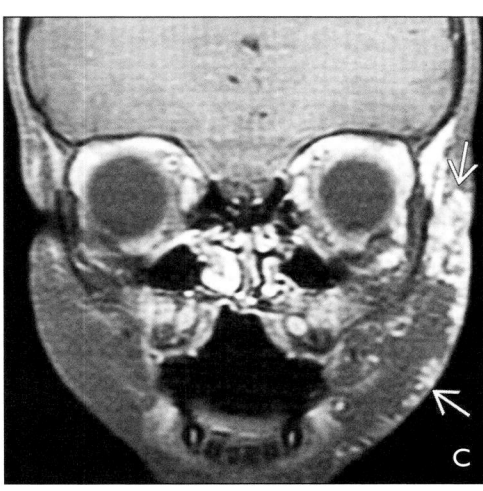

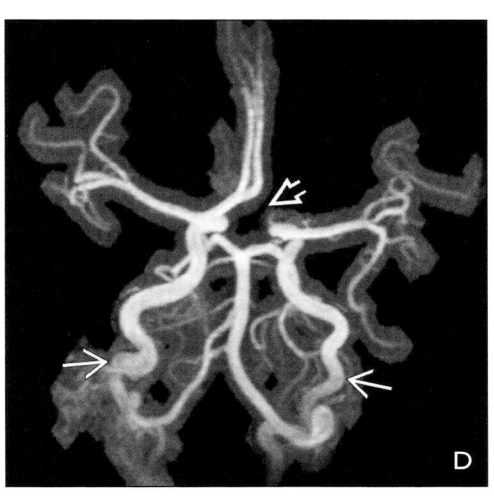

40-15C. Coronal T1 C+ FS scan shows enhancing residual facial hemangioma ➡. 40-15D. MRA shows absent A1 ➡, moderately tortuous ectatic cervical internal carotid arteries ➡.

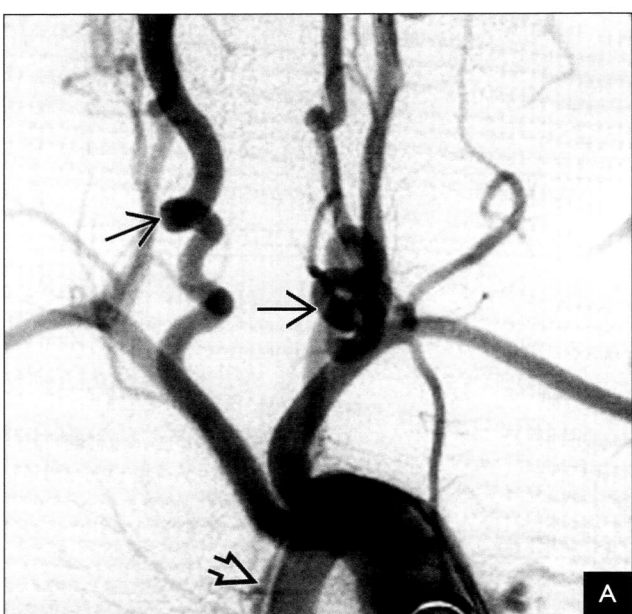

40-16A. *AP DSA demonstrates extracranial vasculopathy in a patient with PHACES with right aortic arch ⊳ and tortuous, ectatic common carotid arteries ⇒. (Courtesy C. Robson, MBChB.)*

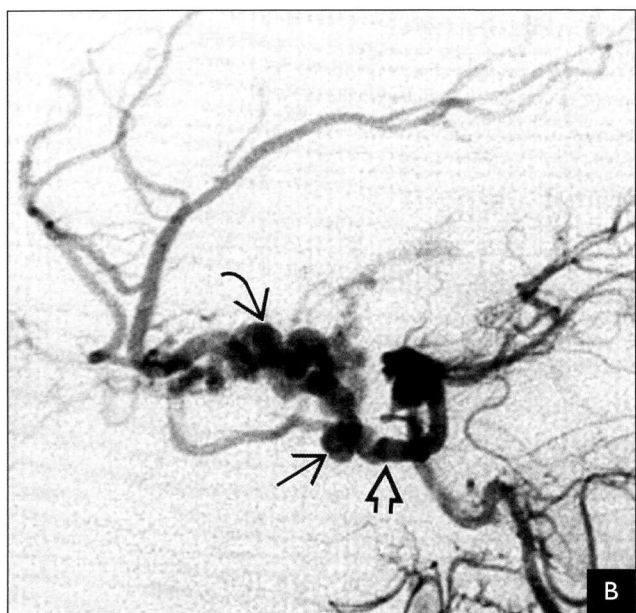

40-16B. *PHACES vasculopathy with absent internal carotid artery, persistent trigeminal artery ⊳ with saccular aneurysm ⇒, and tortuous, ectatic ACA ⇒. (Courtesy C. Robson, MBChB.)*

PRESENTATION. The cutaneous hemangiomas in PHACES are typically bulky, plaque-like geographic lesions **(40-13)**. Unlike the nevus flammeus of Sturge-Weber syndrome, PHACES-related hemangiomas are not always confined to a specific dermatome and are often transspatial.

NATURAL HISTORY. The prognosis in PHACES typically depends on the type and severity of the associated anomalies, not the hemangioma itself. Hemangiomas generally proliferate during the first year of life and then involute spontaneously over the next five to seven years (or more). Most remain asymptomatic and are managed by close observation. Occasionally hemangiomas behave more aggressively, causing visual impairment, skeletal deformities, airway obstruction, high-output cardiac failure, bleeding, or ulceration.

TREATMENT OPTIONS. Treatment options for symptomatic hemangiomas include steroids or propranolol and pulsed dye laser. Saccular aneurysms can be treated by coiling or clipping whereas progressive stenoocclusive disease is sometimes treated with neurosurgical revascularization.

Imaging

CT FINDINGS. NECT may demonstrate soft tissue masses in the orbit, face, and neck as well as cerebellar hypoplasia. CECT depicts hemangiomas as lobulated or plaque-like, intensely enhancing, infiltrating masses. Bone CT may show a small or absent carotid canal.

MR FINDINGS. MR is the best technique to evaluate the presence and extent of craniofacial hemangiomas and to delineate coexisting intracranial malformations **(40-14)**.

T1 scans depict callosal dysgenesis and cerebellar anomalies **(40-15)**. Gray matter heterotopias are best seen on T2WI. Proliferating hemangiomas appear hyperintense on T2WI and may exhibit prominent internal "flow voids." Intense homogeneous enhancement following contrast administration is typical.

ANGIOGRAPHY. Angiography (CTA, MRA, and DSA) detects vessel anomalies and is especially important for identifying saccular aneurysms and stenoocclusive disease **(40-16)**.

Various anomalies of the craniofacial vasculature occur in PHACES patients. These include hypoplasia or aplasia of the internal carotid or vertebral arteries, aberrant origin and/or course of cranial arteries, persistent embryonic vascular anastomoses (typically persistent trigeminal artery), kinking and/or ectasia of major arteries, saccular aneurysms, and progressive arterial stenoses.

Differential Diagnosis

The major differential diagnosis of PHACES is **Sturge-Weber syndrome** (SWS). The facial hemangioma can be (and often is) mistaken for the port-wine stain (nevus flammeus) of SWS. Patients with SWS lack the noncutaneous systemic manifestations of PHACES. The leptomeningeal angioma of SWS appears relatively thin and serpentine, covering the pial surface of the underlying dystrophic cortex, which is shrunken and contains linear

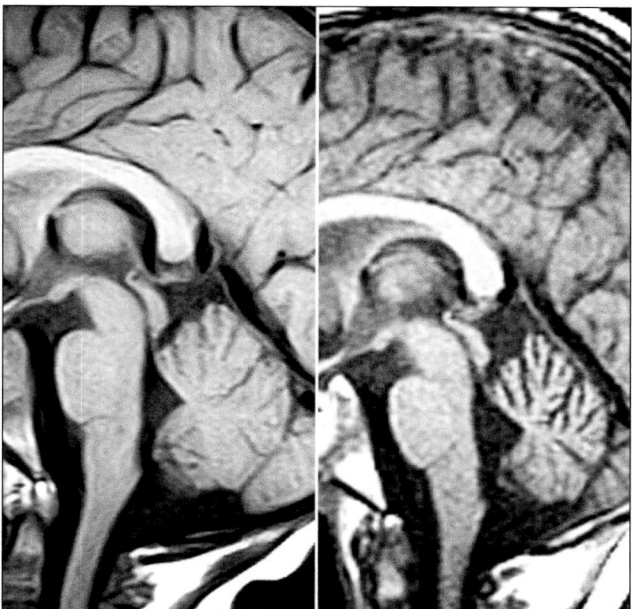

40-17. (Left) Baseline scan in an 18-month-old boy with AT is normal. (Right) Marked vermian atrophy at 4.5 years. (Courtesy S. Blaser, MD.)

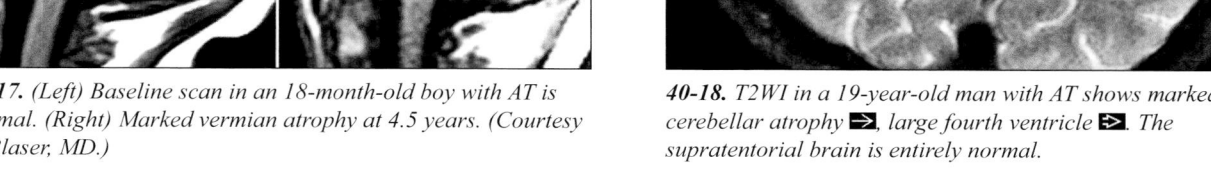

40-18. T2WI in a 19-year-old man with AT shows marked cerebellar atrophy ➔, large fourth ventricle ➔. The supratentorial brain is entirely normal.

calcifications. The intracranial hemangioma of PHACES usually involves the cavernous sinus and/or cerebello-pontine angle, appearing more focal and mass-like.

PHACES SYNDROME

Terminology
- **P**osterior fossa malformations
- **H**emangioma
- **A**rterial cerebrovascular anomalies
- **C**oarctation of the aorta and cardiac defects
- **E**ye abnormalities
- **S**ternal clefting or supraumbilical raphe

Pathology
- Hemangiomas (vascular neoplasm, not malformation)
- Ipsilateral cerebellar hypoplasia
- Arterial stenoses/occlusions, saccular aneurysms, aberrant vessels

Clinical Issues
- Hemangiomas proliferate, then involute

Imaging
- T1 C+ FS MR to delineate hemangiomas
- CTA/MRA to evaluate for vascular anomalies

Ataxia-Telangiectasia

Terminology and Etiology

Ataxia-telangiectasia (AT), also known as Louis-Bar syndrome, is a rare autosomal recessive disorder characterized by oculocutaneous telangiectasias and ataxia. AT is caused by a mutation in chromosome 11q22-23 that encodes a particular nuclear kinase (i.e., ATM) needed to detect damaged DNA.

Pathology

The major neuropathologic findings of AT occur in the cerebellum. The cerebellar hemispheres and vermis show marked atrophy, reflecting the pronounced loss of Purkinje and granule cells that is the pathologic marker of this disease.

At least one-third of all AT patients develop malignancies. Acute lymphoblastic leukemia and lymphoma predominate in younger patients. Nonlymphoid epithelial tumors, mainly carcinomas, represent 15-25% of AT-related neoplasms and develop primarily in adults.

Clinical Issues

AT patients demonstrate heterogeneous clinical manifestations. Mucocutaneous telangiectasis usually begin to appear in early childhood but may be minimal or absent. Neurologic findings include hyperkinesia, cerebellar ataxia, dysarthria, and progressive neurodegeneration. AT patients also exhibit variable humoral and cellular immunodeficiency with recurrent infections as well as acute sensitivity to ionizing radiation.

Imaging and Differential Diagnosis

Imaging studies show mild to moderate nonspecific cerebellar atrophy **(40-17), (40-18)**. Multiple capillary telangiectasias in the cerebral hemispheres, cerebellum, and brainstem can be seen as faint brush-like enhancing foci on T1 C+ scans or multifocal "blooming black dots" on T2* (GRE, SWI) sequences. MRS may show increased Cho in the cerebellum.

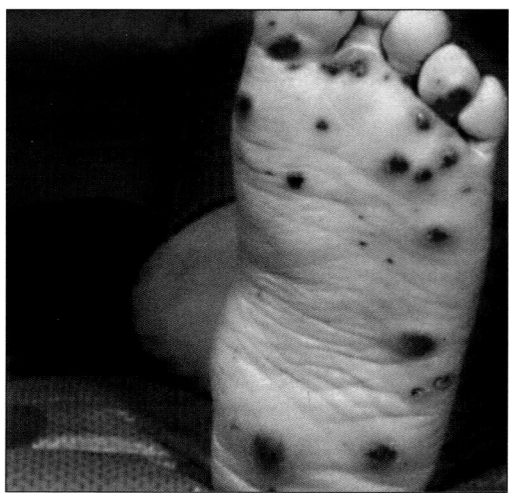

40-19. *Photo of patient with BRBNS shows multiple elevated, bluish skin "blebs" on the foot. (Courtesy AFIP Archives.)*

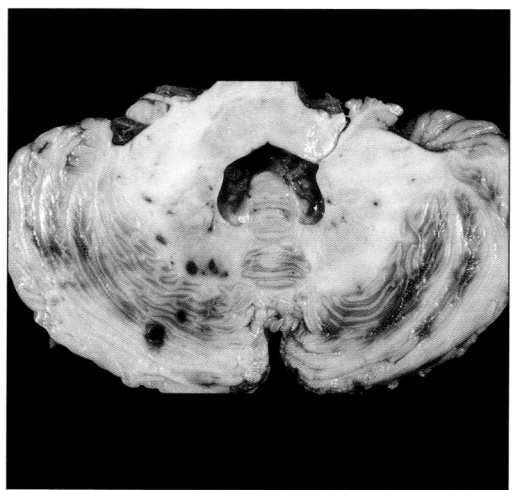

40-20. *Axial cut section through the cerebellum. Multiple developmental venous anomalies (DVAs) characteristic of BRBNS. (R. Hewlett, MD.)*

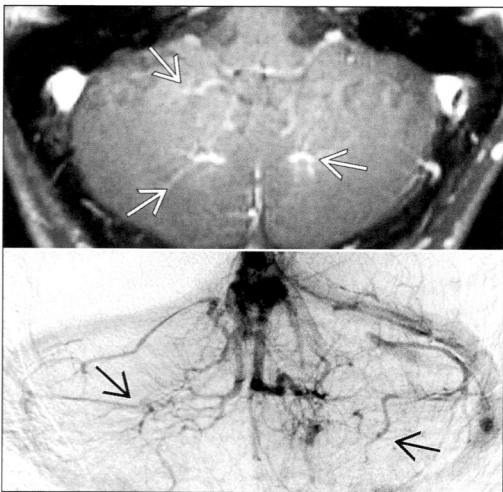

40-21. *(Top) T1 C+ FS scan in a patient with probable BRBNS shows bilateral enhancing DVAs* ⮕. *(Bottom) AP DSA shows bilateral DVAs* ⮕.

The major clinical differential diagnoses of AT are **cerebral palsy** and **Friedrich ataxia**. Serum α-fetoprotein (AFP) is markedly elevated in AT and helps distinguish the disorder.

Unless imaging evidence for multiple cutaneous and/or brain capillary telangiectasias is present, the cerebellar atrophy can be indistinguishable from an ever-growing number of recessive **inherited spinocerebellar degenerations with progressive ataxia**. Elevated Cho on MRS may help distinguish early AT from other forms of ataxia.

Blue Rubber Bleb Nevus Syndrome

Blue rubber bleb nevus syndrome (BRBNS), also known as Bean syndrome, is a rare disorder characterized by multiple venous malformations. BRBNS can be sporadic or inherited as an autosomal dominant disorder associated with chromosome 9p mutation.

BRBNS usually affects the skin, oral cavity, and gastrointestinal tract. The most common presentation is iron deficiency anemia caused by intestinal bleeding. Small, bluish, soft, and compressible ("bleb-like") nevi are the clinical hallmarks of this disorder **(40-19)**.

CNS lesions occur in 15-20% of cases. Reported imaging manifestations include an extensive network of developmental venous anomalies with or without sinus pericranii **(40-20)**, **(40-21)**.

Selected References

Sturge-Weber Syndrome

- Jagtap S et al: Sturge-Weber syndrome: clinical spectrum, disease course, and outcome of 30 patients. J Child Neurol. Epub ahead of print, 2012
- Lo W et al: Updates and future horizons on the understanding, diagnosis, and treatment of Sturge-Weber syndrome brain involvement. Dev Med Child Neurol. 54(3):214-23, 2012
- Watson T et al: Renal lymphangiomatosis, interrupted IVC with persistent primitive hepatic venous plexus and multiple anomalous venous channels: parts of an overlap syndrome? Pediatr Radiol. 42(2):253-6, 2012
- Comi AM: Presentation, diagnosis, pathophysiology, and treatment of the neurological features of Sturge-Weber syndrome. Neurologist. 17(4):179-84, 2011
- Wu J et al: Cortical calcification in Sturge-Weber Syndrome on MRI-SWI: relation to brain perfusion status and seizure severity. J Magn Reson Imaging. 34(4):791-8, 2011
- Puttgen KB et al: Neurocutaneous vascular syndromes. Childs Nerv Syst. 26(10):1407-15, 2010

Other Vascular Phakomatoses

Hereditary Hemorrhagic Telangiectasia

- Bharatha A et al: Brain arteriovenous malformation multiplicity predicts the diagnosis of hereditary hemorrhagic telangiectasia: quantitative assessment. Stroke. 43(1):72-8, 2012
- Eyries M et al: ACVRL1 germinal mosaic with two mutant alleles in hereditary hemorrhagic telangiectasia associated with pulmonary arterial hypertension. Clin Genet. 82(2):173-179, 2012
- Oikonomou A et al: Basal ganglia hyperintensity on T1-weighted MRI in Rendu-Osler-Weber disease. J Magn Reson Imaging. 35(2):426-30, 2012
- McDonald J et al: Hereditary hemorrhagic telangiectasia: an overview of diagnosis, management, and pathogenesis. Genet Med. 13(7):607-16, 2011

PHACES Syndrome

- Hartzell LD et al: Current management of infantile hemangiomas and their common associated conditions. Otolaryngol Clin North Am. 45(3):545-56, vii, 2012
- Mahadi S et al: PHACES syndrome. Arch Dis Child Fetal Neonatal Ed. 97(3):F209-10, 2012
- Rudnick EF et al: PHACES syndrome: otolaryngic considerations in recognition and management. Int J Pediatr Otorhinolaryngol. 73(2):281-8, 2009
- Castillo M: PHACES syndrome: from the brain to the face via the neural crest cells. AJNR Am J Neuroradiol. 29(4):814-5, 2008
- Heyer GL et al: The cerebral vasculopathy of PHACES syndrome. Stroke. 39(2):308-16, 2008

Ataxia-Telangiectasia

- Oza VS et al: PHACES association: a neuroradiologic review of 17 patients. AJNR Am J Neuroradiol. 29(4):807-13, 2008
- Hadjivassiliou M et al: MR spectroscopy and atrophy in Gluten, Friedreich's and SCA6 ataxias. Acta Neurol Scand. 126(2):138-43, 2012
- Wallis LI et al: Proton spectroscopy and imaging at 3T in ataxia-telangiectasia. AJNR Am J Neuroradiol. 28(1):79-83, 2007

Blue Rubber Bleb Nevus Syndrome

- Deng ZH et al: Diagnosis and treatment of blue rubber bleb nevus syndrome in children. World J Pediatr. 4(1):70-3, 2008

41

Anomalies of the
Skull and Meninges

Anomalies of the skull and meninges represent maldevelopment of the embryonic mesenchyme. These include cephaloceles, other skull base defects such as nasal "gliomas" or dermoids, congenital calvarial defects, and other meningeal malformations including lipomas.

We previously discussed how the brain itself develops in Chapter 35. This final chapter of the book focuses on anomalies of the brain coverings, the skull and meninges. We begin with skull base embryology, which is key to understanding the malformations discussed.

Normal Development and Anatomy of the Skull Base

Embryology

The skull base (SB) arises primarily from cartilaginous precursors that ossify in an orderly manner from poste-

rior to anterior and from lateral to medial. More than 100 separate ossification centers participate in developing the definitive SB **(41-1)**.

Forehead and Nose

Prior to the eighth week of gestation, two transient but important spaces are present in the developing forehead and nose: The fonticulus frontalis and prenasal space. The **fonticulus frontalis** lies between the partially ossified frontal bone above and the nasal bones below. The **prenasal space** is a transient dura-filled structure that lies between the nasal bones and the unossified chondrocranium **(41-2A)**.

As the chondrocranium begins to ossify, it leaves some cartilage in front that later becomes the nasal capsule. By this stage, the fonticulus frontalis has closed. The prenasal space then involutes, leaving a small dural diverticulum anterior to the crista galli called the **foramen cecum**. The foramen cecum continues anteroinferiorly as a transient dura-lined channel called the **anterior neuropore**.

The foramen cecum and anterior neuropore establish a temporary connection between the anterior cranial fossa and the nose **(41-2B)**. The anterior neuropore normally regresses completely, leaving a small remnant of the foramen cecum **(41-2C)**. The foramen cecum is approximately four millimeters in diameter at birth and is normally completely ossified by two years of age.

Skull Base

At birth, the *anterior* skull base is composed mostly of cartilage with relatively limited ossification. Ossification of the crista galli and cribriform plate begins at two months and is nearly complete by two years of age. The foramen cecum ossifies last.

The *central* skull base forms from approximately 24 ossification centers. Major named centers include the presphenoid (planum sphenoidale), postsphenoid (basisphenoid with the posterior half of the sella, dorsum sellae, and upper clivus), alisphenoid (greater sphenoid wing), and orbitosphenoid (lesser sphenoid wing). The **inter-sphenoidal synchondrosis** lies between the presphenoid and the postsphenoid (basisphenoid).

The **sphenooccipital synchondrosis** lies between the basisphenoid and basiocciput. It is one of the last sutures to fuse (not completed until age 15-20 years). The embryonic **craniopharyngeal canal**—a Rathke pouch remnant—is a transient tract from the nasopharynx to the pituitary fossa that passes between chondrification centers for the developing pre- and postsphenoid bones. The craniopharyngeal canal is typically obliterated by the twelfth gestational week. It is replaced by the transient **intersphenoidal synchondrosis**, which normally closes around three postnatal months.

The *posterior* skull base consists primarily of the occipital bone, which has four major ossification centers located around the foramen magnum. In contrast to the anterior and central skull base segments, the posterior skull base is almost completely ossified by birth. However, the sutures remain unfused until the second decade. The petrooccipital and occipitomastoid sutures are among the last of all the cranial sutures to close (15-17 years).

Relevant Gross Anatomy

Here we briefly delineate the important aspects of the anterior and central segments of the skull base. A detailed description of cranial nerves—their origins, courses, and imaging appearances—is included in Chapter 23.

Anterior Skull Base

The *endocranial* surface of the anterior skull base (ASB) forms the floor of the anterior cranial fossae. The endocranial surface is composed of the orbital plates of the frontal bones, the ethmoid bone with its cribriform plate and sinus roof, and the lesser sphenoid wing. The *exocranial* surface of the ASB forms the orbital roofs and abuts the nose.

Important bony landmarks of the endocranial ASB are shown in Figure 41-3. In this specimen, the foramen cecum (1) persists as a small bony midline pit immediately in front of the crista galli (2). The olfactory recesses with the sieve-like cribriform plate (3) lie on either side

41-1. Skull base ossification centers shows sphenooccipital synchondrosis ⊳ (between postsphenoid and basiocciput) and craniopharyngeal canal ⊐ (in intersphenoidal synchondrosis, between pre- and postsphenoid). 41-2A. Developing dura (white), unossified chondrocranium (blue). Fonticulus frontalis ⊐ lies between partially ossified frontal, nasal bones. Prenasal space ⊳ is in dura, between nasal bones/cartilage.

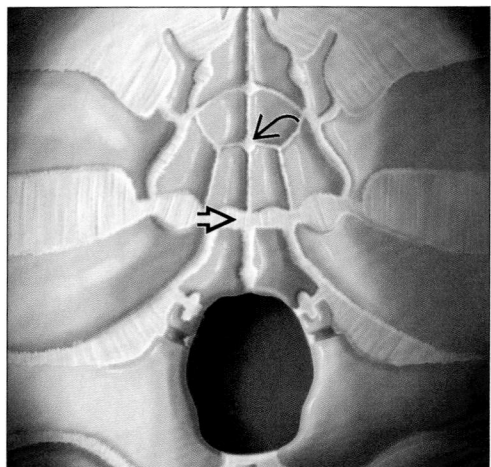
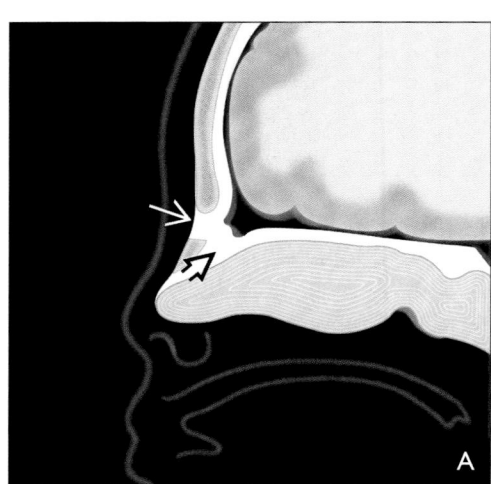

41-2B. Over time, the fonticulus frontalis closes. Chondrocranium is now mostly ossified. Cartilage of developing nasal capsule is shown in blue. Prenasal space, now encased in bone and lined with dura, becomes foramen cecum ⊳. Dura-lined channel ⊐ (anterior neuropore) is open at dorsum of nose ⊐. 41-2C. Graphic depicts a later stage of development, by which point anterior neuropore has regressed. Foramen cecum remnant ⊳, crista galli ⊐ are shown.

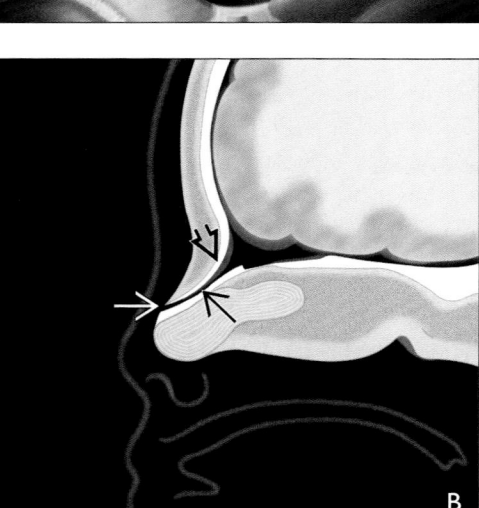
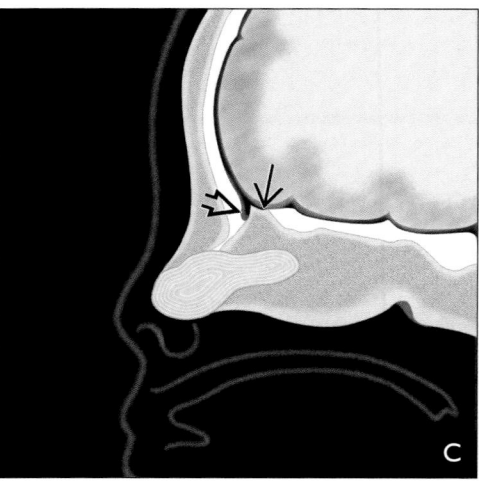

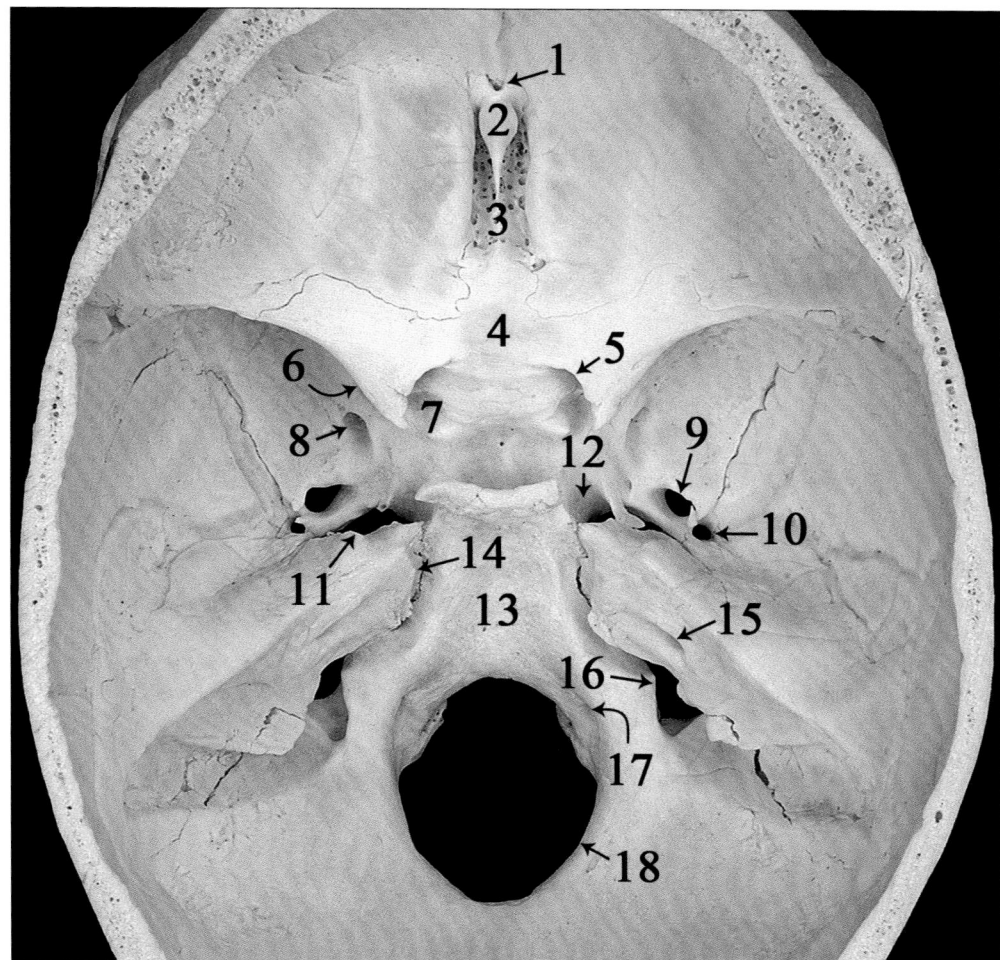

41-3. *Endocranial view, adult skull: Foramen cecum (1), crista galli (2), cribriform plate (3), planum sphenoidale (4), lesser sphenoid wing and optic canal (5), superior orbital fissure (6), endocranial openings of carotid canal (7, 12), foramen rotundum (8), foramen ovale (9), foramen spinosum (10), foramen lacerum (11), clivus (13), petrooccipital fissure (14), IAC (15), jugular foramen (16), jugular tubercle overlying hypoglossal canal (17), foramen magnum (18). (Courtesy M. Nielsen, MS.)*

of the crista galli. A flat bony surface, the planum sphenoidale (4), extends posteriorly from the cribriform plate of the ethmoid bone to the sella turcica.

The lesser wings of the sphenoid bone overhang the optic canals (5), superior orbital fissures (6), and endocranial openings for the internal carotid arteries (7). The optic nerves and ophthalmic arteries pass through the optic canals. The superior orbital fissures transmit the superior orbital veins and oculomotor (CN III) and trochlear (CN IV) nerves, as well as ophthalmic divisions of the trigeminal nerves (CN V_1) and the abducens nerves (CN VI).

Central Skull Base

The endocranial surface of the central skull base (CSB) forms the sella turcica and medial floors of the middle cranial fossae. It is composed of the greater sphenoid wing, the basisphenoid, and the temporal bone anterior to the petrous ridge. A central depression, the sella turcica, is bordered anteriorly by the tuberculum sellae and anterior clinoid processes. The posterior border of the sella is

formed by the dorsum sellae, a prominent bony projection that lies anteromedial to the petrous apices.

Important CSB foramina include the foramen rotundum (8), which transmits the maxillary division of the trigeminal nerve CN V_2, and the foramen ovale (9), which transmits the mandibular nerve CN V_3. The foramen spinosum (10) lies posterolateral to the foramen ovale. The middle meningeal artery enters the cranial cavity through the foramen spinosum.

The foramen lacerum (11) is an irregular cartilage-filled aperture that lies between the sphenoid bone and petrous apex. The internal carotid arteries exit the petrous temporal bone at the endocranial carotid canal (12). The dorsum sellae continues posteroinferiorly as the upper part of a smooth concavity, the clivus (13).

Posterior Skull Base

The posterior skull base (PSB) is formed by the temporal bones posterior to the petrous ridges and the occipi-

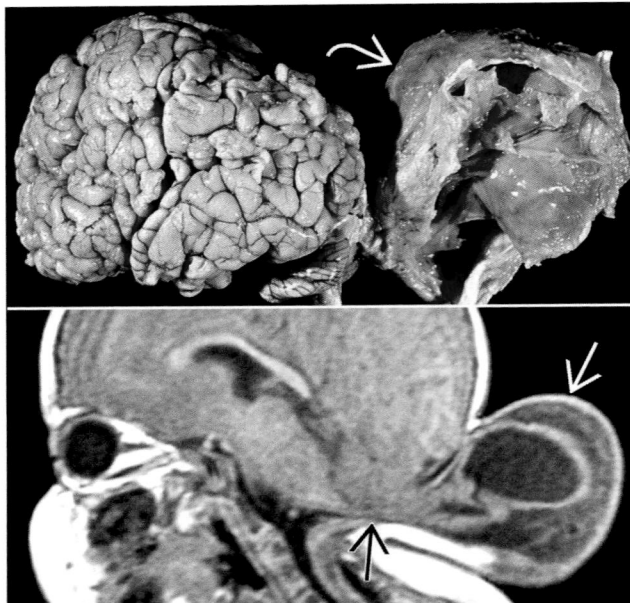

41-4. *(Top) Autopsy shows occipital cephalocele ➘, brain with pachy-/polymicrogyria. (E. T. Hedley-Whyte, MD.) (Bottom) Sagittal T1WI shows occipitocervical meningoencephalocele ➔ with traction of cervicomedullary junction ➔.*

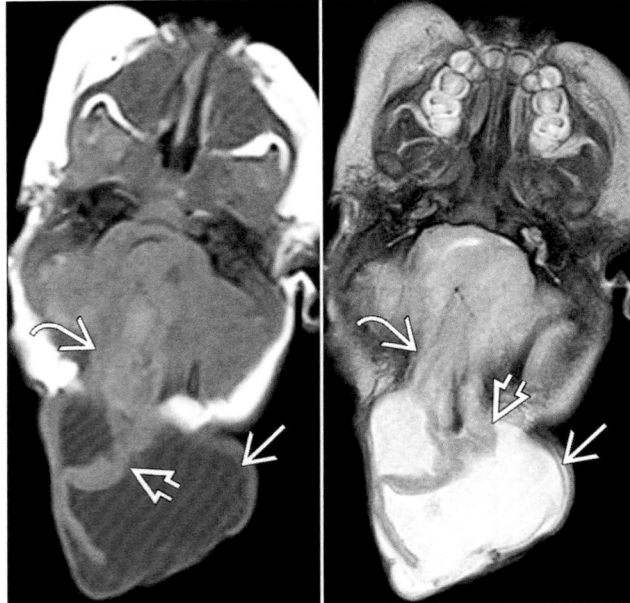

41-5. *(Left) T1WI, (right) T2WI show an occipital cephalocele that contains meninges and CSF ➘, dysplastic brain ➘. Note traction, distortion of the cerebellum ➘.*

tal bone. The petrooccipital fissure (14) lies between the petrous apex and the occipital bone.

The internal acoustic meatus (15) lies along the posterior aspect of the petrous temporal bone and transmits the facial (CN VII) and vestibulocochlear nerves (CN VIII) as well as the labyrinthine artery, which is a small branch of the anterior inferior cerebellar artery.

The jugular foramen (16) lies below the internal acoustic meatus. The jugular foramen transmits CNs IX-XI, the jugular bulb, and the inferior petrosal sinus. The hypoglossal canal (17) transmits CN XII. The foramen magnum (18) contains the medulla, both vertebral arteries, and the spinal segment of CN XI.

Cephaloceles

"Cephalocele" is a generic term for the protrusion of intracranial contents through a calvarial or skull base defect. Cephaloceles that contain herniations of brain tissue, meninges, and CSF are called **meningoencephaloceles**. If the meninges and accompanying CSF are herniated *without* brain tissue, the lesion is termed a **meningocele**. An **atretic cephalocele** is a small defect that contains just dura, fibrous tissue, and degenerated brain tissue. A **gliocele** is a glia-lined pouch that contains only CSF.

Cephaloceles can be congenital or acquired lesions. They are generally classified by location and are named according to the roof and floor of the bone(s) through which they herniate. They can be open or skin-covered. Most congenital cephaloceles have coexisting intracranial abnormalities of varying severity. Cephalocele prevalence and type vary significantly with geographic location and ethnicity.

Cephalocele imaging has four goals: Depict the osseous defect, delineate the sac and define its contents, map the course of adjacent arteries and determine the integrity of the dural venous sinuses, and identify any coexisting anomalies.

We now discuss four of the most common forms of cephalocele: Occipital, frontoethmoidal, parietal, and skull base cephaloceles.

Occipital Cephaloceles

Terminology and Classification

Three subtypes of occipital cephalocele are recognized and identified according to the involved bone(s). From most to least extensive, they are **occipitocervical** (involving the occipital bone, foramen magnum, and neural arches of the upper cervical spine) **(41-4)**, **low occipital** (involving the occipital bone and foramen magnum), and **high occipital** (involving the occipital bone only).

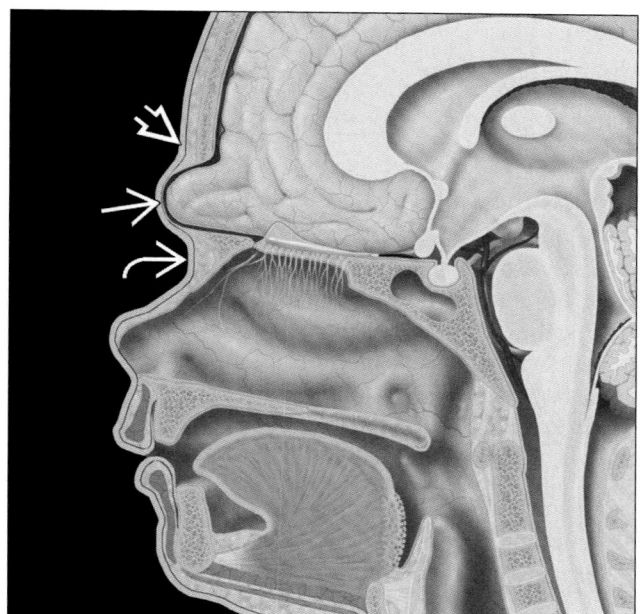

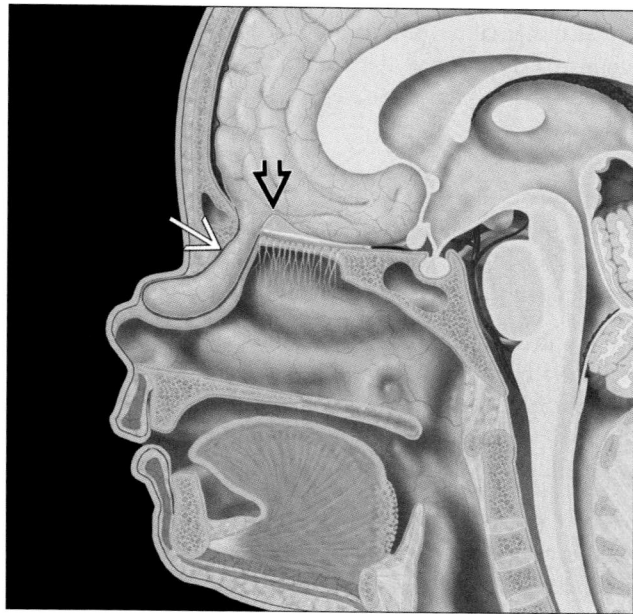

41-6. Graphic depicts frontonasal cephalocele with brain herniating ➡ *through a patent fonticulus frontalis between the frontal bone above* ⧨ *and nasal bone* ⇗ *below.*

41-7. Graphic demonstrates nasoethmoidal cephalocele with brain ➡ *herniating into the nose through a patent foramen cecum in front of the crista galli* ⧨.

Clinical Issues

Occipital cephaloceles account for 75% of cephaloceles in European and North American Caucasians. There is a 2.4:1 male predominance.

Occipital cephaloceles are almost always recognized at birth as a variably sized occipital or suboccipital soft tissue mass. The affected infant is often microcephalic with visible craniofacial disproportion. Neurodevelopmental outcome is related to cephalocele size and contents as well as the presence and type of associated abnormalities.

Imaging

Bone CT with 3D reconstruction delineates the osseous defect well, and multiplanar MR best depicts the sac and its contents. The herniated brain—which can derive from both supra- and infratentorial structures—is always abnormal, appearing dysmorphic, disorganized, and dysplastic (41-5). Depending on the size of the cephalocele, severe traction and distortion of the brainstem and supratentorial structures can be present.

Dura and CSF-filled structures (including the fourth ventricle and sometimes part of the lateral ventricles) are often contained within the sac. In addition to delineating the sac and its contents, identifying the course and integrity of the dural venous sinuses is essential for preoperative planning.

At least half of all patients with occipital cephaloceles have associated abnormalities such as callosal dysgenesis, cerebellar malformations (including Chiari 2 and Dandy-Walker spectrum disorders), and gray matter heterotopias.

Frontoethmoidal Cephaloceles

Terminology and Classification

Frontoethmoidal cephaloceles are also called **sincipital cephaloceles**. In frontoethmoidal cephaloceles, brain parenchyma herniates through a persisting dural projection into the midface, typically the forehead, dorsum of the nose, or orbit.

There are three subtypes of frontoethmoidal cephaloceles. The **frontonasal** subtype is most common, representing 40-60% of frontoethmoidal cephaloceles.

In the **nasoethmoidal** subtype (30%), the sac herniates through a midline foramen cecum defect into the prenasal space.

The least common subtype is **nasoorbital** (10%). Here the cephalocele herniates through the maxilla and lacrimal bone into the inferomedial orbit.

Etiology

Frontonasal cephaloceles protrude through an unobliterated *fonticulus frontalis* into the anterior forehead at the glabella/dorsum of nose (41-6). Nasoethmoidal cephaloceles herniate into the nasal cavity through a *patent foramen cecum* (41-7).

Developmental defects in the lacrimal bones and frontal processes of the maxillary bones result in a nasoorbital cephalocele, which herniates into the orbit.

Clinical Issues

EPIDEMIOLOGY AND DEMOGRAPHICS. Frontoethmoidal cephaloceles represent 10-15% of all cephaloceles and are typically present at birth. There is no gender predilection.

Frontoethmoidal cephaloceles are the most common type of cephalocele seen in southeast Asia and among ethnic southeast Asian immigrants to the United States and Europe, where they are now almost as common as the occipital type.

ASSOCIATED ABNORMALITIES. Associated abnormalities are present in 80% of patients with frontoethmoidal cephaloceles. These include hypertelorism and eye anomalies, corpus callosum dysgenesis and interhemispheric lipomas, hydrocephalus, seizures, neuronal migration anomalies, and microcephaly.

Imaging

NECT scans show a well-demarcated, heterogeneous, mixed-density mass that extends extracranially through a bony defect.

In a **frontonasal cephalocele**, brain herniates into the forehead between the frontal bones above and the nasal bones below **(41-8)**. In the **nasoethmoidal** type, the nasal bone is bowed anteriorly by the cephalocele, and the crista galli is posterior to the defect. The cribriform plate is deficient or absent; the crista galli may be absent or bifid. A **nasoorbital cephalocele** protrudes inferomedially into the orbit through a defect in the lacrimal/frontal process of the maxillary bone.

MR shows a soft tissue mass in direct contiguity with the intracranial parenchyma. The mass is usually heterogeneous in signal intensity but mostly appears isointense with cortex. It does not enhance following contrast administration.

41-8A. 3D CT soft tissue reconstruction in a newborn with a frontonasal encephalocele shows a large mass ➡ protruding anteriorly between the eyes. 41-8B. 3D reformatted bone CT shows a well-delineated frontonasal bony defect ➡ just above the bridge of the nose.

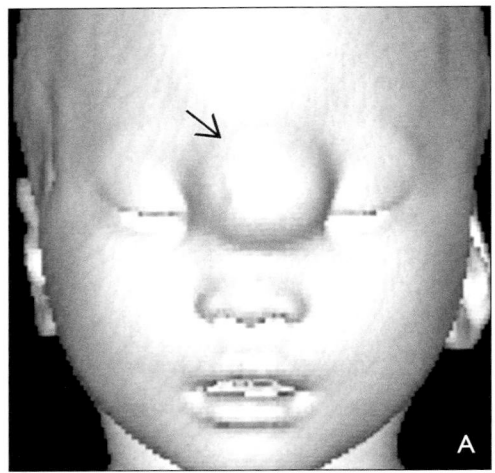

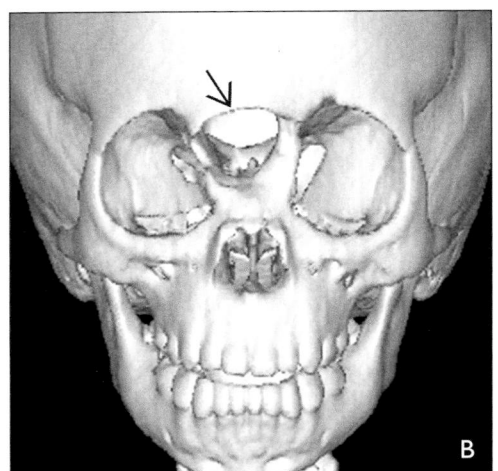

41-8C. Sagittal T1WI in the same patient shows that the skin-covered soft tissue mass ➡ protrudes through a patent fonticulus frontalis ➡. Note absence of corpus callosum with "high-riding" third ventricle, azygous anterior cerebral artery ➡. A Chiari 1 malformation with tonsillar herniation ➡ is also present. 41-8D. T2WI shows that the cephalocele is mostly dysplastic brain ➡. Note arachnoid cyst ➡, polymicrogyria ➡. (Courtesy M. Michel, MD.)

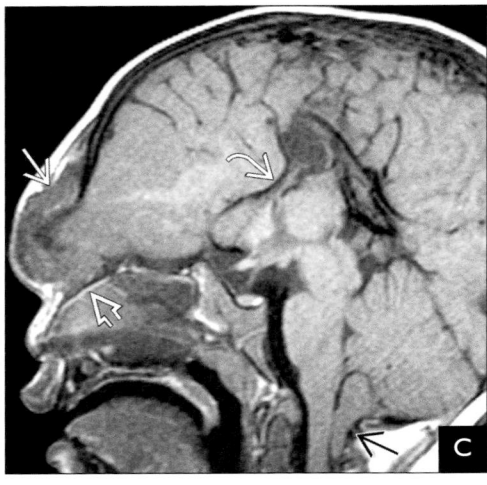

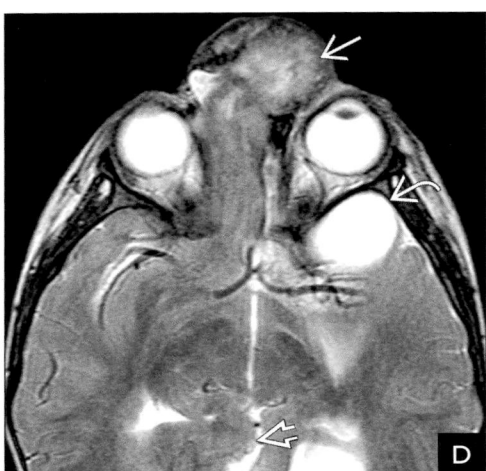

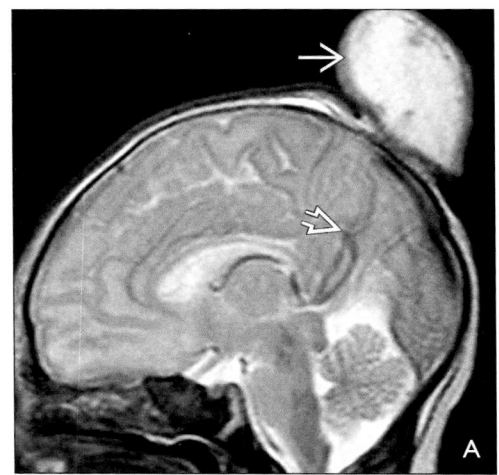

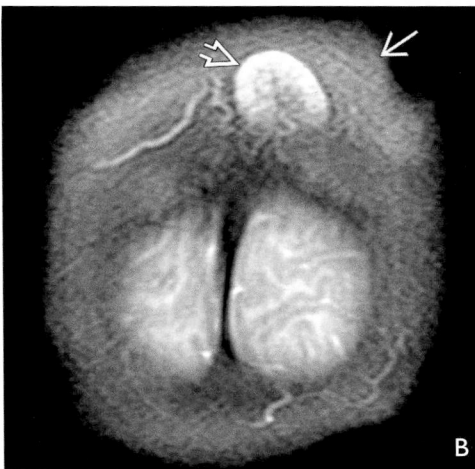

41-9A. Sagittal T2WI shows classic parietal cephalocele ➡️ *in the midline over the posterior vertex. The cephalocele is associated with a falcine sinus* ➡️. *(Courtesy G. Hedlund, DO.) 41-9B. Coronal T2WI in another case shows a scalp mass* ➡️ *with underlying parietal cephalocele* ➡️. *(Courtesy K. Moore, MD.)*

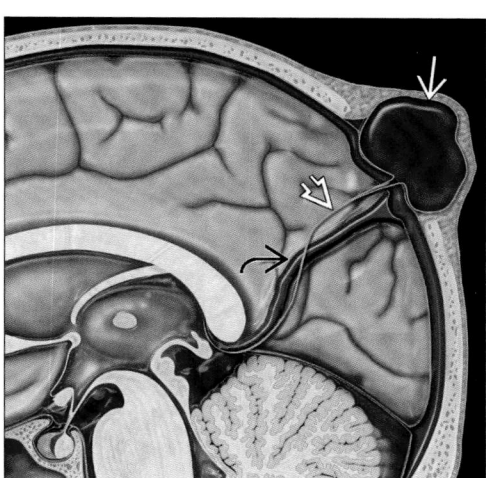

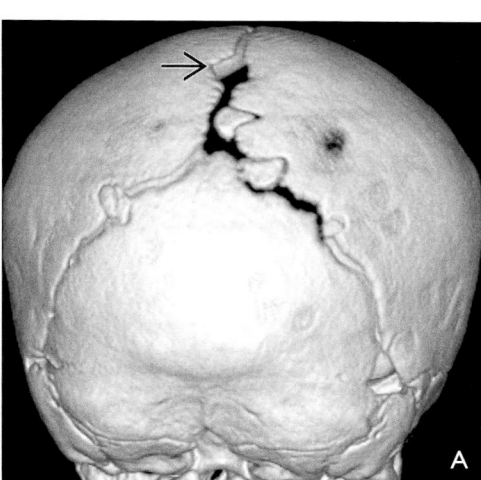

41-10. Sagittal graphic demonstrates a skin-covered atretic parietal cephalocele ➡️ *associated with a dura-lined sinus tract* ➡️ *and a persistent falcine sinus* ➡️. *41-11A. 3D rendered bone CT in a child with an atretic parietal cephalocele demonstrates a small, well-demarcated midline skull defect* ➡️.

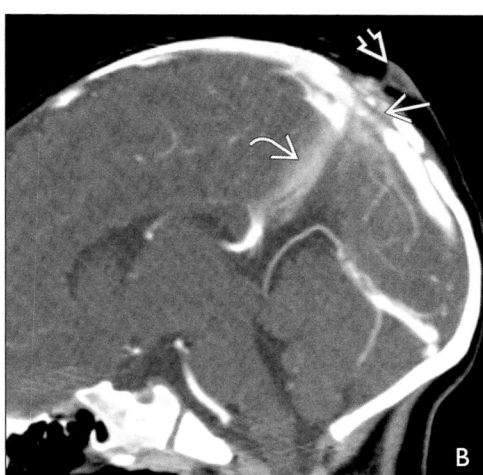

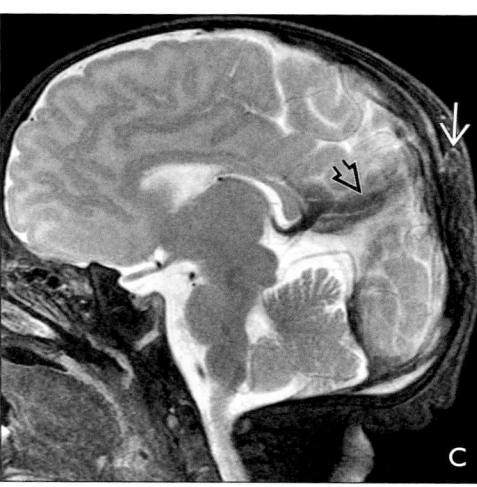

41-11B. CTA in the same patient shows persistent falcine sinus ➡️, *atretic cephalocele* ➡️ *passing between the split superior sagittal sinus* ➡️. *41-11C. Sagittal T2WI in the same patient demonstrates the persistent falcine sinus* ➡️ *and a tiny atretic cephalocele* ➡️. *(Courtesy K. Moore, MD.)*

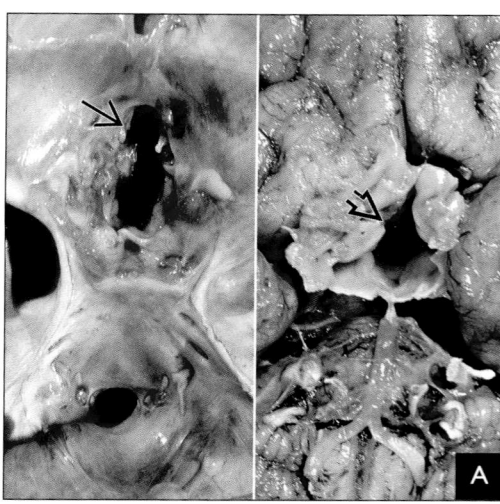

41-12A. Autopsy of sphenoethmoidal cephalocele shows central skull base defect ⮕. Basal view of brain shows the cephalocele sac ⮕.

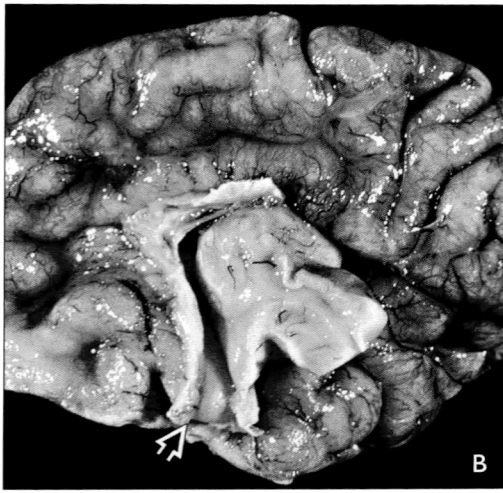

41-12B. Sagittal view shows the cephalocele ⮕, pachygyria, corpus callosum dysplasia. (Courtesy E. T. Hedley-Whyte, MD.)

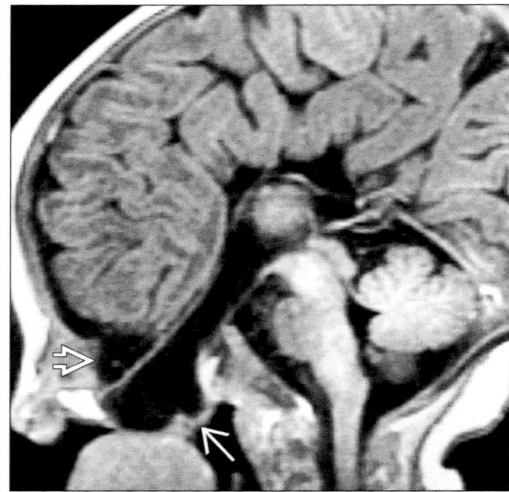

41-13. Sagittal T1WI shows sphenoethmoidal cephalocele ⮕. Hypothalamus, anterior third ventricle ⮕ are retracted into the sac.

Differential Diagnosis

The major differential diagnoses of a frontoethmoidal cephalocele are nasal dermal sinus with or without associated dermoids/epidermoids and nasal cerebral heterotopia (nasal "glioma"). All three lesions present clinically as midline nasal masses. All three have similar embryologic origin (i.e., the dura that normally extends through the embryonic foramen cecum between the developing nasal bone and nasal cartilage fails to regress).

A **nasal dermal sinus** is seen clinically as a small dimple or pit on the nose. It is the opening of a dermal-lined sinus tract that extends intracranially for a variable distance. A dermoid or epidermoid cyst can develop anywhere along the tract. Nasal dermal sinuses have an epithelial lining and do not contain brain parenchyma.

A **nasal "glioma"** is a congenital nonneoplastic heterotopia that consists of dysplastic glial tissue. Most nasal gliomas are extranasal (60%), located along the dorsum of the nose. Approximately one-third are intranasal, lying under the nasal bones. MR scans show no connection between the mass and intracranial contents.

Parietal Cephaloceles

Parietal cephaloceles comprise just 5-10% of all cephaloceles. Most have significant underlying brain and vascular anomalies such as a persistent falcine sinus, sinus pericranii, and/or partial absence of the straight sinus.

MR without and with contrast enhancement is best to delineate parietal cephalocele contents **(41-9)**. Because of the proximity to the superior sagittal sinus, it is important to delineate the position of all dural sinuses and adjacent cortical draining veins with MRV, CTV, or DSA prior to surgery.

A number of parietal cephaloceles are termed **atretic cephaloceles**, small lesions that typically present as midline scalp masses near the posterior vertex **(41-10)**. They are associated with limited defects in the skull that are best visualized on 3D bone CT. They are often associated with a falcine sinus and frequently split the superior sagittal sinus **(41-11)**.

Skull Base Cephaloceles

Skull base (SB) cephaloceles account for 10% of all cephaloceles. They result from developmental failure of proper skull base ossification, which in turn allows migration of neural crest cells and their derivatives through the bony defect.

Skull base cephaloceles can be midline or off-midline (lateral) and are subtyped according to which bony component(s) they involve. There are three types of midline SB cephaloceles. **Sphenopharyngeal** cephaloceles involve just the sphenoid body whereas **sphenoethmoidal** lesions affect both the sphenoid and ethmoid bones **(41-12)**. **Transethmoidal** cephaloceles herniate through the cribriform plate.

Lateral basal cephaloceles can be **sphenomaxillary** (orbital fissure plus maxillary sinus with herniation into the pterygopalatine fossa) or **sphenoorbital** (through the sphenoid bone into the orbit).

Occasionally, **middle cranial fossa arachnoid granulations** are seen as multiple focal outpouchings (arachnoid "pits") in the greater sphenoid ala. These skull base defects can be associated with CSF leak or SB cephalocele.

Imaging of SB cephaloceles is essential to delineate the sac contents completely. The pituitary gland, optic nerves and chiasm, hypothalamus, and third ventricle can all be displaced inferiorly into the cephalocele **(41-13)**.

Intracranial anomalies are frequent findings in association with skull base cephaloceles. Midline anomalies such as corpus callosum dysgenesis and an azygous anterior cerebral artery are common.

Persistent Craniopharyngeal Canal

Terminology

Persistent craniopharyngeal canal (PCPC) is also known as persistent hypophyseal or basipharyngeal canal.

Etiology and Clinical Issues

PCPC is a developmental anomaly with a persistent tract in the interspheniodal synchondrosis **(41-1)** that extends from the nasopharynx to the bottom of the pituitary fossa **(41-14)**, **(41-15)**. It is usually small, uncomplicated, and noted incidentally on imaging studies or at autopsy **(41-16)**. However, occasionally PCPCs can present as large complex skull base lesions with cysts, cephaloceles, midline craniofacial malformations, or pituitary anomalies.

PCPCs are seen in 0.4-0.5% of the population.

Imaging

High-resolution bone CT with 3D reformatted images best delineates the skull base abnormality. Most PCPCs are small, typically < 1.5 mm in diameter. A larger lesion appears as a smoothly marginated cylindrical or ovoid midline bony "canal" extending obliquely downward from the sellar floor to the nasopharynx.

MR findings depend on the contents within the canal. Small, uncomplicated PCPCs may be difficult to identify. Larger lesions show variable signal intensity within the canal itself. Coronal images sometimes show the adeno-

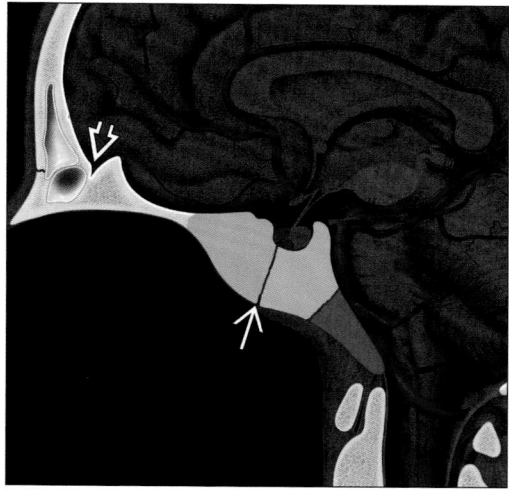

41-14. Presphenoid (green), postsphenoid/ basisphenoid (yellow), basiocciput (red), foramen cecum ➡, intersphenoid synchondrosis ➡.

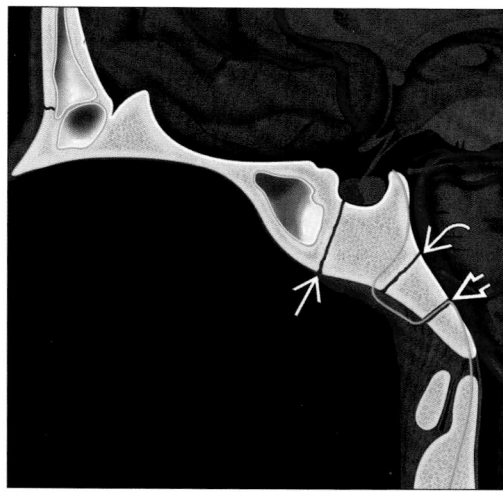

41-15. Intersphenoid ➡ and sphenooccipital synchondroses ➡, notochord migration path (green) forming medial basal canal ➡.

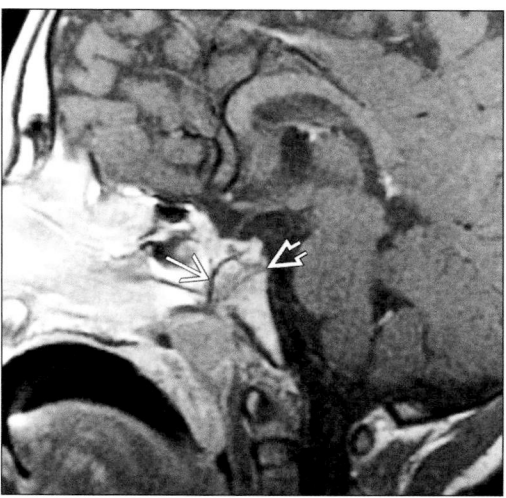

41-16. Sagittal T1WI shows persistent craniopharyngeal canal ➡, sphenooccipital synchondrosis ➡ posterior to the PCPC.

41-17A. Axial bone CT in a 22-year-old woman with chronic diabetes insipidus and headaches demonstrates a persistent craniopharyngeal canal (PCPC), seen here as a smoothly marginated, well-demarcated defect in the central basisphenoid ➡. **41-17B.** 3D reformatted image nicely shows the PCPC ➡ and its relationship to other structures in the central skull base.

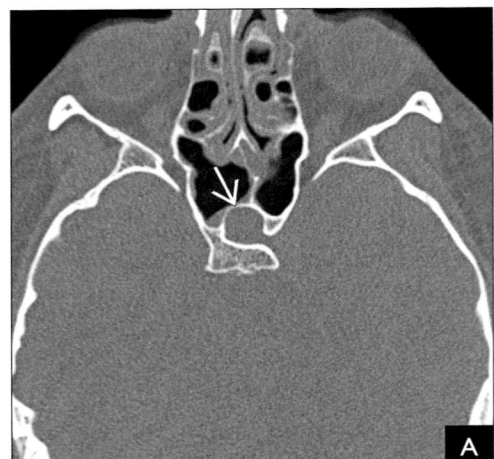

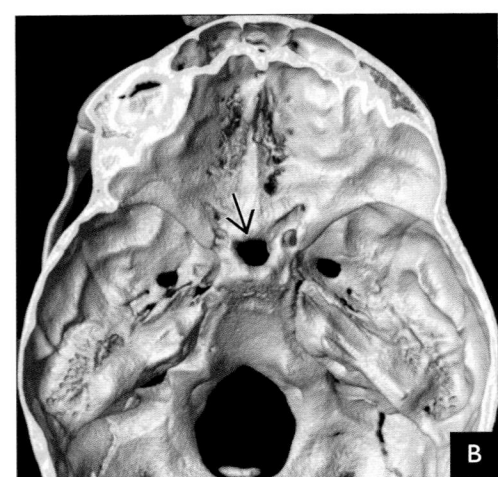

41-17C. Coronal bone CT shows the enlarged PCPC appearing as an elongated tube ➡ that connects the sella with the nasopharynx. **41-17D.** Coronal 3D bone CT elegantly demonstrates the cylindrical shape of the PCPC ➡.

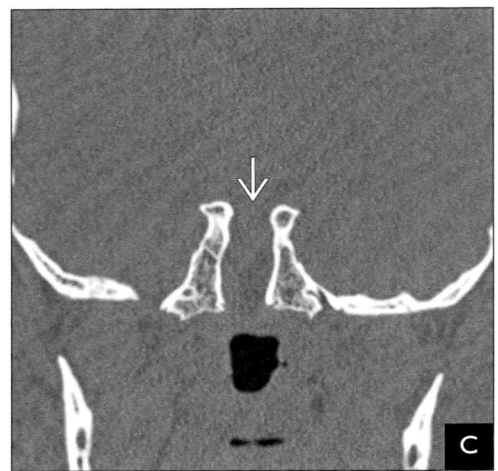

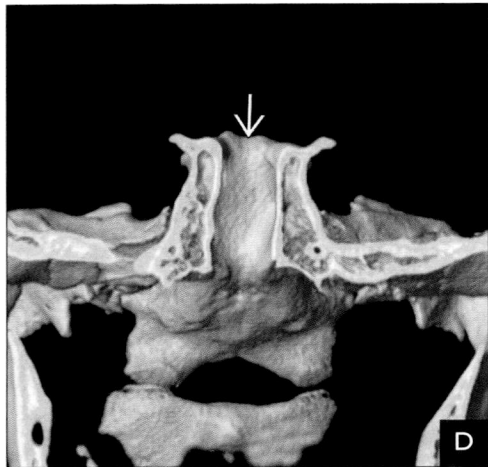

41-17E. Sagittal 3D rendering of the bone CT shows that the PCPC appears to widen slightly ➤ as it approaches the upper aerodigestive tract. **41-17F.** Sagittal T1-weighted MR shows a sphenoidal cephalocele ➡ traversing the PCPC and bulging into the roof of the nasopharynx ➡. (Courtesy P. Chapman, MD.)

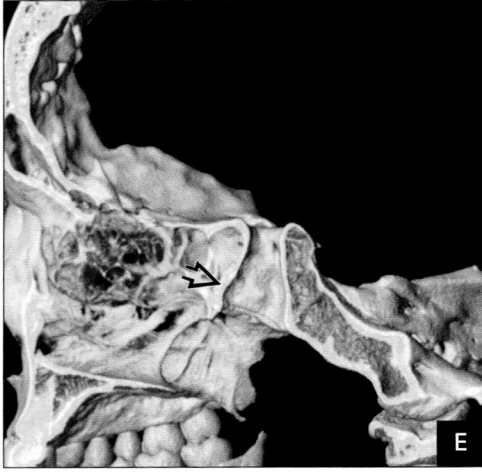

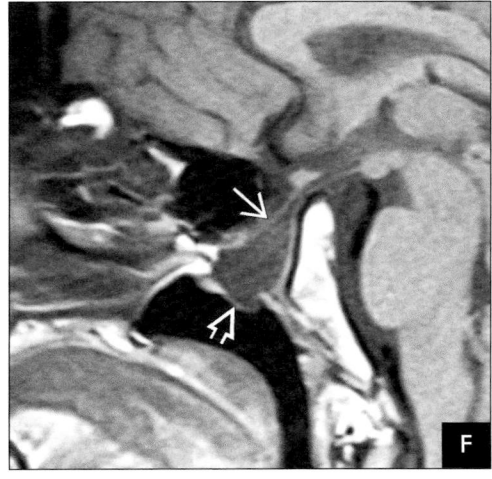

hypophysis sitting on the top of the PCPC, resembling a "golf ball on a tee."

Associated anomalies of the midface (e.g., hypertelorism, cleft palate) and pituitary gland/stalk (e.g., duplicated gland, ectopic adenoma) are common in complex PCPCs. Sphenopharyngeal cephaloceles **(41-17)** and hypothalamic hamartomas are other frequent associations. Reported complications include CSF leaks and recurrent meningitis.

Differential Diagnosis

The major differential diagnosis of PCPC is a **sphenooccipital synchondrosis**, a linear developmental cleft between the basisphenoid and basiocciput. The sphenooccipital synchondrosis gradually decreases in size with increasing age and usually disappears by adulthood. It lies *behind* the dorsum sellae; a PCPC lies *in front of* the dorsum **(41-16)**.

A **persistent medial basal canal** is a developmental variant of the lower clivus and occurs posteroinferior to the sphenooccipital synchondrosis **(41-15)**.

CEPHALOCELES

Occipital Cephaloceles
- Most common in European/North American Caucasians
- 75% of cephaloceles, M:F = 2.4:1
- Typically contains dysplastic brain

Frontoethmoidal Cephaloceles
- 10-15% of cephaloceles
- Southeast Asian predominance
- Frontonasal (40-60%)
  - Through fonticulus frontalis into forehead
- Nasoethmoidal (30%)
  - Through patent foramen cecum into nose
- Nasoorbital (10%)
  - Through lacrimal bone/maxilla into orbit

Parietal Cephaloceles
- 5-10% of cephaloceles
- Most are "atretic"
  - Associated with falcine sinus, sinus pericranii

Skull Base Cephaloceles
- 10% of cephaloceles
- Brain anomalies common (e.g., callosal dysgenesis)

Persistent Craniopharyngeal Canal
- < 1%, usually incidental finding
- Large complex lesions rare
  - Associated with pituitary anomalies
  - May have sphenoidal cephalocele

Craniosynostoses

Craniosynostosis Overview

Terminology

Craniosynostosis is also known as **craniostenosis**, **sutural synostosis**, and **cranial dysostosis**. The craniosynostoses are a heterogeneous group of disorders characterized by abnormal head shape.

Etiology

The calvaria normally expands during infancy and early childhood to accommodate the growing brain. This mostly occurs at narrow seams of undifferentiated mesenchyme—the cranial sutures—that lie between adjacent bones. Compared to most major embryonic structures such as the brain and cardiovascular systems, the cranial sutures form relatively late (at around 16 weeks gestation).

Normal sutures permit skull growth perpendicular to their long axis. As long as the brain grows rapidly, the calvaria expands. As brain growth slows, the sutures close.

The normal order of closure is metopic first, followed by the coronal and then the lambdoid sutures. The sagittal suture normally closes last. Craniostenosis occurs when osseous obliteration of one or more sutures occurs prematurely.

Skull distortion occurs from a combination of (1) insufficient growth perpendicular to the prematurely fused suture and (2) compensatory overgrowth at the nonfused sutures.

Clinical Issues

Craniosynostosis can be associated with neurological and vascular compromise and is therefore important to recognize. Severe deformities can be cosmetically disfiguring and socially stigmatizing.

Precisely when the anatomical and functional anomalies become clinically relevant varies from patient to patient and thus requires a tailored approach to treatment.

Imaging

Imaging plays an essential role in recognition of craniosynostoses, identification of coexisting brain anomalies, preoperative treatment planning, and postoperative follow-up.

Craniosynostoses can be nonsyndromic or syndromic and may affect a single suture or multiple sutures. In this section, we discuss representative examples of each type.

Nonsyndromic Craniosynostosis

Terminology and Etiology

Nonsyndromic synostoses are genetically determined lesions that occur in the absence of a recognizable syndrome.

Gain of function mutations in the *FGF7*, *VCAM1*, and *SFRP4* genes have been identified in osteoblasts derived from cases of single-suture synostosis. *FGF7* is expressed in loose mesenchyme surrounding the mesenchymal condensations in sutures and preferentially activates the fibroblast growth factor receptor 2 gene (*FGFR2*). Upregulation signaling factors such as *FGF7* may lead to inappropriate ligand-receptor binding, increase mitogenic activity, and contribute to skeletal abnormalities related to craniosynostosis.

Pathology

LOCATION. Approximately 60% of all single-suture craniosynostosis cases involve premature fusion of the sagittal suture, followed in frequency by those that involve the coronal (22%) and metopic (15%) sutures. Lambdoid craniosynostosis is very rare, causing just 2% of all cases.

CLASSIFICATION. Craniosynostosis is generally classified by head shape as **scaphocephaly** or dolichocephaly (long and narrow) **(41-18)**, **brachycephaly** (broad and flattened) **(41-21)**, **trigonocephaly** (triangular at the front) **(41-19)**, or **plagiocephaly** (skewed) **(41-20)**.

GROSS PATHOLOGY. Gross examination shows fibrous or bony sutural "bridging." Focal synostosis or diffuse bony "beaking" along the affected suture are typical findings.

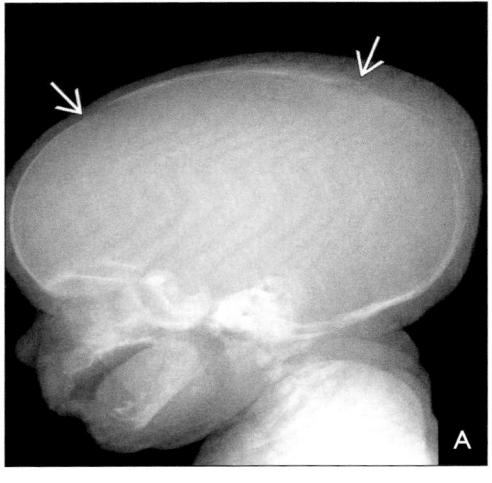
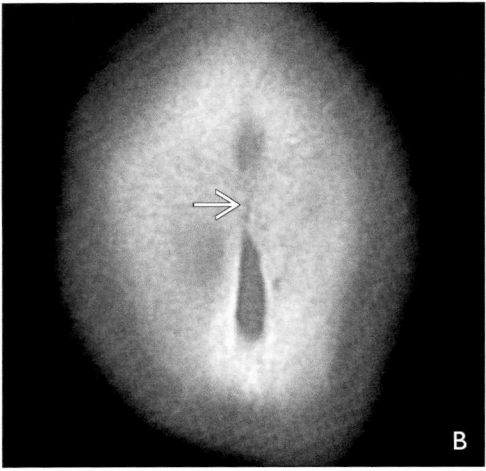

41-18A. Lateral radiograph of a newborn shows pronounced scaphocephaly with unusually severe elongation of the calvaria in the anteroposterior plane ➡. 41-18B. Bone CT in the same patient shows the elongated configuration of the skull. Note severe narrowing with almost complete obliteration of the superior sagittal suture ➡.

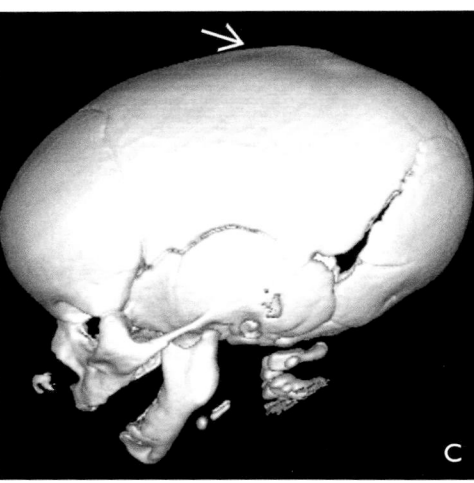
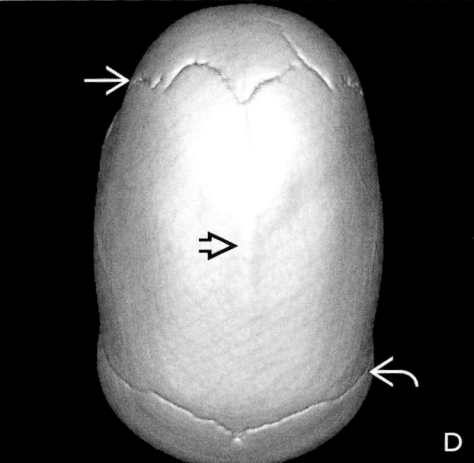

41-18C. Bone CT with 3D shaded surface display (SSD) in the same patient shows the pronounced elongation of the skull. Note ridge of bone along the vertex ➡ that resembles the keel of a ship. (Courtesy K. Moore, MD.) 41-18D. Coronal 3D SSD in the same patient shows normal-appearing coronal ➡, lambdoid ➡ sutures. The sagittal suture is completely fused and demonstrates the elevated midline ridge of bone ➡ characteristic of scaphocephaly.

Clinical Issues

EPIDEMIOLOGY. The overall prevalence of craniosynostosis is estimated at 1:2,000-2,500 live births.

Sporadic craniosynostoses are more common than syndrome-associated cases, accounting for 85% of all craniosynostoses. Between 85-90% of these involve only a single suture whereas 5-15% are multisuture synostoses.

DEMOGRAPHICS. Gender varies with craniostenosis type. Both scaphocephaly and trigonocephaly have a moderate male predominance (M:F = 3.1:1 and M:F = 2:1, respectively).

PRESENTATION. Most craniosynostoses—even syndromic ones—are not detected during pregnancy. Affected infants generally present during the first year of life. The most common presentation is unusual head shape with craniofacial asymmetry.

NATURAL HISTORY. Severe deformities may lead to hydrocephalus, elevated intracranial pressure, compromised cerebral blood flow, and airway obstruction.

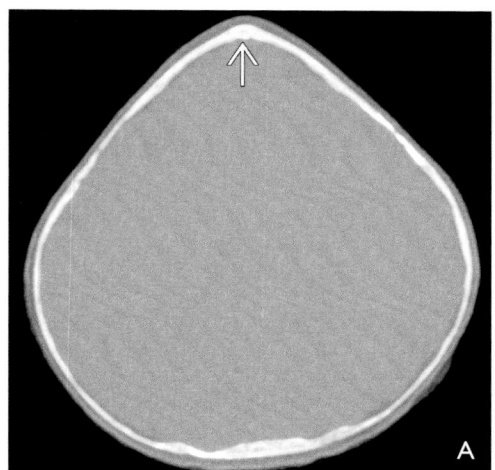

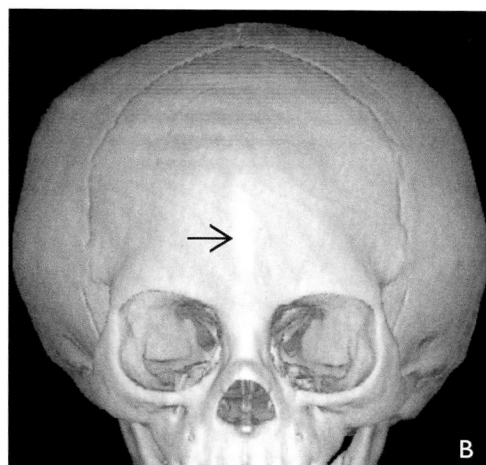

41-19A. Axial NECT in an 18 month old with trigonocephaly shows triangular anterior pointing of the skull ➡. The calvaria appears widened in the transverse plane. 41-19B. AP projection of the 3D SSD in the same patient shows premature metopic suture synostosis with a distinct vertical ridge of bone ➡.

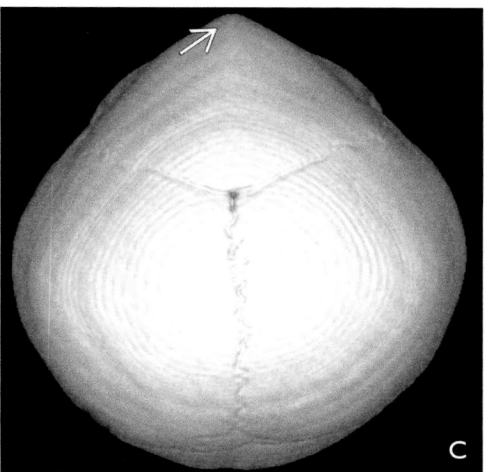

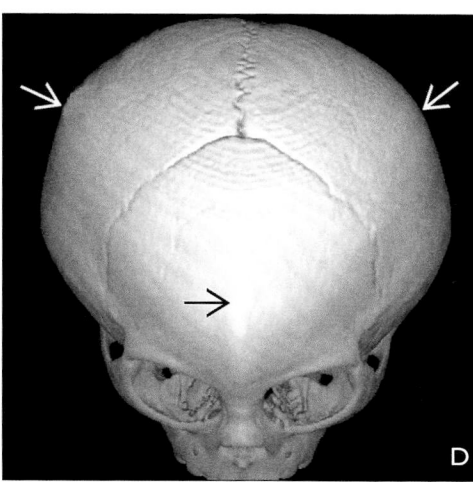

41-19C. Vertex view of the SSD demonstrates the distinct triangular shape of the forehead ➡ characteristic of trigonocephaly secondary to metopic suture synostosis. 41-19D. Angled view shows the widened transverse diameter of the calvaria ➡ and the midline elevated bony ridge along the obliterated metopic suture ➡. (Courtesy K. Moore, MD.)

TREATMENT OPTIONS. Mild deformities are sometimes treated with physiotherapy and head repositioning or orthotic helmet. Severe skull deformities may require one or more surgeries to remodel the cranial vault.

Imaging

GENERAL FEATURES. Digital radiographs are sufficient to identify simple single-suture craniosynostoses. However, in addition to identifying the deformity and affected suture, preoperative planning requires careful imaging assessment of calvarial and dural venous sinus anatomy. Delineating associated intra- and extracranial abnormalities is especially important in evaluating patients with multiple or syndromic synostoses.

CT FINDINGS. While the diagnosis of cranial synostosis can be made clinically or on plain film radiographs, thin-section CT scans with multiplanar reconstruction and 3D shaded surface display (SSD) are invaluable for detailed evaluation and preoperative planning. Head shape generally predicts which suture(s) will be abnormal, but CT is required to determine whether part or all of the affected suture(s) is fused.

Scaphocephaly. Scaphocephaly, also known as dolichocephaly, is caused by sagittal suture synostosis. Patients with scaphocephaly demonstrate an elongated skull with decreased transverse and increased AP measurements. Forehead bossing is common. In severe cases, the sagittal suture is elevated, and the elongated ridge of bone resembles the keel of a ship **(41-18)**.

Brachycephaly. Brachycephaly is caused by bicoronal or bilambdoid synostosis. In such cases, the skull appears widened in the transverse dimension while shortened from front to back **(41-21)**. Craniofacial deformities such as bilateral "harlequin" orbits—peculiar bony deformities seen as elevation/elongation of the superolateral orbit walls—are common.

Trigonocephaly. Trigonocephaly is caused by synostosis of the metopic suture. The forehead appears wedge- or triangle-shaped **(41-19)**. Hypotelorism is common.

Plagiocephaly. In plagiocephaly, the calvaria is very asymmetric. Unilateral single or asymmetric multiple sutural fusions can produce this appearance. In unilateral coronal synostosis, the hemicalvaria is shortened and

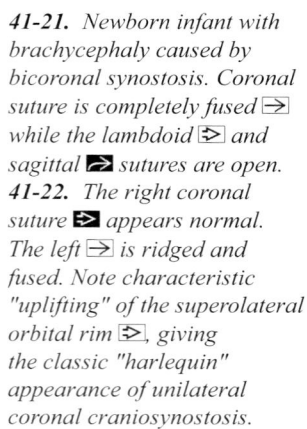

41-20A. NECT scan in a 6-month-old boy with plagiocephaly shows an asymmetric, flattened posterior skull shows bulging in the left posterior parietooccipital area ➘. *41-20B. 3D shaded surface display in the same patient shows synostosis of the left lambdoid suture* ➔ *with posterior bulging of the calvaria* ➘. *The right lambdoid suture* ➘ *appears normal.*

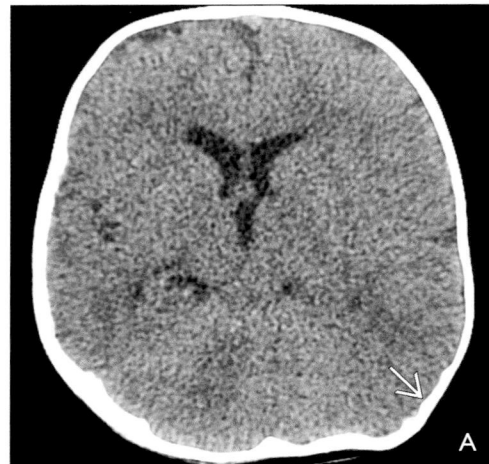

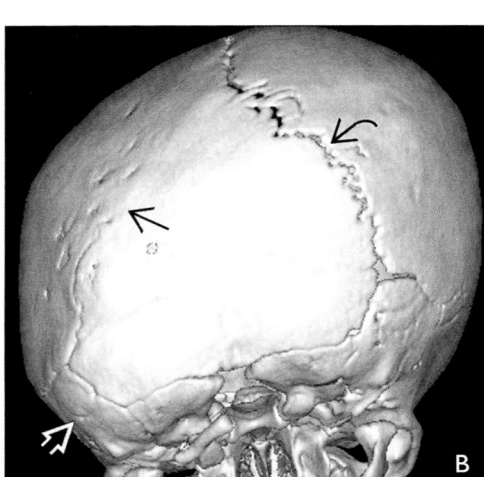

41-21. Newborn infant with brachycephaly caused by bicoronal synostosis. Coronal suture is completely fused ➔ *while the lambdoid* ➘ *and sagittal* ➘ *sutures are open.*
41-22. The right coronal suture ➘ *appears normal. The left* ➔ *is ridged and fused. Note characteristic "uplifting" of the superolateral orbital rim* ➘, *giving the classic "harlequin" appearance of unilateral coronal craniosynostosis.*

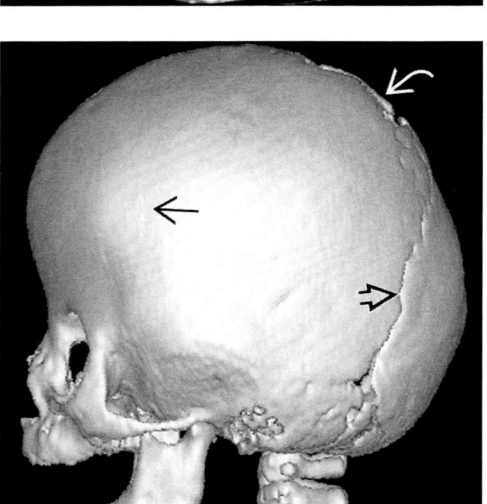

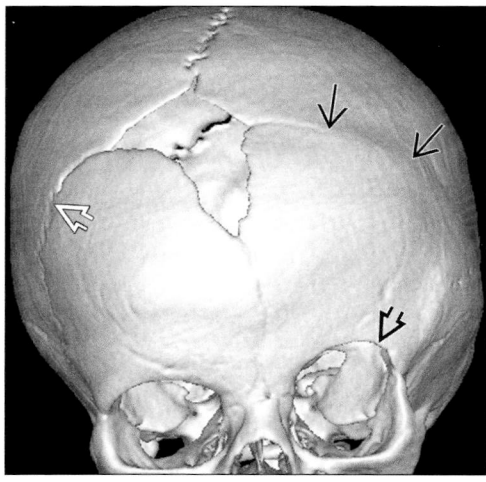

pointed; it may be associated with a unilateral "harlequin" eye (41-22). If the lambdoid suture is fused, the skull assumes a more trapezoid appearance with occipital flattening and posterior ear displacement (41-20).

Turricephaly. Turricephaly or "towering" skull is a more extreme deformity caused by bicoronal or bilambdoid synostosis.

Oxycephaly. The coronal, sagittal, and lambdoid sutures are all fused in oxycephaly.

Kleeblattschädel. Kleeblattschädel is also known as "cloverleaf" skull. Bicoronal and bilambdoid synostoses cause an unusual pattern of bulging temporal bones, towering skull, and shallow orbits (41-23).

MR FINDINGS. MR is helpful to rule out coexisting anomalies. Hydrocephalus, corpus callosum dysgenesis, and gray matter abnormalities may be present but are more common in syndromic craniosynostoses. MRA or CTA is useful to delineate venous sinus drainage prior to surgical intervention.

CRANIOSYNOSTOSIS: IMAGING

Scaphocephaly
- Most common type
- Sagittal suture synostosis
- Elongated "dolichocephalic" skull with midline bony ridge

Brachycephaly
- Bicoronal or bilambdoid synostosis
- Coronal → widened transverse dimension ± "harlequin" orbit
- Lambdoid → flattened occiput

Trigonocephaly
- Metopic suture synostosis
- Wedge- or triangle-shaped forehead

Plagiocephaly
- Usually multiple sutures or unilateral coronal
- Skull very asymmetric

"Cloverleaf" Skull
- Bicoronal + bilambdoid synostoses
- Temporal fossae bulge outward, "towering" skull

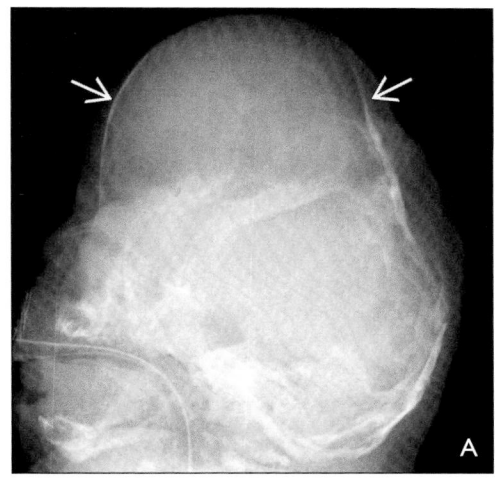

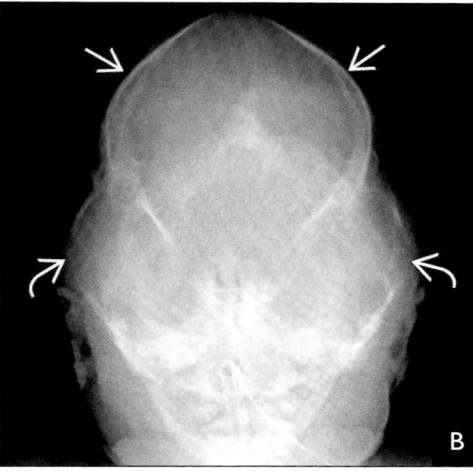

41-23A. Syndromic craniosynostosis is demonstrated by this lateral radiograph in a newborn with Pfeiffer syndrome. Note the unusual "towering" configuration ⇒ of the calvaria. 41-23B. AP radiograph shows the "towering" skull ⇒ especially well. Also note the symmetrically protruding temporal fossae ⇒, which create the classic "cloverleaf" appearance of Kleeblattschädel skull.

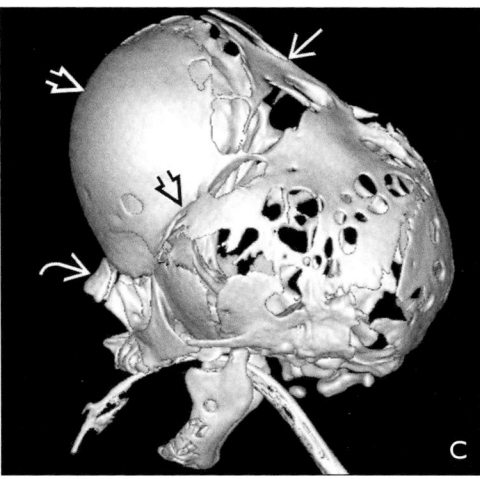

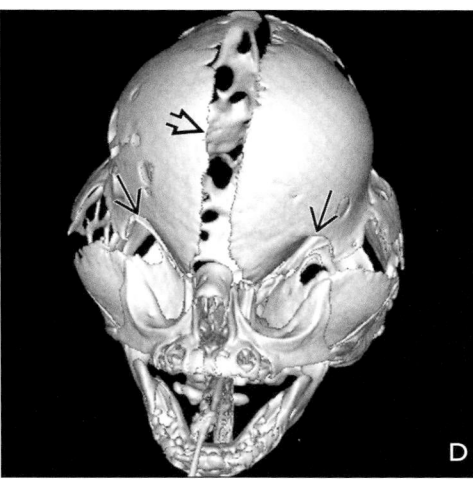

41-23C. Sagittal 3D SSD shows the abnormal head shape with "towering" skull ⇒, frontal bossing ⇒, mandibular and facial hypoplasia ⇒, and protruding temporal fossae ⇒. Premature closure of the squamosal, coronal, lambdoid, and sagittal sutures is present. Multiple "holes" are foci of thinned calvaria. 41-23D. Frontal SSD shows a markedly widened metopic suture ⇒, "harlequin" orbits with superolaterally pointed rims ⇒. (Courtesy K. Moore, MD.)

Syndromic Craniosynostoses

Syndromic craniosynostoses account for just 10-15% of all cranial synostoses. They are much more likely to be associated with other craniofacial and skeletal anomalies than their nonsyndromic counterparts. In addition, brain malformations are common and developmental delay is more frequent. In contrast to sporadic craniosynostoses (in which the sagittal suture is most often affected), bilateral coronal synostosis is the more common pattern in these patients.

Nearly 200 inherited syndromes have been described in conjunction with craniosynostosis. More than 60 different mutations have been identified, the majority of which occur in *FGFR2*.

A few of the more important syndromic craniostenoses are delineated below. We first discuss acrocephalosyndactyly types 1-5, using the eponyms by which these syndromes are most commonly known. We then mention some of the rare acrocephalopolysyndactylys.

Apert Syndrome

Apert syndrome is also known as **acrocephalosyndactyly type 1**. Craniosynostosis with hypertelorism, midface hypoplasia, and cervical spine anomalies is common. Severe symmetric hand and foot syndactyly is present in most patients. Bilateral coronal synostosis is the most common calvarial anomaly.

Of all the syndromic craniosynostoses, patients with Apert syndrome are most severely affected in terms of intellectual disability, developmental delay, CNS malformations, hearing loss, and limb anomalies.

Intracranial anomalies occur in more than half of all Apert cases and include hydrocephalus, callosal dysgenesis, and abnormalities of the septi pellucidi (25-30% each). Cavum vergae and arachnoid cysts are seen in 10-12% of cases. Venous anomalies and Chiari 1 malformation are less common associations.

Acrocephalosyndactyly type 2, also known as Apert-Crouzon or Crouzon syndrome, shows many of the same features seen in Apert syndrome. However, affected individuals more commonly have multiple suture calvarial involvement. Hypertelorism and exophthalmos are prominent features. Both types 1 and 2 acrocephalosyndactyly are associated with *FGFR2* mutations.

Saethre-Chotzen Syndrome

Saethre-Chotzen syndrome is also known as **acrocephalosyndactyly type 3**. A specific mutation in *TWIST* has been associated with this disorder. Duplicated distal phalanges, cone-shaped hallux epiphysis, and syndactyly of the second and third digits are characteristic findings in the extremities.

Waardenburg Syndrome

Waardenburg syndrome (WS) is also known as **acrocephalosyndactyly type 4**. WS is characterized by pigmentation abnormalities and sensorineural hearing loss. Depigmented patches of skin and hair and vivid blue eyes or heterochromia irides are common.

At least six genes are involved in WS, including *SOX10*; mutations in these genes affect myelination. Central myelin deficiency with cerebral and cerebellar hypoplasia is common in the neurological variant of WS. Peripheral demyelinating neuropathy can result in Hirschsprung disease.

Pfeiffer Syndrome

Pfeiffer syndrome is formally known as **acrocephalosyndactyly type 5**. Multiple sutures are typically affected, and severe deformities such as a "cloverleaf" skull are common **(41-23)**.

Carpenter Syndrome

Carpenter syndrome is an autosomal recessive **acrocephalopolysyndactyly** caused by biallelic mutations in *RAB23*. Craniosynostosis is a consistent and severe component. As the name implies, both polydactyly and syndactyly are often present. Umbilical hernia, malformed ears, mental retardation, and hypogenitalism in males are all common associations.

Greig Syndrome

Greig **cephalopolysyndactyly** syndrome (GCPS) is characterized by multiple limb and craniofacial anomalies. GCPS is an autosomal dominant inherited disorder caused by heterozygous mutation or deletion of *GLI3*.

Trigonocephaly with metopic or sagittal synostosis is a distinctive presenting feature of GCPS. Pre- and postaxial polydactyly and cutaneous syndactyly of hands and feet are common. Corpus callosal dysgenesis and mild cerebral ventriculomegaly are recognized associations.

Meningeal Anomalies

Anomalies of the cranial meninges commonly accompany other congenital malformations such as Chiari 2 malformation. **Lipomas** and **arachnoid cysts** are two important intracranial abnormalities with meningeal origin. Arachnoid cysts were considered in detail in Chapter 28. We therefore conclude our discussion of congenital anomalies by focusing on lipomas.

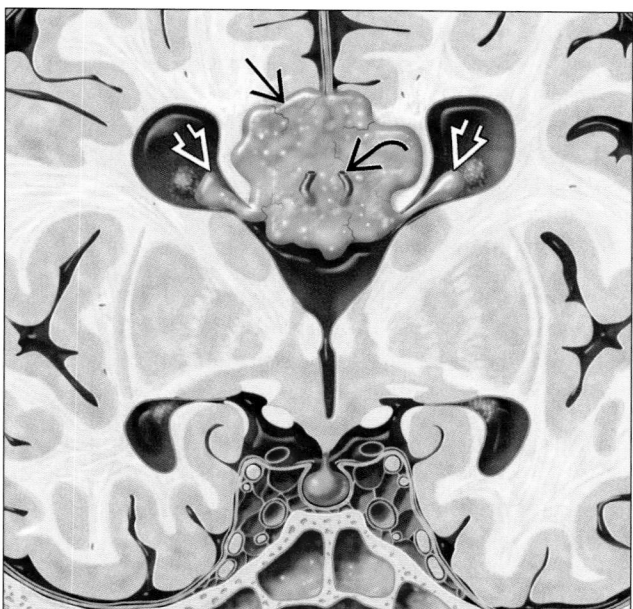

41-24. Graphic depicts corpus callosum agenesis with interhemispheric lipoma ⊡ encasing anterior cerebral arteries ⊡ and extending through choroidal fissure into both lateral ventricles ⊡.

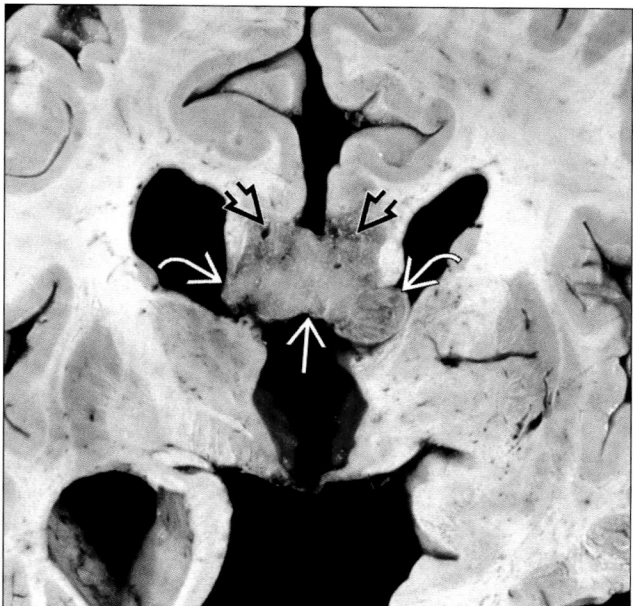

41-25. Autopsy case shows an interhemispheric lipoma ⊡ encasing both anterior cerebral arteries ⊡, extending through choroidal fissure into lateral ventricles ⊡ (Courtesy AFIP Archives.)

Lipomas

Lipomas are sometimes considered benign mesenchymal tumors ("adipositic neoplasms"). Whether they are true neoplasms or congenital malformations is debated. We include lipomas in this chapter rather than in the discussion of intracranial neoplasms because of their frequent association with other congenital malformations.

Fat—adipose tissue—is not normally found inside the arachnoid. Therefore, any fatty tissue inside the skull or spine is abnormal. Because fat deposits commonly accompany congenital malformations such as callosal dysgenesis **(41-24)** or tethered spinal cord, imaging studies should be closely scrutinized for the presence of additional abnormalities.

Terminology

So-called ordinary lipoma is the most common of all soft tissue tumors and is composed of mature adipose tissue.

Etiology

Intracranial lipomas are uncommon lesions whose etiology remains poorly understood. Two explanations have been offered.

Lipomas were once thought to be congenital anomalies. This theory postulates that lipomas arise as malformations of the **embryonic meninx primitiva** (the mesenchymal anlage of the meninges). The primitive meninx normally differentiates into the cranial meninges, invaginating along the choroid fissure of the lateral ventricle.

Maldifferentiation and persistence of the meninx was thought to result in deposits of mature adipose tissue, i.e., fat, along the subpial surface of the brain and spinal cord and within the lateral ventricles.

Current thinking suggests that lipomas represent a genetic aberration. Recent fluorescence in situ hybridization (FISH) and comparative genomic hybridization (CGH) studies have identified clonal cytogenetic aberrations in nearly 60% of ordinary lipomas. The 12q13-15 region is the most commonly involved site. Between 15-20% of lipomas show rearrangements or deletions of the long arm of chromosome 13, particularly 13q12-22.

Pathology

LOCATION. Nonsyndromic lipomas are usually solitary lesions that can be found in virtually any location in the body, including the CNS. Nearly 80% of intracranial lipomas are supratentorial, and most occur in or near the midline. The interhemispheric fissure is the most common overall site (40-50%) **(41-25)**. Lipomas curve over the dorsal corpus callosum, often extending through the choroidal fissures into the lateral ventricles or choroid plexus.

Between 15-25% are located in the quadrigeminal region, usually attached to the inferior colliculi or superior vermis **(41-26)**. Approximately 15% are suprasellar, attached to the undersurface of the hypothalamus or infundibular stalk **(41-27)**. About 5% of lipomas are found in the sylvian fissure.

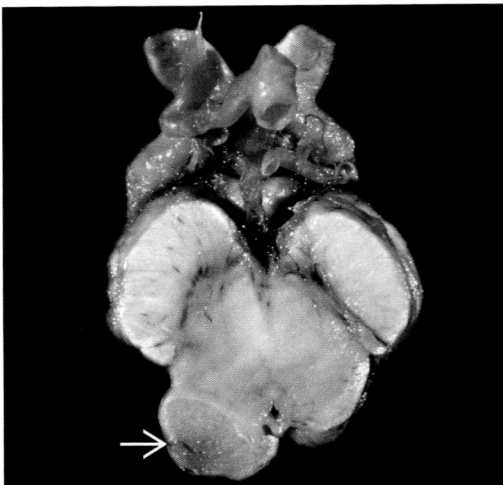

41-26. Autopsy case demonstrates subpial lipoma ➤ attached to quadrigeminal plate. (Courtesy E. T. Hedley-Whyte, MD.)

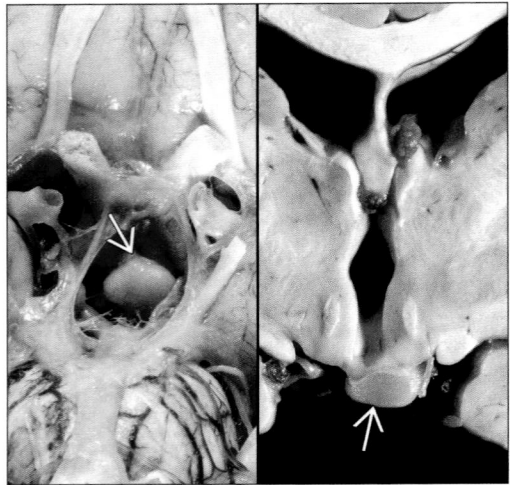

41-27. (Left) Autopsy shows suprasellar lipoma ➤. (Right) Coronal section shows lipoma ➤ attached to hypothalamus. (Courtesy J. Townsend, MD.)

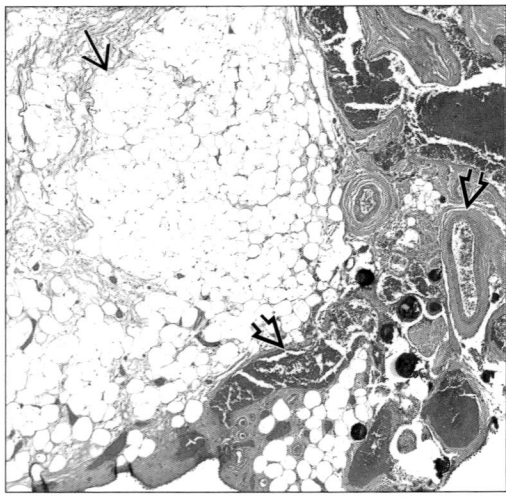

41-28. Low-power photomicrograph shows normal fat cells ➤. Prominent vessels ⧨ course through lesion. (Courtesy E. Rushing, MD.)

Approximately 20% of lipomas are infratentorial. The cerebellopontine angle (CPA) cistern is the most common posterior fossa site (10%).

SIZE AND NUMBER. Lipomas are generally solitary lesions that vary from tiny, barely perceptible fatty collections to huge bulky masses. Most are less than five centimeters in diameter.

GROSS PATHOLOGY. Lipomas appear as bright yellow, lobulated soft masses. They usually adhere to the pia and underlying parenchyma. At least one-third encase adjacent vessels and/or cranial nerves (41-25).

MICROSCOPIC FEATURES. Lipomas are composed of mature, nonneoplastic-appearing adipose tissue with relatively uniform fat cells (41-28). Patchy hyalinization and calcification can be present.

Clinical Issues

EPIDEMIOLOGY AND DEMOGRAPHICS. Lipomas are relatively rare, accounting for less than 0.5% of intracranial masses. They can be found in patients of all ages. There is a slight female predominance.

PRESENTATION. Lipomas are rarely symptomatic and are usually incidental findings on imaging studies. Headache, seizure, hypothalamic disturbances, and cranial nerve deficits have been reported in a few cases.

Syndromic intracranial lipomas occur in encephalocraniocutaneous lipomatosis (see Chapter 39) and Pai syndrome (cutaneous lipomas and facial clefts).

NATURAL HISTORY. Lipomas are benign lesions that remain stable in size. Some may expand with corticosteroid use.

TREATMENT OPTIONS. Lipomas are generally considered "leave me alone" lesions. Because they encase vessels and nerves, surgery has high morbidity and mortality.

Imaging

GENERAL FEATURES. Lipomas are seen as well-delineated, somewhat lobulated extraaxial masses that exhibit fat density/signal intensity.

Two morphologic configurations of interhemispheric fissure lipomas are recognized on imaging studies: A **curvilinear** type (a thin, pencil-like mass that curves around the corpus callosum body and splenium) and a **tubulonodular** type (a large interhemispheric fatty mass). Dystrophic calcification occurs in both types but is more common in bulky tubulonodular lesions.

CT FINDINGS. NECT scans show a hypodense mass that measures -50 to -100 HU. Calcification varies from extensive—nearly two-thirds of bulky tubulonodu-

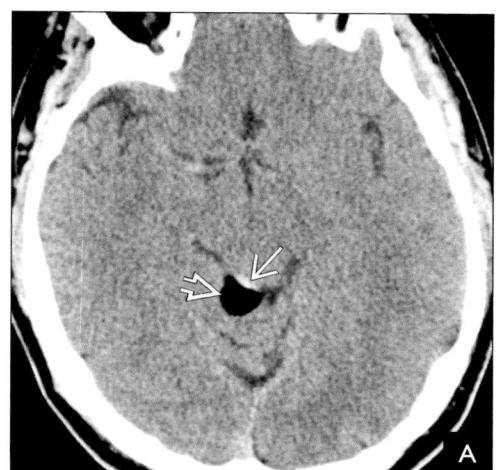

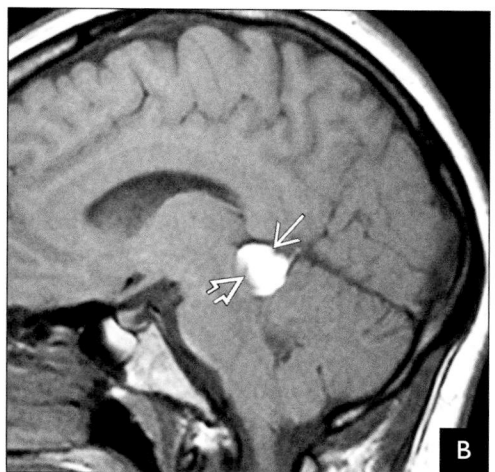

41-29A. Axial NECT scan shows well-delineated, hypodense (-75 HU) lipoma ⇉ attached to the quadrigeminal plate. Some calcification is present ➔. *41-29B.* Sagittal T1WI shows typical hyperintensity of quadrigeminal lipoma ➔. The lesion is in the subpial space. The deep margin is less sharply delineated where it abuts the glia limitans of the tectum ➔.

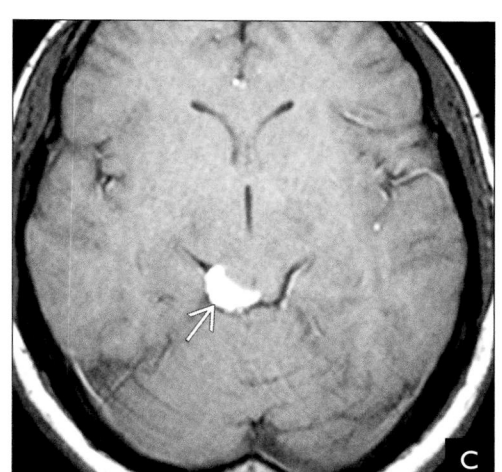

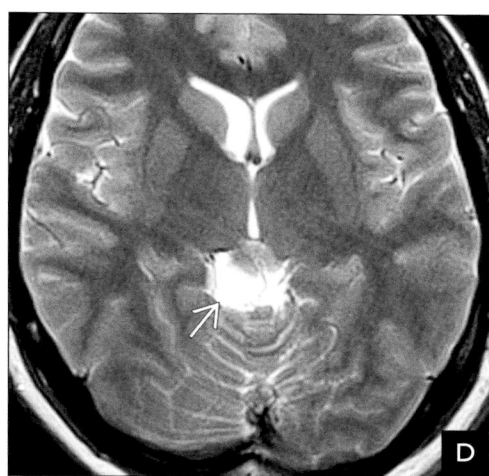

41-29C. Axial T1WI shows that the hyperintense lipoma ➔ is attached to the quadrigeminal plate without a distinct medial border. *41-29D.* FSE T2WI shows that the lipoma ➔ remains hyperintense (because of J-coupling) and cannot be distinguished from the adjacent CSF in the quadrigeminal cistern.

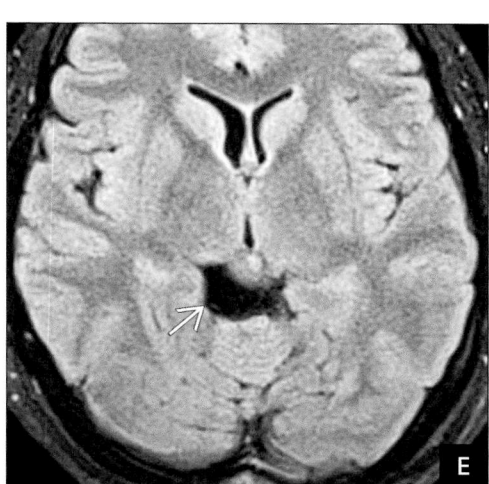

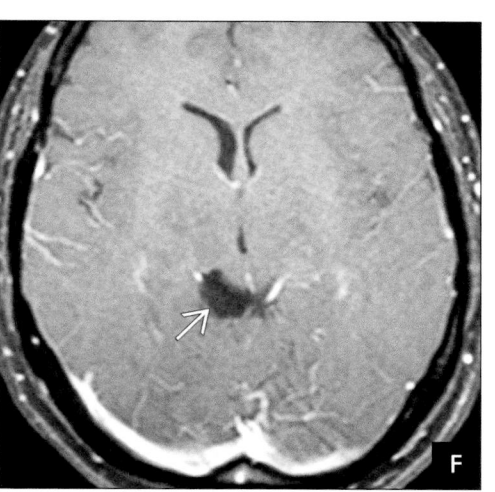

41-29E. The lipoma ➔ is hypointense on STIR. *41-29F.* T1 C+ FS demonstrates that the lipoma ➔ suppresses completely and does not enhance.

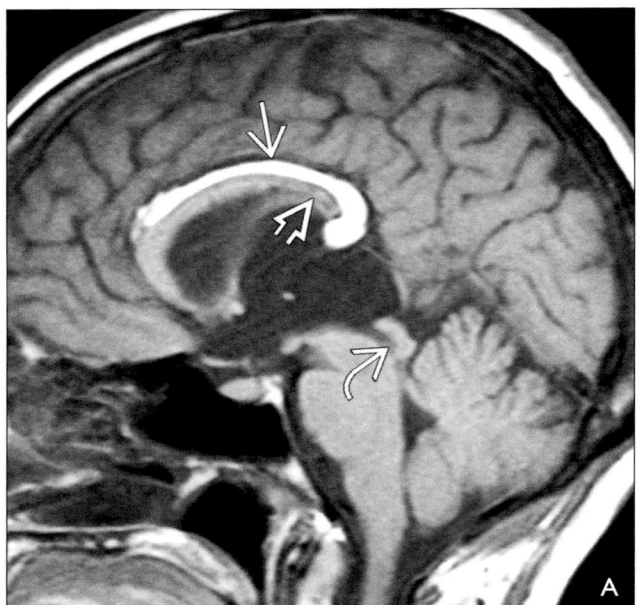

41-30A. Sagittal T1WI shows aqueductal stenosis ➔, curvilinear lipoma ➔ with thin posterior body, absent splenium of corpus callosum ➔.

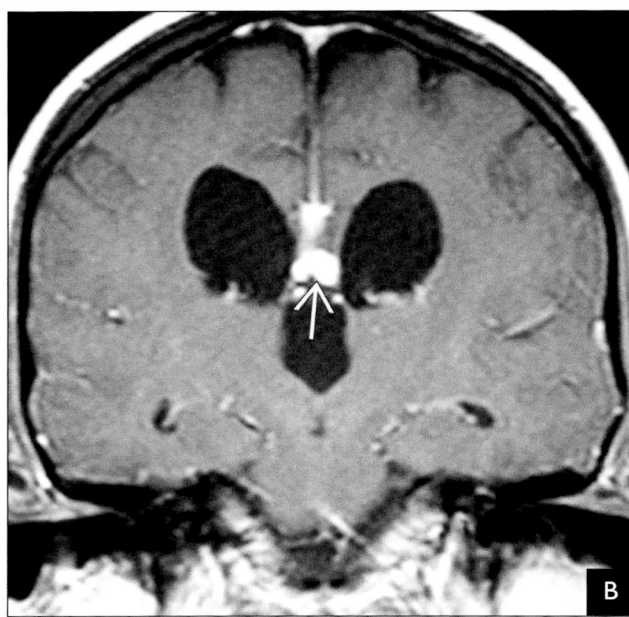

41-30B. Coronal T1 C+ scan shows the interhemispheric lipoma ➔. (Courtesy A. Maydell, MD.)

lar interhemispheric lipomas are partially calcified—to none, generally seen in small lesions in other locations (41-29A), (41-31A), (41-31B). Lipomas do not enhance on CECT scans.

MR FINDINGS. Lipomas follow fat signal on all imaging sequences. They appear homogeneously hyperintense on T1WI and become hypointense with fat suppression (41-29).

Signal on T2WI varies. Fat becomes hypointense on standard T2WI but remains moderately hyperintense on fast spin echo studies because of J-coupling. Fat is hypointense on STIR and appears hyperintense on FLAIR. No enhancement is seen following contrast administration.

Other CNS malformations are common. The most frequent are corpus callosum anomalies. These range from mild dysgenesis (usually with curvilinear lipomas) (41-30) to agenesis (with bulky tubulonodular lipomas) (41-31).

ANGIOGRAPHY. If callosal agenesis is present, CTA or DSA may demonstrate an azygous internal carotid artery or aberrant pericallosal artery course.

Differential Diagnosis

While fat does not appear inside the normal CNS, it *can* be found within the dura and cavernous sinus. Small fatty deposits are sometimes identified within the cavernous sinus and are a normal finding. **Metaplastic falx ossification** is a normal variant that can resemble an inter-

hemispheric lipoma. Dense cortical bone surrounding T1 hyperintense, fatty marrow is the typical finding.

The major differential diagnosis of an intracranial lipoma is an unruptured **dermoid cyst**. Dermoids generally measure 20-40 HU, often calcify, and demonstrate more heterogeneous signal intensity on MR.

INTRACRANIAL LIPOMAS

Etiology
- 2 theories
  - Maldifferentiation of embryonic meninx primitiva
  - Genetic aberration

Pathology
- Usually solitary
- Supratentorial (80%)
  - Interhemispheric fissure (40-50%)
  - Quadrigeminal (15-25%)
  - Suprasellar (15%)
- Infratentorial (20%)
- Gross appearance: Lobulated, yellow
- Microscopic: Mature, nonneoplastic adipose tissue

Clinical Issues
- < 0.5% of intracranial masses
- Usually found incidentally, "leave me alone" lesions

Imaging
- NECT: -50 to -100 HU
  - Ca++ rare except in tubulonodular lesions
- MR: "Just like fat"
  - Other intracranial malformations common
  - Often surrounds, encases vessels/nerves

Differential Diagnosis
- Dermoid cyst
- Falx ossification

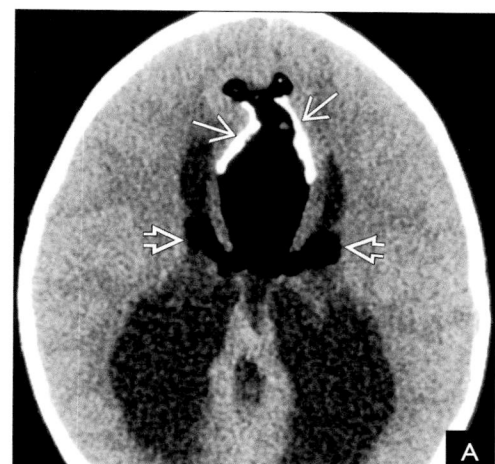 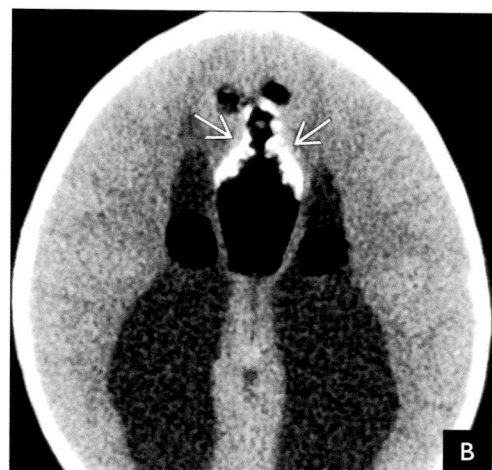

41-31A. Axial NECT scan shows corpus callosum agenesis with parallel, nonconverging lateral ventricles. Large, partially calcified ➡ tubulonodular interhemispheric lipoma extends into both lateral ventricles ⧨ through the choroidal fissures. 41-31B. More cephalad scan in the same patient shows prominent curvilinear calcifications ➡ along the lateral aspects of the interhemispheric lipoma.

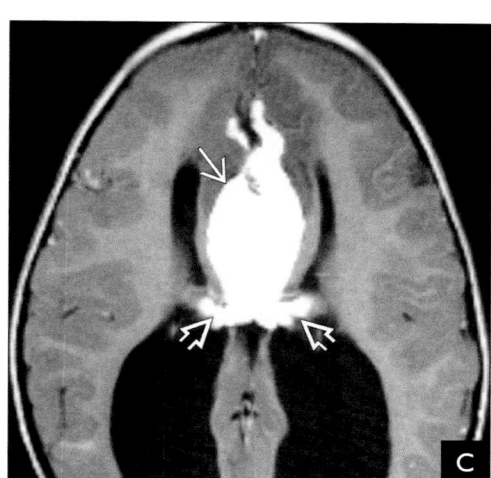 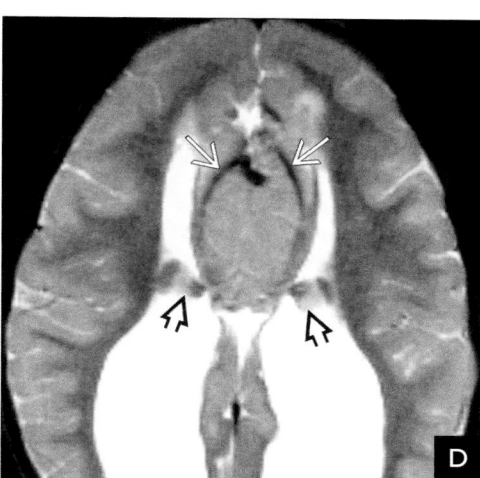

41-31C. Axial T1WI shows the hyperintense lipoma ➡ between the nonconverging lateral ventricles. Extension into the lateral ventricles through the choroid fissures ⧨ is especially well-demonstrated. 41-31D. Standard T2WI shows that the lipoma is hypointense with the calcifications showing as curvilinear hypointensities ➡. Note extension into lateral ventricles ⧨.

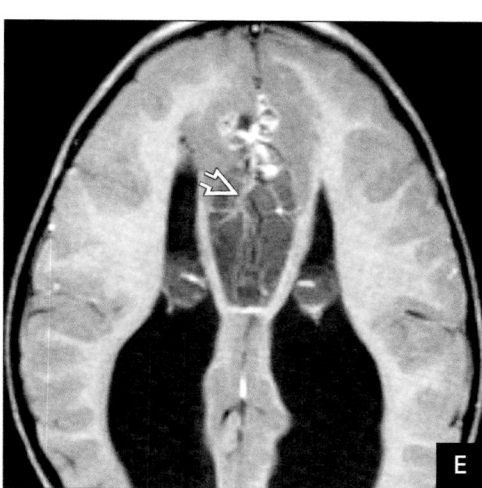 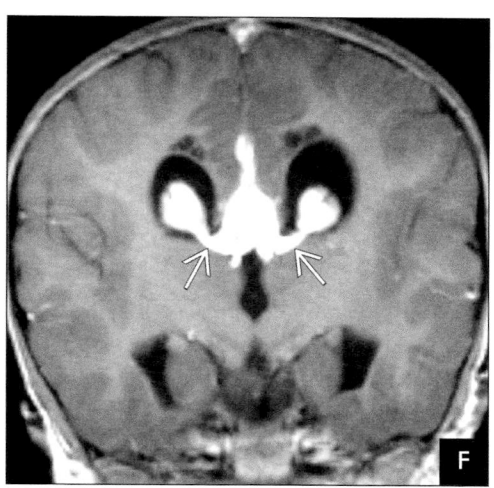

41-31E. Axial T1 C+ FS scan shows that the lipoma becomes profoundly hypointense. Note enhancing vessels ⧨ coursing through the lipoma. 41-31F. Coronal T1 C+ scan without fat saturation elegantly demonstrates the lipoma and its extension through the choroidal fissures into both lateral ventricles ➡ and the choroid plexuses.

Selected References

Normal Development and Anatomy of the Skull Base

Embryology

- Harnsberger HR: Skull base overview. In Diagnostic Imaging: Head and Neck. 2nd ed. Salt Lake City: Amirsys Publishing. V.1.2-7, 2011
- Phillips CD: Persistent craniopharyngeal canal. In Harnsberger HR et al: Diagnostic Imaging: Head and Neck. 2nd ed. Salt Lake City: Amirsys Publishing. V.1.16-17, 2011

Relevant Gross Anatomy

- Harnsberger HR: Skull base overview. In Harnsberger HR: Diagnostic Imaging: Head and Neck. 2nd ed. Salt Lake City: Amirsys Publishing. V.1.2-7, 2011

Cephaloceles

Occipital Cephaloceles

- Menezes AH: Craniovertebral junction abnormalities with hindbrain herniation and syringomyelia: regression of syringomyelia after removal of ventral craniovertebral junction compression. J Neurosurg. 116(2):301-9, 2012

Frontoethmoidal Cephaloceles

- Oucheng N et al: Frontoethmoidal meningoencephalocele: appraisal of 200 operated cases. J Neurosurg Pediatr. 6(6):541-9, 2010

Parietal Cephaloceles

- Hsu SW et al: Atretic parietal cephalocele associated with sinus pericranii: embryological consideration. Brain Dev. 34(4):325-8, 2012

Skull Base Cephaloceles

- Hwang K et al: Congenital orbital encephalocele, orbital dystopia, and exophthalmos. J Craniofac Surg. 23(4):e343-4, 2012

Persistent Craniopharyngeal Canal

- Phillips CD: Persistent craniopharyngeal canal. In Harnsberger HR et al: Diagnostic Imaging: Head and Neck. 2nd ed. Salt Lake City: Amirsys Publishing. V.1.16-17, 2011
- Hughes ML et al: Persistent hypophyseal (craniopharyngeal) canal. Br J Radiol. 72(854):204-6, 1999

Craniosynostoses

Craniosynostosis Overview

- Levi B et al: Cranial suture biology: from pathways to patient care. J Craniofac Surg. 23(1):13-9, 2012
- Tamburrini G et al: Complex craniosynostoses: a review of the prominent clinical features and the related management strategies. Childs Nerv Syst. 28(9):1511-23, 2012

Nonsyndromic Craniosynostosis

- Vinchon M et al: Non-syndromic oxycephaly and brachycephaly: a review. Childs Nerv Syst. 28(9):1439-46, 2012
- Johnson D et al: Craniosynostosis. Eur J Hum Genet. 19(4):369-76, 2011
- Stamper BD et al: Differential expression of extracellular matrix-mediated pathways in single-suture craniosynostosis. PLoS One. 6(10):e26557, 2011

Syndromic Craniosynostoses

- Agochukwu NB et al: Impact of genetics on the diagnosis and clinical management of syndromic craniosynostoses. Childs Nerv Syst. 28(9):1447-63, 2012
- Parthey K et al: SOX10 mutation with peripheral amyelination and developmental disturbance of axons. Muscle Nerve. 45(2):284-90, 2012
- Hurst JA et al: Metopic and sagittal synostosis in Greig cephalopolysyndactyly syndrome: five cases with intragenic mutations or complete deletions of GLI3. Eur J Hum Genet. 19(7):757-62, 2011
- Pingault V et al: Review and update of mutations causing Waardenburg syndrome. Hum Mutat. 31(4):391-406, 2010
- Tokumaru AM et al: Skull base and calvarial deformities: association with intracranial changes in craniofacial syndromes. AJNR Am J Neuroradiol. 17(4):619-30, 1996

Meningeal Anomalies

Lipomas

- Rajan DS et al: Corpus callosum lipoma. Neurology. 78(17):1366, 2012
- Nishio J: Contributions of cytogenetics and molecular cytogenetics to the diagnosis of adipocytic tumors. J Biomed Biotechnol. 2011:524067, 2011
- Truwit CL et al: Pathogenesis of intracranial lipoma: an MR study in 42 patients. AJR Am J Roentgenol. 155(4):855-64; discussion 865, 1990

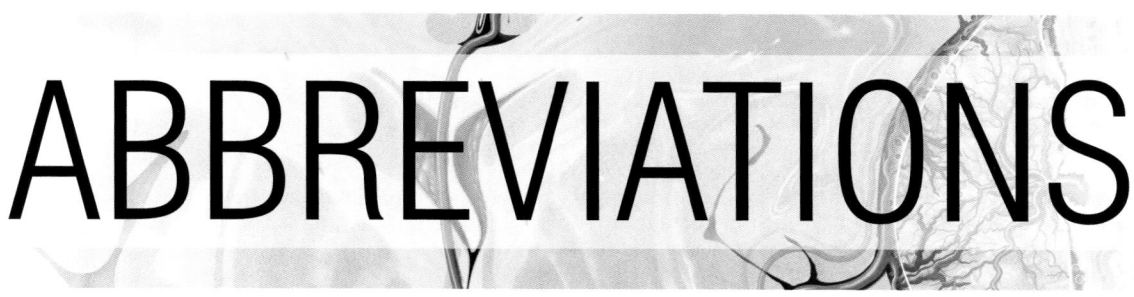

ABBREVIATIONS

A

AA	anaplastic astrocytoma
AA	aortic arch
AAV	ANCA-associated vasculitis
ABC	aneurysmal bone cyst
AbICA	aberrant internal carotid artery
ABRA	amyloid β-related angiitis
Ac	*Acanthamoeba*
AC	anterior commissure
AC	arachnoid cyst
ACA	anterior cerebral artery
ACAS	Asymptomatic Carotid Atherosclerosis Group
AChA	anterior choroidal artery
ACoA	anterior communicating artery
aCPP	atypical choroid plexus papilloma
ACR	American College of Radiology
ACR	American College of Rheumatology
ACTH	adrenocorticotrophic hormone
AD	Alzheimer disease
ADC	apparent diffusion coefficient
ADEM	acute disseminated encephalomyelitis
ADH	antidiuretic hormone
ADNI	Alzheimer Disease Neuroimaging Initiative
AE	anaplastic ependymoma
AED	antiepileptic drug
AFP	α-fetoprotein
AG	angiocentric glioma
AG	arachnoid granulation
AH	adenohypophysis
AHA/ASA	American Heart Association/American Stroke Association
AHE	acute hepatic encephalopathy
AHEM	acute hemorrhagic encephalomyelitis
AHLE	acute hemorrhagic leukoencephalitis
AHO	Albright hereditary osteodystrophy
aHPE	alobar holoprosencephaly
AHT	abusive head trauma
AICA	anterior inferior cerebellar artery
AIDS	acquired immunodeficiency syndrome
aIVOH	acute IVOH
AJCC	American Joint Committee on Cancer
Ala	alanine
ALD	adrenoleukodystrophy
ALK	anaplastic lymphoma kinase
ALL	acute lymphoblastic leukemia
ALS	amyotrophic lateral sclerosis
ALS/MND	amyotrophic lateral sclerosis/motor neuron disease
AM	atypical meningioma
AMB	anaplastic medulloblastoma
AML	acute myeloid leukemia
AMN	adrenomyeloneuropathy
ANCA	antineutrophil cytoplasmic autoantibodies
ANE	acute necrotizing encephalopathy
ANET	angiocentric neuroepithelial tumor
AO	anaplastic oligodendroglioma
AOP	artery of Percheron
AP	aprosencephaly
APMV	anterior pontomesencephalic vein
ApoE	apolipoprotein E
APS	antiphospholipid syndrome

AQP	aquaporin
ARR	arrhinencephaly
ARVS	acute retroviral syndrome
aSAH	aneurysmal subarachnoid hemorrhage
ASB	anterior skull base
ASCO	atherosclerotic, small vessel disease, cardioembolic, other strokes
aSDH	acute subdural hematoma
ASVD	atherosclerotic vascular disease
AT	ataxia-telangiectasia
AT	atelencephaly
AT/RT	atypical teratoid/rhabdoid tumor
ATH	ascending transtentorial herniation
AV	arteriovenous
AVF	arteriovenous fistula
AVM	arteriovenous malformation
AxD	Alexander disease
Aβ	amyloid-β

B

BA	basilar artery
BAVM	brain arteriovenous malformation
BBA	blood blister-like aneurysm
BCNS	basal cell nevus syndrome
BCS	Balo concentric sclerosis
BCT	brachiocephalic trunk
BCT	brain capillary telangiectasia
BD	Behçet disease
BD	brain death
BG	basal ganglia
BIND	bilirubin-induced neurologic dysfunction
BLL-HIV	benign lymphoepithelial lesions of HIV
BMT	benign mesenchymal tumor
BOL	basion-opisthion line
BRBNS	blue rubber bleb nevus syndrome
BRE	bilirubin encephalopathy
BSG	brainstem glioma
bvFTD	behavioral-variant frontotemporal dementia
BVR	basal vein of Rosenthal
BWS	Beckwith-Wiedemann syndrome

C

Ca++	calcium, calcification
CAA	cerebral amyloid angiopathy
CACH	childhood ataxia with CNS hypomyelination
CAD	craniocervical arterial dissection
CADASIL	cerebral autosomal dominant arteriopathy without subcortical infarcts and leukoencephalopathy
CAG	cystosine-adenine-guanine
CAM	cell adhesion molecule
CAMS	cerebrofacial arteriovenous metameric syndrome
CAPNON	calcifying pseudoneoplasm of the neuraxis
CARASIL	cerebral autosomal recessive arteriopathy with subcortical infarcts and leukoencephalopathy
cART	combination antiretroviral therapy
CBD	corticobasal degeneration
CBF	cerebral blood flow
CBS	corticobasal syndrome
CBSC	cobblestone complex
CBV	cerebral blood volume
CC	colloid cyst
CC	corpus callosum
CCA	common carotid artery
CCF	carotid-cavernous fistula
CCh	clival chordoma
CCIS	corpus callosum impingement syndrome
CCM	cerebral canverous malformation
CCSVI	chronic cerebrospinal venous insufficiency
CD	Canavan disease
CDC	Centers for Disease Control and Prevention

CEA	carotid endarterectomy
CECT	contrast-enhanced CT
CERAD	Consortium to Establish a Registry for Alzheimer Disease
CFE	cerebral fat emboli
CG	chordoid glioma
CGH	comparative genomic hybridization
CH	congenital hypothyroidism
CHARGE	coloboma, heart malformations, choanal atresia, developmental retardation, genital anomalies, ear anomalies
CHCC	Chapel Hill Consensus Conference
CHCR	Canadian Head CT Rule
CHE	chronic hepatic encephalopathy
CHI	closed head injury
Cho	choline
CHS	cerebral hyperperfusion syndrome
CHtnE	chronic hypertensive encephalopathy
CIDP	chronic inflammatory demyelinating polyneuropathy
CIN	cervical intraepithelial neoplasia
cIVOH	chronic intraventricular obstructive hydrocephalus
CJD	Creutzfeldt-Jakob disease
CLH	cystic lymphoid hyperplasia
cLIS	classic lissencephaly
CLL	chronic lymphocytic leukemia
CLOVE	congenital lipomatous overgrowth, vascular malformations, epidermal nevi
CM	cerebral malaria
CM1	Chiari 1
CM1.5	Chiari 1.5
CM2	Chiari 2
CM3	Chiari 3
CMB	cerebral microbleed
CMB	classic medulloblastoma
CMD	congenital muscular dystrophy
CML	chronic myelocytic leukemia
CMV	Cytomegalovirus
CN	cranial nerve
CN	cyanide
CNC	central neurocytoma
CNPAS	congenital nasal pyriform aperture stenosis
CNS	central nervous system
CNS SLE	CNS lupus
CNuc	caudate nucleus
CO	carbon monoxide
COACH	cerebellar vermis hypoplasia, oligophrenia, ataxia, ocular coloboma, hepatic fibrosis
CO-Hgb	carboxyhemoglobin
COLD	Cowden-Lhermitte-Duclos syndrome
CORS	cerebello-oculo-renal syndrome
CoVT	cortical vein thrombosis
COW	circle of Willis
CP	cerebral palsy
CP	choroid plexus
CP	craniopharyngioma
CPA	cerebellopontine angle
CPA	cerebral proliferative angiopathy
CPC	choroid plexus cyst
CPCa	choroid plexus carcinoma
cPML	classic PML
CPP	choroid plexus papilloma
CPX	choroid plexus xanthogranuloma
Cr	creatine
CRD	chronic renal disease
CRS	congenital rubella syndrome
CRV	cerebroretinal vasculopathy
crypto	Cryptococcus neoformans
CS	cavernous sinus
CS	congenital syphilis
CS	Cowden syndrome
cSAH	convexal subarachnoid hemorrhage
CSB	central skull base
cSDH	chronic subdural hematoma
CSF	cerebrospinal fluid

CSP	cavum septi pellucidi
CST	cavernous sinus thrombosis
CST	corticospinal tract
CT	computed tomography
CTA	CT angiography
CTE	chronic traumatic encephalopathy
CTM	CT myelography
CTV	CT venography
CV	cavum vergae
CVA	cerebrovascular accident
CVD	cortical venous drainage
CVI	cavum velum interpositum
CVJ	craniovertebral junction
CVM	cerebrovascular malformation
CVP	clival venous plexus
CVS	cerebral vasospasm

D

DAA	double aortic arch
DAI	diffuse axonal injury
DAT	dopamine transporter
dAVF	dural arterivenous fistula
DBS	deep brain stimulator/stimulation
DC	dermoid cyst
DCI	delayed cerebral ischemia
DDMS	Dyke-Davidoff-Masson syndrome
deoxy-Hgb	deoxyhemoblogin
DIA	desmoplastic infantile astrocytoma
DIC	disseminated intravascular coagulopathy
DIG	desmoplastic infantile ganglioglioma
DKA	diabetes ketoacidosis
DLB	dementia with Lewy bodies
DLBCL	diffuse large B-cell lymphoma
DLBD	diffuse Lewy body disease
DM	diabetes mellitus
DM	dural metastasis
DM1	diabetes type 1
DM2	diabetes type 2
DMB	desmoplastic nodular medulloblastoma
DMCV	deep middle cerebral vein
DN	dentate nucleus
DNET	dysembryoplastic neuroepithelial tumor
DSA	digital subtraction angiography
DST	dural sinus thrombosis
DTH	descending transtentorial herniation
DTI	diffusion tensor imaging
DVA	developmental venous anomaly
DVHCP	diffuse villous hyperplasia of the choroid plexus
DVI	diffuse vascular injury
DVST	dural venous sinus thrombosis
DW	Dandy-Walker
DWM	Dandy-Walker malformation
DWS	Dandy-Walker spectrum
DWV	Dandy-Walker variant

E

EBV	Epstein-Barr virus
EC	epidermoid cyst
ECA	external carotid artery
ECCL	encephalocraniocutaneous lipomatosis
ECD	Erdheim-Chester disease
ECM	extracellular matrix
ECST	European Carotid Surgery Trial
EDE	epidural empyema
EDH	epidural hematoma
EDV	end diastolic velocity
EG	*Echinococcus granulosis*
EGF	epidermal growth factor
ELST	endolymphatic sac tumor

EM/EA	*Echinococcus multilocularis/E. alveolaris*
EMA	epithelial membrane antigen
EMH	extramedullary hematopoiesis
EML	extramedullary leukemia
EMP	extramedullary plasmacytoma
EN	epidermal nevus
ENB	esthesioneuroblastoma
EP	ecchordosis physaliphora
ES	empty sella
ETANTR	embryonal tumor with abundant neuropil and true rosettes
EtOH	ethanol
EVD	external ventricular drain
EVNCT	extraventricular neurocytoma
EVOH	extraventricular obstructive hydrocephalus

F

FA	fractional anisotropy
FA	fusiform aneurysm
FASI	focus of abnormal signal
FCD	focal cortical dysplasia
FCMD	Fukuyama congenital muscular dystrophy
FD	fibrous dysplasia
FDG	fluorodeoxyglucose
FES	fat embolism syndrome
FFI	fatal familial insomnia
FGF-23	fibroblast growth factor 23
FIA	familial intracranial aneurysm
FIPA	familial isolated pituitary adenoma syndrome
FISH	fluorescent in situ hybridization
FLAIR	fluid attenuation inversion recovery
FM	foramen magnum
FMD	fibromuscular dysplasia
fMRI	functional MRI
FNS	facial nerve schwannoma
FOS	foscarnet
FS	foramen spinosum
FSH	follicle-stimulating hormone
FSPGR	fast spoiled gradient echo (sequences)
FTD	frontotemporal dementia
FTLD	frontotemporal lobar degeneration
FTLD-FUS	FTLD with tau/TDP-negative and fused-in sarcoma (FUS)-positiive inclusions
FTLD-TAU	tau-positive frontotemporal lobar degeneration; FTLD with tau inclusions
FTLD-TDP	FTLD with tau-negative and TDP-43-positive inclusions
FTLD-UPS	FTLD with positive immunohistochemistry against proteins of the ubiquitin proteasome system

G

GA1	glutaric aciduria type 1
GA2	glutaric aciduria type 2
GAE	granulomatous amebic encephalitis
GAG	glycosaminoglycan
GBM	glioblastoma multiforme
GC	gliomatosis cerebri
GCDH	glutaryl-coenzyme A dehydrogenase
GCPS	Greig cephalopolysyndactyly syndrome
GCS	Glasgow Coma Scale/Score
GCT	germ cell tumor
GCV	ganciclovir
GCyt	gangliocytoma
GFAP	glial fibrillary acidic protein
GG	ganglioglioma
GH	granulomatous hypophysitis
GH	growth hormone
GLD	globoid cell leukodystrophy
Glx	glutamate-glutamine
GM	gray matter
GMH	germinal matrix hemorrhage
GNPC	granule neuron precursor cell
GP	globus pallidus

GRE	gradient recall(ed) (refocused) echo
GS	gliosarcoma
GSF	"growing" skull fracture
GSH	glutathione
GSPN	greater superficial petrosal nerve
GSS	Gerstmann-Sträussler-Schenker disease
GSW	greater sphenoid wing

H

HAART	highly active antiretroviral therapy
HAD	HIV-associated dementia
HAND	HIV-associated neurocognitive disorders
HAS	hereditary systemic angiopathy
HC	hippocampal commissure
HC	hydatid cyst
HCSR	hippocampal sulcus remnants
HD	Huntington disease
HE	hepatic encephalopathy
HELLP	hemolysis, elevated liver enzymes, low platelets
HERNS	hereditary endotheliopathy, retinopathy, nephropathy, and stroke
Hg	mercury
Hgb	hemoglobin
HGBL	hemangioblastoma
HH	hypothalamic hamartoma
HHcy	hyperhomocysteinemia
HHS	hyperglycemic hyperosmolar state
HHT	hereditary hemorrhagic telangiectasia
HHV-6	human herpesvirus 6
hICH	hypertensive intracranial hemorrhage
HIE	hypoxic-ischemic encephalopathy
HIHH	hyperglycemia-induced hemichorea-hemiballismus
HII	hypoxic-ischemic injury
HIV	human immunodeficiency virus
HIVE	HIV encephalitis
HIVL	HIV leukoencephalopathy
HIV-V	HIV vasculopathy
HL	Hodgkin-type lymphoma
HLH	hemophagocytic lymphohistiocytosis
HMEG	hemimegaloencephaly
HOD	hypertrophic olivary degeneration
HP	hypoparathyroidism
HPC	hemangiopericytoma
HPE	holoprosencephaly
HPF	high-power field
HPTH	hyperparathyroidism
HSE	herpes simplex encephalitis
HSV	herpes simplex virus
HT	Hashimoto thyroiditis
HT	hemorrhagic transformation
HTN	hypertension
HU	Hounsfield unit
HUS	hemolytic-uremic syndrome
HVR	hereditary vascular retinopathy

I

IAC	internal auditory canal
IAE	influenza-associated encephalitis/encephalopathy
IASVD	intracranial atherosclerotic vascular disease
ICA	internal carotid artery
ICD-O	International Classification of Diseases for Oncology
ICE	ifosfamide, carboplatin, etoposide
ICH	intracranial hemorrhage
ICP	intracranial pressure
ICV	internal cerebral vein
IEL	internal elastic lamina
IGHD	isolated growth hormone deficiency
IHF	interhemispheric fissure
IIDD	idiopathic inflammatory demyelinating disorder
IIDL	idiopathic inflammatory demyelinating lesion

IIH	idiopathic intracranial hypertension
IIP	idiopathic inflammatory pseudotumor
IJV	internal jugular vein
IL1-β	interleukin-1-β
ILAE	International League Against Epilepsy
ILT	inferolateral trunk
IMD	inherited metabolic disorder
INAD	infantile neuroaxonal dystrophy
iNPH	idiopathic normal pressure hydrocephalus
ION	inferior olivary nucleus
iPML	inflammatory progressive multifocal leukoencephalopathy
IPS	inferior petrosal sinus
IR	inversion recovery
IRIS	immune reconstitution inflammatory syndrome
ISF	interstitial fluid
ISS	inferior sagittal sinus
ISS	International Staging System (for myeloma)
IVH	intraventricular hemorrhage
IVL	intravascular lymphoma
IVOH	intraventricular obstructive hydrocephalus
IVRBA	intraventricular rupture of a brain abscess

J

JCE	JCV encephalopathy
JCM	JC meningitis
JCV	JC virus
JF	jugular foramen
JS	Joubert syndrome
JSRD	Joubert syndrome and related disorders
JXG	juvenile xanthogranuloma

K

KOT	keratocystic odontogenic tumor
KS	Kaposi sarcoma
KSS	Kearns-Sayre syndrome
KTWS	Klippel-Trenaunay-Weber syndrome

L

LAICOD	large artery intracranial occlusive disease
LB	Lewy body
LBD	Lewy body disorder
LBSL	leukoencephalopathy with brainstem/spinal cord involvement and high lactate
LBV	Lewy body variant (of Alzheimer disease)
LCAMB	large cell/anaplastic medulloblastoma
LCH	Langerhans cell histiocytosis
LCM	lymphocytic choriomeningitis
LCMB	large cell medulloblastoma
LD	Leigh disease
LD	Lyme disease
LDD	Lhermitte-Duclos disease
LDL	low-density lipoprotein
LEC	lyphoepithelial cyst
LELPE	lobar extralimbic paraneoplastic encephalopathy
LESA	lymphoepithelial sialadenitis
LFS	Li-Fraumeni syndrome
LGA	low-grade astrocytoma
LGB	lateral geniculate body
LH	luteinizing hormone
LH	lymphocytic hypophysitis
LHON	Leber hereditary optic neuropathy
LINH	lymphocytic infundibuloneurohypophysitis
LIS	lissencephaly
LM	leptomeningeal metastasis
LMN	lower motor neuron
LNB	Lyme neuroborreliosis
LOC	loss of consciousness
LOLA	L-ornithine L-aspartate

LSA	lenticulostriate artery
LYG	lymphomatoid granulomatosis

M

MA	meningioangiomatosis
MA	methamphetamine
MAIC	M. avium-intracellulare complex
MALT	mucosa-associated lymphoid tissue
MAS	macrophage activation syndrome
MAS	McCune-Albright syndrome
MB	medulloblastoma
MBD	Marchiafava-Bignami disease
MBEN	medulloblastoma with extensive nodularity
MCA	middle cerebral artery
MCD	malformation of cortical development
MCI	minimal cognitive impairment
MCM	mega cisterna magna
MCP	middle cerebellar peduncle
MCPH	microcephaly
MD	Marburg disease
MD	mean diffusivity
MD	Menkes disease
MD-CMD	merosin-deficient congenital muscular dystrophy
MDCT	multidetector row CT
MDR TB	multidrug-resistant tuberculosis
MDS	Miller-Dieker syndrome
ME	medulloepithelioma
MEB	muscle-eye-brain disease
MEG	magnetoencephalography
MELAS	mitochondrial encephalomyopathy with lactic acidosis and stroke-like episodes
MEN	multiple endocrine neoplasia
Merlin	moesin-erzin-radixin-like protein
MERRF	myoclonic epilepsy with ragged red fibers
met-Hgb	methemoglobin
MFH	malignant fibrous histiocytoma
MGMT	methylguanine-methyltransferase
MHC	major histocompatibility complex
mHTN	malignant hypertension
mI	myoinositol
MIBG	metaiodobenzylguanidine
MIP	maximum-intensity projection
mivHPE	middle interhemispheric variant of holoprosencephaly
MLC	megaloencephalic leukodystrophy with subcortical cysts
MLD	metachromatic leukodystrophy
MM	multiple myeloma
MMA	methylmalonic acidemia
MMA	middle meningeal artery
MMD	moyamoya disease
MMen	malignant meningioma
MMP	matrix metaloproteinase
MMT	malignant mesenchymal tumor
MPNST	malignant peripheral nerve sheath tumor
MPS	mucopolysaccharidosis
MPV	median prosencephalic vein
MRA	MR angiography
MRI	magnetic resonance imaging
MRSA	methicillin-resistant Staphylococcus aureus
MRT	malignant rhabdoid tumor
MS	multiple sclerosis
MSA	multiple system atrophy
MSA-A	multiple system atrophy of the autonomic type
MSA-C	multiple system atrophy of the cerebellar type
MSA-P	multiple system atrophy of the parkinsonian type
mSDH	mixed-age subdural hematoma
MSG	microcephaly with simplified gyral pattern
MSUD	maple syrup urine disease
mtDNA	mitochondrial DNA
MTI	magnetization transfer imaging
MtOH	methanol

mTOR	mammalian target of rapamycin
MTR	magnetization transfer ratio
MTS	mesial temporal sclerosis
MTT	mean transit time
MVC	motor vehicle collision

N

N₂O	nitrous oxide
NAA	N-acetyl-L-aspartate
NAG	nonastrocytic glioma
NAI	nonaccidental injury
NASCET	North American Symptomatic Carotid Endarectomy Trial
nASVD FA	nonatherosclerotic fusiform aneurysm
NAT	nonaccidental trauma
NB	neuroblastoma
NBD	neuro-Behçet disease
NBIA	neurodegeneration with brain iron accumulation
N-CAM	neural cell adhesion molecule
NCC	neural crest cell
NCC	neurocysticercosis
NCL	neuronal ceroid lipofuscinosis
NCM	neurocutaneous melanosis
NE	neurenteric
NECT	nonenhanced CT
NF	neurofibroma
NF1	neurofibromatosis type 1
NF2	neurofibromatosis type 2
NFT	neurofibrillary tangle
NGC	neuroglial cyst
NGMGCT	nongerminomatous malignant germ cell tumors
NH	neurohypophysis
NINCDS-ADRA	National Institute of Neurological Disorders and Stroke-Alzheimer Disease and Related Disorders
NK cells	natural killer cells
NMO	neuromyelitis optica
NOC	New Orleans Criteria
NPH	normal pressure hydrocephalus
NPSLE	neuropsychiatric systemic lupus erythematosus
NS	neurosarcoid
NS	neurosyphilis
NSC	neural stem cell
NTM	nontuberculous mycobacteria
ntSAH	nontraumatic subarachnoid hemorrhage
NVS	nonvestibular schwannoma

O

OA	oligoastrocytoma
OA	ophthalmic artery
ODS	osmotic demyelination syndrome
OEC	olfactory ensheathing cell
OF	ossifying fibroma
OFC	occipitofrontal head circumference
OFD-6	oro-facial-digital syndrome type 6
OG	oligodendroglioma
OH	obstructive hydrocephalus
OHS	occipital horn syndrome
OP	organophosphate
OPG	optic pathway glioma
OS	osteosarcoma
OXPHOS	oxidative phosphorylation
oxy-Hgb	fully oxygenated hemoglobin

P

PA	pilocytic astrcytoma
PA	pituitary adenoma
PaD	Paget disease

PALE	post-transplant acute limbic encephalitis
PAM	primary amebic meningoencephalitis
PAN	polyarteritis nodosa
PAP	pituitary apoplexy
pAVF	pial arteriovenous fistula
Pb	lead
PB	pineoblastoma
PBD	peroxisomal biogenesis disorder
PC	pineal cyst
PC	posterior commissure
PCa	pituitary carcinoma
PCA	posterior cerebral artery
PCA	posterior cortical atrophy
PCBA	persistent carotid-basilar anastomosis
PCD	paraneoplastic cerebellar degeneration
PChA	posterior choroidal artery
PCNSL	primary central nervous system lymphoma
PCoA	posterior communicating artery
PCPC	persistent craniopharyngeal canal
pCT	CT perfusion
PCV	precentral cerebellar vein
PCV regimen	procarbazine, lomustine, and vincristine
PD	Parkinson disease
PDD	Parkinson disease dementia
PENS	papular epidermal nevus syndrome
PET	positron emission tomography
PF	posterior fossa
pGH	primary granulomatous hypophysitis
PGNT	papillary glioneuronal tumor
PHA	persistent hypoglossal artery
PHACES	posterior fossa malformations, hemangioma, arterial cerebrovascular anomalies, coarctation of the aorta and cardiac defects, eye abnormalities, and sternal clefting or supraumbilical raphe
Phe	phenylalanine
PHP	pseudohypoparathyroidism
PHS	Pallister-Hall syndrome
PHTS	PTEN hamartoma tumor syndrome
PI	pars intermedia
PIA	proatlantal intersegmental artery
PICA	posterior inferior cerebellar artery
PICCC	primary intracranial choriocarcinoma
pICH	primary intracranial hemorrhage
PKAN	pantothenate kinase-associated neurodegeneration
PKU	phenylketonuria
PLE	paraneoplastic limbic encephalitis
PLEX/IA	plasmapheresis/immunoadsorption
PLS	primary lateral sclerosis
PMA	pilomyxoid astrocytoma
PMD	Pelizaeus-Merzbacher disease
PMG	polymicrogyria
PML	progressive multifocal leukoencephalopathy
pMR	MR perfusion
PNET	primitive neuroectodermal tumor
PNET-MB	medulloblastoma
PNF	pelxiform neurofibroma
PNFA	progressive nonfluent aphasia
PNS	paraneoplastic neurologic syndrome
pnSAH	perimesencephalic nonaneurysmal subarachnoid hemorrhage
PNT	perineural tumor
POA	persistent otic artery
PP MS	primary-progressive multiple sclerosis
PPA	propionic acidemia
PPAD9	Poly Pathology AD Assessment 9
PPBS	posterior pituitary "bright spot"
PPCA	postpartum cerebral angiopathy
PPHP	pseudo-pseudohypoparathyroidism
PPOA	persistent primitive olfactory artery
PPT	pineal parenchymal tumor
PPTID	pineal parenchymal tumor of intermediate differentiation
PRES	posterior reversible encephalopathy syndrome
PRL	prolactin

PSA	persistent stapedial artery
PSB	posterior skull base
PSP	progressive supranuclear palsy
PSP-P	parkinsonian-type progressive supranuclear palsy
PSP-RS	Richardson syndrome, richardsonian-type progressive supranuclear palsy
PSV	peak systolic velocity
PTA	persistent trigeminal artery
PTH	parathyroid hormone
PTLD	post-transplant lymphoproliferative disease
PTPF	pterygopalatine fossa
PTPR	papillary tumor of the pineal region
PTV	post-traumatic vasospasm
PV	petrosal vein
PVHI	periventricular hemorrhagic infarction
pVHL	VHL protein
PVL	periventricular leukomalacia
PVNH	periventricular nodular heterotopia
PVS	perivascular space
PWB	port-wine birthmark
PWI	perfusion-weighted imaging
PXA	pleomorphic xanthoastrocytoma

Q

qMRI	quantitative MR

R

RBC	red blood cell
rCBF	relative cerebral blood flow
RCC	Rathke cleft cyst
RCC	renal cell carcinoma
RCH	remote cerebellar hemorrhage
RCVS	reversible cerebral vasoconstriction syndrome
RDD	Rosai-Dorfman disease
RE	Rasmussen encephalitis
RED-M	retinopathy, encephalopathy, and deafness-associated microangiopathy
RF	relapsing fever
RF	Rosenthal fiber
RGC	radial glial cell
RGNT	rosette-forming glioneuronal tumor
RII	radiation-induced injury
RIS	radiologically isolated syndrome
RIVM	radiation-induced vascular malformation
RN	red nucleus
ROI	region of interest
RPLS	reversible posterior leukoencephalopathy syndrome
RR MS	relapsing-remitting multiple sclerosis
RSS	Rotterdam Scan Study
rTPA	recombinant tissue plasminogen activator
RTPS	rhabdoid tumor predisposition syndrome
RTT	Rett syndrome

S

SA	saccular aneurysm
SAE	subcortical arteriosclerotic encephalopathy
SAS	subarachnoid space
SB	skull base
SBP	solitary bone plasmacytoma
SBS	shaken-baby syndrome
SCA	subclavian artery
SCA	superior cerebellar artery
SCCa	squamous cell carcinoma
SCD	sickle cell disease
SCI	subcortical injury
sCJD	sporadic Creutkzfeldt-Jakob disease
SCNSL	secondary CNS lymphoma
SCO	spindle cell oncocytoma
SCVT	supervicial cerebral vein thrombosis

SD	Schilder disease
SD	semantic dementia
SDE	subdural empyema
SDH	subdural hematoma
SE	status epilepticus
SE	subependymoma
SEGA	subependymal giant cell astrocytoma
SEN	subependymal nodule
SFH	subfalcine herniation
SFT	solitary fibrous tumor
sGH	secondary granulomatous hypophysitis
SGNE	specific glioneuronal element
sHPE	semilobar holoprosencephaly
sICH	spontaneous intracranial hemorrhage
SICRET	small infarcts of cochlear, retinal, and encephalic tissue
SIH	spontaneous intracranial hypotension
SILPAH	syndrome of inappropriately low-pressure acute hydrocephalus
SIS	second-impact syndrome
SLE	systemic lupus erythematosus
SMART	stroke-like migraine attacks after radiation therapy
SMCV	superficial middle cerebral vein
SMMCI	solitary median maxillary central incisor syndrome
SN	substantia nigra
SNALE	seronegative autoimmune limbic encephalitis
SNHL	sensorineural hearing loss
SNP	single nucleotide polymorphism
SNPc	substantia nigra pars compacta
SOD	septooptic dysplasia
SOF	superior orbital fissure
SOV	superior ophthalmic vein
SP	senile plaque
SP	solitary plasmacytoma
SP	status pericranii
SP MS	secondary-progressive multiple sclerosis
SphPS	sphenoparietal sinus
SPS	superior petrosal sinus
SS	Sheehan syndrome
SS	straight sinus
SS	superficial siderosis
SS	Susac syndrome
SSAC	suprasellar arachnoid cyst
SSD	shaded surface displays
sSDH	subacute subdural hematoma
SSFS	sinking skin flap syndrome
SS-GRE	steady-state gradient-recalled-echo
SSPE	subacute sclerosing panencephalitis
SSS	superior sagittal sinus
STIR	short inversion time inversion recovery
STN	subthalamic nucleus
SVR	systolic velocity ratio
SVS	slit ventricle syndrome
SWI	susceptibility-weighted imaging
SWS	Sturge-Weber syndrome

T

TAC	tumor-associated cyst
TB	tuberculosis
TBI	traumatic brain injury
TBM	TB meningitis
TC	trichilemmal cyst
TC	tuber cinereum
Tc-99m	technetium-99m
TGA	transient global amnesia
TGA	trigeminal artery
TGF-β	transforming growth factor β
TI	inversion time
TIA	transient ischemic attacks
TIO	tumor-induced osteomalacia
TLE	temporal lobe epilepsy
TM	typical meningioma

TMA	thrombotic microangiopathy
TMZ	temozolomide
TNF-α	tumor necrosis factor-α
TOAST	Trial of Org 10172 in Acute Stroke Treatment
TOF	time of flight
TORCH	toxoplasmosis, rubella, Cytomegalovirus, and herpes
toxo	toxoplasmosis
TR	repetition time
TS	Terson syndrome
TS	transverse sinus
TS	Turcot syndrome
tSAH	traumatic subarachnoid hemorrhage
TSC	tuberous sclerosis complex
TSE	transmissible spongiform encephalopathies
TSH	thyroid-stimulating hormone
TSL	transient splenial lesion
TTD	time to drain
TTM	tumor-to-tumor metastasis
TTP	thrombotic thrombocytopenic purpura
TTP	time to peak

U

UMN	upper motor neuron
US	ultrasound

V

VA	vertebral artery
VACTERL	vertebral anomalies, anal atresia, cardiovascular anomalies, tracheoesophageal fistulas, renal anomalies, and limb defects
VaD	vascular dementia
VBD	vertebrobasilar dolichoectasia
vCJD	variant Creutzfeldt-Jakob disease
VEGF	vascular endothelial growth factor
VGAM	vein of Galen aneurysmal malformation
VGKC	voltage-gated potassium channel complex
VGVC	valganciclovir
VHL	von Hippel-Lindau syndrome
VI	velum interpositum
VLCFA	very long chain fatty acid
vLIS	variant lissencephaly
VofG	vein of Galen
VRE	vancomycin-resistant *Enterococcus*
VS	vestibular schwannoma
VTA	ventral tegmental area
VWM	vanishing white matter disease
VZV	varicella-zoster virus

W

WaD	wallerian degeneration
WD	Wilson disease
WE	Wernicke encephalopathy
WFNS	World Federation of Neurological Societies
WG	Wegener granulomatosis
WHO	World Health Organization
WM	white matter
WMH	white matter hyperintensity
WMIP	white matter injury of prematurity
WNV	West Nile virus
WS	Waardenburg syndrome
WS	watershed
WS	Williams syndrome
WWS	Walker-Warburg syndrome

X

X-ALD	X-linked adrenoleukodystrophy
XDR TB	extensively drug-resistant tuberculosis
XRT	radiation therapy

Z

ZF	zinc-finger (transcription factor)
ZI	zona incerta
ZS	Zellweger syndrome
ZSS	Zellweger syndrome spectrum

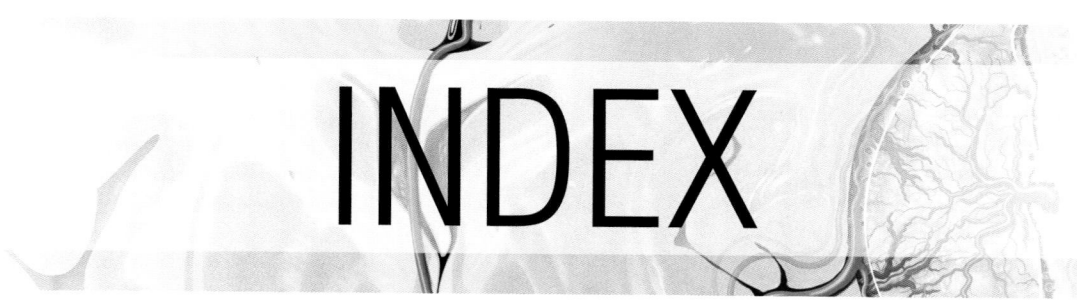